# STROKE

## Pathophysiology, Diagnosis, and Management

*Second Edition*

# STROKE

## Pathophysiology, Diagnosis, and Management

*Second Edition*


EDITED BY

**Henry J.M. Barnett, O.C., M.D., F.R.C.P.(C), F.A.C.P., F.R.C.P.**
Professor
Division of Neurology
Department of Clinical Neurological Sciences
University of Western Ontario Faculty of Medicine
Scientific Director
John P. Robarts Research Institute
London, Ontario, Canada

**J.P. Mohr, M.D.**
Sciarra Professor
Department of Neurology
Columbia University College of Physicians and Surgeons
Director
Division of Cerebrovascular Research
Department of Neurology
Neurological Institute
Columbia Presbyterian Medical Center
New York, New York

**Bennett M. Stein, M.D.**
Byron Stookey Professor and Chairman
Department of Neurological Surgery
Columbia University College of Physicians and Surgeons
Director
Department of Neurological Surgery
Neurological Institute
Columbia Presbyterian Medical Center
New York, New York

**Frank M. Yatsu, M.D.**
Professor and Chairman
Department of Neurology
University of Texas Medical School at Houston
Houston, Texas



**CHURCHILL LIVINGSTONE**
New York, Edinburgh, London, Melbourne, Tokyo

**Library of Congress Cataloging-in-Publication Data**

Stroke : pathophysiology, diagnosis, and management / edited by Henry J.M. Barnett ... [et al.]. — 2nd ed.
p. cm.
Includes bibliographical references and index.
ISBN 0-443-08732-6
1. Cerebrovascular disease. I. Barnett, H. J. M. (Henry J. M.)
[DNLM: 1. Cerebrovascular Disorders. WL 355 S92134]
RC388.5.S8528 1992
616.8'1—dc20
DNLM/DL
for Library of Congress 92-17477
CIP



Distributed in the United Kingdom by Churchill Livingstone, Robert Stevenson House, 1–3 Baxter's Place, Leith Walk, Edinburgh EH1 3AF, and by associated companies, branches, and representatives throughout the world.

Accurate indications, adverse reactions, and dosage schedules for drugs are provided in this book, but it is possible that they may change. The reader is urged to review the package information data of the manufacturers of the medications mentioned.

The Publishers have made every effort to trace the copyright holders for borrowed material. If they have inadvertently overlooked any, they will be pleased to make the necessary arrangements at the first opportunity.

Acquisitions Editor: *Nancy Mullins*
Assistant Editor: *Ann Ruzycka*
Copy Editor: *David Terry*
Production Designer: *Patricia McFadden*
Production Supervisor: *Sharon Tuder*
Production services provided by Bermedica Productions, Ltd.
Cover design by Regina Dahir

Printed in the United States of America

First published in 1992 7 6 5 4 3 2 1

To our wives

Kathleen B., Joan M., Bonita S., and Mich Y.

whose forbearance is here
acknowledged with gratitude.

# *CONTRIBUTORS*

**Harold P. Adams, Jr., M.D.**
Professor and Director, Division of Cerebrovascular Diseases, Department of Neurology, University of Iowa College of Medicine, Iowa City, Iowa

**Henry J.M. Barnett, O.C., M.D., F.R.C.P.(C), F.A.C.P., F.R.C.P.**
Professor, Division of Neurology, Department of Clinical Neurological Sciences, University of Western Ontario Faculty of Medicine; Scientific Director, John P. Robarts Research Institute, London, Ontario, Canada

**J.C. Baron, M.D.**
Director, Unit 320, Institut National de la Santé et de la Recherche Médicale, Caen, France

**Julien Bogousslavsky, M.D.**
Professor Agrégé, Department of Neurology, Centre Hospitalier, Universitaire Vaudois; Assistant Physician, Neurology Service, Centre Hospitalier, Lausanne, Switzerland

**Marie-Germaine Bousser, M.D.**
Clinical Professor, Department of Neurology, Pavillon Lemierre; Head, Department of Neurology, Hôpital Saint-Antoine, Paris, France

**Thomas Brott, M.D.**
Associate Professor, Department of Neurology, University of Cincinnati College of Medicine, Cincinnati, Ohio

**John C.M. Brust, M.D.**
Professor, Department of Neurology, Columbia University College of Physicians and Surgeons; Director, Neurology Service, Harlem Hospital Center, New York, New York

**Dario V. Caccamo, M.D.**
Senior Staff Member, Department of Pathology, Henry Ford Hospital, Detroit, Michigan

**Louis R. Caplan, M.D.**
Professor and Chairman, Department of Neurology, Tufts University School of Medicine; Neurologist-in-Chief, New England Medical Center Hospitals, Boston, Massachusetts

**Janet L. Cobb, M.P.H.**
Statistical Programmer, Statistics and Consulting Unit, Department of Mathematics, Boston University College of Liberal Arts, Boston, Massachusetts

**Bruce M. Coull, M.D.**
Professor, Department of Neurology, Oregon Health Sciences University School of Medicine, Portland, Oregon

**Robert M. Crowell, M.D.**
Associate Professor, Department of Surgery, Harvard Medical School; Director, Division of Cerebrovascular Surgery, Department of Neurosurgery, Massachusetts General Hospital, Boston, Massachusetts

**Ralph B. D'Agostino, Ph.D.**
Professor of Mathematics and Statistics, Division of Statistics, and Director, Statistics and Consulting Unit, Department of Mathematics, Boston University College of Liberal Arts, Boston, Massachusetts

**Thomas J. DeGraba, M.D.**
Assistant Professor, Department of Neurology, University of Texas Medical School at Houston, Houston, Texas

**Henry B. Dinsdale, M.D., F.R.C.P.(C), F.A.C.P.**
Professor and Head, Department of Medicine, Queens University Faculty of Medicine; Physician-in-Chief, Kingston General Hospital; Physician-in-Chief, Hôtel Dieu, Kingston, Ontario, Canada

**J. Donald Easton, M.D.**
Professor and Chairman, Department of Clinical Neurosciences, Brown University Program in Medicine; Neurologist-in-Chief, Rhode Island Hospital, Providence, Rhode Island

**M.E. Fink, M.D.**
Associate Professor, Departments of Neurology and Neurological Surgery, Columbia University College of Physicians and Surgeons; Director, Gavin K. MacBain Neuro-Intensive Care Unit, Division of Critical Care Neurology, Department of Neurology, Columbia Presbyterian Medical Center, New York, New York

**Marc Fisher, M.D.**
Professor, Department of Neurology, University of Massachusetts Medical School; Chief, Department of Neurology, Medical Center of Central Massachusetts, Worcester, Massachusetts

**Robert A. Fishman, M.D.**
Professor, Department of Neurology, University of California, San Francisco, School of Medicine, San Francisco, California

**Allan J. Fox, M.D., F.R.C.P.(C)**
Professor, Departments of Diagnostic Radiology and Clinical Neurological Sciences, University of Western Ontario Faculty of Medicine; Director, Department of Neuroradiology, University Hospital, London, Ontario, Canada

**Anthony J. Furlan, M.D.**
Assistant Clinical Professor, Department of Neurology, Case Western Reserve University School of Medicine, Cleveland, Ohio; Assistant Clinical Professor, Department of Neurology, Pennsylvania State University College of Medicine, Hershey, Pennsylvania; Medical Director, Cerebral Vascular Center, Department of Neurology, Cleveland Clinic Foundation, Cleveland, Ohio

**Julio H. Garcia, M.D.**
Head, Division of Neuropathology, Department of Pathology, Henry Ford Hospital, Detroit, Michigan

**J.C. Gautier, M.D.**
Professor, Department of Neurology, University of Paris Faculty of Medicine; Chief of Service, Cerebrovascular Emergencies, Groupe Hospitalier Pitie-Salpêtriere, Paris, France

**Scott H. Goodnight, M.D.**
Professor, Departments of Pathology and Medicine, Oregon Health Sciences University School of Medicine, Portland, Oregon

**Yasunobu Goto, M.D.**
Department of Neurosurgery, National Cardiovascular Center, Osaka, Japan

**Glen E. Gresham, M.D.**
Professor and Chairman, Department of Rehabilitation Medicine, State University of New York at Buffalo School of Medicine and Biomedical Sciences; Director, Department of Rehabilitation Medicine, Erie County Medical Center, Buffalo, New York

**Marina Grisoli, M.D.**
Assistant Neuroradiologist, Department of Neuroradiology, Istituto Nazionale Neurologico "Carlo Besta," Milan, Italy

**James C. Grotta, M.D.**
Professor, Department of Neurology, University of Texas Medical School at Houston, Houston, Texas

**Vladimir C. Hachinski, M.D., D.Sc.**
Professor and Chairman, Department of Clinical Neurological Sciences, University of Western Ontario Faculty of Medicine, London, Ontario, Canada

**Sandra Hanson, M.D.**
Instructor, Department of Neurology, University of Texas Medical School at Houston, Houston, Texas

**Robert G. Hart, M.D.**
Associate Professor, Department of Medicine, University of Texas Medical School at San Antonio, San Antonio, Texas

**Shirish M. Hastak, M.D., D.M.**
Fellow, Department of Clinical Neurological Sciences, University of Western Ontario Faculty of Medicine; Fellow, Department of Clinical Neurological Sciences, University Hospital, London, Ontario, Canada

**Edward B. Healton, M.D.**
Associate Clinical Professor, Department of Neurology, and Associate Dean, Columbia University College of Physicians and Surgeons, New York, New York

**Michael Hennerici, M.D.**
Professor and Chairman, Department of Neurology, Mannheim Medical School of the University of Heidelberg, Heidelberg, Germany

**Daniel B. Hier, M.D.**
Professor and Chairman, Department of Neurology, University of Illinois College of Medicine, Chicago, Illinois

**S.K. Hilal, M.D., Ph.D.**
Professor, Department of Radiology, Columbia University College of Physicians and Surgeons; Director, Department of Neuroradiology, Neurological Institute, Columbia Presbyterian Medical Center, New York, New York

**Jack Hirsh, M.D.**
Professor, Department of Medicine, McMaster University School of Medicine; Director, Hamilton Civic Hospitals Research Centre, Hamilton, Ontario, Canada

**Khang-Loon Ho, M.D.**
Senior Staff Member, Department of Pathology, Henry Ford Hospital, Detroit, Michigan

**Michael Jacewicz, M.D.**
Assistant Professor, Department of Neurology, University of Tennessee, Memphis, College of Medicine; Chief, Neurology Service, Regional Medical Center at Memphis, Memphis, Tennessee

**Carlos S. Kase, M.D.**
Professor, Department of Neurology, Boston University School of Medicine, Boston, Massachusetts

**Hiroyuki Kato, M.D., D.M., Sc.**
Department of Neurology, Institute of Brain Diseases, Tohoku University School of Medicine, Sendai, Japan

**J. Philip Kistler, M.D.**
Associate Professor, Department of Neurology, Harvard Medical School; Associate Neurologist, Neurology Service, Massachusetts General Hospital, Boston, Massachusetts

**Kyuya Kogure, M.D., D.M., Sc.**
Professor and Chairman, Department of Neurology, Institute of Brain Diseases, Tohoku University School of Medicine, Sendai, Japan

**Donald H. Lee, M.D., F.R.C.P.(C)**
Assistant Professor, Departments of Diagnostic Radiology and Clinical Neurological Sciences, University of Western Ontario Faculty of Medicine, London, Ontario, Canada

**Betsy B. Love, M.D.**
Fellow, Department of Neurology, University of Iowa College of Medicine, Iowa City, Iowa

**Stephen P. Lownie, M.D., F.R.C.S.C.**
Assistant Professor, Department of Clinical Neurological Sciences, University of Western Ontario Faculty of Medicine, London, Ontario, Canada

**Paul C. McCormick, M.D.**
Assistant Professor, Department of Neurosurgery, Columbia University College of Physicians and Surgeons; Assistant Attending Neurosurgeon, Department of Neurology, Neurological Institute, Columbia Presbyterian Medical Center, New York, New York

**J.P. Mohr, M.D.**
Sciarra Professor, Department of Neurology, Columbia University College of Physicians and Surgeons; Director, Division of Cerebrovascular Research, Department of Neurology, Neurological Institute, Columbia Presbyterian Medical Center, New York, New York

**J.W. Norris, M.D., F.R.C.P.**
Professor, Division of Neurology, Department of Medicine, University of Toronto Faculty of Medicine; Director, Stroke Research Unit, Sunnybrook Health Science Center, Toronto, Ontario, Canada

**Nobuyoshi Ogata, M.D.**
Department of Neurosurgery, National Cardiovascular Center, Osaka, Japan

**Christopher S. Ogilvy, M.D.**
Assistant Professor, Department of Surgery, Harvard Medical School; Assistant Visiting Neurosurgeon, Department of Neurosurgery, Massachusetts General Hospital, Boston, Massachusetts

**Robert G. Ojemann, M.D.**
Professor, Department of Surgery, Harvard Medical School; Visiting Neurosurgeon, Department of Neurosurgery, Massachusetts General Hospital, Boston, Masschusetts

**David M. Pelz, M.D., F.R.C.P.(C)**
Associate Professor, Departments of Diagnostic Radiology and Clinical Neurological Sciences, University of Western Ontario Faculty of Medicine, London, Ontario, Canada

**Michael S. Pessin, M.D.**
Professor, Department of Neurology, Tufts University School of Medicine; Senior Neurologist, New England Medical Center Hospitals, Boston, Massachusetts

**George W. Petty, M.D.**
Assistant Professor, Department of Neurology, Mayo Medical School; Senior Associate Consultant, Department of Neurology, Mayo Clinic, Rochester, Minnesota

**William A. Pulsinelli, M.D., Ph.D.**
Professor and Chairman, Department of Neurology, University of Tennessee, Memphis, College of Medicine; Chief, Department of Neurology, Semmes-Murphey Clinic, Memphis, Tennessee

**Wolfgang Rautenberg, M.D.**
Associate Professor, Department of Neurology, Mannheim Medical School of the University of Heidelberg, Heidelberg, Germany

**James T. Robertson, M.D.**
Professor and Chairman, Department of Neurosurgery, University of Tennessee, Memphis, College of Medicine, Memphis, Tennessee

**R.L. Sacco, M.D.**
Assistant Professor, Departments of Neurology and Public Health (Epidemiology), Columbia University College of Physicians and Surgeons, New York, New York

**Jeffrey L. Saver, M.D.**
Clinical Instructor, Department of Clinical Neurosciences, Brown University Program in Medicine; Assistant Neurologist, Department of Neurology, Rhode Island Hospital, Providence, Rhode Island

**Mario Savoiardo, M.D.**
Associate Chief, Department of Neuroradiology, Istituto Nazionale Neurologico "Carlo Besta," Milan, Italy

**Robert F. Spetzler, M.D.**
Professor and Chairman, Division of Neurosurgery, Department of Surgery, University of Arizona College of Medicine; J.N. Harber Chairman of Neurological Surgery and Director, Barrow Neurological Institute, Phoenix, Arizona

**Bennett M. Stein, M.D.**
Byron Stookey Professor and Chairman, Department of Neurological Surgery, Columbia University College of Physicians and Surgeons; Director, Department of Neurological Surgery, Neurological Institute, Columbia Presbyterian Medical Center, New York, New York

**Wolfgang Steinke, M.D.**
Department of Neurology, Mannheim Medical School of the University of Heidelberg, Heidelberg, Germany

**Jonathan Y. Streifler, M.D.**
Department of Neurology, Petah Tikva and the Sackler Faculty of Medicine, Tel Aviv University, Tel Aviv, Israel

**Thomas K. Tatemichi, M.D.**
Associate Professor, Department of Neurology, Neurological Institute, Columbia Presbyterian Medical Center, New York, New York

**Harry V. Vinters, M.D., F.R.C.P.(C)**
Associate Professor, Division of Neuropathology, Department of Pathology, University of California, Los Angeles, UCLA School of Medicine; Member, Brain Research Institute, UCLA Medical Center, Los Angeles, California

**Fernando Viñuela, M.D.**
Professor, Department of Radiology, University of California, Los Angeles, UCLA School of Medicine; Director, Endovascular Therapy Service, Division of Neuroradiology, Department of Radiological Sciences, UCLA Medical Center, Los Angeles, California

**Babette B. Weksler, M.D.**
Professor, Department of Medicine, Cornell University Medical College, New York, New York

**Philip A. Wolf, M.D.**
Professor, Department of Neurology, and Research Professor of Preventive Medicine and Epidemiology, Department of Medicine, Boston University School of Medicine; Senior Visiting Physician, Department of Neurology, University Hospital, Boston, Massachusetts

**Frank M. Yatsu, M.D.**
Professor and Chairman, Department of Neurology, University of Texas Medical School at Houston, Houston, Texas

**Yasuhiro Yonekawa, M.D.**
Professor and Chairman, Department of Neurosurgery, National Cardiovascular Center, Osaka, Japan

**Joseph M. Zabramski, M.D.**
Clinical Assistant Professor, Division of Neurosurgery, Department of Surgery, University of Arizona College of Medicine; Chairman, Section of Cerebrovascular Surgery, and Director, Neurosurgical Laboratory, Barrow Neurological Institute, Phoenix, Arizona

# PREFACE

The first edition of *Stroke* reflected the rapidly advancing knowledge in diagnostic techniques, research, and interventional therapies, which promised to lead to the discarding of past nihilisms toward stroke treatment. This second edition "stands on the shoulders of those previous observations" in reflecting the flourishing advances in pathophysiologic insights, diagnostic accuracies, and effective therapies to both reduce brain damage from strokes and minimize stroke recurrences. Progress in neuroimaging techniques for cerebral vascular changes and in the understanding of brain metabolism have redefined the nature of cerebrovascular diseases as a dynamic and evolving process. This knowledge has ignited the quest for greater diagnostic accuracy and precise therapies. Interventional neuroradiology has also made substantial inroads in improving diagnostic precision and in therapy, particularly for aneurysms and arteriovenous malformations. Finally, the development and refinement of modern, sophisticated clinical trial designs to achieve scientifically valid and statistically meaningful conclusions have resulted in a number of important and definitive studies on stroke, such as those on carotid endarterectomy for transient ischemic attacks (TIAs), anticoagulation for atrial fibrillation, and the use of ticlopidine for TIAs, to mention but a few. Thus, by culling from the first edition, refining and enhancing where necessary, we are able to present a comprehensive body of work in a clinically useful single volume.

As we stated in the Preface to the first edition and now reiterate with conviction and a sense of achievement, "We have organized the book to provide practical and ready access to the conventional approaches to stroke syndromes, but have also examined viable future options in stroke therapy and prevention. More importantly, we hope we have conveyed a sense of the excitement of stroke research, the enthusiasm for which is fueled by the certain knowledge that stroke occurrences can be further curtailed to an irreducible minimum."

*Henry J.M. Barnett,* M.D.
*J.P. Mohr,* M.D.
*Bennett M. Stein,* M.D.
*Frank M. Yatsu,* M.D.

# *ACKNOWLEDGMENTS*

The editors are grateful to the following organizations and foundations, whose interest and support helped make this contribution on stroke a reality.

The Adriana Blood Endowment, Houston, Texas
The Clayton Foundation for Research, Houston, Texas
The Cullen Trust for Healthcare, Houston, Texas
The Horace B. Goldsmith Foundation, New York, New York
The Richard Ivey Foundation, London, Ontario, Canada
National Institutes of Neurological Disease and Stroke, Bethesda, Maryland
The Sciarra Research Fund of New York, New York, New York
The Byron Stookey Professorship of Neurological Surgery, Columbia University College of Physicians and Surgeons, New York, New York

# CONTENTS

# STROKE

## Pathophysiology, Diagnosis, and Management

*Second Edition*

# *COLOR PLATES*

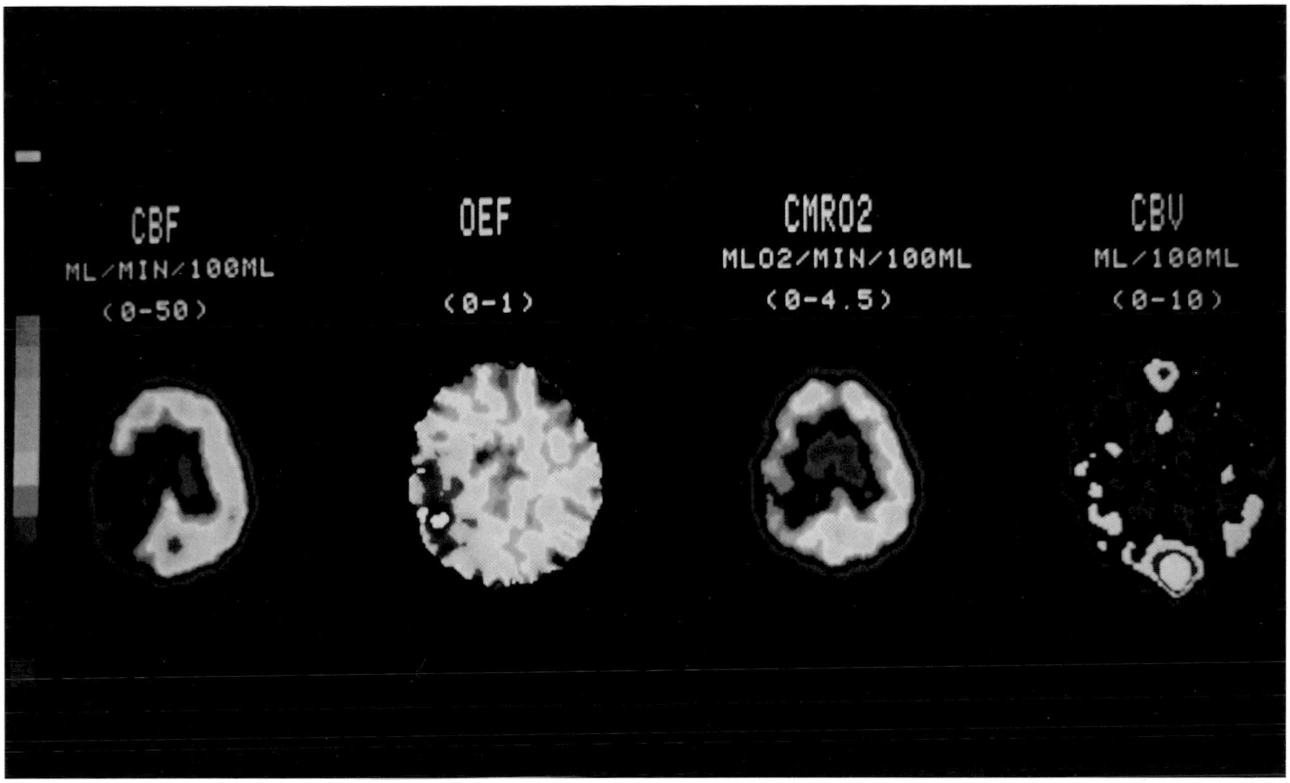


**Plate 6-1**

**Plate 6-1.** Quantitative positron emission tomographic (PET) images showing cerebral blood flow (CBF), oxygen extraction fraction (OEF), cerebral metabolic rate of oxygen ($CMRO_2$), and cerebral blood volume (CBV) according to a pseudocolor scale ranging from 0 to a maximum pixel value of 50 ml/100 ml/min, unity, 4.5 ml/100 ml/min, and 10 ml/100 ml, respectively. The data were obtained using the $^{15}O$ continuous inhalation technique at a level 60 mm above and parallel to the orbitomeatal line in a 76-year-old patient 30 hours after the abrupt onset of right hemiparesis and global aphasia due to middle cerebral artery embolism from a cardiac source; at the time of the PET study, clinical recovery was rapid. On these images, the left side of the brain is to the reader's left, and anterior is at the top. There is a marked reduction of CBF in the left parietorolandic cortex (minimum value: 13 ml/100 ml/min) associated with a markedly increased OEF (maximum value: 1.90 ml/100 ml/min) and a marginally increased CBF. This pattern of critical cerebral ischemia (?"penumbra") still present 30 hours after the onset of stroke was associated with an excellent clinical outcome and normal corresponding computed tomographic scan at follow-up, suggesting potentially viable tissue.

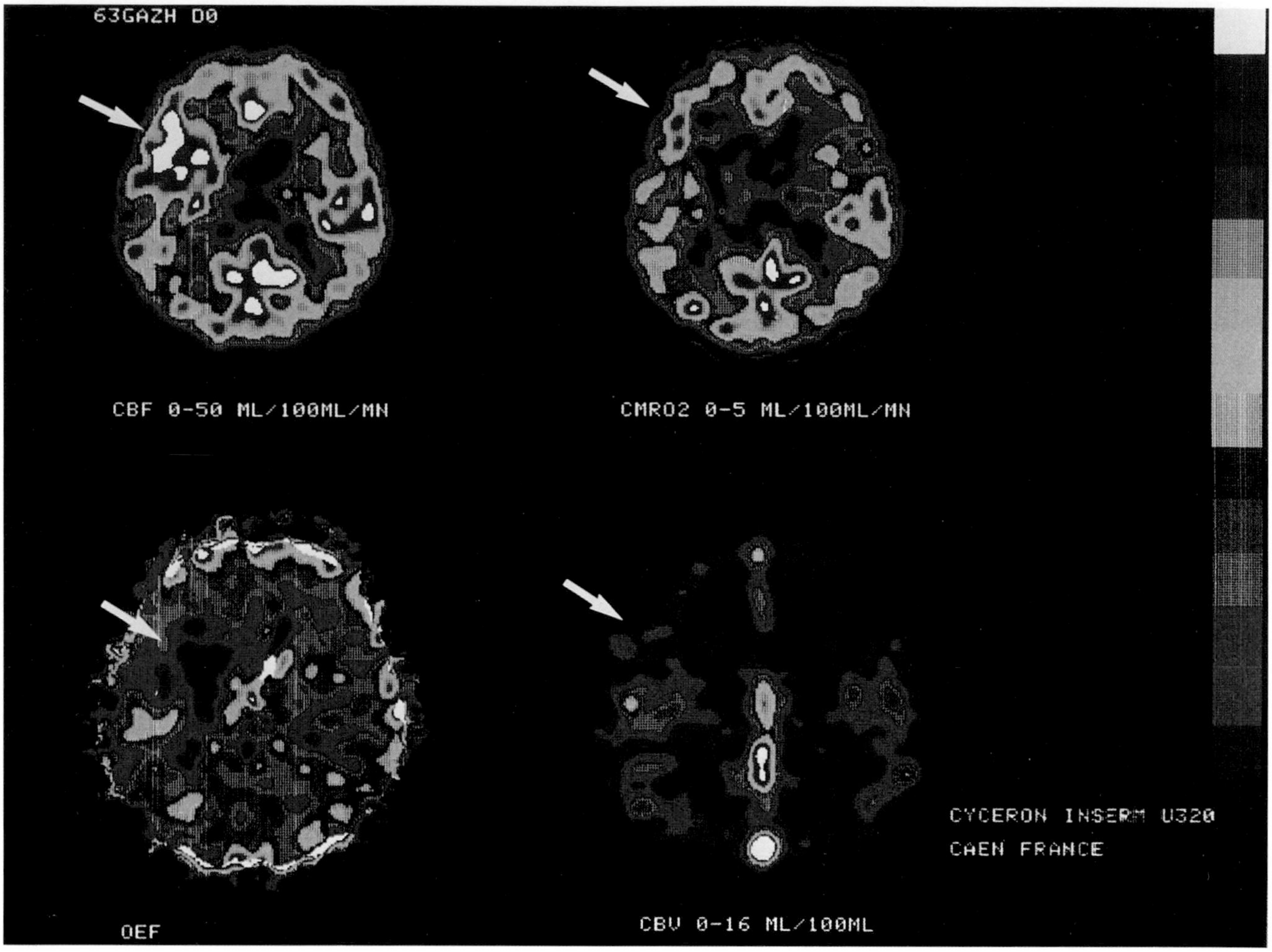


**Plate 6-2**

**Plate 6-2.** Quantitative positron emission tomographic (PET) images of cerebral blood flow (CBF), cerebral metabolic rate of oxygen ($CMRO_2$), oxygen extraction fraction (OEF), and cerebral blood volume (CBV) obtained at the level of the basal ganglia in a 61-year-old patient 16 hours after onset of left hemiparesis presumably due to right-middle cerebral artery embolism of cardiac origin. The images are shown according to a pseudocolor scale ranging from 0 to a maximum pixel value of 50 ml/100 ml/min, 5 ml/100 ml/min, unity, and 16 ml/100 ml for CBF, $CMRO_2$, OEF, and CBV, respectively; the right side of the brain is on the reader's left side. The data demonstrate an area of increased CBF in the right perisylvian, insula, and basal ganglia regions, associated with an increased CBF and a decreased OEF ("luxury-perfusion" with absolute hyperemia, documenting early reperfusion of previously ischemic tissue). The $CMRO_2$ is preserved in the cortical ribbon, which was morphologically intact at follow-up computed tomographic scan (obtained at day 62 post-stroke).

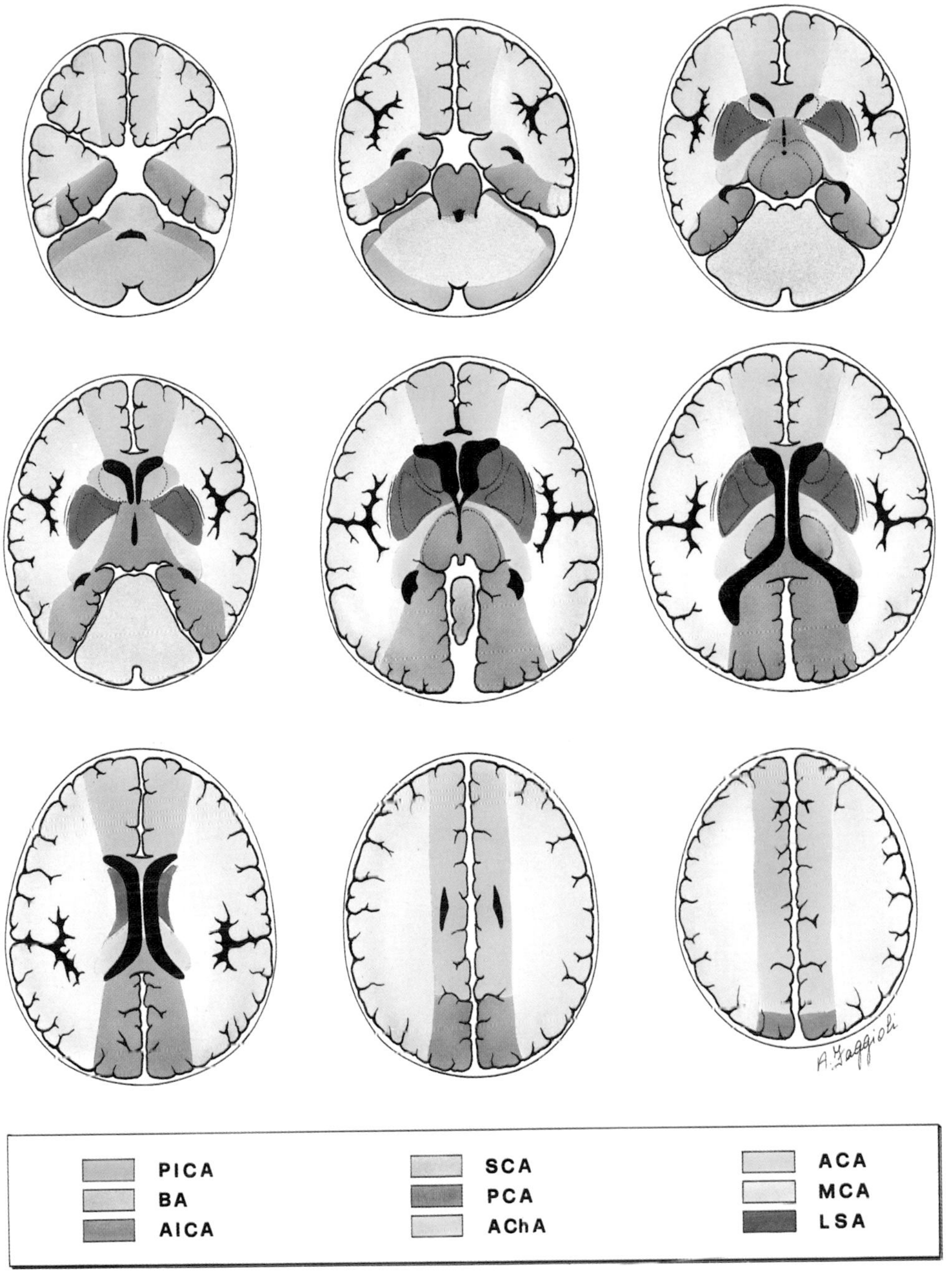


**Plate 9-1**

**Plate 9-1.** Vascular territories. Territory of perforating lenticulostriate arteries (LSA) of the middle cerebral artery (MCA) is indicated separately. Posterior cerebral artery (PCA) territory includes that of the perforating branches of the posterior communicating artery. Variations and overlapping of territories are frequent, particularly in posterior fossa, between the posterior inferior cerebellar artery (PICA) and the anterior inferior cerebellar artery (AICA), and at the genu of the internal capsule. BA, basilar artery; SCA, superior cerebellar artery; AChA, anterior choroidal artery; ACA, anterior cerebral artery. (From Savoiardo M: The vascular territories of the carotid and vertebrobasilar system. Diagrams based on CT studies. Ital J Neurol Sci 7:405, 1986, with permission.)

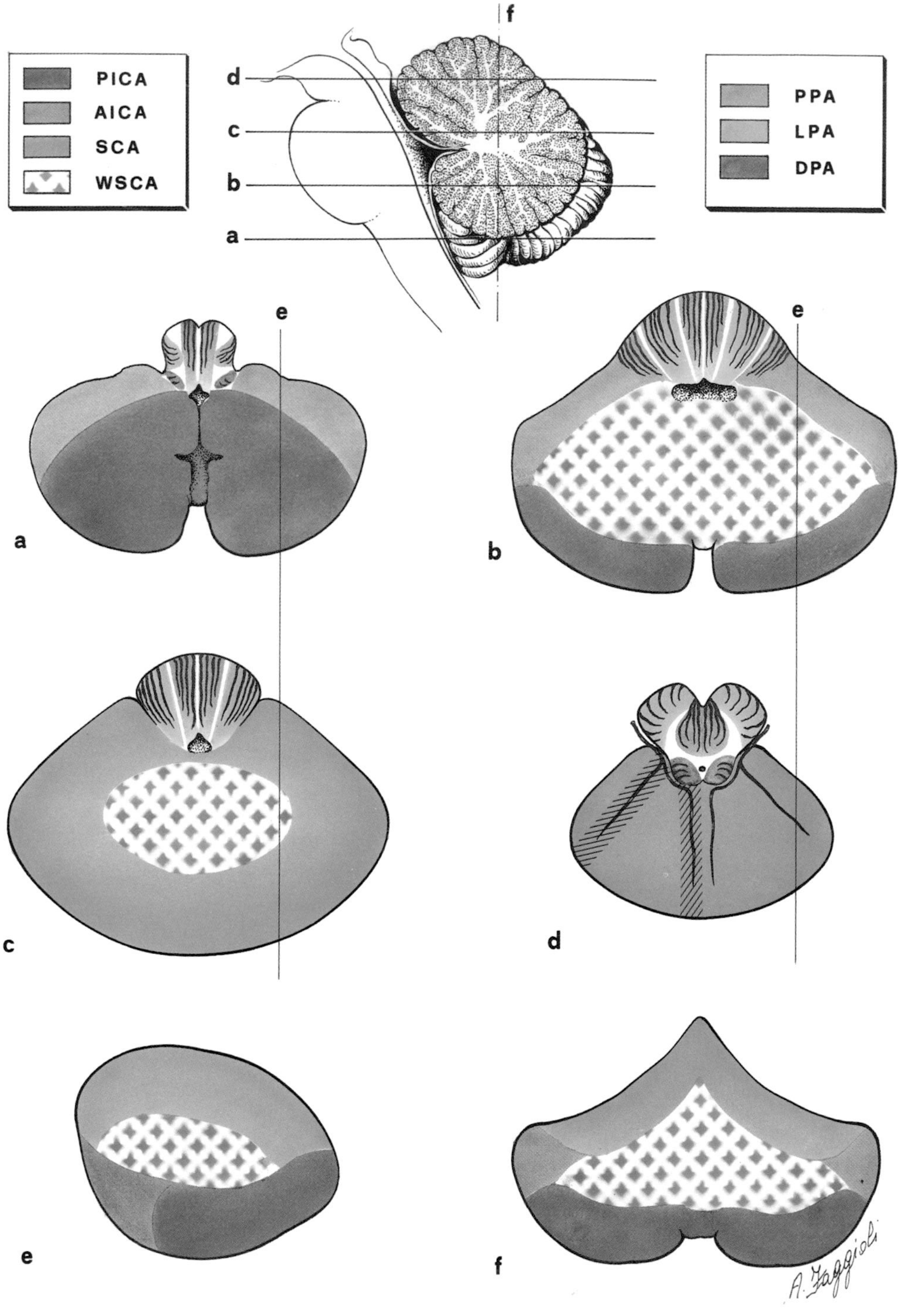


**Plate 9-2**

**Plate 9-2.** Detailed schematic drawing of vascular territories in cerebellum and brain stem obtained from computed tomography and magnetic resonance imaging studies. (**A–D**) Axial, (**E**) sagittal paramedian, and (**F**) coronal sections are shown. Course of penetrating branches of the brain stem is superimposed on territories. Orientation of vermian and hemispheric branches of the superior cerebellar artery (SCA) is indicated in Fig. D; distribution of infarcts in these territories is indicated by shading. PICA, posterior inferior cerebellar artery; AICA, anterior inferior cerebellar artery; WSCA, watershed area in deep white matter mostly supplied by SCA; PPA, paramedian penetrating arteries; LPA, lateral penetrating arteries; DPA, dorsal penetrating arteries. (From Savoiardo M, Bracchi M, Passerini A, Visciani A: The vascular territories in the cerebellum and brainstem: CT and MR study. AJNR 8:199, 1987, with permission.)

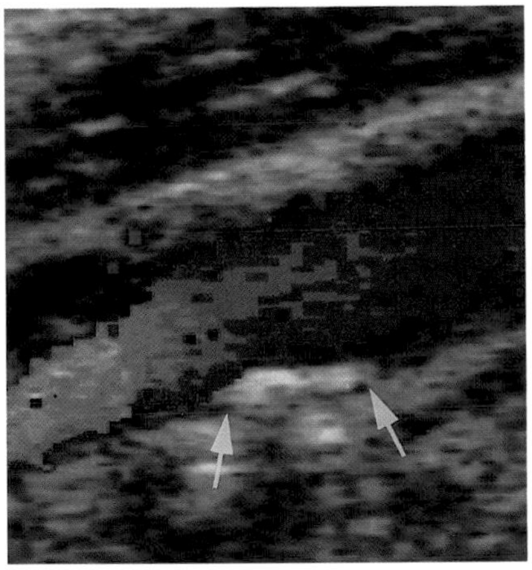

**Plate 12-1A**

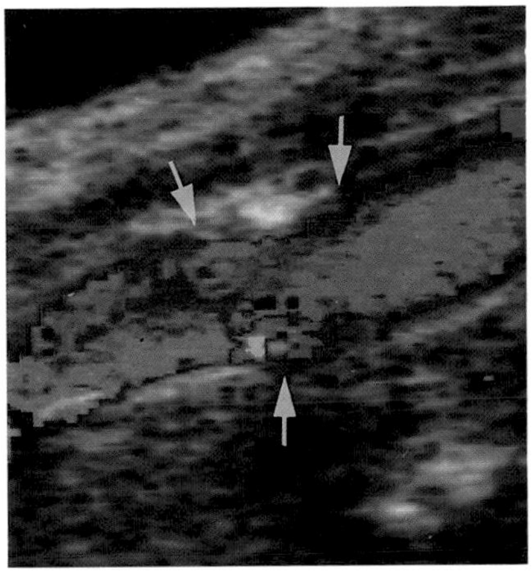

**Plate 12-1B**

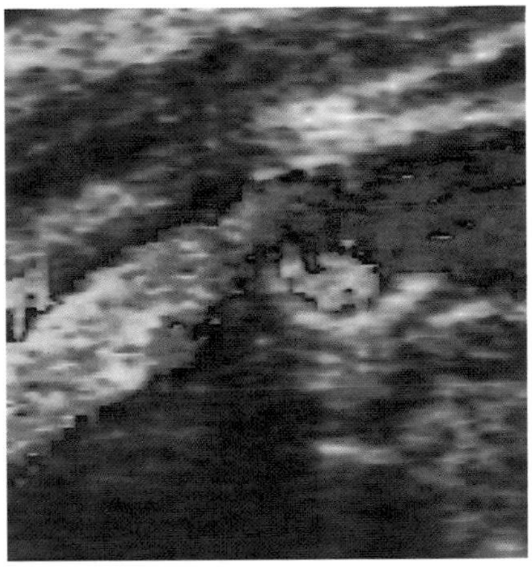

**Plate 12-1C**

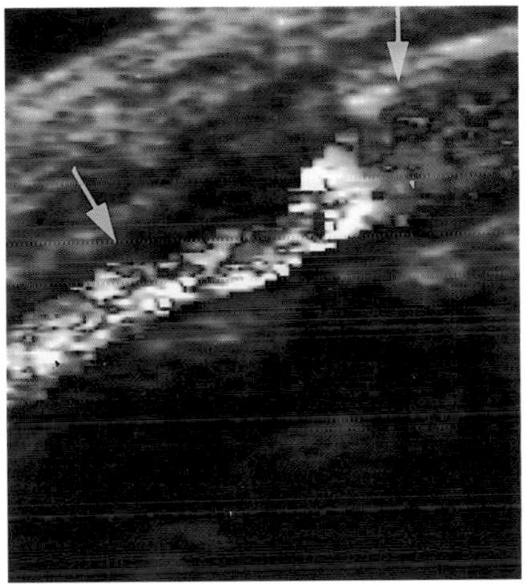

**Plate 12-2A**

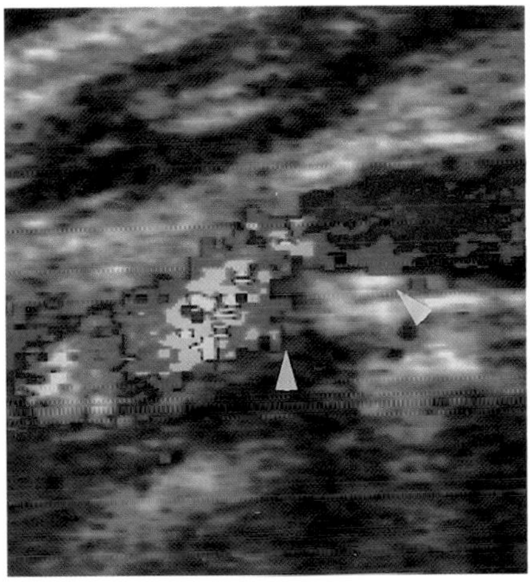

**Plate 12-2B**

**Plate 12-1.** Color Doppler flow imaging of nonstenotic carotid artery plaques (arrows indicate plaque extent). (**A**) Undisturbed flow dynamics at the site of a smooth homogeneous bifurcation plaque. (**B**) Smooth, homogeneous plaque at the anterior wall of the bifurcation; small plaque with adjacent minor turbulence at the opposite vessel wall. (**C**) Central ulcer crater with blue coded turbulence in a partially calcified plaque.

**Plate 12-2.** Color Doppler flow imaging of internal carotid artery (ICA) stenoses (arrows indicate plaque extent). (**A**) Moderate smooth ICA stenosis with a long segment of color fading and minor turbulence (blue). (**B**) Wedge-shaped plaque at the origin of the ICA producing a high-grade stenosis. Poststenotic mixed hemodynamic pattern with aliasing, flow reversal, and scattered turbulence.

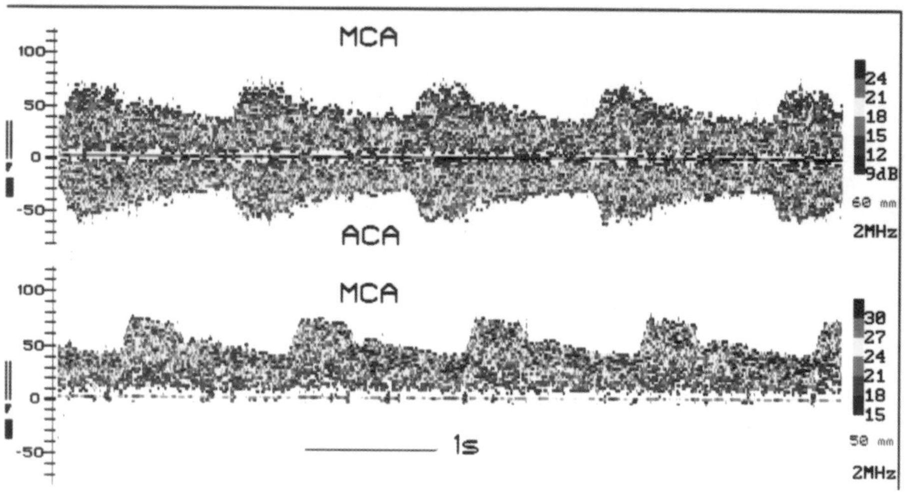


Plate 12-3

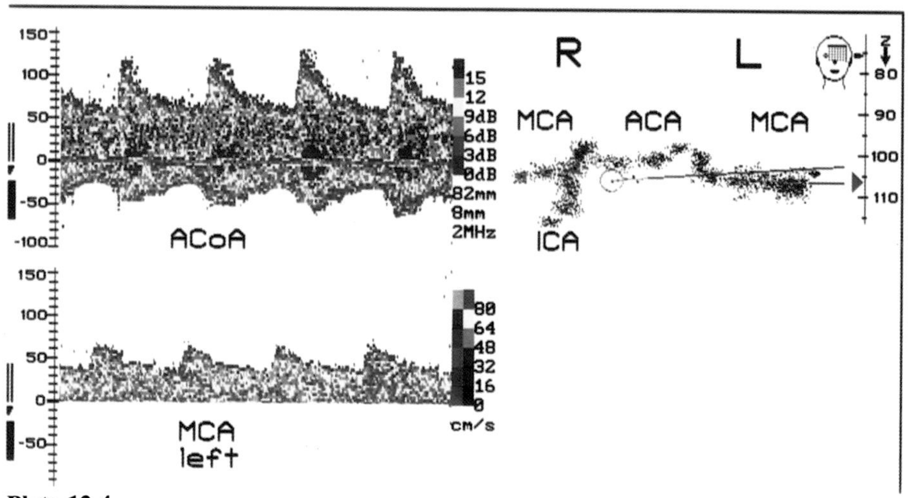


Plate 12-4

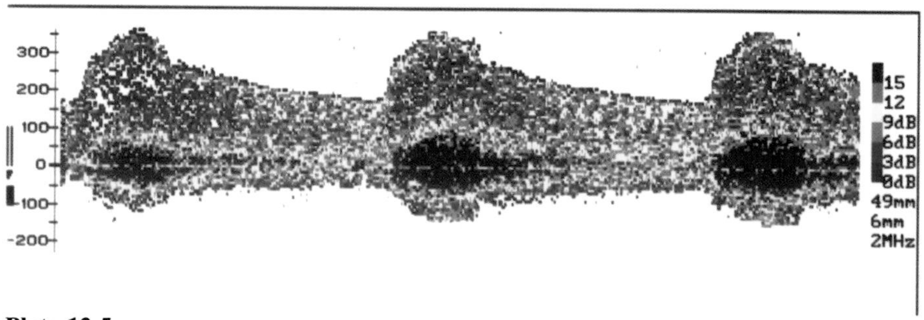


Plate 12-5

**Plate 12-3.** Doppler spectra of the middle cerebral artery (MCA) and anterior cerebral artery (ACA).

**Plate 12-4.** (Left) Doppler spectra of anterior communicating artery (ACoA) (increased velocities, low frequency signals) and left middle cerebral artery (MCA) (normal velocities) are shown in a patient with internal carotid artery (ICA) occlusion. (Right) A frontal view of the basal cerebral arteries as recorded from selected positions of the sample volume in the same patient.

**Plate 12-5.** High-grade stenosis of the left middle cerebral artery shown by transcranial Doppler examination (increased velocities, low frequency signals) and magnetic resonance angiography (anteroposterior and axial views).

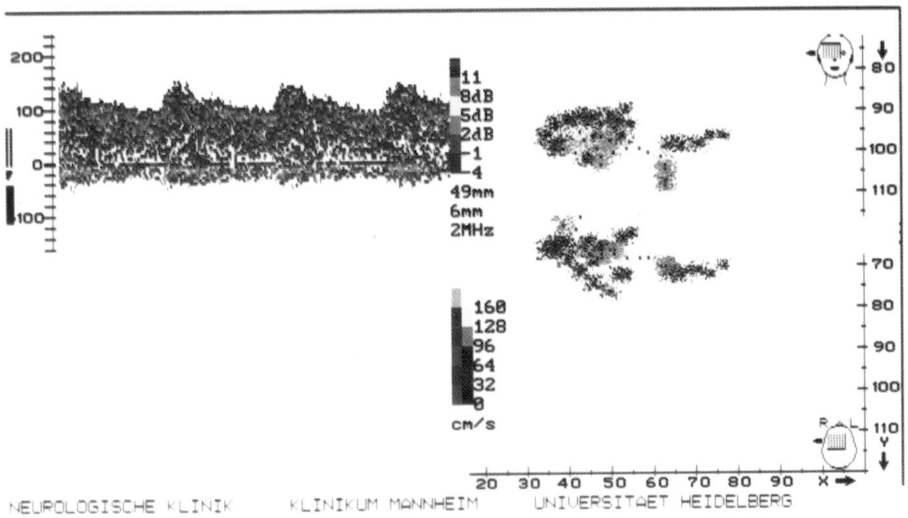


**Plate 12-6**

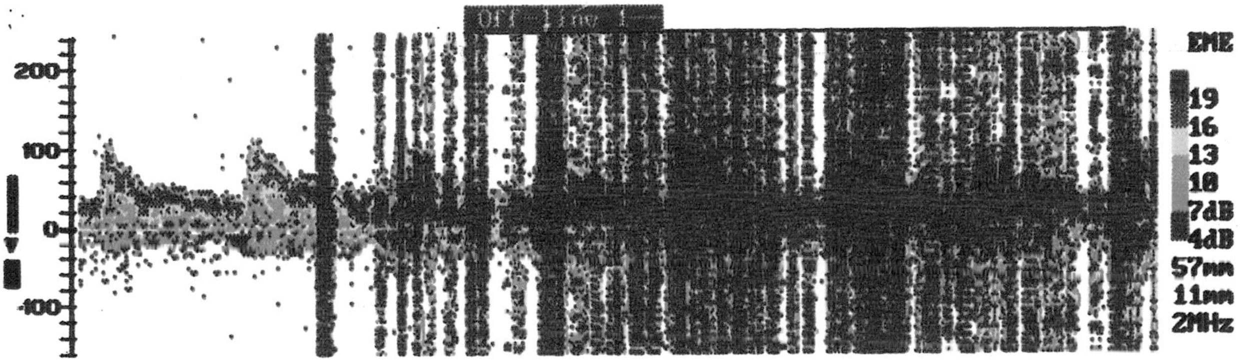


**Plate 12-7**

**Plate 12-6.** Two-dimensional transcranial Doppler investigation of arteriovenous malformation on the right side, illustrating the extent of the lesion and offering detailed hemodynamic information within distinct areas of the lesion.

**Plate 12-7.** Transcranial Doppler image showing sudden appearance of a bolus of microbubbles in the middle cerebral artery.

# I

# *PATHOPHYSIOLOGY OF STROKE*

## Frank M. Yatsu, Section Editor

A literal explosion of information, to use an old cliche, accurately describes the dramatic increase in sophisticated and promising research in strokes, largely attributable to the use of reproducible animal models of strokes and the application of modern investigative tools, such as those of molecular and cellular biology. This unprecedented growth in knowledge about stroke pathophysiology and insights into therapy are being pursued globally, as reflected by contributions on positron emission tomography (PET) from France and on the neurobiology of brain ischemia from Japan. The exciting leap forward was signaled and palpably intensified by knowledge that ischemically impaired brain cells undergo infarction by a series of defined neurochemical events, such as the action of excitotoxins or the influx of channel ions, which can be modified to avert infarction. In addition to leads from basic studies, now being translated into clinical trials, such as the use of excitotoxin inhibitors or calcium channel blockers, greater insight into the pathogenesis of atherosclerosis causing strokes promises to provide more specific strategies for stroke prevention, the ultimate treatment of strokes due to atherosclerosis. The various pathophysiologic updates on strokes that impact the bedside care of stroke patients is reviewed comprehensively by experienced and respected investigators and include epidemiology, atherosclerosis, animal models, neurochemistry/neurobiology of brain ischemia, cerebral spinal fluid (CSF), positron emission tomography (PET), and neuropathology.

# 1

# *EPIDEMIOLOGY OF STROKE*

Philip A. Wolf
Janet L. Cobb
Ralph B. D'Agostino

Stroke is the most common life-threatening neurologic disease and is the third leading cause of death in the United States, after heart disease and cancer. Although stroke is more often disabling than lethal, 150,300 deaths were attributed to stroke in 1988.[6] In the elderly, the segment of the population where most stroke occurs, it was also a major source of disability leading to institutionalization. The American Heart Association estimates there were 2,020,000 stroke survivors in the United States in 1986, many of whom required chronic care.[6]

Epidemiology is "the study of the distribution and determinants of disease frequency" in human populations.[52] Any consideration of the epidemiology of stroke, therefore, needs to include both elements: distribution—disease incidence, prevalence, and secular trends—and determinants—predisposing conditions and risk factors. Since stroke results from a number of pathologic processes, the distribution and determinants of specific stroke subtypes must be considered as well. Recent studies have provided new insights into risk factors for embolic stroke, and for intracerebral and subarachnoid hemorrhage, and these are reviewed in detail in this chapter.

While medical and surgical therapies to reduce the damage from impending or recent-onset stroke must be pursued, it seems likely that prevention will be the most effective strategy in reducing the ravages of cerebrovascular disease. Prevention will be facilitated by an understanding of predisposing host and environmental factors, which have been identified and defined in recent years, chiefly through prospective epidemiologic study. The relative impact of each of these risk factors is becoming clearer and controlled clinical trials have demonstrated the efficacy of risk factor modification in stroke prevention.

In addition to relying on a review of the pertinent literature, in this chapter we utilize, when appropriate, 36-year follow-up data from the Framingham Study. This prospective study of a general population sample is ideal for the examination of the determinants, incidence, and manifestations of stroke as they evolved over 36 years of follow-up. Assessment of risk factors, which were measured systematically and prospectively, many years prior to the appearance of clinical disease, provides the least distorted picture of the evolution of these host and environmental factors into clinical disease.

## INCIDENCE OF STROKE

The American Heart Association estimates that there were 500,000 new cases of stroke in the United States in 1986, and approximately 400,000 stroke patients are discharged annually from acute-care hospitals in the United States, three-fourths after an initial stroke and the remainder following recurrence.[6] Inci-

This work was supported in part by grants 2-RO1-NS-17950-09 (National Institute of Neurological Disorders and Stroke), R01-HL40423 (National Institute on Aging, National Heart, Lung, and Blood Institute), and Contract NIH-NO1-HC-38038 (National Heart, Lung, and Blood Institute).

dence of stroke was determined over 36 years of follow-up of 5,070 men and women, aged 30 to 62, who were free of cardiovascular disease (CVD) at entry to the study in 1950. The population was examined every 2 years, and follow-up was quite satisfactory.

Since 1968, study subjects suspected of stroke have been evaluated neurologically in the hospital at the time of the stroke. During the past 10 years at least one computed tomography (CT) scan of the brain was performed on approximately 85 percent of cases, and stroke type was confirmed by CT scan in 54 percent of all strokes. Over 36 years, since the study began, the neurologic deficit of the stroke was confirmed by a Framingham Study neurologist in 40 percent of cases; since 1981 when surveillance was intensified, nearly two-thirds of stroke cases have been confirmed in this way. Follow-up of the population has been satisfactory; less than 10 percent were completely lost to follow-up by death after 36 years.

After 36 years of follow-up in the Framingham Study, there were 693 cases of stroke and transient ischemic attacks (TIAs). The average annual incidence of all strokes combined increased with age and doubled in successive decades (Table 1-1). Perspective concerning incidence of coronary heart disease (CHD) and stroke may be gained by comparing analogous manifestations: myocardial infarction (MI) and stroke resulting from atherothrombotic brain infarction (ABI) (Fig. 1-1). Comparing these two major manifestations of atherosclerotic disease, age-adjusted average annual incidence rate of MI was three times that of ABI; in women MI incidence was approximately twice that of ABI. Comparing incidence by gender, MI developed 2.75 times more often in men than in women, while ABI was approximately 1.3 times more frequent in men. In both sexes, rates rose with age; however, the 20-year lag in MI incidence experienced by women was not seen for ABI, where age-specific rates were similar in both men and women. Comparing MI to ABI, in men the age-adjusted average annual incidence rate of MI was three times that of ABI; in women MI incidence was approximately twice that of ABI. Comparing incidence by gender, MI developed 2.75 times more often in men than in women, while ABI was approximately 1.3 times more frequent in men.

## FREQUENCY OF STROKE BY TYPE

The in-hospital assessment of stroke at Framingham by a study neurologist has helped document the stroke and determine stroke subtype as well as to differentiate stroke from other neurologic disease. Utilizing these data it was usually possible to determine if the stroke mechanism was hemorrhage or infarction and to distinguish subarachnoid from intraparenchymatous hemorrhage. Diagnosis of lacunar infarction was based on clinical and CT scan findings, while criteria for embolic infarction required a definite cardiac source for embolism. Distinguishing extracranial from intracranial cerebral infarction was made on clinical grounds, including noninvasive carotid studies; angiography was performed by the study subjects' personal physicians rather infrequently. The relative frequency of stroke by type shows there to be no substantial difference in stroke manifestation by sex (Fig. 1-2). Atherothrombotic brain infarction, including infarction secondary to large vessel atherothrombosis as well as lacunar infarction, occurred most frequently in 44 percent of the total. TIAs alone accounted for approximately 21 percent of all stroke events and were more frequent in men, while cerebral embolism (CE), 21 percent overall, was marginally more frequent in women (23 percent) than men (18 percent). Intracranial hemorrhage, accounted for 12 percent of all stroke events. Subarachnoid hemorrhage (SAH) was more frequent in women (7.2 percent) than men (5.9 percent) and was also slightly more prevalent (6.6 percent) than intracerebral hemorrhage (IH) (5.1 percent). SAH was invariably confirmed, by neurologic workup including angiography, to result from a ruptured berry aneurysm, while hemorrhage was verified by CT scan of

**TABLE 1-1. Two-Year Incidence of ABI and Stroke[a]**

| | Men | | | | Women | | | |
|---|---|---|---|---|---|---|---|---|
| | ABI | | Stroke | | ABI | | Stroke | |
| Age Group | Rate/1,000 | No. Cases | Rate/1,000 | No. Cases | Rate/1,000 | No. Cases | Rate/1,000 | No. Cases |
| 35–44 | 0.0 | 0 | 0.4 | 2 | 0.0 | 0 | 0.7 | 4 |
| 45–54 | 1.6 | 13 | 4.3 | 34 | 1.3 | 13 | 2.4 | 24 |
| 55–64 | 4.2 | 39 | 9.1 | 84 | 2.4 | 29 | 5.6 | 67 |
| 65–74 | 9.1 | 54 | 19.6 | 117 | 7.6 | 66 | 16.7 | 145 |
| 75–84 | 18.7 | 35 | 42.3 | 79 | 14.8 | 48 | 33.4 | 108 |
| 85–94 | 0.0 | 0 | 11.6 | 2 | 15.8 | 8 | 53.4 | 27 |
| Total | 4.8 | 141 | 10.7 | 318 | 4.1 | 164 | 9.4 | 375 |

*Abbreviation*: ABI, atherothrombotic brain infarction.
[a] All types combined in men and women.
(Data from the Framingham Study: 36-year follow-up.)

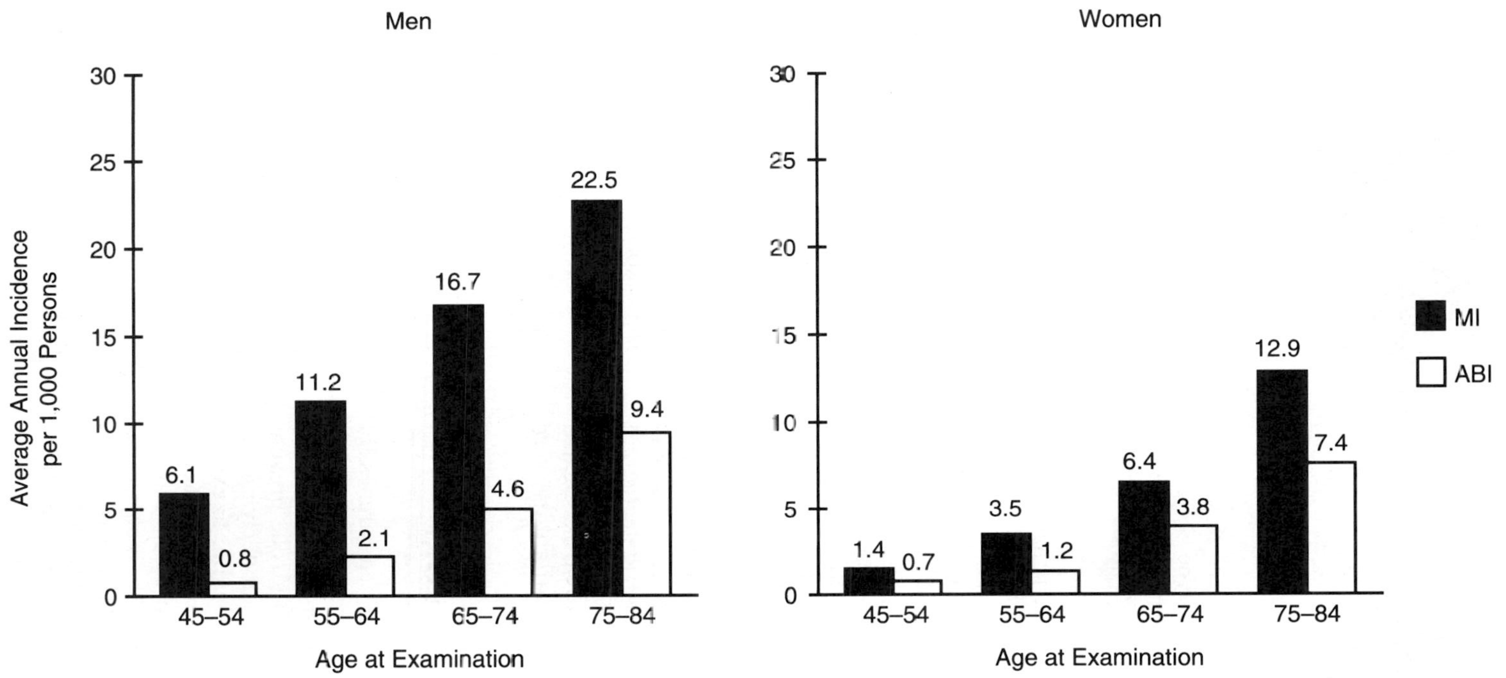


**Fig. 1-1.** Incidence of myocardial and brain infarction in men and women according to age categories: 36-year follow-up. (Data from the Framingham Study.)

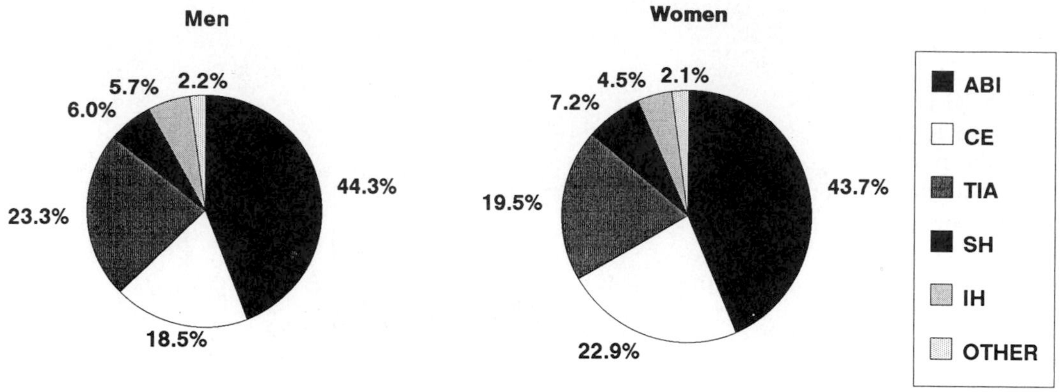


**Fig. 1-2.** Frequency of stroke by type in men and women: 36-year follow-up. ABI, atherothrombotic brain infarction; CE, cerebral embolism; TIA, transient ischemic attacks; SH, subarachnoid hemorrhage; IH, intracerebral hemorrhage. (Data from the Framingham Study.)

the brain. In other populations, in contrast to these Framingham findings, IH has been found to occur more frequently than SAH. For example, in Rochester, Minnesota between 1945 and 1976 primary IH was five times more frequent than SAH,[23] and most stroke registries have reported a higher prevalence of IH. In the Harvard Cooperative Stroke Registry, however, IH and SAH occurred with equal frequency (12 percent) among strokes hospitalized in two Boston hospitals.[56] In the National Survey of Stroke, a sample of hospitalized strokes in the United States from 1971 to 1976, rates were more like those in Framingham with 5.9 percent of stroke due to SAH and 6.3 percent attributed to IH.[63] The use of CT scan to distinguish between stroke types will detect small IHs previously counted as ABIs and probably not as SAHs. It is estimated that 24 percent of strokes called infarcts in decades prior to CT scan availability were probably IHs.[18]

## RISK FACTORS FOR STROKE

Identification of risk factors for stroke, awareness of its relative importance and of its interaction with other precursors, may yield important clues concerning pathogenesis and thereby lead to stroke prevention. Since the pathogenetic process underlying the various stroke types differ, it is reasonable to expect that risk factors for infarction differ from risk factors for hemorrhage. Furthermore, precursors of intraparenchymatous bleeding need not be identical to those for subarachnoid hemorrhage. There is reason to believe that risk factors for stroke from atherosclerosis of the carotid and vertebral arteries may differ in their impact when compared to stroke resulting from lacunar infarction, and precursors of embolic stroke are also likely to be different. Nevertheless, certain predisposing factors, particularly elevated blood pressure, seem common to most stroke types.

### Atherogenic Host Factors

Assessment of the importance of each of the major atherogenic risk factors was made specifically in that stroke type resulting most directly from atherothrombosis, ABI. The relative impact of each of these risk factors can be assessed in each sex, by comparing the size of the multivariate regression coefficients (Table 1-2). These coefficients were standardized for the varied units and scales, and take into account the contribution made by other risk factors. The larger the standardized multivariate regression coefficient the greater the impact on ABI incidence. Statistical significance indicates the risk factor made a significant independent contribution to risk in that age category even after the other cardiovascular risk factors were

**TABLE 1-2. Risk Factors for ABI: Standardized Multivariate Regression Coefficients[a]**

| Risk Factor | Standardized Multivariate Regression Coefficients | | | |
|---|---|---|---|---|
| | Men (Ages) | | Women (Ages) | |
| | 35–64 | 65–94 | 35–64 | 65–94 |
| Hypertension | 0.761*** | 0.426*** | 0.814*** | 0.477*** |
| Systolic BP | 0.613*** | 0.395*** | 0.629*** | 0.396*** |
| Diastolic BP | 0.642*** | 0.228* | 0.615*** | 0.369*** |
| LVH by ECG | 0.113 | 0.192** | 0.130* | 0.228*** |
| Cigarettes | 0.468*** | 0.197* | 0.090 | 0.274*** |
| Total chol. | −0.060 | −0.114 | 0.096 | −0.097 |
| Glucose intol. | 0.108 | 0.115 | 0.054 | 0.156* |
| Rel. weight | 0.266* | 0.009 | 0.157 | 0.195* |
| Hematocrit | 0.324* | 0.105 | 0.051 | −0.098 |

*Abbreviations*: ABI, atherothrombotic brain infarction; BP, blood pressure; LVH, left ventricular hypertrophy; ECG, electrocardiogram; chol., cholesterol; intol., intolerance; rel., relative.

* $P < 0.05$; ** $P < 0.01$; *** $P < 0.001$.

[a] Multivariate contains systolic blood pressure, LVH by ECG, cigarette smoking, glucose intolerance, total serum cholesterol, and the other appropriate variable.

(Data from the Framingham Study: 36-year follow-up.)

taken into account. These risk factors included definite hypertension, systolic blood pressure, diastolic blood pressure, left ventricular hypertrophy by electrocardiogram (ECG-LVH), cigarette smoking, total cholesterol, glucose intolerance, Metropolitan Relative Weight, and hematocrit. In addition, comparing the size of the coefficients in men and women and in younger and older age groups gives a clearer picture of the relative impact of each risk factor on brain infarction incidence.

## Hypertension

Hypertension is the paramount risk factor for stroke. The standardized multivariate regression coefficient of definite hypertension as a categorical variable for levels of blood pressure 160/95 mmHg or greater, is large in both men and women, denoting the powerful and independent contribution of definite hypertension to incidence of brain infarction. Normotension is considered to be present when pressures are less than 140/90; levels between 140/90 and 160/95 or greater are considered to represent borderline or mild hypertension (Fig. 1-3). It is noteworthy that the coefficient for hypertension is smaller in the older age group, corresponding to a reduced, but still statistically significant effect.

Overall, the age-adjusted relative risk of stroke among definite hypertensive persons, compared to normotensive persons, is 3.1 in men and 2.9 in women, and even borderline levels carry a 50 percent increased stroke risk (Table 1-3). By comparing relative risk of stroke in each age category it is apparent the impact of hypertension decreases with advancing age. However, definite hypertension still confers a significant increased risk of stroke in men and women aged 75 to 84 years. Risk of stroke is related to the level of the pressure throughout its range with no critical value of pressure, systolic or diastolic, below which stroke does not occur. For stroke generally, and for ABI specifically, there is no evidence that women tolerate hypertension better than men.

A substantial portion of stroke incidence is directly attributable to hypertension, and a portion of stroke in the population would be eliminated if hypertension were effectively treated.[16] This portion, the *population attributable fraction*, was estimated to be 56.4 percent of strokes in men and 66.1 percent in women based on an analysis of 26-year follow-up of Framingham data.

## Systolic versus Diastolic Pressure Level

Both systolic and diastolic blood pressure level are strongly and independently related to ABI incidence. Both components of blood pressure have the largest coefficients even in the oldest age group when compared with the other risk factors (Table 1-2). When compared to other components of blood pressure by means of average standardized regression coefficients (Table 1-4), it is apparent that neither pulse pressure, nor mean arterial pressure, nor diastolic blood pressure exerts more of an impact on ABI incidence than systolic blood pressure, although all are highly correlated and statistically significant. At each level of diastolic blood pressure, incidence of stroke rises as systolic blood pressure rises, in both men and women, and at normal, borderline, and hypertensive systolic blood pressure levels (Table 1-5). Furthermore, among persons with systolic blood pressures 160 mmHg or greater, stroke risk does not increase with increasing levels of diastolic blood pressure (Fig. 1-4). On the other hand, among persons with diastolic hypertension, incidence of stroke increases steadily as the level of systolic blood pressure rises (Fig. 1-4).

Diastolic blood pressure has been thought to be of greater importance than systolic pressure. Clinical trials of antihypertensive treatment and disease prevention, principally stroke, have used diastolic blood pressure as the basis for categorization of subjects. However, evidence for the ascendancy of diastolic blood pressure over systolic is lacking.[65] Diastolic blood pressure is difficult to measure accurately, varies within a narrower range than hypertension, and seems to offer no advantages in predicting cardiovas-

**TABLE 1-3. Relative Risk[a] of Stroke Among Hypertensive Patients by Age and Sex**

| Hypertensive Status | Age (years) 45–54 | 55–64 | 65–74 | 75–84 | Total Rate[b] Crude | Age-Adjusted |
|---|---|---|---|---|---|---|
| Men | | | | | | |
| Borderline | 3.1 | 2.3 | 1.8 | 0.7 | 1.9 | 1.5 |
| Definite | 4.6 | 5.1 | 3.2 | 1.9 | 3.8 | 3.1 |
| Women | | | | | | |
| Borderline | 2.4 | 1.5 | 2.0 | 1.1 | 2.5 | 1.5 |
| Definite | 3.6 | 3.6 | 4.4 | 1.4 | 5.2 | 2.9 |

[a] Relative to normotensive subjects.
[b] Total rate, both crude and age-adjusted, includes the age group 35–44.
(Data from the Framingham Study: 36-year follow-up.)

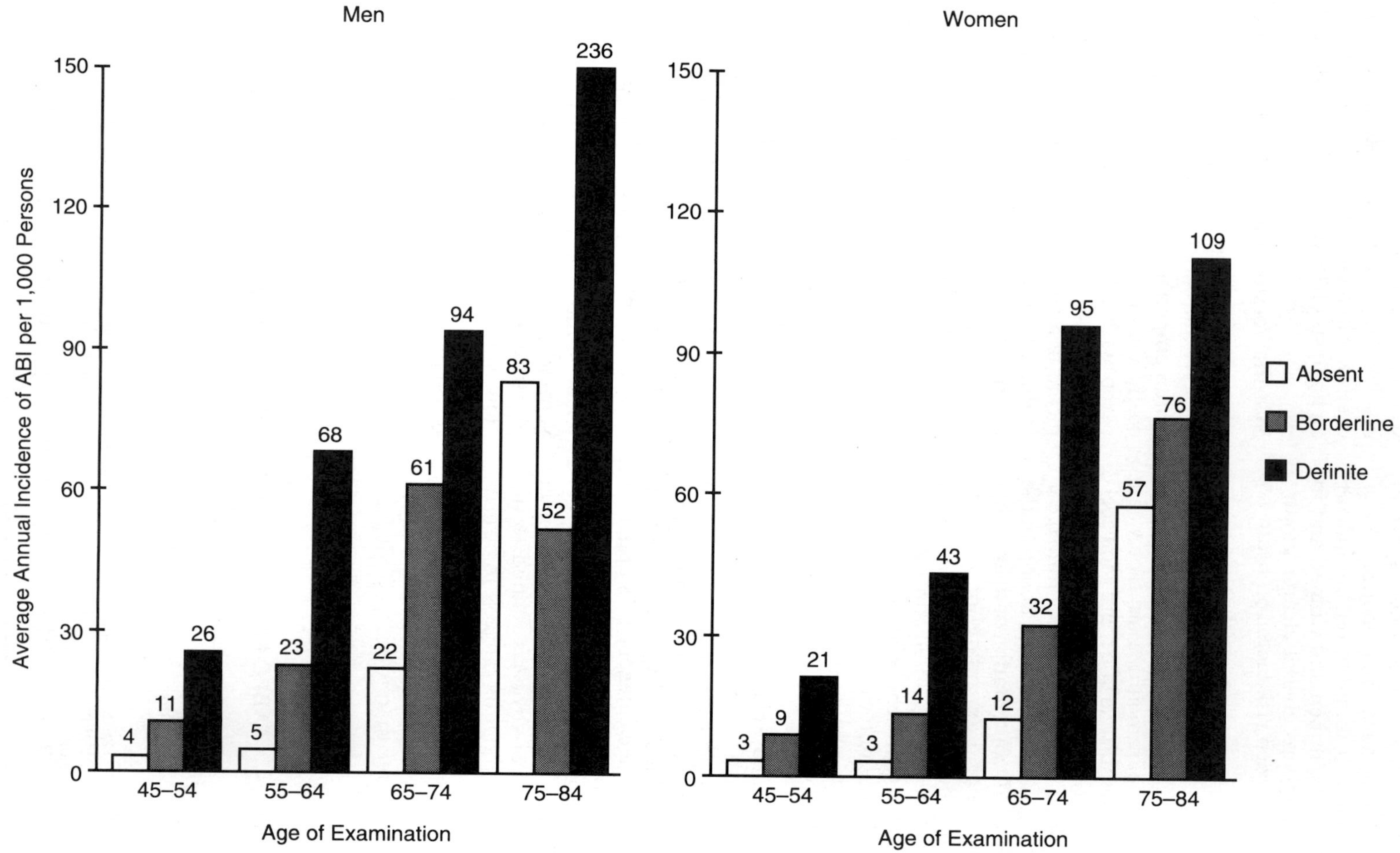


**Fig. 1-3.** Incidence of atherothrombotic brain infarction according to hypertensive status and age, in men and women: 36-year follow-up. (Data from the Framingham Study.)

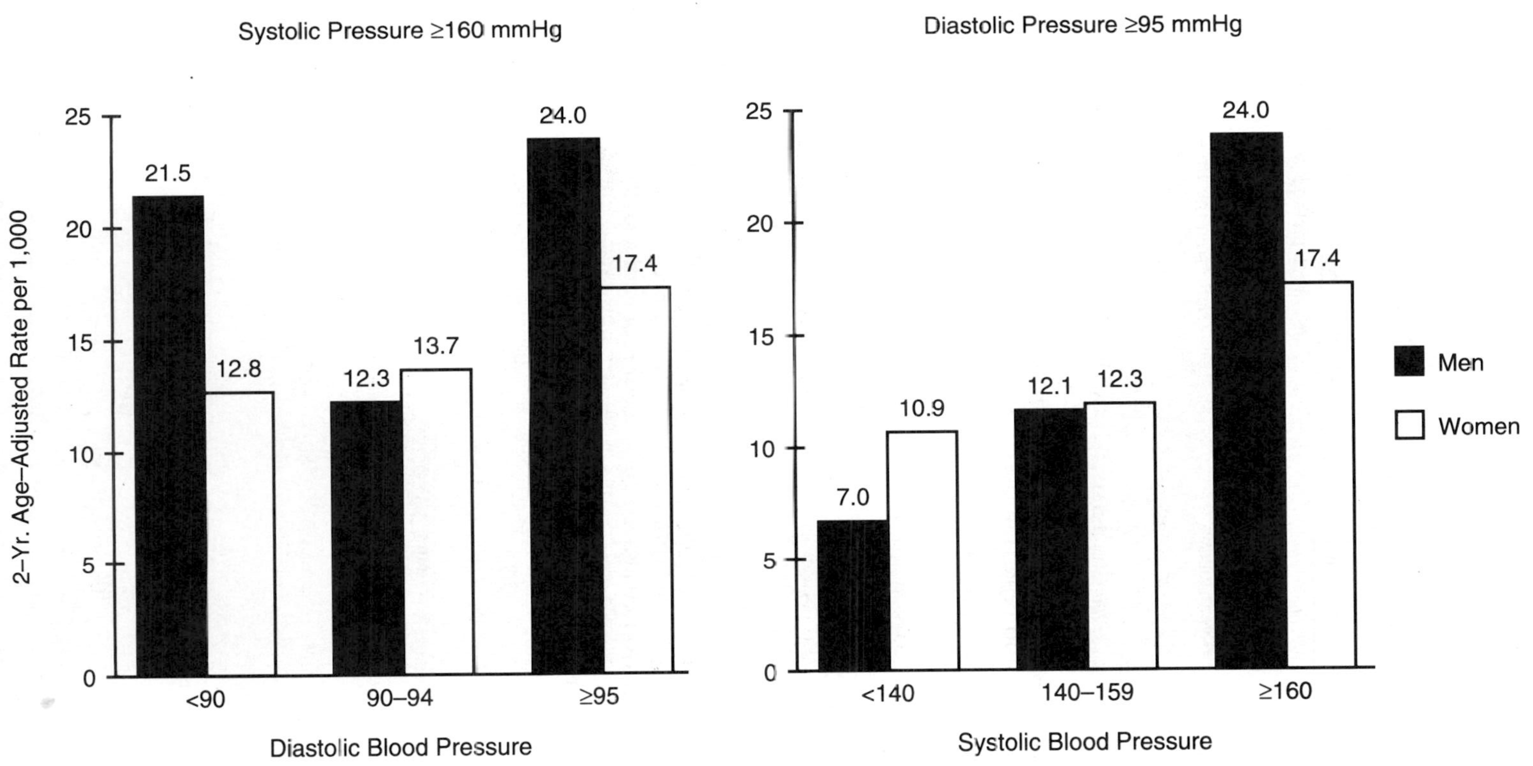


**Fig. 1-4.** Incidence of stroke in systolic and diastolic hypertensive patients according to diastolic and systolic blood pressure levels, men and women, ages 35 to 84 years: 36-year follow-up. (Data from the Framingham Study.)

**TABLE 1-4. Gradients of Risk of Brain Infarction[a]**

| Component of Blood Pressure | Average Standardized Regression Coefficients | |
|---|---|---|
| | Men | Women |
| Pulse pressure | 0.4667* | 0.4787 |
| Mean arterial pressure | 0.5678 | 0.6628 |
| Systolic blood pressure | 0.5721 | 0.6250 |
| Diastolic blood pressure | 0.4789 | 0.6026 |

* $P < 0.0001$ for all.
[a] According to component of blood pressure; subjects 45–84 years old.
(Data from the Framingham Study: 36-year follow-up.)

**TABLE 1-5. Two-Year Age-Adjusted Rate[a] of Stroke per 1,000[b]**

| | Systolic Pressure | Diastolic Pressure <90 | 90–94 | 95+ |
|---|---|---|---|---|
| Men | <140 | 7.3 | 6.6 | 7.0 |
| | 140–159 | 11.3 | 8.1 | 12.1 |
| | 160+ | 21.5 | 12.3 | 24.0 |
| Women | <140 | 6.0 | 5.5 | 10.9 |
| | 140–159 | 8.7 | 8.6 | 12.3 |
| | 160+ | 12.8 | 13.7 | 17.4 |

[a] Direct method using entire (sex-specific) population as standard.
[b] By sex and level of systolic and diastolic blood pressure (mmHg), men and women ages 35–84 years.
(Data from the Framingham Study: 36-year follow-up.)

cular complications of hypertension. On this basis, once aortic valvular disease has been excluded, a leading stroke neurologist has reported discontinuing the practice of routinely measuring and reporting the diastolic pressure.[20]

## Isolated Systolic Hypertension

With advancing age, there is a disproportionate rise in systolic blood pressure while the diastolic pressure levels off and then begins to decline. In the elderly, this isolated elevation of systolic pressure becomes highly prevalent (Fig. 1-5). Isolated systolic hypertension, systolic pressure above 160 mmHg and diastolic pressure below 95 mmHg, is present in approximately 20 percent of men and 30 percent of women above age 80.[37] This isolated elevation of the systolic pressure results from decreased arterial wall elasticity, which is a consequence of arteriosclerotic changes, was considered to be a consequence rather than a precursor of cardiovascular disease. However, it has been demonstrated in Framingham and in other epidemiologic studies, that stroke and cardiovascular disease incidence was significantly increased in persons with isolated systolic hypertension.[12] Risk was proportionately related to the level of systolic pressure even after diastolic pressure, age, and digital pulse-wave configuration (an index of arterial rigidity) were taken into account.[41] It is apparent from these 36-year follow-up data from Framingham that incidence of stroke is increased in the elderly with isolated systolic hypertension (Fig. 1-6). In addition, it is clear that incidence of stroke generally, and ABI specifically, is related to level of systolic pressure among persons with diastolic blood pressure below 95 mmHg (Fig. 1-7). The recent report of a striking beneficial effect of blood pressure reduction in isolated systolic hypertensive patients give these data added significance,[69] and will be emphasized below.

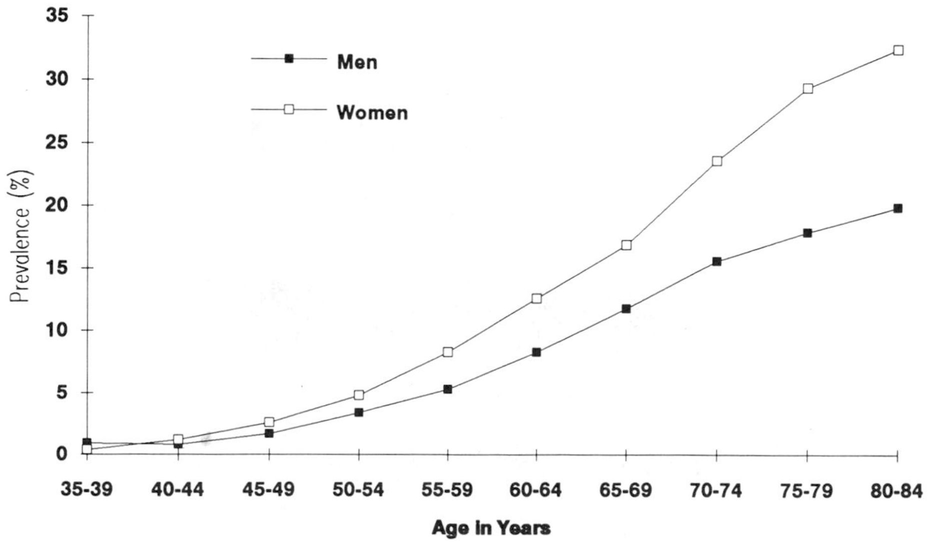


**Fig. 1-5.** Prevalence of isolated systolic hypertension in men and women, ages 35 to 84 years: 36-year follow-up. (Data from the Framingham Study.)

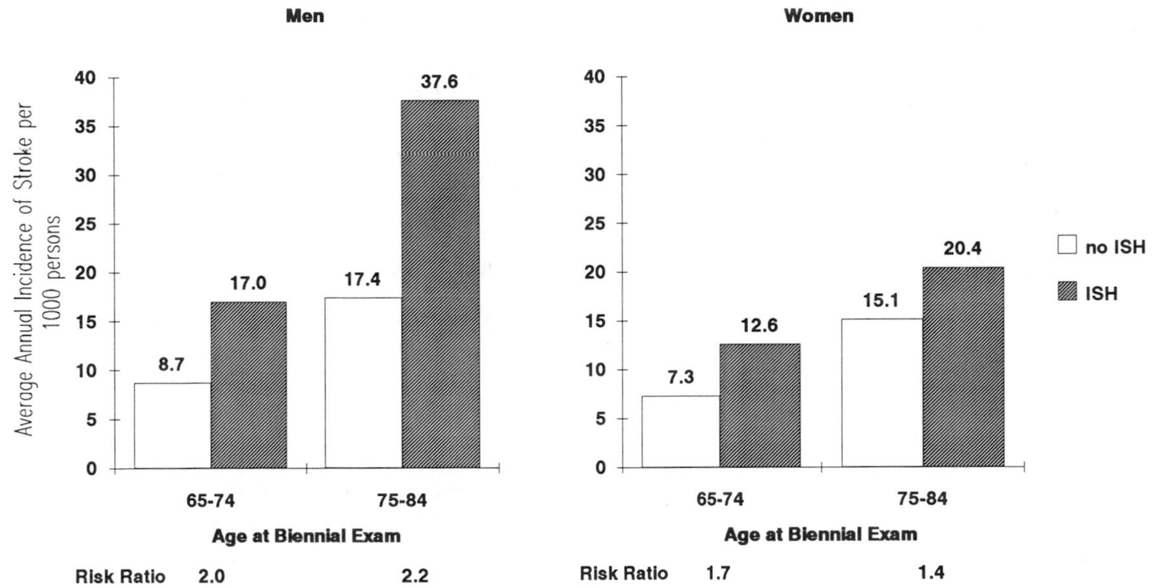


**Fig. 1-6.** Incidence of stroke in men and women with isolated systolic hypertension (ISH) in the elderly (ages 65 to 84 years): 36-year follow-up. (Data from the Framingham Study.)

## Stroke and Coronary Heart Disease Incidence According to Severity of Hypertension

It is often asserted that at mild or borderline elevations of blood pressure CHD is the chief cardiovascular outcome, while at higher levels of pressure, stroke is more likely. This was corroborated by computing the ratio of MI to ABI with increasing severity of hypertension (Table 1-6). There is a clear trend, in both men and women, with MI:ABI ratios falling as severity of hypertension increased. Stroke was also more likely to be the initial manifestation of cardiovascular disease among those with definite hypertension, compared with normotensives, and represented the first CVD event in 19 percent of men and 26 percent of women with definite hypertension.

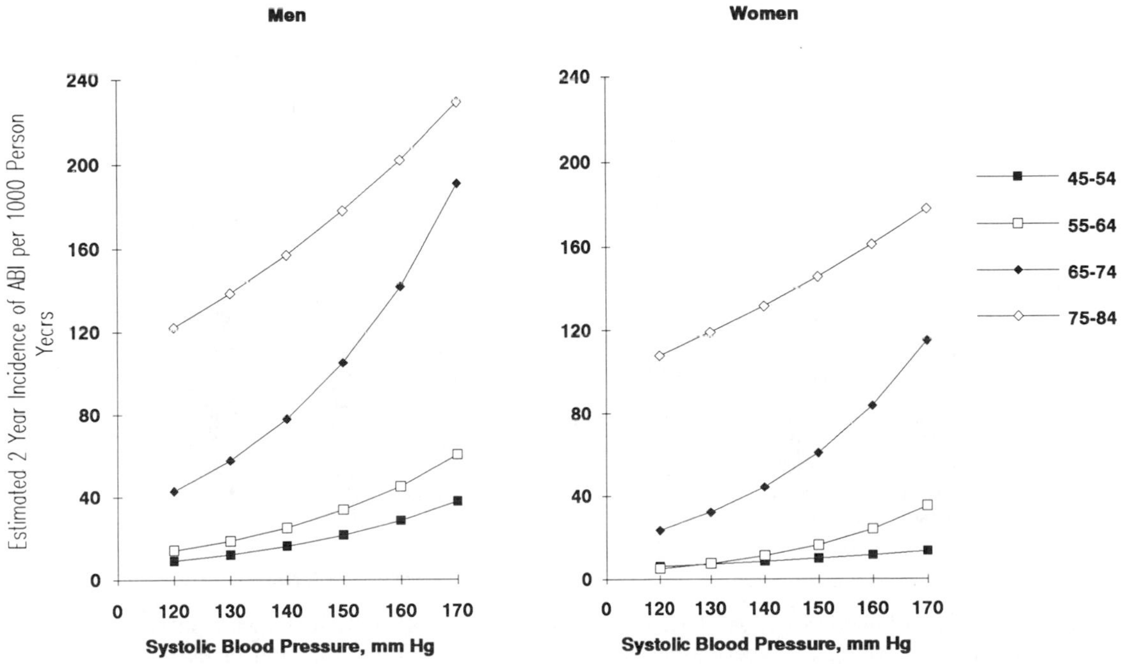


**Fig. 1-7.** Incidence of brain infarction according to systolic blood pressure in men and women, ages 45 to 84 years, whose diastolic pressure is below 95 mmHg: 36-year follow-up. ABI, atherothrombotic brain infarction. (Data from the Framingham Study.)

**TABLE 1-6. Ratio of MI to ABI According to Hypertensive Status**

| Hypertensive Status | Ratio of Age-Adjusted Average Annual Incidence of MI and ABI | |
|---|---|---|
| | Men[a] | Women[a] |
| Normotension | 5.2 | 3.4 |
| Borderline hypertension | 4.8 | 2.0 |
| Definite hypertension | 2.2 | 1.1 |

*Abbreviations*: MI, myocardial infarction; ABI, atherothrombotic brain infarction.

[a] Ages 35–94.

(Data from the Framingham Study: 30-year follow-up.)

## Heart Disease and Impaired Cardiac Function

Cardiac diseases and impaired cardiac function are not properly considered risk factors but are rather disease or organ dysfunction that predisposes to stroke. Although hypertension is the preeminent risk factor for stroke of all types, at each blood pressure level, persons with impaired cardiac function have a significantly increased stroke risk (Fig. 1-8). The prevalence of these cardiac contributors to stroke increases with age (Fig. 1-9). CVD is highly prevalent among stroke cases: 80.8 percent were hypertensive; 32.7 percent had prior CHD; 14.5 percent had cardiac failure; 14.5 percent had atrial fibrillation (AF); and only 13.6 percent had none of these. Cardiac disease is an important precursor of stroke (Fig. 1-10) and is dealt with in detail elsewhere in this volume.

## Coronary Heart Disease

In Framingham, CHD was ascertained prospectively on biennial examination as well as by monitoring hospitalizations over 36 years of follow-up. Acute MI predisposes to stroke, particularly in the days and weeks following the event, and stroke incidence may be reduced by antiplatelet and antithrombotic therapy.[72] Among transmural MIs, anterior wall infarcts are more likely to lead to stroke than transmural infarcts at other sites. The mechanism is presumed to be cerebral embolism from an intracardiac mural thrombus. Often, however, the mechanism of stroke in persons with CHD is less apparent. Persons with uncomplicated angina pectoris (AP), non-Q wave infarction, and clinically silent MI also had an increased incidence of ischemic stroke.[42] Recent data from Framingham suggest that silent or unrecognized MI survivors had a 10-year incidence of stroke of 17.8 percent in men and 17.3 percent in women, an inci-

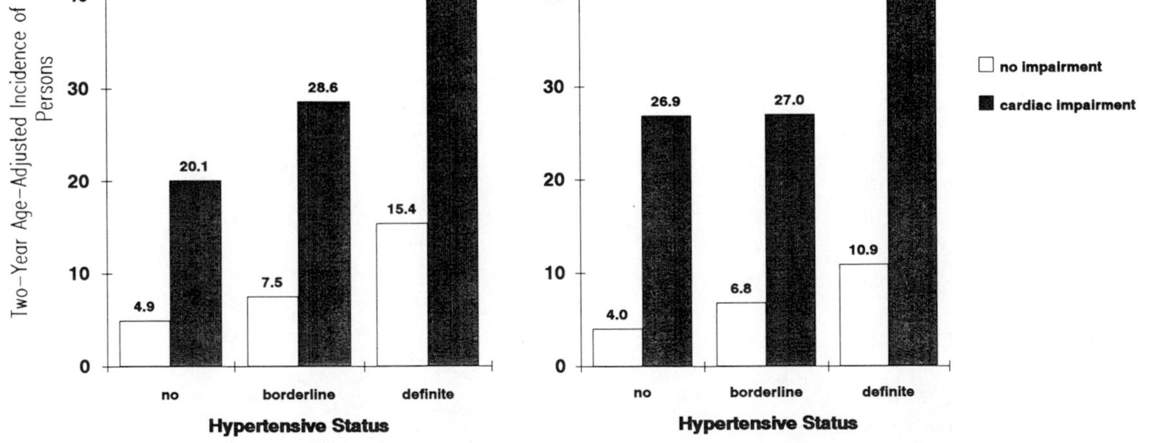


**Fig. 1-8.** Age-adjusted incidence of stroke in men and women, ages 45 to 84 years, with and without impaired cardiac function, according to hypertensive category. Impaired cardiac function includes coronary heart disease, congestive heart failure, left ventricular hypertrophy, by electrocardiogram, or heart enlargement on x-ray: 36-year follow-up. (Data from the Framingham Study.)

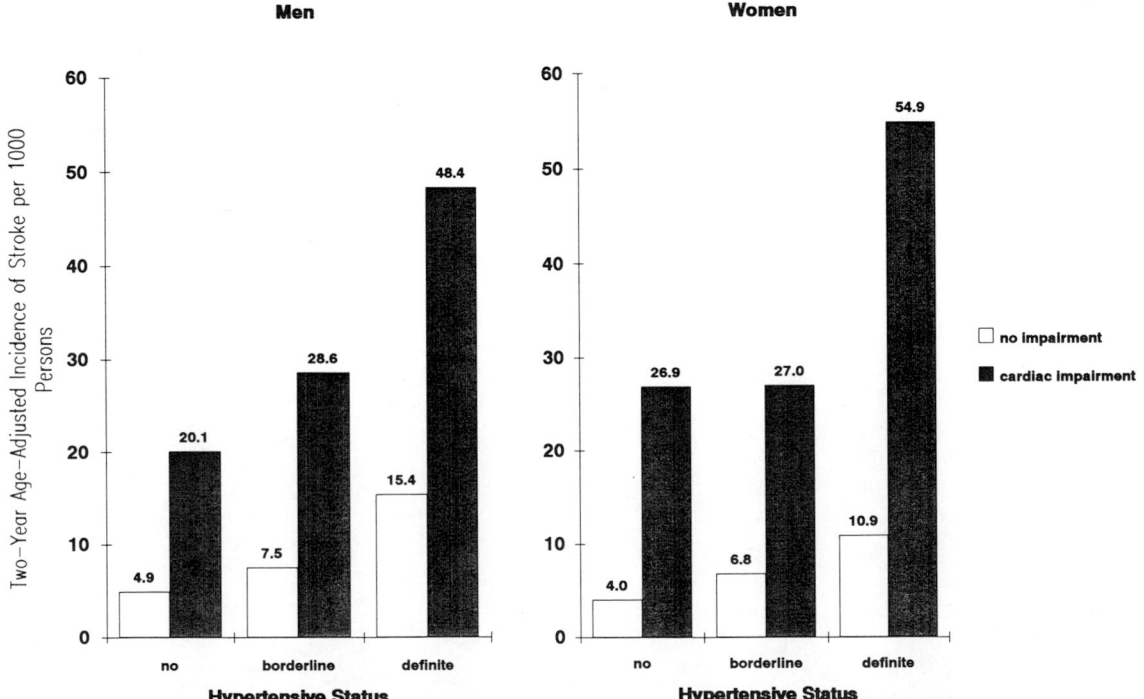

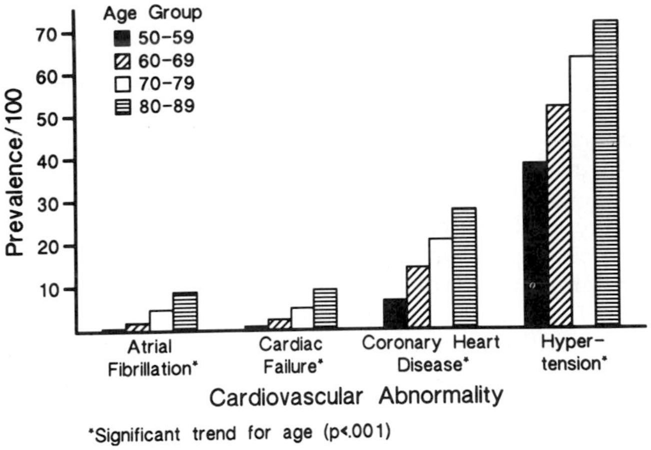


**Fig. 1-9.** Prevalence of cardiovascular abnormality with increasing age, men and women combined: 34-year follow-up. (Data from the Framingham Study.)

**TABLE 1-7. Two-Year Stroke Incidence in Subjects With and Without Chronic Nonrheumatic Atrial Fibrillation, Men and Women Combined**

| Age Group (years) | No. With Strokes | Strokes With Atrial Fibrillation (%) |
|---|---|---|
| 30–39 | 4 | 0.0 |
| 40–49 | 11 | 0.0 |
| 50–59 | 89 | 6.7 |
| 60–69 | 161 | 8.1 |
| 70–79 | 150 | 21.3 |
| 80–89 | 47 | 36.2 |
| Total | 462 | 14.7 |

dence not that much less than the 19.5 percent and 29.3 percent in men and women, respectively, that is seen following recognized MI.

## Atrial Fibrillation

In association with rheumatic heart disease and mitral stenosis, atrial fibrillation is acknowledged to predispose to stroke. In recent years, chronic AF without valvular heart disease, previously considered to be innocuous, has been associated with a 5.6 increased incidence of stroke. AF is also the most prevalent cardiac arrhythmia in the elderly. In the Framingham Study AF incidence more than doubled in successive decades and rose from 0.2 per 1,000 for ages 30 to 39 to 39.0 per 1,000 for ages 80 to 89 years. Atrial fibrillation was particularly important in the elderly since the proportion of total strokes associated with this arrhythmia increased steadily with age reaching 36.2 percent for ages 80 to 89 years (Table 1-7).[85] Although the prevalence of other cardiac contributors to stroke also increased with age, the increased incidence of stroke in persons with AF was probably a consequence of the AF and not the associated CHD or cardiac failure. This becomes apparent when age trends in risk of stroke are examined (Fig. 1-11). While attributable risk of stroke increased with age for AF, risk of stroke attributable to cardiac failure, CHD, and hypertension declined with age.[86] Of interest, in this age group 23.5 percent of stroke was attributable to AF, which approached that of hypertension (33.4 percent), a much more prevalent disorder.

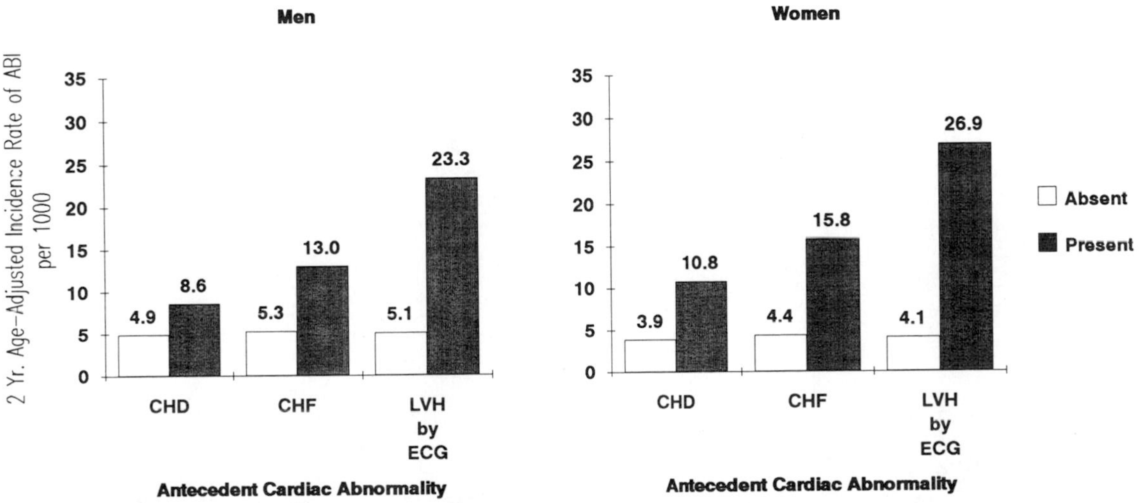


**Fig. 1-10.** Incidence of atherothrombotic brain infarction (ABI) in the presence of cardiac diseases or impairment: coronary heart disease (CHD), congestive heart failure (CHF), left ventricular hypertrophy by electrocardiogram (LVH by ECG), in men and women ages 45 to 84 years: 36-year follow-up. (Data from the Framingham Study.)

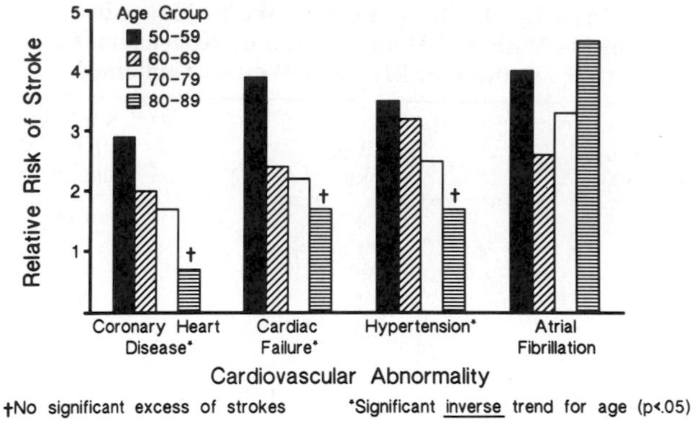


**Fig. 1-11.** Estimated relative risk of stroke with advancing age according to the presence of coronary heart disease, cardiac failure, hypertension, and atrial fibrillation: 34-year follow-up. (Data from the Framingham Study.)

Although most persons with nonrheumatic atrial fibrillation do not sustain a stroke, and stroke prevention with chronic warfarin anticoagulation is not innocuous, recent clinical trial findings strongly support low-intensity Coumadin therapy, which has more than 85 percent effectiveness in stroke prevention, when prothrombin time prolongation was in the therapeutic range.

## Left Ventricular Hypertrophy by Electrocardiogram

Left ventricular hypertrophy by electrocardiogram (LVH by ECG), increases in prevalence with age and blood pressure. Risk of ABI increased by more than fourfold in men and sixfold in women with this abnormal ECG pattern (Fig. 1-10). This increased risk persisted even after the influence of age and other atherogenic precursors, including systolic blood pressure, were taken into account (Table 1-2).

## Blood Lipids

Total serum cholesterol is significantly and independently related to the development of coronary heart disease in men and women, but the impact seems to diminish beyond age 60, particularly in men. However, when the components of cholesterol, high-, low-, and very low-density lipoprotein cholesterol, are related to incidence of CHD, even in persons over age 60, a relationship reemerges. High-density lipoprotein-cholesterol (HDL) has an inverse association and low-density lipoprotein-cholesterol (LDL) a direct relationship to incidence of CHD. A significant impact on CHD incidence can be shown by blood lipids using the total cholesterol/HDL-cholesterol ratio up to age 80. For example, in persons aged 75 to 79 years the risk ratio for elevated total cholesterol/HDL-cholesterol ratio is 1.6 for men and 1.8 for women. For stroke generally, and for ABI in particular, the relationship of total serum cholesterol and incidence of disease is neither clear nor consistent (Table 1-2). Using 36-year follow-up data, no clear influence of total cholesterol to ABI is apparent (Fig. 1-12). Relating the total cholesterol/HDL-cholesterol ratio, measured on the tenth to twelfth biennial examinations, to ABI, and to MI for comparison, over the ensuing 14 to 18 years a significant direct relationship to MI is shown in both men and women (Fig. 1-11). However, for ABI a nonsignificant inverse relationship is seen in men. A U-shaped or quadratic pattern occurs in women where a modest significant trend is seen (Fig. 1-13).

A surprisingly consistent finding has been the relationship between *low* total serum cholesterol and *increased* incidence of intracerebral hemorrhage. When initially noted in Japanese, who generally had low serum cholesterol levels by western standards, no cause and effect relationship was seriously considered. However, an etiologic link has been suggested

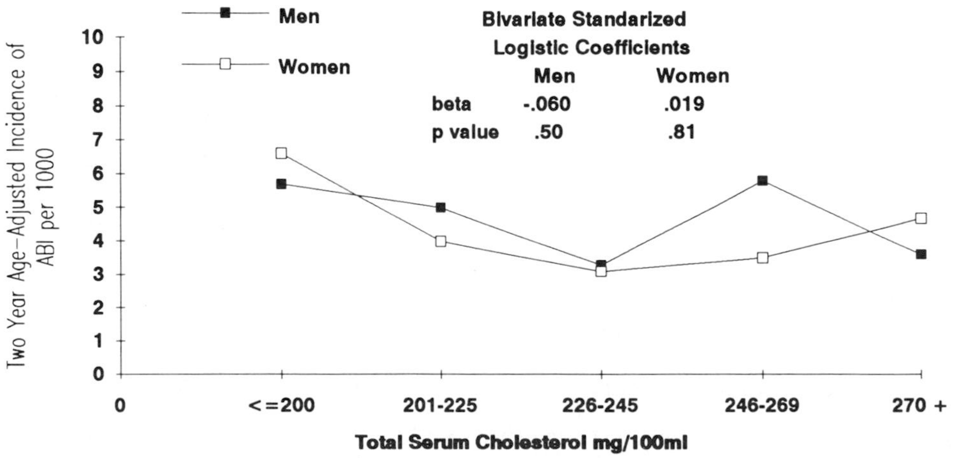


**Fig. 1-12.** Incidence of brain infarction according to total serum cholesterol, in men and women, ages 35 to 84 years: 36-year follow-up. ABI, atherothrombotic brain infarction. (Data from the Framingham Study.)

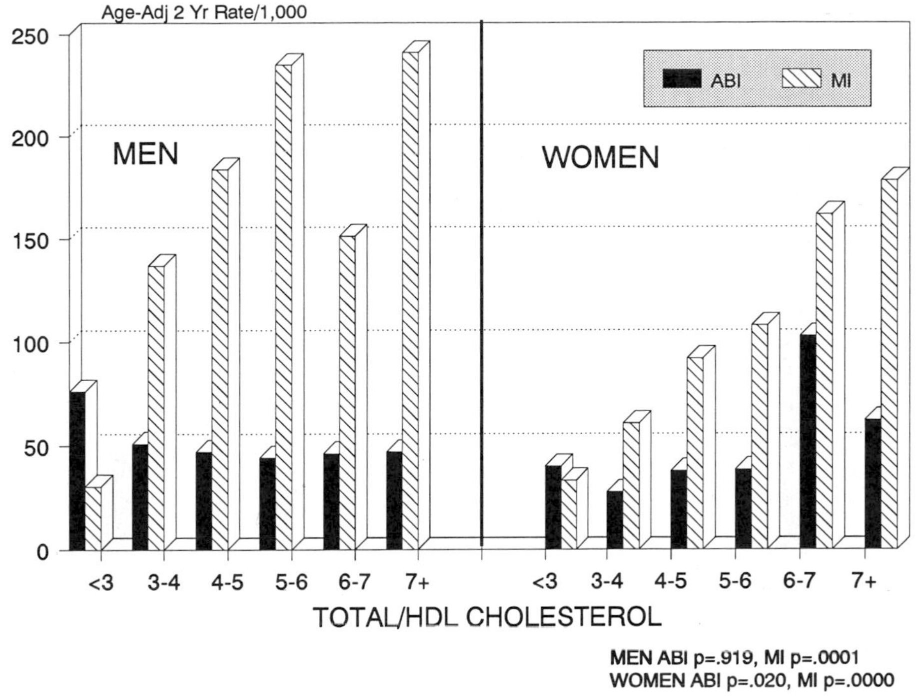


**Fig. 1-13.** Incidence of brain and myocardial infarction according to total cholesterol/HDL-cholesterol ratio, in men and women, ages 35 to 84 years: 36-year follow-up. ABI, atherothrombotic brain infarction; MI, myocardial infarction; HDL, high-density lipoprotein. (Data from the Framingham Study.)

by the recent confirmation of this relationship in other oriental populations, in Hawaiian-Japanese, and in 1989 in Multiple Risk Factor Intervention Trial (MRFIT) screenees in men in the United States. Prospective epidemiologic study of Japanese men and women in Japan have shown this relationship, which has also been confirmed in Hawaiian-Japanese men.[76,89]

Evidence that the low cholesterol-high intracerebral hemorrhage relationship is not restricted to Orientals has recently emerged from follow-up in the United States of MRFIT screenees, 90 percent of whom were whites. Despite the large size of the study group of 350,977 men, aged 35 to 57 years at screening, followed for 6 years for mortality, only 83 deaths from intracerebral hemorrhage and 55 deaths from subarachnoid hemorrhage occurred. In the lowest serum cholesterol category, less than 160 mg/dl, the risk factor-adjusted relative risk of intracranial hemorrhage was 1.0, and relative risk at all higher levels of serum cholesterol was approximately 0.32 (Fig. 1-14). When deaths from intracranial hemorrhage were examined by entry diastolic blood pressure the age-adjusted rate of death was significant only in persons with pressures above 90 mmHg. The death rate was 23.07 per 10,000 in the lowest serum cholesterol category, below 160 mg/dl, and ranged from 3.09 to 4.83 in the four higher categories. The interaction of high diastolic blood pressure and low serum cholesterol in promoting intracerebral hemorrhage suggested to some investigators "that very low serum cholesterol levels weaken the endothelium of intracerebral arteries, resulting in hemorrhagic stroke in the presence of hypertension."[35] They also suggest alcohol consumption, dietary protein deficiency, and a higher intake of polyunsaturated fatty acids, both linoleic acid derived from vegetable oils and eicosapentanoic acid from fish oil acting to reduce platelet aggregability.[29]

These data also provide evidence for a direct relationship between high levels of total serum cholesterol and ischemic stroke, particularly in hypertensives in this predominantly United States white males sample (Fig. 1-12). Despite the limitations of death certificate diagnoses, the findings are quite persuasive as a result of the large sample-size and the prospective nature of the study.

Although the relationship between blood lipids and stroke is unclear, serum lipid levels have been related to carotid artery atherosclerosis in a number of studies using the ultrasonographic evidence of extracranial carotid artery atherosclerosis or internal carotid artery wall thickness as an indicator of atherosclerosis.[57,68] It seems clear that atherosclerosis of the carotid artery, and of the circle of Willis in autopsy studies, is related to levels of blood lipids. On the other hand, the relationship to stroke generally may be obscured by the differing influence of lipids on the varying vascular pathologies underlying stroke. As

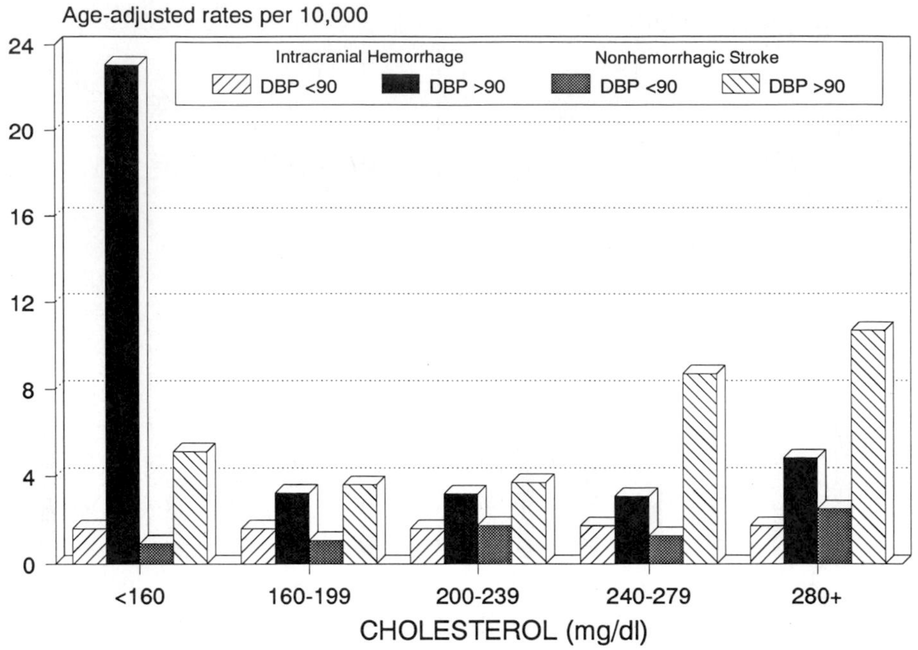


**Fig. 1-14.** Ischemic stroke and intracerebral hemorrhage death rates in men with normal and elevated diastolic blood pressure (DBP) according to screening serum cholesterol level. Multiple Risk Factor Intervention Trial screenees; 6-year follow-up. (Data from Iso et al.[35])

was seen in the MRFIT data (Fig. 1-12) low levels of serum cholesterol, less than 180 mg/dl, and particularly less than 160 mg/dl, seem to promote IH and perhaps SAH, while elevated levels foster large vessel atherothrombosis. There is no apparent influence on lacunar infarcts or on strokes secondary to cerebral embolism.

The high rates of hemorrhage and stroke generally and low rates of CHD in Japanese in Japan and Hawaii, have occurred in persons with low total serum cholesterol levels, by western standards, and in the presence of a high prevalence of hypertension.[62]

## Diabetes

Diabetics are known to have an increased susceptibility to coronary, femoral, and cerebral artery atherosclerosis. Surveys of stroke patients and prospective study have confirmed the increased risk of stroke in diabetics. In the United States, in the period 1976 to 1980, a medical history of stroke was 2.5 to 4 times more common in diabetics than in persons with normal glucose tolerance.[47] The Honolulu Heart Program of Japanese men living in Hawaii found diabetes conferred a twofold increased risk of thromboembolic stroke that was independent of other risk factors.[1] Evaluation of the impact of diabetes on stroke in a population-based cohort in Rancho Bernardo disclosed a relative risk of stroke that was 1.8 in men and 2.2 in women, even after adjusting for the effect of other pertinent risk factors.[9]

In Framingham, peripheral arterial disease with intermittent claudication occurs more than four times as often in diabetics. The coronary and cerebral arteries are also affected, but to a lesser extent.[39] For atherothrombotic brain infarction, the impact of glucose intolerance, that is, physician-diagnosed diabetes, glycosuria, or a blood sugar above 150 mg/100 ml, is greater in women than men and was significant as an independent contributor to incidence only in older women (Table 1-2). However, at all ages both men and women with glucose intolerance have approximately double the risk of ABI as nondiabetics (Fig. 1-15).

## Obesity

Obese persons have higher levels of blood pressure, blood glucose, and atherogenic serum lipids, and on that account alone could be expected to increase stroke incidence. Obesity, as expressed as a Metropolitan Relative Weight that is more than 30 percent above average, is a significant independent contributor to ABI incidence in men aged 35 to 64 and women 65 to 94 years (Table 1-2). However, even in the other two age-sex groups, obesity exerts an adverse influence on health status that is probably mediated through elevated blood pressure, impaired glucose tolerance, and other mechanisms. Recent studies have suggested that the pattern of obesity is also important, with central obesity and abdominal deposition of fat more strongly associated with atherosclerotic disease.[22]

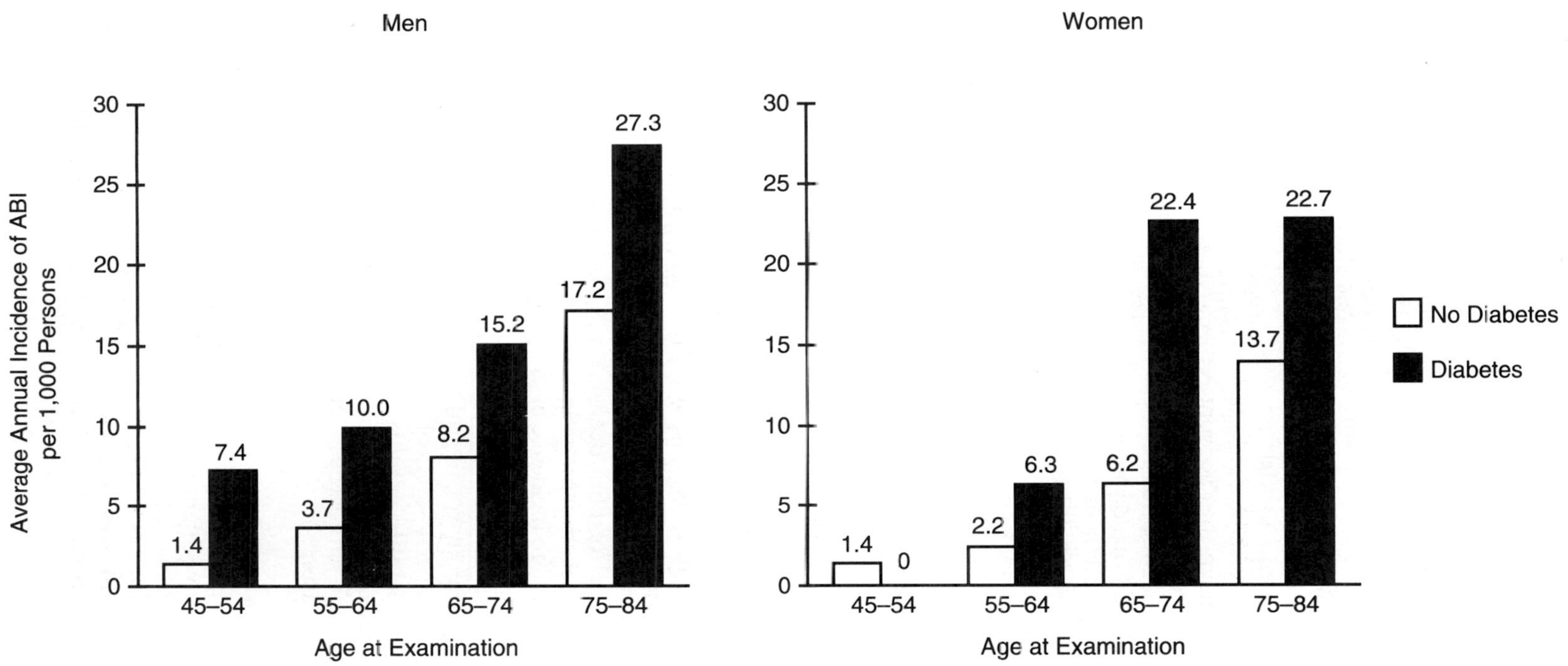


**Fig. 1-15.** Diabetes and incidence of atherothrombotic brain infarction according to age category, men and women: 36-year follow-up. (Data from the Framingham Study.)

## Hematocrit

Some studies, including Framingham, have demonstrated a relationship between high-normal hematocrit level and incidence of cerebral infarction.[38] Confirmation of this relationship has come from an autopsy study of Japanese stroke patients and from several clinical and radiologic studies of patients with stroke.[77,78] In these 36-year follow-up data, elevated blood hematocrit, within the normal range, and generally not pathologically elevated red cell mass, is significantly and independently associated with ABI in men aged 35 to 64, but not in the other three age-sex categories. This significant relationship to ABI persisted even after the confounding effects of cigarette smoking and hypertension were taken into account (Table 1-2). The reason for the different impact in the two sexes is unclear. Increased concentration of red cells in combination with high blood fibrinogen levels raises blood viscosity.[61] This interaction may reach pathologic significance in narrowed small penetrating arteries, and in high-grade stenosis of a major cerebral artery. Reduction of high-normal hematocrit by venesection has decreased blood viscosity and correspondingly increased cerebral blood flow.

## Fibrinogen

Serum fibrinogen has been implicated in atherogenesis and in arterial thrombus formation. A number of epidemiologic studies have shown a substantial and significant independent impact of fibrinogen on cardiovascular disease incidence, including stroke.[83] In this prospective study, fibrinogen in combination with elevated systolic blood pressure, was found to be a potent risk factor for stroke in a sample of 54 Swedish men followed for 13 years. Level of fibrinogen, measured on the tenth biennial examination in Framingham, was significantly related to incidence of cardiovascular disease including stroke.[40]

However, fibrinogen was also positively associated with most of the major risk factors for stroke, including age, hypertensive status, hematocrit level, obesity, and diabetes. There is considerable optimism that further study of fibrinogen and other clotting factors will yield important clues to the pathogenesis of atherosclerotic cardiovascular disease.

## Race

Compared with whites, blacks have higher death rates from stroke. Age-adjusted incidence rates are 1.5 times higher for black men and 2.3 times higher for black women than for whites.[27] In the National Health and Nutrition Examination Survey I: Epidemiologic Follow-up Study (NHEFS), age-adjusted mortality for blacks from stroke was 1.98 times that of whites.[58] Of interest, 31 percent of excess mortality could be accounted for by six key risk factors for cardiovascular disease. A further 38 percent of the excess deaths could be accounted for by family income, leaving 31 percent of the excess black total mortality unexplained. Blacks had higher hospitalization rates, a higher prevalence of hypertension and diabetes, and more IH and less extracranial and large artery atherosclerotic disease than whites.[27,43] The epidemiology of stroke in blacks and Hispanics is being investigated with increased intensity in a number of multiracial populations in the United States.[66]

Orientals have been known to have a low rate of CHD and a high prevalence of stroke. A high incidence and prevalence of stroke in the Chinese was found in a survey of six mainland cities with rates that were comparable to those of native Japanese in Japan.[50] The disparity between the stroke and CHD death rates, and presumably a similar disparity in incidence rates, is usually attributed to the high prevalence of hypertension and the low levels of blood lipids in Orientals.[62] Hypertension is generally related to high salt intake and perhaps to genetic factors, while the low serum lipids are related to the low levels of animal fat and protein in the Oriental. Cerebrovascular disease was the most frequently certified cause of death in Japan during the 3 decades following World War II, and the mechanism of stroke was most frequently thought to be IH. By 1980, as stroke death rates fell, cancer became the leading cause of death. In Japanese men in Hawaii and San Francisco, deaths attributed to stroke also fell relative to those attributed to CHD and cancer. In 1985 heart disease became the second leading cause of death in Japan (114.8 per 100,000), following cancer (156.4 per 100,000), and stroke fell to the third position (110.6 per 100,000).[36]

It is now well established that infarction, not hemorrhage, is the most frequent stroke mechanism in Japanese and accounts for two-thirds of stroke events in Japanese, be they resident in Japan or Hawaii. However, IH does occur several times more frequently in Japanese than in United States whites or blacks. There is also a difference in the site of the atherosclerotic arterial pathology with a predominance of intracranial disease in Japanese in contrast to the pattern in white Americans where the extracranial arteries are the focus of most of the atherosclerotic occlusive disease. In Japan, including rural Japan, substantial changes have occurred in the diet since World War II. These include an increase in animal fat and animal protein and a reduction in the amount of sodium chloride in the diet.[70]

## Family History of Stroke

Although family history of stroke is perceived to be an important marker of increased stroke risk, confirmation by epidemiologic study has been lacking. In a recent report, maternal history of death from stroke was significantly related to stroke incidence in a cohort of Swedish men born in 1913.[81] Other significant risk factors included hypertension, abdominal pattern of obesity, and fibrinogen level; however, maternal history of fatal stroke was independently related to stroke even after these variables were taken into account. It seems ironic that family history of stroke, a frequently mentioned, and nearly universally acknowledged, predisposing factor has been so infrequently documented in epidemiologic studies.

## Environmental Factors

### Cigarette Smoking

Cigarette smoking, a powerful risk factor for MI and sudden death has been clearly linked to brain infarction, as well as to IH and SAH (Table 1-2).[13,88] A similar relationship between cigarette smoking and stroke has been seen in Hawaiian Japanese men after 10 years of follow-up in the Honolulu Heart Study, where cigarette smoking made a significant independent contribution to cerebral infarction and intracranial hemorrhage risk.[2]

In the late 1970s, several studies of oral contraceptives and stroke in young women identified cigarette smoking as an important risk factor. Surprisingly, the association between cigarette smoking, oral contraceptives, and stroke was primarily related to subarachnoid hemorrhage. In the Royal College of General Practitioners Study of oral contraceptive use, the increased risk of subarachnoid hemorrhage occurred principally in women above age 35, who were current or former oral contraceptive users, and who smoked cigarettes.[80] In the Nurses' Health Study, a cohort of nearly 120,000 women were followed prospectively for 8 years for the development of stroke. There was an increased risk of subarachnoid hemorrhage as well as thrombotic stroke in cigarette smokers. Relative risk of subarachnoid hemorrhage showed a dose-response relationship from 4-fold in light smokers to 9.8-fold in smokers of 25 or more cigarettes daily.[13] Of note, in each smoking category the relative risk of subarachnoid hemorrhage, whether or not other associated risk factors were taken into account, was twice as great as for thromboembolic stroke.

The association between cigarette smoking and subarachnoid hemorrhage from aneurysm was also found in men (as well as women), in Framingham[67] and in New Zealand[10] in case-control analyses. In a case-control study of 114 patients with subarachnoid hemorrhage in a defined region in Finland, cigarette smokers were significantly more prevalent in cases than in controls matched for age, sex, and domicile.[21] Relative risk of subarachnoid hemorrhage in smokers, as compared with nonsmokers, was 2.7 in men and 3.0 in women. The authors suggested that smoking promoted a temporary increase in blood pressure, which, acting in concert with the "metastatic emphysema effect," was responsible for subarachnoid hemorrhage from cerebral aneurysm. No more reasonable hypothesis has been promulgated to explain this powerful relationship.

That cigarette smoking increases risk of thrombotic stroke and subarachnoid hemorrhage is generally accepted; the relationship of cigarette smoking to intracerebral hemorrhage is less well established. Data from the Honolulu Heart Program firmly links cigarette smoking in Hawaiian men of Japanese ancestry to stroke both "thromboembolic and hemorrhagic."[2]

Risk of "hemorrhagic" stroke was significantly greater (relative risk 2.5) in cigarette smokers than in nonsmokers; this excess risk of stroke was independent and persisted at a relative risk of 2.8 even after the other associated risk factors of age, diastolic blood pressure, serum cholesterol, alcohol consumption, hematocrit, and body mass.

In a meta-analysis of 32 separate studies, including those cited above, cigarette smoking was a significant independent contributor to stroke incidence in both sexes and at all ages, and was associated with an approximately 50 percent increased risk overall when compared with nonsmokers.[71] The risk of stroke generally, and of ABI specifically, rose as number of cigarettes smoked per day increased, in both men and women.[88]

### Oral Contraceptives

An increased risk of stroke was reported in users of oral contraceptives (OCs), particularly in older women, that is, above age 35, and predominantly in those with other cardiovascular risk factors, particularly hypertension and cigarette smoking.[73] The relative risk of stroke was estimated to be increased fivefold in OC users and former users with risk concentrated in cigarette smokers above age 35. However, the mechanism of stroke in OC users is unclear. Cerebral infarction is more likely to be due to thrombotic disease than to atherosclerosis; it is known that clotting is enhanced by the OC-induced increased platelet aggregability and by its alteration of clotting factors to favor thrombogenesis. In young women with unexplained ischemic stroke, use of OCs is presumed to be the "cause" of the infarct; however the stroke was attributed to OC use in no more than 10 percent of a series of carefully studied patients.[3] Although there have been few systematic investigations of OCs and stroke in the 1980s, in case-control studies of stroke in OC users conducted in the 1970s, "thromboembolism" was the type of stroke said to occur most frequently in OC users. However, women in the case group often experienced transient episodes of neurologic dysfunction, "TIAs," or stroke events categorized as being due to "ill-defined and uncertain" causes. Risk of stroke was highest in women who took OCs containing higher levels of estrogen; the lower levels of estrogen in the newer OC formulations seem to have substantially reduced the hazard, and former users seem to be at no increased risk of stroke.[75]

Of particular interest is the interaction between OCs, cigarette smoking, and subarachnoid hemorrhage.[51] Prospective observation of over 40,000 women, half of whom were taking OCs, showed an increased risk of fatal subarachnoid hemorrhage (not cerebral infarction) in women taking OCs.[64] Risk was increased fourfold in cigarette smokers above age 35 with most cases confined to this group.

## Alcohol Consumption

As in myocardial infarction, impact of alcohol consumption on stroke risk is related to the amount of alcohol consumed.[31] Heavy alcohol use, either habitual daily heavy alcohol consumption or binge drinking, seems to be related to an excess of stroke and stroke deaths. Light or moderate alcohol consumption, on the other hand, is convincingly associated with a reduced incidence of CHD.[74] Light and moderate alcohol use tends to raise the HDL-cholesterol and may be associated with a reduction in CHD incidence, while high levels of alcohol intake are linked to hypertension and hypertriglyceridemia and may, in this way, by associated with an increased rate of CHD.

The relationship of alcohol consumption to stroke occurrence is less clearly elucidated. Available evidence rather uniformly demonstrates an adverse effect of heavy alcohol consumption on stroke occurrence.[30] Stroke incidence has been positively associated with heavy alcohol consumption in prospective studies in Yugoslavia.[46] There was a powerful dose-response relationship, in the Honolulu Heart Study of men of Japanese ancestry, between alcohol consumption and incidence of IH and SAH, even after taking other pertinent risk factors, particularly blood pressure, into account.[17] However, there was no significant relationship to thromboembolic stroke. Data from the Framingham study also suggest an increased incidence of brain infarction and stroke with increased levels of alcohol use, but only in men.

There are a number of mechanisms by which heavy alcohol consumption may predispose to and moderate alcohol consumption protect from stroke.[48] Cigarette smoking is more frequent in heavy drinkers, and there is attendant hemoconcentration. Alcohol and cigarette smoking have been shown to increase both blood hematocrit and viscosity, and rebound thrombocytosis during abstinence has been observed. Cardiac rhythm disturbances, particularly AF, occur with alcohol intoxication, producing what has been termed "holiday heart."[19] Acute alcohol intoxication has been named as a precipitating factor in stroke in young people, both in thrombotic stroke and in SAH.[32]

Increased incidence of intracerebral hemorrhage has been related to alcohol consumption in the Honolulu Heart Program with a strong dose-response relationship. Increases in alcohol consumption were related to increasing levels of blood pressure, cigarette smoking, and to lower serum cholesterol levels, all risk factors for intracerebral hemorrhage.[17] However, even after taking these factors into account, alcohol consumption was independently related to incidence of intracranial hemorrhage, both subarachnoid and intracerebral; no significant relationship was found between alcohol and thromboembolic stroke. Age-adjusted, estimated relative risk of intracerebral hemorrhage for light drinkers (1 to 14 oz per month), as compared to nondrinkers, was 2.1, for moderate drinkers (15 to 39 oz per month) 2.4, and for heavy drinkers (40+ oz per month) 4.0. After adjustment was made for the other associated risk factors, intracerebral hemorrhage was 2.0, 2.0, and 2.4 times as frequent, respectively, in these alcohol consumption categories.

Heavy alcohol use, 3+ drinks daily, was associated with higher rates (relative risk 3.64) of hospitalization for intracerebral hemorrhage.[45] Age, higher blood pressure, and black race (but not heavy alcohol consumption after these factors were taken into account), were independent predictors of intracerebral hemorrhage. The authors suggest the effect of heavy alcohol consumption on "hemorrhagic" stroke is mediated by raised blood pressure. A lower incidence of "occlusive stroke" hospitalizations were seen among heavy drinkers; the relative risk of 0.62 was not statistically significant (95 percent confidence index 0.29 to 1.31).

## Physical Activity

Leisure-time and work-associated vigorous physical activity has been linked to lower CHD incidence. More physically active longshoremen had lower rates of myocardial infarction, but had no reduction in stroke incidence.[59] In a study of 17,000 former Harvard students, those who were more physically active had about half the risk of fatal CHD and one-third the mortality rate of their least active fellow alumni.[60] No such data exist demonstrating a reduction in stroke occurrence from vigorous habitual leisure-time physical activity.

Vigorous exercise may exert a beneficial influence on risk factors for atherosclerotic disease by reducing elevated blood pressure as a result of weight loss and by reducing the pulse rate, raising the HDL- and lowering the LDL-cholesterol, improving glucose tolerance, and by promoting a lifestyle conducive to favorably changing detrimental health habits such as cigarette smoking.[48,49] These salutary effects have not been uniformly demonstrated to result in reduced stroke incidence. Furthermore, there are substantial limitations to studies of physical activity and disease, the principal potential pitfall being the self-selection of different levels of activity at work or leisure.

## SECULAR TRENDS IN STROKE INCIDENCE AND MORTALITY

In the past 20 years a dramatic decline in death from stroke has occurred in most industrialized nations. In the United States the decline of 53 percent in stroke mortality, a 5 percent annual decrement, represents an acceleration of the 1 percent annual decline from 1915 to 1970 (Fig. 1-16). This accelerated decline supports the influence of modifiable environmental factors in stroke occurrence. Reduction in stroke mortality occurred in both sexes, in blacks and whites, and in all regions of the United States. Furthermore, death rates attributable to stroke have declined in the face of falling total death rates. In fact, the diminution in stroke death has been a major contributor to the decline in total cardiovascular diseases, providing further substantiation that the stroke decline is real and not an artifact of death certification or coding practices (Fig. 1-17).

The decline was initially noted in hospital admissions for intracerebral hemorrhage in Goteberg, Sweden by clinicians who identified a decreased frequency of hemorrhage and a 10-year "delay" in onset of this disease, both of which they attributed to more effective treatment of severe hypertension.[8] Declining incidence of hemorrhage and of ischemic stroke was documented in the population-based study in Rochester, Minnesota. The accelerated decline in stroke mortality has been attributed to the realization of the importance of hypertension as the premier risk factor for stroke, whether the stroke mechanism was hemorrhage or infarction, and the demonstration that treatment will reduce stroke and stroke death.[11] Controlled clinical trials of treatment of severe and moderately severe diastolic hypertension conducted in the late 1960s demonstrated the efficacy of blood pressure

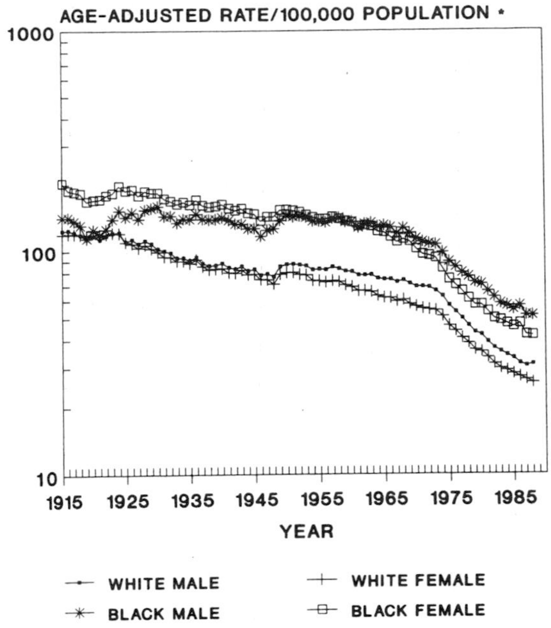


• Adjusted to U.S. population, 1940.

**Fig. 1-16.** Trends in death rates for cerebrovascular disease by sex and race, United States, 1915–1988.

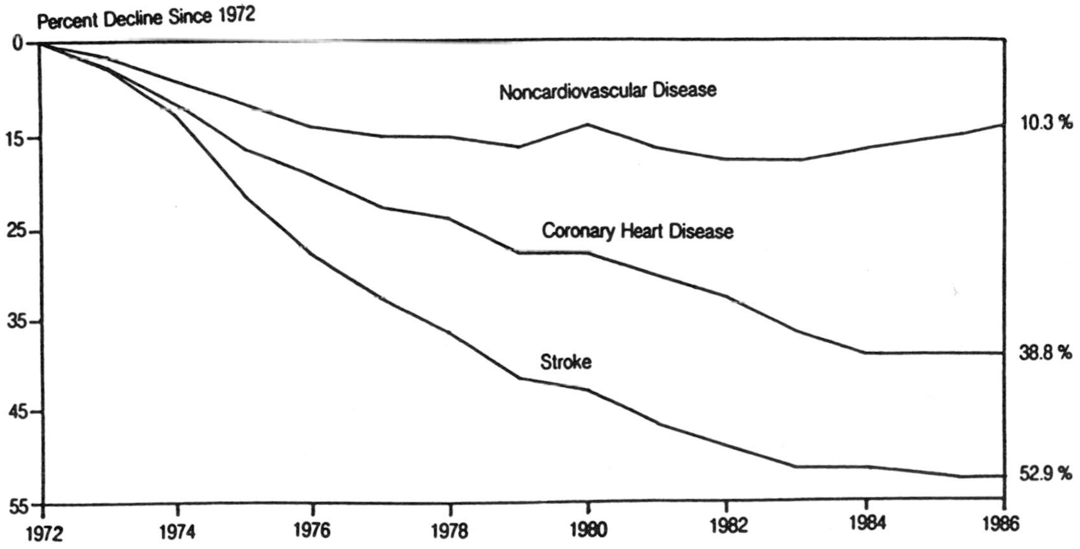


*Source: Vital Statistics of the U.S. NCHS (Provisional for 1986).*

**Fig. 1-17.** Decline in age-adjusted mortality rates for cardiovascular diseases, United States, 1972 to 1986. (From White,[82] with permission.)

lowering in stroke prevention. In the past decade, trials of control of mild hypertension, diastolic blood pressure 90 to 109 mmHg, has demonstrated the efficacy of treatment of this most prevalent level of elevated blood pressure in stroke prevention.[54] In controlled clinical trials, blood pressure control has rather uniformly been followed by a reduction in stroke occurrence and death, the benefit of treatment occurred in a surprisingly short period of time following blood pressure reduction.[14]

This momentous decline in death rates from stroke could come from either decreased incidence of stroke, improved survival of stroke patients, or from a combination of these effects.[17] Evidence supporting the role of declining incidence of stroke came from the community-based study of Rochester, Minnesota, where stroke incidence declined over time coincident with improved control of hypertension[24] (Fig. 1-18). However, in a critical review of available studies of geographic and secular trends in stroke mortality and incidence the authors concluded that most studies of stroke incidence were neither adequate or comparable.[55] They concluded, "the only firm evidence we have that stroke incidence is decreasing comes from Rochester, Minnesota, where rates reflect stroke risk among white rural Americans. This important but isolated finding needs confirmation."

Evidence to support improved survival following stroke was found in the National Hospital Discharge Survey, which showed a decreasing case-fatality rate from stroke from 1970 to 1983.[26] There are three possible explanations for the reduced case-fatality rates for stroke: (1) improved acute stroke care has prolonged survival, (2) stroke events in recent years are less severe and life-threatening than formerly, or (3) stroke cases that previously went undetected, and were milder in severity, are now routinely diagnosed. Improved acute stroke care may be responsible for some degree of improvement in stroke survival, although the data are conflicting.[25] Considerable evidence is accumulating that the severity of strokes is decreasing.[28] Hospital case-fatality rates in Allegheny County, Pennsylvania decreased significantly from 19.6 percent to 11 percent from 1971 to 1980.[4] This decline in death rates coincided with a reduction in the severity of stroke. Fewer stroke patients were comatose, and this reduction in prevalence of coma was thought to be responsible for more than 80 percent of the decline in the case-fatality rate.

It is quite likely that small cerebral infarctions or hemorrhages, with mild or minimal neurologic deficits, which would not have been accurately diagnosed in the past, are now identified as definite strokes through the routine use of CT.[11] The widespread availability of a diagnostic test for stroke, particularly for stroke in the elderly, may be particularly important here. The increase in diagnostic sensitivity afforded by the CT scan, and in the 1990s by MR scan, may counterbalance the impact of declining mortality and incidence.[15] In Rochester, Minnesota incidence rates have leveled off and perhaps even started to rise coincident with the availability the CT scan.[49] In Allegheny County the advent of CT was accompanied by a twofold increase in survivorship of stroke patients.[48] The evidence is that both declining case-fatality rates and reduced incidence are contributing to the decline

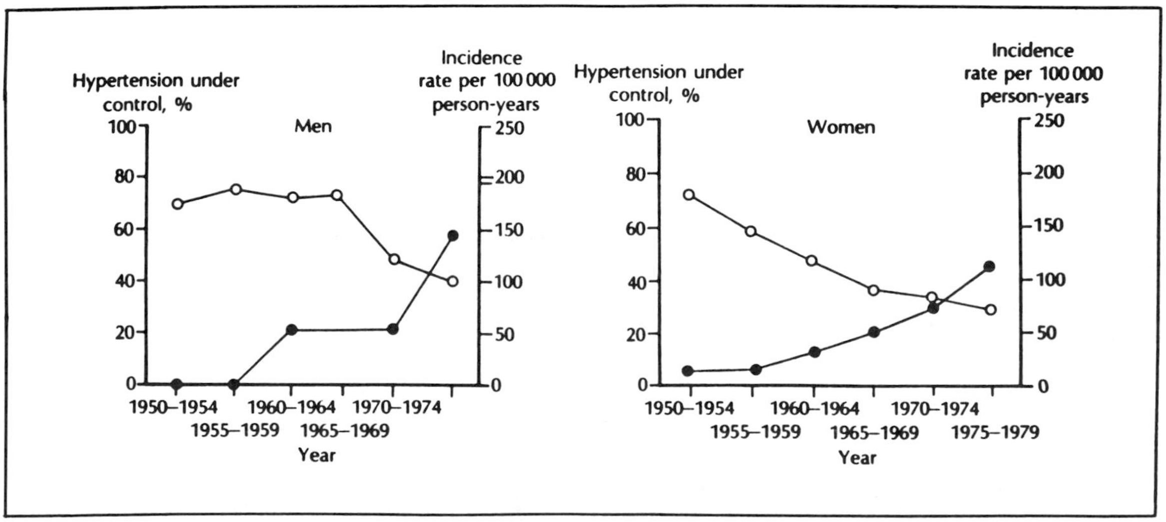


**Fig. 1-18.** Average annual incidence rates (adjusted for age to 1950 United States white population) for stroke in Rochester, Minnesota, and percentage of persons with hypertension under control (diastolic blood pressure below 95 mmHg) in various periods, in men and women. (From Garraway and Whisnant,[24] with permission.)

in death rates from stroke in the United States[33] and in other western nations.[5]

Stroke severity has fallen dramatically in Rochester, Minnesota, where there was a significant ($P < 0.001$) reduction in 30-day case-fatality rates from 33 percent during 1945 to 1949 to 17 percent during 1980 to 1984;[54] the 1980 to 1984 quinquennium coincided with the availability of head CT scan. This trend of falling stroke severity has also been noted in other populations. In a study of stroke outcome in Allegheny County, Pennsylvania, age-adjusted mortality rates declined significantly from 1971 to 1980 for four sex-race groups, while hospital case-fatality rates also fell from 19.6 percent to 11 percent between 1971 and 1980.[48] The decline in death rates corresponded to a reduction in the severity of stroke with fewer patients in coma. The authors found reduced severity of stroke events was responsible for more than 80 percent of the decline in case-fatality rates. Survival following stroke also improved from 49 to 62 percent in a five-county rural area of North Carolina between 1970 to 1973 and 1979 to 1980.[44] The decline in death rates corresponded to United States vital statistics and census data reports for the same five-county area, where a 24 percent decline from 1970 to 1980 had occurred, and these reports concluded the decrease in deaths from stroke mortality resulted not solely from a decrease in incidence but in substantial measure from improved survival following stroke.[44]

There are a number of possible mechanisms contributing to the decline in stroke severity. First, increased awareness and recognition of transient ischemic attacks on the part of the general population and physicians must explain some portion of the increase in prevalence of these events. This increased recognition would tend to increase the incidence of total cerebrovascular events while reducing the case-fatality rate. Second, reduction in severity might result from a differential decline in the incidence of specific stroke subtypes with high case-fatality rates such as intracerebral and subarachnoid hemorrhage. In the Rochester, Minnesota population a decline in intracerebral hemorrhage incidence occurred over 25 years, 1945 to 1979;[18] it was estimated that 24 percent of hemorrhages in the years prior to the advent of the CT scan had incorrectly been attributed to cerebral infarction and that these hemorrhages tended to be smaller and less severe.

There has been a clear decline in case-fatality rates for intracerebral hemorrhage in Hisayama, Japan due in part to a decrease in the incidence of massive ganglionic hemorrhages from 1961 to 1983 in the two cohorts studied in that area of Japan.[79] In addition, decreased case-fatality rates following subarachnoid hemorrhage have been reported in the period 1975 to 1984 in Rochester, Minnesota and for white men and women in the United States.[34]

## STROKE PREVENTION THROUGH RISK FACTOR MANAGEMENT

There has been rapid decline in death rates from stroke in the United States and in most other industrialized nations since 1968.[44] In the United States this decline of more than 50 percent in mortality rates in a 20-year span supports the notion that modifiable environmental influences are operating in stroke and cardiovascular disease occurrence. At least part of the decline results from a reduction in the incidence and severity of stroke that most clinicians attribute to improved detection and treatment of hypertension.[24] Prevention of stroke, and perhaps stroke recurrence, may be accomplished by reduction of elevated blood pressure, prevention and treatment of predisposing cardiac diseases, and probably by encouraging cessation of cigarette smoking. While CHD incidence and recurrence can be reduced by cholesterol lowering, there is little evidence that such an effort would reduce stroke directly. Of course, CHD is a major precursor of stroke and is the principal cause of death of stroke and TIA survivors, and on that account CHD prevention is certainly worthwhile.

### Control of Hypertension and Stroke Prevention

Following clinical observation of patients with treated and untreated hypertension with prospective epidemiologic study, it is apparent that level of blood pressure is related to incidence of stroke, and this is true for severe, moderate, and even mild hypertensive persons.[53] From a combined analysis of nine major prospective studies, including 420,000 individuals with a mean 10-year follow-up, there was clear evidence of a graded relationship between diastolic pressure and stroke and CHD incidence.[79] There was no threshold level below which risk gradients were flat. For every 7.5 mmHg diastolic pressure increase there was a 46 percent increase in stroke incidence and a 29 percent increase in CHD. Relating these findings from prospective observational study to randomized trials of blood pressure reduction demonstrated that treatment prevented stroke. The findings should put to rest the concern that reduction of blood pressure in hypertensive persons serves to precipitate stroke. From a statistical analysis of 14 treatment trials with a total of 37,000 hypertensive subjects, it was clear that reduction of blood pressure in the hypertensive subjects reduced stroke incidence.[46] There was an average blood pressure reduction of 5.8 mmHg and a corresponding reduction in stroke incidence of 42 percent. This observed reduction in stroke closely approximated that expected on the basis of prospective observational studies. Unfortunately, the 14 percent decrease in CHD rates was considerably lower than expected. The explanation for the lesser effect on CHD incidence is being sought. It may relate to the adverse influence on electrolyte, glucose, and lipid metabolism of the thiazide diuretics that were the mainstay of treatment in most of the trials.[48] It is important to note that these substantial and significant reductions in stroke incidence occurred during the course of the trials. In these studies, the duration of blood pressure reduction was brief, from 2 to 5 years, suggesting interruption of a precipitating factor rather than interfering with atherogenesis.[49] Presumably, more prolonged blood pressure control would have both effects.

Emphasis has been placed on the diastolic component in virtually all treatment trials, although stroke risk is clearly no less directly related to systolic pressure levels (Table 1-2). In the elderly, where isolated elevation of the systolic pressure is common, treatment was thought to be ineffective in reducing pressure, hazardous in terms of side effects, and unwarranted on the basis of availability epidemiologic data. In 4,736 persons above age 60, with systolic blood pressure levels above 160 mmHg and diastolic pressures below 90 mmHg, blood pressure reduction was associated with a 36 percent reduction in stroke and a 27 percent reduction in MI and coronary death after 4.5 years of follow-up.[69] These findings have enormous importance, since two-thirds of all individuals with hypertension, between the ages of 65 and 89 years, have isolated systolic hypertension. The bulk of strokes occur in this age group.[84] It is clear from the SHEP Trial and from the European Working Party on Hypertension in the Elderly (EWPHE) study, that antihypertensive medication was well tolerated by the elderly.[7] SHEP demonstrated that reduction of pressure was accomplished with relative ease, approximately half were controlled with chlorthalidone alone, and was well tolerated as evidenced by a 90 percent compliance rate in the active treatment group at 5 years. Since increased blood pressure is the most powerful risk factor for stroke, and since the benefits of treatment occur so promptly, control of increased blood pressure, systolic as well as diastolic levels, is the cornerstone of stroke prevention.

### Cessation of Cigarette Smoking

Based on data from the Nurses Health Study and from Framingham, it seems clear that stopping smoking is followed by a reduction in stroke risk, in a remarkably short time. Risk of CHD decreases by approximately 50 percent within 1 year of smoking cessation and reaches the level of those who never smoked within 5 years. In Framingham, in both men and women, risk of stroke in former cigarette smokers did not differ from that of persons who never smoked by the end of 5 years. There was no age effect, suggesting that cigarette smoking exerted a precipitating effect on stroke (and on MI and sudden death), which was reversed with smoking cessation. Since smoking confers an increase in stroke risk of 40 percent in men and 60 percent in women, after all other pertinent risk factors have been taken into account, cessation may be expected to significantly reduce risk of stroke.

### Prevention and Treatment of Heart Disease, Including Atrial Fibrillation

Since CHD, cardiac failure, and AF predispose to stroke, prevention of these cardiovascular contributors can be anticipated to reduce incidence of stroke.[18] On the basis of current knowledge of the epidemiology of cardiac failure, prevention of obesity and treatment of hypertension may be beneficial. Reduction of CHD risk requires, in addition to hypertension control and smoking cessation, dietary or pharmacologic treatment to reduce elevated total and LDL-cholesterol and to try to increase the HDL-cholesterol fraction. Prevention of AF might best be accomplished by preventing the appearance of the major precursor of AF, which is heart disease.

### Identification of High-Risk Candidates for Stroke Prevention

Each physician can identify "prime" candidates for stroke among his asymptomatic patients. Control of severe and moderately severe hypertension will definitely prevent stroke. Patients with these levels of blood pressure require vigorous and sustained therapy to maintain normotension. However, the bulk of hypertensive persons are those with borderline elevations of blood pressure, accounting for 70 percent of all hypertensives. Treatment of this large population with mild and borderline blood pressure elevation with drugs would be an extraordinary therapeutic and financial effort. While the rewards of such an effort may be correspondingly great, it seems more likely that many persons whose risk of developing atherosclerotic disease is low, will be exposed to costly drugs with dangerous or unpleasant side effects. What is needed is a way of selecting persons at substantially increased risk of stroke and other cardiovascular disease for intensive preventive intervention, including pharmacologic treatment of hypertension. For the remainder, whose risk of stroke is average or only mildly increased, hygienic measures should be prescribed. These include weight loss, reduction of salt (as well as calories and fat) in the diet, cigarette smoking cessation, and moderate physical activity, all measures that can be advocated for most people.

A stroke risk profile has been developed, utilizing data from 36 years of follow-up from Framingham, which allows the physician to determine a patient's probability of stroke.[87] This can be done based on information collected during the course of taking a comprehensive medical history and conducting a physical examination, plus obtaining an ECG. Using a table that is sex-specific, probability is determined by a point system depending on

1. Age
2. Systolic blood pressure
3. Antihypertensive therapy use
4. Presence of diabetes
5. Cigarette smoking
6. History of cardiovascular disease (CHD or cardiac failure)
7. ECG abnormalities (LVH or AF)

Risk is distributed over a wide range and permits the physician to rapidly relate a particular patient's probability of stroke to that of an average person of the same age and sex.

The stroke risk profile will help the physician to identify which borderline hypertensive patients warrant pharmacologic treatment by virtue of an increased probability of stroke usually attributable to the presence of several other risk factor abnormalities. By restricting drug treatment to persons with a systolic blood pressure level, who have two or more other risk factor abnormalities, (not including age and male sex), it is possible to identify a group consisting of 22 percent of the men and 14 percent of the women at high risk. In this group approximately 40 percent of strokes will occur within the subsequent 10 years.[87] Clearly there are other situations not considered here when a patient can be identified to be at substantially increased risk of stroke: recent TIA, recent-onset AF, recent MI, during and immediately following cardiac surgery, and others that are dealt with elsewhere.

## REFERENCES


1. Abbott RD, Donahue RP, MacMahon SW et al: Diabetes and the risk of stroke: the Honolulu Heart Program. JAMA 257:949, 1987
2. Abbott RD, Yin Yin MA, Reed DM, Yano K: Risk of stroke in male cigarette smokers. N Engl J Med 315:717, 1986
3. Adams HP, Butler MJ, Biller J, Toffol GJ: Nonhemorrhagic cerebral infarction in young adults. Arch Neurol 43:793, 1986
4. Ahmed OI, Orchard TJ, Sharma R et al: Declining mortality from stroke in Allegheny county, Pennsylvania: trends in case fatality and severity of disease, 1971–1980. Stroke 19:181, 1988
5. Alfredsson L, von Arbin M, de Faire U: Mortality from and incidence of stroke in Stockholm. Br Med J 1:292:1299, 1986
6. American Heart Association: 1991 Heart and Stroke Facts. Dallas, 1991
7. Amery A, Birkenhager W, Brixko P et al: Mortality and morbidity results from the European Working Party on High Blood Pressure in the Elderly Trial. Lancet 1:1349, 1985
8. Aurell M, Hood B: Cerebral hemorrhage in population after a decade of active anti-hypertensive treatment. Acta Med Scand 176:377, 1964
9. Barrett-Connor E, Khaw K: Diabetes mellitus: an independent risk factor for stroke. Am J Epidemiol 128:116, 1988
10. Bonita R: Cigarette smoking, hypertension and the risk of subarachnoid hemorrhage: a population-based case-control study. Stroke 17:831, 1986
11. Broderick JP, Phillips SJ, Whisnant JP et al: Incidence rates of stroke in the eighties: the end of the decline in stroke? Stroke 20:577, 1989
12. Colandrea MA, Friedman GD, Nichaman MZ et al: Systolic hypertension in the elderly: an epidemiologic assessment. Circulation 41:239, 1970
13. Colditz GA, Bonita R, Stampfer MJ et al: Cigarette smoking and risk of stroke in middle-aged women. N Engl J Med 318:937, 1988
14. Collins R, Peto R, MacMahon S et al: Blood pressure, stroke and coronary heart disease. II. Short-term reductions in blood pressure: overview randomised drug trials in their epidemiological context. Lancet 335:827, 1990
15. Cooper R, Sempos C, Hsieh S-C, Kovar MG: Slowdown in the decline of stroke mortality in the United States, 1978–1986. Stroke 21:1274, 1990
16. Deubner DC, Tyroler HA, Cassel JC et al: Attributable risk, population attributable risk, and population attributable fraction of death associated with hypertension in a biracial population. Circulation 52:901, 1975
17. Donahue RP, Abbott RD, Reed DM, Yano K: Alcohol and hemorrhagic stroke: The Honolulu Heart Program. JAMA 255:2311, 1986
18. Drury I, Whisnant JP, Garraway WM: Primary intracerebral hemorrhage: impact of CT on incidence. Neurology (NY) 34:653, 1984
19. Ettinger PO, Wu CF, DeLaCruz C, Jr et al: Arrhythmias and the "holiday heart": alcohol-associated cardiac rhythm disorders. Am Heart J 95:55, 1985
20. Fisher CM: The ascendancy of diastolic blood pressure over systolic. Lancet 2:1349, 1985
21. Fogelholm R, Murros K: Cigarette smoking and subarachnoid hemorrhage: a population-based case-control study. J Neurol Neurosurg Psychiatry 50:70, 1987
22. Folsom AR, Prineas RJ, Kaye SA, Munger RG: Incidence of hypertension and stroke in relation to body fat distribution and other risk factors in older women. Stroke 21:701, 1990
23. Furlan AJ, Whisnant JP, Elveback LR: The decreasing incidence of primary intracerebral hemorrhage: a population study. Ann Neurol 5:367, 1979
24. Garraway WM, Whisnant JP: The changing pattern of hypertension and the declining incidence of stroke. JAMA 258:214, 1987
25. Garraway WM, Whisnant JP, Drury I: The changing pattern of survival following stroke. Stroke 14:699, 1983
26. Gillum RF: Cerebrovascular disease morbidity in the United States, 1970–1983: age, sex, region, and vascular surgery. Stroke 17:656, 1986

27. Gillum RF: Stroke in blacks. Stroke 19:1, 1988
28. Gillum RF, Gomez-Marin O, Kottke TE et al: Acute stroke in a metropolitan area. 1970 and 1980: The Minnesota Heart Survey. J Chronic Dis 11:891, 1985
29. Goodnight SH, Jr, Harris WS, Connor WE, Illingworth DR: Polyunsaturated fatty acids, hyperlipidemia and thrombosis. Artheriosclerosis 2:87, 1982
30. Gorelick PB: The status of alcohol as a risk factor for stroke. Stroke 12:1607, 1989
31. Hennekens CH: Alcohol. p. 130. In Kaplan NM, Stamler J (eds): Prevention of Coronary Heart Disease, Practical Management of the Risk Factors. WB Saunders, Philadelphia, 1983
32. Hillbom M, Kaste M: Does ethanol intoxication promote brain infarction in young adults? Lancet 2:1181, 1978
33. Howard G, Toole JF, Becker C et al: Changes in survival following stroke in five North Carolina counties observed during two different periods. Stroke 20:345, 1989
34. Ingall TJ, Whisnant JP, Wiebers DO, O'Fallon WM: Has there been a decline in subarachnoid hemorrhage mortality? Stroke 20:718, 1989
35. Iso H, Jacobs DR, Wentworth D et al: Serum cholesterol levels and six-year mortality from stroke in 350,977 men screened for the multiple risk factor intervention trial. N Engl J Med 320:904, 1989
36. Japanese Health and Welfare Ministry: AMA Med News 17:12, 1986
37. Kannel WB, Gordon T: Evaluation of cardiovascular risk in the elderly: the Framingham Study. Bull NY Acad Med 54:573, 1978
38. Kannel WB, Gordon T, Wolf PA et al: Hemoglobin and the risk of cerebral infarction: the Framingham Study. Stroke 3:409, 1972
39. Kannel WB, McGee DL: Diabetes and cardiovascular disease: the Framingham Study. JAMA 241:2035, 1979
40. Kannel WB, Wolf PA, Castelli WP et al: Fibrinogen and risk of cardiovascular disease: the Framingham Study. JAMA 258:1183, 1987
41. Kannel WB, Wolf PA, McGee DL et al: Systolic blood pressure, arterial rigidity, and risk of stroke: the Framingham Study. JAMA 245:1225, 1981
42. Kannel WB, Wolf PA, Verter J: Manifestations of coronary disease predisposing to stroke: the Framingham Study. JAMA 250:2942, 1983
43. Kittner SJ, White LR, Losonczy KG et al: Black-white differences in stroke incidence in a national sample: the contribution of hypertension and diabetes mellitus. JAMA 264:1267, 1990
44. Klag MJ, Whelton PK, Seidler AJ: Decline in US stroke mortality, demographic trends and antihypertensive treatment. Stroke 20:14, 1989
45. Klatsky AL, Armstrong MA, Friedman GD: Alcohol use and subsequent cerebrovascular disease hospitalizations. Stroke 20:741, 1989
46. Kozarevic DJ, McGee D, Vojvodic N et al: Frequency of alcohol consumption and morbidity and mortality: the Yugoslavia Cardiovascular Disease Study. Lancet 1:613, 1980
47. Kuller LH, Dorman JS, Wolf PA: Cerebrovascular diseases and diabetes. p. 1. In National Diabetes Data Group: Diabetes in America, Diabetes Data Compiled for 1984. Vol. 18. Department of Health and Human Services, NIH Publication No. 85-1468, August 1985
48. Leon AS, Blackburn H: Physical inactivity. p. 86. In Kaplan NM, Stamler J (eds): Prevention of Coronary Heart Disease, Practical Management of the Risk Factors. WB Saunders, Philadelphia, 1983
49. Leon AS, Connett J, Jacobs DR, Rauramaa R: Leisure-time physical activity levels and risk of coronary heart disease and death: the Multiple Risk Factor Intervention Trial. JAMA 258:2388, 1987
50. Li S, Schoenberg BS, Wang C et al: Cerebrovascular disease in the People's Republic of China: epidemiologic and clinical features. Neurology (Cleveland) 35:1708, 1985
51. Longstreth WT, Koepsell TD, Yerby MS, van Belle G: Risk factors for subarachnoid hemorrhage. Stroke 16:377, 1985
52. MacMahon B, Pugh TF: Epidemiology: Principles and Methods. Little, Brown, Boston, 1970
53. MacMahon S, Cutler JA, Stamler J: Antihypertensive drug treatment: potential, expected and observed effects on stroke and on coronary heart disease. Hypertension, suppl I. 13:I-45, 1989
54. MacMahon S, Peto R, Cutler J et al: Blood pressure, stroke and coronary heart disease. I. Prolonged differences in blood pressure: prospective observational studies corrected for the regression dilution bias. Lancet 335:765, 1990
55. Malmgren R, Warlow C, Bamford J, Sandercock P: Geographical and secular trends in stroke incidence. Lancet 2:1196, 1987
56. Mohr JP, Caplan LR, Melski JW et al: The Harvard Cooperative Stroke Registry: a prospective registry of cases hospitalized with stroke. Neurology (NY) 28:754, 1978
57. O'Leary DH, Anderson KM, Wolf PA et al: Cholesterol and carotid atherosclerosis in older persons: the Framingham Study. Ann Epidemiol 2:147, 1992
58. Otten MW, Teutsch SM, Williamson DF, Marks JS: The effect of known risk factors on the excess mortality of black adults in the United States. JAMA 263:845, 1990
59. Paffenbarger RS, Laughlin ME, Gina AS et al: Work activity of longshoremen as related to death from coronary heart disease and stroke. N Engl J Med 282:1109, 1970
60. Paffenbarger RS, Wing AL, Hyde RT: Physical activity as an index of heart attack risk in college alumni. Am J Epidemiol 108:161, 1978
61. Pearson TC, Thomas DJ: Physiological and pharmacological factors influencing blood viscosity and cerebral blood flow. p. 33. In Tognomi G, Gerattinin S (eds): Drug Treatment and Prevention in Cerebrovascular Disorders. Elsevier North-Holland, Amsterdam, 1979
62. Reed DM: The paradox of high risk of stroke in populations with low risk of coronary heart disease. Am J Epidemiol 131:579, 1990

63. Robbins M, Baum HM: Incidence: the National Survey on Stroke, suppl 1. 12:45, 1981
64. Royal College of General Practitioners' Oral Contraception Study: further analyses of mortality in oral contraceptive users. Lancet 1:541, 1981
65. Rutan GH, McDonald RH, Kuller LH: A historical perspective of elevated systolic vs diastolic blood pressure from an epidemiological and clinical trial viewpoint. J Clin Epidemiol 42:663, 1989
66. Sacco RL, Hauser WA, Mohr JP, Foulkes MA: One-year outcome after cerebral infarction in whites, blacks and hispanics. Stroke 22:305, 1991
67. Sacco RL, Wolf PA, Bharucha NE et al: Subarachnoid and intracerebral hemorrhage: natural history, prognosis, and precursive factors in the Framingham Study. Neurology (NY) 34:847, 1984
68. Salonen R, Seppanen K, Rauramaa R, Salonen JT: Prevalence of carotid atherosclerosis and serum cholesterol levels in eastern Finland. Atherosclerosis 8:788, 1988
69. SHEP Cooperative Research Group: Prevention of stroke by antihypertensive drug treatment in older persons with isolated systolic hypertension: final results of the Systolic Hypertension in the Elderly Program (SHEP). JAMA 265:3255, 1991
70. Shimamoto T, Komachi Y, Inada H et al: Trends for coronary heart disease and stroke and their risk factors in Japan. Circulation 79:503, 1989
71. Shinton R, Beevers G: Meta-analysis of relation between cigarette smoking and stroke. Br Med J 298:789, 1989
72. Smith P, Arnesen H, Holme I: The effect of warfarin on mortality and reinfarction after myocardial infarction. N Engl J Med 323:147, 1990
73. Stadel BV: Oral contraceptives and cardiovascular disease. N Engl J Med 288:672, 1981
74. Stampfer MJ, Colditz GA, Willett WC et al: A prospective study of moderate alcohol consumption and the risk of coronary disease and stroke in women. N Engl J Med 319:267, 1988
75. Stampfer MJ, Willett WC, Colditz GA et al: A Prospective study of past use of oral contraceptive agents and risk of cardiovascular diseases. N Engl J Med 319:1313, 1988
76. Tanaka H, Ueda Y, Hayashi M et al: Risk factors for cerebral hemorrhage and cerebral infarction in a Japanese rural community. Stroke 13:62, 1982
77. Thomas DJ, Marshal J, Ross Russell RW et al: Effect of haematocrit on cerebral blood flow in man. Lancet 2:1163, 1966
78. Tohgi H, Yamanouchi H, Murakami M et al: Importance of the hematocrit as a risk factor in cerebral infarction. Stroke 9:369, 1978
79. Ueda K, Hasuo Y, Kiyohara Y et al: Intracerebral hemorrhage in a Japanese community, Hisayama: incidence, changing pattern during long-term follow-up, and related factors. Stroke 19:48, 1988
80. Vessey MP, Lawless M, Yeates D: Oral contraceptives and stroke: findings in a large prospective study. Br Med J 289:530, 1984
81. Welin I, Svardsudd K, Wilhelmsen L et al: Analysis of risk factors for stroke in a cohort of men born in 1913. N Engl J Med 317:521, 1987
82. White, MF: Reducing cardiovascular risk factors in the United States—an overview of the National Educational Programs. Cardiovasc Risk Factors 1:277, 1991
83. Wilhelmsen L, Svardsudd K, Korban-Bengsten K et al: Fibrinogen as a risk factor for stroke and myocardial infarction. N Engl J Med 311:501, 1984
84. Wilking SVB, Belanger A, Kannel WB et al: Determinants of isolated systolic hypertension. JAMA 260:3451, 1988
85. Wolf PA, Abbott RD, Kannel WB: Atrial fibrillation: a major contributor to stroke in the elderly; the Framingham Study. Arch Interna Med 147:1561, 1987
86. Wolf PA, Abbott RD, Kannel WB: Atrial fibrillation, an independent risk factor for stroke in the elderly: the Framingham Study. Stroke 22:983, 1991
87. Wolf PA, D'Agostino RB, Belanger AJ, Kannel WB: Probability of stroke: a risk profile from the Framingham Study. Stroke 22:312, 1991
88. Wolf PA, D'Agostino RB, Kannel WB et al: Cigarette smoking as a risk factor for stroke: the Framingham Study. JAMA 259:1025, 1988
89. Yano K, Reed DM, MacLean CJ: Serum cholesterol and hemorrhagic stroke in the Honolulu Heart Program. Stroke 20:1460, 1989

# 2
# ATHEROGENESIS AND STROKES

Thomas J. DeGraba
Marc Fisher
Frank M. Yatsu

Strokes due to atherosclerosis or so-called atherothrombotic brain infarction (ABI) remain numerically the most common neurologic disorder among adults in America and the third major cause of death and disability behind coronary heart disease and cancer.[106] Similar findings continue in other industrialized countries, but with stroke risk-factor intervention, particularly hypertension control, a gratifying reduction has occurred over the last several decades.[106] While more effective means of reducing stroke risk factors must be developed, such as educational and motivational techniques to discontinue smoking or taking needed medication, greater precision in identifying stroke-prone individuals, as opposed to collective risks, will require further insights into the metabolic and molecular biologic underpinnings in ABIs. Galvanized by important pathophysiologic findings in coronary artery disease, with therapeutic implications and subsequent clinical trials resulting in disease reduction, similar efforts are now being considered with ABIs whose basic pathogenetic mechanisms are similar to coronary artery disease. By defining precise metabolic and molecular biologic abnormalities in ABIs, their correction or modification should provide the ultimate cure for strokes, namely, prevention.

Support for this work was provided by the Clayton Foundation for Research, Houston; the Cullen Trust for Health Care of Houston; the U.S. Public Health Service, and the Roy M. and Phyllis Gough Huffington Chair.

Since publication of the first edition of *Stroke* in 1986, a proliferation of basic and clinical information has been published on ABIs. In this chapter, newer and more exciting studies are emphasized primarily, while providing a broad overview. We review the epidemiology, pathogenesis, and therapy of ABIs; the latter two receive special attention because of their practical and potential therapeutic implications in averting ABIs. For studies on the pathogenesis of atherosclerosis, the two dominant theories, namely, injury healing and the lipid hypotheses, are discussed, especially interventional strategies modifying the process.

## EPIDEMIOLOGY

Since the topic of epidemiology is reviewed extensively by Dr. Philip A. Wolf in Chapter 1, only a few salient features relevant to ABIs will be commented upon as they relate to atherogenesis. Risk factors for ABIs are similar to coronary heart disease (CHD), as demonstrated in the Framingham Study by Kannel et al.[57,58] By the twenty-fourth biennial examination of the Framingham, Massachusetts population, 334 strokes occurred, and analysis of risk factors confirmed that the five major risks for CHD were identical, namely, hypertension, clinical symptoms of CHD, cardiac failure, electrocardiographic (ECG) or radiographic evidences of CHD, and atrial fibrillation. Because atherosclerosis is a diffuse vascular disease, and

ABI and CHD are virtually inseparable pathologic entities, efforts to reduce atherosclerosis should be beneficial in impacting both ABI and CHD. In addition to these five, other prominent risk factors common to both CHD and ABI are diabetes mellitus, smoking and perhaps stress, obesity, and sedentary life.[106] Although lipid abnormalities, namely, elevated low-density lipoprotein (LDL) and reduced high-density lipoprotein (HDL), are consistent risk factors for CHD, that is not uniformly the case with ABI, although the majority of the reported series show a relationship between elevated total cholesterol, increased LDL, or reduced HDL with ABIs, as extensively reviewed by Tell et al.[103]

Of controllable risk factors, hypertension and smoking have yielded to public education campaigns but the recidivism rate for the latter remains high.[106] More effective means of identifying hypertensives and monitoring their therapies are needed as are interventions to discontinue smoking.[18] That hypertension is unambiguously associated with increased risk for stroke has been amply demonstrated recently and has been shown to be cost-effective.[82,84] For example, Cutler et al.[22] reviewed 17 large-scale, controlled, clinical trials on drug treatment for hypertension and found a salutary effect in reducing mortality and morbidity. Of nine similarly analyzable trials with an aggregate 43,000 patients followed for an average of nearly 6 years, a 6 mmHg reduction in mean diastolic blood pressure conveyed an 11 percent decrease in mortality, largely attributable to a 38 percent decline in fatal strokes. Nonfatal strokes were also decreased, although inexplicably coronary heart disease mortality was not significantly affected; use of thiazidelike diuretic drugs to control hypertension may, however, be less beneficial for CHD. In a further analysis of collective studies from nine centers involving 430,000 individuals followed for a mean of 10 years and experiencing 843 strokes and 4,856 CHD events, MacMahon et al.[69] found that, by correcting for random fluctuations in diastolic blood pressure by "regression dilution," a parallel reduction of both ABI and CHD was seen with decreasing diastolic blood pressures. Metanalyses of a number of dissimilar series may provide data supporting our preconceived notions, such as lower blood pressures reducing ABIs. To avoid biases, prospective studies are required to answer this question. However, until these data are forthcoming, the conventional view that hypertension control averts both CHD and ABI remains a prudent one.

In a large self-reporting study by Fiebach et al.[28] of 119,963 nurses, aged 30 to 55 years, questioned initially in 1976 and then again in 1982, both ABI and CHD were significantly more common with relative risks of 3.5 and 2.6, respectively, for those reporting hypertension. The number of strokes in follow-up was 175 (50 fatal and 125 nonfatal) and 308 CHD (66 fatal and 242 nonfatal myocardial infarctions). Although self-reporting, the medically sophisticated and knowledgeable nature of the respondents make the results creditable. Medical knowledge did not, inexplicably, translate to therapy of hypertension.

In North Karelia, Finland, where the CHD rate was virtually the highest in the world, considered epidemic, and provoking concerns by the public and politicians to intervene, the cost-benefit issue of treating hypertension was analyzed.[106] Analysis was based primarily on the number of reduced ABI and CHD attributable to treated hypertension and comparing medication costs to medical care costs for ABI and CHD if they were to occur without treatment. Nissinen et al.[84] conclude that therapy of hypertension is cost-beneficial but note that less expensive medications would improve that ratio substantially, since they account for 86 percent of the costs.

As noted above, the role of cigarette smoking in provoking ABI has been substantiated repeatedly,[78,80] but as with other "habits" that have addictive potential, more effective alternatives or interventions are required, particularly for vulnerable persons. Whether moderate amounts of alcohol are beneficial is uncertain.[26,36] In the Honolulu Heart Program, which followed more than 8,000 men over 12 years, 197 drinkers and 93 nondrinkers had strokes; no relationship could be established between alcohol consumption and ABIs, but an association exists with hemorrhagic strokes due to aneurysms. On the other hand, "light" drinking may convey protection against strokes as opposed to teetotalers.[37] Whether genetic or racial factors play a role is uncertain and requires further investigation.[51,88]

## PATHOLOGY

Expanding knowledge about the pathogenesis of atherosclerotic plaque development and the cellular contributors to the process are important from a pathophysiologic and potentially therapeutic perspective. Therefore, it is appropriate to review the basic pathology of atherosclerosis and the cellular contributors to atherosclerotic plaque development. The earliest lesion of atherosclerosis is the fatty streak.[99] Fatty streaks can be seen as early as late childhood or early adolescence. The fatty streak is widely distributed throughout the arterial vasculature without predilection for foci seen in more advanced lesions. Fatty streaks are grossly visible as areas of yellowish discoloration of the intimal surface of large to medium-sized arteries, and they are readily apparent when fat staining techniques are employed. On a microscopic level, fatty streaks are noted to consist primarily of lipid-laden macrophages known as foam cells.[81] A small percentage of the foam cells are smooth muscle cells in origin. Extracellular lipid is also apparent in fatty streaks. The macrophages that become foam cells are primarily derived from circulating monocytes, which gain entry into the arterial

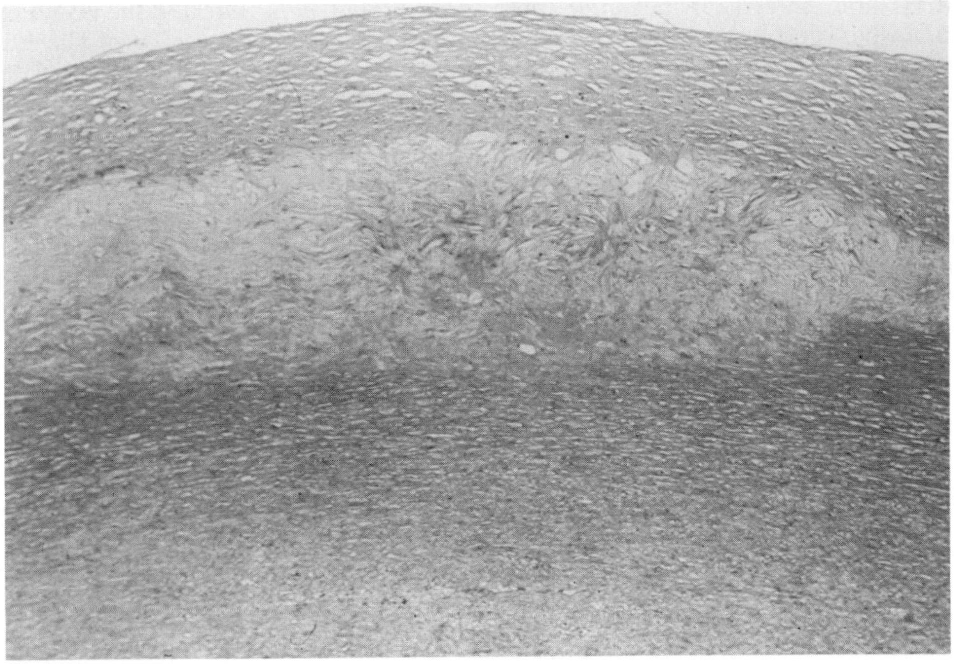

**Fig. 2-1.** A fibrous plaque from a human aorta. (From Fisher,[30] with permission.)

wall at very early stages in the atherogenic process.[72,95] T-lymphocytes are also present in early plaques.

As fatty streaks progress, typically over many years, fibrosis plaques (Fig. 2-1) begin to develop in middle-aged and older adults.[75] The sites where these fibrous plaques develop are more localized than fatty streaks, typically occurring at arterial branch points or opposite arterial bifurcations. The fibrous plaque consists of an intact endothelial lining, which overlays a fibrous cap. The fibrous cap contains foam cells, transformed smooth muscle cells, lymphocytes, a connec-

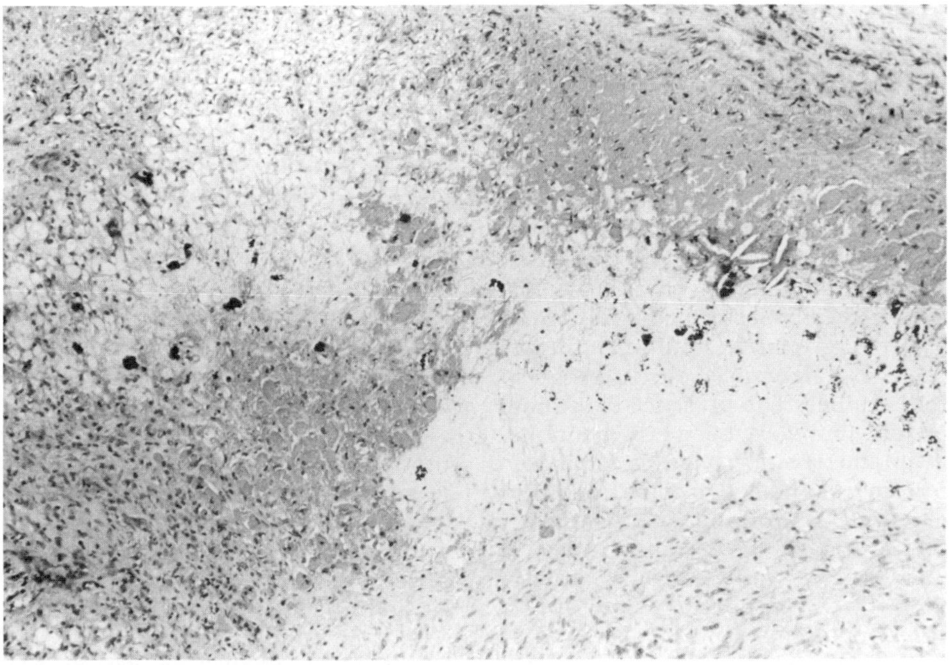

**Fig. 2-2.** A complicated plaque containing calcification and hemosiderin. (From Norris and Hachinski,[85] with permission.)

tive tissue matrix and a central necrotic core, including cellular debris, and free extracellular lipid and cholesterol crystals. The percentage of the plaque derived from each of these constituents may vary, and this will influence the consistency of the plaque for soft versus hard characteristics. Small arterioles are commonly observed at the periphery of the plaque and engender the possibility of hemorrhagic transformation in some fibrous plaques. The complicated plaque represents the most advanced stage of atherogenesis, and these plaques are similar to fibrous plaques. However, they commonly contain hemosiderin, areas of intraplaque calcification, and disruption of the endothelial lining[75] (Fig. 2-2).

## SYMPTOM DEVELOPMENT

Plaques usually enlarge insidiously over decades. It is only when the plaque burden reaches a substantial percentage of the arterial luminal diameter that symptoms typically occur. Plaque destabilization leading to symptom development is an important consideration concerning potential prevention of atherosclerotic complications, such as ischemic stroke or myocardial infarction (MI). Studies of patients with acute MI have demonstrated that disruption of the plaque luminal surface is a common feature associated with coronary thrombosis and symptoms development.[27] Luminal thrombi are typically associated with disruption or ulceration of the endothelial lining, leading to arterial obstruction. Blood within the plaque or intraplaque hemorrhage appears to be secondary to the luminal disruption, with dissection of luminal blood into the plaque.[23] Primary intraplaque hemorrhage has only occasionally been hypothesized as an initiator for coronary artery plaque destabilization and symptom development.

It has been proposed that a similar mechanism, primary luminal surface disruption, is responsible for the development of symptoms in large-vessel extracranial arteries such as the carotid and vertebral basilar arteries.[31] Pathologic studies of symptomatic extracranial arteries are usually performed after carotid endarterectomy.[53] The presence of luminal surface disruption has been less vigorously pursued than in the coronary artery studies. The presence of luminal surface disruption has, therefore, been less commonly documented. Intraplaque hemorrhage is commonly seen both in symptomatic and asymptomatic carotid arteries.[3,64] Failure to detect luminal surface disruption frequently in carotid artery specimens may be secondary to the less precise evaluation of these arteries in comparison to the coronary artery studies. Two recent autopsy series of patients expiring acutely after carotid artery occlusion have been reported.[71,86] These studies, in which the carotid arteries were carefully evaluated, demonstrated the presence of luminal surface disruption in every case. They appear to support the hypothesis that extracranial arterial thrombi frequently develop secondary to luminal surface disruption in a similar fashion to that observed in the coronary arteries. It is important to distinguish whether symptoms develop secondary to luminal surface disruption or primary intraplaque hemorrhage because these concepts have potential impacts upon preventative therapy. If luminal surface disruption is the primary mechanism, then antithrombotic or antiplatelet therapy should have a role in the prevention of secondary thrombi, which could lead to symptom development.

## SMALL-ARTERY ATHEROSCLEROSIS

Small arteries, such as the lenticulostriate arteries, basilar penetrating arteries, and medullary arteries supplying deep cerebral white matter, appear to have differences in the nature of atherosclerosis in comparison to the large extracranial arteries (Fig. 2-3). These arteries and their degenerative processes are important because they are associated with the development of lacunar strokes and diffuse white matter changes associated with dementia. Therefore, understanding the nature of their degenerative changes may be important. In the lenticulostriate arteries, lipohylanosis and microatheromata have been observed in patients suffering small-vessel lacunar infarction.[29] In medullary arteries from patients with diffuse white matter disease, the most prominent finding observed was concentric lamellar arrangements of collagen fibers with the deposition of a fibrohyaline substance in the adventitia.[35] Cellular constituents were few, and the presence of lipid was limited. These observations concerning the degenerative changes in small arteries imply differences in comparison to those described in larger arteries. Therefore, the underlying pathogenetic process may be different.

## CELLULAR CONTRIBUTORS

As previously described, the major cellular contributors to large-vessel atherosclerosis appear to be monocytes/macrophages, smooth muscle cells, and endothelial cells. These three cell types interact with each other and the plaque milieu in a variety of complex ways. Study of the cellular aspects of atherogenesis dates back to the work of Virchow and other nineteenth century pathologists. Recently, Russel Ross and colleagues have updated earlier work concerning the cellular aspects of atherosclerosis and incorpo-

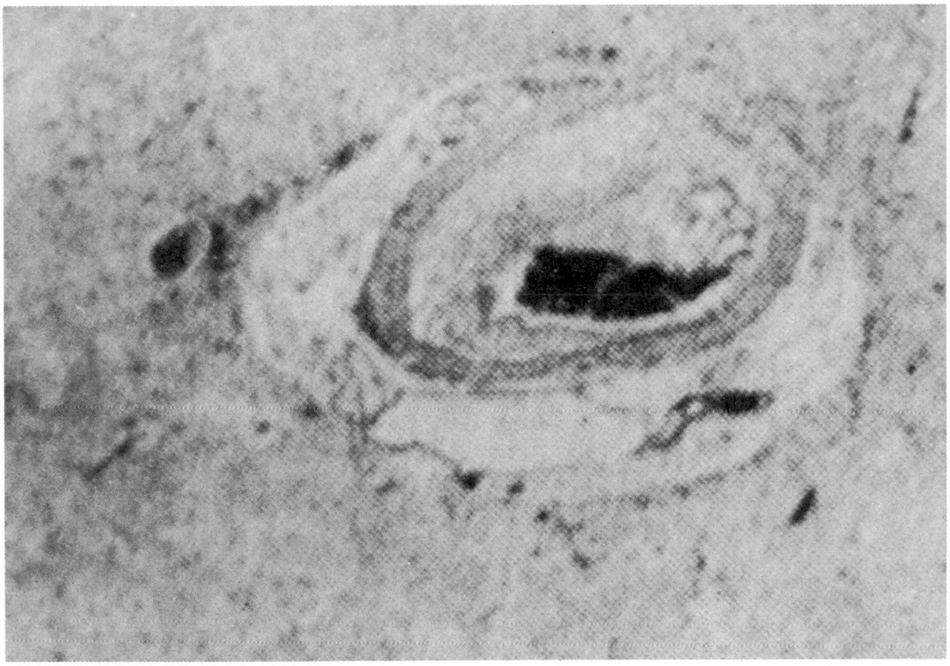

**Fig. 2-3.** An example of small-vessel degenerative changes in a patient with lacunar stroke.

rated these concepts into the "response to injury" hypothesis of atherogenesis[94] (Fig. 2-4). This hypothesis and its corollaries have been studied in a variety of animal atherosclerosis models and also in human atherosclerotic plaques. This hypothesis suggests that the earliest initiating event for atherogenesis is functional or morphologic injury to the endothelial lining of large to medium-sized arteries. Endothelial injury can be mediated by a number of processes, including hypertension, hyperlipidemia, cigarette smoke,

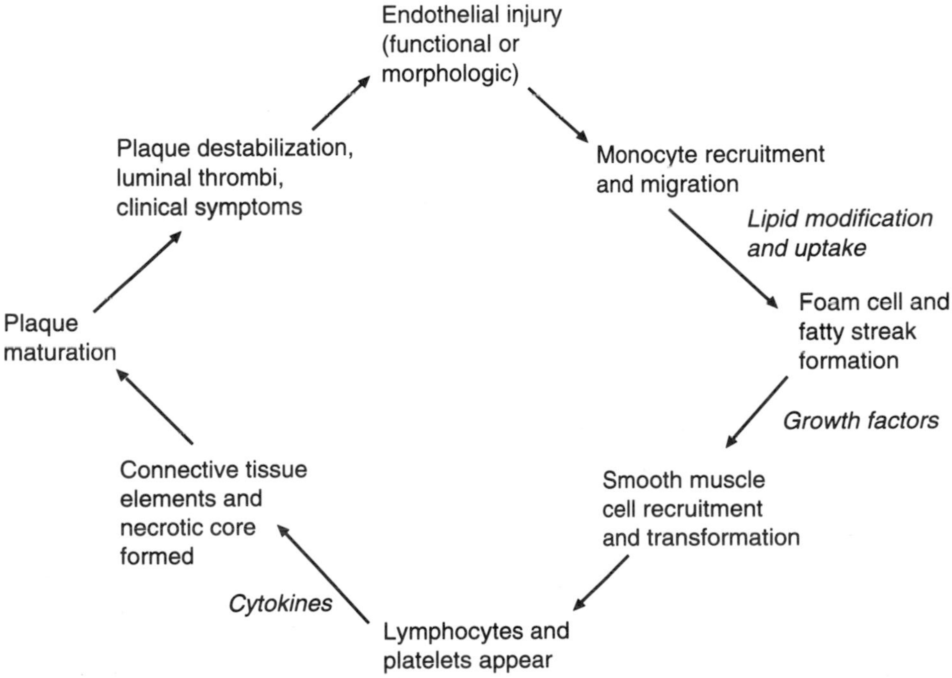


**Fig. 2-4.** The cellular events of atherosclerosis in schematic form. (From Fisher,[30] with permission.)

homocysteine, and radiation.[94] The endothelial injury is, in most cases, functional and not morphologic. This leads to the early adhesion and then intimal migration of circulating blood monocytes into the vessel wall.[94] Lipids enter the vessel wall via the endothelial cells in a complex fashion involving both active and passive transport.[54] Vessel wall monocyte-derived macrophages imbibe LDL cholesterol to form foam cells, a hallmark of early plaque development. Additionally, intercellular messengers such as platelet-derived growth factor (PDGF) and others are released by macrophages, endothelial cells, and, to a lesser degree, platelets to promote smooth muscle cell migration from the adventitia into the intima.[83] The smooth muscle cells are also apparently transformed from a contractile state into a more synthetic state.[13] Cytokines released by the macrophages, smooth muscle cells, endothelial cells and, perhaps, T-lymphocytes, which are also present in early atherosclerotic plaques, may play a role in cellular interactions as well. Synthesis of the connective tissue elements by smooth muscle cells leads to further plaque development and matrix formation. Cell necrosis and death of lipid-laden cells generates the lipid core associated with more advanced lesions. As this dynamic and complex process proceeds over decades, the plaque slowly enlarges, leading to luminal compromise and ultimately symptom development, as previously discussed. The "response to injury" hypothesis and the subsequent cellular events imply that atherogenesis is an ongoing and dynamic process, which potentially could be interrupted at various points.

## LOW-DENSITY LIPOPROTEIN-OXIDATION AND CELLULAR ASPECTS OF ATHEROGENESIS

It is clear that lipids play an important role in atherosclerotic plaque development, as do the cellular contributors. Linking the interaction between the cellular contributors of atherogenesis to the lipid aspects has been a vexing problem, but recent work appears to have clarified potential interactions between these important aspects of atherogenesis. LDL is taken up by vessel wall macrophages and smooth cells to form foam cells as an important early part of atherosclerotic plaque development. Native LDL is taken up at a relatively slow rate by its receptor.[11] However, modified LDL is taken up much more rapidly by the "scavenger receptor." Modification of LDL appears to be important, and this modification may occur primarily via oxidation[100] (Fig. 2-5). LDL-oxidation can be induced by free radicals produced by macrophages, smooth muscle cells, or endothelial cells. All three cell types have been observed to induce LDL-oxidation in vitro. Oxidized LDL has been demonstrated in human and experimental animal atherosclerotic plaques.[108] Oxidized LDL may contribute to atherogenesis in other ways besides LDL accumulation within foam cells. Oxidized LDL has cytotoxic properties and could promote endothelial injury and its propagation. Oxidized LDL appears to have chemoattractant properties for circulating monocytes and may contribute

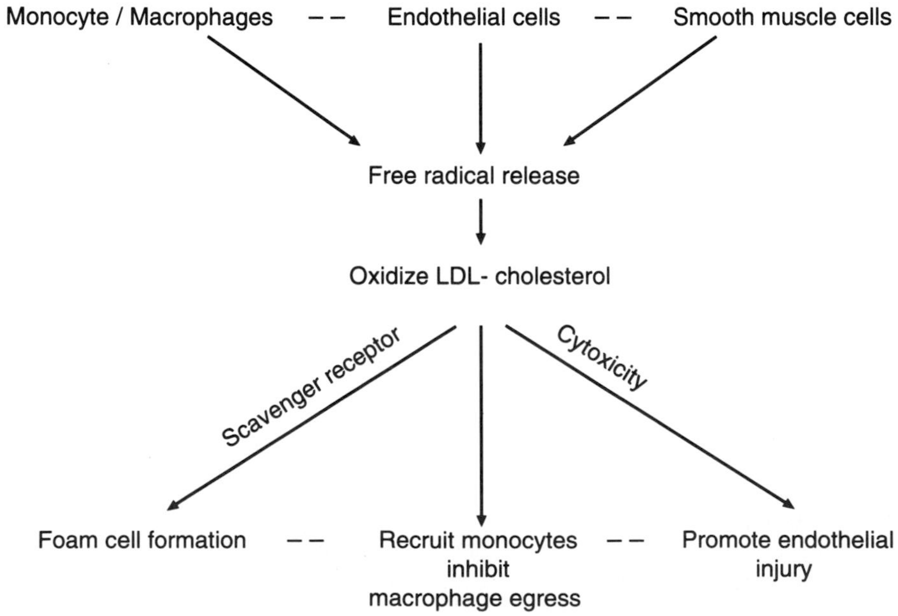


**Fig. 2-5.** A representation of how oxidized low density lipoprotein (LDL)-cholesterol is formed and its significance. (From Fisher,[30] with permission.)

to monocyte accumulation within plaques. Paradoxically, oxidized LDL inhibits egress of plaque macrophages and may therefore enhance accumulation of monocyte-derived macrophages within plaques. All of these mechanisms suggest that oxidized LDL may have an important role in atherogenesis and help to unify the cellular components of plaque development with the lipid contributors. Certainly the cellular and lipid contributors to atherogenesis must interact with one another, and LDL oxidation may be an important link.

The reported contribution of oxidized LDL to atherosclerotic plaque development suggests that inhibiting LDL-oxidation might reduce atherosclerotic plaque formation. Probucol is a lipid-lowering medication with modest effects on LDL-cholesterol level, but it has been shown to substantially inhibit experimental atherogenesis.[15] In an animal hyperlipidemic model of atherosclerosis, probucol was noted to have beneficial effects despite the maintenance of high LDL and total cholesterol levels. Probucol has antioxidant effects and has been observed to reduce endothelial cell and copper-induced LDL-oxidation.[91] It is likely that the effects of Probucol on atherogenesis are primarily mediated through its antioxidant effects. Human trials with probucol to inhibit femoral and coronary artery atherosclerosis are in progress, and results should be available in the near future.

## THERAPEUTIC IMPLICATIONS OF CELLULAR PROLIFERATION

Important advances have been made toward the reduction of atherosclerosis and associated clinical disorders by the treatment of risk factors such as hyperlipidemia, smoking, and hypertension. A great amount of effort in regard to patient education and medical intervention has been expended. There may, however, be inherent limits regarding risk factor intervention regarding both patient compliance with medication and ability to change lifestyle and dietary habits. The interaction of risk factors with the cellular aspects of atherogenesis suggests that treating at a cellular level may impact upon the final common pathway for atherosclerotic plaque formation when risk-factor modification is not tenable. As knowledge increases about the cellular aspects of atherogenesis, interventional approaches at this level become more apparent.

Epidemiologic studies revealed that populations consuming large quantities of marine mammals and fish have a reduced rate of ischemic stroke and cardiovascular disease. In both Japanese and Eskimo populations, the dietary consumption of marine mammals and fish was associated with increased blood and cellular levels of *n*-3 fatty acids.[39] Experimental studies have demonstrated that *n*-3 fatty acids have a wide variety of cellular effects that would appear to be beneficial with regard to the atherosclerotic process.[32] It has been observed that monocyte production of free radicals, interleukin-1, leukotriene-$B_4$, tumor necrosis factor, and platelet-activating factor are all diminished in association with the exposure of these cells to *n*-3 fatty acids. Monocyte chemotaxis is also inhibited in association with *n*-3 fatty acids, and endothelial cell production of PDGF is similarly reduced. Serum lipid levels do not appear to be significantly affected by dietary supplementation with *n*-3 fatty acids. It is likely that *n*-3 fatty acids exert their beneficial effects on atherosclerosis by a variety of cellular mechanisms, which favor impending plaque development.

The potential beneficial effects of *n*-3 fatty acids have been evaluated in animal atherosclerosis models. Two studies of dietary *n*-3 fatty acids supplementation in swine have demonstrated a significant reduction in the extent of coronary atherosclerosis in treated animals as compared to control animals who were maintained on a hyperlipidemic diet alone.[62,104] Additionally, another study in primates demonstrated that dietary substitution with *n*-3 fatty acids was also effective in reducing the extent of aortic, femoral, and carotid atherosclerosis.[24] It was observed that the number of vessel wall macrophages was diminished in the carotid atherosclerotic lesions of the treated group as compared to the controls, supportive of the cellular effects as previously outlined.

Two studies of *n*-3 fatty acid dietary supplementation have been reported in humans after coronary angioplasty.[25,92] One study demonstrated benefit in reducing the restenosis rate after angioplasty, while the second study of a similar design did not show benefit. Both of these studies included only relatively small numbers of patients, and a large multicenter trial with an adequate sample size is now being conducted. Restenosis after coronary angioplasty is not the same process as primary atherogenesis, and even if *n*-3 fatty acids are not effective in this setting, trials in native atherosclerosis are probably warranted. A trial involving the treatment of early carotid atherosclerosis with *n*-3 fatty acids would appear to be an ideal location, as the intervention can be followed with noninvasive technology as compared to invasive angiography necessary at present in coronary artery studies.

Other potential cellular level interventions for atherosclerosis have been suggested. As mentioned previously, LDL-oxidation and its inhibition offers a novel therapeutic intervention. Probucol has been evaluated in animal models and human trials are proceeding. Other antioxidants potentially may be of interest as antiatherogenic agents. The 21-aminosteroids, derived from methylprednisolone, have substantial antioxidant qualities.[7,33] They have been observed to inhibit monocyte free radical production and also monocyte-induced LDL-oxidation.[7] The 21-aminosteroids lack glucocorticoid and mineralocorticoid side effects and therefore should be evaluated in animal models of atherosclerosis and, if effective, should be considered for human trial.

Voltage-regulated calcium channel blockers have been widely evaluated in animal models of atherosclerosis.[34] The results have been conflicting, but agents such as diltiazem, verapamil, and flunarizine appear to have beneficial effects independent of lipid lowering of blood pressure qualities. Nifedipine has been evaluated in humans with coronary atherosclerosis. The INTACT trial evaluated the effect of nifedipine, 80 mg daily for 3 years, in patients with angiographically documented coronary artery disease.[67] Repeat angiography 3 years later demonstrated a significant reduction in the number of angiographically documented new lesions in the treatment group as compared to the controls. However, no difference was observed in the rate of progression of preexistent lesions. A similar result was observed in a smaller Italian trial. Isradipine is presently being evaluated in patients with mild to moderate carotid atherosclerosis.

Heparin has effects on smooth muscle cell proliferation and is another drug being studied to inhibit atherogenesis, primarily because of cellular effects.[19] One can anticipate further advances concerning cellular intervention for atherosclerosis as knowledge about the cellular cascade of atherogenesis increases. A potential therapy will need to be taken for many years, and therefore safety as well as efficacy will be paramount.

## ATHEROGENESIS: THE LIPID HYPOTHESIS

Although the two separate theories of atherogenesis—(1) the injury healing hypothesis and (2) the lipid hypothesis—dominate investigative inquiries, the two mechanisms likely operate synergistically. To pursue this likelihood, we are conducting laboratory studies assessing the probability that lipoprotein receptor activity will more vigorously amplify growth factor genes in susceptible individuals via transducing agents. Despite this likely synergism, discussing each hypothesis separately simplifies the understanding of pathogenesis as well as therapeutic implications for atheroma regression.

The role of the lipids, cholesterol, and saturated fats in inducing atherosclerosis has had initial and sustained support from epidemiologic and experimental investigations.[106] Simply stated, an increase of these lipids in diet, and subsequently in serum, parallels the association of lipids with atherosclerosis, primarily coronary heart disease (CHD). For atherosclerotic brain infarction (ABI), this relationship is less firm, but as reviewed by Tell et al.,[103] the majority of studies on this matter show a correlation, as discussed below.

Insight into the role of cholesterol and saturated fats in promoting atherosclerosis was substantially enhanced by the Nobel Prize-winning studies of Brown and Goldstein,[11] which complement the literal information explosion on atherogenesis published over the past several decades. The molecular biologic studies of Brown and Goldstein, however, provided mechanistic approaches to the problem of atherosclerosis and helped galvanize approaches to therapy, specifically, drugs interfering with cholesterol synthesis and, more recently, antioxidants.[88,91] A crucial process in atherogenesis appears to be the production of oxidized LDL from elevated concentrations of serum LDL. In turn, oxidized LDL is taken up by scavenger macrophages in the arterial wall, an apparent early event in atherogenesis.[54]

Under normal circumstances and homeostasis, cholesterol intake and efflux are in equilibrium. Cholesterol influx meets the continuing body need for (1) constantly turning over cells whose membrane has an obligate requirement for cholesterol, (2) bile formation in liver, necessary for its detergent action that emulsifies and absorbs dietary fats, and (3) hormone synthesis, requiring the cholesterol structure as backbone. Dietary cholesterol is packaged in chylomicrons in the gut and delivers fats to adipose tissue and muscle by the action of capillary lipoprotein lipase. Meanwhile cholesterol is taken to the liver, where it merges with endogenous cholesterol synthesis (Fig. 2-6). The protein package for plasma solubility is of relatively low density, by convention, very low density lipoprotein (VLDL), because of its relative buoyancy to other lipoproteins. Dietary cholesterol in the United States averages between 500 and 750 mg/day (each egg yolk containing approximately 250 mg cholesterol), and endogenous hepatic synthesis is approximately 1,000 mg/day.[106] Although dietary cholesterol does not "add on" to the serum lipid concentration because it causes end-product inhibition, and multiple factors affect cholesterol uptake, distribution, and excretion, nonetheless, certain individuals are "high responders" in whom dietary increases in cholesterol is paralleled by similar elevations in serum, particularly of LDL, the atherogenic cholesterol-carrying lipoprotein.[35,106] Although the precise mechanism of elevated LDL in provoking atherosclerosis is uncertain, its oxidation or acetylation may play a role.[108] The complex relationship between dietary cholesterol and serum levels is also affected substantially by dietary saturated fats, which further increase LDL levels by interfering with LDL receptor uptake by cells. In addition to saturated fats, the trans, as opposed to cis, monounsaturated fatty acids are particularly hypercholesterolemic.[80]

Research on the relationship between lipid alterations and atherosclerosis has paralleled increasing investigative sophistication and technological advances, as in protein chemistry and molecular biol-

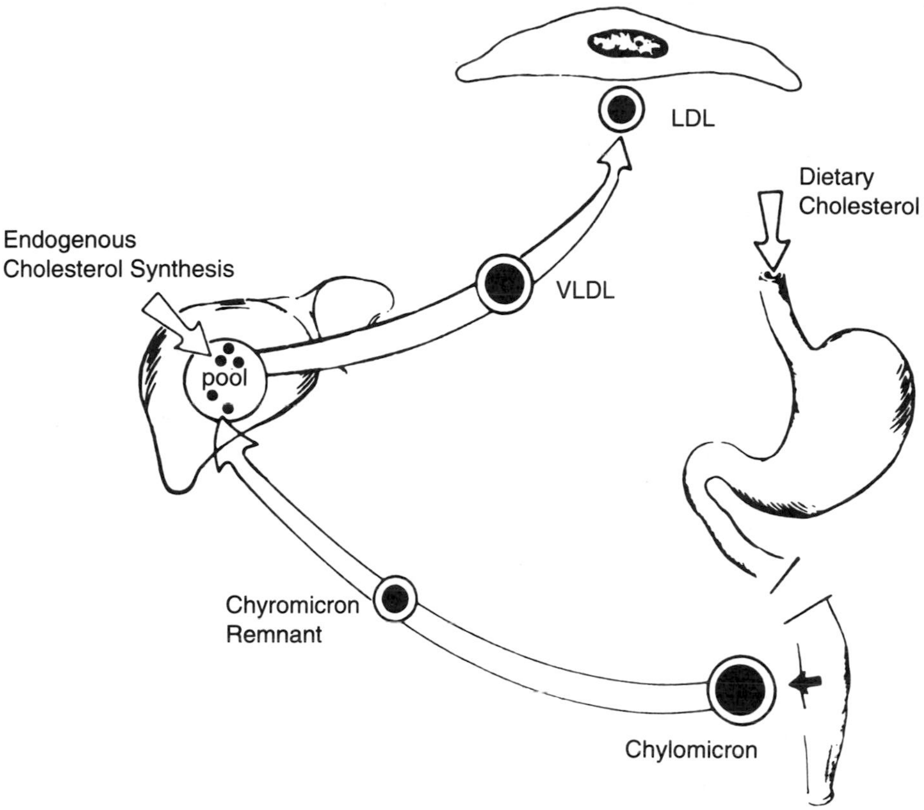


**Fig. 2-6.** Cholesterol influx into body tissues results from dietary source and endogenous cholesterol synthesis. Dietary cholesterol is packaged in a protein envelope of chylomicrons and enters the circulation through the thoracic duct. In the circulation, plasma enzymes serially alter chylomicrons to form chylomicron remnants, which are ultimately taken up by the liver, where they are pooled with endogenously synthesized cholesterol. The half-life of chylomicrons, which measure up to 5,000 Å, is several minutes. In the liver both endogenous and exogenous cholesterol is packaged for plasma solubility in a protein resulting in very low density relative to plasma density, hence the term very low density lipoprotein (VLDL). VLDL, which measures between 500 and 800 Å, has a half-life of several hours, releasing large quantities of triglycerides at adipose tissue and muscle, is serially altered in serum by enzymes to form first an intermediate-density lipoprotein (IDL; not shown in the diagram), and finally, low-density lipoprotein (LDL). LDL has the single surface apoprotein B, which binds with LDL receptors for cellular uptake (receptor-mediated endocytosis). LDL accounts for two-thirds of the plasma lipid, measures 200 Å, and has a half-life of several days. Each molecule of LDL has 1,500 molecules of cholesterol-ester in its core. (From Yatsu and Fisher,[106] with permission.)

ogy, and the development of analytic techniques such as high performance liquid chromatography. The powerful observations of Brown and Goldstein, which catalyzed their sequencing the LDL receptor, was the lack of any cellular downregulation of endogenous cholesterol synthesis by familial hypercholesterolemic fibroblasts in the presence of increasing amounts of extracellular LDL, unlike normal cells. They deduced that there must exist a receptor at the membrane that is defective for familial hypercholesterolemia (FH). In addition to an absence of cholesterol synthesis downregulation, the other normal responses were absent, namely, downregulation of LDL receptor synthesis and upregulation of acylcholesterol acyltransferase (ACAT) (Fig. 2-7).

Sequencing of the receptor identified five major components: (1) binding site, (2) epidermal growth factor (EGF) precursor homologous portion, (3) *O*-linked sugars segment, (4) transmembrane spanning sequence, which is hydrophobic because of the lipid nature of the membrane, and (5) the intracytoplasmic portion (Fig. 2-7). The intact receptor, after binding to LDL, will undergo endocytosis after reaching a specialized section of the membrane called "coated pits." When defective receptor structures exist, such as the variety of familial ones identified with altered cytoplasmic domains due to genetic alterations (Figs. 2-8 and 2-9), these patients cannot incorporate LDL by endocytosis, resulting in elevated serum LDL that is atherogenic.

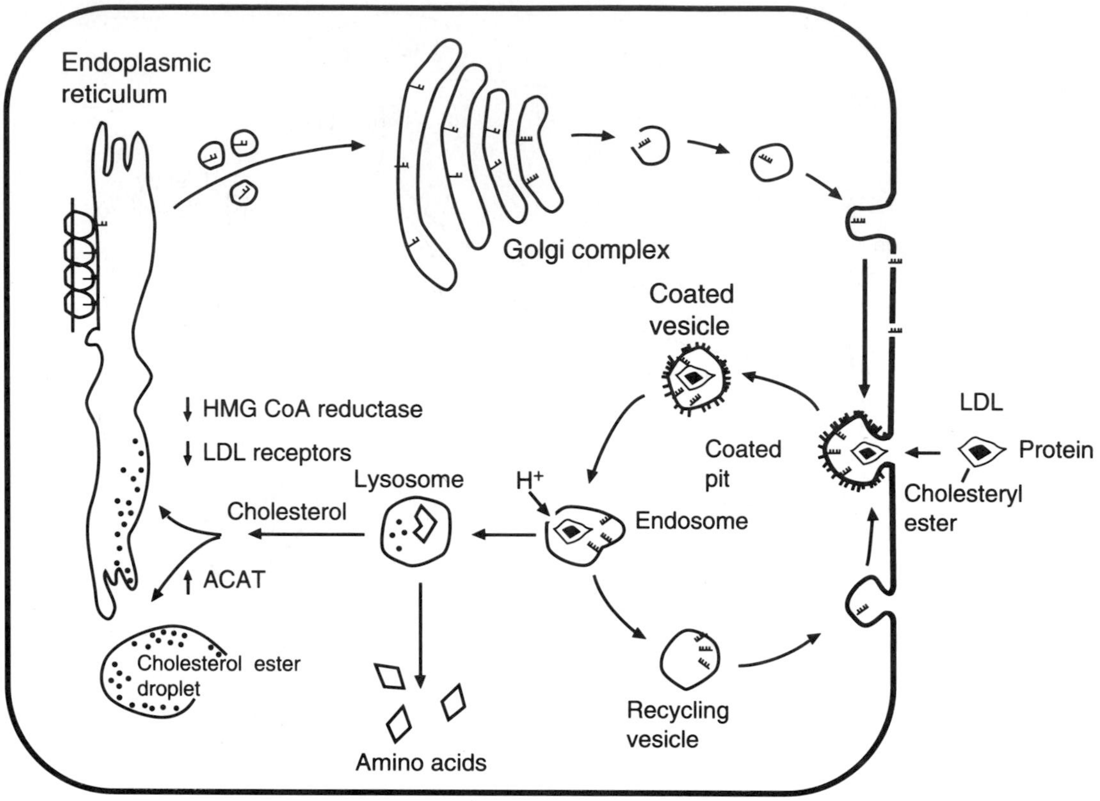


**Fig. 2-7.** Low-density lipoprotein (LDL) and its receptor binding, uptake (endocytosis or internalization), degradation, and metabolic consequences. LDL receptors are synthesized in the endoplasmic reticulum, travel to the Golgi complex, and then reach the plasma membrane. Plasma LDL as protein cholesterol-ester complex binds with the LDL receptor, migrates to the coated pits from where LDL is endocytosed as a coated vesicle. The LDL receptor is recycled from the endosome to the cell surface, while LDL is transferred to the lysosome where hydrolytic enzymes degrade the complex to release from cholesterol and amino acids. Free cholesterol provokes three important intracellular processes: (1) downregulation of 3-hydroxy-3-methylglutaryl-CoA reductase (HMG-CoA reductase), (2) downregulation of LDL receptors, and (3) upregulation of acyl-CoA-cholesterol acyltransferase (ACAT). End-product inhibition for the first mechanisms regulates the quantity of intracellular cholesterol, while the last of substrate activation provokes intracellular storage. (Reproduced by permission from Brown MS, Goldstein JL, copyright, 1986 by the Nobel Foundation, Science 1986; 232:34.)

Although correlation of elevated low-density lipoprotein (LDL) and reduced high density lipoprotein (HDL) with CHD is accepted, such a consistent lipoprotein abnormality has not been reported with ABI. In a comprehensive review of the more than two dozen studies reporting plasma lipids in strokes, Tell et al.[103] find that 23 of 26 studies found abnormalities with lipids and/or lipoproteins. However, differences in techniques, study design, population, and other factors make it impossible to perform metanalyses to merge all studies. They conclude that further prospective studies, using similar methods, are needed to answer this question definitively. For lipoproteins, when analyzed, only two studies report correlations of strokes with elevated LDL, while five show an inverse relationship between HDL and strokes. The timing of the blood analyses after stroke may be important, as Mendez et al.[77] suggest, although the long-term effect of lipoproteins on atherogenesis imply that acute changes may be less meaningful. In more recent studies analyzing the various blood lipids, including LDL and HDL, reduced HDL or elevated LDL is a consistent finding. For example, in the report of Shieh et al.,[98] in which rigorous attempts to fractionate the lipoproteins are made, reduction of HDL2 correlated inversely with strokes, a finding supported by Adams et al.[1] and Giubilei et al.,[47] although the last authors found that elevated LDL was contributory as did Grotta et al.[41] Since more recent studies using conventional analytic techniques continue to show varying findings with respect to either LDL or HDL changes with strokes, more dynamic studies on LDL and HDL metabolism demonstrating their in vivo synthesis and fractional catabolic rates may clarify more precisely the abnormality occurring with ABI.

In our own studies on LDL and HDL metabolism in

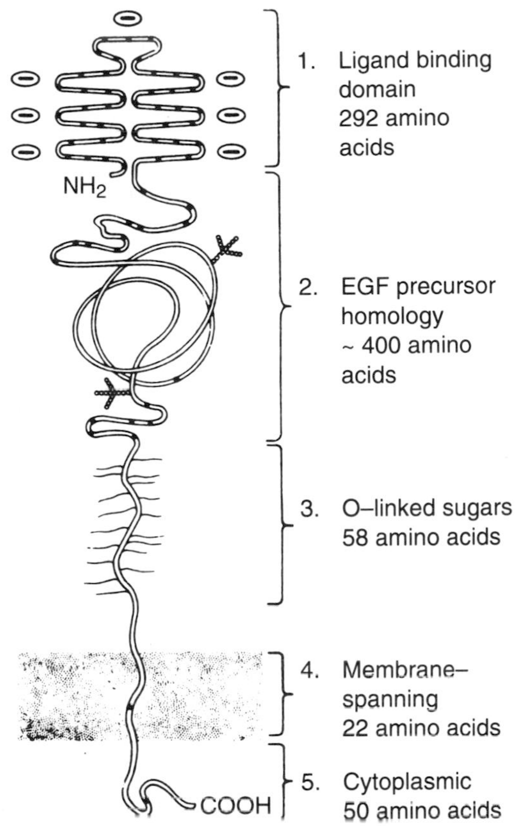


**Fig. 2-8.** The low-density lipoprotein (LDL) receptor. The LDL receptor gene and chromosome 19 spans 45 kilobases, is made up of 18 exons and 17 introns, and has 5 domains. The first (*1*) is the site for LDL binding, is made up of 292 amino acids and contains highly negatively charged amino acids. The second (*2*) domain has a high homology to the epidermal growth factor (EGF) precursor and contains approximately 400 amino acids. The third (*3*) domain has *O*-linked sugars and 58 amino acids. The fourth (*4*) domain is intramembranous and contains 22 hydrophobic amino acids. The fifth (*5*) domain is the intracytoplasmic portion and contains 50 amino acids. (Reproduced by permission from Brown MS, Goldstein JL, copyright 1986 by the Nobel Foundation, Science 1986; 232:34.)

vivo in 22 ABI and controls, autologously purified LDL and HDL3, obtained by ultracentrifugation and labeled with iodine-125, show significant differences in metabolism between ABI and normal controls. For HDL3, the fractional catabolic rate is faster in ABI, and for LDL, it is slower. This finding showing a reciprocal relationship between HDL and LDL metabolism corresponds to an increased LDL/HDL ratio but suggests that impaired "reverse cholesterol transport," mediated in part by HDL may be a significant factor in ABI pathogenesis. Since HDL metabolism is complex due to the action of multiple enzymes, especially cholesterol transfer protein, and LDL plays a dominant role in delivering cholesterol to liver for bile formation, reverse cholesterol transport cannot be reduced to but one factor. Nonetheless, the importance of HDL's role in this pathway provides an operational model.

A finding of interest and requiring confirmation, reported by Zenker et al.,[109] is an association of ABI with elevated lipoprotein (a) (Lp(a)); Lp(a) is a LDL molecule linked to a long-chain polypeptide attached by sulfhydryl bonds to apoprotein B. In their studies, they find no abnormalities in any other lipids, such as total cholesterol, LDL-cholesterol, HDL-cholesterol, or triglycerides—only with Lp(a). Whether their population is genetically different to display these findings will require further investigation. Meanwhile, the majority of world reports indicate that the major lipoprotein abnormality with ABIs is either a reduced HDL or elevated LDL or both.[103] Current investigations must go beyond quantitative studies on plasma concentrations and perform more dynamic metabolic studies on synthesis and catabolic rates to determine their impact on atheroma formation and regression.

## DIETARY ASPECTS OF PLASMA LIPIDS

Dietary intake of cholesterol and saturated fatty acids is implicated in producing high levels of total cholesterol and LDL in the population at risk for atherosclerotic disease,[45] although dissenting opinions exist on this causal relationship,[44] Mattson et al.[73] report an approximate 10 mg/dl increase in total plasma cholesterol for every 100 mg of dietary cholesterol per 1,000 calories. While the debate continues as to whether the relationship of diet cholesterol to plasma cholesterol is linear[48,73] or logarithmic,[61] convincing evidence exists for the reverse phenomenon that lowering cholesterol intake significantly reduces total plasma cholesterol.[45]

Poor regulation of dietary fat consumption by Americans has placed this population at risk for premature atherosclerosis. Stephen and Wald[101] report that dietary fat consumption peaked in the 1950s and mid-1960s at 40 to 42 percent of total caloric intake. Since that time, it declined to approximately 36 percent of total energy intake by 1984, although the percent of saturated fatty acid intake is 15 to 20 percent of the American diet.[93] The strategy for dietary control by the American Heart Association[45] and the National Cholesterol Education Program (NCEP)[93] is aimed at establishing criteria for the population at risk, instituting a diet that decreases dietary cholesterol, saturated fatty acids, and calories, and includes public education of dietary management.[65]

Initial treatment of elevated cholesterol and LDL levels should begin with dietary therapy. The NCEP[93] recommended target goal for patients with coronary heart disease or with at least two coronary heart disease risk factors should be aimed at lowering the LDL

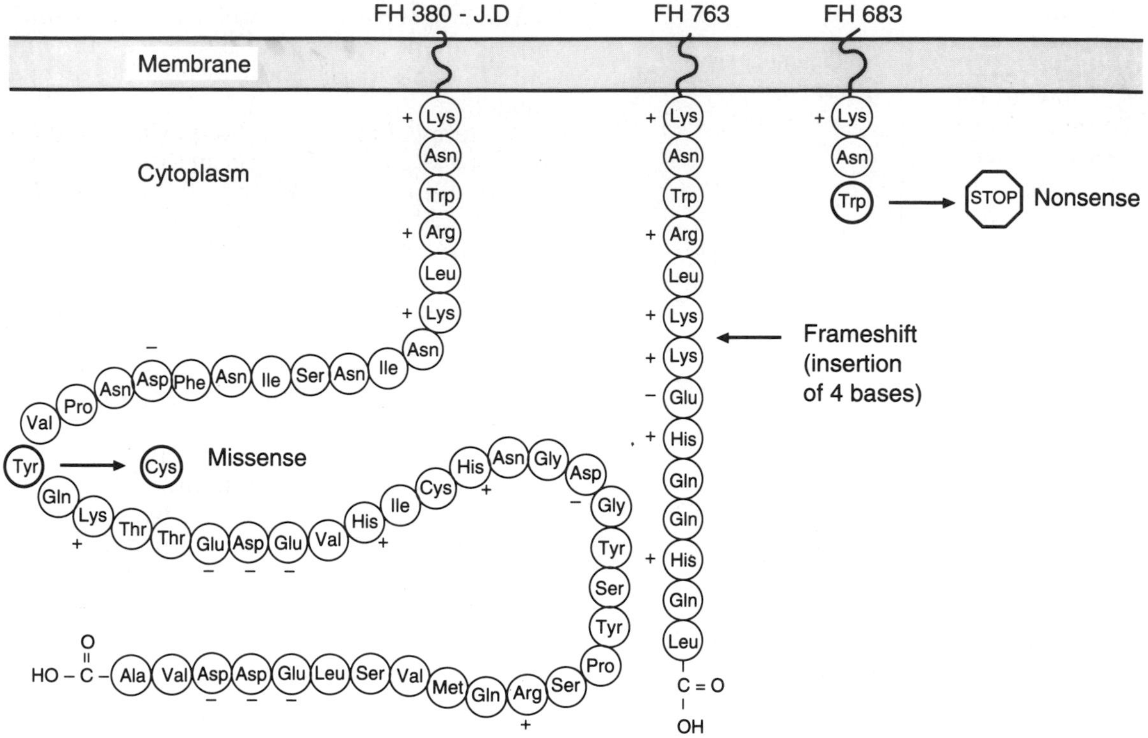


**Fig. 2-9.** Gene mutations of the intracytoplasmic domains of the low-density lipoprotein receptor and displaying three familial abnormalities associated with hypercholesterolemia. The gene mutations occur in exons 17 and 18. Familial hypercholesterolemia (FH) 380-JD is characterized by a single base change of cysteine for tyrosine at position 807. High FH 763, a frameshift is present with the insertion of four bases due to the duplication of four nucleotides following the codon for the sixth amino acid of the cytoplasmic tail. In FH 683, the tryptophan codon is converted to a nonsense or stop codon.

cholesterol to under 130 mg/dl, and those without coronary heart disease or risk factors should have a goal of less than 160 mg/dl. Initiation of dietary therapy should begin when those goal levels are exceeded.

**Step-One and Step-Two Diets.** Dietary therapy is aimed at reducing cholesterol level while maintaining good nutritional status and can be attained in two steps.

The Step-One Diet requires the intake of total fat to be less than 30 percent of total calorie intake, saturated fats less than 10 percent of total calorie intake, and total dietary cholesterol to be less than 300 mg/day. After starting the Step-One Diet, cholesterol levels should be measured at 4 to 6 weeks and then again at 3 months. If strict adherence to the Step-One Diet has been followed without reaching the target levels, the Step-Two Diet (a dietitian is greatly beneficial at this stage) should be employed.

The Step-Two Diet recommends that total fat intake be less than 30 percent of the total caloric intake and that saturated fat intake be less than 7 percent of the total caloric intake, with the dietary cholesterol being less than 200 mg/day. Desired cholesterol levels should be attained at 4 to 6 weeks and in 3 months after the initiation of the Step-Two Diet. Intensive dietary therapy should be pursued for at least 6 months before initiating drug therapy, although for patients having LDL cholesterol levels greater than 225 mg/dl, a slightly shorter duration may be considered before advancing to drug therapy.

Although beneficial to patients' long-term health, low-fat diets may be difficult for patients to tolerate and, thus, may decrease compliance. Therefore, it is prudent to consider the rationale and alternatives for a low saturated fat diet.

**Saturated versus Unsaturated Fatty Acids.** The evidence suggests that replacing saturated fatty acids with polyunsaturated and monounsaturated fatty acids is beneficial in lowering total cholesterol and LDL.[45,93] Originally, polyunsaturated acids alone were believed optimal in reducing cholesterol and LDL levels. However, recent studies indicate that monounsaturated fatty acids, such as oleic acid, reduces LDL and cholesterol levels equally as well as linoleic acid.[74] Ginsberg et al.[38] demonstrated that a modification of the Step-One Diet, by adding an additional 8 percent to the total fat intake in the form of monounsaturated fats, produced a reduction in LDL levels equal to or better than the Step-One Diet alone. In addition, Grundy[42] showed that diets high in monounsaturated fatty acids lowered LDL and total cholesterol as effectively as the low fat diet containing less than 20 percent of the total calories as fatty acids. In a study of coronary heart disease in seven countries, Keys[60] found that coronary heart disease mortality was extremely low in Greece despite the average fat intake of 40 percent of the total calories. However, the diet revealed that only 8 percent of total caloric intake was saturated fat, with the remainder consisting primarily of monounsaturated fatty acids (i.e., oleic acid, found in olive oil). In addition to the monounsaturated fatty acid oleic acid, Bonanome and Grundy[6] demonstrated that stearic acid, a long-chain saturated fatty acid, decreases total cholesterol and LDL. These data suggest that there may be leeway in the amount of fatty acids allowed in a cholesterol-lowering diet, depending on the type of fat. One drawback, however, to the use of a high monounsaturated diet is the difficulty that arises if weight reduction is desired in the patient.

**Unsaturated Fat versus High Carbohydrate Diet.** Reduction of saturated fatty acids in a diet can also be achieved by replacement with a high carbohydrate intake. In addition to lowering cholesterol levels, this diet also promotes weight reduction and provides evidence that supports the theory that a high carbohydrate-lower fat diet decreases risk for breast and colon cancer. Problems may arise with this alternative diet, since Americans may not accept such a low fat diet. In addition, diets low in fat and high in carbohydrates have been reported to lower HDL cholesterol and elevate triglyceride.[42,79]

**Weight Reduction and Cholesterol Level.** Excess body weight has been associated with high VLDL and moderate LDL increases, as well as low HDL levels.[45] Obesity promotes other atherosclerotic risk factors, such as hypertension and diabetes. Olefsky et al.[87] demonstrated a favorable change in plasma lipid levels in response to weight reduction. It is recommended that weight reduction be supported for patients who substantially exceed their target weight.

**Dietary Modification in the Elderly.** Utilization of dietary modification in the elderly population requires somewhat more individualized attention. In this population, concern arises that a decreased nutritional intake may be imposed by a strict diet. It is clearly recommended with these patients that Step-One Diets be instituted under the supervision of a physician as well as a dietitian and that the use of the Step-Two Diet be used only very cautiously.[97]

**Genetic Regulation of Lipid Metabolism.** Although dietary intake plays a major role in plasma and cholesterol levels, genetic regulation of lipid metabolism also plays a crucial role. The patient's response to dietary therapy may be variable and, indeed, some patients are poor responders to this method of lipid control. The need exists for a reliable biologic marker to identify those patients who respond unfavorably to dietary therapy.[43,107]

**Dietary Management Education.** Success in dietary management in achieving reduction of cholesterol and saturated fatty acid intake as well as reaching ideal body weight is dependent upon an educational process and the patient's understanding of the relationship between blood lipids and atherosclerosis. Crucial to its success is the patient's motivation to intervene, a process requiring the physician's personal concern, and frequently involving the family members, particularly spouses who may prepare meals.

## THERAPY OF ATHEROTHROMBOTIC BRAIN INFARCTIONS FOR PRIMARY AND SECONDARY PREVENTION: REDUCTION OF CHOLESTEROL

With CHD, controversy over whether cholesterol reduction will decrease its incidence continues, but less stridently and less persuasively. Because objective data indicate a beneficial effect in lowering cholesterol (i.e., decreasing LDL while raising HDL) to reduce CHD, this advice, by extension, can be given for ABI prevention and recurrence, despite the absence of objective, prospective, randomized studies assessing this question. While these prospective studies, underpinned with basic studies on lipoprotein metabolism, are needed, the dramatic benefits in CHD make it prudent to recommend these strategies for patients at risk for ABI,[52] since the disease process of atherosclerosis for CHD is fundamentally similar for ABI. Clearly, the disease process is multifactorial, and the variety of other stroke risk factors must be reduced, such as hypertension and smoking, but normalizing LDL and HDL would appear to be a critical factor for the long term.[21,40] To provide background on the evidence supporting cholesterol reduction for CHD, various investigations demonstrating these findings are reviewed briefly here.

The growing interest in and concern for the relationship between elevated cholesterol and CHD prompted authorities and scientists in the United States and Europe to take a position on this issue based upon available clinical data.[93] For example, a major effort to educate the American public regarding the untoward effects of cholesterol was launched in 1987 with the National Cholesterol Education Program (NCEP),[41] sponsored by the National Institutes of Health (NIH) and a number of public and private health organizations.[46,66] One of the first important pieces of evidence linking cholesterol reduction to decreases in CHD was the Lipid Research Clinics Coronary Primary Prevention Trial (1984)[68] in which nearly 4,000 middle-aged men with hypercholesterolemia (above 260 mg/dl) and asymptomatic of CHD were randomly treated with low fat and low cholesterol diet plus either placebo or cholestyramine, a bile sequestrant that will lower blood cholesterol levels. In the more than 7-year follow-up, the cholestryramine-treated group experienced a reduction of total cholesterol and LDL-cholesterol by 9 percent and 12 percent, respectively, and a decrease in CHD events by 19 percent. In other words, a 1 percent reduction in cholesterol was associated with a 2 percent decrease in CHD event rates. The follow-up was sufficiently short to experience any substantial stroke rates, reflecting their occurrence in older individuals. Similarly, in the Helsinski Heart Study,[70] over 4,000 males with elevated cholesterol were randomly treated with gemfibrozil, 600 mg twice daily, or placebo. Gemfibrozil reduced LDL by 11 percent, triglycerides by 35 percent, and raised HDL by 11 percent, while CHD was decreased by 34 percent. Since gemfibrozil raises HDL, it is concluded that the additional reduction of CHD over that found with cholestryramine by an additional one-third is explained on this basis. Because reduced HDL may play a critical role in ABI, as noted above, the use of gemfibrozil with low HDL (below 35 mg/dl) may be warranted.

The benefits of reducing cholesterol with medication and an associated decrease in CHD are shown in several other studies such as the Coronary Drug Project in which nearly 4,000 post-MI patients were treated with either niacin or placebo. Fifteen years after initiation, and 6 years after completion of the study, the treatment group, showing a lower cholesterol level, had an 11 percent reduction in CHD.[14] Similar results were reported by the Stockholm Ischemic Heart Study, in which niacin was combined with clofibrate; the treatment group had 36 percent fewer deaths due to CHD.[20]

Further evidence indicating a benefit of reduced cholesterol in CHD is the Leiden Intervention Trial, in which 39 CHD patients were treated with diets low in cholesterol and saturated fats over a 2-year period and were found to have reduced cholesterol, a reduced cholesterol:HDL ratio, and decreases in both blood pressure and weight. It is of interest that this regimen was associated with lack of atheroma progression, demonstrated by coronary angiography.[2] Similar reduction in CHD with dietary intervention was reported in the Oslo Study Diet and Antismoking Trial in which nearly a 50 percent reduction occurred.[49] Other investigations showing reduction of atherosclerosis by angiography include the Cholesterol Lowering Atherosclerosis Study (CLAS) in which colestipol, a bile sequestrant, plus nicotinic acid, resulted in a 16 percent reduction, compared to 2 percent in controls.[17] Finally, the Familial Atherosclerosis Treatment Study (FATS) studied the effects of niacin plus colestipol, lovastatin plus colestipol, or colestipol alone. The combined therapies both lowered LDL and raised HDL and also showed objective regression of CHD.[9]

Additional studies by others using similar lipid-lowering strategies have augmented the evidence that atheroma regression can be achieved objectively.[5,8,12,16,50,56,89]

## Lipid-Lowering Drugs

### *Bile Sequestrants*

As with other lipid-lowering drugs, bile sequestrants must be used only with dietary interventions to reduce cholesterol and saturated fat intake. Otherwise the lipid-lowering measures are fruitless. For all lipid-lowering agents, the lowest effective dosing of the agent should be sought, to minimize both side effects and costs.

The two primary bile sequestrants, cholestryramine and colestipol, resins that bind intestinal bile, are formed in the liver from cholesterol and excrete bile in the stool. As a result, bile is not recycled in the "enterohepatic cycle" in which bile acts to emulsify dietary fats for absorption. Reduced bile recycling signals the liver to upregulate more LDL receptors to increase bile production, which results in lowered serum LDL-cholesterol concentrations. Coupled to this action of LDL receptor upregulation is the occasional occurrence of increased synthesis of VLDL and of triglycerides. Under these circumstances, niacin can reduce this secondary reaction.

Older patients, who are more prone to ABIs, are frequently unable to tolerate bile sequestrants; these patients are more vulnerable to the side effects of gastrointestinal discomfort and nausea. To minimize these side effects, which may limit the use of these drugs, the dose may be spaced throughout the day and taken with food, especially high-fiber foods. The dose of bile sequestrants, which should be mixed in a fluid such as orange juice, is as follows: cholestryramine, 8 g twice daily, using 4-g packets, or colestipol, 10 g twice daily, using 5-g packets.[55]

### *3-Hydroxy-3-methylglutaryl–Coenzyme A Reductase Inhibitors*

HMG-CoA reductase inhibitors are the most powerful drugs reducing cholesterol synthesis, and at present a variety of analogues exist, although not all have been fully tested in humans. Those available include lovastatin (Mevinolin), mevastatin (Compactin), pravastatin (CS-514, Eptastatin, or SQ 31000) and simvastatin (Synvinolin, MK-733).[50] The drugs, discovered in Japan by scientists investigating molds, achieve their results because of the homologous structure to HMG-CoA. In addition to a reduction of endogenous cholesterol synthesis, the fractional catabolic rate of LDL is increased due to an upregulation of LDL receptors.[4,55] Hepatitis and myopathy can occur with these drugs, which require monitoring of liver function tests and creatine kinase monthly during the first year and then at several monthly intervals thereafter.[55] Myopathy increases with the use of certain drugs, such as cyclosporine, fibric acid derivatives (e.g., gemfibrozil and clofibrate), erythromycin, and niacin; therefore, their concurrent use should be minimized.[55] The starting dose of lovastatin is 20 mg nightly to start, but this dose may need to be increased to 80 mg nightly or twice daily to achieve a cholesterol reduction (primarily LDL) of 15 to 25 percent.

### *Fibric Acid Drugs*

Clofibrate and gemfibrozil are first- and second-generation fibric acid derivatives and have been widely touted to increase HDL, the "good cholesterol," particularly when it is reduced to low levels of less than 35 mg/dl. The ability of gemfibrozil, for example, to raise HDL and to decrease coronary heart disease endpoints was statistically confirmed in the Helsinki Heart Study, which had results similar to those achieved by the Lipid Research Clinic Coronary Primary Prevention Trial (LRC CPPT) in which diet and cholestryramine were used. The value of increasing HDL levels may be to improve the delivery of membrane cholesterol to liver for bile formation, so-called "reverse cholesterol transport."[25,76]

Fibric acid derivatives also inhibit platelet-derived growth factors (PDGF) and function to blunt the proliferative response of smooth muscle cells.[102] Gastrointestinal distress and nausea are common side effects, which are reduced by taking the medication with meals. These drugs can potentiate the action of coumarin and thereby prolong prothombin time, which requires careful monitoring.[55] The starting dose of clofibrate is 500 mg daily and of gemfibrozil is 300 mg twice daily; the maximum dose is 1 g twice daily and 600 mg twice daily, respectively. In our own experience with elderly individuals, the hypolipidemic effects, especially in raising HDL, are not readily achieved. More data are needed on this issue, and especially on the important one of whether the elevation of HDL increases reverse cholesterol transport, causes atheroma regression, and decreases ABI incidence.

### *Niacin*

Niacin is a B vitamin that inhibits the synthesis of VLDL, the precursor of LDL, which results in lower LDL concentrations. As noted above, the drug is effective in combination with bile sequestrants.[55] The drug can be used alone as well. Niacin also increases HDL levels by reducing its catabolic rate. Niacin causes flushing and itching, which can be very annoying, but these side effects can be minimized by starting at very low doses and increasing very slowly. The body not only can accommodate to the effects of niacin, but one aspirin taken a half hour before intake can minimize symptoms by inhibiting the responsible prostaglandin cascade.[55] Liver enzymes should be monitored every several weeks initially, then every several months, and uric acid and blood glucose require periodic checks, since these may increase. The drug should not be used in those with gouty arthritis and diabetes mellitus.[55]

The starting dose of niacin is 100 mg two to three times daily, taken with meals, occasionally requiring antacids; it should be increased slowly to doses of 3 to 7 g daily to achieve a 15 to 15 percent reduction in serum cholesterol.

### *Low-Density Lipoprotein-Antioxidants: Probucol*

Probucol not only inhibits cholesterol synthesis, it increases LDL clearance and bile formation. Importantly, the most significant action of this drug may be to prevent oxidation of LDL, in which form they are scavenged by arterial wall macrophages, which are believed to contribute to atherogenesis.[55,59,110] HDL levels are reduced, but the dense HDL particles involved in reverse cholesterol transport are not affected.[55] Probucol should not be used in patients with prolonged QT intervals on ECG.[55] The dose of probucol is 50 mg twice daily.

## Calcium Channel Blockers and Other Lipid-Lowering Strategies

Calcium channel blockers have been variably successful in retarding or averting atherosclerosis in animal models of atherosclerosis, similar to the human experience. Nonetheless, on the basis of our studies, showing a beneficial result of calcium channel blockade in reducing the endocytosis of negatively charged LDL, its use in hypertensives is warranted because of its dual potential in both reducing blood pressure and in possibly minimizing atherosclerosis.[105]

Drugs affecting Lp(a) may, in the future, prove of value in retarding atherogenesis causing ABIs.[109] Lp(a) is believed to be atherogenic because of its homology to kringle 4 of plasminogen.[102]

### *Atheroma Regression*

Impressive findings exist on the association of reducing dietary and serum lipid levels with atheroma regression.[5,8,10,16,55,89] These studies have been performed on CHD and peripheral vascular disease (PVD), but not yet on ABIs. Since the primary disease process is basically similar for these three, it is anticipated that efforts to reduce serum lipids in ABI-prone individuals should result in stroke reduction due to atheroma regression of cerebral arteries. Relevant to this issue of lowering elevated lipids is the occurrence of ABIs primarily in older individuals whose well-developed disease may not yield to interventions to demonstrate clinical benefit. In addition, the cost: benefit ratio, considering the retired and usually fixed-income nature of these individuals, requires consideration. Nonetheless, as inferred from conclusions drawn from elderly patients with CHD, the benefits are potentially realizable.[40] Similarly, the most inexpensive measures should be used to achieve lipid lowering.[96] Although no definitive data exist on the value of lipid-lowering to prevent ABIs, this approach is warranted until definitive information is forthcoming, especially in those who are at increased risk of ABIs due to multiple risk factors, including abnormal lipid profiles.

### *PDAY Study on the Relationship of Blood Lipids to Atherosclerosis: Preliminary Report*

A revealing and sobering ongoing study on the relationship of blood lipids to atherosclerosis is from the Pathobiological Determinants of Atherosclerosis in Youth (PDAY) Research Group.[76] Eight centers in the United States participate in analyzing aortas, coronary arteries, blood, and other relevant information from young people aged 15 to 34 years, who died violently. In their preliminary report in 1990, of 728 cases, an analysis of 390 males showed a positive correlation between the degree of atherosclerosis and VLDL and LDL levels and a negative association with HDL. Furthermore, a strong, independent relationship existed with smoking, determined at postmortem by the serum thiocyanate concentrations. These striking findings support not only a relationship between risk factors and atherosclerosis as one which begins early in life, but clearly its multifactorial character, including blood flow and hemodynamic parameters.

### *Other Antihypertensive Agents*

Greater insight into the selection of antihypertensive agents, as alluded to above for calcium channel blockers, may prove to be important for their effects of the lipid profile. For example, beta blockers change the prolife of LDL to smaller, more dense and more atherogenic particles, without affecting the total cholesterol concentration.[102] Thus, the apparent benefits of beta blockade on flow-related aspects of atherogenesis may be negated by its altering the lipid profile. Further longitudinal studies are clearly needed to determine the significance of these findings, but bear close attention in the future.

### *Lipoprotein-Apheresis*

Lipoprotein-apheresis may become a therapeutic option for patients resistant to dietary and drug interventions.[63] In addition, extraction of both LDL and fibrinogen results in improved hemorrheologic parameters and an increase in HDL. These findings suggest that for individuals prone to ABIs and who are not surgical candidates for endarterectomy, apheresis may provide a relatively rapid means of provoking atheroma regression.

## PRACTICAL DIETARY MANAGEMENT OF ABNORMAL LIPID PROFILES IN ATHEROTHROMBOTIC BRAIN INFARCTION-PRONE INDIVIDUALS

Elevation of serum cholesterol, particularly the profile of increased LDL and reduced HDL, likely causes atherosclerosis of cerebral and extracerebral vessels, the primary etiology of thrombotic stroke or atherothrombotic brain infarction (ABI). Reduction of cholesterol to prevent primary or secondary ABIs has not, however, been scientifically proven in randomized, prospective, placebo-controlled studies. Nonetheless, extension of arguments on the usefulness of hypolipidemic strategies for coronary heart disease (CHD) to ABIs is logical, since brain vascular territory is contiguous with all arteries and similarly susceptible to processes causing atherosclerosis. Critical differences and concerns exist between those prone to ABI and those prone to CHD: the former is a more elderly population, and whether realizable gains can occur as measured by atheroma regression, ABI reduction, or cost effectiveness is unknown. Despite the absence of these data, extension of the value in reducing serum cholesterol in CHD to prevent primary and secondary cardiac endpoints is sufficiently powerful to justify its application to those who are ABI-prone. Until prospective studies can document the value of cholesterol-lowering strategies in averting ABIs, we believe it prudent to following this regimen in patients at risk for ABIs. Overriding considerations in elderly patients are issues of cost, especially for the majority who are on fixed incomes, and therefore the most conservative and least costly means of achieving cholesterol reduction should be sought. The least costly, of course, is dietary modification, which reduces the daily quantity of cholesterol and saturated fats.

This discussion focuses on dietary therapies, but physicians must individualize their approach. As a rule, if dietary interventions fail after a reasonable trial of perhaps 6 months or more, drug therapy is warranted, provided it does not cause a fiscal hardship to the patient.

### Dietary Guidelines: American Heart Association

Successful dietary management of elevated serum lipids requires both reduction of cholesterol and saturated fat intake but also to achieve an ideal weight.[21,55] Success in achieving both goals is dependent upon an educational process for the patient, to promote understanding of the relationship between blood lipids and atherosclerosis. Crucial to its success is the patient's motivation to intervene, a process requiring the physician's personal concern and frequently the involvement of family members, especially the spouse who prepares meals.

The guidelines of the American Heart Association are prudent ones for reducing cholesterol and saturated fats by emphasizing the foods to avoid. For example, specific foods to avoid are (1) red meats, which are high in cholesterol and saturated fats, (2) eggs (each egg yolk contains approximately 250 mg cholesterol), (3) whole milk, and (4) butter. If the source of meat flies (e.g., chicken) or swims (e.g., fish), it is relatively low in cholesterol. Certain fish provide omega-3 fatty acids, which may blunt the atherogenic process by minimizing the inflammatory process seen in atheromas.

When simple guidelines for dietary intervention do not improve an abnormal lipid profile nor cause weight reduction to achieve and maintain their ideal body weight, consultation with a trained dietitian, who can develop an educational relationship with the patient, is warranted.

### Dietary Consultation

Dietitians can be immensely helpful in translating the sometimes abstract nature of food content and their quantities to their practical application. A change in the lifestyle of a person's lifelong pattern of eating will frequently require a professional dietician to educate the patient and family on the choice of foods and the cholesterol, fat, and caloric content, as well as the use of innovative menus that present food artfully and tastefully.

### "Rule of 3" on Dietary Restrictions to Lower Cholesterol and Fat Intake

A simple means of having patients remember the recommended quantity of dietary cholesterol and fat is by the "Rule of 3" as noted below:

1. Reduce daily cholesterol to less than 3 × 100 or 300 mg.
2. Reduce daily fat intake to less than 3 × 10 or 30 percent of calories.
3. Reduce daily saturated fats to less than 3 × 10 or 30 percent of total fat intake (i.e., increase polyunsaturated fatty acids).

## SUMMARY AND CONCLUSIONS

Strokes due to atherosclerosis remain numerically the most prominent neurologic disease affecting adults, and despite substantial gains in stroke reduction, further decreases are anticipated as greater insights into pathogenesis are uncovered. Mechanisms related to alterations in cholesterol metabolism and in the abnormal proliferation of smooth muscle cells were reviewed, especially as they related to potential interventional therapies for reducing atherothrombotic brain infarction (ABI), both primarily and secondarily, after either transient ischemic attacks (TIAs) or small strokes. Beneficial results from therapeutic interventions in coronary heart disease, as reviewed in this chapter and elsewhere in this volume, offer the hope and expectation that similar results can be achieved in reducing ABIs. Prospective, randomized, placebo-controlled studies are needed to determine the effectiveness of therapies affecting both cholesterol metabolism and smooth muscle proliferation, but until these are available, efforts to normalize all risk factors is warranted.

## REFERENCES

1. Adams RJ, Carroll RM, Nichols FT et al: Plasma lipoproteins in cortical versus lacunar infarction. Stroke 20:448, 1989
2. Arntzenius AC, Krombout D, Barth JD et al: Diet, lipoproteins, and the progression of coronary atherosclerosis: the Leiden Intervention Trial. N Engl J Med 312:805, 1985
3. Bassiouny HS, Davis H, Massawa N et al: Critical carotid stenosis: morphologic and chemical similarity between symptomatic and asymptomatic plaques. J Vasc Surg 9:202, 1989
4. Bilheimer DW, Grundy SM, Brown MS et al: Mevinolin and colestipol stimulate receptor-mediated clearance of low density lipoprotein from plasma in familial hypercholesterolemia heterozygotes. Proc Natl Acad Sci USA 80:4124, 1983
5. Blankenhorn DHG, Nessim SA, Johnson RL et al: Beneficial effects of combined colestipol-niacin therapy on coronary atherosclerosis and coronary venous bypass grafts. JAMA 257:3233, 1987
6. Bonanome A, Grundy SM: Effects of dietary stearic acid on plasma cholesterol and lipoprotein levels. N Engl J Med 318:1244, 1989
7. Braughler JM, Hall ED, Jocobson EJ et al: The 21-aminosteroids: potent inhibitors of lipid peroxidation for the treatment of central nervous system trauma and ischemia. Drugs Future 14:14, 1989
8. Brensike JF, Levy RI, Kelsey SF et al: Effects of therapy with cholestyramine on progression of coronary arteriosclerosis: results of the NHLBI Type II Coronary Intervention Study. Circulation 69:313, 1984
9. Brown BG, Lin JT, Schaefer SM et al: Niacin or lovastatin, combine with colestipol, repress coronary atherosclerosis and prevent clinical events in men with elevated apolipoprotein B. Circulation 40:266, 1989
10. Brown G, Albers JJ, Fisher LD et al: Progression of coronary artery disease as a result of intensive lipid-lowering therapy in men with high levels

of apolipoprotein B. N Engl J Med 323:1289, 1990
11. Brown MS, Kovanen PT, Goldstein JL: Regulation of plasma cholesterol by lipoprotein receptors. Science 212:628, 1981
12. Buchwald H, Varco RL, Matts JP et al: Effects of partial ileal bypass surgery on mortality and morbidity from coronary heart disease on patients with hypercholesterolemia: report of the Program on the Surgical Control of the Hyperlipidemias (POSCH). N Engl J Med 323:946, 1990
13. Campbell GR, Chamley-Campbell JH: The cellular pathology of atherosclerosis. Pathology 13:423, 1981
14. Canner PL, Berge KG, Wenger NK et al: Fifteen year mortality in Coronary Drug Project patients: long-term benefit with niacin. J Am Coll Cardiol 8:1245, 1986
15. Carew TE, Schwenke DC, Steinberg D: Antiatherogenic effect of probucol unrelated to its hypocholesterolemic effect. Proc Natl Acad Sci USA 84:7725, 1987
16. Cashin-Hemphill L, Mack WJ, Pogoda J et al: Beneficial effects of colestipol-niacin on coronary atherosclerosis: a 4-year follow-up. JAMA 264:3013, 1990
17. Cashin-Hemphill L, Sanmarco ME, Blankenhorn DH: Augmented beneficial effects of colestipol-niacin therapy at four years in the CLAS trial. Circulation 80:II–381, 1989
18. Castelli WP, Wilson WP, Levy D et al: Cardiovascular risk factors in the elderly. Am J Cardiol 63:12H, 1989
19. Castellot JJ, Beeler DL, Rosenberg RD, Karnovsky MJ: Structural determinants of the capacity of heparin to inhibit the proliferation of vascular smooth muscle cells. J Cell Physiol 120:315, 1984
20. Clarson LA, Rosenhamer G: Reduction of mortality in the Stockholm Ischaemic Heart Disease Secondary Prevention Study by combined treatment with clofibrate and nicotinic acid. Acta Med Scand 223:405, 1988
21. Connor WE, Connor SL: The dietary treatment of hyperlipidemia. Med Clin North Am 66:485, 1982
22. Cutler JA, MacMahon SW, Furberg CD: Controlled clinical trials of drugs treatment for hypertension: a review. Hypertension 13:136, 1989
23. Davies MJ, Thomas AC: Plaque fissuring: the cause of acute myocardial infarction, sudden ischemic death, and crescendo angina. Br Heart J 53:363, 1985
24. Davis HR, Bridenstine RT, Vesselinovitch D, Wissler RW: Fish oil inhibits development of atherosclerosis in rhesus monkeys. Arteriosclerosis 7:441, 1987
25. Dehmer GJ, Popma JJ, Egerton K et al: Reduction in the rate of early restenosis after coronary angioplasty by a diet supplemented with n-3 fatty acids. N Engl J Med 139:733, 1988
26. Donahue RP, Abbott RD, Reed DM, Yano K: Alcohol and hemorrhagic stroke: the Honolulu Heart Program. JAMA 255:2311, 1986
27. Falk E: Plaque rupture with severe pre-existing stenosis precipitates coronary thrombosis. Br Heart J 50:127, 1983
28. Fiebach NH, Hebert PR, Stampfer MJ et al: A prospective study of high blood pressure and cardiovascular disease in women. Am J Epidemiol 130:646, 1989
29. Fisher CM: Capsular infarcts, with underlying vascular lesions. Arch Neurol 36:65, 1979
30. Fisher M: Atherosclerosis, cellular aspects and potential interventions. Cerebrovasc Brain Metab Rev 3:114, 1991
31. Fisher M, Blumenfeld A, Smith TW: The importance of carotid plaque disruption and hemorrhage. Arch Neurol 76:241, 1987
32. Fisher M, Leaf A, Levine PH: n-3 Fatty acids and cellular aspects of atherosclerosis. Arch Intern Med 149:1726, 1989
33. Fisher M, Levine PH, Doyle EM et al: A 21-aminosteroid inhibits oxidation of human low density lipoprotein by human monocytes. Atherosclerosis 90:197, 1991
34. Fronek K: Calcium antagonists and experimental atherosclerosis. Cardiovasc Drug Rev 8:229, 1990
35. Furuta A, Ishii N, Nishihara Y, Horie A: Medullary arteries imaging and dementia. Stroke 22:442, 1991
36. Gianturco SH, Bradley WA: Lipoprotein-mediated cellular mechanisms for atherogenesis in hypertriglyceridemia. Semin Thromb Hemostas 14:165, 1988
37. Gill JS, Shipley MJ, Hornby RH et al: A community case-control study of alcohol consumption in stroke. Int J Epidemiol 17:542, 1988
38. Ginsberg HN, Barr SL, Gilbert A et al: Reduction of plasma cholesterol levels in normal men on an American Heart Association Step-1 diet or a Step-1 diet with added monounsaturated fat. N Engl J Med 322:574, 1990
39. Goodnight SH, Fisher M, Fitzgerald GA, Levine PM: Assessment of the therapeutic use of dietary fish oil in atherosclerotic vascular disease and thrombosis. Chest 95:19S, 1989
40. Gordon DJ, Rifkind BM: Treating high blood cholesterol in the older patient. Am J Cardiol 63:48H, 1989
41. Grotta JC, Yatsu FM, Pettigrew LC et al: Prediction of carotid stenosis progression by lipid and hematologic measurements. Neurology (NY) 39:1325, 1989
42. Grundy SM: Comparison of monounsaturated fatty acid and carbohydrates for lowering plasma cholesterol. N Engl J Med 314:745, 1986
43. Grundy SM: Cholesterol and coronary heart disease: future disease. JAMA 264:3053, 1990
44. Grundy SM, Barret-Connor E, Rudel LL et al: Workshop on the impact of dietary cholesterol on plasma lipoproteins and atherogenesis. Arteriosclerosis 8:95, 1988
45. Grundy SM, Bilheimer D, Blackburn H et al: Rational of the diet-heart statement of the American Heart Association: report of Nutrition Committee. Circulation 65:839a, 1982
46. Grundy SM, Goodman DEW, Rifkind BM,

Cleeman JI: The place of HDL in cholesterol management: a perspective from the National Cholesterol Education Program. Arch Intern Med 149:505, 1989
47. Guibilei F, D'Antona R, Antonini R et al: Serum lipoprotein pattern variations in dementia and ischemic stroke. Acta Neurol Scand 81:84, 1990
48. Hessted DM, McGandy RB, Myers ML, Stare FJ: Quantitative effects of dietary fat on serum cholesterol in man. Am J Clin Nutr 17:281, 1965
49. Hjermann I, Holme I, Leren P: Oslo Study Diet and Antismoking Trial: results after 102 months. Am J Med 80:7, 1986
50. Hoeg JM, Brewer HB, Jr: 3-Hydroxy-3-methylglutaryl-coenzyme A reductase inhibitors in the treatment of hypercholesterolemia. JAMA 258:3522, 1987
51. Howard G, Evans GW, Toole JF et al: Characteristics of stroke victims associated with early cardiovascular mortality in their children. J Clin Epidemiol 43:49, 1990
52. Illingworth DR: Management of hyperlipidemia: goals for the prevention of atherosclerosis. Clin Invest Med 13:211, 1990
53. Imparato AM, Riles RS, Mintzer R et al: The importance of hemorrhage in the relationship between gross morphologic and cerebral symptoms in 376 carotid artery plaques. Ann Surg 197:195, 1983
54. Jaffee EA: Cell biology of endotherlial cells. Hum Pathol 18:234, 1987
55. Kane JP, Malloy MJ: Treatment of hyperlipidemia. Annu Rev Med 41:471, 1990
56. Kane JP, Malloy MJ, Ports TA et al: Regression of coronary atherosclerosis during treatment of familial hypercholesterolemia with combined drug regimen. JAMA 264:3007, 1990
57. Kannel WB, Castelli WP, Gordon T: Cholesterol in the prediction of atherosclerotic disease: new perspectives in the Framingham Study. Ann Intern Med 90:85, 1979
58. Kannel WB, Wolf PA, Verter J: Manifestations of coronary disease predisposing to stroke: the Framingham Study. JAMA 250:2942, 1983
59. Kesaniemi YA, Grundy SM: Influence of probucol on cholesterol metabolism in man. J Lipid Res 25:780, 1984
60. Keys A: Coronary heart disease in seven countries. Circulation, suppl I. 41:1, 1970
61. Keys A, Anderson JT, Grande F: Serum-cholesterol response to changes in diet. II. Effects of cholesterol in the diet. Metabolism 14:759, 1965
62. Kim DN, Ho HT, Lawrence DA et al: Modification of lipoprotein patterns and retardation of atherogenesis by a fish oil; supplement to a hyperlipidemic diet for swine. Atherosclerosis 76:35, 1989
63. Kottke BA, Pineda AA, Case MT et al: Hypercholesterolemia and atherosclerosis: present and future therapy including LDL-apheresis. J Clin Apheresis 4:35, 1988
64. Lennihan L, Kupsky WJ, Mohr JP et al: Lack of association between carotid plaque hematoma and ischemic cerebral symptoms. Stroke 18:879, 1987
65. Lenzant C: A new challenge for America: the National Cholesterol Education Program. Circulation 73:855, 1986
66. Levy RI, Blankenhorn D, Davis CE et al: AHA Conference report on cholesterol: intervention studies. Circulation 80:739, 1989
67. Lichtlen PR, Rafflenbeul W, Jost S et al: Retardation of angiographic progression of coronary artery disease by nifedipine. Lancet 335:1109, 1990
68. Lipid Research Clinics Program: The Lipid Research Clinics' Coronary Primary Prevention Trial (CPPT) results. JAMA 251:351, 1984
69. MacMahon S, Peto R, Cutler J et al: Blood pressure, stroke, and coronary heart disease. 1. Prolonged differences in blood pressure: prospective observational studies corrected for the regression dilution bias. Lancet 335:765, 1990
70. Manninen V, Elo Mo, Frick MH et al: Lipid alterations and decline in the incidence of coronary heart disease in the Helsinki Heart Study. JAMA 260:641, 1988
71. Masawa N, Hoshida Y, Joshita T et al: Three-dimensional morphologic analysis of thrombotic occlusive arteries in autopsies of atherosclerotic cerebral infarction. Stroke 21:1, 1990
72. Masuda J, Ross R: Atherogenesis during low level hypercholesterolemia in the non-human primate. Arteriosclerosis 10:178, 1990
73. Mattson FH, Erickson BA, Klingman AM: Effect of dietary cholesterol on serum cholesterol in man. Am J Clin Nutr 25:589, 1972
74. Mattson FH, Grundy SM: Comparison of effects of dietary saturated, monounsaturated, and polyunsaturated fatty acids on plasma lipids and lipoprotein in man. J Lipid Res 26:194, 1985
75. McGill HC: The pathogenesis of atherosclerosis. Clin Chem 34:833, 1988
76. McGill HC, Jr: Relationship of atherosclerosis in young men to serum lipoprotein cholesterol concentrations and smoking: a preliminary report from the Pathobiological Determinants of Atherosclerosis in Youth (PDAY) Research Group. JAMA 264:3018, 1990
77. Mendez I, Hachinski V, Wolfe B: Serum lipids after stroke. Neurology (NY) 37:507, 1987
78. Menotti A, Mariotti S, Seccareccia S, Giampaoli S: The 25-year estimated probability of death from some specific causes as a function of twelve risk factors in middle-aged men. Eur J Epidemiol 4:60, 1988
79. Mensink RP, Katan MB: Effects of monounsaturated fatty acid versus complex carbohydrates on high density lipoproteins in healthy men and women. Lancet 1:122, 1987
80. Mensink RP, Katan MB: Effect of dietary trans fatty acids on high-density and low-density lipoprotein cholesterol levels in health subjects. N Engl J Med 323:439, 1990
81. Mitchinson MJ, Ball RY: Macrophages and atherogenesis. Lancet 2:146, 1987
82. Nakano KK: An overview of stroke. Epidemiology, classification, risk factors and clinical aspects. Postgrad Med 80:82, 1986

83. Nathan CF: Secretory products of macrophages. J Clin Invest 79:319, 1987
84. Nissinen A, Tuomilehto J, Kottke TE, Puska P: Cost-effectiveness of the North Karelia Hypertension Program. Med Care 24:767, 1986
85. Norris JW, Hachinski VC: Prevention of Stroke. Springer-Verlag, New York, 1991
86. Ogata J, Masuda J, Yutani C et al: Rupture of atheromatous plaque as a cause of thrombotic occlusion of stenotic internal carotid artery. Stroke 21:1740, 1990
87. Olefsky J, Reaven GM, Farquhar JW: Effects of weight reduction in obesity. J Clin Invest 53:64, 1974
88. Ooi WL, Budner NS, Cohen H et al: Impact of race on treatment response and cardiovascular disease among hypertensives. Hypertension 14:227, 1989
89. Ornish D, Brown SE, Scherwitz LW et al: Can lifestyle changes reverse coronary heart disease?—the Lifestyle Heart Trial. Lancet 336:129, 1990
90. Parthasarathy S, Khoo JC, Miller E et al: Low-density lipoprotein rich in oleic acid is protected against oxidative modification: implications for dietary prevention of atherosclerosis. Proc Natl Acad Sci USA 87:3894, 1990
91. Parthasarathy S, Young SG, Witzum JL et al: Probucol inhibits oxidation of low density lipoprotein. J Clin Invest 77:641, 1986
92. Reis GJ, Sipperly ME, McCabe CH et al: Randomized trial of fish oil for prevention of restenosis after coronary angioplasty. Lancet 2:177, 1989
93. Report of the National Cholesterol Education Program Expert Panel on Detection, Evaluation and Treatment of High Blood cholesterol in Adults. Arch Intern Med 148:36, 1988
94. Ross R: The pathogenesis of atherosclerosis: atherogenesis and inflammation. Lab Invest 58:249, 1988
95. Ross R, Wight TN, Strandess E, Thiele B: Human atherosclerosis I. Cell constitution and characteristics of advanced lesions of the superficial femoral artery. Am J Pathol 114:79, 1984
96. Schulman KA, Kinosian B, Jacobson TA et al: Reducing high blood cholesterol level with drugs: cost-effectiveness of pharmacologic management. JAMA 264:3025, 1990
97. Sempos C, Fulwood R, Haimes C et al: The prevalence of high blood cholesterol levels among adults in the United States. JAMA 264:3053, 1990
98. Shieh SM, Shen MM, Tsai WJ et al: Serum lipids and lipoprotein abnormalities in patients with thrombotic stroke—with exploring the protective role of HDL subfractions. Proc Natl Sci Counc Repub China 9:298, 1985
99. Stary HC: Evolution and progression of atherosclerosis in the coronary arteries of children and adults. p. 20. In Bates SR, Gangloff EC (eds): Atherogenesis and Aging. Springer-Verlag, New York, 1987
100. Steinberg D, Parthasarathy S, Carew TE et al: Beyond cholesterol: modifications of low-density lipoprotein that increases its atherogenicity. N Engl J Med 320:915, 1989
101. Stephen AM, Wald NJ: Trends in individual consumption of dietary fat in the United States, 1920–1984. Am J Clin Nutr 52:457, 1990
102. Superko HR: Drug therapy and the prevention of atherosclerosis in humans. Am J Cardiol 64:31G, 1989
103. Tell GS, Crouse JR, Furberg CD: Relation between blood lipids, lipoproteins, and cerebrovascular atherosclerosis: a review. Stroke 19:423, 1988
104. Weiner B, Ockene IS, Levine PH et al: Inhibition of atherosclerosis by cod liver oil in a hyperlipidemic swine model. N Engl J Med 315:841, 1986
105. Yatsu FM, Alam R, Alam SS: Enhancement of cholesterol ester metabolism in cultured human monocyte-derived macrophages by verapamil. Biochem Biophys Acta 847:77, 1985
106. Yatsu FM, Fisher M: Atherosclerosis: current concepts on pathogenesis and interventional therapies. Ann Neurol 26:3, 1989
107. Yatsu FM, Kasturi R, Alam R et al: Molecular biology of atherothrombotic strokes. Stroke, suppl II. 21:131, 1990
108. Yla-Herttuala S, Palinski W, Rosenfeld MR et al: Evidence for the presence of oxidatively modified low density lipoprotein in atherosclerotic lesions of rabbit and man. J Clin Invest 84:1068, 1989
109. Zenker G, Koltringer P, Bone G et al: Lipoprotein(a) as a strong indicator for cerebrovascular disease. Stroke 17:942, 1986
110. Zimetbaum P, Eder H, Frishman W: Probucol: pharmacology and clinical application. J Clin Pharmacol 30:3, 1990

# 3
# ANIMAL MODELS OF BRAIN ISCHEMIA

William A. Pulsinelli
Michael Jacewicz

The pathogenesis of human brain damage from focal (stroke) or global (cardiac arrest) ischemia is influenced by numerous factors, each of which may vary widely. Risk factors such as age, genetics, diet, hypertension, and diabetes mellitus interact to create an overwhelming number of possible combinations in any single individual experiencing a stroke or cardiac arrest. Critics suggest that such complexities thwart the development of any single animal model that reflects accurately all of the risk factors and pathophysiologic events that cause ischemic brain damage.[227] Although correct, such reasoning ignores completely the primary purpose of animal models and fails to recognize the scientific strategy of reductionism invoked in modern-day basic, applied, or clinical research. The goal of reductionism in scientific inquiry is to enhance the homogeneity of the dependent variable by limiting the independent variables, ideally to one. Thus, disease-oriented research, neurologic or otherwise, has evolved to even simpler systems than animal models with the development of tissue slices and cell culture techniques.

The principal strength of animal models of human disease, including those of cardiac arrest and ischemic stroke, is that they eliminate much of the variability associated with the human condition and thereby provide the experimentalist with the degree of control and predictability necessary for hypothesis testing. Thus, while the development of a single animal model that accurately mimics all the complexities of human stroke or cardiac arrest might seem desirable, we suggest that such a model controverts good scientific design and is therefore unnecessary. Instead, the first and most important step in selecting or developing an animal stroke model is the formulation of a thoughtful hypothesis focused on a limited number of variables. Scheinberg[178] said it well: ". . . a stroke model must be appropriate to the type of question which the experiment is asking. A good model is not an art form; it must be able to provide specific information."

Despite many obvious advantages of animal models, their utility in identifying effective pharmacotherapies for clinical brain ischemia has been questioned.[162,227] The failure of drugs that attenuate ischemic-brain damage in animals to modify the outcome of human stroke or cardiac arrest has been used as evidence that the animal models do not adequately simulate the human condition. The lack of a correlation between effective pharmacoprotection in animal versus human brain ischemia, however, has other more likely explanations: (1) erroneous conclusions of neuroprotection in animals because of a failure to vigorously replicate the study and consequentially a type I ($\alpha$) error,[162] (2) drugs identified as neuroprotective against histologic or biochemical injury in animal studies may be insufficiently robust to affect the less sensitive endpoint measures used in clinical trials,[133] and (3) drug therapy in clinical stroke studies has been initiated, with rare exceptions, too late (i.e., hours after the time thresholds for maximal injury).

This chapter identifies and discusses the variables that impact importantly on the neurologic outcome of

This work was supported by NIH grants NS-24302, NS-03346, and NS-07141.

animal models of brain ischemia, reviews the strengths and weaknesses of various cardiac arrest and focal stroke models, and finally emphasizes where possible the relevance of these models to the human condition. A detailed tabulation of available models and a description of their surgical preparation have been presented in a number of reviews[58,62,99,131,133,134,136,218,219] and in the previous version of this chapter.[132]

## DEPENDENT VARIABLES

In the following subsections, we review the important dependent variables that determine the physiologic, histopathologic, and behavioral outcomes of animal models of global and focal brain ischemia. The accuracy and consistency with which animal preparations reproduce the severity plus the spatial and temporal characteristics of clinically defined ischemia largely determine their acceptability as models of the human condition.

### Types of Cerebral Ischemia

#### Global Ischemia

Clinically relevant cerebral ischemia is encountered most frequently as cardiac arrest (global ischemia) or as single or multiple occlusions of intracranial or extracranial cerebral arteries (focal ischemia or stroke). The transient but complete loss of cerebral blood flow (CBF) that accompanies cardiac arrest must last no longer than 5 to 10 minutes[12] if the normothermic patient is to recover in a nonvegetative state. Animal models that simulate human cardiac arrest must therefore cause severe, global, or bihemispheric ischemia that is readily reversible. In animals, if the arrested heart is successfully resuscitated or if mechanical occlusions of cerebral arteries causing global or forebrain ischemia are reversed, CBF rapidly recovers to levels above normal (hyperemia), and 5 to 10 minutes later CBF falls to approximately 50 percent of control values (delayed hypoperfusion).[111,126,168]

The histopathologic consequences of transient global ischemia in humans or animals is irreversible injury to highly vulnerable neurons.[16] The terms *selectively vulnerable neurons* or *selective ischemic necrosis of neurons* are used interchangeably to describe such injury.[157,159] The ischemia-sensitive neurons include, for example, the hippocampal CA1 pyramidal neurons, the cerebellar Purkinje cells, medium-sized striatal neurons, and pyramidal neurons in neocortical layers 3, 5, and 6.[16,157]

#### Focal Ischemia

Focal vascular occlusion (stroke) in humans and animals causes a more moderate and spatially variable reduction of CBF that lasts for hours or, frequently, is permanent. CBF may be moderately or severely reduced in the central zone of the vascular bed fed by the occluded blood vessel, but rarely does CBF fall to zero in focal ischemia (Fig. 3-1).[17] Ischemia becomes progressively less severe toward the periphery of the occluded vascular bed and is often surrounded by a hyperemic zone during the early hours after ischemia onset. CBF eventually normalizes in the vascular territory supplied by surrounding collateral blood vessels. The spatial and temporal dynamics of ischemia in focal vascular occlusion varies considerably both between and within patients[215] and also between and within animal models.[17]

Cerebral vascular occlusions caused by emboli or acute thrombosis in humans may organize and become permanent, but, more commonly, endogenous fibrinolytic mechanisms reopen[19,165,231] the occluded vessels within 6 to 12 hours.[51] Reperfusion of a focal vascular bed after several hours of moderate to severe ischemia causes a less predictable pattern of CBF than reperfusion following transient global ischemia.[97] A brief period of initial reperfusion hyperemia followed by delayed hypoperfusion may or may not develop.

Focal brain ischemia that lasts an hour or longer invariably causes cerebral infarction.[97] Cerebral infarction differs histologically from selective neuronal necrosis in that glial cells and all neurons are killed.[16] The time interval to obtain complete infarction of the compromised vascular bed is approximately 2 to 3 hours in rodents[97] and 4 to 8 hours in anesthetized primates,[33,90] but the interval may be shorter in awake primates. The time window for maximal infarction in humans is unknown but presumably is similar to that of primates.

The apparent discrepancy between global brain ischemia where the complete loss of CBF kills only a fraction of brain neurons, that is, highly vulnerable neurons, and focal brain ischemia where more moderate blood flow loss kills all brain cell types (cerebral infarction) is readily explained by differences in the duration of ischemia. Clinically defined global brain ischemia lasts only minutes, while focal brain ischemia lasts hours or permanently. Thus the combined duration and degree of ischemia (see later discussion in this chapter) is more important to the histopathologic outcome of global and focal ischemia than is the anatomic distribution of blood flow loss.

### Severity of Cerebral Ischemia

The degree and duration of reduced blood flow to brain, that is, the severity of ischemia, are the two most important variables that determine the neurologic outcome of humans and animals. Provided that modifying factors, such as brain temperature (see later sections in this chapter) are held constant, the degree and duration of CBF loss interact to determine whether the brain develops only reversible dysfunction, irreversible damage to selectively vulnerable neurons, or the death of all cell types (cerebral infarction).

The large variance of available data that depicts the correlation between brain injury and the degree of ischemia precludes an accurate quantitative description of this relationship. Nevertheless, by segregating the degree and duration of ischemia into broad categories, the interactive effects of these two variables on brain injury can be illustrated in a semiquantitative manner (Table 3-1).

Cerebral ischemia sufficiently severe to cause persistent anoxic depolarization for more than a few minutes causes some degree of ischemic brain damage in all species. Despite data that show that brain injury may evolve in areas of ischemia without persistent anoxic depolarization,[4,200] the CBF threshold for anoxic depolarization (loss of ionic homeostasis) remains a useful index of the severity of ischemia. Although the absolute CBF (ml/100 g tissue/min) for anoxic depolarization differs among species, reduction of CBF for more than a few minutes below 35 to 40 percent of normal values in rats[204] and below 25 to 30 percent in larger species[4,75,199] usually causes anoxic depolarization.

Ischemia lasting for a few minutes and approaching but not falling below the CBF threshold for anoxic depolarization causes only reversible cellular dysfunction (Table 3-1). If such ischemia persists for an hour or longer, especially if associated with recurrent depolarization potentials, selective ischemic necrosis of neurons or even cerebral infarction may develop. Ischemia severe enough to cause anoxic depolarization is poorly tolerated by brain. A few minutes of this degree of ischemia causes selective necrosis of neurons and only slightly longer durations lead to cerebral infarction.

**TABLE 3-1. The Effect of the Severity of Ischemia on Brain Injury**

| Duration of Ischemia (min) | Degree of Ischemia[a] (as % of Control CBF) | |
|---|---|---|
| | 35–40% | <35–40% |
| 0–30 | Reversible dysfunction | Selective neuronal necrosis |
| ~60 | Selective neuronal necrosis | Infarction |
| >60 | Infarction | Infarction |

[a] The degrees of ischemia presented in this table are taken from microregional cerebral blood flow (CBF) measurements using the $^{14}C$-iodoantipyrine indicator-fractionation method in Spontaneously Hypertensive rats subjected to middle cerebral artery occlusion.[86,204] Persistent anoxic depolarization developed proximal to neocortical tissue in which CBF fell below 35–40% of control values. The CBF threshold for anoxic depolarization in larger animals is reported to be nearer 25–30% of control levels, but such values were obtained with hydrogen clearance methods, which may underestimate CBF.

Variability in behavioral, neurochemical, and histopathologic results between and within laboratories using seemingly identical animal models of cerebral ischemia is a frequent and troublesome problem. Many factors may contribute to such variance, but the most common and important cause is the failure to adopt measures to eliminate, reduce, or standardize the variability in the severity of the ischemic insult. The principal cause of the inconsistency in cerebral ischemia, especially in animal models that produce incomplete or partial ischemia, is a marked difference among animals in the size and number of cervical blood vessels that may provide collateral blood flow to brain. Such differences in the collateral blood supply exist between and within species and even within the same animal strain.[154,167] To control for interanimal variance, and to improve the reproducibility of the ischemic insult, the severity of blood flow loss should be examined in every animal subjected to ischemia. Behavioral (loss of righting response), electrophysiologic (electroencephalogram, sensory evoked potentials, depolarization potentials), and minimally invasive CBF techniques (hydrogen clearance, laser Doppler flowmetry) are well-proven methods for monitoring the severity of cerebral ischemia in animals that are designated for either acute or long-term experiments.

Frequently it is impractical or technically impossible to monitor the severity of ischemia in every animal. In such instances, investigators who adopt well-established animal models should demonstrate that the severity of ischemia achieved in their laboratory is similar to that published by the laboratory(ies) that developed the model. Those who decide to develop new animals models of focal or global brain ischemia are obliged to make a detailed study of the severity, reproducibility, and temporal profile of CBF during ischemia and during cerebral reperfusion.

The severity of cerebral ischemia can be modified greatly by alterations of arterial blood pressure, arterial oxygen and carbon dioxide tensions, glucose, and hematocrit. Each of these variables must be measured and regulated within narrow limits if the animal model is to recreate the desired ischemic insult in a reproducible manner. Placement of small catheters in peripheral arteries of animals as small as gerbils facilitates serial sampling of arterial blood. Except in rare circumstances, the absence of such measurements seriously weaken any conclusions concerning pathophysiologic events or the effectiveness of the pharmacologic treatment under study.

## Perfusion (Arterial) Pressure

CBF is normally maintained relatively constant over a wide range of cerebral perfusion pressures.[153] Cerebral perfusion pressure is the difference between mean arterial blood pressure and intracranial pressure. Since the latter is relatively constant and small compared to arterial pressure it is common practice to correlate CBF versus mean arterial blood pressure. The phenomenon of preserved CBF over a wide range of mean arterial blood pressures in normal brain is termed *autoregulation.* As the mean arterial pressure falls below limits that differ somewhat among species (e.g., in humans 50 to 60 mmHg, in rats 70 to 80 mmHg), CBF falls proportionally to changes in arterial blood pressure. Autoregulation of CBF is lost gradually in areas of brain with mild to moderate ischemia,[47] but as blood flow falls below 30 percent of normal values, autoregulation is completely lost.[47,153]

### Carbon Dioxide and Oxygen Tensions

The arterial tensions of $CO_2$ and $O_2$ directly alter the severity of cerebral ischemia, and consequently both variables must be measured and regulated carefully in animal models. Cerebral vasodilation or vasoconstriction associated in normal brain with hypercapnia and hypocapnia, respectively, are only slightly diminished in mild to moderate ischemia.[89,181] However, as with autoregulation, all vascular reactivity to $CO_2$ is lost in severe ischemia.[89,181]

Small reductions of arterial oxygen tension are immediately compensated by increased CBF in normal brain.[157] Such compensation is not possible in ischemic brain, and therefore even mild degrees of hypoxia can magnify the severity of ischemia.

### Hematocrit

The blood hematocrit influences the severity of ischemia through its effects on serum viscosity and through its hemoglobin content, which determines oxygen-carrying capacity.[69] The cellular components of blood, that is, its hematocrit, cause it to behave as a non-Newtonian fluid with a viscosity that varies inversely with CBF.[69] Thus maintaining the hematocrit within the normal range assures adequate oxygen-carrying capacity and prevents blood flow changes caused by altered plasma viscosity.

## Brain Temperature

Brain temperature during cerebral ischemia and recirculation is second only to the severity of blood flow loss in its importance to the final pathophysiologic outcome. Experimental animal studies in the 1950s established that hypothermia of 5 to 10°C markedly attenuates ischemic injury to brain.[171] Clinically, such information has been long exploited in cardiopulmonary bypass surgery and other types of surgery that may compromise the cerebral circulation. Despite earlier experimental studies to suggest that even mild hypothermia might be neuroprotective,[8,213] a clear demonstration that a 3 to 4°C reduction of brain temperature significantly reduced ischemic brain damage was first presented by Busto et al.[22] Since then, multiple laboratories have confirmed that a few degrees increase[44] or decrease[27,106,128,226] of brain temperature during cerebral ischemia significantly accentuates or reduces brain injury, respectively. Furthermore, it has been shown that both elevated or depressed brain temperatures during the early period of cerebral recirculation also modify the histopathologic outcome from ischemia.[20,104]

Several factors greatly affect the rate and degree of heat loss from brain. The loss of a heat source normally provided by warm circulating blood and the depression of cerebral metabolism, both of which accompany global brain ischemia, cause a more rapid and larger heat loss with global than with focal brain ischemia. Anesthesia, likewise, may markedly reduce CBF and the metabolic rate, thereby enhancing the decline in brain temperature in animals subjected to cerebral ischemia. Insulating tissues such as hair, skin, subcutaneous fat, and the skull bone all retard heat loss from the brain. In regions where these insulating tissues are removed for experimental purposes, local heat loss is greatly increased. Finally, the size of the brain has a substantial impact on the rate of the heat loss with smaller brains losing temperature more rapidly than larger ones.

There is no consensus on how best to monitor the brain's temperature in animals subjected to cerebral ischemia. Some have recommended that temperature probes be placed beneath the temporalis muscle and adjacent to the calvarium,[22] while others have suggested that accurate monitoring of brain temperature can only be achieved with probes placed either in the brain substance or in the epidural space.[129] Whatever the method selected, it is clear that the rectal temperature does not adequately reflect brain temperature during periods of more than a few minutes of global ischemia; within 15 to 20 minutes of global ischemia, the rectal temperature can underestimate brain temperature by as much as 5 or 6°C.[22] During cerebral recirculation, however, in animals that are neither anesthetized nor in which the insulating tissues overlying the brain are disturbed, the rectal temperature usually lies within ±1.0°C of brain temperature (Ko et al., unpublished observations). Monitoring and maintaining the rectal temperature may therefore be an adequate method to control brain temperature during cerebral recirculation.

## Brain Glucose

Despite considerable experimental and clinical evidence that the plasma/brain glucose concentrations are important determinants of the severity of ischemic brain damage, the complex pathophysiologic relationships between these variables remain to be clarified. Myers and Yamaguchi[139] first reported that hyperglycemic monkeys developed greater brain damage and more extensive neurologic deficits from brief cardiac arrest than normoglycemic control animals. Confirmatory studies have shown consistently that hyperglycemia augments brain damage in animals subjected to transient global/forebrain (cardiac arrest-like) ischemia.[60,93,113,166,185,216] However, in focal brain ischemia (stroke) elevated plasma/brain glucose concentrations were reported to increase,[36,37,49,143–145,232] decrease,[63,102,235] or have no effect[158] on the volume of cerebral infarction. The apparent discrepancy of these latter data probably reflects a complex interaction between the temporal pattern of hyperglycemia and the severity of cerebral ischemia on ischemic brain injury. A detailed discussion of these relationships is beyond the scope of this chapter, but suffice it to say that the plasma/brain glucose concentrations greatly modify ischemic brain injury. Accordingly, this dependent variable must be monitored and controlled within limits that are defined by the experimental hypothesis.

Glucose enters brain from blood via facilitated diffusion on a carrier molecular with a $K_m$ for glucose of 5 to 6 mM.[64,105] Since the normal blood glucose concentration in most animals is slightly below the transport $K_m$, the entry of glucose into brain is highly dependent upon its concentration in the blood. The brain glucose concentration is approximately one-third that of blood and varies linearly with the blood glucose concentration over a wide range of values.[64] Since the brain glucose concentration during ischemia is a critical determining factor in the histopathologic and neurologic outcome from ischemia, it is important that the blood glucose concentration be measured shortly *before* and *during* ischemia.

## Species Considerations

The selection of an ideal species and method for modeling human global or focal brain ischemia might, at first glance, appear straightforward. Artificially induced cardiac arrest plus cardiopulmonary resuscitation or the surgical occlusion of a cerebral blood vessel in a subhuman primate are unquestionably the most anthropomorphically appropriate models. Such rationale, however, must be tempered by current dictates of animal ethics and more practical considerations such as expenditures of time and money. The purchase price of subhuman primates plus the costs of appropriate around-the-clock intensive care following transient global or focal brain ischemia in this species are prohibitively expensive for all except a few stringently designed experiments.

Several methods are available for producing well-controlled and reproducible global/forebrain or focal ischemia (see later sections) in a variety of animal species from small rodents up to large subhuman primates. Although much useful scientific and clinical information has come from studies in cats, dogs, and subhuman primates over the past 30 years, there are compelling scientific and ethical reasons for limiting most future studies on cerebral ischemia to rodents. The financial advantages of working with rodent models span the full range of cost accounting from purchase, maintenance, surgery, and endpoint analysis. Lower costs, however, do not alone justify the use of rodents to the exclusion of other species. More important considerations are (1) the scientific knowledge base defining the pathophysiology of cerebral ischemia is many times greater for rodents than for other species; (2) the methods for producing global/forebrain ischemia are similar for all species, and CBF is more easily controlled and monitored in rodents than in larger species; and (3) important pathophysiologic factors, including the vascular anatomy, temporal and spatial changes in blood flow during ischemia, ischemic and postischemic metabolism, and histopathologic changes, are either very similar or identical for rodents and larger species.

Brain ischemia research in species larger than rodents should be limited to specific experimental conditions, questions, or hypotheses that justify the use of these animals. Selected examples of acceptable reasons for using cats, dogs, or subhuman primates include (1) computerized tomographic, positron emission tomographic, or magnetic resonance imaging studies of cerebral circulation, metabolism, or brain injury that require large brains for satisfactory images; (2) specific questions concerning behavioral effects of global or focal brain ischemia that require the more developed brains of larger animals or subhuman primates; (3) experiments to verify the species relevance of a hypothesis that has been *exhaustively* tested in rodents and has been found to have substantial pathophysiologic importance; and (4) the testing of pharmacologic or other therapeutic measures that have been proved to be *unequivocally* effective in rodents and that require testing in subhuman primates before the therapy is subjected to a clinical trial. Finally, laboratories that have invested considerable money and years of research to develop and standardize large animal models of focal or global brain ischemia should be permitted to continue most of their studies. It is important to protect these repositories of knowledge concerning the complex methods necessary to achieve reproducible results in large animal models of brain ischemia.

## Effects of Anesthesia

Because of their complex and often unpredictable effect on brain metabolism and blood flow,[185] anesthetics complicate the study of ischemia pathophysiology. It is naive, however, to consider anesthetics as generically alike and therefore interchangeable in animal modeling. While some anesthetics act primarily by CNS "depression" (e.g., halothane, barbiturates), others (e.g., nitrous oxide, ketamine, enfluorane) cause cortical and subcortical "excitation," which interferes with neural networks responsible for awareness of pain. Not all anesthetics depress cerebral metabolism (e.g., nitrous oxide, fentanyl, and ketamine),[149,186] but when they do, blood flow may or may not be similarly affected. For example, barbiturates and halothane both decrease cerebral metabolism in a dose-dependent manner, but barbiturates (vasoconstrictors) also reduce basal CBF ( by as much as 50 percent),[149] whereas halothane (a vasodilator) in low doses increases CBF (by up to 30 percent).[118] Furthermore, anesthesia can also mask (e.g., MK-801)[147,151] or unmask (e.g., nimodipine)[95] the action of certain vasoactive drugs.

Anesthesia can lower blood pressure and body temperature, and if the animal is not mechanically ventilated, can cause hypercarbia and respiratory acidosis. By avoiding deep anesthesia and by monitoring blood pressure, the investigator can minimize hypotension and its deleterious effects on ischemic regions with lost autoregulation.[47,153] In the absence of mechanical ventilation, anesthesia causes the arterial $PCO_2$ to rise (to very high levels if anesthesia is deep or prolonged). CBF in normal brain rises markedly in response to hypercarbia, and the potential exists for an "intravascular steal" of blood from regions of marginal ischemia. Furthermore, as the intracerebral blood volume increases, so does intracranial pressure, which can further aggravate ischemia. Finally, a fall in blood pH (severe respiratory acidosis) predisposes the animal to cardiac arrhythmias (triggered by ischemic brain injury or by toxic levels of anesthetic), and the compromised cardiac output can worsen brain (and cardiac) ischemia and end in death. All these systemic complications of anesthesia can be minimized or controlled by careful monitoring of physiologic variables.

Some critics have pointed to the profound impact of anesthesia on the pathophysiology of ischemia in questioning the relevance of animal stroke models to human stroke.[227] It should be noted, however, that anesthetized animals experiencing cerebral ischemia directly mimic the unfortunate patients who suffer intraoperative stroke (e.g., after cardiac arrest, severe blood loss). It should also be reemphasized that the purpose of animal stroke models is not to simulate the complexities of the human condition but to test hypotheses that are relevant to human disease. For ethical and legal reasons, the use of anesthetics in animal models is usually unavoidable, but it should be stressed that their side effects can be identified, studied, and controlled.

## MEASURABLE ENDPOINTS IN ISCHEMIA MODELS

The behavioral, anatomic, biochemical, and physiologic endpoints available for analysis in experimental stroke are numerous, and their selection, like the choice of a stroke model, should depend on the hypothesis to be tested. Several endpoints, however, deserve special comment. *Mortality,* although simple to measure in experimental stroke, offers very limited insight into mechanisms of ischemic brain injury. *Neurologic deficits,* sought because of their relevance to human stroke, are often variable despite identical vascular manipulation and treatment. Motor impairment after middle cerebral artery (MCA) occlusion, for example, depends more on internal capsule ischemia than on the overall size of the infarct in both primates[196] and rats (Jacewicz et al., unpublished observations). More complex behaviors require specialized training of both animal and investigator and are more difficult to assess in small animals. Thus, most investigators choose endpoints that are "objective" and more easily quantified than behavioral deficits. However, these objective measures (e.g., CBF, cerebral glucose metabolism, histology) can still show marked regional (and microregional) heterogeneity after ischemia, which presents its own problems (e.g., requiring simultaneous "'multiparametric" analysis with techniques of sufficient resolving power to avoid errors of tissue averaging). However, among all endpoints, the "gold standard" to which animal stroke models must be subjected (and to which the other endpoints must ultimately be compared) is *histopathology.* Does a particular vascular manipulation cause ischemic damage, and, if so, where and how much? Is the histopathology similar to that seen in human stroke or cardiac arrest? These basic questions precede all others because they define the stroke model, and, pending the discovery of earlier molecular or physiologic events that unambiguously doom the brain cell, histopathology remains the criterion by which ischemic injury and animal models are judged. Finally, before any stroke model is to be considered standardized, the reproducibility and relationship between changes in *cerebral blood flow* (i.e., the degree and duration of cerebral ischemia) and histologic outcome should be characterized. Only then will the stroke model offer meaningful interpretations of changes in a multitude of biochemical, physiologic, and other molecular endpoints.

## GLOBAL/FOREBRAIN ISCHEMIA MODELS

The following subsections review briefly the advantages and disadvantages of available methods to produce experimental global and forebrain ischemia. No special consideration is given to species, since the methods available for producing global/forebrain ischemia are usually applicable to both small and large animals. Rodent models of global/forebrain ischemia are covered in slightly greater detail for reasons cited above and because rodent models are by far the most commonly used.

The hallmarks of all animal models that simulate human brain ischemia caused by cardiac arrest are *transient, bihemispheric,* or *global* ischemia that is either *complete* or *severe*. Such models can be separated into two categories: those that cause the complete loss of blood flow to the entire brain (global models) and those that cause severe but incomplete ischemia of the forebrain (forebrain models) (Table 3-2). The latter models also cause mild to moderate ischemia of the brain stem and the cerebellum. In clinically relevant forebrain models, severe ischemia is defined as the loss of blood flow sufficient to cause persistent anoxic depolarization of forebrain structures. The duration of ischemia in either type of model is usually 5 to 15 minutes, but in some, ischemia is maintained for 30 to 60 minutes before circulation is returned to the brain. The histopathologic outcome of both global and forebrain models is necrosis of selectively vulnerable neurons unless modifying factors, such as hyperthermia or hyperglycemia, escalate the injury to cerebral infarction.

Important differences between global and forebrain ischemia models must be considered when designing a study to test a specific hypothesis. Hypotheses that concern the pathophysiology of hindbrain ischemia must be examined in a global ischemia model, since the reduction of blood flow to the brain stem and cerebellum in forebrain models is quite mild and variable. In contrast, the pathophysiology of forebrain ischemia may be studied equally well with either a global or a forebrain model provided that forebrain ischemia is sufficiently severe to rapidly cause persistent an-oxic depolarization of the forebrain structures. Few differences have been reported in the neurochemical or histopathologic responses of the rodent forebrain subjected to the severe but incomplete ischemia produced by forebrain methods versus the complete ischemia achieved with global methods.[11,113,160,163,164,179,185,233]

Practical considerations in selecting a global versus a forebrain model are (1) a lower survival rate in global models, presumably caused by severe hindbrain ischemia and injury to critical brain stem respiratory and/or cardiovascular regulatory centers and (2) global models must be artificially ventilated until brain stem respiratory centers recover after cerebral recirculation. Spontaneous respiration is maintained in the forebrain models, and unless the animals are paralyzed and mechanically ventilated, hyperventilation develops. The mild hyperoxia and hypocarbic alkalosis caused by hyperventilation in these models is short-lived, and within 5 to 10 minutes of cerebral recirculation, arterial blood gases return to normal.[167] Differences in the respiratory physiology between global and forebrain models has led to few differences in either neurochemistry or histopathology.[11,113,160,163,164,179,185]

**TABLE 3-2. Methods for Producing Global/Forebrain Ischemia**

| Methods | Global Ischemia[a] | Forebrain Ischemia[a] |
|---|---|---|
| Cardiac arrest | Primate[139]<br>Dog[24,177]<br>Cat[208]<br>Rat[11,38,217] | |
| Artificially raise intracranial pressure | Dog[66,146]<br>Rabbit[116,180]<br>Rat[113] | |
| Occlude ascending aorta and/or intrathoracic branches | Primate[80,127]<br>Dog[18,87,191]<br>Cat[3,88]<br>Rabbit[1]<br>Rat[39] | Rat[39] |
| Neck tourniquet plus occlude vertebral/basilar arteries | Primate[92]<br>Dog[42]<br>Rabbit[101] | Dog[50,91] |
| Neck tourniquet plus hypotension | Primate[148,193]<br>Rat[185] | Rat[185] |
| Occlude carotids and vertebral/basilar arteries | | Primate[228]<br>Cat[61]<br>Rat[94,167,179] |
| Occlude carotids plus hypotension | | Rat[190] |
| Occlude carotids | | Rat[55,154]<br>Gerbil[82] |
| Profound hypotension | | Primate[15]<br>Rat[230] |

[a] Most references represent the original description of a particular method in a species and/or important modifications of the original method.

## Cardiac Arrest

Ventricular fibrillation caused by electric shock of the myocardium,[177,208] apnea,[139] or the intravenous injection of KCl,[11] are standard methods for arresting the heart in small and large animals. Although the induction of cardiac arrest is relatively simple, rapid and effective resuscitation procedures require skill, and consequently such models are used in only a few well-experienced laboratories.[177,208]

The influence of systemic organ (heart, lung, kidney, etc.) ischemia on the pathogenesis of clinical brain ischemia is best studied in animal models that employ cardiac arrest. Ischemic injury to the heart, lungs, kidneys, or other systemic organs may profoundly alter the recoverability of brain from transient, complete ischemia. Clarification of the interactions between systemic organ and brain ischemia are important for the development of effective treatments for cardiac arrest. Nevertheless, the principal strength of cardiac arrest models, that is, the capacity to simulate whole-body ischemia, rapidly becomes its Achilles heel, if, as is frequently the case, the hypothesis being tested requires the elimination of variables caused by systemic organ ischemia. Moreover, when testing drugs for their ability to directly protect neurons in cardiac arrest models, the possibility that drug-related improvement in systemic organ function may expedite neurologic recovery must be considered. An additional weakness of experimental cardiac arrest is the variability of resuscitation time and, consequently, brain injury. Early difficulties in resuscitating the heart and the high mortality, immediate and late, due to brain stem ischemia have been largely but not completely overcome with improved resuscitation protocols.[24,177,208]

### Elevation of Intracranial Pressure

Raising intracranial pressure above arterial pressure by the injection of artificial cerebral spinal fluid into the subarachnoid space is a simple and effective method for eliminating blood flow to the entire brain.[66,113,116,146,180] The procedure has been criticized by some as being nonphysiologic, since it produces a bloodless brain. Other disadvantages of the procedure are that hypotensive drugs are required to prevent reflex arterial hypertension.

### Occlusion of the Ascending Aorta and/or Intrathoracic Branches

Occlusion of the ascending aorta alone and/or in conjunction with its main intrathoracic branches is an effective method for producing total-body ischemia in all species.[3,18,39,41,80,191] Global or forebrain ischemia may be achieved by occluding all or only selected arteries. Early problems with injury to the lungs and myocardium have been largely overcome by the Brockman and Jude[18] modification, which allows continued oxygenation and perfusion of the lungs and heart. Disadvantages of the method include the trauma of thoracic surgery and the impact that systemic organ ischemia may have on survival or on ischemic brain injury.

### Cervical Tourniquet

Inflation of a pneumatic cuff placed around the neck is an effective, noninvasive method to occlude the common carotid and cervical collateral arteries supplying the brain.[42,92] However, perfusion of the hindbrain is unaltered by cervical compression alone, since the vertebrals and anterior spinal arteries are protected from compression by the vertebral bones. Surgical laminectomy at the C2 level[92] exposes both the vertebrals and anterior spinal arteries to the occluding pressure gradients generated by the inflated neck tourniquet. Alternatively, cervical cuff compression may be combined with either hypotension[148,193] and/or surgical occlusion of the vertebral or basilar arteries[50,101] to obtain global brain ischemia. The patency of the trachea is maintained during cervical compression by inserting a ridged orotracheal tube. Occlusion of jugular venous drainage and cerebral venous stasis are disadvantages of this method.

### Occlusion of Cervical Arteries

Occlusion of the common carotid arteries in the neck combined with either vertebral[161,163,167,179,209] or basilar artery occlusion[61,94] and/or hypotension[190] are used frequently to produce severe forebrain ischemia, especially in rodents. Bilateral occlusion of the common carotid and vertebral arteries (four-vessel occlusion)[161,163,167] and bilateral common carotid artery occlusion combined with hypotension[190] in rodents are the most widely used models of transient forebrain ischemia. Both models behave similarly with regard to neurochemical, behavioral, and histopathologic changes following 5 to 15 minutes of severe forebrain ischemia. Each model's advantages and disadvantages have been discussed in detail by Ginsberg and Busto.[62]

Bilateral carotid artery occlusion in the gerbil is another frequently used model of transient forebrain ischemia.[82] An incomplete circle of Willis in the majority of gerbils eliminates the need to occlude collateral blood flow provided by the vertebral-basilar arteries. Disadvantages of this model include a propensity to develop seizures in animals subjected to ischemia for longer than 5 minutes and the difficulty with monitoring important systemic variables in such small animals.[62]

### Profound Hypotension

Profound hypotension has been used to produce global brain ischemia.[15,230] The distribution and severity of blood flow loss, however, differ considerably from that produced by the previously described models. Ischemia caused by profound hypotension is most severe in arterial boundary zones that lie between major intracranial arteries. Consequently, the distribution of brain injury differs considerably from that caused by models that produce uniformly severe global or forebrain ischemia. Hypotension models are appropriate for the study of shock in humans but are not well suited for simulating the conditions of cardiac arrest ischemia.

## FOCAL ISCHEMIA MODELS

While Flourens[53] first described the effects of emboli introduced into the cerebral vascular system in 1847, almost a century elapsed before focal infarcts were achieved by an external occlusion of one of the major intracranial arteries in monkeys and dogs.[23,156,224] Over the next 50 years, numerous methods to induce focal cerebral ischemia were developed (Table 3-3), but only a few models were standardized. Rarely was the ischemic insult systematically characterized with neuropathologic and CBF studies, and the technical pitfalls (Table 3-4) worked out to optimize reproducibility. Of these, the most relevant to the human condition has been middle cerebral artery occlusion (MCAO), and MCAO experiments involving several species have contributed greatly to our current knowledge of ischemia pathophysiology.[4,58,62,165]

**TABLE 3-3. Methods to Achieve Focal Cerebral Ischemia**

| Method | Potentially Reversible | Species |
|---|---|---|
| Extrinsic MCA occlusion | | |
| Ligature | Yes | Primate,[34] dog,[2] cat,[73] rabbit,[188] rat[170,183] |
| Aneurysm clip | Yes | Primate,[150,196,198] dog,[196] cat,[196] rabbit,[120] rat[21,205,206] |
| Miniature hook | Yes | Cat,[112] rat[17,97] |
| Electrocautery | No | Primate,[81] cat,[71,72,79] rat,[17,211] gerbil[234] |
| Inflatable balloon | Yes | Primate,[41,192] cat[225] |
| Embolic intravascular occlusion | | |
| Microsphere(s) | No | Primate,[14,221] dogs,[155] rat[100,184] |
| Rubber cylinder | No | Dogs,[130] rat[210] |
| Autologous clot | Yes | Primates,[77] dog,[135] rabbit,[114,236] rat[103] |
| Platelet aggregates | Yes | Primates,[54] rabbit,[152] rat[56,57] |
| Nylon thread | Yes | Rat[67,140] |
| In situ MCA thrombosis | Yes | Primate,[78] rat[142] |
| Cortical photocoagulation | No | Rat[45,222,223] |
| Carotid occlusion | Yes | Rat,[107,119] gerbil[9,108,109,229] |

*Abbreviation:* MCA, middle cerebral artery.

Early experiments performed mostly in cats and primates have contributed a number of important findings regarding MCAO.[43,121–124,196,220] First, blood flow did not cease but reversed direction in the distal MCA segment after MCAO.[35] Second, the site of MCAO (proximal vs distal) affected the topography of ischemic damage. Occlusion distal to the lenticulostriate branches of the MCA spared the basal ganglia, while more proximal MCA occlusions allowed a variable amount of retrograde flow to reach the lenticulostriates and led to variable infarction.[131] Regardless of the MCAO site, however, ischemia topography, severity, and accompanying neurologic deficits were not induced with any consistency, even after less traumatic orbital approaches were developed to minimize the artifacts of extensive craniotomy, blood loss, and retraction ischemia.[10,33–35,43,70,81,95,121,123,137,150,196,198] The chief cause of the interspecies and intraspecies differences in lesion production was attributed to vascular collaterals.[123,124,214] For example, cats and rhesus macaques,[121] in contrast to squirrel monkeys,[220] suffered little infarction unless hypotension was added to MCAO so as to obliterate the collateral blood flow.

Once a region of *dense* focal ischemia was attained, a more or less similar sequence of cortical events ensued.[43,123,220] Venous blood darkened (oxygen desaturation) and was followed by particulate flow ("venous sludging") and formation of platelet thrombi, which was preventable with heparin in cats and macaques[122] but not in squirrel monkeys that suffered larger infarcts.[197] Small foci of pallor coalesced, and after a brief initial dilatation, arteries constricted. The vasoconstriction could be reversed by topical saline irrigation or by application of papavarine, but not by raising blood pressure. Blood flow became segmented in the pale "core" areas, while vasodilatation persisted in "marginal zones."[220] Cortical pallor, once established, was not easily reversed with recirculation and suggested that the process of cerebral infarction was under way with infarct inception requiring approximately 1 hour of ischemia.[169] Up to 1 cm away from the ischemic core, a border hyperemia developed with independent fluctuations resembling the spreading depression of Leão.[124] When infarctions were very large, the potential for cerebral edema to exacerbate ischemia in a confined, unyielding cranium[73,74] was directly visualized through a cranial window against which pial vessels became flattened and their blood supply obliterated within hours after MCAO.[121]

Later experiments, taking advantage of new quantitative CBF techniques (hydrogen clearance, autora-

**TABLE 3-4. Factors That May Influence the Consistency of Ischemic Damage After MCAO**

| Factor[a] | Predisposes to More Damage | Predisposes to Less Damage |
|---|---|---|
| Species and strain | SHR,[17,30,49] SHRSP,[29,31] squirrel monkeys[220] | Wistar rats,[17,29,31,171] Sprague-Dawley rats,[30] macaques,[123] cats[123] |
| Model | Closed skull (raised intracranial pressure)[73] | Open skull (pressure reduced by craniotomy)[73] |
| | Sympathetic denervation[6,175,176] (? also caused by injury to MCA nerve plexus) | |
| Site of MCAO | Proximal (plus distal to isolate lenticulostriate arteries)[131,182,205] | Distal[7,28,30,182,205] |
| Surgical technique | MCA trauma and vasospasm,[81] retraction ischemia[81] | Incomplete MCA occlusion |
| | Brain hyperthermia[25]: temporal muscle removal by electrocautery, burr hole drilling without irrigation | Brain hypothermia: craniotomy irrigation at room temperature |
| | Infection, post-op fever, hypotension,[123] anesthesia,[212] hemorrhage, drug effect, hyperglycemia[143,158,232] | Anesthetic effect: inactivity (gerbils), drug effect[20] |
| Anesthesia | Hypercarbia: intravascular steal,[202,203] raised intracranial pressure | ?Depress CNS metabolic needs[186] |

*Abbreviations:* CNS, central nervous system; MCA, middle cerebral artery; MCAO, MCA occlusion; SHR, Spontaneously hypertensive rat; SHRSP, SHR stroke prone.

[a] Other factors: Inadequate numbers of animals causing type II errors[17,83,162] or type I errors.[189]

diography) revealed that regional CBF in open skull preparations underwent relatively little fluctuation during the critical early hours after MCAO[72,79,195] unless complicated by hypotension or hypercarbia. With hypercarbia, CBF fell further (intravascular steal) in ischemic regions with CBF already less than 40 percent of baseline.[202,203] Finally, separate blood flow thresholds were identified for cerebral electrical (synaptic) failure (CBF = 15 to 18 ml/100 g/min or 35 to 40 percent of baseline) and for the loss of potassium and calcium ionic homeostasis (CBF = 8 to 12 ml/100 g/min).[5,13,68] Brain tissue perfused between these two thresholds formed an "ischemic penumbra" in which ischemically threatened cortex was electrically dysfunctional but still viable.[4,75] However, blood flows of 35 to 40 percent of baseline triggered anaerobic glycolysis,[207] edema formation,[117] and loss of autoregulation,[201] and within 1 to 2 hours hampered neuronal firing recovery[76] and caused scattered (sometimes laminar) ischemic neuronal necrosis.[194,207] If 3 or more hours in duration, the CBF less than 35 to 40 percent of baseline led to infarction[90,137] and a peri-infarct region of graded neuronal loss.[125] The sequential ultrastructural changes during the first hour after MCAO included swelling of neuronal mitochondria, condensation of the cytoplasm, and swelling of astrocytes.[59] Despite the productive research conducted in cats and primates, use of primates, dogs, and cats has waned, and rodent models have become more prevalent.

## Single Common Carotid Occlusion in Gerbils

Early attempts to induce focal stroke in rats by a unilateral common carotid occlusion were unsuccessful unless hypoxia[107] or hypotension[119] were added. In contrast, about 20 percent of gerbils subjected to a similar occlusion developed fatal hemispheric ischemia.[108] Because the posterior communicating arteries are absent in the circle of Willis, a high proportion (30 to 60 percent) of gerbils develop signs of hemispheric ischemia upon (reversible) occlusion of a common carotid artery.[109,110] The resulting ischemic damage depends on the ischemic interval prior to recirculation: 5 minutes of ischemia provokes CA1 neuronal lesions,[229] whereas 1 hour or more can cause fatal hemispheric infarction, especially if the anterior vascular anastomoses between the hemispheres is small.[9] Since the surgical procedure is easy, large numbers of animals have been used for drug screening purposes. Unfortunately, as many as half the animals (depending on the supplier, gerbil colony, and shipment) develop convulsions[98] (clonic and "running" fits) after ischemia, altering the pathophysiology of the ischemic insult and undermining "intent to treat" drug strategies. Furthermore, the body temperature is all too easily lowered by stroke, drugs, and inactivity. Cannulating the tiny gerbil tail (or femoral) artery is not only technically heroic, but more importantly, serial blood sampling is impossible without risking hemorrhagic hypotension. Thus, monitoring physiologic variables (other than body temperature, which is mandatory) in gerbils is impractical, and the exclusion of convulsing animals from data analysis can inadvertently introduce bias. Consequently, experiments employing gerbils must always be repeated in other species before any findings can be judged as "definitive."

## Middle Cerebral Artery Occlusion in Rats

MCAO in the rat was first reported in 1975,[170] but did not constitute a standardized model until 1981, when Tamura and his colleagues described a subtemporal approach to the proximal MCA in the Sprague-Dawley rat and compared CBF changes after MCAO to histologic outcome.[205,206,211] The CBF threshold for consistent histopathologic damage in the striatum and cortex was found to be higher in rats (25 ml/100 g/min at 4 hours after MCAO) than in cats and primates.[211] Because the CBF gradation between normal and ischemic tissue was steep, the model offered a rather narrow "penumbra" for salvage by therapeutic intervention. Subsequently, the precise placement and extent of the occlusion site along the MCA was recognized as an important factor for consistent lesion production: the lenticulostriate arteries had to be isolated from both the proximal and distal supply of CBF for consistent infarction of the basal ganglia.[7] Distal MCAO (above the lenticulostriates) in Wistar rats produced no infarction in the basal ganglia and little or highly variable infarction in the cortex,[28,182] which prompted additional vascular manipulations to accentuate the severity of ischemia. Ipsilateral common carotid occlusion was added to MCAO[17,85] and coupled with temporary (1 hour) occlusion of the contralateral carotid artery,[26] the latter superimposing transient forebrain ischemia onto MCAO. Occlusion of individual branches of the MCA further characterized the patterns of collateral blood flow and suggested that the frontopyriform branch of the MCA behaved as an end artery.[174]

Various attempts to improve lesion reproducibility met with only limited success until the Spontaneously Hypertensive rat (SHR) and its stroke-prone cohort (SHRSP) were shown to suffer larger and much less variable infarcts following MCAO than most other animal models of focal stroke (Fig. 3-1).[17,29,30,31,49,65] This permitted pathophysiologic investigations and drug testing to be conducted with greater statistical power and more manageable numbers of inexpensive animals, as well as the study of the relationship of hypertension to stroke. As in cats and primates, a CBF of 35 to 40 percent of baseline (which in rats is three times greater than in cats and primates) was shown to trigger cerebral acidosis,[141] induce heat shock proteins and globally to inhibit pro-

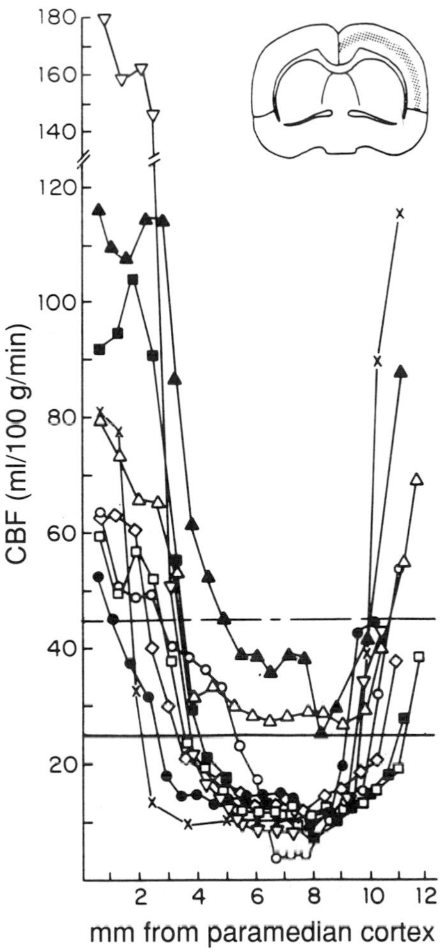


**Fig. 3-1.** Serial cerebral blood flow measurements in eight Spontaneously Hypertensive rats subjected to 2.5 hours of middle cerebral artery occlusion plus ipsilateral common carotid occlusion. The measurements were taken along a central cortical band stretching from the paramedian cortex to the rhinal sulcus (stippled region in inset) at the level of basal ganglia. Blood flow drops with variable steepness from the paramedian region supplied by the anterior cerebral artery. The solid line indicates the cerebral blood flow threshold for early (4 hours after middle cerebral artery occlusion) neuropathologic change[164], while the dotted line shows the cerebral blood flow threshold for a variety of injurious biochemical and physiologic changes.[86] (Adapted from Jacewicz et al,[84] with permission.)

tein synthesis,[85] and, more recently, to depolarize the cortex,[204] which results in infarction if sustained beyond 3 hours.[86,97]

Why do hypertensive rats suffer larger, more consistent infarcts after MCAO than their closely related normotensive counterparts? It had been believed that the thickening of the arterial wall (induced by chronic hypertension) encroached on the vascular lumen and reduced the vessel's distensibility, thereby hampering the compensatory vasodilator response to ischemia and accentuating the infarct process. However, more recent experimental work has suggested that cerebrovascular hypertrophy may not explain the more severe ischemia suffered by hypertensive rats, and in fact hypertrophy may actually counteract stroke: chronic sympathetic denervation in SHRSP suppresses hypertrophy, but the incidence of spontaneous cerebral hemorrhages and infarction actually increases.[6,175,176] What then predisposes the hypertensive rat to infarction?

Initial work with the SHR and SHRSP subjected to MCAO yielded some surprising relationships between hypertension and infarct susceptibility.[29,30] First, very young (5 weeks of age) SHR and SHRSP developed large infarcts before either hypertension or vascular pathology became established. Second, infarct vulnerability in SHRSP was due to smaller caliber vascular anastomoses (between the MCA and anterior cerebral artery) which was inherited via an autosomal recessive gene locus.[32] That hypertension per se was of secondary importance to the vascular collaterals was strengthened by other observations. First, approximately 10 percent of young[30] and adult (Jacewicz et al., unpublished observations) SHR suffered small infarcts or no infarct at all after MCAO, and the correlation between preocclusion blood pressure and infarct magnitude was poor.[30,83] Second, induced hypertension (by deoxycorticosterone-acetate and salt administration) in normotensive strains failed to provoke large infarcts after MCAO.[29] Third, adult SHR treated with antihypertensive agents suffer infarcts (after tandem MCA and common carotid occlusion) that are only 20 percent smaller than the very large infarcts in untreated controls.[187] These data suggest that infarct susceptibility in SHR stems from a lack of vascular collateral blood flow that is genetically related (but not directly linked) to hypertension. Since very large infarcts after MCAO (presumably due to inadequate collateral blood flow) also occur with highly variable (usually low) frequency in normotensive rats,[17,49] the gene (or set of genes) governing infarct susceptibility can be dissociated from hypertension, and, presumably, is extant in normotensive populations of rats (and in other species as well). If so, this would explain much of the inconsistency in ischemic brain damage in focal stroke models and perhaps in the human condition as well. One can hypothesize that, while hypertension may produce extensive atherosclerotic disease and compromise blood flow through a major cerebral artery (e.g., the MCA), only the patient with inherited small-caliber collaterals suffers a catastrophic stroke. Other patients can remain asymptomatic because what actually determines outcome is some as yet unidentified autosomal recessive gene (or set of genes) governing the availability of vascular collaterals.

One criticism of SHR subjected to MCAO, however, is that the ischemia is too severe for otherwise useful therapies to be effective.[62,172,173] However, focal cortical infarct volume has been reduced by 15 to 25 percent in SHR treated with hydralazine,[187] nimodipine,[83] MK-801,[48] and idazoxan.[115] A 15 to 25 percent decrement in infarct volume may appear modest, but it is the equivalent of a 30 to 50 percent infarct reduction in nonhypertensive rats that generate infarct volumes half as large as in SHR. The investigator, however, should observe certain caveats when using SHR in drug testing. Therapy should be instituted before the infarct process becomes irreversible (approximately 3 hours after ischemia onset)[97] and should match the duration of ischemic conditions (i.e., continue as long as the process of injury is active).[48,83,84] The numbers of animals (determined by power analysis) should be adequate to avoid a type II error,[17,83,162] and the experiments should be replicated to avoid a type I error.[189] Within these qualifications, the SHR subjected to MCAO provide a stringent test for any drug purporting to protect against focal ischemic stroke. While a negative result should not deter the investigator from repeating the experiments, using a model offering less severe ischemia, a positive result suggests a genuinely potent therapeutic effect and should act as a stimulus to continue with further experimental (and perhaps clinical) testing.

## Intravascular Occlusion Models

Intravascular occlusion of the MCA can be achieved by in situ thrombosis (via a catheterized copper coil in dogs),[78] by intravascular infusion of platelet proaggregants (e.g., arachidonic acid)[52] or by embolism of a preformed thrombus[138] or other thrombogenic material (see review of del Zoppo and associates[40]). Photoactive gents, such as rose bengal, have been given systemically and followed by focal illumination to produce carotid platelet thrombi that embolize and cause small cerebral infarcts resembling hypertensive *lacunes* in humans.[56,57] Alternatively, following dye administration, precisely localized brain regions (with the skull intact) can be illuminated to induce endothelial damage, intravascular platelet aggregation, thrombosis, and infarction.[46,62,222] These models of intravascular occlusion are ideally suited for the evaluation of thrombolytic therapy in ischemic stroke.[40,223] In addition, the ischemic stroke can be studied within the intact skull, free of alterations in cerebrospinal fluid dynamics introduced by craniectomy and without the damage caused to the nerve plexus coursing along the MCA. Among those models featuring multiple emboli, a major disadvantage is that the number and size of cerebral lesions are often difficult to control for statistical comparisons, and they may cause excessive brain edema as well.

A siliconized rubber cylinder (made from a nylon filament) has been threaded up the internal carotid artery into the circle of Willis to reversibly obstruct both the middle and anterior cerebral arteries in the Wistar rat.[140] A 3-hour temporary occlusion causes massive hemispheric ischemia that proves universally fatal within a day.[67] This model presents a striking contrast to the trivial infarction usually produced by MCAO in the Wistar rat, and it suggests that the (1) collateral blood flow from the anterior cerebral artery is essential for salvaging the MCA territory, (2) endothelial injury and secondary thrombosis in the cerebral vasculature may occur (this remains to be proved) and thwart the recovery of circulation, and (3) the effects of an intact skull on ischemia are not to be minimized in rodents (e.g., SHR that undergo a small craniectomy for MCAO may suffer massive hemispheric infarctions but still survive the insult).[17]

Animal models have and will continue to contribute importantly to our understanding of the pathophysiology of human neurologic disease and its treatment. Although neurology was well served before the latter half of this century by purely observational and descriptive methods, technological developments over the last 20 years, particularly in the fields of neuroradiology and molecular biology, have enhanced the clinician's ability to explore the nature of human disease. Nevertheless, ethical considerations associated with human experimentation and physical limitations of even our most advanced technologies seriously restrict hypotheses testing in humans at the cellular and molecular levels. Animal models of central nervous system disease singularly provide the means for examining such hypotheses and for the testing of new pharmacologic agents.

## REFERENCES


1. Ames A, Wright R, Kowada M: Ischemia. II. The no-reflow phenomenon. Am J Pathol 52:437, 1968
2. Anthony L, Goldring S, O'Leary JL, Schwartz HG: Experimental cerebrovascular occlusion in dog. Arch Neurol 8:515, 1963
3. Arsenio-Nunes ML, Hossmann K-A, Farkas-Bargeton E: Ultrastructural and histochemical investigation of the cerebral cortex of cat during and after complete ischaemia. Acta Neuropathol (Berl) 26:329, 1973
4. Astrup J, Siesjo B, Symon L: Thresholds in cerebral ischemia—the ischemic penumbra. (Editorial.) Stroke 12:723, 1981
5. Astrup J, Symon L, Branston NM, Lassen NA: Cortical evoked potential and extracellular $K^+$ and $H^+$ at critical levels of brain ischemia. Stroke 8:51, 1977
6. Baumbach GL, Heistad DD: Cerebral circulation in chronic arterial hypertension. Hypertension 12:89, 1988
7. Bederson J, Pitts L, Tsuji M et al: Rat middle cerebral artery occlusion: evaluation of the model and development of a neurologic examination. Stroke 17:472, 1986
8. Berntman L, Welsh FA, Harp JR: Cerebral pro-

tective effect of low-grade hypothermia. Anesthesiology 55:495, 1981
9. Berry K, Wisniewski HM, Svarzbein L, Baez S: On the relationship of brain vasculature to production of neurological deficit and morphological changes following acute unilateral common carotid artery ligation in gerbils. J Neurol Sci 25:75, 1975
10. Blair RDG, Waltz AG: Regional cerebral blood flow during acute ischemia. Neurology (NY) 20:802, 1970
11. Blomqvist P, Wieloch T: Ischemic brain damage in rats following cardiac arrest using a long-term recovery model. J Cereb Blood Flow Metab 5:420, 1985
12. Brain Resuscitation Clinical Trial I Study Group: Randomized clinical study of thiopental loading in comatose survivors of cardiac arrest. N Engl J Med 314:397, 1986
13. Branston NM, Strong AJ, Symon L: Extracellular potassium activity, evoked potential and tissue blood flow. J Neurol Sci 32:305, 1977
14. Bremer AM, Watanabe O, Bourke RS: Artificial embolization of the middle cerebral artery in primates: description of an experimental model with extracranial technique. Stroke 6:334, 1975
15. Brierley JB, Brown AW, Excell BJ, Meldrum BS: Brain damage in the rhesus monkey resulting from profound arterial hypotension. I. Its nature, distribution and general physiological correlates. Brain Res 13:68, 1969
16. Brierley JB, Graham DI: Hypoxia and vascular disorders of the central system, p. 125. In Adams JH, Corsellis JAN, Duchen LW (eds): Greenfield's Neuropathology. Wiley, New York, 1984
17. Brint S, Jacewicz M, Kiessling M et al: Focal brain ischemia in the rat: methods for reproducible infarction using tandem occlusion of the distal middle cerebral and ipsilateral common carotid arteries. J Cereb Blood Flow Metab 8:474, 1988
18. Brockman SK, Jude JR: The tolerance of the dog brain to total arrest of circulation. Bull Johns Hopkins Hosp 106:74, 1960
19. Buchan A, Gates P, Pelz D, Barnett H: Intraluminal thrombus in the cerebral circulation: implications for surgical management. Stroke 19:681, 1988
20. Buchan A, Pulsinelli W: Hypothermia but not the N-methyl-D-aspartate antagonist, MK-801, attenuates neuronal damage in gerbils subjected to transient global ischemia. J Neurosci 10:311, 1990
21. Buchan AM, Xue D, Slivka A: A new model of focal stroke in the rat. Stroke 23:273, 1992
22. Busto R, Dietrich W, Mordecal G et al: Small differences in intraischemic brain temperature critically determines the extent of neuronal injury. J Cereb Blood Flow Metab 7:729, 1987
23. Campbell JB, Forster FM: The anterior cerebral artery in the macaque monkey. J Nerv Ment Dis 99:229, 1944
24. Cerchiari EL, Hoel TM, Safar P, Sclabassi RJ: Protective effects of combined superoxide dismutase and deferoxamine on recovery of cerebral blood flow and function after cardiac arrest in dogs. Stroke 18:869, 1987
25. Chen H, Chopp M, Welch KMA: Effect of mild hyperthermia on the ischemic infarct volume after middle cerebral artery occlusion in the rat. Neurology (NY) 41:1133, 1991
26. Chen ST, Hsu CY, Hogan EL et al: A model of focal ischemic stroke in the rat: reproducible extensive cortical infarction. Stroke 17:738, 1986
27. Chopp M, Knight R, Tidwell C et al: The metabolic effects of mild hypothermia on global cerebral ischemia and recirculation in the cat: comparison to normothermia and hyperthermia. J Cereb Blood Flow Metab 9:141, 1989
28. Coyle P: Middle cerebral artery occlusion in the young rat. Stroke 13:855, 1982
29. Coyle P: Outcomes to middle cerebral artery occlusion in hypertensive and normotensive rats. Hypertension 6:169, 1984
30. Coyle P: Different susceptibilities to cerebral infarction in spontaneously hypertensive (SHR) and normotensive Sprague-Dawley rats. Stroke 17:520, 1986
31. Coyle P, Jokelainen PT: Differential outcome to middle cerebral artery occlusion in spontaneously hypertensive stroke-prone rats (SHRSP) and Wistar Kyoto (WKY) rats. Stroke 14:605, 1983
32. Coyle P, Odenheimer DJ, Sing CF: Cerebral infarction after middle cerebral artery occlusion in progenies of spontaneously stroke prone and normal rats. Stroke 15:711, 1984
33. Crowell R, Olsson Y, Klatzo I, Ommaya A: Temporary occlusion of the middle cerebral artery in the monkey: clinical and pathological observations. Stroke 1:439, 1970
34. Crowell RM, Marcoux FW, DeGirolami U: Variability and reversibility of focal cerebral ischemia in unanesthetized monkeys. Neurology (NY) 31:1295, 1981
35. Crowell RM, Olsson Y, Ommaya AK: Angiographic and microangiographic observations in experimental cerebral infarction. Neurology (NY) 21:710, 1971
36. de Courten-Myers G, Kleinholz M, Wagner K, Myers R: Fatal strokes in hyperglycemic cats. Stroke 20:1707, 1989
37. de Courten-Myers G, Myers R, Schoofield L: Hyperglycemia enlarges infarct size in cerebrovascular occlusion in cats. Stroke 19:623, 1988
38. De Garavilla L, Babbs CF, Tacker WA: An experimental circulatory arrest model in the rat to evaluate calcium antagonists in cerebral resuscitation. Am J Emerg Med 2:321, 1984
39. de la Torre JC, Fortin T: Partial or global rat brain ischemia: the SCOT model. Brain Res Bull 26:365, 1991
40. del Zoppo GJ: Relevance of focal cerebral ischemia models experience with fibrinolytic agents. Stroke 21:IV155, 1990
41. del Zoppo GJ, Copeland BR, Waltz TA et al: The beneficial effect of intracarotid urokinase of acute stroke in a baboon model. Stroke 17:638, 1986

42. Dennis C, Kabat H: Behavior of dogs after complete temporary arrest of the cephalic circulation. Proc Soc Exp Biol Med 40:559, 1939
43. Denny-Brown D, Meyer JS: The cerebral collateral circulation. II. Production of cerebral infarction by ischemic anoxia and its reversibility in early states. Neurology (NY) 7:567, 1957
44. Dietrich WD, Busto R, Valdes I, Loor Y: Effects of normothermic versus mild hyperthermic forebrain ischemia in rats. Stroke 21:1318, 1990
45. Dietrich WD, Ginsberg MD, Busto R, Watson BD: Photochemically induced cortical infarction in the rat. 1. Time course of hemodynamic consequences. J Cereb Blood Flow Metab 6:184, 1986
46. Dietrich WD, Ginsberg MD, Busto R, Watson BD: Photochemically induced cortical infarction in the rat. 2. Acute and subacute alterations in local glucose utilization. J Cereb Blood Flow Metab 6:195, 1986
47. Dirnagl U, Pulsinelli W: Autoregulation of cerebral blood flow in experimental focal brain ischemia. J Cereb Blood Flow Metab 10:327, 1990
48. Dirnagl U, Tanabe J, Pulsinelli W: Pre- and post-treatment with MK-801 but not pretreatment alone reduces neocortical damage after focal cerebral ischemia in the rat. Brain Res 527:62, 1990
49. Duverger D, MacKenzie ET: The quantification of cerebral infarction following focal ischemia in the rat: influence of strain, arterial pressure, blood glucose concentration, and age. J Cereb Blood Flow Metab 8:449, 1988
50. Eleff SM, Maruki Y, Monsein LH et al: Sodium, ATP, and intracellular pH transients during reversible complete ischemia of dog cerebrum. Stroke 22:233, 1991
51. Fieschi C, Argentino C, Lenzi GL et al: Clinical and instrumental evaluation of patients with ischemic stroke within the first six hours. J Neurol Sci 91:311, 1989
52. Fieschi C, Battistini N, Volanto F et al: An experimental study with intracarotid ADP infusion in rabbits. Science 6:617, 1975
53. Flourens JP: Note touchant l'action de divers substances injectées dans les artères. Acad Sci 24:905, 1847
54. Fritz VU, Levien LJ: Pathogenesis of transient ischemic attacks and stroke in baboons. Stroke 20:386, 1989
55. Fujishima M, Nakatomi Y, Tamaki K et al: Cerebral ischaemia induced by bilateral carotid occlusion in spontaneously hypertensive rats. J Neurol Sci 33:1, 1977
56. Futrell N: Embolic stroke from a carotid arterial source in the rat: pathology and clinical implications. Neurology (NY) 39:1050, 1989
57. Futrell N, Watson BD, Dietrich WD et al: A new model of embolic stroke produced by photochemical injury to the carotid artery in the rat. Ann Neurol 23:251, 1988
58. Garcia JH: Experimental ischemic stroke: a review. Stroke 15:5, 1984
59. Garcia JH, Kalimo H, Kamijyo Y, Trump BF: Cellular events during partial cerebral ischemia. I. Electron microscopy of feline cerebral cortex after middle-cerebral-artery occlusion. Virchows Arch [Cell Pathol] 25:191, 1977
60. Ginsberg M, Welsh F, Budd W: Deleterious effect of glucose pretreatment on recovery from diffuse cerebral ischemia in the cat. Stroke 11:347, 1980
61. Ginsberg MD, Budd WW, Welsh FA: Diffuse cerebral ischemia in the cat. I. Local blood flow during severe ischemia and recirculation. Ann Neurol 3:482, 1978
62. Ginsberg MD, Busto R: Rodent models of cerebral ischemia. Stroke 20:1627, 1989
63. Ginsberg MD, Prado R, Dietrich WD et al: Hyperglycemia reduces the extent of cerebral infarction in rats. Stroke 18:570, 1987
64. Gjedde A, Crone C: Blood-brain glucose transfer: repression in chronic hyperglycemia. Science 214:456, 1981
65. Graham DI: Focal cerebral ischemia. (Editorial.) J Cereb Blood Flow Metab 8:769, 1988
66. Hallenbeck JM, Bradley ME: Experimental model for systematic study of impaired microvascular reperfusion. Stroke 8:238, 1977
67. Hara H, Nagasawa H, Kogure K: Nimodipine prevents postischemic brain damage in the early phase of focal cerebral ischemia. Stroke 21:102, 1990
68. Harris RJ, Symon L, Branston NM, Bayhan M: Changes in extracellular calcium activity in cerebral ischaemia. J Cereb Blood Flow Metab 1:203, 1981
69. Harrison M: Influence of haematocrit in the cerebral circulation. Cerebrovasc Brain Metab Rev 1:55, 1989
70. Harvey J, Rasmussen T: Occlusion of the middle cerebral artery: an experimental study. Arch Neurol Psychiatry 66:20, 1951
71. Hatashita S, Hoff JT: Cortical tissue pressure gradients in early ischemic brain edema. J Cereb Blood Flow Metab 6:1, 1986
72. Hatashita S, Hoff JT: Biomechanics of brain edema in acute cerebral ischemia in cats. Stroke 19:91, 1988
73. Hayakawa T, Waltz AG: Immediate effects of cerebral ischemia: evolution and resolution of neurological deficits after experimental occlusion of one middle cerebral artery in conscious cats. Stroke 6:321, 1975
74. Hayakawa T, Waltz AG, Hansen T: Relationships among intracranial pressure, blood pressure and superficial cerebral vasculature after experimental occlusion of one middle cerebral artery. Stroke 8:426, 1977
75. Heiss WD: Flow thresholds of functional and morphological damage of brain tissue. Stroke 14:329, 1983
76. Heiss WD, Rosner G: Functional recovery of cortical neurons as related to degree and duration of ischemia. Ann Neurol 14:294, 1983
77. Hill ND, Millikan CH, Walkin KG: Studies in cerebrovascular disease: experimental production of cerebral infarction by intracarotid injection of homologous blood clot. Mayo Clin Proc 30:625, 1955
78. Hirschberg M, Hofferberth B: New model of in

situ cerebral thrombosis in dogs. Stroke 19:741, 1988
79. Hossmann KA, Schuier FJ: Experimental brain infarcts in cats. I. Pathophysiological observations. Stroke 11:583, 1980
80. Hossmann KA, Zimmermann V: Resuscitation of the monkey brain after 1 h complete ischemia. I. Physiological and morphological observations. Brain Res 81:59, 1974
81. Hudgins WR, Garcia JH: The effect of electrocautery, atmospheric exposure, and surgical retraction on the permeability of the blood-brain barrier. Stroke 1:375, 1970
82. Ito U, Spatz M, Walker JT Jr, Klatzo I: Experimental ischemia in Mongolian gerbils. I. Light microscopic observations. Acta Neuropathol (Berl) 32:209, 1975
83. Jacewicz M, Brint S, Tanabe J, Pulsinelli WA: Continuous nimodipine treatment attenuates cortical infarction in rat subjected to 24 hours of focal cerebral ischemia. J Cereb Blood Flow Metab 10:89, 1990
84. Jacewicz M, Brint S, Tanabe J et al: Nimodipine pretreatment improves cerebral blood flow and reduces brain edema in conscious rats subject to focal cerebral ischemia. J Cereb Blood Flow Metab 10:903, 1990
85. Jacewicz M, Kiessling M, Pulsinelli WA: Selective gene expression in focal cerebral ischemia. J Cereb Blood Flow Metab 6:263, 1986
86. Jacewicz M, Tanabe J, Pulsinella WA: The CBF threshold and dynamics for focal cerebral infarction in spontaneously hypertensive rats. J Cereb Blood Flow Metab. (In Press)
87. Jackson DL, Dole WP: Total cerebral ischemia: a new model system for the study of post-cardiac arrest brain damage. Stroke 10:38, 1979
88. Jenkins LW, Povlishock JT, Becker D et al: Complete cerebral ischemia: an ultrastructural study. Acta Neuropathol (Berl) 48:113, 1979
89. Jones SC, Bose B, Furlan AJ et al: $CO_2$ reactivity and heterogeneity of cerebral blood flow in ischemic, border zone, and normal cortex. Am J Physiol 257:H473, 1989
90. Jones T, Morawetz R, Crowell R et al: Thresholds of focal cerebral ischemia in awake monkeys. J Neurosurg 54:773, 1981
91. Kabat H, Dennis C: Decerebration in the dog by complete temporary arrest of the cephalic circulation. Proc Soc Exp Biol Med 38:864, 1938
92. Kabat H, Dennis C, Baker AB: Recovery of function following arrest of the brain circulation. Am J Physiol 132:737, 1941
93. Kalimo H, Rehncrona S, Soderfeldt B et al: Brain lactic acidosis and ischemic cell damage. 2. Histopathology. J Cereb Blood Flow Metab 1:313, 1981
94. Kameyama M, Suzuki J, Shirane R, Ogawa A: A new model of bilateral hemispheric ischemia in the rat: three-vessel occlusion model. Stroke 16:489, 1985
95. Kamijyo Y, Garcia JH: Carotid arterial supply of the feline brain. I. Applications to the study of regional cerebral ischemia. Stroke 6:361, 1975
96. Kanda K, Flaim SF: Effects of nimodipine on cerebral blood flow in conscious rat. J Pharmacol Exp Ther 236:41, 1986
97. Kaplan B, Brint S, Tanabe J et al: Temporal thresholds for neocortical infarction in rats subjected to reversible focal cerebral ischemia. Stroke 22:1032, 1991
98. Kaplan H, Miezejeski C: Development of seizures in the Mongolian gerbil. J Comp Physiol Psychol 81:267, 1972
99. Katzman R, Clasen R, Klatzo I et al: Report of Joint Committee for Stroke Resources. IV. Brain edema in stroke. Stroke 8:512, 1977
100. Kogure K, Busto R, Scheinberg P, Reinmuth OM: Energy metabolites and water content in rat brain during the early stage of development of cerebral infarction. Brain 97:103, 1974
101. Kowada M, Ames A III, Majno G, Wright RL: Cerebral ischemia. I. An improved experimental method for study: cardiovascular effects and demonstration of an early vascular lesion in the rabbit. J Neurosurg 28:150, 1968
102. Kraft S, Larson P Jr, Shuer L et al: Effect of hyperglycemia on neuronal changes in a rabbit model of focal cerebral ischemia. Stroke 21:447, 1990
103. Kudo M, Aoyama A, Ichimori S, Fukunaga N: An animal model of cerebral infarction: homologous blood clot emboli in rats. Stroke 13:505, 1982
104. Kuroiwa T, Bonnekoh P, Hossmann K-A: Prevention of postischemic hyperthermia prevents ischemic injury of CA1 neurons in gerbils. J Cereb Blood Flow Metab 10:550, 1990
105. LaManna J, Harik S: Regional comparisons of brain glucose influx. Brain Res 326:299, 1985
106. Leonov Y, Sterz F, Safar P et al: Mild cerebral hypothermia during and after cardiac arrest improves neurologic outcome in dogs. J Cereb Blood Flow Metab 10:57, 1990
107. Levine S: Anoxic-ischemic encephalopathy in rats. Am J Pathol 36:1, 1960
108. Levine S, Payan HI: Effects of ischemia and other procedures on the brain and retina of the gerbil. Exp Neurol 16:255, 1966
109. Levine S, Sohn D: Cerebral ischemia in infant and adult gerbils: relation to incomplete circle of Willis. Arch Pathol 87:315, 1969
110. Levy DE, Brierley JB: Communications between vertebro-basilar and carotid arterial circulations in the gerbil. Exp Neurol 45:503, 1974
111. Levy D, Van Uitert R, Pike C: Delayed postischemic hypoperfusion: a potentially damaging consequence of stroke. Neurology (NY) 295:1245, 1979
112. Little JR: Implanted device for middle cerebral artery occlusion in conscious cats. Stroke 8:258, 1977
113. Ljunggren B, Norberg K, Siesjo BK: Influence of tissue acidosis upon restitution of brain energy metabolism following total ischemia. Brain Res 77:173, 1974
114. Lyden PD, Zivin JA, Soll M et al: Intracerebral hemorrhage after experimental embolic infarction. Arch Neurol 44:848, 1987
115. Maiese K, Pek L, Berger S, Reis D: Protection of

focal ischemic infarction by idazoxan and rilmenidine: a role for central imidazole receptors in stroke? J Cereb Blood Flow Metab 11:S427, 1991
116. Marshall LF, Durity F, Lounsbury R et al: Experimental cerebral oligemia and ischemia produced by intracranial hypertension. 1. Pathophysiology, electroencephalography, cerebral blood flow, blood-brain barrier, and neurological function. J Neurosurg 43:308, 1975
117. Matsuoka Y, Hossmann KA: Cortical impedance and extracellular volume changes following middle cerebral artery occlusion in cats. J Cereb Blood Flow Metab 2:466, 1982
118. McDowall G: The effect of clinical concentrations of halothane on the blood flow and oxygen uptake of the cerebral cortex. Br J Anaesth 39:186, 1967
119. Mendelow AD, Graham DI, McCulloch J, Mohamed A: The distribution of ischaemic damage and cerebral blood flow after unilateral carotid occlusion and hypotension in the rat. Stroke 15:704, 1984
120. Meyer FB, Anderson RE, Sundt TM: Intracellular brain pH, indicator tissue perfusion, electroencephalography and histology in severe and moderate focal cortical ischemia in the rabbit. J Cereb Blood Flow Metab 6:71, 1986
121. Meyer JS: Circulatory changes following occlusion of the middle cerebral artery and their relation to function. Neurosurgery 15:653, 1958
122. Meyer JS: Localized changes in properties of the blood and effects of anticoagulant drugs in experimental cerebral infarction. N Engl J Med 258:151, 1958
123. Meyer JS, Denny-Brown D: The cerebral collateral circulation. I. Factors influencing collateral blood flow. Neurology (NY) 7:447, 1957
124. Meyer JS, Fang HC, Denny-Brown D: A polarographic study of the cerebral collateral circulation. Arch Neurol Psychiatry 72:296, 1954
125. Mies G, Auer LM, Ebhardt G et al: Flow and neuronal density in tissue surrounding chronic infarction. Stroke 14:22, 1983
126. Miller C, Lampard D, Alexander K, Brown W: Local cerebral blood flow following transient cerebral ischemia. Stroke 11:534, 1980
127. Miller J, Myers R: Neurological effects of systemic circulatory arrest in the monkey. Neurology (NY) 20:715, 1970
128. Minamisawa H, Nordstrom C-H, Smith M-L, Siesjo BK: The influence of mild body and brain hypothermia on ischemic brain damage. J Cereb Blood Flow Metab 10:365, 1990
129. Miyazawa T, Hossman K-A: Changes in brain temperature during global forebrain ischemia in rats are underestimated by measurements in temporal muscle. J Cereb Blood Flow Metab 11:S125, 1991
130. Molinari GF: Experimental cerebral infarction. I. Selective segmental occlusion of intracranial arteries in the dog. Stroke 1:224, 1970
131. Molinari GF: Clinical relevance of experimental stroke models. p. 19. In Price TR, Nelson E (eds): Cerebrovascular Diseases. Raven Press, New York, 1979
132. Molinari GF: Experimental models of ischemic stroke. p. 57. In Barnett HJM, Stein BM, Mohr JP, Yatsu FM (eds): Stroke: Pathophysiology, Diagnosis, and Management. Vol 1. Churchill Livingstone, New York, 1986
133. Molinari GF: Why model strokes? (Editorial.) Stroke 19:1195, 1988
134. Molinari GF, Laurent JP: A classification of experimental models of brain ischemia. Stroke 7:14, 1976
135. Molinari GF, Rajjoub R, Lightfoote WE: Experimental transient ischemic attacks, neurologically silent infarctions and completed strokes caused by blood clot embolism, abstracted. Neurology (NY) 28:379, 1978
136. Moossy J: Morphological validation of ischemic stroke models. p 3. In Price TR, Nelson E (eds): Cerebrovascular Diseases. Raven Press, New York, 1979
137. Morawetz RB, DeGirolami U, Ojemann RG et al: Cerebral blood flow determined by hydrogen clearance during middle cerebral artery occlusion in unanesthetized monkeys. Stroke 9:143, 1978
138. Muller TH, Koch V, Righter B, Eisert WG: Reperfusion of the carotid artery in rabbits: a new in vivo model of thrombolysis. Fibrinolysis 2:701, 1988
139. Myers R, Yamaguchi S: Nervous system effects of cardiac arrest in monkeys. Arch Neurol 34:65, 1977
140. Nagasawa H, Kogure K: Correlation between cerebral blood flow and histologic changes in a new rat model of middle cerebral artery occlusion. Stroke 20:1037, 1989
141. Nakai H, Yamamoto YL, Diksic M et al: Tripletracer autoradiography demonstrates effects of hyperglycemic on cerebral blood flow, pH, and glucose utilization in cerebral ischemia of rats. Stroke 19:764, 1988
142. Nakayama H, Dietrich WD, Watson BD et al: Photothrombotic occlusion of rat middle cerebral artery: histopathological and hemodynamic sequelae of acute recanalization. J Cereb Blood Flow Metab 8:357, 1988
143. Nedergaard M: Transient focal ischemia in hyperglycemic rats is associated with increased cerebral infarction. Brain Res 408:79, 1987
144. Nedergaard M, Astrup J: Infarct rim: effect of hyperglycemia on direct current potential and ($^{14}$C)2-deoxyglucose phosphorylation. J Cereb Blood Flow Metab 6:607, 1986
145. Nedergaard M, Diemer NH: Focal ischemia of the rat brain, with special reference to the influence of plasma glucose concentration. Acta Neuropathol (Berl) 73:131, 1987
146. Neely W, Youmans J: Anoxia of canine brain without damage. JAMA 183:1085, 1963
147. Nehls DG, Park CK, MacCormack AG, McCulloch J: The effects of N-methyl-D-aspartate receptor blockade with MK-801 upon the relationship between cerebral blood flow and glucose utilisation. Brain Res 511:271, 1990
148. Nemoto E, Bleyaert A, Stezoski SW et al: Global brain ischemia: a reproducible monkey model. Stroke 8:558, 1977

149. Nilsson L, Siesjo BK: The effect of phenobarbitone anaesthesia on blood flow and oxygen consumption in the rat brain. Acta Anaesthesiol Scand [Suppl] 57:18, 1975
150. O'Brien MD, Waltz AG: Transorbital approach for occluding the middle cerebral artery without craniectomy. Stroke 4:201, 1973
151. Park CK, Nehls DG, Teasdale GM, McCulloch J: Effect of the NMDA antagonist MK-801 on local cerebral blood flow in focal cerebral ischaemia in the rat. J Cereb Blood Flow Metab 9:617, 1989
152. Passero S, Battistini N, Fieschi C: Platelet embolism in rabbit brain. Stroke 12:781, 1981
153. Paulson O, Strandgaard S, Edvinsson L: Cerebral autoregulation. Cerebrovasc Brain Metab Rev 2:161, 1990
154. Payan HM, Levine S, Strebel R: Effects of cerebral ischemia in various strains in rats. Proc Soc Exp Biol Med 120:208, 1965
155. Penry JK, Netsky MG: Experimental embolic occlusion of a single leptomeningeal artery. Arch Neurol 3:57/391, 1960
156. Petersen JN, Evans JP: The anatomical end results of cerebral arterial occlusion: experimental and clinical correlation. Trans Am Neurol Assoc 63:88, 1937
157. Plum F, Pulsinelli W: Cerebral metabolism and hypoxic-ischemic brain injury. p. 1086. In Asbury A, McKhann G, McDonald A (eds): Diseases of the Nervous System. WB Saunders, Philadelphia, 1986
158. Prado R, Ginsberg M, Dietrich WD et al: Hyperglycemia increases infarct size in collaterally perfused but not end-arterial vascular territories. J Cereb Blood Flow Metab 8:186, 1988
159. Pulsinelli W: Selective neuronal vulnerability: morphological and molecular characteristics. p. 29. In Kogure K et al (eds): Mechanisms of Ischemic Brain Damage. Prog Brain Res, vol 63. Elsevier, New York, 1985
160. Pulsinelli W, Brierley J, Plum F: Temporal profile of neuronal damage in a model of transient forebrain ischemia. Ann Neurol 11:491, 1982
161. Pulsinelli W, Buchan A: The four-vessel occlusion rat model: methods for complete occlusion of vertebral arteries and control of collateral circulation. Stroke 19:913, 1988
162. Pulsinelli W, Buchan A: The utility of animal ischemia models in predicting pharmacotherapeutic response in the clinical setting. p. 87. In Ginsberg M (ed): Cerebrovascular Diseases. Sixteenth Research (Princeton) Conference. Raven Press, New York, 1989
163. Pulsinelli W, Duffy T: Regional energy balance in rat brain after transient forebrain ischemia. J Neurochem 40:1500, 1983
164. Pulsinelli W, Duffy T, Levy D et al: Ischemic injury to selectively vulnerable neurons in the rat. p. 35. In Bes A, Braquet P, Paoletti R, Siesjo BK (eds): Cerebral Ischemia. Excerpta Medica, Amsterdam, 1984
165. Pulsinelli W, Jacewicz M, Buchan A: Hypoxic-ischemic disorders and stroke. Principles of Drug Therapy in Neurology. In Johnston M et al (eds): FA Davis, Philadelphia, 1992
166. Pulsinelli W, Waldman S, Rawlinson D: Moderate hyperglycemia augments ischemic brain damage: a neuropathological study in the rat. Neurology (NY) 32:1239, 1982
167. Pulsinelli WA, Brierley JB: A new model of bilateral hemispheric ischemia in the unanesthetized rat. Stroke 10:267, 1979
168. Pulsinelli WA, Levy DE, Duffy TE: Regional cerebral blood flow and glucose metabolism following transient forebrain ischemia. Ann Neurol 11:499, 1982
169. Ralston B, Rasmussen T, Kennedy T: Occlusion of the middle cerebral artery under normotension, and anemically induced and chemically induced hypotension. Neurosurgery 12:26, 1953
170. Robinson RG, Shoemaker WJ, Schlumpf M et al: Effect of experimental cerebral infarction in rat brain on catecholamines and behaviour. Nature 255:332, 1975
171. Rosomoff H: Hypothermia and cerebral vascular lesions. Arch Neurol Psychiatry 78:454,1957
172. Roussel S, Pinard E, Seylaz J: Kynurenate does not reduce infarct size after middle cerebral artery occlusion in spontaneously hypertensive rats. Brain Res 518:353, 1990
173. Roussel S, Pinard E, Seylaz J: Focal cerebral ischemia in chronic hypertension: no protection by R-phenyl-isopropyl-adenosine. Brain Res 545:171, 1991
174. Rubino GJ, Young W: Ischemic cortical lesions after permanent occlusion of individual middle cerebral artery branches in rats. Stroke 19:870, 1988
175. Sadoshima S, Busija D, Brody M, Heistad D: Sympathetic nerves protect against stroke in stroke-prone hypertensive rats. Hypertension 3:I124I126, 1981
176. Sadoshima S, Busija DW, Heistad DD: Mechanisms of protection against stroke in stroke-prone spontaneously hypertensive rats. Am J Physiol 244:H406, 1983
177. Safar P, Stezoski W, Nemoto EM: Amelioration of brain damage after 12 minutes' cardiac arrest in dogs. Arch Neurol 33:91, 1976
178. Scheinberg P: Discussion. p. 35. In Price TR, Nelson E (eds): Cerebrovascular Diseases. Raven Press, New York, 1979
179. Schmidt-Kastner R, Paschen W, Grosse Ophoff B, Hossman K-A: A modified four-vessel occlusion model for inducing incomplete forebrain ischemia in rats. Stroke 20:938, 1989
180. Schutz H, Silverstein PR, Vapalahti M et al: Brain mitochondrial function after ischemia and hypoxia. I. Ischemia induced by increased intracranial pressure. Arch Neurol 29:408, 1973
181. Seki H, Yoshimoto T, Ogawa A, Suzuki J: The $CO_2$ response in focal cerebral ischemia—sequential changes following recirculation. Stroke 15:699, 1984
182. Shigeno T, McCulloch J, Graham DI et al: Pure cortical ischemia versus striatal ischemia. Surg Neurol 24:47, 1985
183. Shigeno T, Teasdale GM, McCulloch J, Graham DI: Recirculation model following MCA occlusion in rats. I. Cerebral blood flow, cerebrovascular permeability, and brain edema. J Neurosurg 63:272, 1985

184. Siegel BA, Meidinger R, Elliott AJ et al: Experimental cerebral microembolism: multiple tracer assessment of brain edema. Arch Neurol 26:73, 1972
185. Siemkowicz E, Hansen AJ: Clinical restitution following cerebral ischemia in hypo-, normo-, and hyperglycemic rats. Acta Neurol Scand 58:1, 1978
186. Siesjo BK: Brain Energy Metabolism. Wiley, Chichester, England, 1978
187. Slivka A: Effect of antihypertensive therapy on focal stroke in spontaneously hypertensive rats. Stroke 22:884, 1991
188. Slivka A, Pulsinelli W: Hemorrhagic complications of thrombolytic therapy in experimental stroke. Stroke 18:1148, 1987
189. Slivka A, Silbersweig D, Pulsinelli W: Carnitine treatment for stroke in rats. Stroke 21:808, 1990
190. Smith ML, Auer RN, Siesjo BK: The density and distribution of ischemic brain injury in the rat following 2–10 min of forebrain ischemia. Acta Neuropathol (Berl) 64:319, 1984
191. Snyder JV, Nemoto EM, Carroll RG, Safar P: Global ischemia in dogs: intracranial pressures, brain blood flow and metabolism. Stroke 6:21, 1975
192. Spetzler RF, Selman WR: New design for an implantable vessel occluder. Surg Neurol 13:317, 1979
193. Steen P, Gisvold S, Milde J et al: Nimodipine improves outcome when given after complete cerebral ischemia in primates. Anesthesiology 62:406, 1985
194. Strong AJ, Tomlinson BE, Venables GS et al: The cortical ischaemic penumbra associated with occlusion of the middle cerebral artery in the cat. 2. Studies of histopathology, water content, and in vitro neurotransmitter uptake. J Cereb Blood Flow Metab 3:97, 1983
195. Strong AJ, Venables GS, Gibson G: The cortical ischaemic penumbra associated with occlusion of the middle cerebral artery in the cat. I. Topography of changes in blood flow, potassium ion activity, and EEG. J Cereb Blood Flow Metab 3:86, 1983
196. Sundt TM Jr, Waltz AG: Experimental cerebral infarction: retro-orbital, extradural approach for occluding the middle cerebral artery. Mayo Clin Proc 41:159, 1966
197. Sundt TM, Waltz AG: Hemodilution and anticoagulation. I. Effects of the microvasculature and microcirculation of the cerebral cortex after arterial occlusion. Neurology (NY) 17:230, 1967
198. Symon L: Experimental model of stroke in the baboon. Adv Neurol 10:199, 1975
199. Symon L: Flow thresholds in brain ischaemia and the effects of drugs. Br J Anaesth 57:34, 1985
200. Symon L, Branston N, Harris R, Wang A: The current status of ischaemic thresholds. p. 63. In Bes A, Braquet P, Paoletti R, Siesjo BK (eds): Cerebral Ischemia. Elsevier, Amsterdam, 1984
201. Symon L, Branston NM, Strong AJ: Autoregulation in acute focal ischemia. I. An experimental study. Stroke 7:547, 1976
202. Symon L, Khodadad G, Montoya G: Effect of carbon dioxide inhalation on the pattern of gaseous metabolism in ischaemic zones of the primate cortex1. I. An experimental study of the 'intracerebral steal' phenomenon in baboons. J Neurol Neurosurg Psychiatry 34:481, 1971
203. Symon L, Pasztor E, Branston NM: The distribution and density of reduced cerebral blood flow following acute middle cerebral artery occlusion: an experimental study by the technique of hydrogen clearance in Baboons. Stroke 5:355, 1974
204. Takeda Y, Jacewicz M, Pulsinelli W: Blood flow threshold for ischemic depolarizaiton of rat neocortex. Soc Neurosci Abs 17: 1991
205. Tamura A, Graham DI, McCulloch J, Teasdale GM: Focal cerebral ischaemia in the rat. 1. Description of technique and early neuropathological consequences following middle cerebral artery occlusion. J Cereb Blood Flow Metab 1:53, 1981
206. Tamura A, Graham DI, McCulloch J, Teasdale G: Focal cerebral ischaemia in the rat. 2. Regional cerebral blood flow determined by [$^{14}$C]iodoantipyrine autoradiography following middle cerebral artery occlusion. J Cereb Blood Flow Metab 1:61, 1981
207. Tanaka K, Greenberg JH, Gonatas NK, Reivich M: Regional flow-metabolism couple following middle cerebral artery occlusion in cats. J Cereb Blood Flow Metab 5:241, 1985
208. Todd MM, Dunlop B, Shapiro HM et al: Ventricular fibrillation in the cat: a model for global cerebral ischemia. Stroke 12:808, 1981
209. Todd NV, Picozzi P, Crockard HA, Russell RWR: Recirculation after cerebral ischemia: simultaneous measurement of cerebral blood flow, brain edema, cerebrovascular permeability and cortical EEG in the rat. Acta Neurol Scand 74:269, 1986
210. Turner JH: Brain scan in cerebral ischemia. Stroke 6:703, 1975
211. Tyson G, Teasdale G, Graham D, McCulloch J: Focal cerebral ischemia in the rat: topography of hemodynamic and histopathological changes. Ann Neurol 15:559, 1984
212. Tyson GW, Teasdale GM, Graham DI, McCulloch J: Cerebrovascular permeability following MCA occlusion in the rat: the effect of halothane-induced hypotension. J Neurosurg 57:186, 1982
213. Vacanti FX, Ames A III: Mild hypothermia and $Mg^{++}$ protect against irreversible damage during CNS ischemia. Stroke 15:695, 1984
214. Vander Eecken HM, Adams RD: The anatomy and functional significance of the meningeal arterial anastomoses of the human brain. Neuropathol Exp Neurol 12:132, 1953
215. van der Zwan A, Hillen B: Review of the variability of the territories of the major cerebral arteries. Stroke 22:1078, 1991
216. Vasquez-Cruz J, Marti-Vilalta JL, Ferrer I et al: Progressing cerebral infarction in relation to plasma glucose in gerbils. Stroke 21:1621, 1990
217. von Planta I, Weil MH, von Planta M et al: Cardiopulmonary resuscitation in the rat. J Appl Physiol 65:2641, 1988

218. Waltz AG: Clinical relevance of models of cerebral ischemia. Stroke 10:211, 1979
219. Waltz AG: Comparative pathophysiology of ischemic stroke models: an evaluation. p. 11. In Price TR, Nelson E (eds): Cerebrovascular Diseases. Raven Press, New York, 1979
220. Waltz AG, Sundt TM: The microvasculature and microcirculation of the cerebral cortex after arterial occlusion. Brain Res 90:681, 1967
221. Watanabe O, Bremer A, West CR: Experimental regional ischemia in the middle cerebral artery territory in primates. I. Angio-anatomy and description of an experimental model with selective embolization of the internal carotid artery bifurcation. Stroke 8:61, 1977
222. Watson BD, Dietrich WD, Watchel M, Ginsberg MD: Induction of reproducible brain infarction by photochemically initiated thrombosis. Ann Neurol 17:497, 1985
223. Watson BD, Prado R, Dietrich WD et al: Mitigation of evolving cortical infarction in rats by recombinant tissue plasminogen activator following photochemically induced thrombosis. p. 317. In Powers WJ, Raichle ME (eds): Cerebrovascular Diseases. Fifteenth Research (Princeton) Conference. Raven Press, New York, 1987
224. Watts JW: Ligation of the anterior cerebral artery in monkeys. Nerv Ment Dis 79:153, 1934
225. Weinstein PR, Anderson GG, Telles DA: Neurological deficit and cerebral infarction after temporary middle cerebral artery occlusion in unanesthetized cats. Stroke 17:318, 1986
226. Welsh F, Sims R, Harris V: Mild hypothermia prevents ischemic injury in gerbil hippocampus. J Cereb Blood Flow Metab 10:557, 1990
227. Wiebers DO, Adams HP Jr, Whisnant JP: Animal models of stroke: are they relevant to human disease? Stroke 21:1, 1990
228. Wolin LR, Massopust LC Jr, Taslitz N: Tolerance to arrest of cerebral circulation in the rhesus monkey. Exp Neurol 30:103, 1971
229. Yamamoto K, Morimoto K, Yanagihara T: Cerebral ischemia in the gerbil: transmission electron microscopic and immunoelectron microscopic investigation. Brain Res 384:1, 1986
230. Yamauchi Y, Kato H, Kogure K: Brain damage in a new hemorrhagic shock model in the rat using long-term recovery. J Cereb Blood Flow Metab 10:207, 1990
231. Yarnell P, Earnest M, Kelly G, Sanders B: Disappearing carotid defects. Stroke 9:258, 1978
232. Yip PK, He YY, Hsu CY et al: Effect of plasma glucose on infarct size in focal cerebral ischemia-reperfusion. Neurology (NY) 41:899, 1991
233. Yoshida S, Busto R, Martinez E et al: Regional brain energy metabolism after complete versus incomplete ischemia in the rat in the absence of severe lactic acidosis. J Cereb Blood Flow Metab 5:490, 1985
234. Yoshimine T, Yanagihara T: Regional cerebral ischemia by occlusion of the posterior communicating artery and the middle cerebral artery in gerbils. J Neurosurg 58:362, 1983
235. Zasslow MA, Pearl RG, Shuer LM et al: Hyperglycemia decreases acute neuronal ischemic changes after middle cerebral artery occlusion in cats. Stroke 20:519, 1989
236. Zivin JA, Lyden PD, DeGirolami U et al: Tissue plasminogen activator: reduction of neurologic damage after experimental embolic stroke. Arch Neurol 45:387, 1988

# 4
# NEUROCHEMISTRY OF STROKE

Kyuya Kogure
Hiroyuki Kato

## ISCHEMIA-INDUCED PANNECROSIS OF BRAIN CELLS

### Energy Failure

The diversity of mechanisms causing brain cell damage from ischemia has been gradually clarified by recent studies. For nearly 40 years, from the late 1940s to the early 1980s, ischemia-induced death of brain cells was ascribed simply to energy failure.[29] A summary of this theory is that cell viability depends upon its intact homeostasis. Mechanisms that maintain the cellular homeostasis, such as operation of ion pumps, active transport, and scheduled turnover of functional and constitutional molecules, are energy-dependent; any impairment of cellular respiration due to ischemia results in a disruption of homeostasis and death of the cell. This type of brain cell death is generally referred to as "death by energy failure" and is characterized by pannecrosis—death of affected neurons, glia cells, and vascular wall. The temporal evolution for ischemic infarction can usually take minutes to hours, and focal damage is almost always associated with brain edema. Experiments of fundamental importance concerning energy failure (energy theory) were completed in the early 1980s.[30,75,78,87] Effects of ischemia on cerebral energy state were studied early by Lowry et al.[90] Atkinson's "energy charge" of tissue,[10] which is equal to one-half the average number of anhydride-bound phosphate groups per adenosine moiety, has also been adopted frequently by many investigators working in the field of energy metabolism in ischemic brain tissue. Following these studies, Kogure et al.[79] estimated the rate of high-energy phosphate use in rat brain, using a decapitation model (Fig. 4-1), and pointed out that the electroencephalogram (EEG) became isoelectric approximately 12 seconds after decapitation, while the level of brain adenosine triphosphate (ATP) was still more than one-third control values (1.2 mmol/kg compared to 2.8 mmol/kg).

For more clinically oriented studies, effects of ischemia on the functional and structural integrity of brain were investigated by Astrup et al.[9] They proposed that a condition for the brain, called "penumbra," lies between the upper threshold of electrical failure and the lower threshold of energy failure, that is, ion pump failure. Such an area is now referred to as "misery perfusion." According to their observations, electrical activity of brain diminishes below cerebral blood flow (CBF) of 17 ml/100 g/min while the ion pump is still operating. Relevant to this particular point are the early studies on the relationship between cortical impedance, size of the extracellular space, and excitability of cortex during total ischemia of cat brain.[47] We recommend a review by Siesjö,[152] which is a standard reference book for the early investigations on brain ischemia and energy metabolism.

### Putative Bloodborne Chemical Mediators

In ischemia-induced pannecrosis of brain tissue, Shiga et al.[151] reported suppression of brain edema in rats with the use of antineutrophil monoclonal antibody. Utilizing a transient middle cerebral artery occlusion model, they studied changes in brain water

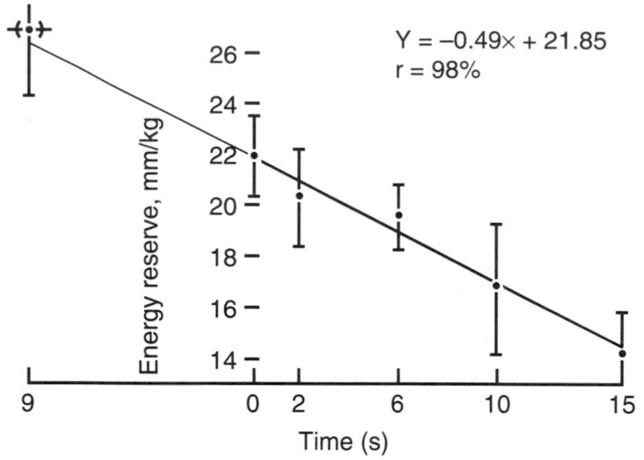


**Fig. 4-1.** Energy charge calculated at short increments of time following decapitation. The lighter line represents back-extrapolation of the curve to demonstrate that the theoretical assumption of an approximate 8- to 10-second delay in freezing, under the circumstances of the decapitation experiment, allows close agreement with the near-ideal data obtained in freezing in situ while maintaining the steady-state conditions. The latter data are plotted on the back-extrapolation line and the time of −9 second agrees with the predicted time deviation. (From Kogure et al.[79] with permission.)

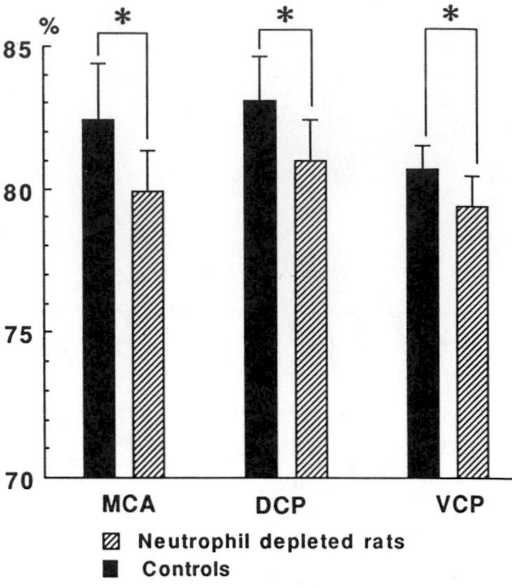


**Fig. 4-2.** Brain water contents of neutrophil-depleted rats in the middle cerebral artery territory cortex (MCA), the dorsal caudate-putamen (DCP), and the ventral caudate-putamen (VCP) were significantly reduced compared to those of control animals 1 day after 1 hour of MCA occlusion. $^*P < 0.05$. (From Shiga et al.,[151] with permission.)

content in the distribution of the middle cerebral artery area of antibody-treated animals and compared this to saline-treated control rats. In the antineutrophil monoclonal antibody-treated rats, neutrophils in the peripheral blood were depleted during ischemia and throughout the reperfusion period. Results of the study suggest that the suppression of ischemic brain edema was due to a depletion of neutrophils (Fig. 4-2).

This phenomenon was reproducible under the same experimental conditions when the animals were treated with colchicine. Colchicine inhibits accumulation of neutrophils at the site of ischemic injury, phagocytosis of invading mononuclear phagocytes, reactive microglia, and interleukin-1 (IL-1) production. It is of interest to note that known chemical mediators that increase vascular permeability, such as bradykinin,[171] serotonin,[179] histamine,[28] arachidonic acid,[15,172] and free radicals[114] are produced by reactive microglias, bloodborne neutrophils, and macrophages, which infiltrate areas injured by ischemia. The depletion of circulating neutrophils and the suppression of their functions is presumed to result in a reduced release of chemical mediators in the ischemic blood-parenchymal cell border of brain, which results in suppressed postischemic edema formation. On the other hand, pannecrosis of brain tissue caused by focal ischemia may, at least in part, result from indiscriminate injury of tissue due to neutrophil-derived active oxygen and free radicals as secondary products. The role of intercellular adhesion molecule-1 (ICAM-1) or endothelial leukocyte adhesion molecule (ELAM), produced in the endothelium, and IL-1 or IL-8, products of ischemia-induced brain parenchyma, as chemotactic factors for neutrophil invasion must be clarified in this regard.

## POSTISCHEMIC, SELECTIVELY VULNERABLE NEURONS

No cell can survive a prolonged ischemic state. Any possible recovery from ischemic cell injury can result only where blood flow has been restored. The ischemic core in the brain usually occurs while collateral circulation is developing and opening up. Thus, the marginal zone, lying between the ischemic core and the surrounding, normally perfused tissue, may receive restored blood flow and have a chance of surviving postischemic injury. If the postischemic blood flow restores energy to the brain before the critical period, most of the affected cells, except the so-called selectively vulnerable neurons, can survivc after a short time. The selectively vulnerable neurons, whose distribution in the central nervous system was clarified by $^{45}Ca$-autoradiography[8] (Fig. 4-3), may die hours to days after transient ischemic insults, while exhibiting normal blood flow, energy state, and osmotic homeostasis, such as $H^+$, $Na^+$, $K^+$, and water. This well-known phenomenon was first reported by Kirino[68] and Pulsinelli et al.[133] as "delayed neuronal death."

Among selectively vulnerable neurons, a hierarchy exists of susceptibility to ischemia. Following ischemia of only 5 minutes duration in the gerbil brain, selective neuronal damage is recognized only in the

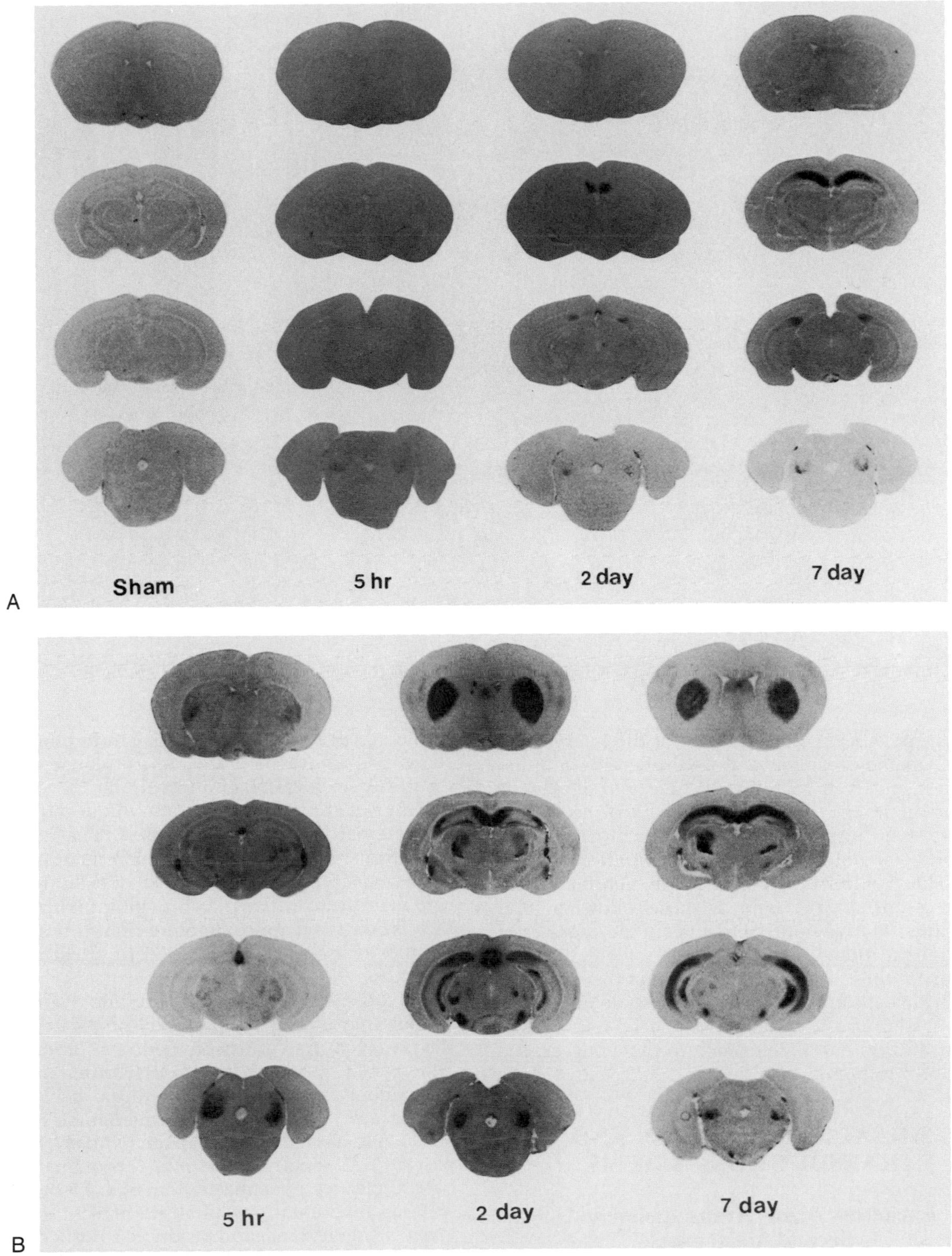


**Fig. 4-3.** Representative $^{45}Ca$ autoradiographs after (**A**) 5, (**B**) 10, and (**C**) 15 minutes of ischemia. The animals were killed at 5 hours, 2 days, and 7 days of reperfusion. Areas of abnormal calcium accumulation (blackening of the autoradiographs) correspond to areas of histopathologic neuronal damage. Note that neuronal damage is produced in specific regions, depending on both severity of ischemia and duration of reperfusion. (From Araki et al.,[8] with permission.) (*Figure continues.*)

C

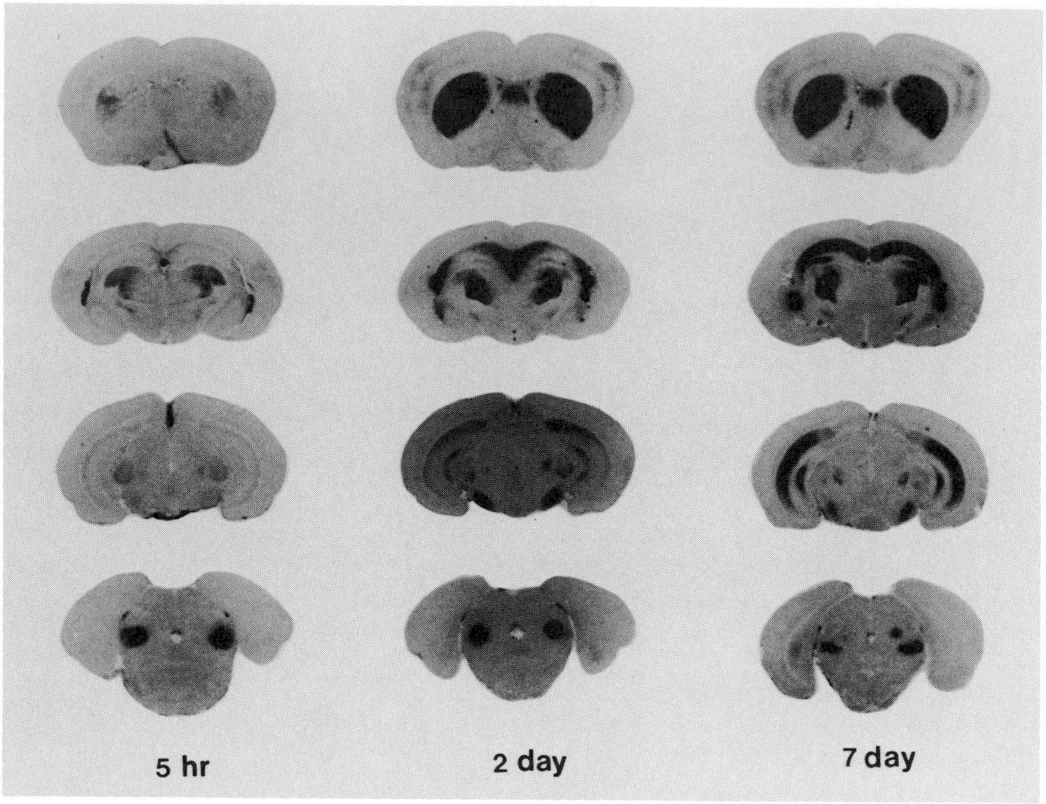


**Fig. 4-3** (*Continued*). **C**

hippocampal CA1 sector and part of the inferior colliculus. On the other hand, if the ischemic condition continues for 10 to 15 minutes, neuronal damage is widespread in the 3rd and 5th layers of neocortex, striatum, septum, CA3 sector of the hippocampus, thalamus, medial geniculate body, and substantia nigra. These patterns of postischemic neuronal damage are essentially the same as those following 10 to 30 minutes of transient ischemia in the four-vessel occlusion rat model. The important information emerging from these studies is that most of the ischemia-labile brain cells are located either in structures of the limbic system or the basal ganglia. This finding is of interest and potential relevance to dementia caused by cerebral ischemia.

## SIGNAL TRANSMISSION AND TRANSDUCTION SYSTEMS

### Excitatory Signal Transmission and Second Messengers

Interestingly, most of the ischemia-susceptible neurons are innervated by glutamatergic fibers. This evidence suggests that there is a definite relationship between glutamate-mediated neurotransmission and postischemic neuronal injury. The essential sequence in the evolution of this process can be illustrated as shown in Figures 4-4 and 4-5. Prolonged ischemia results in an elevation of intracellular $Ca^{2+}$ activity,[153] and an elevation of the $Ca^{2+}$ activity in the presynaptic terminal leads to an increased release of various neurotransmitters, depending upon the various types of neurons. For example, release of excitatory amino acid neurotransmitters, such as glutamate and aspartate, is enhanced approximately eight times during 10 minutes of ischemia, compared to preischemic concentration.[13]

Increased concentration of excitatory amino acids at the synaptic clefts causes excitotoxic action[20,23] on the postsynaptic vulnerable neurons. Besides the excitatory amino acids, if an agonist stimulates the corresponding metabotropic receptors, such as muscarinic acetylcholine, alpha-1, histamine $H_1$, 5-$HT_{1c}$, 5-$HT_2$, and *N*-methyl-D-aspartate (NMDA), phospholipase C (PLC) is activated via the G protein. Phospholipase C cleaves phosphatidylinositol 4,5-diphosphate ($PIP_2$), a functional phospholipid present in the postsynaptic membrane, and produces so-called phospholipid-derived second messengers: inositol 1,4,5-triphosphate ($IP_3$) and 1,2-diacylglycerol (DG).[33]

If the cerebral cortex is directly affected by ischemia, Abe et al.[2] estimated that the ischemia-induced agonist-mediated activation of the phospholipase C and breakdown of the polyphosphoinositides (PPIs)

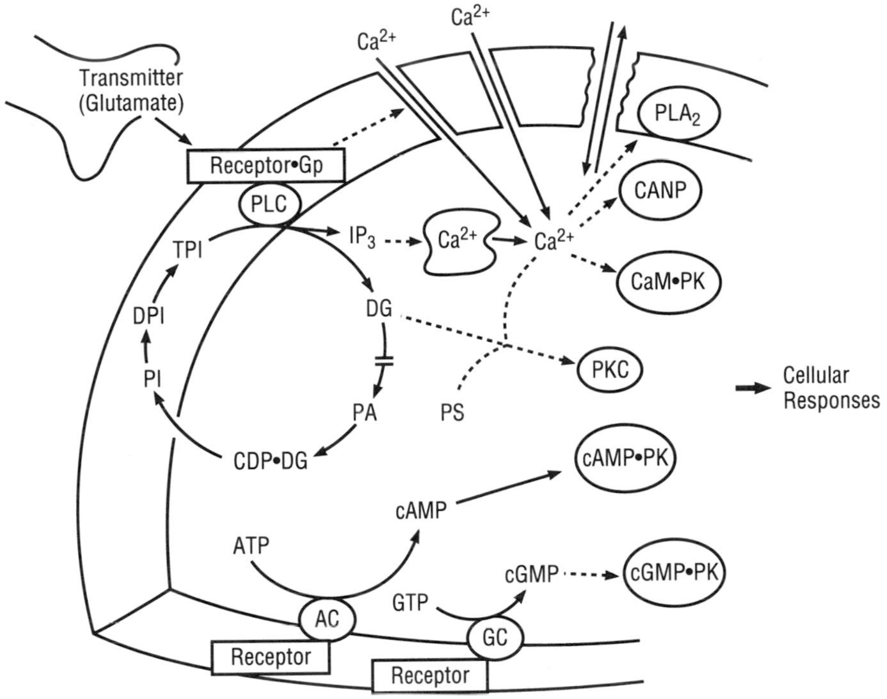


**Fig. 4-4.** A schematic diagram illustrating the intracellular signal transducing system, which is considered to be related to the postischemic neuronal injury in the selectively vulnerable neurons. The disruption of membrane on the right top is the hypothetical membrane perturbation (see text for details). (From Kogure et al.,[81] with permission.)

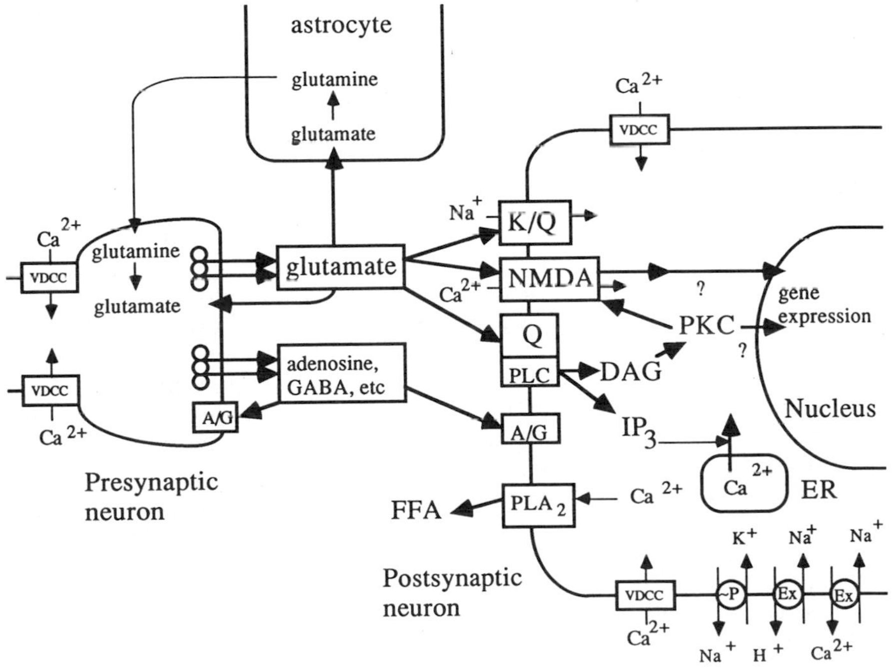


**Fig. 4-5.** A schematic diagram illustrating the relations between neurotransmitters, receptors, calcium channels, and intracellular signal transducing system in postsynaptic cells (see text for details). PKC, protein kinase C; DAG, diacylglycerol; $IP_3$, inositol triphosphate; GABA, γ-aminobutyric acid; PLC, phospholipase C; NMDA, *N*-methyl-D-aspartate receptor; $PLA_2$, phospholipase $A_2$; FFA, free fatty acids; A/G, adenosine/GABA receptor; ER, endoplasmic reticulum; VDCC voltage-dependent calcium channel; K/Q, kainate/quisqualate receptor; Q, quisqualate receptor.

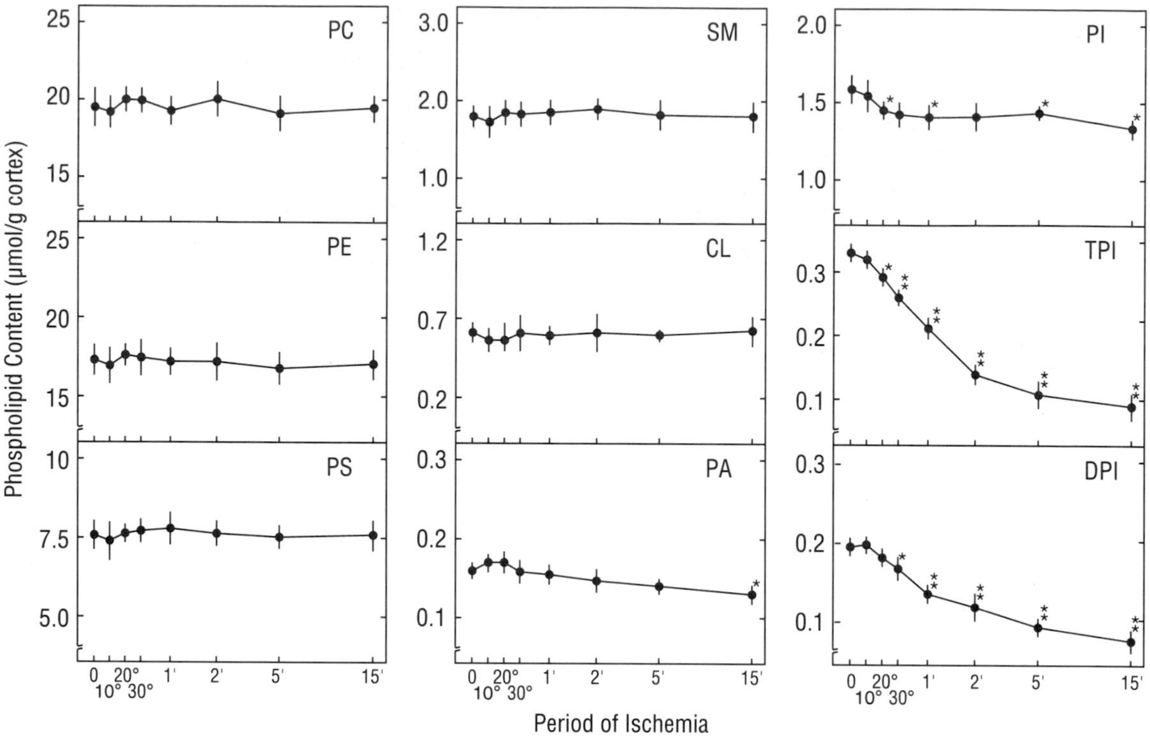


**Fig. 4-6.** Changes in the amounts of phospholipids during ischemia in gerbil cerebral frontoparietal cortexes. Periods of ischemia were 0 (control), 10 seconds, 20 seconds, 30 seconds, 1 minute, 2 minutes, 5 minutes, and 15 minutes. $N = 5$. The amounts of phosphatidylcholine (PC), phosphatidylethanolamine (PE), phosphatidylserine (PS), sphingomyelin (SM), and cardiolipin (CL) did not show significant changes throughout 15 minutes of ischemia. The amount of phosphatidic acid (PA) showed a significant decrease at 15 minutes of ischemia ($*P < 0.05$). The amount of inositol-containing phospholipids (PI and PPI) began to decrease as early as 20 seconds or 30 seconds ($*P < 0.05$; $**P < 0.01$). (From Abe et al.,[2] with permission.)

may begin in less than 30 seconds (Fig. 4-6). Simultaneously, activated ionotropic receptor opens $Ca^{2+}$ gates independently from the altered membrane potential. This type of gate opening, even though the molecular mechanism is not known, is described as agonist-mediated or receptor-operated gate opening. $IP_3$ binds to the $Ca^{2+}$ endostore and mobilizes endogenous $Ca^{2+}$. Together with the exogenous $Ca^{2+}$, accessed through the voltage-dependent and voltage-independent agonist-mediated $Ca^{2+}$ gates, the intracellular $Ca^{2+}$ activity is markedly increased at this time.[154] A portion of $IP_3$ is converted to $IP_4$ by $IP_3$ kinase, and $IP_4$ also potentiates calcium influx into cells from extracellular spaces.[14] From the time of $Ca^{2+}$-dependent activation of calmodulin-dependent protein kinase (CaM/PK) occurs, elevation of intracellular $Ca^{2+}$ activity begins less than 60 seconds after induction of ischemia.[22]

DG can activate protein kinase C (PKC) if phosphatidylserine (PS) exists and $Ca^{2+}$ activity is elevated.[111] Thus, the phosphatidylinositol (PI) response, which is stimulated mainly by glutamatergic, cholinergic, and noradrenergic neurotransmitters, involves the production of DG and $IP_3$ from triphosphoinositides, and results in the activation of PKC. DG can also be produced from phosphatidylcholine (PC) by choline phosphotransferase. However, at the onset of ischemia, DG may be produced by phospholipase C, predominantly from PPIs, because the fatty acid composition of DG, increased at the onset of ischemia, is similar to inositol phospholipids and not that of PC or other phospholipids (Table 4-1). PC-derived DG may play an important role for so-called suspended activation of PKC, which is discussed in a later section of this chapter. On the other hand, the possibility exists that membrane-derived arachidonic acids from DG, PE, and PC, also activate PKC.[66,99,112]

## Secondary Effector Enzymes and Regulators

Excitability of hippocampal CA1 pyramidal cells, cited here as an example of selectively vulnerable neurons, is regulated mainly by potassium currents across the plasma membrane. The pyramidal cells in the rat have a voltage-dependent chloride current, which is active at resting potentials and is inhibited either by membrane depolarization or activation of PKC. Thus, blockade of this chloride current by activation of PKC potentiates transmission of dendritic excitatory events.[100] PKC may also play a major role in the long-term potentiation of hippocampal pyrami-

**TABLE 4-1. Changes in the Amount and the Fatty Acid Composition of 1,2-Diacylglycerol During Ischemia in Gerbil Cerebral Frontoparietal Cortex[a]**

| Acyl Group | Control | Period of Ischemia | | | | | | |
|---|---|---|---|---|---|---|---|---|
| | | 10 s | 20 s | 30 s | 1 min | 2 min | 5 min | 15 min |
| DG[b] | 74.5 ± 6.1 | 73.8 ± 6.0 | 73.9 ± 6.2 | 84.2 ± 7.0 | 102.3 ± 6.7* | 125.1 ± 8.8** | 144.8 ± 8.9** | 161.7 ± 9.6** |
| C16:0 | 60.5 ± 3.9 | 61.1 ± 4.2 | 59.7 ± 4.0 | 61.6 ± 3.5 | 67.1 ± 3.6* | 75.4 ± 4.1** | 83.7 ± 4.2** | 94.7 ± 4.9** |
| C16:1 | 5.2 ± 0.5 | 5.1 ± 0.4 | 5.2 ± 0.5 | 5.0 ± 0.5 | 5.1 ± 0.5 | 5.3 ± 0.5 | 5.3 ± 0.4 | 5.6 ± 0.5 |
| C18:0 | 25.1 ± 2.3 | 25.1 ± 2.0 | 25.7 ± 2.5 | 34.2 ± 3.1* | 49.2 ± 2.9** | 59.3 ± 4.2** | 65.3 ± 3.8** | 72.4 ± 4.3** |
| C18:1 | 24.9 ± 2.2 | 23.7 ± 2.1 | 24.0 ± 2.2 | 24.1 ± 2.3 | 24.6 ± 2.0 | 35.1 ± 2.9* | 45.6 ± 3.5** | 50.1 ± 3.8** |
| C18:2 | 4.7 ± 0.3 | 4.4 ± 0.4 | 4.6 ± 0.3 | 4.6 ± 0.3 | 4.8 ± 0.4 | 5.7 ± 0.4* | 6.7 ± 0.4** | 7.4 ± 0.3** |
| C20:4 | 16.7 ± 2.0 | 16.3 ± 1.8 | 16.9 ± 1.9 | 26.5 ± 3.0* | 41.8 ± 3.1** | 53.2 ± 4.3** | 60.1 ± 3.8** | 65.7 ± 4.0** |
| C22:4 | 0.4 ± 0.0 | 0.4 ± 0.0 | 0.4 ± 0.1 | 0.5 ± 0.1 | 0.4 ± 0.0 | 0.5 ± 0.0 | 0.5 ± 0.1 | 0.6 ± 0.1* |
| C22:6 | 11.5 ± 0.9 | 11.5 ± 1.0 | 11.3 ± 0.9 | 11.8 ± 1.1 | 11.6 ± 1.0 | 15.7 ± 1.1* | 22.3 ± 1.6** | 26.9 ± 1.3** |

[a] Values are means ± SD, expressed as nmol/g wet weight; $N = 5$.
[b] 1,2-Diacylglycerol.
* $P < 0.05$; ** $P < 0.01$.
(From Abe et al.,[2] with permission.)

dal cells[93] by playing a key role in the regulation of neuronal excitability of CA1 cells under normal and pathologic conditions. In fact, blockade of PKC ameliorated selective neuronal damage in the CA1 sector.

The carefully designed experiments conducted by Hara et al.[45] revealed that inhibition of protein kinase C activity by staurosporine markedly reduced pyramidal cell death in the CA1 sector of rat hippocampus after transient ischemia. Blockade of other protein kinases did not preserve the CA1 neurons in similar experiments (Table 4-2). An obvious conclusion deduced from these data is that the protein kinase C is a pivotal enzyme for delayed neuronal death; further studies are required to clarify the mechanism of action of PKC.

The increased intracellular $Ca^{2+}$ activity may act upon PI-specific calcium-sensitive phospholipase C, but under ischemic circumstances PPIs are already precipitated (Fig. 4-6), and no method is available to prove the ischemia-induced $Ca^{2+}$-dependent activation of this enzyme. Meanwhile, increased cytosolic $Ca^{2+}$ activity does activate various $Ca^{2+}$-dependent enzymes in a nonspecific fashion. For example, alteration of free fatty acid composition by 2 minutes of ischemia (Fig. 4-7) may reflect activation of phospholipase $A_2$, plasmalogenase, and other phospholipases. However, increased docosahexaenoic acid 2 minutes after the onset of ischemia indicates decomposition of the plasma membrane lipid bilayer.

Degradation of ribonucleoside 5′-phosphates by ischemia elevates the level of xanthine derivatives and activates the cyclic nucleotidase. Therefore, besides the various receptors that react to the corresponding agonists, increased $Ca^{2+}$ activity, xanthine derivatives, and activated $Ca^{2+}$-dependent calmodu-

**TABLE 4-2. Effects of Various Protein Kinase Inhibitors on Delayed Neuronal Death of Hippocampal CA1 Neurons in Gerbils[a]**

| Treatment | Dose (ng) | *N* | Neuronal Density (n/mm) |
|---|---|---|---|
| Sham operation | — | 12 | 246 ± 23* |
| Vehicle | — | 13 | 81 ± 47 |
| Staurosporine | 0.1 | 7 | 117 ± 55 |
| | 1 | 10 | 166 ± 78* |
| | 10 | 10 | 201 ± 95* |
| KT5720 | 10 | 9 | 91 ± 69 |
| KT5822 | 10 | 10 | 109 ± 78 |
| W-7 | 10 | 9 | 111 ± 82 |

[a] Various protein kinase inhibitors were injected topically into the CA1 subfield of the hippocampus 30 min prior to 5-minute forebrain ischemia. Values are means ± SD.
* $P < 0.01$ vs vehicle (Kruskal-Wallis test and two-tailed Mann-Whitney U test).
(From Hara et al.,[45] with permission.)

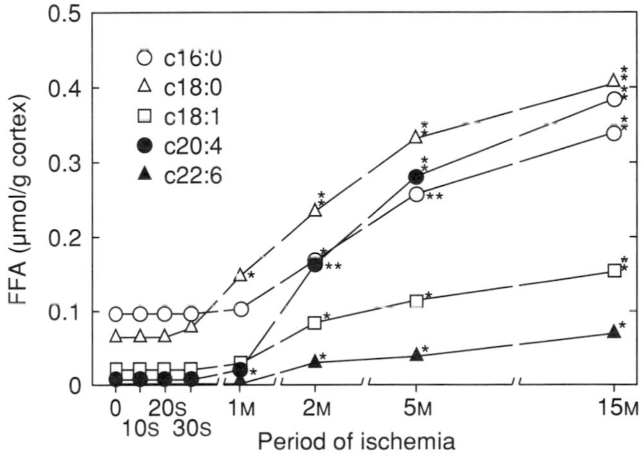


**Fig. 4-7.** Changes in the contents of free fatty acids during ischemia in gerbil cerebral frontoparietal cortexes. Periods of ischemia were 0 (sham control), 10 seconds, 20 seconds, 30 seconds, 1 minute, 2 minutes, 5 minutes, and 15 minutes. $N = 5$. Standard deviations are within 15 percent of mean values. Amounts of palmitic acid, stearic acid, oleic acid, arachidonic acid, and docosahexaenoic acid significantly increased during 15 minutes of ischemia (*$P < 0.05$, **$P < 0.01$). (From Abe et al.,[2] with permission.)

lin[18,74,138] may also participate in ischemia-induced activation of adenylate cyclase and guanylate cyclase and the generation of cyclic adenosine monophosphate (cAMP) and cyclic guanosine monophosphate (cGMP). cAMP and cGMP kinases are also activated. At the onset of ischemia, activation of secondary effector enzymes and phosphorylation of corresponding secondary regulators occur within a few minutes. In addition, the lining proteins of plasma membrane and cytoskeleton begin to decompose within a few minutes after the onset of ischemia.[70]

## Membrane Perturbation and Protein Synthesis

Loss of structural, and thus functional integrity of plasma membrane[39,160] results in a loss of the cell's osmotic barrier, creating serious problems for the maintenance of homeostasis. Thus, severe and prolonged ischemia may cause greater damage of membranes, as contrasted with the effects of brief ischemia, which may destroy the affected cells instantaneously. On the other hand, if the brain cells can restore their energy level following recirculation, various ion pumps will counteract the passive ionic movement along concentration gradients and normalize osmotic homeostasis. However, homeostasis of $Ca^{2+}$ and other divalent cations in affected neurons are not readily achieved, even within 24 hours of the insult[170] (Table 4-3).

In selectively vulnerable neurons, protein synthesis is markedly suppressed throughout the postischemic period.[16,83] In Araki's experiment[7] on the Mongolian gerbil, incorporation of L-[methyl-$^{14}$C] methionine into the protein fraction in postischemic brain was impaired not only in the CA1 sector but also in the histopathologically intact neocortex, striatum, and thalamus, even with nonlethal 2 minutes of ischemia (Table 4-4). This inhibition was found at the early stages of recirculation following ischemia. Extensive recovery of protein synthesis in these areas occurred at 5 to 48 hours of recirculation, but its recovery was markedly delayed in the CA1 sector. On the other hand, 1-minute ischemia did not produce any significant neuronal damage nor inhibition of protein synthesis in the CA1 sector, which is most vulnerable to ischemia.

Gerbils subjected to 3 minutes of ischemia also revealed severe impairment of protein synthesis in the above-cited regions, and the whole hippocampus during the early stage of recirculation. Although extensive recovery of protein synthesis in these structures gradually occurred, observed at 5 to 48 hours following recirculation, persistent inhibition of protein synthesis occurred in the majority of the histologically vulnerable hippocampal CA1 sector. Yosidomi et al.,[191] utilizing the same experimental setup, studied the effects of 5 minutes of forebrain ischemia. Protein synthesis at 1 hour following recirculation was almost completely suppressed throughout the brain except for the diencephalon (Fig. 4-8). Conversely, a slight increase in amino acid incorporation was observed in the medial hypothalamus and thalamus after 2 hours of recirculation. Reduced protein synthesis tended to recover following 2 hours of recirculation, although recovery in cortical layer 3 and CA1 of the hippocampus remained poor even at 4 hours following recirculation. Protein synthesis in all brain regions, except for the CA1 subfield, recovered fully 24 hours after recirculation. Suppression of L-[methyl-$^{14}$C]methionine incorporation into the CA1 subfield persisted even at 72 hours following recirculation.

These studies indicate that even a brief, so-called nonlethal, ischemia can produce severe inhibition of protein synthesis in selectively vulnerable regions during the early stage of recirculation. Mechanisms underlying the transient, slight increase in protein synthesis in the medial thalamus and hypothalamus have not been elucidated at present. It is an interesting finding (Fig. 4-8) that in some animals treated with either a calcium channel blocker, 1-[bis-(4-fluorophenyl)methyl]-4-(2,3,4-trimethoxybenzyl)-piperazine dihydrochloride (KB-2796), or pentobarbi-

**TABLE 4-3. Postischemic Changes of $Mg^{2+}$ and $Ca^{2+}$ Content Following 20-minute Forebrain Ischemic in Several Brain Regions of Rats[a]**

| | Sham Operation | 20 min + 2 h | 6 h | 12 h | 24 h | 48 h | 72 h |
|---|---|---|---|---|---|---|---|
| Cerebral cortex | | | | | | | |
| $Mg^{2+}$ | 634 ± 37(7) | 638 ± 33(8) | 619 ± 19(8) | 667 ± 24(7) | 697 ± 31**(7) | 720 ± 38**(8) | 659 ± 30(8) |
| $Ca^{2+}$ | 201 ± 50(6) | 189 ± 8(8) | 182 ± 7(7) | 192 ± 13(8) | 211 ± 13(7) | 229 ± 37(7) | 252 ± 49*(8) |
| Hippocampus | | | | | | | |
| $Mg^{2}$ | 626 ± 50(6) | 675 ± 48(8) | 635 ± 28(7) | 666 ± 29(7) | 804 ± 58**(8) | 745 ± 100*(8) | 724 ± 87*(8) |
| $Ca^{2+}$ | 243 ± 37(6) | 241 ± 24(8) | 227 ± 19(8) | 224 ± 17(7) | 279 ± 24(8) | 528 ± 207**(8) | 600 ± 248**(8) |
| Striatum | | | | | | | |
| $Mg^{2+}$ | 624 ± 22(7) | 675 ± 43(8) | 645 ± 14(8) | 670 ± 28(8) | 756 ± 64**(8) | 712 ± 71**(7) | 650 ± 26(8) |
| $Ca^{2+}$ | 219 ± 36(7) | 225 ± 10(7) | 221 ± 20(8) | 238 ± 41(8) | 292 ± 73(8) | 386 ± 153(8) | 560 ± 353**(8) |

[a] The unit of data is μg/g dry tissue wt, and data are expressed as mean value ± SD of six to eight experiments. Number of subjects is shown in parentheses. Significant difference from the values in sham-operated animals is denoted by $*P < 0.05$, $**P < 0.01$ (Dunnett's test).
(From Tsuda et al.,[170] with permission.)

**TABLE 4-4. Incidence and Distribution of Postischemic Inhibition of Protein Synthesis in the Gerbil Brain[a] After Recirculation Following 1-, 2-, or 3-Minute Ischemia**

| | | Recirculation after Ischemia | | | | | | | | | | |
|---|---|---|---|---|---|---|---|---|---|---|---|---|
| | | 1-min Ischemia | | | 2-min Ischemia | | | | 3-min Ischemia | | | |
| Region | S | 1 h | 5 h | 24 h | 1 h | 5 h | 24 h | 48 h | 1 h | 5 h | 24 h | 48 h |
| Neocortex | 0/10 | 0/10 | 0/10 | 0/8 | 8/9 | 2/10 | 0/12 | 0/6 | 9/10 | 4/10 | 2/10 | 0/6 |
| Striatum | 0/10 | 0/10 | 0/10 | 0/8 | 7/9 | 4/10 | 0/12 | 0/6 | 10/10 | 4/10 | 2/10 | 0/6 |
| Septum | 0/10 | 0/10 | 0/10 | 0/8 | 0/9 | 0/10 | 0/12 | 0/6 | 0/10 | 0/10 | 0/10 | 0/6 |
| Hippocampus | | | | | | | | | | | | |
| CA1 | 0/10 | 0/10 | 0/10 | 0/8 | 7/9 | 3/10 | 2/12 | 0/6 | 9/10 | 8/10 | 7/10 | 5/6 |
| CA3 | 0/10 | 0/10 | 0/10 | 0/8 | 0/9 | 0/10 | 0/12 | 0/6 | 6/10 | 0/10 | 0/10 | 0/6 |
| CA4 | 0/10 | 0/10 | 0/10 | 0/8 | 0/9 | 0/10 | 0/12 | 0/6 | 6/10 | 0/10 | 0/10 | 0/6 |
| DG | 0/10 | 0/10 | 0/10 | 0/8 | 0/9 | 0/10 | 0/12 | 0/6 | 6/10 | 0/10 | 0/10 | 0/6 |
| Thalamus | 0/10 | 0/10 | 0/10 | 0/8 | 7/9 | 2/10 | 0/12 | 0/6 | 8/10 | 2/10 | 0/10 | 0/6 |

Abbreviations: S, sham-operated group; DG, dentate gyrus.
[a] $N = 6$–12 hemispheres.
(From Araki et al.,[7] with permission.)

tal, restoration of impaired protein synthesis was observed at 72 hours following recirculation. In this regard, two different types of calcium channel blockers, a dihydropyridine (nicardipine) and a piperazinyl ethanol derivative (NC-1100), have already been reported to inhibit delayed neuronal death in gerbils.[6,52] Flunarizine has also been reported to inhibit delayed neuronal death induced by ischemia resulting from combined bilateral carotid occlusion and hypotension in rats,[26,177] even though flunarizine failed to protect against cell loss in the gerbil model experiencing severe ischemia.

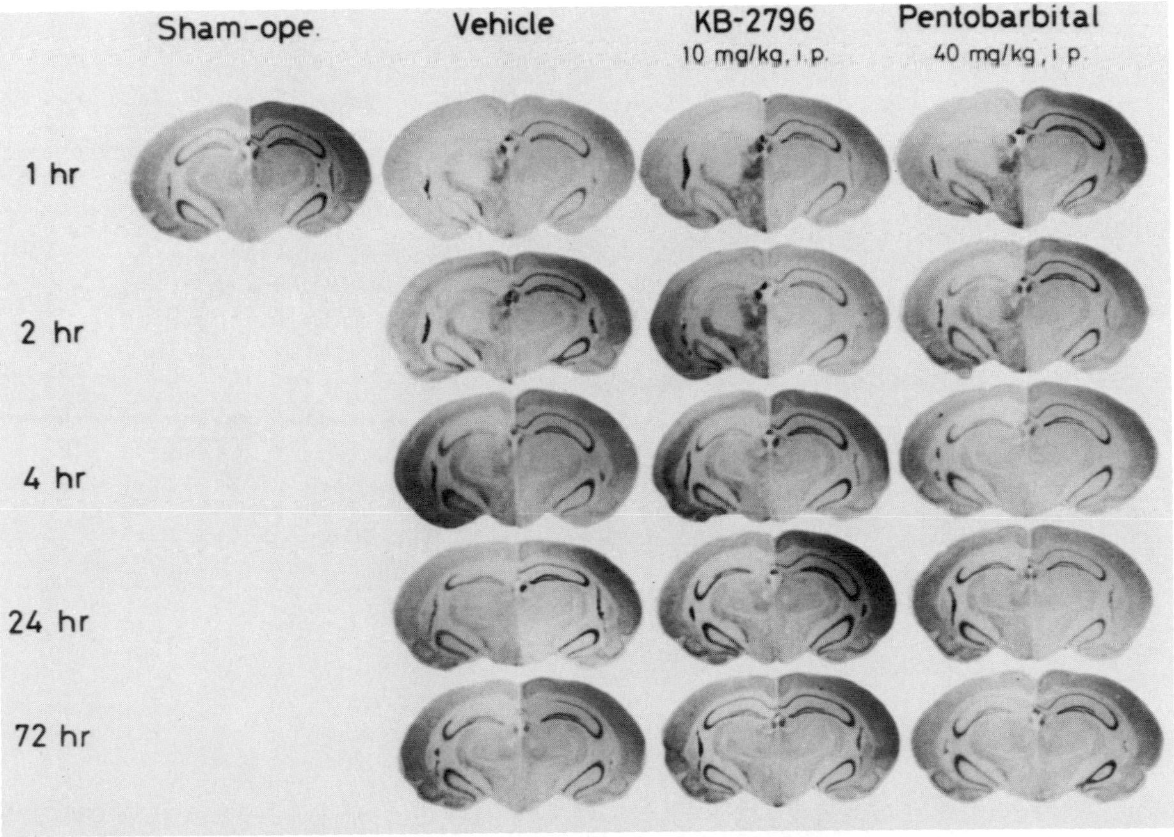


**Fig. 4-8.** Effects of KB-2796 (see text) and pentobarbital on protein synthesis and cell preservation in postischemic gerbil brains. Left half: autoradiograms of L-[methyl-$^{14}$C]methionine (protein synthesis). Right half: histologic staining with toluidine blue. (From Yoshidomi et al.,[191] with permission.)

It is presumed that postischemic suppression of protein synthesis is partly caused by $Ca^{2+}$-dependent events. We hypothesize the suppression to occur from (1) disturbed amino acid transport across the perturbed plasma membrane (Fig. 4-8), (2) abnormalities in gene expression and postischemic DNA damage, and (3) polyribosomal disaggregation and deranged protein synthesis. Another factor is the lowered microtopical availability of adenosine triphosphate (ATP) for the protein synthesis (4), as discussed previously; ATP molecules are preferentially consumed by ion pumps in the face of osmotic barrier disruption.

It can be deduced from the above-mentioned experimental data and discussions that ischemically affected neurons can survive only with the restoration of essential protein molecules, normal energy state, and normal osmotic homeostasis. At the end of the cellular and molecular events in the cells' survival, proteins fail to complete their turnover with de novo molecules, which results in a loss of structural and functional integrity, homeostasis, and cell viability. We consider these mechanisms crucial in accounting for delayed neuronal death.

## POSTISCHEMIC MATURATION

Death of selectively vulnerable neurons does not occur at the time of membrane perturbation but rather hours to days after the loss of the osmotic barrier.[142] Other examples, illustrated in Figure 4-9, are the chronological autoradiogram obtained by Tanaka.[82] Forebrain ischemia in the gerbil led to no acute postischemic changes in hematoxylin and eosin morphologic sections and the examination of $^{45}Ca$-autoradiogram following ischemia of 5- to 15-minute duration. Inspections of coronal sections, however, shows that ischemia of only 5 minutes duration results in delayed necrosis of pyramidal cells in the hippocampal CA1 region. If ischemia continues for 10 minutes, cells in the thalamus and the third, fifth and sixth layers of the cortex will exhibit delayed necrosis. Although not shown in the photograph, these changes are also shared by cells in the nucleus amygdalae.

If the ischemic condition is maintained for a longer period of 15 minutes, these same neurons will display maturational necrosis,[51] and if the ischemia is protracted, these cells will exhibit acute necrosis. The

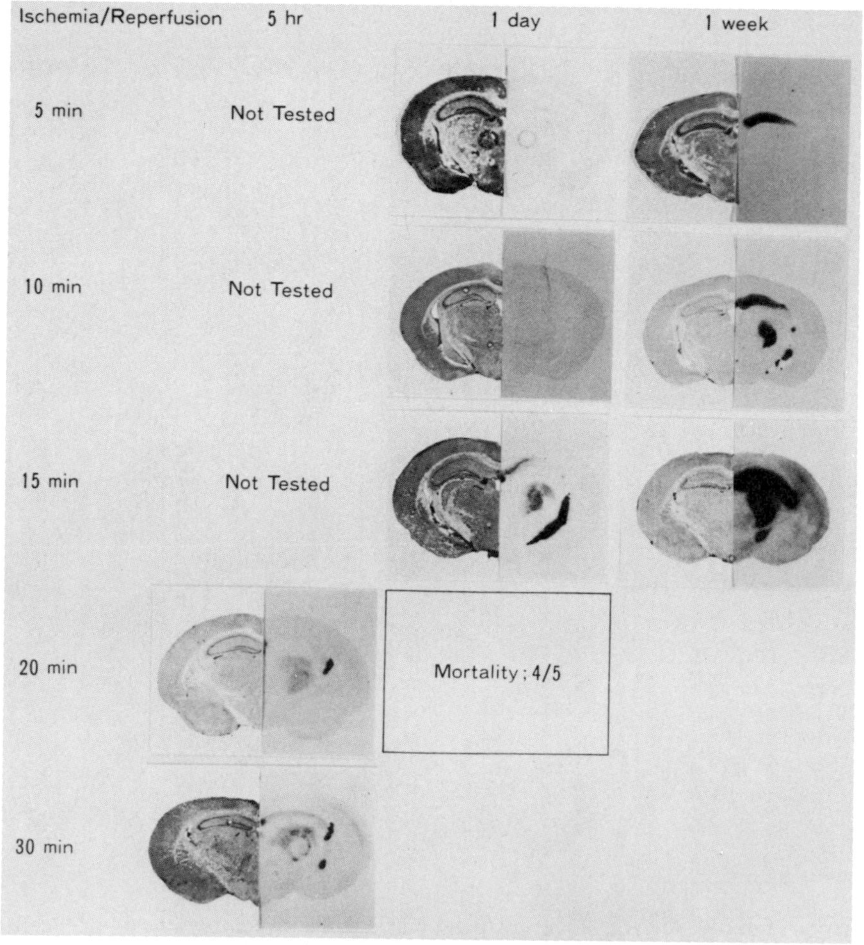


**Fig. 4-9.** Representative $^{45}Ca$-autoradiograms (right half) and hematoxylin-eosin stainings (left half) in the brain slices of the Mongolian gerbil following ischemia. (From Kagure et al.,[82] with permission.)

experimental evidence, therefore, clearly indicates that the fate of these cells is not determined by the specific nature of the cells, but simply depends on the severity of the ischemic insults. Moreover, a continuum of transitions or changes exists between acute cell death and tardy, delayed neuronal necrosis, and between the latter and survival without any abrupt differences in the mechanisms of these alternative outcomes. It is clear, therefore, that the distinctions between the above-noted ischemically induced cellular changes of so-called acute, maturational, and delayed necrosis are essentially artificial. Furthermore, distinctions between death due to energy failure and to membrane perturbation may not be made in cases of severe ischemia.

## INTRANUCLEAR EVENTS

### Immediate Early Gene Effects and Transcription Factors

Ischemia induces abrupt agonist discharges, resulting in elevated cytosolic $Ca^{2+}$, activation of secondary effector enzymes and secondary regulators, and release of various membrane-derived lipids products, such as arachidonic acid and platelet-activating factor (PAF), which can alter intranuclear events despite restoration of the energy state. For example, induction of an immediate early gene upregulation, such as c-fos and c-jun, were reduced by a PAF antagonist in rodent hippocampus and in cultured cells.[12] Treatment with PAF also induces expression of the cell cycle regulatory genes, such as calcyclin. Thus, in the face of a restored energy state, following ischemia, a relationship between membrane phospholipid metabolism and immediate early gene expression has been demonstrated.

Onodera et al.[121] reported a transient and dramatic induction of c-fos mRNA in the cerebral cortex after transient forebrain ischemia (Fig. 4-10). Under the same conditions, mRNA of c-myc was not reliably detectable in the cerebral cortex of either control or postischemic animal. Thus, the increase in the c-fos mRNA levels observed 30 to 90 minutes after recirculation may be specific and reflect an increased rate of c-fos transcription during recirculation. However, Ruppert and Wille[141] reported no elevation of c-fos mRNA levels in the cerebellum after ischemia without reperfusion.

Induction of nuclear proto-oncogenes may be involved in the cellular processes that modulate genomic events and neuronal activity associated with ischemia, although the significance of increased c-fos expression is still unknown. The product of c-fos forms a complex that associates with transcriptional control elements containing AP-1 sites and mediates long-term responses to signals that regulate differentiation;[136] c-fos may serve as a master switch to upregulate other genes in response to exogenous stimuli.[96] During the recirculation period, other short-lived proteins accumulate inspite of depressed synthesis of most proteins, suggesting preferential production of proteins required for the recovery process. By the same token, Abe et al.[1] detected induction of the zinc finger gene, an immediate early gene which utilizes the zinc-finger motif to bind DNA in contrast to Fos/Jun, which utilizes the leucine zipper motif to bind the AP-1 site of DNA after transient focal ischemia in rat cerebral cortex (Fig. 4-11). A previous study of Kingston et al.[67] suggests a possible relationship between induction of a transcription factor gene and heat shock protein (HSP) 70 gene. Transient cerebral ischemia is a simple model to provide stress to the central nervous system and change signal transduction, growth regulation and neuronal differentiation, which should induce not only early inducible gene families and transcription factors but also stress response proteins such as HSP70.[3,55,121,158] Therefore, Abe and colleagues examined possible inductions of

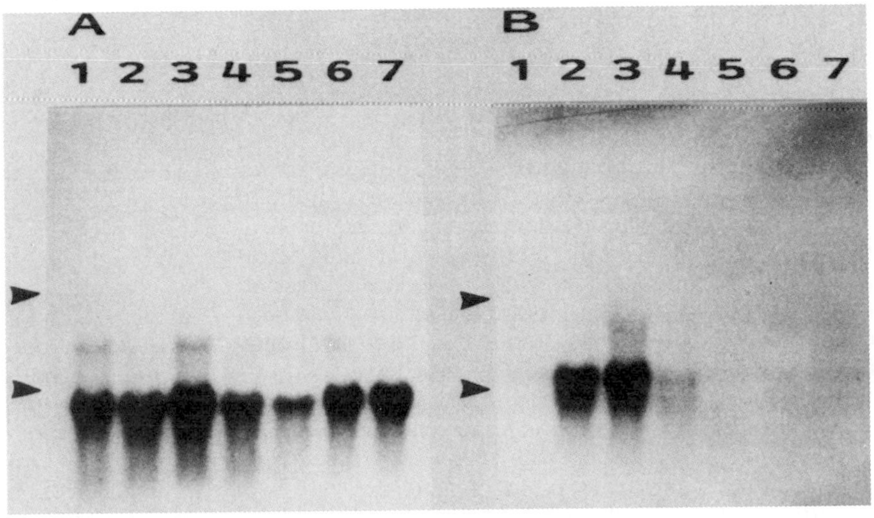


**Fig. 4-10.** Time course of c-fos expression in the rat cerebral cortex after transient forebrain ischemia (20 minutes). The arrowheads indicate the migration of 18S and 28S ribosomal RNAs. Northern filters were probed either for (**A**) human $\beta$-actin and (**B**) v-fos. Lane *1*, control; lanes *2* to *7*, recirculation (*2*, 0.5 hour; *3*, 1.5 hours; *4*, 3 hours; *5*, 6 hours; *6*, 14 hours; *7*, 24 hours after ischemia). (From Onodera et al.,[121] with permission.)

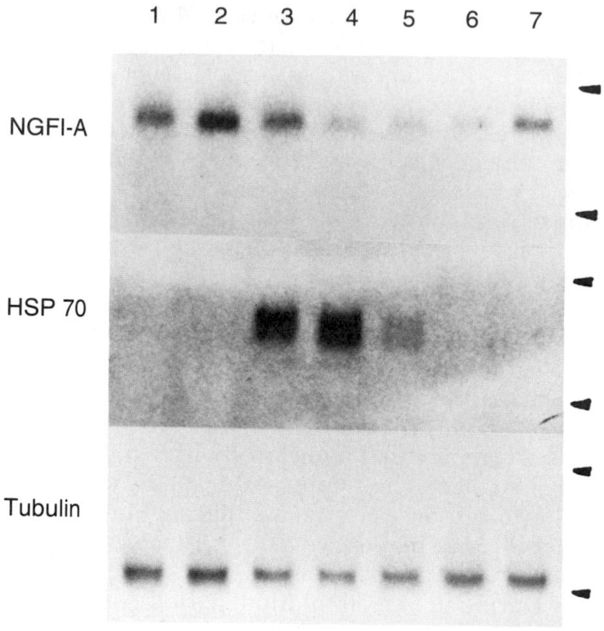


**Fig. 4-11.** Autoradiograms of Northern blot analyses show changes of gene expression of zinc finger (NGFI-A), HSP70, and tubulin. Lanes *1, 2, 3, 4, 5, 6,* and *7* represent the case of sham control, 1, 3, 8 hours, 1, 2, and 7 days of reperfusion, respectively, after 30 minutes of transient focal ischemia of rat cerebral cortex. Each lane contains 15 μg of total RNA, and arrowheads indicate 28S and 18S ribosomal RNA. (From Abe et al.,[1] with permission.)

the zinc finger gene and HSP70 gene after transient focal ischemia in rat cerebral cortex by Northern blot analysis.

The level of mRNA in cells is regulated by the balance of its synthesis and degradation. Transient increase of zinc finger-coding mRNA may be due to increased synthesis or posttranscriptional regulation, that is, decreased degradation or both. Even though Abe et al.'s result did not show which mechanism contributed the transient increase of this mRNA, it is of interest that the level of this mRNA transiently increased at 1 hour and decreased for a longer duration (from 8 hours at the earliest to 2 days of reperfusion). Recent findings on the zinc finger gene indicate that its deregulated expression contributes to retroviral-mediated malignant transformation of cells[184] and that this gene is homozygously deleted in Wilms tumor, which is an autosomal recessive childhood nephroblastoma.[40] These data suggest a crucial role of this gene in cell growth regulation and differentiation. Neurons may need alterations of gene expression in the recovery process from an ischemic insult in order to adapt metabolic responses of neuronal cells after ischemia[76] or to achieve a specific neuronal plasticity to integrate a postischemic neuronal network.[150] The transient increase of zinc finger-coding mRNA after ischemia observed in this study may reflect one aspect of such rearrangement of gene expression of neuronal cells in the brain.

Transcriptional programs were investigated by Szekely et al.,[162,163] who reported that activation of NMDA receptors in primary cultures of cerebellar granule cells by glutamate induces c-fos, c-jun, jun-B, zif/268 (zinc finger) gene. This effect of glutamate was blocked by MK-801, a NMDA receptor antagonist, but was not blocked by CNQX, an AMPA/KA-type receptor antagonist. These data suggest the possibility that glutamate itself induces groups of transcription factors.

## Heat Shock Protein 70 Messenger Ribonucleic Acid

In our studies, HSP70 mRNA is not detected in brains of sham controls, but it is induced by transient ischemia, reaching a maximum at 8 hours after reperfusion. The amount of HSP70 mRNA becomes undetectable by 2 days after reperfusion. At present, no report has shown the zinc finger gene to regulate HSP70 gene expression, and our results do not support a relationship, although gene expression of zinc finger occurred earlier than the induction of HSP mRNA.

Heat shock induces cellular changes such as the following: loss of DNA polymerase a and b activities, blockade of RNA splicing, loss of translational activity, movement of HSP70 into and out of the nucleus, and changes in nucleolar morphology.[132] Similar types of changes have also reported with cerebral ischemia.[16,68] HSP70 is essential for the restoration of normal ribosome assembly, promotion of new ribosomal synthesis, and acceleration of the recovery of nucleolar morphology after heat shock[89,131] by ATP-dependent mechanisms.[88] Therefore, if HSP70 is produced in sufficient amounts in affected brain cells after ischemia, this protein may potentially protect against cell death.

An immunohistochemical examination recently showed that HSP70 protein staining is much lower in the CA1 neurons than in cortical or CA3 neurons following transient ischemia.[178] As discussed previously, HSP70 is induced when cells are subjected to various stressful conditions and may play a cell-protective role. The so-called heat shock response may also partly regulate expression of the amyloid precursor protein (APP) gene.[144] Amyloid protein derived from APP enhances the survival of hippocampal neurons in vitro.[180] Therefore, induction of HSP70 mRNA and APP mRNA within parietal cortex and hippocampal CA1 region in gerbil brains was examined at 1 hour to 7 days after 10 minutes of bilateral common carotid artery occlusion, utilizing the level of tubulin mRNA as an internal standard[3] (Fig. 4-12). Northern blot analysis revealed hybridization of the HSP70 probe to two sizes of mRNA corresponding to HSP70 and heat shock cognate protein 70 (HSC70). With reperfusion, both HSP70 mRNA and HSC70 mRNA were induced. The levels of both HSP70 and HSC70 mRNAs reached maximum at 8 hours, and then declined. The amount

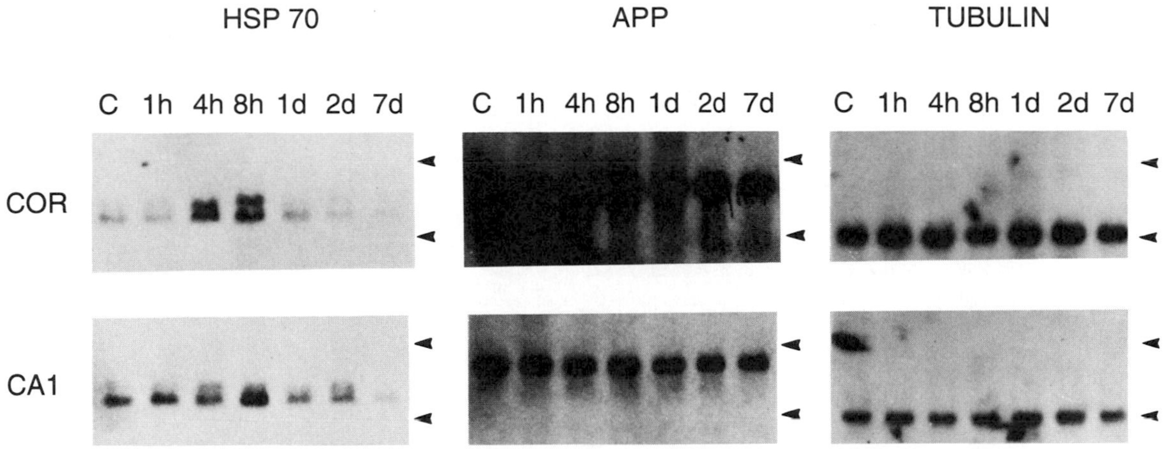


**Fig. 4-12.** Northern blot analyses of heat shock protein 70, amyloid precursor protein, and tubulin mRNAs in hippocampal CA1 and parietal cortex after 1 to 8 hours and 1 to 7 days of reperfusion after 10 minutes of ischemia. Each lane contains 15 $\mu g$ of total RNA. C represents the sham control. Arrowheads represent the ribosomal RNAs. (From Abe et al.,[3] with permission.)

of increase of HSP70 mRNA was relatively smaller in the CA1 cells than in the parietal cortical cells at 8 hours after the reperfusion. The induction of HSP70 mRNA continued up to 2 days in CA1 cells when the amount of the message in cortical cells already decreased below the level in CA1 cells. No significant induction was observed in the amount of APP mRNA or tubulin mRNA after ischemia. The relatively high level of HSC70 mRNA expression found normally in the hippocampal CA1 region suggests an active turnover of clathrin in this area. Clathrin forms a coat for pinocytotic vesicles in cells.[34] HSC70 has a role to disassemble the clathrin cage and involves intracellular transportation. Induction of HSC70 mRNA found in this experiment may relate to the induction of immunoreactive clathrin in this area,[192] suggesting a role of clathrin in the selective damage of CA1 neurons. Continuous elevation of HSP70 mRNA in CA1 cells suggests that CA1 cells are under persistently stressful conditions after reperfusion.[181] However, lower mRNA levels at 4 and 8 hours in CA1 cells than in cortical cells suggests a limitation of mRNA induction in these cells.[166] Impaired synthesis of the protein ubiquitin has also been shown immunohistochemically in rat hippocampal CA1 neurons after an ischemic insult.[91] Taken together with our results, these findings indicate that CA1 cells do not produce enough HSP mRNA and ubiquitin after ischemia, although both are essential for stress responses.

## Amyloid Precursor Protein Messenger Ribonucleic Acid

Although the promotor region of the APP gene has a similar base-pair sequence to the shock consensus element,[144] our data indicate that APP gene may not simply be regulated by heat shock response. In fact, the APP gene promotor sequence showed that at least four mechanisms could regulate the APP gene expression: the stress response; Jun/Fos response; the putative protein binding at the GC-rich element; and the possible methylation of the CpG region.[144] APP is not a homogeneous single molecule, but is composed of several isoforms.[165] APPs with the Kunitz type protease inhibitor (KPI) domain (APP 770, APP 751, and APP 563, encoding 770, 751 or 563 amino acid precursors, respectively) may have a different biologic function from APP without the KPI domain (APP 695). However, according to Abe's unpublished data, no change was observed in the level of KPI domain-containing APP mRNA in the cortex of the same experimental model using a cDNA probe which selectively recognizes the KPI domain.

In contrast to the above-cited transient ischemia model in gerbils, selective induction of Kunitz-type protease inhibitor domain-containing amyloid precursor protein mRNA was evident utilizing Northern blot analysis in a middle cerebral artery occlusion model of rats.[4] As shown in Figure 4-13, APP mRNA, which encodes the KPI domain (KPI in Fig. 4-13) was induced in the cerebral cortex, while the total amount of APP did not change. APP mRNA which encodes the KPI domain began to increase at 1 day, reaching a maximum at 4 days, and then decreased, but remained elevated for as long as 21 days. Because the amount of APP 695 mRNA is much higher than APP 751/770 mRNA in the brain,[109,165] induction of APP 751/770 mRNAs does not contribute significantly to the total APP mRNA. The amount of total APP and KPI-containing APP mRNA did not show significant changes in the cerebellum, which was not affected by the insult. No changes were seen in the level of tubulin mRNAs, both in the cerebral cortex and the cerebellum. These results indicate that APP mRNA, which encodes the KPI domain, is inducible after cerebral ischemia, while mRNA for APP 695 is not.

A recent study showed that APP 751 and/or APP 770 is protease nexin-II (PN-II), a protease inhibitor that

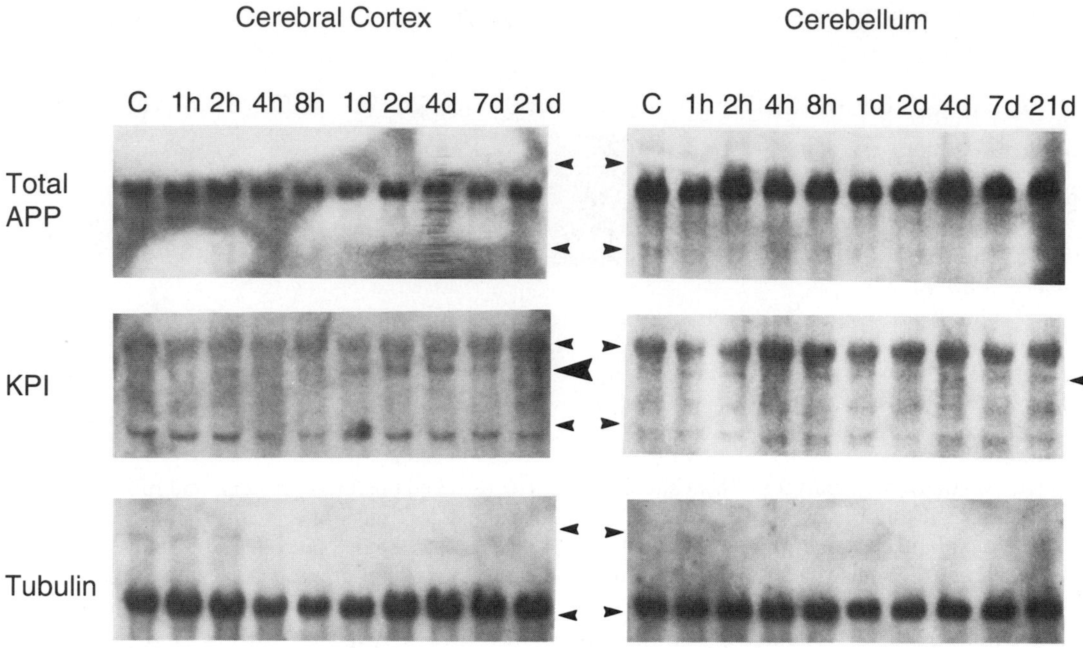


**Fig. 4-13.** Northern blot analyses of amyloid precursor protein (APP) and tubulin mRNAs in the rat cerebral cortex (the territory of the occluded middle cerebral artery) and cerebellum at 1 to 8 hours and 1 to 21 days after the occlusion of unilateral middle cerebral artery. The cDNA probe FB68L recognizes total amounts of APP mRNA (Total APP). The KunBS probe recognizes APP751/770 mRNAs (KPI). Each lane contains 15 $\mu$g of total RNA. C represents the sham control. Small arrowheads represent ribosomal RNAs. The large arrowheads represent APP mRNAs, which contain the KPI domain. The weak bands just below the 18S ribosomal RNA in KPI are the remaining signals of a former probe. (From Abe et al.,[4] with permission.)

is synthesized and secreted by the cell.[175] It forms SDS-resistant complexes with the epidermal growth factor (EGF) binding protein, the gamma-subunit of nerve growth factor and trypsin; the complexes then bind back to the cells and are rapidly internalized and degraded.[175,176] It is now suggested that the physiologic function of PN-II/APP, a potent antichymotrypsin, is the regulation of a chymotrypsinlike protease, which could generate amyloid $\beta$-protein and other peptides that contribute to the formation of neuritic plaques.[176] Thus, KPI-containing APP may have a role in the regulation of certain proteases in the extracellular environment. Cerebral ischemia, on the other hand, involves activation of various proteases. Therefore, our results suggest a selective role for APP species containing the KPI domain, which may be involved in the regulation of chymotrypsinlike protease in the integrative process of rat brain cells after focal cerebral ischemia.

## Deoxyribonucleic Acid

Ischemia injures DNA.[167] Adult male Mongolian gerbils were subjected for 15 minutes of forebrain ischemia and sacrificed at 0, 1, and 4 hours after recirculation. Cryotome sections of the brain were then subjected to the in situ nick translation procedure according to a modification of previously described methods.[50] In the control group, the number of autoradiographic grains, both in the cortex and the CA1 sector of the hippocampus was 0 to 2 per nucleus, suggesting that single-strand breaks occurred at low rates under normal conditions. In the cortex, no significant changes were seen with 15 minutes of ischemia or in the postischemic recirculation periods. The number of grains in the CA1 sector of hippocampus was similar to that of controls with 15 minutes of ischemia. However, 1 hour after the recirculation, the grains increased three to five times compared to controls, indicating that DNA single-strand breaks were accelerated by ischemic and postischemic insults. Four hours after recirculation, the number of the grains returned to control levels, suggesting that structural damage of DNA was repaired. The results demonstrate that ischemic and postischemic insults injure DNA structures in selectively vulnerable CA1 sector of the hippocampus. Although DNA single-strand breaks were rapidly repaired within 4 hours after recirculation, it is possible that transient DNA damage aggravates postischemic disturbances in protein synthesis or RNA metabolism.

## POSTISCHEMIC DISINTEGRATION OF BRAIN CELLS

### Brain Edema and Disorders in Microcirculation

When reperfusion takes place after a relatively brief period of ischemia, both the phosphocreatine levels and the adenylate energy charge are rapidly and completely restored to normal ranges. However, recovery of ATP levels may be only 70 to 80 percent of control.[118,134] Reperfusion following protracted ischemia does not ensure substantial recovery of energy levels, presumably due to injured energy-producing systems.

Ischemia leads to accumulation of various osmolal substances such as $Na^+$, lactate and other organic acids that facilitate edema formation upon recirculation.[48] Theoretically, no brain edema takes place during complete cerebral ischemia: "no flow, no edema."[25,77] On the other hand, focal cerebral ischemia is usually accompanied by brain edema[41,77] because of the presence of residual or collateral circulation, which supplies edema fluid to the ischemic region. This small amount of perfusion is not sufficient to maintain energy production, but is sufficient to supply edema constituents (water and sodium) to the lesion and to remove $K^+$ from the lesion (Fig. 4-14). Obviously, this channel comes from the nonischemic area through the peripheral region of the ischemic focus. Thus, development of cerebral edema initially and predominantly occurs in the periphery of focal cerebral ischemia due to its accessibility to edema constituents in this cross-talking region.[62,77] A possible contribution of neutrophils to edema formation is discussed in the section on pannecrosis in this chapter.

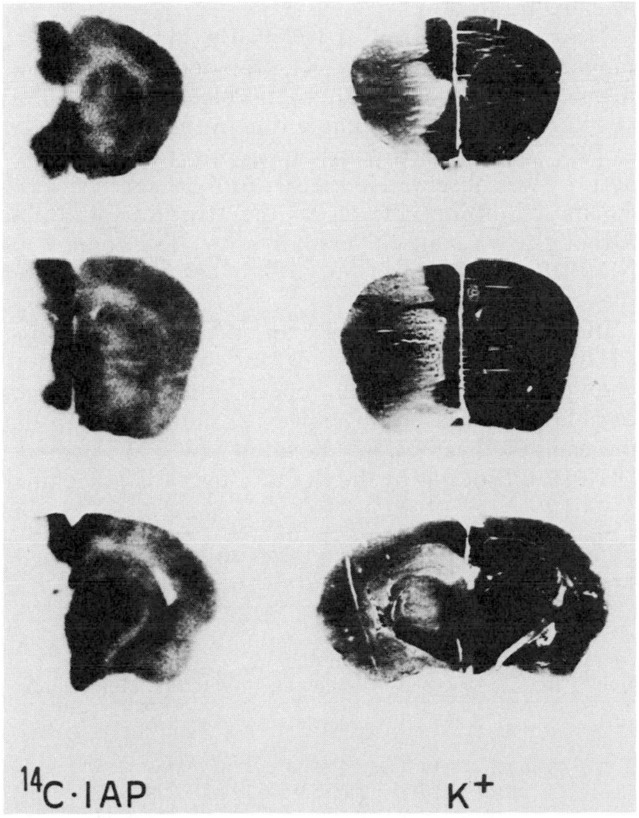


**Fig. 4-14.** Iodo[$^{14}$C]antipyrine (IAP) autoradiographs and $K^+$ pictures of a gerbil brain that had suffered 2 hours hemispheric ischemia (*left on the pictures*). Note greater $K^+$ depletion in the periphery of ischemia. (From Kato et al.,[62] with permission.)

Hemorheologically, hematocrit (Hct) of this marginal zone increases markedly with developing ischemia. When a brain artery is occluded, the intravascular pressure distal to the occlusion decreases markedly, resulting in an hydrostatic pressure gradient generated between the peripheral patent arteries and the ischemic focus. As a result, an ischemic lesion in a richly vascularized area is rapidly shrunk by developing collateral channels. Such spontaneous postischemic tissue perfusion is characterized by a columnar or moth-eaten pattern of perfused regions,[80] with areas of reactive hyperemia juxtaposed between hypoperfused areas. A combined study of red corpuscle flow and fluid element flow of the blood is required to elucidate their pathophysiologic characteristics. Izumiyama et al.[53] have reported that a limited distribution of red blood cells (RBCs), compared with plasma, is observed in the penumbral area (Fig. 4-15). The systemic Hct of those experimental animals was 45.1 percent, whereas the brain tissue Hct was approximately 32 percent. Such a difference has been observed by other authors,[32,86] and is considered to be due, in part, to differences in the velocity of blood flow that segregate plasma and RBCs, as small blood vessels bifurcate from the main trunks. In addition, the relative proportion of RBCs and plasma is less in small vessels than in larger vessels. It is assumed that when RBCs are sufficiently elastic to pass through the ischemic boundary, the outer high Hct zone will decrease, and the collateral channel will improve to carry oxygen and glucose inward and carry metabolic waste outward.

### Decomposition of the Membrane

During reperfusion, disintegration of ischemically susceptible and dying neurons progress in a systematic fashion. Morphologic changes in ribosomal assembly were mentioned earlier.[16,68] Decomposition of cytoplasmic membranes also affects the functional and perhaps structural integrity of membrane bound receptors. For instance, binding activity of [$^3$H]quinuclidinyl benzilate ([$^3$H]QNB) to muscarinic cholinergic receptors[120] (Table 4-5) in the CA1 sector of rat hippocampus decreased significantly at only 60 minutes following recirculation after 20 minutes of forebrain ischemia. Early after recirculation, [$^3$H]PN 200-

**TABLE 4-5. Time Course of [$^3$H]Quinuclidinyl Benzilate Binding in Rat Hippocampus After 20 Minutes of Transient Forebrain Ischemia (Four-Vessel Occlusion Model)[a]**

| | | CA1 Subfield | | | CA3 Subfield | | |
|---|---|---|---|---|---|---|---|
| Time (h) | *N* | Stratum Oriens | Stratum Radiatum | Stratum Lacunosum-Moleculare | Stratum Oriens | Stratum Radiatum | Dentate Gyrus (Stratum Moleculare) |
| Control | 8 | 444 ± 6 | 458 ± 7 | 319 ± 6 | 351 ± 8 | 382 ± 6 | 436 ± 4 |
| 1 | 7 | 404 ± 11* | 442 ± 6 | 328 ± 8 | 347 ± 14 | 360 ± 14 | 427 ± 6 |
| 3 | 7 | 404 ± 11* | 442 ± 6 | 328 ± 8 | 347 ± 14 | 360 ± 14 | 428 ± 6 |
| 6 | 8 | 415 ± 9* | 442 ± 7 | 333 ± 10 | 336 ± 8 | 370 ± 6 | 430 ± 9 |
| 12 | 7 | 390 ± 11** | 407 ± 14* | 296 ± 9 | 326 ± 14 | 352 ± 15 | 399 ± 14 |
| 24 | 6 | 373 ± 16** | 385 ± 15** | 283 ± 24 | 312 ± 14 | 325 ± 14** | 394 ± 11* |
| 48 | 6 | 357 ± 25* | 401 ± 15* | 279 ± 25 | 324 ± 28 | 327 ± 11** | 388 ± 24 |
| 168 | 8 | 280 ± 17** | 350 ± 13** | 240 ± 17** | 327 ± 13 | 341 ± 10** | 400 ± 10* |

[a] Data are mean ± SEM fmol/cm$^2$.
* $P < 0.05$, **$P < 0.01$, respectively, different from control by Mann-Whitney U test.
(From Onodera and Kogure,[120] with permission of the American Heart Association, Inc.)

110, a dihydropyridine $Ca^{2+}$ channel blocker ([$^3$H]PN) binding in the CA1 subfield decreased when there were no microscopic abnormalities of the CA1 pyramidal cells. The postischemic change in adenosine A1 receptor began 12 hours after recirculation (Table 4-6). The diterpene compound forskolin is a potent activator of adenylate cyclase, binding with high affinity to the catalytic subunit of the enzyme.[145,146] This compound also labels glucose transport protein[148,149] and to certain extent directly alters the gating of voltage-dependent potassium channels.[46] Therefore, forskolin binding should be another marker for the integrity of cytoplasmic membranes. Postischemic alteration of [$^3$H]forskolin binding sites were obvious by only 1 hour after recirculation (Table 4-7), when a significant decrease in binding activity was noticed in the CA1 subfield.[119]

On the other hand, [$^3$H]phorbol 12,13-dibutyrate ([$^3$H]PDBu) autoradiography revealed that the hippocampus contains the highest concentration of PKC molecules in the brain.[183] The time course of [$^3$H]PBDu binding in rat hippocampus after 20 minutes of forebrain ischemia was studied to elucidate the progression of changes associated with postischemic neuronal damage.[116] [$^3$H]PDBu binding activity in postischemic hippocampus changed not only in the CA1 subfield, where selective pyramidal cell necrosis was noticed, but also in the histologically intact CA3 and dentate gyrus (Fig. 4-16). The CA1 sector showed gradual increase in binding during early recirculation (1 to 12 hours after reperfusion) when no microscopic damage of CA1 pyramidal cells was seen. Binding activity in CA1 reached maximum 3 hours after recirculation.

Transient increases in [$^3$H]PDBu binding in CA1 may presumably reflect PKC translocation to membrane. It is likely that glutamate released during and/or after ischemia may play a role in the translocation of PKC.[173] In CA3, a transient depression of binding activity was observed in the stratum oriens, in spite of constant binding activity in the stratum radiatum. Although we cannot explain the discrepancy of [$^3$H]PDBu binding in CA3, differences in innervation may play a role.

In the molecular layer of the dentate gyrus, [$^3$H]PDBu binding sites exhibited no significant change during the early reperfusion period. Seven days after recirculation, however, the binding in the molecular layer was elevated by 33 percent. [$^3$H]PDBu binding in the dentate gyrus is associated

**TABLE 4-6. Time Course of [$^3$H]Cyclohexyladenosine Binding in Rat Hippocampus After 20 Minutes of Transient Forebrain Ischemia (Four-Vessel Occlusion Model)[a]**

| | | CA1 Subfield | | | CA3 Subfield | | |
|---|---|---|---|---|---|---|---|
| Time (h) | *N* | Stratum Oriens | Stratum Radiatum | Stratum Lacunosum-Moleculare | Stratum Oriens | Stratum Radiatum | Dentate Gyrus (Stratum Moleculare) |
| Control | 8 | 268 ± 9 | 312 ± 5 | 162 ± 10 | 173 ± 9 | 236 ± 9 | 236 ± 5 |
| 1 | 7 | 246 ± 11 | 310 ± 14 | 170 ± 7 | 182 ± 14 | 240 ± 8 | 227 ± 7 |
| 3 | 7 | 243 ± 10 | 297 ± 12 | 152 ± 7 | 167 ± 10 | 222 ± 14 | 224 ± 7 |
| 6 | 8 | 235 ± 13 | 274 ± 12 | 153 ± 12 | 161 ± 10 | 200 ± 9 | 220 ± 9 |
| 12 | 7 | 186 ± 11* | 256 ± 18** | 122 ± 8** | 127 ± 16 | 176 ± 19** | 179 ± 11** |
| 24 | 6 | 230 ± 11** | 276 ± 11** | 158 ± 9 | 171 ± 8 | 212 ± 15 | 208 ± 9** |
| 48 | 6 | 184 ± 14* | 231 ± 10* | 131 ± 5** | 143 ± 4** | 181 ± 6* | 195 ± 7* |
| 168 | 8 | 80 ± 11* | 121 ± 18* | 72 ± 8* | 130 ± 11** | 160 ± 16* | 168 ± 9* |

[a] Data are mean ± SEM fmol/cm$^2$.
* $P < 0.01$, **$P < 0.05$, respectively, different from control by Mann-Whitney U test.
(From Onodera and Kogure,[120] with permission of the American Heart Association, Inc.)

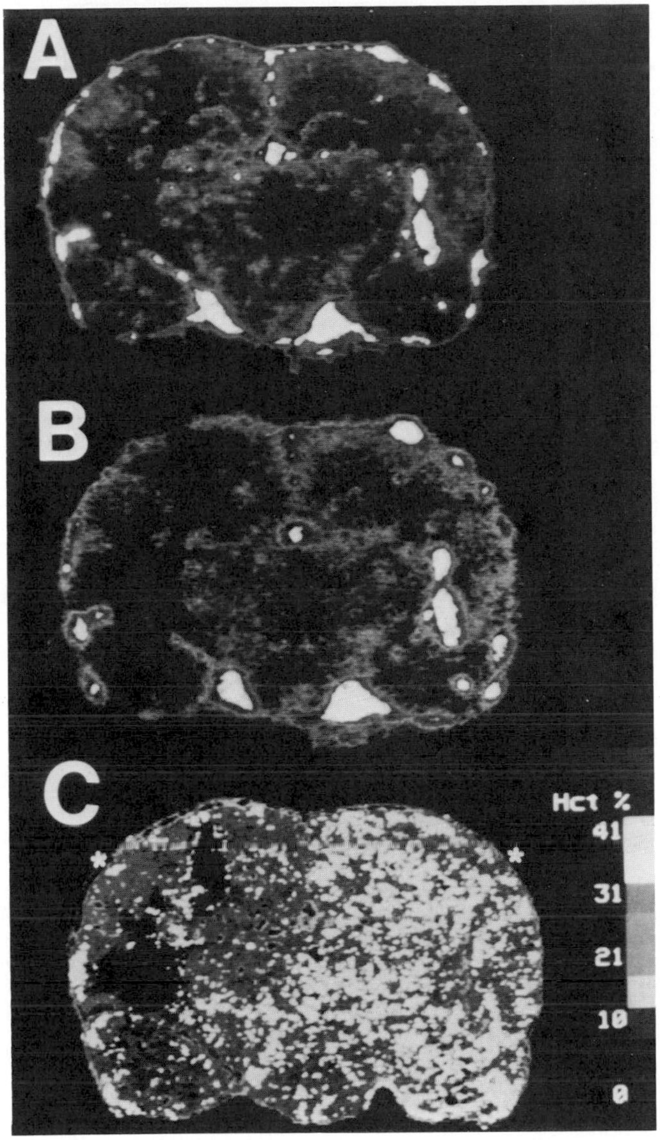


**Fig. 4-15.** A pair of autoradiograms taken with a single brain section showing the right hemisphere (*left on the pictures*) as the side affected by microsphere emboli. (**A**) Coronal section at the level of the midthalamus, showing the distribution of $^{125}$I-bovine serum albumin. The ipsilateral poorly perfused areas are thought to be the ischemic penumbra adjacent to the core. (**B**) Distribution of [$^{18}$F]2-fluoro-2-deoxy-D-glucose-labeled red blood cells. Limited penetration of red blood cells into the circumscribed boundary zone was observed. (**C**) Hematocrit mapping generated by pixel-by-pixel calculation. The mean tissue hematocrit in the contralateral hemisphere to emboli was 31.9 percent, and a global reduction was noted on the ipsilateral side. In the intraischemic zone, a relatively low hematocrit area is observed, surrounded by an outer high hematocrit area where plasma skimming is considered to be developed. (From Izumiyama et al.,[53] with permission.)

**TABLE 4-7. Time Course of [$^3$H]Forskolin Binding in the Rat Hippocampus After Various Periods of Recirculation (Ligand Concentration 10 nM)[a]**

| | $CA_1$ (Average) | $CA_3$ (Stratum Lucidum) | Hilus | Dentate Gyrus |
|---|---|---|---|---|
| Control | 22 ± 1.4 | 98 ± 14.9 | 168 ± 5.6 | 58 ± 2.0 |
| Recirculation | | | | |
| 1 h | 20 ± 1.7** | 95 ± 6.8 | 157 ± 6.2 | 56 ± 1.6 |
| 3 h | 16 ± 1.4** | 92 ± 8.7 | 160 ± 12.8 | 54 ± 1.3** |
| 6 h | 16 ± 0.6** | 109 ± 4.8 | 162 ± 5.5 | 49 ± 1.1* |
| 12 h | 14 ± 1.3** | 97 ± 4.5 | 165 ± 8.1 | 49 ± 3.2 |
| 1 day | 15 ± 1.0** | 109 ± 7.8 | 165 ± 8.1 | 51 ± 2.4 |
| 3 days | 12 ± 1.0** | 112 ± 12.1 | 154 ± 3.8 | 56 ± 3.5 |
| 7 days | 11 ± 1.3** | 105 ± 8.0 | 139 ± 3.7** | 53 ± 2.1 |

[a] Optical densities were converted to fmol/cm$^2$ tissue using the [$^3$H]microscale (Amersham). Results are expressed as means ± SEM from 6 to 10 animals.

(From Onodera and Kogure,[119] with permission)

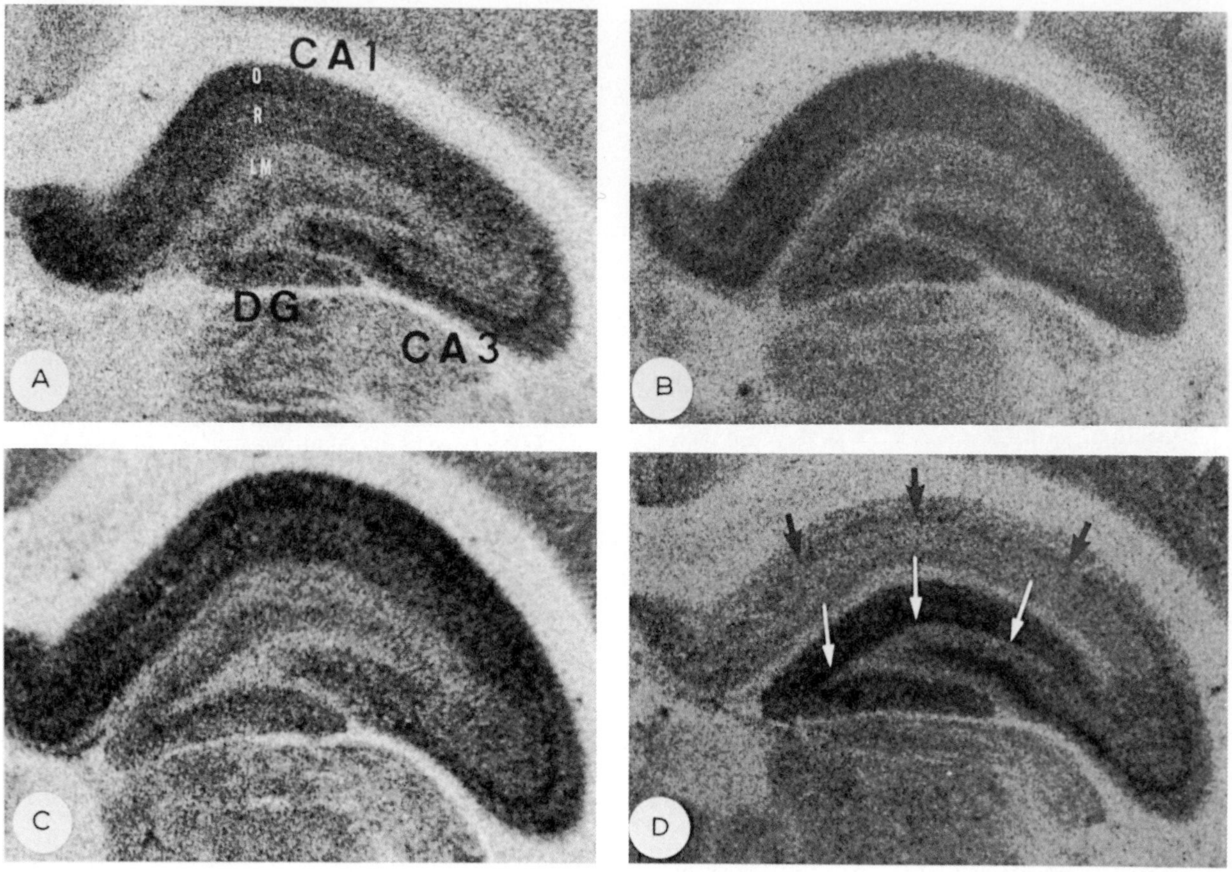


**Fig. 4-16.** [$^3$H]Phorbol 12,13-dibutyrate ([$^3$H]PDBu) autoradiograms from a control animal and animals rendered ischemic. Hippocampal formation of the (**A**) control animal and (**B**) animals killed 6 hours, (**C**) 2 days, and (**D**) 7 days after ischemia. Marked enhancement of [$^3$H]PDBu binding in the CA1 was noticed 6 hours after ischemia. Seven days after ischemia, grain density in the strata oriens, radiatum, and lacunosum-moleculare exhibited decreased [$^3$H]PDBu binding sites in accordance with CA1 pyramidal cell loss. However, binding sites in the stratum pyramidale of the CA1 were preserved (*black arrows*). Note the increase in grain density in the dentate gyrus (molecular layer), with higher [$^3$H]inositol 1,4,5-triphosphate ([$^3$H]$IP_3$) binding in the supragranular layer (*white arrows*). DG, dentate gyrus; LM, stratum lacunosum-moleculare; O, stratum oriens; R, stratum radiatum. (From Onodera et al.,[116] with permission.)

with the afferent terminals but not with dentate granule cells. Interestingly, the inner region of the stratum moleculare (supragranular layer), which receives inputs from commissural and association fibers and septal neurons, displayed higher activity compared to the outer region of the stratum moleculare, where the perforant path from the entorhinal cortex terminates. We also found this elevation of binding activity to be suspended more than 3 months after the insult.

## Decomposition of Microorganels

[$^3$H]inositol 1,4,5-trisphosphate ([$^3$H]$IP_3$) binding in the hippocampal formation was strikingly heterogeneous and was highest in the CA1 subfield.[119,182] The strata oriens, pyramidale, and radiatum had higher binding activity than the stratum lacunosum-moleculare in the CA1 subfield (Fig. 4-17). The CA3 exhibited very low [$^3$H]$IP_3$ binding. In the dentate gyrus, the stratum moleculare has higher binding activity than the stratum granulosum. Early in the recirculation period, the time course of [$^3$H]$IP_3$ binding activity of the dendritic fields in CA1 was quite distinct from that of the stratum pyramidale. The strata oriens, radiatum, and lacunosum-moleculare showed significant reduction in the binding activity 3 hours after ischemia, followed by marked loss of binding sites 7 days after ischemia. However, in the stratum pyramidale, significant reductions in [$^3$H]$IP_3$ binding activity was not observed until 2 days after recirculation, when neuronal damage was observed. The alteration of [$^3$H]$IP_3$ binding sites in the CA3 and dentate gyrus was minimal.

The role of $Ca^{2+}$-dependent calmodulin-dependent protein kinase II (CaM kinase II) is implicated in a variety of neuronal functions.[65,186–188] Since CaM kinase II is a major protein for postsynaptic density,[43] the enzyme may play a pivotal role in synaptic plas-

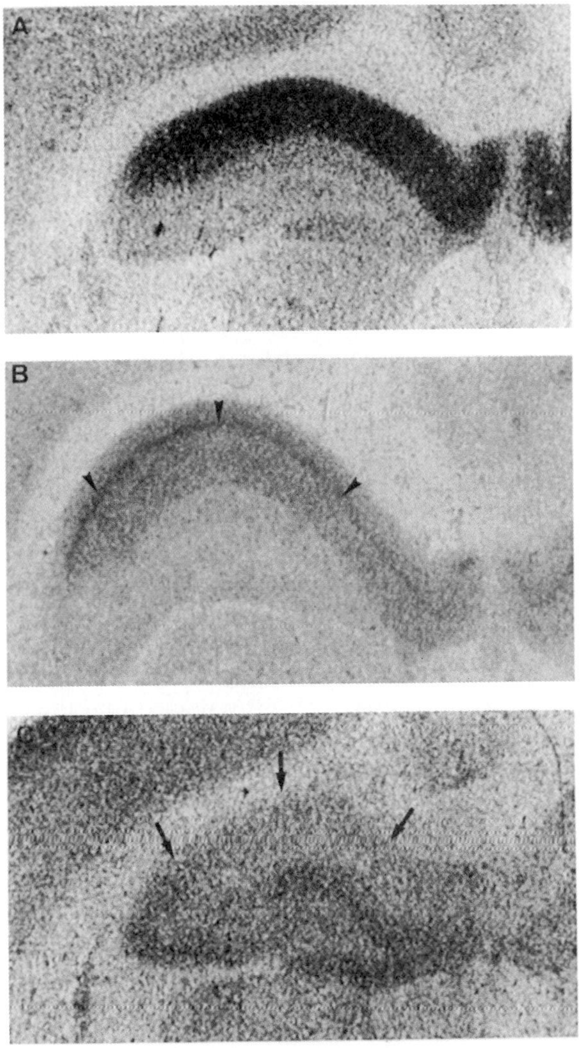


**Fig. 4-17.** [$^3$H]Inositol 1,4,5-triphosphate ([$^3$H]$IP_3$) autoradiograms from (**A**) a control animal, and animals killed (**B**) 6 hours and (**C**) 7 days after ischemia. [$^3$H]$IP_3$ binding sites were highly concentrated in the CA1 subfield. Note reduced binding in the strata oriens, radiatum, and lacunosum-moleculare 6 hours after ischemia, while binding in the stratum pyramidale (*arrowheads*) was not altered. Grain density in the CA1 was markedly reduced and no stratal difference is visible 7 days after ischemia (*arrows*), when CA1 pyramidal cells were depleted. (From Onodera and Kogure,[119] with permission.)

ticity.[92,94] According to Onodera et al.,[117] CA1 pyramidal cells and dentate granule cells exhibited strong immunoreactivity in somata and neurites, whereas little staining was observed in the nuclei.[38] The CA3 pyramidal cells exhibited moderate immunoreactivity, and the stratum lucidum in the CA3 subfield was also immunopositive. Sections incubated without primary antibody or with preimmune serum showed no significant staining throughout the experiments. Six hours after ischemia, CA1 and CA3 pyramidal cells and dentate granule cells lost CaM kinase II immunoreactivity in neuronal perikarya. However, immunoreactivity in the dendritic fields, such as the strata oriens and radiatum of CA1 and CA3 and the stratum moleculare of the dentate gyrus, was preserved, and the decrease of immunoreactivity in the CA3 stratum lucidum was minimal. A similar immunohistochemical pattern was observed 1 day after ischemia. In contrast to the recovery of immunoreactivity of CA3 pyramidal cells and dentate granule cells, immunoreactivity in CA1 remained depressed 3 days after recirculation. Seven days after ischemia, immunoreactivity was greatly reduced in the CA1 subfield, indicating that CaM kinase II molecules in the CA1 subfield are preferentially located on CA1 pyramidal cells. The CA3 and dentate gyrus regained near-normal immunoreactivity at this point.

Since this enzyme phosphorylates components of neuronal cytoskeletal protein, such as tubulin, microtubule-associated protein 2 (MAP 2), and tau factor,[186,188] the disruption of CaM kinase II systems after ischemia could affect transport of materials through neuronal processes, the shape of neurites, and/or membrane bound-receptor signaling. Resurrection of CaM kinase II in the ischemia-resistant neurons may play a critical role in the reconstruction of neuronal networks damaged by ischemic insult.

The data discussed above suggest that postischemic disintegration of vulnerable neurons becomes biochemically detectable as early as 1 to 3 hours after recirculation. According to the time course of changes observed in calcium-effector mechanism, such as the calcium channel (indicated by [$^3$H]PN binding activity), calcium endostore (indicated by [$^3$H]$IP_3$ binding activity), protein kinase C (indicated by [$^3$H]PDBu binding activity), and CaM kinase II (indicated by a polyclonal antibody immunohistochemistry), it is assumed that the detrimental postischemic cascade becomes irreversible when the affected neurons lose their ability to control calcium homeostasis. From the therapeutic point of view, this situation appears difficult to ameliorate because of its multifarious nature, unless a pivotal and treatable enzyme is identified at the cross-talk point in the transduction pathways.

## REPEATED ISCHEMIA

Recent experiments disclosed unique sequential events of neuronal damage and protection following repeated ischemic insults;[61,71,168] these findings may have important clinical implications and may contribute to the elucidation of mechanisms and dynamics involved in ischemic brain damage. When the brain is exposed to a brief period of ischemia that is short enough to permit recovery without any appreciable morphologic damage, but is sufficiently long to induce cellular responses, the selective vulnerability of the neurons in the brain is drastically altered. The response of brain to secondary ischemic insults, following preconditioning with sublethal ischemia, is time-dependent.[63] The vulnerability of brain to ischemia is emphasized, and damage is cumulative after shorter intervals between ischemia; however, protection (tolerance) is induced and damage is attenuated after longer intervals between ischemia (Fig. 4-18).

The brain is most vulnerable to succeeding ischemic insults 1 hour after preconditioning with 2 minutes of ischemia in gerbils[60] or 3 minutes of ischemia in rats,[105] as compared to shorter or longer intervals. Neuronal damage in brain following secondary global ischemia is emphasized in selectively vulnerable regions, such as the hippocampal CA1 subfield, caudate/putamen, and ventral thalamus. As a result, neuronal damage from 3 minutes of global ischemia in gerbils induced 1 hour after pretreatment with 2 minutes of ischemia is greater than damage from single 3 minutes of ischemia or damage from 3 minutes of ischemia induced 5 minutes or 6 hours after pretreatment.[63] Furthermore, three such sublethal ischemic insults repeated at 1-hour intervals in gerbils (2 minutes) or in rats (3 minutes) produce consistent neuronal damage to selectively vulnerable regions, which is greater than damage after equivalent single periods of ischemia (6 minutes and 9 minutes, respectively), or than damage after ischemic insults repeated at 5 minutes or 4- to 6-hour intervals.[60,105]

## The Cumulative Effect

The mechanisms of cumulative brain damage following repeated ischemia may be severalfold: (1) regional cerebral blood flow decreases after global ischemia, known as postischemic hypoperfusion, and is most pronounced 1 hour after the insult;[59,168] (2) protein synthesis in the vulnerable brain areas is severely depressed for several hours, even after sublethal ischemia,[7] (3) the excitotoxic mechanism is involved in the same way as in transient cerebral ischemia[58] without alterations in the amount of neurotransmitters released during each ischemic insult,[108] but with alterations in receptor sensitivity and second-messenger system activity.[56,57] The degree of vulnerability occurs depending upon the stage of impaired circulation, metabolism, and signal-transducing systems.

## Polyamine Metabolism

It has been known that transient cerebral ischemia causes remarkable changes in the synthesis of putrescine, spermidine, and spermine, namely, a sharp increase in the activity of the first key enzyme ornithine decarboxylase (ODC)[125,126] and a prolonged precipitation in the activity of *S*-adenosylmethionine decarboxylase (SAMDC): the second key enzyme.[27,73] Increased activity in ODC increases the level of putrescine,[124,128] together with suppressed conversion of putrescine into spermidine and spermine via SAMDC. Paschen et al.[125,127,129] reported that the postischemic putrescine levels correlate closely with the duration of ischemia and with the density of neurons.

Paschen et al.[130] recently studied regional changes in polyamine profiles that differ after 5 or 15 minutes of ischemia or three 5-minute periods of ischemia with 60-minute intervals between occlusion. Spermine levels were significantly reduced in the hippocampal CA1 subfield after 5 minutes of ischemia and, in addition, in the striatum and thalamus after three

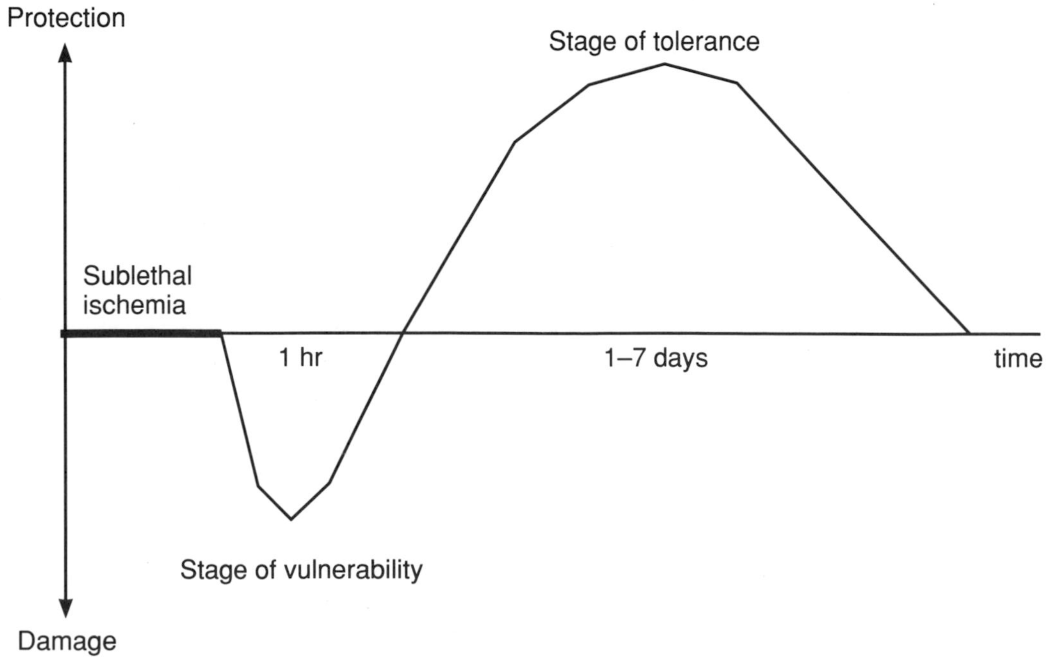


**Fig. 4-18.** A schematic diagram illustrating the temporal profile of altered vulnerability of neurons in the brain following pretreatment with sublethal ischemia.

times 5 minutes of ischemia. The half-life of polyamine in brain is about 12 to 14 days,[147] and the level is quite stable for several days, even after decapitation. The marked reduction in spermine levels (and, to a lesser extent, putrescine and spermidine) in brain regions, known to be most vulnerable to repetitive ischemia, was therefore an unexpected finding. A possible explanation for these changes is, according to Paschen et al.,[130] a release of polyamines from intracellular compartments into the extracellular space and their clearance into the circulating blood. Increased putrescine level in the cytosol may also facilitate calcium influx.[17,49,84,129] Increased putrescine levels in the extracellular compartment may also activate glial proliferation.[194] On the other hand, decrease in spermine levels may affect the calcium-buffering capacity of mitochondria.[54,110,140] In addition, polyamines released from dying neurons may diffuse into their vicinity and bind to polyamine recognition sites at the NMDA receptor and enhance their receptor-mediated intracellular response.[42,135,155,156]

In summary, postischemic steep rise in ODC activity and the resultant polyamine dysmetabolism may contribute to the postischemic brain injury and to the mechanism of cumulative brain damage following repeated ischemia.

### Tolerance

In contrast to increased neuronal damage with shorter intervals between ischemia, tolerance is induced when secondary insults are rendered 1 to 7 days after pretreatment with sublethal ischemia; ischemic neuronal damage from secondary ischemic insults is significantly ameliorated.[69,71] Global cerebral ischemia rendered 3 to 5 minutes in gerbils consistently produce destruction of hippocampal CA1 pyramidal cells, but do not when such ischemia is rendered 1 to 7 days after preconditioning the brain with sublethal 2-minutes ischemia. However, the tolerance disappears by 14 days after preliminary ischemia.[63]

The mechanism of tolerance induction to ischemia is not fully understood, but a role for the stress response is suggested. The stage at which tolerance takes place coincides with heat shock/stress protein induction in the surviving neurons.[69] Reports showing that preliminary exposure to hyperthermia induces tolerance to succeeding ischemic insults also support this view.[21,72] Experimental evidence indicates that sublethal ischemia induces conspicuous gene expression of HSP70 and c-fos in CA1 neurons.[113] These evidences suggest that tolerance is induced through altered gene expression to synthesize a protective protein. Elucidation of this mechanism awaits further study, but its clarification may help develop strategies for protection against ischemic brain damage.

At present, no rational explanation exists that elucidates both the mechanism for cumulative brain damage or induction of tolerance to ischemia following repeated ischemia, but clues are available. For example, Nakano et al.[106] studied the time course of changes in the amount and composition of free fatty acids (FFAs) accumulated during 5 minutes of ischemia and after various postischemic recirculation durations (3 minutes, 1 hour, 24 hours, 3 days, and 6 days) in the gerbil cerebral cortex. Liberated FFAs in response to the second 5-minute ischemia, at various recirculation intervals (3 minutes, 1 hour, 3 days, and 6 days) following the initial insult, were also measured to evaluate changes in cellular responses. The former study (Fig. 4-19) disclosed that the FFA levels transiently returned to control levels at 1 hour recirculation, increased again a few days after the onset of recirculation, followed by a final return to control levels after 6 days recirculation. The delayed increase in all FFA levels was clearly observed 3 days after recir-

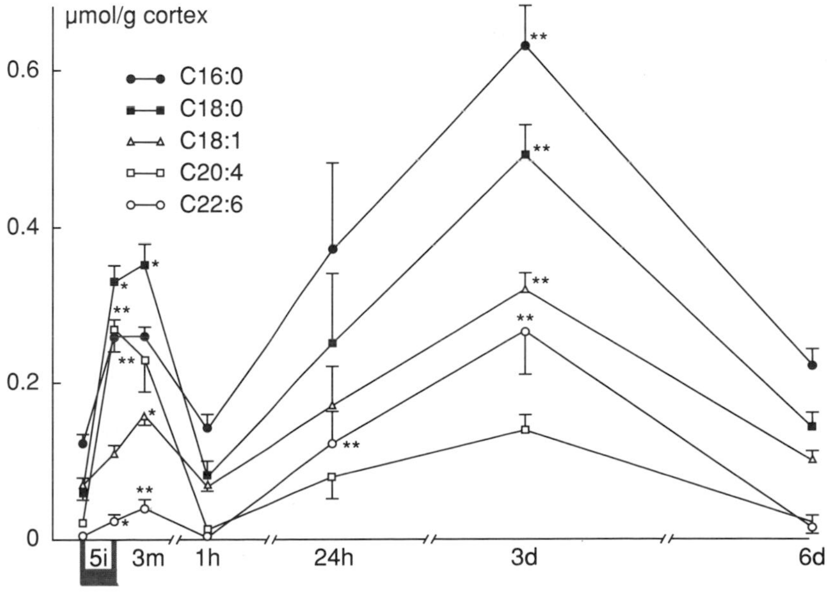


**Fig. 4-19.** Time course of changes in the free fatty acid levels accumulated during 5 minutes of ischemia (5i) and after various recirculation durations (3m, 3 minutes; 1 h and 24 h, 1 and 24 hours; 3 d and 6 d, 3 and 6 days). The free fatty acid levels increased during ischemia and the early period of recirculation and returned to the control levels in 1 hour. However, they increased again a few days after the onset of recirculation. (*$P < 0.05$, **$P < 0.01$ compared with sham control.) (From Nakano et al.,[106] with permission.)

**TABLE 4-8. Changes in Amount of Free Fatty Acids Liberated During the Initial or the Second 5-Minute Ischemia Following at Various Intervals[a]**

| | 5i ($N$ = 5) | 5i-3m-5i ($N$ = 8) | 5i-1h-5i ($N$ = 6) | 5i-3d-5i ($N$ = 6) | 5i-6d-5i ($N$ = 6) |
|---|---|---|---|---|---|
| Total | 0.71 ± 0.05 | 1.79 ± 0.21 | 0.40 ± 0.03 | 10.78 ± 1.22* | 1.89 ± 0.28 |
| C16:0 | 0.14 ± 0.02 | 0.56 ± 0.08 | 0.01 ± 0.01 | 3.80 ± 0.37* | 0.60 ± 0.12 |
| C18:0 | 0.27 ± 0.02 | 0.54 ± 0.06 | 0.14 ± 0.02 | 2.78 ± 0.35* | 0.48 ± 0.09 |
| C18:1 | 0.04 ± 0.01 | 0.25 ± 0.04 | 0.04 ± 0.01 | 1.65 ± 0.19* | 0.26 ± 0.04 |
| C20:4 | 0.25 ± 0.01 | 0.30 ± 0.03 | 0.21 ± 0.02 | 1.06 ± 0.14** | 0.31 ± 0.06 |
| C22:6 | 0.02 ± 0.00 | 0.14 ± 0.04 | 0.01 ± 0.00 | 1.50 ± 0.25* | 0.26 ± 0.06 |

[a] Each free fatty acid (FFA) concentration was calculated by subtracting the prior mean accumulated FFA concentration from the individual FFA concentration at the end of the respective 5-minute ischemia (5i). The changes in FFA concentrations at the end of the single 5-minute ischemia served as control.

* $P < 0.01$; ** $P < 0.05$.

Abbreviations: 3m, 3-minute recirculation; 1h, 1-hour recirculation; 3d and 6d, 3- and 6-day recirculation.

(From Nakano et al.,[106] with permission.)

culation. At this stage, the total amount of accumulated FFAs was no less than about seven times the amount for controls. Taking vascular washout and reacylation mechanisms into consideration, the amount of liberated FFAs is considerable. Furthermore, the increased FFAs contained a large amount, C16:0, C18:1, and C22:6, suggesting that the main source of these liberated FFAs are the membrane structural lipids, other than PPIs, which are only minor sources of free C16:0, and their contribution to the production of free C18:1 is negligible. Phosphatidylcholine or phosphatidylethanolamine may be decomposed by the combined actions of phospholipase A2 and lysophospholipase.[11,31,95,159]

Surprisingly, despite the liberation of such a large amount of FFAs, PPIs were maintained at control levels.[5] If this delayed increase in FFA levels reflects the process of cell death or the result of epileptic seizures, PPI levels could not be maintained at control values. Histopathologic[24] and palmitate incorporation[169] studies have also demonstrated that the cerebral cortex is almost intact during this period. Since the cellular and subcellular origin of liberated FFAs at this time period is not clear, the significance of the delayed increase in FFA levels remain unknown.

The latter study (Table 4-8) disclosed that the cellular response to the second ischemia was quite different from the initial one, even 6 days after recirculation, suggesting that membrane lipid metabolism had not yet recovered, even at such a late period.

## POSTISCHEMIC EXOFOCAL NEURONAL DEATH

Recently, Nagasawa et al.[101] have found that a retarded neuronal death phenomenon occurs in ipsilateral remote areas of the brain outside the ischemic areas of rat brain after transient focal ischemia. In their model, transient focal ischemia was induced by embolization of the right middle cerebral artery (MCA), and after 15, 30, 60, and 90 minutes of MCA occlusion, recirculation was achieved by removal of the embolus. Chronological changes in the distribution of neuronal damages were determined by using the $^{45}Ca$-autoradiography and histologic methods. To assess a possible mechanism involved, local cerebral glucose metabolism measurements were investigated.

It was evident from the studies that $^{45}Ca$ accumulated not only in the lateral segment of the caudate/putamen and the cerebral cortex, which were directly affected by the ischemic insult (Fig. 4-20), but also in the ipsilateral ventral posterior nucleus of the thalamus and the pars reticularis of the substantia nigra, which lay outside the ischemic areas. In the cerebral cortex and the lateral segment of the caudate/putamen, which were supplied by the occluded MCA, after 60 minutes of MCA occlusion, the level of regional cerebral blood flow (rCBF) was reduced to approximately 12 percent and 3 percent, respectively, as compared to the corresponding regions of control rats. Acute necrosis of neurons and neuroglial cells observed in these ischemic foci is attributed to energy failure. Histologic examination revealed, however, very little edema in this model.

In the thalamus and the substantia nigra, in which $^{45}Ca$ accumulation was detected after 3 days of recirculation following transient MCA occlusion, no significant reduction in CBF was found even after 60 minutes of MCA occlusion, as compared to corresponding regions of sham-operated rats. The mechanism of injury in both remote areas cannot be attributed either to energy failure or complications of edema formation. On the other hand, both of the remotely affected areas have transsynaptic connections with the cerebral cortex and the caudate putamen, respectively.[44,174] Because the observed neuronal changes in the ipsilateral thalamus and subsantia nigra were not

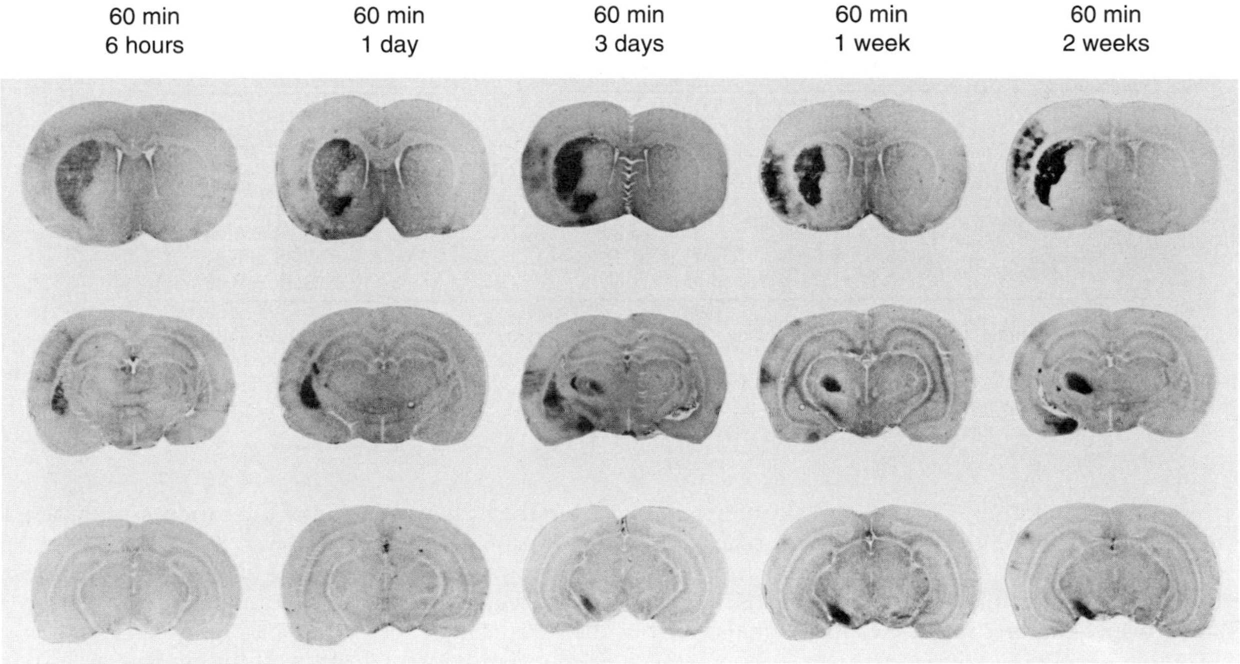


**Fig. 4-20.** $^{45}Ca$-autoradiograms of rat brain obtained after 60 minutes of middle cerebral artery occlusion followed by 6 hours, 1 day, 3 days, 1 week, and 2 weeks recirculation. Representative autoradiograms show coronal sections at the level of caudate putamen (*top*), thalamus (*middle*), and substantia nigra (*bottom*). (From Nagasawa and Kogure,[101a] with permission.)

apparent in histologic studies until 3 days after ischemia, it is suggested that these findings regarding both remote areas are consistent with secondary neuronal degeneration of cells that send axons to the ischemic areas.

### Dying-Back Injury in the Thalamus

In the thalamus, histologic damage was limited to the ventral posterior nuclei (VPM, VPL), and selective neuronal death in this area may be explained as a process of retrograde degeneration resulting from thalamocortical fiber damage caused by the preceding ischemic insult in the postcentral gyrus of the central cortex, which forms anatomically close fiber connections with this area.[97] The phenomenon of dying-back injuries is well known in experiments on head trauma.[123,157] It is also known that the ablation of cerebral cortical fibers reduces glutamate uptake in the synaptic terminals of the corticostriatal and corticothalamic fibers, and it is believed that these fibers are glutamatergic.[36,189] The nonphysiologic release of large quantities of neurotransmitters could occur at axon terminals of the thalamus when cortical neuronal cells are damaged by an ischemic insult. This phenomenon could induce a collapse of homeostasis, related to postsynaptic membrane ion permeability, and could possibly lead to cell death in the thalamus.[139]

Moreover, from 2-[$^{14}C$]deoxyglucose autoradiograms obtained after 90 minutes of MCA occlusion, followed by 1 week of recirculation, regional cerebral glucose utilization (rCGU) in the thalamus showed a tendency to decrease, to a variable extent, as compared to corresponding regions in the contralateral hemisphere (Table 4-9). These data suggest that the mechanism of selective neuronal death observed in the thalamus is not the same as that observed in the substantia nigra. Although the data cannot be interpreted at present, [$^3H$]$IP_3$ and [$^3H$]forskolin binding

**TABLE 4-9. Local Cerebral Glucose Utilization Measured After 90 Minutes of Middle Cerebral Artery Occlusion Followed by 1 Week Recirculation**

| Structure | Ischemic Side | Nonischemic Side |
|---|---|---|
| Thalamus (ventral posterior nucleus) | 7.20 ± 0.29 | 8.20 ± 0.88 |
| Substantia nigra | 10.12 ± 0.76* | 7.68 ± 0.64 |

[a] Values are given in mean ± SD mg/100 g/min. Five animals.
*$P < 0.01$, compared with value in the same row using a t-test.
(From Nagasawa and Kogure,[101] with permission.)

**TABLE 4-10. [$^3$H]IP$_3$ and [$^3$H]Forskolin Binding in the Frontoparietal Cortex Lateral Caudate Putamen, Thalamus, and Substantia Nigra 4 Weeks after 90 Minutes of Middle Cerebral Artery[a]**

| | [$^3$H]IP$_3$ Binding | | [$^3$H]Forskolin Binding | |
|---|---|---|---|---|
| Ischemic Side | Control ($N$ = 6) | 4 Weeks ($N$ = 6) | Control ($N$ = 6) | 4 Weeks ($N$ = 6) |
| FrPaSS | 110.59 ± 12.35 | 63.53 ± 4.11* | 44.21 ± 6.32 | 21.84 ± 2.89* |
| CPu(L) | 158.82 ± 12.35 | 67.65 ± 5.88* | 228.42 ± 22.10 | 22.63 ± 1.84* |
| Thalamus | 77.06 ± 3.53 | 239.41 ± 51.18* | 34.21 ± 3.68 | 37.89 ± 6.84 |
| SN | 81.18 ± 13.53 | 63.53 ± 1.17* | 75.53 ± 8.68 | 23.16 ± 3.42* |

Abbreviations: IP$_3$, inositol triphosphate; FrPaSS, frontoparietal cortex CPu(L), lateral caudate putamen; SN, substantia nigra

[a] Values are given in means ± SD fmol/mg tissue using the [$^3$H]microscale. Significant difference from control values: $*P < 0.01$ (t-test).

(Data from Nagasawa and Kogure,[103a] with permission.)

activities in the thalamus and substantia nigra exhibit remarkable differences 4 weeks after recirculation[102,103] (Table 4-10). Different mechanisms may have been responsible for the exofocal postischemic delayed neuronal changes in the two individual areas.

### Disinhibitory Overexcitation in the Substantia Nigra

The mechanisms of retarded neuronal death and increased glucose uptake in the substantia nigra are less easily explained. We speculate that the phenomenon may be explained by abnormal functioning of neurotransmitters in the transsynaptic process associated with this ischemic foci. It has been shown, for example, that the pars reticularis of the substantia nigra consists of fibrous connections originating in the caudate/putamen and projecting over the globus pallidus, forming the striatonigral pathway.[161] The caudate nucleus of the rat contains high concentrations of several neurotransmitters, such as acetylcholine, dopamine, glutamate, substance-P and γ-aminobutyric acid (GABA). The neuroinhibitory transmitter GABA plays an important functional role in the striatonigral pathway.[35,98,104,190] Moreover, on the ischemic side, glucose metabolism was increased approximately 30 percent in the substantia nigra, compared with the corresponding region in the contralateral hemisphere, after 90 minutes of MCA occlusion followed by 1 week of recirculation. Increase in rCGU may be explained by altered neuronal function, hypermetabolism, and diminished inhibitory output from the caudate/putamen, affected by the preceding ischemia. Onodera et al.,[122] using a receptor autoradiographic method, reported that the benzodiazepine receptor density in the pars reticularis of the substantia nigra increased approximately twice as much as the control group after ischemic neuronal death of the lateral part of the caudate/putamen. They deduced that this phenomen reflected denervation hypersensitivity in the substantia nigra, resulting from suppression of the GABAergic output from the ischemic lesion of the caudate/putamen. Disinhibition can induce postsynaptic long-term potentiation or a continuous excitatory state in the substantia nigra. As a result, it could lead to a collapse of homeostasis of the cell and to neuronal death.

Chronologically, [$^3$H]forskolin binding activity was markedly decreased in the lateral segment of the caudate/putamen supplied by the occluded MCA after 90 minutes of ischemia, with no recirculation, and remained low, following various periods of recirculation (Fig. 4-21). On the other hand, no alteration of the activity was seen on day 1, but a marked decrease of [$^3$H]forskolin binding activity was observed 3 days after the ischemic insult in the ipsilateral substantia nigra (Fig. 4-21). This delayed decrease in binding activity in the substantia nigra strongly suggests that striatonigral terminal degeneration at presynaptic sites is caused by preceding ischemic damage of the ipsilateral caudate/putamen and that exofocal postischemic neuronal damage in the substantia nigra is caused by a transsynaptic process associated with the ischemic foci. Tamura et al.,[164] using an MCA occlusion model with no recirculation, observed postischemic hyperemia in the ispilateral substantia nigra of the rat brain and speculated that this hyperemia was related to the hyperactivity of the substantia nigra, which resulted from disinhibition of the striatonigral pathway.

## SLOWLY PROGRESSIVE NEURONAL DAMAGE

Ischemia-induced death of neurons, either death by energy failure or by delayed neuronal death, features of loss of calcium homeostasis, which rapidly progresses, taking at most a few days, even in delayed neuronal death. However, recently we have found another type of postischemic neuronal death in which the evolving process takes weeks to several months to complete: no detectable increase is observed in intracellular calcium content. Degeneration is initiated by

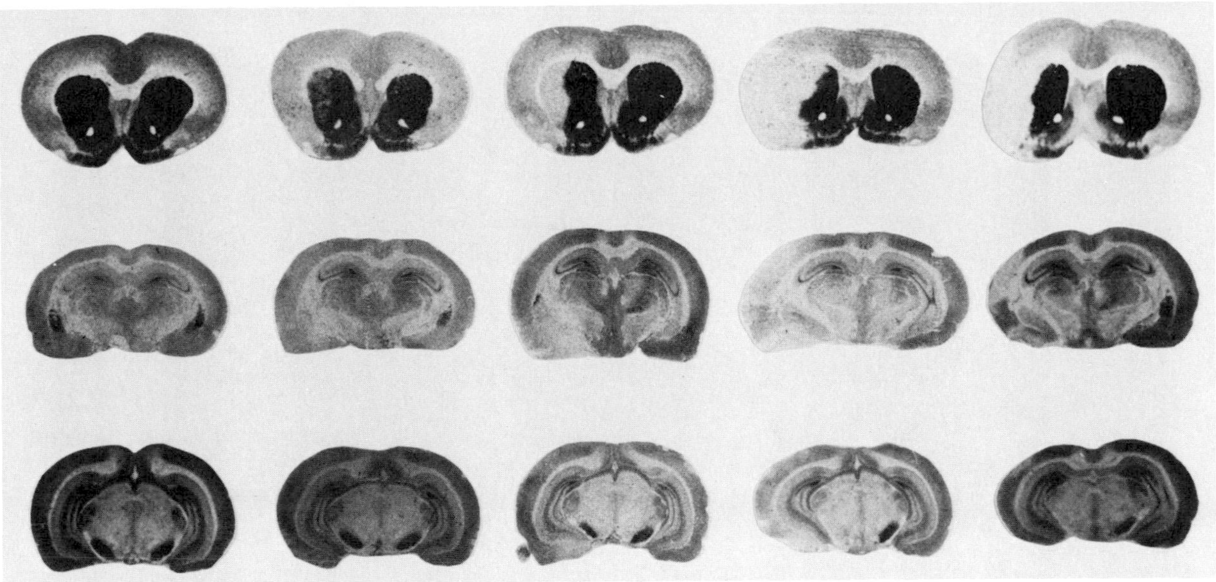


**Fig. 4-21.** [$^3$H]Forskolin binding of rat brain obtained after 90 minutes of middle cerebral artery occlusion followed by 0 hours, 1 day, 3 days, and 4 weeks circulation. Representative autoradiograms show coronal sections at the level of caudate/putamen (*top*), thalamus (*middle*), and substantia nigra (*bottom*). (From Nagasawa and Kogure,[103] with permission.)

a brief, so-called "nonlethal" ischemia, and the outcome is modulated by reactive changes occurring in the surrounding glial processes.

Slowly progressive neuronal death, originally described by Nakano et al.,[107] occurs in the dorsal portion of the caudate nucleus of rat after 15 minutes of middle cerebral artery occlusion. The change, characterized by eosinophilic and pyknotic cells, staining of affected neurons, becomes visible in hematoxylin and eosin (H-E)-stained sections within a few days after the ischemic insult. Those neurons are intimately surrounded by numerous reactive astrocytes (glial fibrillary acidic protein (GFAP)-positive astrocytes) and markedly express the specific binding protein to basic fibroblast growth factor (bFGF) on the eosinophilic neuron[64] (Fig. 4-22).

From the chronological point of view, the density of bFGF binding sites on the pyknotic, eosinophilic neuron becomes maximal 2 weeks after the insult. Affected neurons do not disappear in this model. One month after the insult, those neurons are still acidophilic, but a marked decrease in the density of the bFGF binding sites is observed. Noteworthy is the almost total disappearance of reactive astrocytes from the site. The affected area appears normal at the end of the 3-month observation period.

Pretreatment of tissue sections with bFGF prior to anti-bFGF immunostaining (bFGF-anti-bFGF procedures) intensely labeled many small cells in the ischemic lesions in this study. The most likely explanation for it is that bFGF was bound to these cells; this finding was more directly verified by the labeling of the cells with biotinylated bFGF. That their staining intensity with biotinylated bFGF was markedly reduced by adding excess unlabeled bFGF indicates that the competition occurred between biotinylated and unlabeled bFGF for bFGF-binding sites of these cells.

To clarify what type of cells was labeled with bFGF, sequential stainings with H-E and then bFGF-anti-bFGF procedures were performed; these studies demonstrated that bFGF-labeled cells were exclusively ischemic neurons characterized by pyknotic nuclei and homogeneously eosinophilic cytoplasm in H-E preparations. The possibility that these ischemic cells were derived from astrocytes, microglia, or blood cells is unlikely because these cells were negative for GFAP, Ricinus communis agglutinin 1 (RCA 1) binding, and leukocyte-common antigen (LCA).

In order to reveal the chemical substrate for bFGF binding, the tissue sections were incubated with heparinase or heparitinase, which degrades heparin or heparan sulfate, respectively, before the bFGF-anti-bFGF procedures, because bFGF is known to have an affinity for heparin and heparan sulfate.[143] While pretreatment of tissue sections with heparinase did not affect the binding of bFGF to ischemic cells, heparitinase pretreatment markedly reduced its binding, suggesting that heparan sulfate is the chemical substrate for bFGF binding to the cells.

In vivo, heparan sulfate is bound to a core protein in the form of heparan sulfate proteoglycan (HSPG), which is a major proteoglycan in brain.[37] Recently, it

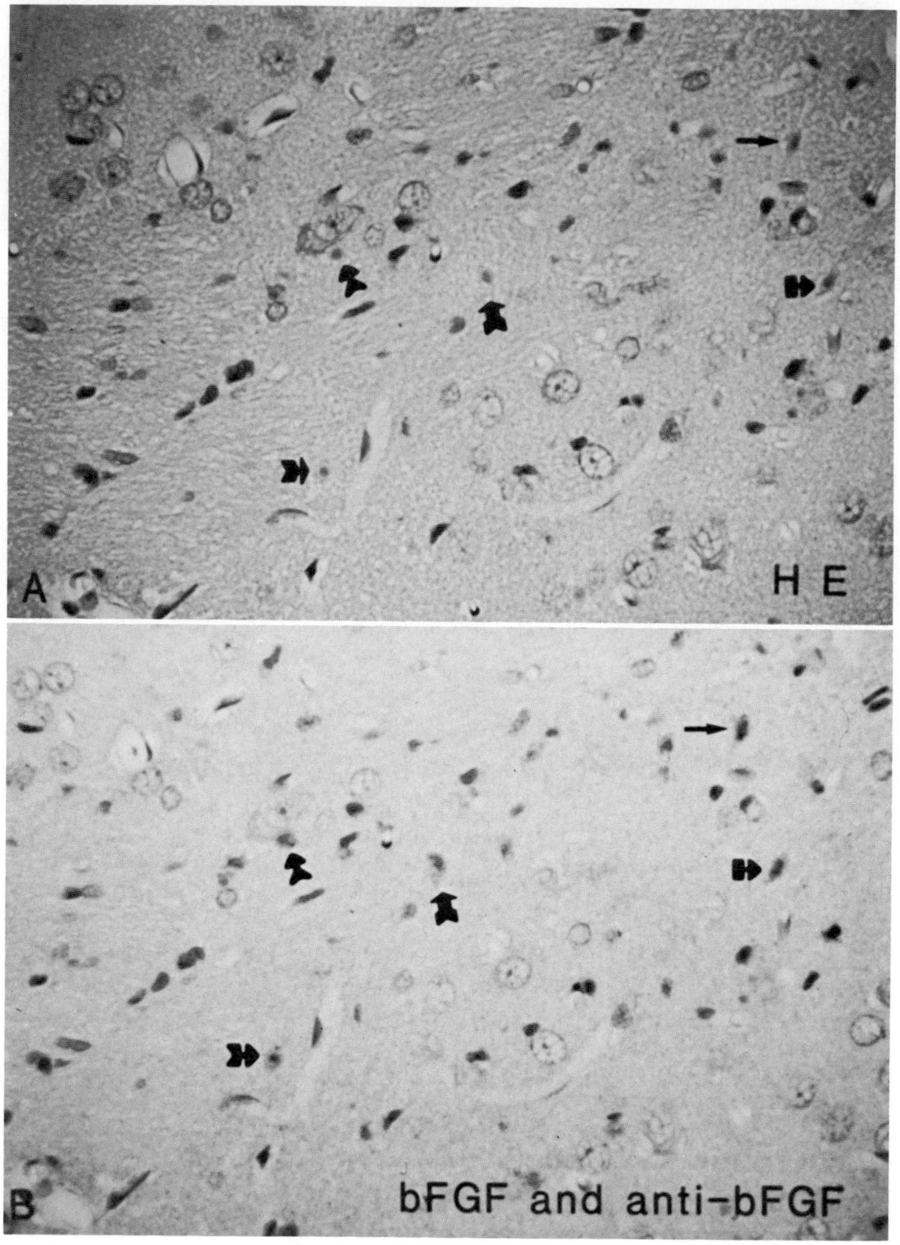


**Fig. 4-22.** (**A & B**) Ischemic neurons with pyknotic nuclei and eosinophilic cytoplasm are seen to have bFGF-binding sites in the rat striatum 14 days after 1 hour of middle cerebral artery occlusion. (Fig. A: H & E; Fig. B: immunostained with anti-bFGF antibody. Both Fig. A and Fig. B are of the same brain section.) (From Kato et al.,[64] with permission.)

has been reported that bFGF bound to HSPG becomes resistant to various proteases[143] and that these bFGF-HSPG complexes have the ability to bind to specific receptors present in the cell membrane and produce their biologic effects.[137,143] Thus, HSPG appears to play an important role in the interaction between bFGF and its specific receptor. Furthermore, HSPG has been reported to have trophic effects on neurons[19,85,185] The appearance of abundant bFGF-binding sites, probably HSPG, in or on the ischemic neurons in the present study may contribute to the repair process, successful or abortive, of insulted neurons. However, the alternate explanation that the accumulation of HSPG is a pathologic response of dying neurons could not be ruled out.

To clarify the slowly progressive neuronal changes, Onodera et al.[115] studied 20 minutes of forbrain ischemia in the rat and showed that a total loss of CA1 pyramidal cells of the hippocampus was associated with no changes in the thickness of the sector 7 days after the ictus. Marked atrophy of the CA1 subsector and approximately 40 percent pyramidal cell loss in the CA3 cells were observed 3 months after the ischemic insult. In addition to this postischemic, slowly progressive cell loss in both the glia cells surrounding the affected CA1 neurons and the pyramidal neurons in the CA3 subfield, marked ectopic sprouting of mossy fibers from the granular cell in the dentate gyrus to the supragranular layer of the dentate gyrus and the infrapyramidal layer of the CA3 was evident.

A similar type of marked mossy fiber sprouting was seen after selective lesioning of hippocampal CA3 neurons with kainic acid.[193] If fetal hippocampal neurons were grafted into lesioned CA1 or CA3, mossy fibers invaded the transplants and eventually prevented the posttraumatic aberrant sprouting of mossy fibers.

Presumably, such slowly progressive postischemic and/or posttraumatic processes, including the aberrant mossy fiber sprouting, are possibly only with trauma-mediated expression of specific genes, including groups of guide-RNA, or changes in the DNA sequence itself. Prevention of sprouting by hippocampal graft strongly suggests the the grafts and recipient tissue start an avid intercellular membrane communication in an organized fashion to promote reconstruction processes of lost neuronal network.

## CONCLUSION

In conclusion, ischemia must be considered a cytohazard to the brain. As with other harmful stress to the brain, ischemia becomes lethal to the brain cells when maintainence of structural and functional homeostasis is affected. Below such a threshold, ischemia rouses a variety of stress responses in the affected area.

The stress response is provoked through agonist-mediated membrane-borne second messengers and the resultant activation of the intracellular signal transduction system. We have learned recently from a neat, well-controlled experiment[63] that the amount of agonist released into the synaptic cleft by ischemia may be important only to the initiation of the abrupt and nonphysiologic intracellular response, and that the fate of the affected cells after the triggering is modified by a variety of factors interacting with the progression of the cascade reaction along the signal transduction system.

Injured brain cells can recover their structural and functional integrity if the proper environment for the reconstruction process can be reestablished. Intracellular transmembrane signaling may play an important role in reestablishing such an environment in the affected brain tissue. If the cells in the vicinity of the injury fail to respond to intracellular transmembrane signaling, the affected brain cells may become necrotic, degenerate, and eventually disappear from the site.

If this occurs, one can probably ameliorate the ischemic outcome by many means, including pharmacologic approaches. A means of estimating the width of the therapeutic window and determining the pivotal steps to be modified involves the use of a cascade algorithm. It seems likely that membrane perturbation causes(1) loss of osmotic barrier to the cytosol, (2) derangement of the transport system across the membrane (e.g., ions and water, and amino acids), and (3) overproduction of phospholipid-derived messengers to the gene expression. We conclude that, at present, protecting the membrane from avid lipolysis is the best way to minimize the ischemic brain cell injury.

## ACKNOWLEDGMENT

We would like to acknowledge our colleagues, especially Drs. H. Nagasawa, M. Izumiyama, H. Onodera, K. Abe, Y. Shiga, H. Aoki, T. Araki, M. Yoshidomi, H. Hara, and Y. Yamasaki of our department, for their effort and advice in preparing the manuscript.

## REFERENCES

1. Abe K, Kawagoe J, Sato S et al: Induction of the "zinc finger" gene after transient focal ischemia in rat cerebral cortex. Neurosci Lett 123:248, 1991
2. Abe K, Kogure K, Yamamoto H et al: Mechanism of arachidonic acid liberation during ischemia in gerbil cerebral cortex. J Neurochem 48:503, 1987
3. Abe K, Tanzi RE, Kogure K: Induction of HSP70 mRNA after transient ischemia in gerbil brain. Neurosci Lett 125:166, 1991
4. Abe K, Tanzi RE, Kogure K: Selective induction of Kunitz-type protease inhibitor domain-containing amyloid precursor protein mRNA after persistent focal ischemia in rat cerebral cortex. Neurosci Lett 125:172, 1991
5. Abe K, Yoshidomi M, Kogure K: Arachidonic acid metabolism in ischemic neuronal damage. Ann NY Acad Sci 559:259, 1989
6. Alps BJ, Calder C, Wilson AD: Comparative protective effects of nicardipine, flunarizine, lidoflazine and nimodipine against ischemic injury in the hippocampus of the Mongolian gerbils. Br J Pharmacol 93:877, 1988
7. Araki T, Kato H, Inoue T, Kogure K: Regional impairment of protein synthesis following brief cerebral ischemia in the gerbil. Acta Neuropathol 79:501, 1990
8. Araki T, Kato H, Kogure K: Selective neuronal vulnerability following transient cerebral ischemia in the gerbil: distribution and time course. Acta Neurol Scand 80:548, 1989
9. Astrup J, Siesjo BK, Symon L: Threshold in cerebral ischemia: the ischemic penumbra. Stroke 12:723, 1981
10. Atkinson DE: The energy charge of the adenylate pool as a regulatory parameter. Biochemistry 7:4030, 1966

11. Aveldano M, Bazan NG: Differential lipid deacylation during brain ischemia in a homeotherm and a poikilotherm: content and composition of free fatty acids and triglycerols. Brain Res 100:99, 1975
12. Bazan N: Significance of phospholipase A2 activation and second messengers in brain damage. In Kogure K, Siesjö BK (eds): Proceedings of Sendai Forum '91, in press.
13. Benveniste H, Drejer J, Schousboe A, Diemer NH: Elevation of the extracellular concentrations of glutamate and aspartate in rat hippocampus during transient cerebral ischemia monitored by intracerebral microdialysis. J Neurochem 43:1369, 1984
14. Berridge MJ, Irvine RF: Inositol triphosphate, a novel second messenger in cellular signal transduction. Nature 312:315, 1984
15. Black KL, Hoff JT: Leukotrienes increase blood-brain barrier permeability following intraparenchymal injections in rats. Ann Neurol 18:349, 1985
16. Bodsch W, Takahashi K, Barbier B et al: Cerebral proteins and ischemia. Prog Brain Res 63:197, 1985
17. Bondy SC, Walker CH: Polyamines contribute to calcium-stimulated release of aspartate from brain particulate fraction. Brain Res 371:96, 1986
18. Broston CO, Huang YC, Breckenridge BM et al: Identification of a calcium-binding protein as a calcium-dependent regulation of brain adenylate cyclase. Proc Natl Acad Sci USA 72:64, 1975
19. Chernoff EAG: The role of endogenous heparan sulfate proteoglycan in adhesion and neurite outgrowth from dorsal root ganglia. Tissue Cell 20:165, 1988
20. Choi DW, Maulucci-Gedde M, Kriegstein AR: Glutamate neurotoxicity in cortical cell culture. J Neurosci 7:357, 1987
21. Chopp M, Chen H, Ho KL et al: Transient hyperthermia protects against subsequent forebrain ischemic cell damage in the rat. Neurology (NY) 39:1396, 1989
22. Churn SB, Taft WC, DeLorenzo RJ: Effects of ischemia on multifunctional calcium/calmodulin-dependent protein kinase type II in the gerbil. Stroke, suppl 3. 21:III-112, 1990
23. Coyle JT, Bird SJ, Evans RH et al: Excitatory amino acid neurotoxins: selectivity, specificity, and mechanisms of action. Neurosci Res Prog Bull 19:331, 1981
24. Crain BJ, Westerkam WD, Harrison AH, Nadler JV: Selective neuronal death after transient forebrain ischemia in the Mongolian gerbil: a silver impregnation study. Neuroscience 27:387, 1988
25. Crockard A, Iannotti F, Hunstock AT et al: Cerebral blood flow and edema following carotid occlusion in the gerbil. Stroke 11:494, 1980
26. Deshpande JK, Wieloch T: Ameriolation of ischaemic brain damage by postischaemic treatment with flunarizine. Neurol Res 7:27, 1985
27. Dienel GA, Cruz NF, Rosenfeld SJ: Temporal profiles of proteins responsive to transient ischemia. J Neurochem 44:600, 1985
28. Domer FR, Bortje SB, Bing EG, Raddix I: Histamine and acetylcholine induced changes in the permeability of the blood-brain barrier of normotensive and spontaneously hypertensive rats. Neuropharmacology 22:615, 1983
29. Duffy TE, Nelson SR, Lowry OH: Cerebral carbohydrate metabolism during acute hypoxia and recovery. J Neurochem 19:959, 1972
30. Duffy TE, Levy DE, Pulsinelli WA: Cerebral hypoxia-ischemia and the metabolic rate. p. 352. In Passoneau JV et al (eds): Cerebral Metabolism and Neural Function. Williams & Wilkins, Baltimore, 1980
31. Edgar AD, Strosznajder J, Horrocks LA: Activation of ethanolamine phospholipase A2 in brain during ischemia. J Neurochem 39:1111, 1982
32. Everett NB, Simmonds B, Lasher EP: Distribution of blood (Fe-59) and plasma (I-131) volumes of rats determined by liquid nitrogen freezing. Circ Res 4:419, 1956
33. Fisher SK, Agranoff BW: Receptor activation and inositol lipid hydrolysis in neural tissues. J Neurochem 48:999, 1987
34. Flaherty KM, DeLuca-Flaherty C, McKay DB: Three-dimensional structure of the ATPase fragment of a 70K heat shock cognate protein. Nature 346:623, 1990
35. Fonnum F, Gottesfeld Z, Grofova I: I. Distribution of glutamate decarboxylase, choline acetyltransferase and aromatic amino acid decarboxylase in the basal ganglia of normal and operated rats: evidence for striatopallidal, striatopeduncular, and striatonigral GABAergic fibers. Brain Res 143:125, 1978
36. Fonnum F, Storm-Mathisen J, Divac I: Biochemical evidence for glutamate as neurotransmitter in corticostriatal and corticothalamic fibers in rat brain. Neuroscience 6:863, 1981
37. Fransson L-A: Structure and function of cell-associated proteoglycans. Trends Biochem Sci 12:406, 1987
38. Fukunaga K, Goto S, Miyamoto E: Immunohistochemical localization of $Ca^{2+}$/calmodulin-dependent protein kinase II in rat brain and various tissues. J Neurochem 51:1070, 1988
39. Furukawa K, Yamana K, Kogure K: Post-ischemic alterations of spontaneous activities in rat hippocampal CA1 neurons. Brain Res 530:257, 1990
40. Gessler M, Poustka A, Cavenee W et al: Homozygous deletion in Wilms tumors of a zinc-finger gene identified by chromosome jumping. Nature 343:774, 1990
41. Gotoh O, Asano T, Koide T et al: Ischemic brain edema following occlusion of the middle cerebral artery in the rat. I. The time course of the brain water, sodium, and potassium contents and blood-brain barrier permeability to $^{125}I$-albumin. Stroke 16:101, 1985
42. Gotti B, Duverger D, Bertin J et al: Ifenprodil and SL 82.0715 as cerebral anti-ischemic agents. I. Evidence for efficacy in models of focal cerebral ischemia. J Pharmacol Exp Ther 247:1211, 1988
43. Grab DJ, Carlin RK, Siekevitz P: Function of calmodulin in postsynaptic densities. II. Pres-

ence of a calmodulin-activatable protein kinase activity. J Cell Biol 89:440, 1981
44. Grofova I, Rinvik E: An experimental electron microscopic study on the striato-nigral projection in the cat. Exp Brain Res 11:249, 1970
45. Hara H, Onodera H, Yoshidomi M et al: Staurosporine, a novel protein kinase C inhibitor, prevents postischemic neuronal damage in the gerbil and rat. J Cereb Blood Flow Metabol 10:646, 1990
46. Hoshi T, Garber SS, Aldrich RW: Effect of forskolin on voltage-gated $K^+$ channels is independent of adenylate cyclase activation. Science 240:1652, 1988
47. Hossmann K-A: Cortical steady potential, impedance and excitability changes during and after total ischemia of cat brain. Exp Neurol 28:389, 1971
48. Hossmann K-A, Zimmerman V: Resuscitation of the monkey brain after 1 hour's complete ischemia. I. Physiological and morphological observations. Brain Res 81:59, 1974
49. Iqbal Z, Koenig NH: Polyamines appear to be second messengers in mediating $Ca^{2+}$-fluxes and neurotransmitter release in potassium-stimulated synaptosomes. Biochem Biophys Res Commun 133:563, 1985
50. Iseki S: DNA strand breaks in rat tissues as detected by in situ nick translation. Exp Cell Res 167:311, 1986
51. Ito U, Spatz M, Walker JT, Klatzo I: Experimental cerebral ischemia in Mongolian gerbils. I. Light microscopic observations. Acta Neuropathol (Berl) 32:209, 1975
52. Izumiyama K, Kogure K: Prevention of delayed neuronal death in gerbil hippocampus by ion channel blockers. Stroke 19:1003, 1988
53. Izumiyama M, Kogure K, Lockwood AH et al: Penetration of red blood cells into the ischemic boundary in the early phase of cerebral embolism. p. 55. In Tomita M, Sawada T, Naritomi H, Heiss W-D (eds): Cerebral Hyperemia and Ischemia: From the Standpoint of Cerebral Blood Volume. Elsevier, Amsterdam, 1988
54. Jensen JR, Lynch G, Baudry M: Polyamines stimulate mitochondrial calcium transport in rat brain. J Neurochem 48:765, 1987
55. Jorgensen MB, Deckert J, Wright DC, Gehlert DR: Delayed c-fos proto-oncogene expression in the rat hippocampus induced by transient global ischemia: an in situ hybridization study. Brain Res 484:393, 1989
56. Kato H, Araki T, Hara H, Kogure K: Sequential changes in muscarinic acetylcholine, adenosine A1 and calcium antagonist binding sites in the gerbil hippocampus following repeated brief ischemia. Brain Res 553:33, 1991
57. Kato H, Araki T, Hara H, Kogure K: Autoradiographic analysis of second-messenger systems in the gerbil hippocampus following repeated brief ischemic insults. Brain Res Bull 27:759, 1991
58. Kato H, Araki T, Kogure K: Role of the excitotoxic mechanism in the development of neuronal damage following repeated brief cerebral ischemia in the gerbil: protective effects of MK-801 and pentobarbital. Brain Res 516:175, 1990
59. Kato H, Araki T, Kogure K et al: Sequential cerebral blood flow changes in short-term cerebral ischemia in gerbils. Stroke 21:1346, 1990
60. Kato H, Kogure K: Neuronal damage following non-lethal but repeated cerebral ischemia in the gerbil. Acta Neuropathol 79:494, 1990
61. Kato H, Kogure K, Nakano S: Neuronal damage following repeated brief ischemia in the gerbil. Brain Res 479:366, 1989
62. Kato H, Kogure K, Sakamoto N, Watanabe T: Greater disturbance of water and ion homeostasis in the periphery of experimental focal cerebral ischemia. Exp Neurol 96:118, 1987
63. Kato H, Liu Y, Araki T, Kogure K: Temporal profile of the effects of pretreatment with brief cerebral ischemia on the neuronal damage following secondary ischemic insult in the gerbil: cumulative damage and protective effects. Brain Res 553:238, 1991
64. Kato T, Nakano S, Kogure K et al: The binding of basic fibroblast growth factor to rat ischemic neurons. Neuropathol Appl Neurobiol 1992, in press.
65. Kennedy MB, McGuinness T, Greengard P: A calcium/calmodulin-dependent protein kinase from mammalian brain that phosphorylates synapsin I: partial purification and characterization. J Neurosci 3:818, 1983
66. Kikkawa U, Kishimoto A, Nishizuka Y: The protein kinase C family: heterogeneity and its implications. Annu Rev Biochem 58:31, 1989
67. Kingston RE, Baldwin AS, Jr, Sharp PA: Regulation of heat shock protein 70 gene expression by c-myc. Nature 312:280, 1984
68. Kirino T: Delayed neuronal death in the gerbil hippocampus following ischemia. Brain Res 239:57, 1982
69. Kirino T, Tsujita Y, Tamura A: Induced tolerance to ischemia in gerbil hippocampal neurons. J Cereb Blood Flow Metab 11:299, 1991
70. Kitagawa K, Matsumoto M, Niinobe M et al: Microtubule-associated protein 2 as a sensitive marker for cerebral ischemic damage—immunohistochemical investigation of dendritic damage. Neuroscience 31:401, 1989
71. Kitagawa K, Matsumoto M, Tagaya M et al: "Ischemic tolerance" phenomenon found in the brain. Brain Res 528:21, 1990
72. Kitagawa K, Matsumoto M, Tagaya M et al: Hyperthermia-induced neuronal protection against ischemic injury in gerbils. J Cereb Blood Flow Metabol 11:449, 1991
73. Kleihues P, Hossmann K-A, Pegg AE et al: Resuscitation of the monkey brain after one hour complete ischemia. III. Indications of metabolic recovery. Brain Res 95:61, 1975
74. Klumpp S, Guerini D, Krebs J, Schultz JE: Effect of tryptic calmodulin fragments on guanylate cyclase activity from *Paramecium tetraurelia.* Biochem Biophys Res Commun 142:857, 1987
75. Kogure K: Lack of oxygen in cerebral energy metabolism. Japan J Neuropsychopharmacol 14:277, 1982
76. Kogure K: Signal transducing system in postischemic death of selectively vulnerable brain

cells. p. 95. In Kanazawa I (ed): Neurotransmitters. Focus on excitatory amino acids. Excerpta Medica, Amsterdam, 1988
77. Kogure K, Busto R, Scheinberg P: The role of hydrostatic pressure in ischemic brain edema. Ann Neurol 9:273, 1981
78. Kogure A, Busto R, Schwartzman RJ: The dissociation of cerebral blood flow, metabolism, and function in the early stages of developing cerebral infarction. Ann Neurol 8:278, 1980
79. Kogure K, Busto R, Scheinberg P et al.: Dynamics of cerebral metabolism during moderate hypercapnia. J Neurochem 24:471, 1975
80. Kogure K, Busto R, Scheinberg P, Reinmuth OM: Energy metabolism and water content in rat brain during the early stage of development of cerebral infarction. Brain 97:103, 1974
81. Kogure K, Onodera H, Tsuda T, Araki T, Nishioka K: Roles of calcium-activated enzymic reactions in ischemia-induced neuronal injury. p. 240. In Hartmann A, Kuschinsky W (eds): Cerebral Ischemia and Calcium. Springer-Verlag, Berlin, 1989
82. Kogure K, Tanaka J, Araki T: The mechanism of ischemia-induced brain cell injury: the membrane theory. Neurochem Pathol 9:145, 1988
83. Kogure K, Tobita M, Sato H, Onodera H: Impairment of protein synthesis in selectively vulnerable neurons. p. 119. In Raichle ME, Powers WJ (eds): Cerebrovascular Diseases. Raven Press, New York, 1987
84. Komulainen H, Bondy SC: Transient elevation of intrasynaptosomal free calcium by putrescine. Brain Res 401:50, 1987
85. Lander AD, Fujii DK, Gospodarowicz D, Reichardt LF: Characterization of a factor that promotes neurite outgrowth: evidence linking activity to a heparan sulfate proteoglycan. J Cell Biol 94:574, 1982
86. Levin VA, Ausman JI: Relationship of peripheral venous hematocrit to brain hematocrit. J Appl Physiol 26:433, 1969
87. Levy DE, Duffy TE: Cerebral energy metabolism during transient ischemia and recovery in the gerbil. J Neurochem 28:63, 1977
88. Lewis MT, Pelham HB: Involvement of ATP in the nuclear and nucleolar functions of the 70 kd heat shock protein. EMBO J 4:3137, 1985
89. Lowe DG, Moran LA: Molecular cloning and analysis of DNA complementary to three mouse Mr=68000 heat shock protein mRNA. J Biol Chem 261:2102, 1986
90. Lowry OH, Passonneau JV, Hasselberger FX et al: Effect of ischemia on known substrates and cofactors of the glycolytic pathway in the brain. J Biol Chem 239:18, 1964
91. Magnussen KG, Wieloch TW: Impairment of protein ubiquitination may cause delayed neuronal death. Neurosci Lett 96:264, 1989
92. Malenka RC, Kauer JA, Perkel DJ et al: An essential role for postsynaptic calmodulin and protein kinase activity in long-term potentiation. Nature 340:554, 1989
93. Malenka RC, Madison DV, Nicoll RA: Potentiation of synaptic transmission in the hippocampus by phorbol esters. Nature 321:175, 1986
94. Manilow R, Schulman H, Tsien RW: Inhibition of postsynaptic PCK or CaMKII blocks induction but not expression of LTP. Science 245:862, 1989
95. Marion J, Wolfe LS: Origin of the arachidonic acid released post-mortem in rat forebrain. Biochim Biophys Acta 574:25, 1979
96. Marx JL: The fos gene as "master switch." Science 237:854, 1987
97. Matthews MA: Death of the central neuron: an electron microscopic study of thalamic retrograde degeneration following cortical ablation. J Neurocytol 2:265, 1973
98. McNair J, Sutin J, Tsubokawa T: Supression of cell firing in the substantia nigra by caudate nucleus stimulation. Exp Neurol 37:395, 1972
99. McPhail LC, Clayton CC, Synderman R: A potential second messenger role for unsaturated fatty acids: activation of $Ca^{2+}$-dependent protein kinase. Science 224:622, 1984
100. Miller R: Protein kinase C: a key regulator of neuronal excitability? Trends Neurosci 9:538, 1986
101. Nagasawa H, Kogure K: Exo-focal postischemic neuronal death in the rat brain. Brain Res 524:196, 1990
101a. Nagasawa H, Kogure K: Multi-focal delayed neuronal damage after transient regional ischemia. Mechanism of vascular dementia. Clin Neurol 30:396, 1990
102. Nagasawa H, Kogure K: Alterations of [$^3$H]inositol 1,4,5-triphosphate binding in the postischemic rat brain. Neurosci Lett 133:129, 1991
103. Nagasawa H, Kogure K: Exo-focal postischemic neuronal damage in the rat brain: alteration of [$^3$H]forskolin binding using in vitro autoradiography. Brain Res 563:7, 1991
103a. Nagasawa H, Kogure K: Mapping second messenger systems in exo-focal postischemic brain areas of the rat: in vitro [$^3$H]inositol 1,4,5-triphosphate and [$^3$H]forskolin binding. J Cereb Blood Flow Metabol 11(Suppl 2):S8, 1991
104. Nagy J, Carter D, Fibiger H: Anterior striatal projections to the globus pallidus, entopeduncular nucleus and substantia nigra in the rat: the GABA connection. Brain Res 158:15, 1978
105. Nakano S, Kato H, Kogure K: Neuronal damage in the rat hippocampus in a new model of repeated reversible transient cerebral ischemia. Brain Res 490:178, 1989
106. Nakano S, Kogure K, Abe K, Yae T: Ischemia-induced alterations in lipid metabolism of the gerbil cerebral cortex. I. Changes in free fatty acid liberation. J Neurochem 54:1911, 1990
107. Nakano S, Kogure K, Fujikura H: Ischemia-induced slowly progressive neuronal damage in the rat brain. Neuroscience 38:115, 1990
108. Nakata N, Kato H, Liu Y, Kogure K: Effects of repeated cerebral ischemia on extracellular glutamate concentration in the gerbil hippocampus. Neurosci Lett 1992, in press.
109. Neve RL: Genetic studies support a neuronal origin for the beta amyloid polypeptide. Neurobiol Aging 10:400, 1989
110. Nicchitta C, Williamson JR: Spermine: a regula-

tor of mitochondria; calcium cycling. J Biol Chem 259:12978, 1984
111. Nishizuka Y: The role of protein kinase C in cell surface signal transduction and tumor promotion. Nature 308:693, 1984
112. Nishizuka Y: The molecular heterogeneity of protein kinase C and its implications for cellular regulation. Nature 334:601, 1988
113. Nowak TS Jr, Ikeda J, Nakajima T: 70-kDa heat shock protein and c-fos gene expression after transient ischemia. Stroke, suppl 3. 21:III-107, 1990
114. Olsen SP: Free oxygen radicals decrease electrical resistance of microvascular endothelium in brain. Acta Physiol Scand 129:181, 1987
115. Onodera H, Aoki H, Yae T, Kogure K: Post-ischemic synaptic plasticity in the rat hippocampus after long-term survival: histochemical and autoradiographic study. Neuroscience 38:125, 1990
116. Onodera H, Araki T, Kogure K: Protein kinase C activity in the rat hippocampus after forebrain ischemia: autoradiographic analysis by [$^3$H]phorbol 12,13-dibutyrate. Brain Res 481:1, 1989
117. Onodera H, Hara H, Kogure K et al: $Ca^{2+}$/calmodulin-dependent protein kinase II immunoreactivity in the rat hippocampus after forebrain ischemia. Neurosci Lett 113:134, 1990
118. Onodera H, Iijima K, Kogure K: Mononucleotide metabolism in the rat brain after transient ischemia. J Neurochem 46:1704, 1986
119. Onodera H, Kogure K: Mapping second messenger systems in the rat hippocampus after transient forebrain ischemia: in vitro [$^3$H]forskolin and [$^3$H]inositol 1,4,5-trisphosphate binding. Brain Res 487:343, 1989
120. Onodera H, Kogure K: Calcium antagonist, adenosine A1, and muscarinic binding in rat hippocampus after transient ischemia. Stroke 21:771, 1990
121. Onodera H, Kogure K, Ono Y et al: Proto-onocogene c-fos is transiently induced in the rat cerebral cortex after forebrain ischemia. Neurosci Lett 98:101, 1989
122. Onodera H, Sato G, Kogure K: GABA and benzodiazepine receptors in the gerbil brain after transient ischemia: demonstration by quantitative receptor autoradiography. J Cereb Blood Flow Metab 7:82, 1987
123. Parson LC, Guthrie MD: Nerve fiber degeneration following a single experimental cerebral concussion in the rat. Neurosci Lett 24:199, 1981
124. Paschen W, Hallmayer J, Mies G: Regional profiles of polyamines in reversible cerebral ischemia of Mongolian gerbils. Neurochem Pathol 7:143, 1987
125. Paschen W, Hallmayer J, Mies G, Rohn G: Ornithine decarboxylase activity and putrescine levels in reversible cerebral ischemia of Mongolian gerbils: effect of barbiturate. J Cereb Blood Flow Metabol 10:236, 1990
126. Paschen W, Hallmayer J, Rohn G: Regional changes of polyamine profiles after reversible cerebral ischemia in Mongolian gerbils: effects of nimodipine and barbiturate. Neurochem Pathol 8:27, 1988
127. Paschen W, Rohn G, Meese Co et al: Poliamine metabolism in reversible cerebral ischemia: effect of $\alpha$-difluoromethylornithine. Brain Res 453:9, 1988
128. Paschen W, Schmidt-Kastner R, Djuricic B et al: Polyamine changes in reversible cerebral ischemia. J Neurochem 49:35, 1987
129. Paschen W, Schmidt-Kastner R, Hallmayer J, Djuricic B: Polyamines in cerebral ischemia. Neurochem Pathol 9:1, 1988
130. Paschen W, Widmann R, Weber C: Changes in regional polyamine profiled in transient cerebral ischemia (single versus repetitive ischemia): evidence for release of polyamines from injured neurons. Neurosci Lett 135:121, 1992
131. Pelham HRB: HSP70 accelerates the recovery of nucleolar morphology after heat shock. EMBO J 3:3095, 1984
132. Pelham HRB: Heat shock and the sorting of luminal ER protein. EMBO J 8:3171, 1989
133. Pulsinelli WA, Brierley JB, Plum F: Temporal profile of neuronal damage in a model of transient forebrain ischemia. Ann Neurol 11:491, 1982
134. Pulsinelli WA, Duffy TE: Regional energy balance in rat brain after transient forebrain ischemia. J Neurochem 40:1500, 1983
135. Ransom RW, Stec NL: Cooperaive modulation of [$^3$H]MK-801 binding to the *N*-methyl-D-aspartate receptor-ion complex by L-glutamate, glycine and polyamines. J Neurochem 51:830, 1988
136. Rauscher FJ, Cohen DR, Curran T et al: Fos-associated protein p39 is the product of the jun proto-oncogene. Science 240:1010, 1988
137. Rifkin DB, Moscatelli D: Recent developments in the cell biology of basic fibroblast growth factor. J Cell Biol 109:1, 1989
138. Rosenberg GB, Minocherhomjee AM, Storm DR: Reconstitution of calmodulin-sensitive adenylate cyclase from bovine brain with phospholipids, calmodulin, and beta-adrenergic receptors. Methods Enzymol 139:776, 1987
139. Rothman SM, Olney JW: Glutamate and the pathophysiology of hypoxic-ischemic brain damage. Ann Neurol 19:105, 1986
140. Rottenberg H, Marbach M: Regulation of $Ca^{2+}$ transport in brain mitochondria. I. The mechanism of spermine enhancement of $Ca^{2+}$ uptake and retention. Biochim Biophys Acta 1016:77, 1990
141. Ruppert C, Wille W: Proto-oncogene c-fos is highly induced by disruption of neonatal but not of mature brain tissue. Mol Brain Res 2:51, 1987
142. Sakamoto N, Kogure K, Kato H, Ohtomo H: Disturbed $Ca^{2+}$ homeostasis in the gerbil hippocampus following brief transient ischemia. Brain Res 364:372, 1986
143. Saksela O, Moscatelli D, Sommer A, Rifkin DB: Endothelial cell-derived heparan sulfate binds basic fibroblast growth factor and protects it from proteolytic degradation. J Cell Biol 107:743, 1988
144. Salbaum JM, Weidermann A, Lemaire HG: The

promotor of Alzheimer's disease amyloid A4 precursor gene. EMBO J 7:2807, 1988

145. Seamon KB, Daly JW: High-affinity binding of forskolin to rat brain membranes. Adv Cyclic Nucleotide Res 19:125, 1985
146. Seamon KB, Padgett W, Daly JW: Forskolin: unique diterpene activator of adenylate cyclase in membranes and intact cells. Proc Natl Acad Sci USA 78:3363, 1981
147. Seiler N, Bolkenius FN: Polyamine reutilization and turnover in brain. Neurochem Res 10:529, 1985
148. Sergate S, Kim HD: Inhibition of 3-*O*-methylglucose transport in human erythrocytes by forskolin. J Biol Chem 260:14677, 1985
149. Shanahan MF, Morris DP, Edwards BM: [$^3$H]Forskolin: direct photoaffinity labeling of the erythrocyte D-glucose transporter. J Biol Chem 262:5978, 1987
150. Sheng M, Greenberg ME: The regulation and function of c-fos and other immediate early genes in the nervous system. Neuron 4:477, 1990
151. Shiga Y, Onodera H, Kogure K et al: Neutrophil as a mediator of ischemic edema formation in the brain. Neurosci Lett 125:110, 1991
152. Siesjö BK: Brain Energy Metabolism. Wiley, New York, 1978
153. Siesjö BK: Historical overview, calcium, ischemia, and death of brain cells. Ann NY Acad Sci 522:638, 1988
154. Siesjö BK: Bengtsson F: Calciumfluxes, calcium antagonists, and calcium-related pathology in brain ischemia, hypoglycemia, and spreading depression: a unifying hypothesis. J Cereb Blood Flow Metabol 9:127, 1989
155. Singh L, Oles R, Woodruff G: In vivo interaction of a polyamine with the NMDA receptor. Eur J Pharmacol 180:391, 1990
156. Sprosen TM, Woodruff G: Polyamines potentiate NMDA whole-cell currents in cultured striatal neurons. Eur J Pharmacol 179:477, 1990
157. Steward O: Reorganization of neuronal connections following CNS trauma: principles and experimental paradigms. J Neurotrauma 6:99, 1989
158. Sukhatme VP, Kartha S, Toback et al: A novel early growth response gene rapidly induced by fibroblast, epithelial cells and lymphocyte mitogenes. Oncogene Res 1:343, 1987
159. Sun GY, Foudin LL: On the status of lysolecithin in rat cerebral cortex during ischemia. J Neurochem 43:1081, 1984
160. Suzuki R, Yamaguchi T, Li C-L, Klatzo I: The effects of 5-minute ischemia in Mongolian gerbils. II. Changes of spontaneous neuronal activity in cerbral cortex and CA1 sector of hippocampus. Acta Neuropathol (Berl) 60:217, 1983
161. Szabo J: Projections from the body of the caudate nucleus in the rhesus monkey. Exp Neurol 27:1, 1970
162. Szekely AM, Barbaccia ML, Alho H, Costa E: In primary cultures of cerebellar granule cells the activation of *N*-methyl-D-aspartate-sensitive glutamate receptors induces c-fos mRNA expression. Mol Pharmacol 35:401, 1989
163. Szekely AM, Costa E, Grayson DR: Transcriptional program coordination by *N*-methyl-D-aspartate-sensitive glutamate receptor stimulation in primary cultures of cerebellar neurons. Mol Pharmacol 38:624, 1990
164. Tamura A, Nakayama H, Kirino T et al: Remote disinhibition hyperemia after focal cerebral ischemia. p. 195. In Tomita M, Sawada T, Naritomi H, Heiss WD (eds): Cerebral Hyperemia and Ischemia: From the Standpoint of Cerebral Blood Volume. Elsevier, Amsterdam, 1988
165. Tanzi RE, McClatchey AI, Lamperti ED et al: Protease inhibitor domain encoded by an amyloid protein precursor mRNA associated with Alzheimer's disease. Nature 331:528, 1988
166. Theodorakis NG, Morimoto RI: Posttranscriptional regulation of HSP70 expression in human cells. Mol Cell Biol 7:4357, 1987
167. Tobita M, Nagano I, Nakamura S, Kogure K: DNA single-strand breaks in postischemic gerbil brain detected by in situ nick translation. J Cereb Blood Flow Metab suppl 2 11:S361, 1991
168. Tomida S, Nowak TS, Jr, Vass K et al: Experimental model for repetitive ischemic attack in the gerbil: the cumulative effect of repeated ischemic insults. J Cereb Blood Flow Metab 7:773, 1987
169. Tone O, Miller JC, Bell JM, Rapoport SI: Regional cerebral palmitate incorporation following transient bilateral carotid occlusion in awake gerbils. Stroke 18:1120, 1987
170. Tsuda T, Nishioka K, Kogure K: Prevention against ischemic injury of the CA1 neurons in the rat hippocampus at 24 hr reperfusion by $Mg^{2+}$. Neuroscience 44:335, 1991
171. Unterberg A, Baethmann A: The kallikrein-kinin system as mediator in vasogenic brain edema. 1. Cerebral exposure to bradykinin and plasma. J Neurosurg 61:87, 1984
172. Unterberg A, Wahl M, Hammersen F, Baethmann A: Permeability and vasomotor response of cerebral vessels during exposure to arachidonic acid. Acta Neuropathol 73:209, 1987
173. Vaccarino F, Guidotti A, Costa E: Ganglioside inhibition of glutamate-mediated protein kinase C translocation in primary cultures of cerebellar neurons. Proc Natl Acad Sci USA 84:8707, 1987
174. Van Buren JM, Borke RC: Variations and Connections of Human Thalamus. 2nd Ed. Springer-Verlag, Berlin, 1972
175. Van Nostrand WE, Cunningham DD: Purification of protease nexin II from human fibroblasts. J Biol Chem 262:8508, 1987
176. Van Nostrand WE, Wagner SL, Suzuki M et al: Protease nexin-II, a potent antichymotrypsin, shows identity to amyloid $\beta$-protein precursor. Nature 341:546, 1989
177. Van Reempts J, Haseldonckx M, Van Deuren B et al: Structural damage of the ischemic brain: involvement of calcium and effects of postischemic treatment with calcium entry blockers. Drug Dev Res 8:387, 1986
178. Vass K, Welck WJ, Nowak TS, Jr: Localization of

70-kDa stress protein induction in gerbil brain after ischemia. Acta Neuropathol 77:128, 1988
179. Westergaard E: The blood-brain barrier to hoseradish peroxidase under normal and experimental conditions. Acta Neuropathol 39:181, 1977
180. Whitson JS, Selkoe DJ, Cotman CW: Amyloid β-protein enhances the survival of hippocampal neurons in vitro. Science 243:1488, 1989
181. Wielock T: Neurochemical correlates to selective neuronal vulnerability. Prog Brain Res 63:69, 1985
182. Worley PF, Baraban JM, Colvin JS, Snyder SH: Inositol triphosphate receptor localization in brain: variable stoichiometry with protein kinase C. Nature 325:159, 1987
183. Worley PF, Baraban JM, Snyder SH: Heterogeneous localization of protein kinase C in rat brain: autoradiographic analysis of phorbol ester receptor binding. J Neurosci 8:199, 1986
184. Wright JJ, Gunter KC, Mitsuya H et al: Expression of a zinc finger gene in HTLV-1- and HTLV-II-transformed cells. Science 248:588, 1990
185. Wujek JR, Akeson RA: Extracellular matrix derived from astrocytes stimulates neuritic outgrowth from PC12 cells in vitro. Dev Brain Res 34:87, 1987
186. Yamamoto H, Hukunaga K, Tanaka E, Miyamoto E: $Ca^{2+}$- and calmodulin-dependent phosphorylation of microtubule-associated protein 2 and tau factor, and inhibition of microtubule assembly. J Neurochem 41:1119, 1983
187. Yamauchi T, Fujisawa H: Tyrosine 3-monooxygenase is phosphorylated by $Ca^{2+}$-, calmodulin-dependent protein kinase, followed by activation by activator protein. Biochem Biophys Res Commun 100:807, 1981
188. Yamauchi T, Fujisawa H: Phosphorylation of microtubule-associated protein 2 by calmodulin-dependent protein kinase (kinase II), which occurs only in the brain tissue. Biochem Biophys Res Commun 109:975, 1982
189. Yong AB, Bromberg MB, Penney JB, Jr: Decreased glutamate uptake in subcortical areas deafferented by sensorimotor cortical ablation in the cat. J Neurosci 1:241, 1981
190. Yoshida M, Rabin A, Anderson M: Monosynaptic inhibition of neurons of the substantia nigra by caudate-nigral fibers. Brain Res 32:225, 1971
191. Yoshidomi M, Hayashi T, Abe K, Kogure K: Effects of a new calcium channel blocker, KB-2796, on protein synthesis of the CA1 pyramidal cell and delayed neuronal death following transient forebrain ischemia. J Neurochem 53:1589, 1989
192. Yoshimi K, Kudo T, Iwata N, Nishimura K: Change of clathrin precedes delayed neuronal death of CA1 cells after ischemia. Jap J Neurochem 29:456, 1990
193. Zheng J, Onodera H, Kogure K: Hippocampal grafts prevent mossy fiber sprouting in the kainic acid-lesioned hippocampal formation. J Cereb Blood Flow Metab, suppl 2. 11:S765, 1991
194. Zini I, Zoli M, Grimaldi R et al: Evidence for a role of neosynthetized putrescine in the increase of glial fibrillary acidic protein immunoreactivity induced by a mechanical lesion in the rat brain. Neurosci Lett 120:13, 1990

# 5
# *CEREBROSPINAL FLUID IN CEREBROVASCULAR DISORDERS*

Robert A. Fishman

This chapter deals with the diagnostic role of cerebrospinal fluid in cerebrovascular disorders and the pathophysiology of the changes involved. Examination of the cerebrospinal fluid (CSF), long established as a useful aid in neurologic diagnosis, may be indicated in some patients with acute stroke for the following reasons: (1) to establish the presence of subarachnoid hemorrhage (the relative reliability of lumbar puncture and computed tomography in this regard is discussed below); (2) to exclude the presence of inflammation in the CSF of patients whose apparent stroke is a manifestation of infection (particularly meningovascular syphilis) or immunologic disorders, including the various forms of vasculitis, granulomatous angiitis, cranial arteritis, and lupus; and, rarely, (3) for CSF cytology in patients with meningeal malignancies whose illness may simulate an ischemic disorder.

## LABORATORY EXAMINATION

Normal CSF contains no more than 5 lymphocytes or mononuclear cells/mm$^3$. A higher white cell count is pathognomonic of disease in the central nervous system or meninges. A stained smear of the sediment is necessary for an accurate differential cell count. In cases of bloody CSF due to a traumatic puncture, the white count is elevated by the cells contributed by the blood. A useful approximation of a true white cell count can be obtained by using the following correction for the presence of the added blood: if the patient has a normal hemogram, subtract from the total white cell count (per mm$^3$) 1 white cell for each 1,000 red blood cells (RBC) present. Thus, if bloody fluid contains 10,000 red cells and 100 white cells/mm$^3$, 10 white cells would be accounted for by the added blood and the corrected leukocyte count would be 90/mm$^3$. If the patient's hemogram reveals significant anemia or leukocytosis, the following formula may be used to determine more accurately the number of white cells (W) in the spinal fluid before the blood was added[4]:

$$W = \frac{\text{blood WBC} \times \text{CSF RBC}}{\text{blood RBC}} \times 100$$

The presence of blood in the subarachnoid space produces a secondary inflammatory response, which leads to a disproportionate increase in the number of white cells. This elevation in the white cell count is most marked about 48 hours after an acute subarachnoid hemorrhage, at a time when meningeal signs are most striking.[24]

To correct CSF protein values for the presence of added blood in the fluid, subtract 1 mg for every 1,000 red blood cells. Thus, if the red cell count is 10,000/

mm$^3$ and the total protein is 110 mg/dl, the corrected protein level would be about 100 mg/dl. The corrections are reliable only if the cell count and total protein are both measured from the same tube of fluid.

## Blood in the Cerebrospinal Fluid: Differential Diagnosis and the Three-Tube Test

Several observations are required to differentiate between a traumatic spinal puncture and preexisting subarachnoid hemorrhage (Table 5-1). At the time of puncture, the fluid should be collected in at least three separate tubes (the *three-tube test*). In traumatic punctures, the fluid generally clears between the first and the third collections. This is detectable by the naked eye and should be confirmed by cell count. In subarachnoid bleeding, the blood is generally evenly admixed in the three tubes. A sample, preferably 1 ml, of the bloody fluid should be centrifuged and the supernatant fluid compared with tap water to exclude the presence of pigment. Spectrophotometry is more sensitive than the eye in detecting low concentrations of pigment, and its use has been advocated by some groups.[22]

In a sample from a traumatic puncture, the supernatant fluid is clear if the red count is less than about 100,000 cells/mm$^3$. With bloody contamination of greater magnitude, plasma proteins are sufficiently present to cause minimal xanthochromia; this requires enough serum to raise the protein concentration about 100 mg/dl above the initial level. Following subarachnoid bleeding the supernatant fluid becomes pigmented, indicating that the blood has been present long enough to permit lysis of red cells. This probably requires at least 2 to 4 hours, although the average life of the red cell in the peripheral blood is about 120 days. The rapid lysis of red cells in CSF has not been well explained. It is not due to any osmotic difference between plasma and CSF since the osmolarity of both fluids is essentially the same. It appears likely that the absence from the CSF of sufficient plasma proteins, which stabilize the red cell membrane, is largely responsible for the rapid lysis of red cells.

It is important to note that the supernatant fluid usually remains clear for 2 to 12 hours after the onset of subarachnoid bleeding. (This may mislead the physician to erroneously conclude that the observed blood is due to needle trauma in patients who have received a lumbar puncture within the early hours following aneurysmal rupture.) Walton[24] reviewed the CSF findings in 286 cases of subarachnoid hemorrhage and found that 10 percent of patients with bloody fluid had clear supernatant fluid 12 hours after the presumed onset while all the fluids were xanthochromic thereafter. After an especially traumatic puncture, some blood and xanthochromia may be present for as long as 2 to 5 days following the initial puncture. In pathologic states associated with a CSF protein greater than 150 mg/dl, and in the absence of bleeding, a faint degree of xanthochromia may be detected. When the protein is elevated to much higher levels (as in spinal block, polyneutritis, and meningitis), the xanthochromia may be considerable. A xanthochromic fluid with a normal protein level or an elevation to less than 150 mg/dl usually indicates a previous subarachnoid or intracerebral hemorrhage (although, the xanthochromia is rarely due to severe jaundice).[4]

Xanthochromia due to carotenoids has been observed in food faddists with dietary hypercarotenemia, whose CSF actually looks orange. A faintly brown or dark color of the fluid has been noted rarely in patients with malignant melanomatosis of the meninges.[4]

## Pigments

Three major pigments derived from red cells may be detected in the fluid: oxyhemoglobin, bilirubin, and methemoglobin. These have been identified quantitatively by absorption spectrophotometry and by calculations based on absorbance at specific wave-

**TABLE 5-1. Differential Features of Subarachnoid Hemorrhage and Traumatic Puncture: The Three-Tube Test**

| CSF Finding | Subarachnoid Hemorrhage | Traumatic Puncture |
|---|---|---|
| Pressure | Increased or normal | Normal |
| Appearance | Equal blood in all tubes | First or last tube is bloodier, others are clearer |
| Supernatant fluid color | Pigment in excess of protein level | Clear |
| RBC count and hematocrit | Essentially similar in all three tubes | Variable in different tubes |
| WBC count | Proportional to RBC count in earliest stages, relatively increased later | Proportional to RBC count |
| Clot formation | Absent | Occurs rarely |
| Repeat puncture at higher interspace | Findings similar to those at initial tap | Usually clear |

*Abbreviations*: CFF, cerebrospinal fluid, RBC, red blood cells; WBC, white blood cells.
(From Fishman,[4] with permission.)

lengths.[9] However, usually the eye can readily differentiate the color changes, although spectrophotometry has greater sensitivity.[22]

Oxyhemoglobin is red, but after dilution it appears pink or orange. It is released with lysis of red cells and may be detected in the supernatant fluid within 2 hours after the release of blood in the subarachnoid space. It reaches a maximum level in about the first 36 hours and gradually disappears over the next 7 to 10 days. Its presence may also be detected with the benzidine test.

Bilirubin is a yellow, iron-free derivative of hemoglobin produced in vivo following the hemolysis of red cells. Free bilirubin is conjugated with glucuronic acid in the liver to form bilirubin glucuronide. Both free and conjugated bilirubin are albumin-bound, although conjugated bilirubin dissociates readily to enter the urine. With severe jaundice, both free and conjugated bilirubin are detected in the CSF, and the degree of bilirubin pigmentation is increased when the CSF protein is elevated. Xanthochromia, by definition, means yellow color, but it has been customary to use the term to describe pink or yellow coloration of the fluid. In view of the significance of the different pigments, it is more useful to describe the color specifically as yellow, pink, or orange.

Bilirubin formation in the CSF is considered to depend on the ability of macrophages and other cells in the leptomeninges to degrade hemoglobin. Roost et al.[16] studied the conversion of hemoglobin heme to bilirubin in a rat model of subarachnoid hemorrhage. The enzyme responsible for the conversion, hemeoxygenase, was found in the choroid plexus, arachnoid, and cortex. Its activity was increased fourfold after a delay of about 12 hours, analogously to the delay in the appearance of bilirubin observed in humans. The delay may depend upon the migration of sufficient macrophages into the leptomeninges.

Bilirubin is first detected about 10 hours after the onset of subarachnoid bleeding. It reaches a maximum at 48 hours and may persist for 2 to 4 weeks after extensive bleeding.[24] The severity of the meningeal signs associated with subarachnoid bleeding correlates with the inflammatory response, that is, with the maximal pleocytosis. It may be roughly correlated with the level of bilirubin in the spinal fluid, although bilirubin itself does not cause meningeal irritation (in severe jaundice, the CSF is bilirubin stained without a pleocytosis). The usual temporal pattern of these changes following subarachnoid hemorrhage is shown[4] in Figure 5-1. Bilirubin is also the major pigment responsible for the xanthochromia associated with a high level of protein in spinal fluid. The presence of bilirubin may be also demonstrated spectrophotometrically and with the van den Bergh reaction.[9]

Methemoglobin, a brown pigment that is dark yellow in dilution, is a reduction product of hemoglobin characteristically found in encapsulated subdural hematomas and in old, loculated intracerebral hemorrhages. It may be detected by spectrophotometry of the spinal fluid in patients with such encapsulations of large size, but the pigment is not generally observed in other xanthochromic spinal fluids.[9] The presence of methemoglobin may be confirmed with the potassium cyanide test.

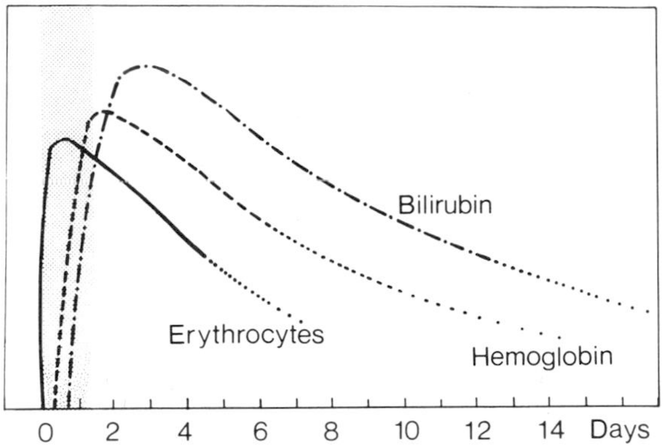


**Fig. 5-1.** Subarachnoid bleeding: the pigmentary changes in cerebrospinal fluid (CSF) following a single subarachnoid hemorrhage. The red blood cell count is usually maximal within the first 24 hours and is usually apparent in the supernatant CSF within the first 4 to 10 hours after bleeding. The pink color is usually maximal within the first 24 to 48 hours, then gradually disappears. Bilirubin appears after the detection of hemoglobin. Its yellow color usually appears 9 to 15 hours after bleeding (excluding the bilirubin that enters from the serum) as hemoglobin is degraded by the leptomeningeal cellular infiltrates. The meningeal signs are usually maximal at about the same time that the CSF bilirubin is at its height. This coincides with the time of maximal leukocytic pleocytosis. The bilirubin disappears slowly from the CSF, often after 10 to 14 or more days. (From Fishman RA,[4] with permission.)

It is useful to note the degree of CSF pigmentation in relation to the protein level. The presence of xanthochromia out of proportion to the total protein content, and in the absence of jaundice or hypercarotenemia, indicates previous bleeding into the CSF or into the brain or spinal cord adjacent to the CSF.

## RELIABILITY OF LUMBAR PUNCTURE AND COMPUTED TOMOGRAPHY IN DETECTING HEMORRHAGIC CEREBROSPINAL FLUID

Computed tomography (CT) or magnetic resonance imaging (MRI) are the initial investigations of choice in most patients suspected of having intracerebral or subarachnoid hemorrhage, and, if these are promptly available, lumbar puncture (LP) generally should be deferred.[3] MRI has not been systematically evaluated in the early diagnosis of hemorrhagic stroke and subarachnoid hemorrhage. Its sensitivity to the detection of methemoglobin and to patterns of vascular flow are noteworthy. However, in most emergency settings, CT is the more readily available, and therefore, the preferred technique.

Prior to starting anticoagulant therapy in patients with presumed stroke in evolution or transient ischemic attacks (TIAs), it long has been common practice to examine the CSF to exclude the presence of unsuspected intracranial and/or subarachnoid bleeding due to ruptured aneurysm or arteriovenous malformation. More recently it was suggested that CT is the only procedure required to evaluate patients prior to their undergoing anticoagulation. However, when the diagnostic reliability of CT and LP was compared,[17] CT was shown to be superior to LP in detecting intracerebral hemorrhage, but LP was more accurate in diagnosing subarachnoid hemorrhage per se because of the artifacts imposed by the adjacent skull. The presence of xanthochromia is a good index of a previous subarachnoid hemorrhage, but MacDonald and Mendelow[12] have emphasized that blood staining in the absence of xanthochromia was found in about half their patients with ruptured aneurysm. They conclude that, in suspected subarachnoid hemorrhage, CT is the primary investigation and lumbar puncture is necessary in those patients with a normal CT scan.

Patients with an acute stroke should be evaluated with CT before receiving anticoagulant therapy. If this is not available, then diagnostic lumbar puncture generally is indicated. Following LP, heparin anticoagulation should not be started for at least 1 hour to reduce the risk of spinal hematoma, which is a complication of the procedure. Ruff and Dougherty[17] have reported an increase in the occurrence of spinal epidural and subdural hematoma, causing paraplegia or radiculopathy as well as subarachnoid hemorrhage if anticoagulation was started within 1 hour of the LP.

## PROTEINS AND ENZYMES IN CEREBROSPINAL FLUID AS MARKERS OF THE CAUSE AND SEVERITY OF STROKE

An elevation in total CSF protein content occurs as a consequence of breakdown of the blood-brain barrier. Such elevations occur with ischemic infarction in the absence of hemorrhagic lesions and corelate roughly with size and location of the infarct. Infarctions close to the ventricular or pial surfaces favor increases in protein level. The CSF protein level tends to be the greatest 2 to 3 weeks after occult infarction. This correlates with the time of maximal contrast enhancement with CT; the delay may be related to new endothelial cell formation occurring in the ischemic penumbra.

Many investigators have sought more specific proteins and enzymes that might better correlate with the extent and severity of ischemic brain lesions than total protein. These have included the following CSF enzymes: glutamic oxaloacetic transaminase, lactic dehydrogenase, creatine phosphokinase, aldolase, and adenylate kinase. Almost every enzyme that has been studied in blood has also been studied in CSF.[1] Enzymes in CSF might be derived from the plasma, from the damaged brain, or from cellular elements present in CSF. Many reports have been deficient in analyzing which of these sources might be responsible for an elevated enzyme level. No single enzyme assay has yet proved to be sufficiently sensitive or specific a measure to warrant its routine use in clinical practice for the differential diagnosis of stroke.

Various CSF protein fractions have been investigated following stroke in a search for specific markers of cerebral damage, including myelin basic protein (MBP), tau fraction, transferrin, and IgG. Strand et al.[20] found increases of MBP most evident 4 to 5 days after cerebral infarction. Following hemorrhagic stroke, the increases were greatest during the first day. The concentration of MBP correlated with the size of the infarct observed with CT. Changes in none of these protein fractions have been shown to have diagnostic specificity apart from the immunoglobulins. An elevated IgG index and the presence of multiple CSF oligoclonal bands (absent from the serum) serve as indicators of increased immunoglobulin formation within the CNS and of an immune-mediated tissue response. Such changes are characteristic of meningovascular syphilis and may be seen in other cerebral vasculitides, including lupus erythematosus, periarteritis, giant-cell arteritis, and granulomatous angiitis. In evaluating such change, other causes must be excluded, such as demyelinating disorders, inflammatory disorders (including bacterial, viral, and parasitic diseases), paraneoplastic syndromes, and even carcinomatous meningitis, all of which conditions may be associated with abnormal CSF immunoglobulins.

## DIFFERENTIAL DIAGNOSIS OF CEREBROVASCULAR DISEASES

The CSF examination is useful in the differential diagnosis of the various forms of cerebrovascular disease.[2] The changes in the CSF associated with stroke are well illustrated by Merritt and Fremont-Smith's[13] analysis of 121 autopsy-proven cases, including 70 of cerebral hemorrhage and 51 of cerebral thrombosis. Known embolic lesions originating in the heart were excluded, although some of the patients probably had emboli originating in the carotid system. Patients with evidence of neurosyphilis were also excluded from the analysis. Sornas et al.[19] studied the cytologic changes following stroke in 116 patients. Lumbar punctures were performed within 3 days of onset, and the tap was repeated at 2- to 3-day intervals for a week and at weekly intervals thereafter. Many of these patients survived the stroke and thus differ from the fatal cases documented by Merritt and Fremont-Smith.[13] The results of these studies are as follows.

## Cerebral Hemorrhage

In 70 fatal cases of cerebral hemorrhage, the CSF pressure at first puncture was increased above 200 mm in 57 percent, above 300 mm in 38 percent, and above 400 mm in 19 percent of these cases. In almost half these fatal cases, the patients had a normal level of intracranial pressure, which indicates that this is a poor index of prognosis. It is of special interest that 20 percent of the patients had a clear fluid and the rest had varying degrees of pigmentation attributable to blood and its products. Fluids appearing grossly bloody to the naked eye contained several thousand to many hundreds of thousands of red cells/mm$^3$. Although the initial proportion of white cells to red cells was the same as in blood, there was a progressive increase in the absolute number of white cells and their proportion to the red cells, reflecting the meningeal reaction induced by blood. The precise temporal relationships between the number of red cells and the relative increase in white cell count was not described. In addition, with necrosis of the ventricular wall secondary to hemorrhage adjacent to the ventricle, an even greater leukocytic response was introduced. Cell counts as high as 1,900 and 3,600 leukocytes/mm$^3$ (largely polymorphonuclear cells) were observed in such cases. The blood fluids had an increase in protein content initially proportional to the red cell count but then elevated out of proportion to the cell count, reflecting an increased influx of serum proteins across the disrupted blood-brain barrier. The protein levels varied between 40 and 2,200 mg/d.[13]

In the series of Sornas et al.[19] 16 patients with intracerebral hematoma were studied. They also showed a polymorphonuclear response greater than that observed with ischemic strokes. Four patients had a mild pleocytosis, and four others had a marked pleocytosis (700, 900, 4,600, and 21,000 polymorphonuclear leukocytes, respectively). The maximal granulocytic response occurred on the third or fourth day after onset. A polymorphonuclear reaction on the first day pointed to the presence of an intracerebral hematoma.

Lee et al.[11] found that 25 percent of 16 patients with autopsy-verified intracerebral hemorrhage had a clear fluid. However, the lumbar punctures were performed within 24 hours in three cases and within 48 hours in the fourth. Thus, a delayed appearance of blood in the lumbar sac with intracerebral hemorrhage might explain the clear fluid in such cases. MR and CT imaging commonly demonstrate small intracerebral hemorrhages that in many cases would be considered as ischemic syndromes on clinical grounds. A clear CSF certainly does not exclude such small intracerebral bleeds.

A low CSF glucose level may also be noted in bloody spinal fluid due to subarachnoid hemorrhage of whatever cause. The precise incidence of this finding is not established because often the CSF glucose has not been systematically analyzed in patients with obvious subarachnoid hemorrhage. Merritt and Fremont-Smith[13] reported that most patients with subarachnoid hemorrhage had normal CSF glucose levels, but 4 of 21 cases had a glucose level below 40 mg/dl. In a small group of patients, Troost et al.[21] observed that low CSF glucose levels occurred most frequently 4 to 8 days after the hemorrhage. Sambrook et al.[18] studied the CSF glucose during the first 10 days after subarachnoid hemorrhage or stroke, reporting a glucose level below 40 mg/dl in 4 of 24 patients with subarachnoid hemorrhage. The maximum fall occurred between the first and sixth day and appeared to depend upon the extent of rebleeding. No other specific changes were noted in the CSF glucose level in subarachnoid hemorrhage or stroke. The mechanism of the low glucose is considered to depend upon increased rates of glycolysis in tissue immediately adjacent to the CSF, including leptomeninges and neuropil.[4] The depression in glucose level is associated with increased lactate levels.

## Cerebral Thrombosis

The intracranial pressure was usually normal or only slightly elevated in the 51 patients with cerebral thrombosis reported by Merritt and Fremont-Smith.[13] These pressures were greater than 200 mm in 21 percent of these autopsy-proven cases; in 4 percent the pressure was between 300 and 400 mm. The occurrence of intracranial hypertension in these fatal cases reflected extensive cerebral infarction and edema. In 51 fatal cases, 46 patients had a clear fluid, 4 had a xanthochromic fluid, and 1 had a blood-tinged fluid. Thus, about 10 percent of the cases were associated with hemorrhagic infarction, which was reflected in the fluid. The white cell count in 7 of the 51 patients was between 6 and 67 cells/mm$^3$; counts in the rest were normal. The relationship between the degree of pleocytosis and the time after the onset of the stroke was not worked out, nor were other forms of arteritis (cranial arteritis or granulomatous angiitis), apart from neurosyphilis, excluded. The protein content was normal in half the patients, and only in two patients was it over 100 mg/dl. (It is not clear whether other causes of increased CSF protein, such as myxedema or diabetic polyneuropathy, were excluded in these patients.) In the series of Sornas et al.,[19] serial punctures after ischemic stroke revealed a minor leukocytic response, which was maximal during the first 7 days. The white count was usually normal by the end of the second week.

## Cerebral Embolism

The CSF changes associated with cerebral embolism generally cannot be differentiated from those associated with cerebral thrombosis. In 13 patients with nonseptic embolism, the cell count was normal in 10; in 3 there was a slight pleocytosis with a high of 45 white cells/mm³.[13] It is very likely that these autopsy-proven cases of cerebral thrombosis included patients with emboli from the carotid system. (The carotid arteries in the neck were not examined at autopsy in the 1930s.) The CSF findings associated with septic embolism due to subacute bacterial endocarditis are discussed below.

In summary, the use of the CSF findings in the differential diagnosis of cerebral thrombosis, embolism, and hemorrhage is limited. In the Boston series,[13] 20 percent of the patients with cerebral hemorrhage had a clear fluid at the first puncture, and 10 percent of the patients with cerebral thrombosis had a xanthochromic or slightly bloody fluid. The fact that a clear CSF does not exclude a cerebral hemorrhage or a hemorrhagic infarction must be considered in the decision to institute anticoagulant therapy. Computed tomography or MR imaging are better indicators of the presence of intrahemispheric blood and should be obtained before starting anticoagulation.

## Giant-Cell (Temporal) Arteritis

The neurologic manifestations of giant-cell (temporal) arteritis are diverse, and the CSF findings are also variable.[7] The CSF is usually normal in patients when the disease is manifested chiefly in the external carotid arteries. However, when the cerebral vasculature is involved, abnormalities of the CSF have been noted, which is not surprising. The pressure is usually normal. Occasionally, pleocytosis has been reported with counts as high as 650 white cells/mm³, including both lymphocytes and polymorphonuclear granulocytes. The CSF protein may be increased to a level as high as several hundred mg/dl with few if any cells. The CSF glucose levels have been normal in the available reports.[7]

## Granulomatous Angiitis

Granulomatous angiitis is an uncommon necrotizing vasculitis confined primarily to the central nervous system. Koo and Massey[10] reported an increased CSF pressure (greater than 220 mm) in 6 of 18 published cases. Younger et al.[25] have summarized the CSF findings in 55 reported cases. The CSF protein was elevated in 80 percent of cases, as high as 600 mg/dl, most often less than 200 mg/dl. The cell count was increased in 75 percent, varying between 10 and 250 mononucular cells per mm³. Evidence for mild subarachnoid bleeding was observed in a few cases; decreased CSF glucose levels were seen in these. The CSF gamma globulin level was increased in some patients, but this was not reported by most authors. Oligoclonal bands may be observed in well-documented cases of granulomatous arteritis. The observation that about 20 percent of patients have a normal CSF indicates the difficulty in diagnosis.[23]

## Bacterial Endocarditis

The incidence of neurologic complications in bacterial endocarditis was 39 percent in the review by Pruitt et al.[14] The neurologic manifestations were diverse and included cerebral embolism, subarachnoid and intracerebral hemorrhage, and seizures. There were a wide variety of infectious agents, including streptococci, staphylococci, *Hemophilus*, enterobacteria, and *Candida*. The CSF findings in 69 patients were also diverse. In 21 of the 69 patients (30 percent) the CSF was normal, but in 19 patients (28 percent) the fluid was purulent (demonstrating a polymorphonuclear leukocytic pleocytosis) with a high protein content and a reduced glucose content. In 17 patients (25 percent) the fluid was aseptic (predominantly lymphocytic pleocytosis) with a normal glucose level and a normal or slightly elevated protein level. In 9 patients (13 percent) the fluid was hemorrhagic (more than 200 red cells/mm³ in all tubes). Cultures were positive in only 11 of the 69 patients, and in each of these the fluid was purulent. There was a close correlation between the CSF findings and the infecting organism. Virulent organisms such as *Staphylococcus aureus, Streptococcus pneumoniae,* and enteric gram-negative rods were frequently associated with a purulent fluid. Conversely, a relatively nonvirulent organism such as *Streptococcus viridans* was usually associated with a normal or aseptic CSF.

## Venous Thrombosis

Occlusion of the intracranial venous sinuses and the cerebral veins occurs in diverse conditions, including infection, head injury, tumor, dehydration, hypercoagulable states, and also as a primary or idiopathic disorder.[5] The occlusion may involve the superior longitudinal sinus and bridging veins, the lateral sinuses, and cavernous sinuses. The occlusions may be rapid or gradual in onset and variable in extent. The CSF findings in these heterogeneous disorders are highly variable. The CSF pressures are greatly elevated with acute and extensive thrombosis involving the superior longitudinal and lateral sinuses, but normal pressures may occur with gradual occlusions despite extensive involvement. Sinus occlusion may cause a pseudotumor syndrome with severe intracranial hypertension but an otherwise normal CSF. The fluid is usually clear and cell-free unless associated with hemorrhagic venous infarction of adjacent brain that results in subarachnoid hemorrhage, minor or massive in degree. In such cases, the CSF reveals the spectrum of changes seen with subarachnoid hemorrhage. In patients with septic thrombophlebitis, an inflammatory CSF may be observed with a variable degree of pleocytosis and protein elevation; the CSF glucose is normal in the absence of diffuse inflammation of the leptomeninges.

## Migraine

The CSF is normal between migrainous episodes. However, a low-grade inflammatory response is not uncommon during episodes of complicated migraine, for example, hemiplegic migraine or basilar migraine. In such cases a leukocytic response as high as 350/mm$^3$, with a predominance of granulocytes, has been reported. In one report,[15] CSF protein concentration was as high as 217 mg/dl. Lumbar puncture is rarely performed in patients with typical migraine attacks, and therefore the frequency of CSF pleocytosis is not known. Raskin[15] describes a CSF pleocytosis of 15 to 100 lymphocytes/mm$^3$ in 10 patients with severe but uncomplicated migraine. The mechanism of these low-grade inflammatory changes is not known.

## Congestive Heart Failure

The intracranial pressure is characteristically elevated in cases of severe congestive heart failure. Harrison[8] and Friedfeld and Fishberg[6] studied the venous pressure and CSF pressure in such cases; they showed that the intracranial hypertension was secondary to increased central venous pressure and that both returned toward normal with the administration of digitalis. Merritt and Fremont-Smith[13] reported a series of 32 patients with congestive heart failure with CSF pressures ranging between 185 and 500 mm; about 50 percent of the patients had a pressure of 300 mm or greater. While the increased intracranial pressure in these cases was attributable to increased central venous pressure, additional contributing factors were the severity of the respiratory acidosis and the degree of cerebral hypoxia associated with heart failure. Both acidosis and hypoxia cause acute cerebral vasodilation and increased cerebral blood flow and thereby intracranial hypertension. However, the quantitative importance of each of the three factors—central venous pressure, acidosis, and hypoxia—in such cases has not been delineated. The CSF cell count and total protein content were normal in these patients.

In summary, CSF examination has a small but well-defined role in the diagnosis and management of some patients with cerebrovascular disease.

## REFERENCES

1. Banik NL, Hogan EL: Cerebrospinal fluid enzymes in neurological disease. p. 205. In Wood JH (ed): Neurobiology of Cerebrospinal Fluid. Plenum, New York, 1983
2. Britton M, Hultman E, Murray V, Sjöhlm H: The diagnostic accuracy of CSF analysis in stroke. Acta Med Scand 214:3, 1983
3. Duffy GP: Lumbar puncture in spontaneous subarachnoid hemorrhage. Br Med J 285:1163, 1982
4. Fishman RA: Cerebrospinal Fluid in Diseases of the Nervous System. 2nd Ed. WB Saunders, Philadelphia, 1992
5. Fishman RA: Cerebral veins and sinuses. p. 204. In Rowland LP (ed): Merritt's Textbook of Neurology. 8th Ed. Lea and Febiger, Philadelphia, 1989
6. Friedfeld L, Fishberg AM: The relation of cerebrospinal and venous pressures in heart failure. J Clin Invest 13:495, 1934
7. Hamilton CR, Shelley WM, Tumulty PA: Giant cell arteritis: including temporal arteritis and polymyalgia rheumatica. Medicine (Baltimore) 50:1, 1971
8. Harrison WG: Cerebrospinal fluid pressure and venous pressure in cardiac failure and the effect of spinal drainage in the treatment of cardiac decompensation. Arch Intern Med 53:782, 1934
9. Kjellin KG, Soderstrom CE: Diagnostic significance of CSF spectrophotometry in cerebrovascular diseases. J Neurol Sci 23:359, 1974
10. Koo EH, Massey EW: Granulomatous angiitis of the central nervous system: protean manifestations and response to treatment. J Neurol Neurosurg Psychiatry 51:1126, 1988
11. Lee MC, Heaney LM, Jacobson RL et al: Cerebrospinal fluid in cerebral hemorrhage and infarction. Stroke 6:648, 1975
12. MacDonald A, Mendelow AD: Xanthochromia revisited: a re-evaluation of lumbar puncture and CT scanning in the diagnosis of subarachnoid. J Neurol Neurosurg Psychiatry 51:342, 1988
13. Merritt HH, Fremont-Smith F: The Cerebrospinal Fluid. WB Saunders, Philadelphia, 1938
14. Pruitt AA, Rubin RH, Karchmer AW et al: Neurologic complications of bacterial endocarditis. Medicine (Baltimore) 57:329, 1978
15. Raskin NG: Headache. 2nd Ed. pp. 68, 81. Churchill Livingstone, New York, 1988
16. Roost KT, Pimstone NR, Diamond I et al: The formation of cerebrospinal fluid xanthochromia after subarachnoid hemorrhage: enzymatic conversion of hemoglobin to bilirubin by the arachnoid and choroid plexus. Neurology (NY) 22:973, 1972
17. Ruff RL, Dougherty JH: Evaluation of acute cerebral ischemia for anticoagulant therapy: com-

puted tomography or lumbar puncture. Neurology (NY) 31:736, 1981
18. Sambrook MA, Hutchison EC, Aber GM: Metabolic studies in subarachnoid hemorrhage and strokes. I. Serial changes in acid-base values in blood and cerebrospinal fluid. Brain 96:171, 1973
19. Sornas R, Ostlund H, Muller R: Cerebrospinal fluid cytology after stroke. Arch Neurol 26:489, 1972
20. Strand T, Alling C, Karlsson B et al: Brain and plasma proteins in spinal fluid as markers for brain damage and severity of stroke. Stroke 15:138, 1984
21. Troost BT, Walker JE, Cherington M: Hypoglycorrhachia associated with subarachnoid hemorrhage. Arch Neurol 19:438, 1968
22. Vermeulen M, Hasan D, Blijenberg BG et al. Xanthochromia after subarachnoid hemorrhage needs no revisitation. J Neurol Neurosurg Psychiatry 52:826, 1989
23. Vincent FM: Granulomatous angiitis. N Engl J Med 296:452, 1977
24. Walton JN: Subarachnoid Hemorrhage. Livingstone, Edinburgh, 1956
25. Younger DS, Hags AP, Brust J, Rowland LP: Granulomatous angiitis of the brain: an inflammatory reaction of diverse etiology. Arch Neurol 45:514, 1988

# 6
# POSITRON EMISSION TOMOGRAPHY STUDIES IN ISCHEMIC STROKE

J.C. Baron

By allowing quantitative tomographic maps of cerebral blood flow (CBF), cerebral blood volume (CBV), cerebral metabolic rate of oxygen ($CMRO_2$), brain glucose utilization (CMRGlu), and intracellular pH ($pH_i$) in humans, positron emission tomography (PET) provides better delineation of pathophysiologic mechanisms contributing to ischemic strokes. In addition, PET has allowed the development of new functional concepts on the therapy of acute brain ischemia and on mechanisms of functional recovery.[3,5,27,28]

Although several of the above-mentioned physiologic variables are accessible by other investigative methods (e.g., xenon CBF and Kety-Schmidt $N_2O$ techniques), it is the concomitant measurement, in absolute quantitative terms, of several of these variables in the same subject with high-resolution axial images that characterizes the power of PET. In addition, access to CBF and CBV allows computation of the CBV/CBF ratio, which represents the local circulatory mean transit time ($t$) and its corollary, the CBF/CBV ratio, which is quasi-linearly proportional to the local cerebral perfusion pressure (CPP). Likewise, measurement of CBF and $CMRO_2$ allows quantitative mapping of both oxygen extraction fraction (OEF) and the end-capillary partial oxygen tension, which reflects the partial tissue oxygen tension ($PtO_2$), while the CMRGlu/$CMRO_2$ reflects the stoichiometric relationship between glucose use and oxygen consumption. Finally, with selective plasma and red cell markers, quantitation of local cerebral plasma and erythrocyte volumes, and hence local cerebral hematocrit can be accomplished. In Table 6-1 are listed the main physiologic variables quantifiable with PET, together with the most accepted and best validated methods allowing their measurement, and the average value measured in regions of interest predominantly containing normal gray matter. The reader is referred to technical articles published elsewhere for further details and methodologic references.[10,13,37] A point worthy of mention relates to the quantitation of these variables in absolute terms, which necessitates obtaining arterial blood for radioactivity counting (input function). Although this is achieved safely using fine catheters inserted in the radial artery (with which no complications have been reported thus far), its performance has medical contraindications and is not always possible to perform. Attempts to obtain accurate quantitation using, for example, arterialized (heated hand) venous blood, expired air radioactivity levels, reflecting pulmonary circulation or external cardiac radioactivity monitoring, have not been successful. However, the only example where such alternatives for arterial blood radioactivity is acceptable is with CMRGlu measurement ("in vivo autoradiographic approach") using [$^{18}$F]2-fluoro-2-deoxy-D-glucose ($^{18}$F-FDG) and the heated-hand method.[13,62] Nevertheless, nonquantitative imaging of CBF, CBV, OEF, or CMRGlu remains of interest in situations where

**TABLE 6-1. Physiologic Variables Measured by Positron Emission Tomography**

| Physiologic Variable | Abbreviation | Normal Values (Gray Matter) | Main Radiotracers | Method |
|---|---|---|---|---|
| Cerebral blood flow | CBF | 50 ml 100 ml$^{-1}$ min$^{-1}$ | $^{15}$O-$CO_2$<br>$^{15}$O-$H_2O$<br>$^{11}$C or [$^{15}$O]Butanol<br>[$^{18}$F] or [$^{11}$C]Fluoromethane | Bolus or steady-state<br>Bolus or steady-state<br>Bolus<br>Bolus |
| Cerebral blood volume | CBV | 4 ml 100 ml$^{-1}$ | $^{15}$O-CO<br>$^{11}$C-CO | Bolus or steady-state<br>Bolus to equilibrium |
| Cerebral metabolic rate of oxygen | $CMRO_2^a$ | 4 ml 100 ml$^{-1}$ min$^{-1}$ | $^{15}$O-$O_2$ | Bolus or steady-state |
| Cerebral metabolic rate of glucose | CMRGlu$^a$ | 8 mg 100 ml$^{-1}$ min$^{-1}$ | [$^{18}$F]Fluoro-2-deoxy-D-glucose<br>[$^{11}$C]2-Deoxy-D-glucose<br>[$^{11}$C]1-D-glucose | Bolus<br>Bolus<br>Bolus |
| Tissular pH | pHt | 7.04 | $^{11}$C-DMO (intracellular pH)<br>$^{11}$C-$CO_2$ | Bolus<br>Continuous inhalation |
| Oxygen extraction fraction | OEF | 0.40 | $^{15}$O-$CO_2$ (or $^{15}$O-$H_2O$) and $^{15}$O-$O_2$ | From CBF and $^{15}O_2$ distribution |
| Mean transit time | $t$ | 0.08 min | — | Ratio CBV/CBF (inversely proportional to the cerebral perfusion pressure) |
| Tissue partial $O_2$ tension | $ptO_2$ | 31.2 mmHg | — | From CBF and $CMRO_2$ |
| Local tissue hematocrit | tHt | 0.28 | [$^{11}$C]Albumin + $^{11}$C-CO | Bolus to equilibrium |

[a] The conversion factors to obtain $CMRO_2$ and CMRGlu in micromolar (μM) units are 44.6 μmol/ml and 5.56 μmol/mg, respectively.

interpretation can be adequate without absolute numbers. In most instances, qualitative images of radioactivity distribution so obtained are not linearly proportional to corresponding functional parameters so that quantitation is always necessary for research purposes. Furthermore, qualitative imaging can be misleading because it does not reflect global alterations of brain physiology.

In addition to the above "nonspecific" physiologic variables, PET also allows investigation of specific binding sites/receptors. For example, preliminary results of studies of changes in specific glial and neuronal markers (using $^{11}$C-PK 11195 and $^{11}$C-flumazenil, respectively) after brain infarction have recently appeared.[38,75]

The instrumentation characteristics of PET cameras as well as the description and problems related to cyclotron use, radiochemistry and computer science are outside the scope of this chapter. The interested reader is referred to specialized articles and books.[29] Present-day PET cameras are capable of acquiring 7 to 31 brain slices simultaneously, which allows true three-dimensional (3-D) imaging with practical spatial resolution in the order of 5 mm and a temporal resolution less than 5 seconds. However, the complexity of computer PET science has advanced rapidly recently with, for example, development of 3-D volume reconstruction, stereotaxic localization/normalization, and multiparameter nonlinear, compartmental analysis of dynamic PET data.[29]

Although the problem of the partial volume effect is diminishing with new PET cameras, with increasingly better spatial resolution, it is likely to remain a limitation of PET measurements and must be considered in the interpretation of published results. Because of the difficulty in analyzing pure tissue compartments, absolute gray matter values for several of the physiologic variable listed in Table 6-1 appear lower than expected from older techniques, particularly CBF, $CMRO_2$ and CMRGlu. Also, the partial volume effect makes it theoretically difficult to detect narrow borderzones with intermediate values, such as the *ischemic penumbra*.[68]

## NORMAL COUPLING OF CEREBRAL BLOOD FLOW, CEREBRAL METABOLIC RATES OF OXYGEN AND GLUCOSE, AND CEREBRAL BLOOD VOLUME

With physiological conditions, there exists in each subject a matching of local values of CBF, $CMRO_2$, and CBV, according to linearly proportional relationships.[48,74] The CBF-$CMRO_2$ matching is such that local CBF values are highest in areas of highest $CMRO_2$ and vice versa; this describes the metabolic regulation of the cerebral circulation and explains why the distribution of CBF, as demonstrated in PET images, is superimposable on that of $CMRO_2$ while the OEF image is uniform. Thus, in the normal resting human brain, the local CBF reliably reflects the prevailing $CMRO_2$, although this coupling phenomenon may be altered during focal brain activation.

In individual normal subjects, there also exists a coupling between local CBF and CBV, which indicates that the degree of local vasodilatation in brain is strictly proportional to local tissue perfusion.[74] Since CBV, as measured by PET, reflects mainly the resistance (arteriolar) and capacitance (venular) blood volume, PET is able to evaluate the flow-to-resistance relationships. Studies in normal subjects also demonstrate a linear relationship between local CBV and $CMRO_2$ values.[74] Overall, the coupling among CBF, CBV, and $CMRO_2$ observed by PET reflects the metabolic regulation of cerebrovascular resistance and, in turn, of tissue perfusion, which operates at the local level in the normal brain.

Investigations of the relationships between CBF and CMRGlu have shown that in normal subjects the perfusion-metabolism coupling also applies to CMRGlu.[14,18] Likewise, excellent linear correlations between local $CMRO_2$ and CMRGlu values exist in control subjects, indicating coupling between oxygen consumption and glucose utilization in "resting" (but perhaps not during the "activated") human gray matter. The calculated stoichiometric relationship ($CMRO_2$/CMRGlu ratio) is close to the expected value of 6, indicating that glucose metabolism in the brain is almost exclusively oxidative.[18]

## THE INTERRELATIONSHIPS OF CEREBRAL BLOOD FLOW, CEREBRAL BLOOD VOLUME, CEREBRAL METABOLIC RATE OF OXYGEN, AND BRAIN GLUCOSE UTILIZATION IN STROKE

Studies in stroke have allowed delineation of diversely altered interplay among local CBF, CBV, $CMRO_2$, and CMRGlu values, thereby allowing clearly defined patterns of changes in physiologic coupling that distinguish widely different pathophysiologic situations. Three main types of patterns have been described: primary metabolic depression, hemodynamic failure, and luxury-perfusion.

### Primary Metabolic Depression

This pattern is defined as a matched decrease in CBF and $CMRO_2$ without alteration in the OEF, indicating that the normal perfusion-metabolism coupling is preserved in these hypometabolic areas.[6,9] Recent studies have demonstrated that CBV is also proportionally reduced in such areas, further documenting preserved coupling,[74] while the limited available data suggest a matched reduction in CMRGlu and $CMRO_2$, indicating a physiologic oxidative use of glucose.[18] Overall, primary metabolic depression appears as a global reduction in synaptic activity in an otherwise normally regulated tissue. Following stroke, primary metabolic depression is prone to widely affect both cortical and subcortical structures, as a result of disconnection (see the section Remote Metabolic Effects of Stroke in this chapter).

### Hemodynamic Failure

Hemodynamic failure, defined by a fall in the cerebral perfusion pressure (CPP) below the lower threshold of CBF autoregulation, is characterized by a reduction in CBF unaccompanied by a proportional reduction in $CMRO_2$—a disruption in the physiologic flow-metabolism coupling. Such a state of uncoupling, immediately detectable on the PET images as a focal increase in the OEF, has been termed *misery perfusion*.[7,9] This increase in the OEF above the normal value of 0.40, up to values approaching the theoretical maximum of 100, draws on the wide reserve of oxygen extraction that allows the brain, despite a reduced CBF, to maintain a normal $CMRO_2$—albeit at the expense of a threateningly reduced $PtO_2$. This initial phase where $CMRO_2$ is fully preserved is called *oligemia*. Beyond this phase, if CPP drops further, $CMRO_2$ begins to fall precipitously, characterizing the phase of *true ischemia* where tissue function is definitely impaired. Thus, misery perfusion spans from simple oligemia to true ischemia, since CBF is reduced and OEF elevated across the whole continuum of hemodynamic failure (Plate 6-1). In addition to CBF, OEF, and $CMRO_2$, PET allows mapping of CBV. Since the phenomenon of autoregulation is based on vasodilation of resistance vessels to counteract any reduction in CPP, it was postulated that imaging of CBV could help detect such changes in cerebrovascular resistance. Clear-cut increases in cortical blood volume were demonstrated during both oligemia and ischemia,[30,66] maximal in the former but returning toward normal values in the latter as a result of vascular collapse and metabolic depression.[74] Furthermore, CBV imaging was also able to identify the initial phase of vasodilatation which efficiently maintains CBF—the phase of autoregulation characterized by normal CBF, OEF, and $CMRO_2$, but elevated CBV, that is, a CBF-CBV uncoupling (see Table 6-2). A further application of the combined measurement of CBV and CBF is the use of CBV/CBF ratio and its converse, the CBF/CBV ratio. The former ratio has a unit of time and represents the local mean circulatory transit time, $t$, a physiologic parameter indicative of flow velocity. With PET, $t$ is obtained by dividing, pixel by pixel, the CBV parametric map (in ml/100 $ml^{-1}$) by the corresponding CBF map (in ml/100 $ml^{-1}$ $min^{-1}$). It indicates the "coupling" between blood flow and velocity in a given block of tissue and therefore increases as soon as CBF autoregulation is called upon. The converse ratio (CBF/CBV) has a unit of $min^{-1}$ and is a reliable index of the local CPP to which it is probably quasi-linearly proportional. The use of this ratio for small brain regions in single patients[74] has allowed demonstration in the living human brain of the successive stages of declining CPP from autoregulation to overt ischemia (Fig. 6-1). These studies have delineated a threshold value of the CBF/CBV ratio of about 7 $min^{-1}$ (normal value in controls 10 to 12 $min^{-1}$),

**TABLE 6-2. Patterns of Multiparameter Relationships as Revealed by Positron Emission Tomography in Acute Stroke**

| Pattern | CBF | CBV | OEF | $CMRO_2$ | Mechanism |
|---|---|---|---|---|---|
| Autoregulatory range | N | + | N | N | Vasodilatation (hemodynamic) reserve |
| Misery-perfusion | | | | | |
| Oligemia | – | ++ | + to ++ | N | Oxygen extraction reserve |
| Ischemia | – – | + | ++ | – | Metabolic depression (neuronal shutdown) |
| Luxury-perfusion | | | | | |
| Relative | – or N | + | – | – – | Ischemic necrosis |
| Absolute | + | + | – – | N to – – | Reactive hyperemia or necrosis |
| Pure metabolic depression | – | – | N | – | Synaptic hypofunction (neuronal death, diaschisis) |

N, normal; +, increased; ++, extremely increased; –, reduced; – –, extremely reduced.
*Abbreviations*: CBF, cerebral blood flow; CBV, cerebral blood volume; OEF, oxygen extraction fraction; $CMRO_2$, cerebral metabolic rate of oxygen.

below which the CBF falls and the OEF rises corresponding to the lower limit of autoregulation;[30,74] this, however, is not a sharp change but, rather, a smooth threshold. The OEF value at which the CBV is maximally elevated (lower limit of the vasodilatory reserve) has been recorded at 0.53.[39] The CBF/CBV ratio below which the $CMRO_2$ begins to fall, signaling ischemia, is not well defined as yet, but Sette et al.[74] reported a value of approximately 4 $min^{-1}$. These observations demonstrate the power of PET in evaluating in single subjects the local brain response to hemodynamic failure by allowing measurement at the local level not only of CBF, CBV, OEF, and $CMRO_2$, but also of the local CPP, a parameter that had previously been extrapolated from knowledge of systemic arterial pressure.

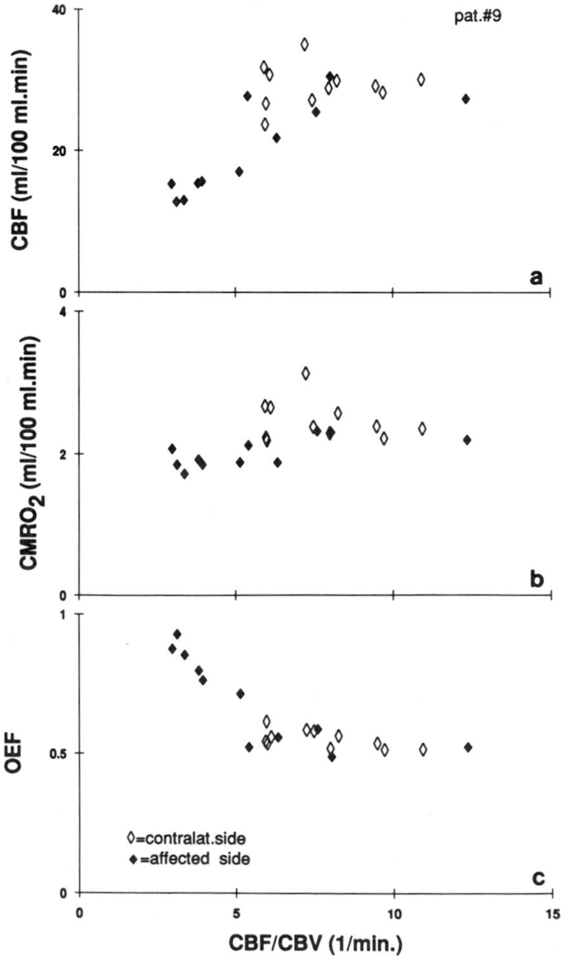


**Fig. 6-1.** Local values of cortical cerebral blood flow (CBF), oxygen extraction fraction (OEF), and cerebral metabolic rate of oxygen ($CMRO_2$) obtained in the patient described in Plate 6-1 from various areas of the hemispheres ipsilateral and contralateral to the left middle cerebral artery embolism, plotted as a function of corresponding local cerebral blood flow/cerebral blood volume (CBF/CBV) ratios. The data show the theoretically expected behavior of CBF, $CMRO_2$, and OEF as the local cerebral perfusion pressure (CPP), which is reflected in the CBF/CBV ratios, fall from normal to extremely low values. The data demonstrate efficient CBF autoegulation down to CBF/CBV ratios around 7 $min^{-1}$, followed by a fall in CBF in proportion to that of CPP; at this stage, the OEF rises (*top*) to values close to 100 percent; the $CMRO_2$ is well maintained for moderately low CPP (oligemia) but falls at lower CPP (true ischemia). These data demonstrate the capability of positron emission tomography to estimate in vivo local CPP and to relate brain hemodynamics and oxygen metabolism to the effects of arterial occlusion in a single patient. (From Sette et al.,[74] with permission.)

### Luxury Perfusion

Luxury perfusion was recognized by Lassen, long before the advent of PET, as the cause of both the *red vein syndrome* described by neurosurgeons and the early angiographic *blush* of recanalized brain infarction.[45] It is characterized by an oxygen supply in excess of demand, and its hallmark in PET studies is a focal reduction of the OEF.[1,9,10,49] This type of uncoupling, the converse of misery perfusion, indicates a reestablishment of perfusion and hence of the CPP in a previously ischemic tissue. PET studies have clearly demonstrated that luxury perfusion can have diverse appearances as well as mechanisms. Thus, CBF may be increased (hyperfusion), normal or even decreased (relative luxury perfusion), but is consistently in excess of prevailing $CMRO_2$. $CMRO_2$ may be either close to normal, as in the *reactive hyperemia* that immediately takes place in reperfused ischemic but nonnecrotic tissue, or reduced, depending on the severity of the damage incurred during ischemia. Although CBV has rarely been studied in this context, unpublished reports indicate that it is increased (true hyperemia) when there is hyperperfusion, revealing a state of *vasoparalysis* with abnormal vasodilatation (Plate 6-2 and Fig. 6-2).

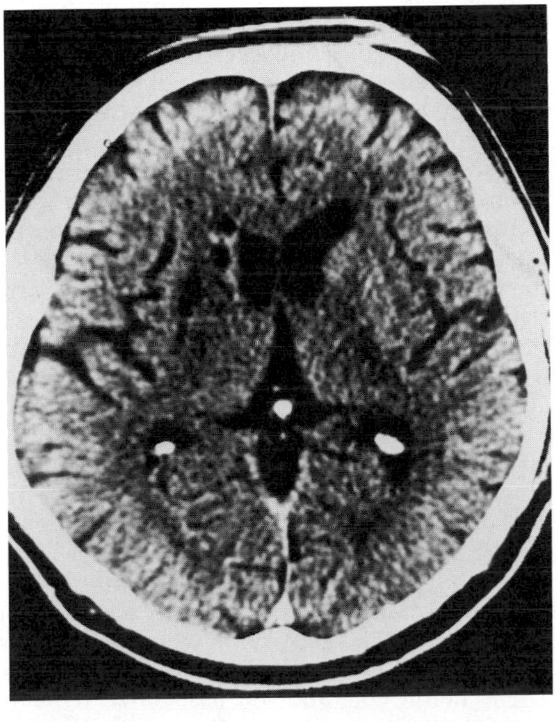

**Fig. 6-2.** Follow-up computed tomography scan (obtained at day 62 poststroke) of the 61-year-old patient described in Plate 6-1. Actually cerebral metabolic rate of oxygen was markedly reduced in the basal ganglia area, which demonstrated infarction at late CT scan. Clinically, functional recovery was excellent. (For quantitative positron emission tomography images, see Plate 6.1.)

The various patterns of altered physiologic variables that are encountered in stroke are summarized in Table 6-2. It shows that PET allows not only delineation of widely different pathophysiologic situations but also differentiation of the three conditions with reduced CBF (namely, misery perfusion, pure metabolic depression, and relative luxury perfusion). In addition, PET reveals abnormal hemodynamic changes despite normal CBF (i.e., during autoregulatory challenge and luxury perfusion), which emphasizes how misleading isolated CBF measurements may be. This capacity of multiparametric PET imaging also justifies its use in drug trials in stroke[24,33] as the therapeutic strategy would obviously depend on the type of pathophysiologic pattern observed.

#### *Cerebral Metabolic Rate of Oxygen and Cerebral Metabolic Rate of Glucose Uncoupling in Cerebrovascular Disease*

Because of the logistics involved in performing both $^{15}O$ and $^{18}FDG$ studies in the same setting, only a few reports have appeared on the relationships of $CMRO_2$ and CMRGlu in stroke. In addition, problems exist with the use of the $^{18}FDG$ model to evaluate CMRGlu in acutely ischemic tissue.[13] Hence both the FDG rate constants and the "lumped constant" can be grossly altered in this model, resulting in spurious values for CMRGlu. Studies that have attempted to overcome these problems have demonstrated clear-cut $CMRO_2$-CMRGlu uncoupling.[18,82] In acutely ischemic or necrotic tissue, CMRGlu is better preserved than $CMRO_2$, indicating anaerobic shift of glycolysis.[18,34,82] The reverse uncoupling has also been observed, mainly in tissues surrounding the actual infarct, suggesting the oxidative use of substrates other than glucose.[18]

## THE ISCHEMIC AND INFARCTED AREAS

### Studies of Cerebral Blood Flow, Cerebral Blood Volume, Oxygen Extraction Fraction, and Cerebral Metabolic Rate of Oxygen

Flow metabolism uncoupling, as evidenced by focally increased or decreased OEF, is present in over 90 percent of cases studied acutely[3,8,9] with both the misery perfusion and luxury perfusion types of uncoupling observed.

### Focal Misery Perfusion

Focal misery perfusion has been reported in 35 to 45 percent of patients studied within 3 to 4 days of onset, in 57 percent of cases studied within 24 hours, in 83 percent of patients studied within 12 hours and in 100 percent of those studied within 9 hours.[2,8,9,80] The findings indicate that, contrary to previously held belief, the phase of oligemia-ischemia is still ongoing in most cases studied up to 9 hours poststroke onset, and in more than one-third of those studied within 4 days, while reperfusion has taken place in the remaining. However, true ischemia with very high OEF (greater than 0.80) and reduced $CMRO_2$ has been observed almost exclusively within 12 hours after onset, affecting predominantly the cortical ribbon after middle cerebral artery (MCA) occlusion.[80] Oligemia characterized by very high OEF (greater than 0.80), but preserved $CMRO_2$ can be observed until the 4th day, while, in the remaining cases, reduced $CMRO_2$ with mildly elevated OEF prevails.[9,16,19]

Follow-up PET studies of the areas showing definite ischemia in the acute phase has been possible in a few cases only.[2,17,19,49,51,64,80] There are two main types of metabolic evolution: in the first, a profound fall in $CMRO_2$ occurs, associated with infarction and a variably evolving CBF (either further fall or marked increase). The second type of evolution also associated with ultimate infarction is characterized by an increase in CBF without any change in the reduced $CMRO_2$. Thus, in all cases, the initially elevated OEF uniformly falls with a second study because of either a further reduction in $CMRO_2$ or an increase in CBF or both; this fall in the OEF characterizes the transition from ischemia to infarction.[80] However, a few cases have been reported in which a similar situation of initial ischemia (in one patient still present as late as 30 hours after clinical onset) did not lead to actual infarction.[19,64] This variable final outcome of ischemia as viewed by PET may represent a potentially reversible "ischemic penumbra" in humans. Wise et al.,[80] and more recently Ackerman et al.,[2] pointed out that, even when patients are studied hyperacutely (less than 9 hours after onset), a core of ischemia exists, particularly involving the deep MCA territory, where CBF and $CMRO_2$ are already extremely low and OEF less increased than in the surrounding tissue, indicating an already established infarction. Wise et al.[80] suggested that, because of poor collaterals, the deep MCA territory suffers necrosis hours before the cortical ribbon; the latter thus has the potential to sustain several hours of critical ischemia (penumbra) and yet recover function in some instances.

Baron et al.[19] reported that the oligemic areas with very high OEF and essentially unchanged $CMRO_2$ had a good outcome at follow-up PET scan and CT study, while the areas exhibiting mildly elevated OEF with markedly reduced $CMRO_2$ consistently went on to frank necrosis. Lenzi et al.[49] attempted to relate the $CMRO_2$ values measured in the core of infarction to the qualitative clinical outcomes and claimed that in the early phase (first 2 weeks) values below 1.25 ml/100 g/min were always associated with poor outcome. Above that threshold value, outcome could be either good or bad; at later times after onset, this relationship was no longer apparent. Baron et al.[16] studied 25 patients and related the values measured to the tissue outcome as assessed by serial CT scans; in areas with misery-perfusion, well-defined thresholds separated viable from necrotic areas, demonstrating values of 11 and 1.7 ml/100 g/min for CBF and $CMRO_2$, respectively (55 and 70 percent of contralateral values, respectively). Powers et al.[65] classified 50 patients according to their clinical outcome and measured the minimum values for focal CBF, $CMRO_2$, CBV, and OEF. The minimum values for $CMRO_2$ in patients with good outcome was 1.3 ml/100 g/min, while the $CMRO_2$ value in the infarcted areas were below this threshold in 80 percent of the cases; corresponding analysis of CBF, CBV, and OEF did not reveal definable thresholds. In expanding their initial study to 17 patients studied 30 hours to 12 days poststroke, Baron et al.[19] were able to confirm previously published threshold values, but indicated the presence of some overlap of viable, partly necrotic, and necrotic brain areas about these thresholds. Recently, Ackerman et al.[2] reported on five patients studied within 2 to 6 hours of onset and found that areas with $CMRO_2$ below 1.5 ml/100 g/min always went on to infarction on late CT scan, while those with $CMRO_2$ above 2.5 ml/100 g/min were always intact; values with intermediate $CMRO_2$ displayed either infarcted or intact tissue. Overall, the above studies indicate a threshold for $CMRO_2$ at about 1.5 ml/100 g/min, below which, when measured more than 2 to 6 hours after onset, necrosis is constantly observed; above that value, there may well exist a "gray zone" for $CMRO_2$, in which tissue outcome is uncertain, corresponding to the concept of *penumbra* and therefore justifying prompt therapeutic interventions. Whether therapeutic interventions could prevent infarction in those areas remains to be proved, but could be tested by experimental models adapted to PET research.[23,79,83,84]

Pharmacologic increase of the systemic arterial pressure (SAP) has been reported in two patients with marked misery perfusion. Wise et al.[80] reported a patient studied at day 4 poststroke, in whom the increase in SAP resulted in a marked elevation of the CBF in the affected area but was associated with an inverse change in the OEF of the same magnitude, without improvement either in the $CMRO_2$ or in the clinical deficit. However, the $CMRO_2$ already was well below the above-mentioned infarction threshold, and the tissue outcome at day 4 was presumably already settled. Ackerman et al.[2] reported a patient investigated 2 to 6 hours poststroke, in whom an increase in SAP for 3 hours increased CBF in the zone surrounding the ischemic core and was associated with an improvement in oxygen metabolism and clinical outcome.

## Luxury Perfusion in Acute Stroke

Absolute luxury perfusion (i.e., with hyperperfusion) indicating recanalization of the occluded artery, has been recorded in the surround of the infarct in only one of 11 patients studied within 16 hours of clinical onset, but in 7 of 12 stroke patients studied in the interval between 16 and 30 hours after onset. After 48 hours, Baron et al.[16] noted that hyperperfusion may affect not only the irreversibly damaged area (as defined by serial CT scans), but also its surroundings, which are differentiated by profoundly reduced $CMRO_2$ in the infarct and essentially preserved $CMRO_2$ in the latter zone (Fig. 6-1). *Relative* luxury perfusion, however, appears the most frequent pattern during this period;[16] it indicates partial reperfusion in an already necrotic tissue, presumably through collateral channels. In addition to the patterns of misery-perfusion and luxury-perfusion, a matched reduction in residual CBF and $CMRO_2$ in the infarct core has also been reported in the acute stage,[9,16] presumably indicating partial reperfusion with fortuitously matching flow-metabolism. Finally, in the subacute phase of ischemic strokes, neighboring areas of brain tissue may occasionally show the coexistence of mild misery perfusion, relative luxury-perfusion, and matched CBF-$CMRO_2$ depression.[9]

## Prognostic and Therapeutic Implications of Positron Emission Tomography Findings in Acute Stroke

The data reviewed above indicate that the pattern of CBF-$CMRO_2$ uncoupling, as visualized by OEF images, carries no specific inference regarding tissue outcome. The absolute values for CBF and $CMRO_2$ appear to have closer relationships to final outcome, although the dynamics of ischemia, a key factor in addition to severity in the early hours after stroke, remain largely unknown because PET studies only provide a discontinuous "snapshot" of changes in a given patient. Although $CMRO_2$ values below 1.5 ml/100 ml/min seem to predict ultimate infarction, it is not known whether immediate therapeutic action could prevent this ominous outlook; conversely, moderately reduced $CMRO_2$ values (between 1.5 and 2.5 ml/100 ml/min) appear to be associated with variable tissue outcome (?"penumbra"). A better understanding of these issues will certainly accrue from PET studies of focal experimental cerebral ischemia in nonhuman primates.[83,84] Despite these uncertainties, however, PET findings already suggest that therapeutic enhancement of CBF would be of no use, or could even be deleterious, if luxury perfusion is at play, while the use of neuroprotectors would make little sense if $CMRO_2$ is already profoundly depressed. One of the uses of PET, therefore, could be to help select into drug trials only those patients whose CBF-$CMRO_2$ pattern would most closely match the drug's presumed mechanism of action.

Another implication of PET studies for management of the acute ischemic stroke patient relates to the issue of management of arterial hypertension. Demonstration of misery perfusion in a given patient implies that any lowering of the systemic blood pressure may have potentially damaging effects, since it will further reduce the CPP and, in turn, will also affect CBF because loss of autoregulation makes flow directly pressure-dependent. Conversely, if absolute luxury perfusion is present, cautious reduction of arterial hypertension may be warranted, particularly if early edema is demonstrated by computed tomography (CT) scanning or magnetic resonance imaging (MRI), since experimental studies show that hyperperfusion is a critical factor in the development of malignant poststroke brain swelling. Studies are needed to assess this possibility.

## Long-Term Evolution of Findings

Evolution of the hemodynamic and metabolic parameters following the acute phase of stroke has been studied almost exclusively within the infarct core. The salient finding is the constant phase of luxury perfusion in the necrotic tissue, starting at about the 2nd or 3rd day (see above) and lasting several weeks.[1,9] during this phase, CBF increases progressively to often reach normal or above-normal values around the 8th to 12th day; focal OEF varies in a mirror fashion, falling to very low values around the 10th day. This rise in CBF takes place without any significant increase in $CMRO_2$,[17] indicating purposeless reperfusion in an already necrotic tissue. These events presumably reflect the development of neovascularization, with a loss of the normal flow-metabolism regulation. In established infarction, a positive linear correlation exists between local CBF and the magnitude of CT contrast enhancement,[12] indicating leakage of proteins through a damaged blood-brain barrier.

In areas surrounding the infarct, mild physiologic changes are seen in the subacute phase in over 75 percent of the cases.[16] Thus luxury perfusion may persist over several days in the areas surrounding the final infarct, associated with either normal or only mildly decreased $CMRO_2$. Misery perfusion may be seen in ultimately viable areas until the 12th day.[16] In a number of instances, $CMRO_2$ was reduced despite a mildly increased OEF, suggesting the superimposition of mild oligemia on a background of synaptic depression presumably reflecting selective neuronal loss or deafferentation (see the section Remote Metabolic Effects of Stroke in this chapter).

Following this subacute phase, the infarcted area progressively takes on its final appearance of an area with close-to-zero CBF and $CMRO_2$. The process of cavitation lasts about 2 months, during which CBF slowly falls while the OEF returns to baseline. The surrounding tissue often exhibits normal CBF and $CMRO_2$ values; however, in many cases, a matched decrease in CBF and $CMRO_2$ affects a widespread area of brain tissue (see the section Remote Metabolic Effects of Stroke). Finally, in a small proportion of patients with minor strokes or chronic carotid or middle cerebral artery occlusions, protracted hemodynamic impairment persists, as repeatedly demonstrated by PET, taking the form of either reduced hemodynamic reserve or frank misery perfusion and affecting preferentially the borderzone cortical areas.[7,30,47,69,70,72,76] Because these changes suggest an increased susceptibility for further ipsilateral ischemic events, they have led to the performance of the now abandoned superficial temporal artery to MCA bypass surgery.[7,31,46,67,72]

### Studies of Tissue pH

Using $^{11}$C-DMO as a marker of intracellular pH, Syrota et al.[77] found markedly increased $^{11}$C uptake in four of nine recent (10 to 34 days) carotid artery infarcts, suggesting that local alkalosis was operative. Since combined $^{15}$O studies revealed prominent luxury perfusion in the affected brain area in these four patients, the results exclude tissue acidosis as the causal factor for luxury perfusion. Because $^{11}$C-DMO linearly correlated with decreases in local OEF, the hypothesis was advanced that perfusion in excess to local metabolic demand could have triggered tissue alkalosis by removing metabolically produced $CO_2$ and, in turn, decreasing local $H^+$ content. These findings were confirmed and expanded in a further study measuring intracellular pH in absolute units.[78] The intracellular alkalosis observed within the necrotic area could also be due to infiltration of phagocytic cells, using glycolysis to synthesize hydrogen peroxide. Hakim et al.[34] reported normal pH in the core of reperfused infarction, but these results may have reflected the more acutely studied nature of the patients or that the $^{11}$C-DMO method used provided only whole-tissue pH. In patients with hypoperfusion, Hakim et al.[34] reported reduced pH, indicating tissue acidosis unrelated to enhanced anaerobic glycolysis, which was ruled out by a normal CMRGlu/$CMRO_2$ ratio. Using the $^{11}CO_2$-whole tissue pH method, Senda et al.[73] also observed tissue acidosis in hypoperfused, acutely ischemic tissue; in less acute conditions, and in the setting of hyperperfusion and lowered OEF, these authors also found an increased pH, in agreement with earlier findings.

### Studies of Cerebral Blood flow, Cerebral Metabolic Rate of Oxygen, and Brain Glucose Utilization

Using $^{13}NH_3$ as a perfusion tracer and $^{18}$FDG to measure CMRGlu, Kuhl et al.[42] found two opposite patterns of uncoupling among these two variables in early infarcts. Initially, $^{13}$N uptake was low, but $^{18}$F uptake relatively preserved, suggesting persistent ischemia with enhanced anaerobic glycolysis, while later the data suggested reperfusion within the hypometabolic tissue. However, uncertainties concerning possible alterations in the $^{18}$FDG kinetic constant ($k{*}s$) and lumped-constant within recent infarcts[32] precluded any firm conclusion from such data. In three studies[18,34,82] both $CMRO_2$ and CMRGlu were measured. Preservation of CMRGlu relative to $CMRO_2$ was observed within the core of the infarct, implying enhanced anaerobic glycolysis; as luxury perfusion was constant, "anaerobic" glycolysis occurred in the face of tissue hyperoxia, inferring that mechanisms other than hypoxia were at play. On the other hand, Hakim et al.[34] observed preserved CMRGlu/$CMRO_2$ coupling in acutely ischemic tissue, despite local acidosis. Finally, zones of depressed CMRGlu, but preserved $CMRO_2$, immediately surrounding the area of tissue damage have been reported,[18] suggesting that substrates other than bloodborne glucose were oxidized for energy production in this tissue. This evidence for a disruption of the CMRGlu/$CMRO_2$ coupling indicates that the measurement of glucose utilization does not reliably reflect the tissue's synaptic activity during a recent stroke. These findings explain, in part, the weak correlation between neurologic outcome and ipsilateral hemisphere CMRGlu.[44]

## REMOTE METABOLIC EFFECTS OF STROKE

The occurrence of metabolic depression (see the section on the interrelationships of CBF, CBV, $CMRO_2$ and CMRGlu for a definition of terms) in morphologically intact brain areas distant from the site of stroke has been clearly documented by PET (for review, see ref. 5). These unexpected effects have been subjected to extensive investigations regarding their topographic, neuroanatomic, morphologic, and clinical correlates in order to provide a better understanding of the biologic mechanisms underlying the clinical expression of, and recovery from, stroke.[4,26,35]

### Contralateral Cerebellar Hypometabolism

Contralateral cerebellar hypometabolism (CCH), first described by Baron et al.,[6] who coined the terms "crossed cerebellar diaschisis," consists of metabolic depression of the cerebellar hemisphere contralateral to supratentorial stroke (Fig. 6-3). It occurs in about 50 percent of patients with either a cortical or subcortical stroke[58] but is more frequent with large frontoparietal infarcts and with subcortical lesions affecting the internal capsule, including posterior limb lacunes.[49,52,58,59] These topographic correlations suggest that CCH results from damage to the descending corticopontocerebellar system and reflects transneuronal functional depression.[6] Although CCH is correlated with the severity of hemiparesis,[6,58] this association is not systematic, indicating that damage to the pyramidal system is neither necessary nor sufficient to induce CCH, but rather the proximity of the pyramidal and corticopontine fibers causes this association. In the vast majority of patients, CCH exhibits no tendency to recover and may actually evolve into transneuronal degeneration. However, the fact that CCH can be observed within the first hours of stroke,

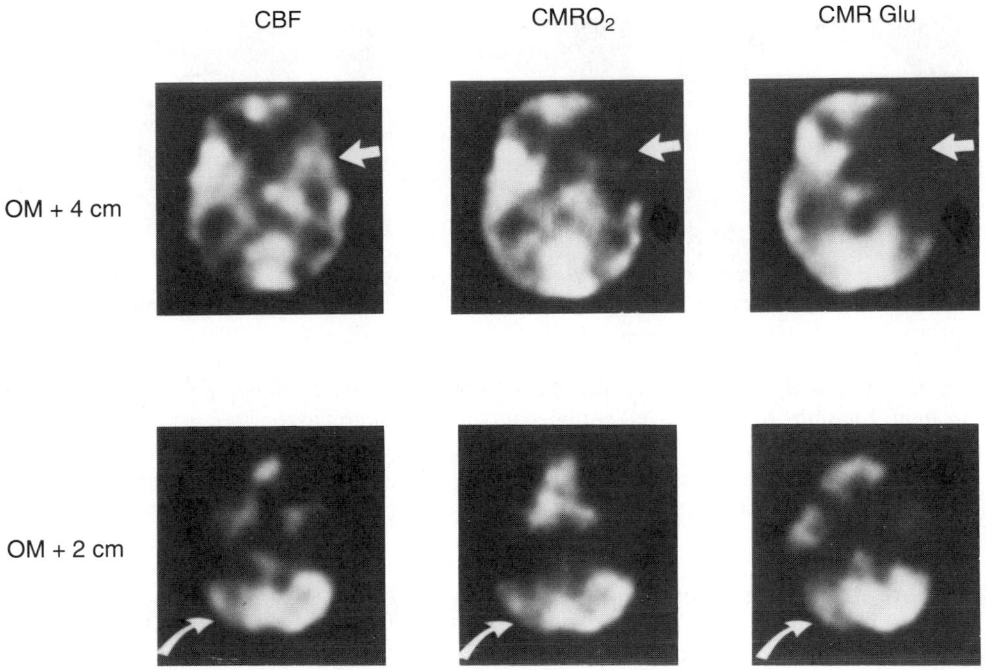


**Fig. 6-3.** Quantitative images of cerebral blood flow, cerebral metabolic rate of oxygen, and cerebral metabolic rate of glucose obtained at two brain levels in a 37-year-old patient 6 days after massive right MCA infarction due to cardiac embolism. On these images, the right side of the brain is on the reader's right. The data show on level OM +4 cm a profoundly reduced cereral metabolic rate of oxygen and cerebral metabolic rate of glucose in the infarcted area associated with a heterogeneous CBF showing combined areas of markedly reduced, moderately reduced, and increased flow (luxury-perfusion, *straight arrows*); on level OM +2 cm, a proportional reduction in flow, oxygen consumption, and glucose utilization in the entire left cerebellar hemisphere (crossed cerebellar diaschisis) demonstrating primary metabolic depression, is seen, a remote transneuronal effect of right MCA infarction, which damages the crossed corticopontocerebellar pathway. (Adapted from Baron et al.,[18] with permission.)

and sometimes disappears within a few days, indicate that it is a manifestation of acute deafferentation and not necessarily the forerunner of degeneration.[43,58] Finally, CCH can be a manifestation of a secondary effect of functional depression of the cerebral cortex, as shown both during unilateral carotid infusion of barbiturates in epileptic patients and as a result of cortical hypometabolism in thalamic stroke patients.[5,59]

The clinical correlates, if any, of CCH remain as yet unsettled. An occurrence of both CCH and ipsilateral ataxia has been anecdotically reported in two patients,[20,71] but was not confirmed by Pappata et al.[59]

## Thalamocortical Diaschisis

PET studies have demonstrated that unilateral thalamic or thalamocapsular strokes frequently induce depression of energy metabolism involving the entire ipsilateral cortical mantle.[11,60] This effect occurs regardless of the size, exact nuclear topography, or side of the thalamic lesion, and is independent of involvement of the adjacent internal capsule (Fig. 6-4). One exception to this rule are ventroposterolateral (VPL) thalamus infarcts, which do not induce this phenomenon.[22] Although diffuse over the whole cortex, the metabolic effect often predominates in the projection area corresponding to the nuclear topography of the thalamic lesion, supporting the view that the so-called "nonspecific" thalamocortical systems are implicated.[11] In addition to involving the ipsilateral cortex, metabolic depression also affects, albeit to a lesser degree, the contralateral cortical ribbon.[11,15] It is also more profound early after stroke and tends to recover gradually over the ensuing months, according to a monoexponential model with a half-recovery time in the range of 8 to 10 months.[15,21] These findings suggest that initial metabolic depression reflects a transsynaptic hypofunction of the cortical neurons, while subsequent recovery reveals a considerable potential for postdeafferentation reorganization. The metabolic asymmetry recovers more rapidly, but plateaus at a value slightly below normal, a "metabolic scar," which may reflect actual anterograde degeneration of the thalamocortical fibers.[15] The cortical metabolic effects of unilateral thalamic stroke, and its subsequent recovery, are significantly associated with the presence of neuropsychological impairment,[15] while patients who are spared neuropsychological impairment (e.g., VPL stroke) exhibit no cortical hypometabolism.[22] These results indicate that cortical

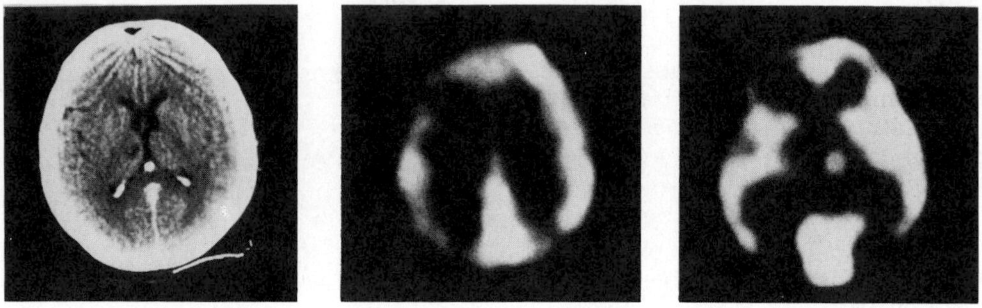

A B C

**Fig. 6-4.** (**A**) Computed tomography scan and (**B & C**) positron emission tomography images obtained in a 57-year-old woman, 2 months following a left paramedian thalamic infarct associated with persistent impairment in verbal fluency and memory. The PET images of cerebral glucose utilization, obtained at the levels of the corona radiata (B) and of the basal ganglia (C) show significant metabolic depression affecting the entire cortical mantle on the side of the thalamic infarct. (The left side of the images corresponds to the left side of the brain.)

hypometabolism is linked to the neuropsychological expression of thalamic infarction as well as to its recovery. These results may have important therapeutic implications for interventional manipulation of the deafferented cortical fields. Patients with bilateral paramedian thalamic infarction syndrome, including memory impairment and apathy, display a clear-cut reduction in cortical oxygen consumption that affects the entire cerebral cortex without significant regional preponderance, suggesting that cortical deafferentation may play a role in the development of "thalamic dementia."[50]

## White Matter Damage

Damage to the optic radiations as a result of MCA infarction induces a significant reduction in glucose utilization in the disconnected part of the ipsilateral primary visual cortex, sometimes spreading to the visual association areas.[63] While lacunes of the posterior limb of the internal capsule without neuropsychological sequelae are likely to induce CCH, they do not alter cortical metabolism to any significant extent.[59] In one patient with fluctuating intellectual dysfunction and multiple lacunes, Metter et al.[54] observed a left frontal cortex hypometabolism attributed to a lacune in the anterior limb of the left internal capsule, probably interrupting the thalamocortical fibers from the dorsomedial nucleus. Herholz et al.[36] reported that subcortical white matter infarcts induce hypoperfusion of the overlying cerebral cortex, presumably due to disconnection.

## Subcortical Aphasia

Metter et al.[55–57] investigated the relationships between cortical hypometabolism and language impairment in 47 patients with subcortical aphasia. They reported that, although the subcortical lesion itself did have a direct relationship to the aphasia measures, left frontal and temporal hypometabolism also affected verbal fluency and comprehension tasks, respectively. Similarly, Karbe et al.[40] found an excellent correlation between the loss of verbal comprehension and left parietotemporal hypometabolism in patients with subcortical stroke and aphasia; furthermore, they also demonstrated an inverse relationship between left prefrontal hypometabolism and verbal comprehension impairment.

## Effects of Cortical Lesions on Subcortical Metabolism

PET studies have clearly demonstrated the frequent occurrence of significant hypometabolism affecting the striatum and thalamus ipsilateral to cortical strokes.[9,42,61,80] Striatal hypometabolism resulted preferentially from prerolandic cortical lesions. Published data also suggest the association of deep nuclear hypometabolism with specific measures for impaired cognitive and language performance;[55,56] for example, left caudate and thalamic hypometabolism is significantly more prominent in Broca's than in Wernicke's and conduction aphasias.[53]

Experimental studies in rats revealed that the metabolic depression affecting the ipsilateral thalamus partly reflects a process of active retrograde degeneration of the damaged thalamocortical neurons; however, striatal hypometabolism is not associated with clear-cut neuronal death.[26]

## Intracortical Effects

PET studies of corticosubcortical strokes have frequently demonstrated a reduction in CBF and/or metabolism, affecting large areas of morphologically normal ipsilateral cerebral cortex, a phenomenon that occasionally persists to the chronic stage.[9,42,57] However, these effects have proved difficult to interpret. Thus a rim of cortical metabolic depression around an acute infarct may either represent the "ischemic penumbra," or may be the result of spreading edema, or, finally, represent selective neuronal damage. In the chronic stage, hypometabolism may reflect not only the latter, but also damage to the subcortical afferents in cases with lesions involving the white matter ("undercutting"), especially from the basal ganglia or the thalamus (see above). Regardless of its exact mechanisms, the extent and magnitude of cortical hypometabolism with left-sided (dominant) corticosubcortical strokes are strongly correlated with both the severity and type of aphasia.[40,53,56]

## Contralateral (?Transcallocal) Cortical Effects

The phenomenon of contralateral cortical effects is of great clinical interest, since it may explain some of the "diffuse" symptoms associated with supratentorial strokes such as agitation, confusion, and coma.[4,26] Initial PET studies of cerebral oxygen consumption in a heterogeneous group of stroke patients were inconsistent in demonstrating this effect,[49,81] presumably because a number of factors were not considered, such as subject's age, delay of the investigation since stroke onset, lesion topography, and underlying large-vessel occlusion. In patients with unilateral thalamic strokes, Baron et al.[11,15] demonstrated a significant reduction in contralateral cortical glucose utilization, which tended to recover monoexponentially. These results are consistent with PET studies of cortical CMRGlu in baboons subjected to unilateral lesion of the nucleus basalis of Meynert.[41] Recently, Dobkin et al.[25] reported on the occurrence of contralateral hemispheric diaschisis wherein most of the above-mentioned confounding factors were taken into account; they found a significantly reduced contralateral CBF in recent strokes, which correlated to the subject's age but not with the degree of lethargy.

## REFERENCES

1. Ackerman RH, Correia JA, Alpert NM, Baron JC et al: Positron imaging in ischemic stroke disease using compounds labelled with oxygen-15. Arch Neurol 38:537, 1981
2. Ackerman RH, Lev MH, Mackay BC et al: PET studies in acute stroke: findings and relevance to therapy. J Cereb Blood Flow Metab, suppl 1. 9:S359, 1989
3. Baron JC: Positron tomography in cerebral ischemia. Neuroradiology 2:509, 1985
4. Baron JC: Remote metabolic effects of stroke. p. 91. In Wade J et al (eds): Impact of Functional Imaging in Neurology and Psychiatry. J. Libbey, Paris, 1987
5. Baron JC: Depression of energy metabolism in distant brain structures: studies with PET in stroke patients. Semin Neurol 9:281 1989
6. Baron JC, Bousser MG, Comar D, Castaigne P: Crossed cerebellar diaschisis in human supratentorial brain infarction. Trans Am Neurol Assoc 105:459, 1980
7. Baron JC, Bousser MG, Rey A et al: Reversal of focal "misery-perfusion syndrome" by extra-intracranial arterial bypass in hemodynamic cerebral ischemia: a case study with $^{15}O$ positron tomography. Stroke 12:454, 1981
8. Baron JC, Bousser MG, Comar D et al: Apport de la tomographie par émission de positrons dans l'étude physiopathologique de l'ischémie cérébrale chez l'homme. Presse Med 12:3066, 1983
9. Baron JC, Bousser MG, Comar D et al: Noninvasive tomographic study of cereral blood flow and oxygen metabolism in vivo: potentials, limitations and clinical applications in cerebral ischemic disorders. Eur Neurol 20:273, 1981
10. Baron JC, Comar D, Bousser MG et al: Etude tomographique chez l'homme du débit sanguin et de la consommation d'oxygène du cerveau par inhalation continue d'oxygène 15. Rev Neurol (Paris) 134:545, 1978
11. Baron JC, D'Antona R, Pantano P et al: Effects of thalamic stroke on energy metabolism of the cerebral cortex. Brain 109:1243, 1986
12. Baron JC, Delattre JY, Chiras J et al: Comparison study of CT and positron emission tomographic data in recent cerebral infarction. AJNR 4:536, 1983
13. Baron JC, Frackowiak RSJ, Herholz K et al: Use of positron emission tomography in the investigation of cerebral hemodynamics and energy metabolism in cerebrovascular disease. J Cereb Blood Flow Metabol 9:723, 1989
14. Baron JC, Lebrun P, Collard P et al: Non-invasive measurement of blood flow, oxygen consumption and glucose utilization in the same brain regions in man by positron emission tomography: concise communication. J Nucl Med 23:391, 1982
15. Baron JC, Levasseur M, Mazoyer B et al: The link between cortical hypometabolism and neuropsychological deficit after thalamic lesions: a PET study. J Cereb Blood Flow Metabol, suppl. 9:740, 1989
16. Baron JC, Rougemont D, Bousser MG et al: Local CBF, oxygen extraction fraction and $CMRO_2$: prognostic relevance in recent cerebral infarction in humans. J Cereb Blood Flow Metab, suppl 3:1, 1983
17. Baron JC, Rougemont D, Lebrun-Grandie P et al: Measurement of local blood flow and oxygen consumption in evolving irreversible cerebral infarction: an in vivo study in man. p. 205. In Meyer JS, Lechner E, Reivich M (eds): Cerebral Vascular Disease. Vol. 4. Excerpta Medica, Amsterdam, 1983
18. Baron JC, Rougemont D, Soussaline F et al: Local interrelationship of cerebral oxygen consumption and glucose utilization in normal subjects and in ischemic stroke patients: a positron tomography study. J Cereb Blood Flow Metab 4:140, 1984
19. Baron JC, Samson Y, Pantano P et al: Interrelationships of local CBF, OEF and $CMRO_2$ in ischemic areas with variable outcome: further PET studies in humans. J Cereb Blood Flow Metabol, suppl 1. 7:41, 1987

20. Bogousslavsky J, Regli F, Delaloye B et al: Hemiataxie et déficit sensitif ipsilateral: infarctus du territoire de l'artère choroïdienne antérieure, diaschisis cérébelleux croisé. Rev neurol (Paris) 142:671, 1986
21. Cambon H, Baron JC, Pappata S et al: Recovery of cortical metabolism after thalamic lesions in humans: a manifestation of plasticity. J Cereb Blood Flow Metabol, suppl. 7:194, 1987
22. Chabriat H, Levasseur M, Pappata S et al: PET studies of cortical metabolism in patients with postero-lateral thalamic stroke. Neurology (NY), suppl 1. 40:213, 1990
23. De Ley G, Weyne J, Demeester G et al: Experimental thromboembolic stroke studied by positron emission tomography: immediate versus delayed reperfusion by fibrinolysis. J Cereb Blood Flow Metab 8:539, 1988
24. Depresseux JC, Franck G, Van Cauwenberge H: Evaluation métabolique et circulatoire de l'accident cérébral ischémique aigu chez l'homme par tomographie d'émmission positonique. Presse Med 16:1145, 1987
25. Dobkin JA, Levine RL, Lagoze HL et al: Evidence for transhemispheric diaschisis in unilateral stroke. Arch Neurol 46:1333, 1989
26. Feeney D, Baron JC: Diaschisis. Stroke 17:817, 1986
27. Fieschi C, Di Piero V, Lenzi GL et al: Pathophysiology of ischemic brain disease. Stroke, suppl 4. 21:IV-9, 1990
28. Frackowiak RSJ: The pathophysiology of human cerebral ischaemia: a new perspective obtained with positron tomography. Q J Med 223:713, 1985
29. Frost JJ, Wagner HN: Quantitative Imaging: Neuroreceptors, Neurotransmitters and Enzymes. Raven Press, New York, 1990
30. Gibbs JM, Wise RJS, Leenders KL et al: Cerebral haemodynamics in occlusive carotid-artery disease. Lancet 1:933, 1984
31. Gibbs JM, Wise RJS, Thomas DJ et al: Cerebral haemodynamic changes after extracranial-intracranial bypass surgery. J Neurol Neurosurg Psychiatry 50:140, 1987
32. Gjedde A, Wienhard K, Heiss WD et al: Comparative regional analysis of 2-fluorodeoxyglucose and methylglucose uptake in brain of four stroke patients, with special reference to the regional estimation of the lumped constant. J Cereb Blood Flow Metab 5:163, 1985
33. Hakim AM, Evans AC, Berger L et al: The effect of nimodipine on the evolution of human cerebral infarction studied by PET. J Cereb Blood Flow Metab 9:523, 1989
34. Hakim AM, Pokrupa RP, Villaneuva J et al: The effects of spontaneous reperfusion on metabolic function in early human cerebral infarcts. Ann Neurol 21:279, 1987
35. Heiss WD, Pawlik G, Hebold I et al: Can positron emission tomography be used to gauge the brain's capacity for functional recovery following ischemic stroke? p. 345. In Ginsberg MD et al (ed): Cerebrovascular Disease. Raven Press, New York, 1989
36. Herholz K, Heindel W, Rackl A et al: Regional cerebral blood flow in patients with leukoaraiosis and atherosclerosic carotid artery disease. Arch Neurol 47:392, 1990
37. Herscovitch P: Measurement of regional cerebral hemodynamics and metabolism by positron emission tomography. p. 179. In Neuromethods. Vol. 8. Humana Press, Clifton, NJ, 1988
38. Junck L, Jewett DM, Kilbourn MR et al: PET imaging of cerebral infarcts using a ligand for the peripheral benzodiazepine binding site. Neurology (NY), suppl 1. 40:265, 1990
39. Kanno I, Uemura K, Higano S: Oxygen extraction fraction at maximally vasodilated tissue in the ischemic brain estimated from the regional $CO_2$ responsiveness measured by positron emission tomography. J Cereb Blood Flow Metab 8:227, 1988
40. Karbe H, Herholz K, Szelies B: Regional metabolic correlates of token test results in cortical and subcortical left hemispheric infarction. Neurology (NY) 39:1087, 1989
41. Kiyosawa M, Baron JC, Hamel E: Time course of efects of unilateral lesions of the nucleus basalis of Meynert on glucose utilization of the cerebral cortex: positron tomography in baboons. Brain 112:435, 1989
42. Kuhl DE, Phelps ME, Kowell AP et al: Effects of stroke on local cerebral metabolism and perfusion: mapping by emission computed tomography of $^{18}$FDG and $^{13}NH_3$. Ann Neurol 8:47, 1980
43. Kushner M, Alair A, Reivich M et al: Contralateral cerebellar hypometabolism following cerebral insult: a positron emission tomographic study. Ann Neurol 15:425, 1984
44. Kushner M, Reivich M, Fieschi C et al: Metabolic and clinical correlates of acute ischemic infarction. Neurology (NY) 37:1103, 1987
45. Lassen NA: The luxury perfusion syndrome and its possible relation to acute metabolic acidosis localized within the brain. Lancet 2:1113, 1966
46. Leblanc R, Tyler JL, Mohr G et al: Hemodynamic and metabolic effects of cerebral revascularization. J Neurosurg 66:529, 1987
47. Leblanc R, Yamamoto YL, Tyler JL et al: Borderzone ischemia. Ann Neurol 22:707, 1987
48. Lebrun-Grandie P, Baron JC, Soussaline F et al: Coupling between regional cerebral blood flow and oxygen consumption in the normal human brain: a study with positron tomography and oxygen 15. Arch Neurol 40:230, 1983
49. Lenzi GL, Frackowiak RSJ, Jones T: Cerebral oxygen metabolism and blood flow in human cerebral ischemic infarction. J Cereb Blood Flow Metab 2:231, 1982
50. Levasseur M, Baron JC, Sette G et al: Brain energy metabolism in bilateral paramedian thalamic infarcts: a positron tomography study. Brain, 1992 (in press)
51. Marchal G, Evans A, Dagher A et al: The evolution of cerebral infarction with time: a PET study of the ischemic penumbra. J Cereb Blood Flow Metabol, suppl 1. 7:S99, 1987
52. Martin WR, Raichle ME: Cerebellar blood flow and metabolism in cerebral hemisphere infarction. Ann Neurol 14:168, 1983

53. Metter EJ, Kempler D, Jackson C et al: Cerebral glucose metabolism in Wernicke's, Broca's, and conduction aphasia. Arch Neurol 46:27, 1989
54. Metter EJ, Mazziotta JC, Itabaschi HA et al: Comparison of glucose metabolism, x-ray CT and postmortem data in a patient with multiple cerebral infarcts. Neurology (NY) 35:1695, 1985
55. Metter EJ, Riege WH, Hanson WR et al: Comparison of metabolic rates, language and memory in subcortical aphasia. Brain Lang 19:33, 1983
56. Metter EJ, Riege WH, Hanson WR et al: Subcortical structures in aphasia. Arch Neurol 45:1229, 1988
57. Metter EJ, Wasterlain CG, Kuhl DE et al: $^{18}$FDG positron emission tomography in a study of aphasia. Ann Neurol 10:173, 1981
58. Pantano P, Baron JC, Samson Y: Crossed cerebellar diaschisis: further studies. Brain 109:677, 1986
59. Pappata S, Mazoyer B, Tran Dinh S et al: Cortical and cerebellar hypometabolic effects of capsular, thalamo-capsular, and thalamic stroke: a positron tomography study. Stroke 21:519, 1990
60. Pappata S, Tran Dinh JC, Samson Y et al: Remote metabolic effects of cerebrovascular lesions: magnetic resonance and positron tomography imaging. Neuroradiology 29:1, 1987
61. Pawlik G, Herholz K, Beil C et al: Remote effects of focal lesions on cerebral blood flow and metabolism. p. 59. In Heiss WD (ed): Functional Mapping of the Brain in Vascular Disorders. Springer-Verlag, Berlin, 1985
62. Phelps ME, Huang SC, Hoffman EJ et al: Tomographic measurement of local glucose metabolic rate in humans with (F-18) 2-fluoro-2-deoxy-D-glucose: validation of method. Ann Neurol 6:371, 1979
63. Phelps ME, Mazziotta JC, Kuhl DE et al: Tomographic mapping of human cerebral metabolism: visual stimulation and deprivation. Neurology 31:517, 1981
64. Powers WJ, Grubb RL, Baker RP et al: Regional cerebral blood flow and metabolism in reversible ischemia due to vasospasm. J Neurosurg 62:539, 1986
65. Powers WJ, Grubb RL, Jr, Darriet D, Raichle ME: Cerebral blood flow and cerebral metabolic rate of oxygen requirements for cerebral function and viability in humans. J Cereb Blood Flow Metab 5:600, 1985
66. Powers WJ, Grubb RL, Raichle ME: Physiological response to focal cerebral ischemia in humans. Ann Neurol 16:546, 1984
67. Powers WJ, Martin WRW, Herscovitch P et al: Extracranial-intracranial bypass surgery: hemodynamic and metabolic effects. Neurology (NY) 34:1168, 1984
68. Powers WJ, Mintun A: Role of positron emission tomography in identification of the ischemic penumbra. p. 273. In Raichle M, Powers J (eds): Cerebrovascular Disease. Raven Press, New York, 1987
69. Powers WJ, Press GA, Grubb RL et al: The effect of hemodynamically significant carotid artery disease on the hemodynamic status of the cerebral circulation. Ann Intern Med 106:27, 1987
70. Pozzilli C, Itoh M, Matsuzawa T et al: Positron emission tomography in minor ischemic stroke using oxygen-15 steady-state technique. J Cereb Blood Flow Metab 7:137, 1987
71. Sakai F, Aoki S, Kan S et al: Ataxic hemiparesis with reduction of ipsilateral cerebellar blood flow. Stroke 17:1016, 1986
72. Samson Y, Baron JC, Bousser MG et al: Effects of extra-intracranial arterial bypass on cerebral blood flow and oxygen metabolism in humans. Stroke 16:609, 1985
73. Senda M, Alpert NM, Mackay BC et al: Evaluation of the $^{11}CO_2$ positron emission tomographic method for measuring brain pH. II. Quantitative pH mapping in patients with ischemic cerebrovascular diseases. J Cereb Blood Flow Metab 9:859, 1989
74. Sette G, Baron JC, Mazoyer B et al: Local brain hemodynamics and oxygen metabolism in cerebro-vascular disease: positron emission tomography. Brain 112:931, 1989
75. Sette G, Baron JC, Young AR et al: Changes in the distribution of $^{11}$C-PK 11195 and $^{11}$C-flumazenil in the infarcted brain following temporary middle cerebral artery occlusion (MCAO) in anaesthetized baboons: a PET analysis. J Cereb Blood Flow and Metab, suppl 2. 11:S12, 1991
76. Sgouropoulos P, Baron JC, Samson Y et al: Sténoses et occlusions persistantes de l'artère cérébrale moyenne; conséquences hémodynamiques et métaboliques étudiées par tomographie à positrons. Rev Neurol (Paris) 141:698, 1985
77. Syrota A, Castaing M, Rougemont D et al: Tissue acid base balance and oxygen metabolism in human cerebral infarction studied with PET. Ann Neurol 14:419, 1983
78. Syrota A, Samson Y, Boullais C et al: Tomographic mapping of brain intracellular pH and extracellular water space in stroke patients. J Cereb Blood Flow Metab 5:358, 1985
79. Weine J, DeLey G, Demeester G et al: PET studies of changes in cerebral blood flow and oxygen metabolism after unilateral microembolization of brain in anesthetized dogs. Stroke 18:128, 1987
80. Wise RJS, Bernardi S, Frackowiak RSJ et al: The transition from ischemia to infarction as reflected in regional oxygen extraction. Brain 106:197, 1983
81. Wise RJS, Gibbs J, Frackowiak RSJ et al: No evidence for transhemispheric diaschisis after human cerebral infarction. Stroke 17:853, 1986
82. Wise RJS, Rhodes CG, Gibbs JM et al: Disturbances of oxidative metabolism of glucose in recent human cerebral infarcts. Ann Neurol 14:627, 1983
83. Wong DG, Villemagne V, Goldman S et al: Cerebral blood flow and metabolism measured by PET in jeopardized cerebrum after experimental stroke. J Cereb Blood Flow Metab, suppl 1. 9:S262, 1989
84. Young AR, Sette G, Derlon JM et al: Middle cerebral artery occlusion in the baboon: validation studies for the therapy of cortical ischaemic damage. J Cereb Blood Flow Metab, suppl 2. 11:S554, 1991

# 7
# PATHOLOGY OF STROKE

Julio H. Garcia
Khang-Loon Ho
Dario V. Caccamo

The development of a focal neurologic deficit is designated *stroke* if the cause of the deficit is thought to be the consequence of a local disturbance in the cerebral circulation. The main causes of these, frequently abrupt, changes in brain circulation are a reflection of either obstruction of the cerebral blood flow or rupture of the wall of a vessel supplying the brain or spinal cord.

In this chapter we have assembled material that describes, in sequence, the nature of the main vascular diseases and the structural deformities affecting the brain as a consequence of either ischemic or hemorrhagic events.

## VASCULAR DISEASES (ANGIOPATHIES)

*Atherosclerosis* as a source of brain infarcts, particularly in the territory of the basilar and internal carotid arteries, is discussed in Chapter 2.

### Anatomic Variations

Anatomic variations and persistent anastomotic channels in the arteries located at the base of the brain are relatively common; especially frequent are asymmetry in the caliber of the vertebral arteries and a posterior cerebral artery originating from the ipsilateral internal carotid.[46]

### Aneurysms

Aneurysms are localized segmental dilatations of the arterial wall; depending on their shape and etiology, intracranial aneurysms can be classified into saccular (berry), dissecting, traumatic, fusiform (atherosclerotic), inflammatory (mycotic), and neoplastic (oncotic) aneurysms.

*Saccular* (berry) aneurysms are discussed in detail in Chapter 31.

*Dissecting and traumatic aneurysms:* Dissections and effects of trauma on the cervicocerebral arteries are discussed in Chapter 38.

#### Fusiform Aneurysm

Fusiform (atherosclerotic) aneurysms are considerably less frequent than saccular aneurysms. They are large, fusiform-shaped, associated with severe atherosclerosis, and occur mostly after the age of 60.[26] These deformities commonly involve the basilar and internal carotid arteries, in particular, the cavernous segment of the latter. Fusiform aneurysms can enlarge and reach enormous size, compressing and distorting neighboring cranial nerves and brain parenchyma. Bleeding originating from these vascular deformities is uncommon. Infarcts involving the brain stem or diencephalon are the most common complications of atherosclerotic aneurysms.

#### Inflammatory (Mycotic) Aneurysm

Cerebral aneurysms of inflammatory origin are divided into infectious, usually referred to as mycotic, aneurysms, and noninfectious aneurysms that are associated with connective tissue diseases such as polyarteritis nodosa or giant-cell arteritis. Aneurysms at the site of bacterial lodgings are often associated with subacute bacterial endocarditis, and most commonly they coexist with cardiac valvular disease secondary to infections with gram-positive cocci.[117] True mycotic aneurysms (secondary to fungal infection) are less common than bacterial ones; they may be caused by *Aspergillus, Candida,* and *Mucor* infections.[66] Destruction of the elastic lamina and tunica media by the infectious agents constitutes the basis for the aneurysmal formation. Most bacterial aneurysms are small, less than 1.0 cm in diameter, and involve peripheral arterial branches, in particular, the small branches of the middle cerebral artery located over the convexity of the cerebral hemispheres.[8,77] Fungal aneurysms tend to involve the large arteries at the base of the brain.[55] The thinned arterial wall at the aneurysmal site may rupture easily, and this event results in a clinical picture similar to that provided by a ruptured saccular aneurysm, that is, subarachnoid or intracerebral hemorrhages.

### Neoplastic (Oncotic) Aneurysms

Intracranial neoplastic aneurysms secondary to tumor embolism to cerebral arteries are rare, but their role in producing massive intracranial hemorrhage has been well recognized. The two most common neoplasms associated with neoplastic aneurysms are cardiac myxoma and choriocarcinoma.[16,67] Like mycotic aneurysms, most neoplastic aneurysms are small and involve peripheral, small branches of the cerebral arteries that are often buried in the cortical sulci.

## Vascular Malformations

Many vascular malformations (angiomas) of the central nervous system result from the failure of the normal maturation of the vessels or persistence of vascular patterns normally present in the embryo.[74] Despite their designation as angiomas, these lesions are not neoplastic. Vascular malformations of the central nervous system (CNS) are traditionally classified into capillary telangiectasis, venous angioma, cavernous hemangioma, and arteriovenous malformation, including the varix of the vein of Galen. There is a good correlation between the morphologic appearance of the malformation and the natural history of each major type. Most vascular malformations are small, less than 2 or 3 cm in diameter, and 90 percent are clinically silent.

### Capillary Telangiectases

A capillary telangiectasis is typically a small (0.3 to 1.0 cm) lesion that cannot be visualized by angiography. They are anatomic curiosities discovered at autopsy. Telangiectases are commonly found in the pontine base; they are less frequent in the cerebral white matter, where they look like clusters of petechiae. Telangiectases are aggregates of small capillaries with an open lumen, each lined by a single flat endothelial cell layer. The vascular channels are separated from each other by normal brain parenchyma.[95] Gliosis, mineralization, and significant hemorrhage are very rare. Transitional forms between capillary telangiectasis and other types of vascular malformations similar to capillary telangiectases have been observed in the cerebrum, cerebellum, and pons in patients with hereditary hemorrhagic telangiectasis or Osler-Weber-Rendu disease.[63,108]

### Venous Angiomas

These are the most frequently recognized type of vascular malformation found at autopsy; they are composed of groups of abnormal veins separated by either normal neural parenchyma or brain tissue with gliosis and ischemic injury. One or more large varicose veins are often present in the angioma. Thickening and sclerosis of the vessel wall are common, but mineralization of the walls is rare. Venous angiomas are not visualized during the arterial phase of angiography[17] and are more frequent in the spinal cord and spinal meninges than in the brain.[21]

### Cavernous Hemangioma

A cavernous hemangioma is a well-circumscribed dark red to black compact mass composed of closely apposed sinusoidal-type vessels that lack intervening neural parenchyma. Marked hyalinization and thickening of the component vessel walls are common. Calcification or even ossification can occur in some of the large cavernous hemangiomas that are more commonly found in deep-seated structures like the thalamus.[94] Gross or microscopic hemorrhages and gliosis of the adjacent neural parenchyma are common.

### Arteriovenous Malformation

Arteriovenous malformations (AVM) are the most significant vascular malformations of the central nervous system. Ninety-three percent of the arteriovenous malformations are located supratentorially, the rest may involve cerebellum, brain stem, or spinal cord.[124,125] The characteristic shape of a cerebral AVM consists of a lesion with a broad base on the cerebral convexity and an apex pointing toward the ventricular cavity. Microscopically, AVM are composed of many large arteries, arterialized veins, and veins intermingled with islands of gliotic neural parenchyma and old hemorrhagic lesions. There is no recognizable capillary component in most AVM. Sclerosis, thickening, and mineralization of the vessel's wall is common. Amyloid deposits in the vascular wall as well as thrombosis with recanalization are common. Segmental dilatations of the component vessels similar to those found in saccular aneurysms are frequently associated with AVM.[124,125]

## Arteriolosclerosis

The designation arteriolosclerosis applies to structural alterations involving small penetrating arteries (such as the lenticulostriate vessels) and arterioles or vessels with an outer diameter less than 50 $\mu$m and a tunica media devoid of internal elastic lamina. The best-known causes of small blood vessel disease (or arteriolosclerosis) are arterial hypertension, diabetes mellitus, and aging. Perforating arteries develop accelerated atheromatosis or subintimal deposits of fibroblasts and lipid-laden macrophages (microatheroma), usually in arteries measuring 100 to 400 $\mu$m in diameter[36,37,39,40] (Fig. 7-1).

The degenerative process in arterioles involves the tunica media where the smooth muscle fibers are progressively replaced by type IV collagen and plasma deposits. The resulting structural abnormality is called hyalinization (or glassy appearance). Fisher[35] introduced the term *lipohyalinosis* to describe the combination of hyaline and lipid deposits at the same site of the same vessel. The identity of the involved vessel is masked by the disease process, but most involved vessels are probably small arteries at the transition point where they lose their internal elastica and become arterioles (Fig. 7-2).

Other changes of arteriolosclerosis include fibrinoid necrosis,[121,135] which designates a brightly eosinophilic, finely granular deposit of plasma proteins and necrotic smooth muscle cells that is visible in the tunica media of large arterioles in the basal ganglia and thalami. Microaneurysms affecting intraparenchymal blood vessels have been classified by Fisher[38] into four types: (1) miliary saccular aneurysms (300 to 1,100 $\mu$m) involve arteries with a diameter of 40 to 160 $\mu$m (Fig. 7-3); (2) miliary aneurysms in lipohyalinosis can measure as much as 0.5 to 1.5 mm in diameter and are not connected to the vascular lumen; (3) fusiform miliary aneurysms, and (4) pseudoaneurysms or "bleeding globes" that are formed by masses of erythrocytes and platelets held together by the fibers of the tunica adventitia. The application of new methods of examining the intracerebral vessels utilized by Challa et al.[22] has brought into question the accuracy of traditional descriptions of small blood vessel disease.

## Cerebral Amyloid Angiopathy

Cerebral amyloid angiopathy (CAA) is a characteristic acellular mural thickening secondary to the deposition of an amorphous eosinophilic amyloid material stainable by Congo red (yellow-green birefringence under polarized light), and thioflavin S or T (fluorescent under ultraviolet light).[109,126] In CAA, amyloid infiltrates the tunicae media and adventitia of small blood vessels of the cerebral neocortex and adjacent leptomeninges; arterioles, small arteries, venules, and capillaries may all show amyloid deposits. Topographically CAA is patchy and asymmetrical, but vascular deposits are more common in the parietal and occipital lobes than in the rest of the brain.[137] The involved blood vessels, particularly those located in the leptomeninges, frequently show additional deformities such as microaneurysm formation, double-barrel lumen, fibrinoid necrosis, and obliterative intimal changes.[89] Ultrastructurally, CAA

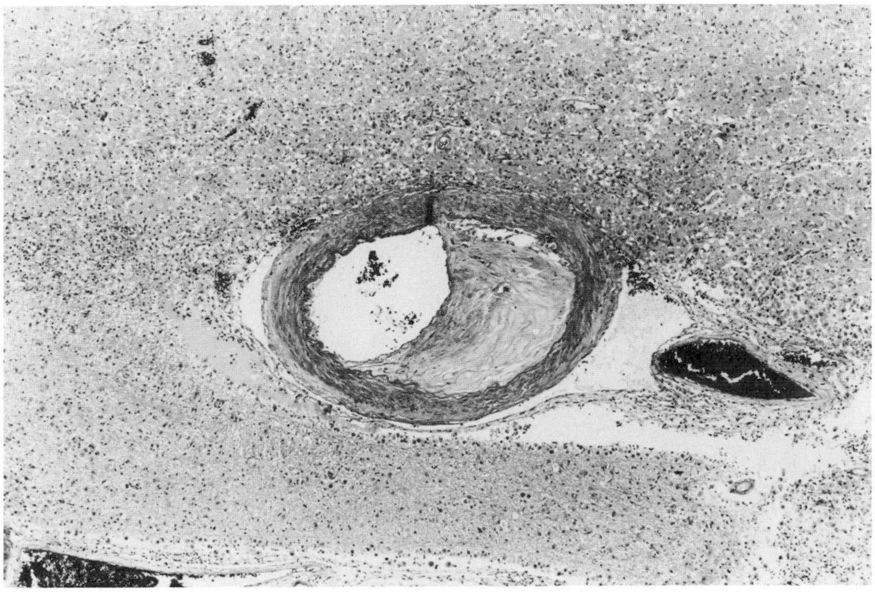

**Fig. 7-1.** Microatheroma in a penetrating small artery; the subintimal fibrosis results in eccentric narrowing of the lumen. (Hematoxylin & eosin; × 13.)

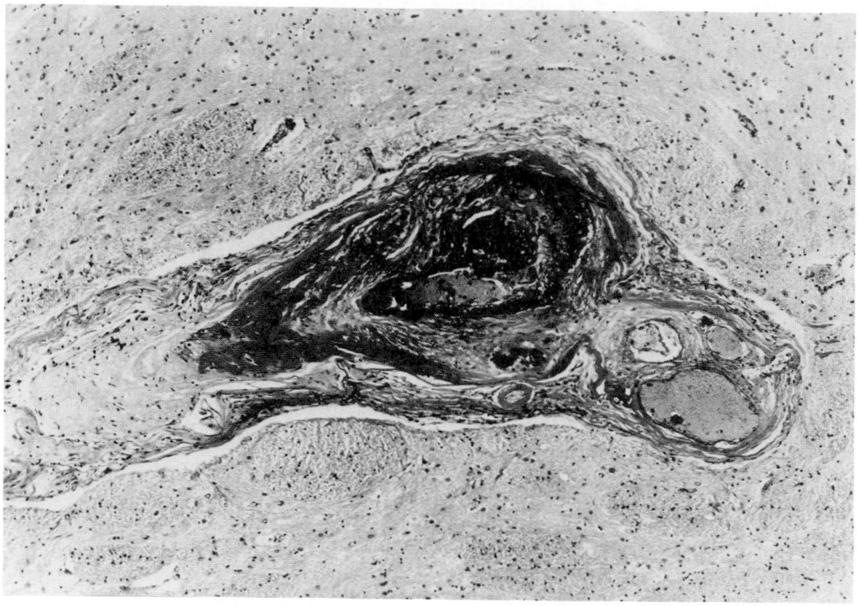

**Fig. 7-2.** Lipohyalinosis and fibrinoid necrosis in a penetrating vessel, probably an artery. The patient suffered from severe arterial hypertension. (Hematoxylin & eosin; × 20.)

consists of randomly arranged, nonbranching, nonparallel filaments, each having a diameter of 7 to 9 nm; the bulk of the amyloid deposits replaces the smooth muscle cells in the media. The origin of amyloid and the mechanism by which it is deposited in the vessel wall remain unknown.

CAA is associated with several clinicopathologic entities: cerebral hemorrhage,[68,70,90] Alzheimer's disease,[53,88,133] Down's syndrome,[54] dementia pugilistica,[11] cerebral microinfarcts,[51,70] vasculitis,[56,99] periventricular leukoencephalopathy,[69,86] late postirradiation encephalopathy,[91] spongiform encephalopathy (especially the Gerstmann-Sträussler syndrome),[1] and vascular malformations.[62] Tumorlike amyloid deposits (amyloidoma) in the brain have been reported in a few cases.[120]

CAA has been recognized as an important cause of nontraumatic intracerebral hemorrhage in aged persons with or without Alzheimer's disease.[70,132] CAA-related intracerebral hemorrhage is a disease of the elderly with a mean age of 73 for women and 71 for men. Thirty percent of these patients have a "mixed microangiopathy" (with both hypertensive and CAA changes). Over 40 percent of patients with CAA-related intracerebral hemorrhage have some degree of dementia and a similar proportion show neuropathologic change of Alzheimer's disease at autopsy. Intracerebral hemorrhages in CAA patients are usually lo-

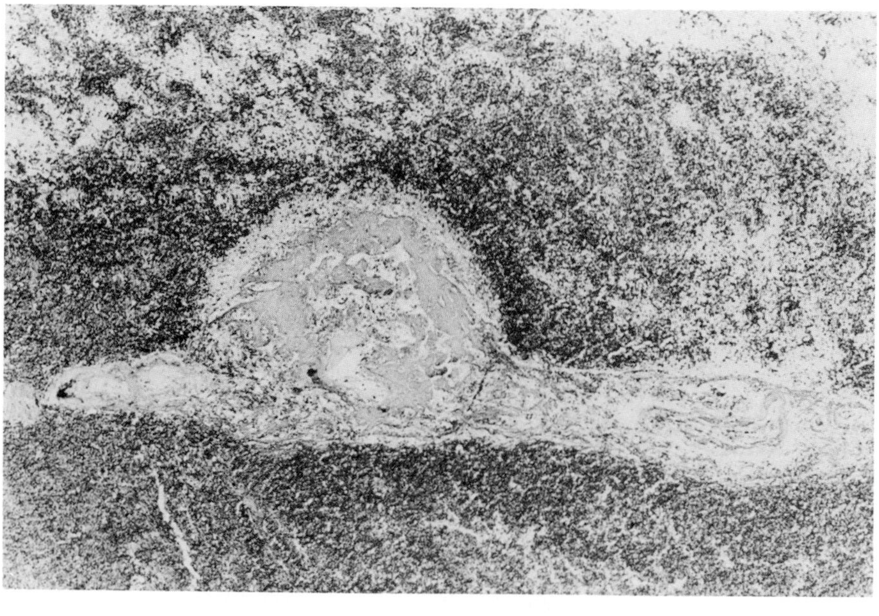

**Fig. 7-3.** Miliary saccular aneurysm in a brain vessel from a hypertensive patient; recently extravasated red blood cells are also visible. (Hematoxylin & eosin; × 20.)

bar hemorrhages, often involving the frontal and parietal lobes, and rarely involving deep ganglionic structures or cerebellum.[68,132] Multiple, old, microscopic hemorrhages and microscopic infarcts are common in CAA, but subarachnoid and subdural hemorrhages are rare.

Two important hereditary syndromes of CAA have been recognized.[51,87,136] Icelandic familial cerebral hemorrhage, recognized in 1935, is an important cause of morbidity and mortality among families in northwest Iceland. Inheritance is by autosomal dominant transmission. Patients usually die at age 20 to 40 years from intracerebral hemorrhage; most are not demented. The diagnosis of this type of CAA can be made by demonstrating decreased content of cystatin C in the CSF.[71] Hereditary cerebral hemorrhage with amyloidosis HCHWA-Dutch type has an autosomal dominant inheritance, is often associated with both dementia and periventricular leukoencephalopathy.[58] The amyloid in HCHWA-Dutch type is a $\beta$-amyloid (or A4) protein, which is similar to the amyloid found in the brain of patients with Alzheimer's disease.

## Cerebral Angiitis

The terms arteritis, vasculitis, and angiitis are used interchangeably because, in addition to arteries, veins and capillaries may be involved in some of the inflammatory conditions. Angiitis does not involve cerebral vessels alone. These diseases are systemic and are invariably accompanied by prominent clinical manifestations and laboratory findings. Granulomatous angiitis is the exception. Cerebral angiitis may be caused by infectious agents, mechanical trauma, radiation, and toxins. In bacterial and fungal infection, the wall of cerebral arteries may be directly involved by hematogenous lodgment of infectious organisms or from contiguous invasion by bacteria from infected leptomeninges. Cerebral angiitis may be associated with viral infections, in particular, herpes simplex, herpes zoster, cytomegalovirus, and papovavirus. The most important angiitides, however, are the noninfectious systemic necrotizing angiitis affecting multiple organ systems. Many of these inflammatory processes appear to have an immunologic basis.[73]

Temporal (giant-cell) arteritis and granulomatous angiitis are discussed in Chapter 25.

### Polyarteritis Nodosa

Classic polyarteritis nodosa (PAN) is a disease affecting small or medium-sized muscular arteries that characteristically involves the renal and visceral arteries but spares the pulmonary vessels. PAN affects young men more frequently than women; PAN is characterized by nonspecific systemic complaints such as low-grade fever, malaise, weakness, leukocytosis, hypertension, and hematuria. The etiology of PAN is unknown. Many patients with PAN have serologic evidence of hepatitis B antigen and antineutrophil antibodies.[116] The involved arteries show extensive leukocytic infiltration, including neutrophils, eosinophils, and mononuclear cells, as well as fibrinoid necrosis of the wall. Neurologic syndromes associated with PAN include polymyositis, peripheral neuropathy, mononeuritis multiplex, and "stroke," which is usually the result of either intracranial thrombosis or hemorrhage. A syndrome characterized by keratitis and deafness was described by Cogan in nonsyphilitic individuals; this disease may represent one of the clinical expressions of PAN.[5]

### Hypersensitivity (Leukocytoclastic) Angiitis

Hypersensitivity or leukocytoclastic argiitis, also called *microscopic polyarteritis,* is differentiated from classic polyarteritis nodosa by the involvement of small vessels (arterioles, venules, and capillaries). The disease may involve the skin, mucous membranes, lungs, heart, gastrointestinal tract, brain, and skeletal muscles. The affected vessels show fibrinoid necrosis and infiltration of neutrophils. Hypersensitivity angiitis may be associated with Henoch-Schönlein purpura, cryoglobulinemia, or angiitis associated with malignancy and connective tissue disease. As is true of polyarteritis nodosa, the neurologic expressions are those of either hemorrhage or thrombosis.

### Takayasu's Disease

Takayasu's disease, a form of granulomatous angiitis of medium and large arteries, involves primarily the aortic arch and its branches; it is less common in the thoracic and abdominal aorta. The disease is most common in the Orient and predominates in women in the 15- to 45-year-old group.[59] Microscopically, the lesion is characterized by mononuclear cell infiltration of the adventitia, perivascular cuffing of vasa vasora, granulomatous changes with multinucleated giant cells (Langhans cells) in the tunica media with foci of fibrinoid necrosis. At a later stage obliteration may occur secondary to thickening and fibrosis of the wall. The luminal narrowing and obliteration are the morphologic basis for the clinical manifestations of the disease: patients exhibit no arterial pulsation and no marked drop in blood pressure in the upper extremities; visual field defects, retinal hemorrhages, blindness, and variable neurologic syndromes such as dizziness and stroke are also common.

### Systemic Lupus Erythematosus

Systemic lupus erythematosus (SLE), a multisystem disease of autoimmune origin, is a chronic, remitting, and relapsing illness characterized by injury to the skin, joints, kidney, and serosal membranes.[130] Like most autoimmune diseases, SLE predominates among women in the second or third decades of life. SLE appears to be a heterogeneous disorder resulting from complex interactions among genetic, hormonal, and environmental factors. The morphologic changes in SLE are extremely variable, reflecting the variability of the clinical manifestations in individual patients. The acute necrotizing vasculitis involving small arteries may involve almost any tissue. The arterial lesion is characterized in the early stage by fibrinoid necrosis and in the late stage by fibrous thickening of the wall and narrowing of the lumen. Deposits of immunoglobulins, DNA and C3 protein have been demonstrated in the vessel walls, supporting the theory that the inflammation may be mediated by immune complexes. Neurologic manifestations of SLE patients include psychiatric disorders, seizures, dementia, cerebral blindness, long tract signs, and several others. The morphologic basis for the CNS symptoms is unclear; the symptoms have been attributed to angiitis with thrombosis and multiple petechiae. However, a recent autopsy study revealed no significant angiitis among SLE patients with neuropsychiatric disorders.[7] Instead, most cerebral lesions were attributed to brain infarcts of probable embolic origin.[29,32]

### Miscellaneous Vascular Disorders

*Fibromuscular dysplasia* is discussed in Chapter 27. *Moyamoya disease* is discussed in Chapter 26.

### Sturge-Weber Syndrome

Sturge-Weber syndrome, also termed *encephalotrigeminal angiomatosis,* is characterized by an extensive capillary-venous malformation affecting a cerebral hemisphere. Skull x-ray examination gives a typical "tramlike" appearance produced by calcifications in the cortex. A homolateral facial nevus or "port-wine" stain is visible in the distribution of the trigeminal nerve. Most patients have contralateral hemiparesis, Jacksonian seizures, mental retardation, and glaucoma.[138] The capillary-venous angiomatosis predominantly involves the pia mater, but the subjacent cortex is also frequently involved. The abnormal vessels are often thickened by hyaline collagenous tissue and by confluent deposits of small calcospherites. The neighboring brain parenchyma is atrophic and gliotic. Sturge-Weber syndrome may be associated with other vascular malformations in intracranial and extracranial locations.[102]

### Thrombotic Thrombocytopenic Purpura

The primary process of thrombotic thrombocytopenic purpura (TTP) is intravascular platelet aggregation with fibrin deposition involving arterioles and capillaries but not venules. Signs of inflammation are lacking in the involved vessels. Thrombi may be covered by endothelial cells and appear to be intramural. TTP in adults has a hexad of clinical findings: neurologic changes, renal dysfunction, microangiopathic changes, hemolytic anemia, thrombocytopenia, and fever. Neurologic manifestations occur in 74 to 90 percent of the cases and include headache, confusion, seizures, paresis, and coma.[2,110] These findings may change rapidly and may be transient, reflecting the fleeting nature of the microvascular lesions. The diagnosis of TTP is based on the recognition of the clinical manifestations. Histologic confirmation of the diagnosis may include blood smear for demonstrating schistocytes and gingival biopsy to look for thrombotic microangiopathy.[20]

## ISCHEMIC LESIONS

### Lesions of Hypotensive (or Hemodynamic) Origin

Ischemia or decreased blood flow, below the levels of autoregulatory compensation (60 mmHg MABP) can be the consequence of (1) hypotensive or hemodynamic crises and (2) occlusive vascular disease involving any of the blood vessel types.

Ischemic lesions of the CNS having a hemodynamic origin are the consequence of episodic cardiac arrest, abrupt drops in systemic blood pressure, shock, peripheral vascular collapse, and, less frequently, cardiac dysrhythmias. The resulting parenchymal lesions can be of a very diverse nature and principally involve the cerebral cortical mantle, the basal ganglia, the cerebellar cortex, the cerebral white matter, the brain stem, the spinal cord, and various combinations of different sites at these components of the CNS.

Systemic injuries of the type produced by an episode of cardiac arrest, as an example, are said to *selectively* involve specific sites of the CNS such as the arterial border (or boundary) zones of the cerebral hemispheres (Fig. 7-4), the cerebellum, and the spinal cord. This is attributed to the precarious circulation existing at sites located at the end of an arterial territory. Further selective vulnerability has been noted in the involvement of various cell types located at these sites; thus, the pyramidal cells of the hippocampus and the Purkinje cell layer of the cerebellum are two types of neurons that are most susceptible to an ischemic crisis. In the cerebral cortex, layers III to V are more likely to be injured by ischemia than the rest of the cortical layers. Likewise in the basal ganglia, the globus pallidus is more susceptible to the ischemic injury than the striatum and small neurons become necrotic before large neurons[44,101,122] (Fig. 7-5).

After a cardiac arrest or a hypotensive crisis, the extent of the brain injury is influenced by the duration and severity (measured by the blood pressure level upon recovery) of the ischemic event; additional factors influencing the outcome of a hypotensive ischemic injury include age of the patient (the younger the

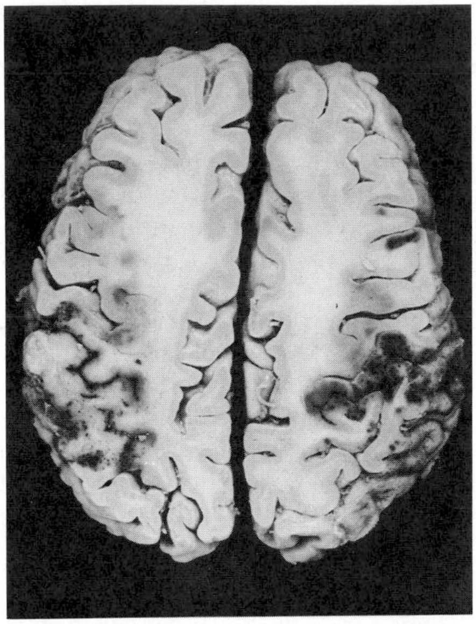

**Fig. 7-4.** Bilateral hemorrhagic infarcts (especially prominent at the arterial boundary zones) in a patient who survived 5 days an episode of cardiac arrest, secondary to myocardial infarct. There was no occlusion of any intracranial vessel.

individual the longer the tolerance for ischemia); body temperature (hypothermia protects neurons from the ischemic injury, whereas hyperthermia may have the opposite effect),[118] and serum glucose content (hypoglycemia at the time of the ischemic event is said to protect the ischemic brain by limiting the rate of production of lactic acid).[46] Some investigators[106] have suggested that length of survival, after the cardiac arrest, may be an additional factor in determining the extent of brain injury.

The neurologic expressions of ischemic injuries caused by systemic abnormalities, such as cardiac arrest and arterial hypotension, are discussed in Chapters 36 and 37. As seen in imaging studies, the brain lesions attributed to ischemia of hypotensive origin are almost always bilateral and relatively symmetrical regardless of their location in the CNS. Some hypotensive ischemic lesions may have a *hemorrhagic* character (Fig. 7-4). This is explained by the presence, in the involved segment of the brain, of numerous petechiae that almost always remain confined to the gray matter structures. This grossly visible hemorrhagic quality of some ischemic lesions is attributed to the effects of reperfusing a previously ischemic territory at a time when necrosis of the microvasculature may be at its peak; alternatively, the nonocclusive nature of the ischemic event may be such that a trickle of blood flow is retained into the injured area.[46]

Systemic hypoperfusion of the brain has also been proposed as one of several mechanisms that may induce a diffuse lesion in the periventricular white matter of the cerebral hemispheres. Leuko-araiosis, or areas of decreased density on either CT scanning or MR imaging of the head, is a common finding among persons older than 65 years. The clinical significance of this abnormality is a subject of much controversy; prospective neuropsychological studies in aged patients with leuko-araiosis have concluded that the condition is asymptomatic. Numerous explanations have been offered as being the cause of this periventri-

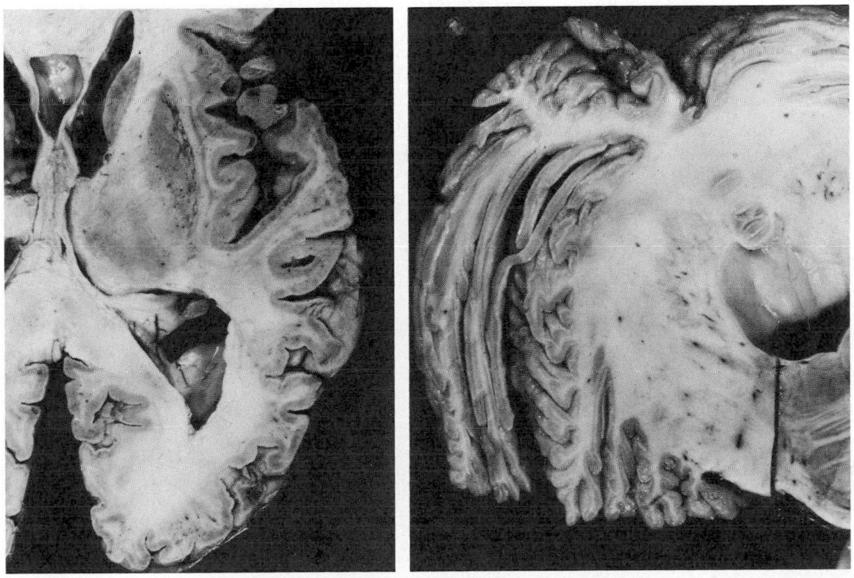


**Fig. 7-5. (A)** Atrophic scarring of gray matter (cortex and striatum) in a patient who survived, several weeks, a severe hypotensive crisis. **(B)** Atrophic scarring of cerebellar cortex in the same patient as described in Fig. A.

cular image; these include a normal anatomic structure (subcallosal fasciculus), an expression of multiple sclerosis, cerebral amyloid angiopathy, chronic arterial hypertension, hypoperfusion as a result of congestive heart failure, delayed effects of radiotherapy, and several others. Among premature newborns, the condition of periventricular leukomalacia, or areas of necrosis involving the corona radiata is generally thought to be secondary to the effects of hypoxemia (caused by pulmonary immaturity) and ischemia (caused by systemic hypotension and cardiac failure).[47]

## Brain Infarcts Secondary to Focal Ischemia

Brain infarcts may be the consequence of either embolism or thrombosis. The latter is thought to be secondary to local vascular disease; in a significant percentage of cases, the causes of intracranial vascular occlusions responsible for brain infarcts remain undetected.[115] Many patients with vascular occlusion of unknown etiology may have hematologic abnormalities that promote intravascular coagulation, such as antiphospholipid antibodies.[12,82]

### Embolic Brain Infarcts

Two common sources of embolism to the brain are the left-sided chambers of the heart (especially after a transmural myocardial infarct) and the origin of the internal carotid artery (ICA). The mitral and aortic valves can be the sites where vegetations form in patients who have hypercoagulable states, the classical example being a patient with an adenocarcinoma of the pancreas who develops multiple thrombi in both veins and cardiac valves. Valvular vegetations in these patients are usually made of fibrin and are sometimes called *marantic vegetations.* "Marantic" endocarditis is an inappropriate designation because marasmus does not influence the formation of vegetations and because there is no inflammatory component as the ending *itis* implies. The preferred name is *nonbacterial thrombotic vegetations* (Fig. 7-6). Patients with SLE are prone to develope vegetations of a similar type that are sometimes called *Libman-Sacks vegetations.* Congenital valvular defects and systemic infections can also be the precipitating factors for the formation of bacterial-infected vegetations; this results in the classical condition of bacterial endocarditis (subacute or acute depending upon the microorganism involved). The origin of cerebral emboli among patients with atrial fibrillation is disputed; postmortem studies of these patients seldom show mural thrombi in the atrial appendages of the heart. Nevertheless, it is well established that patients with atrial fibrillation have a 33 percent increased risk of developing brain infarcts that are presumed to be of embolic origin.[139]

Artery-to-artery embolism frequently results from the detachment of mural thrombi from the ICA, at the site of an ulcerated atheromatous plaque. In such cases, the material occluding small branches of the ophthalmic or middle cerebral arteries is composed primarily of platelets and fibrin. Examination of the retina shortly after the embolic event sometimes allows visualization of the embolic material thanks to

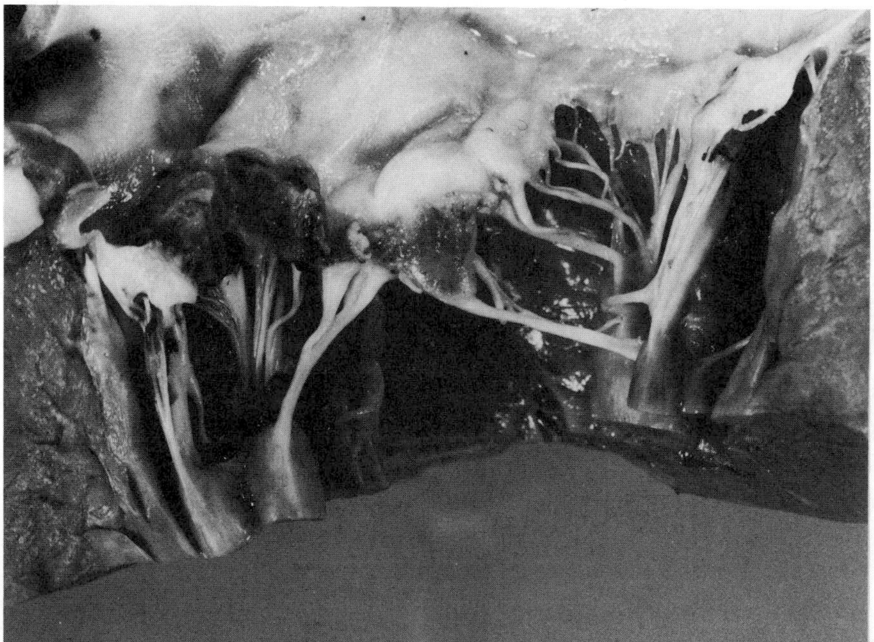

**Fig. 7-6.** Mitral valve with rheumatic changes and nonbacterial vegetations on the atrial surface of the anterior leaflet.

the bright yellow color of the cholesterol crystals. Within the cerebral hemispheres most emboli are distributed in the territory of the middle cerebral artery (MCA), which is the main and most direct branch of the ICA. Emboli to the cerebral hemispheres commonly lodge at the junction between cortex and white matter and preferentially involve the bottom of the sulcus rather than the crest of the gyrus. Many brain infarcts of embolic origin are hemorrhagic, presumably because the ischemic tissue is often reperfused when the embolizing material lyses and the occluded vessel is reopened. Another common feature of embolic infarcts is their relatively small size (usually less than 2.0 cm in diameter) and their multiplicity within a single arterial territory. The inflammatory response by polymorphonuclear leukocytes at the site of an embolic infarct is usually more pronounced than it is at sites of thrombotic infarcts; this is reflected in a relatively high increase in the neutrophil count in the cerebral spinal fluid, which, in addition, may also contain numerous erythrocytes.

Observations made in an animal model of carotid embolism[42] suggest that there may be at least three types of tissue responses to cerebral embolism. The most conspicuous one consists of sharply circumscribed areas of coagulation necrosis that convert into fluid-filled cavities; most features of these lesions are essentially identical to those of *lacunar infarcts* (discussed later in this chapter). A second type of tissue response observed at the site of an embolic occlusion consists of neuronal necrosis with proliferation of astroglial cells and formation of small (less than 1.5 cm in average diameter) retracted scars. The third type of lesion observed in animals with experimental brain embolism consists of selective neuronal necrosis without either astroglial or macrophage reaction in what might be called a miniature example of *incomplete brain infarct,* as defined in the following section.

## Thrombotic Arterial Infarcts

The classical example of thrombotic arterial brain infarct is seen in the hypertensive, diabetic patient who has severe atherosclerosis of the basilar artery; at the site of extreme narrowing the vessel develops a thrombus that completely occludes the artery; a similar set of circumstances may lead to the thrombotic occlusion of a middle cerebral artery. As studied serially in experimental animals, occluding an intracranial artery results in an instantaneous drop in the local cerebral blood flow and loss of function of the tissues supplied by the occluded vessel. For the next several minutes, perhaps hours, the tissue changes induced by this type of ischemia can be detected only with the microscope; some of these changes may be of a reversible nature. One of the methods to reverse the effects of ischemia might include perfusion of the ischemic territory; dramatic reversals of ischemic deficits have been documented among persons who suffer transient neurologic deficits during carotid endarterectomy.[127]

Reperfusion can be complicated by massive intracerebral bleeding at the site of an incipient brain infarct. This phenomenon probably explains one of the well-documented complications of carotid endarterectomy; in a few patients undergoing this operation, the postoperative period is complicated by a massive, usually fatal, intracerebral hemorrhage. There are no experimental data to identify the time when endarterectomy is most likely to result in massive intracerebral bleeding.[13,19]

In many experimental situations it is said that approximately 2 to 3 hours after the occlusion of an artery, the brain lesion becomes irreversible.[27] This needs verification in a large series of animals; the sharply demarcated areas of coagulation necrosis that occur after occluding a major brain artery are not visible even in autopsy specimens before 12 to 24 hours after the occurrence of the neurologic deficit. In rats with middle cerebral artery occlusion, Dereski et al.[28] report that coagulation necrosis or pan-necrosis in the territory of the occluded atery does not become visible before 48 to 72 hours, and Swanson et al.[128] have noted that 3 to 7 days after the arterial occlusion is the optimal time to see the gross lesion (Fig. 7-7).

The microscopic events in the area destined to become necrotic have been well documented in experimental animals. Selected neuronal perikarya become dense and shrunken, while astrocytic nuclei increase in diameter and the neuropil adopts a markedly spongy appearance as a reflection of swelling involving the dendritic tree and the astrocytic processes.[49,50] An initial wave of infiltration by neutrophils begins about 1 to 4 hours after the arterial occlusion; this is followed some 8 hours later by a second massive increase in the number of neutrophils

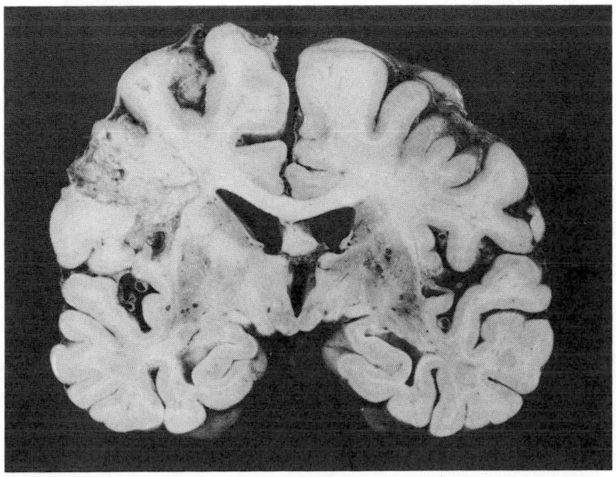

**Fig. 7-7.** Brain infarct (subacute: about 2 to 3 weeks old by clinical history) in the territory of one of the middle cerebral artery branches.

visible within the ischemic territory. Coincidental with the presence of the neutrophils, neuronal perikarya in increasing numbers show signs of necrosis as suggested by cytoplasmic eosinophilia and pyknosis. The presence of macrophages, first noted on the fourth day, becomes more obvious by the end of the tenth day when the lesion consists almost exclusively of regenerated microvessels and lipid-laden macrophages. Despite the extensive structural changes affecting the vascular tree, leakage of circulating macromolecules within the territory of the occluded artery is minimal. These statements are based on observations made in experimental animals; comparable studies on humans are not feasible.

Brain infarcts that are reperfused at some critical, but as yet undefined, time period adopt a hemorrhagic character; these lesions are sometimes called *red infarcts* (Fig. 7-8), as opposed to the *pale, bland,* or *anemic infarcts* lacking a grossly visible hemorrhagic component. Two types of hemorrhages have been described in brain infarcts: type I consists of numerous punctate hemorrhages that generally remain confined to the gray matter structures and do not result in either tissue swelling or added deterioration of the neurologic deficit; type II hemorrhage in an arterial brain infarct is a large collection of blood frequently involving the white matter structures and dissecting the surrounding tissues in an unpredictable fashion.[10] This type of hemorrhage frequently extends into the ventricular cavities; the extension of the subarachnoid space through the cortical mantle occurs less frequently. The occurrence of type II hemorrhage is reflected in an abrupt added deterioration of the neurologic deficit; and the abrupt extension of the bleeding into the ventricles can be lethal.

The ultimate fate of brain tissues made necrotic by an arterial occlusion is the reabsorption of the dead cells by macrophages leading to the formation of a fluid-filled cavity at the site of the original brain infarct. The time necessary for a brain infarct to become a cavity cannot be predicted accurately; it is assumed that the larger the lesion the longer it will take for cavitation to develop. Large infarcts in the territory of the middle cerebral artery may take several months before they convert into a cavity (Fig. 7-9).

As is true of embolic infarcts, the tissue responses visible at sites where large arteries become occluded are not always predictable. Tissue responses are primarily dependent on the severity of the ischemic event.[81] Severity can be influenced by two main factors: the level to which the local cerebral blood flow (CBF) falls and duration of the ischemic event. Both factors are influenced by blood pressure changes (since autoregulation is lost at the site of the infarct) and by the local conditions dependent on the collateral vessels. Marcoux et al.[92] described two patterns of local CBF change in a group of 27 subhuman primates with middle cerebral artery occlusion: in group A the local CBF values dropped to less than 10 ml/100 g/min, whereas local CBF values in group B oscillated between 15 and 20 ml/100 g/min. All brain lesions in animals in group A proceeded to coagulation necrosis and beginning of cavitation by the end of the fourth week; in contrast, brain lesions in animals in group B consisted of selective neuronal destruction with preservation of astroglia and without cavity formation.

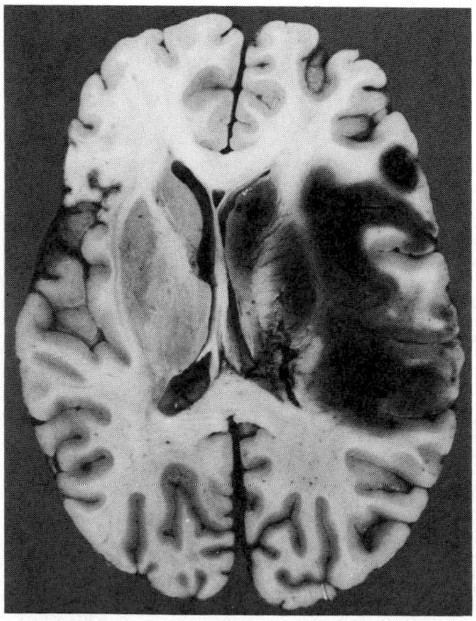

**Fig. 7-8.** Hemorrhagic infarct in the territory of the middle cerebral artery.

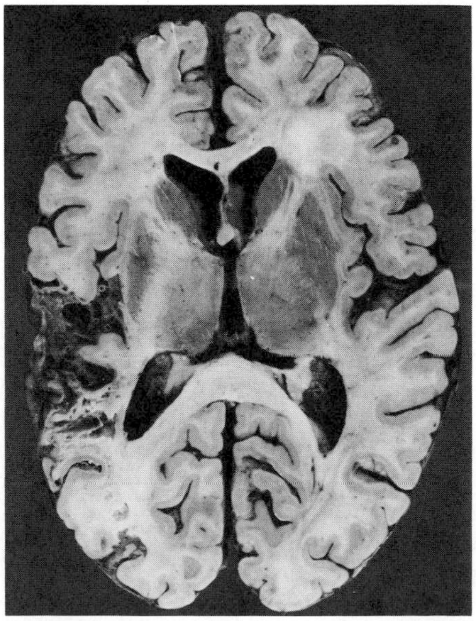

**Fig. 7-9.** Infarct, cavitary, in the territory of the middle cerebral artery.

The name *incomplete cerebral infarct* has been suggested for this second type of lesion,[80] and Garcia et al.[48] reported the case of a young patient who suffered an embolic occlusion of a middle cerebral artery several years before death; at autopsy the artery had recanalized and the brain lesion was that of incomplete cerebral infarct of the type described by Lassen[80] in vivo in humans and by Marcoux et al.[92] in subhuman primates.

## Lacunar Infarcts

The designation lacunar infarcts is applied to destructive brain lesions of presumed ischemic origin having a maximum diameter of 1.5 cm (Fig. 7-10); the vessels whose occlusion is thought to be responsible for the lacunar infarct (or lacune) are penetrating arteries or arterioles generally having a caliber of less than 200 $\mu$m.[39] The name *lacune* is derived from an astronomical term (lacuna) meaning a black hole in outer space. Because of their small size lacunar infarcts are not detectable by in vivo imaging studies until the time when they become cavitary. Lacunes are most commmonly found at these anatomic sites: the basal ganglia, thalamic nuclei, base of the pons, centrum semiovale, and, less frequently, cerebral and cerebellar cortices. The etiology of the vascular disease associated with lacunes is generally attributed to the consequences of arterial hypertension and diabetes mellitus on small penetrating vessels; these are thought to become occluded as a result of progressive mural thickening and hyalinization. A second possible mechanism for the development of lacunes is embolism from the internal carotid artery.[43] The histologic features of lacunes are thought to be comparable to those of other brain infarcts, but a detailed analysis of this topic has not been published.

## Brain Lesions Secondary to Sinus/Venous Thrombosis

Occlusion of an intracranial vein may have disastrous effects because there are no collateral connections among cerebral veins and because close to 70 percent of the intracranial blood is contained within the veins and sinuses of the brain.

Three varieties of lesions have been recognized among patients with intracranial sinus thrombosis. The first and most common lesion is the development of subarachnoid hemorrhage accompanied by massive swelling of the cerebral hemispheres that may lead to compression of the cerebral ventricles; this type of lesion has been observed among children with superior sagittal sinus thrombosis. The condition of sinus thrombosis constitutes an emergency that requires prompt medical treatment with agents that prevent additional thrombus formation[31]; surgical intervention to attempt recanalization of the sinus has not been successful. The second type of lesion consists of a localized area of brain softening (or infarct) (Fig. 7-11) having a topographic distribution that overlaps two or more arterial territories; characteristically the lesion is markedly edematous and accompanied by large hemorrhages that are profuse in the white mat-

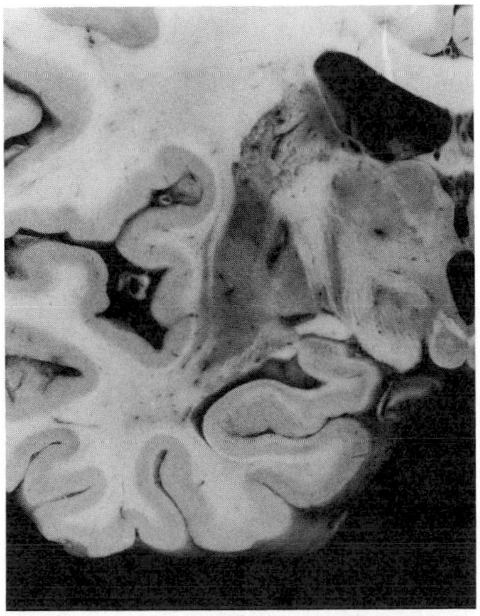

**Fig. 7-10.** Small lacunar infarct (about 2 weeks old by clinical history) in the territory of one of the lenticulostriate arteries.

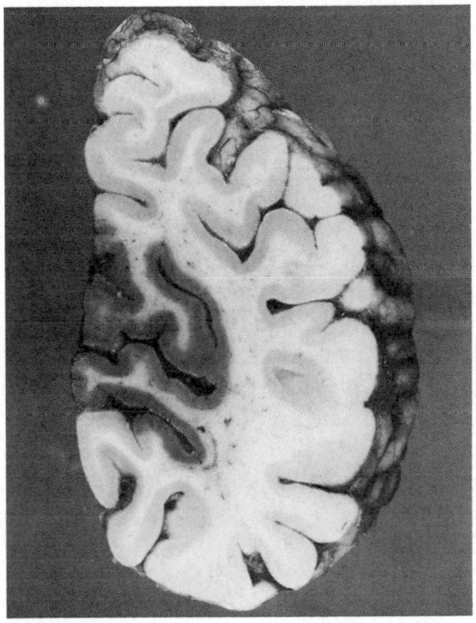

**Fig. 7-11.** Hemorrhagic infarct, secondary to cortical vein thrombosis.

ter as well as in the cortex or basal ganglia. Occlusion of a midline sinus, such as the sinus rectus, induces hemorrhagic infarct on both sides of the midline with extensive involvement of the thalamic nuclei. A third type of brain lesion is more diffuse, multifocal, and subtle; its detection usually requires microscopic evaluation of the involved tissues. It consists of the plugging of numerous capillaries and venules by thrombi composed of platelets, fibrin, and erythrocytes. This type of event has been observed in patients dying during acute sickle cell crises.[45]

At the microscopic level four features differentiate venous lesions from infarcts of arterial origin. First, venous infarcts have abundant signs of cellular and extracellular edema, including frequent "plasma lakes." Second, a common feature of venous infarcts is the presence of abundant neutrophils distributed in sheets, instead of the perivascular cuffs commonly seen in lesions secondary to arterial embolism. Third, characteristic of venous infarcts is the relative preservation of the neuronal morphology, even in areas where extensive edema and neutrophil accumulation, as well as hemorrhage, may be present. Fourth, coagulation necrosis[45] is absent in venous infarcts.

Before the parenchymal lesions develop, sinus/venous thromboses are best demonstrated by CT scanning and angiography.

## Subcortical Leukoencephalopathy; Hypertensive Encephalopathy

Structural alterations involving the white matter that surrounds the lateral ventricles are seen on CT scans with increasing frequency after the age of 65. The combination of a dementing syndrome and the existence of subcortical leukoencephalopathy is designated by some authors as *Binswanger's disease*[111]; this designation is not universally accepted, among other reasons because it is unclear whether Binswanger described one or more diseases in his original publication.[104] The designation of *subcortical leukoencephalopathy* seems preferable because it does not imply a specific or single etiologic mechanism. It has been suggested that the structural alterations of the long, penetrating, radial arteries that supply the white matter, commonly known as *arteriolosclerosis*, are the most frequent etiologic cause for subcortical leukoencephalopathy. Arteriolosclerosis is common among persons with arterial hypertension, diabetes mellitus, and advanced age. The concentric narrowing of the lumen of these radial vessels is thought to result in a "low-grade" or "chronic" ischemia that eventually affects the integrity of the white matter fibers. Other mechanisms invoked to explain the changes in tissue structure include chronic hypoperfusion (as a result of cardiac failure) and miscellaneous angiopathies such as cerebral amyloid angiopathy.

At the microscopic level a variety of structural alterations have been described under the designation of subcortical leukoencephalopathy. These include loss of myelin sheaths, loss of axons, proliferation of astrocytes, infiltration by lipid-laden macrophages, cavitation, and various degrees of disappearance of oligodendrocytes.[3]

## Brain Swelling Associated with Infarcts; Herniations

Retention of protein-free fluid in the intracellular glial compartment is one of the earliest consequences of acute brain ischemia. Postischemic brain edema peaks at 48 to 72 hours after the beginning of symptoms; after this acme the tissue swelling disappears at a rapid pace comparable to that observed during the period of edema formation. Postischemic brain edema is a potential cause of death through the induction of brain herniations.[103] Brain edema and herniations are particularly significant causes of death among patients with large infarcts in the territory of the ICA, MCA, and the large arterial branches supplying the cerebellum. Some authors[129] have recommended surgical excision of swollen infarcted cerebellar tissues as a means to decrease the high mortality that may accompany this condition.

Several types of herniations or displacements of brain tissue into an adjoining anatomic compartment have been described under these names: *cingulate, uncinate, sphenoidal, tonsillar, vermal,* and *central herniations.* Two of these are associated with mechanisms that cause death: uncinate herniation is the result of massive swelling of the temporal lobe or nearby structures; the displacement of the uncus in a medial direction stretches the third nerve fibers, compresses the

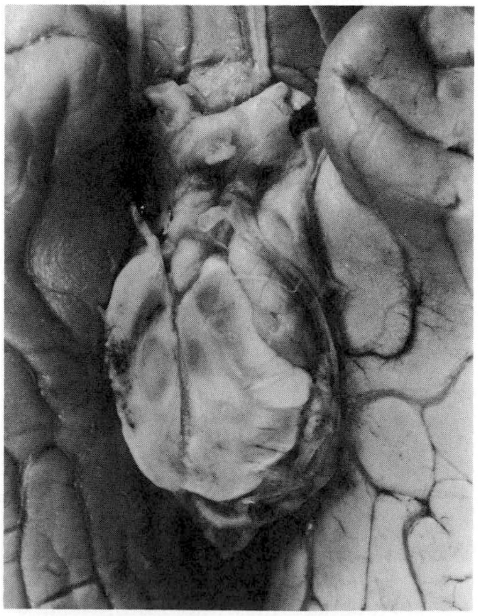

**Fig. 7-12.** Unilateral herniation of the uncus showing compression of ipsilateral cerebral peduncle and stretching of the posterior cerebral artery.

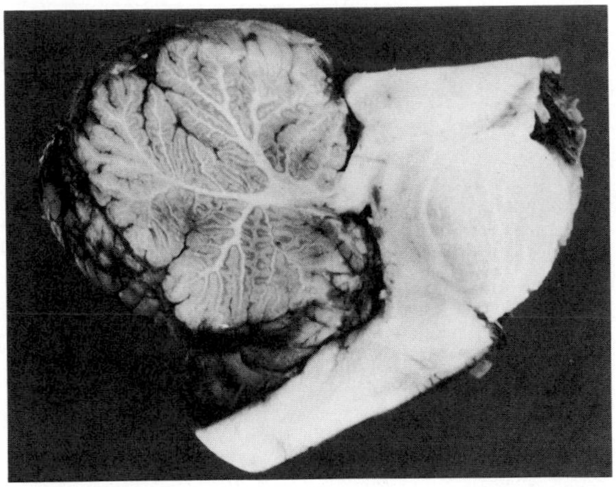

**Fig. 7-13.** Cerebellar herniation; there is narrowing and displacement of the fourth ventricle as well as compression of the lower medulla and the upper spinal cord.

ipsilateral cerebral peduncle, and pinches the initial segment of the posterior cerebral artery (Fig. 7-12). The latter effect may be complicated by the development of a second, hemorrhagic infarct in the ipsilateral temporal-occipital lobes. Uncinate herniation also induces stretching of the mesencephalic branches of the posterior cerebral artery that supply the tegmentum of the midbrain and pons. Through this mechanism uncinate herniation may cause secondary infarcts and hemorrhages (sometimes called *Duret's hemorrhages)* in the midline of the upper brain stem.[100]

The second type of herniation that may cause death develops at the level of the foramen magnum where swollen cerebellar tissues may escape the posterior fossa into the upper cervical spinal canal; the presence of swollen tissues at this site can induce mechanical compression and thus inhibit the cardiorespiratory centers located in the lower medulla (Fig. 7-13). This mechanism explains instances of sudden death following the abrupt removal of spinal fluid from the lumbar area in patients who have large posterior fossa "tumors," including swollen, infarcted tissues.

## INTRACEREBRAL HEMORRHAGE

### Definition

Spontaneous hemorrhage is a phenomenon particularly important in the central nervous system and its coverings. Primary intracerebral hemorrhage (ICH) is defined as a nontraumatic hemorrhage within the parenchyma of the brain. This definition includes lobar, ganglionic, thalamic, cerebellar, and brain stem hemorrhages. Some authors have attempted to differentiate brain hemorrhage from brain "hematoma," the hemorrhage being a deep-seated, poorly circumscribed accumulation of blood extending to the ventricles. A "cerebral hematoma," in contrast, would be a superficial and more localized accumulation of blood, that reaches the cerebral surface, but does not extend to the ventricles.[137] However, there are many exceptions to these broad categories and the terms "cerebral hemorrhage" and "cerebral hematoma" are used interchangeably.

### Etiology and Pathogenesis

Hypertension is the principal risk factor for primary ICH. The risk of ICH parallels the increase in blood pressure, and is related to elevations of both systolic and diastolic pressures. The availability of CT scanning has changed some of the traditional concepts on the frequency of hemorrhages. About 25 percent of ICHs were diagnosed as ischemic "strokes" in the pre-CT era. Small hemorrhages, both in normotensive and hypertensive patients, went many times undetected (Fig. 7-14).

Primary ICH associated with arterial hypertension occurs most frequently in selected sites. Approximately 70 percent of primary ICH occur in the basal ganglia and thalamus, 13 percent in the brain stem, 10 percent in the cerebral lobes, and 9 percent in the cerebellum. The putamen, the most common location for ICH, is the site of approximately one-third to one-half of all brain bleeding.[97,105,123]

Mechanisms that may explain the ICH, associated with hypertension, include rupture of microaneurysms, arteriolosclerosis, necrosis of vessels, and rupture of veins or dissecting aneurysms. The prevalent view is that ICH results from the rupture of small arterial or arteriolar aneurysms. Originally described by Charcot and Bouchard,[23] microaneurysms are found in small vessels primarily in the striate arteries. These aneurysms measure between 300 and 900 $\mu$m in diameter and usually arise at the site of branching, especially at the bifurcation sites of the proximal branches of the striate arteries in the putamen, thalamus, and pallidum.[113] Hemosiderin-containing macrophages and hyperplastic astrocytes can be found near these aneurysms. In many instances, the aneurysmal wall shows a smudgy bright red appearance, that is called fibrinoid necrosis. Charcot-Bouchard aneurysms are found with greater frequency in hypertensive patients (approximately 50 percent) compared to normotensive individuals (5 to 8 percent).[25] The incidence of aneurysms is greatest in the brains of hypertensive patients with either large or small ICH. In hypertensive patients over the age of 65, aneurysms are more common than in younger hypertensive patients. Microaneurysms are almost never found in normotensive individuals under the age of 65.[25,112] In addition to aneurysms, degenerative changes are also common in the small penetrating arteries of hypertensives. These changes include a peculiar intramural accumulation of lipid and hyaline material often called *lipohyalinosis*.[37]

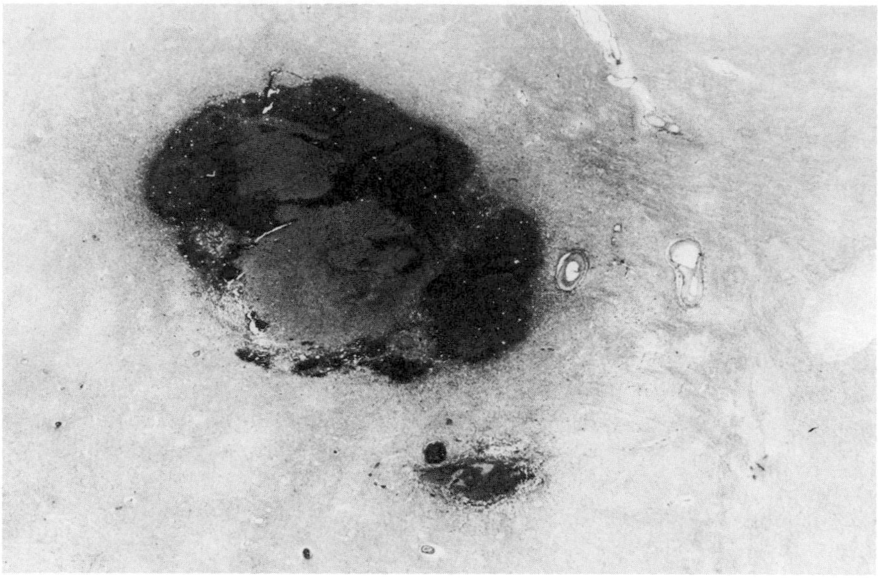

**Fig. 7-14.** Recent intracerebral (ganglionic) hemorrhage in a chronic hypertensive; two nearby arteries show hyalinization. (Hematoxylin & eosin; × 2.5.)

## Miscellaneous Causes of Intracerebral Hemorrhage

Arterial hypertension is the major cause of primary ICH; but, in recent years several other conditions have been linked to the development of ICH. Most of these have been listed by Kase[75] in a recent review. Some of the very rare conditions include exposure to cold weather, severe dental pain, correction of congenital heart defects in children, and as a consequence of carotid endarterectomy. The mechanisms responsible for the hemorrhages in these apparently unrelated conditions are complex, but probably include acute rises in blood pressure with an acute increase in local cerebral blood flow at the site of a previously poorly perfused or overtly ischemic area ("reperfusion").[18]

## Morphology

At autopsy, external inspection of a brain with a large ICH may disclose localized flattening of the gyri, uni- or bilateral herniations, either uncinate or cerebellar.

The gross characteristics of the hematoma vary according to the time elapsed since the start of the hemorrhage. Most patients usually survive the ICH for a few hours or days; the exception might be primary ICH in the pons; some of these patients may die within minutes of the bleed (Fig. 7-15). As a result of early hemolysis, the change of color may become apparent in the blood clot. Large ICH may rupture into the lateral ventricles where blood may fill the ventricular cavities and spill to the subarachnoid space through the 4th ventricle outlets (Fig. 7-16). Rupture

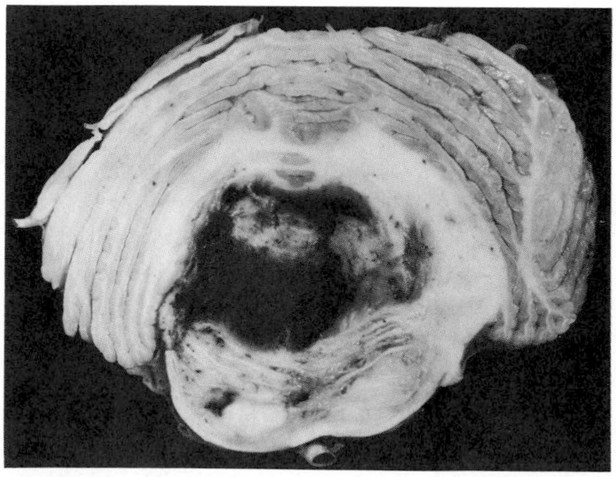

**Fig. 7-15.** Recent primary pontine hemorrhage in a hypertensive patient. There are also small infarcts (healed) in the base of the pons.

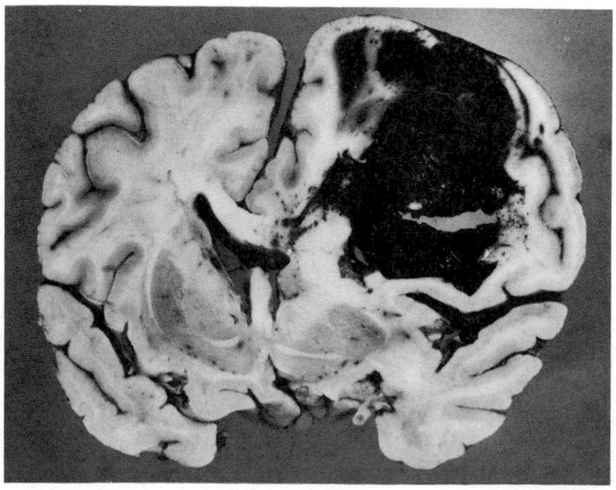

**Fig. 7-16.** Recent lobar hemorrhage in a hypertensive patient.

through the cerebral cortex is less common. There are very few publications documenting the time-dependent changes that occur in or around an ICH. The following generalizations are a reflection of our personal experiences. After a few days or weeks, ICH is transformed into a semiliquid red-brown mass. Brown and yellow pigmentation can be seen in the adjacent parenchyma, as a consequence of the metabolic changes affecting the hemoglobin pigment. Hemosiderin-laden macrophages, astrocytosis, and vascular proliferation can be seen at the edges of the hemorrhage. After several months, and depending on the size, an ICH can be completely reabsorbed, and the lesion is eventually replaced by a cavity with rusty brown walls (apoplectic cyst). Large ICHs may sometimes take years to be completely reabsorbed.

## Lobar Hemorrhages

Lobar hemorrhages occur in the subcortical white matter of the cerebral hemispheres or in the centrum ovale. Most ICHs associated with hypertension occur in the region of the basal ganglia. The association between hypertension and lobar hemorrhage is not as definite as with ICH of the basal ganglia. Approximately 30 percent of lobar ICHs are believed to be secondary to hypertension; other causes, such as eclampsia or amyloid angiopathy, may induce ICH in this location at a more frequent rate than hypertension.

## Primary or Metastatic Tumors

Lobar ICH may be the initial manifestation of a brain tumor, either primary or metastatic. Autopsy studies, have demonstrated tumors in 1 to 2 percent of spontaneous ICH.[114] Up to 10 percent of patients with ICH have an associated neoplasm that is demonstrable in CT scans.[84] Among gliomas, glioblastoma multiforme and oligodendroglioma are characteristically associated with sudden, spontaneous large intracerebral hemorrhages. Bleeding in these types of gliomas may reflect the abnormal structure of the blood vessels located in the tumor stroma.[141] Spontaneous ICH is much less common in astrocytomas and ependymomas compared to other gliomas. Germ-cell tumors of the pineal gland or the suprasellar region may also be associated with an increased frequency of spontaneous intracerebral bleeding.[141]

Metastatic brain tumors may also become manifest as ICH, usually of the lobar type. In some instances, cerebral bleeding may be the first manifestation of a tumor, the primary site being clinically occult.[52,119] Choriocarcinoma and melanoma are associated with an increased risk of spontaneous brain bleeding. Hemorrhage at the site of a brain metastasis from bronchogenic carcinoma or renal cell carcinoma is also relatively common.

## Hematologic Disorders

Coagulopathies and myeloproliferative disorders are also associated with spontaneous ICH. ICH can occur in patients with disseminated intravascular coagulation (DIC). In this condition, ICHs are a manifestation of a systemic bleeding disorder and the hemorrhages are seldom restricted to the brain. ICH also occurs in hemophiliacs, especially in patients who have very low levels of circulating factor VIII.[6,93]

ICHs are important complications of leukemia; ICH can occur in any phase of the disease, and a hemorrhagic "stroke" can be the initial manifestation of the leukemia. ICHs are especially common in children with acute leukemia and evidence of ICH can be found in as many as 50 percent of leukemic brains examined at autopsy.[57] A significant reduction in the incidence of this complication has been attributed to the effects of chemotherapy and the availability of platelet transfusions.

The morphologic findings in the brains of leukemics include multifocal hemorrhages, mostly petechial and located in the white matter; large brain hematomas can also be found in leukemics. Infiltrates of leukemic cells are common at the site of bleeding. However, direct infiltration of vessel walls by leukemic cells is probably not the mechanism responsible for the bleeding; thrombocytopenia and DIC also play a significant role.[107]

## Delayed Posttraumatic Intracerebral Hematomas ("Spät-Apoplexie")

The condition known as delayed posttraumatic ICH was first described by Bollinger,[9] and refers to intracerebral or intraventricular bleeding that occurs several days after an episode of closed head trauma. Most affected patients are young and asymptomatic, until ICH occurs unexpectedly; the bleeding may result in death. ICH in these patients occurs predominantly in the white matter of the centrum ovale, and there is no predilection for the basal ganglia. The pathogenesis is unknown, and, in fact, the existence of the condition remains disputed.[98] A few well-documented cases, have been reported as late as 1990.[33]

## Cerebral Hemorrhages in the Newborn

Intracranial hemorrhages that occur during the newborn period may be subdural, subarachnoid, intraparenchymatous and periventricular/intraventricular in location.

Subdural hemorrhages are related to obstetric trauma, and, with improved obstetric care, those hemorrhages have become uncommon. Subarachnoid hemorrhages, although relatively common, are usually self-limited and of not great clinical importance. Intraparenchymal hemorrhages often originate in the cerebellum.

The incidence of subependymal and intraventricular hemorrhages varies according to birthweight of premature infants. Infants who weigh 1,500 g have an incidence of 40 to 50 percent, while newborns weighing less than 1,250 g have an incidence of approximately 60 percent.[30] In infants weighing 500 to 750 g, the incidence is as high as 73 percent.[65] Subependymal and intraventricular hemorrhages are essentially conditions of the premature infants, although they can sometimes be seen in the full-term newborn. There is an inverse relationship between gestational age and the incidence of subependymal and intraventricular hemorrhages.[30]

Although subependymal and intraventricular hemorrhages can occur pre- or intrapartum, most bleeding develop between 5 and 25 hours after birth.[34,41] Hemorrhages usually arise in the subependymal germinal matrix in the thalamostriate groove, at the site of the foramen of Monro, although in very premature neonates it may occur more posteriorly and in mature neonates it may arise within the choroid plexus. In most cases, the hemorrhage extends into the ventricles and then spreads to the ventricular system, and through Luschka's foramina and Magendie's foramen to the subarachnoid space, where an obliterative arachnoiditis can lead to obstructive hydrocephalus. In 15 percent of cases, intraventricular hemorrhage may be complicated by periventricular hemorrhagic infarction, which consists of a large area of hemorrhagic necrosis of periventricular white matter. This lesion should not be confused with periventricular leukomalacia, which is also very common in premature infants and consists of ischemic nonhemorrhagic symmetric areas of necrosis of periventricular white matter. The presence of periventricular hemorrhagic infarction is indicative of poor neurologic outcome.[134]

The pathogenesis of subependymal and intraventricular hemorrhages in the newborn is complex and multifactorial. Intravascular (decrease or increase in cerebral blood flow), vascular (integrity of the capillary wall), and extravascular factors (such as deficient vascular support and fibrinolytic activity) appear to participate in the pathogenesis of subependymal bleeding. The complex interrelationship of these factors has been recently reviewed by Volpe.[134]

## SUBARACHNOID HEMORRHAGE

Nontraumatic subarachnoid hemorrhage (SAH) constitutes approximately 6 to 8 percent of all strokes (or abrupt focal neurologic deficit).[79] The prevalence of SAH varies depending on case selection and method of study. In autopsy series, the major cause of spontaneous SAH, ruptured saccular aneurysm, constitute about 55 percent of all cases,[85] while in neuroradiologic series, aneurysms may represent a much larger proportion of SAH.[131] The most common causes of SAH are as follows:

1. Traumatic
2. Aneurysm rupture (saccular, atherosclerotic, mycotic)
3. Vascular malformation (arteriovenous, cavernous, angioma)
4. Bleeding disorders (leukemia, anticoagulation treatment, DIC)
5. Vasculitis (polyarteritis nodosa, SLE, granulomatous arteritis)
6. Drug abuse (cocaine, amphetamines)
7. Infections (sepsis, bacterial meningitis)
8. Thrombosis of cerebral sinus
9. Secondary to intraparenchymatous bleeding

In spite of thorough radiologic and postmortem examinations, the cause of SAH may remain undetected in as many as 20 percent of the cases.[15,64]

### Pathology of Subarachnoid Hemorrhage

Subarachnoid hemorrhage describes bleeding into the subarachnoid space where the blood comes in direct contact with the cerebrospinal fluid. In most patients who die shortly after an episode of SAH, the ventral surface of the base of the brain is covered by a layer of red liquid and clotted blood. The extent and site of the hemorrhage depends on the cause of the bleeding. In most cases of ruptured aneurysms, the bulk of the hemorrhage is collected at the base of the brain, where the hemorrhage may fill the subarachnoid cisterns and may even enter, through Luschka's foramina and Magendie's foramen, the ventricular system. Subarachnoid hemorrhages localized to the cerebral convexity are more common in cases of ruptured arteriovenous malformations.

The arachnoid membrane is very resistant to the pressure of spinal fluid or blood and large collections of blood are necessary to produce arachnoidal rupture and extension of the blood into the subdural space. Large collections of blood in the subarachnoid space may produce intracerebral hemorrhages that appear primary at first glance. Thus, rupture of anterior communicating artery aneurysms often produces large ICHs in the frontal lobes, that may spread to the frontal horn of the lateral ventricle.

The presence of blood in the subarachnoid space elicits an inflammatory and fibrotic reaction. Approximately 4 to 16 hours after the hemorrhage, an inflammatory reaction consisting mainly of neutrophils becomes evident in the meninges. The inflammatory reaction reaches a peak at 36 hours, and after 24 hours the lining cells of the subarachnoid space undergo hyperplasia, become detached from the arachnoid membrane, and become phagocytic. After 3 or 4 days, hemosiderin granules can be detected in the cytoplasm of macrophages. Fibrosis of the pia mater progressively develops and may obliterate the subarachnoid space.[60]

### Complications of Subarachnoid Hemorrhage

Increased intracranial pressure may be the result of obstruction to the CSF circulation (secondary to adhesions between pia and arachnoid membranes), dysfunction of arachnoidal granulations, and brain edema. Severe and sustained elevations of the CSF pressure may result in transtentorial (uncinate) and tonsillar (cerebellar) herniations.

Cerebral infarction after SAH is a major cause of death and of permanent disability among patients who survive the acute stage. Causes for cerebral infarction after SAH include a reduction in cerebral blood flow due to increased intracranial pressure, impaired autoregulation, and vasospasm.[96]

Vasospasm is one of the major complications of SAH, and it probably is the leading cause of ischemia and cerebral infarction.[76] The morphologic substrate of vasospasm has not been clearly defined. Arterial vessels near the ruptured aneurysm and distal to this site may show obliterative changes, such as subintimal concentrical fibrosis, reduction in the caliber of the lumen, and even thrombosis. However, these changes are more likely the consequences rather than the cause of vasospasm; such vascular changes have been found in patients who survive days or weeks after the episode of SAH; the same changes are rare in patients who die a few days after the hemorrhage.

## DRUGS AND STROKES

### Opiates

Opiates can be linked to stroke by several direct and indirect mechanisms. Indirectly, stroke may be the result of cerebral embolism in drug abusers who inject intravenously and in whom infectious endocarditis develops, or among those who have "mycotic" aneurysms. A hemorrhagic stroke may develop in drug addicts afflicted with severe hepatitis and deranged clotting. More directly, opiate overdose may produce respiratory depression and hypotension, leading to ischemic stroke. A direct toxic injury on the vessels may be produced by heroin or other substances mixed with the opiate, such as quinidine or lactose. Embolization of foreign material, such as talc or starch is also known to produce cerebral embolism. A syndrome of heroin myelopathy has been described in patients who develop acute paraparesis, sensory loss, and urinary retention shortly after an injection of heroin. The symptoms are believed to reflect the effects of an infarct in the territory of the anterior spinal artery.[72]

### Amphetamines

Amphetamines can produce uncontrolled hypertension resulting in either intracerebral or subarachnoid hemorrhage.[61] In addition, a pattern of "vasculitis" has been observed in cerebral angiograms of amphetamine users.[140] Pathologic studies in these patients have shown a necrotizing vasculitis affecting small cerebral blood vessels.[24]

### Phenylpropanolamine

Phenylpropanolamine is a widely available, over-the-counter medication in many nasal decongestants; occasional hemorrhagic strokes have been attributed to the use of this drug.[78]

### Cocaine, "Crack"

Cocaine has been linked with a high incidence of hemorrhagic stroke. The hemorrhagic complication has been related to the intranasal or parenteral intake or the smoking of "crack." Saccular aneurysms were demonstrated in 7 and arteriovenous malformations in 6 of 25 patients who had both cocaine abuse and stroke.[14] Postulated mechanisms responsible for the occurrence of stroke include acute hypertension and sympathicomimetic vasospasm.[83]

### Phencyclidine

Strokes have also been associated with the use (intake) of phencyclidine (PCP) and LSD. The former produces intracranial hemorrhage probably because of acute rises in arterial blood pressure; focal neurologic deficits have been attributed to the effects of vasoconstriction.[4]

## ACKNOWLEDGMENT

We thank Ms. Barbara Caracciolo for her valuable secretarial support.

## REFERENCES

1. Adam J, Crow TJ, Duchen LW et al: Familial cerebral amyloidosis and spongiform encephalopathy. J Neurol Neurosurg Psychiatry 45:37, 1982
2. Amorosi EL, Ultmann JE: Thrombotic thrombocytopenic purpura report of 16 cases and review of the literature. Medicine (Baltimore) 45:139, 1966
3. Babikian V, Ropper AH: Binswanger's disease: a review. Stroke 18:2, 1987
4. Bessen H: Intracranial hemorrhage associated with phencyclidine abuse. JAMA 248:585, 1982
5. Bicknell JM, Holland JV: Neurogenic manifesta-

tions of Cogan syndrome. Neurology (NY) 28:278, 1978
6. Biggs R: Haemophilia treatment in the United Kingdom from 1969 to 1974. Br J Haematol 35:484, 1974
7. Blaustein HG: Neuropsychiatric manifestations of systemic lupus erythematosus. N Engl J Med 318:218, 1987
8. Bohmfalk GL, Story JL, Wissinger JP et al: Bacterial intracranial aneurysms. J Neurosurg 48:369, 1978
9. Bollinger O: Über traumatische Spät-Apoplexie: ein Beitrag zur Lehre von der Hirnerschüterung. p. 457. In Internationale Beitrage zur wissenschlaftlichen Medizin. Festschrift, Rudolf Virchow. Hirschwald, Berlin, 1891
10. Bougouslavsky J, Regli F, Uské A et al: Early spontaneous hematoma in cerebral infarct: is primary cerebral hemorrhage overdiagnosed? Neurology (NY) 41:837, 1991
11. Brandenberg W, Hallervorden J: Dementia pugilistica mit anatomischem Befund. Virchows Arch [A] 325:680, 1954
12. Briley DP, Coull BM, Goodnight SH: Neurological disease associated with antiphospholipid antibodies. Ann Neurol 25:221, 1989
13. Bruetman ME, Field WS, Crawford ES et al: Cerebral hemorrhage in carotid artery surgery. Arch Neurol 9:458, 1963
14. Brust JCM: Stroke and drugs. p. 517. In Handbook of Clinical Neurology. Vinken PJ, Bruyn GW, Klawans HL, Toole JF (eds): Vol. 55 (revised series 11). Vascular Diseases Part III. Elsevier, New York, 1989
15. Burrows EH, Leeds NE: Neuroradiology. Churchill Livingstone, London, 1981
16. Burton E, Johnson J: Multiple cerebral aneurysms and cardiac myxoma. N Engl J Med 282:35, 1970
17. Cabanes J, Blasco R, Garcia M et al: Cerebral venous angiomas. Surg Neurol 11:385, 1979
18. Caplan LR: Intracerebral hemorrhage revisited. Neurology (NY) 38:624, 1988
19. Caplan LR, Skillman J, Ojemann R et al: Intracerebral hemorrhage following carotid endarterectomy: a hypertensive complication? Stroke 9:457, 1978
20. Case Records of the Massachusetts General Hospital: Case 30—1991. N Engl J Med 325:265, 1991
21. Cawthorn DF, Cacayorin ED, Modesti LM et al: Spinal vascular tumors: dilemmas and diagnosis and management. Neurosurgery 16:625, 1985
22. Challa VK, Moody DM, Bell MA: The Charcot-Bouchard aneurysm controversy: impact of a new histologic technique, abstracted. J Neuropathol Exp Neurol 50:354, 1991
23. Charcot JM, Bouchard CH: Nouvelles recherches sur la pathogénie de l'hémorrhage cérébrale. Arch Physiol Norm Pathol 1:110, 1868
24. Citron BP, Halpern M, McCarron M et al: Necrotizing angiitis associated with drug abuse. New Engl J Med 283:1003, 1970
25. Cole FM, Yates PO: The occurrence and significance of intracerebral microaneurysm. J Pathol Bacteriol 93:393, 1967
26. Courville CB: Arteriosclerotic aneurysms of the circle of Willis. Bull Los Angeles Neurol Soc 27:1, 1962
27. Crowell RM, Marcoux FW, De Girolami U: Variability and reversibility of focal cerebral ischemia in unanesthetized monkeys. Neurology (NY) 31:1295, 1981
28. Dereski MO, Chopp M, Garcia JH et al: Focal cerebral ischemia in the rat: evolution of histopathologic abnormalities. 1991
29. Devinsky O, Petito CK, Alonso DR: Clinical and neuropathological findings in systemic lupus erythematosus: the role of vasculitis, heart emboli and thrombotic thrombocytopenic purpura. Ann Neurol 23:380, 1988
30. Editorial: Ischemia and haemorrhage in the premature brain. Lancet 2:847, 1984
31. Einhäupl KM, Villringer A, Haberl RL et al: Clinical spectrum of sinus venous thrombosis. p. 149. In Einhäupl K, Kempski O, Baethmann A (eds): Cerebral Sinus Thrombosis. Plenum Press, New York, 1990
32. Ellis SG, Verity MA: Central nervous system involvement in systemic lupus erythematosus: a review of neuropathologic findings in 57 cases, 1955–1977. Semin Arthritis Rheum 8:212, 1979
33. Elsner H, Rigamonti D, Corradino G et al: Delayed traumatic intracerebral hematoma: "Spät-Apoplexie": report of two cases. J Neurosurg 72:813, 1990
34. Emerson P, Fujimura M, Howat P et al: Timing of intraventricular hemorrhage. Arch Dis Child 52:183, 1977
35. Fisher CM: Lacunes, small deep cerebral infarcts. Neurology (NY) 15:774, 1965
36. Fisher CM: The arterial lesions underlying lacunes. Acta Neuropathol 12:1, 1969
37. Fisher CM: Pathological observations in hypertensive cerebral hemorrhage. J Neuropathol Exp Neurol 30:536, 1971
38. Fisher CM: Cerebral miliary aneurysms in hypertension. Am J Pathol 66:313, 1972
39. Fisher CM: Lacunar strokes and infarcts: a review. Neurology (NY) 332:871, 1982
40. Fisher CM, Karnes WE, Kubik CS et al: Lateral medullary infarction—the pattern of vascular occlusions. J Neuropathol Exp Neurol 20:323, 1961
41. Friede RL: Hemorrhages in asphyxiated premature infants. p. 44. In: Developmental Neuropathology. 2nd Ed. Springer-Verlag, New York, 1989
42. Futrell N, Garcia JH, Millikan C: Morphology of evolving microinfarctions in the rat brain, abstracted. J Neuropathol Exp Neurol 49:301, 1991
43. Futrell N, Millikan C: The fallacy of the lacune hypothesis. Stroke 21:1251, 1990
44. Garcia JH: Morphology of global cerebral ischemia: a review. Crit Care Med 16:979, 1988
45. Garcia JH: Thrombosis of cranial veins and sinuses: brain parenchymal effects. p. 27. In Ein-

häupl K, Kempski O, Baethmann A (eds): Cerebral Sinus Thrombosis. Plenum Press, New York, 1990
46. Garcia JH, Anderson ML: Circulatory disorders and their effects on the brain. p. 621. In Davis RL, Robertson DM (eds): Textbook of Neuropathology. 2nd Ed. Williams & Wilkins, Baltimore, 1991
47. Garcia JH, Brown GG: Vascular dementia: analysis of neuropathologic changes and metabolic alterations. J Neurol Sci 1992 (in press)
48. Garcia JH, Conger KA, Hudetz AG: Patterns of ischemic injury to the brain: the influence of local hemodynamic factors. p. 68. In Hartmann A, Kuschinsky W (eds): Cerebral Ischemia and Hemorrheology. Springer-Verlag, Berlin, 1988
49. Garcia JH, Kamijyo Y: Cerebral infarction: evolution of histopathological changes after occlusion of a middle cerebral artery in primates. J Neuropathol Exp Neurol 33:409, 1974
50. Garcia JH, Lossinsky A, Conger KA et al: Neuronal ischemic injury: light microscopy, ultrastructure and biochemistry. Acta Neuropathol 43:85, 1978
51. Gilbert JJ, Vinters HV: Cerebral amyloid angiopathy: incidence and complications in the aging brain. I. Cerebral hemorrhage. Stroke 14:915, 1983
52. Gildersleeve N, Koo AH, McDonald CJ: Metastatic tumor presenting as intracerebral hemorrhage. Radiology 124:109, 1977
53. Glenner GG: Alzheimer's disease: the commonest form of amyloidosis. Arch Pathol Lab Med 107:281, 1988
54. Glenner GG, Wong CW: Alzheimer's disease and Down's syndrome: sharing of a unique cerebrovascular amyloid fibril protein. Biochem Biophys Res Commun 122:1131, 1984
55. Goldman JA, Fleischer AS, Leifer W et al: *Candida albicans* aneurysm associated with systemic lupus erythematosus. Neurosurgery 4:325, 1979
56. Gray F, Vinters HV, Le Noan H et al: Cerebral amyloid angiopathy and granulomatous angiitis: immunohistochemical study using antibodies to the Alzheimer A4 peptide. Hum Pathol 21:1290, 1990
57. Groch SN, Sayre GP, Heck FJ et al: Cerebral hemorrhage in leukemia. Arch Neurol 2:439, 1960
58. Haan J, Algra PR, Roos RAC: Hereditary cerebral hemorrhage with amyloidosis—Dutch type: clinical and computed tomographic analysis of 24 cases. Arch Neurol 47:649, 1990
59. Hall S, Barr W, Lie JT et al: Takayasu arteritis: a study of 32 North American patients. Medicine (Baltimore) 64:89, 1985
60. Hammes EM: Reaction of the meninges to blood. Arch Neurol Psychiatry 52:505, 1944
61. Harrington H, Heller MA, Dawson D: Intracerebral hemorrhage and oral amphetamine. Arch Neurol 40:503, 1983
62. Hart MN, Merz P, Bennet-Gray J et al: β-Amyloid protein of Alzheimer's disease is found in cerebral and spinal cord vascular malformations. Am J Pathol 132:167, 1988
63. Heffner RR, Solitaire GB: Hereditary hemorrhagic telangiectasis: neuropathological observation. J Neurol Neurosurg Psychiatry 32:274, 1969
64. Heidrich R: Subarachnoid hemorrhage. p. 68. In Vinken PJ, Bruyn GW (eds): Handbook of Clinical Neurology: Vascular Diseases of the Nervous System. Part II. North-Holland Publishing, Amsterdam, 1972
65. Hill A, Volpe JJ: Seizures, hypoxic-ischemic brain injury and intraventricular hemorrhage in the newborn. Ann Neurol 10:109, 1981
66. Ho KL: Acute subdural hematoma and intracerebral hemorrhage: rare complications of rhinocerebral mucormycosis. Arch Otolaryngol 105:279, 1979
67. Ho KL: Neoplastic aneurysm and intracranial hemorrhage. Cancer 46:1442, 1982
68. Ishii N, Nishihara Y, Horie A: Amyloid angiopathy and lobar cerebral hemorrhage. J Neurol Neurosurg Psychiatry 47:1203, 1984
69. Janota I, Mirsen TR, Hachinski VC et al: Neuropathologic correlates of leukoaraiosis. Arch Neurol 46:1124, 1989
70. Jellinger K: Cerebrovascular amyloidosis with cerebral hemorrhage. J Neurol 214:195, 1977
71. Jensson O, Gudmundsson G, Arnason A et al: Hereditary cystatin C (gamma-trace) amyloid angiopathy of the CNS causing cerebral hemorrhage. Acta Neurol Scand 76:102, 1987
72. Judice DJ, Leblanc HJ, McGarry PA: Spinal cord vasculitis presenting as spinal cord tumor in a heroin addict. J Neurosurg 48:131, 1978
73. Kadison P, Haynes BF: Vasculitis: mechanism of vessel damage. p. 703. In Gallin J et al (eds): Inflammation: Basic Principles and Clinical Correlation. Raven Press, New York, 1988
74. Kaplan HA, Aronson SM, Browder EJ et al: Vascular malformations of the brain; an anatomical study. J Neurosurg 27:630, 1961
75. Kase CS: Intracerebral hemorrhage: non-hypertensive causes. Stroke 17:590, 1986
76. Kassell NF, Boarini DJ: Patients with ruptured aneurysms: pre- and postoperative management. p. 1367. In Wilkins RH, Rengachary SS (eds): Neurosurgery. Vol. 2. McGraw-Hill, New York, 1985
77. Katz RI, Goldberg HI, Selzer ME: Mycotic aneurysm. Arch Intern Med 134:939, 1974
78. King J: Hypertension and cerebral hemorrhage after trimolets ingestion. Med J Aust 2:258, 1979
79. Kurtzke JF: Epidemiology of cerebrovascular disease. In McDowell F, Caplan L (eds): Cerebrovascular Survey Report 1985 for the National Institute of Neurological and Communicative Disorders and Stroke. Bethesda, MD, 1985
80. Lassen NA: Incomplete cerebral infarction—focal incomplete ischemic necrosis not leading to emollision. Stroke 13:522, 1982
81. Lassen NA, Ingvar DH, Skinhoj E: Brain functions and blood flow. Sci Am 239:62, 1978
82. Levine SR, Welch KMA: The spectrum of neuro-

logic disease associated with antiphospholipid antibodies lupus anticoagulants, and anti-cardiolipin antibodies. Arch Neurol 44:876, 1987
83. Levine SR, Welch KMA: Cocaine and stroke. Stroke 19:779, 1988
84. Little JR, Dial B, Belanger G et al: Brain hemorrhage from intracranial tumor. Stroke 10:283, 1979
85. Locksley HB: Report on the cooperative study of intracranial aneurysms and subarachnoid hemorrhage. Section V, Part I. Natural History of subarachnoid hemorrhage, intracranial aneurysms and arteriovenous malformations: based on 6368 cases in the cooperative study. J Neurosurg 25:219, 1966
86. Loes DJ, Biller J, Yuh WTC et al: Leukoencephalopathy in cerebral amyloid angiopathy: MR imaging in four cases. AJNR 11:485, 1990
87. Luyendijk W, Bots GTAM, Vegter-van der Vlis M et al: Hereditary cerebral hemorrhage caused by cortical amyloid angiopathy. J Neurol Sci 85:267, 1988
88. Mandybur TI: The incidence of cerebral amyloid angiopathy in Alzheimer's disease. Neurology (NY) 25:120, 1975
89. Mandybur TI: Cerebral amyloid angiopathy: the vascular pathology and complications. J Neuropathol Exp Neurol 45:79, 1986
90. Mandybur TI, Bates SRD: Fatal massive intracerebral hemorrhage complicating cerebral amyloid angiopathy. Arch Neurol 35:246, 1978
91. Mandybur TI, Gore I: Amyloid in late post-irradiation necrosis of brain. Neurology (NY) 19:983, 1969
92. Marcoux FW, Morawetz RB, Crowell MD et al: Differential regional vulnerability in transient focal cerebral ischemia. Stroke 13:339, 1982
93. Martinowitz U, Heim M, Tadmor R et al: Intracranial hemorrhage in patients with hemophilia. Neurosurgery 18:858, 1986
94. McCormick WF: The pathology of vascular "arteriovenous" malformations. J Neurosurg 24:807, 1966
95. McCormick WF, Nofzinger JD: "Cryptic" vascular malformations of the central nervous system. J Neurosurg 24:865, 1966
96. Meyer CHA, Lowe D, Meyer M et al: Progressive change in cerebral blood flow during the first three weeks after subarachnoid hemorrhage. Neurosurgery 12:58, 1983
97. Mohr JP, Caplan LR, Melshi JW et al: The Harvard Cooperative Stroke Registry: a prospective registry. Neurology (NY) 28:754, 1978
98. Morin MA, Pitts FW: Delayed apoplexy following head injury ("traumatische Spät-Apoplexie"). J Neurosurg 33:542, 1970
99. Murphy MN, Sima AAF: Cerebral amyloid angiopathy associated with giant cell arteritis: a case report. Stroke 16:514, 1985
100. Nedergaard M, Klinken L, Paulson OB et al: Secondary brainstem hemorrhage in stroke. Stroke 14:501, 1983
101. Neubuerger KT: Lesions of the human brain following circulatory arrest. J Neuropathol Exp Neurol 13:144, 1954
102. Newton TH, Troost BT, Moseley I: Angiography of arteriovenous malformations and fistulas. p. 64. In Wilson CB, Stein BM (eds): Intracranial Arteriovenous Malformations. Williams & Wilkins, Baltimore, 1984
103. Ng LKY, Nimmannitya J: Massive cerebral infarction with severe brain swellings: a clinicopathological study. Stroke 1:158, 1970
104. Olszewski J: Subcortical arteriosclerotic encephalopathy: review of the literature on so-called Binswanger's disease and presentation of two cases. World Neurol 3:362, 1962
105. Omae T, Ueda K, Ogata J, Yagamuchi T: Parenchymatous hemorrhage: etiology, pathology and clinical aspects. p. 287. In Vinken PJ, Bruyn GW, Klawans HL et al (eds): Handbook of Clinical Neurology. Vol. 54 (revised series 10). Vascular Diseases: Part II. Elsevier, New York, 1989
106. Petito CK, Feldmann E, Pulsinelli WA et al: Delayed hippocampal damage in humans following cardiorespiratory arrest. Neurology (NY) 37:1281, 1987
107. Pochedly C: Neurologic manifestations in acute leukemia: symptoms due to increased cerebrospinal fluid pressure and hemorrhage. NY State J Med 75:575, 1975
108. Reagan TJ, Bloom WH: The brain in hereditary hemorrhagic telangiectasia. Stroke 2:361, 1971
109. Richardson EP, Jr: Amyloid in the human brain. West J Med 143:518, 1985
110. Ridolfi RL, Bell WR: Thrombotic thrombocytopenic purpura. Medicine (Baltimore) 60:413, 1981
111. Román GC: Senile dementia of the Binswanger's type: vascular form of dementia in the elderly. JAMA 258:1782, 1987
112. Rosenblum WI: Miliary aneurysms and "fibrinoid" degeneration of blood vessels. Hum Pathol 8:133, 1977
113. Ross-Russell RW: Observations on intracerebral aneurysms. Brain 86:425, 1963
114. Russell DB: The pathology of spontaneous intracranial hemorrhages. Proc R Soc Med 47:689, 1954
115. Sacco RL, Ellenberg JH, Mohr JP et al: Infarcts of undetermined cause: The NINCDS Stroke Data Bank. Ann Neurol 25:382, 1989
116. Savage COS, Ng YC: The etiology and pathogenesis of major systemic vasculitides. Postgrad Med J 62:627, 1988
117. Schold C, Earnest MP: Cerebral hemorrhage from a mycotic aneurysm developing during appropriate antibiotic therapy. Stroke 9:207, 1978
118. Sekar TS MacDonnell K-F, Namsirikul P et al: Survival after prolonged submersion in cold water without neurologic sequelae: report of two cases. Arch Intern Med 140:775, 1980
119. Shuangshoti S, Panyathanya R, Wichienkur P: Intracranial metastases from unsuspected choriocarcinoma. Neurology (NY) 24:649, 1974
120. Spaar FW, Goebel HH, Volles E, Wickboldt J: Tumor-like amyloid formation (amyloidoma) in the brain. J Neurol 224:171, 1981
121. Spiro D, Lattes RG, Wiener J: The cellular pathology of experimental hypertension. I. Hyper-

tension arteriolarsclerosis. Am J Pathol 47:19, 1965

122. Steegmann AT: The neuropathology of cardiac arrest. p. 1005. In Minckler J (ed): Pathology of the Nervous System. Vol. I. McGraw-Hill, New York, 1968
123. Stehbens WE: Intracerebral and intraventricular hemorrhages. p. 284. In: Pathology of the Cerebral Blood Vessels. CV Mosby, St. Louis, 1972
124. Stein BM, Wolpert SM: Arteriovenous malformations of the brain. I. Current concepts and treatment. Arch Neurol 37:1, 1980
125. Stein BM, Wolpert SM: Arteriovenous malformations of the brain. II. Current concepts and treatment. Arch Neurol 37:69, 1980
126. Stokes MI, Trickey RJ: Screening for neurofibrillary tangles and argyrophilic plaques with congo red and polarized light. J Clin Pathol 20:241, 1973
127. Sundt TM, Sharbrough FW, Piepgras DG et al: Correlation of cerebral blood flow and carotid endarterectomy with results of surgery and hemodynamics of cerebral ischemia. Mayo Clin Proc 56:533, 1981
128. Swanson RA, Morton MT, Tsao-Wu G et al: A semi-automated method for measuring brain infarct volume. J Cereb Blood Flow Metab 10:290, 1990
129. Sypert GW, Alvord EC, Jr: Cerebellar infarction: a clinicopathological study. Arch Neurol 32:357, 1975
130. Tan EM, Cohen AS, Fries J-F et al: The revised criteria for the classification of systemic lupus erythematosus. Arthritis Rheum 25:1271, 1982
131. Toole JF, Robinson MK, Mercuri M: Primary subarachnoid hemorrhage. p. 1. In Vinken PJ, Bruyn GW, Klawans HL (eds): Handbook of Clinical Neurology. Vol. 55 (revised series 11). Vascular Diseases: Part III. Elsevier, Amsterdam, 1989
132. Vinters HV: Cerebral amyloid angiopathy: a critical review. Stroke 18:311, 1987
133. Vinters HV, Miller BL, Pardridge WM: Brain amyloid and Alzheimer disease. Ann Intern Med 109:41, 1988
134. Volpe JJ: Intraventricular hemorrhage and brain injury in the premature infant. Clin Perinatol 16:361, 1989
135. Watanabe J: Ultrastructure of the retinal arterioles in spontaneously hypertensive rats. Acta Soc Ophthalmol Jpn 74:999, 1970
136. Wattendorff AR, Bots GThAM, Went LN, Endtz LJ: Familial cerebral amyloid angiopathy presenting as recurrent cerebral hemorrhage. J Neurol Sci 55:121, 1982
137. Weisberg LA, Stazio A, Shamsnia M et al: Nontraumatic parenchymal brain hemorrhages. Medicine (Baltimore) 69:277, 1990
138. Wilkins RH, Brody IA: Sturge-Weber syndrome. Arch Neurol 21:554, 1969
139. Wolf PA, Dawser TR, Thomas HE Jr et al: Epidemiologic assessment of chronic atrial fibrillation and risk of stroke: the Framingham study. Neurology (NY) 28:973, 1978
140. Yo YJ, Cooper DR, Wellenstein DE et al: Cerebral angiitis and intracerebral hemorrhage associated with methamphetamine abuse: case report. J Neurosurg 58:109, 1983
141. Zülch KH: Neuropathology of intracranial hemorrhage. Prog Brain Res 30:151, 1968

# II

# *DIAGNOSTIC STUDIES FOR STROKE*

## J.P. Mohr, Section Editor

This section discusses the role of the major diagnostic tests, in conjunction with other technologies, such as lumbar puncture and clinical neurophysiologic tests, in the detection and assessment of the severity and outcome of stroke. These techniques are described sufficiently to make accessible the scientific basis of the methods and also to show how the tests are performed. The chapters are predominantly concerned with the application and findings of these diagnostic techniques in each of the major settings of stroke: the asymptomatic population, after transient ischemic attacks, in acute stroke, and over time. The first chapter in this section discusses how recent advances in the application of diagnosis algorithms have increased our competence in understanding and coping with the problems in this field.

Digital venous angiography, in its heyday at the time of the first edition, has been superseded to such an extent that full treatment in a chapter of its own is no longer justified.

On the other hand, magnetic resonance imaging, which was just getting under way in 1984, has developed so remarkably that it now requires two chapters, one describing techniques of brain imaging, and the other scrutinizing the rapidly developing field of angiography.

Noninvasive evaluation has also undergone immense refinements. Phonangiography has all but disappeared as duplex Doppler has strengthened its position and now offers the advantages of imaging of the bifurcation as well as analysis of the velocity profiles. The introduction of color-coded duplex methods has led to the inclusion of color images. Transcranial Doppler was introduced in 1982, and in the years since the first edition, it has become a widely used technology that has earned its prominent position in the chapter on Doppler techniques.

Because there are numerous reproductions of brain images in acute stroke throughout the book, such illustrations are less numerous in this section.

# 8
# *OVERVIEW OF LABORATORY STUDIES IN STROKE*

J.P. Mohr

## ACUTE STROKE

Faced with an acute stroke, the physician must determine the cause, estimate the severity, consider the possibility it may progress or recur, and seek ways of stabilizing or reversing it. Because the possibility of worsening or recurrence is paramount, speedy efforts should be made to arrive at a diagnosis of stroke mechanism.

### Brain Imaging

In most hospitals the first step taken with laboratory tests is to try to image the injured site by computerized tomography (CT) or magnetic resonance (MR) image. If neither is available, estimates of risk factor analysis and clinical assessments of syndrome greatly help but cannot substitute with certainty for brain imaging.

The initial scan should separate hemorrhage from ischemia or infarction. For the CT scan, high-density signal attenuation (about 80 HU) points to hemorrhage, low-density to ischemia, the reverse the case for MR scanning using the most frequent method of the long T2 sequence. In CT scanning, the high-density abnormality from parenchymatous hemorrhage is usually rather circumscribed in the acute stage, and gradually loses its density over a week in the smaller hemorrhages, persisting as long as months for the larger or more intense hemorrhage. Infarction followed by hemorrhagic transformation is more easily recognized when it is confined to the cerebral surface,[3] but it may mimic the findings of hematoma, making a certain differential diagnosis difficult.[24] One exception, a finding that seems specific for hemorrhage, is the pooling of blood found in some lobar hemorrhages.[61] Although hemorrhagic infarction is uncommon in the first hours after stroke, no certain rule can be claimed. Hemorrhagic infarction can be inferred when the lesion lies in the territory of a single surface branch or is limited to the cortex in ribbonlike fashion, but even these findings have been mimicked in lobar hemorrhage. MR scanning shows the same uniform density as does CT for hematomas, but suffers the same problem as CT in failing to separate dense hemorrhagic infarction from hematoma in all cases. MR is even more sensitive than CT in showing minor examples of hemorrhagic infarction. In some instances, autopsy-documented hemorrhagic infarction has appeared isodense or even hypodense on CT scan and has been seen as scattered flecks of very low signal peppered through the infarct site.

On CT scan, infarction appearing as a low-density focus occurs as early as 3 hours,[20] but more often does not make an appearance before 6 hours. After 12 hours almost half the cases are positive,[39] and certainly after 48 hours,[55] reaching a plateau within 3 days in more than 60 percent of cases. Recently completed studies suggest both CT and MR are comparable for detecting the lesion in the earliest hours, and neither have much success before about 3 to 4 hours from onset.[39] On CT, the low-density abnormality is seen early more often with embolic infarction, where the infarcts have more complete tissue necrosis and edema, and seen later with perfusion failure from thrombosis of large arteries, where the necrosis may be more patchy and edema less obvious.

In the cerebrum, the topography of the CT or MR abnormality may assist in differentiating distal infarction due to large-artery thrombosis from infarction attributed to embolism: the former is higher over the convexity and usually spares the sylvian region, while the latter conforms more to the territory supplied by one or more cerebral surface branches. Small surface infarcts are not always easily visualized on CT scan, since they may be hidden in the gyral pattern of the convexity; MR is a better tool. In late CT scanning, some low-density lesions are the late effect of parenchymatous hematoma, a diagnosis more easily made by MR where the residual methemoglobin leaves a permanent signal change. A high-density mass in the stem of the middle cerebral artery strongly suggests embolism,[49,60] but this occurs infrequently.

MR scanning offers a clear advantage over CT for imaging flowing blood, which appears black on the MR, allowing a diagnosis with a high degree of accuracy.[43] This physiologic effect allows the diagnosis of arteriovenous malformation in ways difficult for CT scan, which relies on hemorrhage, calcification, or contrast enhancement to suggest the diagnosis, even though it is positive in up to 80 percent of cases.[29] MR has also become the tool of choice for the demonstration of cavernous angiomas, which have a low signal center and high signal rim commonly called a "tiger eye." These small angiographically occult lesions may cause brain hemorrhage. MR also may demonstrate the thrombosed dome of a recently ruptured aneurysm, a difficult imaging feat rarely achieved by CT scan.

Both CT and MR can document deep infarcts,[51] MR imaging smaller lesions than those seen by CT, especially in the basal ganglia and thalamus.[37] MR is preferred over CT for the smaller infarcts deep in the brain and for those in the brain stem.[49] Yet the mere imaging of these smaller lesions does not settle the mechanism, whether thrombotic or embolic.[38] However, when a core of very low signal is seen on MR, the uncommon deep lesions from old hemorrhage can be differentiated from those of infarction. Coexisting surface infarcts often confound attempts to attribute aphasiologic abnormalities to deep infarcts seen on CT scan.[6,58] Many of the larger deep infarcts are not due to microatheroma in the lenticulostriates but have had an associated cerebral surface component that reflects their embolic origin. No findings on CT or MR reliably separate a deep lesion due to thrombosis of a small feeding artery from one occluded by embolism.

## Duplex and Transcranial Doppler

In experienced hands, the duplex and transcranial Doppler methods may provide useful information within minutes, adding to the assessment of acute stroke. In a setting of occlusion, in the early hours after stroke, before brain imaging can demonstrate the changes of infarction, duplex Doppler may disclose high-grade stenosis of a carotid or vertebral artery. Transcranial Doppler may infer extracranial carotid occlusion[23] or high-grade stenosis by collateral across the circle of Willis to the affected side, inferred by reversal of flow in the ipsilateral anterior cerebral, or by blunted waveforms in the cerebral vessels ipsilateral to a hemodynamically significant lesion.[54]

Intracranial disease may also be documented by stenosis of the basilar or a major cerebral artery. When the middle cerebral velocity signal is missing ipsilateral to symptomatic hemispheral dysfunction, a good correlation has been found for angiographic evidence of occlusion.[27] Proof of occlusion of a major cerebral artery is difficult to demonstrate directly, but increased velocity in an adjacent cerebral artery may indicate augmentation flow bearing collateral.[4] Recanalization has been demonstrated.[41] When the Doppler waveforms indicate greatly reduced resistance to flow, an arteriovenous shunt may be suspected, helping to suggest arteriovenous malformation in some instances of brain hemorrhage. Although vasospasm after acute aneurysm rupture is not usually found in the first day or so, transcranial Doppler has proved it is a useful tool for the early detection of vasospasm and as a means of following its course.[32]

## Lumbar Puncture

Long the mainstay of diagnosis, lumbar puncture has been relegated to a minor role where high-quality brain imaging is available. Widespread subarachnoid hemorrhage or local subarachnoid collections can usually be detected by CT scan and MR can image most of the larger aneurysms and all of the arteriovenous malformations and cavernous angiomas, obviating the purpose of lumbar puncture, which simply proves the existence of subarachnoid hemorrhage but not the cause. Where imaging is not available, lumbar puncture is distinctive for subarachnoid hemorrhage; it usually shows blood and high-protein and xanthochromic fluid in the major syndrome caused by parenchymatous brain hemorrhage, but may appear normal in small brain hemorrhage. It is in this last setting where a diagnosis of hemorrhage versus infarction is important, and treatment with anticoagulants must be decided; therefore in this case lumbar puncture alone is not sufficient to rule out hemorrhage when the spinal fluid is clear. In the rare instance of arteritis, lumbar puncture may show elevated white cell counts and elevated protein, findings also encountered in large infarcts.

## Angiography

Angiography remains the preferred tool for demonstrating aneurysms and vasospasm,[32] for easily diagnosing arteriovenous malformation, and for separating embolism from large artery thrombosis. Recent evidence suggests many embolic occlusions are quite transient, forcing a plan for prompt angiography if a diagnosis of occlusion due to embolism is to be confirmed.[9,21] Thrombosis is expected to persist. The search for a source of embolism is a separate issue from documenting the occurrence of brain embolism. In the case of the former, conventional monitoring of arrhythmias, blood cultures, echocardiography, and the like usually take days. If delayed until the results of these tests are complete, angiography could yield a negative study. *Digital subtraction angiography,* a technique which underwent rapid development in the last decade, is fast being eclipsed in some centers by *magnetic resonance angiography,* which has almost matched conventional angiography in estimation of disease at the carotid bifurcation,[34] and is rapidly developing the potential to estimate blood flow and other time-based changes.[53] In both digital and MR angiography,[7] the circle of Willis and the basilar artery, their main branches, and many of the large surface vessels can be imaged well enough to determine if some are occluded.

Both digital and MR angiography demonstrate arteriovenous malformations, but neither method is as yet the equal of *cut-film angiography* in demonstrating vasospasm and the widespread stenoses found in arteritis.

## Studies of Blood Flow and Metabolism

### *Xenon Computed Tomography and Single Photon Emission Computed Tomography*

Xenon computed tomography blood flow imaging is gaining acceptance[28] and has now been supplemented by single photon emission computed tomography (SPECT).[18] Both demonstrate both local and distant functional effects after stroke, and some have shown effects on resting flows remote from the site of infarction. Applied quickly after infarction, the deficit in local flow may be evident before the tissue signal changes appear on CT or MR scan. Neither technique separates hemorrhage from infarction. It remains uncertain if these methods will predict the potential for clinical recovery.[10] A combination of transcranial Doppler and cerebral blood flow has been helpful in tracking the course of vasospasm in subarachnoid hemorrhage.[22]

### *Positron Emission Tomography*

Positron emission tomography (PET) scanning[13] has demonstrated its power in documenting the functional metabolic response of the brain to focal infarction, but its availability remains limited. It remains the best method for demonstrating viable tissue in carotid occlusive disease[59] and has been able to demonstrate the remote effects of infarction, some spread over wide areas[26] and some explained as transsynaptic depression or diaschesis.[1] Tissue cubes, some 10 to 15 mm to a side, are being resolved.[46]

## Transient Ischemic Attacks

It is only after the symptoms have faded that a diagnosis of transient ischemic attack (TIA) is justified. In the acute symptomatic phase, the approach is that of an acute stroke. Symptoms may fade or entirely disappear, yet brain imaging demonstrates a recent ischemic lesion. The old definition of TIA as any neurologic deficit resolving in 24 hours is now out of date. The actual duration of a brief ischemic event is typically measured in minutes, not hours. When symptoms have lasted longer than 1 hour, there has been a higher frequency of brain lesions found than when the symptoms have lasted for minutes.

After it is certain all symptoms have disappeared, investigation of a TIA is directed at underlying disease, which may predict the risk of recurrence in the same or different vascular territory.

By habit and because of a surgical option for therapy, TIAs are often equated with the surgically correctable disease in the neck at the carotid bifurcation. However, TIAs may occur in territories remote from the carotid. For those affecting the carotid territory, duplex and transcranial Doppler should suffice to demonstrate whether high-grade stenosis or occlusion exists and whether there is indication of the development of some vascular collateral. Embolism may account for many transient ischemic attacks, yet some may be explained by "distal insufficiency" in the far fields of the middle cerebral artery or in the borderzone between the middle and anterior cerebral arteries.[45] This suprasylvian location would be expected to produce a clinical deficit involving the forearm and hand. There has been a high frequency of stereotypic neurologic deficits in a given patient suffering repeated TIAs.[44] Even in single attacks, distal brachial sensorimotor syndromes lead all others in frequency. *Positron emission tomography* and *single photon emission computed tomography* can determine whether the brain supplied through the stenosis or by collaterals around the stenosis or occlusion suffers from inadequate flow[1] or *"misery perfusion syndrome,"*[2] which has been shown to be surgically reversible in some instances. In the even more severe state of distal intracranial internal carotid artery stenosis with abundant collaterals associated with the moyamoya disorder,[52] hyperventilation has been shown to precipitate focal symptoms. The demonstration of such extreme degree of sensitivity of cerebral flow to alterations in $PCO_2$ suggests "cerebral claudication"[37] may even occur.

*Angiography, venous bolus angiography,*[12] *digital subtraction angiography,*[15] and *magnetic resonance angiography* have all become popular for demonstrating stenosis or occlusion of the carotid, but *duplex and transcranial Doppler* are now almost their equal. In experienced centers, the combination Doppler to demonstrate high-grade stenosis and the degree of collateral, and MR angiography for anatomy, threaten to replace all invasive angiography in the evaluation of extracranial occlusive disease. Even though the risks are small, angiographic complications in direct injection studies remain a risk to be avoided where possible. However, conventional angiography is still the tool of choice to show ulceration, a component of carotid disease that may still explain many forms of stroke. When Doppler fails to indicate high-grade stenosis, reliance on MR angiography, digital angiography, or venous bolus angiography may not be fully justified.

## ASYMPTOMATIC DISEASE

Asymptomatic disease usually is manifest by a bruit discovered on routine office evaluation or stenosis on a Doppler done as a screening test. The bruit of carotid stenosis and from radiated heart murmurs are difficult to distinguish clinically. The improvement in Doppler technology has been so great that a bruit is no longer considered a sign of stenosis of the carotid artery,[16] but only as an indication for a Doppler study.

*Doppler studies* of the flow velocities through arteries have been available for years.[62] Some of the devices using Doppler signals display the different velocities encountered along an artery in different colors according to velocity, allowing the clinician to see the stenosis in one color, the normal flow in another. Like spectral analysis, Doppler studies can be useful to follow the course of a stenosis.[42] Although impressive, the information from conventional continuous-wave Doppler analysis adds little to that available from other methods, and has its own sources of error.[62] Pulsed-wave, range-gated Doppler techniques[15] have been developed that can scan the lumen from wall to wall in tiny steps. Newer devices that allow color-coded displays permit better characterization of the flow patterns. Despite such improved characterizations, it has not yet become evident that the extra information obtained relates to stroke risk.[19] To date, it has been the rate of progression of the extracranial carotid stenosis, not the specific characteristics of the velocity profiles, that predict subsequent symptoms. Virtually nothing is known of the prognosis for asymptomatic stenosis of the intracranial vessels.

Brain imaging may demonstrate prior stroke. In roughly 20 percent of patients with high-grade carotid stenosis, and in a similar number of patients seen for their first symptomatic stroke, CT scan shows evidence of prior brain infarction. Most of the lesions are small and are in brain regions not likely to cause major symptoms, but a small percentage have been as large as a portion of a cerebral lobe, a finding not easily dismissed, although not in any way explained.

Asymptomatic aneurysms, arteriovenous malformations, cavernous angiomas, and dural fistulas have also been reported by brain imaging. Little is known of the prognostic significance of such findings, except for aneurysms, where a few studies have indicated a higher risk of hemorrhage from those 8 to 15 mm in size.

## REFERENCES


1. Baron JC, Bousser MG, Comar D, Castaigne P: "Crossed cerebellar diaschesis": a remote functional depression secondary to supratentorial infarction of man. J Cereb Blood Flow Metab, suppl 1. 1:500, 1981
2. Baron JC, Bousser MG, Rey A et al: Reversal of focal "misery-perfusion syndrome" by extra-intracranial arterial bypass in hemodynamic cerebral ischemia. Stroke 12:454, 1981
3. Brahme FJ: CT diagnosis of cerebrovascular disorders: a review. Comput Tomogr 2:173, 1978
4. Brass LM, Duterte DL, Mohr JP: Anterior cerebral artery velocity changes in disease of the middle cerebral artery stem. Stroke 20:1737, 1989
5. Buonanno FS, Kistler JP et al: Proton ($^1$H) nuclear magnetic resonance (NMR) imaging in stroke syndromes. Neurol Clin North Am 1:243, 1983
6. Castaigne P, Lhermitte F, Buge A et al: Paramedian thalamic and midbrain infarcts :clinical and neuropathological study. Ann Neurol 10:127, 1981
7. Cline HE, Lorensen WE, Souza SP et al: 3D surface rendered MR images of the brain and its vasculature. J Comput Assist Tomogr 15:344, 1991
8. Comerota AJ, Cranley JJ, Cook SE: Real-time B-mode carotid imaging in diagnosis of cerebrovascular disease. Surgery 6:718, 1981
9. Delal PM, Shah PM, Aiyar RR: Arteriographic study of cerebral embolism. Lancet 2:358, 1961
10. Demeurisse M, Verhas M, Capon A, Paternot J: Lack of evolution of the cerebral blood flow during clinical recovery of a stroke. Stroke 14:77, 1983
11. Donaldson RM, Emanuel RW, Earl CJ: The role of two-dimensional echocardiography in the detection of potentially embolic intracardiac masses in patients with cerebral ischemia. J Neurol Neurosurg Psychiatry 44:803, 1981
12. Ducos de Lahitte M, Marc-Vergnes JP, Rascol A et al: Intravenous angiography of the external cerebral arteries. Radiology 137:705, 1980
13. Frackowiak RSJ, Wise RJS: Positron tomography in ischemic cerebrovascular disease. Neurol Clin North Am 1:183, 1983
14. Frisen L, Kjällman L, Lindberg B, Svendsen P: Detection of extracranial carotid stenosis by computed tomography. Lancet 1:1319, 1979

15. Furlan AJ, Weinstein MA, Little JR, Modic MT: Digital subtraction angiography in the evaluation of cerebrovascular disease. Neurol Clin North Am 1:55, 1983
16. Gautier JC, Rosa A, Lhermitte F: Auscultation carotidienne: correlations chez 200 patients avec 332 angiographies. Rev Neurol 131:175, 1975
17. Gross CR, Kase CS, Mohr JP et al: Stroke in south Alabama: incidence and diagnostic features: a population-based study. Stroke 15:249, 1984
18. Hanyu H, Arai H, Kobayashi Y et al: Remote effects in cerebral infarction—123I-IMP SPECT study. Kaku Igaku 27:629, 1990
19. Hennerici M, Steinke W, Rautenberg W, Mohr JP: Symptomatic and asymptomatic high-grade carotid stenosis in Doppler color flow imaging. Neurology (NY) 42:131, 1992
20. Inoue Y, Takemoto K, Miyamoto T et al: Sequential computed tomography scans in acute cerebral infarction. Radiology 135:655, 1980
21. Irino T, Tandea M, Minami T: Angiographic manifestations in postrecanalized cerebral infarction. Neurology 27:471, 1977
22. Jakobsen M, Enevoldsen E, Dalager T: Spasm index in subarachnoid haemorrhage: consequences of vasospasm upon cerebral blood flow and oxygen extraction. Acta Neurol Scand 82:311, 1990
23. Kaps M, Damian MS, Teschendorf U, Dorndorf W: Transcranial Doppler ultrasound findings in middle cerebral artery occlusion. Stroke 21:532, 1990
24. Kase CS, Williams JP, Mohr JP: Lobar intracerebral hematomas. Neurology (NY) 32:1146, 1982
25. Kistler JP, Buonanno FS, Dewitt LD et al: Vertebral basilar posterior cerebral territory stroke—delineation by proton nuclear magnetic resonance imaging. Stroke 15:417, 1984
26. Kiyosawa M, Bosley TM, Kushner M et al: Middle cerebral artery strokes causing homonymous hemianopia: positron emission tomography. Ann Neurol 28:180, 1990
27. Kushner MJ, Zanette EM, Bastianello S et al: Transcranial Doppler in acute hemispheric brain infarction. Neurology (NY) 41:109, 1990
28. Lassen N, Ingvar DH, Skinhoj E: Brain function and blood flow: changes in the amount of blood flowing in areas of the human cerebral cortex, reflecting changes in the activity of those areas, are graphically revealed with the aid of radioactive isotope. Sci Am 239:62, 1978
29. Leblanc R, Ethier R, Little JR: Computerized tomography findings in arteriovenous malformations of the brain. J Neurosurg 51:765, 1979
30. Lees RS, Lees AM, Strauss WH: External imaging of human atherosclerosis. J Nucl Med 24:154, 1983
31. Lennihan L, Petty GW, Mohr JP et al. Transcranial Doppler detection of anterior cerebral artery vasospasm. Stroke 20:151, 1989
32. Liliequist B, Lindqvist M, Valdimarsson E: Computed tomography and subarachnoid hemorrhage. Neuroradiology 14:21, 1977
33. Ludwig JW, Verhoeven LHJ, Engels PHC: Digital video subtraction angiography (DVSA) equipment: angiographic technique in comparison with conventional angiography in different vascular areas. Br J Radiol 55:545, 1982
34. Mattle HP, Kent KC, Edelman RR et al: Evaluation of the extracranial carotid arteries: correlation of magnetic resonance angiography, duplex ultrasonography, and conventional angiography. J Vasc Surg 13:838, 1991
35. McCullough EC, Baker HL, Jr: Nuclear magnetic resonance. Radiol Clin North Am 20:3, 1982
36. Mohr JP: Asymptomatic carotid artery disease. Stroke 13:431, 1982
37. Mohr JP: Discussion. In Reivich M (ed): Cerebrovascular Disease. Proceedings of the Thirteenth Princeton Conference in Cerebrovascular Disease. Raven Press, New York, 1983
38. Mohr JP: Lacunes. Neurol Clin North Am 1:201, 1983
39. Mohr JP, Biller J, Hilal SK et al: MR vs CT imaging in acute stroke: 18th Joint International Conference on Stroke. Stroke 1992
40. Mohr JP, Caplan LR, Melski JW et al: The Harvard Cooperative Stroke Registry: a prospective registry of cases hospitalized with stroke. Neurology (NY) 28:754, 1978
41. Mohr JP, Duterte DI, Oliveira VR et al. Recanalization of acute middle cerebral artery occlusion. Neurology (NY) 38:215, 1988
42. Norrving B, Nilsson B, Olsson J: Progression of carotid disease after endarterectomy: a Doppler ultrasound study. Ann Neurol 12:548, 1982
43. Nussel F, Wegmuller H, Huber P: Comparison of magnetic resonance angiography, magnetic resonance imaging and conventional angiography in cerebral arteriovenous malformation. Neuroradiology 33:56, 1991
44. Pessin MS, Duncan GW, Mohr JP, Poskanzer DC: Carotid artery territory transient ischemic attacks. N Engl J Med 296:358, 1977
45. Pessin MS, Hinton RC, Davis KR et al: Mechanisms of acute carotid stroke: a clinicoangiographic study. Ann Neurol 6:245, 1979
46. Phelps ME, Mazziotta JC, Kuhl DE et al: Tomographic mapping of human cerebral metabolism: visual stimulation and deprivation. Neurology (NY) 31:517, 1981
47. Powers WJ, Martin ERW, Herscovitch P et al: Extracranial-intracranial bypass surgery: hemodynamic and metabolic effects. Neurology (NY) 34:1168, 1984
48. Rascol A, Clanet M, Manelfe: Pure motor hemiplegia: CT study of 30 cases. Stroke 13:11, 1982
49. Savoiardo M, Bracchi M, Passerini A, Visciani A: The vascular territories in the cerebellum and brainstem: CT and MR study. AJNR 8:199, 1987
50. Schuknecht B, Ratzka M, Hofmann E: The "dense artery sign"—major cerebral artery thromboembolism demonstrated by computed tomography. Neuroradiology 32:98, 1990
51. Sipponen JT, Kaste M, Sepponen RE et al: Nuclear magnetic resonance imaging in reversible cerebral ischaemia. Lancet 1:294, 1983
52. Suzuki J, Kodama N: Moyamoya disease—a review. Stroke 14:104, 1983
53. Tarnawski M, Padayachee S, Graves MJ et al: Measurement of time-averaged flow in the middle

cerebral artery by magnetic resonance imaging. Br J Radiol 64:178, 1991
54. Tatemichi TK, Chamorro A, Petty GW et al. Hemodynamic role of ophthalmic artery collateral in internal carotid artery occlusion. Neurology (NY) 40:461, 1990
55. Tatemichi TK, Mohr JP, Rubinstein LV et al: CT findings and clinical course in acute stroke: the NINCDS stroke data bank. Presented at the Tenth International Joint Conference on Stroke and Cerebral Circulation. 22 February 1985, New Orleans, LA
56. Tatemichi TK, Oropeza LA, Sacco RL et al. Doppler diagnosis of vertebral artery occlusion: role of runoff into the posterior inferior cerebellar artery. Ann Neurol 26:158, 1989
57. Wallesch CW, Kornhuber HH, Kunz T, Brunner RJ: Neuropsychological deficits associated with small unilateral thalamic lesions. Brain 106:141, 1983
58. Weaver RG, Jr, Howard G, McKinney WM et al: Comparison of Doppler ultrasonography with arteriography of the carotid bifurcation. Stroke 4:402, 1980
59. Yamauchi H, Fukuyama H, Kimura J et al: Hemodyamics in internal carotid artery occlusion examined by positron emission tomography. Stroke 21:1400, 1990
60. Yock DH Jr: CT demonstration of cerebral emboli. J Comput Assist Tomogr 5:190, 1981
61. Zilkha A: Intraparenchymal fluid-blood level: a CT sign of recent intracerebral hemorrhage. J Comput Assist Tomogr 7:301, 1983
62. Zwiebel WJ, Crummy AB: Sources of error in Doppler diagnosis of carotid occlusive disease. AJNR 2:231, 1982

# 9
# COMPUTED TOMOGRAPHY SCANNING

Mario Savoiardo
Marina Grisoli

In the first clinical paper devoted to computed tomography (CT) published in 1973 by Ambrose,[3] the author concludes that "in the overall investigation of cerebrovascular disease, computerized transverse axial scanning will, without doubt, come to be an invaluable means of distinguishing between hemorrhage and infarction." The following year, Paxton and Ambrose[108] reported positive CT studies in 66 of 66 intracranial hemorrhages and in 27 of 55 patients with occlusive cerebrovascular disease and observed density changes in the evolution of the infarction.

In the following years, numerous papers dealing with different aspects of cerebrovascular disease clarified most of the CT features that can be encountered in patients with transient ischemic attack (TIA), ischemic or hemorrhagic infarction, and intracranial hemorrhage. About 10 years ago, magnetic resonance imaging (MRI) appeared, and has since integrated, and sometimes substituted, CT in neuroimaging. CT, however, still retains an important role in the diagnosis of cerebrovascular disease. The sum of the knowledge about CT scanning in the different aspects of cerebrovascular disease will be outlined in this chapter.

## TRANSIENT ISCHEMIC ATTACKS

Before CT was available, transient ischemic attacks (TIAs) were not usually considered to be associated with permanent focal lesions of the brain. However, CT demonstrated that small infarcts may sometimes manifest clinically as TIAs, and pathologic reports also support this view.[9] Even small hematomas or other lesions such as vascular malformations or tumors may rarely be found (Fig. 9-1). If the occasional unexpected pathologic change is excluded, there is much disagreement about the interpretation of findings in TIAs.

In a few instances of TIA, normal plain CT with postcontrast cortical enhancement, corresponding to capillary blush and early filling veins on angiography, is observed.[18,20,75] This finding is clearly correlated with the preceding TIA; however, postcontrast enhancement may represent a transient phenomenon, but it may also be associated with a small cortical infarct, even if this is hardly demonstrable by CT (Fig. 9-2). Permanent tiny cortical changes may be more easily demonstrated with MRI.

Small infarcts and atrophy are also a fairly frequent observation; in some series, however, they were considered unrelated to the presenting TIA;[19] however, other authors pointed out that, being on the appropriate side, they were related to the TIAs. Perrone et al.[110] reported small infarcts, mainly in the basal ganglia, in 34 percent of their patients with TIAs; they also pointed out that lateralized atrophy, which is a fairly common finding in patients with occlusion or severe stenosis of the homolateral internal corotid artery, was probably due to insufficient vascular supply to that hemisphere.

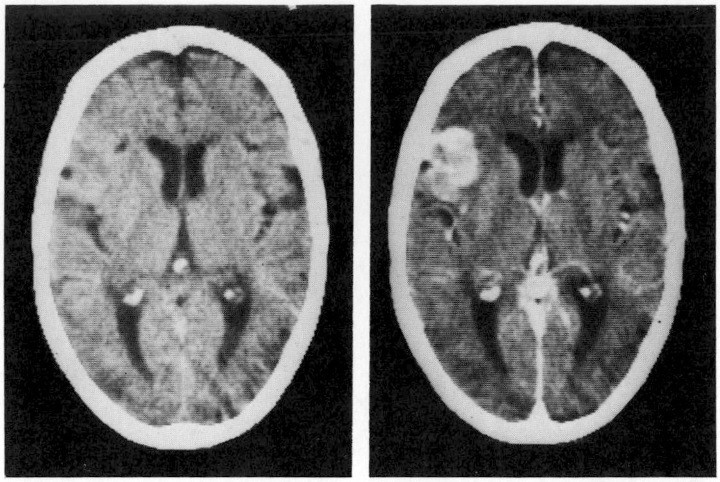

A B

**Fig. 9-1.** Metastases from unknown primary tumor presenting as TIAs. Patient had repeated, transient episodes of expressive aphasia and/or right hemiparesis for 20 days. (**A**) Plain computed tomography scan only shows minimal compression of left sylvian fissure. (**B**) Postcontrast computed tomography scan shows an enhancing nodule in frontal operculum. A second nodule, not shown, was present in the left motor cortex (left side is on reader's left).

The importance of a small infarction in determining permanent or transient neurologic symptoms and signs depends on its strategic location. A small infarction far away from crucial areas may even be completely asymptomatic.[4] Therefore when, in a patient with recent TIAs, CT detects a small recent infarct in the appropriate area, the correlation is obvious. Nevertheless, in most of the cases, a clear correlation between age of the infarct and previous TIAs is not possible, and a small infarct in the basal ganglia has to be regarded as a coincidental finding, an expression, however, of the same cerebrovascular disease that also causes TIAs.

In TIAs occurring in the vertebrobasilar system, CT findings are almost always normal;[74,110] only when the TIA presents as transient global amnesia are a significant number of infarcts found in the territory of the left posterior cerebral artery.[80]

In summary, in patients with TIAs, CT demonstrates a significant number of small infarctions only in the carotid system or in the territory of the posterior cerebral arteries, but never, or very rarely, in the posterior fossa. TIAs without infarction certainly exist but should be differentiated from the new category suggested by Waxman and Toole[155] of cerebral infarction with transient neurologic signs. CT and other di-

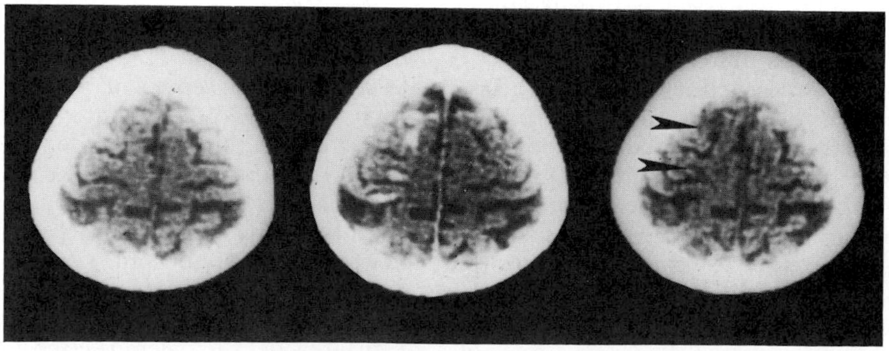

A B C

**Fig. 9-2.** Small infarcts in a patient with TIA manifested by proximal right arm and leg weakness. (**A**) Plain computed tomography scan, 10 days after TIA, is normal except for cortical atrophy. (**B**) Postcontrast computed tomography scan shows enhancement in the watershed area between left anterior cerebral artery and middle cerebral artery territories. (**C**) Repeat computed tomography scan, 10 months later, shows small cortical infarcts corresponding to the areas of previous enhancement (*arrowheads*). (Left side is on reader's left.)

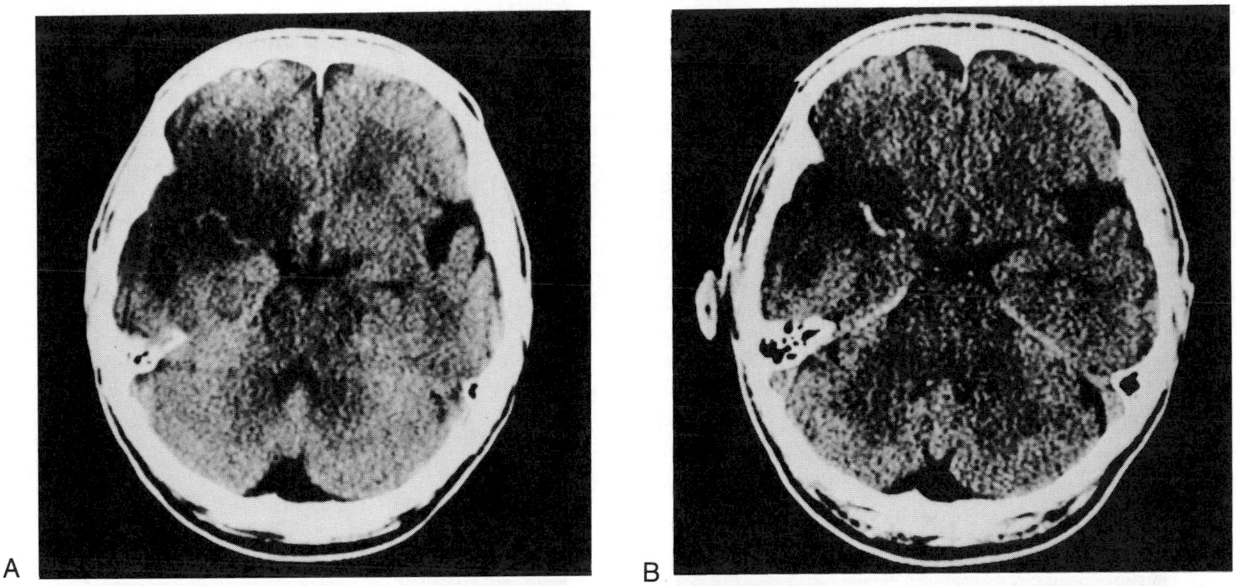


**Fig. 9-3.** Two-day infarction in right middle cerebral artery distribution. The occluded initial segment of the middle cerebral artery is hyperdense. (**A**) The hyperdense acute thrombus is visible on the 10-mm-thick section. (**B**) The thrombus is better demonstrated in the thin, 3-mm-thick section.

agnostic tools demonstrate that such cases occur more frequently than previously thought.

In our opinion, it must be borne in mind that TIA is a clinical concept that is perhaps becoming outdated,[27] and that the main role of CT in patients with TIAs is to rule out an unexpected pathologic change. Whether a normal scan or a small infarct is found, this result does not change the investigative approach, which is based on other laboratory and neuroradiologic studies.

## INFARCTION

### General Aspects

The possibility of recognizing ischemic cerebral infarction has greatly increased since the early CT studies because of both the higher resolution of currently available CT machines and the knowledge of the density changes of the infarctions in their stages of evolution. Apart from clinical criteria, several CT aspects have to be considered to define that a certain lesion is an infarction: location and distribution of the lesion, density changes and their evolution in serial scans, and modifications of the lesion after intravenous contrast administration.

### Location

The infarction within a vascular territory may involve all or part of the territory. One or more territories of the major arteries may be involved, or, on the contrary, the borderzones between different vascular territories may be affected. The location of the lesion is, therefore, an important diagnostic element: a lesion straddling different vascular territories is not likely to be an infarction.

The different vascular territories as seen on CT have been studied and have also been correlated with func-

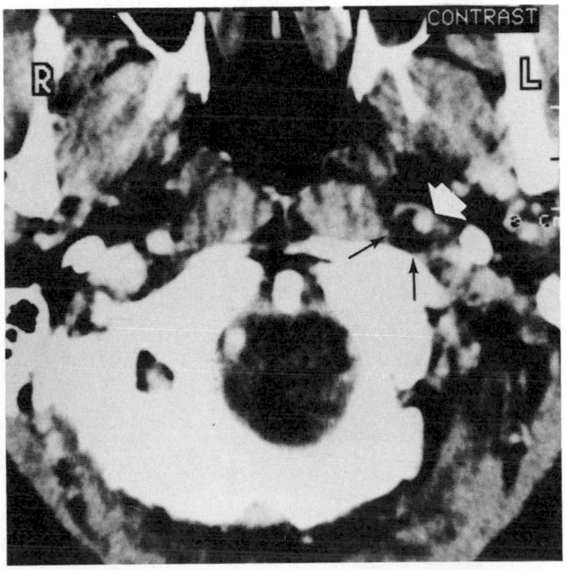


**Fig. 9-4.** Postcontrast computed tomography scan in a patient with extracranial left internal carotid artery dissection. The patent lumen is hyperdense (*white arrow*), while the subacute intramural hematoma (*black arrows*) is hypodense. The dissection was confirmed by magnetic resonance imaging and angiography.

tional areas[14,31,56,125,141,142] (Plate 9-1). In posterior fossa, the vascular territories have been defined also with the help of MRI, which, particularly in the lower part of posterior fossa, is much more useful than CT because of greater contrast sensitivity and lack of bony artifacts[125] (Plate 9-2).

The frequency of infarctions in the areas of the major arterial territories is similar in the series observed in our clinic (the Besta Neurologic Institute) and in various reported series.[16,29,114,124] The middle cerebral artery territory is the most frequently involved (62 percent in our early series of about 500 cases), followed by the posterior cerebral artery (14 percent), and the anterior cerebral artery (5 percent). Infarcts in the posterior fossa were observed in 5 percent of our cases, while multiple territories or watershed areas accounted for the remaining 14 percent.

Localization of an infarct in a certain territory has only a modest value in indicating the occluded or stenotic artery; for this purpose, other studies (ultrasonography, angiography, MR angiography) are necessary. However, occasionally the occluded intracranial vessel can be visualized (see the following section, Density Changes) (Fig. 9-3), and direct or reformatted CT images of the extracranial carotid arteries may be demonstrative[61,64,148] (Fig. 9-4).

## Density Changes

The infarcted area appears as a hypodense lesion generally 24 to 48 hours after the stroke, but occasional positive CT scans are observed even 3 hours after onset.[66] The hypodensity is initially mild and poorly defined; in middle cerebral artery infarct, the

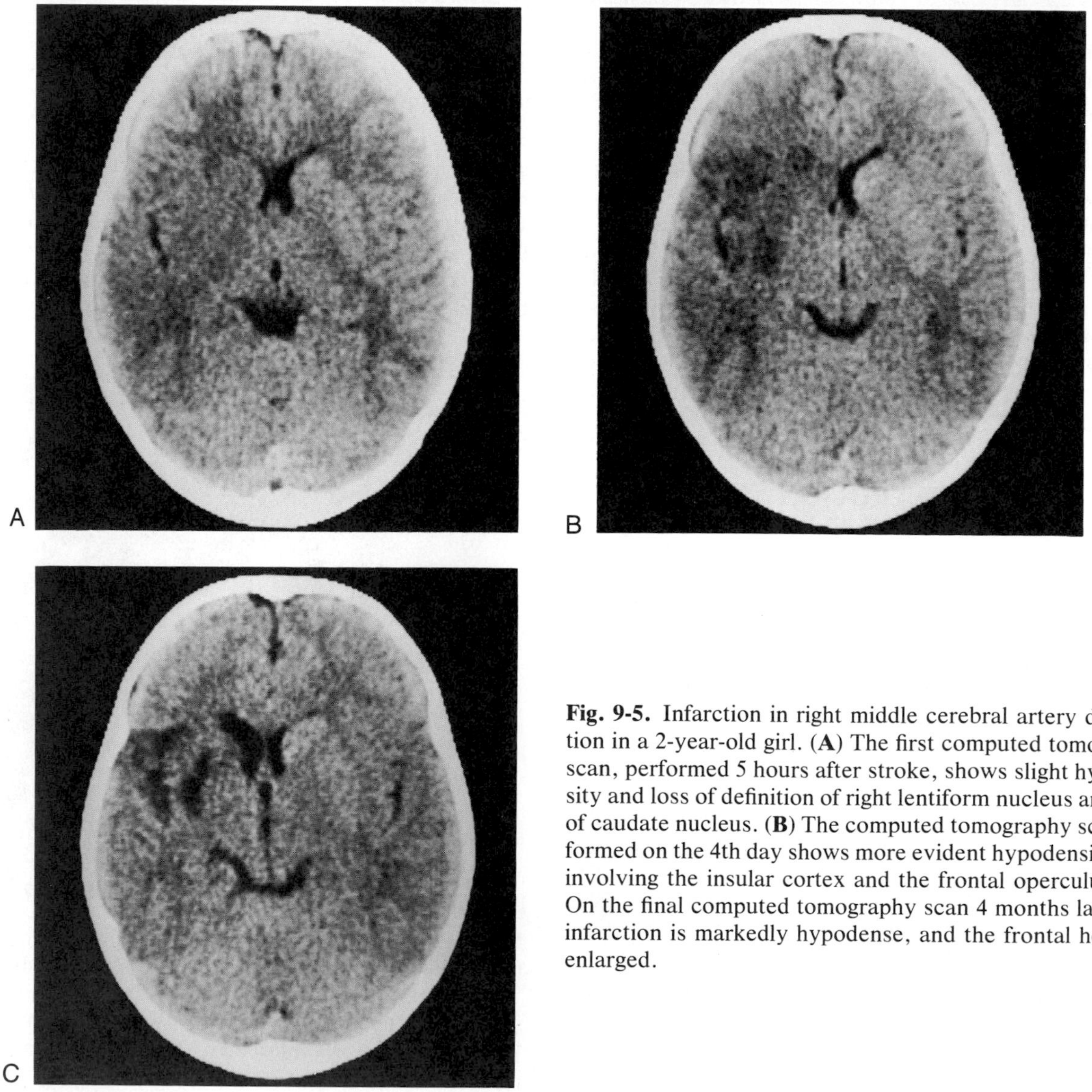


**Fig. 9-5.** Infarction in right middle cerebral artery distribution in a 2-year-old girl. (**A**) The first computed tomography scan, performed 5 hours after stroke, shows slight hypodensity and loss of definition of right lentiform nucleus and head of caudate nucleus. (**B**) The computed tomography scan performed on the 4th day shows more evident hypodensity, also involving the insular cortex and the frontal operculum. (**C**) On the final computed tomography scan 4 months later, the infarction is markedly hypodense, and the frontal horn has enlarged.

insular cortex may lose its gray matter density.[149] In proximal occlusion of this artery, slight hypodensity of the lentiform nucleus and loss of definition of its margins may also be visible on CT scans performed within 4 hours after stroke.[17,146] These have been reported as early, subtle signs of middle cerebral artery infarction (Fig. 9-5). Within 2 or 3 days the attenuation values become lower, the margins of the lesion become better defined, and the lesion clearly appears to involve both gray and white matter. The best evidence of the lesion in this early phase is, therefore, on the 3rd and 4th day after the stroke. In addition, in this period of edema and necrosis, there is often evidence of mass effect.

Occasionally, the segment of the artery occluded by an embolus or a thrombus may appear hyperdense in early studies.[46,113,162] This sign has been reported particularly in the main trunk of the middle cerebral artery where it has been observed in up to 50 percent of the patients with recent infarction in this vessel territory[8,130,145] (Fig. 9-3).

The edema and mass effect of the infarction gradually subside, and the hypodensity becomes less evident in the following days. The hypodensity may almost completely disappear and the infarcted area may become nearly indistinguishable from the normal surrounding brain.

This phenomenon occurs in the 2nd or 3rd week and corresponds to the period in which invasion of macrophages and proliferation of capillaries are observed on pathologic specimens. The rate of this occurrence varies in different series. On scans performed 10 days after stroke, Skriver and Olsen[135] found disappearance of hypodensity in 54 percent of their 50 cases. Becker et al.[11] named this phenomenon the "fogging effect," observing it at some time in all the cases of their smaller series examined with six consecutive CT scans within 42 days after stroke. However, with the high-resolution CT scans now available, some mottling of the infarcted area is usually recognizable.

In large infarcts, the fogging effect is usually partial and appears as isodense superficial curvilinear bands; they correspond to the gray matter of the cortical mantle (Fig. 9-6), where the cellular reaction is more marked than in the white matter and where petechial hemorrhages may occur[66,160] (see Fig. 9-16B). This phenomenon has to be kept in mind when one is judging the size of the infarct: a scan performed in the 2nd or 3rd week after stroke may lead one to underestimate the size of the infarct or even to fail to recognize the infarct itself. As the process of tissue breakdown and phagocytosis continues, the infarcted area gradually becomes replaced by cystic spaces filled with fluid; on CT scan, therefore, the hypodensity again becomes more evident, with attenuation values now in the range of cerebrospinal fluid (CSF). The margins of the infarct also become sharply demarcated. Dilatation of the homolateral ventricle and of the adjacent cisterns and even retraction of the midline structures may become evident.

## Edema and Mass Effect

In ischemic infarcts, the edema seen in the early stage involves both gray and white matter and is present only in the area affected by ischemia; swelling

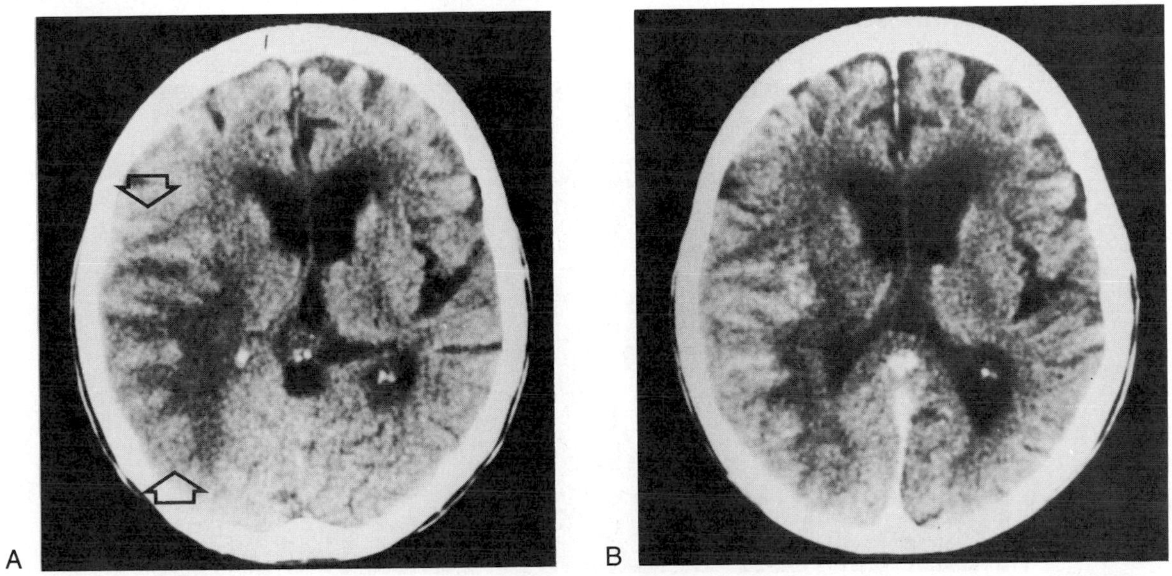

**Fig. 9-6.** Right middle cerebral artery infarction 6 days after stroke. (**A**) On plain computed tomography scan, the "fogging effect" brings the attenuation values of the involved posterior sylvian cortex to normal levels (*arrows*). The underlying white matter remains hypodense. (**B**) On postcontrast computed tomography scan, the infarcted cortical mantle presents slight enhancement.

of the infarcted gray and white matter is actually the first sign visible with the naked eye on the pathologic specimens.[160] This is an important element for the differential diagnosis from tumors; in tumors, the vasogenic edema is confined to the white matter and tends to track along white matter pathways, such as the internal and external capsule; involvement of the subcortical regions gives the characteristic digitate pattern (Fig. 9-7). There are very few exceptions to this general rule: Monajati and Heggeness[100] found that only 4 of their 339 patients with infarct presented edema in the white matter pathways, while only 2 of 155 supratentorial tumors showed edema not only in the white matter but also in the overlying gray matter.

In the phase of the "fogging," the gray matter tends to become isodense, while the white matter may remain hypodense; the plain CT features of infarcts and tumors may be similar, but decrease of mass effect in infarcts and patterns of enhancement help in the differentiation[89] (Fig. 9-6).

Obviously, the extent of mass effect in the early phase of the edema is proportional to the size of the infarct.[66] Mass effect may therefore be life-threatening in large infarcts involving the whole territory of the middle cerebral artery or in the posterior fossa. In the posterior fossa, large cerebellar infarcts may compress the brain stem and occlude the 4th ventricle, causing acute triventricular hydrocephalus; in these cases, suboccipital decompression may be a life-saving procedure.[132,144]

Some reports suggested that there is a relationship between hyperglycemia in acute stroke and extent of edema, size of the infarct as documented by CT, and clinical outcome.[12,26] This association would require careful measures to control serum glucose levels in early stroke to limit edema and infarct size and improve outcome. However, other series did not confirm the correlation between hyperglycemia and size of the infarct at final CT, even if clinical recovery was significantly poorer.[79]

## Contrast Enhancement

Another major aspect to consider in CT scans of infarcts is the pattern observed after intravenous contrast administration.

Variable responses of the infarcted area to administration of contrast medium in different stages have been noted since early CT studies.[36,158] In the first 5 or 6 days after stroke, intravenous contrast administration usually does not modify the attenuation values of the infarcted area or modifies them very little.

After the first week, contrast enhancement of the infarcted area is prominent in the great majority of the cases; contrast enhancement is particularly evident in the 2nd and 3rd week after stroke and may last up to a month or even longer.[11,25,66,114,158] Contrast enhancement coincides with radioisotope uptake.[34,158]

After this stage, contrast enhancement diminishes and on late CT scans the attenuation values of the infarcted area remain unmodified after administration of contrast medium.

The contrast enhancement may appear in different patterns, from small, patchy, scattered areas or long curvilinear bands to large compact areas of intense elevation of attenuation values. The distribution is mostly in the gray matter, either of the cortical mantle or of the basal ganglia[120] (Figs. 9-8, 9-9, and 9-10). However, delayed CT scans demonstrate a diffuse spreading of the enhancement, also involving the white matter in the infarcted area.[66]

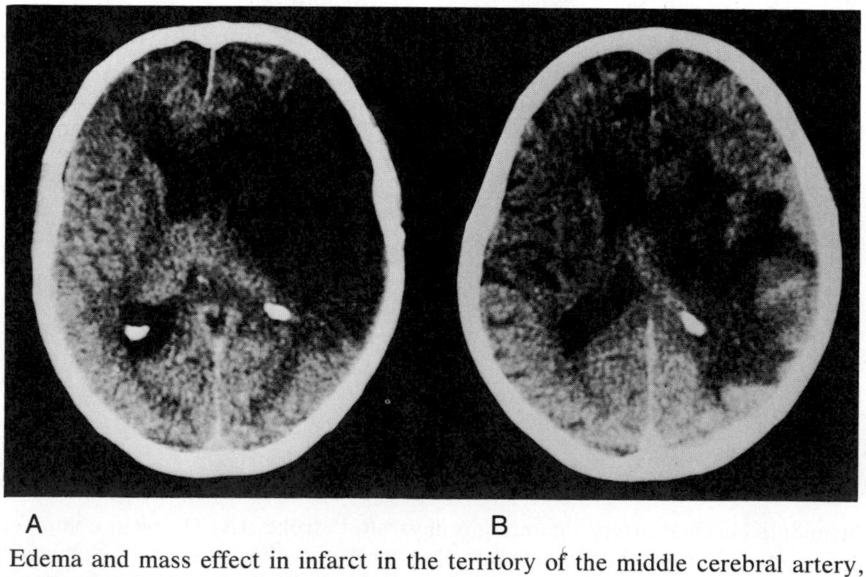

A B

**Fig. 9-7.** (**A**) Edema and mass effect in infarct in the territory of the middle cerebral artery, 3 days after stroke. The hypodensity also involves the gray matter. (**B**) In tumor, the vasogenic edema tracks along white matter pathways and does not involve gray matter.

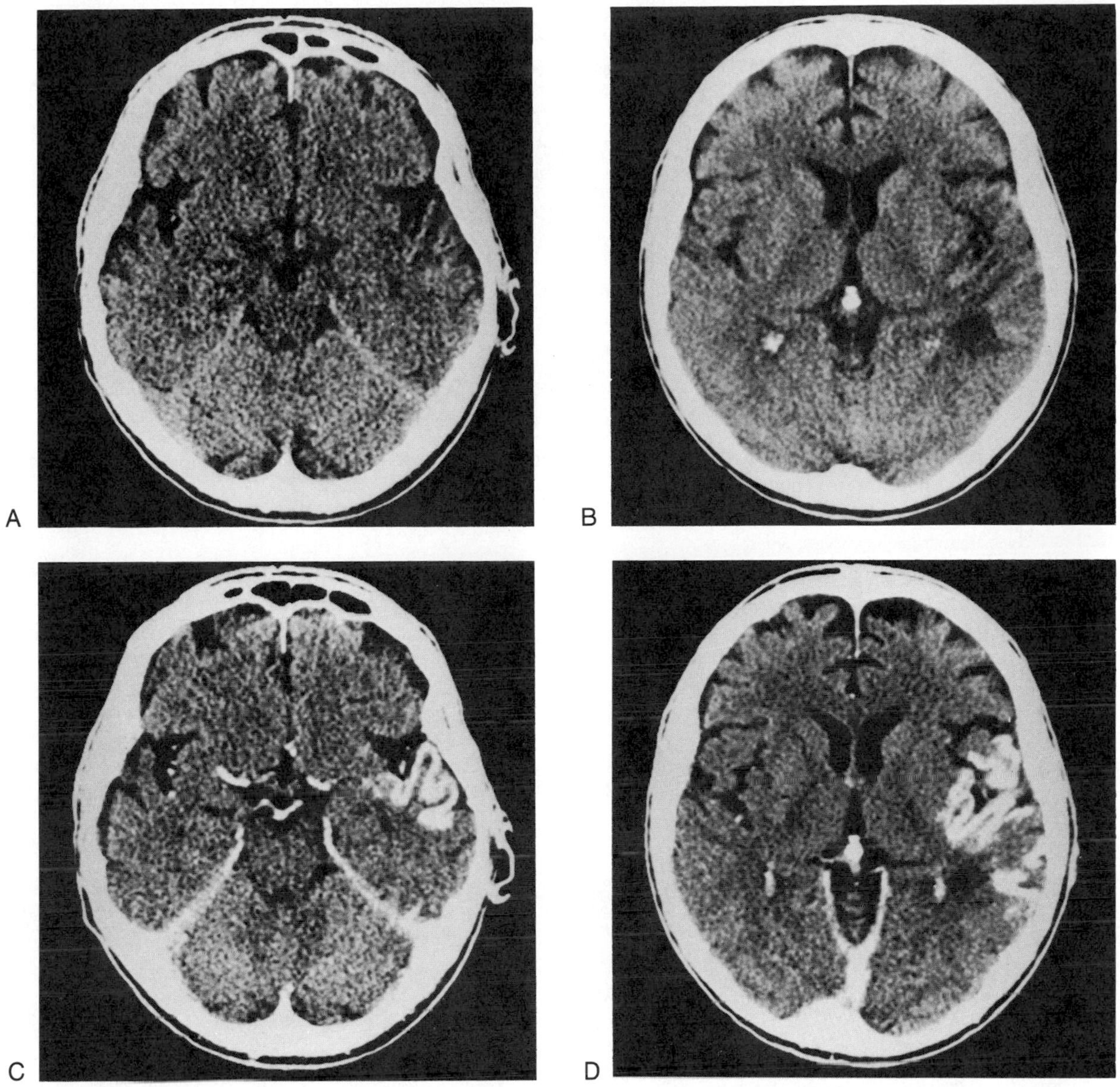


**Fig. 9-8.** Infarction in left middle cerebral artery territory 13 days after stroke. (**A & B**) In the "fogging" phase the plain computed tomography scans only show minimal white matter hypodensity. (**C & D**) Postcontrast computed tomography scans show marked cortical enhancement.

A coincidence both in distribution and time between enhancement and the fogging effect has been noted by Skriver and Olsen.[136] This coincidence is an important element in understanding the pathophysiologic mechanism of contrast enhancement in infarcts.

Dysautoregulation with hyperemia and alteration of the blood-brain barrier, vascular necrosis, and vascular proliferation of capillaries with abnormally permeable endothelium have been considered as explanations for contrast enhancement.[25,66,158] It is likely that all these factors may play a role in the contrast enhancement of infarcts;[120] however, dysautoregulation or "luxury perfusion," which may explain a more transient, early, and peripheral gray matter enhancement,[75] usually disappears in a few days.[66] Vascular necrosis involving hemorrhages might explain only a minority of the cases, since hemorrhagic infarctions represent probably about 20 percent of cerebral infarcts,[30,34,42] while contrast enhancement is a much more frequent phenomenon. Nevertheless, it is not necessary for vascular necrosis to occur in order to explain extravascular passage of contrast medium; this simply requires an abnormality of the blood-brain barrier.

Therefore, both the progressive accumulation of iodine in extravascular spaces demonstrated by CT

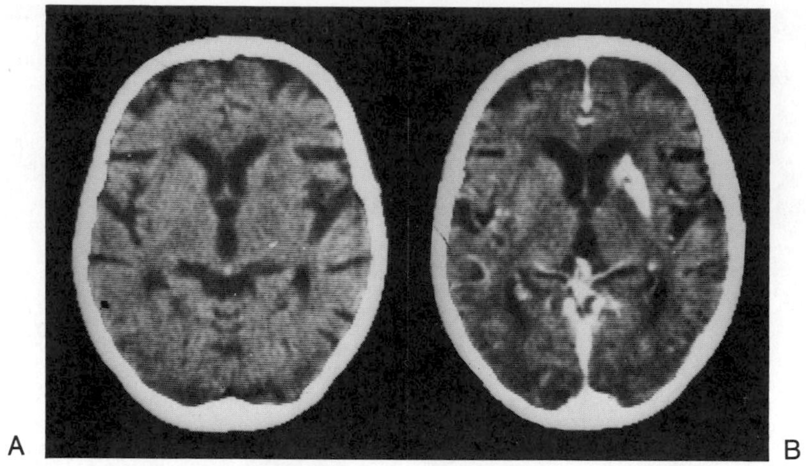


**Fig. 9-9.** (**A**) Barely visible hypodensity in anterior limb of left internal capsule and putamen, 14 days after stroke. (**B**) Intense, homogeneous enhancement is seen on postcontrast scan.

scans[121] and the peak of this phenomenon in the 2nd to 3rd week after stroke (a period coinciding with the peak of new capillary growth) demonstrate that contrast enhancement in infarcts mostly depends on leakage of contrast medium through the abnormally permeable endothelium of new capillaries[25,59,66] (Fig. 9-11).

Frequency of contrast enhancement in the appropriate stage of evolution in the infarct is different in various series, ranging from about 50 percent to almost 100 percent of the cases.[11,25,66,83,114,136]

Contrast enhancement generally parallels the fogging effect and, similarly to it, is transient, and therefore may not be visible on a single CT study performed in the "appropriate" period. This fact, together with the time interval between injection and CT scan and the improved resolution of CT machines, explains the different frequencies reported. On serial

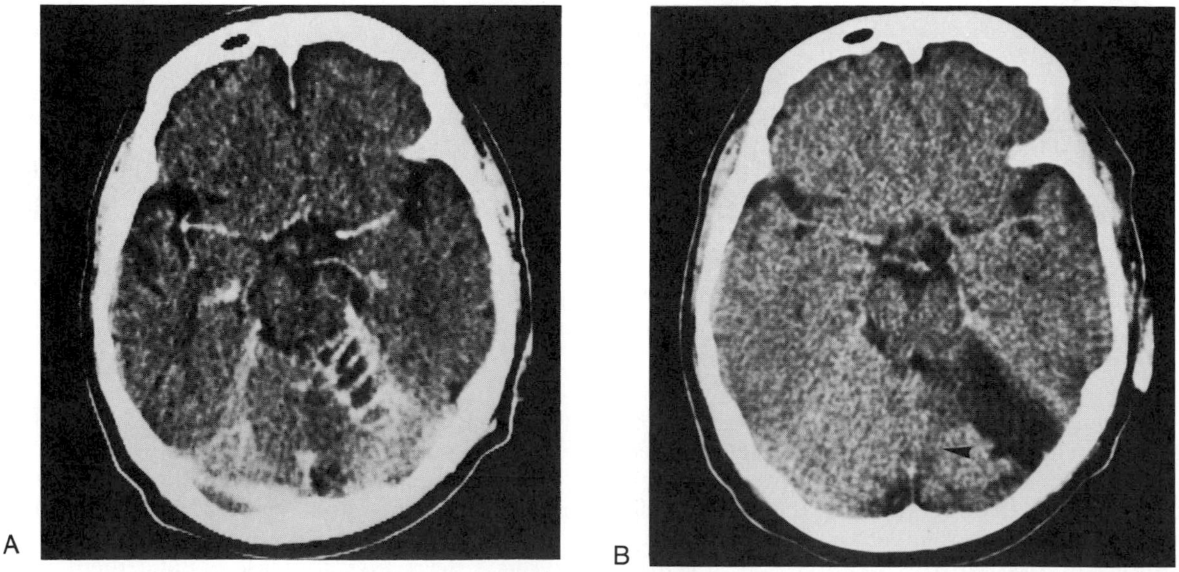


**Fig. 9-10.** Infarction in the territory of the left superior cerebellar artery. (**A**) Postcontrast computed tomography scan 8 days after stroke shows cortical enhancement; observe the pattern of orientation of the cerebellar folia, separated by edematous underlying white matter. (**B**) Plain computed tomography scan 6 months later shows marked hypodensity of the infarct in the territory of central and lateral hemispheric branches of the superior cerebellar artery. Minimal hypodensity (*arrowhead*) probably indicates incomplete infarction in the territory of the superior vermian branch (see Plate 9-2C).

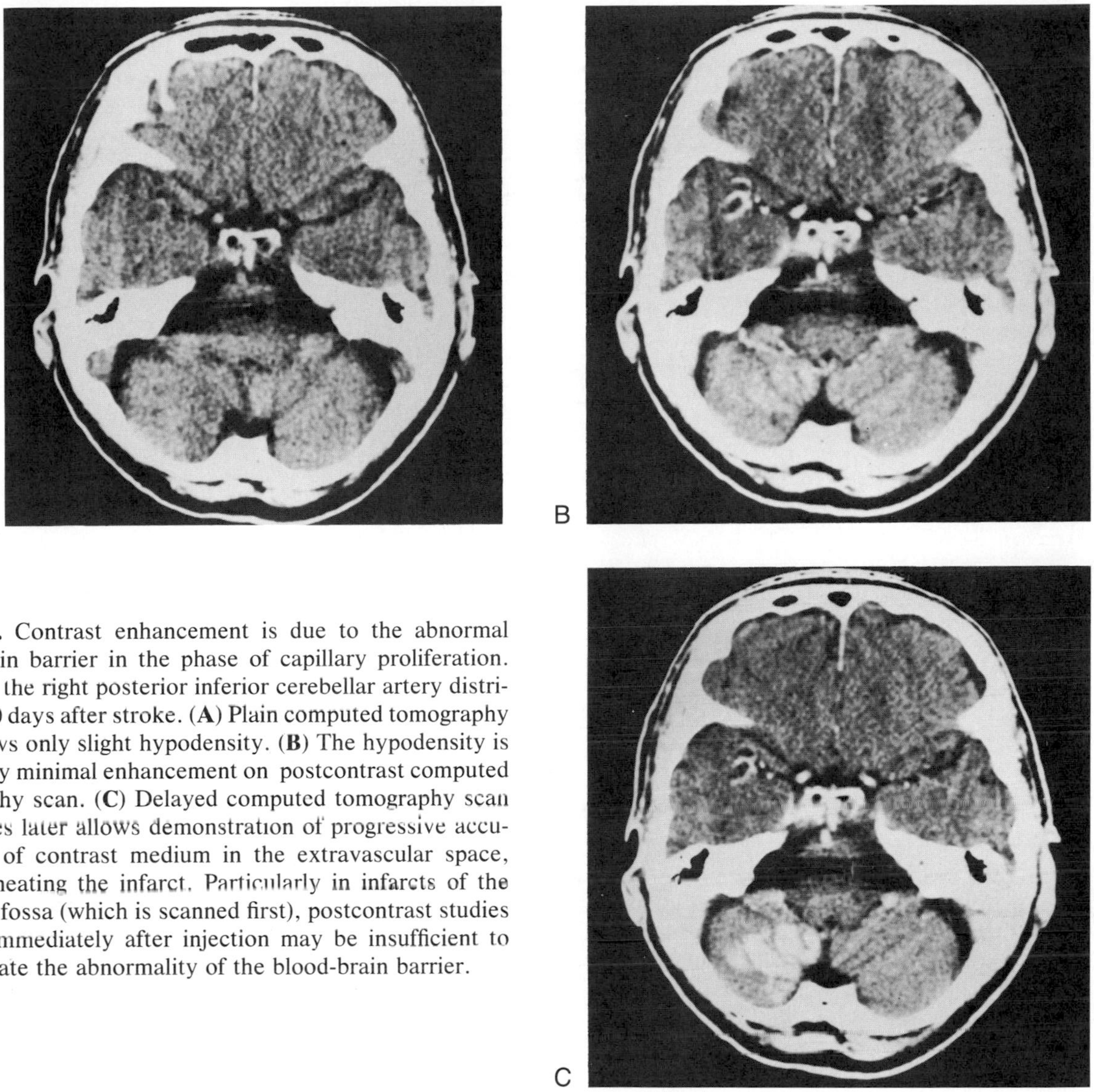

A B C

**Fig. 9-11.** Contrast enhancement is due to the abnormal blood-brain barrier in the phase of capillary proliferation. Infarct in the right posterior inferior cerebellar artery distribution, 10 days after stroke. (**A**) Plain computed tomography scan shows only slight hypodensity. (**B**) The hypodensity is masked by minimal enhancement on postcontrast computed tomography scan. (**C**) Delayed computed tomography scan 15 minutes later allows demonstration of progressive accumulation of contrast medium in the extravascular space, thus delineating the infarct. Particularly in infarcts of the posterior fossa (which is scanned first), postcontrast studies starting immediately after injection may be insufficient to demonstrate the abnormality of the blood-brain barrier.

scans repeated at short intervals, contrast enhancement is constantly observed at some time during the evolution of the infarct, particularly if a hyperosmolar medium is injected.[11,25] Contrast enhancement of the infarcted area improves the possibility of recognizing the infarct when the fogging effect is present. However, the elevation of attenuation values by contrast medium in a hypodense area may bring them up to the normal range. The infarct may not be visible and may be overlooked if only postcontrast study is performed. This event, which may be called a "masking effect," was observed in 5 percent of the cases in the series reported by Wing et al.[158]

Another point, stressed by Skriver and Olsen,[136] is that the infarct demonstrated by contrast enhancement is usually smaller than that demonstrated by late plain scans; the best correlation with the late scan is seen on the plain CT on the 3rd or 4th day after stroke.

In conclusion, the visibility of an infarct on CT scan fluctuates in the different phases, being good in the phase of edema, sometimes poor in the phase of proliferation of capillaries and invasion of macrophages, and excellent in the stage of glial scar and cyst formation. Contrast enhancement may be helpful in the second phase, when it can obviate the fogging effect (Fig. 9-12).

The need for contrast medium administration in infarcts has been questioned. Serial scans may resolve the doubtful cases, and, moreover, warnings about risks of contrast medium administration have been expressed.[25,71,114]

In particular, Kendall and Pullicino[71] found that the prognosis of patients with infarct who had re-

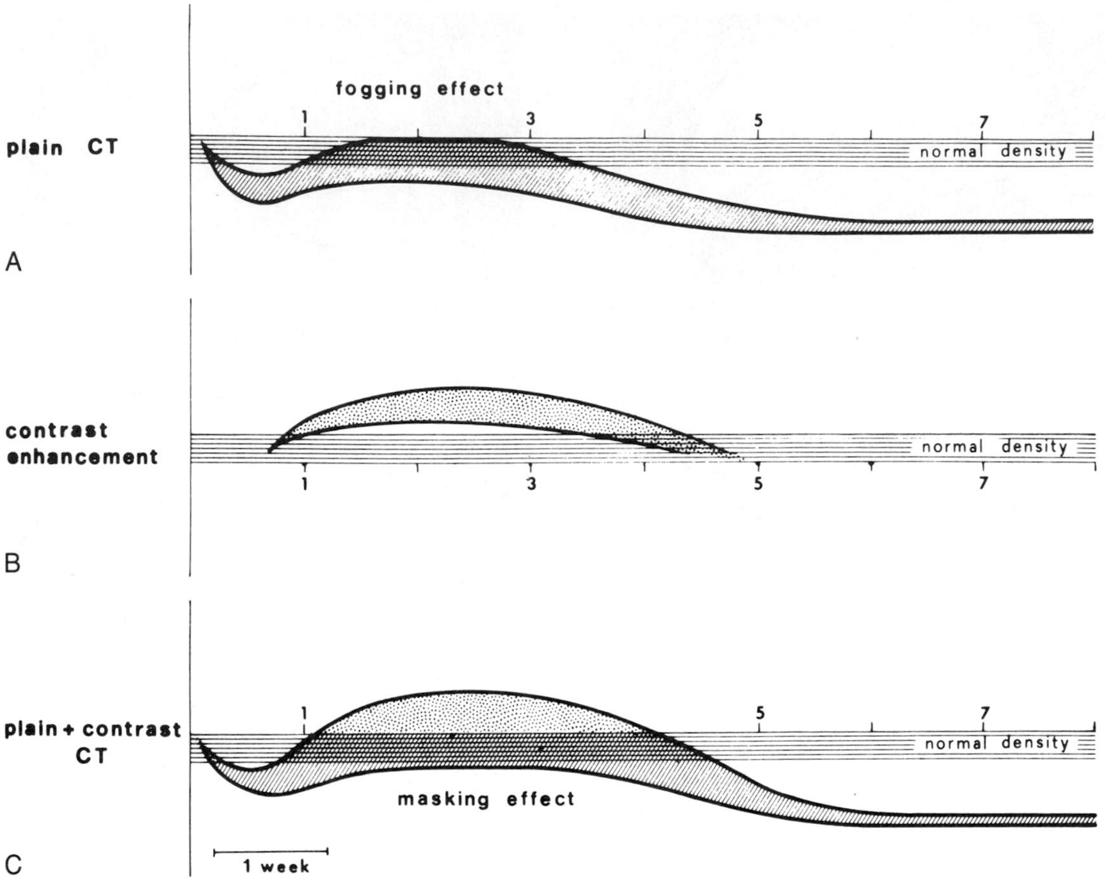


**Fig. 9-12.** (**A**) Schematic representation of density changes of infarcted area on plain computed tomography scan; in the 2nd and 3rd week the density may return to normal level. (**B**) In this period contrast enhancement is most evident. (**C**) Combination of plain computed tomography and contrast-enhanced computed tomography scans improves the possibility of detecting infarcts, but contrast enhancement may mask a hypodense area.

ceived contrast medium was poorer than that of the patients who had not received contrast. The difference was not statistically significant; however, it is conceivable that the neurotoxicity of the contrast agents which extravasate through the abnormal blood-brain barrier may adversely affect borderline viable neurons, thus influencing negatively the outcome of these patients.[121] The nonionic contrast media currently used are probably less hazardous for the patients than the ionic ones used a few years ago; still, the use of contrast medium in patients with stroke has progressively declined.

An important observation has been made by Hayman et al.[57] In a group of patients examined within 28 hours after stroke with delayed CT and high-dosage contrast medium, seven cases were found to present massive extravasation of contrast medium indicating severe vasogenic edema. Of these seven patients, four subsequently developed large hemorrhagic infarctions. The massive enhancement was regarded as an indicator of patients who are prone to develop hemorrhagic infarction. However, in view of the possible hazard of contrast medium in infarcts, administration of high dosages is hardly recommendable.

## Limitations to Recognizability: Artifacts and Size

Other limitations to the visibility of an infarct, besides its own density changes, are related to its location and size. Infarcts near the skull base, such as in the middle and posterior fossa, may escape detection because of bone-related artifacts. In the posterior fossa, only cerebellar infarctions are easily recognized, particularly in the territory of the superior cerebellar arteries (Fig. 9-10); brain stem infarcts, however, are less easily visible. Even when they are clinically devastating because of their strategic location, brain stem infarcts are relatively small. Therefore, CT demonstration of infarcts in the lower pons and medulla is exceptional because of the combination of small size and artifacts, while, at the level of

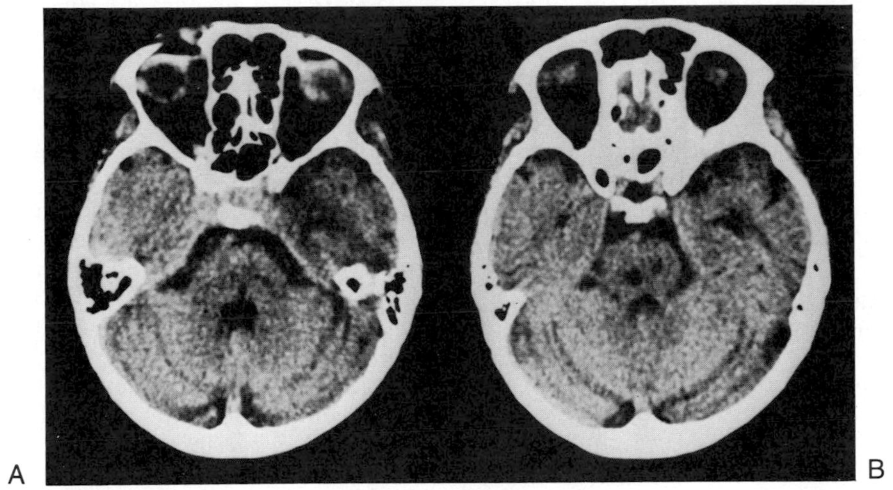


**Fig. 9-13. (A & B)** Bilateral infarcts in central and upper pons in a patient with emboli of cardiac origin. The distribution is in the territory of paramedian penetrating arteries.

upper pons and midbrain, infarcts can be more frequently recognized.[62,74,139,150] (Fig. 9-13). In the case of lacunar infarcts, the difficulty in recognizing them is directly related to their size.

In suspected posterior fossa infarct, MRI becomes a mandatory examination; it can demonstrate even the small lateral medullary infarction, almost never demonstrated by CT.[125]

## Lacunar Infarcts

Lacunar infarcts usually occur in the distribution of the penetrating small branches of the middle cerebral, posterior cerebral, anterior choroidal, and basilar arteries and may result in a large number of characteristic syndromes.[41,98] There is a high incidence of hypertension in these patients.[41,96,99]

The lacunes of very few millimeters in diameter may escape detection not only in the brain stem; larger lacunes measuring 0.5 to 1.5 cm diameter are recognized (Fig. 9-14), and their location has helped in reassessing the anatomic basis for the clinical syndromes for which they are responsible.[39,67,88,109,117,122,138,139,147]

Although the occlusion of the penetrating arteries is most often the result of lipohyalinosis, fibrinoid necrosis, or microatheroma,[41,98] occlusion of small arteries may be caused by emboli of cardiac or carotid

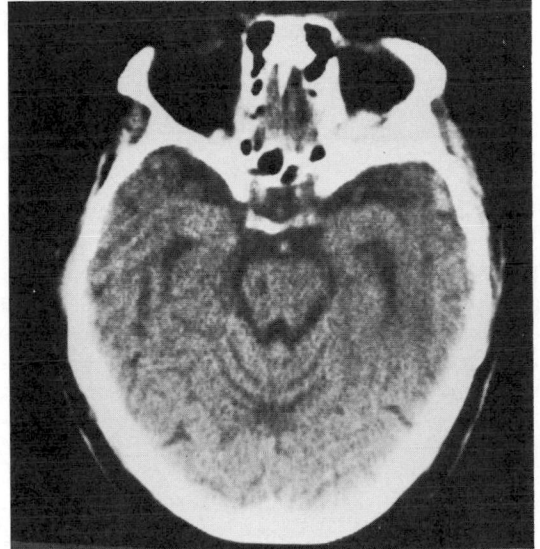

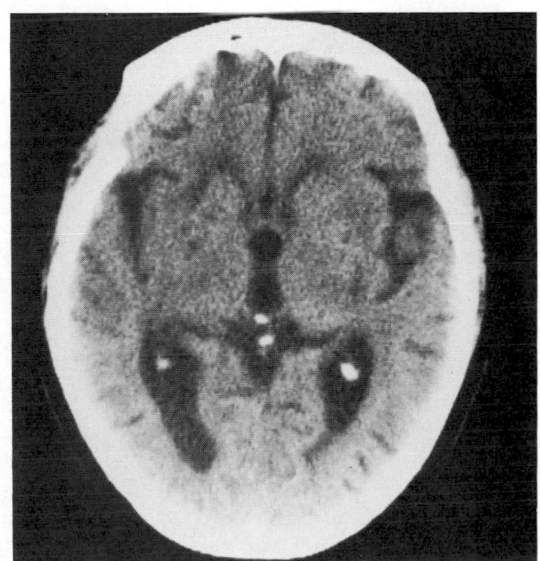


**Fig. 9-14.** Computed tomography scans in a hypertensive patient. (**A**) Lacunar infarct in right upper pons. (**B**) Lacunar infarcts in both thalami and both lentiform nuclei.

origin.[115,117] In patients presenting clinically with a lacunar syndrome, large infarcts can be found at CT in a significant number of cases.[103,153]

It can be concluded, therefore, that CT is essential in establishing that a clinical lacunar syndrome is really due to a lacunar infarct; even in that case, however, CT should not be the final study, but, in selected cases, further investigation is needed to search for possible sources of emboli.[103,115]

## Subcortical Arteriosclerotic Encephalopathy (Binswanger's Disease)

Subcortical arteriosclerotic encephalopathy was first described by Binswanger in 1894, and the subject was reviewed by Olszewski[107] in 1962. In the past years, the availability of CT studies, and then of MRI, has revived interest in this disease.

The disease affects elderly, usually hypertensive persons, causing progressive dementia and transient, recurrent neurologic deficits that may lead to a pseudobulbar paralysis. Arteriosclerotic changes in the basal arteries and thickening and hyalinosis of the long medullary arteries are prominent. These changes result in lacunar infarcts in the basal ganglia and mostly in extensive demyelination of the periventricular white matter and of the centrum semiovale with relative sparing of the subcortical arcuate fibers. The density of the white matter is therefore the point of interest on CT studies of patients with Binswanger's disease.

Mild changes of white matter density occurring with age have been documented.[5,165] However, in old, hypertensive patients, with the clinical picture of subcortical arteriosclerotic encephalopathy, striking changes of the white matter with low density, either

A
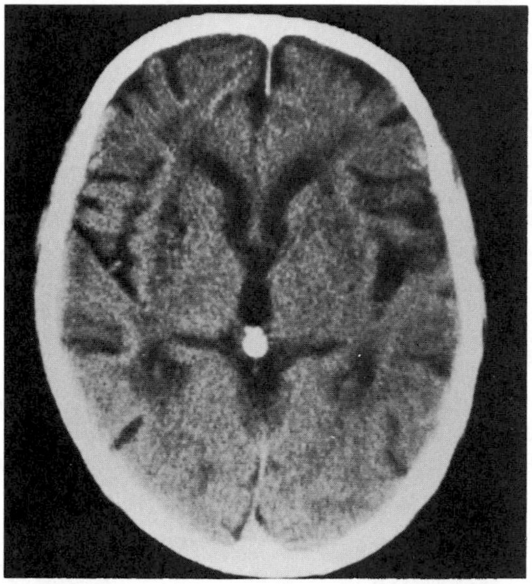

B
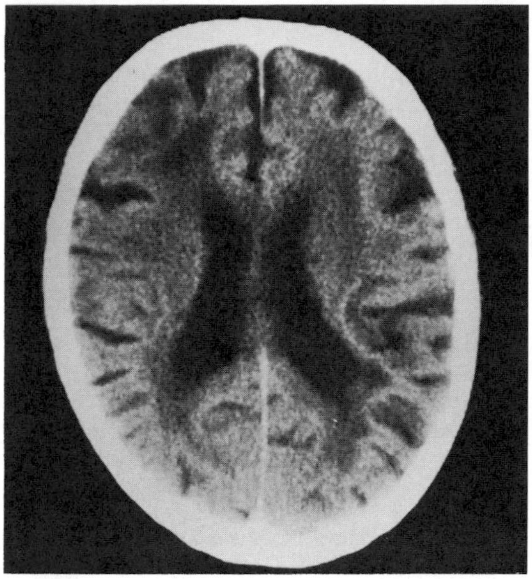

C
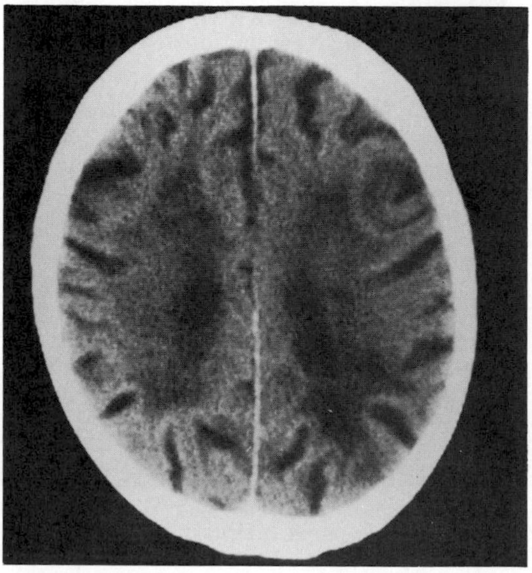

**Fig. 9-15.** Computed tomography scans showing subcortical arteriosclerotic encephalopathy in a 70-year-old hypertensive patient. (**A**) Lacunar infarcts in the basal ganglia. (**B & C**) Hypodensity of periventricular and subcortical white matter; dilated ventricles and sulci.

diffuse to the whole centrum semiovale or limited to the periventricular region, mostly around the frontal horns, are often observed. The ventricles are dilated, with ragged margins; cortical sulci may be dilated. Lacunar infarcts are also part of the CT picture (Fig. 9-15). Pathologic correlation has been obtained in a number of cases and strict correspondence between CT and pathologic findings has been observed.[50,85,166]

Similar clinical pictures may be observed in patients with pseudobulbar palsy, corresponding to the "état lacunaire," and in multiinfarct dementia. A more steady progression of neurologic deficits and the presence on CT scan of the white matter hypodensities without cortical infarcts favor the diagnosis of subcortical arteriosclerotic encephalopathy.

Loizou et al.[85] pointed out that the location of the white matter changes corresponds to the deep paraventricular watershed area between the deep, perforating branches and the cortical medullary arteries.[159] Therefore, the anatomic picture of the disease can be considered the result of chronic ischemia in this watershed area, secondary to arteriosclerotic, hypertensive vasculopathy with a peculiar distribution.

Other conditions, such as amyloid angiopathy,[51] leukodystrophies, demyelinating diseases, and cerebral syphilis may cause white matter hypodensity.[47,60] Even excluding these other disorders, white matter hypodensity in elderly patients is much more common than the clinical diagnosis of Binswanger's disease. In these patients, MRI often demonstrates even more dramatically the white matter changes. Dementia and other neurologic disturbances are often absent; therefore, the significance of these changes has been questioned. Hachinski et al.[53] proposed a new, neutral, and general term, "leukoaraiosis" (=white matter rarefaction), to label these white matter changes.

Recent positron emission tomography (PET) studies and local cerebral blood flow measurements obtained by the stable xenon CT method demonstrated that diffuse cerebral hypoperfusion, particularly in combination with the poor collateral circulation of the periventricular white matter, is responsible for leukoaraiosis.[77,92] We also observed cases of asymmetric white matter changes on MRI in which the side more affected corresponded to the side of the more severely stenotic carotid artery.

In conclusion, there is probably a spectrum of white matter changes in elderly people, generally caused by hypoperfusion, that can be called leukoaraiosis. CT and MRI may detect these abnormalities even when they do not cause symptoms and signs. Only when the changes are severe enough and are accompanied by the appropriate neurologic symptomatology, are we justified in using the term Binswanger's disease or subcortical arteriosclerotic encephalopathy.

### Hemorrhagic Infarcts

Cerebral ischemic infarcts become hemorrhagic when the blood reenters the capillary bed either through the collateral circulation or after fragmentation of the original embolus. Anticoagulant therapy may also convert an ischemic infarction to a hemorrhagic one.[40] In hemorrhagic infarcts of arterial origin, hemorrhages occur only in the gray matter, and are almost constant, provided that the ischemia has lasted long enough to damage the capillary walls and that the systemic blood pressure has remained above 60 mmHg.[160]

The infarcted gray matter may become entirely

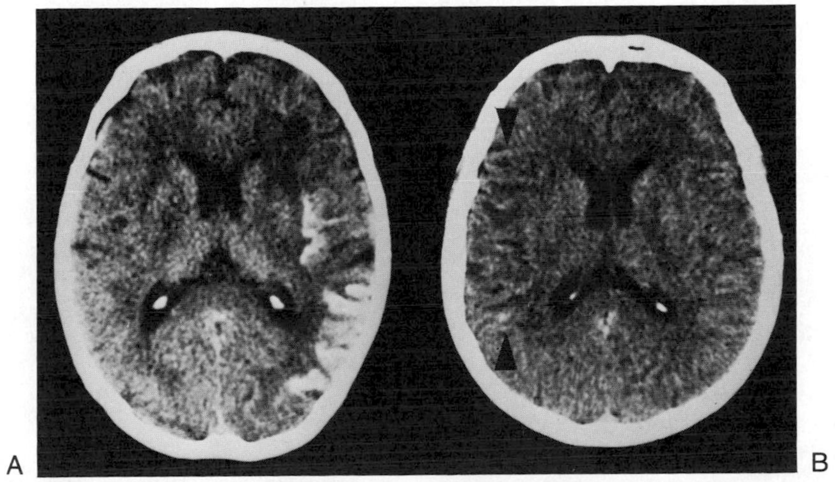

**Fig. 9-16.** Hemorrhagic infarcts in middle cerebral artery distribution: two different cases. (**A**) Marked cortical hyperdensity on plain computed tomography scan 15 days after a stroke indicates diffuse petechial hemorrhages. (**B**) In the second case, the findings are subtle, consistent with rare and smaller petechiae (*arrowheads.*).

hemorrhagic, but, in large infarcts, only the periphery may be affected while the center remains pale.[160] Small and rare petechial hemorrhages are, therefore, an extremely frequent microscopic finding in all infarcts; however, diapedesis of red blood cells significant enough to make an infarct red or hemorrhagic, is observed in about 20 percent of cases.[21,34,42,57]

In spite of this reported frequency, CT observations of hemorrhagic infarcts are rare.[16] The reason for this is twofold: small petechiae are not detected because of volume averaging[2] and because the time of increased density due to the extravasated blood (see the section on intracerebral hemorrhages later in this chapter) may be so short as to escape detection if serial scans are not performed. Tiny petechiae contribute to the "fogging effect" of ischemic infarcts. MRI demonstrates hemorrhagic infarction better than CT, and for a longer time. On CT scan, observation of a single area of high density within an infarction several days after stroke leaves the possibility either of hemorrhagic infarction or of a resolving hematoma within the area of infarction. A peripheral location and a patchy distribution suggest hemorrhagic infarction.[21] Early spontaneous hematoma within a cerebral infarct may occur even in the first 24 hours and may be mistaken for a primary cerebral hemorrhage if a previous CT scan had not been performed. Rapid clinical worsening usually accompanies the intervening hematoma.[15]

The usual CT appearance of hemorrhagic infarction is that of mixed hypodense and hyperdense areas in the cortical or deep gray matter. In cases with large confluent petechiae, the hyperdensity may involve the whole infarcted area (Figs. 9-16 and 9-17). Contrast enhancement may be minimal, barely detectable, or massive.[34,66,154,164] When massive bleeding occurs, the enhancement may assume a ring shape as in primary intracerebral hematomas (see the sections on hemorrhages later in this chapter) (Fig. 9-17).

Hemorrhagic infarcts or even hematomas may also result from dural sinus thrombosis; in venous pathologic conditions they more frequently involve the subcortical white matter.[154]

## Dural Sinus Thrombosis

In dural sinus thrombosis, the clinical presentation may be consistent with a stroke, but more often epileptic seizures, lethargy, and signs of increased intracranial pressure are present.[116] In fact, focal, lateralized CT signs are less frequently observed than are small ventricles and direct signs of thrombosed sinus.[44,116] The ventricles may subsequently enlarge.[73]

The focal signs in the brain tissue include hemorrhagic infarctions, hematomas, low-density areas of edema or infarctions, and areas of gyral enhancement. The hemorrhagic infarctions may be single or multiple, unilateral or bilateral; when they occur on both sides in the supraventricular regions, mostly in the parasagittal areas, in a nontraumatized patient, they should suggest superior sagittal sinus thrombosis.[23]

The "direct" sign of recent sinus thrombosis consists of a small hyperdensity within the sinus representing the clot (Fig. 9-18); more frequently, however, the thrombus, particularly the old thrombus, is only

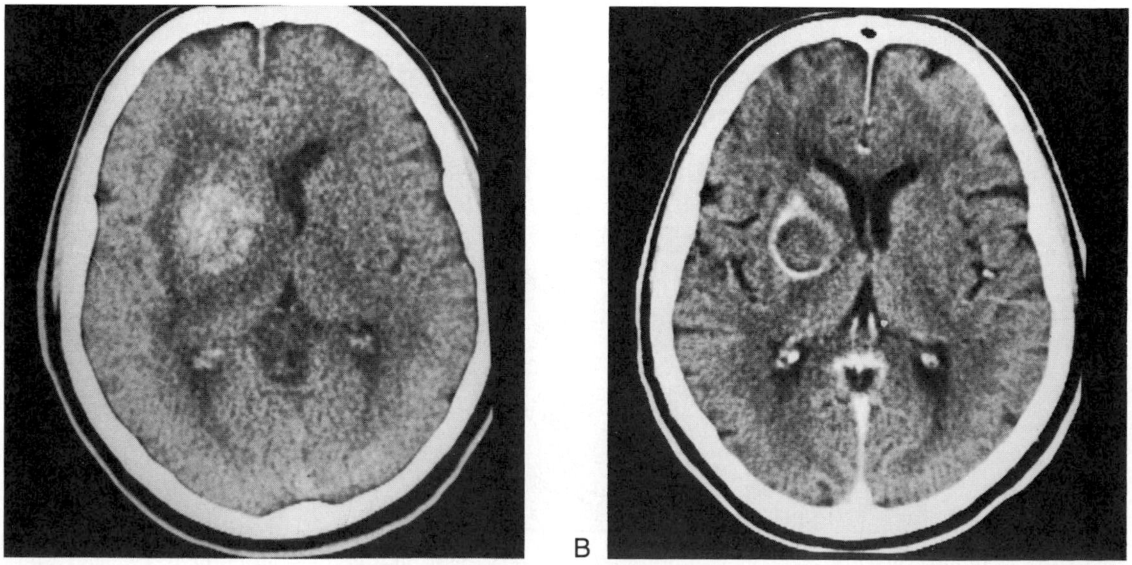

A B

**Fig. 9-17.** (**A**) Plain computed tomography scan 6 days after stroke shows massive bleeding in infarction in the territory of the right lenticulostriate arteries. (**B**) Postcontrast computed tomography scan 6 weeks later shows ring-shaped enhancement.

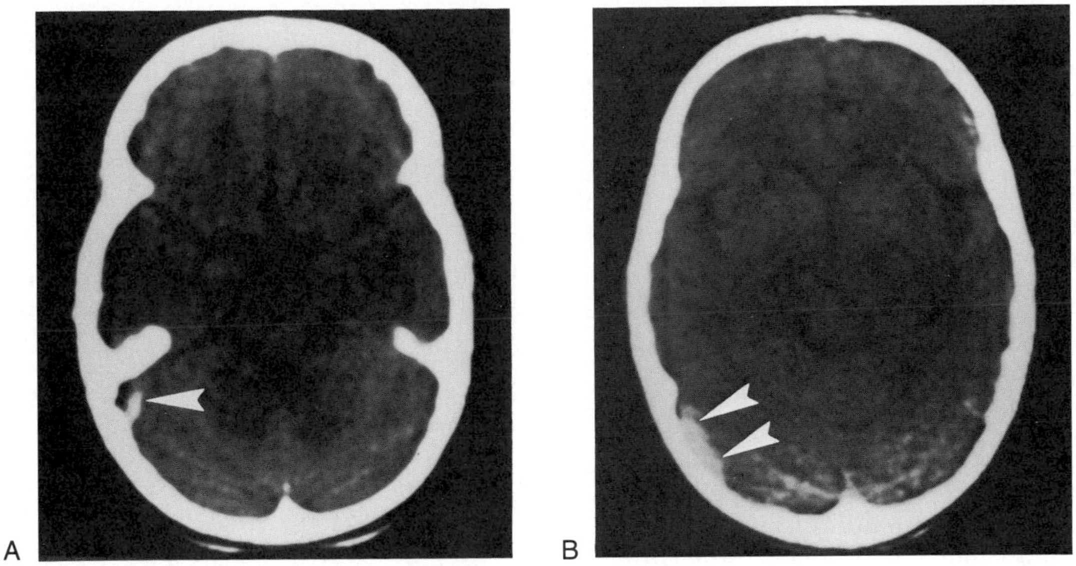


**Fig. 9-18.** (**A & B**) Acute thrombosis of the right transverse sinus (*arrowheads*) in a 5-year-old girl. The recent clot is hyperdense on the plain computed tomography scan.

recognized as a nonenhancing area within the sinus on postcontrast CT scan. The "empty triangle" has been called the "delta sign"[24,44,116] (Fig. 9-19).

The "cord sign," which is a hyperdense streak converging on the superior sagittal sinus seen on plain scan, represents an extension of the thrombosis to a cortical vein and, although rare, is considered a pathognomonic sign.[24,116]

Recognizing the delta sign is often difficult; it is usually not visible with the standard window setting, but requires a higher window level and more extended window width. In addition, a subtle line of apparent filling defect at the base of the triangle of the superior sagittal sinus is usually a bone-related artifact,[133] and a delta sign with short extension may be caused by splitting or duplication of the sinus.[24,116] One must, therefore, be very cautious about diagnosing sinus thrombosis based on subtle CT signs; the use of angiography is fully justified to investigate such cases further. MRI may also solve, noninvasively, the diagnostic problem and should be the first examination in a case of suspected dural sinus thrombosis.

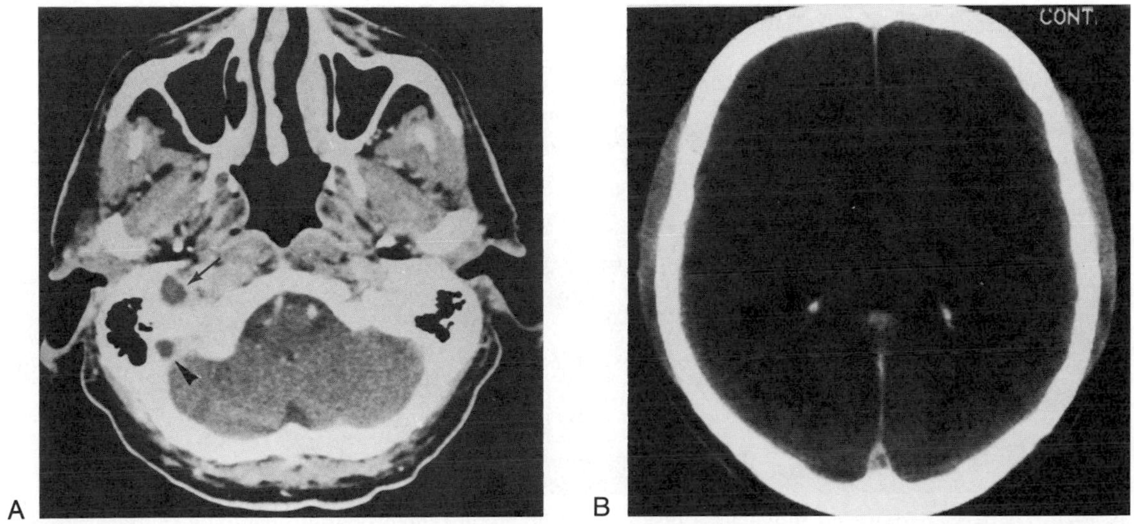


**Fig. 9-19.** Dural sinus thrombosis of more than a month duration in two different cases; postcontrast computed tomography studies. (**A**) The hypodense thrombus of the right sigmoid sinus is delineated by the enhancing dura (*arrowhead*). Thrombosis extends to the internal jugular vein (*arrow*). (**B**) Demonstration of the "delta sign" in a thrombosed superior sagittal sinus may require appropriate window setting.

## Stroke in Children

Stroke in children has a widespread range of causes.[168] The problems of perinatal pathologic changes and of intracerebral bleeding or ischemic infarcts occurring as a complication of known underlying diseases such as leukemia, intracranial infections, or trauma will not be analyzed here. Stroke in children, usually manifesting with acute hemiplegia, differs from that of adults in several respects: it is a single event, TIA does not exist (except in moyamoya), heart disease is the most frequent predisposing condition, but usually no predisposing factors are found.[128] The high frequency of nasopharyngeal and tonsillar infections reported in other series[55] was not observed in our cases.[124]

While the abnormalities observed on angiography are often peculiar, and different from those observed in adults, there are not unusual features in CT findings except for extreme rarity of localization in vertebrobasilar territory, absence of lacunar infarcts, and discrepancy between frequent extensive parenchymal damage and good functional recovery.

One disease, however, has more distinctive although nonspecific features: moyamoya.

## Moyamoya

Moyamoya is by no means limited to children, but is the cause of stroke in 10 to 15 percent of children with cerebrovascular disease and is almost the only cause of bilateral disease in children.[55]

Diagnosis of moyamoya is made by angiography, but CT findings are highly suggestive when bilateral infarcts are demonstrated in a child or young adult. Other angiodysplasias or arteritides may cause the same CT picture; however, they are less frequent than moyamoya, or, as in cases of postmeningitic vasculitis, they are easily diagnosed on the basis of clinical history.

In moyamoya, infarcts in different phases of their evolution, but usually old, cortical, and preferably in distal or watershed areas, are the most common finding, followed in frequency by atrophy with ventricular dilatation[54,143] (Fig. 9-20). Occasionally, intracerebral or subarachnoid bleeding may be observed. However, we found this only in one young adult who also presented with a basilar artery aneurysm.

Since in old infarcts there is no rupture of the blood-brain barrier, it is not surprising that postcontrast examination is negative and that demonstration of the tiny vessels that form the typical basal network is obtained only in a minority of cases, sometimes only with high-dosage bolus injection.[143] Scanning on a modified coronal plane, parallel to the long axis of the supraclinoid segment of the carotid siphons and of the vessels forming the basal network, has been advocated. All five patients examined with this technique showed a "nebulalike" hyperdensity, corresponding perfectly to the angiographic picture.[6]

Lack of CT demonstration of the basal network may be related to its actual disappearance during the evolution of the disease;[140] however, monitoring the progression of the disease with repeated angiograms is unjustified.

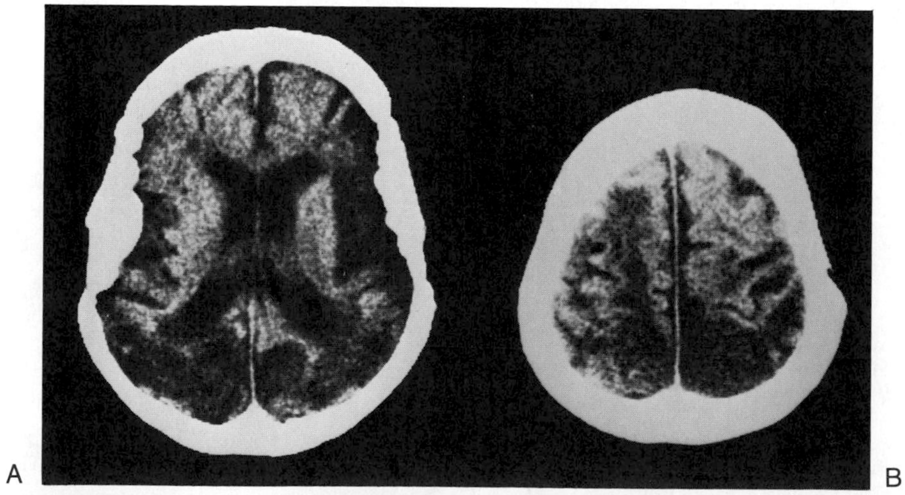


**Fig. 9-20. (A & B)** Advanced moyamoya disease with bilateral temporoparieto-occipital (middle cerebral arteries and posterior cerebral arteries), right frontal (middle cerebral artery), and left frontoparietal parasagittal (anterior cerebral artery and watershed anterior cerebral artery-middle cerebral artery) infarcts. Irregularities of bone on both sides indicate the site of previous external-internal carotid artery bypasses. (Left side is on reader's left.)

## INTRACEREBRAL HEMORRHAGES

CT has brilliantly solved the problem of recognizing intracerebral hematomas: in the first study by Paxton and Ambrose,[108] hemorrhages were recognized in 100 percent of the cases.

Prior to the availability of CT, intracerebral hematomas were diagnosed on the basis of clinical presentation, evidence of avascular lesion with mass effect on angiography, and occasional ring uptake of radioisotope around the hematoma. Presence of blood in the CSF at lumbar puncture was diagnostic, but it only occurred when the hematoma had ruptured into the ventricles or toward the subarachnoid spaces; in deep-seated hematomas, however, this evidence was lacking.

### General Aspects

CT studies demonstrate that the intracerebral hematoma appears as a high-density lesion that is immediately recognizable when the bleeding occurs. The circulating blood is also hyperdense with respect to the brain tissue, as is demonstrated by the higher attenuation values observed in large pools of blood such as in giant nonthrombosed aneurysms and arteriovenous malformations (see Fig. 9-31A).

In vitro studies demonstrated that the whole blood with normal hematocrit and normal hemoglobin level has an attenuation value of 55 to 60 Hounsfield units (HU); the freshly extravasated blood is, therefore, immediately demonstrable. Packed red cells at an hematocrit of 90 percent, representative of clotted blood, and actual retracted clot measure about 80 to 85 HU. The attenuation values depend on the hemoglobin content, while iron has a low influence and the contribution of calcium is negligible.[104,105]

That the attenuation values of circulating blood depend on the hematocrit is also demonstrated by CT scans of patients with polycythemia, which mimic postcontrast examinations because of the high density of all arterial and venous vessels (Fig. 9-21).

At very low hemoglobin levels, therefore, a hematoma may appear with attenuation values similar or even inferior to those of the normal brain tissue (24 to 46 HU). In fact, decreased absorption values were described in a cerebellar hematoma occurring in a severely anemic patient.[68]

### Density Changes and Evolution

In clinical situations, it is extremely rare to observe a hematoma in the first minutes; however, cases of continuing intracerebral hemorrhage have been observed and a density of 54 HU, which corresponds exactly to the expected data, was reported.[86,90]

In a very short period of time (about 3 hours) the process of clot formation and clot retraction takes place. The first CT scan, therefore, usually demonstrates a homogeneous, well-defined area of high density, with attenuation values around 80 HU. The spontaneous intracerebral hematoma presents a rounded or oval or, sometimes, a more irregular shape depending on its size and location; spontaneous intracerebral hemorrhages tend to dissect along the fiber tracts with less disruption of the brain tissue than occurs with posttraumatic lacerations.[37,160]

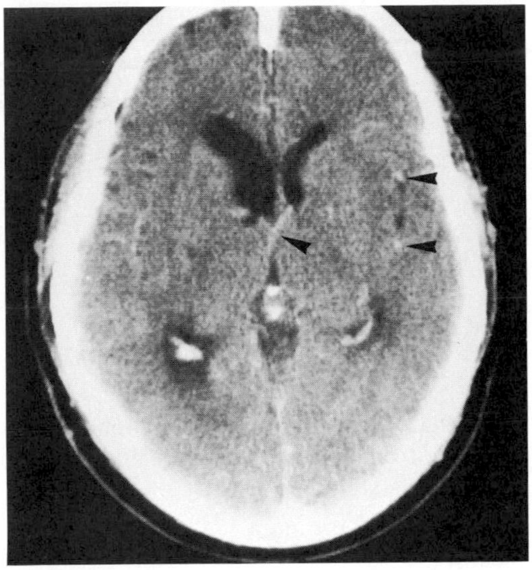

**Fig. 9-21.** Plain computed tomography scan of a patient with secondary polycythemia and hematocrit of 70 percent; high attenuation values in arteries and veins (*arrowheads*) simulate a postcontrast study.

The evolution of intracerebral hematomas has been reviewed by several authors.[13,37,38,52,72,94,102] The hematoma exerts a mass effect that is proportional to its size: extensive surrounding edema is not seen, but a faint, thin rim of low density appears early at the periphery of the hematoma. This peripheral rim may be attributable to a combination of serum separation in clot retraction with edema and ischemic necrosis of the surrounding compressed brain.[29,38,72] The peripheral low-density rim of the serum expressed by the retracted clot was clearly demonstrated in phantom studies by Bergström et al.[13] and Kendall and Radue.[72]

Intracerebral fluid-blood level is rarely seen in recent hemorrhages; a fluid-blood level observed in a few cases at CT by Zilkha[167] was not found to be associated with bleeding in a cyst, but, at operation or postmortem examination, only layering of clotted and unclotted blood was demonstrated. Since the smaller, nondependent part of the fluid-blood interface was of low density and no cyst cavity was found, separation of serum with subsequent resorption is likely.[167] This phenomenon is transient, as it was observed only in very recent hemorrhages; one should be aware of this in order to avoid making a hasty judgment of bleeding in a preexisting tumoral cyst.

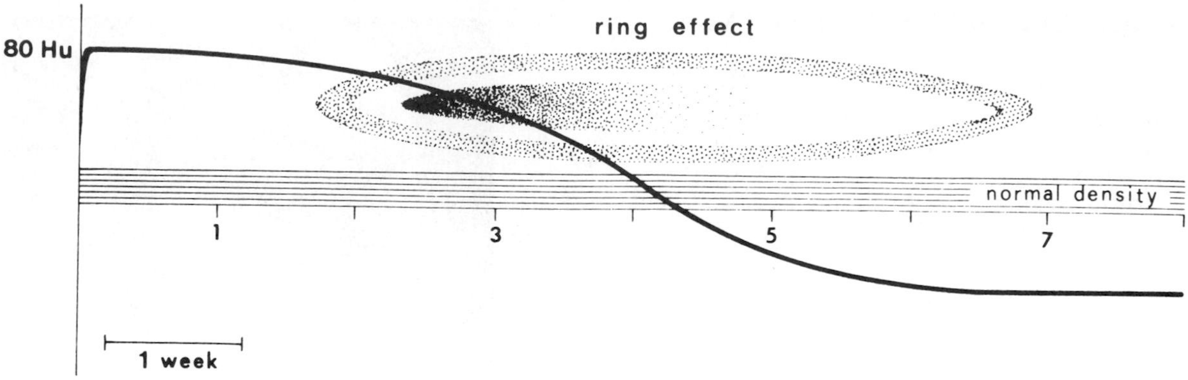


**Fig. 9-22.** Schematic representation of density changes in intracerebral hematoma. Ring enhancement is present from approximately the 10th day to the 7th week.

After reaching the plateau of about 80 HU in a few hours, the hematoma appears as a well-defined, homogeneous, hyperdense mass lesion with negligible or absent postural changes,[72] even though a mixture of clotted and unclotted blood is found at surgery in virtually all cases. The density of the hematoma then begins to decline because of the breakdown of hemoglobin, progressing concentrically, with consequent enlargement of the peripheral zone of hypodensity. The central area of hyperdensity also fades progressively, but it remains the last to change to normal and then to low-attenuation values.

Dolinskas et al.[37] calculated the rate of the density changes both in terms of attenuation values and size: they found an average decrease in density of 1.4 HU/day and of 0.65 mm/day. It follows, therefore, that the central hyperdensity reaches values similar to the normal brain in 3 to 4 weeks and then becomes totally hypodense. Disappearance of the hyperdensity is obviously more rapid in small than in large hematomas (Fig. 9-22). The mass effect, however, remains present because the hematoma has simply changed its density values[94] (Fig. 9-23); the process of resorption with reduction of mass effect and reduction of the hematoma to a slit cavity containing a yellowish fluid takes much longer. After months, therefore, the CT scan may demonstrate only a narrow streak of hypodensity with attenuation values similar to those of CSF, and an enlarged homolateral ventricle. In small hematomas, the residual cavity may even become unrecognizable.

This is a considerable difference between intracerebral hematomas and infarctions. In infarctions, the size of the involved area changes very little with time

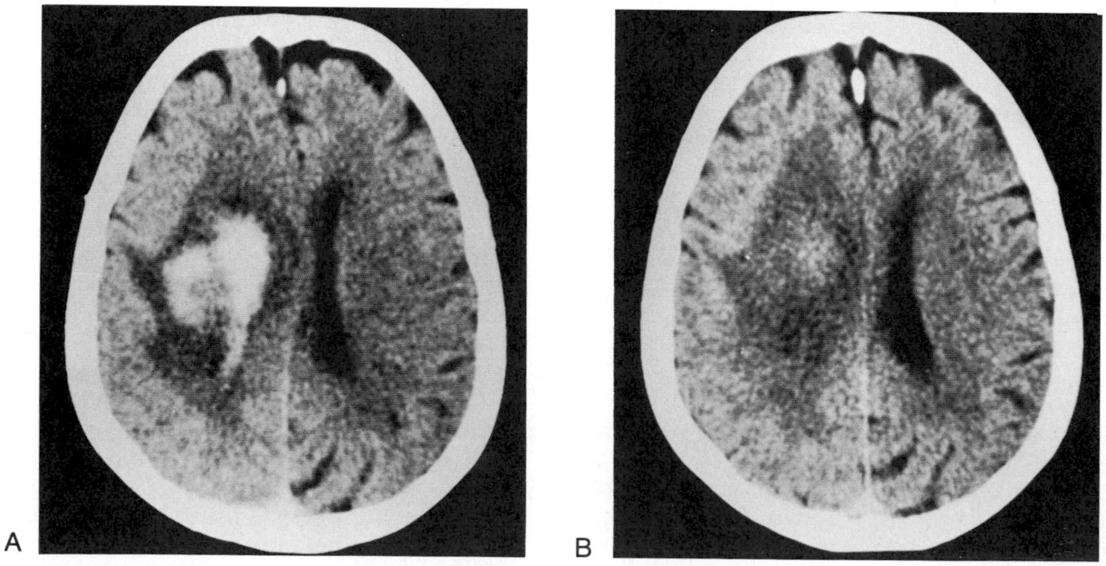


**Fig. 9-23.** (**A**) Hematoma 6 days after stroke. (**B**) Same hematoma 30 days after stroke. Despite the density changes, the size of the hematoma and its mass effect are unchanged.

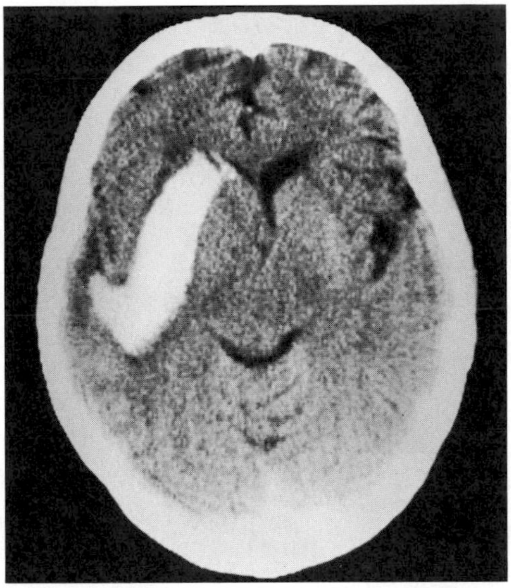

**Fig. 9-24.** Acute hematoma of the right external capsule. The hematoma dissects the brain tissue along the white matter of the capsule, displacing the insular cortex outward and the lentiform nucleus inward, and tracks around the posterior end of the sylvian fissure.

because there is destruction of the brain tissue, while in spontaneous intracerebral hematomas the reduction in size of the cavity is sometimes surprising because the brain tissue was mainly dissected without much destruction (Figs. 9-24 and 9-25). Therefore, the observation on late scans of a narrow streak of hypodensity in an appropriate site, such as in the external capsule or in the lobar white matter in a patient with previous stroke, indicates previous hematoma rather than infarction. Confirmation may be exquisitely obtained by MRI through demonstration of the rim of decreased signal intensity in T2-weighted images due to hemosiderin.

## Contrast Enhancement

Administration of intravenous contrast medium is usually unnecessary in cases of intracerebral hemorrhages, at least in the early stages. However, when the plain CT scan demonstrates white matter edema around the acute hematoma or abnormal densities adjacent to, or surrounding, the hematoma, postcontrast examination is required because of possible bleeding in a tumor or in a vascular malformation (Fig. 9-26).

In any case, in the first few days after hypertensive spontaneous hemorrhage, no significant changes are observed after contrast enhancement. After 1 week or 10 days, a ring enhancement is observed around the hematoma, at the periphery of the enlarging low-density area. This ring enhancement surrounds the central hyperdensity, which has begun to reduce in size and intensity, forming a targetlike image (Fig. 9-27).

The ring of enhancement corresponds to the area of granulation tissue with neovascularity, phagocytosis, and gliosis that surrounds the hematoma. In this zone, the newly formed capillaries have an abnormal blood-brain barrier that allows extravasation of contrast medium or of radioisotopes. The phenomenon is very similar to that observed in infarcts, and it is visible on serial scans for up to 6 to 8 weeks.[38,72,169] If the clinical history is unknown, this pattern of enhancement may be misleading, since it is also seen in abscesses and tumors; follow-up CT scans or MRI studies may be necessary in doubtful cases (Fig. 9-26). On the other hand, a bleeding tumor or vascular malformation may be completely masked by the hyperdensity of the hematoma and its surrounding, enhancing ring. Particularly in cases of lobar hematomas, even if angiography does not show a vascular malformation, in young, nonhypertensive patients, we recommend late CT scans, because of the possibility of detecting the nodule of a cryptic vascular malformation[127] (Fig. 9-28). Also in these cases, early MRI may demonstrate the vascular malformation undetected by CT.

## Location

The well-established concept that spontaneous intracerebral bleeding occurs overwhelmingly in the basal ganglia region has come into question. Prognosis is poorer and mortality is higher in deep-seated hematomas, particularly if they are large and rupture into the ventricles.[72] It is obvious, therefore, that autopsy series counted more basal ganglia than lobar hematomas. With the in vivo diagnosis offered by CT, frequency of basal ganglia hemorrhages has been found lower than that of more peripheral bleedings.[29,72,101] Our early series of 150 spontaneous hematomas also supports this view: spontaneous hematomas occurred in the cerebral lobes in 52 percent of the cases, in the basal ganglia in 37 percent, and in the posterior fossa in 11 percent.[124] However, a different selection of patients can play an important role in determining discrepancies.

Cerebellar hematomas occur more frequently in elderly patients; while in the general population frequency of cerebellar hematomas is about 10 percent, Moseley and Olney[101] reported a frequency of 18 percent in a series of patients over 70 years of age.

It remains true that hypertension is more frequent in persons with basal ganglia and pontine lesions than lobar hematomas, although hypertension is frequently observed also in persons with the latter.[72]

Rupture into the ventricular system is obviously an aggravating factor; however, CT studies demonstrate that intraventricular rupture, which occurred in 32 percent of the hematomas reviewed by Kendall and Radue,[72] is not an ominous sign as previously

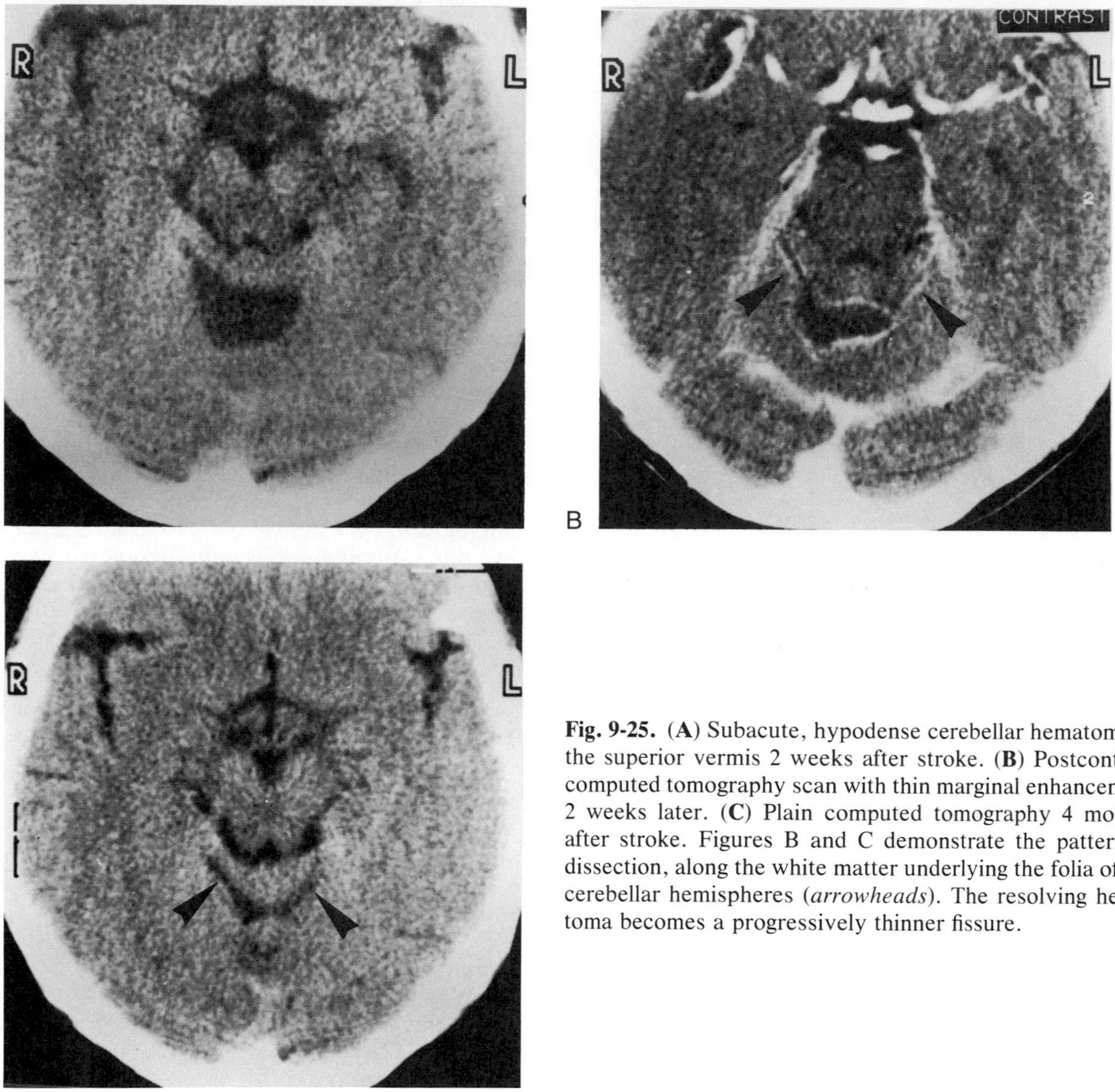


**Fig. 9-25.** (**A**) Subacute, hypodense cerebellar hematoma in the superior vermis 2 weeks after stroke. (**B**) Postcontrast computed tomography scan with thin marginal enhancement 2 weeks later. (**C**) Plain computed tomography 4 months after stroke. Figures B and C demonstrate the pattern of dissection, along the white matter underlying the folia of the cerebellar hemispheres (*arrowheads*). The resolving hematoma becomes a progressively thinner fissure.

thought.[28] Communication of the hematomas with the ventricles may lead to a porencephalic cyst.

In conclusion, CT studies in intracerebral hemorrhages are always diagnostic when performed in the early stage. When clinical presentation or plain CT raise the possibility of bleeding in a tumor or from a vascular malformation, postcontrast examination or MRI and angiography are necessary. Postcontrast examination on late CT scan or MRI may demonstrate the nodule of an angiographically occult vascular malformation. Late CT scans are also helpful in monitoring possible late complications of intraventricular or subarachnoid rupture, such as hydrocephalus or expanding porencephalic cysts.

## SUBARACHNOID HEMORRHAGE: ANEURYSMS

The blood that extravasates into the subarachnoid spaces from a ruptured aneurysm elevates the attenuation values of these spaces above those of the brain tissue. Therefore, blood in the subarachnoid space is usually easily demonstrated by CT, provided that the examination is performed in the first few days after the hemorrhage (Fig. 9-29). When CT is obtained within 4 or 5 days, a positive scan is found in about 90 percent of cases.[1,65,131] The high density rapidly declines, and blood may usually be demonstrated for no

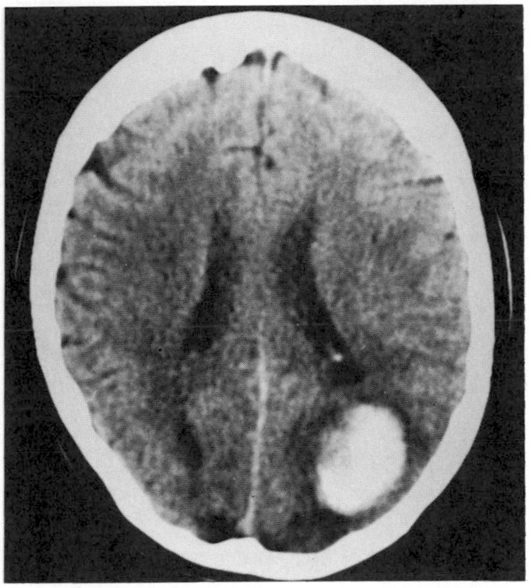
A

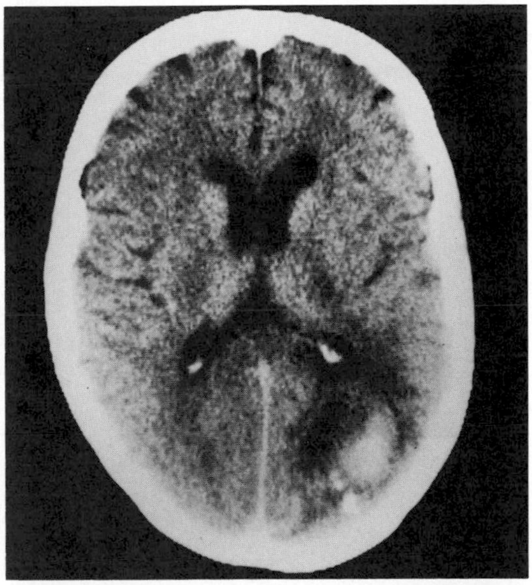
B

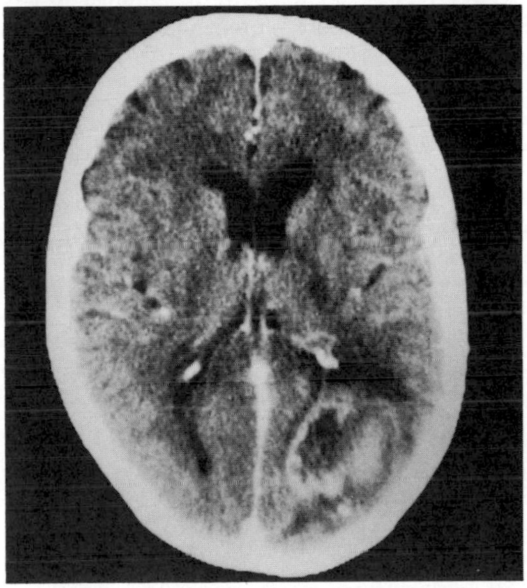
C

**Fig. 9-26.** (**A**) Acute lobar hematoma in a 64-year-old woman. (**B**) On plain computed tomography scan 16 days later, decrease in density allows easy recognition of calcifications. (**C**) Postcontrast computed tomography demonstrates irregular marginal enhancement. Magnetic resonance imaging confirmed hematoma in tumor, glioblastoma multiforme at histologic examination.

more than 8 to 10 days. Obviously, the amount of blood in the cerebral cisterns is the key factor determining its recognizability; however, there is no correlation between the amount of blood detected by CT and by lumbar puncture.[33] Moreover, with unquestionable bleeding verified by lumbar puncture, an occasional negative CT scan may be obtained even 1 day after the hemorrhage. Therefore, CT cannot be a complete substitute for lumbar puncture, and an early negative CT scan cannot rule out a subarachnoid hemorrhage (SAH). However, much more information can be obtained by CT in patients with SAH.

First, CT can exclude the possibility that the SAH is due to the rupture into the subarachnoid spaces of an intracerebral hematoma or to bleeding from a silent tumor, which would orient differently both the angiographic study and the management of the patient.[22,112] Second, CT can localize the aneurysm that has bled. Localization can be based either on an uneven distribution of blood in the cisterns or on the presence of a localized hematoma around the aneurysm, which may also rupture into the brain tissue (Fig. 9-30). The most easily predictable aneurysm is that of the anterior communicating artery, which shows a greater amount of blood in the frontal interhemispheric fissure and may cause either a midline hematoma, which extends through the lamina terminalis into the septum, or a lateralized frontal lobe hematoma.

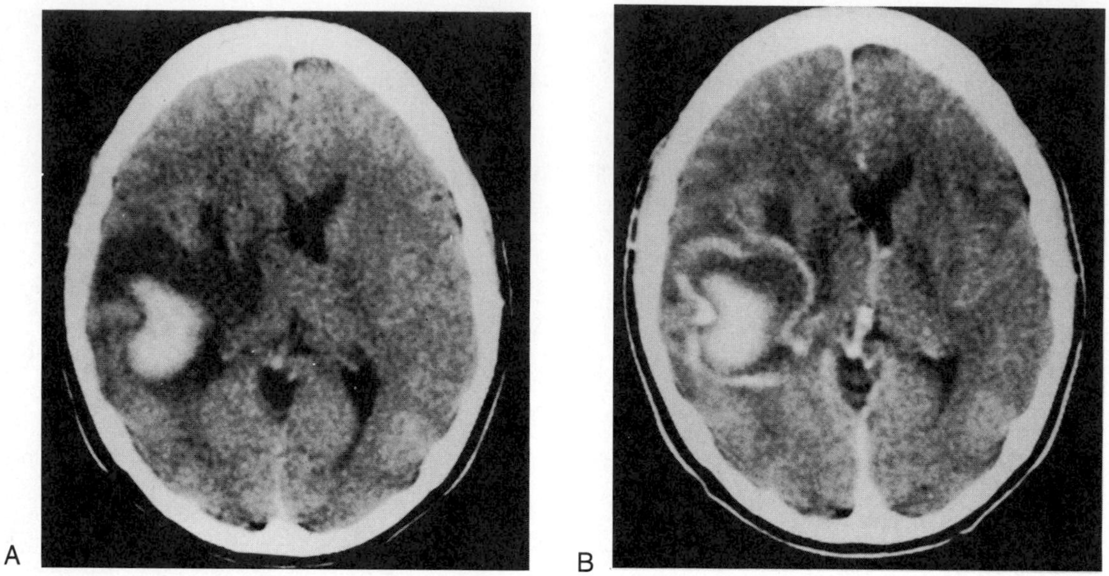

**Fig. 9-27.** Posterior temporal hematoma, 10 days after stroke. (**A**) Plain computed tomography scan. (**B**) Postcontrast computed tomography scan. The ring enhancement delineates exactly the hematoma, hypodense at the periphery.

In both cases the blood may rupture into the ventricles.

The second most predictable aneurysm is that of the middle cerebral artery, which shows more blood in the homolateral sylvian fissure and may form a hematoma extending all along the fissure, with rare rupture into the opercula.

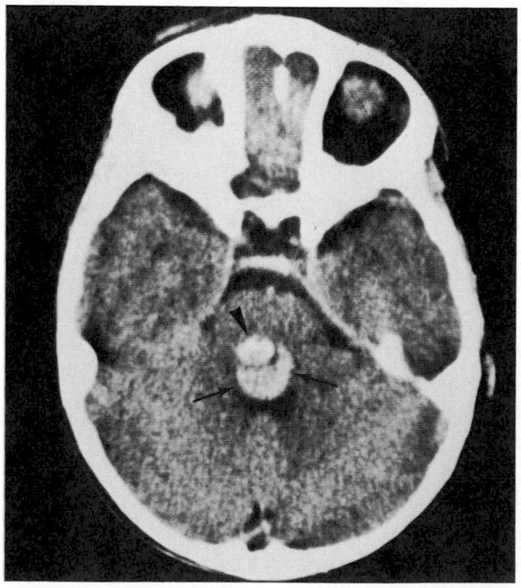

**Fig. 9-28.** Hematoma from cavernous hemangioma of the pons. Eight days after the bleeding, the decrease in density of the hematoma (*arrows*) allows recognition of the nodule of the hemangioma (*arrowhead*). The diagnosis was confirmed by magnetic resonance imaging and proved by operation.

In aneurysm of the carotid bifurcation or at the origin of the posterior communicating artery, there is usually a more even distribution of blood in the cisterns. Aneurysms of the carotid bifurcation may cause frontal hematomas similar to those of the anterior communicating artery. Prevalence of blood in the posterior fossa points to aneurysms of the vertebrobasilar system.

Finally, a confusing picture may be offered by the rare cases of subdural hematoma caused by aneurysms bleeding into the subdural space through a breached arachnoid and arachnoidal adhesions.[45]

There is, in conclusion, a fairly frequent overlapping of the CT patterns, so that a prediction of the site of the aneurysm is made with a high degree of confidence only if there is a localized hematoma or a well-defined difference in the distribution of the cisternal blood. Only in aneurysm of the anterior communicating artery is the accuracy of localization high,[65,131] in spite of the presence of a "typical" septal hematoma in the minority of cases.[163] However, the much rarer pericallosal aneurysm causes a very similar blood distribution; angiography is always necessary to define the aneurysm.[84]

CT localization of the bleeding aneurysm would seem futile, since angiography demonstrates the aneurysm; in these cases, CT is able, at most, to guide the angiographic study. Localization becomes important when multiple aneurysms are found, which happens in about 15 percent of the cases. Kendall et al.,[70] however, contend that CT localization of the bleeding aneurysm is always essential and that the angiographic study should be limited to the region of bleeding. In their series of multiple aneurysms, there is no

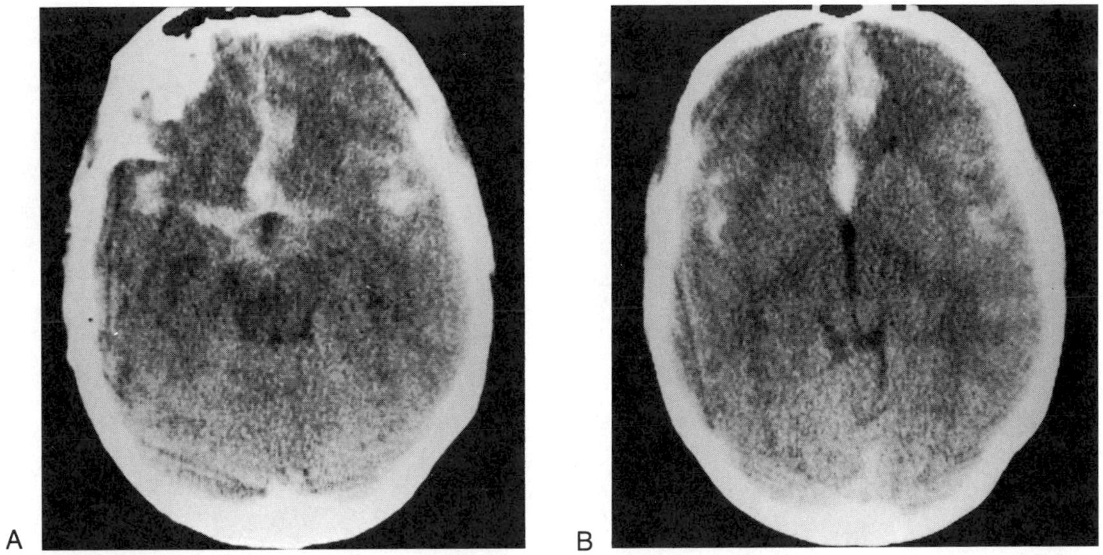

**Fig. 9-29.** (**A & B**) Computed tomography scan performed a few hours after subarachnoid hemorrhage; the distribution of blood in the cisterns suggests bleeding from anterior communicating artery aneurysm that was confirmed by angiography and surgery.

evidence that incidental aneurysms carry a significant risk; therefore, they should be ignored. However, this view is not shared by all the neurosurgeons and, when elective surgery for incidental aneurysms is considered, precise CT localization is important only for determining the priority of treatment.

CT without intravenous contrast administration is able to detect giant aneurysms because of their high density and is particularly useful in partially thrombosed, calcified aneurysms. Depending on their location, such aneurysms sometimes must be differentiated from craniopharyngiomas, pituitary adenomas, meningiomas, or other lesions that may calcify. Calcifications and thrombosis, however, are not the rule in giant aneurysms and all the patterns may be encountered, from nonthrombosed to completely thrombosed aneurysms (Fig. 9-31 and 9-32). MRI, of course, is usually very demonstrative.

The thrombosed parts of the aneurysm may have variable densities, sometimes lower than the part

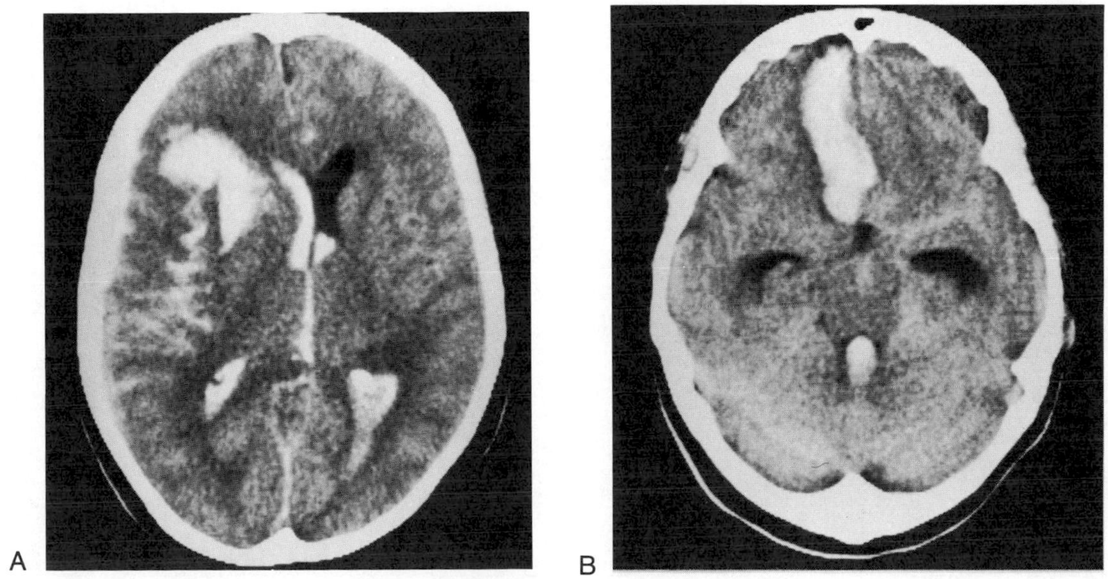

**Fig. 9-30.** Bleeding aneurysms with subarachnoid and intraventricular hemorrhages and intracerebral hematomas. Two different cases. (**A**) Aneurysm of the right middle cerebral artery bifurcation. (**B**) Aneurysm of the anterior communicating artery. The blood filling the 4th ventricle causes acute hydrocephalus.

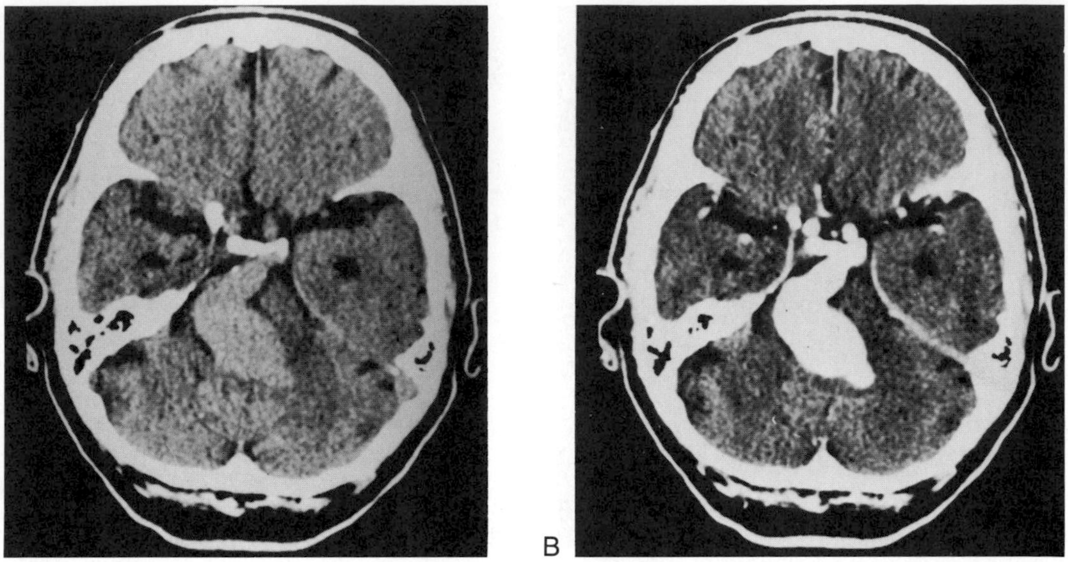

**Fig. 9-31.** Giant, fusiform basilar artery aneurysm, with compression of the brain stem. (**A**) The circulating blood is normally hyperdense. Tiny calcifications are visible in the aneurysmal wall. (**B**) Postcontrast computed tomography scan with uniform, complete enhancement confirms absence of thrombosis.

where blood is circulating. Comparison of plain with postcontrast CT scan or with angiography demonstrates the relationship of the two parts. Contrast enhancement may also be observed in the thick fibrous layer at the periphery of the thrombus,[111] which may rarely be the source of emboli and thus the cause of distal infarction. The partially thrombosed aneurysm therefore presents a fairly characteristic pattern with a central or eccentric enhancing area (i.e., the patent lumen), a peripheral isodense or slightly hyperdense area (i.e., the thrombus), and a surrounding, hyperdense, enhancing rim. This "target sign," in appropriate situations, is highly specific for giant, partially thrombosed aneurysms[111,129] (Fig. 9-32).

Contrast administration is always necessary to demonstrate the smaller-sized aneurysms; MRI or MR angiography, however, may become the examination of choice. On CT scan, possibility of detection

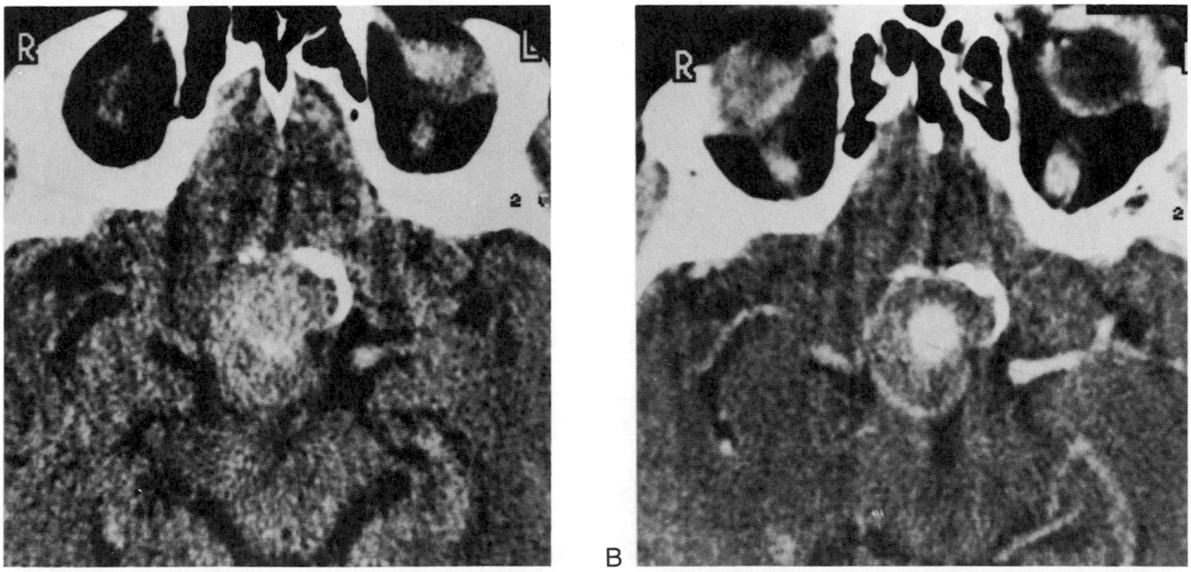

**Fig. 9-32.** Giant, partially thrombosed aneurysm of the anterior communicating artery. (**A**) Plain computed tomography scan. (**B**) Postcontrast computed tomography scan. Comparison of plain with postcontrast study allows recognition of thrombosed peripheral part and of central patent lumen.

after enhancement is good for anterior communicating and middle cerebral artery aneurysms, while it is poorer for those of the internal carotid and posterior communicating arteries.[48] However, it is our policy to avoid injection of contrast medium in patients with SAH, who are going to be subjected, in any case, to angiography. Only if angiography is negative might one expect to demonstrate on postcontrast CT a lesion that was unsuspected on plain CT and missed by angiography. This is only a theoretical possibility, while more emphasis should be placed on the possibility of a bleeding lesion in the spinal canal, mimicking a ruptured intracranial aneurysm. In patients with SAH, we never found a positive postcontrast CT scan with both normal plain CT and angiography, while we have found two neurinomas of the cauda equina and a spinal cord arteriovenous malformation presenting only with SAH, which were diagnosed by myelography after negative results on a four-vessel study. MRI may now demonstrate noninvasively the spinal pathology responsible for bleeding.

Intravenous contrast administration has been found to cause diffuse enhancement in the subarachnoid spaces in a considerable number of patients with SAH, particularly when it was performed in the first few days.[32,63,65,163] The enhancement is usually found in all the basal cisterns and may extend over the convexity. It does not help, therefore, in localizing the aneurysm but seems valuable for predicting vasospasm and cerebral infarcts.[63] The mechanism of subarachnoid enhancement in SAH has not been clearly established; the hypothesis that subarachnoid enhancement is related to thickening of the leptomeninges is unlikely, since this is a local, late reactive change. The most likely explanation is leakage of contrast medium from the vessels whose blood-CSF interface has been altered by the irritating effect of the surrounding blood.[65,137] If this is so, one has to consider the potential risk of adding a neurotoxic contrast agent in the CSF to the blood already present. In patients in poor equilibrium, even if nonionic, less neurotoxic contrast media are now used, it seems safer to rely upon the demonstration of blood in the cisterns for predicting vasospasm. Retrospective and prospective studies have demonstrated that development of symptomatic cerebral vasospasm is predicted with good accuracy on the basis of the presence of clots or thick layers of blood in the cisterns in the first few days after SAH.[32,43,76]

If clinical deterioration occurs, CT easily demonstrates whether it is due to rebleeding, infarction, or development of hydrocephalus. Frequency of hydrocephalus is variable in different series; ventricular dilatation is approximately present in one-third of the cases with SAH.[1,35,93,134] Many cases show spontaneous regression after 1 or 2 weeks.[93] The main factor determining the development of hydrocephalus is the amount of blood present in the cisterns and mostly in the ventricles (Fig. 9-30): all patients with intraventricular hemorrhage have some degree of ventricular dilatation and carry a poor prognosis.[97,134] Periventricular hypodensity, which indicates transependymal passage of CSF, also points to progression of hydrocephalus.[134]

Hydrocephalus is also associated with reduced cerebral blood flow and clinical deterioration.[93] Therefore, many factors, interfering with each other, are involved in determining the clinical evolution of the patients with SAH. CT is the main tool for monitoring these patients and serial CT studies are often needed in the pre- and postoperative period.

## INTRACRANIAL HEMORRHAGES: VASCULAR MALFORMATIONS

Cerebral vascular malformations may cause hemorrhages in the brain with rupture into the subarachnoid space or the ventricles. However, they may present with seizure disorder or, more rarely, with focal neurologic signs. Different types of vascular malformations have different tendencies to bleed and have different appearances on CT.

Cerebral vascular malformations are classified as (1) arteriovenous malformations, (2) venous angiomas, (3) cavernous hemangiomas, and (4) capillary angiomas or telangiectases.[119] Some authors also add varices as a separate entity.

Arteriovenous malformations had long been considered the most frequent cerebral vascular malformation;[91] however, a prospective autopsy series of more than 4,000 consecutive brains challenges previous reported frequences of cerebral vascular malformations. In this series of 177 vascular malformations in 165 brains, the most frequently encountered malformation was the venous angioma (59 percent), followed by telangiectasis (16 percent), arteriovenous malformation (14 percent), cavernous hemangioma (9 percent), and varix (2 percent).[123] These findings simply mean that small venous angiomas and telangiectases, which are most often not relevant from the clinical point of view, have also been overlooked in autopsy series.

The relative frequency with which cerebral vascular malformations are observed at CT or MRI has yet to be established.

### Arteriovenous Malformations

Arteriovenous malformations (AVMs) are probably the most commonly diagnosed type of cerebral vascular malformation and have the greatest tendency to bleed. Frequency of bleeding is quite variable both in neurosurgical series and in necropsy studies;[157] one-third to one-half of patients with AVM present at CT scan with intracranial hemorrhage.[69,82,156]

CT findings in nonbleeding AVMs are often diagnostic: AVMs usually appear as slightly hyperdense, well-defined lesions with sometimes irregular or multilobular but sharp margins; occasional thin hypodense areas at the periphery or within the lesion are seen; the lesions rarely exhibit mass effect, but are associated instead with dilatation of the homolateral ventricle and of the adjacent sulci. Calcifications are rarely seen, but microcalcifications may contribute to the high density of the lesion.

The low-density areas are sometimes the result of previous hematomas or infarctions or may represent surrounding atrophy or demyelination. Plain CT abnormalities, often suggestive of AVM, are seen in about 80 percent of the cases.[58,82] However, contrast medium administration is usually crucial for a specific diagnosis: the lesion strongly enhances, and tortuous vascular channels, representing the feeding arteries, but mostly the larger draining veins, are often demonstrated (Fig. 9-33).

Sometimes the features of the lesion are not so typical; MRI usually answers the question.

CT features are less evident when bleeding occurs: the hematoma may mask part of the lesion, and presence of mass effect and edema may lead one to include bleeding tumor in the differential diagnosis, but again MRI and angiography are usually diagnostic.

AVMs are more frequently lobar rather than deep; therefore, a spontaneous lobar hematoma in a young or middle-aged, nonhypertensive person should make one suspect vascular malformation. If angiography gives negative results, CT (or MRI) should, in any case, be repeated after resolution of the hematoma because of the possibility of detecting the nodule of the vascular malformation on late postcontrast CT scan. AVMs may, in fact, be occult on angiography either transiently when the bleeding occurs or permanently if they are thrombosed. CT (like MRI) is able to detect these lesions, which accounted for 11 percent of the cases reported by Leblanc et al.[82] However, in these cases, definite correct diagnosis is sometimes obtained only at histologic examination, and glioma or other tumors are a possible misdiagnosis.[10,78,81]

## Venous Angiomas

Of all cerebral vascular malformations, venous angiomas probably have the lowest tendency to bleed. We observed only two hematomas associated with venous angiomas, while demonstration of venuos angiomas at angiography or CT or MRI is an incidental, not rare, occurrence in studies performed for unrelated reasons. The venous angioma is composed of a tuft of venous channels converging on a larger venous collector, interspersed in normal brain tissue. For this reason and because of reduced tendency to bleed, preventive surgery is not indicated and therefore pathologic demonstration is often lacking. The diagnosis, however, must be considered sufficiently proved when angiography demonstrates a group of veins in a medusa or umbrellalike pattern in normal venous phase, and when CT demonstrates the venous channels crossing the brain to reach a subependymal or a superficial vein without any nodule or other abnormalities of the surrounding brain tissue[152] (Fig. 9-34). The umbrellalike pattern reflects the embryologic development of these venous anomalies;[151] unfortunately, it is difficult to demonstrate with either CT or MRI.

A few cases with small nodular component seen on postcontrast CT scan have been reported.[87,95] It is

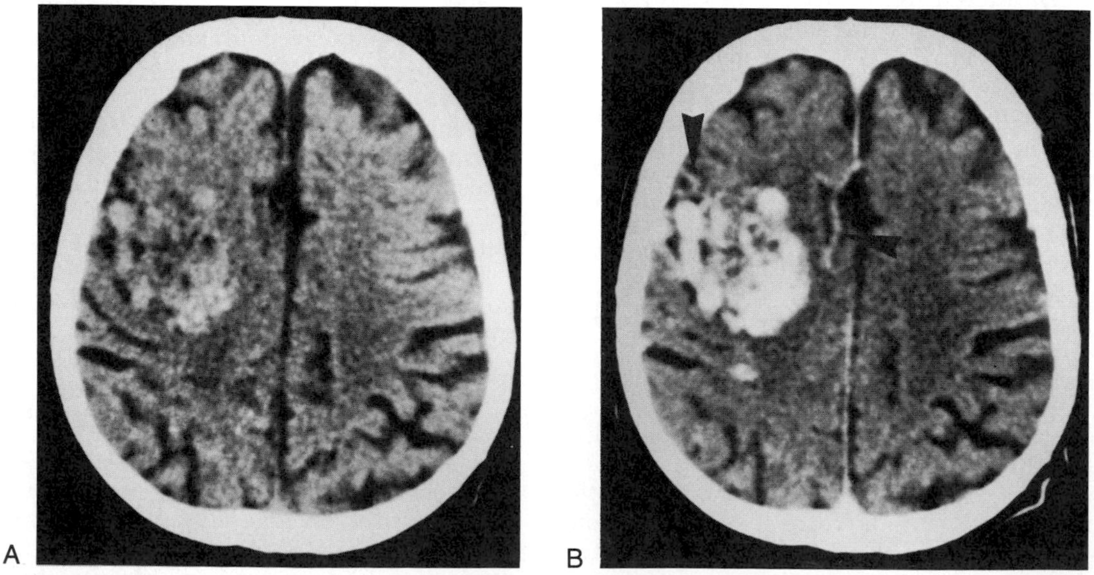


**Fig. 9-33.** Arteriovenous malformation. (**A**) Plain computed tomography scan. (**B**) Postcontrast computed tomography scan. Postcontrast study also demonstrates feeding arteries (*arrowheads*).

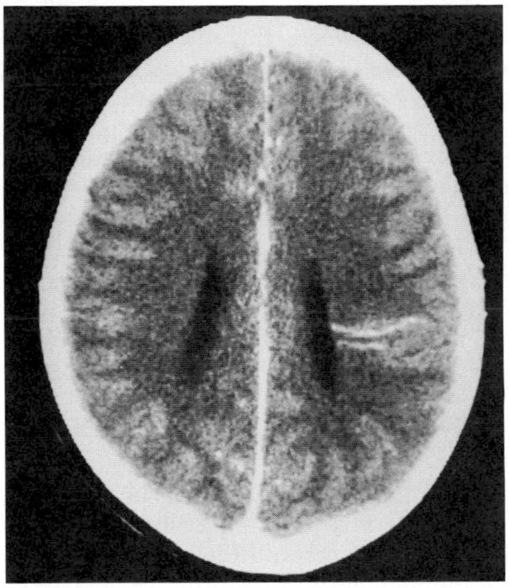

**Fig. 9-34.** Venous angioma. Only postcontrast computed tomography scan shows the anomalous venous channels crossing normal brain tissue.

likely that the nodular component represents the point of convergence of the venous channels combined with tortuosity of the large draining vein. Otherwise, a nodular component on CT scan associated with a large draining vein points more to a cavernous hemangioma; MRI is helpful in defining these cases. Mixed angiomas, arteriovenous and venous, telangiectatic and cavernous, are also sometimes observed on histologic examination.

## Cavernous Hemangiomas

Cavernous hemangiomas are peculiar vascular malformations because they have no intervening brain tissue among the thin-walled sinusoidal spaces of which they are composed. Even if they do not have a true capsule, cavernous hemangiomas are well circumscribed and are therefore easily removed at surgery.[49] Cavernous hemangiomas are the second most relevant cerebral vascular malformation after AVMs, and MRI demonstrates them with increased frequency. Their frequency of bleeding is uncertain: before CT became available, it seemed high, because cavernous hemangiomas were diagnosed mostly when they had bled. After CT, cavernous hemangiomas presenting only with focal epilepsy were more frequently recognized.[126] However, even in these cases MRI demonstrates that microhemorrhages not detectable by CT are almost the rule.

The most frequent CT pattern consists of a well-defined, slightly inhomogeneous hyperdense area without mass effect (Fig. 9-35). Hypodense areas at the periphery or in the center of the nodule are rarely seen, while calcifications are most frequently observed. In four cases we observed, the cavernous hemangioma was isodense, recognizable only after contrast enhancement. Contrast enhancement is a constant feature.[127]

In our experience, cavernous hemangiomas were the most common angiographically occult vascular malformation. Pathologic circulation or early draining veins were found in only a minority of cases. Therefore, in the appropriate clinical setting, a combination of an avascular area in the capillary phase of

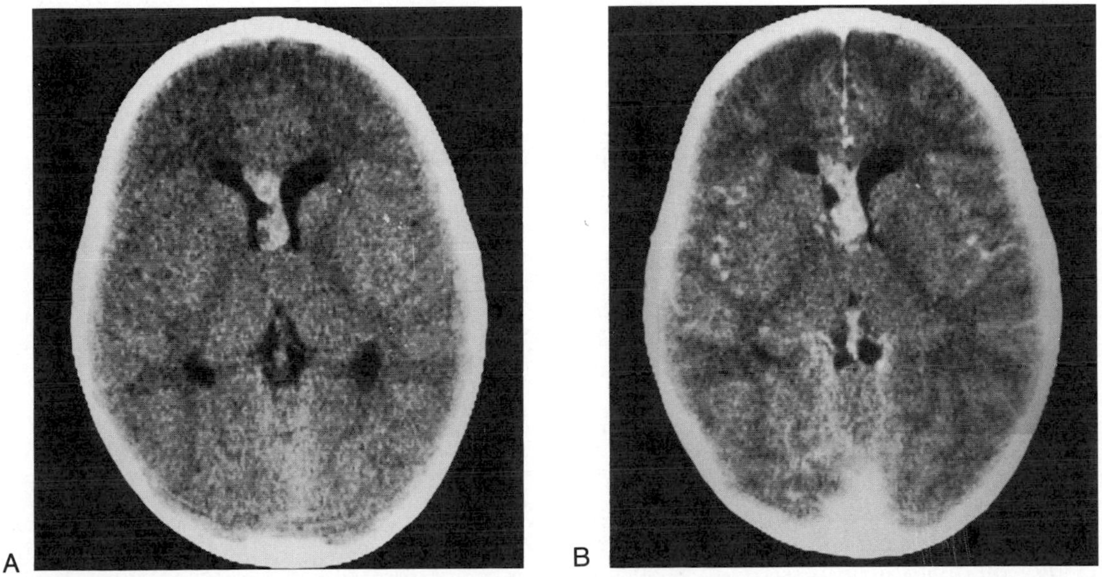

**Fig. 9-35.** Cavernous hemangioma, surgically verified, in unusual, septal location. (**A**) Plain computed tomography scan shows well-defined, hyperdense lesion. (**B**) Lesion slightly enhances on postcontrast study. Magnetic resonance imaging yielded higher diagnostic specificity.

the angiogram, with an enhancing nodule without mass effect on CT scan, suggests the possibility of cavernous hemangioma.[7,127] MRI demonstrates cavernous hemangiomas better than CT and may eliminate the necessity of angiography.

### Capillary Angiomas or Telangiectases

Capillary angiomas seem to be the second most frequently occurring cerebral vascular malformation.[123] However, similar to venous angiomas, they are usually not clinically relevant. In addition, telangiectases are not demonstrated by angiography: to our knowledge, the only case in which pathologic circulation was reported was a mixed angioma, with telangiectases, cavernous angioma, and dilated venous channels.[118] Since the most frequent location of telangiectases is in the pons,[91,119] it is reasonable to suppose that spontaneous hematomas in nonhypertensive patients occurring in the pons are due, at least in part, to ruptured telangiectases. CT easily detects pontine hematomas; less frequently, it is able to demonstrate the underlying vascular malformation. However, in patients without hemorrhage, with symptoms and signs referable to a brain stem lesion, CT may occasionally demonstrate a hyperdense, sometimes calcified, enhancing lesion, without significant mass effect and without growth, consistent with a cryptic vascular malformation. Results of angiography are usually negative.[161] MRI in a few cases may suggest a cavernous hemangioma, but sometimes only a chronic hematoma is recognizable. Pathologic proof is almost always lacking; even in hemorrhagic cases, at evacuation of the hematoma, histologic diagnosis is usually not obtained.[106]

## SUMMARY

CT is by no means the only neuroradiologic examination that has to be performed in patients with cerebrovascular disease, and has largely been substituted for or complemented by MRI; but it is safe, noninvasive, and, in some instances, can conclude the neuroradiologic workup. CT studies may also be complemented with dynamic CT and with xenon enhancement to monitor the pathophysiologic changes that occur in cerebrovascular occlusive disease. However, these studies are not routinely performed and have not been included in this chapter.

CT, performed without contrast medium and sometimes with contrast enhancement (using iodine), is usually the first examination in patients with cerebrovascular disease, whether ischemic or hemorrhagic, and is extremely valuable in orienting the subsequent diagnostic and therapeutic approach. In suspected posterior fossa lesions, however, MRI should be the examination of choice. In patients with TIAs and infarcts, CT scan excludes the presence of unexpected lesions and the presence of bleeding, but other investigations are necessary if the site of the stenotic or occluded artery has to be determined. In patients with intracerebral bleeding, CT may be the only examination; but, if a vascular malformation is suspected, angiography becomes necessary. Angiography is always needed in subarachnoid hemorrhage, provided that the patient's condition does not contraindicate the examination. In general, one should always consider the patient's condition and the medical or surgical therapeutic implications expected from the various studies to avoid unnecessary or risky procedures.

## ACKNOWLEDGMENTS

We would like to thank Dr. Carla Carollo and Dr. Luciano De Lorenzi for their collaboration in selecting CT scans, Ms. Luciana Caposio, x-ray technician, and Mr. Paolo Tinelli for photographic assistance.

## REFERENCES

1. Adams HP, Jr, Kassel NF, Torner JC, Sahs AL: CT and clinical correlations in recent aneurysmal subarachnoid hemorrhage: a preliminary report of the Cooperative Aneurysm Study. Neurology (NY) 33:981, 1983
2. Alcalà H, Gado M, Torack RM: The effect of size, histologic elements, and water content on the visualization of cerebral infarcts: a computerized cranial tomographic study. Arch Neurol 35:1, 1978
3. Ambrose J: Computerized transverse axial scanning (tomography). 2. Clinical application. Br J Radiol 46:1023, 1973
4. Araki G, Mihara H, Shizuka M et al: CT and arteriographic comparison of patients with transient ischemic attacks: correlation with small infarction of basal ganglia. Stroke 14:276, 1983
5. Arimitsu T, Di Chiro G, Brooks RA, Smith PB: White-grey matter differentiation in computed tomography. J Comput Assist Tomogr 1:437, 1977
6. Asari S, Satoh T, Sakurai M et al: The advantage of coronal scanning in cerebral computed angiotomography for diagnosis of moyamoya disease. Radiology 145:709, 1982
7. Bartlett JE, Kishore PRS: Intracranial cavernous angioma. AJR 128:653, 1977
8. Bastianello S, Pierallini A, Colonnese C et al: Hyperdense middle cerebral artery CT sign: comparison with angiography in the acute phase of ischemic supratentorial infarction. Neuroradiology 33:207, 1991
9. Beal MF, Williams RS, Richardson EP, Jr, Fisher CM: Cholesterol embolism as a cause of transient ischemic attacks and cerebral infarction. Neurology (NY) 31:860, 1981
10. Becker DH, Townsend JJ, Kramer RA, Newton TH: Occult cerebrovascular malformations: a

series of 18 histologically verified cases with negative angiography. Brain 102:249, 1979
11. Becker H, Desch H, Hacker H, Pencz A: CT fogging effect with ischemic cerebral infarcts. Neuroradiology 18:185, 1979
12. Berger L, Hakim AM: The association of hyperglycemia with cerebral edema in stroke. Stroke 17:865, 1986
13. Bergström M, Ericson K, Levander B et al: Variation with time of the attenuation values of intracranial hematomas. J Comput Assist Tomogr 1:57, 1977
14. Berman SA, Hayman LA, Hinck VC: Correlation of CT cerebral vascular territories with function. I. Anterior cerebral artery. AJR 135:253, 1980
15. Bogousslavsky J, Regli F, Uské A, Maeder P: Early spontaneous hematoma in cerebral infarct: is primary cerebral hemorrhage overdiagnosed? Neurology (NY) 41:837, 1991
16. Bogousslavsky J, Van Melle G, Regli F: The Lausanne Stroke Registry: analysis of 1,000 consecutive patients with first stroke. Stroke 19:1083, 1988
17. Bozzao L, Bastianello S, Fantozzi LM et al: Correlation of angiographic and sequential CT findings in patients with evolving cerebral infarction. AJNR 10:1215, 1989
18. Bradac GB: CT and angiography in the diagnosis of cerebrovascular occlusive diseases, p. 199. In Cecchini A, Nappi G, Arrigo A (eds): Cerebral Pathology in Old Age. Neuroradiological and Neurophysiological Correlations. Emiras, Pavia, 1982
19. Bradac GB, Oberson R: CT and angiography in cases with occlusive disease of supratentorial cerebral vessels. Neuroradiology 19:193, 1980
20. Bradac GB, Oberson R: Angiography and Computed Tomography in Cerebro-Arterial Occlusive Disease. 2nd Ed. Springer-Verlag, New York, 1983
21. Brahme FJ: CT diagnosis of cerebrovascular disorders: a review. Comput Tomogr 2:173, 1978
22. Brismar J: Computer tomography as the primary radiologic procedure in acute subarachnoid hemorrhage. Acta Radiol [Diagn] (Stockh) 20:849, 1979
23. Brismar J: Computer tomography in superior sagittal sinus thrombosis. Acta Radiol [Diagn] (Stockh) 21:321, 1980
24. Buonanno FS, Moody DM, Ball MR, Laster DW: Computed cranial tomographic findings in cerebral sinovenous occlusion. J Comput Assist Tomogr 2:281, 1978
25. Caillé JM, Guibert F, Bidabé AM et al: Enhancement of cerebral infarcts with CT. Comput Tomogr 4:73, 1980
26. Candelise L, Landi G, Orazio EN, Boccardi E: Prognostic significance of hyperglycemia in acute stroke. Arch Neurol 42:661, 1985
27. Caplan LR: Are terms such as completed stroke or RIND of continued usefulness? Stroke 14:431, 1983
28. Caplan LR, Mohr JP: Intracerebral hemorrhage: an update. Geriatrics 33:42, 1978
29. Cecchini A, Cosi V: TC: indicazioni diagnostiche, risultati e limiti nelle malattie cerebro-vascolari. Ital J Neurol Sci, suppl. 1:37, 1979
30. Constant P, Renou AM Caillé JM et al: Aspects tomodensitométriques des accidents ischémiques cérébraux. J Neuroradiol 4:291, 1977
31. Damasio H: A computed tomographic guide to the identification of cerebral vascular territories. Arch Neurol 40:138, 1983
32. Davis JM, Davis KR, Crowell RM: Subarachnoid hemorrhage secondary to ruptured intracranial aneurysm: prognostic significance of cranial CT. AJNR 1:17, 1980
33. Davis JM, Ploetz J, Davis KR et al: Cranial computed tomography in subarachnoid hemorrhage: relationship between blood detected by CT and lumbar puncture. J Comput Assist Tomogr 4:794, 1980
34. Davis KR, Ackerman RH, Kistler JP, Mohr JP: Computed tomography of cerebral infarction: hemorrhagic, contrast enhancement, and time of appearance. Comput Tomogr 1:71, 1977
35. Davis KR, New PFJ, Ojemann RG et al: Computed tomographic evaluation of hemorrhage secondary to intracranial aneurysm. AJR 127:143, 1976
36. Davis KR, Taveras JM, New PFJ et al: Cerebral infarction diagnosis by computerized tomography: analysis and evaluation of findings. AJR 124:643, 1975
37. Dolinskas CA, Bilaniuk LT, Zimmerman RA, Kuhl DE: Computed tomography of intracerebral hematomas. I. Transmission CT observations on hematoma resolution. AJR 129:681, 1977
38. Dolinskas CA, Bilaniuk LT, Zimmerman RA et al: Computed tomography of intracerebral hematomas. II. Radionuclide and transmission CT studies of the perihematoma region. AJR 129:689, 1977
39. Donnan GA, Tress BM, Bladin PF: A prospective study of lacunar infarction using computerized tomography. Neurology (NY) 32:49, 1982
40. Drake ME Jr, Shin C: Conversion of ischemic to hemorrhagic infarction by anticoagulant administration: report of two cases with evidence from serial computed tomographic brain scans. Arch Neurol 40:44, 1983
41. Fisher CM: Lacunar strokes and infarcts: a review. Neurology (NY) 32:871, 1982
42. Fisher CM, Adams RD: Observations on brain embolism with special reference to the mechanism of hemorrhagic infarction. J Neuropathol Exp Neurol 10:92, 1951
43. Fisher CM, Kistler JP, Davis JM: Relation of cerebral vasospasm to subarachnoid hemorrhage visualized by computerized tomographic scanning. Neurosurgery 6:1, 1980
44. Ford K, Sarwar M: Computed tomography of dural sinus thrombosis. AJNR 2:539, 1981
45. Friedman MB, Brant-Zawadzki M: Interhemispheric subdural hematoma from ruptured aneurysm. Comput Radiol 7:129, 1983
46. Gács G, Fox AJ, Barnett HJM, Viñuela F: CT visualization of intracranial arterial thromboembolism. Stroke 14:756, 1983

47. Ganti SR, Cohen M, Sane P, Hilal SK: Computed tomography of cerebral syphilis. J Comput Assist Tomogr 5:345, 1981
48. Ghoshhajra K, Scotti L, Marasco J, Baghai-Naiini P: CT detection of intracranial aneurysms in subarachnoid hemorrhage. AJR 132:613, 1979
49. Giombini S, Morello G: Cavernous angiomas of the brain: account of fourteen personal cases and review of the literature. Acta Neurochir (Wien) 40:61, 1978
50. Goto K, Ishii N, Fukasawa H: Diffuse white-matter disease in the geriatric population: a clinical, neuropathological, and CT study. Radiology 141:687, 1981
51. Gray F, Dubas F, Roullet E, Escourolle R: Leukoencephalopathy in diffuse hemorrhagic cerebral amyloid angiopathy. Ann Neurol 18:54, 1985
52. Grumme T, Lanksch W, Wende S: Diagnosis of spontaneous intracerebral hemorrhage by computerized tomography. p. 284. In Lanksch W, Kazner E (eds): Cranial Computerized Tomography. Springer-Verlag, Berlin, 1976
53. Hachinski VC, Potter P, Merskey H: Leuko-araiosis. Arch Neurol 44:21, 1987
54. Handa J, Nakano Y, Okuno T et al: Computerized tomography in moyamoya syndrome. Surg Neurol 7:315, 1977
55. Harwood-Nash DC, Fitz CR: Neuroradiology in Infants and Children. CV Mosby, St Louis, 1976
56. Hayman LA, Berman SA, Hinck VC: Correlation of CT cerebral vascular territories with function. II. Posterior cerebral artery. AJNR 2:219, 1981
57. Hayman LA, Evans RA, Bastion FO, Hinck VC: Delayed high dose contrast CT: identifying patients at risk of massive hemorrhagic infarction. AJNR 2:139, 1981
58. Hayman LA, Fox AJ, Evans RA: Effectiveness of contrast regimens in CT detection of vascular malformations of the brain. AJNR 2:421, 1981
59. Hayman LA, Sakai F, Meyer JS et al: Iodine-enhanced CT patterns after cerebral arterial embolization in baboons. AJNR 1:233, 1980
60. Heinz ER, Drayer BP, Haenggeli CA et al: Computed tomography in white-matter disease. Radiology 130:371, 1979
61. Heinz ER, Pizer SM, Fuchs H et al: Examination of the extracranial carotid bifurcation by thin-section dynamic CT: direct visualization of intimal atheroma in man (Part 1). AJNR 5:355, 1984
62. Hinshaw DB Jr, Thompson JR, Hasso AN, Casselman ES: Infarctions of the brainstem and cerebellum: a correlation of computed tomography and angiography. Radiology 137:105, 1980
63. Hirata Y, Matsukado Y, Fukumura A: Subarachnoid enhancement secondary to subarachnoid hemorrhage with special reference to the clinical significance and pathogenesis. Neurosurgery 11:367, 1982
64. Hodge CJ, Leeson M, Cacayorin E et al: Computed tomographic evaluation of extracranial carotid artery disease. Neurosurgery 21:167, 1987
65. Inoue Y, Saiwai S, Miyamoto T et al: Postcontrast computed tomography in subarachnoid hemorrhage from ruptured aneurysms. J Comput Assist Tomogr 5:341, 1981
66. Inoue Y, Takemoto K, Miyamoto T et al: Sequential computed tomography scans in acute cerebral infarction. Radiology 135:655, 1980
67. Iragui VJ, McCutchen CB: Capsular ataxic hemiparesis. Arch Neurol 39:528, 1982
68. Kasdon DL, Scott RM, Adelman LS, Wolpert SM: Cerebellar hemorrhage with decreased absorption values on computed tomography: a case report. Neuroradiology 13:265, 1977
69. Kendall BE, Claveria LE: The use of computed axial tomography (CAT) for the diagnosis and management of intracranial angiomas. Neuroradiology 12:141, 1976
70. Kendall BE, Lee BCP, Claveria E: Computerized tomography and angiography in subarachnoid hemorrhage. Br J Radiol 49:483, 1976
71. Kendall BE, Pullicino P: Intravascular contrast injection in ischaemic lesions. II. Effect on prognosis. Neuroradiology 19:241, 1980
72. Kendall BE, Radue EW: Computed tomography in spontaneous intracerebral haematoma. Br J Radiol 51:563, 1978
73. Kingsley DPE, Kendall BE, Moseley IF: Superior sagittal sinus thrombosis: an evaluation of the changes demonstrated on computed tomography. J Neurol Neurosurg Psychiatry 41:1065, 1978
74. Kingsley DPE, Radue EW, Du Boulay EPGH: Evaluation of computed tomography in vascular lesions of the vertebrobasilar territory. J Neurol Neurosurg Psychiatry 43:193, 1980
75. Kinkel WR, Jacobs L, Kinkel PR: Gray matter enhancement: a computerized tomographic sign of cerebral hypoxia. Neurology (NY) 30:810, 1980
76. Kistler JP, Crowell RM, Davis KR et al: The relation of cerebral vasospasm to the extent and location of subarachnoid blood visualized by CT scan: a prospective study. Neurology (NY) 33:424, 1983
77. Kobari M, Meyer JS, Ichijo M, Oravez WT: Leukoaraiosis: correlation of MR and CT findings with blood flow, atrophy, and cognition. AJNR 11:273, 1990
78. Kramer RA, Wing SD: Computed tomography of angiographically occult cerebral vascular malformations. Radiology 123:649, 1977
79. Kushner M, Nencini P, Reivich M et al: Relation of hyperglycemia early in ischemic brain infarction to cerebral anatomy, metabolism, and clinical outcome. Ann Neurol 28:129, 1990
80. Ladurner G, Skvarc A, Sager WD: Computer tomography in transient global amnesia. Eur Neurol 21:34, 1982
81. Leblanc R, Ethier R: The computerized tomographic appearance of angiographically occult arteriovenous malformations of the brain. Can J Neurol Sci 8:7, 1981
82. Leblanc R, Ethier R, Little JR: Computerized tomography findings in arteriovenous malformations of the brain. J Neurosurg 51:765, 1979
83. Lee KF, Chambers RA, Diamond C et al: Evaluation of cerebral infarctions by computed tomog-

raphy with special emphasis on microinfarction. Neuroradiology 16:156, 1978
84. Liliequist B, Lindqvist M, Valdimarsson E: Computed tomography and subarachnoid hemorrhage. Neuroradiology 14:21, 1977
85. Loizou LA, Kendall BE, Marshall J: Subcortical arteriosclerotic encephalopathy: a clinical and radiological investigation. J Neurol Neurosurg Psychiatry 44:294, 1981
86. Longo M, Fiumara F, Pandolfo I, D'Avella N: CT observation of an ongoing intracerebral hemorrhage. J Comput Assist Tomogr 7:362, 1983
87. Maehara T, Tasaka A: Cerebral venous angioma: computerized tomography and angiographic diagnosis. Neuroradiology 16:296, 1978
88. Manelfe C, Clanet M, Gigaud M et al: Internal capsule: normal anatomy and ischemic changes demonstrated by computed tomography. AJNR 2:149, 1981
89. Masdeu JC: Enhancing mass on CT: neoplasm or recent infarction? Neurology (NY) 33:836, 1983
90. Mason WG Jr, Latchaw RE, Yock DH, Jr: Spontaneous hemorrhage during cranial computed tomography. AJR 135:181, 1980
91. McCormick WF, Hardman JM, Boulter TR: Vascular malformations ("angiomas") of the brain, with special reference to those occurring in the posterior fossa. J Neurosurg 28:241, 1968
92. Meguro K, Hatazawa J, Yamaguchi T et al: Cerebral circulation and oxygen metabolism associated with subclinical periventricular hyperintensity as shown by magnetic resonance imaging. Ann Neurol 28:378, 1990
93. Menon D, Weir B, Overton T: Ventricular size and cerebral blood flow following subarachnoid hemorrhage. J Comput Assist Tomogr 5:328, 1981
94. Messina AV, Chernik NL: Computed tomography: the "resolving" intracerebral hemorrhage. Radiology 118:609, 1975
95. Michels LG, Bentson JR, Winter J: Computed tomography of cerebral venous angiomas. J Comput Assist Tomogr 1:149, 1977
96. Miller VT: Lacunar stroke: a reassessment. Arch Neurol 40:129, 1983
97. Mohr G, Ferguson G, Khan M et al: Intraventricular hemorrhage from ruptured aneurysm: retrospective analysis of 91 cases. J Neurosurg 58:482, 1983
98. Mohr JP: Lacunes. Stroke 13:3, 1982
99. Mohr JP, Caplan LR, Melski JW et al: The Harvard Cooperative Stroke Registry: a prospective registry. Neurology (NY) 28:754, 1978
100. Monajati A, Heggeness L: Patterns of edema in tumors vs. infarcts: visualization of white matter pathways. AJNR 3:251, 1982
101. Moseley IF, Olney J: Intracranial hemorrhage in the elderly: neuroradiology. p. 215. In Cecchini A, Nappi G, Arrigo A (eds): Cerebral Pathology in Old Age. Neuroradiological and Neurophysiological Correlations. Emiras, Pavia, 1982
102. Müller HR, Wiggli U: Cerebral, cerebellar and pontine hemorrhages. p. 249. In Du Boulay GH, Moseley IF (eds): CAT in Clinical Practice. Springer-Verlag, Berlin, 1977
103. Nelson RF, Pullicino P, Kendall BE, Marshall J: Computed tomography in patients presenting with lacunar syndromes. Stroke 11:256, 1980
104. New PFJ, Aronow S: Attenuation measurements of whole blood and blood fractions in computed tomography. Radiology 121:635, 1976
105. Norman D, Price D, Boyd D et al: Quantitative aspects of computed tomography of the blood and cerebrospinal fluid. Radiology 123:335, 1977
106. O'Laoire SA, Crockard A, Thomas DGT, Gordon DS: Brain-stem hematoma: a report of six surgically treated cases. J Neurosurg 56:222, 1982
107. Olszewski J: Subcortical arteriosclerotic encephalopathy: review of the literature on the so-called Binswanger's disease and presentation of two cases. World Neurol 3:359, 1962
108. Paxton R, Ambrose J: The EMI scanner: a brief review of the first 650 patients. Br J Radiol 47:530, 1974
109. Perman GP, Racy A: Homolateral ataxia and crural paresis: case report. Neurology (NY) 30:1013, 1980
110. Perrone P, Candelise L, Scotti G et al: CT evaluation in patients with transient ischemic attack. Correlation between clinical and angiographic findings. Eur Neurol 18:217, 1979
111. Pinto RS, Kricheff II, Butler AR, Murali R: Correlation of computed tomographic, angiographic and neuropathological changes in giant cerebral aneurysms. Radiology 132:85, 1979
112. Pluchino F, Lodrini S, Savoiardo M: Subarachnoid hemorrhage and meningioma: report of two cases. Acta Neurochir (Wien) 68:45, 1983
113. Pressman BD, Tourje EJ, Thomson JR: Early CT sign of ischemic infarction: increased density in a cerebral artery. AJNR 8:645, 1987
114. Pullicino P, Kendall BE: Contrast enhancement in ischemic lesions. I. Relationship to prognosis. Neuroradiology 19:235, 1980
115. Pullicino P, Nelson RF, Kendall BE, Marshall J: Small deep infarcts diagnosed on computed tomography. Neurology (NY) 30:1090, 1980
116. Rao KCVG, Knipp HC, Wagner EJ: Computed tomographic findings in cerebral sinus and venous thrombosis. Radiology 140:391, 1981
117. Rascol A, Clanet M, Manelfe C et al: Pure motor hemiplegia: CT study of 30 cases. Stroke 13:11, 1982
118. Roberson GH, Kase CS, Wolpow ER: Telangiectases and cavernous angiomas of the brain stem: "cryptic" vascular malformations: report of a case. Neuroradiology 8:83, 1974
119. Russell DS, Rubinstein LJ: Pathology of Tumours of the Nervous System. 3rd Ed. Edward Arnold, London, 1971
120. Sage MR: Blood-brain barrier: phenomenon of increasing importance to the imaging clinician. AJNR 3:127, 1982
121. Sage MR: Kinetics of water-soluble contrast media in the central nervous system. AJNR 4:897, 1983
122. Saris S: Chorea caused by caudate infarction. Arch Neurol 40:590, 1983
123. Sarwar M, McCormick WF: Intracerebral ve-

nous angioma: case report and review. Arch Neurol 35:323, 1978
124. Savoiardo M, Bracchi M: Neuroradiology of stroke. p. 94. In Callaghan N, Galvin R (eds): Recent Research in Neurology. Pitman, London, 1984
125. Savoiardo M, Bracchi M, Passerini A, Visciani A: The vascular territories in the cerebellum and brainstem: CT and MR study. AJNR 8:199, 1987
126. Savoiardo M, Passerini A: CT, angiography, and RN scans in intracranial cavernous hemangiomas. Neuroradiology 16:256,1978
127. Savoiardo M, Strada L, Passerini A: Intracranial cavernous hemangiomas: neuroradiologic review of 36 operated cases. AJNR 4:945, 1983
128. Schoenberg BS, Mellinger JF, Schoenberg DG: Cerebrovascular disease in infants and children: a study of incidence, clinical features, and survival. Neurology (NY) 28:763, 1978
129. Schubiger O, Valavanis A, Hayek J: Computed tomography in cerebral aneurysms with special emphasis on giant intracranial aneurysms. J Comput Assist Tomogr 4:24, 1980
130. Schuknecht B, Ratzka M, Hofmann E: The "dense artery sign"—major cerebral artery thromboembolism demonstrated by computed tomography. Neuroradiology 32:98, 1990
131. Scotti G, Ethier R, Melançon D: Computed tomography in the evaluation of intracranial aneurysms and subarachnoid hemorrhage. Radiology 123:85, 1977
132. Scotti G, Spinnler H, Sterzi R, Vallar G: Cerebellar softening. Ann Neurol 8:133, 1980
133. Segall HD, Ahmadi J, McComb JG et al: Computed tomographic observations pertinent to intracranial venous thrombotic and occlusive disease in childhood: state of the art, some new data, and hypotheses. Radiology 143:441, 1982
134. Silver AJ, Pederson ME Jr, Ganti SR et al: CT of subarachnoid hemorrhage due to ruptured aneurysms. AJNR 2:13, 1981
135. Skriver EB, Olsen TS: Transient disappearance of cerebral infarcts on CT scan, the so-called fogging effect. Neuroradiology 22:61, 1981
136. Skriver EB, Olsen TS: Contrast enhancement of cerebral infarcts: incidence and clinical value in different states of cerebral infarction. Neuroradiology 23:259, 1982
137. Sobel DF, Li FC, Norman D, Newton TH: Cisternal enhancement following subarachnoid hemorrhage, abstracted. AJNR 1:374, 1980
138. Soisson T, Cabanis EA, Iba-Zizen MT et al: Pure motor hemiplegia and computed tomography: 19 cases. J Neuroradiol 9:304, 1982
139. Stiller J, Shanzer S, Yang W: Brainstem lesions with pure motor hemiparesis: computed tomographic demonstration. Arch Neurol 39:660, 1982
140. Suzuki J, Takaku A: Cerebrovascular "moyamoya" disease; disease showing abnormal net-like vessels in the base of the brain. Arch Neurol 20:288, 1969
141. Takahashi S, Goto K, Fukasawa H et al: Computed tomography of cerebral infarction along the distribution of the basal perforating arteries. I. Striate arterial group. Radiology 155:107, 1985
142. Takahashi S, Goto K, Fukasawa H et al: Computed tomography of cerebral infarction along the distribution of the basal perforating arteries. II. Thalamic arterial group. Radiology 155:119, 1985
143. Takeuchi S, Kobayashi K, Tsuchida T et al: Computed tomography in moyamoya disease. J Comput Assist Tomogr 6:24, 1982
144. Taneda M, Ozaki K, Wakayama A et al: Cerebellar infarction with obstructive hydrocephalus. J Neurosurg 57:83, 1982
145. Tomsick TA, Brott TG, Chambers AA et al: Hyperdense middle cerebral artery sign on CT: efficacy in detecting middle cerebral artery thrombosis. AJNR 11:473, 1990
146. Tomura N, Uemura K, Inugami A et al: Early CT finding in cerebral infarction: obscuration of the lentiform nucleus. Radiology 168:463, 1988
147. Tredici G, Pizzini G, Bogliun G, Tagliabue M: The site of motor corticospinal fibres in the internal capsule of man: a computerized tomographic study of restricted lesions. J Anat 134:199, 1982
148. Tress BM, Davis S, Lavain J et al: Incremental dynamic computed tomography: practical method of imaging the carotid bifurcation. AJNR 7:49, 1986
149. Truwit C, Barkovich AJ, Gean-Marton A et al: Loss of the insular ribbon: another early CT sign of acute middle cerebral artery infarction. Radiology 176:801, 1990
150. Tsai FY, Teal JS, Heishima GB, et al: Computed tomography in acute posterior fossa infarcts. AJNR 3:149, 1982
151. Valavanis A, Schefer S, Wichmann W: Cavernomas and venous angiomas of the brain. Riv Neuroradiol, suppl 2. 3:89, 1990
152. Valavanis A, Wellauer J, Yasargil MG: The radiological diagnosis of cerebral venous angioma: cerebral angiography and computed tomography. Neuroradiology 24:193, 1983
153. Van Gijn J, Kraaijeveld CL: Blood pressure does not predict lacunar infarction. J Neurol Neurosurg Psychiatry 45:147, 1982
154. Vonofakos D, Artmann H: CT findings in hemorrhagic cerebral infarct. Comput Radiol 7:75, 1983
155. Waxman SG, Toole JF: Temporal profile resembling TIA in the setting of cerebral infarction. Stroke 14:433, 1983
156. Weisberg LA: Computed tomography in the diagnosis of intracranial vascular malformations. Comput Tomogr 3:125, 1979
157. Weisberg LA, Nice C, Katz M: Cerebral Computed Tomography. A Text-Atlas. WB Saunders, Philadelphia, 1978
158. Wing SD, Norman D, Pollock JA, Newton TH: Contrast enhancement of cerebral infarcts in computed tomography. Radiology 121:89, 1976
159. Wodarz R: Watershed infarctions and computed tomography: a topographical study in cases with stenosis or occlusion of the carotid artery. Neuroradiology 19:245, 1980

160. Yates PO: Vascular disease of the central nervous system. p. 86. In Blackwood W, Corsellis JAN (eds): Greenfield's Neuropathology. 3rd Ed. Edward Arnold, London, 1976
161. Yeates A, Enzmann D: Cryptic vascular malformations involving the brainstem. Radiology 146:71, 1983
162. Yock DH, Jr: CT demonstration of cerebral emboli. J Comput Assist Tomogr 5:190, 1981
163. Yock DH, Jr, Larson DA: Computed tomography of hemorrhage from anterior communicating artery aneurysms, with angiographic correlation. Radiology 134:399, 1980
164. Yock DH Jr, Marshall WH Jr: Recent ischemic brain infarcts at computed tomography: appearances pre- and postcontrast infusion. Radiology 117:599, 1975
165. Zatz LM, Jernigan TL, Ahumada AJ, Jr: White matter changes in cerebral computed tomography related to aging. J Comput Assist Tomogr 6:19, 1982
166. Zeumer H, Schonsky B, Sturm KW: Predominant white matter involvement in subcortical arteriosclerotic encephalopathy (Binswanger disease). J Comput Assist Tomogr 4:14, 1980
167. Zilkha A: Intraparenchymal fluid-blood level: a CT sign of recent intracerebral hemorrhage. J Comput Assist Tomogr 7:301, 1983
168. Zimmerman RA, Bilaniuk LT, Packer RJ et al: Computed tomographic-arteriographic correlates in acute basal ganglionic infarction of childhood. Neuroradiology 24:241, 1983
169. Zimmerman RD, Leeds NE, Naidich TP: Ring blush associated with intracerebral hematoma. Radiology 122:707, 1977

# 10

# *MAGNETIC RESONANCE SCANNING*

S.K. Hilal
J.P. Mohr

Magnetic resonance imaging (MRI) has become, for many, the preferred technique of brain imaging because of the wealth of information it offers. It is limited, however, by a longer imaging time, which may not be tolerated by patients with acute cerebrovascular accidents. The diminished sensitivity for the detection of subarachnoid hemorrhage is another limiting factor of MRI. Computed tomography (CT) is usually more readily accessible and has the advantage of lower cost. Magnetic resonance technology is expensive and requires substantial technical expertise in the proper operation and maintenance of the facility. The manufacturers of the equipment have made major strides in standardizing the instrumentation and making its operation within the grasp of most technologists with reasonable training. Also, recent techniques have remarkably shortened imaging time and have become capable of selectively depicting the vascular anatomy and tissue perfusion. MR spectroscopy is making major inroads and is permitting in vivo biochemical characterization of ischemic/infarcted brain, thereby opening the possibility of evaluating the reversibility of an infarction.

MRI is based on the interaction between radio waves and certain nuclei of the body tissues, in the presence of a powerful magnetic field. Hydrogen (protons) is the most common nuclear magnetic resonance (NMR)-observable nucleus within the human body. It enters into the composition of water, fats, and almost every other organic molecule normally present in tissue. Water protons and fat protons are the most extensively imaged nuclei clinically. Besides hydrogen (protons), sodium and phosphorus in the human body were imaged, using 1.5 tesla magnets. These nuclei are much less abundant than hydrogen, thus producing images of much less spatial resolution than is possible with protons. Sodium and phosphorus, however, offer the potential of biochemical characterization of the tissues such as assessing the extent of tissue damage, grade of malignancy, and/or response to treatment. Similarly, proton spectroscopy has made important progress by becoming clinically available for depicting the distribution of important biochemical compounds in the brain such as *N*-acetylaspartate, lactate, creatine, choline, and inositol. The significance of these compounds in cerebral ischemia and/or infarction is under study at this moment. Experience will permit the judicious use of this information.

When the human body is positioned in a strong magnetic field, its MRI-observable nuclei become susceptible to excitation by intermittent radiofrequency pulses. The energy from the radiofrequency pulses is absorbed and then released until the tissue being scanned has completely reemitted the energy absorbed and has undergone complete relaxation. The energy released from the excited tissue occurs over a short period of time according to two relaxation constants known as T1 and T2. The contrast in a given MR image will depend on which of these two constants is dominant in the imaging technique used. In clinical practice, three types of images are generated: (1) T1-weighted, in which the cerebrospinal fluid has a low-signal intensity relative to the brain, while fat has a high-signal intensity; (2) T2-weighted, where cerebrospinal fluid has increased signal relative to brain, and fat has almost no signal; and finally, (3) images with a balanced T1- and T2-weighting, often called "spin density"-weighted images, where brain and cerebrospinal fluid are comparable in signal intensity. The image contrast in this last type is primarily dependent on the abundance of protons in a given pixel.

Other forms of images include T2*-weighted images that tend to emphasize blood products and are useful in detecting small amounts of hemorrhage. T2* images are obtained by using a high field (1.5 T) and a long echo time with a spin-echo sequence (TR 2,500 ms or more, and TE 80 ms or more). A gradient echo technique emphasizes the T2* effect of paramagnetic blood products and is often used as an additional sequence for the study of patients with stroke to evaluate the presence of hemorrhage. Finally, the use of flow-sensitive imaging techniques has permitted the depiction of the extracranial and intracranial blood vessels in a totally noninvasive fashion. Arteries and veins can be imaged separately. Also, images depicting cerebral perfusion and diffusion of water molecules have been improving in quality and precision. These techniques are relatively new and require further evaluation to establish the true clinical utility.

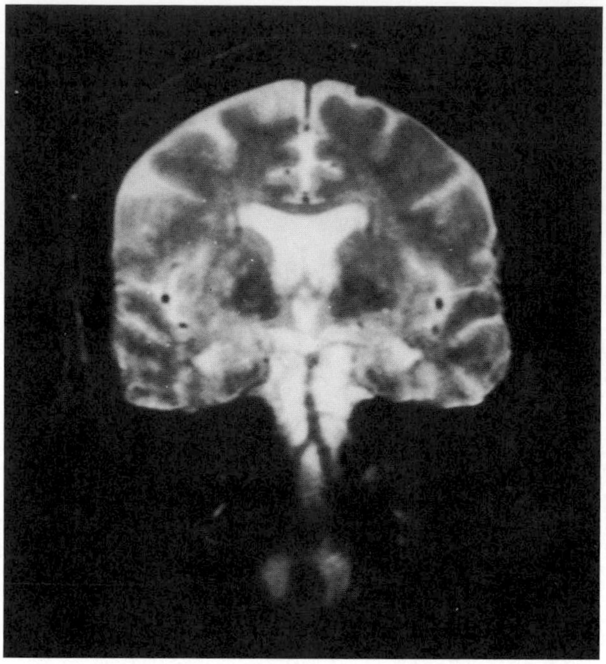

**Fig. 10-1.** Coronal T2-weighted MR showing basilar stenosis shown independently by angiogram and insonated by transcranial Doppler.

## INFARCTION

### Technique

A standard protocol for the study of a patient with stroke includes images with T1-weighted, T2-weighted, and spin-density images. The T1-weighted images (TR 600 to 800 ms and TE of 20 to 30 ms) provide good anatomic definition and are most useful for the detection of hemorrhage or vascular thrombosis. Gyral swelling can often be appreciated. T2-weighted images (TR 2,500 ms or more, and TE 80 ms) are best suited for the demonstration of cerebral parenchymal damage and the associated increase in tissue water encountered in brain edema and infarctions. This pulse sequence is also helpful in depicting the normal signal void from arteries and veins. Occluded or stenotic vessels can often be demonstrated on these images (Fig. 10-1). The long T2-weighted images have become the preferred pulse sequence for the demonstration of the site and extent of increased tissue water accompanying edema or infarction. The study of the appearance and response of an infarction to treatment is best documented by T2-weighted images. Many lesions well below the size detected on CT are found by MR. Gradient echoes with a short flip angle and a long TE are recommended for the detection of small amounts of blood. A spin-density weighted image (TR 2,500 ms, TE 30 ms) helps in depicting infarctions close to the ventricle and in the detection of ischemic changes in the very early 5 phase of stroke. It is believed that the slight increase of water in the brain may be seen early using this pulse sequence.

The use of paramagnetic contrast agents, such as gadolinium, may help to define areas of blood-brain barrier breakdown. It will aid in the differential diagnosis and helps to visualize flow abnormalities within the larger vessels.

Hemorrhage is easily diagnosed by both T2 and T1 images. The paramagnetic effect of methemoglobin and hemosiderin permits dating of hematomas and helps separate hematomas from hemorrhagic infarction.[9] Flowing blood helps diagnose arteriovenous malformations and a characteristic appearance permits a diagnosis of cavernous angioma as never before. Subdural and epidural hemorrhages are easily demonstrated, often when asymptomatic, because of their age or small size. MRI is the most sensitive imaging modality for the detection of cavernous angiomas because of the paramagnetic effect of old blood. Also, small subdural hematomas and epidural hematomas often missed on CT can be readily detected by MR imaging.

Magnetic resonance angiography (MRA) is rapidly gaining acceptance for the diagnosis of extracranial vascular disease. Each of the carotid vessels or the vertebral arteries can be depicted individually in multiple projections, providing an accurate assessment of the profile of the vessel, which is quire comparable to angiography. Carotid stenoses between 50 and 100 percent are diagnosed by MRA with almost the same sensitivity and specificity as conventional angiography. At present, the limitation lies in the inability of MRA to image highly stenotic vessels with a minute residual open lumen. Intracranial aneurysms and arteriovenous malformations can be detected by a variety of imaging techniques, including conventional T2-weighted images and MRA pulse sequences.

## Early Changes

Experimental stroke models in cats showed parenchymal signal changes as early as 30 minutes, using T2-weighted technique, and in all cases by 4 hours.[4] The increased MR signal image was correlated with histochemical studies documenting increase in brain water, in which brain edema occurred and increased before structural changes occurred.[25] Some areas of viable but ischemic tissue were found to be normal, or at least structurally unaltered, even when the MRI signal showed an abnormality in the hyperacute stage. This stage lasted "a few hours."[25] Although brain water increased before structural damage was evident,[4] the image data did not permit easy separation of brain edema from surrounding brain water. Early hopes that the paramagnetic substances could separate ischemia from infarction have been somewhat frustrated to date.[32]

The sequence of signal changes in clinical studies have been similar to those of animal studies, but the time course has been more prolonged. The earliest MRI observations in stroke have been those relating to abnormal vascular dynamics and to morphologic changes resulting from brain swelling (Fig. 10-2). It remains to be seen if different MR pulse sequences can define the different territories of infarction, ischemia, and simple edema.[10] T2-weighted parenchymal signal change in some patients with nonhemorrhagic strokes have been seen as early as 45 minutes,[34] but the first images as late as 10 hours have been negative in other cases when the follow-up image at 24 hours was positive.

The early MRI changes in acute stroke can be categorized as follows.

### Abnormal Magnetic Resonance Images of the Cerebral Vessels

The restoration of the normal flow void usually seen in the major intracranial arteries is one of the earliest observations in stroke patients. It is best seen on T2-weighted images because of their greater sensitivity to motion and because of the ease with which one can detect the normal flow void against the bright signal of the surrounding cerebrospinal fluid in the basal cisterns and the sylvian fissure. The restoration of the normal flow void is observed in 35 to 40 percent of patients with a stroke who will eventually proceed to have an MR-detectable infarction. It has been observed in the carotid artery, the middle cerebral artery, and the vertebrobasilar systems. The absence of the normal flow void has been seen as early as a few minutes after the ictus.

Another vascular sign is arterial enhancement, which is observed on the T1-weighted images and consists of a conspicuous bright high-intensity appearance of the cortical vessels, which is further accentuated after contrast administration. It is seen in more than half the patients studied with contrast MR in the first 24 hours after the onset of the deficit.[60] These statistics refer to patients who will eventually develop an MRI-observable infarction in the area of the clinical stroke. Transient ischemic attacks are excluded from these statistics. The arterial enhancement sign is due to the markedly slowed flow in either an anterograde or retrograde direction. The slow flow, therefore, could be due to narrowing of the vessel or due to retrograde filling from collaterals (Fig. 10-3). Occlusion of the vessel from thrombosis will also, at some stage, appear as a high-signal vessel wall hemorrhage has also been seen in an artery suffering dissection (Fig. 10-4).

### Local Brain Swelling

Local brain swelling refers to the observation of swollen gyri or mass effects without alteration of the signal characteristics of the brain. This finding is more pronounced in cases of cortical infarction and is seen in the first 24 hours in two-thirds of the patients who will eventually develop an infarction observable on MR. It is particularly prominent with cortical infarctions and can precede by several hours the T2 signal changes.

### Changes in the Parenchymal Signal Intensity

The early experiences with infarction, studied over varying periods of time up to 36 hours by 0.15 T-resistive magnets[14] did not show a major difference between CT and MR. MR also showed a higher frequency of lesions: in a study by Salgado et al.,[44] of patients with transient ischemic attacks (TIAs), 86 percent showed MR changes, compared with 42 percent for CT, while for infarction, a smaller difference was appreciated, although the margins of the lesion were clearer on MR. In some studies, a "fogging effect" has been seen and explained as developing hemorrhagic infarction.[51] In some studies MR seemed to image the infarct lesion earlier than does CT scanning,[46,47] and the lesion topography appeared larger,

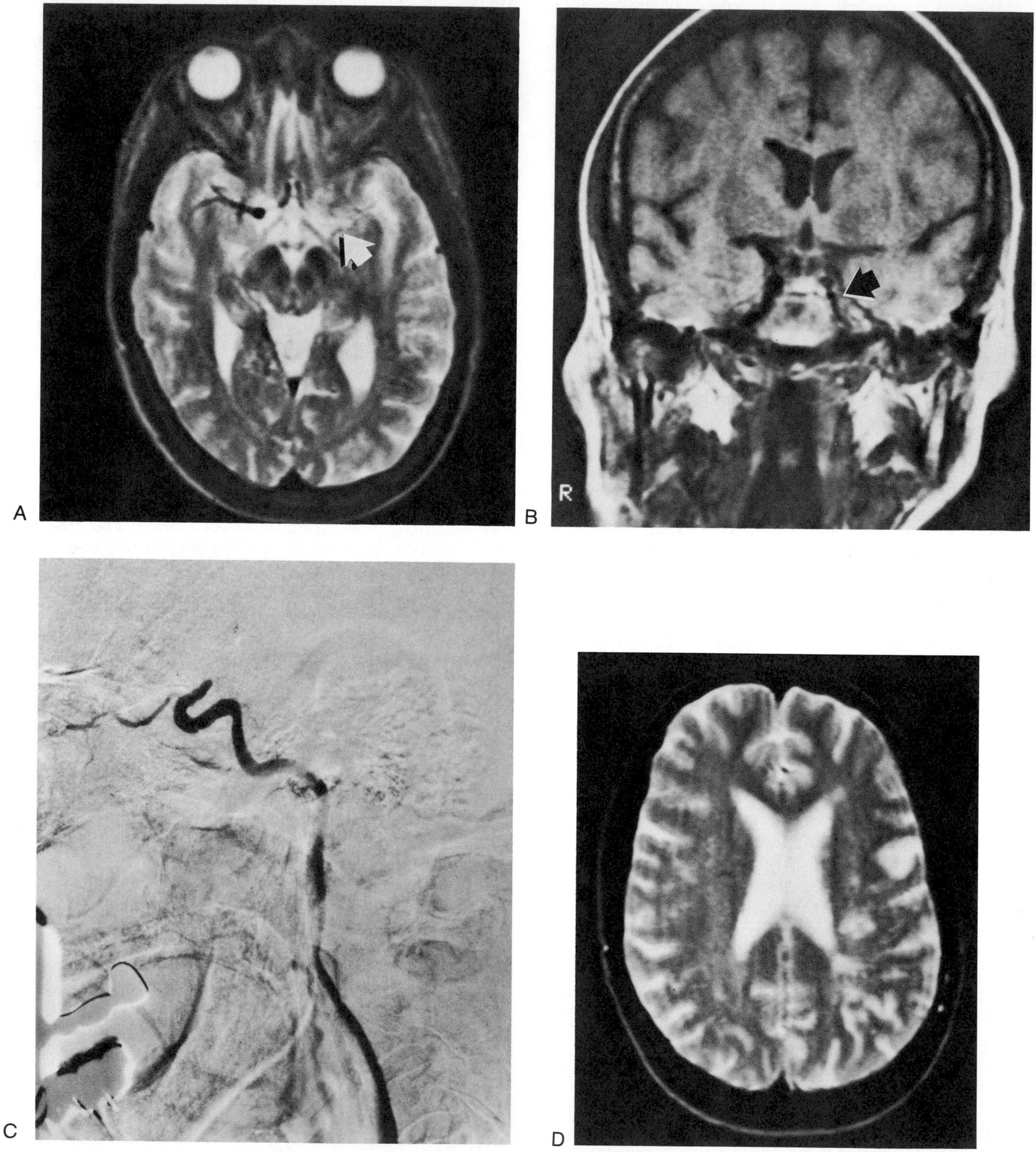


**Fig. 10-2.** **(A)** Axial T2-weighted MR showing absence of the normal flow void in the middle cerebral artery and no signal changes in the brain. **(B)** Coronal T1-weighted MR showing the signal void in the middle cerebral artery and early hemispheral edema. **(C)** Angiogram demonstrating the occluded middle cerebral artery. **(D)** Axial T2-weighted MR showing the high convexity, centrum semiovale ''distal field'' infarction.

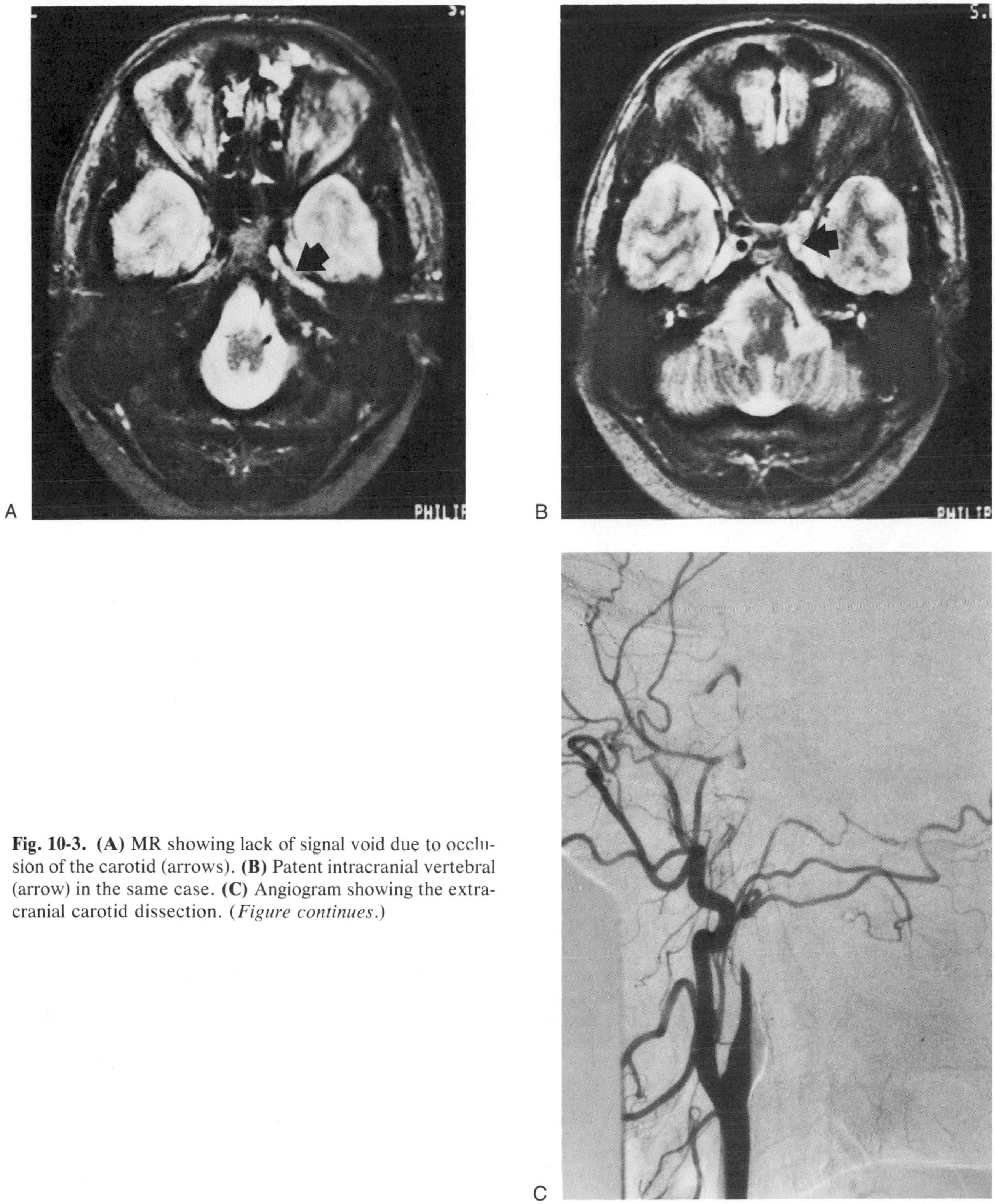


**Fig. 10-3.** **(A)** MR showing lack of signal void due to occlusion of the carotid (arrows). **(B)** Patent intracranial vertebral (arrow) in the same case. **(C)** Angiogram showing the extracranial carotid dissection. (*Figure continues.*)

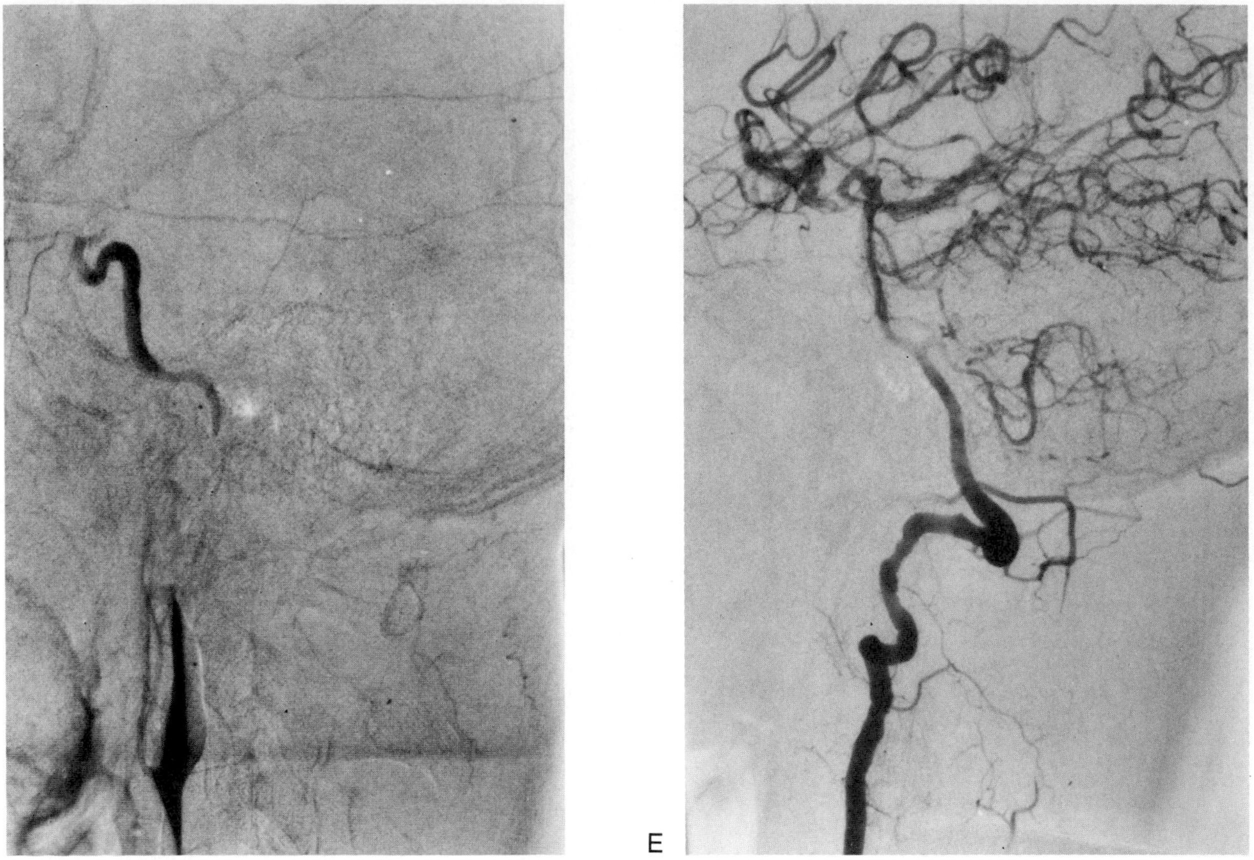

D E

**Fig. 10-3** (*Continued*). **(D)** Angiogram showing the vertebral dissection. **(E)** Angiogram showing the vertebral dissection in the same angiogram.

possibly because of edema.[18] High-signal changes were documented with MRI within 24 hours of onset for many years in humans,[57] but the issue of reversibility of the clinical deficit has not yet been clarified.

In the largest study using resistive magnets, Fukuda et al.[14] reported in Japanese on 16 patients studied within 36 hours from the onset of symptoms, using a resistive magnet (0.15 T), with T1- and T2-weighted images compared with CT. Both CT and MR showed large cortical infarcts better than smaller lesions of the basal ganglia and brain stem. Infarction was seen earlier on MRI than on CT in eight patients, the time ranging from 2, 6, 7, to 10 hours after onset. Fukuda and colleagues were unable to differentiate infarction from perifocal edema by CT or by MR. In two patients the lesions were seen on T2-weighted images earlier than on T1. These investigators found that the size of abnormal findings gradually developed and reached a maximum by days 5 to 7, after which they gradually subsided and reached a stable size after about 2 months.

More recent studies have rarely found changes of brain MR signals in the first few hours. In our study, only 15 percent of the cases examined within 8 hours showed a change in the brain signal on the long TR sequences (proton density or T2-weighted images). At 24 hours almost 90 percent[5,60] of the patients in whom an MR-observable infarction is developing will show a signal change on the long TR sequences. This is to be compared to 50 percent sensitivity to signal changes on the T1-weighted images (Fig. 10-5). The decreased sensitivity of the T1-weighted images is due to the negative mix of the T1 effect and proton density characteristic of the infarction. T2-weighted images and proton density images seem equally sensitive to the detection of infarction, with the observation that proton density images may occasionally show the lesion more conspicuously than the T2-weighted images, particularly in the early course of the process and for lesions close to the ventricles and subarachnoid spaces where the high signal of the cerebrospinal fluid can mask the detection of the adjacent infarction.

The time course of the parenchymal signal changes on T2-weighted sequences followed the morphologic evidence of brain swelling by several hours. These findings raise interesting questions about the significance of the brain signal changes. The appearance of the high signal on the T2-weighted image coincides

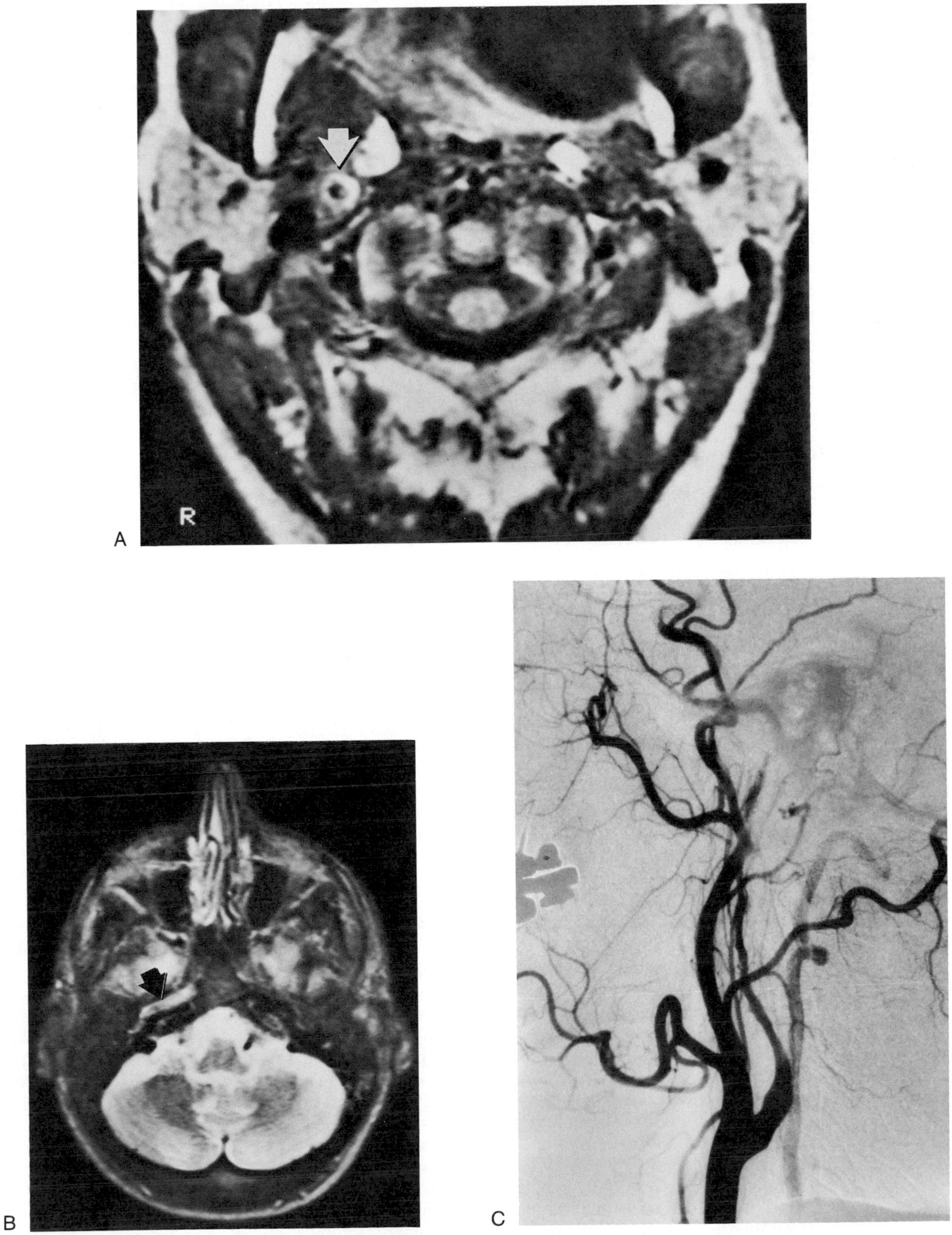


**Fig. 10-4.** **(A)** T2-weighted MR showing carotid dissection with hematoma in the extracranial carotid vessel wall (arrow). **(B)** T2-weighted MR showing high signal from slowed arterial flow in the petrous portion of the internal carotid. **(C)** The angiogram shows the dissection in the extracranial portion of the internal carotid.

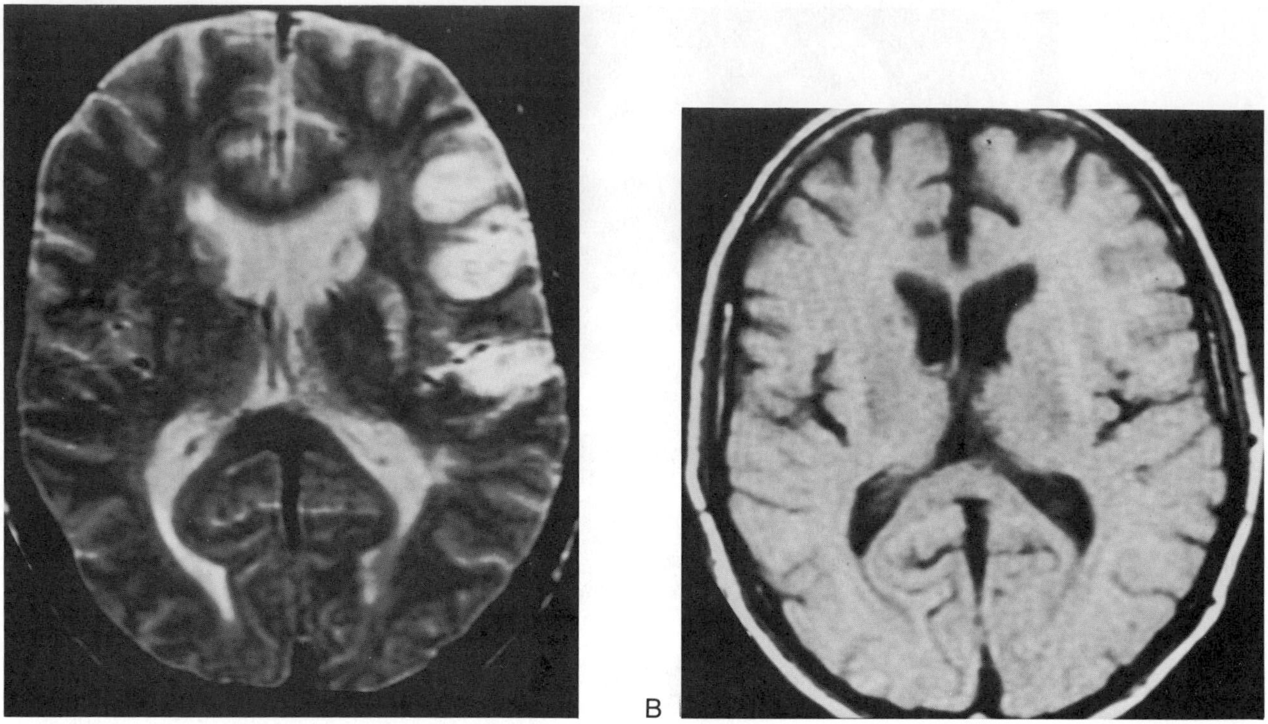

A B

**Fig. 10-5. (A)** T2-weighted MR 27 hours after stroke showing acute hemispheral convexity infarction. **(B)** T1-weighted MR at 27 hours showing faint changes over the same site showing prominent changes on T2.

with the appearance and course of vasogenic edema, which results from the blood-brain barrier damage. The initial brain swelling is presumed to coincide with the cytotoxic edema phase, where small amounts of water (about 3 percent of tissue volume) are believed to enter the intracellular space as a consequence of the failure of the sodium-potassium adenosine triphosphate (ATP) pump. Such a small change of tissue water may not be sufficient to change the T2 characteristic of brain tissue. Also, in the early stage of infarction, tissue water, particularly intracellular water of cytotoxic edema, may be bound and less available for MRI observation.

Signal changes more than 24 hours after the onset of ischemic stroke are seen in the majority of cases (Fig. 10-6). Further, 30 percent of patients with an infarction visualized in the first 24 hours show an increase in size on the follow-up scan.[5] This time course of the development of lesions on T2-weighted images suggests that MR, in its current stage of development, cannot depict the entire region of brain that is at risk of infarction, and areas that fall in the penumbra zone of the infarction are not identified in the early stages of the process. The question arises, therefore, as to whether the T2 signal changes of the brain mean that an irreversible damage has occurred. Further research, and perhaps the use of chemical shift imaging and spectroscopy in conjunction with conventional imaging, could elucidate the significance of the signal changes on MRI infarction. Sodium imaging[20] has shown, in a few cases, very early infarctions before any signal changes were observed on proton imaging. The experience with sodium imaging is still limited, and further work will improve our understanding of the early events taking place in the process of cerebral infarction and perhaps help to establish the point at which the lesion becomes irreversible.

## Contrast Enhancement

Several recent studies on the use of MRI contrast agents have revealed interesting insights into the mechanism of enhancement in cerebral infarctions.[7,56,21,23,33,35] Gadopentate dimeglumine was the first clinically approved contrast medium for MRI, and is currently still the most widely used agent. It is a paramagnetic substance shortening the T1 relaxation of hydrogen nuclei in unbound water molecules. In most infarctions (more than 80 percent of the cases) the typical sequence of parenchymal enhancement goes as follows: contrast enhancement is not seen before 6 days, is most visible in the subacute phase (7 to 30 days), slowly fades away in the chronic phase (more than 30 days), and may persist for 6 weeks.[19] In a recent review, Crain et al.[7] observed this sequence of enhancement in 67 of 82 lesions studied. They called it the "progressive enhancement pattern." In this group the enhancement is seen later than the T2 signal changes, which are observed by 24 hours of the onset of stroke. Furthermore, the enhanced area is smaller than that depicted on the T2 weighted images. In other words, in this group of patients the enhancement trails the T2 signal changes. In the remaining 15 patients of their series Crain and colleagues observed a pattern of early and/or intense enhancement in the first 7 days after the onset of the stroke. In these cases the gadolinium enhancement appeared at the same time as the T2 changes and covered the same area. Also, clinically, this second group of patients with early enhancement had a better neurologic outcome. Crain et al. attributed the two types of enhancement pattern to a difference in the underlying pathologic processes in each case. In the "progressive enhancement" group it is believed that the arterial occlusion is complete and that there is insufficient collateral circulation to transport enough contrast

A

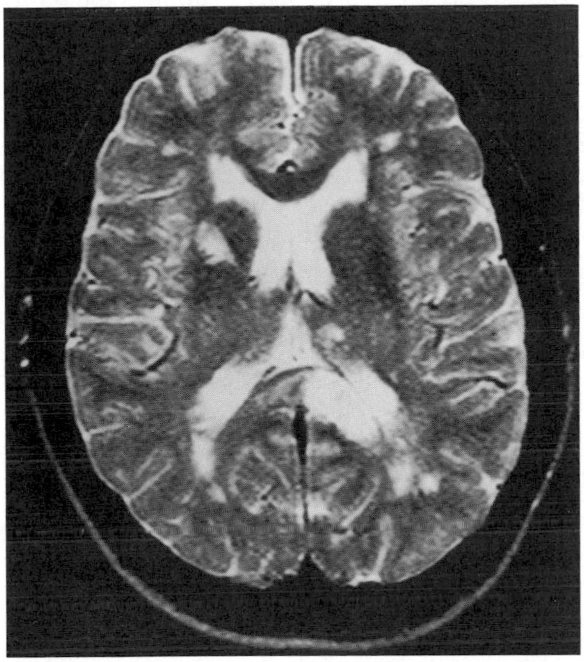

B

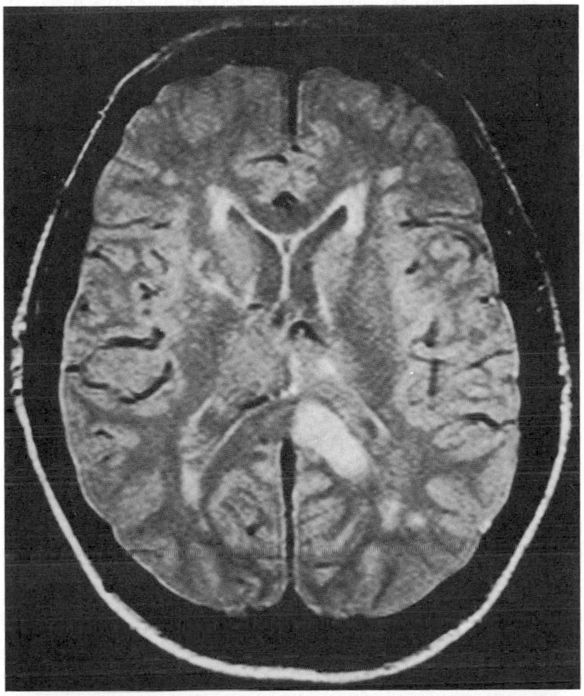

C

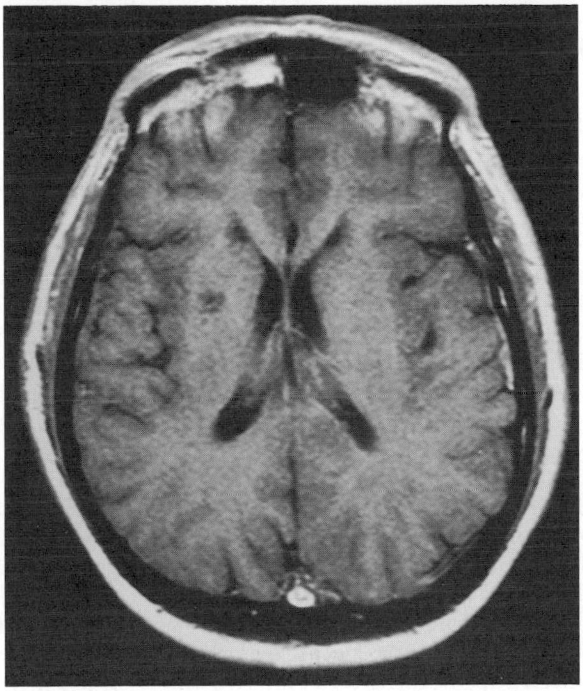

**Fig. 10-6. (A)** T2-weighted MR 3 weeks after acute stroke showing the clinically recent occipital and callosal infarction, and the old contralateral capsular infarction. **(B)** Balanced MR at the same time. **(C)** T1-weighted MR at the same time showing only faint signs of the recent infarction and the well-established signs of old infarction.

agent to the site of infarction. In the "early and/or intense enhancement" it is believed that either the occlusion is incomplete or that there is sufficient collateral circulation to transport the contrast agent to the infarction. In other words, the ischemia in this second group is partial. This reasoning would also explain the more favorable clinical outcome obtained in these cases.

Another type of contrast enhancement in stroke patients is the enhancement of arteries. This is an accentuation of the image of the arteries, which normally show a signal void. There is not only restoration of the signal of the artery, but there is further enhancement of these vessels. It is seen in the arteries supplying the region of infarctions where there is substantial slowing of the circulation. It is most commonly observed in association with cortical parenchymal enhancement of the "progressive" type with late onset; that is, in those cases with complete ischemia.

## Appearance of Cerebral Infarction

A distinctive diagnostic aspect of infarctions is their appearance, which depends on the vascular territory involved. The conformity of an infarction to a vascular territory is an important element in the diagnosis that helps to distinguish these lesions from brain tumors, brain inflammation, and brain trauma. Besides conforming to a known vascular territory, infarctions tend to have less mass effect for their size than neoplasms, particularly rapid-growing neoplasms. Cortical enhancement and cortical hemorrhage also favor the diagnosis of infarction. A brief discussion of the various vascular territories is helpful as a background for the diagnosis of cerebral infarctions.

### Supratentorial Vascular Territories

Lesions due to vascular occlusions of the anterior, middle, or posterior cerebral arteries or their branches in their course in the subarachnoid space usually result in the characteristic distribution of the infarction.

The anterior cerebral artery gives a few perforators (including the recurrent artery of Heubner), which enter the anterior perforated substance supplying the anterior portion of the caudate nucleus and the anterior limb of the internal capsule. These perforators arise from the initial segment of the anterior cerebral artery; more distally, the anterior cerebral artery supplies the orbital surface of the frontal lobe and the frontal pole, the medial aspect of the frontal lobe, a small strip on the convexity aspect of the frontal and parietal lobes, the genu and the anterior two-thirds of the corpus callosum, the fornix, and the septum pellucidum.

The middle cerebral artery provides perforating branches through the anterior perforated substance, which supplied the anterior two-thirds of the internal capsule, most of the globus pallidus, and nearly all the putamen. Distally, the middle cerebral artery supplies the insula, almost 80 percent of the convexity surface of the frontal and parietal lobes, the entire lateral aspect of the temporal lobe, the tip of the temporal lobe, and a small strip on the inferior surface of the temporal lobe. It receives collaterals from the anterior cerebral artery and posterior cerebral arteries along a strip on the convexity surface of the brain only a few centimeters lateral to the superior sagittal sinus.

The posterior cerebral artery supplies the posterior thalamus and midbrain through its perforating thalamic and thalamogeniculate branches. Its peripheral branches supply the medial aspect of the entire occipital and parietal lobes and extends over the convexity aspect of these two lobes to anastomose with middle cerebral branches. The posterior cerebral supplies also the tentorial surface of the occipital lobe and the posterior two-thirds of the temporal lobe (Fig. 10-7).

The anterior choroidal artery supplies the optic tract anteriorly, the choroid plexus of the lateral ventricle, the hippocampal formation, the lateral thalamic nuclei, a large portion of the posterior limb of the internal capsule, and the optic radiation (Fig. 10-8).

### Posterior Fossa Vascular Territories

Infarctions of the brain stem and cerebral hemispheres are notoriously difficult to appreciate on CT because of the bone artifacts from the skull. MRI is by far the preferred modality for imaging these lesions. The practical problem, however, is that patients with brain stem lesions are often uncooperative and unable to hold still during the MR examination. This problem is decreasing because of the availability of the fast imaging sequence (fast spin-echo techniques), which remarkably reduce examination time and are better tolerated by the sick patient.

Ischemic lesions in the pons are usually due to occlusion of the basilar artery or its perforating vessels. Characteristically, they involve one side of the pons and seem to stop abruptly at the midline. Its appearance is due to the very characteristic distribution of the median perforating arteries of the basilar artery.

The cerebellum is supplied by three artery territories. The posterior inferior cerebellar artery territory (PICA) covers the posterior lateral part of the medulla, the cerebellar tonsils, and the inferior lateral aspects of the cerebellar hemispheres and the inferior vermis. Occlusions of various segments of this vessel will produce a characteristic infarction in the territory described above. The territory of the anterior inferior cerebellar artery (AICA) will produce infarctions in the brachium pontis and the anterior inferior aspect of the cerebellar hemisphere. A small segment of the posterior medulla is also supplied by the AICA. The superior cerebellar artery territory includes the

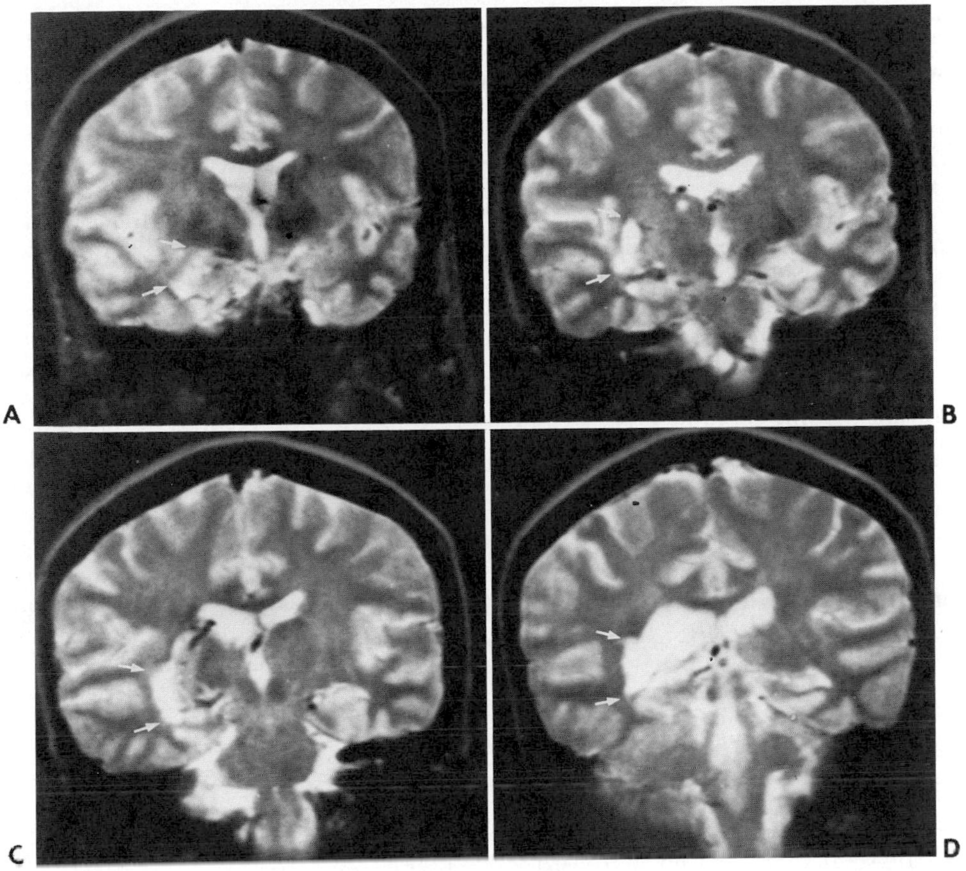


**Fig. 10-7.** Four coronal views of the brain on T2-weighted MR showing infarction in the territory of the anterior choroidal artery territory. (From Mohr et al.,[34] with permission.)

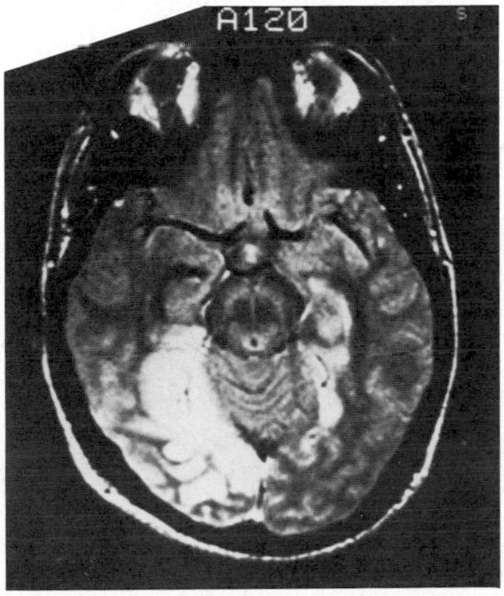


**Fig. 10-8.** Axial T2-weighted MR showing bilateral posterior cerebral artery territory infarction.

mesencephalon, the quadrigeminal plate, the superior cerebellar peduncle, the superior medullary velum, the superior vermis, and the posterior part of the cerebellar hemispheres. While the collateral anastomoses over the cerebellar hemispheres are generous between the superior cerebellar, the anterior inferior cerebellar, and the posterior inferior cerebellar arteries, the brain stem vascular supply is primarily from end arteries with no significant collateral channels, making it more vulnerable to occlusive vascular disease than the cerebellar hemispheres.

## White Matter Lesions

The great sensitivity of MR to changes in water protons has created images that, in some instances, may not be safely assumed to represent the products of infarction, that is, tissue loss alone. Other possibilities include edema, enlarged vascular spaces, transudation of spinal fluid across incompetent ventricular walls, and even thinning of tissue from atrophy and transsynaptic fiber degeneration.[41] The most important is the possibility that patchy white matter signal changes is a sign of arteriolosclerosis. Van Swieten et al.[55] found periventricular images of increased signal of T2-weighted images in 10 percent of those in their sixties, and in 50 percent of those in their eighties among their 40 subjects. Whole-brain sections in 19 patients showed a correlation with the histologic severity of demyelination and astrocytic gliosis. They noted that demyelination was related to an increased wall thickness of the arterioles up to 150 μm. Axonal loss was present to varying degrees in the white matter showing demyelination. They concluded that arteriolosclerosis was the primary factor in the pathogenesis of diffuse white matter lesions in the elderly, setting in train demyelination and axonal loss. It may well be that MR has properly directed attention to what was dismissed as staining artifacts in earlier neuropathology studies. Brains showing these lesions have shown poor blood flow in the white matter as tested by single photon emission computed tomography (SPECT).[8]

The perivascular spaces are seen most frequently in association with the anterior perforated substance near the anterior commissure, occasionally in the midbrain, and frequently in the subcortical white matter in the high convexity lesion.

### Late Changes

The shrinkage of tissue after infarction is a well-known effect. Less well known is the distant effect on pathways and target organs as the degenerating fiber pathways cause tissue shrinkage. Uchino et al.[54] studied presumed Wallerian degeneration of the corticospinal tract through the brain in 25 patients who had suffered supratentorial infarction. Within 3 months some signal hyperintensities were seen on T2-weighted images ipsilaterally in the brain stem and at 6 months the ipsilateral brain stem had become smaller ipsilaterally.

MR is just beginning to be used to track the course of therapy on lesions. Koppensteiner et al.[27] reported a patient with polyarteritis nodosa in whom multiple cerebral lesions were seen on the first MR, but the majority of which had disappeared completely on follow-up studies. Autopsy showed no abnormalities in the brain save for the single area seen on MR. Other examples will doubtless be documented.

## DURAL SINUS THROMBOSIS

MRI is the preferred modality for the diagnosis of venous sinus thrombosis clinically. The collateral venous channels on the surface of the brain are quite abundant and have enough capacity to compensate for a slow sinus occlusion, and in these cases no clinical symptoms may be observed. If the sinus occlusion is rapid and/or involves a large sinus, such as the superior sagittal sinus or the lateral sinus, the process may cause hemorrhagic venous infarction in the affected territory.

In the case of the superior sagittal sinus thrombosis one sees parasagittal hemorrhagic infarctions commonly bilaterally, but not always. The infarction will not leave the characteristic vascular territory distribution and tends to occur at the gray-white matter junction. Hemorrhagic transformation within the infarction is seen as a high signal on the T1-weighted image or a signal void on the T2-weighted image, depending on the age of the hemorrhagic changes. Besides hemorrhagic infarction, there is absence of the signal void in the superior sagittal sinus seen on the T1 images, and one may see the hyperintensity of the sinus on the T1 images because of the methemoglobin phase. The T2-weighted images may show what appears to be a signal void in the sinus, which is due to the paramagnetic effect of the blood product, such as the intracellular methemoglobin phase or the intracellular deoxyhemoglobin. The most reliable sign therefore is a high signal from the sinus on the T1-weighted images. The MR image might be confusing in some cases when there is a partial thrombosis of the sinus or recanalization of the previously occluded sinus. In such cases only a fraction of the cross-section of the sinus may be blocked by the clot and the associated infarction may not be hemorrhagic.

## ARTERIAL OCCLUSION

The signal void of occlusion has been found in many instances of large-artery intracranial occlusion. A recent report from the Japanese literature by Uchino et al.[53] indicated all 10 angiographically proven examples of middle cerebral artery stem occlusion with stroke were identified by the absence of flow void on MR, demonstrated as an isodense or hypodense structure on T2-weighted images. Absence of the expected flow void was also found in the sylvian fissure in eight cases on T2-weighted images.

## NONOCCLUSIVE INFARCTION

Cerebral infarctions result from a variety of mechanisms not requiring a vascular occlusion. Examples are hypotension, anemia, hypoxemia (open heart surgery), hypoglycemia, or metabolic enzymatic deficiencies such as mitochondrial encephalopathies. In most cases in children, the gray matter, particularly that of the basal ganglia, seems to be more affective than any other part of the brain. Also, typically in cases of severe hypotension, there may be involvement of the borderzones and adjacent distal arterial territories of the major cerebral arteries. This state is also observed in occlusions of the cervical carotid artery with diminished perfusion to the cerebral hemisphere. Other lesions include the changes brought about by occlusive disease of small vessels, such as in

Binswanger's disease with diffuse increased signal intensity in the subcortical white matter.

Another condition that deserves mention is the transient hyperintensity of white matter in patients with hypertensive encephalopathy or preeclampsia and eclampsia. In these cases there is a reversible increase in the white matter signal in the para-atrial regions and often also in the cerebellar white matter.

## HEMORRHAGIC INFARCTION

Hemorrhagic transformation of ischemic brain infarction was found at autopsy to occur more often in embolic strokes than in thrombotic strokes. The rate of hemorrhagic infarctions was reported to vary from 54[12] to 78 percent.[24] It is believed that the hemorrhagic transformation of a pale infarction results from a two-step process: (1) an ischemic insult that causes damage to the endothelial vascular wall, and (2) restoration of blood flow to the injured vascular territory. The reperfusion may be due to either a recanalization of the occluded vessel or the establishment of collateral blood supply to the infarction or both. In recent studies by CT scans and angiography Bozzao et al.[3] found that hemorrhagic infarction developed in 18 of 36 stroke patients with middle cerebral artery occlusion within 7 days after onset, while no hemorrhagic infarction was present on the initial CT obtained at 4 hours. Pessin et al.[40] comment that "hemorrhagic infarction is a natural and common tissue accompaniment of cerebral embolic infarction. Its clinical significance may have been exaggerated as a consequence of its association with the neurologic effects of the infarct itself." Hemorrhagic transformation is more common in cortical infarction. It was observed in all patients with a cortical hypointensity seen on CT (10/10) reported by Bozzao et al.,[3] while they found hemorrhagic changes in only 11 out of 24 patients with basal ganglia infarctions. The preponderance of hemorrhagic changes in cortical lesions is due to the collateral blood supply in the cortex. Mechanisms of hemorrhage in deep strokes depend only on the recanalization of the middle cerebral artery (MCA) stem and its perforating branches, since there is no potential for establishing a collateral circulation to the deep infarction.

It is important to distinguish between hemorrhagic infarction and parenchymatous hematoma in the assessment of intracranial bleeding, and both should not be casually grouped together. There are undoubtedly some parenchymatous hematomas that arise from severe multicentric bleeding after reperfusion of capillaries injured by ischemia. These cases cannot be distinguished from the rupture of one or more small arterioles without the ischemic insult. Parenchymatous hematomas are known to be associated with clinical worsening, unlike hemorrhagic infarctions. Parenchymatous hematomas on CT generally show a more homogeneous high-density, well-demarcated region with a prominent mass effect and frequently intraventricular bleeding. Hemorrhagic infarctions, on the other hand, are more inhomogeneous, patchy, and gyriform in distribution.

On MRI, hemorrhagic infarctions are recognized by a high-signal intensity on T1-weighted images and patchy signal void in the midst of the high-signal region of T2-weighted images (Fig. 10-9). Cortical hemorrhagic infarctions may show a serpiginous signal void of the cortical zone of the affected gyri. The changes in signal intensity of hemorrhagic infarction differ from that of the usual hematoma in that it is not associated with the pronounced signal void on T2-weighted images or on gradient echo sequences. Also, the appearance of the high signal due to methemoglobin occurs very early after the ischemic episode (1st or 2nd day) and is not in keeping with the usual 3 to 4 days needed for the oxidation process of hemoglobin to methemoglobin.[17] Compared to CT, MR is more sensitive to detection of intraparenchymal blood, while subarachnoid hemorrhage is better detected by CT.

## CEREBRAL HEMATOMA

In the early days of MRI, CT was deemed more sensitive than MR for the detection of cerebral hemorrhage.[26] With the early, smaller (0.15 tesla) magnets available, Bydder et al.[6] found very low intensity areas (black signals) in 11 of 12 cases involving central regions (three cases), and a peripheral rim (seven cases), or more diffuse patterns (two cases). The central low-intensity regions were found in all stages from the acute to the chronic phases.

This was at the time when the MR characteristics of blood were little understood and when the available magnet systems had a relatively low field (0.15 tesla) that did not permit the detection of the full spectrum of signal changes from each of the blood products. It was the work of Gomori and his collaborators[15,16] that laid down the foundation of our understanding of the MR characteristics of cerebral hematomas at different fields. For descriptive purposes, the MRI appearance of cerebral hematoma can be classified into four stages: hyperacute, acute, subacute, and late.

### Hyperacute Hematoma

It is rare that a cerebral hematoma is imaged in the hyperacute stage in the actual clinical setting. This stage lasts only a few hours and it is uncommon that a patient can actually be imaged so soon after a stroke. Hyperacute hematomas consist of freshly extravasated red blood cells containing oxyhemoglobin. There are no paramagnetic properties of oxyhemoglobin, which has no unpaired electrons. MRI signal characteristics of oxyhemoglobin are similar to those

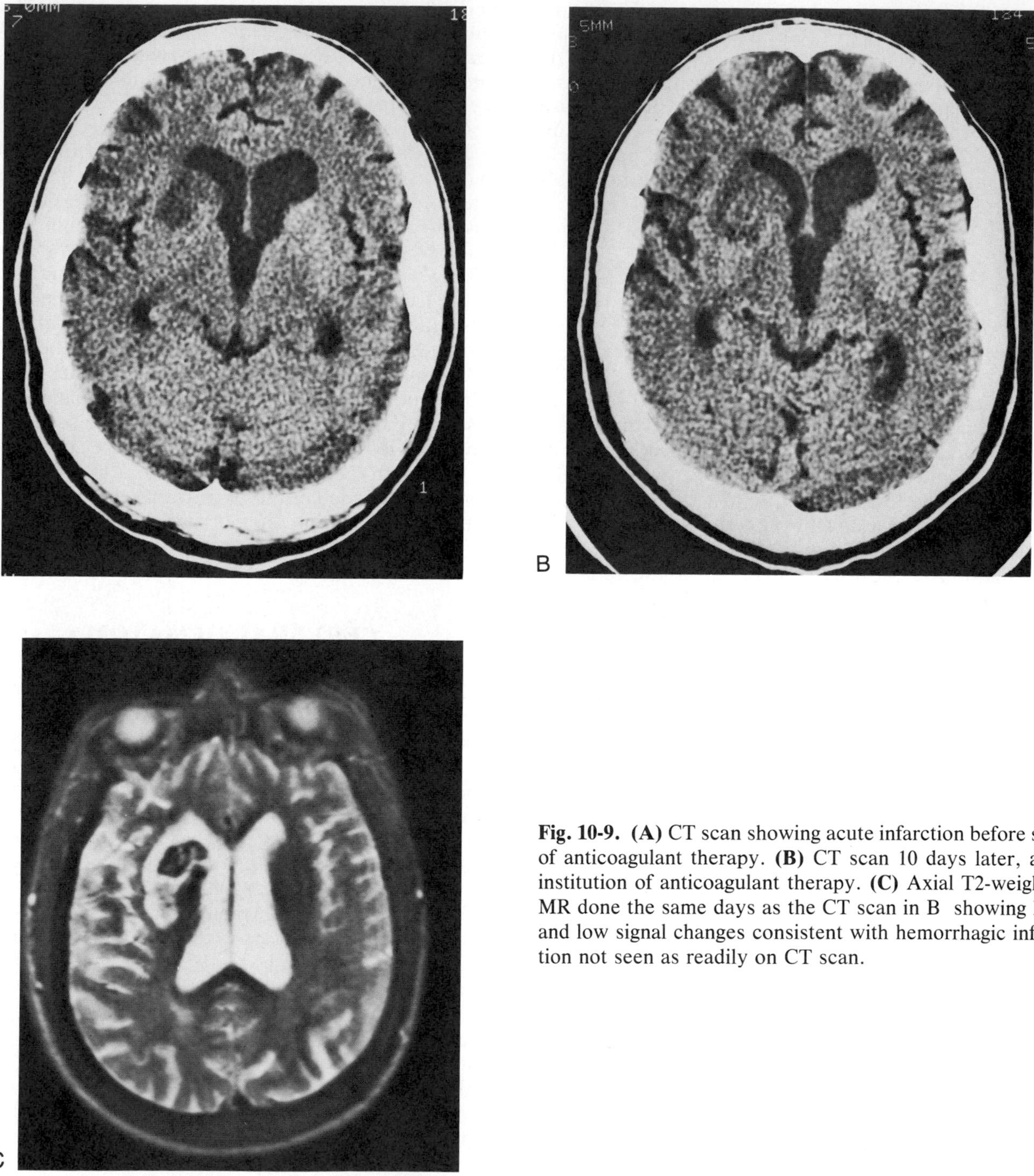

A B C

**Fig. 10-9.** **(A)** CT scan showing acute infarction before start of anticoagulant therapy. **(B)** CT scan 10 days later, after institution of anticoagulant therapy. **(C)** Axial T2-weighted MR done the same days as the CT scan in B showing high and low signal changes consistent with hemorrhagic infarction not seen as readily on CT scan.

of any other brain lesion, being slightly hypointense on T1-weighted images and bright on T2-weighted images because of the higher water content increasing the spin density. The hematoma is very sharply demarcated with a hypointense rim on T1-weighted images representing a serum pocket surrounding the retracted clot. On T2-weighted images this rim is bright and is surrounded by a zone of brain edema.

Weingarten et al.[58] studied experimental animals and showed that neither T1- nor T2-weighted sequences can reliably detect small hematomas in the hyperacute stage, but that hypointense signals could often be obtained. Zyed et al.[62] documented hypointense signals in 45 of 46 cases studied. Using a very high field magnet (2.35 tesla), Zuerrer et al.[61] studied the course of hematomas in 28 pediatric patients. Hematomas less than 3 days old showed an isointense to mildly hypointense appearance on T1-weighted images and were strikingly hypointense on long T2-weighted images. After about a week, the hematoma signal also became hyperintense on T1-weighted images. The changes were evident on the periphery first, spreading centripetally. The hematomas became uniformly hyperintense by the end of the 2nd week. Gomori et al.[15] compared the appearance of hemorrhage in the 1st week from that in the 1st month from that after a year. In all studies, the disappearance of the central hypointensity helped establish the time of onset of hemorrhage retrospectively.

## Acute Hematoma

During the acute stage, which starts several hours after bleeding, oxyhemoglobin, a diamagnetic molecule, is reduced to deoxyhemoglobin, which has four unpaired electrons and is paramagnetic (Fig. 10-10). The iron atom in this molecule is shielded by the surrounding globin protein from the close approach of water molecules. Consequently, deoxyhemoglobin cannot affect the relaxivity of water protons by dipole-dipole interaction, precluding a shortening of the T1 of water. No bright signal therefore should be expected on the T1-weighted images from deoxyhemoglobin. The packaging of the paramagnetic deoxyhemoglobin in the red cells, on the other hand, will cause a focal distortion of the magnetic field, leading to a significant T2* effect, which reduces the signal on the T2-weighted images. In short, the acute hematoma signal characteristics appear around 24 hours from the bleed, and they consist primarily of a slightly hypointense signal on T1-weighted images and a markedly hypointense region on the T2-weighted signal. The hypointensity on the T1 is due to the pronounced shortening of the T2 relaxation. The signal void on the T2-weighted images is better appreciated on a higher field magnet and with longer echo times (TE = 80 ms or longer).

## Subacute Hematoma

The subacute stage occurs at 2 to 7 days after the bleeding and is marked by methemoglobin formation as a result of the oxidation of oxyhemoglobin and/or deoxyhemoglobin. At the beginning of the subacute stage the methemoglobin is contained within intact red blood corpuscles, and toward the end of this stage the red blood cells lyse, freeing methemoglobin, which diffuses throughout the hematoma. At this stage the hematoma is a proteinaceous water solution. At the same time there is an inflammatory repair

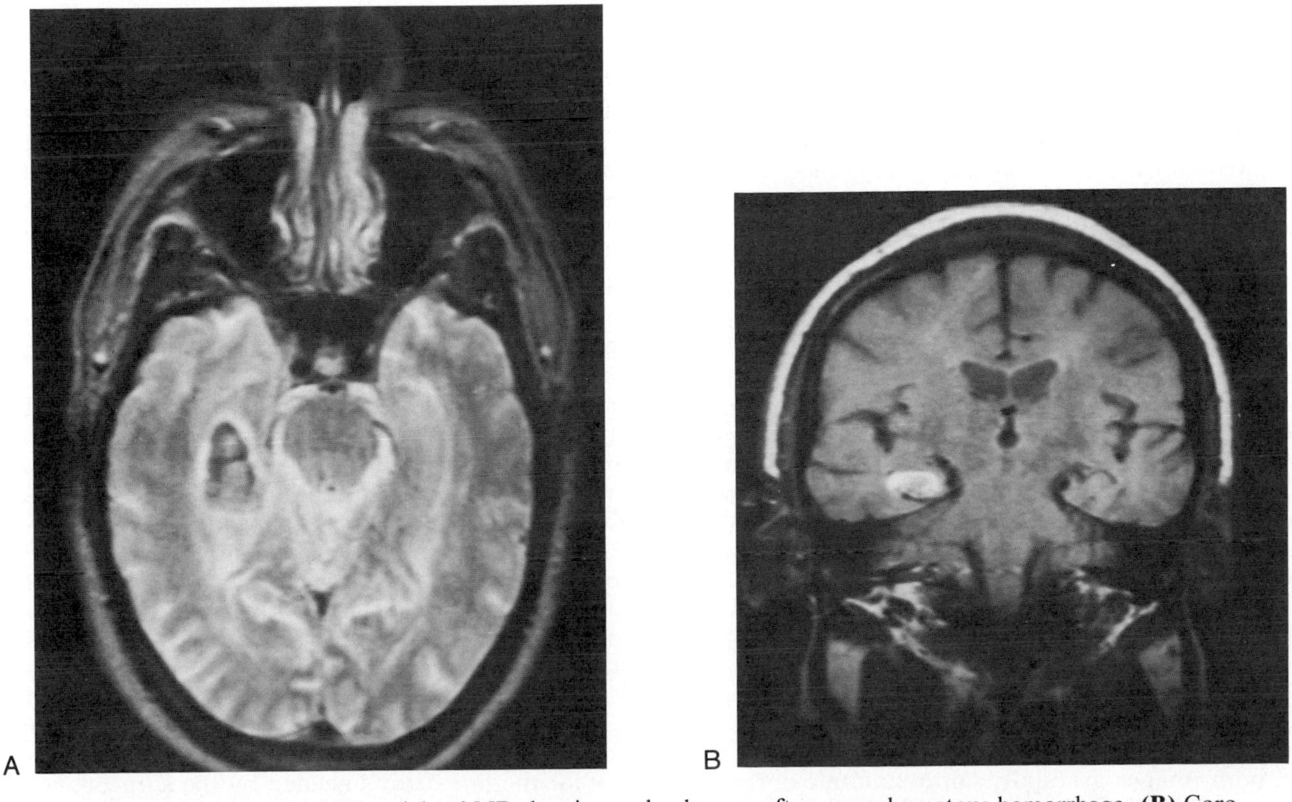

**Fig. 10-10.** **(A)** Axial T2-weighted MR showing early changes after parenchymatous hemorrhage. **(B)** Coronal T1-weighted MR at the same time showing predominantly bright signal from the recent hemorrhage.

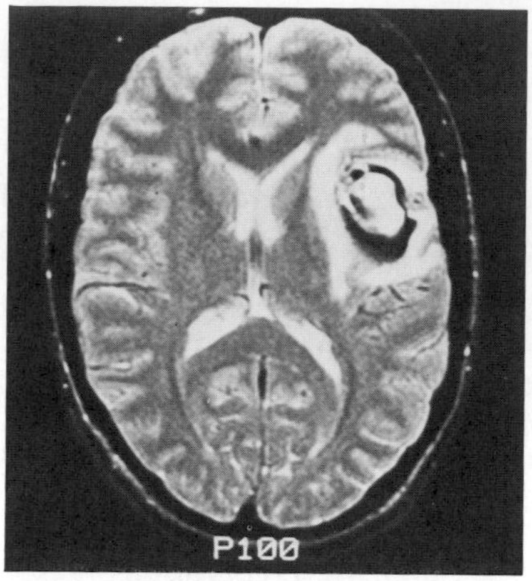


**Fig. 10-11.** Axial T2-weighted MR showing rim of edema, external ring of low signal and central high signal.

response within the tissue surrounding the hematoma with phagocytes and macrophages infiltrating the boundary of the hematoma (Fig. 10-11).

This process results in storage of iron products in the periphery of the hematoma. The MRI image characteristic of the subacute phase depends on (1) the presence of methemoglobin, (2) whether the methemoglobin is still packaged in the red blood cells (RBCs), and (3) on the extent of the phagocytic activities in the periphery of the hematoma.

In the early subacute phase on the T1-weighted image the methemoglobin will produce a bright signal at the periphery of the hematoma and gradually spreads to within the clot because the oxidation of methemoglobin starts at the periphery. On the T2-weighted image in the early subacute phase, there is a signal void at the site of the hematoma as long as there are intact red blood cells containing the methemoglobin. The periphery of the hematoma has a dark zone due to the signal void from the T2* effect of the macrophages (perhaps hemosiderin form). In the late subacute phase the hematoma is bright on both T1 and T2. The high signal on T1 is due to the shortening of the T1 of water by dipole-dipole interaction with methemoglobin, and the bright signal on T2 is due to the increased water spin-density in the proteinaceous watery solution of the hematoma. Again, at this stage, there is a black rim surrounding the hematoma due to ferrous iron stored, such as in hemosiderin form.

## Intermediate Changes

After the first week, the hypointense T2-weighted images gradually become hyperintense, while T1-weighted images also become progressively hyperintense, both images gradually approximating one another (Fig. 10-12).[17] The changes occur first at the periphery of the hematoma toward the center. The signal changes reflect the increasing concentration of methemoglobin, which replaces the deoxyhemoglobin.

## Late Changes

In the late stages, beyond 1 month, the T2-weighted images become even more hypointense.[15] These changes reflect the conversion of methemoglobin to hemosiderin, most of which is found in macrophages. The location of macrophages broadly throughout the hematoma makes the hypointensity rather diffuse—the later in the course, the more diffuse. T1-weighted images also show similar findings. Thulborn et al.[50] studied changes in rat hemorrhage and found both ferritin and hemosiderin, iron-storage substances in chronic hematomas. These changes have been recently summarized by Williams et al.[59]

The existence of chronic changes in the rim of the lesion was used by Nakajima et al.[37] to document the frequency of hemorrhages in a group of clinically asymptomatic patients. The authors reported in Japanese their detection of 17 patients with asymptomatic hemorrhages among 2,757 who had brain MR using a 1.0-T unit. These 17 patients represented a 1.5 percent frequency among patients with stroke and 9.5 percent among those with hemorrhage. No other estimates of frequency have yet appeared to our knowledge as of late 1991.

## Arteriovenous Malformations

Only in recent years has attention been paid to the ability of MRI to document flowing blood. The very low intensity signal characteristic of blood flowing through vessels through an area of hemorrhage helps demonstrate arteriovenous malformation (AVM) as the underlying cause. A special program has been developed by General Electric, using their 1.5 tesla MRI to stall the flowing blood image, leaving behind the images indicative of previous hemorrhage alone, a program we have also reproduced at our institution for use on a Phillips MR device.

As opposed to angiogram, which reveals nothing of the brain parenchyma, MR shows the relationships to surrounding brain well and has proved superior to angiography in defining the nidus[38] and the margins of the lesion.[22] Evidence of prior hemorrhage and its source,[31] the size of the nidus, the source of flow to the lesion, the course of draining veins, and the relation of the malformation to normal brain structures are now regularly shown (Fig. 10-13). The nidus of the AVM is best seen by MR compared with CT or angiogram.[38]

In the last 5 years, this technique has almost eclipsed angiogram and far surpassed CT scanning for the diagnosis of AVM.[28] MR has yet to replace angiography for the fine details needed by the surgeon, but for routine diagnosis and management planning, MR can now be relied upon as the first line of diagnosis

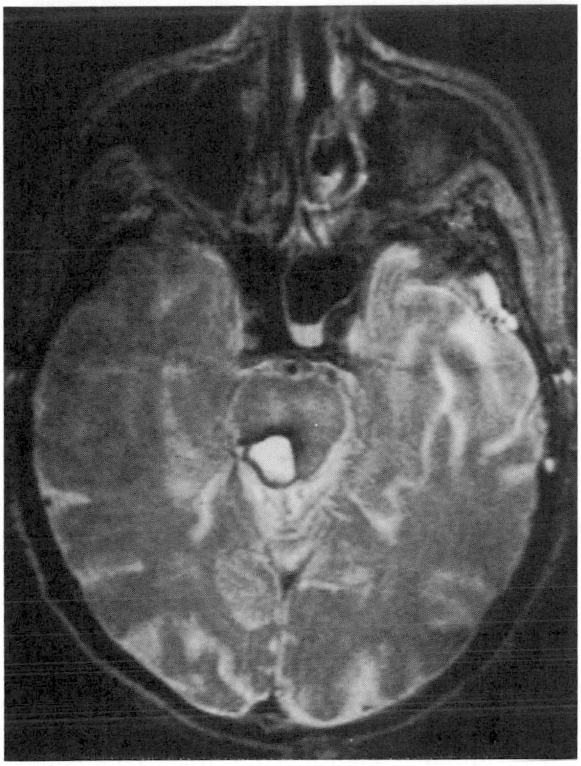

A

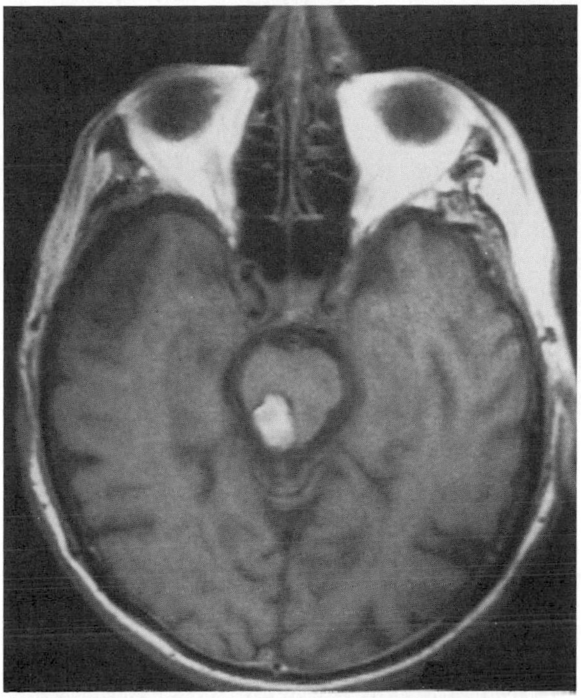

B

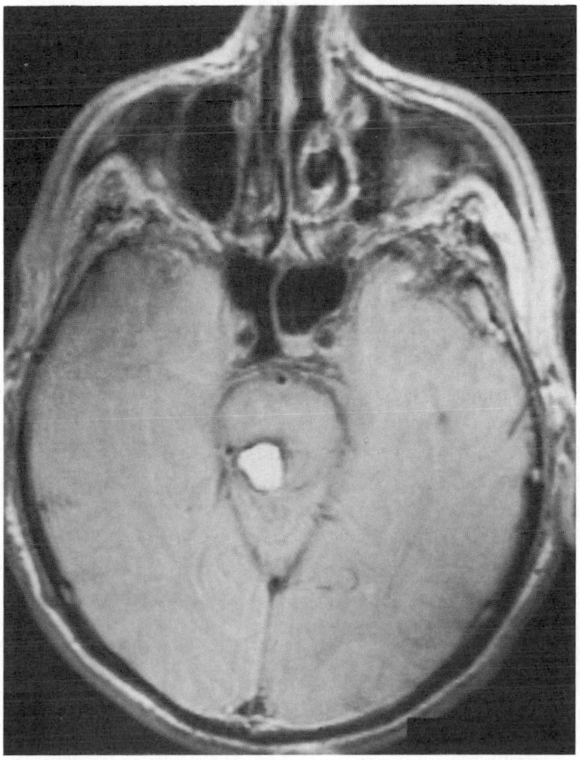

C

**Fig. 10-12. (A)** Axial T2-weighted MR showing changes several weeks after parenchymatous hemorrhage. **(B)** Axial balanced MR at the same time showing similar changes. **(C)** Axial T1-weighted MR at the same time showing similar changes.

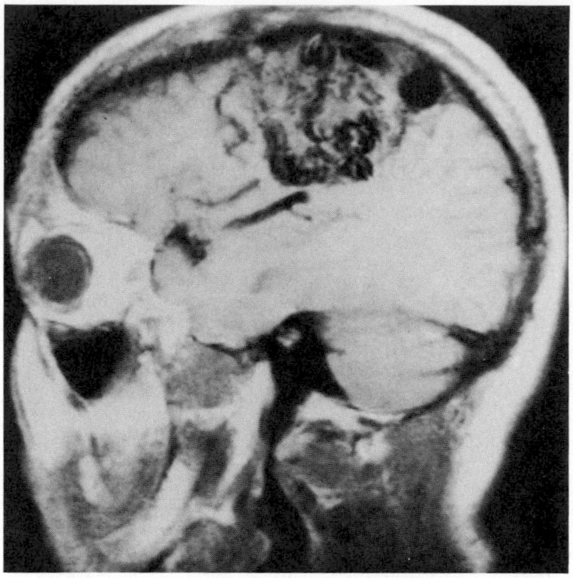


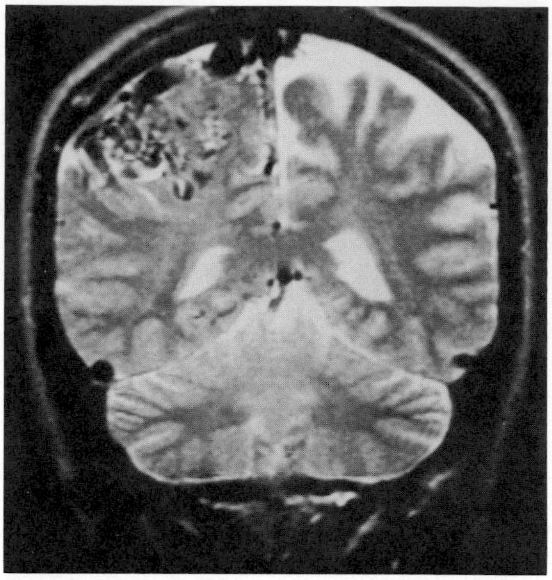


**Fig. 10-13. (A)** Sagittal T1-weighted MR of a large convexity AVM. **(B)** Coronal T2-weighted MR of the same AVM.

(Fig. 10-14). Early reports with low field magnets[28,45] showed the high-flow vascular channels of an AVM as dark areas or regions of "reduced signal." The intensity of the signal void is related to the flow rates, a finding that offers the opportunity to calculate blood flow noninvasively.

It has even become possible to combine techniques: in a study of 35 patients with AVM imaged by MR, the epileptogenic AVM seems more superficial in the cortex, had bled before, and was somewhat larger than the nonepileptogenic.[52]

## Cavernous Malformations

The small angiomas known as cavernous malformations have been readily identified by MR. The flow through these lesions is minimal, and therefore they are rarely seen on angiograms. The distinctive central focus of high signal surrounded by hypointensity seen on MR, the so-called "cat's eye," makes the diagnosis more frequent since the introduction of MR scanning. This appearance, once considered pathognomonic for cavernous angiomas, is so no longer, as it has also been found in AVM[42] and even in tumor.[49] Even so, the distinctive finding has been used by several authors to explain small hematomas found in unusual locations, such as the brain stem (Fig. 10-15).[13] The margins of the lesions are often smoother than those found in AVMs.[22]

Magnetic resonance imaging has allowed study of family members, which in a small series of cases have suggested a hereditary basis for some instances of multiple cavernous malformations.[43] Through this method, multiple foci have been seen in the same patient, one quite remote from the other (Fig. 10-16).

## Aneurysm

At first, any value for MR in acute subarachnoid hemorrhage was doubted. However, improved magnets and computer programs now makes it possible to separate the blood and aneurysm from surrounding brain and spinal fluid, and MR has been found as useful as CT for the diagnosis of subarachnoid hemorrhage.[30] Spickler et al.[48] studied acute subarachnoid hemorrhage in *Macaca* monkeys and made similar correlations in patients hours to weeks later. It was possible to demonstrate acute subarachnoid hemorrhage as an isointense signal in place of the normally hypointense cerebrospinal fluid spaces on T1-weighted images (Fig. 10-17). This signal changes after 4 days to a hyperintense signal on T1-weighted images, which was attributed to methemoglobin formation within the clot matrix.

MR has now come into general use as a means of diagnosing vascular causes of large compressive intracranial lesions, including cavernous aneurysms, dolicoectatic basilar arteries, (Fig. 10-17) and large basilar aneurysms.[2,29] A few striking examples have been described in which the dome or base of the aneurysm has been visualized by MR when it was not found by angiography.[39] Nagata et al.[36] reported in Japanese on 12 giant aneurysms studied by MR in which intraluminal thrombosis was found in 9. They noted thrombosis was more frequent in the larger aneurysms. The finding that thrombi were more prevalent posteriorly and inferiorly near the neck prompted the suggestion that it might be explained by stagnation of blood flow. This technique could benefit from further development.

Postoperatively, the use of ferromagnetic clips ini-

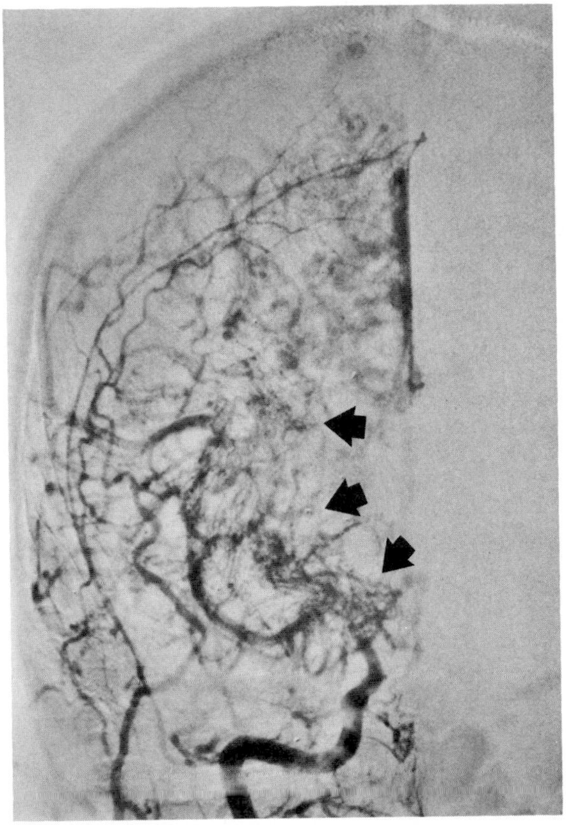

A

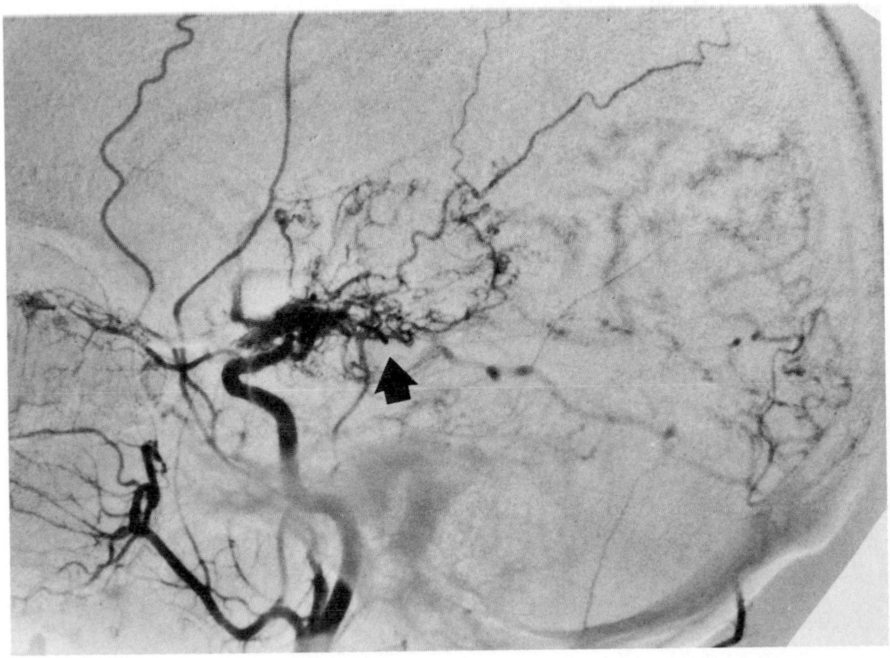

B

**Fig. 10-14. (A & B)** Angiograms showing both moyamoya changes and an arteriovenous malformation, the resistance to flow from the carotid stenosis and associated moyamoya preventing adequate visualization of the arteriovenous malformation. (*Figure continues.*)

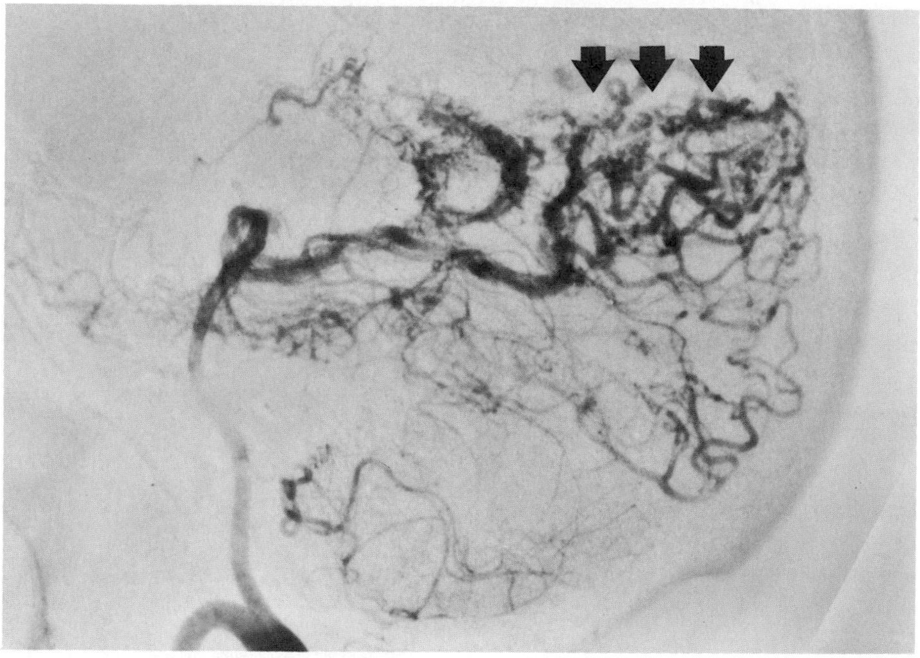

C

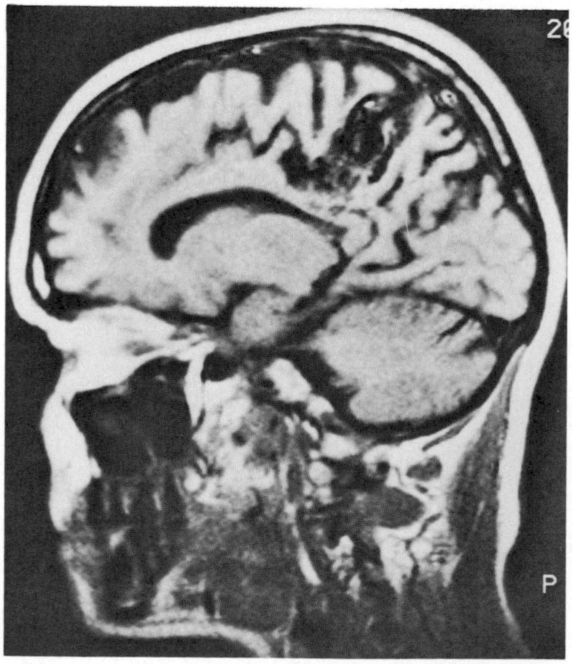


D

**Fig. 10-14** (*Continued*). **(C & D)** T1-weighted sagittal MR and gradient-recalled echo imaging sequence MR showing the presence and extent of an arteriovenous malformation better than that seen by angiogram. (*Figure continues*.)

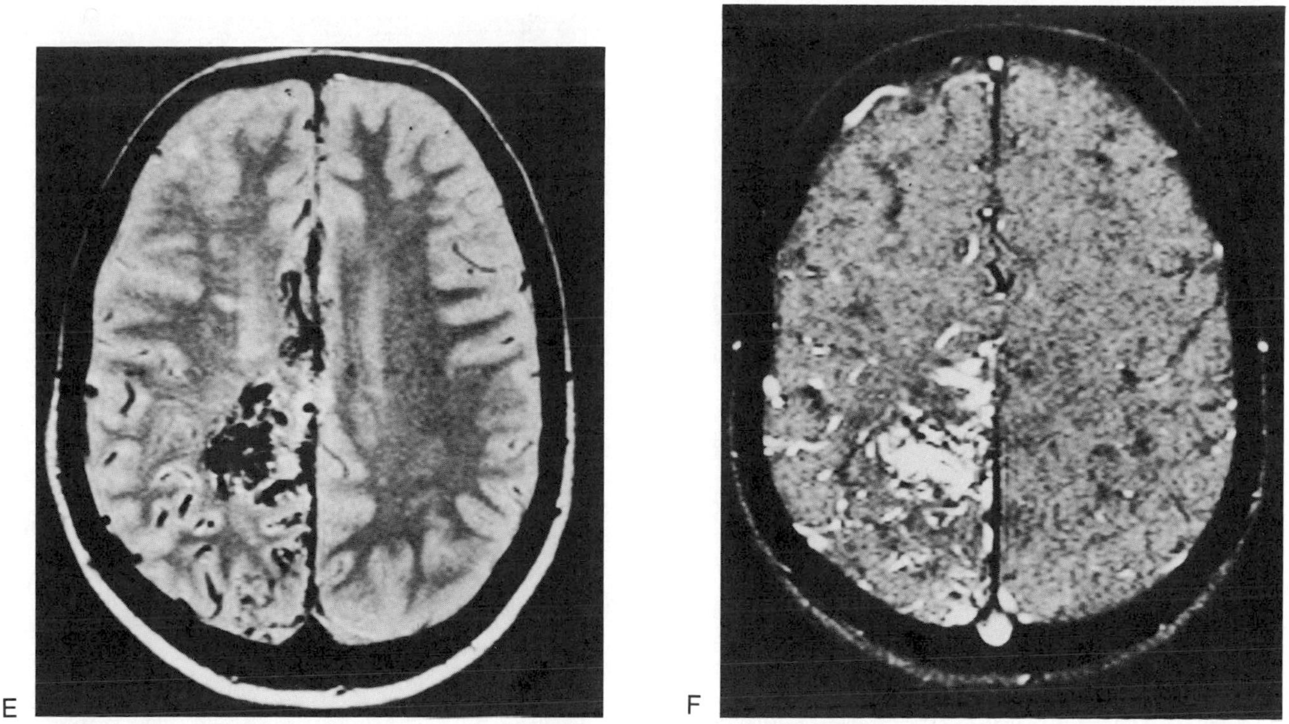


**Fig. 10-14** (*Continued*). **(E)** Axial T2-weighted MR and gradient-recalled echo imaging sequence MR **(F)** showing the presence and extent of an arteriovenous malformation better than seen by angiogram.

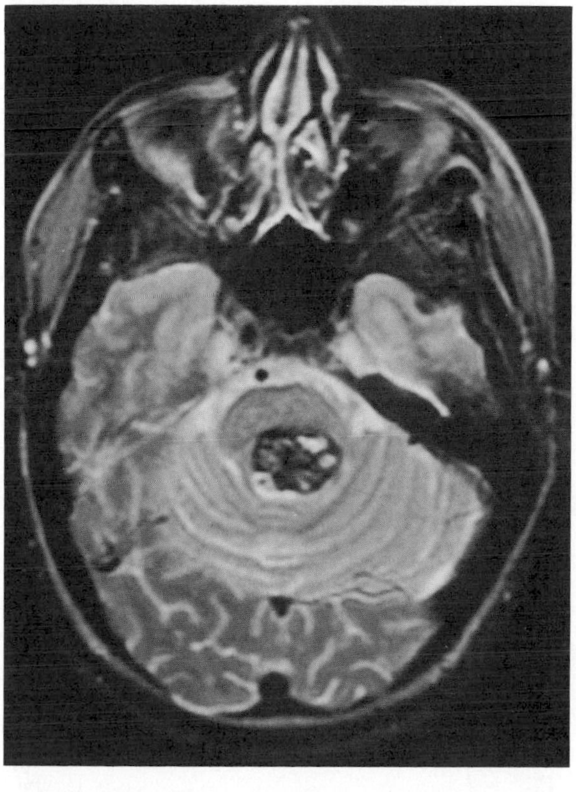

**Fig. 10-15.** Axial T2-weighted MR of a large cavernous angioma of the brainstem, later removed surgically.

tially made MR imaging a risk for postoperative evaluations, but these risks have subsided considerably with the introduction of nonferromagnetic materials. The main current problems are the major changes induced in the MR signal by the presence of the magnetic artifact.[11]

## COMPARISON OF MAGNETIC RESONANCE IMAGING AND COMPUTED TOMOGRAPHY SCANNING

MR offers a number of advantages over CT scanning. Multiplanar imaging is easily achieved by MR, more so than by CT. The gray and white matter differentiation is more conspicuous on MR images than by CT. The lack of signal from bone gives MR imaging an advantage over CT for the detection of infarction in the posterior fossa, particularly in the brain stem. The intrapetrous artifact, which is almost always present in CT, crossing the image of the brain stem, is absent on MRI. Indicative of these observations was an early study by Kertesz et al.[26] with 87 patients with infarction studied within a week by CT and MR: 40 patients were studied from 1 week to 4 months, and 25 were studied a year after onset. MR was found more sensitive than CT for the detection of infarction as well as TIA.[1]

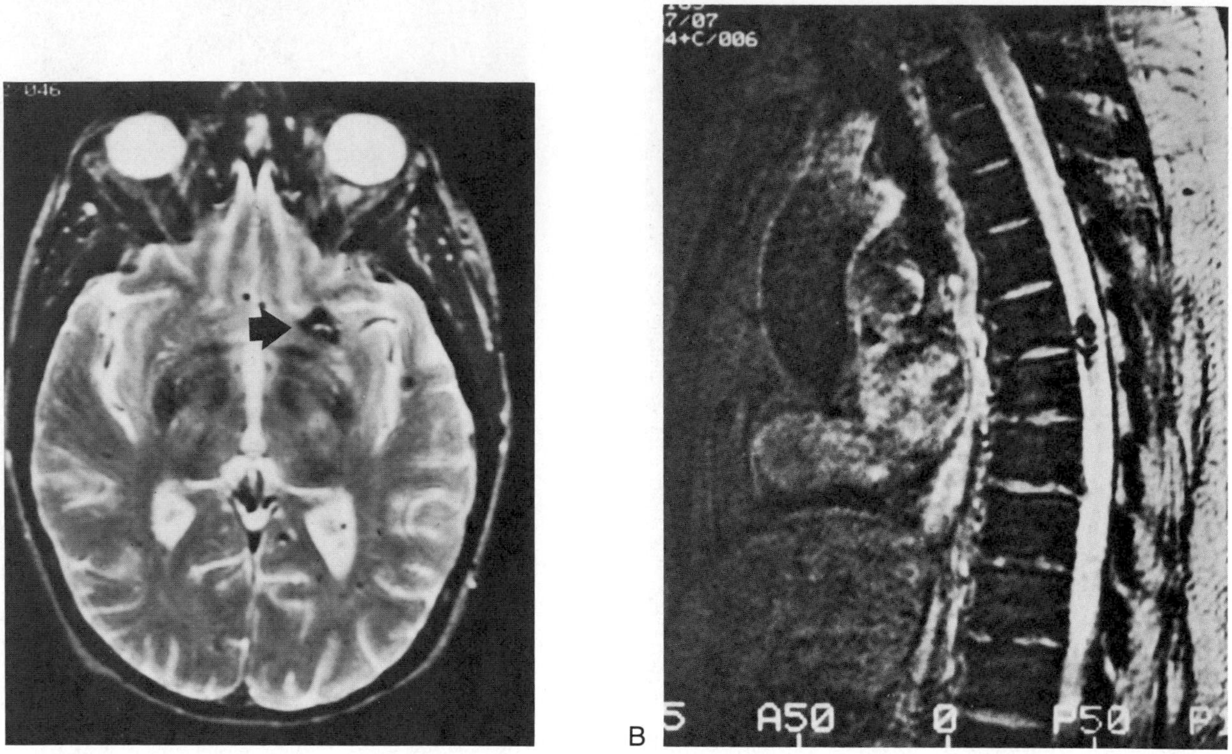


A B

**Fig. 10-16.** **(A & B)** T2-weighted MR images showing a cavernous angioma in the temporal lobe **(A)** and the spinal cord **(B)** in the same patient.

We had the opportunity to perform both MRI and CT within minutes of each other or MRI minutes to weeks after an initial stroke event.[34] The findings have not always been easily explained. Within 3 hours of acute stroke, 78 patients were recruited for brain imaging to compare the sensitivity of CT versus MR scans in detecting the first signs of hematoma or bland or hemorrhagic infarction. Follow-up scans were performed at 24 hours, 3 to 10 days, and 3 months. The mean time to first scan was 192 minutes (SD 122). Although infarction was detected as early as 1 hour, the fraction of positive first scans approached an asymptote at 5 hours. Overall, neither CT not MR proved superior in the early detection of hematoma or infarction. However, MR showed deep or brain stem infarction more frequently than did CT scan (14 vs 9 of 23), while CT scanning was at least as good as MR for convexity infarction (19 vs 18 of 36) and showed the lesions earlier. After 24 hours, MR more conspicuously defined the lesion limits.

Bryan et al.[5] found that by the end of the first 24 hours the long TR sequences of MRI are significantly more sensitive to the detection of infarction than CT, which can reveal only 58 percent of the lesions. On follow-up studies these workers found that CT is positive in 82 percent of the patients, while MR is positive in 95 percent of the cases that will eventually develop a detectable infarction corresponding to the site of the

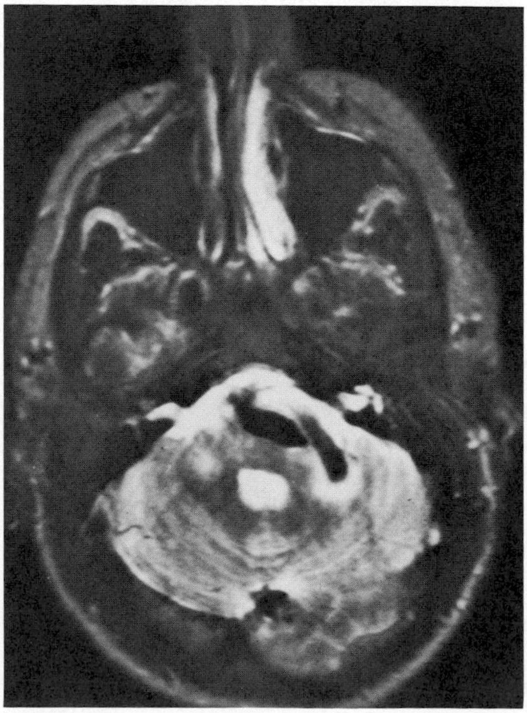

A

**Fig. 10-17.** **(A & B)** Axial T2-weighted **(A)** and sagittal T1-weighted. (*Figure continues.*)

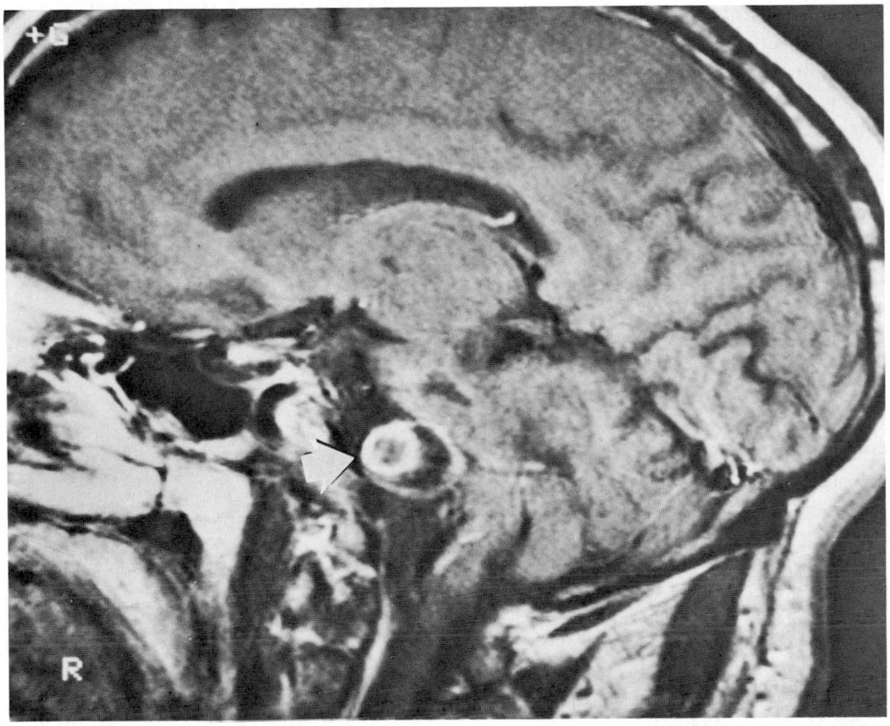

B

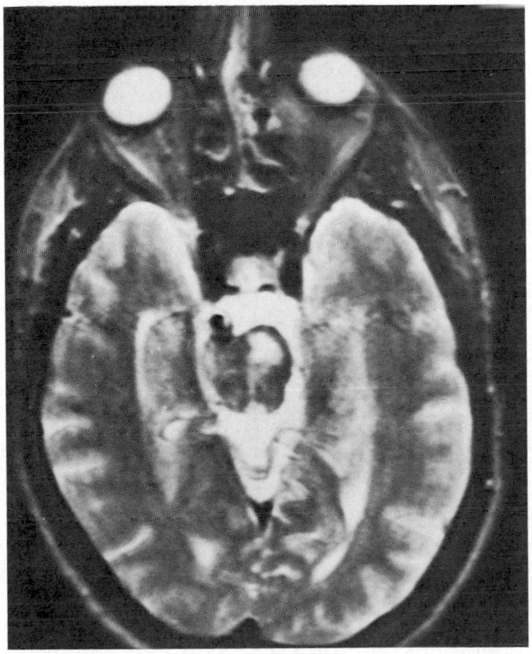

C

**Fig. 10-17** (*Continued*). **(B)** MR showing the thickened basilar in a case of dolico-ectasia with pontine infarction **(C)** in a plane above those showing the dolico-ectasia.

clinical stroke. The follow-up studies revealed new lesions that were not detected on the first examination, and lesions already seen appeared to be larger and more conspicuous on the follow-up studies.

CT is not only less sensitive than MR for the detection of acute infarction (58 percent vs 90 percent), but those lesions that are detected on CT are often difficult to identify, leading to only a tentative diagnosis. Imakita et al.[21] found MR more reliably positive than CT, with contrast enhancement helping the MR to show the lesion better. Bozzoa et al.[3] studied 36 patients with MCA infarction with CT within 4 hours of stroke and found 70 percent scans. This somewhat higher sensitivity is mostly due to the exclusion of posterior fossa infarctions and particularly brain stem lesions, which are very difficult to detect on CT due to the notorious intrapetrous artifact. Bozzoa and colleagues have also shown that early hypodensity on the initial CT, obtained within 4 hours after the ictus, predicted a hemorrhagic outcome in 72 percent of the patients. On the other hand, none of the patients who developed their CT hypodensity later than 24 hours developed hemorrhagic lesions. All patients with early CT hypodensity in the cortex developed hemorrhagic lesions, while the deep hemispheric infarctions were less prone to develop hemorrhage than cortical lesions.

## REFERENCES


1. Awad I, Modic M, Little JR et al: Focal parenchymal lesions in transient ischemic attacks: correlation of computed tomography and magnetic resonance imaging. Stroke 17:399, 1986
2. Bollensen E, Buzanoski JH, Prange HW: Brainstem compression by basilar artery anomalies as visualized by MRI. J Neurol 238:49, 1991
3. Bozzao L, Angeloni U, Bastianello S et al: Early angiographic and CT findings in patients with hemorrhagic infarction in the distribution of the middle cerebral artery. Am J Neuroradiol 12:1115, 1991
4. Brant-Zawadski M, Pereira B, Weinstein P et al: MR imaging of acute experimental ischemia in cats. AJNR 7:7, 1986
5. Bryan RN, Levy LM, Whitlow WD et al: Diagnosis of acute cerebral infarction: comparison of CT and MR imaging. AJNR 12:611, 1991
6. Bydder GM, Pennock JM, Porteous R et al: MRI of intracerebral haematoma at low field (0.15T) using T2 dependent partial saturation sequences. Neuroradiology 30:367, 1988
7. Crain MR, Yuh WTC, Greene GM et al: Cerebral ischemia: evaluation with contrast-enhanced MR imaging. AJNR 12:631,
8. De Cristofaro MT, Mascalchi M, Pupi A et al: Subcortical arteriosclerotic encephalopathy: single photon emission computed tomography magnetic resonance imaging correlation. Am J Physiol Imaging 5:68, 1990
9. Demaerel P, Van Hecke P, Marchal G et al: MRI of intraparenchymal hematoma: responsible mechanisms. J Belge Radiol 73:279, 1990
10. DeWitt LD: Clinical use of NMR imaging in stroke. Stroke 17:328, 1986
11. Doyon D, David P, Halimi P: Les clips vasculaires cérébraux en IRM: contre indication absolue où relative. J Radiol 70:123, 1989
12. Fisher CM, Adams RD: Observations on brain embolism with special reference to the mechanism of hemorrhagic infarction. J Neuropathol Exp Neurol 10:92, 1951
13. Froment JC, Bascoulergue Y, Crouzet G et al: Apparently isolated, spontaneous haematomas of the brain stem: seven cases explored by CT and MRI. J Neuroradiol 16:38, 1989
14. Fukuda O, Sato S, Suzuki T et al: MRI of acute cerebral infarction. No Shinkei Geka 17:31, 1989
15. Gomori JM, Grossman RI, Goldberg HI et al: Intracranial hematomas: imaging by high-field MR. Radiology 157:87, 1985
16. Gomeri JM, Grossman RI, Hackney DB et al: Variable appearances of subacute intracranial hematomas on high field spin echo MR. AJR 150:171, 1988
17. Gomori JM, Grossman RI, Yu IC, Asakura T: NMR relaxation times of blood: dependence on field strength, oxidation state, and cell integrity. J Comput Assist Tomogr 11:684, 1987
18. Heiss W-D, Herholz K, Boecher-Schwarz HG et al: PET, CT, and MR imaging in cerebrovascular disease. J Comp Tomogr 10:903, 1986
19. Hesselink JR, Press GA: MR contrast enhancement of intracranial lesions with Gd DTPA. Radiol Clin North Am 26:873, 1988
20. Hilal SK, Maudsley AA et al: In vivo imaging of sodium-23 in the human head. J Comput Asst Tomogr 9:1, 1985
21. Imakita S, Nishimura T, Yamada N et al: Magnetic resonance imaging of cerebral infarction: time course of Gd DTPA enhancement and CT comparison. Neuroradiology 30:372, 1988
22. Imakita S, Nishimura T, Yamada N et al: Cerebral vascular malformations: applications of magnetic resonance imaging to differential diagnosis. Neuroradiology 31:320, 1989
23. Imakita S, Yamada N, Nishimura T et al: Magnetic resonance imaging of cerebrovascular disorders: cerebral infarction. Rinsho-Hoshasen 34:657, 1989
24. Jorgensen L, Rorvik A: Ischemic cerebrovascular disease in an autopsy series. I. Prevalence, location and predisposing factors in verified thromboembolic occlusions, and their significance in the pathogenesis of cerebral infarction. J Neurol Sci 3:490, 1966
25. Kato H, Kogure K, Ohtomo H et al: Correlations between proton nuclear magnetic resonance imaging and retrospective histochemical images in experimental cerebral infarction. J Cereb Blood Flow Metabol 5:267, 1985
26. Kertesz A, Black SE, Nicholson L, Carr T: The sensitivity and specificity of MRI in stroke. Neurology (NY) 37:1580, 1987
27. Koppensteiner R, Base W, Bognar H et al: Course of cerebral lesions in a patient with periarteritis

nodosa studied by magnetic resonance imaging. Klin Wochenschr 67:398, 1989
28. Leblanc R, Levesque M, Comair Y, Ethier R: Magnetic resonance imaging of cerebral arteriovenous malformations. Neurosurgery 21:15, 1987
29. Maruyama K, Tanaka M, Ikeda S et al: A case report of quadriparesis due to compression of the medulla oblongata by the elongated left vertebral artery. Rhinsho Shinkeigaku 29:108, 1989
30. Matsumura K, Matsuda M, Handa J, Todo G: Magnetic resonance imaging with aneurysmal subarachnoid hemorrhage: comparison with computed tomography scan. Surg Neurol 34:71, 1990
31. Mawad ME, Hilal SK, Silver AJ, Sane P: High resolution, high field MR imaging of cerebral arteriovenous malformations. Radiology 153:143, 1984
32. McNamara MT, Brant-Zawadski M, Berry I et al: Acute experimental cerebral ischemia: MR enhancement using Gd-DTPA. Radiology 158:701, 1986
33. Miyashita K, Naritomi H, Sawada T et al: Identification of recent lacunar lesions in cases of multiple small infarctions by magnetic resonance imaging. Stroke 19:834, 1988
34. Mohr JP, Biller J, Hilal SK et al: MR vs CT imaging in acute stroke. Proceedings of the International Conference on Stroke and the Cerebral Circulation. Phoenix, Arizona, 1992
35. Muller W, Kramer G, Roder RG, Kuhnert A: Balance of T1-weighted images before and after application of a paramagnetic substance (Gd DTPA). Neurosurg Rev 10:117, 1987
36. Nagata I, Kikuchi H, Yamagata S et al: Intraluminal thrombosis and growth mechanism of giant intracranial aneurysms. No Shinkei Geka 18:1115, 1990
37. Nakajima Y, Ohsuga H, Yamamoto M, Shinohara Y: Asymptomatic cerebral hemorrhage detected by MRI. Rinsho Shinkeigaku 31:270, 1991
38. Nussel F, Wegmuller H, Huber P: Comparison of magnetic resonance angiography, magnetic resonance imaging and conventional angiography in cerebral arteriovenous malformation. Neuroradiology 33:56, 1991
39. Pertuiset B, Haisa T, Bordi L et al: Detection of a ruptured aneurysmal sac by MRI in a case of negative angiogram: successful clipping of an anterior communicating artery aneurysm—case report. Acta Neurochir (Wien) 100:84, 1989
40. Pessin MS, Teal PA, Caplan LR: Hemorrhagic infarction: guilt by association. AJNR 12:1123, 1991
41. Prencipe M, Marini C: Leuko-araiosis: definition and clinical correlates—an overview. Eur Neurol 29:27, 1989
42. Rapacki TF, Brantley MJ, Furlow TW, Jr et al: Heterogeneity of cerebral cavernous hemangiomas diagnosed by MR imaging. J Comput Assist Tomogr 14:18, 1990
43. Rigamonti D et al: Cerebral cavernous malformations: incidence and familial occurrence. N Engl J Med 319:343, 1988
44. Salgado ED, Weinstein M, Furlan AJ et al: Proton magnetic resonance imaging in ischemic cerebrovascular disease. Ann Neurol 20:502, 1986
45. Schoerner W, Bradac GB, Treisch J et al: Magnetic resonance imaging (MRI) in the diagnosis of cerebral arteriovenous angiomas. Neuroradiology 28:313, 1986
46. Sipponen JT, Kaste M, Ketonen L: Serial nuclear magnetic resonance (NMR) imaging in patients with cerebral infarction. Comput Assist Tomogr 7:585, 1983
47. Spetzler RF, Zabramski JM, Kaufman B, Yeung HN: Acute NMR changes during MCA occlusions: a preliminary study in primates. Stroke 14:185, 1983
48. Spickler E, Lufkin R, Teresi L et al: MR imaging of acute subarachnoid hemorrhage. Comput Med Imaging Graph 14:67, 1990
49. Sze G, Harper PS, Galicich JH et al: Hemorrhagic neoplasms: MR mimics of occult vascular malformations. Am Soc Neuroradiol 10–15 May: 125, 1987
50. Thulborn KR, Sorensen AG, Kowall NW et al: The role of ferritin and hemosiderin in the MR appearance of cerebral hemorrhage: a histopathologic biochemical study in rats. AJNR 11:291, 1990
51. Toriga S: (personal communication)
52. Trussart V, Berry I, Manelfe C et al: Epileptogenic cerebral vascular malformations and MRI. J Neuroradiol 16:273, 1989
53. Uchino A, Ohnari N, Ohno M: MRI of middle cerebral artery occlusion. Nippon Igaku Hoshasen Gakkai Zasshi 49:1355, 1989
54. Uchino A, Onomura K, Ohno M: Wallerian degeneration of the corticospinal tract in the brain stem: MR imaging. Radiat Med 7:74, 1989
55. van Swieten JC, van den Hout JH, van Ketel BA et al: Periventricular lesions in the white matter on magnetic resonance imaging in the elderly: a morphometric correlation with arteriolosclerosis and dilated perivascular spaces. Brain 114:761, 1991
56. Virapongse C, Mancuso A, Quisling R: Human brain infarcts: Gd-DTPA-enhanced MR imaging. Radiology 161:785, 1986
57. Wall SD, Brant-Zawadski M, Jeffrey RB, Barnes B: High frequency CT findings within 24 hours after cerebral infarction. AJR 138:307, 1982
58. Weingarten K, Zimmerman RD, Deo-Narine V et al: MR imaging of acute intracranial hemorrhage: findings on sequential spin-echo and gradient-echo images in a dog model. AJNR 12:457, 1991
59. Williams KD, Drayer BP, Bird CR: Mengetic resonance imaging in the diagnosis of intracerebral hematoma. BNI 5:16, 1989
60. Yuh WTC, Crainb MR, Loes DJ et al: MR imaging of acute cerebral ischemia: findings in the first 24 hours. AJNR 12:621, 1991
61. Zuerrer M, Martin E, Boltshauser E: MR imaging of intracranial hemorrhage in neonates and infants at 2.35 Tesla. Neuroradiology 33:223, 1991
62. Zyed A, Hayman LA, Bryan RN: MR imaging of intracerebral blood: diversity in the temporal pattern at 0.5 and 1.0 T. AJNR 12:469, 1991

# 11
# *CEREBRAL ANGIOGRAPHY*

Stephen P. Lownie
Donald H. Lee
Allan J. Fox
David M. Pelz

This chapter begins with a discussion of the safety and technical aspects of diagnostic cerebral angiography. The angiographic indicators of pathology are outlined, including the findings seen in cerebral infarction, the significance of the collateral circulation, the hemodynamic effects of arterial stenosis, and the correlation of angiographic changes with disease processes. The findings seen in specific pathologies are reviewed. Lastly, magnetic resonance angiography is briefly discussed.

## SAFETY AND TECHNICAL ASPECTS

Refinements in cerebral angiography have been geared toward either increasing patient safety or improving diagnostic accuracy. The two goals do not necessarily go hand in hand. For example, intravenous digital subtraction angiography (IV-DSA) eliminates the risk of procedure-related stroke,[102] but its tendency to overlap vessels and lack of spatial resolution have prevented it from replacing intraarterial methods. Intraarterial DSA, which compromises on spatial resolution compared to conventional (film screen) angiography, is gradually replacing the latter, because of advantages in patient comfort, contrast sensitivity, and (possibly) patient safety.[20,27,102]

### Patient Safety

From the time of its introduction in 1927[73] until the 1950s to 1960s, virtually all cerebral angiography was performed by direct needle puncture of the carotid and vertebral arteries. As early as 1941 Farinas[33] cannulated the femoral artery with a catheter using an open approach, passing it up to the abdominal aorta to perform angiography. Ten years later Bierman and colleagues[9] used a catheter technique to perform carotid angiography in two cancer chemotherapy patients. In 1953 the era of percutaneous angiography was ushered in by Seldinger.[96] He used a needle with a stylet to puncture the artery, through which a flexible metal guidewire was inserted, whereupon the needle was removed and a polyethylene catheter having the same diameter as the needle was advanced over the wire. He and his colleagues performed 35 aortograms without complications.

In 1963 Lang[57] conducted a survey of 204 physicians who were using the Seldinger technique. There were 89 serious or fatal complications in 11,402 procedures. Local arterial thrombosis accounted for 53 percent of these, arterial embolism 10 percent, and remote arterial thrombosis 10 percent. Thus, thromboembolic phenomena were the cause of three-quarters of all of the serious or fatal complications.

Two potential solutions to the problem of catheter-related thrombosis were considered.[31,37] One was to systemically heparinize the patient. Nejad et al.[78] found that a small systemic dose of heparin (30 units/kg) was sufficient to eliminate 95 percent of the surface clot on indwelling catheters in dogs. Clinical trials comparing systemic heparinization with controls (in which heparin was used in the catheter flushing solution only) showed a significantly lower incidence of thromboembolic complications and catheter thrombus.[5,111] However, heparinized patients showed a higher incidence of local hematoma and had longer arterial compression times.[5,111] The second solution to the problem of thrombosis was to coat the catheters with heparin to make them less thrombogenic.[37] In a controlled study in which heparinized catheters were used, Eldh and Jacobsson[31] detected no catheter thrombus in 26 patients, compared to an 80 percent detection rate in controls.

At the present time, most centers do not systemically heparinize patients for routine diagnostic cerebral angiography. Neuroradiologists either intermittently flush the catheter with heparinized saline or run a heparinized infusion into the catheter between contrast injections. As a result, a delayed mild systemic anticoagulation usually occurs.[112] It is not known whether routine systemic anticoagulation[21] results in a decreased risk of stroke during (or after) the procedure. The risk appears similar whether systemic heparin is used or not.[23,24]

Besides using either local or systemic heparin to prevent thrombosis, other factors associated with the formation of catheter thrombus have been identified. Mani[67] found the most significant factor to be the ratio of the diameter of the catheter to the diameter of the artery. In a prospective study of 176 femoral catheterizations, using either 5 French (1.6 mm) or 7 French (2.4 mm) diameter catheters, the 9 cases of catheter thrombus all occurred with the use of the larger catheter. Formerly, large-bore catheters were required to allow adequate injection rates of contrast agent to perform arch aortograms. Improvements in catheter material strength have allowed 6 French[29] and more recently 5 French[45] catheters to be used for arch studies instead.

In summary, the use of heparin-impregnated catheters (with or without systemic heparinization), the practice of catheter flushing or catheter infusion with heparinized saline, the progressive reductions in catheter diameter, and the heparin coating of guidewires have all contributed to angiography that is safer for the patient. An indication of the safety of cerebral angiography today is furnished by two recent prospective studies. Earnest et al.[24] reported the complications of 1,517 angiograms in 1983. The incidence of stroke was 0.33 percent. In patients with cerebrovascular disease, the figure rose to 0.63 percent. There was one death (0.07 percent). Permanent deficits were associated with advanced age, elevated serum creatinine (greater than 1.2 mg/dl), and the use of more than one catheter. Higher volumes of contrast agent and lengthier procedures were not associated with neurologic complications, although local hematomas were more common in such situations. In 1987 Dion et al.[23] studied 1,002 procedures. There were no deaths. Stroke occurred in 0.4 percent. In cerebrovascular patients, 0.7 percent sustained permanent neurologic events. A procedure time greater than 60 minutes and the presence of hypertension were both associated with central nervous system (CNS) complications occurring within 24 hours of the procedure. Subacute (24- to 72-hour) neurologic events were associated with the volume of contrast injected, advanced age, and diabetes mellitus. These prospective studies have borne out the conventional wisdom of performing safe cerebral angiography. Patients should be well hydrated prior to the procedure. Blood pressure should be under good control if the patient is hypertensive. The procedure should be of reasonably short duration. Excessive volumes of contrast (more than 200 ml) should be avoided. The risk factors of advanced age, cerebrovascular disease, elevated creatinine, and diabetes mellitus cannot be modified, but should enter into the primary decision to perform cerebral angiography in a particular patient.

## Technical Aspects

As the percutaneous methods became more widely used, most angiographers recognized that selective cannulation of the great vessels was mandatory for adequate intracranial angiography. Modified catheters and guidewires were developed to aid in the negotiation of tortuous atherosclerotic vessels. During retrograde passage up the aorta, the J-shaped guidewire was found to prevent inadvertent vessel injury.[77] Certain catheter configurations, either preshaped by the manufacturer or shaped by the angiographer, facilitated selective cannulation of the origins of the innominate, left common carotid, and left subclavian arteries.[46,107]

In the evaluation of cerebrovascular disease, the angiographer determines from the clinical history and neurologic examination the major arterial territory (i.e., carotid or vertebral, right or left) suspected to be causing the patient's symptoms. That territory is studied first. Extracranial (cervical) and intracranial views in anteroposterior (AP) and lateral projections are obtained. Arterial, capillary, and venous phases are visualized intracranially. If the major vessel is occluded or intracranial flow is compromised, the contralateral artery is studied in order to evaluate the intracranial collateral circulation. In addition, any potential extracranial source of vessel reconstitution is also studied (e.g., the carotid artery in the case of vertebral artery occlusion, since muscular collaterals from the carotid system may reconstitute a proximally occluded vertebral, or vice versa). With symptoms in one carotid territory, both carotid arteries are usually studied. Selective vertebral injections are generally not performed unless the intracranial collateral circulation needs to be seen. In vertebrobasilar disease, however, the carotids are usually injected in addition to the vertebrals.

The arch aortogram, performed in the right posterior oblique (RPO) projection to open up the arch of the aorta, provides a survey of the great vessel origins, including the vertebral arteries. Often a routine part of the study of atherosclerotic patients, its diagnostic yield is rather low. In Akers' series of 1,000 patients who had arch aortograms, only 18 had significant intrathoracic pathology.[1] Some angiographers only perform an arch aortogram if symptoms remain unexplained after selective carotid and subclavian and/or vertebral injections—about 10 percent of patients ultimately requiring it.[52]

The advent of digital computer technology has allowed immediate subtraction images to be obtained by digitizing the radiologic image into a matrix before and after the injection of radiographic contrast.[20,27] The spatial resolution of this method depends on the size of the matrix, which is 512 for most systems currently in use, although systems with 1,024 matrices are available. Such spatial resolution is less than that obtained with conventional film screen methods, but contrast sensitivity is superior with the digital techniques.[20] The advantages of intraarterial digital subtraction angiography (DSA) include the ability to use smaller doses of contrast agent, and thus smaller catheters.[20,27] Because images are computerized immediately and can be replayed, there is no time lost in developing, checking, or changing film as there is with conventional methods. The overall procedure time is shortened, decreasing patient discomfort. These advantages have led to a gradual adoption of intraarterial DSA by most centers. Whether the advantages of DSA translate into increased patient safety is not certain. In one study,[102] the incidence of procedure-related stroke following intraarterial DSA was 0.7 percent, as compared to 0.8 percent for conventional film screen angiography. However, both of these figures are higher than were seen in the aforementioned prospective studies by Earnest et al.[24] and Dion et al.,[23] which involved conventional methods.

## ANGIOGRAPHIC INDICATORS OF PATHOLOGY

### Angiography of Cerebral Infarction

Computed tomography (CT) and magnetic resonance (MR) imaging have supplanted cerebral angiography in the primary diagnosis of cerebral infarction. However, because angiography remains important in elucidating the cause of infarction, the primary findings should be appreciated.

Arterial branch occlusion is the most frequent angiographic finding in stroke.[58,105] In descending order, the middle, posterior, and anterior cerebral arteries and their branches are affected.[58] A local region of avascularity may be seen during the capillary phase of the angiogram. As a result of the obstruction, regional arteries may take a long time to empty themselves of contrast, and as a result they may still be seen during the capillary or venous phases of the angiogram.[105] Another phenomenon commonly seen with arterial branch occlusion is late filling of the occluded vessel in a retrograde manner from distal collateral branches.[58]

When contrast passes rapidly into local cerebral veins, the terms arteriovenous shunting or early venous filling are used.[35] The cause may be either local vasodilatation or a bypass of the occluded capillary bed. The finding is common in the first 2 weeks following infarction. An associated capillary blush in the infarcted region may also occur.[91]

Ultimately, recanalization of occluded cerebral vessels usually takes place. Almost half recanalize within 1 week.[49] Some residual vessel narrowing or local stenosis is typical. Distal cerebral branches may occlude in the interim. The only remaining signs of infarction in this subacute stage may be the evidence of mass effect or capillary blush.

### The Collateral Circulation

The collateral circulation of the brain, although well studied anatomically, remains poorly understood physiologically. Collateral blood flow is most frequently invoked in the preservation of blood flow to an area of brain which would otherwise be rendered ischemic. In addition, collateral circulation is seen in situations not necessarily preserving blood flow. Arteriovenous malformations are the paradigm of this situation. Finally, inappropriate collateral has been postulated to actually cause ischemia by diverting blood away from the brain (the so-called "steal effect"), as in the subclavian steal phenomenon.

Collateral pathways are conveniently divided into intracranial and extracranial types.[61,69,76,97,114] The most physiologically important is the circle of Willis (Fig. 11-12D). Leptomeningeal anastomoses, the connections between superficial cortical branches of the major arterial territories, are less effective than the circle of Willis in maintaining flow (Fig. 11-1). Extracranial pathways include extracranial-to-intracranial and extracranial-to-extracranial anastomoses. The former comprise numerous branches of the external carotid artery (ECA), which by various routes anastomose with either the petrous, cavernous, or supraclinoid (ophthalmic) segments of the internal carotid artery (ICA) (Fig. 11-2). Also among this group are the unusual transdural anastomoses (rete mirabile) between dural arteries and superficial cortical vessels.[59,113] The extracranial-to-extracranial group includes reconstitution of the carotid system by the vertebral artery (or vice versa) through muscular collaterals, in the event of more proximal occlusion of the artery (Fig. 11-2). Anatomic variations may also permit such collateral to arise.[87]

In a review of 573 angiograms (445 patients) done on our unit in 1990, collateral circulation was observed in 24 percent of cases (unpublished data); 52 cases involved atherosclerotic disease. Among these, the circle of Willis collateral was seen in 86 percent, and was the exclusive form of collateral in 44 percent.

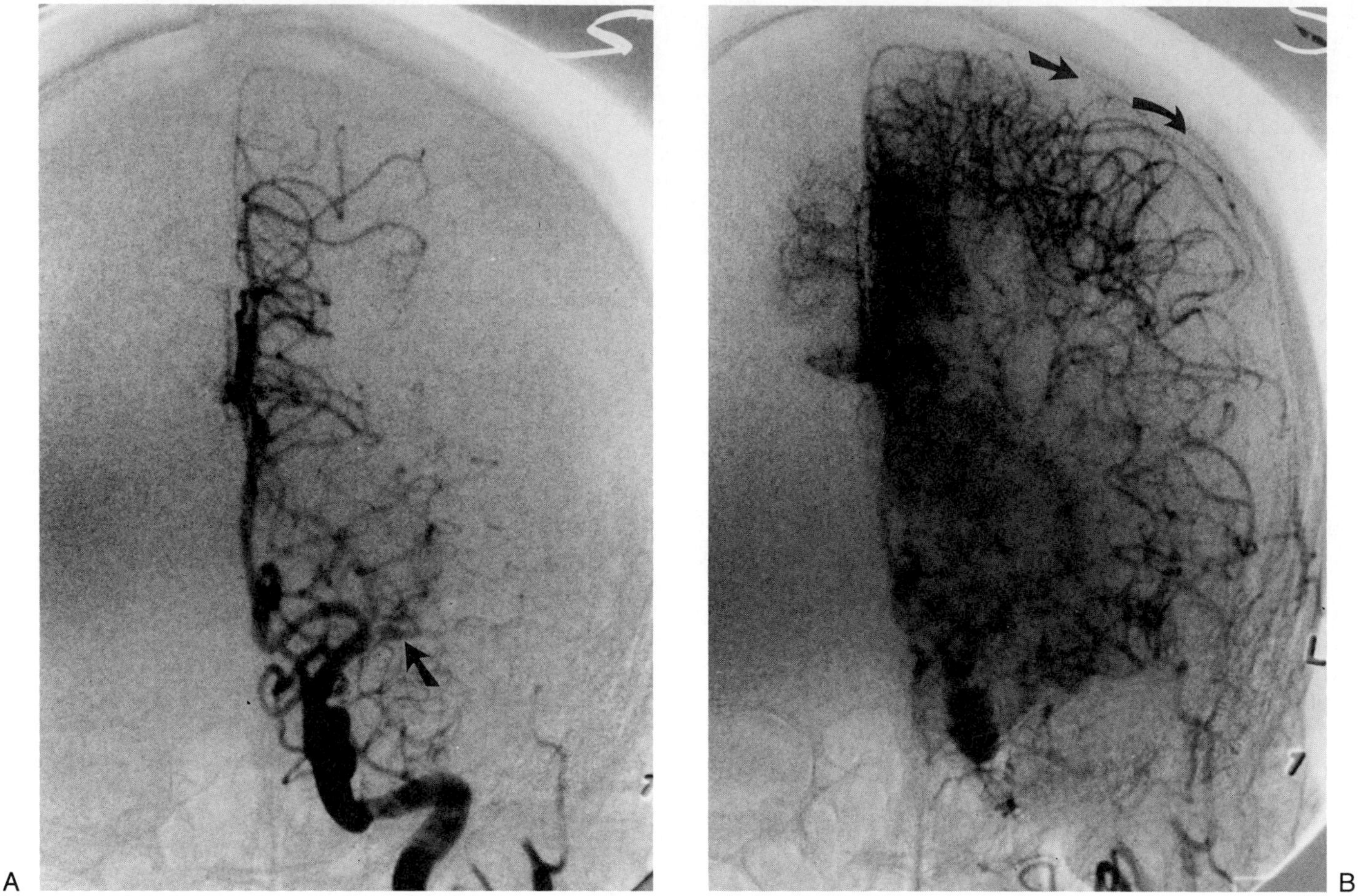

**Fig. 11-1.** A 55-year-old man presenting with right-sided weakness and dysarthria. (**A**) Left carotid angiogram, anteroposterior (Towne) projection, early arterial phase, shows a tapered occlusion of the left middle cerebral artery (*arrow*). (**B**) Late arterial phase shows leptomeningeal collateral from anterior to middle cerebral territories across convexity (*arrows*).

Circle of Willis plus ECA-to-ICA collateral accounted for a further 25 percent of observed collateral. In the atherosclerotic carotid occlusions, the ophthalmic artery was the most frequent (74 percent) and the most hemodynamically significant form of ECA-to-ICA collateral.

One potential consequence of the preservation of cerebral blood flow by the circle of Willis is that poorly developed circles may be more common in cases of cerebral infarction. There is pathologic evidence to substantiate this. "Normal" circles are considered to have all of their constituent vessels at least 1 mm in diameter. In a series comparing 194 infarcted brains with 350 normal ones, the normals had 52 percent normal circles, while the infarcts had only 33 percent.[3] Tiny posterior communicating and tiny proximal anterior cerebral arteries were more frequent in the infarcted brains. Another study, comparing 49 infarcted brains with 88 controls, substantiated these findings.[7]

Collateral blood flow to the brain may present a devious route for cerebral emboli. This could occur if atheromatous disease affected the collateral artery itself. Alternatively, the "stump" of an occluded ICA may act as the source of emboli passing through ECA collateral.[6]

Inappropriate collateral, as in the subclavian steal phenomenon, may be overrated as a cause of neurologic symptoms. In a Doppler study of 324 patients with reversed vertebral artery flow, 64 percent had no neurologic symptoms at all, while 31 percent had hemispheric events due to concomitant carotid stenosis.[44] The 5 percent who clinically had brain stem events all had bilateral flow reversal in the vertebral arteries. Thus, although angiographically striking (Fig. 11-3), careful clinical and ultrasound evaluation is warranted to establish true brain stem ischemia in such patients.

## Hemodynamic Effects of Stenosis

As the diameter of a rigid tube decreases, the rate of fluid flowing through it also declines. The relationship is not linear. In fact, the flow decreases as a func-

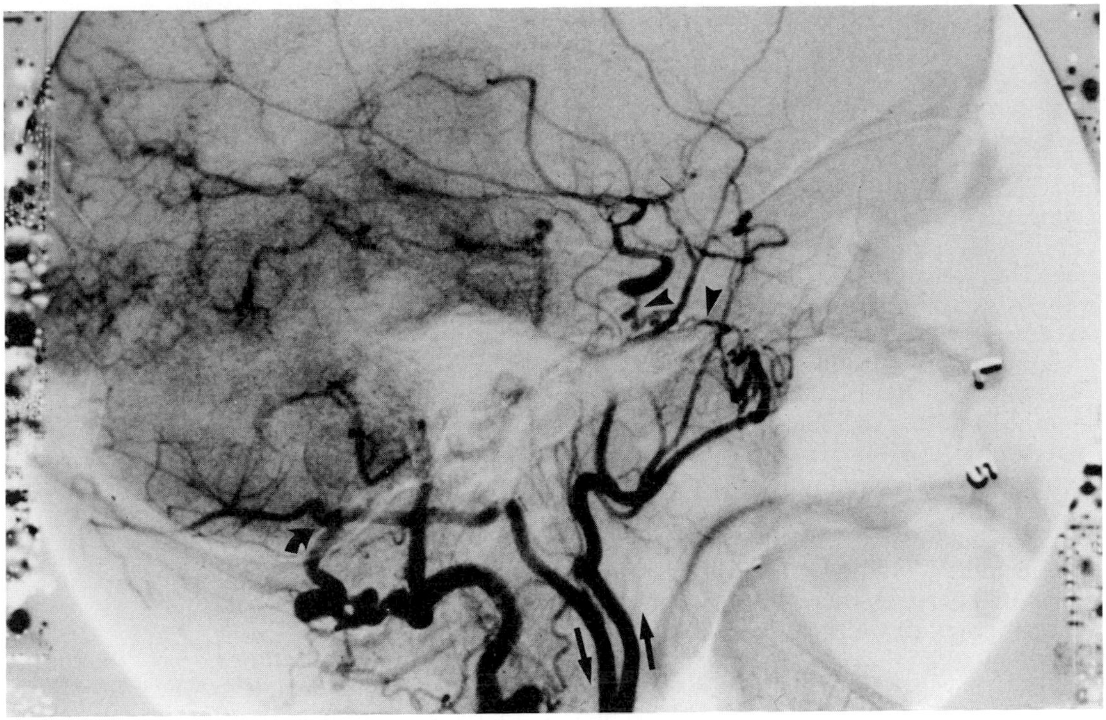

**Fig. 11-2.** Patient with left common carotid occlusion (not shown). Left vertebral angiogram, lateral view. Enlarged muscular branch of the vertebral artery (*curved arrow*) retrogradely fills the occipital branch of the external carotid artery (*arrow downward*) to reconstitute the external (*arrow upward*), which then reconstitutes the cavernous and supraclinoid internal carotid artery via branches including the artery of the foramen rotundum (*arrowheads*).

**Fig. 11-3.** A 55-year-old man with symptoms of vertebrobasilar insufficiency and absent left radial pulse. Right vertebral injection, anteroposterior view, shows retrograde flow down the left vertebral artery (*arrow downward*), which reconstitutes the left subclavian artery (*smaller arrow*). Arch aortography showed complete occlusion of left subclavian artery 3 cm from its origin.

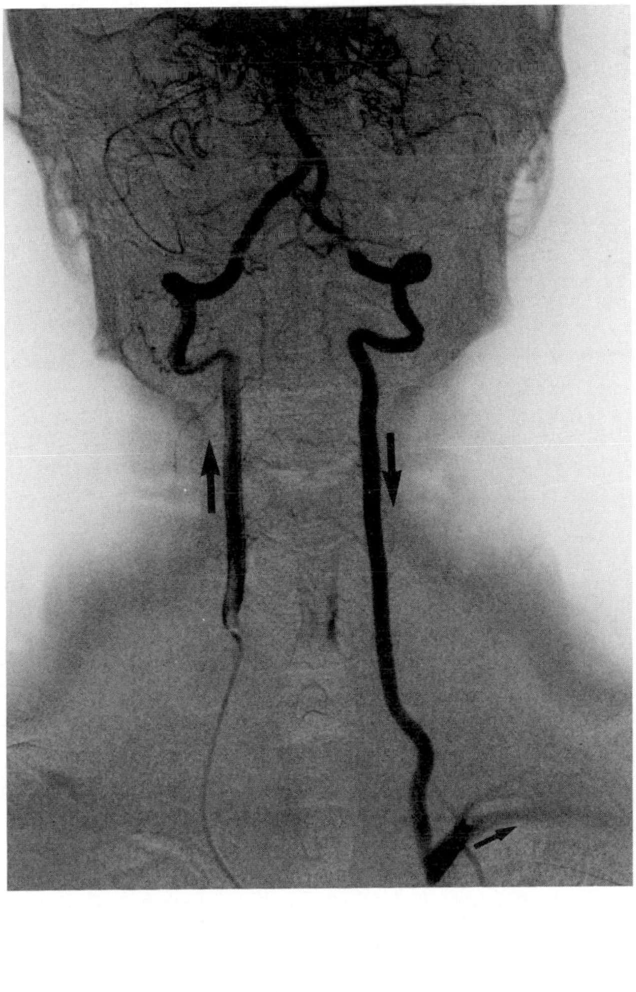

tion of the fourth power of the radius, a very steep rate of decline.

In living systems the above relationship only partially applies. In two canine studies arterial blood flow did not decrease until the cross-sectional area was reduced by 80 percent.[68,72] This corresponds to a reduction in arterial diameter of 50 to 60 percent.

Studies in humans have yielded comparable results. In two studies in which patients underwent application of an external carotid clamp, there was no significant change in pressure or flow until the cross-sectional area was reduced by 70 percent to 90 percent.[14,106] Another study of 61 patients with atherosclerotic narrowing showed that a reduction of luminal diameter by 63 percent uniformly resulted in a significant distal pressure drop.[22] Stenosis of 48 to 62 percent had variable effects.

In short, when the diameter of an artery is decreased by up to 50 percent, there is little or no measurable effect on flow. Above this, flow declines rapidly in proportion to the decrease in the diameter of the radius. Also, the degree of the stenosis is more important than its length. Doubling the length of a 1.5-cm stenosis reduces flow by only 5 to 8 percent.[109] With tandem stenoses, the combined effect is not additive, but corresponds approximately to the effect of the more severe stenosis alone.[109]

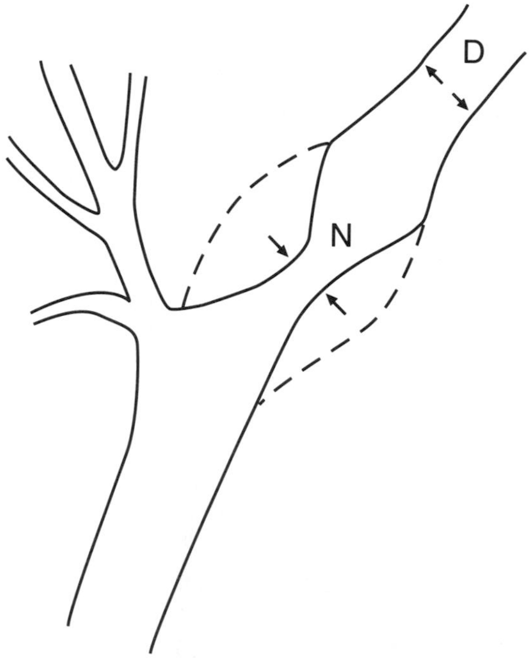


**Fig. 11-4.** Percent stenosis is calculated by subtracting the numerator N (the width in millimeters of the lumen at the greatest region of stenosis) from the denominator D (the width of the artery distal to the carotid bulb or any poststenotic dilatation), dividing by the denominator, and multiplying by 100:

$$\% \text{ stenosis} = \frac{D - N}{D} \times 100$$

Although flow is more closely related to luminal area than luminal diameter, conventional angiographic measurements of stenosis are based on the latter. In the Joint Study of Extracranial Arterial Occlusion (1969), the segment of arterial stenosis was compared to the lumen of normal-appearing artery above the normally dilated carotid bulb.[11] Others have used the width proximal to the stenosis as the denominator.[4] The clinical significance of high-grade carotid stenosis, and the beneficial effect of surgically relieving it, have been recently demonstrated.[81] In that study, the percent luminal narrowing was calculated based on the artery distal to the bulb (Fig. 11-4).[82]

### Differential Diagnosis of Specific Diseases

Generally, the findings seen at cerebral angiography allow for a straightforward radiologic diagnosis. In the case of arterial stenosis, the location is one point of differentiation. Atherosclerosis characteristically involves the proximal internal carotid artery, while dissection and fibromuscular dysplasia typically occur in the upper cervical part of the vessel.

The string sign of a long, tapered stenosis of the internal carotid artery is most often due to atheromatous disease, either near-occlusion or partial thrombosis.[74] The other causes are dissection and radiation-induced fibrosis.

The findings associated with various disease processes are summarized in Table 11-1. In certain instances, the distinction between two or more conditions cannot be made. Arterial occlusion due to atherosclerotic thrombosis versus embolism is one example. Another is the long, smooth stenosis of the upper cervical internal carotid artery, which occurs in both dissection and intimal fibroplasia. In such situations, repeat angiography may help make the distinction. Embolism recanalizes often without a trace, and dissection usually heals with restoration of the lumen—in contrast to atherosclerosis and intimal fibroplasia.

## ANGIOGRAPHIC FINDINGS IN SPECIFIC PATHOLOGIES

### Atherosclerosis

There have been numerous angiographic studies of the topography of atherosclerosis causing cerebrovascular disease.[8,43,79] Comparison is troublesome because of differences in patient demographics and differences in disease severity (stroke vs transient ischemia vs no symptoms). However, certain generalizations may be made. The common carotid bifurca-

**TABLE 11-1. Principal Angiographic Findings and Their Occurrence in Disease**

| Finding | Disease(s) | Fig. | Ref. |
|---|---|---|---|
| Occlusion | | | |
| Abrupt | Embolism | 11-9 | 80 |
| | Atherosclerosis | | 68 |
| Tapered | Atherosclerosis | | 68 |
| | Dissection | | 84 |
| | Embolism (unusual) | | 81 |
| Stenosis | | | |
| Smooth, short | Atherosclerosis | 11-8 | |
| Smooth, long | Intimal fibroplasia | | 94 |
| | Dissection | | |
| Irregular | Atherosclerosis | 11-7 | 62 |
| | Dissection | 11-11 | 84 |
| | Fibromuscular dysplasia | | 92 |
| | Arteritis | 11-17 | 96 |
| String sign | Dissection | | 84 |
| | Atherosclerosis | | 72 |
| | Radiation fibrosis | | 53 |
| Multiple (intracranial) | Arteritis | 11-17 | 96 |
| | Atherosclerosis | | 99 |
| | Moyamoya | 11-18 | 101 |
| With aneurysm | Dissection | 11-13 | 86 |
| Ulceration | Atherosclerosis | 11-6, 11-7 | 62 |
| Dilatation | Dolichoectasia | 11-20 | 106 |
| | Poststenotic | | |
| String of beads | Fibromuscular dysplasia | | 91 |
| Intimal flap | Dissection | 11-14 | 87 |
| Double density | Ulceration (en face) | 11-6 | 61 |
| Two bands of contrast | Dissection (en face) | 11-15 | 88 |
| Puff of smoke | Moyamoya | 11-18 | 101 |

tion/proximal internal carotid artery is by far the commonest site of involvement, being affected in 50 to 80 percent of patients presenting with cerebrovascular disease. At this location, stenosis (greater than 50 percent) is about two to three times more common than complete arterial occlusion. The next most frequent site of involvement is the vertebral artery. Here, unlike the carotid system, stenosis and occlusion are about equal in occurrence. The origin of the vertebral artery is most commonly involved. The proximal subclavian arteries are third most frequently affected, the left side two to three times more often than the right. Intracranially, stenosis (greater than 50 percent) or occlusion is uncommon. Individually, the basilar (Fig. 11-5), intracranial carotid, and proximal circle of Willis arteries are each involved in 1 to 4 percent of patients.

The pathologic features of cervicocranial atherosclerosis include stenosis, ulceration, hemorrhage into a plaque, intraluminal thrombus formation, and occlusion.[100] Stenotic changes at the common carotid bifurcation are most prominent along the posterior wall of the common and internal carotid arteries. Thus the lateral projection often best depicts the most severe narrowing. Internal carotid stenosis is generally classified as severe (70 to 99 percent, Fig. 11-6), moderate (30 to 69 percent, Fig. 11-7), or mild (less than 30 percent). Markedly severe stenosis causes slowing of internal carotid blood flow, resulting in delayed filling of intracranial branches as compared to extracranial ones (Fig. 11-8).

Atheromatous ulceration was first recognized surgically during carotid endarterectomy, platelet thrombi being seen within the base of the ulcer craters.[50] Ulcer-related debris was invoked as a cause of embolic stroke, even in the absence of hemodynamically significant stenosis.[75] Angiographically, ulcers are often best seen in the lateral projection, although oblique views may be superior.[66] The internal carotid artery is the commonest site of ulceration, while external carotid ulceration occurs rarely.[115] Virtually all ulcers are within 2.5 cm of the bifurcation. The best radiographic criterion of ulceration is the so-called penetrating niche, simply the crater of contrast material seen below overhanging edges of atheroma (Figs. 11-6 and 11-7). The ulcer cavity is contained within the atheroma, not extending beyond the projected line of normal artery wall. Irregularity of the vessel wall is a less reliable criterion of ulceration, since tandem plaque formation may cause such an appearance.[12] If the ulcer is partly or completely superimposed on the artery, a circumscribed double density may be seen, which is another criterion for ulceration, but which warrants a film at 90 degrees to show the crater (Fig. 11-6).[115]

Reports of the accuracy of the angiographic detection of ulceration, as correlated with the findings at surgery, vary from 50 to 86 percent.[12,28] Very severe or

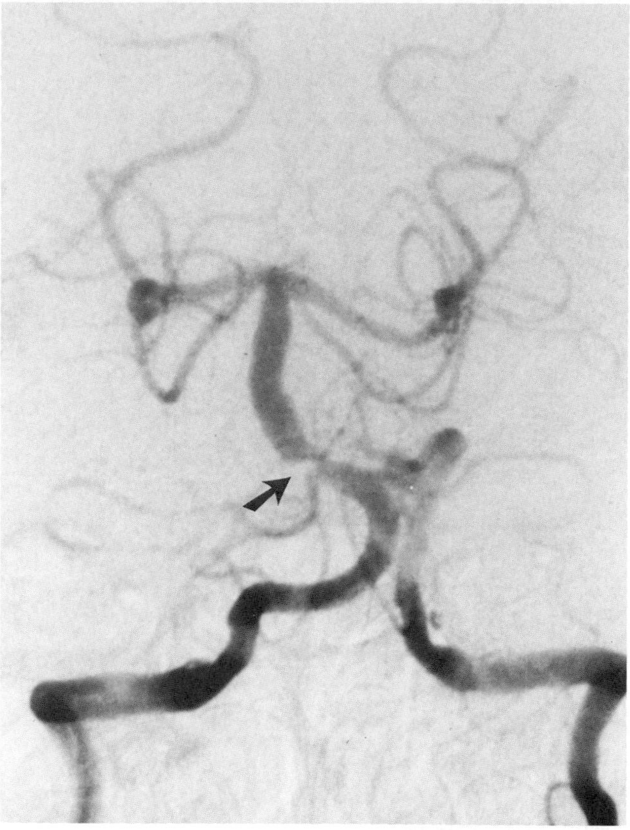

**Fig. 11-5.** Left vertebral injection, anteroposterior view. Significant stenosis, proximal basilar artery, just distal to the origin of anterior inferior cerebellar artery (*arrow*).

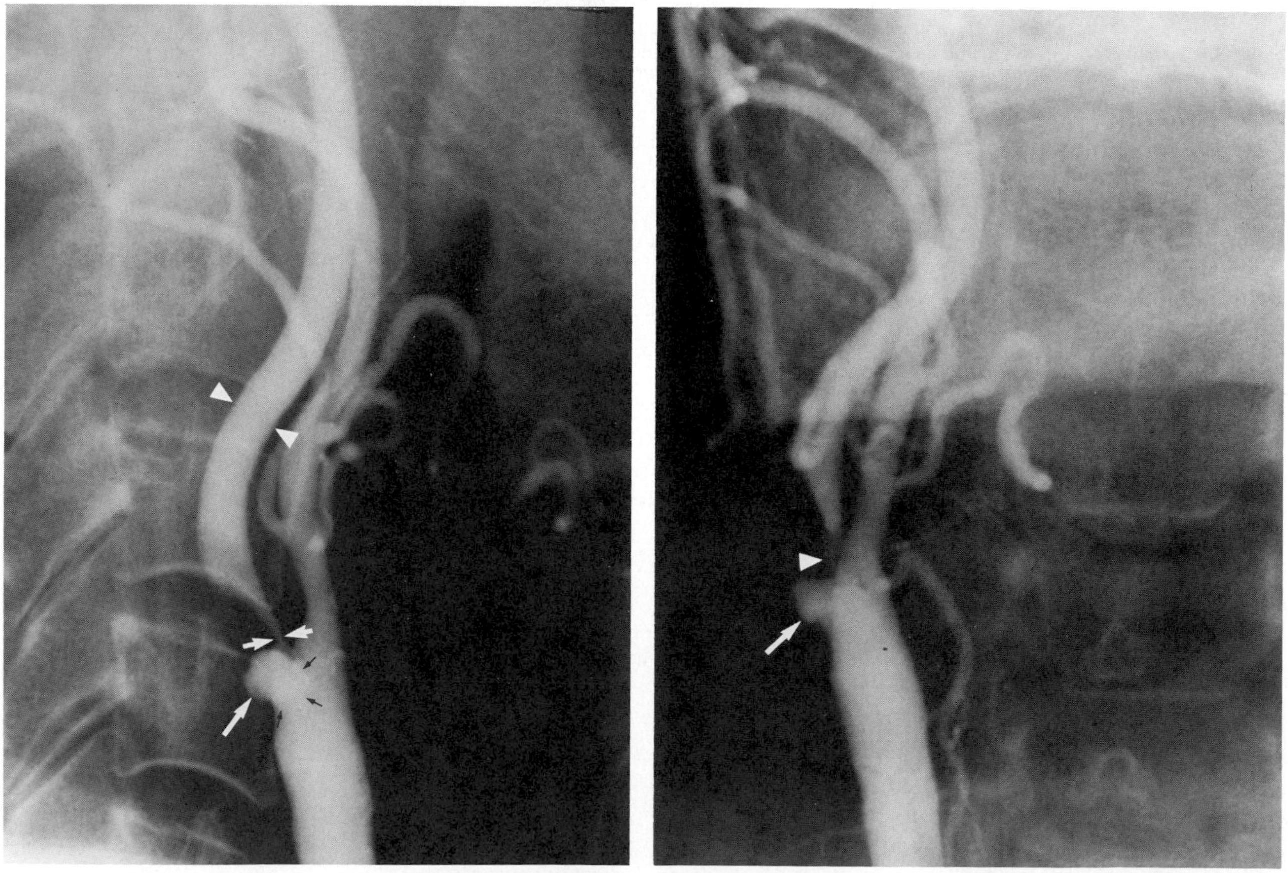

A B

**Fig. 11-6.** A 66-year-old man with right hemisphere TIAs. (**A**) Right common carotid angiogram, lateral view, shows severe stenosis of proximal internal carotid artery (80 percent using width at *small white arrows* as numerator and width at *arrowheads* as denominator). Large area of ulceration also observed (*longer white arrow*). Note the double density (outlined by *small black arrows*) superimposed on the carotid bifurcation. (**B**) Same injection, anteroposterior view, shows area of severe stenosis (*arrowhead*) and the lateral component of the ulcer (*arrow*), which caused the double density.

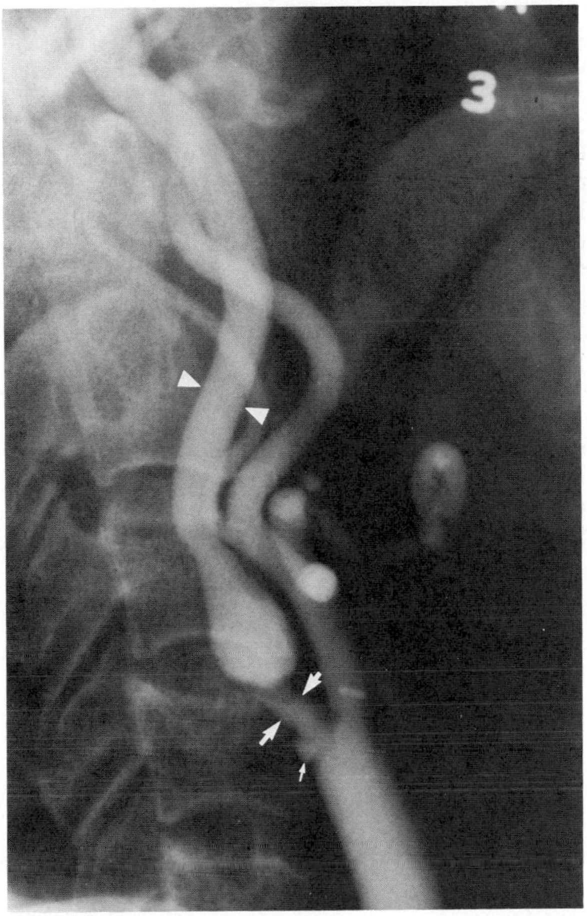


**Fig. 11-7.** Right common carotid injection, lateral view. Width of lumen at narrowest point (*larger arrows*) compared to denominator (*arrowheads*) yields stenosis of 40 percent. Note the small ulcer (*small arrow*).

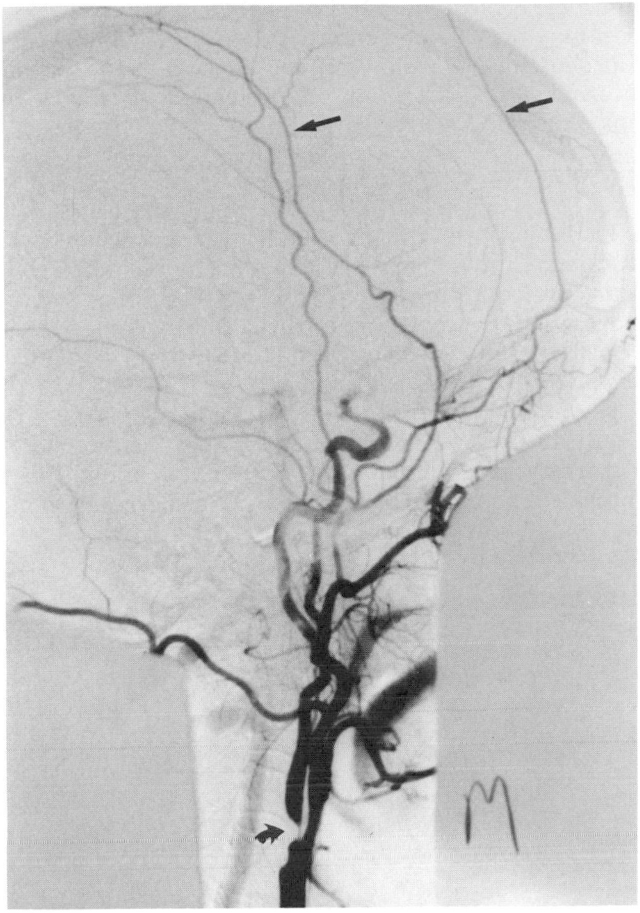

**Fig. 11-8.** A 56-year-old woman with right-sided amaurosis fugax. Right common carotid angiogram, lateral view, shows a near-occlusion of the proximal internal carotid artery (*curved arrow*). Distally, the external carotid branches (*straight arrows*) are well filled, but the distal internal carotid fills only very slowly.

very mild degrees of stenosis tend to reduce the accuracy of detection. False positive interpretations are due to vessel wall irregularities, plaque hemorrhage, and flow phenomena.[26,66] This relative inaccuracy of angiography in ulcer detection has hindered clinical trials in determining the pathogenic importance of ulceration in mild to moderate degrees of carotid stenosis.[82]

Hemorrhage into an atherosclerotic plaque is underrecognized and probably underrated in importance in the production of symptoms. A study of 50 carotid endarterectomies revealed 12 subintimal hematomas and 20 ulcerated plaques.[25] The distinguishing feature at angiography was a more spheroid shape than the smooth atheromatous plaque, with sharper angles with the adjacent vessel wall. Subintimal hematoma has been postulated to cause spontaneous disappearance of carotid stenosis at follow-up angiography.[53]

Another local complication of carotid atherosclerosis, typically associated with severe stenosis and frequently associated with ulceration or irregular atheroma, is the formation of intraluminal thrombus. A luminal filling defect, separated from the vessel wall by contrast material on two or more projections, is considered the best angiographic criterion.[93] Multiple views of the carotid bifurcation may be necessary. The thrombus is typically smooth, but may be of variable shape, including elongated, tubular or ball-like.[86] Radiologic differential diagnosis includes a smooth protruding plaque, dissection, and laminar flow caused by severe stenosis.[86]

Internal carotid occlusion may occur in the setting of an acute stroke,[90] or may occur silently, depending upon the intracranial collateral circulation and the proclivity to distal embolization. The degree to which the collateral pathways can support the intracranial circulation is remarkable; reports exist of occlusion of all four extracranial vessels with minimal neurologic symptoms.[108] It is most important to establish that complete occlusion truly exists. Near-complete occlusion may only be detected with a prolonged imaging run showing very slow antegrade flow.[95] The distal internal carotid artery may exhibit collapse down to a tiny string of contrast.[38]

## Embolism

The majority of intracranial arterial occlusions are embolic. Embolic material, derived either from the heart or from carotid bifurcation atheroma,[42] may lodge virtually anywhere in the cerebrovascular tree, from the high cervical internal carotid artery to the peripheral cerebral arterioles.

The middle cerebral artery (MCA) is the most commonly affected vessel.[62] Emboli typically arrest where the artery tapers beyond its first major branch, the anterior temporal artery (Fig. 11-9).[2,10] Larger emboli may lodge more proximally in the MCA trunk, at the level of the internal carotid bifurcation, or where the ICA narrows in the upper cervical region. The posterior cerebral artery, upper basilar artery and its branches, and anterior cerebral artery are less common or unusual sites.[16,39]

Radiologically, cerebral embolism was first recognized in the setting of complete arterial occlusion, when follow-up angiography revealed recanalization and a normal vessel appearance.[40] Investigators performing serial angiography, beginning in the acute stage, have demonstrated actual migration of embolic fragments.[18] Distal migration occurs within hours to days of the onset of symptoms, although the migration itself may occur over a period of seconds to minutes.

Without the benefit of repeat angiography showing a patent normal artery, or the fortuitous observation of clot migration, the angiographic diagnosis of embolism is not categorical. Intracranial atheromatous

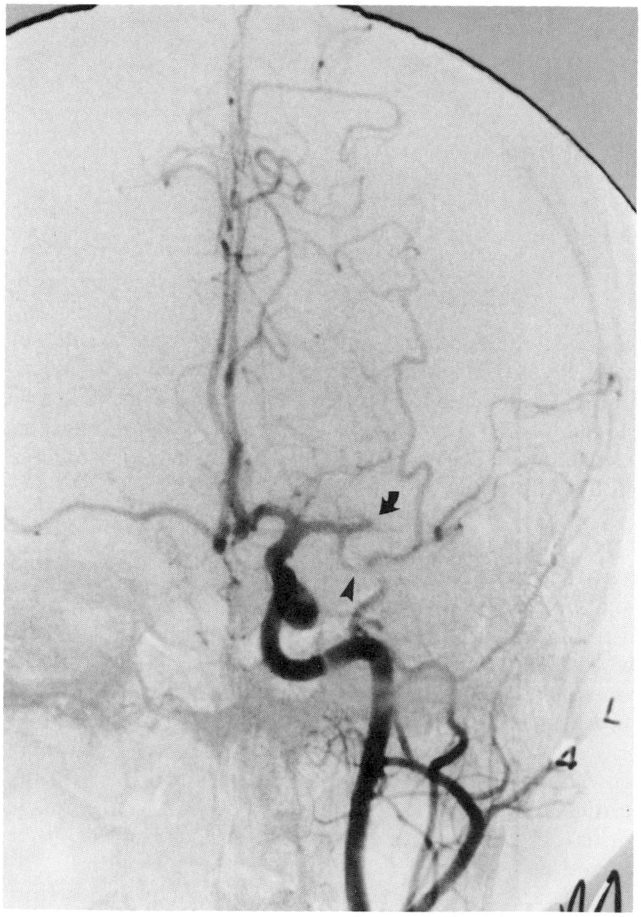

**Fig. 11-9.** A 32-year-old woman with sudden onset of aphasia and right hemiparesis. Left carotid injection, anteroposterior view, shows occlusion of the middle cerebral artery just beyond its first cortical branch (*arrow*). There is also an occlusion of the proximal branch, the anterior temporal artery (*arrowhead*).

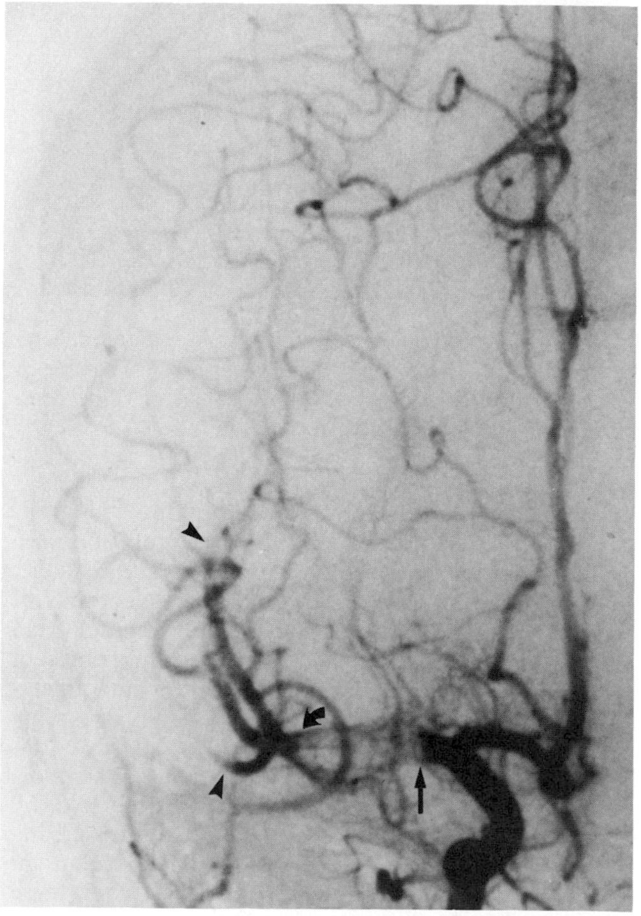

**Fig. 11-10.** Right carotid angiogram, anteroposterior (Towne) projection. Intraluminal filling defect due to clot in middle cerebral artery beginning just distal to the internal carotid bifurcation (*straight arrow*). The artery fills distally (from *curved arrow*), but there are downstream occlusions (*arrowheads*).

disease, that is, stenosis with superimposed thrombosis, must also be considered. The classic appearance of an abrupt arrest of contrast is strongly suggestive of an embolus (Fig. 11-9).[19] A convex proximal edge indicates an intraluminal filling defect. Uncommonly, the clot may be only partially occlusive, and the obstructed artery may fill distally (Fig. 11-10).

## Dissection

Dissections of the craniocervical arteries are traditionally separated according to whether they are extracranial or intracranial, spontaneous or traumatic. Most of the reported carotid territory dissections have been spontaneous (Fig. 11-11).[30,36,83] In the posterior circulation, the extracranial vertebral arteries are often involved due to minor trauma, for example, chiropractic neck manipulation (Fig. 11-12). The majority of basilar artery dissections are spontaneous (Figs. 11-13, 11-14, and 11-16).[65]

Arterial dissection presents a number of appearances angiographically. The most frequent finding is that of irregular, often eccentric, vessel narrowing.[30,83] In the case of internal carotid dissection, the narrowing typically begins distal to the carotid bulb (unlike atherosclerosis) and extends to the level of the skull base, where the vessel resumes its normal caliber (Fig. 11-11). Severe narrowing in such cases has been termed the angiographic *string sign*.[83] In extracranial vertebral artery dissection, the narrowing begins near the level of C2 and extends a variable distance (Fig. 11-12).

Segmental stenosis preceded by luminal outpouching (due to pseudoaneurysm formation) has been described as the pearl and string appearance. Vessel encroachment either proximal or immediately distal to an aneurysm, particularly an aneurysm not related to an arterial bifurcation, strongly favors dissection (Fig. 11-13).[63]

Definitive angiographic diagnosis requires the visualization of the true and false lumens.[41] Seen in pro-

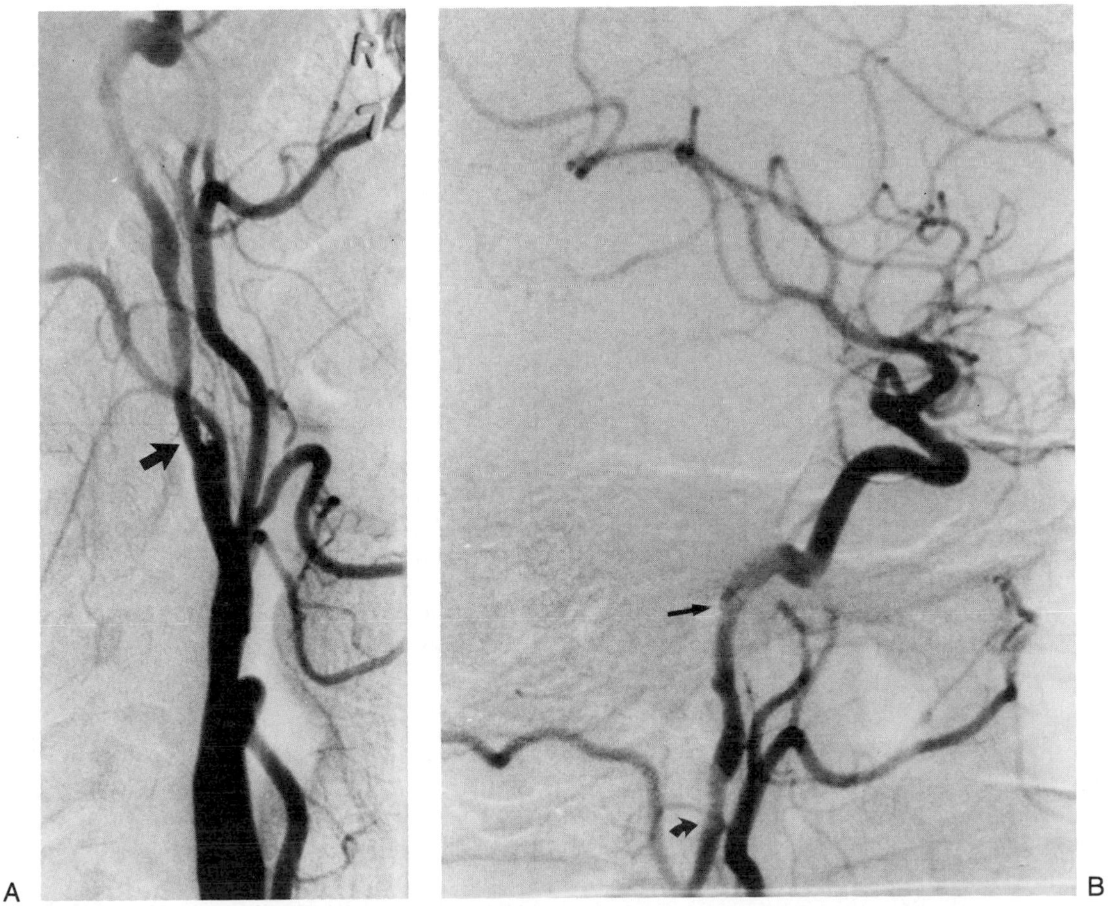


**Fig. 11-11.** A 41-year-old woman with sudden headache and right ptosis. (**A**) Right common carotid injection, lateral view, shows irregular narrowing of the internal carotid artery (*arrow*). (**B**) The irregular narrowing (*curved arrow*) extends to the level of the skull base, where the lumen returns to its normal configuration (*straight arrow*).

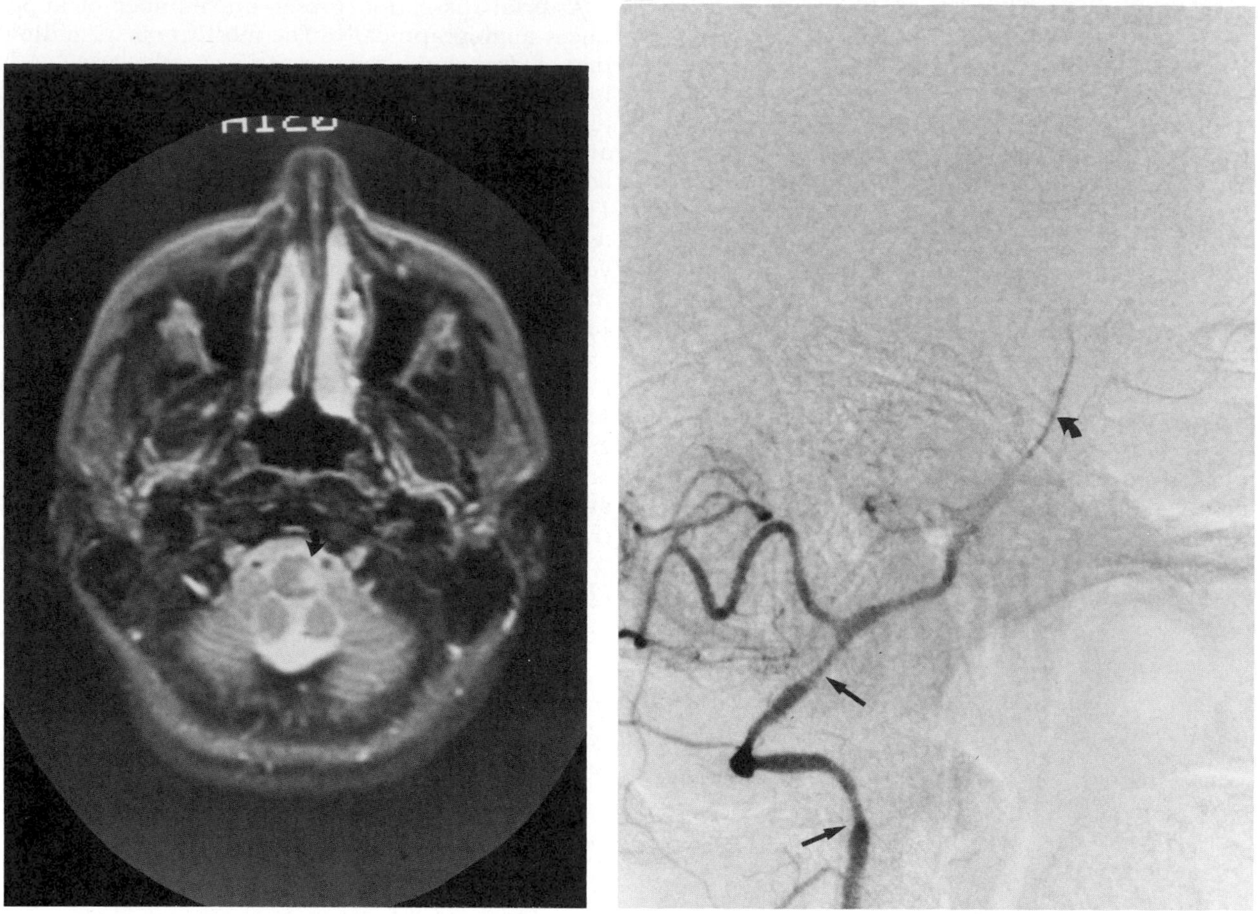

A B

**Fig. 11-12.** A 29-year-old woman who developed ataxia, right hemisensory loss, and left Horner's syndrome 2 hours after chiropractic neck manipulation. (**A**) Axial T2-weighted MRI shows small infarction in left lateral medulla (*arrow*). (**B**) Left vertebral injection, lateral view, shows irregular narrowing of vertebral artery (*straight arrows*) and only a small amount of contrast reaching the basilar artery (*curved arrow*). (*Figure continues.*)

file, the presence of an intimal flap (Fig. 11-14) is pathognomonic. If the two lumens are *en face,* then two strips of contrast, of different densities, may be seen (Fig. 11-15).[56]

Improved diagnostic accuracy is obtained with magnetic resonance (MR) imaging, which can demonstrate eccentric high signal intensity blood within the vessel wall (Fig. 11-16).

## Fibromuscular Dysplasia

Pathologically, arterial fibromuscular dysplasia (FMD) most commonly involves the media of the arterial wall. Originally identified in the renal arteries, since 1964 it has been known to also involve extrarenal vessels, including the internal carotid artery.[85]

In large angiographic series, the incidence of detection of FMD ranges from 0.3 to 0.7 percent.[47,48] Detection is frequently incidental; in one series of 52 patients, over half were not having symptoms attributable to the disease, and less than 20 percent had cerebral ischemia.[48]

The internal carotid artery is affected in 70 to 90 percent of cases, the vertebral arteries less often.[48,84] Bilateral involvement occurs in more than half. The epicenter of the ICA disease is at the level of the C2 vertebra. The proximal 2.5 cm of the ICA is almost never involved.[48,84]

The angiographic hallmark of FMD is the string of beads, contiguous alternating areas of constriction and dilatation, seen in 80 percent of cases.[84] The areas of dilatation widen the vessel to more than its normal caliber, in contrast to atherosclerosis.[48] Less frequent is the appearance of single or multiple areas of tubular stenosis, without intervening dilatation.

Rarely, FMD may involve the intracranial circulation, including the ICA, MCA, and vertebrobasilar system.[92] It may not be possible to differentiate the arterial beading or tubular stenosis from changes due to

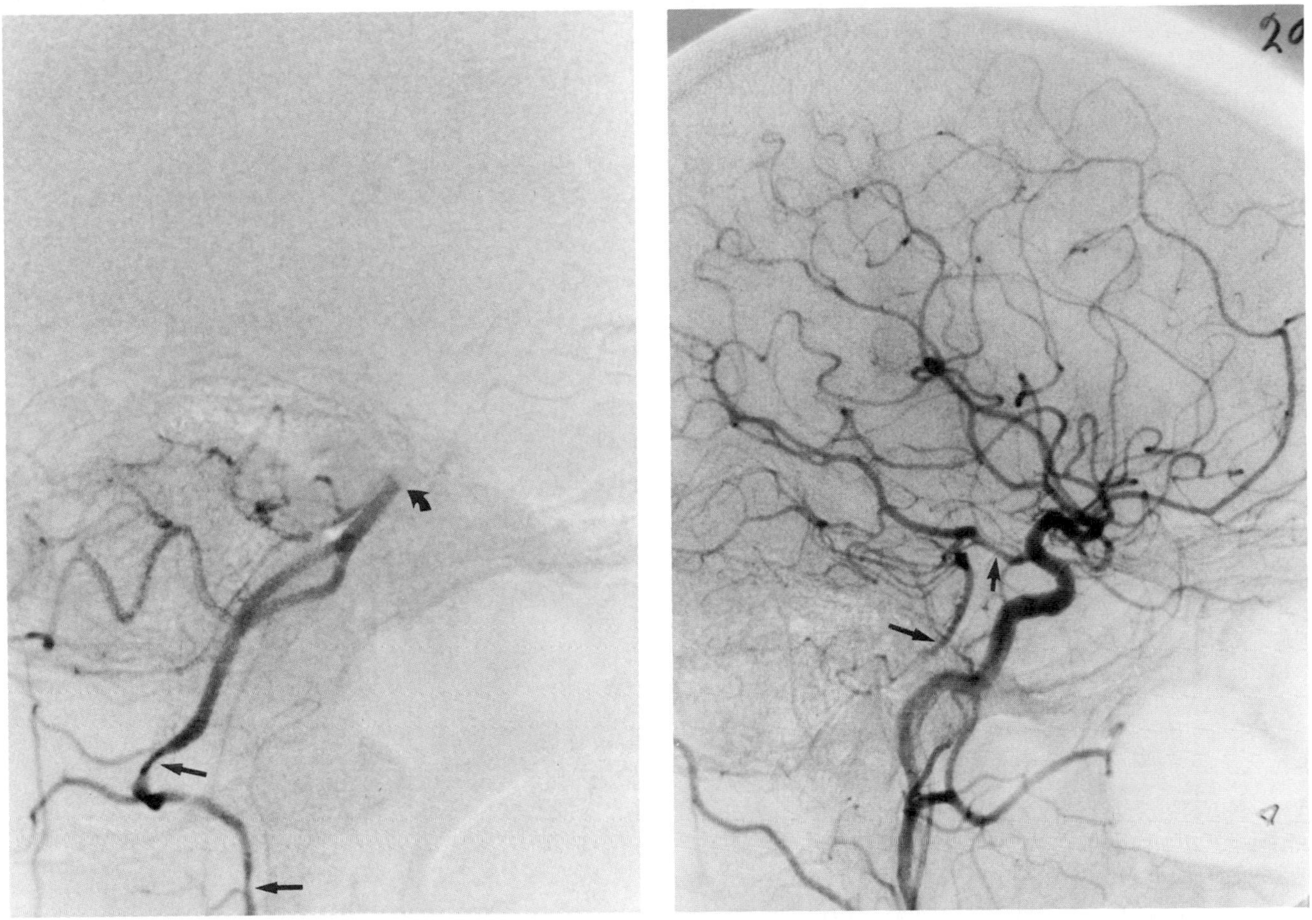

C D

**Fig. 11-12** (*Continued*). (**C**) Right vertebral injection, lateral view, similarly shows irregularly narrowed vertebral artery, consistent with bilateral vertebral dissections (*straight arrows*). Arrest of contrast in the midbasilar artery (*curved arrow*) secondary to flow watershed or embolus. (**D**) Right carotid injection, lateral view, shows circle of Willis collateral through the posterior communicating artery (*shorter arrow*), which fills the basilar and its branches (*longer arrow*).

cerebral arteritis, if the extracranial vessels are unaffected.

When fibroplasia involves the intima rather than the media, segments of smooth stenosis are seen angiographically.[103] Short segments may resemble atherosclerosis. Long areas of severe stenosis may cause a "string sign" similar to arterial dissection, particularly since the proximal internal carotid tends to be spared in both conditions.[103] The string sign usually resolves on follow-up angiography in dissection, but not with intimal fibroplasia.

## Cerebral Arteritis

A myriad of unusual conditions affecting the intracranial vasculature are subsumed under the title *arteritis*. The common denominator is an inflammatory process that affects the entire blood vessel wall. It is convenient to separate these conditions according to their infectious or noninfectious nature. Bacterial, viral, tuberculous, and fungal infections are not frequently assessed by angiography since the advent of computed tomography (CT) and MR imaging. All tend to involve the basal arteries, although pure basal involvement is a particular feature of tuberculosis.[60] Of the viruses, herpes zoster is the only one visible angiographically.[34]

The noninfectious causes are again separated into necrotizing and nonnecrotizing conditions.[15,34] Polyarteritis nodosa causes a necrotizing arteritis, with arterial narrowings and small aneurysms seen both intracranially and extracranially. The nonnecrotizing arteritides include the collagen vascular diseases, neurosarcoidosis, giant-cell arteritis, angiitis associated with Hodgkin's lymphoma, Takayasu's disease, and granulomatous angiitis.[116]

Angiographic findings in cerebral arteritis are nonspecific. The most frequent finding is vessel narrowing (Fig. 11-17). This usually affects longer arterial segments than intracranial atherosclerosis, and is cir-

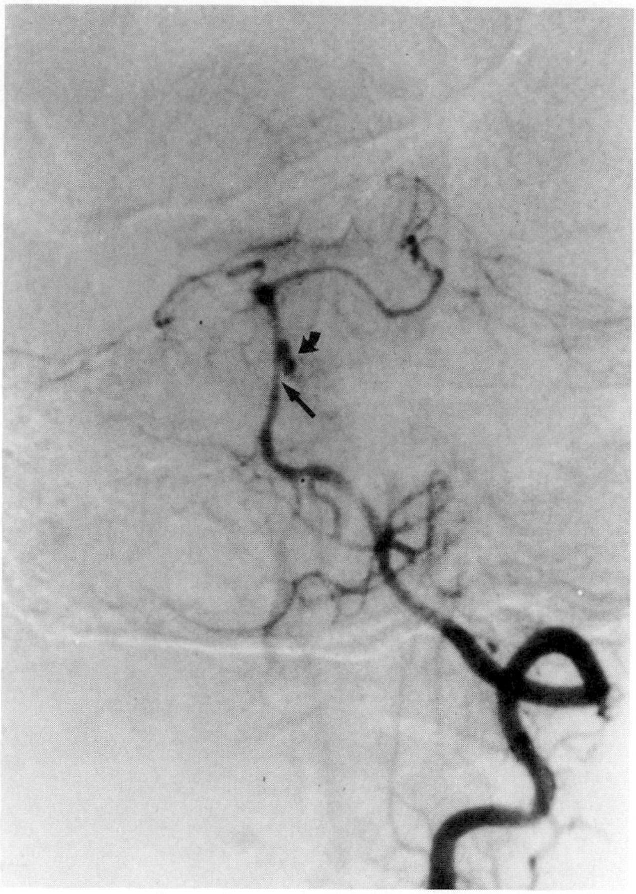

**Fig. 11-13.** Left vertebral angiogram, right posterior oblique view. Aneurysmal outpouching of the midbasilar artery (*curved arrow*). Narrowing of the basilar artery immediately proximal to the aneurysm (*straight arrow*). Surgically and pathologically proven dissection.

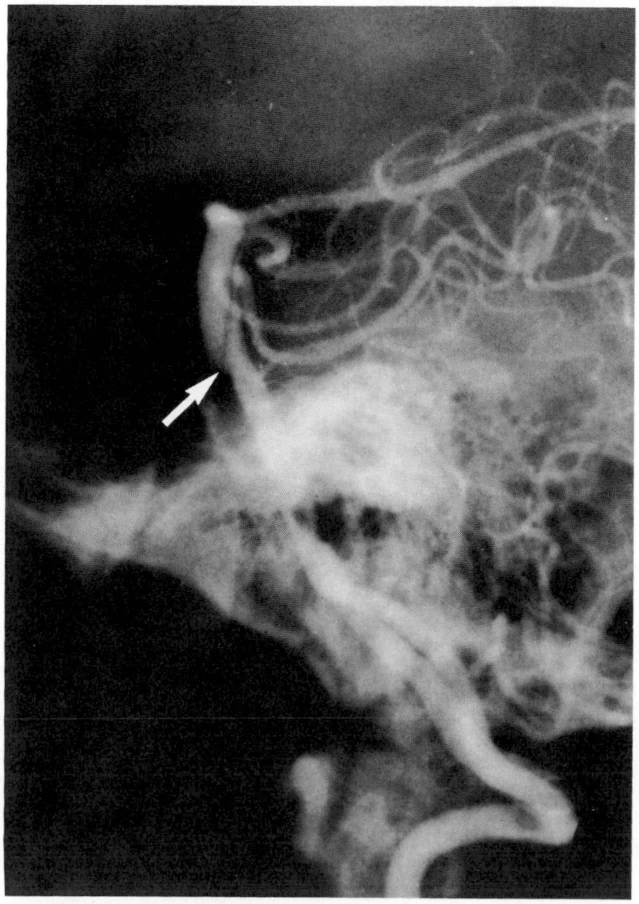

**Fig. 11-14.** Right vertebral injection, lateral view. The upper basilar artery is widened, and an intimal flap is seen (*arrow*), diagnostic of dissection.

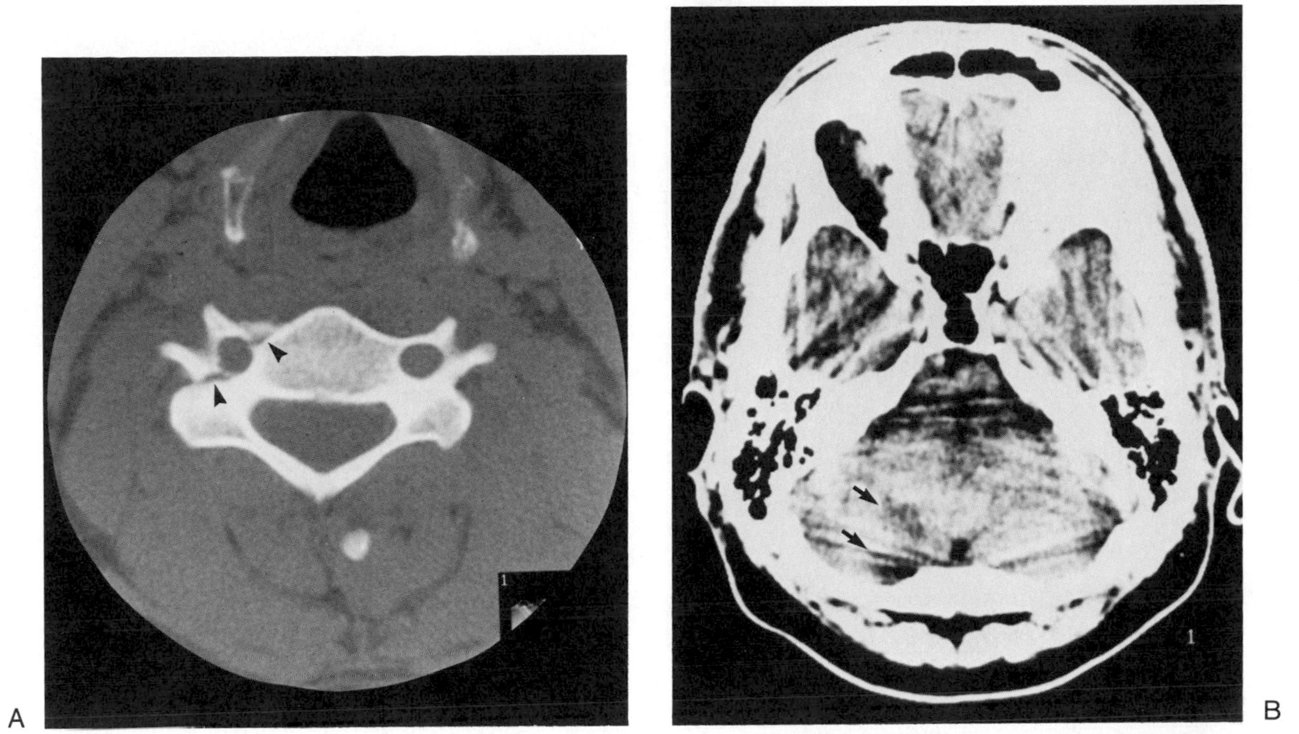

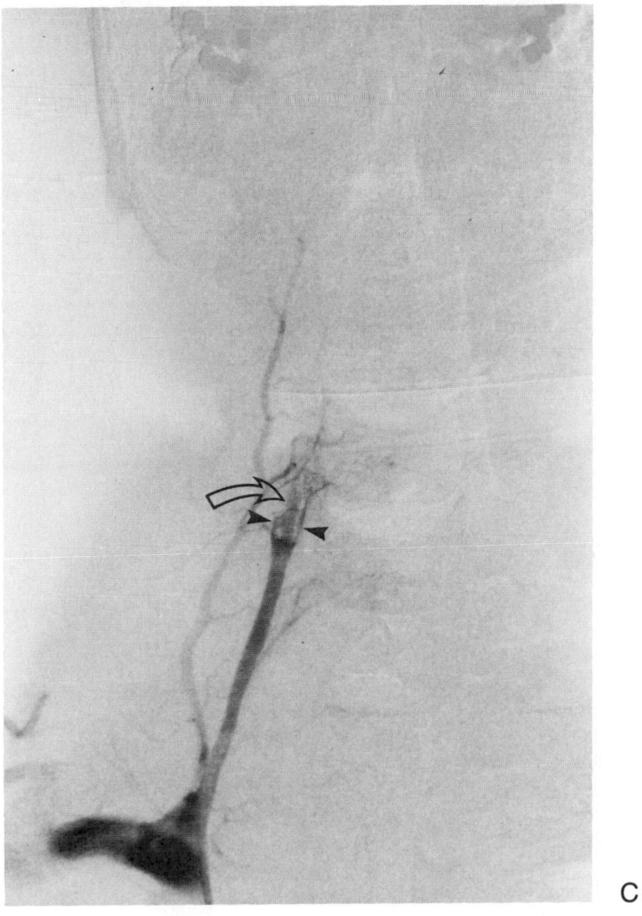

**Fig. 11-15.** A 28-year-old man with a recent C4–C5 fracture dislocation and acute onset of vertigo and facial numbness. (**A**) Axial CT of the cervical spine at the C5 level shows fracture line extending across the foramen transversarium (*arrowheads*). (**B**) CT scan of the head without contrast enhancement shows low densities in right cerebellar hemisphere (*arrows*). (**C**) Right vertebral angiogram, anteroposterior projection, shows occlusion of the artery in the midcervical region. There is widening of the artery (*between arrowheads*) with bands of contrast seen peripherally (*arrowheads*) and centrally (*clear curved arrow*). Diagnosis: traumatic dissection.

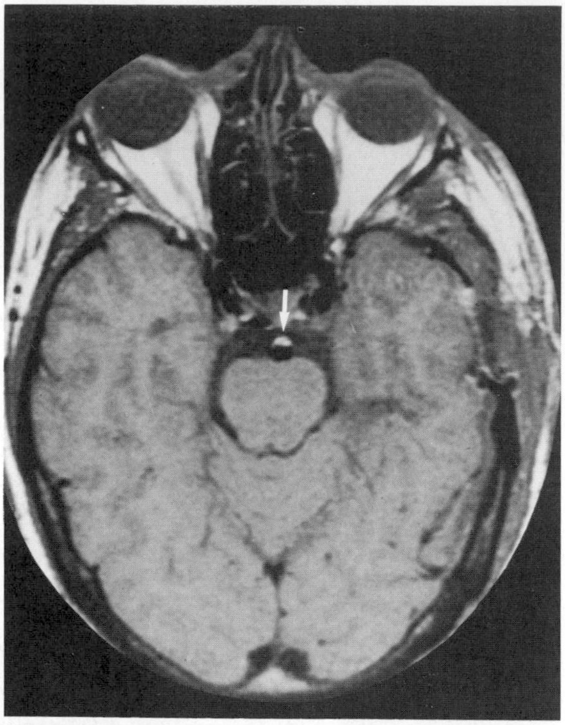

**Fig. 11-16.** Axial T1-weighted MRI showing eccentric high signal in or adjacent to the wall of the basilar artery (*arrow*) consistent with dissection.

A 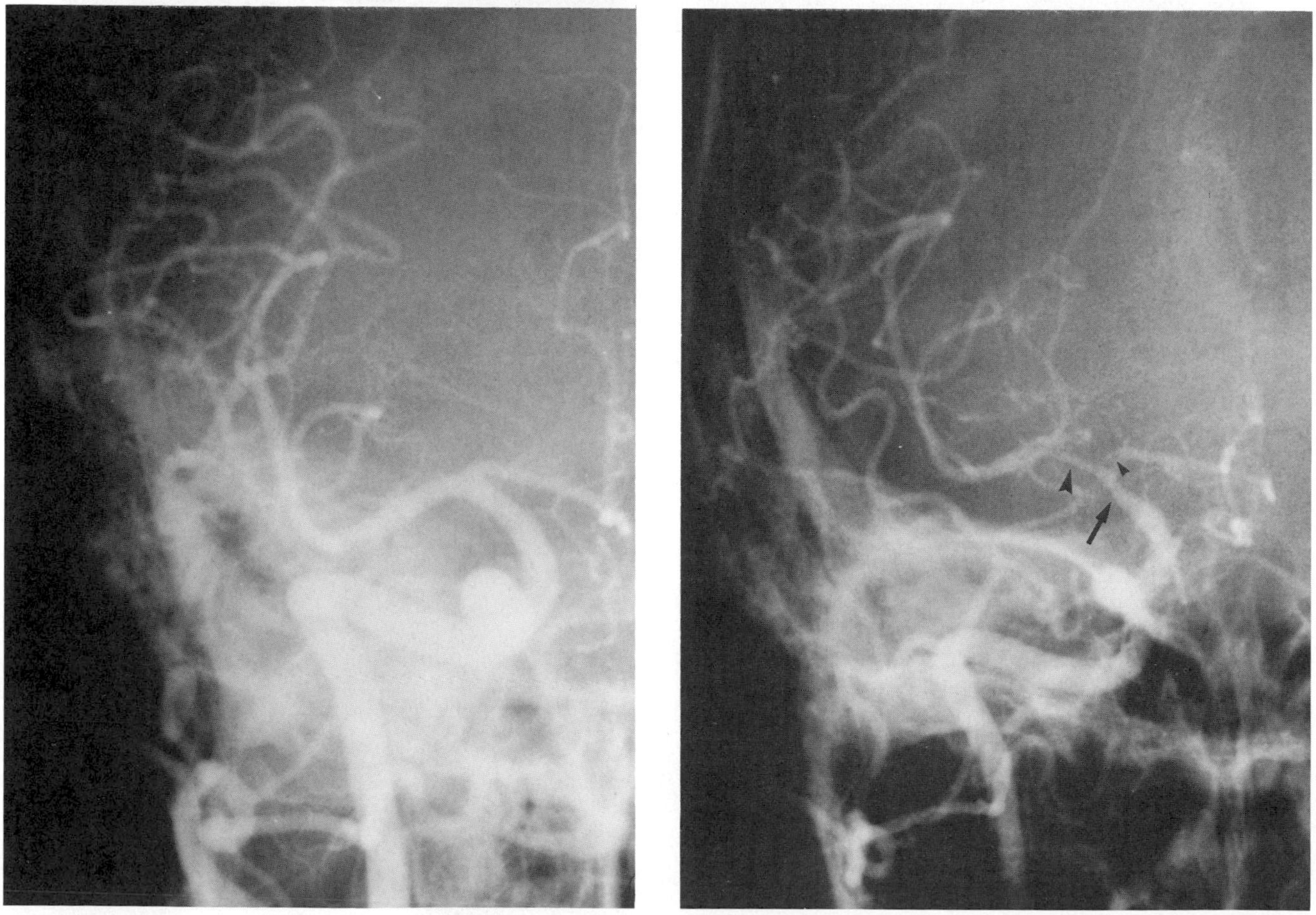 B

**Fig. 11-17.** A 53-year-old woman with subacute progressive illness and multiple cerebral infarctions. (**A**) Right carotid angiogram, anteroposterior (Towne) projection, done during early phase of illness, is essentially normal. (**B**) Repeat injection, 3 months later, shows a progressive arteriopathy with severe narrowing of the supraclinoid carotid artery (*straight arrow*) and middle (*large arrowhead*) and anterior (*small arrowhead*) cerebral arteries. Arteritis of unknown cause.

cumferential as opposed to the frequent eccentric position of the latter.[34] Irregular narrowing or a shaggy appearance is more common with infectious etiologies.[60] "Beading" of the vessels, that is, alternating dilatations and constrictions, is more specific to arteritis, but is also seen in FMD and atherosclerosis intracranially, albeit rarely.[54] Involvement of extracranial arteries may help in distinguishing atherosclerosis, FMD, polyarteritis nodosa, and Takayasu's disease (with its arch involvement) from each other and from other purely cranial diseases such as giant-cell arteritis and granulomatous angiitis.

## Moyamoya Disease

In 1968 Kudo[55] described a progressive condition manifested by spontaneous occlusion of the intracranial segments of the internal carotid arteries. Associated involvement of the other circle of Willis vessels was observed. Suzuki coined the term "moyamoya" (Japanese for hazy, like a puff of cigarette smoke) to describe the development of exuberant collateral through the small perforating branches of the basal arteries commonly seen in the condition.[104] In addition to this collateral, other abnormal anastomoses include the so-called "rete mirabile" between external carotid branches to the dura and superficial cortical arteries.[59,113]

Suzuki and Takaku[104] staged the disease according to the degree of stenosis or occlusion of the ICA and its branches, and the amount of moyamoya. The disease is initially restricted to stenosis of the distal supraclinoid carotid artery. The moyamoya then develops and later intensifies as the anterior and middle cerebral arteries occlude. It diminishes as the disease spreads proximally to the anterior choroidal and posterior communicating arteries, since the basal perforators mainly arise from these vessels (Fig. 11-18). Ultimately the external carotid rete mirabile forms the principal collateral system as the moyamoya disappears.

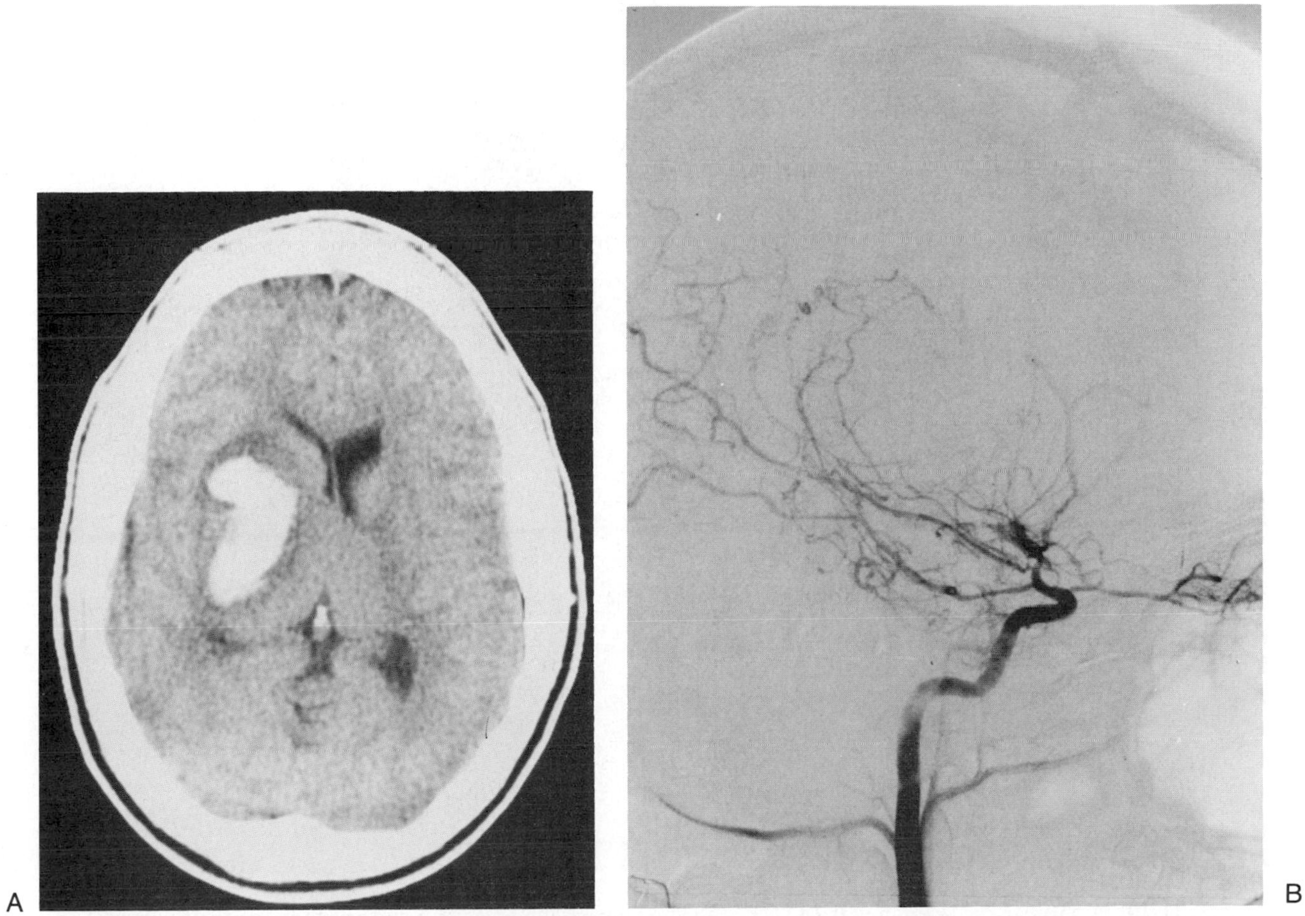


**Fig. 11-18.** A 17-year-old Caucasian man with acute left hemiplegia. (**A**) CT scan without contrast enhancement shows acute hemorrhage in the right putamen. (**B**) Right common carotid injection shows a tight stenosis of the supraclinoid carotid artery, prominent basal perforating vessels (moyamoya), poor filling of the middle cerebral artery, and no filling of the anterior cerebral artery.

## Venous Disease

Cortical venous and dural sinus thrombosis should be considered when the topography of cerebral infarction does not correspond to either an arterial branch or arterial watershed territory.[13,32] Cerebral infarction with patchy areas of hemorrhage can also suggest a venous cause (Fig. 11-19A).

MR scan has emerged as the method of choice for imaging cerebral venous disease. However, cerebral angiography is often performed during the course of investigation of (presumed) arterial occlusive disease. It is important to routinely obtain films of the venous phase. Occasionally, an unsuspected venous thrombosis may be detected.

Partial or complete lack of opacification of one or more of the dural sinuses is the angiographic hallmark of venous occlusion (Fig. 11-19B).[13] Usually other signs are also present, including lack of cortical venous filling, delayed emptying, or abnormal collateral venous drainage.[13]

## Fusiform Aneurysms/Dolichoectasia

Apart from presenting clinically with mass effect[17] or hemorrhage,[98] fusiform aneurysms may produce ischemia, by one of three mechanisms: thrombosis of the aneurysm itself, small perforating artery occlusion, or distal embolization. Thrombosis of vertebrobasilar fusiform aneurysms with massive brain stem infarction is usually fatal.[80,117] Occlusion of a pontine perforator may cause only unilateral pontine infarction.[89] Embolization into the posterior cerebral or middle cerebral territory distal to fusiform aneurysms has been observed.[101]

In a large fusiform sac, thrombus invariably lines the wall, and there is characteristically sluggish blood flow within it (Fig. 11-20). During or after angiography, there is a risk of thromboembolism. In the one case encountered at our institution (unpublished), complete thrombosis of the basilar artery and death occurred 3 days after cerebral angiography. This was probably related to the pre- and postprocedure altera-

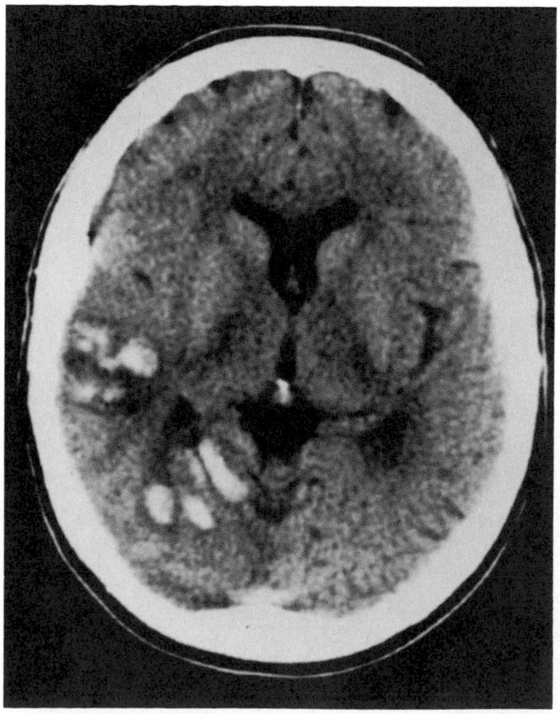

A

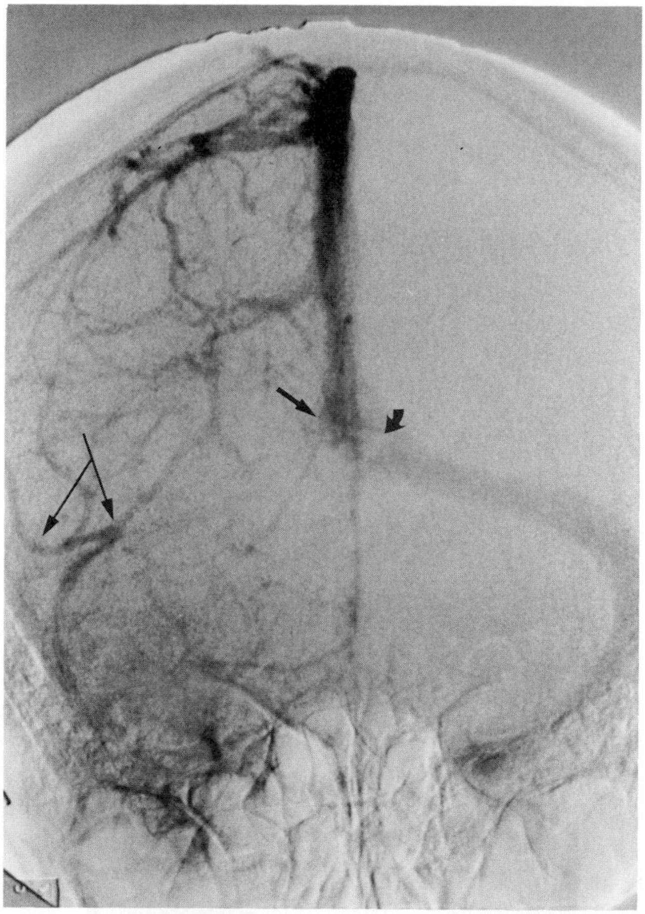

B

**Fig. 11-19.** A 55-year-old woman with (**A**) CT scan showing patchy areas of hemorrhage in the right occipital and temporal lobes. (**B**) Right carotid angiogram, anteroposterior (Towne) projection, showing occlusion of the right transverse sinus at the torcular (*short straight arrow*). Possible filling defect in the left side of the torcular (*curved arrow*). Collateral venous drainage over the right convexity veins into the right transverse sinus (*long straight arrows*).

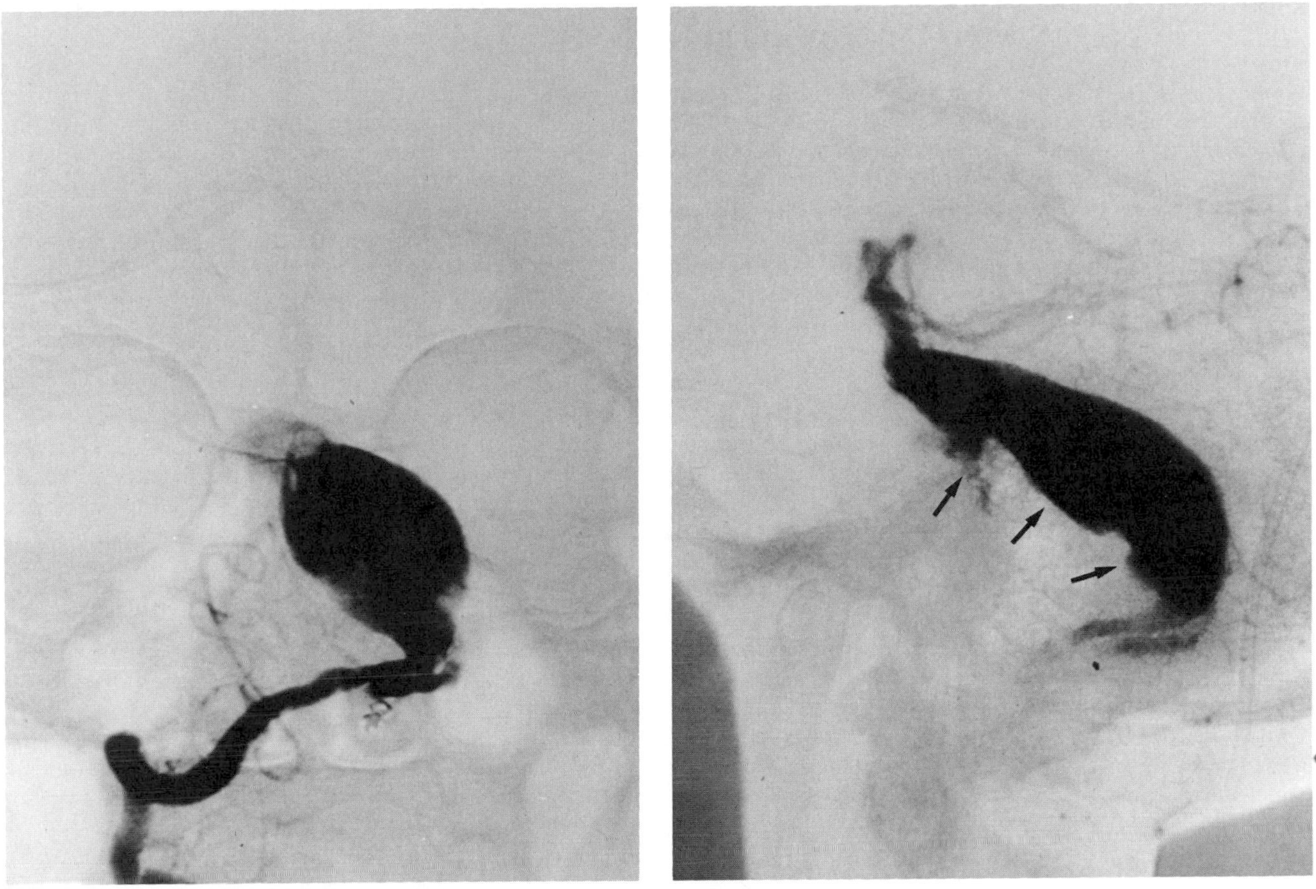

A B

**Fig. 11-20.** A 62-year-old hypertensive man with brain stem transient ischemic attacks and strokes. (**A**) Right vertebral injection, anteroposterior view, showing massively dilated basilar artery with sluggish flow to the basilar apex. (**B**) Same injection, lateral view, showing irregular anterior wall of the aneurysm due to the presence of mural thrombus (*arrows*).

tions in the patient's anticoagulants. Others[99] encountering such complications have postulated that contrast stasis interferes with local blood flow; while this would explain transient ischemia, it would not explain thrombosis. Such untoward events should be considered when diagnostic angiography is contemplated, since CT and MR will secure the diagnosis in most patients.

## MAGNETIC RESONANCE ANGIOGRAPHY

When living tissue is placed in a strong permanent magnetic field, hydrogen protons within the tissue behave like small bar magnets and line up parallel to the lines of the magnetic field. A second (temporary) magnetic field can be created using a short burst of radiofrequency (RF) energy. This pulse of RF energy causes the small bar magnets to swing out of their initial alignment into a temporary new alignment with the RF field. Once the pulse ends, the little magnets switch back to their previous orientation. In doing so, they themselves emit a very small RF signal. The detection of this signal is the basis of MR imaging.

### Time-of-Flight Angiography

There are two ways in which radiofrequency pulses may be applied to a tissue to bring out differences between protons in moving tissue (e.g., blood) and the protons in the surrounding stationary tissue. One way is to apply pulses to a predetermined volume of the tissue. All of the protons inside that volume will be subjected to radiofrequency energy. However, outside protons which flow into the volume (e.g., protons in moving blood) will not be so affected. The resulting differences in relative magnetization between the stationary and the moving protons forms the basis of time-of-flight (TOF) angiography.

Time-of-flight MR angiography is done in either a two-dimensional (2D-TOF)[51] or three-dimensional (3D-TOF)[70,71,110] mode. In the 2D mode, imaging begins with RF excitation of a thin slice of tissue, typically 1.5- to 3-mm thickness. In the case of carotid bifurcation imaging, the slice is usually in the transverse (axial) plane. The two dimensions of the image matrix are in the right-to-left and anterior-to-posterior directions, respectively. Carotid artery blood flow is predominantly in the inferior-to-superior direction. Thus a cross-sectional image is obtained with such a slice. Many axial slices are obtained in this manner, adequate to span the region of interest. A computer program is then used to construct angiographic projections, which may be viewed from multiple angles, including the conventional anteroposterior direction (Fig. 11-21).[51]

In contrast to the 2D approach, the 3D time-of-flight method treats the whole region of interest as one "slice" or volume. Instead of each axial slice being sequentially excited by an RF pulse, the entire volume is exposed at once. The third dimension, in the inferior-superior direction, is spatially "encoded" along its axis by a gradient in the magnetic field.

The quality of the angiogram depends upon two important variables. One is the ability to visualize the difference between flowing blood and stationary tissue, that is, the contrast between the two. The second is the ability to make out the fine details of vessel anatomy. The first is termed the contrast sensitivity; the second is the spatial resolution. 2D time-of-flight has greater contrast sensitivity than the 3D technique.[51] The reason is that the 2D imaging slice is thinner than the 3D volume. Protons moving through a thin slice remain distinctly different from their stationary counterparts, but when passing through a larger volume they gradually lose their magnetization difference. Thus, distal flow or slow flow is not as well seen with 3D-TOF. On the other hand, spatial resolution is superior with the 3D method.[94] There is no gap between slices as with 2D, and 3D allows for thinner slices, 1 mm or less in width. For these and other reasons,[94] 3D-TOF is preferred over 2D for intracranial TOF angiography (Fig. 11-22).

Much of the clinical experience in the use of MR angiography for cerebrovascular disease has been in studies of the carotid bifurcation (Fig. 11-23). The correlation between conventional angiography and 2D-TOF angiography in one study was 56 to 70 percent ($P = 0.0001$).[64] Those patients with severe stenosis (defined as 80 to 99 percent) had the best correlation with angiography, over 90 percent. However, MR angiography was correct in only 25 percent of carotid occlusions—most were misdiagnosed as severe stenosis when a small vessel or artifact was seen distally.[64]

MR angiography tends to overestimate the degree (and length) of a stenosis, due to loss of signal arising from nonlaminar flow patterns.[51,64,71,110] At its present

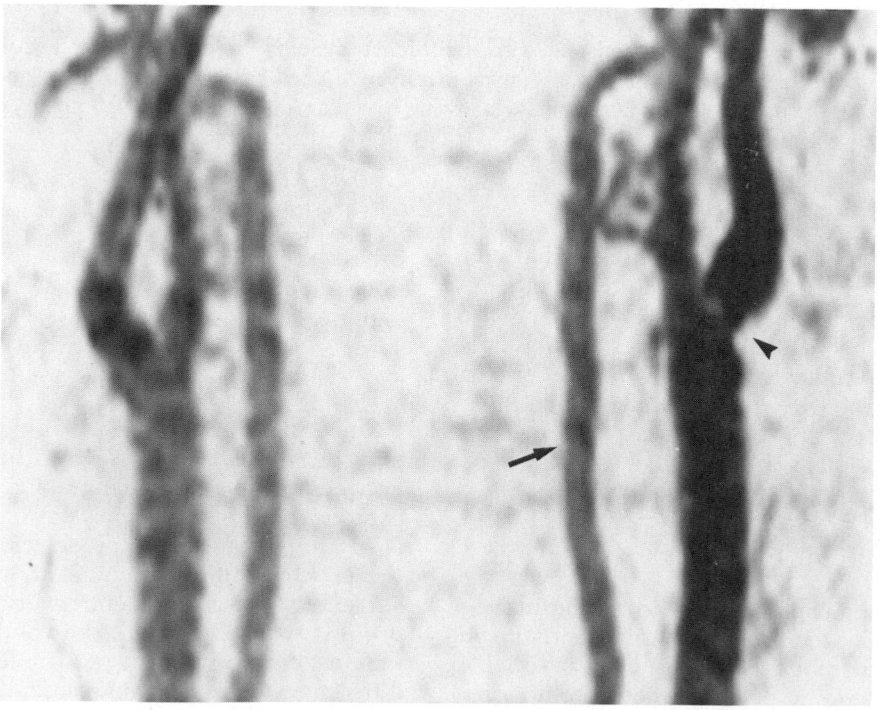

**Fig. 11-21.** MR angiogram using two-dimensional time-of-flight technique. Mild atheromatous changes at left carotid bifurcation (*arrowhead*). Note that with the computer projection algorithm, the vertebral artery (*arrow*) is seen in the same two-dimensional projection as the carotid. (Scan parameters: TR 45 ms, TE 8.7 ms, flip angle 45°, NEX = 1, FOV 19 cm, 256 × 256 matrix. Acquisition time: 12 min 35 s.)

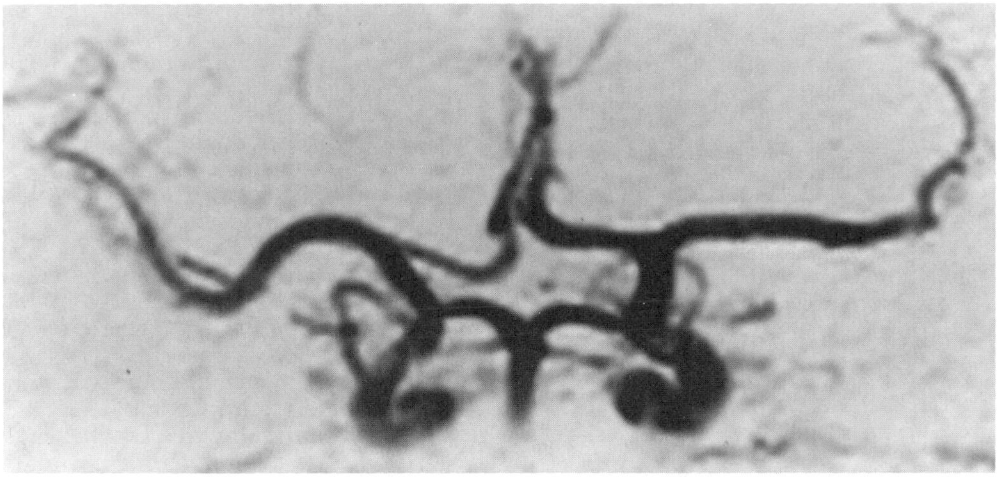

**Fig. 11-22.** 3D time-of-flight angiogram of the circle of Willis. Normal study. (Scan parameters: TR 34 ms, TE 4.7 ms, flip angle 25°, NEX = 1, FOV 20 cm, 256 × 256 matrix. Acquisition time: 9 min 18 s.)

level of development, MR angiography is certainly a reliable screening study to rule out severe carotid stenosis. Differentiating stenosis from occlusion angiographically still warrants a conventional angiogram.

## Phase Contrast Angiography

The second method by which contrast between moving and stationary protons may be obtained with MR is the phase contrast (PC) technique. By applying pulses to the imaging volume in a certain manner, protons in motion can be highlighted while nonmoving protons are not. The pulses cause a change in the phase (or angular orientation about the axis) of moving protons that is dependent on their velocity. The magnitude of the phase change after repeated pulses gives a signal whose direction is related to the initial direction of the applied pulse. Three directions of pulse application yield three dimensions of information.[88]

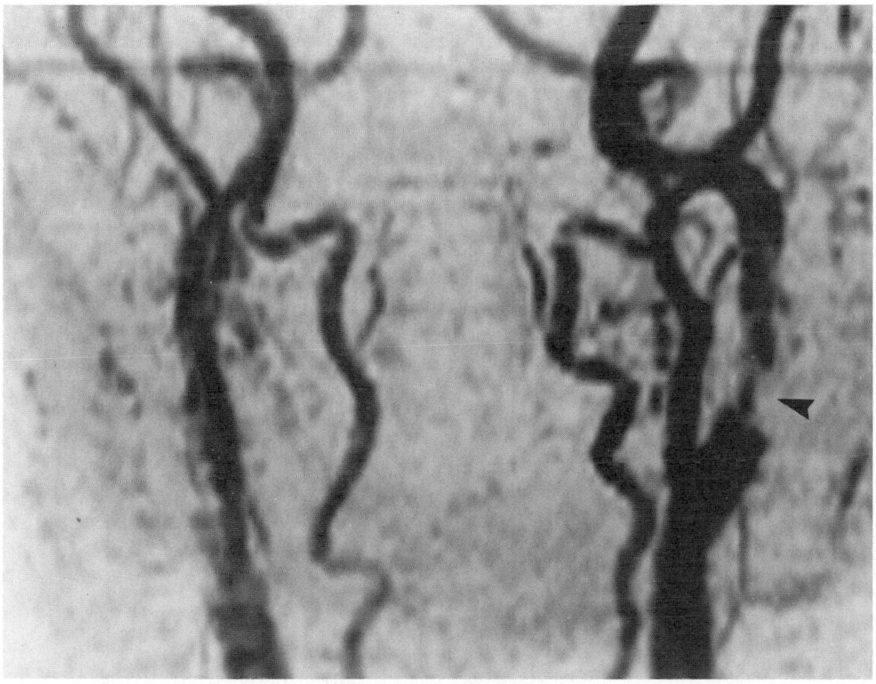

**Fig. 11-23.** 2D time-of-flight angiogram of the cervical region. Moderately severe stenosis of the proximal left internal carotid artery (*arrowhead*). Scan parameters as in Figure 11-21.

Inherent in the phase contrast technique is a greater sensitivity to slow flow than exists with TOF angiography, allowing visualization of venous anatomy.[110] This greater sensitivity also makes PC more prone to signal loss due to nonlaminar flow.[88] PC angiography is more specific than time-of-flight for true flow: with TOF, thrombus may appear similar to flowing blood because both can have high signal intensity.[51]

## REFERENCES


1. Akers DL, Markowitz IA, Kerstein MD: The value of aortic arch study in the evaluation of cerebrovascular insufficiency. Am J Surg 154:230, 1987
2. Allcock JM: Occlusion of the middle cerebral artery: serial angiography as a guide to conservative therapy. J Neurosurg 27:353, 1967
3. Alpers BJ, Berry RG: Circle of Willis in cerebral vascular disorders. Arch Neurol 8:398, 1963
4. Alter M, Kieffer S, Resch J, Ansari K: Cerebral infarction: clinical and angiographic correlations. Neurology (NY) 22:590, 1972
5. Antunovic R, Rosch J, Dotter CT: The value of systemic arterial heparinization in transfemoral angiography: a prospective study. AJR 127:223, 1976
6. Barnett HJM, Peerless SJ, Kaufmann JCE: "Stump" of internal carotid artery—a source for further cerebral embolic ischemia. Stroke 9:448, 1978
7. Battacharji SK, Hutchinson EC, McCall AJ: The circle of Willis—the incidence of developmental abnormalities in normal and infarcted brains. Brain 90:747, 1967
8. Bauer RB, Sheehan S, Wechsler N, Meyer JS: Arteriographic study of sites, incidence, and treatment of arteriosclerotic cerebrovascular lesions. Neurology (NY) 12:698, 1962
9. Bierman HR, Miller ER, Byron RL et al: Intra-arterial catheterization of viscera in man. AJR 66:555, 1951
10. Bladin PF: A radiologic and pathologic study of embolism of the internal carotid–middle cerebral arterial axis. Radiology 82:615, 1964
11. Blaisdell WF, Claus RH, Galbraith JG et al: Joint study of extracranial arterial occlusion. IV. A review of surgical considerations. JAMA 209:1889, 1969
12. Blaisdell FW, Glickman M, Trunkey DD: Ulcerated atheroma of the carotid artery. Arch Surg 108:491, 1974
13. Bousser M-G, Chiras J, Bories J, Castaigne P: Cerebral venous thrombosis—a review of 38 cases. Stroke 16:199, 1985
14. Brice JG, Dowsett DJ, Lowe RD: Haemodynamic effects of carotid artery stenosis. Br Med J 2:1363, 1964
15. Burger PC, Burch JG, Vogel FS: Granulomatous angiitis. An unusual etiology of stroke. Stroke 8:29, 1977
16. Caplan LR: "Top of the basilar" syndrome. Neurology (NY) 30:72, 1980
17. Dandy WE: Intracranial Arterial Aneurysms. Hafner, New York, 1969
18. Dalal PM, Shah PM, Sheth SC, Deshpande CK: Cerebral embolism: angiographic observations on spontaneous clot lysis. Lancet 1:61, 1965
19. Davis DO, Rumbaugh CL, Gilson JM: Angiographic diagnosis of small vessel cerebral emboli. Acta Radiol Diagn 9:264, 1969
20. Davis PC, Hoffman JC: Work in progress: intra-arterial digital subtraction angiography: evaluation in 150 patients. Radiology 148:9, 1983
21. Debrun GM, Vinuela FV, Fox AJ: Aspirin and systemic heparinization in diagnostic and interventional neuroradiology. AJNR 3:337, 1982
22. Deweese JA, May AG, Lipchik EO, Rob CG: Anatomic and hemodynamic correlations in carotid artery stenosis. Stroke 1:149, 1970
23. Dion JE, Gates PC, Fox AJ et al: Clinical events following neuroangiography: a prospective study. Stroke 18:997, 1987
24. Earnest F, Forbes G, Sandok BA et al: Complications of cerebral angiography: prospective assessment of risk. AJNR 4:1191, 1983
25. Edwards JH, Kricheff II, Gorstein F et al: Atherosclerotic subintimal hematoma of the carotid artery. Radiology 133:123, 1979
26. Edwards JH, Kricheff II, Riles T, Imparato A: Angiographically undetected ulceration of the carotid bifurcation as a cause of embolic stroke. Radiology 132:369, 1979
27. Eggers FM, Price AC, Allen JH, James AE: Neuroradiologic applications of intraarterial digital subtraction angiography. AJNR 4:854, 1983
28. Eikelboom BC, Riles TR, Mintzer R et al: Inaccuracy of angiography in the diagnosis of carotid ulceration. Stroke 14:882, 1983
29. Eisenberg RL, Mani RL: The six French catheter in arch aortography. Radiology 125:822, 1977
30. Ehrenfeld WK, Wylie EJ: Spontaneous dissection of the internal carotid artery. Arch Surg 111:1294, 1976
31. Eldh P, Jacobsson B: Heparinized vascular catheters: a clinical trial. Radiology 111:289, 1974
32. Enevoldson TP, Ross Russell RW: Cerebral venous thrombosis: new causes for an old syndrome? Q J Med 77:1255, 1990
33. Farinas PL: New technique for arteriographic examination of abdominal aorta and its branches. AJR 46:641, 1941
34. Ferris EJ, Levine HL: Cerebral arteritis: classification. Radiology 109:327, 1973
35. Ferris EJ, Shapiro JH, Simeone FA: Arteriovenous shunting in cerebrovascular occlusive disease. AJR 98:631, 1966
36. Fisher CM, Ojemann RG, Roberson GH: Spontaneous dissection of the cervico-cerebral arteries. Can J Neurol Sci 5:9, 1978
37. Formanek G, Frech RS, Amplatz K: Arterial thrombus formation during clinical percutaneous catheterization. Circulation 41:833, 1970
38. Gabrielson TO, Seeger JF, Knake JE et al: The

nearly occluded internal carotid artery: a diagnostic trap. Radiology 138:611, 1981
39. Gacs G, Fox AJ, Barnett HJM, Vinuela F: Occurrence and mechanisms of occlusion of the anterior cerebral artery. Stroke 14:952, 1983
40. Gannon WE, Chait A: Occlusion of the middle cerebral artery with recanalization. AJR 88:24, 1962
41. Giedke H, Kriebel J, Sindermann F: Dissecting aneurysm of the petrous portion of the internal carotid artery: case report and review of previous cases. Neuroradiology 10:121, 1975
42. Gunning AJ, Pickering GW, Robb-Smith AHT, Ross Russell R: Mural thrombosis of the internal carotid artery and subsequent embolism. Q J Med 33:155, 1964
43. Hass WK, Fields WS, North RR et al: Joint study of extracranial arterial occlusion. II. Arteriography, techniques, sites, and complications. JAMA 203:159, 1968
44. Hennerici M, Klemm C, Rautenberg W: The subclavian steal phenomenon: a common vascular disorder with rare neurological deficits. Neurology (NY) 38:669, 1988
45. Hinck VC: Single catheter for aortic arch and selective cerebral angiography. AJNR 7:159, 1986
46. Hinck VC, Judkins MP, Paxton HD: Simplified selective femorocerebral angiography. Radiology 89:1048, 1967
47. Houser OW, Baker HL: Fibromuscular dysplasia and other uncommon diseases of the cervical carotid artery: angiographic aspects. AJR 104:201, 1968
48. Houser OW, Baker HL, Sandok BA, Holley KE: Cephalic arterial fibromuscular dysplasia. Radiology 101:605, 1971
49. Irino T, Taneda M, Minami T: Angiographic manifestations in postrecanalized cerebral infarction. Neurology (NY) 27:471, 1977
50. Julian OC, Dye WS, Javid H, Hunter JA: Ulcerative lesions of the carotid artery bifurcation. Arch Surg 86:803, 1963
51. Keller PJ, Drayer BP, Fram EK et al: MR angiography with two-dimensional acquisition and three-dimensional display: work in progress. Radiology 173:527, 1989
52. Kerber CW, Cromwell LD, Drayer BP, Bank WO: Cerebral ischemia. I. Current angiographic techniques, complications, and safety. AJR 130:1097, 1978
53. Kishore PRS, Dick AR: Spontaneous disappearance of carotid stenosis. Radiology 129:721, 1978
54. Knopman DS, Anderson DC, Mastri A, Larson D: Leptomeningeal artery atherosclerosis visualized by angiography: clinical correlates. Stroke 9:262, 1978
55. Kudo T: Spontaneous occlusion of the circle of Willis: a disease apparently confined to Japanese. Neurology (NY) 18:485, 1968
56. Kunze S, Schiefer W: Angiographic demonstration of a dissecting aneurysm of the middle cerebral artery. Neuroradiology 2:201, 1971
57. Lang EK: A survey of the complications of percutaneous retrograde arteriography: Seldinger technic. Radiology 81:257, 1963
58. Lanner LO, Rosengren K: Angiographic diagnosis of intracerebral vascular occlusions. Acta Radiol Diagn 2:129, 1964
59. Leeds NE, Abbott KH: Collateral circulation in cerebrovascular disease in childhood via rete mirabile and perforating branches of anterior choroidal and posterior cerebral arteries. Radiology 85:628, 1965
60. Leeds NE, Goldberg HI: Angiographic manifestations in cerebral inflammatory disease. Radiology 98:595, 1971
61. Lehrer GM: Arteriographic demonstration of collateral circulation in cerebrovascular disease. Neurology (NY) 8:27, 1958
62. Lhermitte F, Gautier JC, Derouesne C: Nature of occlusions of the middle cerebral artery. Neurology (NY) 20:82, 1970
63. Liliequist B: The roentgenologic appearance of spontaneous dissecting aneurysm of the cervical internal carotid artery. Vasc Surg 2:223, 1968
64. Litt AW, Eidelman EM, Pinto RS et al: Diagnosis of carotid artery stenosis: comparison of 2DFT time-of-flight MR angiography with contrast angiography in 50 patients. AJNR 12:149, 1991
65. Lownie SP, Fox AJ, Drake CG: Spontaneous dissections of the basilar artery, abstracted. Presented at the 29th annual meeting of the American Society of Neuroradiology, Washington DC, June 1991.
66. Maddison FE, Moore WS: Ulcerated atheroma of the carotid artery: arteriographic appearance. AJR 107:530, 1969
67. Mani RL: Computer analysis of factors associated with thrombus formation observed on pullout angiograms. Invest Radiol 10:378, 1975
68. Mann FC, Herrick JF, Essex HE, Baldes EJ: The effect on the blood flow of decreasing the lumen of a blood vessel. Surgery 4:249, 1938
69. Margolis MT, Newton TH: Collateral pathways between the cavernous portion of the internal carotid and external carotid arteries. Radiology 93:834, 1969
70. Masaryk TJ, Modic MT, Ross JS et al: Intracranial circulation: preliminary clinical results with three-dimensional (volume) MR angiography. Radiology 171:793, 1989
71. Masaryk TJ, Modic MT, Ruggieri PM et al: Three-dimensional (volume) gradient-echo imaging of the carotid bifurcation: preliminary clinical experience. Radiology 171:801, 1989
72. May AG, Deweese JA, Rob CG: Hemodynamic effects of arterial stenosis. Surgery 53:513, 1963
73. Moniz E: L'Encéphalographie artérielle, son importance dans la localisation des tumeurs cérébrales. Rev Neurol 2:72, 1927
74. Mehigan JT, Olcott C: The carotid "string" sign: differential diagnosis and management. Am J Surg 140:137, 1980
75. Moore WS, Hall AD: Ulcerated atheroma of the carotid artery: a cause of transient cerebral ischemia. Am J Surg 116:237, 1968

76. Mount LA, Taveras JM: Arteriographic demonstration of the collateral circulation of the cerebral hemispheres. Arch Neurol Psychiatry 78:235, 1957
77. Nebesar RA, Pollard JJ: A curved-tip guide wire for thoracic and abdominal angiography. AJR 97:508, 1966
78. Nejad MS, Klaper MA, Steggerda FR, Gianturco C: Clotting on the outer surface of vascular catheters. Radiology 91:248, 1968
79. Newton TH, Adams JE, Wylie EJ: Arteriography of cerebrovascular occlusive disease. N Engl J Med 270:14, 1964
80. Nishizaki T, Tamaki N, Takeda N et al: Dolichoectatic basilar artery: a review of 23 cases. Stroke 17:1277, 1986
81. North American Symptomatic Carotid Endarterectomy Trial Collaborators: Beneficial effect of carotid endarterectomy in symptomatic patients with high-grade carotid stenosis. N Engl J Med 325:445, 1991
82. North American Symptomatic Carotid Endarterectomy Trial (NASCET) Steering Committee: North American Symptomatic Carotid Endarterectomy Trial: methods, patient characteristics, and progress. Stroke 22:711, 1991
83. Ojemann RG, Fisher CM, Rich JC: Spontaneous dissecting aneurysm of the internal carotid artery. Stroke 3:434, 1972
84. Osborn AG, Anderson RE: Angiographic spectrum of cervical and intracranial fibromuscular dysplasia. Stroke 8:617, 1977
85. Palubinskas AJ, Ripley HR: Fibromuscular hyperplasia in extrarenal arteries. Radiology 82:451, 1964
86. Pelz DM, Buchan A, Fox AJ et al: Intraluminal thrombus of the internal carotid arteries: angiographic demonstration of resolution with anticoagulant therapy alone. Radiology 160:369, 1986
87. Pelz DM, Fox AJ, Vinuela F et al: The ascending pharyngeal artery: a collateral pathway in complete occlusion of the internal carotid artery. AJNR 8:177, 1987
88. Pernicone JR, Siebert JE, Potchen EJ et al: Three-dimensional phase-contrast MR angiography in the head and neck: preliminary report. AJNR 11:457, 1990
89. Pessin MS, Chimowitz MI, Levine SR et al: Stroke in patients with fusiform vertebrobasilar aneurysms. Neurology (NY) 39:16, 1989
90. Pessin MS, Duncan GW, Davis KR et al: Angiographic appearance of carotid occlusion in acute stroke. Stroke 11:485, 1980
91. Pitts FW, Haskin ME, Riggs HE, Groff RA: "Tumor-stain" in cerebrovascular disease. J Neurosurg 21:298, 1964
92. Rinaldi I, Harris WO, Kopp JE, Legier J: Intracranial fibromuscular dysplasia: report of two cases, one with autopsy verification. Stroke 7:511, 1976
93. Roberson GH, Scott WR, Rosenbaum AE: Thrombi at the site of carotid stenosis: radiographic diagnosis. Radiology 109:353, 1973
94. Schmalbrock P, Yuan C, Chakeres DW et al: Volume MR angiography: methods to achieve very short echo times. Radiology 175:861, 1990
95. Sekhar LN, Heros RC, Lotz PR, Rosenbaum AE: Atheromatous pseudo-occlusion of the internal carotid artery. J Neurosurg 52:782, 1980
96. Seldinger SI: Catheter replacement of the needle in percutaneous arteriography: a new technique. Acta Radiol 39:368, 1953
97. Shapiro R: Thrombosis of the internal carotid artery. Radiology 58:94, 1952
98. Shokunbi MT, Vinters HV, Kaufmann JCE: Fusiform intracranial aneurysms: clinicopathologic features. Surg Neurol 29:263, 1988
99. Smoker WRK, Corbett JJ, Gentry LR et al: High-resolution computed tomography of the basilar artery. 2. Vertebrobasilar dolichoectasia: clinico-pathologic correlation and review. AJNR 7:61, 1986
100. Special Report from the National Institute of Neurological Disorders and Stroke: Classification of cerebrovascular diseases. III. Stroke 21:637, 1990
101. Steel JG, Thomas HA, Strollo PJ: Fusiform basilar aneurysm as a cause of embolic stroke. Stroke 13:712, 1982
102. Stevens JM, Barter S, Kerslake R et al: Relative safety of intravenous digital subtraction angiography over other methods of carotid angiography and impact on clinical management of cerebrovascular disease. Br J Radiol 62:813, 1989
103. Sukoff MH, Dorsey TJ, Johnson DA et al: Intimal fibroplasia of the internal carotid arteries. Stroke 2:483, 1971
104. Suzuki J, Takaku A: Cerebrovascular "moyamoya" disease. Arch Neurol 20:288, 1969
105. Taveras JM, Gilson JM, Davis DO et al: Angiography in cerebral infarction. Radiology 93:549, 1969
106. Tindall GT, Odom GL, Cupp HB, Dillon ML: Studies on carotid artery flow and pressure: observations in 18 patients during graded occlusion of proximal carotid artery. J Neurosurg 19:917, 1962
107. Vitek JJ: Femoro-cerebral angiography: analysis of 2,000 consecutive examinations, special emphasis on carotid arteries catheterization in older patients. AJR 118:633, 1973
108. Vitek JJ, Halsey JH, McDowell HA: Occlusion of all four extracranial vessels with minimal clinical symptomatology: case report. Stroke 3:462, 1972
109. VonRuden WJ, Blaisdell FW, Hall AD, Thomas AN: Multiple arterial stenoses: effect on blood flow. Arch Surg 89:307, 1964
110. Wagle WA, Dumoulin CL, Souza SP, Cline HE: 3DFT MR angiography of carotid and basilar arteries. AJNR 10:911, 1989
111. Walker WJ, Mundall SL, Broderick HG et al: Systemic heperinization for femoral percutaneous coronary arteriography. N Engl J Med 288:826, 1973
112. Wallace S, Medellin H, DeJongh D, Gianturco C: Systemic heparinization for angiography. AJR 116:204, 1972

113. Weidner W, Hanafee W, Markham CH: Intracranial collateral circulation via leptomeningeal and rete mirabile anastomoses. Neurology (NY) 15:39, 1965
114. Wilson M: Angiography in cerebrovascular occlusive disease. Am J Med Sci 250:554, 1965
115. Wood EH, Correll JW: Atheromatous ulceration in major neck vessels as a cause of cerebral embolism. Acta Radiol Diagn 9:520, 1969
116. Younger DS, Brust JCM, Hays A, Rowland LP: Granulomatous angiitis of the central nervous system: a nonspecific reaction of diverse etiology, abstracted. Ann Neurol 20:157, 1986
117. Yu YL, Moseley IF, Pullicino P, McDonald WI: The clinical picture of ectasia of the intracerebral arteries. J Neurol Neurosurg Psychiatry 45:29, 1982

# 12

# ULTRASOUND IMAGING AND DOPPLER SONOGRAPHY IN THE DIAGNOSIS OF CEREBROVASCULAR DISEASES

Michael Hennerici
J.P. Mohr
Wolfgang Rautenberg
Wolfgang Steinke

## TECHNOLOGY

A variety of noninvasive ultrasound techniques have been developed during recent years for the detection of extracranial and intracranial arterial diseases.[4,24,38,49,100,113,122,130] Some of these, such as continuous-wave (CW) and pulsed-wave (PW) Doppler sonography, assess the hemodynamics according to the Doppler shift. This effect bears Christian Andreas Doppler's name. Doppler's observation[31] "of the colored light of the double stars" was published in Prague in 1842 and provided Satomura and Kameko with the basic tool for their early studies at the end of the 1950s, which resulted in the construction of the first "Doppler rheograph" for noninvasive vascular diagnosis.

The Doppler effect is familiar to anyone who has stood in one place and listened to a source of sound passing by: the rising pitch of the passing movement of sound rushes toward the listener and equally drops as the source leaves him behind. For the examination of vessels, ultrasound frequencies between 1 and 10 MHz are used by means of a transmitter/receiver system according to the following equation:

$$\Delta f = 2 \times f \times v \times \cos\frac{\alpha}{c}$$

where $f$ is the emitting ultrasound frequency, $v$ is the flow velocity in the vessel, $\alpha$ is the angle between ultrasound beam and vessel axis, $c$ is the ultrasound velocity in tissue (approximately 1,500 m/s), and $f$ is the Doppler frequency shift recorded. This frequency is within the audible range (200 to 20,000 Hz) and is proportional to the velocity of the source from which it is reflected, that is, mainly the blood cells in the arterial and venous vessels of the body.

As demonstrated in Figure 12-1, flow directed toward the ultrasound probe results in a negative Doppler frequency shift, while flow in the direction of the probe results in a positive Doppler frequency shift. Since flow velocity changes across the diameter of a vessel, not only a single frequency but a frequency spectrum can regularly be recorded. It ranges from 0.5 to 3.5 kHz in a normal internal carotid artery when the conventional 4-MHz ultrasound emission frequency is used. Low-frequency-range (100 to 400 Hz) reflections of the arterial wall may interfere with the Doppler frequency spectrum analysis because such reflections have an intensity three times greater than that of the moving blood elements. However, they are usually cut off by a high-pass filter applied to the instruments. The amplitude of the Doppler signal is proportional to the number of blood corpuscles reflecting the ultrasound and to the position of the beam axis with respect to the vessel axis: the steeper the angle, the higher the echo reflection and the lower the dispersion of energy that reduces the signal to noise ratio. When the ultrasound probe has a perpendicular position to the vessel axis, the cosine of 90 degrees is zero, and no Doppler signal can be received. Thus,

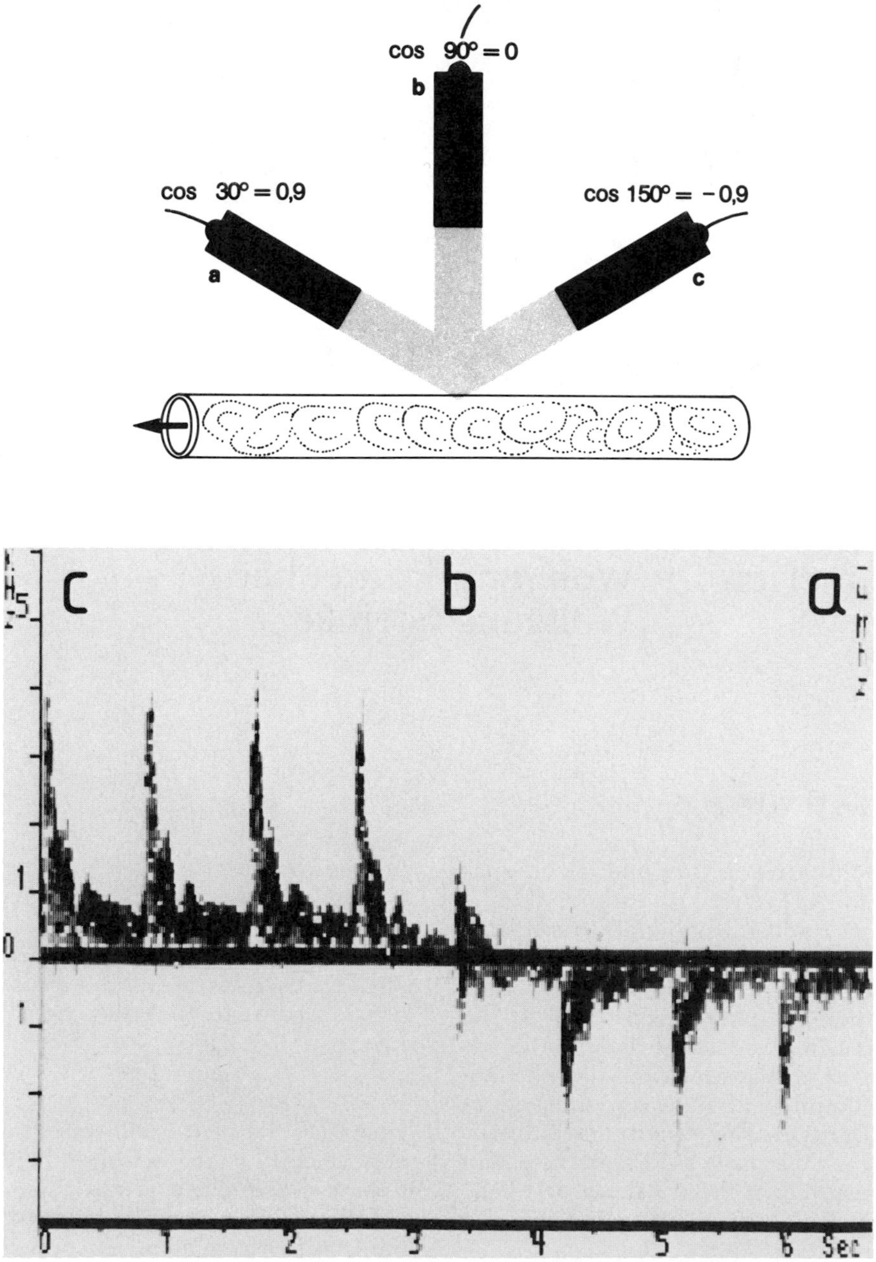


**Fig. 12-1.** Influence of different angles on Doppler shift inside a vessel.

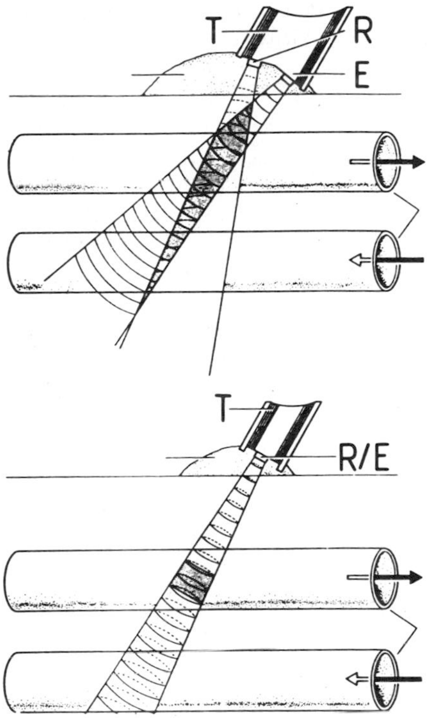


**Fig. 12-2.** Principle of continuous-wave and pulsed-wave Doppler (according to Eden). E, emitting crystal; R, receiving crystal; T, transducer.

both considerations indicate there is an optimal angle between the axis of the vessel and that of the beam. This angle is about 30 degrees for the recording of Doppler signals in the human body.

Both continuous-wave and pulsed-wave Doppler techniques are used for the assessment of blood flow velocities in extracranial vessels. Continuous-wave systems use two transducers, one of which emits while the other receives ultrasound continuously. This system is very useful for the detection of a broad range of flow velocity alterations, including very high blood flow velocities such as occur in severe stenosis. However, it does not provide any information about the topographic origin of the ultrasound-reflecting source in the tissue. To detect the source of the signal, pulsed-wave Doppler systems are used, in which ultrasound is both emitted and received subsequently from a single piezocrystal in the transducer (Fig. 12-2). Pulsed-wave Doppler is the only method useful for the evaluation of intracranial blood flow velocities within the major basal cerebral arteries[1] because the knowledge of the tissue depth from which the signal is derived is crucial for estimating the artery being insonated. The pulsed-wave Doppler technique has been extended for two-dimensional display and three-dimensional reconstruction of the circle of Willis[52] and the major vessels within the posterior fossa. Most recently it has also been introduced for the assessment of intrathoracic, supra-aortic, and submandibular segments of the cranially bound arteries.[95]

While continuous-wave or pulsed-wave Doppler sonography provides information about intravascular hemodynamics, real-time brightness-modulated (B-mode) sonography images tissue and vessel structures in a two-dimensional gray-scale display. The scan is generated from the amplitude of reflected sound waves, which are modified by tissues with different acoustic impedance. Most of the modern B-mode imaging devices for the assessment of extracranial cerebrovascular disease utilize oscillating piezocrystals to produce 7.5 to 10.0 MHz ultrasound emission frequencies, which provide a high resolution of structural details. B-mode echotomography (Fig. 12-3) is based on amplitude-modulated (A-mode) recordings: given a perpendicular insonation, signals of various

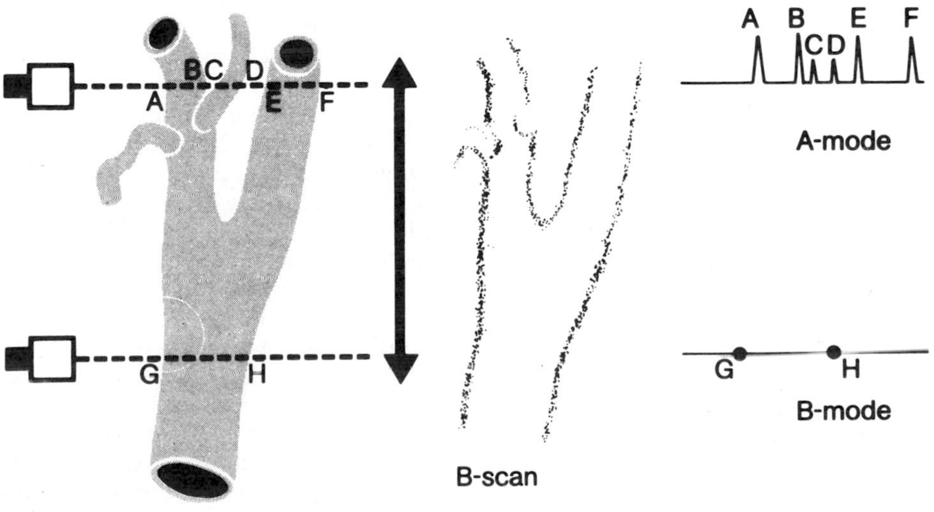


**Fig. 12-3.** Principle of an echotomography: A-mode and B-mode.

amplitudes are recorded according to the different acoustic impedance of the reflecting tissues. On an oscilloscope, the amplitude of these reflections may be brightness-modulated (B-mode), and with a moving transducer a series of such unidimensional recordings can be used to display a two-dimensional grayscale echotomogram. The quality of the B-mode display depends on the lateral and axial resolutions of this ultrasound system.

Both axial resolution and lateral resolution depend on the emitted ultrasound frequency, which has to be selected with respect to the depth of the interesting object. Axial resolution is defined as the smallest distance between two interfaces displayed separately in the beam axis with a range of $\lambda$. The higher the emitted ultrasound frequency, the better the axial resolution. It improves with decreasing spatial pulse length. Lateral resolution reflects the width of this ultrasound beam and describes the smallest distance between two distant side-by-side reflecting interfaces, which can be visualized separately. It depends mainly on the width of the ultrasound beam, which should be as small as possible. Superficial organs are best displayed with high frequencies (7.5 to 10 MHz), whereas deeper ones are better examined using low ultrasound frequencies (1.5 to 5 MHz). This difference stems from the fact that the intensity of the signal is reduced with increasing distance from the ultrasound probe. Thus, the higher the ultrasound frequency, the stronger the attenuation of the intensity.

These ultrasound techniques provide to some extent similar but largely complementary information, which can be used for the diagnosis of different stages of cerebrovascular diseases. The noninvasive nature of all of these techniques has led to their increasing application to the study of the natural history of various cerebrovascular diseases, such as obstructive and dilatative atherosclerosis, inflammatory and degenerative arteriopathies, transient and persistent disorders of the cerebral circulation due to vasospasm, abnormal collateral pathways, and arteriovenous malformations.[47,50,51,74,104,110,111,113]

Combined B-mode and Doppler-mode technologies are used for subsequent or simultaneous imaging of both tissue and flow characteristics in carotid vessels by means of duplex-system or color-coded Doppler flow imaging analysis.[7,30,34,46,63,64,79,99,118,136]

## EXTRACRANIAL APPLICATION

Both CW and PW Doppler devices are used for the examination of the intra- and extracranial brain-supplying arteries. The interpretation of the Doppler signals is based on the analysis of the audio signals, analogue Doppler signal tracings, and frequency spectrum analysis.

The indirect tests, which were all that were available in the initial period of ultrasonography in the study of cerebral atherosclerosis,[5,78] have been all but abandoned today. However, a bidirectional Doppler system using this method can still be useful, as the equipment can almost be carried in the pocket, can be used rapidly, and provides some information regarding movement of blood through vessels even in the hands of a poorly trained examiner. It mainly serves to document the existence of collateral pathways with retrograde blood supply from the external carotid artery via the ophthalmic artery anastomosis in the presence of severe stenosis or total occlusion of the internal carotid artery. If the collateralization from the contralateral carotid artery or the vertebrobasilar systems is sufficient with orthograde perfusion of the ophthalmic artery, this test fails to detect even hemodynamically significant ipsilateral carotid artery obstructions in up to 20 percent. Thus, one should be aware that the detection of a retrograde flow in the fronto-orbital branches of the ophthalmic artery is a strong indicator of a severe underlying pathology within the extracranial carotid artery system. However, if the ophthalmic artery branches are normally perfused, this does not exclude even severe extracranial arterial disease.

Direct tests of the carotid artery system of the neck attempt to detect various parameters of blood flow patterns that indicate abnormalities within, proximal to, or distal to a narrowed arterial segment. The interpretation of these tests provides valuable information on the extent, site, and degree of atherosclerotic lesions of more than 40 percent lumen narrowing. For such processes, the sensitivity (92 to 100 percent) and specificity (93 to 100 percent) of various Doppler techniques have been shown to be similar to arteriography in large series studied, provided the method is used by an experienced examiner.[49,130] The reliability of the diagnosis of carotid artery plaques producing less than 40 percent stenosis is considerably smaller. This is true for both the hand-held CW Doppler technique, which is widespread in Europe, and the conventional PW Doppler analysis incorporated in duplex systems favored in North America, where a moderate-resolution B-mode image mainly assists in the location of a single-gate PW Doppler sample volume. Even after the addition of real-time spectrum analysis and with careful consideration of normal anatomic variations rising within the carotid artery bulb opposite the flow divider, it has not been possible to separate normal conditions from the initial stages of atherosclerosis on the basis of hemodynamic measurements alone. For these circumstances, either simultaneous or complementary use of high-resolution B-mode imaging devices is necessary.

Low-frequency PW Doppler devices are used increasingly to assess the proximal supra-aortic vessel segments (innominate artery, origin of common carotid and vertebral arteries) and distal internal carotid artery (ICA) segments when used with a supraclavicular or submandibular approach.[95]

## Carotid Artery Stenosis and Occlusion

Small plaques producing less than 40 percent lumen narrowing frequently remain undetectable for tests such as Doppler sonography, which rely on the degree of turbulence in flow to estimate the degree of stenosis. Sometimes the audio signal in such cases is altered because of local turbulence or augmented flow, and spectral broadening may be demonstrated in spectrum analysis; however, it is difficult to separate normal conditions from initial stages of atherosclerosis, particularly at the carotid artery bulb.

Several stages of carotid artery stenosis can be separated (Fig. 12-4):

1. A mild stenosis (40 to 60 percent) is characterized by local increase of peak and mean flow velocities (Fig. 12-4A). Peak frequencies range above 4 kHz (4-MHz probe).
2. A moderate stenosis (60 to 80 percent) shows a distortion of the normal pulsatile flow in addition to local increases of peak and mean frequencies (Fig. 12-4B). Peak systolic flow decelerations are found in the poststenotic segment. The peak frequency ranges from 4 to 8 MHz.
3. A severe stenosis (more than 80 percent) produces markedly increased peak velocities exceeding 8 kHz. In addition, pre- and poststenotic spectra are dampened compared with the contralateral unaffected carotid artery (Fig. 12-4C). Retrograde flow direction of the ophthalmic artery may occur.
4. A subtotal stenosis (more than 95 percent) is characterized by a small signal of variable frequencies

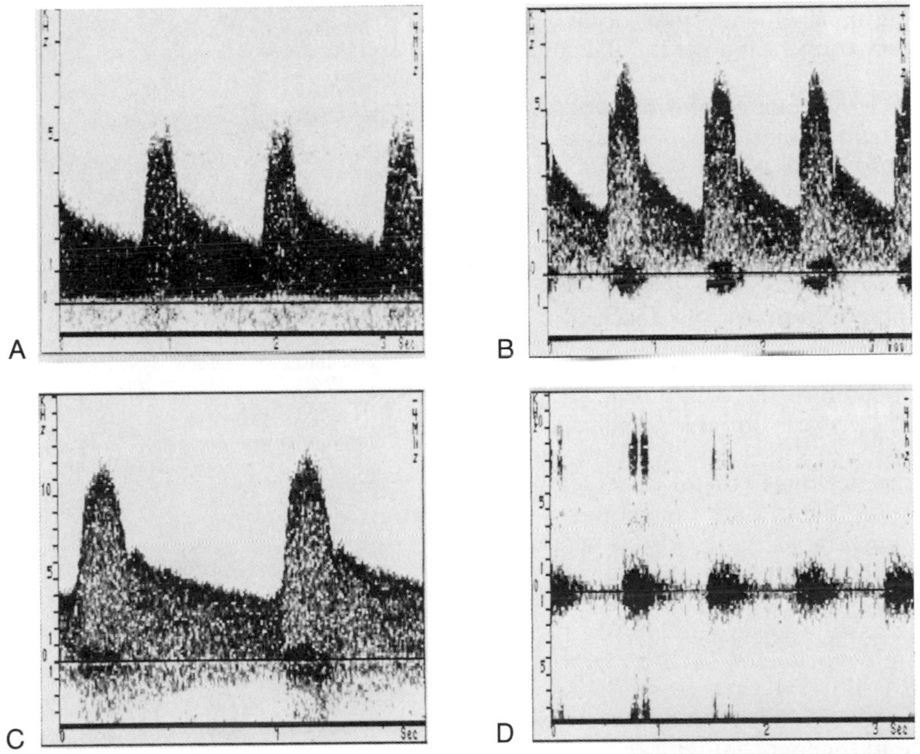

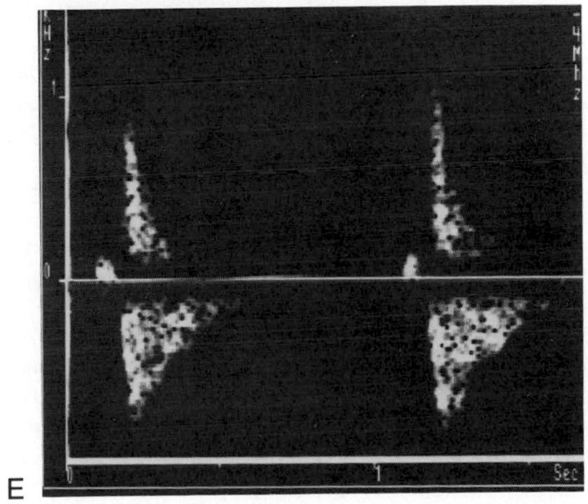

**Fig. 12-4.** Different types of carotid artery stenoses (continuous-wave Doppler). (**A**) Mild stenosis. (**B**) Moderate stenosis. (**C**) Severe stenosis. (**D**) Pseudo-occlusion. (**E**) Carotid artery dissection.

that decrease once a stenosis becomes pseudo-occlusive (Fig. 12-4D). This condition is difficult to separate from complete occlusion and may even be misdiagnosed as complete blockage.

5. With internal carotid artery (ICA) occlusion, in which case no signal is detectable, the spectra of the common carotid artery are damped and retrograde ophthalmic flow may occur.
6. In patients with carotid artery dissections a typical bi- or triphasic "to and fro" signal can be recorded, which may be traced from the bifurcation throughout the course of the ICA to the submandibular region (Fig. 12-4E).
7. Severe intracranial obstructions within the carotid siphon or the middle cerebral artery (MCA) may lead to damped spectra in the ipsilateral extracranial carotid artery. In addition, alterations of flow direction and signal frequency may occur in the ophthalmic artery, depending on the site and degree of the lesion.
8. Intracranial arteriovenous malformations (AVM) and shunts may lead to increased flow velocities in the ipsilateral proximal vessel segments. Therefore, the presence of an AVM can sometimes be assumed by means of extracranial Doppler examinations.

## Vertebral Artery Stenosis and Occlusion

Stenoses in the vertebral artery can be assessed directly if they are located at the origin or at the atlas loop (Fig. 12-5). The criteria for the classification of the degree of the lesion are the same as for the carotid artery system. Severe lesions in distal vessel segments or in intracranial segments and the basilar artery may lead to reduced flow at the locations where the vessel can be recorded. Without additional information from B-mode imaging about the vessel lumen, however, it is not possible to separate obstructive lesions from anatomic variances such as hypoplasia and deep cervical collateral pathways. The same is true for the differentiation between occlusion and a- or hypoplasia. Due to the fact that with the hand-held Doppler technique the vertebral artery can only be recorded at two sites, the sensitivity and specificity for the detection of vertebral artery obstructions producing more than 50 percent lumen narrowing are lower than for similar processes in the carotid artery system.[45,49,128]

## Subclavian and Innominate Arteries: The Subclavian Steal Phenomenon

In patients with severe lesions of the proximal subclavian arteries, Doppler methods are excellent noninvasive tools for the detection of associated flow alterations in the vertebral arteries. Different stages of flow abnormalities can be separated in the most often benign condition of the subclavian steal phenomenon (Fig. 12-6). Severe obstructions of the innominate artery lead to complex hemodynamic alterations within the ipsilateral carotid and vertebral arteries, including reversed-flow signals.[48]

## Advantages and Limitations

Free hand-held Doppler methods are simple, inexpensive, and noninvasive. In experienced hands, it may provide reliable data about lesions producing more than 40 percent lumen narrowing in the carotid

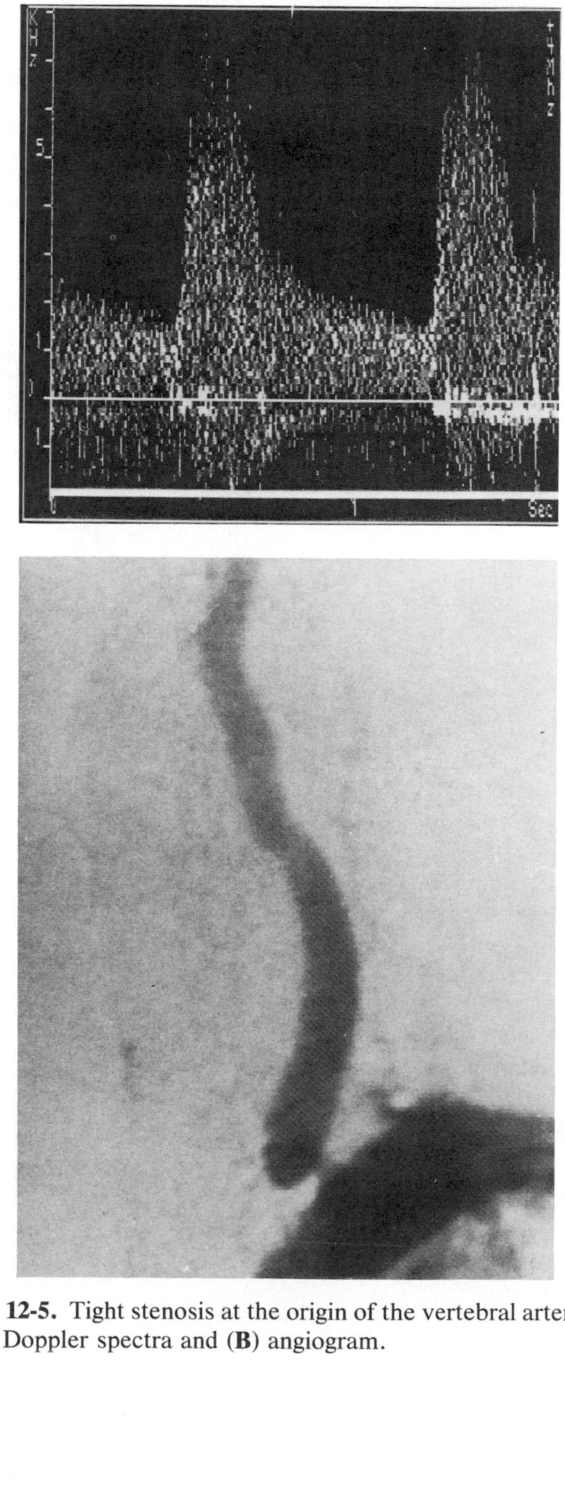

A

B

**Fig. 12-5.** Tight stenosis at the origin of the vertebral artery. (**A**) Doppler spectra and (**B**) angiogram.

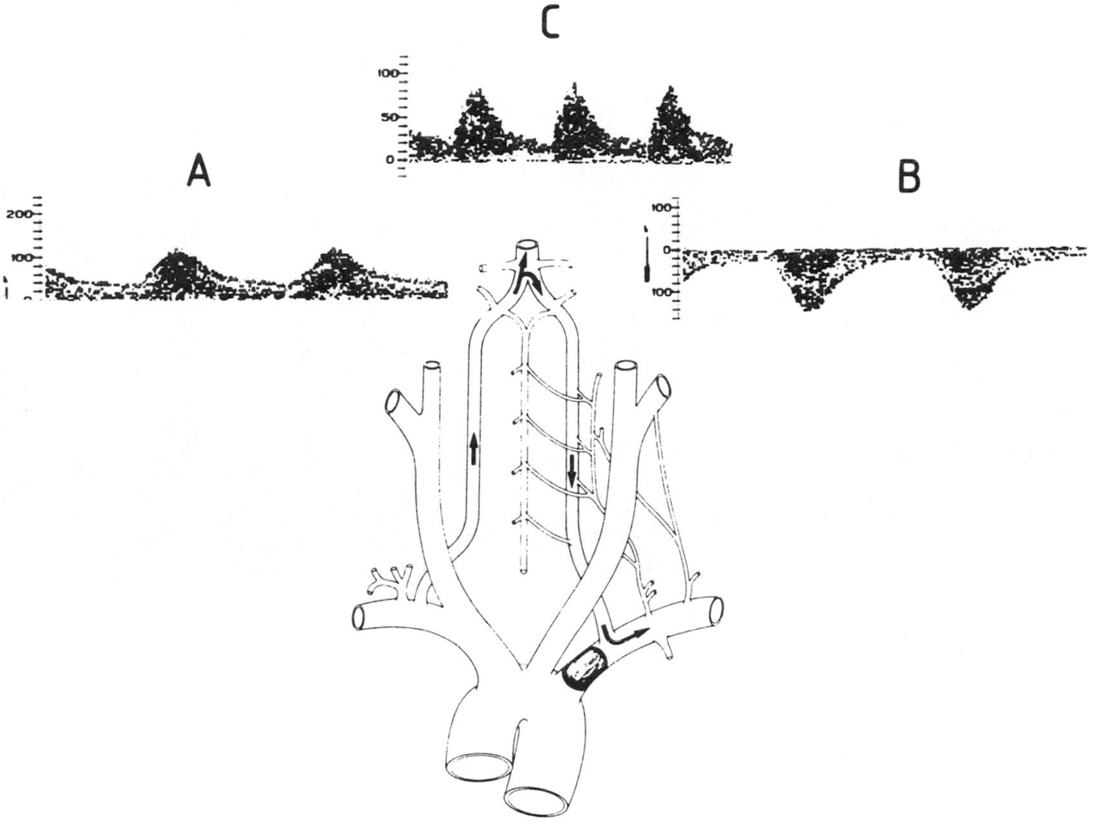


**Fig. 12-6.** Subclavian-steal phenomenon. Schematic drawing and Doppler spectra of (**A**) right vertebral artery (orthograde flow direction); (**B**) left vertebral artery (retrograde flow direction), and (**C**) basilar artery (orthograde flow).

system. All brain-supplying arteries are accessible, including the vertebral arteries. PW Doppler methods, in principle, provide similar results if the Doppler sample volume is adequately positioned. Provided the obstruction of the vessel is small and calcification is absent, the B-mode may be used as a guide for optimal positioning of the sample volume. In the presence of severe stenosis, however, this may be difficult and may lead to misdiagnosis of occlusive lesions, particularly if small sample volumes are used. Lesions of less than 40 percent lumen narrowing and intracranial lesions cannot reliably be detected by Doppler sonography. No information concerning the morphology and surface of a plaque is available. The diagnostic accuracy in the vertebrobasilar system is more limited than in the carotid artery system. The diagnostic validity of the method is dependent on the skill of the operator.

## B-MODE ECHOTOMOGRAPHY

B-mode echotomography allows a clear distinction between normal vessel wall characteristics and abnormal conditions.[53,134] Carotid artery plaque echogenicity, surface structures, and extent can be assessed by sequences of longitudinal and cross sections. They are mandatory to display all aspects of the lesion configuration and to identify correctly the anatomic location of the plaque.

### Echogenicity of Plaque

*Homogeneous* echoes characterize uncomplicated atherosclerotic lesions, consisting of dense fibrotic tissue.[37,54,135] Although these plaques frequently represent early stages of the disease, starting with intimal fibrosis, they are also found in hemodynamically relevant stenoses (Fig. 12-7A). It is consistently reported that ulcerations are rarely seen in homogeneous plaques, and probably no relevant correlation exists with the occurrence of cerebral ischemic events.[69,70,121]

*Heterogeneous* echoes indicate more advanced atherosclerosis with deposition of cholesterol crystals, calcification, inflammation, and intraplaque hemorrhage or necrosis[15,37,88,135] (Fig. 12-7B). Disregarding the variety of components of the atherosclerotic matrix, heterogeneous plaques have controversially been reported to essentially demonstrate intraplaque hemorrhage.[15,88] In particular, a large rounded area of low

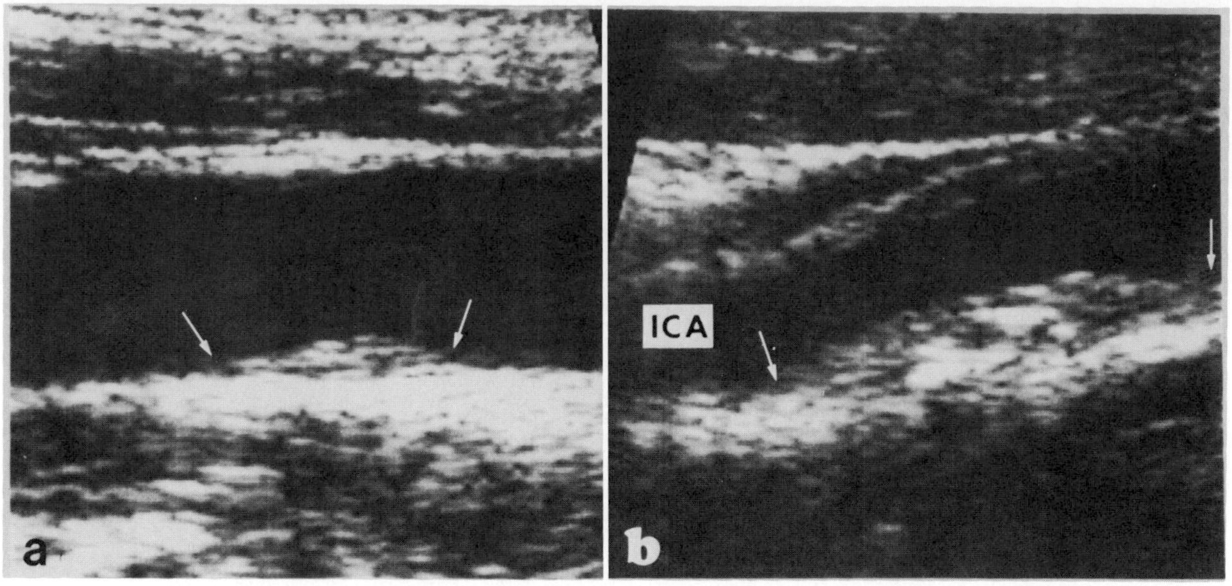


**Fig. 12-7.** (**a**) Flat homogeneous plaque (*arrows*) at the posterior wall of the common carotid artery representing the very early stage of atherosclerosis. (**b**) Large heterogeneous smooth atheroma (*arrows*) at the origin of the internal carotid artery (ICA).

echogenicity in the center of the lesion may be indicative of plaque hemorrhage; however, it may also reflect aggregates of amorphous lipid components.[15,134] Several series reported a correlation between heterogeneous plaque echogenicity and the occurrence of cerebrovascular events.[70,98,121] Several such studies were often based on the pathogenetic concept, which developed from gross morphologic evaluation of carotid endarterectomy specimens and suggested a significant association of plaque hemorrhage with transient ischemic attacks (TIAs) and stroke.[59] However, the validity of this concept seems now a bit out of date.[11,19,71]

*Homogeneous or heterogeneous* echoes may be associated with acoustic shadows, which are mainly due to plaque calcification (Fig. 12-8). Since most of the extended lesions contain various amounts of calcific matrix, adequate visualization of the plaque extent and configuration becomes more difficult with increasing luminal narrowing.[27,134] Echo-intense signals

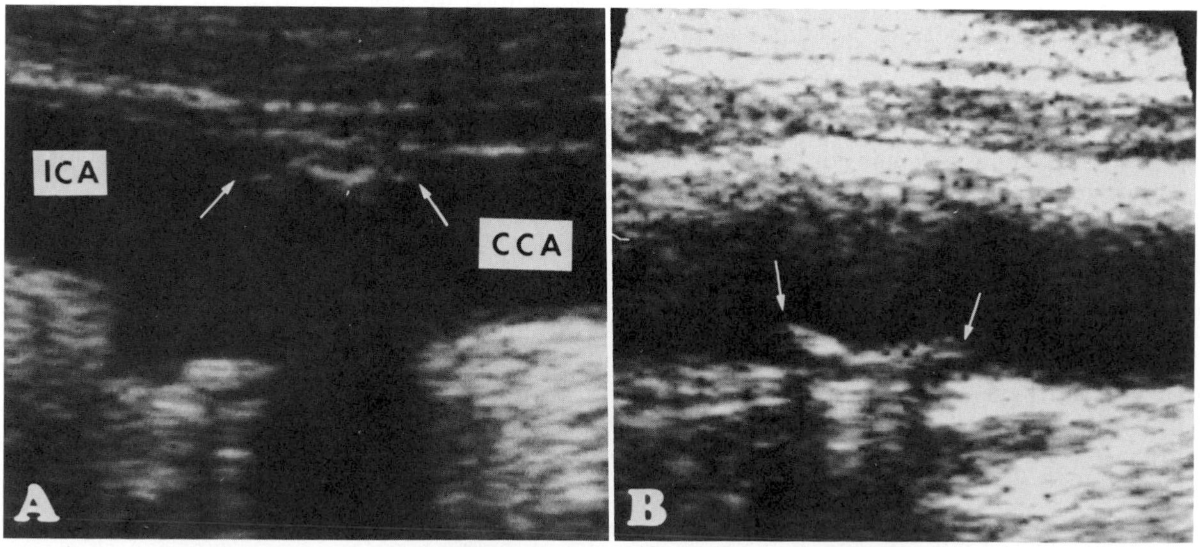


**Fig. 12-8.** Nonstenotic calcified plaques (*arrows*) at the (**A**) anterior and (**B**) posterior vessel wall producing echo shadows. ICA, internal carotid artery; CCC, common carotid artery.

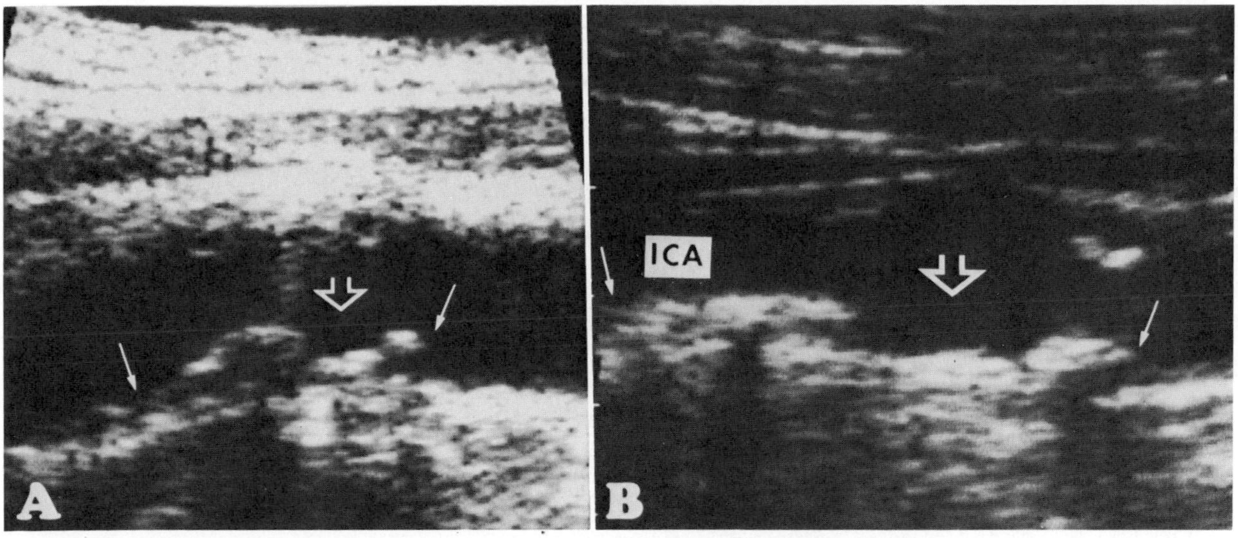


**Fig. 12-9.** Examples of ulcerative plaques. (**A**) Heterogeneous plaque (*thin arrows*) with a small niche in the surface (*open arrow*). (**B**) Long-segment calcified plaque (*thin arrows*) extending from the bifurcation into the internal carotid artery (ICA) with a large central ulcus (*open arrow*).

of small densely calcified plaques located at the anterior vessel wall may also obscure the posterior vascular wall structures.

### Surface Structures of Plaque

Often it is possible to distinguish smooth, irregular, and ulcerative surfaces. In the B-mode image, ulcerations are characterized by a delineated excavation in the plaque (Fig. 12-9). Histologically, the ulcer crater is formed by disruption of the lesion surface due to intraplaque hemorrhage or an extending atherosclerotic matrix. B-mode echotomography is highly accurate in identifying ulcerative carotid artery plaques in anatomic specimens,[37,46] and "healing" of ulcers by covering the niche with a fibrous cap was documented in follow-up examinations.[53] However, B-mode sonography had a lower "in vivo" sensitivity for the detection of ulcerations compared with angiography[9,139] or with carotid endarterectomy specimens.[16] In a more recent comparison of B-mode imaging and angiography with findings of carotid endarterectomy specimens both techniques demonstrated an unsatisfactory diagnostic sensitivity for ulcerations (47 and 53 percent).[28] Thus, the assumed low accuracy of B-mode imaging was confirmed in this study, but it was also evident that angiography could not be the "gold standard" for the detection of ulcerative plaques. Probably because of the discouraging early results[9,139] and the validation problem, no systematic B-mode studies have investigated the significance of ulcerative carotid artery lesions for cerebral embolism.

## Extent of Plaque

Accurate assessment of the plaque extent and luminal narrowing based on B-mode imaging has several limitations and pitfalls (Table 12-1), which were analyzed in detail by Zwiebel et al.[139] and Comerota et al.[27] In a large multicenter B-mode validation study[101] absolute measurements of the lesion width and the minimal residual lumen showed a poor correlation with angiography. The overall accuracy of classifying different degrees of stenosis was 71.8 percent, and B-mode sonography identified correctly only 39 of 96 occlusions (41 percent). In addition, in a subset of the study population, the intra- and interobserver agreement for the quantification of the lesion extent was relatively poor.[89] Comparison of B-mode imaging with the pathology of carotid endarterectomy in the same study demonstrated discrepancies of more than 1 mm in measurements of both the residual vessel

**TABLE 12-1. Limitations of B-mode Sonography of Carotid Atherosclerosis**

| |
|---|
| Limited visualization of vessel structures due to |
| High bifurcation |
| Tortuous vessel |
| Transducer configuration |
| Acoustic shadowing from calcified plaque |
| Identification of ulcerations and echo-poor plaque components |
| Determination of plaque extent without sequential longitudinal and transverse sections |
| Classification of stenosis and diagnosis of occlusion without Doppler information |
| Low inter- and intraobserver reliability |

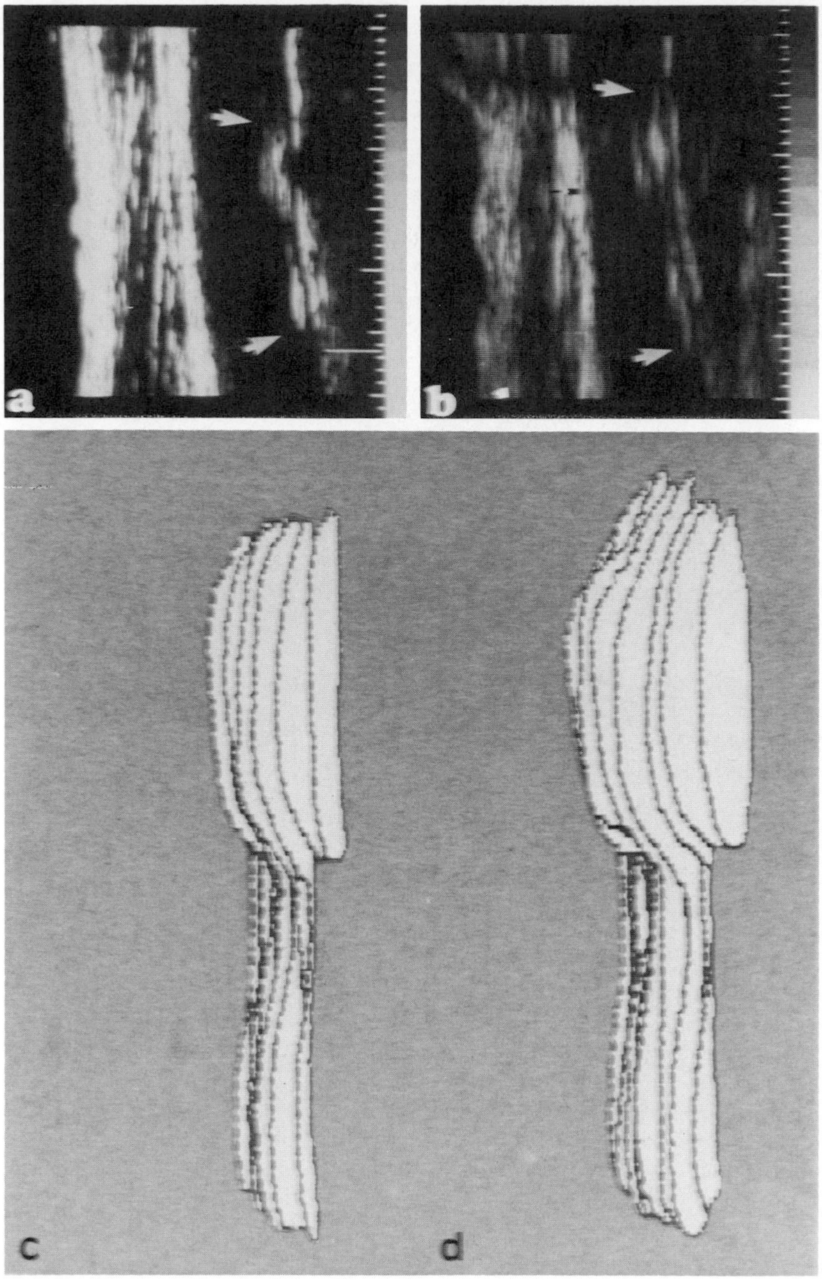

**Fig. 12-10.** (**a**) Heterogeneous, irregular plaque (*arrows*) at the posterior wall of the common carotid artery. (**b**) Increase in lesion size (*arrows*) at follow-up examination 6 months later. (**c & d**) Corresponding three-dimensional reconstructions of the plaque surface from sequential longitudinal sections.

lumen and the lesion extent in 64 percent of the cases.[106] However, quantitative assessment of these studies was limited by considerable heterogeneity in methodology and design of the multicenter trial. In addition, the quantitative assessment of atherosclerotic lesions from endarterectomy specimens poses problems similar to other forms of ultrasound imaging.[36,106] Since two-dimensional studies carry important methodologic limitations, computer-assisted three-dimensional reconstructions of the plaque extent and configuration from sequential longitudinal and transverse B-mode scans have been developed; they are essential for an accurate assessment of progression or regression of carotid artery atherosclerosis in prospective follow-up studies[55,116] (Fig. 12-10).

## DUPLEX SCANNING

### Carotid Artery

The combination of high-resolution B-mode imaging with pulsed-wave Doppler sonography in duplex systems extends the reliability of noninvasive tests and is now widely used for the diagnosis of various degrees of extracranial cerebrovascular disease. As-

**TABLE 12-2. Criteria for the Classification of Carotid Stenosis by Means of Pulsed Wave Doppler Sonography (4 to 5 MHz)**

| Diameter Stenosis (%) | Peak Systolic Frequency (kHz) | Peak Systolic Velocity (cm/s) | End Diastolic Frequency (kHz) | End Diastolic Velocity (cm/s) | Systolic Ratio (ICA/CCA) |
|---|---|---|---|---|---|
| 40–60 | >4.0 | >120 | <1.3 | <40 | <1.8 |
| 61–80 | >4.0 | >120 | >1.3 | >40 | >1.8 |
| 80–90 | >8.0 | >240 | >3.3 | >100 | >3.7 |

*Abbreviations:* ICA, internal carotid artery; CCA, common carotid artery.
Modified from Zwiebel et al.[140]

sessment of the presence and the echomorphologic characterization of small nonstenotic plaques is based on the B-mode echotomogram, since they frequently do not cause flow abnormalities. In addition, the B-mode scan of the arteries serves as a road map for placement of the PW Doppler sample volume. The Doppler spectrum analysis is then used to detect and to categorize carotid artery stenoses with a luminal narrowing greater than 40 percent and to identify the vessel anatomy (Table 12-2; Figs. 12-11 and 12-12).

In early duplex studies, which did not distinguish different degrees of stenosis exceeding 50 percent luminal narrowing,[14,35] the reported sensitivity for the detection of greater than 50 percent stenosis was 95 percent and 81.5 percent. More recent reports classified several grades of carotid artery obstruction

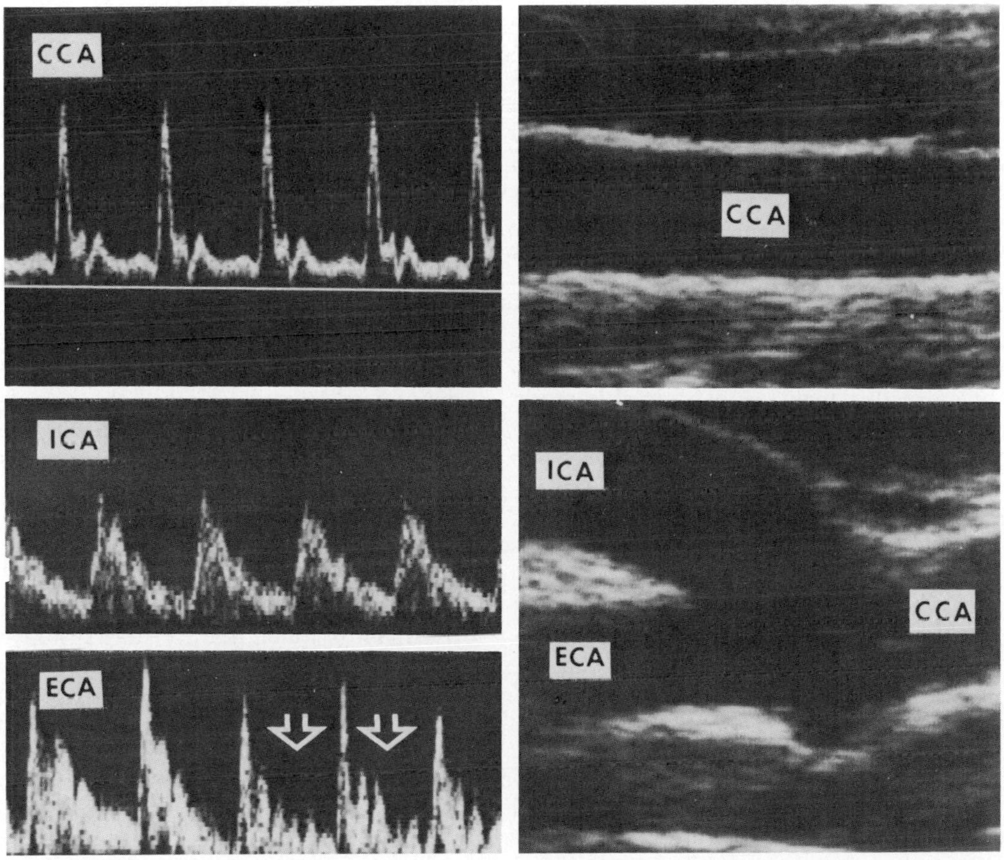


**Fig. 12-11.** Duplex system analysis of a normal carotid artery. Doppler frequency spectra (*left*) and B-mode echotomograms of the common carotid artery (CCA) and the bifurcation with internal carotid artery (ICA) and external carotid artery (ECA). High systolic and low diastolic flow and transmitted oscillation (*open arrows*) from tapping the superficial temporal artery in the ECA. Flow in the ICA is higher in diastole, reflecting a low-resistance pattern. The Doppler waveform in the CCA reflects the two vascular beds it supplies, but it is dominated by the low-resistant flow to the brain.

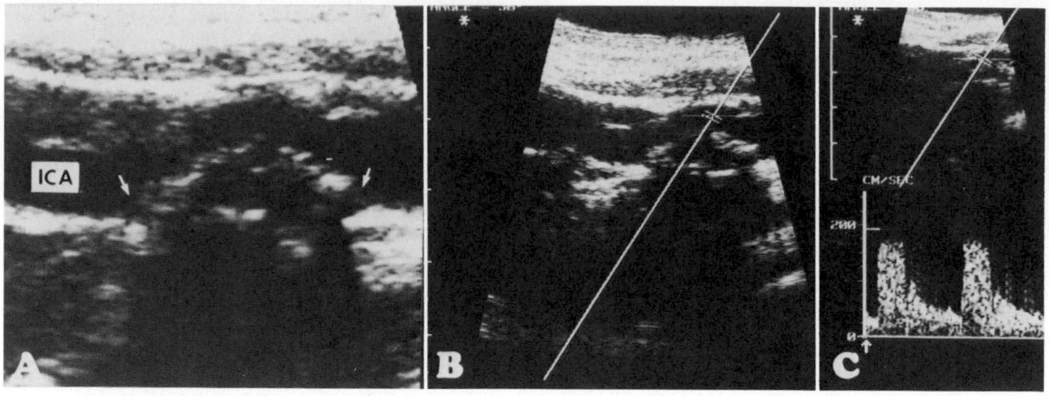


**Fig. 12-12.** Duplex scan of an internal carotid artery stenosis. (**A**) B-mode scan demonstrates a large heterogeneous partially calcified plaque (*arrows*) with a central echolucent core at the origin of the internal carotid artery. (**B**) The Doppler sample volume is placed at the site of stenosis. (**C**) Doppler waveforms demonstrate a peak systolic flow velocity of 190 cm/s, indicating a moderate (60 to 80 percent) stenosis. ICA, internal carotid artery.

greater than 50 percent and correlated the results with angiography; however, comparison of the findings among studies is difficult due to different Doppler criteria used for classification.[60,103,104,125] Jacobs et al.[60] diagnosed 89 percent of the 51 to 90 percent stenoses correctly, using a peak frequency shift of 4 to 8 kHz as the main criterion. Roederer et al.[104] found agreement with angiography in 86 percent of the 50 to 79 percent stenoses that were diagnosed, if the peak frequency exceeded 4 kHz and marked spectral broadening occurred. Accuracy for 80 to 99 percent stenoses was only 71 percent using end-diastolic frequency of greater than 4.5 kHz as an additional criterion. Robinson et al.[103] demonstrated the effect of various threshold values for the diagnostic accuracy of different degrees of carotid artery stenosis. In this study both the sensitivity and specificity was 92 percent for greater than 70 percent cross-sectional area stenoses (50 percent diameter reduction), if a peak systolic velocity exceeding 150 cm/s was used as the diagnostic criterion. Since the reported accuracy of duplex scanning for the diagnosis of carotid artery occlusion varies considerably, the actual reliability of this method in distinguishing severe stenosis from occlusion is controversial.

Duplex scanning has been shown to be very useful for the assessment of carotid artery dissection. It is obvious, even from a small number of case reports, that the sonographic features differ between dissection of the common carotid and the internal carotid arteries. In common carotid artery dissections an intravascular double lumen can typically be visualized with the intimal flap separating both lumina, in which different Doppler flow profiles can be demonstrated. Even retrograde flow direction in one lumen is not unusual.[10,67,138] Depending on the type of internal carotid artery dissection, high-resolution echotomograms of the bifurcation may be unremarkable or may frequently demonstrate a tapering lumen due to the dissecting vessel wall.[120] However, the Doppler spectrum is diagnostic if a characteristic low-frequency high-resistance flow pattern is found with bidirectional or alternating flow components that can be traced along the internal carotid artery in the neck. In a recent study, subsequent follow-up examinations demonstrated improvement or normalization of the Doppler spectrum in the majority of the cases.[56]

## Vertebral Artery

Little has been reported about duplex evaluation of the vertebral arteries, and ultrasound criteria for normal and pathologic conditions have not been well-defined.[6,12] Visualization of the vessel lumen and assessment of intravascular Doppler spectra is limited to the origin of the vertebral artery, its proximal pretransverse course, and the intertransverse segments C3 to C6, while insonation of the atlas loop has not been studied systematically by duplex sonography.

In more than 50 percent of the cases, atherosclerosis of the vertebral artery predominantly involves the ostium. Thus inadequate visualization of the origin in 23 to 38 percent of cases is a major limitation for the assessment of vertebral atherosclerosis.[6,29,126] In one duplex study, 31 of 117 vertebral arteries could not be identified at the ostium. Corresponding angiograms showed that only 9 vessels were occluded and 3 were markedly hypoplastic, but 8 has various degrees of stenosis and 11 were completely normal. Furthermore, in contrast to carotid artery stenosis, Doppler peak frequency and spectral broadening are less reliable criteria for the diagnosis and classification of vertebral stenosis at its ostium.[6,12,29]

Intertransverse segments of the vertebral artery can regularly be displayed, and Doppler spectra are assessed by placing the Doppler sample volume in the

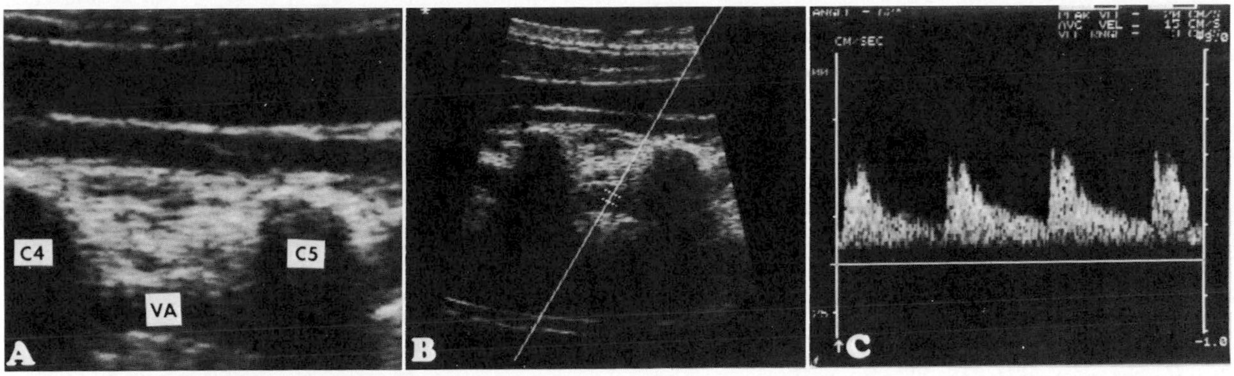


**Fig. 12-13.** Duplex scan of a normal vertebral artery (VA). (**A**) B-mode image of the intertransverse segment of the vertebral artery between the cervical vertebrae C4 and C5. (**B & C**) Doppler waveform recorded from the intertransverse segment demonstrates low-resistant flow pattern.

vessel lumen between two vertebra[12,126] (Fig. 12-13). The normal mean systolic flow velocity ranged from 20 to 40 cm/s in one large series.[12] However, interpretation of flow velocity and pulsatility in vertebral arteries is limited, since proximal and distal atherosclerotic obstructions, dissections, asymmetric vessel diameters of both vertebrals, and other variations in the vertebrobasilar circulation or coexisting significant disease in the carotid artery system may considerably change the flow velocity profiles. However, retrograde or intermediate flow can be interpreted more reliably as a steal phenomenon due to hemodynamically significant disease of the innominate or proximal subclavian arteries (Fig. 12-6). It has also been possible to infer the intracranial vertebral artery status by insonation of the vertebral artery in the neck: a waveform indicating high resistance to flow may be present when an intracranial occlusion of the vertebral artery exists. However, when the occlusion lies cephalad to (above) the posterior inferior cerebellar artery, flow into this branch may suffice to keep the vertebral waveform normal.[124]

## COLOR DOPPLER FLOW IMAGING

The most recent advance of sonographic evaluation of the extracranial brain-supplying arteries is color Doppler flow imaging (CDFI). In addition to conventional duplex systems, CDFI provides color-coded, two-dimensional, real-time information about intravascular blood flow superimposed on the gray-scale image of vessel anatomy. Using linear arrays, the B-mode image is generated from echoamplitude analysis of stationary targets, while the Doppler frequency shift is determined by phase changes between two successive echoes, indicating the velocity and direction of moving targets.[79,137] Blood flow toward or away from the transducer is coded by either red or blue, and the degree of color saturation correlates with the flow velocity, producing decreased saturation with higher velocity. Usually each color pixel represents the mean frequency shift in a given space and time. Since broadening of the Doppler spectrum due to flow disturbance decreases the mean frequency and thus decreases the color-coded frequency shift, the peak frequency is similar to the mean and the color-coded frequency only if blood flow is uniform and not turbulent.[82] Since frequency shifts so great that they exceed equipment competence to display them properly (aliasing) is fundamental to pulsed-wave Doppler sonography, it also occurs with color-coded Doppler signals. In CDFI aliasing is characterized by an abrupt change from pale red to pale blue signals with additional intermediate black lines in some systems. Green or yellow may be admixed to red or blue to indicate spectral broadening or "variance" of frequency shifts, resulting in a "mosaic pattern," if high-frequency turbulence occurs in severe stenosis.

Other CDFI systems use green to display frequency shifts above a selected threshold value ("green tag") to demonstrate the area of highest intrastenotic flow velocity, where the sample volume of the optional PW Doppler system can be placed.

### Carotid Artery

Numerous experimental studies have been performed to investigate the significance of distinct flow phenomena such as flow reversal and boundary layer separation in the normal carotid artery bulb, representing the preferential site of atherogenesis.[76,85,107] Using single- or multigate pulsed-wave Doppler sonography, corresponding findings have been reported; however, the complexity and distribution of secondary flow zones could not be analyzed satisfactorily.[68,87,99] CDFI zones of reversed and separated flow are encoded blue on display. Thus, the spatial and temporal distribution of flow separation can be analyzed.[93] CDFI studies not only confirmed the results from experimental models, that flow reversal mainly occurs at the outer wall of the internal carotid artery,[81,119,137] but also provided additional information: (1) flow separation patterns are more variable than previously assumed and are not restricted to the internal carotid artery bulb;[81,119] and (2) secondary flow may be absent either due to the anatomy of the bifurcation with a missing carotid artery bulb or a plaque filling in the carotid sinus.[57,87]

CDFI increases the capability of conventional ultrasound to detect and characterize small nonstenotic plaques (Plate 12-1):[34,80,118]

1. Plaque extent and the residual vessel lumen can be assessed more accurately due to contrast with color-coded blood flow.
2. Characterization of the plaque surface, especially the detection of ulcerations and differentiation of smooth and irregular surfaces, is improved.
3. Echopoor components of a plaque such as thrombotic material can be identified indirectly by sparing the color-flow signal.

Since CDFI thus identifies potential embolic sources more frequently, the rate of strokes of undetermined origin may decrease by using this technique. Although the degree and distribution of flow disturbance at nonstenotic plaques are variable, typically blue-coded turbulence is seen at irregular surfaces or within ulcerative niches (Plate 12-1C). On the other hand, preliminary evaluation of the morphologic-hemodynamic interaction by CDFI showed that progression of atherosclerosis mainly correlated with the presence of turbulence at the lesion site.[55]

Various methods and criteria are provided by the CDFI technique to classify the degree of carotid stenosis (Fig. 12-14 and Plate 12-2):

1. The point of maximal color-encoded flow velocity—highlighted by the "green tag" function in some systems—can be used to place the PW Doppler sample volume.[93,118] The classification of the grade of stenosis is then based on the Doppler spectrum analysis according to the established criteria for conventional duplex Doppler sonography.
2. The color-coded flow patterns, such as intensity, extent, and duration of color fading, and the presence of poststenotic flow reversal or turbulence ("mosaic pattern") are characteristic for different degrees of stenosis.[39,118]
3. The residual vessel lumen contrasted by color-flow signals ("flow lumen") can be measured in longitudinal or transverse sections.[34,39]

The accuracy of CDFI for the classification of carotid stenosis compared with angiography varied between 71 and 96 percent in the few systematic studies available. It was lowest if flow lumen measurement was the main diagnostic criterion. The capacity of CDFI to separate subtotal stenoses from occlusions has further

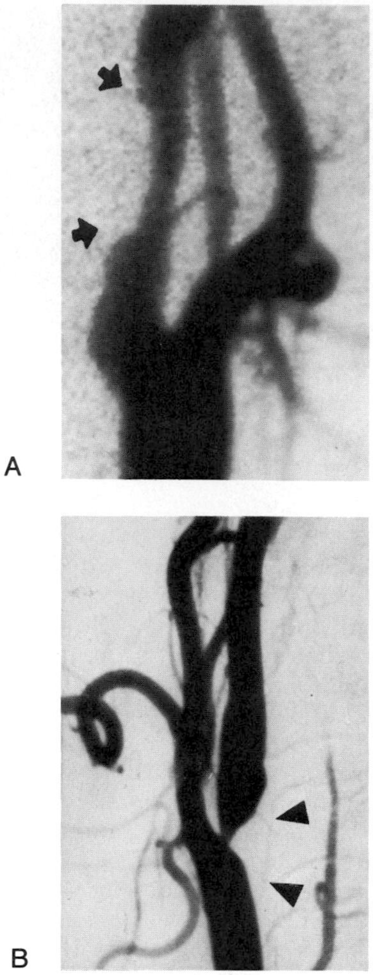

**Fig. 12-14.** (**A**) Angiogram of moderate smooth internal carotid artery stenosis (see Plate 12-2). (**B**) Angiogram of wedge-shaped plaque at the origin of the internal carotid artery, producing a high-grade stenosis (*arrows* indicate plaque extent; see Plate 12-2B).

to be evaluated, since the number of patients studied is yet too small.

CDFI is particularly useful for the diagnosis of rare conditions affecting the carotid artery system. In common carotid artery dissection, which is usually associated with aortic arch dissection, different color-encoded hemodynamic patterns in both the true and false lumen can be visualized, and the site of reentry of the false lumen, producing signs of stenosis in some cases, can be identified.[17,120] Internal carotid artery dissection has a different clinical presentation and probably a different etiology than does dissection of the common carotid artery. In the initial stage CDFI may show the typical finding of a complete occlusion with blue-coded Doppler signals indicating reversed flow in the tapering lumen of the internal carotid artery. On the other hand, even if the vessel anatomy above the bifurcation appears normal on the gray-scale echotomogram, intraluminal color flow signals may be absent. At follow-up examinations CDFI may then demonstrate steadily improving blood flow in the internal carotid artery due to recanalization of the vessel, which is seen in the majority of cases.[56,84] Addition of color-flow signals to conventional duplex sonography also increases the accuracy of the noninvasive evaluation of hypervascular carotid body tumors, since low-flow conditions in small-caliber vessels can be visualized.[112,117]

### Vertebral Artery

Experience with CDFI used for the evaluation of vertebral arteries is still limited. In a series of presumed-normal subjects, not only the origin and the intertransverse segments of the vertebral arteries could be identified in most cases but also the atlas loop.[127] In this study the mean peak systolic flow velocity was 56 cm/s, and the mean resistivity index was 0.69 determined with the integrated PW Doppler system. CDFI is probably superior to conventional duplex sonography for the assessment of normal and pathologic conditions of the vertebral artery; however, no systematic studies are yet available. In one case report the ease of diagnosis of a vertebral pseudoaneurysm with CDFI was emphasized.[133]

### Advantages and Limitations

Compared to conventional duplex scanning CDFI has some advantages for the examination procedure (Table 12-3). Intravascular color-coded blood flow facilitates orientation and vessel identification. Thus the time for a complete examination is significantly reduced,[39,92] and the rate of technically good results of less experienced examiners increases rapidly. Since the site of maximal flow velocity is defined by the color-flow pattern placement of the Doppler sample volume is more reproducible, leading to a high interobserver agreement for the assessment of carotid artery stenosis.[92] In addition, CDFI overcomes time-consuming efforts of PW Doppler sonography in duplex systems to obtain flow information from several sites along the course of the vessel without missing major abnormalities. However, some potential limitations of CDFI for the assessment of carotid artery disease are evident (Table 12-4). Plaque calcification, particularly in high-grade stenosis, may obscure not only the B-mode echotomogram of vascular structures and plaque morphology but may also extinguish the color-flow signals. In one CDFI series the degree of carotid artery stenosis could not be assessed in 12 out of 95 arteries (13 percent) due to calcified plaque.[34] Similar to conventional duplex sonography high location of the bifurcation, deep location of the vessels, and the transducer configuration contributed to 11 percent technically unsatisfactory examinations in another study.[118]

**TABLE 12-3. Advantages of Color Doppler Flow Imaging for Carotid Artery Disease**

| |
|---|
| Simultaneous real-time image of blood flow and vessel anatomy |
| Ease of vessel identification |
| Faster data acquisition and shorter examination time |
| Improved estimation of plaque surface structure and residual vessel lumen |
| Facilitated localization of the point of maximal intrastenotic frequency shift |
| Display of the morphologic-hemodynamic interaction |
| More reliable differential diagnosis of neck masses |
| High intra- and interobserver reproducibility |

**TABLE 12-4. Limitations of Color Doppler Flow Imaging**

| |
|---|
| Variable interpretation of blue-coded signals as |
| Reversed flow |
| Undisturbed flow toward the transducer |
| Turbulence |
| Aliasing phenomenon |
| Suboptimal angle of insonation for B-mode imaging |
| Detection of very slow flow velocity |
| Limited temporal resolution of color-coded flow patterns |
| Shadowing of color signals due to calcified plaque |

## TRANSCRANIAL DOPPLER METHODS

The attenuation of the ultrasonic wave near the skull made recordings of blood flow velocities from intracranial arteries impossible for a long time. In 1982 Aaslid et al.[4] introduced a high-energy bidirectional PW Doppler system operating at low frequencies (1 to 2 MHz), which, for the first time, allowed noninvasive recording of flow velocity from cerebral arteries at the base of the skull.

Low-frequency, high-energy PW Doppler systems are used for transcranial Doppler (TCD) examinations. In addition to hand-held systems, a so-called scan system has been developed.[1] Two probes are incorporated into a helmet. This technique offers the mapping of the recorded velocities as a display of the spectra in horizontal, frontal, and sagittal planes. More recently, transcranial use of color-coded duplex devices through the intact skull has been reported.[18]

Identification of intracranial vessels critically depends on flow direction, depth control of the range-gated Doppler signal, position and tilting of the probe (Table 12-5), and compression tests in selected cases (Table 12-6). Three different approaches allow the recording of intracranial flow velocity: (1) transtemporal (Fig. 12-15 and Plate 12-3), using the temporal "window", (2) transorbital, and (3) nuchal.

Sometimes compression tests are necessary to identify the recorded vessel; in addition, they allow exam-

**TABLE 12-5. Transcranial Doppler Criteria for the Identification of Basal Intracranial Vessels Using the Transtemporal, Transorbital, and Nuchal Approaches**

| Vessel | Probe | Depth (mm) | Flow Direction |
|---|---|---|---|
| *Transtemporal Approach* | | | |
| MCA | Medial | 30–65 | Toward probe |
| ACA | Medial | 55–80 | Away from probe |
| ICA | Caudal | 55–75 | Toward probe |
| PCA, P1 | Posterior | 55–80 | Toward probe |
| PCA, P2 | Posterior | 55–75 | Away from probe |
| *Transorbital Approach* | | | |
| Ophthalmic artery | | 30–60 | Toward the probe |
| ICA, C4, C5 | | 60–80 | Toward the probe |
| ICA, C2, C3 | | 60–80 | Away from the probe |
| *Nuchal Approach* | | | |
| VA | | 50–100 | Away from the probe |
| BA | | 75–120 | Away from the probe |

*Abbreviations:* MCA, middle cerebral artery; ACA, anterior cerebral artery; ICA, internal carotid artery; PCA, posterior cerebral artery; VA, vertebral artery; BA, basilar artery.

ination of the circle of Willis. Before performing a compression test, a duplex scan of the vessel to be compressed should be performed to exclude plaque or stenosis; in addition, the patient should be informed about the potential risk, although the risk of TIA is low if the compression is performed very proximal (Table 12-6).

In general, knowledge of the extracranial noninvasive studies (Doppler, duplex) is essential for the correct interpretation of the transcranial findings. Normal values are given in Table 12-7. The velocities of intracranial vessels vary with age, hematocrit,[21] end-tidal $CO_2$ partial pressure, and other variables.[22]

## Extracranial Arterial Disease

In patients with distal lesions of the ICA (e.g., carotid artery dissections, fibromuscular dysplasia, atypical atherosclerosis, aneurysms) extracranial approach of the low-frequency PW Doppler probe in the submandibular region allows recording of flow velocity in the ICA up to the base of the skull (recording depth: 40 to 80 mm). Figure 12-16 shows an example of a patient with a distal atherosclerotic ICA lesion in 65-mm recording depth indicated by increased velocities and low-frequency signals.

**TABLE 12-6. Transcranial Doppler Criteria for Compression Tests of the Internal Carotid Arteries**

| Vessel Recorded | Vessel Compressed | Effect | Conclusion |
|---|---|---|---|
| MCA | ICA ipsi | Flow ↓ | MCA identified |
| ACA | ICA ipsi | Flow ↓ | ACA identified |
| ACA | ICA ipsi | Flow inversed | ACoA patent |
| ACA | ICA contra | Flow ↑ | ACoA patent |
| PCA, P1 | ICA ipsi | Flow ↑ | PCoA patent |
| PCA, P2 | ICA ipsi | Flow ↓ | Carotid origin of PCA |

*Abbreviations:* MCA, middle cerebral artery; ICA, interior carotid artery; ACA, anterior cerebral artery; ACoA, anterior communicating artery; PCA, posterior cerebral artery; PCoA, posterior communicating artery; ipsi, ipsilateral; contra, contralateral.

**TABLE 12-7. Normal Values of Transcranial Doppler Examination**

| Vessel | Systolic Peak Velocity (cm/s) | Mean Velocity (cm/s) | Diastolic Velocity (cm/s) | Age Group (years) |
|---|---|---|---|---|
| MCA | 94.5 ± 13.6 | 58.4 ± 8.4 | 45.6 ± 6.6 | <40 |
| (50 mm) | 91.0 ± 16.9[a] | 57.7 ± 11.5[a] | 44.3 ± 9.5[a] | 40–60 |
| | 78.1 ± 15.0[a] | 44.7 ± 11.1[a] | 31.9 ± 9.1[a] | >60 |
| ACA | 76.4 ± 16.9 | 47.3 ± 13.6 | 36.0 ± 9.0 | <40 |
| (70 mm) | 86.4 ± 20.1 | 53.1 ± 10.5 | 41.1 ± 7.4[b] | 40–60 |
| | 73.3 ± 20.3 | 45.3 ± 13.5 | 34.2 ± 8.8[b] | >60 |
| PCA | 53.2 ± 11.3 | 34.2 ± 7.8 | 25.9 ± 6.5 | <40 |
| (60 mm) | 60.1 ± 20.6 | 36.6 ± 9.8 | 28.7 ± 7.5[b] | 40–60 |
| | 51.0 ± 11.9 | 29.9 ± 9.3 | 22.0 ± 6.9[b] | >60 |
| VA/BA | 56.3 ± 7.8 | 34.9 ± 7.8 | 27.0 ± 5.3 | <40 |
| (75 mm) | 59.5 ± 17.0 | 36.4 ± 11.7 | 29.2 ± 8.4[b] | 40–60 |
| | 50.9 ± 18.7 | 30.5 ± 12.4 | 21.2 ± 9.2[b] | >60 |
| | Pulsatility Index (All Age Groups) | | | |
| MCA | | 0.92 ± 0.25 | | |
| ACA | | 0.8 ± 0.16 | | |
| PCA | | 0.88 ± 0.21 | | |

*Abbreviations:* MCA, middle cerebral artery; ACA, anterior cerebral artery; PCA, posterior cerebral artery; VA, vertebral artery; BA, basilar artery.
[a] $P < 0.02$.
[b] $P < 0.05$.

## Intracranial Collateralization of Significant Extracranial Lesions

TCD allows noninvasive assessment of the intracranial hemodynamic effects of stenosis or occlusion of the ICA in the neck. The collateral channels can be identified by TCD by various collateral patterns (Table 12-8, Fig. 12-17 and Plate 12-4). The efficacy of collateral flow can usually be assessed. Flow velocities in the middle cerebral artery (MCA) distal to significant stenoses and occlusions vary. It has been shown that asymptomatic patients may have normal peak and mean velocities,[96] indicating adequate collateralization. Schneider et al.[108] described reduced MCA velocities and pulsatile index (PI) values ipsilateral to an occlusion. Symptomatic patients had reduced PI values in the MCA, whereas the PI in asymptomatic patients was normal ipsilateral to an occlusion. Lindegaard et al.[73] found a significant reduction of the pulsatility transmission index ([PTI]; a comparison of the PI of two arteries) of the MCA ipsilateral to an ICA stenosis with 75 percent or greater reduction of the luminal area. Tatemichi et al.[123] showed the main source of collateral to the middle cerebral artery is via the circle of Willis, with the ophthalmic collateral a poor source.

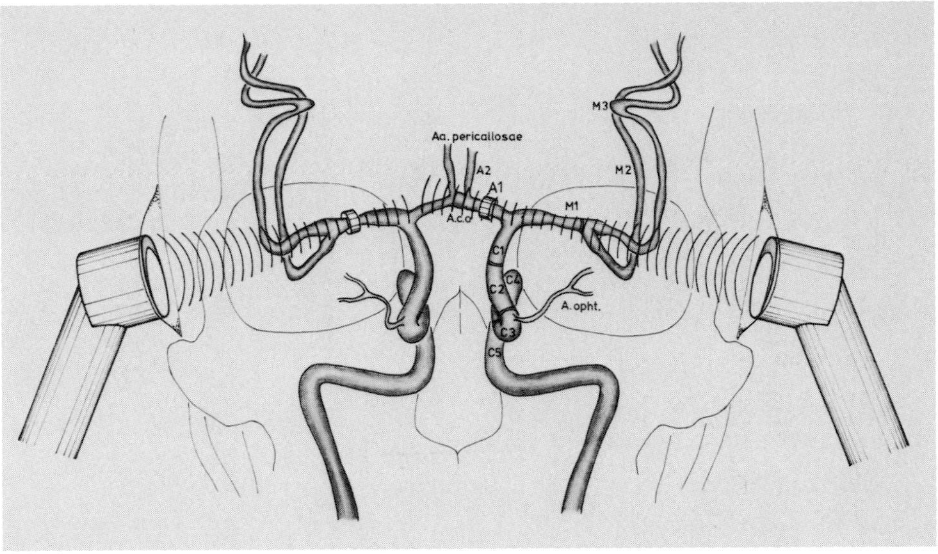


**Fig. 12-15.** Schematic illustration of the position of the sample volume inside the skull, using the transtemporal approach. Aa.pericallosae, pericallosal arteries; A.opht., ophthalmic artery; A.c.a., anterior communicating artery.

## Carbon Dioxide Reactivity

The possibility to assess the intracranial reserve capacity using a $CO_2$ test has long been known.[129] In combination with TCD the $CO_2$ test gives information about the reserve potential of the cerebral circulation.

The method allows the clinician to assess aspects of the cerebral autoregulation, which keeps blood flow constant independent of the systemic pressure. This compensation is based on dilation or constriction of small intracerebral arterioles. The $CO_2$ test assesses the reactivity of the peripheral arterioles to a chemical stimulus. Hypercapnia leads to a vasodilation of the peripheral vessels and to an increased blood flow in the basal arteries at the circle of Willis, which can be recorded by TCD. Since it is known from angiographic studies[58] that the diameter of the large vessels is constant, irrespective of the concentration of $CO_2$ in the blood, changes of blood velocity represent changes of blood flow. Several authors used this method to assess the intracranial reserve capacity in patients with significant extracranial disease.[13,23,102,132] Results have shown that the severity of the extracranial lesion does not predict hemodynamic relevance for intracranial circulation. Patients with carotid artery stenoses and occlusions may show normal or reduced cerebral vasomotor reactivity. This test seems to be useful for the detection of patients at risk for suffering a hemodynamic stroke. However, these patients are rare, and prospective data on larger groups of patients are missing.

**TABLE 12-8. Collateral Channels: Transcranial Doppler Criteria**

| |
|---|
| ACoA |
| Retrograde flow direction in the ipsilateral ACA |
| Increased peak and mean velocities in both ACAs |
| Increased velocities and low-frequency signals in the midline (75–85 mm), ACoA, functional stenosis |
| MCA velocity decrease during contralateral CCA compression |
| PCoA |
| Increased velocities in the ipsilateral PCA (P1) |
| Increased velocities in the basilar artery |
| Low-frequency signals in the region of the PCoA (60–70 mm depth) |
| Leptomeningeal anastomosis |
| Increased velocities in proximal and distal vessel segments (e.g., PCA − P1 and P2) |
| Partly retrograde flow signals in distal vessel segments (e.g., retrograde flow direction in distal MCA branches) |
| Ophthalmic collateral |
| Retrograde flow direction of the ophthalmic artery |

*Abbreviations:* ACA, anterior cerebral artery; ACoA, anterior communicating artery; PCA, posterior cerebral artery; MCA, middle cerebral artery; CCA, common carotid artery; PCoA, posterior communicating artery.

## Orthostatic Reactivity

Monitoring of cerebral hemodynamics during orthostatic maneuvers allows noninvasive assessment of autonomic functions, which is useful in patients with autonomic neuropathy, autonomic failure, and pandysautonomia. In these patients abnormal decreases of flow velocities within the basal cerebral arteries can be detected during orthostatic stress (Fig. 12-18). TCD allows objective assessment of therapeutic effects in this situation. Measurements of intracranial flow velocities during orthostatic stress may be of value in patients with syncope and orthostatic dysregulation.

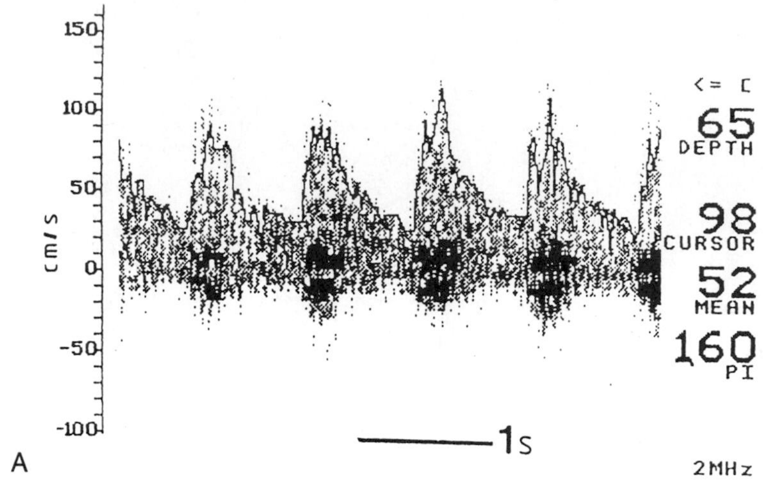


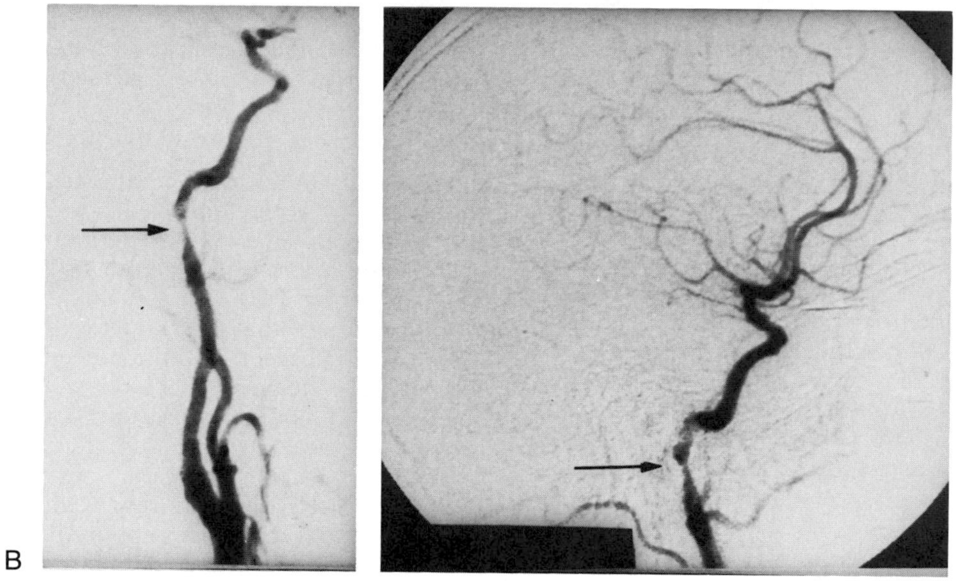


**Fig. 12-16.** (**A**) Doppler spectra (recording depth: 65 mm, increased peak velocities, low-frequency signals). (**B**) Angiogram of a patient with an extracranial distal lesion of the internal carotid artery (*arrows*).

## Carotid Dissections

Whereas extracranial Doppler techniques allow noninvasive diagnosis and follow-up of carotid dissections, TCD enables adequate assessment of the intracranial situation and the dynamic changes during follow-up.[62] In some patients the submandibular approach allows direct recording of a distal ICA stenosis. Sequential TCD recordings are helpful in the detection of hemodynamic changes of intracranial circulation, which in some cases develop within few days.

## Subclavian Steal Phenomenon

TCD for the first time allows noninvasive assessment of blood flow alterations within the basilar artery (BA) in patients with proximal lesions of the subclavian arteries, resulting in steal phenomena of the vertebral arteries.[131] Due to the anatomic variations in this region, the beginning of the basilar artery is difficult to identify by means of TCD.[86] The basilar artery can normally be investigated in recording depths between 75 and 120 mm. In the majority of patients with subclavian steal phenomena, flow direction of the basilar artery is orthograde, about one-third of patients have intermediate stages of flow alterations (Fig. 12-19). Retrograde flow direction of the basilar artery is an extreme rarity and is seen only in patients with multivessel disease and anomalies within the circle of Willis.[65] About 40 percent of patients show alterations of flow velocity in the basilar artery during hyperemia of the ipsilateral arm.

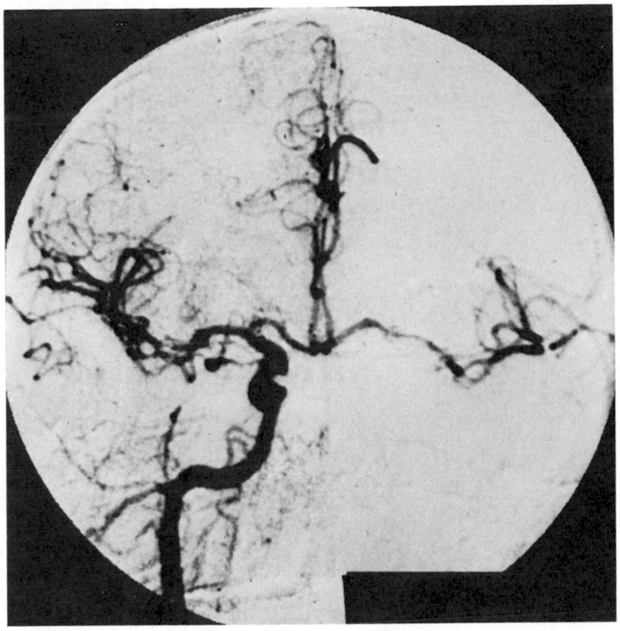

**Fig. 12-17.** Collateral pathway via the anterior communicating artery in a patient with internal carotid artery occlusion on the left side. Display of a two-dimensional transcranial Doppler device (see Plate 12-4).

In patients with obstructions of the innominate artery, TCD is useful in demonstrating complex intracranial hemodynamic alterations. Abnormal flow patterns in these patients are characterized by a damped signal spectrum during early systole, associated with a softly whispering audio signal, which is due mainly to delayed peak blood flow velocity. Latent steal phenomena can be demonstrated in various intracranial vessels during postischemic hyperemia of the upper extremities. In patients with innominate artery obstructive disease, this steal phenomenon seems to be associated with the occurrence of symptoms.[95]

### Intracranial Stenoses and Occlusions

As in extracranial disease, narrowing of intracranial vessels produces various flow abnormalities, such as local increases in mean and peak velocities, low-frequency signals, and disturbed reversed-flow phenomena, depending on the degree of stenosis.[51,73,115] These phenomena allow noninvasive detection of intracranial stenoses of the basal arteries by TCD (Fig. 12-20 and Plate 12-5). In vessel segments distal to severe lesions decreased velocities and damping of the waveform can be seen.[77] Stenoses of more than 50 percent lumen narrowing can reliably be detected within the MCA (M1 segment), carotid siphon, and posterior cerebral artery (PCA) (Table 12-9). Stenoses of distal MCA branches are difficult to detect. So far, no reliable criteria for the exact quantification of intracranial stenoses have been established. Collateral flow via the circle of Willis in cases of severe extracranial lesions sometimes results in functional stenotic signs and may lead to misinterpretations. Occlusion of the M1 segment of the MCA can be assessed if no signal of the MCA can be detected in patients with normal echowindows. This is indicated by detectable signals of the ICA siphon and the anterior cerebral artery (ACA) and by accelerated velocity of the ACA

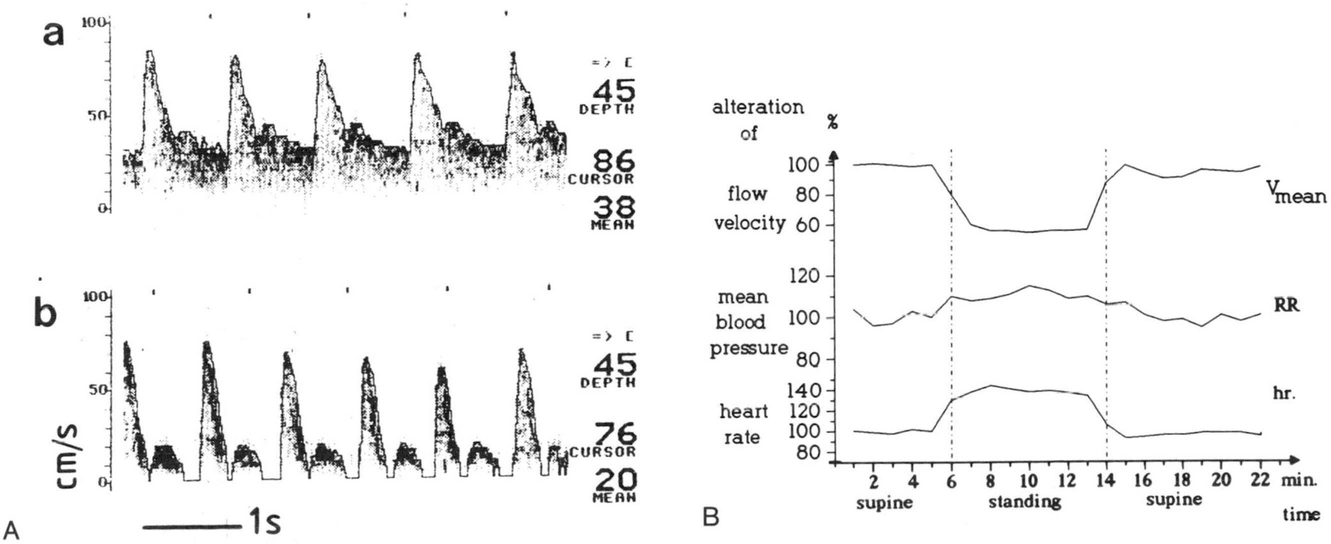


**Fig. 12-18.** (**A**) Dramatic change of flow velocities in a patient with Shy-Drager syndrome investigated in supine (a) and sitting (b) position. (**B**) Simultaneous registration of cardiovascular parameters [mean middle cerebral artery velocity ($V_{mean}$), blood pressure (RR), and heart rate (hr)] reveal an orthostatic flow dysregulation in the middle cerebral artery without cardiovascular dysregulation in a patient with a long history of syncope.

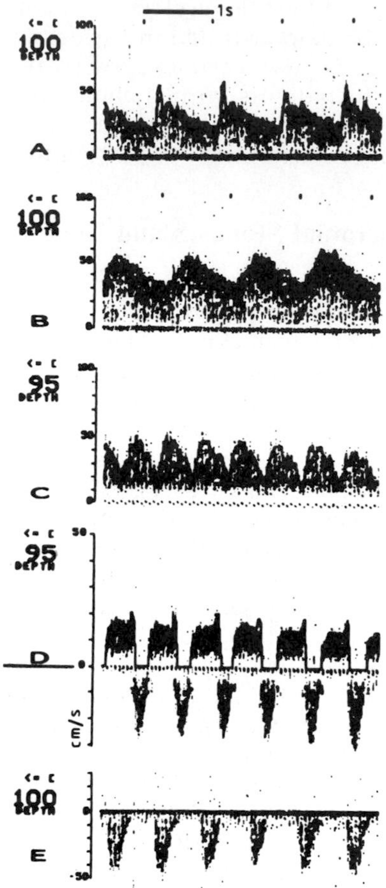

**Fig. 12-19.** Various alterations of flow velocity in basilar arteries in patients with obstructions of the subclavian or innominate arteries. (**A**) Normal. (**B**) Delayed systolic peak. (**C,D**) Intermediate stages. (**E**) Reversal of blood flow.

**TABLE 12-9. Detection of Intracranial Stenoses by Transcranial Doppler in 467 Patients Who Were Investigated Prior to Selective Intra-arterial Angiography**

| | MCA | ICA | PCA | VA | BA |
|---|---|---|---|---|---|
| Right positive | 24 | 21 | 10 | 19 | 9 |
| Right negative | 438 | 445 | 455 | 442 | 453 |
| False positive | 3 | — | — | 1 | — |
| False negative | 2 | 1 | 2 | 5 | 5 |
| Sensitivity (%) | 92 | 91 | 83 | 79 | 64 |
| Specificity (%) | 99 | 100 | 100 | 99 | 100 |
| Test accuracy (%) | 99 | 100 | 100 | 99 | 99 |
| Positive predictive Value (%) | 89 | 100 | 100 | 99 | 100 |
| Negative predictive Value (%) | 99 | 100 | 99 | 98 | 99 |

*Abbreviations:* MCA, middle cerebral artery; ICA, (internal carotid artery) carotid siphon; PCA, posterior cerebral artery; VA, vertebral artery; BA, basilar artery.

when the ACA provides collateral to the MCA over the hemisphere surface.[20,22] In cases of MCA occlusion, damped spectra can be seen in vessel segments proximal to the occlusion, whereas distal MCA branches may show reversed-flow direction.[61] In a series of 467 patients the sensitivity for the detection of MCA occlusion by TCD was 79 percent with a specificity of 100 percent.[97] By continuous monitoring, it was possible for Mohr et al.[83] to document early recanalization of an acute occlusion, one of the few so demonstrated.

TCD results in the vertebrobasilar circulation are less reliable than in the anterior circulation. Due to anatomic variants, the beginning of the basilar artery is difficult to define by TCD criteria alone.[86] The distal basilar artery cannot be acurately investigated through the foramen magnum in two patients due to great distance from the ultrasound probe, resulting in a poor signal to noise ratio. Whereas stenoses of the distal vertebral and basilar arteries can be diagnosed with a sensitivity of 79 percent and 64 percent with a specificity of 99 percent and 100 percent, the sensitivity for the detection of occlusion of the basilar artery was only 36 percent,[97] a finding of major clinical importance. In acute thrombosis of the basilar artery TCD is of limited diagnostic value. The combination of magnetic resonance angiography and TCD may increase the diagnostic accuracy concerning noninvasive detection of intracranial arterial lesions in the future (Fig. 12-20).[33,105]

## Vasospasm in Subarachnoid Hemorrhage

TCD has proven useful in the detection, quantification, and analysis of the time course of vasospasms after subarachnoid hemorrhage (SAH).[3,40,111] It has been found that vasospasms occur at the 4th day after SAH. The maximum of the flow accelerations can be seen between the 11th and 18th days. The normalization of flow velocities occurs within the 3rd and 4th week after SAH. Increased velocities may occur before the appearance of delayed ischemic defects. Rapid increase of velocities during the 4th and 8th days is associated with an increased risk of suffering an ischemic stroke. Therapeutic effects of calcium antagonists can be monitored noninvasively by TCD. Although vasospasm within the territory of the MCA can reliably be detected, spasms of the ACA, in particular the A2 segments, remain a diagnostic problem.[72]

## Dolichoectatic Arteries

In patients with intracranial dolichoectatic arteries, such as the megadolichobasilar artery, significantly reduced peak and mean velocities can be recorded by TCD (Fig. 12-21). This is of clinical importance because in combination with CT or MRI, TCD offers completely noninvasive diagnosis of such an anomaly.[94] A considerable number of patients with

A 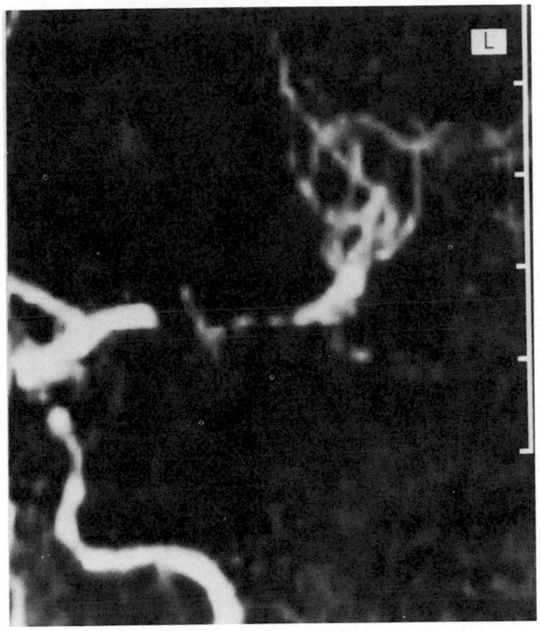 B 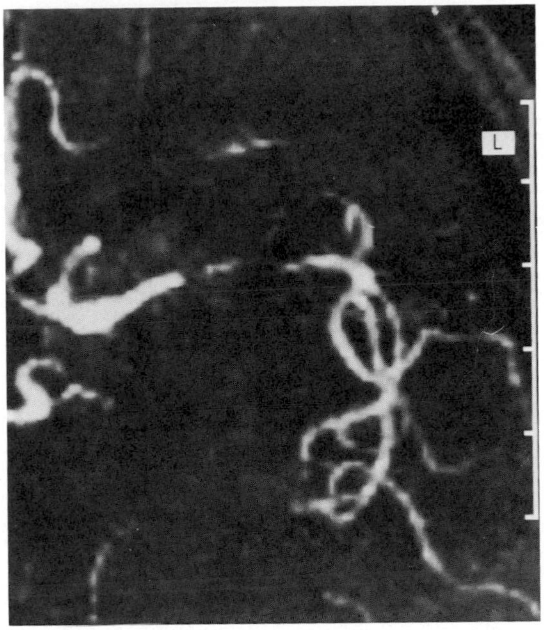

**Fig. 12-20.** MR-angiography. (**A**) AP view; (**B**) axial view of high-grade stenosis of the left middle cerebral artery (see Plate 12-5).

intracranial dolichoectatic arteries suffer from TIAs or stroke. The dramatic reduction of flow velocities, which can often be observed in these patients, suggests a thrombotic source of these ischemic events from slow flow territories.

## Arteriovenous Malformations and Other Fistulas

TCD allows a noninvasive insight into the hemodynamic aspects of intracranial AVMs.[75,90,110] Due to the low peripheral resistance, proximal segments of the feeding vessel show high peak and mean velocities with a low pulsatility index. Feeding vessels can be identified by the lack of $CO_2$ reactivity. A linear relationship between mean velocity, diameter of feeder, and volume of AVM have been reported.[42] Pulsatile flow can be observed in draining veins. Two-dimensional TCD scan allows selective recordings of small-vessel segments within the AVM if the malformation can be investigated directly (Fig. 12-22 and Plate 12-6). Apart from noninvasive diagnosis of the AVM, TCD is particularly useful in the follow-up of patients with and without treatment (e.g., surgery, radiation) and as a monitoring tool during therapeutic intravascular embolization procedures.[90] TCD provides useful information about the changes of velocity in the feeding vessels during intravascular occlusive procedures and helps guide the radiologist. In patients with carotid-cavernous sinus fistulas TCD can detect abnormal velocity patterns, including high velocities and low-frequency signals in the region of the shunt. This is of great diagnostic value when CT and extracranial Doppler studies failed to show any abnormality.

## Patent Cardiac Foramen Ovale

Use of the agitated saline technique, with intravenous injection in the antecubital vein to identify a patent cardiac foramen ovale, can detect the presence of right-to-left shunts from any cause by documentation of the microbubbles reaching the brain. In obvious cases, the distinctive acoustic signal of the microbubbles is not easy to miss (Plate 12-7).

## Intracranial Pressure

Simultaneous measurements of systemic blood pressure, intracranial pressure as monitored by epidural devices, and Doppler signals of the basal cerebral arteries have shown that, with increasing intracranial pressure (ICP), a progressive reduction of diastolic and systolic velocities can be found. Interestingly, different patterns of flow alterations could be demonstrated in different regions of the brain, indicating the existence of different pressure gradients inside the skull.[43] If the intracranial pressure is greater than the diastolic blood pressure, Doppler signals of the basal cerebral arteries are severely altered. Mild and moderate increase of ICP can be compensated by

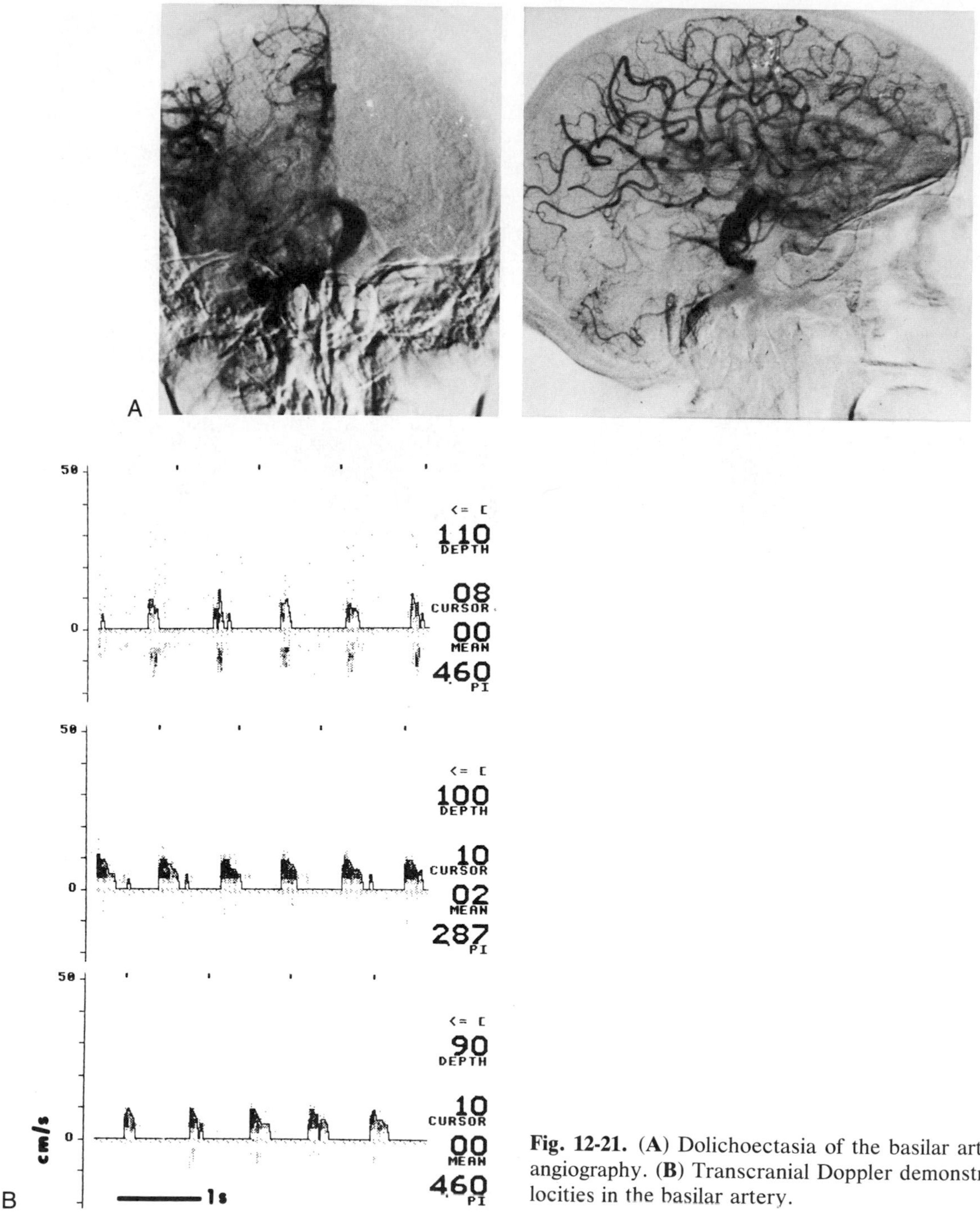


**Fig. 12-21.** (**A**) Dolichoectasia of the basilar artery as shown by angiography. (**B**) Transcranial Doppler demonstrates reduced velocities in the basilar artery.

an increase of the systemic blood pressure; in this situation Doppler signals remain normal.

## Brain Death

In brain-dead patients three different patterns of flow alterations have been reported:[44,91] oscillating flow (Fig. 12-23), systolic spikes, and zero flow. Zero flow is difficult to interpret and may be misleading because insufficient echowindows cannot be excluded if sequential examinations are not available. It has been shown that TCD can be used to confirm brain death if some standards for the performance and interpretation are taken into account.[91] One of these

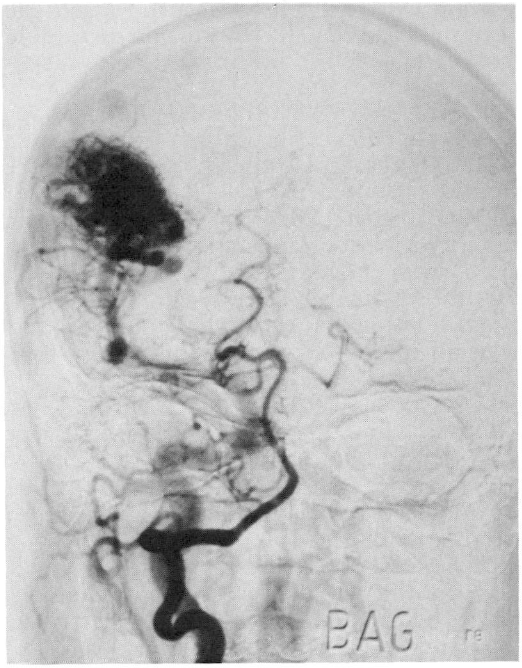


**Fig. 12-22.** Arteriovenous malformation on the right side (see Plate 12-6).

technical standards is that the typical TCD signals suggestive of brain death should be detectable in more than one vessel. With these precautions a sensitivity of 91.3 and a specificity of 100 percent have been reported.[91] These results indicate that TCD is a valid bedside noninvasive method to confirm the diagnosis of brain death if appropriate guidelines for performance and interpretation are taken into account.

## Monitoring

The recording of flow velocities in intracranial arteries provides the means for monitoring circulatory

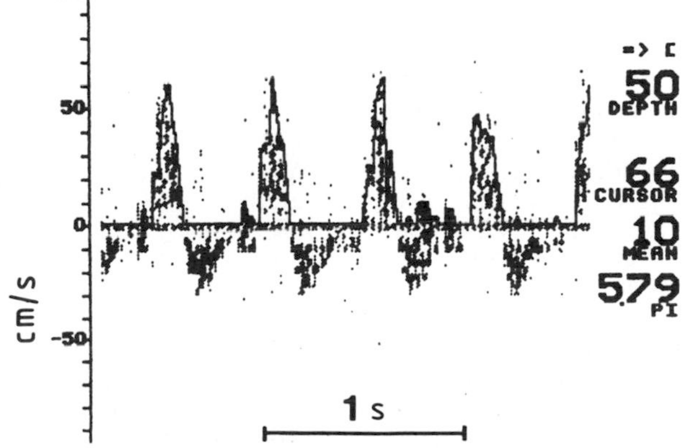


**Fig. 12-23.** Alternating flow profile in the middle cerebral artery in a patient with brain death.

changes during major surgery, interventional neuroradiologic procedures, and in the intensive care unit. The concept of monitoring is the recording of brain function and early detection of transient alterations of brain functions in order to prevent persistent deficits by a rapid therapeutic intervention. Because of its excellent time solution, TCD is an ideal tool for rapid detection of changes of the intracranial circulation. TCD has proven useful in carotid endarterectomy to monitor MCA velocity during ipsilateral ICA clamping. The majority of patients show only a minor decrease of MCA velocity during the clamping phase. This finding questions the routine need for an intraoperative shunt, which seems to be necessary only in a small group of patients.[109] The effect of carotid clamping can be assessed preoperatively, using a carotid compression test. Microemboli have been detected by TCD monitoring during open heart and carotid surgery.[114] Continuous monitoring of patients with migraine may be valuable in clarifying the pathophysiology of the disease. Results reported so far, however, are controversial.

## Functional Investigations

Assessment of changes of blood velocity during neuronal activation by mental activity or light exposure have been reported.[2,32] These findings show that TCD is able to detect, like regional cerebral blood flow methods, changes of blood flow during activation of distinct brain areas[41] (Fig. 12-24).

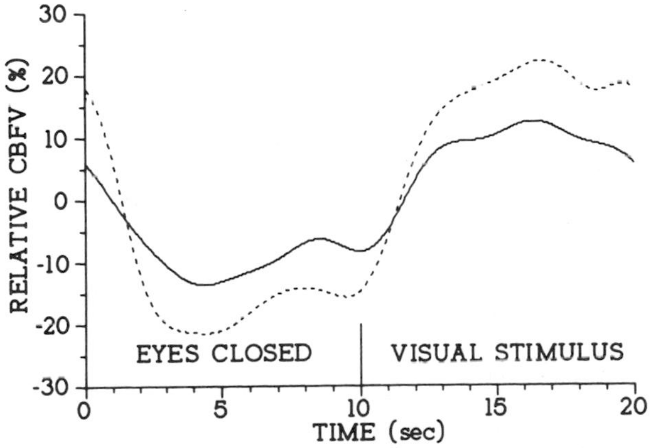


**Fig. 12-24.** Visually evoked posterior cerebral artery response in a patient with a history of migraine. A colored animated cartoon is used as visual stimulus. In normals there is an increase in flow velocity of the posterior cerebral artery of 30 percent above the resting level. Whereas absolute responses are normal for the left (*solid line*) and right side (*dashed line*), there is an abnormal difference (more than 5 SD below normal left/right difference values) between both sides. Scale: percentage deviation from the mean cerebral blood flow velocity (CBFV).

## Advantages and Limitations

TCD is a simple bedside method for recording flow velocities in basal intracranial arteries, and its excellent time solution easily allows monitoring of intracranial circulation. In experienced hands, intracranial occlusive disease can reliably be diagnosed in the anterior circulation. Assessment of intracranial hemodynamics in patients with severe extracranial arterial disease is possible.[8,25] Due to insufficient echowindows not all patients can be investigated. In about 5 percent of patients, predominantly elderly women, the signals recorded from intracranial vessels are insufficient due to ossification. Because of anatomic variations, the diagnostic value in the posterior circulation is limited. This method critically depends on the skill of the examiner. Blood velocity, not blood flow, is measured by TCD.[66]

## REFERENCES


1. Aaslid R: Transcranial Doppler Sonography. Springer-Verlag, New York, 1986
2. Aaslid R: Visually evoked dynamic blood flow response of the human cerebral circulation. Stroke 17:771, 1987
3. Aaslid R, Huber P, Nornes H: Evaluation of cerebrovascular spasm with transcranial Doppler ultrasound. J Neurosurg 60:37, 1984
4. Aaslid R, Markwalder ThM, Nornes H: Noninvasive transcranial Doppler ultrasound recording of flow velocity in basal cerebral arteries. J Neurosurg 57:769, 1982
5. Ackermann RH: A perspective on non-invasive diagnosis of carotid disease. Neurology (NY) 29:615, 1979
6. Ackerstaff RGA, Hoeneveld H, Slowikowski JM et al: Ultrasonic duplex scanning in atherosclerotic disease of the innominate subclavian and vertebral arteries: a comparative study with angiography. Ultrasound Med Biol 10:409, 1984
7. Adiga KR, Fresso SJ, Nayden Y: Noninvasive methods in the diagnosis of extracranial carotid artery disease. Angiology 331, 1984
8. American Academy of Neurology, Therapeutics and Technology Assessment Subcommittee: Assessment: transcranial Doppler. Neurology (NY) 40:680, 1990
9. Anderson DC, Loewenson R, Yock D et al: B-mode, real-time carotid ultrasonic imaging: correlation with angiography. Arch Neurol 40:484, 1983
10. Bashour TT, Crew JP, Dean M et al: Ultrasonic imaging of common carotid artery dissection. J Clin Ultrasound 13:210, 1985
11. Bassiouny HS, Davis H, Massawa N et al: Critical carotid stenoses: morphologic and chemical similarity between symptomatic and asymptomatic plaques. J Vasc Surg 9:202, 1989
12. Bendick PJ, Jackson VP: Evaluation of the vertebral arteries with duplex sonography. J Vasc Surg 3:523, 1986
13. Bishop CCR, Powell S, Insall M et al: Effect of internal carotid artery occlusion on middle cerebral artery blood flow at rest and in response to hypercapnia. Lancet I:710, 1986
14. Blackshear WM, Phillips DJ, Thiele MB et al: Detection of carotid occlusive disease by ultrasonic imaging and pulsed Doppler spectrum analysis. Surgery 86:698, 1979
15. Bluth EI, Kay D, Merritt CRB et al: Sonographic characterization of carotid plaque: detection of hemorrhage. AJR 146:1061, 1986
16. Bluth EI, McVay LV, Merritt CRB et al: The identification of ulcerative plaque with high resolution duplex carotid scanning. J Ultrasound Med 7:73, 1988
17. Bluth EI, Shyn PB, Sullivan MA et al: Doppler color flow imaging of carotid artery dissection. J Ultrasound Med 8:149, 1989
18. Bogdahn U, Becker G, Winkler J et al: Transcranial color-coded real-time sonography in adults. Stroke 21:1680, 1990
19. Bornstein NM, Krajewski A, Lewis AJ et al: Clinical significance of carotid plaque hemorrhage. Arch Neurol 47:958, 1990
20. Brass LM, Duterte DL, Mohr JP: Anterior cerebral artery velocity changes in disease of the middle cerebral artery stem. Stroke 20:1737, 1989
21. Brass LM, Pavlakis SG, De Vivo D et al: Transcranial Doppler measurements of the middle cerebral artery: effect of hematocrit. Stroke 19:1466, 1989
22. Brass LM, Prohovnik I, Pavlakis SG et al: Middle cerebral artery blood velocity and cerebral blood flow in sickle cell disease. Stroke 22:27, 1991
23. Bullock R, Mendelow AD, Bone I et al: Cerebral blood flow and $CO_2$ responsiveness as an indicator of collateral reserve capacity in patients with carotid arterial disease. Br J Surg 72:348, 1985
24. Burns PN: The physical principles of Doppler and spectral analysis. J Clin Ultrasound 15:567, 1987
25. Caplan LR, Brass LM, DeWitt LD et al: Transcranial ultrasound: present status. Neurology (NY) 40:696, 1990
26. Chambers BR, Norris JW: Outcome in patients with asymptomatic neck bruits. N Engl J Med 315:806, 1986
27. Comerota AJ, Cranley JJ, Cook SE: Real-time B-mode carotid imaging in diagnosis of cerebrovascular disease. Surgery 89:718, 1981
28. Comerota AJ, Katz ML, White JV et al: The preoperative diagnosis of the ulcerated carotid atheroma. J Vasc Surg 11:505, 1990
29. Davis PC, Nilsen B, Braun IF et al: A prospective comparison of duplex sonography vs angiography of the vertebral arteries. AJNR 7:1059, 1986
30. Doorly JP, Atkinson PI, Kingston V, Shanik DG: Carotid ultra-sonic arteriography combined with real-time spectral analysis: a comparison with angiography. J Cardiovasc Surg 23:243, 1982
31. Doppler Ch: Über das farbige Licht der Doppelsterne und einiger anderer Gestirne des Him-

mels. Abh Kgl Böhm Ges Wissensch (Prag) p. 465, 1843

32. Droste DW, Harders AG, Rastogi E: A transcranial Doppler study of blood flow velocity in the middle cerebral arteries performed at rest and during mental activities. Stroke 20:1005, 1989
33. Edelman RR, Mattle HP, O'Reilly GV et al: Magnetic resonance imaging of the circle of Willis. Stroke 21:56, 1990
34. Erickson SJ, Mewissen MW, Foley WD et al: Stenosis of the internal carotid artery: assessment using color Doppler imaging compared with angiography. AJR 152:1299, 1989
35. Fell G, Phillips DJ, Chikos PM et al: Ultrasonic duplex scanning for disease of the carotid artery. Circulation 64:1191, 1981
36. Glagov S, Zarins CK: Quantitating atherosclerosis: problems of definition. p. 11. In Bond MG, Insull W, Glagov S et al (eds): Clinical Diagnosis of Atherosclerosis: Quantitative Methods of Evaluation. Springer-Verlag, New York, 1983
37. Goes E, Janssens W, Maillet B et al: Tissue characterization of atheromatous plaques: correlation between ultrasound image and histological findings. J Clin Ultrasound 18:611, 1990
38. Hacke W, Hennerici M, Krämer G, Gelmers HJ: Cerebral Ischemia. Springer-Verlag, New York, 1990
39. Hallam MJ, Reid JM, Cooperberg PL: Color-flow Doppler and conventional duplex scanning of the carotid bifurcation: prospective, double-blind, correlative study. AJR 152:1101, 1989
40. Harders A: Neurosurgical Applications of Transcranial Doppler Sonography. Springer-Verlag, New York, 1986
41. Harders AG, Laborde G, Droste DW, Rastogi E: Brain activity and blood flow velocity changes: a transcranial Doppler study. Int J Neurosci 47:91, 1989
42. Hassler W: Hemodynamic Aspects of Cerebral Angiomas. Springer-Verlag, Vienna, 1986
43. Hassler W, Steinmetz H, Gawlowski J: Transcranial Doppler ultrasonography in raised intracranial pressure and in intracranial circulatory arrest. J Neurosurg 68:745, 1988
44. Hassler W, Steinmetz H, Pirschel J: Transcranial Doppler study of intracranial circulatory arrest. J Neurosurg 71:195, 1989
45. Hennerici M, Aulich A, Sandmann W, Freund HJ: Incidence of asymptomatic extracranial arterial disease. Stroke 12:750, 1981
46. Hennerici M, Freund HJ: Efficacy of CW-Doppler and duplex-system examinations for the evaluation of extracranial carotid disease. J Clin Ultrasound 12:155, 1984
47. Hennerici M, Hülsbömer HB, Hefter H et al: Natural history of asymptomatic extracranial arterial disease. Brain 110:777, 1987
48. Hennerici M, Klemm C, Rautenberg W: The subclavian steal phenomenon: a common vascular disorder with rare neurologic deficits. Neurology (NY) 38:669, 1988
49. Hennerici M, Neuerburg-Heusler D: Gefässdiagnostik mit Ultraschall. Thieme, New York, 1988
50. Hennerici M, Rautenberg W, Mohr S: Stroke risk from symptomless extracranial disease. Lancet, 2:1180, 1982
51. Hennerici M, Rautenberg W, Schwartz A: Transcranial Doppler ultrasound for the assessment of intracranial arterial flow velocity. II. Evaluation of intracranial arterial disease. Surg Neurol 27:523, 1987
52. Hennerici M, Rautenberg W, Sitzer G, Schwartz A: Transcranial Doppler ultrasound for the assessment of intracranial arterial flow velocity. I. Examination technique and normal values. Surg Neurol 27:439, 1987
53. Hennerici M, Rautenberg W, Trockel U et al: Spontaneous progression and regression of small carotid atheroma. Lancet 1:1415, 1985
54. Hennerici M, Reifschneider G, Trockel U et al: Detection of early atherosclerotic lesions by scanning of the carotid artery. J Clin Ultrasound 12:455, 1984
55. Hennerici M, Steinke W: Carotid plaque developments—aspects of hemodynamic and vessel wall interaction. Cerebrovasc Dis 1:142, 1991
56. Hennerici M, Steinke W, Rautenberg W: High-resistance Doppler flow pattern in extracranial carotid dissection. Arch Neurol 46:670, 1989
57. Houi K, Mochio S, Isogai Y et al: Comparison of color flow and 3D image by computer graphics for the evaluation of carotid disease. Angiology 41:305, 1990
58. Huber, P, Handa J: Effect of contrast material, hypercapnea, hyperventilation, hypotonic glucose and papaverine on the diameter of cerebral arteries. Invest Radiol 2:17, 1967
59. Imparato AM, Riles TS, Mintzer R et al: The importance of hemorrhage in the relationship between gross morphologic characteristics and cerebral symptoms in 376 carotid artery plaques. Ann Surg 197:195, 1983
60. Jacobs NM, Grant EG, Schellinger D et al: Duplex carotid sonography: criteria for stenosis, accuracy, and pitfalls. Radiology 154:385, 1985
61. Kaps M, Damian MS, Teschendorf U, Dorndorf W: Transcranial Doppler ultrasound findings in middle cerebral artery occlusion. Stroke 21:532, 1990
62. Kaps M, Dorndorf W, Damian MS, Agnoli L: Intracranial haemodynamics in patients with spontaneous carotid dissection. Eur Arch Psychiatr Neurol Sci 239:246, 1990
63. Keagy BA, Pharr WF, Thomas D, Bowes DE: A quantitative method for the evaluation of spectral analysis: patterns in carotid artery stenosis. Ultrasound Med Biol 8:625, 1982
64. Keller HM, Meier WE, Anliker M, Kumpe DA: Noninvasive measurement of velocity profiles and flow in the common carotid artery by pulsed Doppler ultrasound. Stroke 7:370, 1976
65. Klingelhöfer J, Conrad B, Benecke R, Frank B: Transcranial Doppler ultrasonography of carotid-basilar collateral circulation in subclavian steal. Stroke 19:1036, 1989
66. Kontos HA: Validity of cerebral arterial blood flow calculations from velocity measurements. Stroke 20:1, 1989

67. Kotval PS, Babu SC, Fakhry J et al: Role of the intimal flap in arterial dissection: sonographic demonstration. AJR 150:1181, 1988
68. Ku DN, Giddens DP, Phillips DJ et al: Hemodynamics of the normal carotid bifurcation: in vitro and in vivo studies. Ultrasound Med Biol 11:13, 1985
69. Langsfeld M, Gray-Weale AC, Lusby RJ: The role of plaque morphology and diameter reduction in the development of new symptoms in asymptomatic carotid arteries. J Vasc Surg 9:548, 1989
70. Leahy AL, McCollum PT, Feeley TM: Duplex ultrasonography and selection of patients for carotid endarterectomy: plaque morphology or luminal narrowing? J Vasc Surg 8:558, 1988
71. Lennihan L, Kupsky WJ, Mohr JP et al: Lack of association between carotid plaque hematoma and ischemic cerebral symptoms. Stroke 18:879, 1987
72. Lennihan L, Petty GW, Mohr JP et al: Transcranial Doppler detection of anterior cerebral artery vasospasm. Stroke 20:151, 1989
73. Lindegaard K-F, Bakke SJ, Aaslid R, Nornes H: Doppler diagnosis of intracranial arterial occlusive disorders. J Neurol Neurosurg Psychiatry 49:510, 1986
74. Lindegaard K-F, Bakke SJ, Grolimund P et al: Assessment of intracranial hemodynamics in carotid artery disease by transcranial Doppler ultrasound. J Neurosurg 63:890, 1985
75. Lindegaard KF, Grolimund P, Aaslid R, Nornes H: Evaluation of cerebral AVM's using transcranial Doppler ultrasound. J Neurosurg 65:335, 1986
76. LoGerfo FW, Nowak MD, Quist WC: Structural details of boundary layer separation in a model human carotid bifurcation under steady and pulsatile flow conditions. J Vasc Surg 2:263, 1985
77. Mattle H, Grolimund P, Huber P et al: Transcranial Doppler sonographic findings in middle cerebral artery disease. Arch Neurol 45:289, 1988
78. Melis-Kisman E, Mol JMF: L'application de l'effet Doppler a l'exploration cérébro-vasculaire—rapport préliminaire. Rev neurol 122:470, 1970
79. Merritt CRB: Doppler color flow imaging. J Clin Ultrasound 15:591, 1987
80. Middleton WD, Foley WD, Lawson TL: Color-flow Doppler imaging of carotid artery abnormalities. AJR 150:419, 1988
81. Middleton WD, Foley WD, Lawson TL: Flow reversal in the normal carotid bifurcation: color Doppler flow imaging analysis. Radiology 167:207, 1988
82. Mitchell DG: Color Doppler imaging: principles, limitations, and artifacts. Radiology 177:1, 1990
83. Mohr JP, Duterte DI, Oliveira VR et al: Recanalization of acute middle cerebral artery occlusion. Neurology (NY) 38:215, 1988
84. Mokri B, Sundt TM, Houser OW et al: Spontaneous dissection of the cervical internal carotid artery. Ann Neurol 19:126, 1986
85. Motomiya M, Karino T: Flow patterns in the human carotid artery bifurcation. Stroke 15:50, 1984
86. Mull M, Aulich A, Hennerici M: Transcranial Doppler ultrasonography versus arteriography for assessment of the vertebrobasilar circulation. J Clin Ultrasound 18:539, 1990
87. Nicholls SC, Phillips DJ, Primozich JF et al: Diagnostic significance of flow separation in the carotid bulb. Stroke 20:175, 1989
88. O'Donnell TF, Erdoes L, Mackey WC et al: Correlation of B-mode ultrasound imaging and arteriography with pathologic findings at carotid endarterectomy. Arch Surg 120:443, 1985
89. O'Leary DH, Bryan FA, Goodison MW et al: Measurement variability of carotid atherosclerosis: real-time (B-mode) ultrasonography and angiography. Stroke 18:1011, 1987
90. Petty GW, Massaro AR, Tatemichi TK et al: Transcranial Doppler ultrasonographic changes after treatment for arteriovenous malformations. Stroke 21:260, 1990
91. Petty GW, Mohr JP, Pedley TA et al: The role of transcranial Doppler in confirming brain death: sensitivity, specificity and suggestions for performance and interpretation. Neurology 40:300, 1990
92. Polak JF, Dobkin GR, O'Leary DH et al: Internal carotid artery stenosis: accuracy and reproducibility of color-Doppler-assisted duplex imaging. Radiology 173:793, 1989
93. Polak JF, O'Leary DH, Quist WC et al: Pulsed and color Doppler analysis of normal carotid bifurcation flow dynamics using an in-vitro model. Angiology 41:241, 1990
94. Rautenberg W, Aulich A, Hennerici M: Dolichoectatic intracranial arteries and cerebrovascular events. Stroke 21:I34, 1990
95. Rautenberg W, Hennerici M: Pulsed Doppler assessment of innominate artery obstructive disease. Stroke 19:1514, 1988
96. Rautenberg W, Hennerici M: Intracranial hemodynamic measurements in patients with severe asymptomatic extracranial carotid disease. Cerebrovasc Dis 1:216, 1991
97. Rautenberg W, Schwartz A, Mull M et al: Noninvasive detection of intracranial stenoses and occlusions. Stroke 21:I49, 1990
98. Reilly LM, Lusby RJ, Hughes L et al: Carotid plaque histology using real-time ultrasonography. Am J Surg 146:188, 1983
99. Reneman RS, van Merode T, Hick P et al: Flow velocity patterns in and distensibility of the carotid artery bulb in subjects of various ages. Circulation 71:500, 1985
100. Reneman RS, van Merode T, Hick P, Hoeks APG: Cardiovascular applications of multi-gate pulsed Doppler systems. Ultrasound Med Biol 12:370, 1985
101. Ricotta JJ, Bryan FA, Bond MG et al: Multicenter validation study of real-time (B-model) ultrasound, arteriography, and pathologic examination. J Vasc Surg 6:512, 1987
102. Ringelstein EB, Sievers C, Ecker S et al: Noninvasive assessment of $CO_2$ induced cerebral vasomotor response in normal individuals and patients with internal carotid artery occlusions. Stroke 19:963, 1988

103. Robinson ML, Sacks D, Perlmutter GS et al: Diagnostic criteria for carotid duplex sonography. AJR 151:1045, 1988
104. Roederer GO, Langlois YE, Jager KA et al: The natural history of carotid arterial disease in asymptomatic patients with cervical bruits. Stroke 15:605, 1984
105. Roether J, Wentz KU, Rautenberg W et al: Preliminary results of MR-angiography in vertebrobasilar infarction. J Neurol 238, 124, 1991
106. Schenk EA, Bond MG, Aretz TH et al: Multicenter validation study of real-time ultrasonography, arteriography, and pathology: pathologic evaluation of carotid endarterectomy specimens. Stroke 19:289, 1988
107. Schmid-Schönbein H, Wurzinger J: Vortex transport phenomena of the carotid bifurcation: interaction between fluid-dynamic transport phenomena and hemostatic reactions. p. 64. In Hennerici M, Sitzer G, Weger HD (eds): Carotid Artery Plaques. Karger, Basel, 1988
108. Schneider PA, Rossman ME, Bernstein EF et al: Noninvasive assessment of cerebral collateral blood supply through the ophthalmic artery. Stroke 22:31, 1991
109. Schneider PA, Rossman ME, Torem S et al: Transcranial Doppler in the management of extracranial cerebrovascular disease: implications in diagnosis and monitoring. J Vasc Surg 7:223, 1988
110. Schwartz A, Hennerici M: Non-invasive transcranial Doppler ultrasound in intracranial angiomas. Neurology (NY) 36:626, 1986
111. Seiler RW, Grolimund P, Aaslid R et al: Cerebral vasospasm evaluated by transcranial ultrasound correlated with clinical grade and CT-visualized subarachnoid hemorrhage. J Neurosurg 64:594, 1986
112. Shulak JM, O'Donovan PB, Paushter DM et al: Color flow Doppler of carotid body paraganglioma. J Ultrasound Med 8:519, 1989
113. Spencer M, Reid JM: Quantitation of carotid stenosis with continuous-wave (CW) Doppler ultrasound. Stroke 10:326, 1979
114. Spencer MP, Thomas GI, Nicholls SC, Sauvage LR: Detection of middle cerebral artery emboli during carotid endarterectomy using transcranial Doppler ultrasonography. Stroke 21:415, 1990
115. Spencer MP, Whisler D: Transorbital Doppler diagnosis of intracranial arterial stenosis. Stroke 17:916, 1986
116. Steinke W, Hennerici M: Three-dimensional ultrasound imaging of carotid artery plaques. J Cardiovasc Technol 8:15, 1989
117. Steinke W, Hennerici M, Aulich A: Doppler color flow imaging of carotid body tumors. Stroke 20:1574, 1989
118. Steinke W, Kloetzsch C, Hennerici M: Carotid artery disease assessed by color Doppler flow imaging. AJNR 11:259, 1990
119. Steinke W, Kloetzsch C, Hennerici M: Variability of flow patterns in the normal carotid bifurcation. Atherosclerosis 84:121, 1990
120. Steinke W, Schwartz A, Hennerici M: Doppler color flow imaging of common carotid artery dissection. Neuroradiology 32:502, 1990
121. Sterpetti AV, Schultz RD, Feldhaus RJ et al: Ultrasonographic features of carotid plaque and the risk of subsequent neurologic deficits. Surgery 104:652, 1988
122. Strandness DE: Ultrasound in the study of the atherosclerosis. Ultrasound Med Biol 12:453, 1986
123. Tatemichi TK, Chamorro A, Petty GW et al: Hemodynamic role of ophthalmic artery collateral in internal carotid artery occlusion. Neurology (NY) 40:461, 1990
124. Tatemichi TK, Oropeza LA, Sacco RL et al: Doppler diagnosis of vertebral artery occlusion: role of runoff into the posterior inferior cerebellar artery. Ann Neurol 26:158, 1989
125. Taylor LM, Loboa L, Porter JM: The clinical course of carotid bifurcation stenosis as determined by duplex scanning. J Vasc Surg 8:255, 1988
126. Touboul PJ, Bousser MG, LaPlane D et al: Duplex scanning of normal vertebral arteries. Stroke 71:921, 1986
127. Trattnig S, Hübsch P, Schuster H et al: Color-coded Doppler imaging of normal vertebral arteries. Stroke 21:1222, 1990
128. Trockel U, Hennerici M, Aulich A, Sandmann W: The superiority of combined continuous wave Doppler examination over periorbital Doppler for the detection of extracranial carotid disease. J Neurol Neurosurg Psychiatry 47:43, 1984
129. Tuteur P, Reivich M, Goldberg HI et al: Transient responses of cerebral blood flow and ventilation to changes in $PA_{CO_2}$ in normal subjects and patients with cerebrovascular disease. Stroke 7:584, 1976
130. von Reutern G-M, Büdingen HJ: Ultraschalldiagnostik der hirnversorgenden Arterien. Thieme, Stuttgart, 1989
131. von Reutern G-M, Pourcelot L: Cardiac-cycle dependent alternating flow in vertebral arteries with subclavian artery stenosis. Stroke 9:229, 1978
132. Widder B, Paulat K, Hackspacher J, Mayr E: Transcranial Doppler $CO_2$-test for the detection of hemodynamically critical carotid artery stenoses and occlusions. Eur Arch Psychiatr Neurol Sci 236:162, 1986
133. Wilkinson DL, Polak JF, Grassi CJ et al: Pseudoaneurysm of the vertebral artery: appearance on color-flow Doppler sonography. AJR 151:1051, 1988
134. Wolverson MK, Bashiti HM, Peterson GJ: Ultrasonic tissue characterization of atheromatous plaques using a high resolution real time scanner. Ultrasound Med Biol 9:599, 1983
135. Wolverson MK, Heiberg E, Sundaram M et al: Carotid atherosclerosis: high-resolution real-time sonography correlated with angiography. AJR 140:355, 1983
136. Zbornikova V, Lassvik C, Johansson I: Prospective evaluation of the accuracy of duplex scanning with spectral analysis in carotid artery disease. Clin Physiol 5:257, 1985

137. Zierler RE, Phillips DJ, Beach KW et al: Noninvasive assessment of normal carotid bifurcation hemodynamics with color-flow ultrasound imaging. Ultrasound Med Biol 13:471, 1987
138. Zirkle PK, Wheeler JR, Gregory RT et al: Carotid involvement in aortic dissection diagnosed by duplex scanning. J Vasc Surg 1:700, 1984
139. Zwiebel WJ, Austin CW, Sackett JF et al: Correlation of high-resolution, B-mode and continuous-wave Doppler sonography with arteriography in the diagnosis of carotid stenosis. Radiology 149:523, 1983
140. Zwiebel WJ, Knighton R: Duplex examination of the carotid arteries. Semin Ultrasound CT MRI 11:97, 1990

# III

# *CLINICAL MANIFESTATIONS OF STROKE*

## J.P. Mohr, Section Editor

This section covers the major syndromes of stroke. The overview focuses on the issues involved in differential diagnosis and the use of the laboratory in the application of new research on various subtypes of stroke, including the contentious category of cryptogenic stroke, also known as stroke of undetermined cause.

Because syndromes caused by thrombosis or embolism often mimic one another, these syndromes have been described in detail for each major arterial territory. Those for the extracranial and intracranial carotid arteries have now been combined in one chapter.

Parenchymatous hemorrhage, which was the subject of three chapters in the first edition, is now covered in one chapter. Advances in the diagnosis of cavernous angiomas is documented in the chapters on hemorrhage, arteriovenous malformation, and magnetic resonance imaging. Rapidly developing improvements in interventional radiology have enlarged the field to the extent that this subject now warrants a separate chapter, which in this edition appears as Chapter 49 in the section on Stroke Therapy.

# 13
# CLASSIFICATION OF ISCHEMIC STROKES

J.P. Mohr
R.L. Sacco

The diagnostic accuracy of the classification of ischemic stroke has rapidly evolved with the advancement of technologies to image the brain and blood vessels. Prior determination of infarct subtype were based chiefly on clinical grounds with heavy reliance on clinical syndrome, neurologic examination, and coexisting risk factors. In the unfortunate patient who died, autopsy confirmation was often the basis of the classification. With the widespread application of computed tomography (CT), magnetic resonance imaging (MRI), duplex and transcranial Doppler, single photon emission computed tomography (SPECT), and other diagnostic studies, the clinical impressions have been refined and supported by laboratory confirmation of the infarct subtype.

## FORMS OF INFARCTION

When perfusion pressure falls to critical levels, ischemia develops, progressing to infarction if the effect persists long enough. Ischemic infarction is pathologically divided into bland or hemorrhagic infarction.

When the cause is thrombus, the usual occlusion persists, preventing reperfusion of the infarcted region, resulting in pale, anemic, or *bland infarction*.[3] In regions exposed to circulating blood, such as the edge of a bland infarct, widespread leukocyte infiltration occurs within days. For periods up to several weeks, macrophages invade the infarct and are active for some months until all the products of infarction are carried off. Only scattered red cells are found.

In contrast to the bland form, another type is known as *hemorrhagic infarction*.[9,54] In this variety, varying amounts of red blood cells are found among the necrotic tissues. In some cases, the concentration of red cells is enough to make a high-density appearance consistent with blood on CT or MRI scan, while at autopsy the specimen shows hemorrhagic foci ranging from a few petechiae scattered through the infarct to a mass of confluent petechial foci having almost the appearance of frank hematoma. The timing of hemorrhagic infarction varies widely, as early as a few hours to as late as 2 weeks or longer after an arterial occlusion.

Hemorrhagic infarction has long been explained as a result of reperfusion of the vascular bed of the infarct following relief of the occlusion, such as would occur after fragmentation and distal migration of an embolus[47] or after early reopening of a large vessel occlusion in the setting of an established large infarction.[31,111] Presumably, the full pressure of arterial blood into hypoxic capillaries results in a diapedesis of red cells through their hypoxic walls. The more intense the reperfusion and the more severely damaged the capillary walls, the more confluent the hemorrhagic infarction.

Assuming hemorrhagic infarction reflects restored lumen patency, it should be a consequence of embolization from recanalization or thrombolysis, since the occlusion from thrombus would not be expected to be relieved. This is consistent with greater frequency of hemorrhagic infarction among cardioembolic infarcts.[9,11] Yet in a few cases hemorrhagic infarction develops *distal* to the site of persisting occlusion, that is, in the arterial bed exposed at best only to retrograde collaterals.[86,90] The occurrence of such cases suggests that the process may be related more to the suddenness or severity of the infarction or to surges in arterial blood pressure, rather than to the process of reperfusion per se.[9,90]

## PROBLEMS IN CLINICAL AND LABORATORY DIAGNOSIS OF INFARCTION

Before modern neuroimaging was routinely available, it was the persistent conviction of many neurologists that a definite diagnosis as to stroke mechanism was merely a technical problem awaiting the proper laboratory procedures. For the diagnosis of parenchymatous hemorrhage, especially in the acute phase within days of onset, the development of the CT scan allowed for the definitive distinction between the two. For ischemic stroke, the use of CT scan, MRI, noninvasive vascular imaging and angiography has greatly improved the ability to diagnose stroke, but has still left large areas unresolved.

In most circumstances the clinical features and laboratory data suffice to differentiate acute intracerebral hemorrhage from infarction. Scores that have been developed to help differentiate infarct from hemorrhage when CT is not available, or to help with early mobilization of stroke clinical trial staff, rely on decreased consciousness, headache, and nausea and vomiting as predictors of hemorrhage.[80,91,108,113,121] Small, deep, or lobar hematomas, leading to the presentation of circumscribed focal deficits, can easily mislead those relying on the clinical syndrome alone to mistakenly diagnose infarction. The advent of CT has led to the correction of these misdiagnoses and has resulted in a greater proportion of hemorrhages in stroke series and elimination of the inadvertent use of anticoagulation in the case of a masquerading hemorrhage.[36]

Classification of the ischemic stroke into subtype can now be done well enough to justify the management decisions, but is far from precise. Clinical grounds alone, using age, risk factors, and so on, have been the time-honored means of determining the subtype of infarction, such as separating embolism from thrombosis. Yet, it is often difficult to classify patients into different mechanisms of cerebral infarction solely based on clinical criteria. A thorough diagnostic workup is required, as the presenting clinical syndromes are not often distinctive enough to permit an inference as to the cause of infarction. Even when strenuous efforts are made toward establishing the exact mechanism of infarction, the problem remains difficult. The duplex Doppler, MR angiogram, or conventional angiogram often fail to show either the expected arterial stenosis or occlusion, and the acute findings on the brain image serve only to rule out acute hemorrhage. Even when a significant carotid stenosis is found, judging whether the clinical syndrome arose from an embolic or a hemodynamic mechanism is often difficult.[95] The traditional terms used to classify strokes have had to be supplemented by new ones designed to accommodate the clinically inobvious subtypes of stroke.

Few studies have collected detailed information on the clinical and radiologic characteristics of large homogeneous subsets of patients with acute cerebral infarction. The Stroke Data Bank provided a large collection of prospectively collected information on patients with different subtypes of infarction.[52] A deliberate attempt was made to classify patients into distinct categories and to create new subsets based on presumed mechanism of infarction. This effort resulted in some changes in the large categories of stroke due to infarction. In particular, the group often

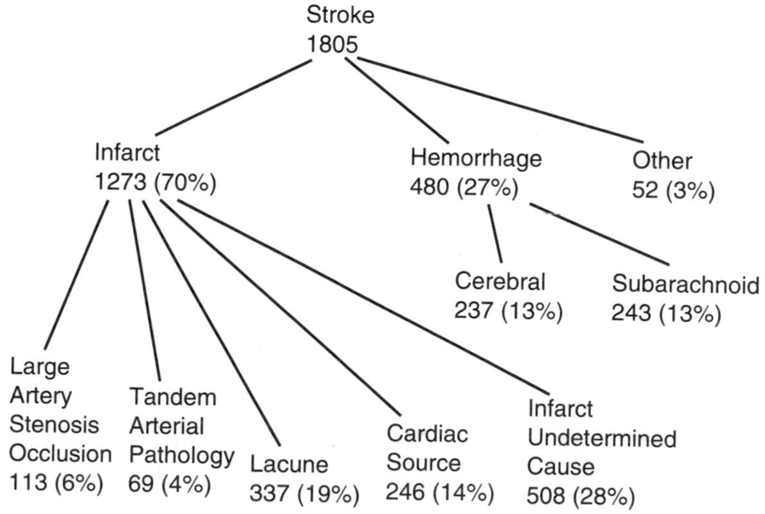


**Fig. 13-1.** Classification of stroke based on data from the NINDS Stroke Data Bank (1983–1986).

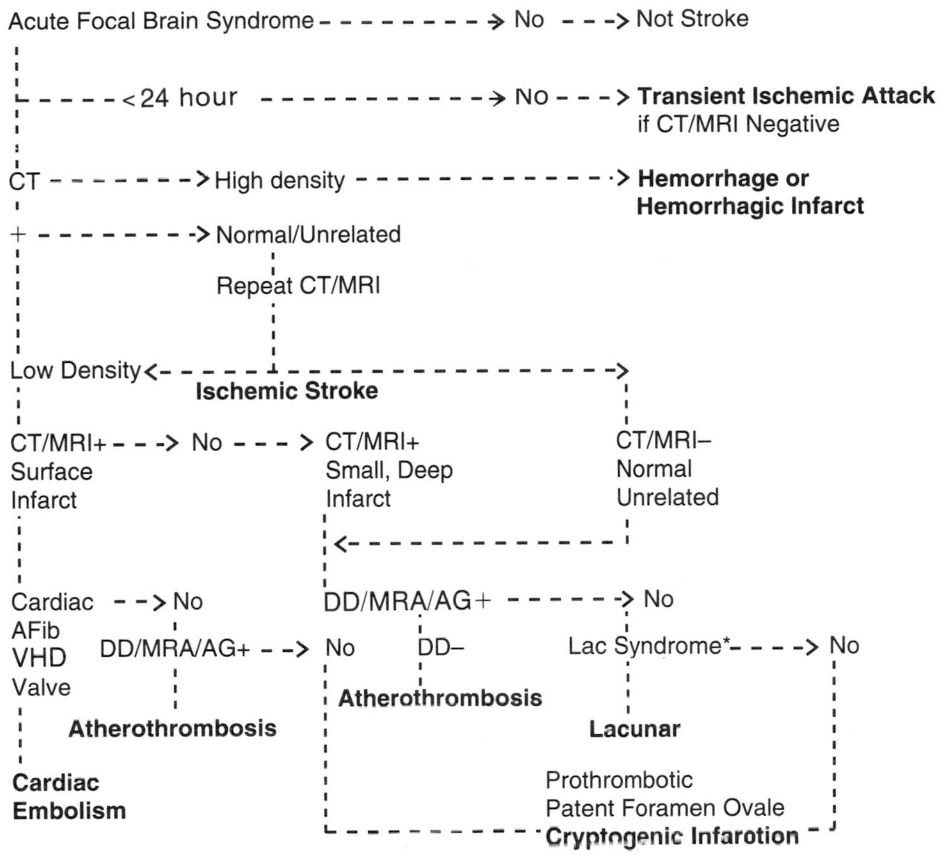


**Fig. 13-2.** Stroke diagnostic algorithm. DD, duplex and transcranial Doppler; MRA, magnetic resonance angiography; AG, cerebral angiogram; CT, computed tomography; MRI, magnetic resonance imaging; *lac syndrome, currently described classic lacunar syndromes, possibly including other syndromes from focal-deep infarction (i.e., cognitive changes from thalamic or caudate infarcts); AFib, atrial fibrillation; MI, myocardal infarction; VHD, valvular heart disease.

labeled as atherothrombosis was divided into two subgroups: large-artery thrombosis with no evidence of embolic infarction and a form of artery-to-artery embolism arising from an atherosclerotic source. A separate category, infarct of undetermined cause, was created to help ensure the homogeneity of the Stroke Data Bank diagnostic groups (Fig. 13-1).

Efforts to establish the diagnosis for the subtype of infarction proved remarkably difficult in a disappointingly high percentage of cases.[105] Despite efforts to arrive at the diagnosis by CT scan or angiogram, it was apparent that the basis for the diagnosis in many of the cases was still a "best clinical guess." Where laboratory data were available, the results indicated that large-artery atherosclerotic occlusive disease was a less frequent cause of stroke, small-vessel or lacunar and cardioembolic infarction were relatively frequent, and the cause for the majority of the cases of infarction could not be classified into these traditional diagnostic categories. The large frequency of surface infarcts in the setting of a normal or distal branch arterial occlusion led most to consider these unexplained cerebral infarcts as examples of embolism where the thrombotic source was undetected. Our findings have forced the creation of a separate diagnostic category for cases whose mechanisms of infarction remain unproven, one known as "infarct of undetermined cause" or "cryptogenic infarction." Apart from a few features they share in common, this category of infarction remains poorly understood and, as yet, has not been successfully characterized as a clinical group (Fig. 13-2).

## SUBTYPES OF ISCHEMIC STROKE

### Infarct with Large-Artery Thrombosis

In review of earlier studies, it appears that thrombosis was a diagnosis of exclusion. In the days of less sophisticated laboratory investigations, the classification of a stroke into one of three major diagnostic categories was as follows: hemorrhage if the spinal fluid were bloody, embolism if atrial fibrillation or rheumatic heart disease were present, and thrombosis if the foregoing were not present. The gradual decline in large-artery thrombosis as a leading diagnosis has resulted from several factors. Leading among them are (1) the more frequent use of duplex and transcranial Doppler in the pursuit of stroke diagnosis, (2) the recognition of several clinical subtypes of thrombosis, especially lacunes,[5,26,84], (3) the documentation that some ischemic strokes associated with large-artery atherothrombosis are produced by artery-to-artery embolism (local embolism),[39,50,64,81] and (4) the discontinuation of the casual classification of a stroke as atherothrombotic in favor of the additional category of an "undetermined" cause.[13,56,71,85,105] Syndromes previously attributed to large-artery atherosclerosis, when more closely evaluated with current technology, have been reclassified.

## Etiology and Mechanism

Many of the descriptions leading to the definition of this subtype stem from the pathologic studies of the past.[4] Atherosclerotic lesions were found at bifurcations and curves of the larger vessels, the more proximal the location in the vascular tree the more severe the atherosclerotic lesions.[49,107] Primary occlusion of the arteries distally located over the cerebral surface was rare.[42,83] Atherosclerotic plaque usually led to progressive stenosis with the final large-artery occlusion due to thrombosis of the narrowed lumen. Intraplaque hemorrhage sometimes led to accelerated occlusion,[89] although the frequency of this is more often a matter of speculation than it is found in pathologic specimens.[73]

The mechanism for stroke in atherothrombus was initially attributed to perfusion failure distal to the site of severe stenosis or occlusion of the major vessel.[12,63,83] In some instances, the major vessel occlusion was rather proximal in the arterial tree, and some degree of collateral flow was interposed between the occlusion and the cerebral territory at risk for infarction.[92,94] Some cases with interposed collateral were spared infarction of any kind, while in others the infarct was located mainly along the most distal brain regions originally supplied by the occluded vessel.[63,83,100,102,119] In the carotid territory, these regions were the suprasylvian frontal, central, and parietal portions of the hemisphere, while in the vertebrobasilar territory, they were the bilateral occipital pole. More recent studies based on positron emission tomography (PET) have not found supportive evidence for selective hemodynamic impairment among patients with transient ischemic attacks (TIAs) with severe carotid stenosis, but the development of borderzone ischemia is probably dependent on multiple factors, not just the degree of stenosis.[20,95,96]

## Clinical Features

Focal cortical syndromes are usually found in this group, but syndromes often attributed to lacunar disease, such as pure motor or sensorimotor stroke, can easily represent the first sign of impending flow failure. Discriminating between infarct subtypes on clinical grounds alone is difficult. In order to determine some of these distinguishing clinical features in the Stroke Data Bank, demographic, stroke risk factors and clinical and radiologic features were compared between the 246 cardioembolic and 113 large-vessel atherosclerotic cerebral infarcts.[117] Stroke Data Bank definitions ensured more transient ischemic attacks in atherosclerotic infarcts and more cardiac disease in cardioembolic infarcts, but the diagnosis was distinguished further. Patients with fractional arm weakness (shoulder different from the hand), hypertension, diabetes, and male gender occurred more frequently in atherosclerotic than cardioembolic infarcts. Atherosclerotic infarcts were more likely to have a fractional arm weakness regardless of infarct size. Clinical features that are observed at stroke onset can help distinguish cerebral infarction subtypes, but are not reliable enough to lead to a definite determination of infarct subtype without confirmatory laboratory data.

## Laboratory Features

In the clinical setting, for a diagnosis of large-artery atherosclerotic occlusive disease, the cerebral angiogram remains the most reliable laboratory test. The occlusion of the internal carotid at its origin or in the siphon has the appearance of a pencil point, blunt end, smooth end, or shoulder, with the intracranial portion of the internal carotid or major cerebral artery stems and branches open.[92] More recently, because of the risks of cerebral angiography,[34,57,74] there has been increased reliance on the duplex and transcranial Doppler to show no or high resistant flow in the extracranial carotid with damped pulsatility in the ipsilateral middle cerebral artery.[18,33,55,115,124,126] MR angiography is quickly becoming a reliable diagnostic tool for the detection of extracranial and intracranial large-artery stenosis and may lead to less reliance on conventional angiography in the future.[79] The usually accepted mechanism of perfusion failure is more readily accepted in occlusive disease, but becomes more difficult to define when, instead, the extracranial vessel is patent, but highly stenotic. Specifying the degree of stenosis that will lead to perfusion difficulty is dependent on multiple factors and is often not distinguishable.[70,95,119,120] Spiral occlusions of the extracranial portion of the internal carotid beyond 2 cm of its origin (a finding consistent with dissection[97]) helps indicate that the carotid lesion may be the source of the stroke, but not by means of perfusion failure.

Intracranial atherosclerotic artery stem stenoses or occlusions may be due to arteriosclerotic thrombosis, but is often difficult to distinguish from an embolism from any extracerebral source.[22,23,120] If one or more appropriate TIAs occurred within the past 30 days, the diagnosis of thrombus may be correct, but the matter can only be settled if a widely patent lumen is subsequently found by serial transcranial Doppler or repeat angiogram.[30] The latter is diagnostic of embolism, while persistence of the occlusion leaves the mechanism unsettled.

Basilar occlusion on angiogram is usually considered the mechanism for brain stem stroke, even though in many such cases the clinical syndrome fits the criteria for lacune,[15,16,21,24] since the territory of infarction, however small, is in the field of supply of a vessel thrombosed by the major basilar atheroma.[45] Similar to the case of the carotid, the finding of stenosis of the basilar prevents a definite diagnosis as to the mechanism of infarction, since infarcts more distal in the vertebrobasilar territory might well be the result of distal embolization.[22] Atheromatous disease of the basilar often affects the vessel at sites where local branches directly supply brain tissue.[17,45,48] In the case of the carotid, the atheroma involves the vessel proximal to the point where its branches supply the brain.[107] In cases where the clinical syndrome of basilar stroke can be localized to the point of the stenosis, infarction may be caused by mural atheroma that only slightly stenoses the basilar, but which totally occludes a small penetrator departing from the basilar at that point. This point, established in a few instances by autopsy, can only be inferred in cases studied by angiogram; CT scanning is usually not of technically high enough quality to detect the small brain stem infarcts. However, MRI scanning has defined the lesion and permitted better delineation of such cases.[68]

The only abnormalities on MRI or CT scan directly attributable to cerebral infarction in the carotid artery territory are abnormalities that can be interpreted to reflect the "distal field" effect along the border-zone between middle and anterior cerebral territories, especially on the middle cerebral side.[12,83,101] This topographic pattern involves the suprasylvian frontal and central regions, shading toward normal in the parieto-occipital region, sparing the region of the sylvian fissure (operculum, insula) and the penetrating territories of the lenticulostriates. The centripetal spread in more severe cases may involve so much of the hemisphere that a differentiation from embolism to the middle cerebral artery stem is impossible. Occlusions involving the territories of the anterior, middle, or posterior cerebral, or basilar artery territory are not distinguishable by brain image between thrombosis and embolism if the scan shows low density only in the proximal fields of the arterial territory. In all cases, any high-density component that suggests hemorrhagic infarction would favor a diagnosis of embolism.

Newer blood flow techniques have also helped confirm the perfusion failure mechanism in cases with atherosclerotic stenosis or occlusive disease through SPECT,[59] xenon CT,[66] regional cerebral blood flow,[88] MRI,[37] and PET.[7,95,110] The more widespread use of these techniques should allow for more accurate distinction between embolism and perfusion failure in the clinical setting.

### Infarct with Tandem Arterial Pathology

In addition to vascular occlusion at the site of atherosclerosis, infarcts are also produced by emboli arising from the proximally situated atheromatous lesions to otherwise healthy branches located more distal in the arterial tree.[50] Nowadays, embolism from a carotid source has become recognized as another, perhaps more common, cause of stroke in a setting of arterial stenosis.[39,64] This mechanism of infarction cuts across most attempts to distinguish thrombus from embolus, and it has earned its own category: tandem arterial pathology.

Embolic fragments may arise from extracranial arteries affected by stenosis or ulcer,[8,28,125] from stenosis of any major cerebral artery stem[1,81] or the basilar artery,[24] from the stump of the occluded internal carotid artery,[6] and even from the intracranial tail of the anterograde thrombus atop an occluded carotid.[103] The frequency of occurrence of embolism of particles large enough to cause stroke and the variety or severity of carotid lesions giving rise to such embolization remain unknown. A variety of mechanisms account for the intracranial stenoses.[78] Embolism from carotid artery dissection[97] is often delayed many days after onset.

## Clinical and Laboratory Features

No satisfactory criteria have yet been developed to certify that a stroke is caused by extracranial arterial disease through the mechanism of embolism. The mechanism is inferred when the clinical syndrome suggests a cortical branch territory, there is no obvious cardioembolic source and the degree of stenosis is less than 80 percent, insufficient to explain the stroke on the grounds of hemodynamic insufficiency, or there is ulcerative plaque imaged by noninvasive duplex Doppler, MR angiography, or cerebral angiogram. The sudden mode of onset usually suggests a diagnosis of embolism. CT and MRI scans are of help only in supporting a diagnosis of embolism, not in inferring its source from the neck. Angiographic evidence of branch occlusion above a carotid stenosis or ulcer is not proof of the source but, when present, serves to classify this type of stroke into the present category.[94]

Comparisons in the NINDS Stroke Data Bank between the 246 cardioembolic and 66 arterial embolic patients with cerebral infarction demonstrated some differences.[117] Even after controlling for differences in the frequency of cardiac disease, transient ischemic attacks, and carotid bruits, the probability of an artery-to-artery embolism was increased by the finding of a superficial infarct alone or by a higher hematocrit. The probability of cardiac embolism was greater with an initial decreased consciousness or with an abnormal first CT. These findings suggested that these two embolic infarct subtypes differed in the location and extent of the cortical infarction. Smaller and more distal infarction in embolism from an arterial source, compared with cardiogenic embolism, suggested a smaller embolic particle size.

## Embolism Attributed to Cardiac or Transcardiac Source

As a cause of stroke, embolism accounts for between 15 and 30 percent of cases,[13,52,71,85] most of which occur from embolism into the territory of the middle cerebral artery. Although the subject of embolism would seem clear enough, in that a particle is swept through the bloodstream until it jams in an artery too small to allow it to pass, the many complexities of the embolic process make it anything but easy to account for on a case by case basis.

The biggest problem is identification of the sources. Given the many possibilities, and given the traditional use of the term "embolism" to refer to a cardiac source,[25,60,76,109] the following discussion is limited to that subject. Embolism was diagnosed in earlier studies mainly when a cardiac source (atrial fibrillation with valvular disease) was obvious.[4] However, the results of more recent studies have shown that emboli, diagnosed angiographically by isolated branch occlusions, may occur despite all efforts to identify the source.[19,85,105]

## Properties of Emboli

The stability of the material is a point of prime importance in clinical and angiographic analysis of cases of embolism. Mural thrombi and platelet aggregates are the most frequent materials embolized to brain. This material is remarkably evanescent, as has been inferred repeatedly by findings on angiogram. Embolic fragments are found in over 75 percent of cases angiogrammed within 48 hours of onset of the stroke, and are then gone when angiogram is repeated later.[14,41,85,112] Embolism is demonstrated in only 11 percent of clinically identical cases when angiogram is delayed beyond 48 hours from clinical onset of the stroke. Persistence of embolic occlusion is the exception rather than the rule. Although it is inferred that the more friable materials will disperse rapidly, no reliable means have been developed thus far to predict which embolic occlusions will persist and which will disappear. Persistence of the occlusion seems to carry a worse functional prognosis.[71]

This evanescant quality of the material may explain the wide variation in the frequency with which embolism is diagnosed in retrospective or prospective studies of stroke. The size of the material embolized determines the site it initially arrests in the circulation, but it does not determine its final point of arrest. Embolic material arrests where the lumen diameter is too small to permit the material to pass. Bifurcations or foci of atheroma at curves in the artery are the two sites where emboli arrest.[2]

Fibrin-platelet complexes and those also laden with bacteria vary considerably in size, some so huge that they have obstructed the stem of the middle cerebral artery,[53] and others have been so small they have lodged asymptomatically in a sensitive region like the rolandic artery (seen in one of our own cases). Calcific plaques have only rarely been described as producing large embolic strokes;[28,125] more often, they seem to produce transient ischemic attacks but not persisting cerebral deficits.[8] For noncompressible objects such as shotgun pellets, the site of embolus can easily be predicted by its size.[67] For the more common fibrin-platelet complexes, however, other factors are involved, especially the poorly understood compressibility of the mass and the time required to transit a certain point of narrowing in the arterial tree. The few cases that document the passage of fibrin-platelet emboli through the arterial tree[77] show considerable alteration in the length and width of the material at different points, indicating it possesses a remarkable elasticity and friability. What is sufficient lumen reduction to arrest the material may not be enough to keep it from changing shape or fragmenting within minutes to hours, leaving the site of the original embolic occlusion widely patent.

Embolic obstruction of an arterial lumen is cleared most commonly by recanalization and fibrinolysis. A column of blood develops between the embolus and the arterial wall, enlarges, and erodes the embolus until the lumen is finally cleared. The exact sequence of the events is not fully understood in human material, but cases documented at different stages during the process make it clear that it is accomplished within periods as short as hours to days.[77,125] The timetable for this process is also poorly understood. In some instances, the erosion takes enough time that noninvasive studies may document stenoses that create turbulence identical to those seen with atheroma. From the angiographic appearance, the gradually eroding embolus is indistinguishable from that found in atherostenosis. During this process, the lumen may appear "stenotic."[65,78]

At the site of occlusion, opportunity exists for thrombus to develop anterogradely throughout the length of the vessel, but this event seems to occur only rarely. Lack of anterograde thrombus implies either that an active flows was proximal to the occlusion or that the occlusion was too short-lived to permit the development of an anterograde thrombus.

At autopsy it is common to find the vessel distended by the embolus. Yet the histologic appearance of the wall at that point usually shows no significant abnormalities. The frequent finding that the vessel wall itself is not significantly injured by the embolus argues against a role for endothelial injury, vasospasm, or necrotizing effects in the pathogenesis of the infarction from embolism.

## Clinical Features

In the past, many syndromes were considered almost specific for embolism, especially pure Wernicke aphasia, isolated hemianopia, and monopareses. In each of these syndromes, it was assumed that the infarct was so focal and so far distal in the arterial tree that local atheroma was not a serious possibility. CT and MRI scanning has shown that any of these syndromes may arise from hematoma, and modern neurologists have become wary of anticoagulation therapy based on clinical syndrome analysis alone.

To these disappointments have been demonstrations that the sudden onset once thought to typify embolism and the non-sudden onset to typify thrombosis may occur in either condition. Non-sudden or fluctuating onset occurs in 5 to 6 percent of documented embolic strokes, the syndrome often requiring 36 hours or so to evolve.[51,85] A clinical diagnosis of multiple transient ischemic attack is often entertained. The reestablishment of flow, presumed further migration of embolic material, and subsequent repeat of these events is thought to be the mechanism involved. Embolic material has even been documented to go to the same site on repeated occasions,[122] the opposite from traditional predictions.

In the Lausanne Stroke Registry, hemianopia without hemiparesis or hemisensory disturbances, Wernicke's aphasia, ideomotor apraxia, and involvement of specific territories (posterior division of middle cerebral artery, anterior cerebral artery, cerebellum, multiple territories) were associated with the presence of a potential cardiac source of embolism.[11]

One syndrome seems to have held its value as a sign of embolism, although it is met only rarely. A spectacular shrinking deficit can occur when the embolus is introduced into the internal carotid, causing a profound full hemisphere syndrome, after which it passes up the internal carotid artery to its final resting place in, say, the angular branch of the middle cerebral artery, leaving only a mild aphasia after a few days or a week.[82] Especially characteristic of the middle cerebral artery migratory embolism is the syndrome of fading hemiparesis with Wernicke's aphasia: the embolus lodges initially at the stem of the middle cerebral artery, occluding the penetrating lenticulostriate branches long enough to produce scattered foci of infarction through the basal ganglia and internal capsule, the involvement of the latter producing the hemiparesis. Distal migration of the embolus then occurs, finally occluding the lower division of the middle cerebral artery at the superior temporal plane and beyond. This infarct yields Wernicke's aphasia. Two separate foci of infarction occur, but both result from the same embolic event.

In the Stroke Data Bank, besides a greater frequency of cardiac disease, patients with cardioembolic infarction more often presented with reduced consciousness.[116,117] Cardioembolic infarcts were more likely to have nonfractional arm weakness, except for those with infarctions less than 20 $cm^3$ where fractional weakness was more frequent. In a separate Stroke Data Bank analysis, history of systemic embolism and an abrupt onset were historical features significantly associated with cardiac sources of embolism.[69] Clinical features observed at stroke onset help distinguish the cardioembolic group from other subtypes, but the diagnosis largely depends on confirmatory laboratory findings suggesting a definite cardiac source of embolism.[98]

## Laboratory Diagnosis

Enough cases and series exist in the literature to preclude simplistic generalizations about the size of the stroke, risk of recurrence, and therapy for embolism of different cause.[25] Unfortunately, the size of the embolic material sufficient to produce a focal stroke is usually small enough to escape detection by echocardiography, and too often eludes all efforts at diagnosis: fully a third or more of such cases fail to show the cause of the embolus despite full use of laboratory investigations.

The role of the CT and MRI scan in the diagnosis of embolism is limited. Only in cases where the infarction is confined to the cerebral surface territory of a single branch can embolism be inferred as the cause. Combinations of infarcts involving branches of different divisions of major cerebral arteries is strongly suggestive that embolism explains at least some of the clinical strokes that have occurred. Embolism is also the leading diagnosis when hemorrhagic infarction is seen on brain image.[9,11] It is inferred by scattered high-density values in the infarct zone. In rare instances, the CT or MRI may show the occlusion itself.[54,79]

A diagnosis of embolism is suggested by a large zone of low density that encompasses what amounts to the entire territory of a major cerebral artery or its main divisions and is larger than one lobe in size. In the presence of a cardiac source, the diagnosis is certain for all practical purposes. Establishing the cardiac source is not always a simple task, but the increasing use of more sensitive cardiac imaging through transthoracic and transesophageal echocardiography has improved the detection of sources of embolism.[27]

Angiography was once considered sufficient to diagnose embolism from any source if the angiogram showed branch occlusion in the absence of other occlusive disease elsewhere.[10,29,30,100] This rule still holds for practical purposes, but isolated branch occlusions may occur in arteritis, and increasing evidence is developing that intracranial atherosclerosis is common enough in some races, especially blacks, that middle cerebral artery stem occlusions may be atheromatous as well as embolic. Recanalizing embolus may mimic all the angiographic features of atherosclerosis.[65] Only when the angiogram is repeated within days of the one demonstrating occlusion, and the initial occlusion is gone, can a diagnosis of embolism be made with confidence. Measures this extreme are impractical for the management of most patients.

## Lacunar Infarction

The special group of cases called lacunar infarction warrant description because they occur as a common set of clinical syndromes, the angiogram is often negative, and the zone of ischemia is confined to the territory of a single vessel, usually quite small. They are understood to reflect arterial disease of the vessels penetrating the brain to supply the capsule, basal ganglia, thalamus, and paramedian regions of the brain stem.[43] Only a handful have been studied by autopsy technique, and an even smaller number have been subjected to serial section to document the lesion.[44] The most frequent such lesion is a tiny focus of microatheroma or lipohyalinosis stenosing one of the deep penetrating arteries. Rare causes include stenosis of the middle cerebral artery stem[3,61] or microembolization to penetrate arterial territories.[44] Lacunes were slow to gain clinical acceptance, but they are now considered to account for between 15 and 20 percent of all cases of stroke.[5,13,52,56,71]

### Clinical Features

Many lacunar strokes are diagnosed by clinical characteristics alone, a practice that has contributed little to their popularity among clinical researchers in the field. The characteristic features of all of these syndromes is their relative purity and their failure to involve higher cerebral functions such as language, praxis, behavior controlled by the nondominant hemisphere, memory, and vision.[87] Efforts to expand the diagnosis into new formulas have shaken the earlier purity of the syndromes,[46] but have both opened up new opportunities for research and confounded the appealing simplicity of the initial syndromes.

### Laboratory Features

CT scanning is positive only for roughly half of even the most common form of lacune, pure motor stroke.[26,84,99] MRI has increased the yield of finding a strategically placed small, deep infarct.[62] The probability that CT or MRI will be positive is roughly a function of the severity of the deficit. The larger deep infarcts, some of which have been called "superlacunes" or "giant lacunes" may be seen by CT or MRI scan as a focal, deep site of infarction without involvement of the cerebral surface.[99] A problem arises in the interpretation of these deep lesions, since an embolus may arrest itself initially in the stem of the middle cerebral artery, causing a large swath of infarction scattered through the lenticulostriate territories. When accompanied by a separate cerebral surface low density, such large, deep infarcts are easily reclassified as examples of embolism, nonthrombotic infarction, or infarction of other cause.

Positive scans in the capsule, adjacent corona radiata, thalamus, or pons have been reported on occasion for the ataxic-hemiparesis, dysarthria-clumsy hand syndrome, and hemiballism.[26,114] Pure sensory strokes have been reported from small thalamic infarcts, some so small as to cause selective proprioceptive loss without pain or temperature deficits.[104] Reports of pure sensory stroke from low densities in the centrum semiovale are probably lacunar, although rarely surface infarction has been demonstrated.[32]

Because the vascular lesion lies in vessels some 200 to 400 $\mu$m in diameter, it is perhaps no surprise the angiogram is normal. Incidental large-vessel disease may be found in some series, but whether etiologically related to the site of infarction is often unclear.[26] Normal angiogram could also be expected if microembolism was the cause of the deep infarction. Whether the outlook for stenosis of the middle cerebral artery stem or the basilar artery differs if the syndrome is lacunar or not remains unsettled.

Because some of the cases of pure motor stroke have been associated with middle cerebral artery stenosis, the mere presence of such a syndrome has not been an indicator of the status of the major artery in question. Transcranial Doppler of the middle cerebral artery stem or basilar artery has helped establish the patency of these large vessels. MR angiography or conventional angiography may be required to settle the matter in some cases and remains our policy in cases where the transcranial Doppler is technically unsatisfactory and the CT or MRI scan shows a large band of low density, one spanning several sections, and one whose abnormality is seen down to the base of the affected basal ganglia.[99] Such a large infarct is not easily accounted for by primary disease in the penetrating artery itself, justifying angiography to seek stenosis of the middle cerebral stem. The prognosis for later hemispherical symptoms in cases with stem stenosis presenting as a lacunar infarct is unknown.

## Infarct of Undetermined Cause or Cryptogenic Infarction

Despite efforts to arrive at a diagnosis, the cause of the infarction in a discouragingly large number of cases remains undetermined. A number of explanations can be offered. The first of the three major reasons for the failure is easily understood: no appropriate laboratory studies are performed. Advanced age, coexisting severe disease with a poor prognosis, and patient or physician unwillingness are only a few of the many reasons for deferring a workup. One reason no longer valid for this approach is that the mechanism of stroke has been diagnosed satisfactorily on clinical grounds alone. Among the syndromes attributed to ischemia, only the Wallenberg syndrome has yet to be reported from hematoma, and causes other than stroke have been so often reported with most of the classical focal brain syndromes that the point need not be labored.

A second common cause for failure is improper timing of the appropriate laboratory studies. Angiograms for embolism over 48 hours after the ictus have a yield as low as 15 percent for evidence of the responsible occlusion.[14] Brain scans performed once only within a few hours of the onset of an ischemic stroke have a similarly low yield. Brain scans performed no matter how often may remain negative in some cases of small lacunar infarction, when the lesion is below the limits of resolution of the scan technique.

As many as 40 percent of the cases of ischemic stroke of undetermined cause fall into the third category, in which normal or ambiguous findings are reached despite appropriate laboratory studies performed at the appropriate time. This last group of cases poses special problems for research in stroke diagnosis. It would be comforting should most of these cases fall among those with the milder deficits, perhaps accounting for the negative laboratory studies by virtue of the relative insensitivity of such tests to smaller lesions. Yet, the scanty data on the subject indicates they are not: they are roughly as severe as ischemic strokes for which a cause is found.

In the Stroke Data Bank, a rigorous diagnostic scheme resulted in a high frequency of infarcts that were difficult to classify into the traditional subtypes, and which were, by default, classified as infarct of undetermined cause.[52,105] The investigators were all aware of the impact of timing on the likelihood of findings on many tests, especially angiography. Despite considerable effort at workup, there remained a large percentage, fully 40 percent, for whom the infarct mechanism escaped explanation and were classified as infarcts of undetermined cause.

## Clinical Features

Cases categorized as ischemic stroke of undetermined cause show no bruit or TIAs ipsilateral to the hemisphere affected by stroke, and have no obvious source of embolism; in short, they do not have the risk factors or prior history that help in suggesting a cardiac embolus or large-artery thrombosis.[71,105]

In the Stroke Data Bank, the mean age at stroke for infarcts of undetermined cause studied by CT and angiogram was 58 years.[104] Of these cases, 27 percent worsened in the hospital, and 41 percent had a moderate to severe weakness score. Hemispheral syndromes predominated in 66 percent; basilar syndromes occurred in 15 percent. Those cryptogenic infarct cases without angiograms differed from those who underwent angiogram by increased age, higher frequency of hypertension, and combined cardiac disease by history, a more severe motor deficit, and a higher 30-day case fatality rate.

## Laboratory Features

The CT or MRI scan performed within 7 days may be normal, may show an infarct limited to a surface branch territory, or may show a large zone of infarction affecting regions larger than that accounted for by a single penetrant arterial territory. In the Stroke Data Bank, among those cryptogenic infarcts fully evaluated, CT demonstrated clinically relevant infarcts in 57 percent; surface infarction was found in 40 percent.[105] Noninvasive vascular imaging fails to demonstrate an underlying large-vessel occlusion or stenosis. No cardiac source of embolism is uncovered by echocardiography, electrocardiography, or Holter monitor.

If an angiogram is performed, the study may be normal and may show a distal branch occlusion or occlusion of a major cerebral artery stem or the top of the basilar artery. Because these latter foci of occlusion can be from thrombotic or embolic cause, their demonstration does not settle the mechanism; only if the extreme effort of repeat angiography is undertaken and occlusion is gone can a diagnosis of embolism be made.

Some examples of the forms of stroke attributed to meningitis, migraine, lupus anticoagulant, arteritis, dissection, hypercoagulable states, and the like may be represented in the cryptogenic subgroup. Efforts should be made in each case to establish the existence of these unusual causes and all such instances so identified and classified as cerebral infarction from other determined causes. Adding together all the estimated frequencies with which such unusual causes present without accompanying evidence of the underlying disease cannot remotely approach the high frequency of the cryptogenic subgroup of stroke documented in the Stroke Data Bank.

## Potential Etiologies

One approach to dealing with this large cohort of cases is their forced reclassification into the traditional categories of atherothrombosis, embolism, or lacune. The presentation of a hemispheral syndrome, a surface infarction by CT and a corresponding branch occlusion documented by angiography or normal angiogram long has been considered suggestive of embolism. *Nonthrombotic ischemia* has been used to describe those cases with normal angiograms. Such findings could be inferred to represent emboli, despite no cardiac source for embolism documented by clinical or laboratory criteria. There is ample evidence for many occult sources of emboli, the difficulty proving their existence, and their role in the first or succeeding ischemic strokes. Reclassification of such cases and others with limited cerebral infarction seen on CT scan as "embolism with inobvious source" would add the majority of the cryptogenic infarct patients to the embolism category, making embolism from all sources the largest subtype of stroke.

Emerging technologies have led to the suggestions that some may be explained by hematologic disorders causing hypercoagulable states from protein C, free protein S, lupus anticoagulant, or anticardiolipin antibody abnormalities.[58,75,106,118] Others have implicated paradoxical emboli through a patent foramen ovale.[35,40,72]

Rather than reclassifying these cases into embolism as the inferred mechanism, we suggest their continued separation as cryptogenic because they represent a sizable cohort of acute strokes for which no mechanism has yet been proved. What remains completely unsettled is the stroke prognosis for cases whose embolus has a readily identifiable presumed "source" as opposed to those cases who have no "source." Lacking a source for embolism and lacking the proof of the nature of the occlusion, classifying such cases as cryptogenic may prove useful eventually to determine if this subgroup of cases differs in some way from those in which the mechanism of stroke is better defined, and to encourage the continued search for causes of brain infarction and precipitants of thromboembolism.

## REFERENCES


1. Adams HP, Gross CE: Embolism distal to stenosis of the middle cerebral artery. Stroke 12:228, 1981
2. Adams RD, Fisher CM: Pathology of cerebral arterial occlusion. In Fields WS (ed): Houston Symposium on Pathogenesis and Treatment of Cerebrovascular Disease. Charles C Thomas, Springfield, IL, 1961
3. Araki G: Small infarctions of the basal ganglia with special reference to transient ischemic attacks. Recent Adv Gerontol 469:161, 1978
4. Aring CD, Merritt HH: Differential diagnosis between cerebral hemorrhage and cerebral thrombosis. Arch Intern Med 56:435, 1935
5. Bamford J, Sandercock P, Jones L, Warlow C: The natural history of lacunar infarction: the Oxfordshire Community Stroke Project. Stroke 18:545, 1987
6. Barnett HJM, Peerless SJ, Kaufmann JCE: "Stump" of internal carotid artery—a source for further cerebral embolic ischemia. Stroke 9:448, 1978
7. Baron JC, Frackowiak RS, Herholz K et al: Use of PET methods for measurement of cerebral energy metabolism and hemodynamics in cerebrovascular disease. J Cereb Blood Flow Metab 9:723, 1989
8. Beal MF, Williams RS, Richardson EP, Fisher CM: Cerebral embolism as a cause of transient ischemic attacks and cerebral infarction. Neurology (NY) 31:860, 1981
9. Beghi E, Bogliun G, Cavaletti G et al: Hemorrhagic infarction: risk factors, clinical and tomographic features, and outcome: a case-control study. Acta Neurol Scand 80:226, 1989
10. Bladin PF: A radiologic and pathologic study of embolism of the internal carotid-middle cerebral arterial axis. Radiology 82:614, 1964
11. Bogousslavsky J, Cachin C, Regli F et al: Cardiac sources of embolism and cerebral infarction-clinical consequences and vascular concomitants: the Lausanne Stroke Registry. Neurology (NY) 41:855, 1991
12. Bogousslavsky J, Regli F: Borderzone infarctions distal to internal carotid artery occlusion: prognostic implications. Ann Neurol 20:346, 1986
13. Bogousslavsky J, Van Melle G, Regli F: The Lausanne Stroke Registry: analysis of 1000 consecutive patients with first stroke. Stroke 19:1083, 1988
14. Bozzao L, Fantozzi LM, Bastianello S et al: Ischaemic supratentorial stroke: angiographic findings in patients examined in the very early phase. J Neurol 236:340, 1989
15. Caplan LR: Occlusion of the vertebral or basilar artery. Follow-up analysis of some patients with benign outcome. Stroke 10:277, 1979
16. Caplan LR: "Top of the basilar" syndrome. Neurology (NY) 30:72, 1980
17. Caplan LR: Intracranial branch atheromatous disease: a neglected, understudied, and underused concept. Neurology (NY) 39:1246, 1989
18. Caplan LR, Brass LM, DeWitt LD et al: Transcranial Doppler ultrasound: present status. Neurology (NY) 40:696, 1990
19. Caplan LR, Hier DB, D'Cruz I: Cerebral embolism in the Michael Reese Stroke Registry. Stroke 14:30, 1983
20. Carpenter DA, Grubb RL, Jr, Powers WJ: Borderzone hemodynamics in cerebrovascular disease. Neurology (NY) 40:1587, 1990
21. Castaigne P, Lhermitte F, Buge A et al: Paramedian thalamic and midbrain infarcts: clinical and neuropathological study. Ann Neurol 10:127, 1981
22. Castaigne P, Lhermitte F, Gautier J: Rôle des lésions artérielles dans les accidents ischémiques cérébraux de l'athérosclérose. Rev Neurol (Paris) 113:1, 1965
23. Castaigne P, Lhermitte F, Gautier JC et al: Internal carotid artery occlusion: a study of 61 instances in 50 patients with post-mortem data. Brain 93:231, 1970
24. Castaigne P, Lhermitte F, Gautier JC et al: Arterial occlusions in the vertebro-basilar system—a study of forty-four patients with post-mortem data. Brain 96:133, 1973
25. Cerebral Embolism Task Force: Second report: cardiogenic brain embolism. Arch Neurol 46:727, 1989
26. Chamorro AM, Sacco RL, Mohr JP et al: Lacunar infarction: clinical-CT correlations in the Stroke Data Bank. Stroke 22:175, 1991
27. Cujec B, Polasek P, Voll C, Shuaib A: Transesophageal echocardiography in the detection of potential cardiac source of embolism in stroke patients. Stroke 22:727, 1991
28. David NJ, Gordon KK, Friedberg SJ et al: Fatal atheromatous cerebral embolism associated

with bright plaques in the retinal arterioles. Neurology (NY) 13:708, 1963
29. Davis DO, Rumbaugh CL, Gilson JM: Angiographic diagnosis of small-vessel cerebral emboli. Acta Radiol (Stockh) 9:264, 1969
30. Delal PM, Shah PM, Aiyar RR: Arteriographic study of cerebral embolism. Lancet 2:358, 1965
31. De Ley G, Weyne J, Demeester G et al: Experimental thromboembolic stroke studied by positron emission tomography: immediate versus delayed reperfusion by fibrinolysis. J Cereb Blood Flow Metab 8:539, 1988
32. Derouesne C, Mas JL, Bolgert AF, Castaigne P: Pure sensory stroke caused by a small cortical infarct in the middle cerebral artery territory. Stroke 15:660, 1984
33. DeWitt LD, Wechsler LR: Transcranial Doppler. Stroke 19:915, 1988
34. Dion JE, Gates PC, Fox AJ et al: Clinical events following neuroangiography: a prospective study. Stroke 18:997, 1987
35. Di Tullio MR, Gopal AS, Sacco RL et al: Prevalence of patent foramen ovale in older cryptogenic stroke patients assessed by contrast echocardiography. J Am Soc Echo 4:294, 1991
36. Drurys I, Whisnant JP, Garraway WM: Primary intracerebral hemorrhage: impact of CT on incidence. Neurology (NY) 34:653, 1984
37. Edelman RR, Mattle HP, Atkinson DJ et al: Cerebral blood flow: assessment with dynamic contrast enhanced T2* weighted MR imaging at 1.5 T. Radiology 176:211, 1990
38. Edelman RR, Mattle HP, Atkinson DJ, Hoogewoud HM: MR angiography. AJR 154:937, 1990
39. Edwards JH, Kricheff II, Riles T, Imparato A: Angiographically undetected ulceration of the carotid bifurcation as a cause of embolic stroke. Radiology 132:369, 1979
40. Falk RH: PFO or UFO?—the role of a patent foramen ovale in cryptogenic stroke. (Editorial.) Am Heart J 121:1264, 1991
41. Fieschi C, Argentino C, Lenzi GL et al: Clinical and instrumental evaluation of patients with ischemic stroke within the first six hours. J Neurol Sci 91:311, 1989
42. Fisher CM: Cerebral thromboangiitis obliterans. Medicine (Baltimore) 36:169, 1957
43. Fisher CM: Lacunes: small deep cerebral infarcts. Neurology (Minneapolis) 15:774, 1965
44. Fisher CM: The arterial lesions underlying lacunes. Acta Neuropathol (Berl) 12:1, 1969
45. Fisher CM: Bilateral occlusion of basilar artery branches. J Neurol Neurosurg Psychiatry 40:1182, 1977
46. Fisher CM: Lacunar strokes and infarcts: a review. Neurology (NY) 32:871, 1982
47. Fisher CM, Adams RD: Observations on brain embolism with special reference to the mechanism of hemorrhagic infarction. J Neuropathol Exp Neurol 10:92, 1951
48. Fisher CM, Caplan LR: Basilar artery branch occlusion: a cause of pontine infarction. Neurology (Minneapolis) 21:900, 1971
49. Fisher CM, Gore I, Okabe N, White PD: Atherosclerosis of the carotid and vertebral arteries—extracranial and intracranial. J Neuropathol Exp Neurol 24:455, 1965
50. Fisher CM, Karnes WE: Local embolism. J Neuropathol Exp Neurol 24:174, 1965
51. Fisher CM, Pearlman A: The non-sudden onset of cerebral embolism. Neurology (Minneapolis) 17:1025, 1967
52. Foulkes MA, Wolf PA, Price TR et al: The Stroke Data Bank: design, methods, and baseline characteristics, Stroke 19:547, 1988
53. Friedlich AL, Castleman B, Mohr JP: Case records of the Massachusetts General Hospital. N Engl J Med 278:1109, 1968
54. Gacs G, Fox AJ, Barnett HJM, Vinuela F: CT visualization of intracranial arterial thromboembolism. Stroke 14:756, 1983
55. Grolimund P, Seiler RW, Aaslid R et al: Evaluation of cerebrovascular disease by combined extracranial and transcranial Doppler sonography: experience in 1,039 patients. Stroke 18:1018, 1987
56. Gross CR, Kase CS, Mohr JP, Cunningham SC: Stroke in south Alabama: incidence and diagnostic features. Stroke 15:249, 1984
57. Hankey GJ, Warlow CP, Sellar RJ: Cerebral angiographic risk in mild cerebrovascular disease. Stroke 21:209, 1990
58. Hart RG, Kanter MC: Hematologic disorders and ischemic stroke: a selective review. Stroke 21:1111, 1990
59. Heiss WD, Herholz K, Podreka I et al: Comparison of $^{99m}$Tc HMPAO SPECT with $^{18}$F fluoromethane PET in cerebrovascular disease. J Cereb Blood Flow Metab 10:687, 1990
60. Hinton RC, Kistler JP, Fallon JT et al: Influence of etiology of atrial fibrillation on incidence of systemic embolism. Am J Cardiol 40:509, 1977
61. Hinton RC, Mohr JP, Ackerman RA et al: Symptomatic middle cerebral artery stem stenosis. Ann Neurol 5:152, 1979
62. Hommel M, Besson G, Le Bas JF et al: Prospective study of lacunar infarction using magnetic resonance imaging. Stroke 21:546, 1990
63. Hulqvist GT: Über Thrombose und Embolie der Arteria carotis und herbei vorkommende Gehirnveränderungen: eine pathologische anatomische Studie. Fischer, Stockholm, 1942
64. Imparato AM, Riles TS, Gorstein F: The carotid bifurcation plaque: pathologic findings associated with cerebral ischemia. Stroke 10:238, 1979
65. Irino T, Tandea M, Minami T: Angiographic manifestations in postrecanalized cerebral infarction. Neurology (NY) 27:471, 1977
66. Johnson DW, Stringer WA, Marks MP et al: Stable xenon CT cerebral blood flow imaging: rationale for and role in clinical decision making. AJNR 12:201, 1991
67. Kase CS, White L, Vinson L, Eichelberger P: Shotgun Pellet Embolus to the middle cerebral artery. Neurology (NY) 31:458, 1981
68. Kistler JP, Buonanno FS, Dewitt LD et al: Vertebral basilar posterior cerebral territory stroke—delineation by proton nuclear magnetic resonance imaging. Stroke 15:417, 1984
69. Kittner SJ, Sharkness CM, Price TR et al: In-

farcts with a cardiac source of embolism in the NINCDS Stroke Data Bank: historical features. Neurology (NY) 40:281, 1990
70. Krayenbuehl HA, Yasargil MG: Cerebral Angiography. (2nd Ed.) Butterworth, London, 1968
71. Kunitz S, Gross CR, Heyman A et al: The pilot stroke data bank: definition, design, data. Stroke 15:740, 1984
72. Lechat P, Mas JL, Lascault G et al: Prevalence of patent foramen ovale in patients with stroke. N Engl J Med 318:1148, 1988
73. Lennihan L, Kupsky WJ, Mohr JP et al: Lack of association between carotid plaque hematoma and ipsilateral cerebral symptoms. Stroke 18:879, 1987
74. Leow K, Murie JA: Cerebral angiography for cerebrovascular disease: the risks. Br J Surg 75:428, 1988
75. Levine Sr, Kim S, Deegan MJ, Welch KMA: Ischemic stroke associated with anti-cardiolipin antibodies. Stroke 18:1101, 1987
76. Lhermitte F, Gautier JC, Derouesne C, Guiraud B: Ischemic accidents in the middle cerebral artery territory (a study of the causes in 122 cases). Arch Neurology (NY) 19:248, 1968
77. Liebeskind A, Chinichian A, Schechter MM: The moving embolus seen during serial cerebral angiography. Stroke 2:440, 1971
78. Little JR, Shawhan B, Weinstein M: Pseudo-tandem stenosis of the internal carotid artery. Neurosurgery 7:574,1980
79. Masaryk TJ, Modic MT, Ross JS et al: Intracranial circulation: preliminary clinical results with three dimensional (volume) MR angiography. Radiology 171:793, 1989
80. Massaro AR, Sacco RL, Timsit SG et al: Early clinical discriminators between cerebral infarction and hemorrhagic stroke. Ann Neurol 30:246, 1991
81. Masuda J, Ogata J, Yutani C et al: Artery to artery embolism from a thrombus formed in stenotic middle cerebral artery: report of an autopsy case. Stroke 18:680, 1987
82. Minematsu K, Yamaguchi T, Omae T: Spectacular shrinking deficit: rapid recovery from a full hemispheral syndrome by migration of an embolus. Neurology (NY), suppl 1. 41:329, 1991
83. Mohr JP: Neurologic complications of cardiac valvular disease and cardiac surgery. p. 143. In Vinken PJ, Bruyn GW (eds): Handbook of Clinical Neurology. Vol. 34: Medical Conditions. North-Holland Publishing, Amsterdam, 1979
84. Mohr JP: Lacunar infarctions. p. 201. In Barnett HJM (ed): Neurological Clinics of North America. WB Saunders, Philadelphia, 1983
85. Mohr JP, Caplan LR, Melski JW et al: The Harvard cooperative stroke registry: a prospective registry of cases hospitalized with stroke. Neurology (NY) 28:754, 1978
86. Mohr JP, Duterte DI, Oliveira VR et al: Recanalization of acute middle cerebral artery occlusion. Neurology (NY), suppl 1. 38:215, 1988
87. Nelson RF, Pullicino P, Kendall BE, Marshall J: Computed tomography on patients presenting with lacunar syndromes. Stroke 11:256, 1980
88. Norrving B, Nilsson B, Risberg J: RCBF in patients with carotid occlusion: resting and hypercapneic flow related to collateral pattern. Stroke 13:155, 1982
89. Ogata J, Masuda J, Yutani C, Yamaguchi T: Rupture of atheromatous plaque as a cause of thrombotic occlusion of stenotic internal carotid artery. Stroke 21:1740, 1990
90. Ogata J, Yutani C, Imakita M et al: Hemorrhagic infarct of the brain without a reopening of the occluded arteries in cardioembolic stroke. Stroke 20:876, 1989
91. Panzer RJ, Feibel JH, Barker WH, Griner PF: Predicting the likelihood of hemorrhage in patients with stroke. Arch Intern Med 14:1800, 1985
92. Perrone P, Candelise L, Scotti G et al: CT evaluation in patients with transient ischemic attack: correlation between clinical and angiographic findings. Eur Neurol 18:217, 1979
93. Pessin MS, Duncan GW, Davis KR et al: Angiographic appearance of carotid occlusion in acute stroke. Stroke 11:485, 1980
94. Pessin MS, Hinton RC, Davis KR et al: Mechanisms of acute carotid stroke: a clinicoangiographic study. Ann Neurol 6:245, 1979
95. Powers WJ. Cerebral hemodynamics in ischemic cerebrovascular disease. Ann Neurol 29:231, 1991
96. Powers WJ, Tempel LW, Grubb RL, Jr: Influence of cerebral hemodynamics on stroke risk: one year follow up of 30 medically treated patients. Ann Neurol 25:325, 1989
97. Quisling RG, Friedman WA, Rhoton AL: High cervical dissection: spontaneous resolution. AJNR 1:463, 1980
98. Ramirez Lassepas M, Cipolle RJ, Bjok RJ et al: Can embolic stroke be diagnosed on the basis of neurologic clinical criteria? Arch Neurol 44:87, 1987
99. Rascol A, Clanet M, Manelfe C: Pure motor hemiplegia: CT study of 30 cases. Stroke 13:11, 1982
100. Ring BA: Diagnosis of embolic occlusions of smaller branches of the intracerebral arteries. AJR 97:575, 1966
101. Ringelstein EB, Zeumer H, Angelou D: The pathogenesis of strokes from internal carotid artery occlusion: diagnostic and therapeutic implications. Stroke 14:867, 1983
102. Romanul FCA, Abramowicz A: Changes in brain and pial vessels in arterial borderzones. Arch Neurol 11:40, 1964
103. Ross Russell, RW: Atheromatous retinal embolism. Lancet 2:1354, 1963
104. Sacco RL, Bello JA, Traub RD, Brust JCM: Selective proprioceptive sensory loss from a thalamic lacunar stroke. Stroke 18:1160, 1987
105. Sacco RL, Ellenberg JA, Mohr JP et al: Infarction of undetermined cause: the NINCDS Stroke Data Bank. Ann Neurol 25:382, 1989
106. Sacco RL, Owen J, Mohr JP, Tatemichi TK: Free protein S deficiency: a possible association with intracranial vascular occlusion. Stroke 1657, 1989

107. Samuel KC: Atherosclerosis and occlusion of the internal carotid artery. J Pathol 71:391, 1956
108. Sandercock PAG, Allen CMC, Corston RN et al: Clinical diagnosis of intracranial haemorrhage using Guy's Hospital Score. Br Med J 291:1675, 1985
109. Santamaria J, Graus F, Rubio F et al: Cerebral infarction of the basal ganglia due to embolism from the heart. Stroke 14:911, 1983
110. Sette G, Baron JC, Mazoyer B et al: Local brain haemodynamics and oxygen metabolism in cerebrovascular disease: positron emission tomography. Brain 112:931, 1989
111. Sloan MA: Thrombolysis and stroke, past and future. Arch Neurol 44:748, 1987
112. Smoker WR, Biller J, Hingtgen WL et al: Angiography of nonhemorrhagic cerebral infarction in young adults. Stroke 18:08, 1987
113. Spitzer K, Thie A, Caplan LR, Kunze K: The MICROSTROKE expert system for stroke type diagnosis. Stroke 20:1353, 1989
114. Sunohara N, Mukoyama M, Mano Y, Satoyoshi E: Action-induced rhythmic dystonia: an autopsy case. Neurology (Cleveland) 34:321, 1984
115. Tatemichi TK, Chamorro A, Petty GW et al: Hemodynamic role of ophthalmic artery collateral in internal carotid artery occlusion. Neurology (NY) 40:461, 1990
116. Timsit S, Sacco RL, Mohr JP et al: Brain infarction severity differs according to cardiac or arterial embolic source: the NINDS Stroke Data Bank. Neurology (NY), suppl 1. 40:417, 1990
117. Timsit S, Sacco RL, Mohr JP et al: Early clinical differentiation of atherosclerotic and cardioembolic infarction: Stroke Data Bank. J Neurol 237:140, 1990
118. Tohgi H, Kawashima M, Tamura K, Suzuki H: Coagulation fibrinolysis abnormalities in acute and chronic phases of cerebral thrombosis and embolism. Stroke 21:1663, 1990
119. Torvick A: The pathogenesis of watershed infarcts in the brain. Stroke 15:221, 1984
120. Torvik A, Jorgensen L: Thrombotic and embolic occlusions of the carotid arteries in an autopsy material. 2. Cerebral lesions and clinical course. J Neurol Sci 3:410, 1966
121. Von Arbin M, Britton M, de Faire U et al: Accuracy of bedside diagnosis in stroke. Stroke 12:288, 1981
122. Whisnant JP: Multiple particles injected may all go to the same cerebral artery branch. Stroke 13:720, 1982
123. Yamaguchi T, Minematsu K, Choki J, Ikeda M: Clinical and neuroradiological analysis of thrombotic and embolic cerebral infarction. Jpn Circ J 48:50, 1984
124. Zanette EM, Fieschi C, Bozzao L et al: Comparison of cerebral angiography and transcranial Doppler sonography in acute stroke. Stroke 20:899, 1989
125. Zatz LM, Iannone AM, Eckman PB, Hecker SP: Observations concerning intracerebral vascular occlusion. Neurology (NY) 15:390, 1965
126. Zierler RE, Kohler TR, Strandness DE, Jr: Duplex scanning of normal or minimally diseased carotid arteries: correlation with arteriography and clinical outcome. J Vasc Surg 12:447, 1990

# 14
# INTERNAL CAROTID ARTERY DISEASE

J.P. Mohr
J.C. Gautier
Michael S. Pessin

The bifurcation of the common carotid artery and the origin of the internal carotid artery (ICA) has been the focus of neurologic attention for many years. The extracranial ICA is by far the commonest site of significant atherosclerotic ICA lesions, while the intracranial ICA is, as a rule, devoid of atherosclerosis beyond its origin to its entry into the skull. The extracranial ICA can be examined clinically and by ultrasound and is easy to approach surgically, and even some of its unusual disorders, such as dissecting aneurysms, are to some extent amenable to conventional surgery. By contrast, the intracranial ICA lends itself poorly to clinical and ultrasound examination, and even angiograms are often difficult to evaluate properly. Only recently has Doppler ultrasonography been applied to the carotid siphon.[191]

## ANATOMY

The cervical segment of the internal carotid artery extends from the common carotid artery bifurcation to the skull base. Intracranially, the internal carotid artery is divided into the petrosal, cavernous, and supraclinoid portions.

### Common Carotid Artery

The right common carotid artery usually arises from the innominate artery and the left, directly from the arch. However, the left common carotid often arises from the innominate artery.[219] The innominate and the left common carotid arteries may appear as a fork from the arch of the aorta, or the left common carotid may rise as high as a few centimeters from the origin of the innominate artery. Rarely, instances of agenesis of a common carotid have been reported.[40,358]

The external and internal carotid arteries are the principal branches of the common carotid artery. The common carotid only rarely gives rise to the branches usually formed from the external carotid artery.

### Bifurcation of the Common Carotid Artery

The bifurcation of the common carotid artery is most often found at the level of the thyroid cartilage. However, anatomic variations are great enough that the bifurcation may be found anywhere within 5 cm of this site.[392] The origin of the internal carotid artery is usually somewhat dilated, extending up to 2 cm from the origin before it assumes a uniform diameter. Although the bifurcation geometry usually places the internal carotid artery posterior to the external carotid, many variants exist, some in which the internal carotid artery wraps around the external carotid to a degree that the positions appear almost reversed.

Measurements of the diameter and angulation of the bifurcation serve to show its modest variation. In their study of 102 normals, Harrison and Marshall[164] found the common carotid artery was 7.6 mm (±1.64 mm) in diameter as it entered the bifurcation, the bulb enlarging to 8.3 mm (±1.95 mm), while the internal carotid artery beyond the bulb narrowed to 5.1

mm (±1.1 mm). At the bifurcation, the angle formed between the external carotid and internal carotid arteries was 36.4 degrees (±18.2 degrees).

The bifurcation area is notable for the presence of the carotid body and the nerve of the carotid sinus. Both receive their blood supply from the external carotid artery. The chemoreceptor function of the carotid body responds to a decrease in arterial $Po_2$, carotid blood flow, and arterial pH and to an increase in arterial $Pco_2$ or blood temperature, in descending order of sensitivity.[72] Its output is mediated by the glossopharyngeal nerve and plays on the nucleus of the tractus solitarius, nucleus ambiguus, paramedian reticular formation, and lateral reticular nucleus. The carotid body has an important regulatory effect on respiration, being the only mediator of hypoxic ventilatory drive, and has additional effects on blood pressure and heart rate. Stimulation of the carotid body produces, among other effects, increased rate and depth of respiration, increased peripheral vascular resistance, with secondary elevation in blood pressure, and bradycardia. Unilateral carotid endarterectomy produces an increase in the $Pco_2$ and failure of response to hypoxia.[361]

An increase in the stretch of the wall of the carotid sinus produces activity of the carotid sinus nerve, which produces reflex hypotension by activating the sympathoinhibitory effect of the nucleus of the tractus solitarius and by activating parasympathetics in the dorsal motor nucleus of the vagus, which slows the heart rate. Hypofunction caused by reducing distension of the carotid sinus or by sectioning of the nerve may produce the opposite effect. Such changes rarely persist beyond 48 hours.[72] Bilateral carotid artery stenosis can be a cause of sustained hypertension.

## External Carotid Artery and Other Ascending Arteries of Interest

The external carotid artery gives rise to the ascending pharyngeal, superior thyroid, lingual, occipital, facial, posterior auricular, internal maxillary, and superficial temporal branches, in that order. These branches rarely arise from the internal carotid artery.[273] The superior laryngeal nerve passes posteriorly near the origin of the ICA, and the hypoglossal nerve courses laterally over the artery. Either of these nerves may be injured in operations on the region of the bifurcation; damage to the hypoglossal nerve causes ipsilateral atrophy of the tongue, occasionally misdiagnosed as a brain stem stroke.

Occlusion of the internal carotid artery at its origin often permits visualization of the ascending pharyngeal artery, which is otherwise often obscured by the contrast in the opacified internal carotid artery. The ascending pharyngeal may anastomose with the middle meningeal and/or occipital arteries.[207]

The occipital artery is an important source of collateral to the extracranial portion of the vertebral artery by means of a small collateral, the proatlantal artery. In cases of occlusion of the common carotid artery below the bifurcation, collateral may arise from the vertebral artery, pass through the proatlantal artery, and, via retrograde flow through the occipital artery to the external carotid artery, reach the bifurcation to supply the internal carotid artery in the usual anterograde manner. Likewise, occlusion of the vertebral artery in the neck may allow flow to the distal extracranial segment of the vertebral artery through the proatlantal artery from the occipital artery.

## Extracranial Internal Carotid Artery

The extracranial ICA extends from the bifurcation to its entry into the carotid canal of the temporal bone without branches or notable change in size[84] (Fig. 14-1). Anomalies are rare.[273] There is considerable variation in the length of the vessel and its degree of tortuosity. In as many as 35 percent of all cases, some form of tortuosity may be encountered,[68] such as undulation, coiling, or kinking of the vessel.[368]

Throughout its course, the internal carotid artery is intimately associated with ascending sympathetic fibers. Near its origin, it is crossed laterally by the hypoglossal nerve. The superior cervical ganglion and the vagus nerve lie immediately behind. Near its entry into the skull, the internal carotid artery is separated from the jugular vein by the glossopharyngeal, vagus, spinal accessory, and hypoglossal nerves.

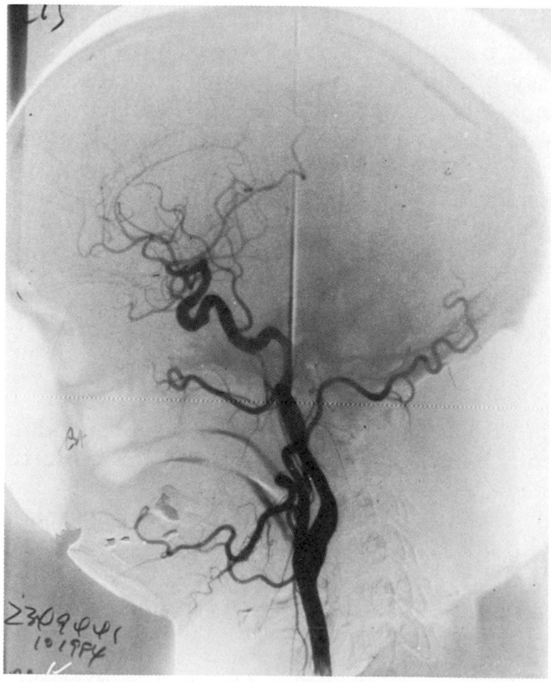

**Fig. 14-1.** Anatomy of the extracranial carotid artery.

## Intracranial Internal Carotid Artery

### Petrosal Portion

The intracranial ICA supplies part of the tympanic cavity and the artery of the pterygoid canal (vidian artery), which may form an anastomosis with the internal maxillary artery.[313]

### Cavernous Portion

The cavernous part of the ICA, approximately 4 to 5 cm in length,[396] enters the cavernous sinus through the foramen lacerum just beneath the gasserian ganglion. It runs rostrally, close to the lateral aspect of the sella turcica. This segment of the vessel becomes progressively more tortuous from infancy to old age, ultimately resulting in the S-shaped carotid siphon that is characteristic of adult humans.[147] The carotid siphon lies within the venous plexus and bears relationships to the 3rd, 4th, 5th, and 6th cranial nerves that run in the lateral wall of the cavernous sinus. A detailed study of the relationship of the ICA to the cavernous sinus has been made by Parkinson.[275]

The carotid siphon gives off a few small branches: the meningeal-hypophyseal trunk, the artery of the inferior cavernous sinus (84 percent of cases),[162] and, less often (28 percent of cases),[162] McConnell's capsular arteries. Rarely (approximately 6 to 8 percent of cases),[162] the ophthalmic and dorsal meningeal arteries arise from the cavernous portion.

The meningeal-hypophyseal trunk is approximately the same size as the ophthalmic artery.[162] It has three tiny branches:[86,219,276] (1) the artery of the tentorium (the artery of Bernasconi and Cassinari),[25] which courses backward to supply the surface of the tentorium; (2) the dorsal meningeal artery, which supplies the wall of the cavernous sinus, the dura of the clivus, and the 6th cranial nerve, and crosses the midline to anastomose with its counterpart; and (3) the inferior hypophyseal artery, which supplies the posterior pituitary gland, resolving into capillaries that enter the pituitary portal system.[350]

The artery of the inferior cavernous sinus supplies the dura of its inferior and lateral wall, and in some cases anastomoses with the middle meningeal artery at the foramen spinosum.[86,162] McConnell's capsular arteries supply the anterior wall of the sella turcica and the anterior lobe of the pituitary, anastomosing with the inferior hypophyseal artery. At this level there are several anastomotic channels between internal and external carotid artery circulations.

### Supraclinoid Portion

The supraclinoid part of the ICA pierces the dura mater medial to the anterior clinoid process. This short stretch, usually less than 1 cm in length,[396] winds upward and slightly laterally,[199] passing over the oculomotor nerve and below the optic nerve. However short, the supraclinoid part of the ICA gives off several important branches and therefore is of great importance for collateral circulation.

Its major branches are well known. The first is the ophthalmic artery, which enters the orbit via the optic foramen. The main branches of the ophthalmic artery are the lacrimal, supraorbital, ethmoidal, and palpebral arteries. The artery of the falx arises from the ethmoidal branch. The ophthalmic artery gives rise to the central retinal artery, not usually seen angiographically, but a capillary blush from the choroid and retina may be visible in the late arterial phase of the angiogram. The many branches of the ophthalmic artery provide rich anastomotic connections with external carotid artery branches and serve as an important collateral channel between the two circulations, offering some protection in the event of internal carotid artery occlusion.

The posterior communicating artery is next, arising from the dorsal aspect of the vessel to run caudally and medially and join the posterior cerebral artery. A slight dilatation, referred to as "junctional dilatation"[330] or infundibulum, may be present. The artery proceeds caudally and medially where it joins the posterior cerebral artery. The posterior communicating artery supplies the anterior and medial parts of the thalamus and walls of the third ventricle by means of severe small branches. When fully developed, keeping the embryonic disposition in the adult, it may serve as an important connection between the carotid and vertebrobasilar circulations. When the posterior cerebral artery arises from the ICA, occlusion of the ICA can cause particularly devastating infarcts. One to three small perforating arteries may arise just distal to the posterior communicating artery and before the origin of the anterior choroidal artery. These vessels supply the anterior perforating substance. When major intracranial occlusive disease affects the circle of Willis, these small branches may be visualized angiographically as prominent collateral pathways.

The anterior choroidal artery usually arises from the internal carotid artery and enters the brain via the choroidal fissure. It is a small branch of the internal carotid artery, arising just distal to the origin of the posterior communicating artery, and it supplies the choroid plexus of the temporal horn, hippocampus, basal ganglia, and lower half of the posterior limb of the internal capsule. Although it is said to arise sometimes from the middle cerebral artery, studies of the anatomy by microdissection show it almost always arises from the internal carotid artery.[146]

The ICA then bifurcates into the anterior and middle cerebral arteries. The middle cerebral artery is the larger and usually is the direct continuation of the ICA. Both the initial segment of the anterior cerebral and the posterior communicating arteries are subject to fairly frequent variations in size that are part of the variations of the circle of Willis.

### Anatomic Anomalies

The main anatomic anomaly of the intracranial ICA is the persistence of the trigeminal artery in the adult. This vessel arises from the ICA as it enters the cavernous sinus and runs caudally either through the sella turcica or the extradural space under the petroclinoid ligament to join the basilar artery, generally between the origins of the superior cerebellar and anterior inferior cerebellar arteries. A full description of this variation and its embryologic, angiographic, and pathologic significance has been given by Lie[219] and Parkinson and Shields.[276]

The other important, if uncommon, variant is that the ophthalmic artery may arise from the middle meningeal artery,[65] with no connection to the intracranial ICA.

### Collateral Branches

Apart from the opthalmic artery and the circle of Willis, there are only a few branches of the intracranial ICA that permit collateral with other vessels. These branches are, at most, very small twigs. They may enlarge and be of great significance under unusual circumstances, such as arteriovenous malformations in the dura mater, but ordinarily they remain too small to play a useful role in ameliorating the effects of thrombotic or embolic intracranial ICA occlusions.

## RELEVANT HISTOLOGY

Extracranial cerebral arteries have the usual structure of elastic or muscular arteries. Intracranial arteries have no external elastic lamina. Although not visible with routine histologic techniques, the elastic lamina may still be stained with special techniques. Generally, arterial cushions, which are often seen as precursors of atherosclerotic lesions, lie at the curvatures and branchings of the arteries.[18] Intracranial arteries are devoid of vasa vasorum.[18]

The extracranial carotid artery shares most of the histology of other limb and trunk vessels of the same size. The intracranial ICA has some unique anatomy. In its initial stretch it lies in a bony encasement, then, in the cavernous sinus, lies within venous blood, two peculiar situations for an artery. It becomes intracranial in the strict sense only in its short supraclinoid segment. We do not know of any histologic study specifically devoted to the intracranial ICA and therefore do not know to what extent the general histologic features of intracranial arteries and their peculiarities bear upon the histologic structure of the intracranial ICA.

## PATHOLOGY

### Atherosclerosis

Atherosclerosis and its complications far exceed all other forms of disease primarily affecting the extracranial and intracranial carotid arteries. Because there are some important differences between the lesions in these two sites, they will be described separately.

### Extracranial Internal Carotid Artery Atherosclerosis

The carotid artery in the neck has proved to be among the favored sites for development of atherosclerosis. The pathologic process in the carotid artery seems similar to that found in other vessels. The fibrous plaques that are considered the hallmark of advancing atherosclerosis occur in the carotid arteries as early as ages 25 to 40, but appear later in the vertebral and intracranial arteries, between ages 40 and 50.[244]

A recurrent injury to the intima is considered to be the important step in the initiation of the atherosclerotic lesion.[266,307] The effects of the injury are influenced by factors such as turbulent flow,[148,265,335,373] hypertension-induced large shearing and vibration forces,[334] chronic hypercholesterolemia,[306] and other less common problems. Platelets adhere to the injured, exposed endothelium,[266] and circulating plasma lipids enter the lesion, especially low-density lipoproteins.[301] Smooth muscle cells migrate from the media to the intima, where they proliferate.[189,386] Views differ as to whether this proliferation occurs from a single cell line[23,287] or as a result of deregulation of proliferation factors from senescence.[237] Whatever the mechanisms involved, the end result is the characteristic histology of the atheroma.[307]

#### *Distribution of Extracranial Lesions*

It is perhaps the functional importance of the eye and brain and their sensitivity to the ischemia that has brought about so many studies on atherosclerosis in its various stages of development in the carotid artery. The disease usually affects the carotid artery in a uni- or multifocal fashion, not diffusely. The intramural lesions occur most frequently at bifurcations and curves[58,128,181,313] (Fig. 14-2). The majority are found in the first 2 cm from the origin of the internal carotid artery.[58,128,181,313] Fewer lesions occur in the intracranial portion in the carotid siphon and intracranially at the stems of the anterior and middle cerebral arteries.[58,128] The occurrence and severity of disease in the carotid siphon appears to be unrelated to that in the carotid sinus, and the results of surgical therapy for carotid sinus disease does not appear to be related to disease in the siphon.[302]

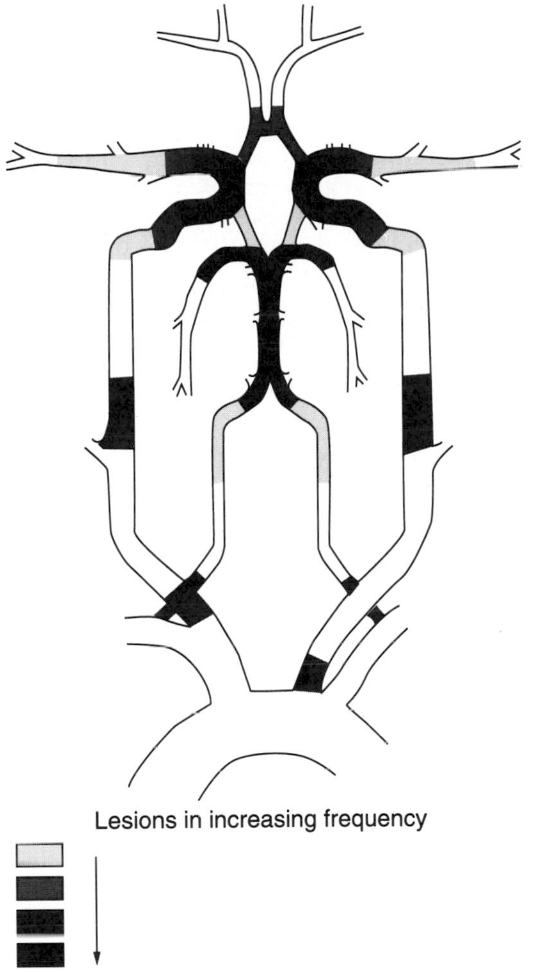


**Fig. 14-2.** Distribution of lesions in the carotid artery territory.

*Carotid Artery Bifurcation Anatomy and Lesion Development*

Attempts have been made to implicate both vessel size and vascular geometry in the development of atheroma at the bifurcation. For the internal carotid artery severely affected by atherosclerosis on one side only, Caplan and Baker[52] found the smaller vessel more frequently involved. Flow separation appears to be another factor. LoGerfo et al.[228,229] used plastic tubing to demonstrate a flow separation effect that occurs at a fork in a tube, and they argued that the extent of the flow separation might play a role in the occurrence and the positioning of an atheroma at the carotid bifurcation. Wood et al.[390] separately demonstrated such boundary separation in human carotid artery bifurcations by painstaking ultrasonic studies. Atheroma opposite the site of the boundary separation was also shown in an autopsy study.[400] Taken together, these findings suggest that the focus of atherosclerosis is determined to some degree by the local flow characteristics, for which the carotid bifurcation seems especially suited. This thesis is becoming more widely accepted, although the findings have been challenged by measurements made of a series of cases studied by angiograms that showed no significant difference between either the size or the angles at the bifurcation in normal or diseased vessels.[164]

*Hemodynamically Significant Stenosis*

The main variables involved in making a stenosis hemodynamically significant are the reduced cross-sectional area,[26,42,325] length of the stenosis,[42] velocity of the blood flow,[398] and blood viscosity.[48] Of these variables, cross-sectional area is the most important. Brice et al.[42] were among the first to define the characteristics of a hemodynamically significant stenosis in vitro. Hemodynamically significant stenosis (i.e., reduced blood flow) occurred in excised human internal carotid arteries when the lumen was constricted along a length of 3 mm to a cross-sectional area of 4 to 5 mm$^2$ (Fig. 14-3). They extended these studies to humans undergoing clamping of the common carotid artery for intracranial aneurysms. The point of sudden fall in pressure distal to the stenosis occurred when the lumen reached 2 mm in diameter at its narrowest point. Little detectable change in flow or pressure developed distal to the stenosis until the critical point was reached, after which any further change produced an even more dramatic fall in pressure and flow. The length of the stenosis was a far less significant factor than was the total cross-sectional area at the narrowest point: over a distance of 4 cm, the resistance increased less than twofold. Lesions in tandem produced cumulative effects only if separated by more than 3 cm (the usual condition that applies to carotid territory stenoses in tandem). The effects of unilateral carotid stenosis were thought not to be influenced by stenoses elsewhere in the system, although the authors did not document this point in their work.[42] This study presented the theory that the carotid stenosis must be 2 mm or tighter to be considered hemodynamically significant. Others have used the method of percentage of reduction in the vascular

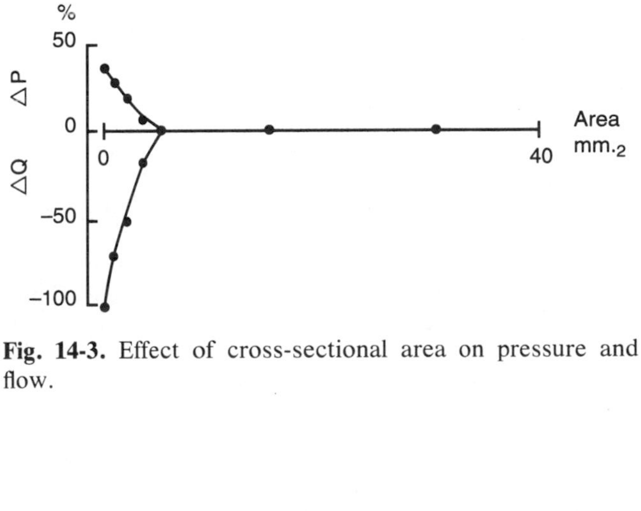


**Fig. 14-3.** Effect of cross-sectional area on pressure and flow.

lumen, noting hemodynamic significance when the diameter is reduced by 50 percent, a figure that corresponds to a cross-sectional reduction of 75 to 80 percent.[26,241]

Archie and Feldtman[10] restudied the original observations by Brice in patients with primary arterial disease, using electromagnetic blood flow measurements in 47 patients before and after carotid endarterectomy. Normal blood flow was still present in up to 60 percent diameter stenosis and 90 percent cross-sectional area stenosis. A 40 percent reduction in blood flow was documented at a 75 percent diameter and 94 percent area stenosis, while a 64 percent reduction of blood flow occurred with 84 percent diameter stenosis and 96 percent area stenosis. These data clearly indicate that these stenoses must be rather severe both in diameter and, especially, in cross-sectional area before significant reductions in blood flow occur. The findings suggested that hemodynamically significant stenosis may not be present until the lumen is even more restricted than the 2-mm lumen diameter suggested by the data of Brice et al.[42]

Although there is copious literature on hemodynamics using a laboratory model, there appears to be a considerable difference in the dynamics of static versus compliant stenosis. Santamore and colleagues[315] found the static stenosis created in a glass rod to be little influenced by changes in perfusion pressure or peripheral resistance. However, the hemodynamics of a stenosis created by a balloon catheter in the dog carotid artery proved somewhat different. The stenotic resistance, computed as the pressure gradient across the stenosis divided by the flow, was sensitive to changes in either perfusion pressure or peripheral resistance. When either was decreased, an increase in stenotic resistance resulted.

### *Tempo of Lesion Development*

Little is known of the tempo of lesion development in the intracranial ICA, so most of the discussion is drawn from experience with extracranial ICA disease. Judging from studies using conventional angiography, digital subtraction methods, or noninvasive techniques, atheromatous stenoses may develop swiftly over months, slowly over years, or even remain static despite being hemodynamically significant.[187] Only a few studies have addressed the fate of asymptomatic lesions. The early study by Javid's group,[186] in which they reangiogrammed 93 patients whose carotid lesion was asymptomatic at the time of the initial angiogram, found that 35 of 93 arteries showed no change in the severity or configuration of the atheroma over 1 to 9 years; 19 had increased their atheroma size by less than 25 percent per year, while 32 had changed more than 25 percent per year; 7 had developed recurrent stenosis or thrombosis. Bauer et al.[21] undertook a similar study of 49 patients by undertaking repeat angiography with a mean interval of 25 months. Some degree of progression of the lesions was found in 17 of the 63 unoperated carotid arteries.

The lower risk of the newer less invasive methods of following the course of internal carotid artery disease has led to the appearance of reports in increasing numbers. These studies indicate that progression of presymptomatic stenosis may be more common than suspected on clinical grounds alone. Norrving et al.[268] followed the course of 64 cases of carotid artery disease over a period of 1 to 13 years, and found a 27 percent rate of progression on the nonoperated, previously asymptomatic side. About 30 percent of the cases with progressing disease became symptomatic with transient ischemic attacks (TIAs) or strokes. By contrast, only 5.5 percent of the vessels showing no progression of the disease process produced symptoms, a highly significant difference ($P < 0.001$).

Roederer et al.[303] studied 167 asymptomatic cases referred to their laboratory, using the noninvasive duplex Doppler technique. Follow-up at 6-month intervals was attempted and was successful for 103 cases at 6 months, 95 cases at 12 months, 64 cases at 24 months, and 17 cases at 36 months. Some degree of progression was documented in 60 percent of cases. Overall, symptoms occurred in 10 cases (TIAs in 6, stroke in 4), accompanied by disease progression in 8. Within 6 months, occlusion occurred in 1 of 5 patients with 80 to 90 percent stenosis; in 7 of 46 cases stenosis increased from initially 50 to 79 percent to 80 to 99 percent; in 4 of 67 cases stenosis increased from initially 16 to 49 percent to 50 to 79 percent. At 24 months, of 33 patients initially 50 to 79 percent stenosed, occlusion occurred in 2, and in 2 stenosis increased to 80 to 99 percent, while of 38 patients initially 16 to 49 percent stenosed, occlusion occurred in 1, 1 became 80 to 99 percent stenosed, and in 7 stenosis increased to 50 to 79 percent. At 3 years, of 11 patients initially 50 to 79 percent stenosed, occlusion occurred in 1, and 2 advanced to 80 to 99 percent stenosis.

Only anecdotal information exists concerning the evolution of lesions already hemodynamically significant when discovered. At times, a dramatic worsening in the degree of stenosis is observed over periods of weeks to months. Other cases, even with pinpoint stenosis, may remain static for years.[186] Of the 183 cases studied by Roederer et al.,[303] 5 had 80 to 99 percent stenosis initially. In 1 case occlusion occurred without symptoms. Of the remaining 4 patients, 1 experienced TIAs, during the first 6 months and underwent endarterectomy. The fate of the others was unreported, but presumably they also underwent surgery, as they were not accounted for in the report at 12 months.

### *Rapid Increase in Stenosis*

That a minor plaque of atherosclerosis could lead to sudden and dramatic increase of the stenosis was explained in some cases by subintimal hemorrhage.[232]

The frequency of such sudden change is not well understood, although estimates ranging over 85 percent have been given.[232] Evidence on this point has been the most difficult to find. Mural thrombus incorporated into the arterial wall may be a cause. Some of the cases may represent arterial dissection, a frequent, if often misdiagnosed, cause of these dramatic sudden lesions; the subject is discussed in more detail below. In the few cases followed, there has been little evidence that sudden worsening occurs. Roederer et al.[303] documented only three instances of disease progression from less than 50 percent stenosis to occlusion between two successive studies. In all three, the planned 6-month interval examinations did not occur, for various reasons. For two of them, the interval between examinations was 12 months and for two others, fully 24 months, in all instances too long a period to determine the rate at which the progression occurred. In all of the cases studied at regular intervals, no instances of dramatic progression were encountered.

## Intracranial Internal Carotid Artery Atherosclerosis

It is well known that most of the significant atherosclerotic lesions of the ICA develop at the origin (carotid sinus) of the ICA and/or at the bifurcation of the common carotid artery. Yet the incidence of such lesions in the intracranial ICA is not negligible. Hulqvist,[179] in a pioneer work, found primary ICA occlusion to occur in a third of the cases near the origin of the ophthalmic artery. Torvik and Jorgensen[352–355] found 14 among 29 recent thrombotic occlusions of the internal carotid artery located in the extracranial as compared with 15 located in the intracranial part of the vessel. Castaigne et al.[57] found that 6 of 27 (22.2 percent) atherosclerotic thrombotic occlusions of the ICA had started in the distal ICA.

Although atherosclerotic lesions have been documented in several pathologic studies, further consideration is given here only to those reports in which the ICA was examined throughout its length. The evaluation of the degree of stenosis of the carotid siphon at autopsy is fraught with difficulties resulting from the marked tendency of this part of the artery to calcification, which often results in fracture when cut, making detailed studies difficult. Samuel[313] reported 85 cases over the age of 45 in which all ICA lesions were atherosclerotic. Atherosclerosis affected the petrous portion in 27 instances, especially in the regions of its two curvatures. The involvement was less extensive than that of the sinus, cavernous, and supraclinoid segments. In one case an occlusion was present only in the petrous portion. The cavernous part was second after the sinus in order of frequency of atherosclerosis, involved in 59 instances, twice very severely. Lesions were mostly situated on the inner curves of the artery.

Such a predilection of lesions for inner curvatures has also been reported by others.[249] However, Fisher et al.[128] found that the outer curve and other parts (of the carotid siphon) were by no means spared, and Zülch[405] depicted lesions on both the outer and inner curvatures of the siphon.

Yates and Hutchinson[396] reported 100 cases in which the clinical picture had suggested ischemia and from which obvious cases of cerebral embolism in young adults with mitral stenosis had been excluded. Lesions of vessels of 0.5 mm or greater in diameter were either atheroma or occlusions by thrombus. Stenoses that reduced the lumen by about half the cross-sectional area ("grade 2") or complete occlusion or severe stenosis where the lumen was less than 1 mm in diameter ("grade 3") were called "significant." Stenoses of the cavernous and supraclinoid ("intradural") parts were found in 3 instances, as compared with 67 instances of such lesions in the carotid sinus. In another 3 cases the primary occlusion by thrombus was found in the petrous portion.

Torvik and Jorgensen[352–355] studied a consecutive series of 994 autopsies and found 15 recent thrombotic occlusions in the intracranial ICA, "the great majority" of which were superimposed upon atherosclerotic stenoses. Other occlusions were either embolic (see below), unclassified, or old. Stenoses found were "roughly averaged" as follows:

Grade 1: reduction of the lumen by less than one-quarter of the square area
Grade 2: reduction of the lumen by one-quarter to one-half the square area
Grade 3: reduction of the lumen by more than one-half the square area

Of the patients with carotid artery occlusion, 29 had grade 2 or grade 3 atherosclerotic stenoses, but 6 of them had embolic occlusions and 8 had unclassified occlusions. Of 25 patients, 10 (40 percent) with extracranial carotid artery occlusion had grade 3 stenoses of the intracranial ICA. Among those 25 extracranial occlusions 1 was embolic, 5 were unclassified, and 6 were old.

Mitchell and Schwartz[249] had 93 cases selected on the criterion of age over 35. They distinguished the "petrous carotid" and the "terminal carotid." Stenoses were graded as follows:

No stenosis: no reduction in the diameter of the arterial lumen
Moderate stenosis: more than one-half the diameter of the original lumen remained
Severe stenosis: less than one-half the diameter of the original lumen remained

A low prevalence of severe stenosis was found in the petrous part. A slightly higher prevalence, about 5 percent, was noted in the terminal carotid. When moderate and severe stenoses were added, percentages were of course higher. Among 186 internal carotid artery stenoses (93 patients), there were 17 stenoses (9 percent) on the petrous part and 50 (26 percent) on the terminal part.

Fisher et al.[128] studied atherosclerosis of the carotid and vertebral arteries in 178 unselected autopsies. Although they acknowledged that their series was not entirely random, they deemed that cases of brain diseases probably had a higher incidence than a completely random series would have had. Grades of stenoses were based visually on the cross-sectional area obliterated:

Grade 0: 0 to 24 percent
Grade 1: 25 to 49 percent
Grade 2: 50 to 75 percent
Grade 3: more than 75 percent but not occluded
Grade 4: total occlusion

There were 15 occlusions in the neck at the carotid sinus. No occlusion was found higher up. All grade 3 stenoses were at the carotid sinus. The second striking site of predilection for atherosclerosis was the region of the carotid siphon. However, in this study stenoses of the intracranial ICA were not graded. Instead, Fisher et al.[129] stressed the difficulties of assessing correctly the degree of stenosis of the calcified siphon, citing the same reasons mentioned earlier.

Lhermitte and colleagues[216] reported 75 cases from a neurologic ward. Atherosclerotic stenoses were graded on the cross-sectional area obliterated:

Grade 0: none or insignificant stenosis
Grade 1: less than 75 percent stenosis
Grade 2: more than 75 percent stenosis
Grade 3: occlusion

The intracranial ICA was divided into petrous and terminal, that is, cavernous + supraclinoid. There were 9 stenoses, all of grade 1 in the petrous stretch and 20 stenoses (18, grade 1; 2, grade 2) in the terminal part. For comparison there were 41 stenoses (28, grade 1; 13, grade 2) in the sinuses. Occlusion was present in 18 instances, always thrombotic. Thrombosis had started 11 times in the sinus, twice in the siphon, and in 5 cases the starting point remained undetermined.

The addition of angiographic evidence sheds further light on the relative prevalence of lesions in the different parts of the intracranial ICA. Marzewski et al.[238] reported 66 patients with 85 greater than 50 percent stenoses of the intracranial ICA: 14 stenoses were petrous, 65 cavernous, and 6 supraclinoid; 19 patients (28 percent) had bilateral intracranial ICA stenoses. Craig et al.[73] reported 58 patients with 58 intracranial ICA stenoses that reduced the lumen by at least a third of its diameter: 9 were petrous, 42 cavernous, and 7 supraclinoid; 4 patients had lesions in two contiguous segments, for example, petrous and cavernous, and 13 patients (22 percent) had bilateral intracranial ICA stenosis. These data confirm that the cavernous stretch of the artery is the most often stenosed part and showed that bilateral intracranial ICA stenoses are by no means rare.

Despite painstaking studies, the problem of the significance of atherosclerotic lesions of the intracranial ICA is still largely unsettled. Discrepancies between studies in which more occlusions occurred in the intracranial ICA than in the extracranial ICA/ICA and those in which no occlusion occurred in the intracranial ICA are obvious. Useful comparisons between some of the series is difficult if not impossible, since grading was different and occlusions were not always separated from stenoses. These studies appeared from 1956 to 1966 when the hemodynamic significance of stenoses may not have been clear to all pathologists. Today terms such as "significant" or "severe" would probably not be applied to stenoses that reduce the lumen by about half. However, two main facts stand out: the intracranial ICA, especially the cavernous part, is the second site of predilection of atherosclerosis, but the extent and severity of the lesions are far behind those of the carotid sinus; and a number (unspecified) of atherosclerotic primary occlusive thromboses occur in the intracranial ICA.

## Histopathology of Internal Carotid Artery Atheroma

### *Extracranial Stenosis or Occlusion*

In the setting of hemodynamically significant atherostenosis, platelet material, possibly mixed with fibrin complexes, have been shown to superimpose themselves on the atheroma, perhaps forming the usual means by which stenosis is converted to thrombotic occlusion of the lumen.[57,124] In Samuel's study[313] the carotid sinus was found to have up to five successive strata of atherosclerosis, which he attributed to the process of layering of mural thrombi.

The carotid lesions found at operation does not always take the form of a thick mound indenting the wall of the artery. In a few instances[224] a thin band of stenosis has been found obstructing cranial or extracranial vessels. The narrow band is thin enough to be invisible on digital subtraction studies and was easily overlooked on the conventional angiogram. Presumably, turbulent flow apparent on Doppler analysis should allow a diagnosis in a patient whose angiogram fails to demonstrate the appropriate lesion.

Hemorrhage into the wall of the atheroma appears to be a common finding in specimens removed at the time of endarterectomy.[125,182,232,261] Fisher and Ojemann[131] found intraplaque hemorrhages in 34 (38 percent) of 90 carotid endarterectomy specimens, but their small size was not sufficient to significantly compromise the arterial lumen (Fig. 14-4). However, the hemorrhage in most instances appears to contribute little to the overall mass effect of the stenosis,[261,271] with a few dramatic exceptions.[232] Standard computed tomography (CT)[174] and magnetic resonance

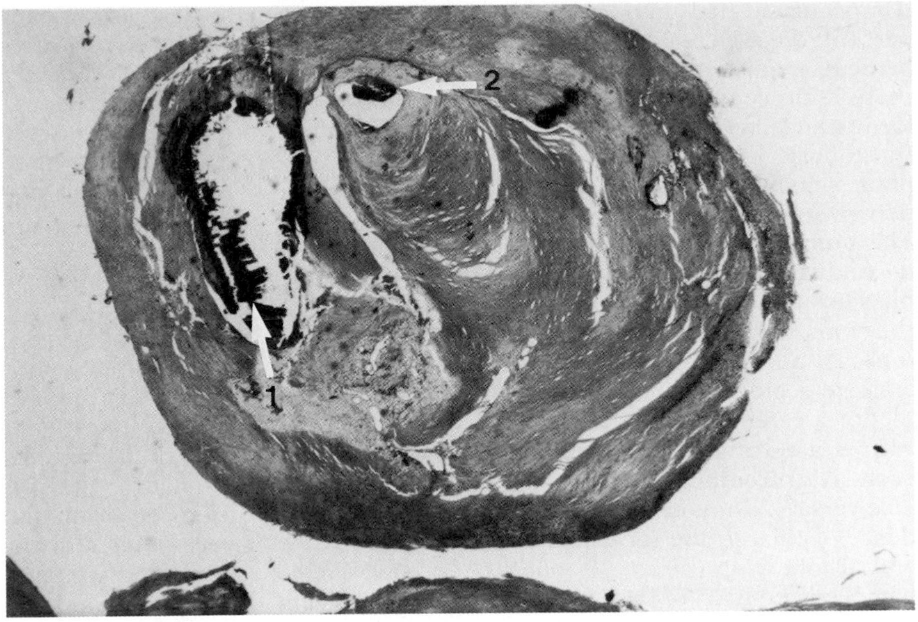


**Fig. 14-4.** Histology of severe stenosis, showing intraplaque hematoma (*1, arrow*) and fibrin-platelet thrombus in lumen (*2, arrow*). (Courtesy of W. Kupsky, MD.)

(MR) imaging[149] at the level of arterial injury has documented intramural carotid hemorrhage, thus providing another method of diagnosis. However, in autopsy series, the subject of intramural hemorrhage has rarely been mentioned.[313] Lennihan et al.[211] found only 2 percent of endarterectomy specimens with wall hemorrhages sufficiently large to explain the stenosis.

### *Intracranial Atherosclerosis*

Atherosclerosis in the intracranial ICA has the same general features as elsewhere in the body.[313] However, one peculiar characteristic is that lesions of the cavernous part very often show a high degree of calcification. Such calcifications account for the dense images seen on radiographs and CT scans; however, calcification of the carotid siphon by no means indicates significant stenosis of the lumen. Mitchell and Schwartz[249] mentioned that medial calcification is seen with particular frequency in the petrous and cavernous parts of the artery. Fisher et al.[129] have given a special and detailed study of calcification of the carotid siphon. They found that calcification increased with age and, in the older age groups, was more pronounced in women. Data about ulceration of plaques are scanty. Mitchell and Schwartz[249] found no ulceration above the carotid sinus, and Fisher et al.[129] mentioned that the intima was not ulcerated.

Occlusion due to "pure" atherosclerosis is uncommon, although pinpoint atherosclerotic stenoses are frequently encountered. Occlusion usually results from superimposed thrombus. Whether there is a relationship between thrombosis and the degree of stenosis is obviously relevant to evaluate the risk of a given stenosis, but there are few data on intracranial ICA stenoses. Castaigne et al.[58] reported 19 unilateral atherosclerotic ICA occlusions, among which 3 had started in the siphon, and 12 bilateral atherosclerotic ICA occlusions, among which 3 had started in both siphons in one patient and one in the siphon and contralateral sinus in another patient. Data suggested differences between unilateral and bilateral occlusions, since among the six primary siphon occlusions two were related to more than 75 percent stenoses, three to 75 to 50 percent stenoses, and one to a less than 50 percent stenosis. Thus 4 of 6 cases of primary occlusive thromboses of the siphon were related to moderate stenoses as compared to only 2 of 21 primary occlusive thrombi of the sinus, all the remaining 19 being related to more than 75 percent stenoses. It may be noted that Yates and Hutchinson[396] mentioned two cases of intracranial ICA primary thrombotic occlusion (case 58: unilateral occlusion of the left ICA; case 93: bilateral ICA occlusion starting in the petrous-cavernous part on the left), in which thrombosis appeared to have been precipitated by a recent hemorrhage into the plaque. A similar case (case 8) was reported by Castaigne and colleagues.[57] It may be that the calcified siphon is brittle and more liable to intramural hemorrhage with subsequent thrombosis.

**Tandem Stenoses.** Stenoses of both the carotid siphon and sinus are another special feature of internal carotid artery atherosclerosis. Craig et al.[73] found only 6 patients (10 percent) with ipsilateral stenoses of siphon and sinus of 33 to 70 percent, but Marzewski et al.,[238] among their 66 patients with an intracranial ICA stenosis of more than 50 percent, found 36 (54 percent) who had 53 extracranial stenoses (24 more than 50 percent; 29 less than 50 percent). In the series of Castaigne et al.[58] only 2 of 6 patients with bilateral

ICA occlusion had tandem stenoses of more than 75 percent; there were 27 patients with one more than 75 percent stenosis, and in every case stenoses of less than 50 percent were present elsewhere on the ICA; for instance, in 16 unilateral ICA occlusions in which thrombosis had started in the sinus, there were siphon stenoses in every case: 60 percent, 1 case; 50 percent, 4 cases; less than 50 percent, eleven cases. The number of reported tandem stenoses of course depends upon the degree of stenosis required for admission in a given series, but concomitant lesions of the sinus and siphon are at least fairly frequent. This makes it all the more difficult, and sometimes impossible, to decide which of the two lesions was responsible for a cerebral ischemic event.

Does a carotid siphon stenosis increase the risk of occlusive thrombosis of a carotid sinus stenosis and vice versa? Castaigne et al.[58] did not find positive evidence of this. In the series from Craig et al.,[73] at the end of follow-up (mean, 30 months), cerebral events had occurred in 25 of the 58 patients (43 percent), and none of these events was in the 6 patients with tandem stenoses. Marzewski et al.[238] followed their 66 patients for a mean of 3.9 years. Eight had isolated TIAs during this period, and seven of the eight had ipsilateral stenoses in their reference angiograms. Among these, 7.5 had tandem stenoses. In the same series 10 strokes in all distributions occurred: 2 were in 30 patients (7 percent) without tandem stenoses on their reference angiograms, while 8 were among 36 patients (22 percent) with tandem stenoses ($P = 0.08$). In five of the eight stroke patients with tandem stenoses the extracranial stenosis was less than 50 percent. Marzewski et al.[238] concluded that patients with extracranial and intracranial ICA disease appear to have the greater stroke risk, which probably reflects more advanced atherosclerotic disease.

It has been stated that tandem stenoses increase the risk of carotid endarterectomy, and this is probably a widely held opinion in many neurologic and surgical circles. However, firm evidence is not available. In a report with a particularly disquieting rate of mortality after carotid endarterectomy a useful comparison between angiographic findings and operative results could not be made.[97] In one report,[319] the outcome from carotid bifurcation endarterectomy was compared in 79 cases with 91 stenoses between the 47 patients with bifurcation disease only and the 44 patients with additional tandem lesions of carotid siphon stenosis. No statistically significant differences were encountered among the strokes occurring in the intraoperative (0 vs 2), perioperative (0 vs 3), or later postoperative (4 vs 2) periods, although the crude figures might seem to suggest otherwise.

In some instances, the intracranial stenosis seems to have been an impersistent finding: Little et al.[226] found two such instances whose "stenosis" had vanished on the postendarterectomy angiogram. The authors raised the possibility that the finding was an artifact of "pseudo-occlusion." Day and colleagues[79] reported two cases of resolving supraclinoid stenosis following endarterectomy of the ICA origin. It was unclear whether the intracranial ICA narrowing was due to atherosclerosis or atherosclerosis plus mural thrombus or embolism. Such data deserve attention for it may be that unknown relationships exist between tandem stenoses, the understanding of which could shed light upon fundamental and therapeutic aspects of atherosclerosis.

**Anterograde and Retrograde Secondary Thrombosis.** Anterograde and retrograde secondary thrombosis of the intracranial ICA is a subject for which only a scanty literature exists. Primary thrombotic occlusion of the carotid sinus is, in most cases, followed by extensive "stagnation" thrombosis. However, occlusions occasionally remain segmental. Pathologically well-studied instances of intracranial ICA thrombotic occlusion are rare. In Yates and Hutchinson's cases[396] 58, 72, 78, and 93, the intracranial ICA was occluded by thrombus, but data are lacking about anterograde and retrograde thrombus. In cases 58 and 93 (case 93 was a bilateral ICA occlusion), the rostral part of the plug remained proximal to the posterior communicating artery, and there was no pericerebral occlusion. In both cases an ipsilateral hemispheral infarct was present. In case 72 there was no cerebral infarct; the occluding material was old. In Torvik and Jorgensen's[352–355] 28 intracranial ICA occlusions, 5 showed anterograde thrombus, 6 retrograde thrombus, 1 both antero- and retrograde thrombus, and 16 showed none. However, these "primary" occlusions were "thromboembolic," and the part of atherosclerotic occlusion cannot be estimated. Nevertheless Torvik and Jorgensen mentioned that all occlusions that were more than a month and a half old were longer than 2 cm and that in three of seven cases with retrograde propagation, the thrombus extended down to the extracranial division of the artery. In the study by Castaigne et al.[58] of six primary occlusions of the carotid siphon, two had no retrograde thrombosis (one of them was a very short occlusion between the origins of the ophthalmic and posterior communicating arteries), in one a retrograde thrombus extended to the cervical part of the artery, and in three the thrombus extended down to the ICA origin. Luessenhop[231] found that when angiography was performed during the first month following the onset of symptoms, 31 percent of the occlusions were in the region of the carotid siphon, but with the passage of time this percentage decreased and became close to zero by 30 months. He thought that this was undoubtedly a consequence of propagation of the thrombi proximally. Most probably, in this series not all occlusions were of atherosclerotic origin.

Based on this literature, it seems reasonable to assume that retrograde thrombi developing down to the ICA origin are not rare. Thus arrest of contrast medium at the sinus on angiograms does not allow firm conclusions as to where the primary occlusion started, inasmuch as the angiographic appearance of the proximal end of carotid occlusion is not of predictive value about the age of the occlusion, at least within the first 6 days from stroke onset.[280]

**Discontinuous Occlusions.** The presence of a patent segment of the ICA between extracranial ICA and intracranial ICA may be found at autopsy, indicating discontinuous occlusion, and it may be difficult or impossible to decide whether the distal plug is thrombotic or embolic.[57,58,352–355] This pathologic situation should be kept in mind as a source of technical difficulties in surgical endarterectomies to remove occlusions of the ICA.

## Associated Atheromatous Lesions and Conditions

Concomitant stenoses or occlusions of the contralateral ICA sinus and of the intracranial arteries are not rare. Besides, in the Mitchell and Schwartz series[249] a strong correlation existed between the degree of carotid and iliac stenosis and the severity of coronary stenosis. The coronary-carotid relationship was present in all age groups in men and in the older age group in women. In men with cardiac infarcts and a high prevalence of severe coronary stenosis the relationship was even more striking. A positive correlation existed also between complicated, that is, ulcerated, calcified, or thrombosed, aortic atherosclerosis and carotid artery stenoses in men. However, in this series the correlation was not specifically studied for the intracranial ICA. In the two recent clinical-angiographic studies of intracranial ICA atherosclerosis by Craig et al.[73] and Marzewski et al.,[238] coronary artery disease was present in 57.6 percent and 48 percent of the patients, peripheral vascular disease in 15.2 percent, hypertension in 39.4 percent and 68 percent, and diabetes mellitus in 50 percent and 39 percent, respectively. In the 58 patients reported by Craig et al.,[73] most had at least two of the above conditions. Thus atherosclerotic disease of the intracranial ICA is part of a widespread atherosclerosis with a high prevalence of the two main risk factors. This accounts in part at least for its poor prognosis.

## Cardiac Embolism

The large series of postmortem cases were often biased toward atherosclerosis. For instance, Fisher et al.[128] did not include embolism to the ICA bifurcation, and Yates and Hutchinson[396] excluded cases of embolism from mitral stenosis in young patients. Torvik and Jorgensen[352–355] found that less than one-fifth of all cerebral emboli were located in the carotid arteries, as emboli tend to lodge in more distal parts of the vessels. Nevertheless, among 43 recent ICA occlusions, 8 were embolic as compared to 27 that were thrombotic, and 8 were unclassified. Blackwood et al.[32] found in 105 patients with infarcts in the ICA territory that cardiac embolism was responsible in 48 (45.7 percent). Among 61 instances of ICA occlusion, Castaigne et al.[58] found 13 cases (21.3 percent) that were due to cardiac embolism.

The true prevalence of ICA embolic occlusion is probably underestimated for three main reasons: first, emboli found at the time of postmortem examination in the pericerebral arteries may well have lodged initially in the ICA and subsequently dislodged and drifted downstream; second, in cases with patent arteries circumstantial evidence is often suggestive of embolism, and at the time of infarction the embolus may well have been for some time lodged in the ICA;[215] and finally, there has always been a tendency to perform fewer angiographies in cases of clinically obvious embolism than in cases presumed to result from atherosclerosis; a recent cooperative study on cerebral embolism did not include angiography in the protocol.[22] This being so, Torvik and Jorgensen[352–355] found at autopsy seven emboli impacted in the intracranial ICA, as compared to one in the carotid sinus. Blackwood et al.[32] mentioned that common sites for lodgement of emboli were at the middle trifurcation and in the distal ICA, in accordance with the findings of Bladin.[33] Castaigne et al.,[58] among 13 embolic ICA occlusions (one from a thrombus of the aortic arch), found 8 instances of block of the intracranial ICA. The emboli were often several centimeters long and patterns of occlusion were complex: one with embolic separate occlusion of extracranial ICA and intracranial ICA, three with occlusions of intracranial ICA, two with an embolus astride the ICA and middle cerebral artery, two astride the ICA, middle cerebral artery, and anterior cerebral artery.

Anterograde thrombus after intracranial ICA embolic occlusion is probably fairly common.[28,58,352–355] Retrograde thrombus may also develop,[352–355] and it has been reported that a "tailing off" appearance of the column of contrast material in the more proximal artery is suggestive of retrograde thrombus extension from occlusion of the supraclinoid ICA where angiography is performed in the first 1 or 2 days.[98] However, Castaigne et al.[58] have reported that a significant retrograde thrombus was not present in any of their cases of embolic intracranial ICA occlusion when autopsied from 18 hours to 3½ months after the stroke. Probably in some of these cases the ophthalmic artery and perhaps the posterior communicating artery remained patent.

The site of impaction of an embolus in a given artery depends on its size and on the configuration of the vessel, branchings being likely sites of arrest of the traveling plug. In some cardiac diseases emboli of a size such as to block the femoral or iliac arteries are not rare. Therefore, embolic ICA occlusion is not unexpected. The bifurcation of the common carotid artery is the first likely site of arrest, then the tortuous intracranial ICA and the bifurcation of its supraclinoid part.

The theories of cardiac embolism have changed during the last decades.[215] Today nonrheumatic atrial fibrillation is likely to be the first responsible condition, followed by postinfarction mural thrombus, although no definite data appear to be available. Conditions like mitral valve prolapse are likely to result in small emboli, which should lodge in pericerebral arteries. In a study of 24 cases of "brain events" (21 cerebral infarcts or TIAs; 1 retinal branch occlusion; 2 seizures) in patients with mitral valve prolapse, angiography being performed in 22 patients, no occlusion of the intracranial ICA was reported.[160] Work emerging on the frequency of patent cardiac foramen ovale indicates that transcardiac emboli are not rare but we do not know yet of an example occluding the carotid artery itself. Permanent intracranial ICA occlusion from such causes is probably not frequent.

## Other Sources of Extracranial Internal Carotid Artery Disease

Apart from atherosclerosis, other causes of carotid artery occlusion include dissection and even embolism from the heart or great vessels. Others approach the status of medical curiosities.

### Arterial Dissection

In recent years, internal carotid artery dissection, either spontaneous or traumatic, has become an important recognized cause of TIAs and stroke within hours or weeks of known trauma,[44,132,234,255,270,271,292,336] warranting its complete presentation elsewhere in this volume.

The pathogenesis of dissection involves the development of a hematoma in the arterial wall either at a subintimal or subadventitial position. A subintimal hematoma may lead to narrowing of the true arterial lumen over a long segment, allowing a stagnation thrombus to completely occlude or serve as an embolic source for distal branch occlusion. Hematoma development in the subadventitial portion may not compromise the true arterial lumen, but an aneurysmal dilatation or pouch may collect thrombus and serve as an embolic source into the distal circulation. The arterial disruption seen with dissection is known to heal with time, as documented by serial angiography. Whether this arteriopathy occurs spontaneously because of an underlying arterial defect and/or in response to trivial trauma such as coughing, sneezing, head-turning, and other normal activities, must be determined on a case-by-case basis.

Hart and Easton[167] have reviewed the major presenting complaints in patients with proven carotid dissection and found that cerebral infarction occurred in 33 percent (23 percent were minor, 10 percent were major or fatal), transient ischemic attacks occurred in 45 percent, head and neck pain in 16 percent, pulsatile tinnitus in 4 percent, and asymptomatic bruits in only 2 percent. Sometimes dissection can be suggested by the clinical presentation if unilateral face or head pain in association with Horner's syndrome and TIAs or stroke is present in a young, otherwise healthy, patient. However, the diagnosis usually rests on angiographic features that include the "string sign,"[132] characterizing a tiny, long segment of contrast in the true lumen of the artery, aneurysmal pouch formation, and the distal location of the arteriopathy compared to atheromatous disease, which tends to accumulate at the bifurcation area. Standard CT[174] and MR imaging[149] at the level of arterial injury has documented intramural carotid hemorrhage, thus providing another method of diagnosis.

The natural history and treatment outcome of carotid dissection has not been studied in a controlled fashion, but the weight of case reports[167] strongly suggests that the outcome is benign in over 90 percent of patients. Surgical treatment either in the form of extracranial carotid thrombectomy or extracranial/intracranial bypass grafting appears unnecessary in the overwhelming majority of patients. The role of anticoagulation and antiplatelet agents is unsettled. A controlled, randomized study will be necessary to establish the efficacy of treatment in those patients with an unstable condition, but would be difficult to mount given the low frequency of the disorder.

### Fibromuscular Dysplasia

A rare condition, fibromuscular dysplasia is encountered in less than 0.6 percent of cases of internal carotid artery disease.[69] It may account for kinks (see below). Intracranial aneurysm occurs in almost 25 percent of cases (see below). Its clinical importance is unclear, but it has often been the subject of publications, and is discussed elsewhere in this volume.

### Arterial Kinks

Kinking of the internal carotid artery may achieve the same hemodynamic effects as atheromatous stenosis. Kinking of the carotid artery is an acquired condition and is not identical with coiling of the carotid, which is believed to be congenital and of no significance clinically.[63,68] Kinking is thought to be caused by atherosclerosis or as a complication of fibromuscular dysplasia.

Its significance arises when positional head changes produce transient cerebral ischemia, a situation in which dramatic reductions in cerebral blood flow have been documented in some cases during intraoperative studies;[333] as yet, the degree of stenosis observed angiographically has not proved to be an adequate basis to determine the need for corrective surgery without the additional studies of the effect of head position change.

Kinking caused by alteration in artery position appears to be a rare cause of transient ischemic attacks. Handa et al.[159] described a case of recurrent transient ischemic attacks following extracranial to intracranial bypass precipitated by yawning. The stretching and kinking of the donor artery by the mouth opening during the yawning was the alleged mechanism.

## Extracranial Internal Carotid Artery Aneurysm

Extracranial ICA aneurysms are very unusual lesions.[68] They are usually the sequelae of a dissecting aneurysm. Only 34 were reported among 8,500 peripheral vascular aneurysms in one large center over a 12-year period.[243] They usually present as a pulsatile mass in the neck. The neurologic symptoms may present with cerebral embolization in addition to the expected syndrome of rupture.[372]

## Complications of Head and Neck Cancer

Primary tumors of the vascular structures are uncommon, usually arising from mesoblastic and neural elements as chemodectomas or paragangliomas.[245] Only 5 percent are bilateral. The mass grows slowly, presenting as dysphagia and hoarseness, although dyspnea, Horner's syndrome, and facial pain may also occur.[161] They produce metastases only in some 2 percent of cases. Local recurrence is uncommon and usually is delayed many years.

Involvement of the extracranial carotid by direct extension of local tumor is distinctly uncommon.[154] However, in hospitals with a large oncology caseload, this complication occurs often enough to warrant consideration. Direct tumor invasion of the arterial wall was described in 37 of 64 carotid arteries taken from patients with head or neck cancer in a study at Memorial Hospital in New York.[182] Three examples of such involvement in the siphon from parasellar tumors were reported by Spallone:[331] two were meningiomas, the third a pituitary adenoma. This complication appears to be extremely rare, having been encountered by Spallone in only three cases among more than 10,000 angiographic examinations surveyed in his institution over a period of approximately 25 years.

Radiation-induced accelerated atherosclerosis has received limited attention but is a recognized complication of radiation given to the head and neck. Huvos et al.[182] found this form of atherosclerosis in 15 of their 64 cases of head and neck tumor with carotid complications. Supervoltage therapy had been given to 24 of the patients, and 45 had had preoperative radiation therapy to the neck. Levinson et al.[214] described three patients with atypical presumably atherosclerotic lesions that developed more than 25 years after external cervical irradiation. The syndromes presented from a variety of inferred mechanisms included cerebral embolization, impaired retinal profusion, and decreased total cerebral profusion. Arterial reconstruction was possible in the stenotic lesions but not in the occluded case.

## Coexisting Intracranial Arterial Aneurysms

Intracranial aneurysms distal to a symptomatic carotid stenosis is uncommonly encountered.[83,110,289,326] The occurrence appears to be entirely coincidental and not causally related. The main issue is whether surgical management of the carotid disease will influence the course of the aneurysm and encourage its rupture or enlargement. In the handful of cases reported, the aneurysm(s) showed no change in size on follow-up angiography postoperative from the carotid endarterectomy at intervals of 1 week,[83] 7 months,[326] and 1 year.[110] The difficulty in predicting the course of an asymptomatic aneurysm is well known,[30,397] and some[289] have recommended prophylactic repair. The scanty data that exist seem to indicate that the carotid lesion can be attacked with no concern for acute aneurysmal rupture.

## Immediate Postoperative Stenosis or Occlusion

It was long assumed that immediate postoperative stenosis or occlusion was uncommon, and deemed not worth the risk of complications from conventional angiography to check on the postoperative status in otherwise asymptomatic patients. Check on the status of the carotid was usually undertaken only in instances of the many and varied focal neurologic deficits apparent postoperatively.[218] Few studies using intraoperative angiography have been reported. Scott et al.[321] found 56 defects, 18 requiring surgical revision, in their series of 137 endarterectomies. This worrisome finding is difficult to interpret, as the authors experienced rates of perioperative stroke (6.8 percent) and death (4.8 percent) that are a bit above the lower rates hoped for in a surgical series. However, the point seemed well taken that intraoperative angiography might help to identify the immediate technical problems.

With the introduction of noninvasive scanning and digital subtraction angiography, the possibilities of morbidity from investigation alone have been reduced to negligible levels. With that reduction has come better documentation of a disappointingly higher incidence of postoperative stenosis and occlusion than was earlier anticipated. Like all clinical series, the incidence of such complications appeared to be inversely proportional to the surgical success, which varies considerably. Among 262 carotid reconstructions studied by digital subtraction angiography, Hertzer et al.[171] documented 5 internal carotid artery occlusions (1.9 percent), 2 of which had neurologic complications, and 2 had more than 30 percent stenosis. Occult carotid artery occlusion was not the only cause for stroke: the angiogram was normal in 4 others with neurologic complications.

Duplex scanning and spectral analysis have shown a higher incidence of postoperative stenosis than is usually appreciated on clinical grounds alone. Ziegler et al.[404] found an overall incidence of persistent high-grade stenosis in fully 19 percent of the cases studied by these methods. Recurrent neurologic symptoms occurred in eight of these cases. The authors believe that the transient nature of some early postoperative stenosis is consistent with proliferation and regression of myointimal lesions in response to arterial injury.

### Recurrence of Stenosis or Occlusion after Endarterectomy

For years, recurrent stenosis after successful endarterectomy was thought to be uncommon. As a treatment, the endarterectomy was considered in most cases to be definitive. In early studies based on recurrent symptoms that led to reangiogram, the incidence of recurrent stenosis varied from 0.6 percent to 9.8 percent.[49] Newer methods of following the course of the postoperative carotid artery have indicated that recurrence and even residual stenosis may be more common than suspected on clinical grounds alone. The 64 cases followed from 1 to 13 years postendarterectomy by Norrving et al.[268] showed occlusion or recurrent stenosis (defined as more than 50 percent) in fully 36 percent of operated cases, which seemed equivalent to the 27 percent rate of progression on the nonoperated, previously asymptomatic, side. About 30 percent of the cases with progressing disease became symptomatic with transient ischemic attacks or strokes. By contrast, only 5.5 percent of the vessels showing no progression of the disease process had symptoms, a highly significant difference ($P < 0.001$).

Two types of recurrence are most frequently recognized: (1) restenosis develops within a few months up to 2 years, and frequently the finding is that of a fibrous hyperplasia reaction;[49] and (2) stenoses occurring beyond 2 years are frequently conventional atheromatous lesions and are sometimes associated with persistent hypertriglyceridemia or hyperlipidemia. The factors contributing to early restenosis include difficulties with surgical technique and hyperlipidemia encouraging severe atherosclerotic formation.

## Miscellaneous Pathologic Disorders of the Intracranial Internal Carotid Artery

In this brief review it is convenient to consider the three anatomic parts of the intracranial ICA separately.

### Petrous Part

The petrous portion of the ICA is separated from the inner ear by bone that is very thin in the infant and child. In addition, the distal part of the cervical ICA is close to the throat, tonsillar fossa, and lymph nodes. Cases with occlusion or stenosis of the intracranial ICA (and in some of the pericerebral branches) have been reported by Shillito[324] and Bickerstaff[29] in children with infection of the ears, throat, nose, or paranasal sinuses, or after tonsillectomy. In some of Shillito's cases and in a comparable case of Banker's,[16] pathologic evidence of acute arteritis was present. When the internal carotid artery erodes the bone it may appear as a red mass in the middle ear when viewed through the tympanic membrane; biopsy in pursuit of a diagnosis can have disastrous consequences.[8] Fractures of the petrous bone can conceivably result in ICA trauma and thus lead to thrombus and/or embolism, but no positive report of that appears to be available.

### Cavernous Part

Stenoses and occlusions of the cavernous segment of the ICA in cavernous sinus infections has been reported in children[29,239,371] and in adults.[31] The intracavernous ICA may also be stenosed by the nonspecific granulomatous arteritis reported by Tolosa.[347] The petrous and cavernous portions can be involved in cranial giant cell arteritis.[380] Meningiomas developed in the sinus can stenose the carotid siphon. Stenosis of the cavernous portion has been described in cluster headache, and it has been speculated that the sympathetic fiber involvement could explain the oculosympathetic paralysis.[106]

### Supraclinoid Part

The supraclinoid part of the artery lies in the spinal fluid space. It may thus be involved by the process of endarteritis obliterans in chronic or subacute meningitides due to syphilis (meningovascular syphilis, Heubner's arteritis), tuberculosis, or pyogenic bacteria, for example, *Pneumococcus.* Stenosis or occlusion results from hyperplasia of subendothelial tissue.[15] Direct invasions of the ICA by hyphae in mucormycosis with infection of the sinus, orbit, and meninges has been reported in a 3-year-old boy.[16] Dissecting aneurysm may involve intracranial arteries, and in 13 of 58 cases the terminal ICA and its branches were affected.[31] Stenosis and occlusion of the intracranial ICA have been reported in drug addicts.[330,391] Thus the supraclinoid siphon is involved in vasospasm, likely due to acute hypertension.[141]

*Moyamoya* is a Japanese word meaning "something hazy like a puff of cigarette smoke drifting in the air."[338] This disorder is the subject of Chapter 26. Here we make only brief mention of those cases involving the intracranial ICA. The condition refers to an angiographic appearance resulting from the enlargement of numerous small collateral channels associated with stenosis or occlusion of the supraclinoid ICA on both sides. It is rare for the stenosis to extend below the level of the 3rd cervical vertebra.[286] Postmortem examinations have been few, and the characteristics of the obstructing arterial process are poorly known but are attributed to subintimal proliferation. An unusual case without intracranial ICA stenoses has been reported.[64] Data supporting congenital and acquired forms have been recorded. Suzuki and Kodama[338] have been impressed by the high prevalence of past inflammations in the head or neck. A stenosis of the carotid siphon with occlusion of the supraclinoid portion and moyamoya have been reported 6 years after irradiation of a pituitary tumor.[24]

### Spontaneous Resolution of Extracranial Disease

Spontaneous resolution of occlusive lesions on the carotid artery may be more common than has been appreciated.[194] Resolving lesions include those due to arterial dissection, fibromuscular dysplasia, and even atheromatous lesions.

## COLLATERAL BLOOD FLOW FOR THE INTERNAL CAROTID ARTERY

When the internal carotid artery is unable to supply its usual territory distally, five major sources of collateral may develop, in a number of variations.[46,204,359]

The most readily recognized extracranial source of collateral is the anastomosis with the internal carotid artery through the orbit. Blood flows anterograde up the external carotid to the orbit where anastomoses occur with the ophthalmic branch of the intracranial internal carotid artery. The anastomoses mainly occur between the maxillary branch of the external carotid artery and the ophthalmic artery in the floor of the orbit (Fig. 14-5). Smaller anastomoses occur over the roof of the orbit between the facial and frontal branches of the external carotid artery and the supratrochlear and supraorbital branches of the ophthalmic artery. From these anastomoses blood flows retrograde in the ophthalmic artery to reach the intracranial portion of the internal carotid artery at the siphon. From there the flow continues distally toward the circle of Willis in the usual anterograde fashion. This collateral is often demonstrated angiographically. Minor variations exist in the anastomosis pattern in the orbit. Collateral to the ophthalmic artery may come from meningeal branches of the external carotid. Rarely, the ophthalmic artery is not a branch of the internal carotid, receiving instead its entire flow from the meningeal artery, a linkage which offers little intracranial supply to the circle of Willis.

The most important source of collateral for a hemisphere comes from the contralateral internal carotid artery via the circle of Willis (Fig. 14-6). In this case, blood flows anterograde up the opposite internal carotid, thence across the circle of Willis at the anterior communicating artery, from which it passes, on the

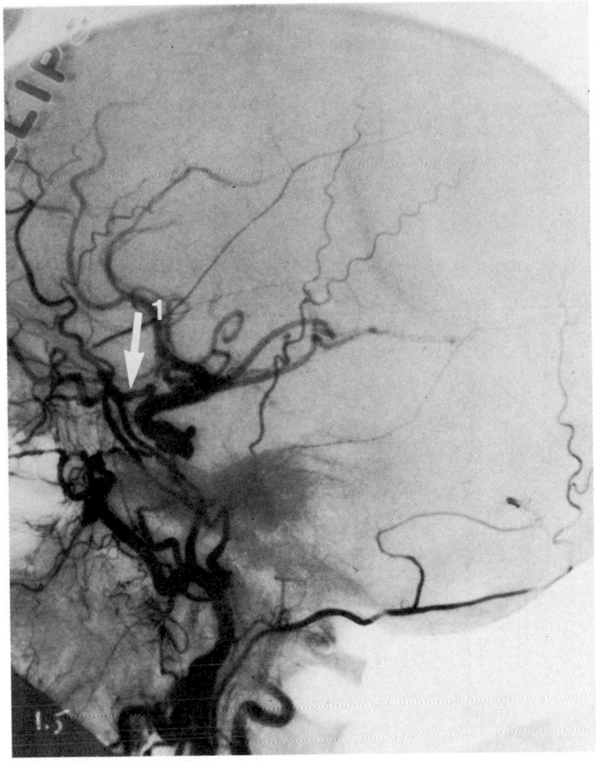


**Fig. 14-5.** Sources of collateral to the internal carotid territory. Ophthalmic artery (*1, arrow*).

one hand, anterograde along the cortical branches of the anterior cerebral artery, and on the other hand, retrograde along the stem of the anterior cerebral artery to the middle cerebral artery stem, and thence distally into the territory of the middle cerebral artery in the usual anterograde fashion. This form of collateral depends on an intact anterior half of the circle of Willis. Many minor variations in the circle of Willis conspire to prevent this collateral from developing, among them an azygous anterior cerebral artery, in which the supply to the anterior cerebral artery arises from a common trunk, with no anterior cerebral artery stem on one side to complete the circle of Willis. In such cases, the two anterior cerebral artery territories may be involved with infarction or spared together, depending on the vascular anatomy.

The vertebrobasilar system may supply the middle and anterior cerebral artery territory by means of collateral through the ipsilateral posterior communicating artery. This collateral is the posterior equivalent of the collateral via the anterior half of the circle of Willis. It depends on a patent posterior communicating artery, which occurs far less commonly than does a patent anterior communicating artery. Rarely, the flow into the internal carotid artery territory from the basilar is by way of a persisting trigeminal artery, which usually reaches the internal carotid near the base of the skull (Fig. 14-7).

Flow retrograde from cerebral arteries through the borderzones over the brain surface may spare some or

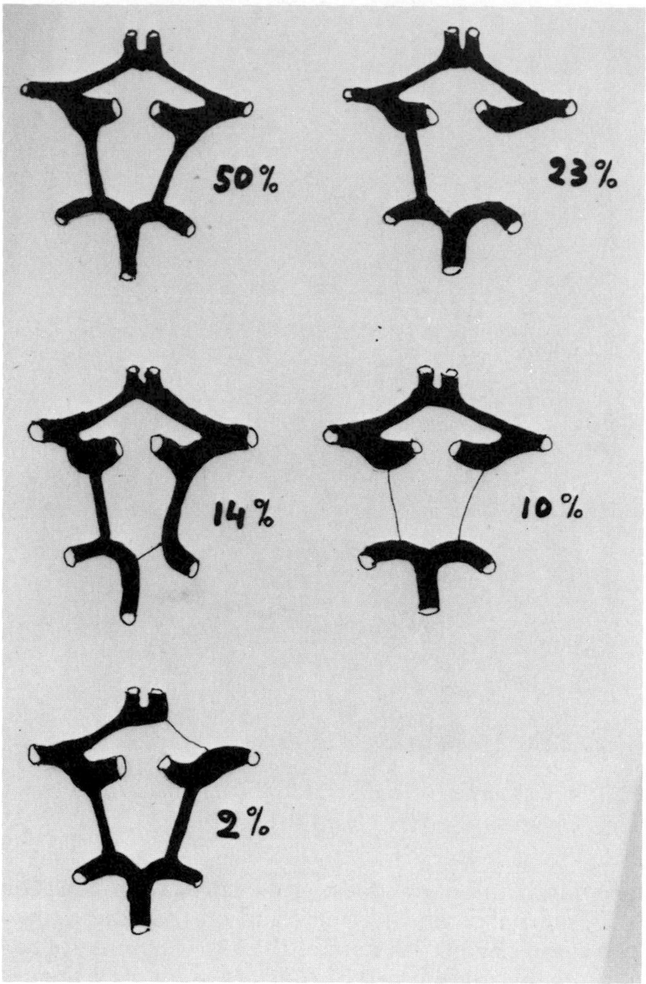


**Fig. 14-6.** Diagram showing the variations in the patterns of the circle of Willis.

all of the cortical surface branches of the endangered arterial territories. In this setting, the anatomy of the circle of Willis plays a vital role: should the posterior communicating artery be too small to carry much collateral, the distal ends of the cortical branches of the posterior cerebral artery may supply collateral to the anterior or middle cerebral artery territories through the borderzone anastomoses over the hemisphere surface; should the stem of the anterior cerebral artery ipsilateral to the occluded internal carotid artery likewise be too small, the anterior cerebral artery may collateralize some or all of the middle cerebral artery surface branches through the borderzone. In such instances, the flow retrograde into the endangered territories varies from full collateral all the way to the stem of the recipient vessel to little more than feeble flow into the distal cortical surface branches.

Other paths of collateral may develop under special circumstances. Cerebral artery surface vessels may anastomose with an extracranial arterial source through a craniotomy site. When the stenosis lies distally, in the intracranial portion of the internal carotid artery, preventing collateral flow via the circle of Willis, not only may cerebral artery surface collaterals develop through the borderzones, but the penetrating arteries (the lenticulostriates) may enlarge within the depths of the brain as well. This condition, met commonly in moyamoya disease has also been encountered in cases of arteriovenous malformations subjected to surgical ligation of the main feeding arteries.[240] Although such anastomoses are rare, they indicate the enormous siphoning effect that may exist in underperfused territories. Their occurrence is also important because they demonstrate the occurrence of fusion of arteries in an adult.

## Clinical Settings for Development of Collateral Blood Flow

In all arterial territories, low perfusion pressure distal to a hemodynamically significant stenosis or occlusion leads to the development of collateral blood flow in the hypoperfused territory. The finding seems to be so familiar to clinicians that few papers on the subject are easily found. Castaigne et al.[58] noted collateral via the ophthalmic artery in every case of in-

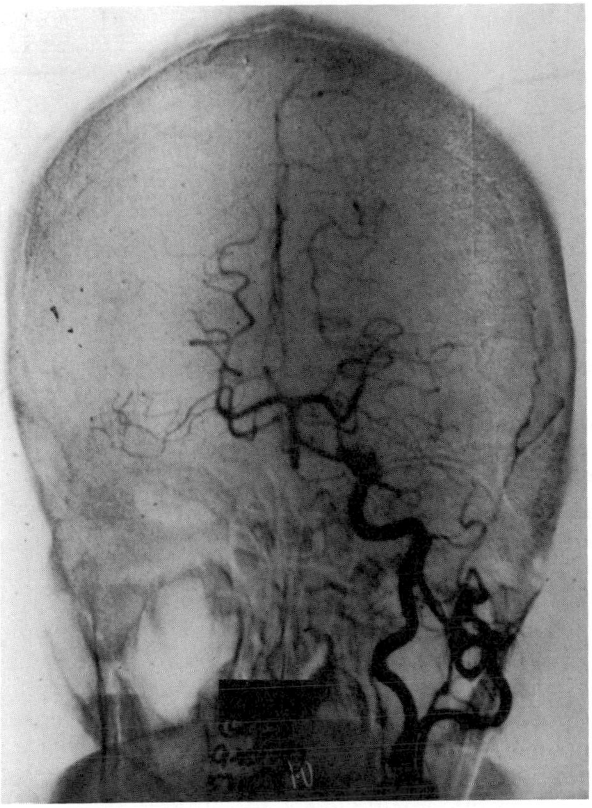

**Fig. 14-7.** Example of a persistent trigeminal artery.

ternal carotid artery occlusion studied, where the carotid artery occlusion lay below the ophthalmic artery. The rate at which such collateral develops is poorly documented. Opinions vary from days to weeks. In our experience, it seems certain that retrograde flow through the orbit can develop rather quickly. However, the speed of development seems almost always insufficient to spare the brain ischemia.

In many instances, when carotid artery stenosis has reached the point of hemodynamic significance, the collateral flow that occurs in response to the flow failure may succeed in preventing major symptoms. Cases of asymptomatic carotid artery occlusion in several autopsy series have shown a patent circle of Willis, inferring that collateral flow has developed to arteries distal to the site of occlusion: five of the internal carotid cases of Fisher et al.[128] and three of Hutchinson and Yates[181] were spared infarction. Although collateralization of an occluded artery would seem sufficient protection against stroke, it is not. Explanation for the continued risk for stroke involves discussion of the mechanism of stroke in carotid artery occlusion.

The role of the development of collaterals in protecting the hemisphere against ischemic events is obviously of great importance. It has long been obvious that the mere demonstration of collateral angiographically bears little relationship to its physiologic effect. Accordingly, investigations using regional cerebral blood flow measurements have been undertaken to clarify the role of collateral evident angiographically. The results have been somewhat disappointing. Awad et al.[12] studied 18 patients with unilateral internal collateral occlusion by both digital subtraction angiography (DSA) and xenon-133 inhalation measurements. They attempted to correlate distribution of the opacification seen on digital subtraction angiography with regional cerebral blood flow determinations by the xenon-133 inhalation method. The nine patients who showed symmetrical filling of the cortical surface branches on DSA showed no significant interhemispheric difference in regional cerebral blood flow. The other nine showed delayed patterns of cortical filling and varying degrees of asymmetry in the regional cerebral blood flow between the two hemispheres. Awad and his colleagues demonstrated that symmetrical filling of the cerebral vessels on DSA correlated with essentially identical regional cerebral blood flow in the two hemispheres. However, they warned that the finding only indicates negligible interhemispheric differences in regional cerebral blood flow, but this did not include normal regional cerebral blood flow. Likewise, since only the larger cortical vessels are seen by DSA, and since the regional cerebral blood flow measurements present total flow in both the larger vessels visualized by DSA and the smaller ones not visualized, the delay in DSA opacification on one side of the brain did not necessarily represent a decrease in regional cerebral blood flow. DSA has not yet reached the point where it can be used as a predictor of regional cerebral blood flow differences bearing on the risk of subsequent stroke.

Nor have other methods been helpful predictors. Using positron emission tomography (PET) measurements (cerebral blood flow, blood volume, oxygen extraction fraction) Powers et al.[290] found that neither the percentage of stenosis nor the residual lumen diameter of the extracranial internal carotid artery was a reliable predictor of the hemodynamic state of cerebral circulation in 19 patients with greater than 66 percent extracranial carotid lumen diameter reduction. Hemodynamic insufficiency of the hemisphere correlated best with angiographic patterns of meningeal and ophthalmic arterial collaterals. These two angiographic collateral patterns, however, were signs of the circulatory inadequacy via the usual carotid artery and circle of Willis routes, observations further corroborated by Tatemichi et al.,[339] using Doppler sonography. These studies indicated that ophthalmic collateral is an insufficient source of supply to the brain and, when present, indicates that the more common sources of collateral are unavailable or incompetent. Prominent ophthalmic collateral is probably a poor, at any rate not a favorable, prognostic sign, findings independently corroborated by Schneider et al.[318]

# PATHOPHYSIOLOGY OF CAROTID ARTERY ISCHEMIA

## General Principles

From disease involving the carotid artery itself, the clinical syndromes that occur result from two basic mechanisms: (1) intracranial arterial occlusion, whether from embolism or from anterograde extension of thrombus across the circle of Willis into the stems of the major cerebral arteries, and (2) perfusion failure due to inadequate collateral distal to hemodynamically significant stenosis or occlusion. Both mechanisms may be operative in the same patient.[37,283]

The problems in diagnosis and management of carotid artery disease lies mainly in clarifying which of these principles is at work in a given case: determining the source of an embolus, determining the severity of the perfusion failure, and predicting future events. The problem is compounded by the need to take into account instances of ischemia in the carotid artery territory from problems unrelated to disease of the carotid artery itself, especially embolism of cardiac origin and lacunar disease. Although some disease is frequently found in the carotid artery, severe disease of this vessel is an uncommon finding: Fisher et al.[128] found arterial thrombosis with infarction in only 18 percent of 57 autopsy-studied cases of stroke among 178 collected cases in 1960 to 1961 at the Massachusetts General Hospital.

Although the majority of cases of carotid artery territory ischemia are broadly attributed to atherosclerosis, a variety of mechanisms seem to be involved. Or, alternately, the atheromatous stenosis may reach the stage of total occlusion of the lumen, and the circulation distally may be inadequate to prevent ischemia. For TIAs, these mechanisms would entail a temporary cessation of flow either in a distal branch artery from embolus, or over the distal territories of the underperfused carotid artery while the carotid artery itself was temporarily blocked. With restoration of blood flow, the ischemic region of the brain quickly recovers and the clinical deficit (TIA) vanishes. For infarction, the processes would presumably be the same, but the effects of the occlusion would persist.

## Embolism

From pathologic studies[4,57,58,125,128,130] it has been determined that carotid artery occlusion results when an atheromatous plaque, already producing high-grade reduction in the arterial lumen, develops superimposed platelet-fibrin thrombus, completing the process. It requires little imagination to envision that as the thrombus accumulates, loose material may be swept into the distal circulation, causing permanent or temporary occlusion of small intracranial arteries and, ultimately, TIAs.

Millikan et al.[248] were the first to report their success using anticoagulants to treat patients with TIAs, a program quickly copied.[272] The rationale for this therapy was their suggestion that fragments of an enlarging thrombus may be swept away by the blood and temporarily occlude cerebral arteries, producing a TIA. This embolic theory of TIA pathogenesis has received support over the years from several studies. Gunning et al.[157] and Castaigne et al.[57] found a loose network of fibrin and platelets in patients at the time of endarterectomy who were recently symptomatic with retinal or hemispheral TIAs. By contrast, patients without recent symptoms have relatively clean atheroma at the time of endarterectomy. Fisher[118] and Ross Russell[308] observed material passing through the retinal circulation during attacks of transient monocular blindness (TMB), documenting that migrating particles could be associated with transient symptoms. Also, evidence has been presented for clinically inobvious cerebral embolization in cases suffering symptomatic transient monocular blindness.[163] However, Fisher and Ojemann's[131] findings in a study of 90 carotid endarterectomy specimens have challenged the embolic theory of TIAs. They found that in three clinical categories—hemispheric TIAs, transient monocular blindness, and asymptomatic, severe carotid artery obstruction producing subocclusion—hemodynamic insufficiency appeared to be the cause for the transient symptoms. Mural thrombus, present in many of the specimens, contributed to the overall obstructive process but had few independent serious consequences beyond this effect.

Proof of this mechanism might be difficult to find, since angiographic[4,78,81,221,298,341,401] and pathologic studies[127] have shown how promptly cerebral emboli fragment and disappear, leaving a patent vessel supplying the clinically affected region.

### Nature of the Embolic Material

Most of the embolic material has been assumed to be platelet aggregates.[2,157,242] Other material has had much less documentation. Beal et al.[22] described a syndrome of multiple foci of cerebral infarction due to cholesterol embolization. The patient was a 69-year-old man who experienced several spells over a period of 3 years, consistent with hemispheral transient cerebral ischemic attacks: numbness and weakness of one or the other hand with a duration of 5 to 8 minutes. Previously, it had been the opinion of many[43] that such crystals were too small to produce focal signs.

### Carotid Artery Sources of the Embolic Material

In a setting of carotid artery occlusion, embolic material may be swept into the brain from the intracranial portion of the thrombus.[308] One patient, described by Countee et al.,[72] experienced transient ischemic attacks 3½ years after an ipsilateral carotid endarterectomy. The apparent source was the occluded stump of the external carotid artery, which was filled with atheromatous debris. The excision of this debris was associated with cessation of the transient ischemic attacks (Fig. 14-8). Rare variations in arterial anatomy may set the stage for an unusual course for the presumed embolic fragments to follow when they leave the ulcerative or stenotic carotid artery lesion. Waller et al.[364] described two cases of transient ischemic attacks involving the brain stem, attributed to microembolization from the carotid artery via a persistent trigeminal artery.

The usual source for the emboli is assumed to be the carotid artery stenosis or ulcerated plaque itself. From the stenosis, loose aggregates of platelet-fibrin complexes presumably might be dislodged.[157] Similar fragments could also occur from associated ulcers (Fig. 14-9). The issue of particle size is obviously of great importance. The size of embolic material sufficient to cause retinal ischemia may be too small to affect or block any but the tiny pial surface branches in the hemisphere and are unlikely to cause symptoms. This point alone may explain the usually asymptomatic state of cases with cholesterol emboli found in retinal vessels. However, once carotid artery

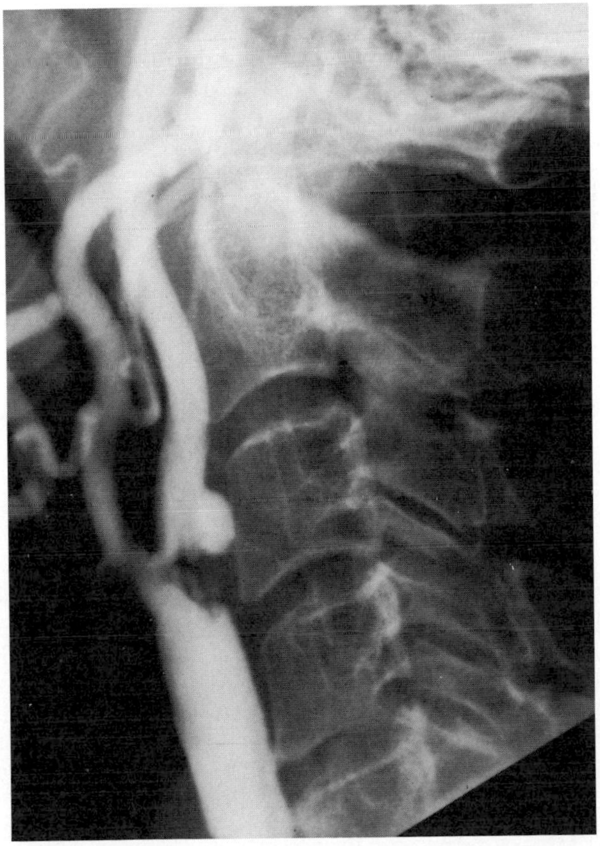

**Fig. 14-8.** Internal carotid artery with combined stenosis and large ulceration.

territory embolism has occurred, no matter how small the particle size, no studies to date permit the inference of continued small-particle embolism; subsequent emboli may be quite a bit larger. A few discouraging cases have been reported. Zatz et al.[401] reported a case (case 5) in which a devastating stroke occurred 17 hours after an angiogram. This study was done for patients with TIAs, and this particular case documented an irregular nonobstructing plaque at the origin of the internal carotid artery. On repeat angiogram 3 hours after the stroke, the plaque was no longer present. Only a minimal irregularity of the wall was seen, and a major occlusion was found in the previously patent stem of the middle cerebral artery above. Zatz and his colleagues concluded that the transient ischemic attacks and major stroke, respectively, were related to embolism from, then of, this atheromatous plaque. In this case, it may be argued that the angiogram itself caused or destabilized the lesion, as may have been the case in another dramatic stroke following angiography.[77]

The possibility of a major stroke in a setting of presumably minor carotid artery disease is the dreaded complication that has dictated many a management decision. The mural hemorrhage thesis of Lusby et al.[232] raised this worry. These authors inferred that the presence of a small ulcer or modest atheroma may suffice to allow a subintimal dissection to develop, usually caused by subintimal hemorrhage. The resultant hemorrhage could thus suddenly convert a modest lesion into a severe stenosis. Worse, the unstable intima atop the subintimal hemorrhage would presumably break down, discharging itself into the arterial lumen as embolic material. The speculation was made that the whole process might be aggravated by the use of aspirin, which might even mask the occurrence of TIAs[55] and help to bring about intramural hemorrhages.[232] If such developments were the result of aspirin therapy, more enthusiasm would be created for elective operative repair of these lesions even in the asymptomatic state. Little evidence has been found to support these claims. Lennihan et al.[211] found only 2 percent with wall hemorrhages large enough to have caused stenosis. They are often induced by the trauma of the surgery and included as part of the specimen. However, those present preoperatively are only rarely large enough to play a role in the stenosis.[124,211,261]

It should be mentioned in passing that the foregoing arguments assume the source of the embolic material is the carotid artery itself.[342] However, it is well recognized that the heart may also be the source.[41,80] Further, it is also possible that platelet coagula develop in the circulating blood.[82,88,365] Thus far, it has not proved possible to separate them on a case by case basis. Until a more reliable method of differentiation becomes available, these unsettling possibilities of carotid artery territory stroke must remain qualitative and not quantitative issues.

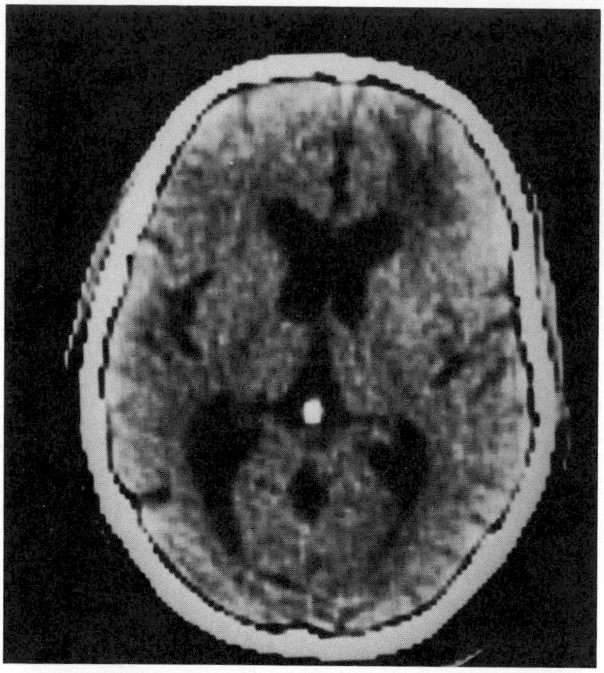
A

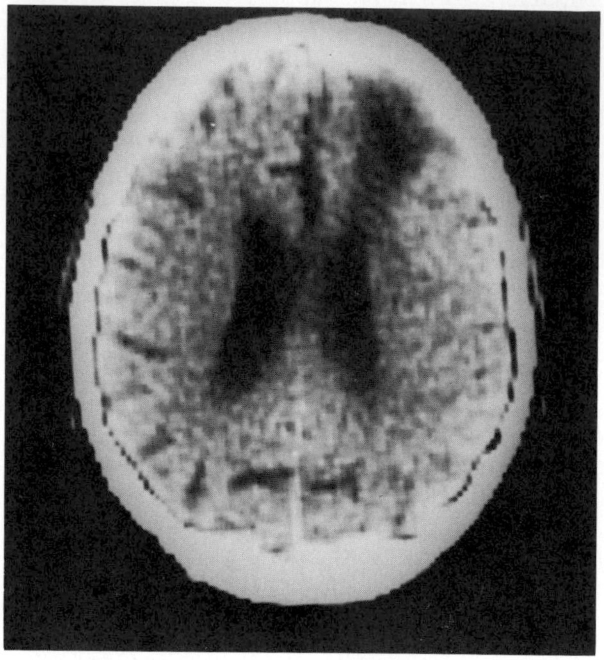
B

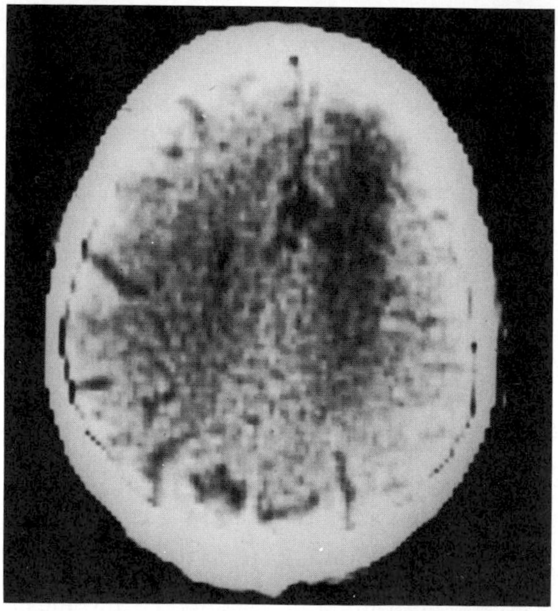
C

**Fig. 14-9.** Computed tomography scan of ''distal field'' or ''borderzone'' infarction.

## Embolic Transient Ischemic Attacks

The embolic theory can account for different types of carotid artery territory TIAs on the basis of separate embolic material occluding different intracranial branches, and probably many TIAs occur as a result of this short-lived embolic mechanism.

The clinical and angiographic details in many of these cases suggest they are a variant—not the usual type of TIA. Duration of the TIA deficit is different in embolic cases: Pessin et al.[281] postulated emboli as the explanation for at least some of the TIAs encountered in their prospective study of 95 consecutively angiogrammed cases of carotid artery TIAs, but in these cases the deficit tended to last far longer than the usual 5 to 7 minutes that characterizes most cases of TIAs associated with severe stenosis of the internal carotid artery. Their findings echoed the earlier work of Acheson and Hutchinson.[1] The findings suggested that many of these cases could be interpreted as examples of clinically short-lived strokes arising from a variety of embolic sources, including cardiac, rather than solely examples of carotid artery stenosis. These cases also showed a high incidence of widely patent carotid arteries. This relatively benign form of embolism has been described as "acceptable minor embolism" (AcME) by Fisher and Ojemann.[131]

Stereotypic transient ischemic attacks are a major problem for the embolic theory. In at least one study, however, artificial emboli injected in the carotid artery circulation gathered in the same vessel.[374] It might be argued that few instances of TIA are truly stereotypic. Exactly repetitive attacks seem rather uncommon.[281] It may be that what seem to be stereotypic attacks are merely attacks with many prominent features that commonly occur in most cases of embolism to branches of the middle cerebral artery. In the published experience with aberrant embolization from Silastic ball therapy for arteriovenous malformations, several cases have been reported in which a similar syndrome occurred from embolism to a variety of different middle cerebral branches: the complaints included focal weakness of the arm,[387] which persisted only a few minutes, and "transient" dysesthesia of the contralateral hand,[260] both common symptoms of TIA.

### Perfusion Failure with Distal Insufficiency

Distal insufficiency is the other major mechanism that may account for cerebral ischemia. This theory has proved attractive because the topography of cerebral infarcts in many cases of carotid artery occlusion closely mimics that found in obvious settings of hypotension, such as cardiac arrest, and because the most reliable correlation with TIAs is severe stenosis.

The "distal insufficiency" concept for ischemia or infarction implies decreased vascular perfusion on those areas of the brain parenchyma located at the greatest distance from the site of stenosis or occlusion.[250] As a consequence, "stagnation thrombus" may develop from local circulatory failure at these distant sites,[116] and infarction follows (Fig. 14-10). The areas at risk include the most distal segments of the cortical branches of the middle cerebral artery, in particular, the superior parietal and posterior temporal-occipital areas.[35,250]

### Distal Field Infarct (Watershed or Borderzone) Topography in Autopsy Studies

Infarction found along the superior frontal, superior parietal, and lateral occipital regions has a long history in the pathology literature.[113,115,222,278,283,299,304,332,352,353,382,383] The topography of the infarction has been better documented than has the mechanism. Several famous cases have been described. Spatz's[332] case showed infarction affecting the left cerebral hemisphere from frontal through posterior parietal regions. All the foci of infarction were suprasylvian, that is, sparing the region of the operculum and the insula. A similar suprasylvian topography was described later by Lindenberg and Spatz[222] as the expected topography in "cerebral Buerger's disease."

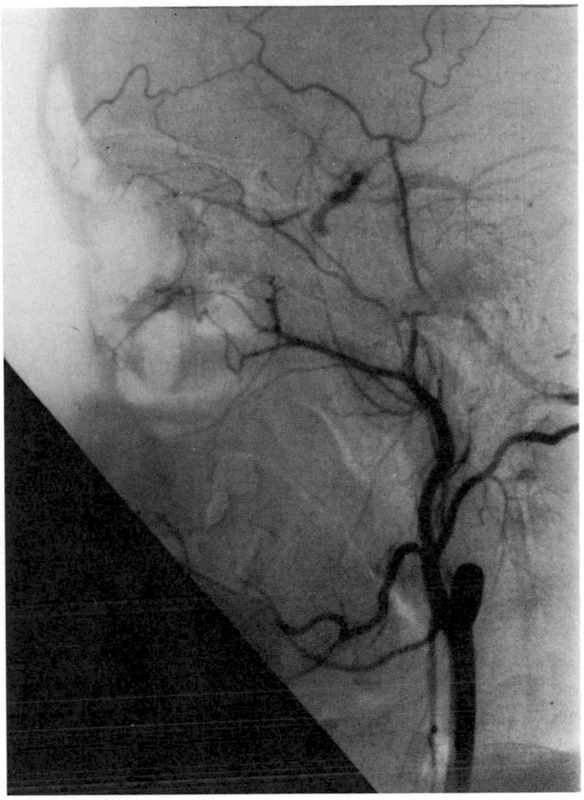

**Fig. 14-10.** Severely stenosed internal carotid artery with a large ulcer.

Interest in the subject became keener after Schneider[317] proposed the thesis of infarction by the process of "distal insufficiency," and many of the autopsy-documented cases with such infarct topography were found associated with a thrombus or severe stenosis of the carotid artery, a condition known before then as infarction at a distance.[58,113,115,116,128,217,304]

### Distal Field Infarct Topography in Radiologic Studies

Studies based on cerebral angiography have attempted to corroborate the findings of radiologic studies of distal field infarct topography, but have had only modest success. In a clinicoangiographic study of acute cerebral infarction from ICA occlusion or tight stenosis, Pessin et al.[283] found a possible mechanism of "low-flow" as the explanation for the infarcts in less than a third of their cases. Angiography revealed a slowing of circulation throughout the entire middle cerebral artery distribution in those cases, as opposed to direct or indirect evidence of intracrancial branch occlusion in those diagnosed as embolic.

CT scanning has been used commonly in settings of carotid territory infarction, but correlations with autopsy findings have only been documented in a few published studies.[383] Ringelstein et al.[299] studied 107 cases of internal carotid occlusion documented by Doppler sonograms, angiograms, and CT criteria and found 44 of 111 infarcts which were attributed to hemodynamic cause, 8 presenting as "watershed" infarction and 44 to "terminal supply area" infarction. Harrison and Marshall[165] also carried out similar studies, this time with CT scan and angiograms, and found the high convexity lesions on CT scan correlated well with those patients who showed poor collateral flow.

Inhalation studies such as xenon and PET scanning has documented the topography of carotid ischemia. Vorstrup et al.[360] showed impaired xenon uptake in suprasylvian areas in a few cases suffering TIAs. Single photon emission computed tomography (SPECT) measurements have found documented increased cerebral blood volume, a sign of dilated collaterals, only in those patients with high-grade carotid stenosis.[356] Positron emission tomography (PET) has uncovered numerous examples of the distal insufficiency perfusion.[293] Known also as the "misery perfusion syndrome,"[20] it has been explained by reduced cerebral metabolism and has proved to be surgically reversible. Low reactivity of middle cerebral blood vessels in a setting of hypercapnia, a sign of fully dilated collaterals, was found by Levine et al.[213] to have a significant relationship ($P = 0.04$) for high-grade carotid stenosis. Leblanc et al.[208] used PET scanning to document the selective vulnerability of the anterior borderzone region with significant reduction in cerebral blood flow and hemodynamic reserve capacity in seven patients (five with TIAs, two asymptomatic) with at least 80 percent internal carotid artery stenosis. Yamauchi et al.[393] demonstrated diminished regional cerebral blood flow, increased oxygen extraction, and a decrease in the ratio of cerebral blood flow to volume consistent with stagnation thrombus occurring in the "borderzone" areas. All these studies point to a state of hemodynamic insufficiency. Yanagihara et al.[395] documented the disappearance of symptoms after endarterectomy but not in those with disease at the carotid siphon, where surgery was not possible. Yet Carpenter et al.,[54] in a study of 32 patients, were unable to document selective borderzone hemodynamic impairment in their cohort of patients with varying degrees of carotid stenosis, the notable exception to the general findings of others.

In the even more severe state of distal intracranial internal carotid artery stenosis with abundant collaterals associated with the moyamoya disorder,[338] hyperventilation has been shown to precipitate focal symptoms. The demonstration of such extreme degrees of sensitivity of cerebral blood flow to alterations in $P_{CO_2}$ may help resurrect interest in notions of "cerebral claudication,"[252] which have been ignored in recent times. The frequency of the misery perfusion syndrome as an explanation for transient ischemic attacks is unknown. The great expense and effort involved in testing even single patients is certain to discourage studies of large groups. However, the demonstration alone is important, since it bears on pathophysiology.

## Perfusion Failure Transient Ischemic Attacks

The principle of distal insufficiency is strongly associated with the high frequency of severe stenosis or occlusion of the carotid[124,271] and for the tendency of TIAs to have the same characteristic from attack to attack.[115,250] The syndromes might vary somewhat from case to case, depending on the collateral arterial pattern for each individual.

The problems of stereotypic TIAs, that is, repetitive in severity and in clinical details, is not easily accounted for by the embolic theory.[126] The data derived from the pathologic study of carotid endarterectomy specimens by Fisher and Ojemann[131] were viewed by the authors as support for the hemodynamic mechanism of TIAs. Severe stenosis (residual lumen less than 1 mm) was present in 33 (98 percent) of 34 cases with hemispheric TIAs, 19 (90 percent) of 21 (no information on 2) cases of transient monocular blindness, but in only 5 (15 percent) of 33 asymptomatic patients. Mural thrombus was present on the atheromatous plaque in 26 (77 percent) of 34 cases of hemispheric TIAs, 22 (96 percent) of 23 cases of transient monocular blindness, and 7 (21 percent) of 33 asymptomatic patients. The absence of mural thrombus, however, in 8 TIA patients as well as the tiny amounts (less than 1 mm) found in an additional 5, together with the absence of TIAs in 7 asymptomatic patients with thrombus makes the stenosis the most important factor underlying TIAs.

In support of the embolic theory, Whisnant[374] showed the original picture of several embolic pellets which had gone to the same cortical branch by "laminar flow." Evidence supporting a hemodynamic insufficiency explanation for repeated stereotyped TIAs has not been forthcoming. It is also argueable whether hemispheral TIAs are ever truly stereotypic.[281]

## Infarction Manifesting as Transient Ischemic Attack

The increase in use of CT evaluation and nuclear magnetic resonance[329] in patients with a clinical picture suggesting transient ischemic attack has demonstrated that a surprisingly large number of such cases already have a focal hypodense area consisting of cerebral infarction in a region clinically related to the symptoms of the transient ischemic attack. Perrone et al.[279] found 34 percent of their 35 patients with TIA showing a positive CT scan consisting of small hypodense areas. These lesions were angiographically correlated with arteriosclerotic abnormalities in the ipsilateral carotid artery. Other investigators[13,35,297,366] have corroborated this observation in a significant number of patients undergoing CT or MRI evaluation, although the duration of TIAs is often not specified or, if noted, is generally longer (hours) than the usual brief (minutes) time frame of more typical carotid TIAs.

## Asymptomatic Carotid Artery Disease

Considering the frightening prospects of stroke in a setting of atheromatous lesions of the carotid artery, it is remarkable that asymptomatic disease of the carotid artery exists at all, let alone seems to be encountered frequently. Perhaps it is the fear of stroke from carotid artery disease that prompts the efforts to detect the disease in its occult state. Whatever the reasons, when the lesion is discovered, the artery is either occluded or stenotic, or the possibility of carotid artery disease is raised by the discovery of a bruit in the neck. The risk for stroke differs in each setting.

### Asymptomatic Carotid Occlusion

The documentation of carotid occlusion by a noninvasive study or angiogram is fairly common. Dyken et al.[94] found a 3 percent incidence of apparent occult severe stenosis or occlusion of the carotid artery in a hospitalized group of cases over 50 years of age. The lesion was documented by reversed flow in the ophthalmic artery determined by directional Doppler ultrasound.

Several studies have addressed the issue of stroke in a setting of common or internal carotid occlusion, but few have broken down the data for the strokes that occurred in the territory of the occlusion. The available data show widely scattered results. Furlan and Whisnant[138] documented 6 cases of stroke ipsilateral to a carotid artery occlusion among their series of 138 angiogrammed cases studied retrospectively, and another 11 which occurred in other vascular territories. The annual stroke rate in their study was 2 percent per year. Grillo and Paterson[153] reviewed the angiographic findings of all patients undergoing aortography or cerebral angiography at their hospital over a 5-year period. They identified 44 patients with occlusion of the internal carotid artery, ranging in age from 45 to 84 years. The incidence of occlusion was essentially the same on both sides. In 3 patients, no symptoms attributable to the carotid occlusion were identified. Fully 23 had had completed stroke before their angiography. An additional 3 cases had their stroke at the time of the angiogram. The 3 otherwise asymptomatic cases had only the nonspecific symptoms of headache and blurred vision; these experienced no neurologic deficits during the 3 years of follow-up. Bogousslavsky et al.[37] found no strokes among 23 cases of carotid occlusion followed for a mean period of 27 months. Sacquegna et al.[312] studied the clinical course of 100 consecutive patients with angiographically proven internal carotid artery occlusion. Of these patients 93 presented with stroke, 7 with TIAs. They followed-up 68 patients from 17 to 69 months; 7 patients developed new stroke, but only 3 were in the territory of the occluded carotid, and 4 patients had TIAs during follow-up. The observed stroke rate was 4.7 percent at 1 year, 12.2 percent at 3 years, and 17.1 percent at 5 years. In a prospective study of patients with asymptomatic bruits, using noninvasive carotid Doppler evaluation, Bernstein and Norris[27] identified 40 patients with unilateral carotid artery occlusion: 19 were occluded at study onset; 21 progressed from stenosis to occlusion. More ischemic events occurred in the group that progressed to occlusion than those already occluded. There were 3 strokes and 9 TIAs in the former group during a mean 30-month follow-up and no strokes and 4 TIAs in the latter group followed for a mean of 48 months. The annual stroke rate was 3.8 percent, indicating the benign course in asymptomatic patients with carotid artery occlusion. Cote et al.,[70] utilizing the data from the Canadian Cooperative Study, found 47 cases with internal carotid artery occlusion who presented either with ipsilateral transient ischemic attack (22 cases), ipsilateral minor infarct (15 cases), or no ipsilateral symptoms (10 cases). The disease affected the origin of the internal carotid artery in 87 percent of cases. Stroke occurred in 11 cases and TIAs in 24 during the follow-up period. The ipsilateral stroke rate was 5 percent per year.

Data culled from the now completed extracranial/intracranial bypass study provided the largest evaluation of patients with angiographically proven bilateral internal carotid artery occlusion.[362] In this study 74 patients were initially identified, of whom 34 were randomized to conservative treatment and followed for a mean of 42 months. Symptoms at initial study entry included nondisabling stroke in 80 percent and/or TIAs in 80 percent; 18 patients had subsequent ischemic events (11 with stroke, 7 with TIAs) with an annual stroke rate of 13 percent per patient year. The survival rate was 71 percent (24 patients), of whom 50 percent were symptom-free or had minor disability. The outcome was better than expected, considering the seriousness of the vascular disease.

It has not yet been established whether there is a critical period of vulnerability for stroke, what role the presence or absence of certain types of collateral plays in the stroke risk, and what risk exists for each of the stroke subtypes—embolism from the stump, the tail, and from other sources, distal insufficiency, and so on. However, these concerns may be excessive, given the low risk for stroke suggested by these studies, even in a setting of occlusion of the internal carotid.

## Asymptomatic Carotid Stenosis

The literature on the risk for stroke in a setting of asymptomatic carotid stenosis remains unsettled[109,212,251,288] but is being addressed by the Asymptomatic Carotid Arteriosclerosis Study. This trial has been organized as a national, multicenter trial currently in progress.[11] All eligible patients with asymptomatic carotid stenosis of 60 percent lumen reduction or greater will receive 325 mg of aspirin daily, and half will be randomly assigned to carotid endarterectomy. All patients will receive appropriate counseling and treatment for risk factor reduction. The endpoints of TIA or stroke in the distribution of the randomized artery will be used to assess the two treatments.

Some earlier studies suggested an enormous risk, others very little, while few addressed the issues of whether the stroke occurs in the territory at risk and by what mechanism. At one end of the spectrum is the study by Podore et al.[288] of the 5-year course for 50 cases more than 50 percent internal carotid artery stenosis: stroke without TIAs developed in 3 cases (4.5 percent), and TIAs occurred in 11 (16.5 percent). In another study, Hennerici and Rautenberg[170] documented the natural history of 122 prospectively selected neurologically asymptomatic patients with extracranial carotid artery disease. Only 3 deaths from stroke occurred in 23 patients who died during the follow-up period of 11 to 36 months. Eight of the living patients experienced transient ischemic attack, one had a stroke, but the others remained asymptomatic. The cumulative stroke rate was 7 percent, which the authors estimated as the same as the average risk of death in a normal population. In 85 percent of the cases there was progression in the extracranial arterial disease, as documented by repeat examination by continuous wave Doppler methods. These studies demonstrated development of lesions in previously normal arteries either alone (25 instances) or in combination with a deterioration of the original stenosis (in 14 cases). Deterioration of the original stenosis alone was seen in nine cases. However, only the occurrence of a combined carotid and vertebral lesion significantly increased the cerebral vascular risk. Under those conditions, the stroke risk was increased sixfold over that for unilateral or bilateral carotid lesions. Durward et al.[93] studied the course of 73 patients with asymptomatic, presumably atheromatous, plaque found at the common carotid bifurcation. Stenosis of more than 50 percent was found in 50 cases and was accompanied by ulceration in an additional 17. Ulceration was found alone in six cases. The observation period averaged up to 4 years, from as short as 6 months to as long as 10 years. Surgical intervention was undertaken only if TIA or minor stroke developed. There was no standard use of antiplatelet or anticoagulant drugs. In the follow-up period, 22 of the patients developed ischemic symptoms. In 12 patients, the symptoms occurred in the territory of the previously asymptomatic carotid artery. Among these 12 patients, 2 experienced stroke with no prior transient ischemic attack. Repeat angiogram in the six patients who developed an ischemic event in the previously asymptomatic territory showed the lesion had progressed significantly in every case, but none had reached complete occlusion. All underwent uneventful endarterectomy. Although symptoms occurred in roughly equal frequency in cases with ulceration alone, stenosis alone, or a combination of stenosis and ulceration, the only instances of infarction occurred in a group with stenosis of more than 50 percent. Ulceration was not associated with infarction. Similar experience was documented by Roederer et al.,[303] who found a 4 percent annual rate of symptoms in their prospective study of 167 cases referred with bruit.

At the extreme benign end of the spectrum is another nonrandomized, noncontrolled study[212] in which 147 cases involving 535 carotid arteries underwent surgery only on the symptomatic side, while the asymptomatic side was left to follow its natural course. No strokes were observed in these patients in a 20-year follow-up period.

While awaiting the outcome of the trial, many still advise prophylactic endarterectomy, others advise platelet inhibitors, some advise no treatment at all. For a surgical option, the risk of endarterectomy[97,343,344] should be lower than the natural history of the disease if the treatment is to have any place as an alternative. Karis[195] recomputed the Jonas and Hass[188] observations to show that a combined morbidity and mortality rate of over 1.4 percent for arteriography, endarterectomy, and the postoperative period for a surgical approach to carotid artery territory TIAs would exceed that of the total morbidity and mortality compared with the medical therapy. Current mortality and morbidity data indicate endarterectomy is being carried out with acceptably low complications in many centers.

## Asymptomatic Ulcerative Disease

Very few studies have been done on the stroke risk for ulcerative disease alone.[251] Dixon et al.[85] followed 153 nonstenotic asymptomatic ulcerative lesions in 141 patients. Over a period up to 10 years hemispheric strokes without antecedent transient ischemic attacks occurred in 19 percent of the deep complicated ulcers, in 21 percent of the deep ulcers, and in 3 percent of those with small shallow ulcers. Because the calculated annual stroke rate for the more complex ulcers was between 4.5 and 7.6 percent, Dixon and associates consider that this rate is comparable to that of the 6 percent annual stroke rate in patients with TIAs, and they recommended prophylactic operation for these cases.

Fisher and Ojemann[131] showed that many ulcers are smooth and thick, that is, they contain no thrombus. The concept of ulcers is mainly based on angiography, where the significance of ulcers may be questioned.

## Asymptomatic Bruit

The widespread availability of Doppler studies have eclipsed much of the earlier anxieties about bruits. A bruit in the neck is commonly encountered in routine clinical examinations. It occurs in 4 to 5 percent of the population aged 45 to 80 years.[173,385] A local cervical bruit can be detected in approximately 70 to 89 percent of patients with a "tight" (75 percent stenosis, or 2 mm or less residual lumen) stenosis of the internal carotid artery.[143,284] The site of maximal intensity of the bruit usually corresponds to the carotid artery bifurcation area, in front of the upper portion of the thyroid cartilage. It can radiate into the ocular region, and its intensity usually decreases with the Valsalva maneuver. The latter point should be useful in differentiating them from bruits originating from the external carotid artery, which should not change with this maneuver, but the finding is disappointingly unreliable.[209] A bruit may be absent in some patients with "tight" stenosis because of a "slow-flow" state through the patent, but severely stenotic, artery.[284]

Auscultation of the orbits may also be useful in the clinical diagnosis of extracranial carotid artery occlusive disease. Fisher[120] noted that an eye bruit may be present on the side contralateral to a carotid artery occlusion, presumably related to augmentation flow through the open carotid system. Others have corroborated this observation,[39,284] while Pessin et al.[284] found this sign to be present with carotid artery occlusion more often than an associated cervical bruit. Ocular bruits have a strong relationship to ipsilateral intracranial carotid siphon stenosis.[178]

Initially, such bruits were assumed to be a sign of internal carotid artery disease[116] and some would agree with one authority[300] that truly asymptomatic bruits are rare. But Doppler and angiographic studies have shown that bruits may arise from many causes other than carotid stenosis, leading among them a radiated noise from aortic stenosis.[143,257] An early method, now abandoned, quantitative phonoangiography, permitted the differentiation of bruits originating locally from atherostenosis from the commonly occurring radiated basal heart murmurs.[202] Modern duplex Doppler techniques have strengthened these findings. Roederer et al.[303] found that bruit alone is not a reliable sign of stenosis: in over half their referral population, the artery with the bruit had a stenosis of less than 50 percent.

Carotid bruit is a frequent finding in patients undergoing other arterial reconstructions. Treimin et al.[357] found 83 such patients among 516 undergoing an elective abdominal aorta operation; they did not pursue the mechanism of the bruit. Four patients had a postoperative stroke. These investigators found no correlation between the stroke and the presence of a carotid bruit, or history of cerebral ischemic symptoms. They questioned the value of prophylactic carotid endarterectomy in patients who undergo abdominal aorta reconstruction. Ropper et al.[305] auscultated the necks of 735 unselected cases undergoing elective surgery and found carotid bruits in 143 (14 percent). Of the 5 cases of perioperative strokes in this group, there was no difference in the incidence of stroke between patients with and without bruits, and 4 strokes occurred in asymptomatic patients without bruits.

Two additional reports[173,385] suggest that the occurrence of a bruit is a better marker for atherosclerosis and coronary artery disease than it is for subsequent TIAs in the vascular territory of the bruit. Both of these studies showed a stroke rate approximately twice that of the control population during a period of 5 to 8 years. However, few of the strokes occurred in the brain ipsilateral to the bruit in the neck. Furthermore, the strokes were of a wide variety of type (including ruptured aneurysm). Finally, the incidence of myocardial infarction was also twice the expected rate. These data suggest that bruit is more a sign of systemic atherosclerosis than it is a predictor of subsequent brain infarction related to a bruit.

It is perhaps no surprise that the reported risk for stroke varies so widely in cases with asymptomatic bruit: few studies have either documented the source of the bruit or agreed on the clinical criteria for stroke and TIA. Some claims have been made that the presence of a bruit is correlated with a stroke rate as high as 15 percent over 2 to 7 years when compared to some 5 percent without bruit.[67] A somewhat lower rate (6.6 percent) was found in another study,[47] carried to only 2.5 years, of patients whose bruit was associated with signs on noninvasive laboratory tests suggesting hemodynamically significant stenosis. However, no strokes occurred in those whose bruit was not judged hemodynamically significant.[47] Similar findings have also been reported in other studies.[197]

Despite calls for angiography and prophylactic endarterectomy,[109,258,344,345] it is worth recalling that at least two studies show a very low risk for stroke: one showed the risk of stroke to be less than 4 percent (2/56) over an average of 3 years;[187,303] others found the risk less than 1 percent (1/168) over an average period of 32 months.[180,193]

## Ocular Bruits with Intracranial Internal Carotid Artery Disease

Auscultation of the eyeball is usually done to detect bruits indicative of intracranial ICA stenoses. However, it has been reported that ocular bruits in relationship with such stenoses are rare.[128,216] Of 100 patients with a unilateral ICA stenosis, 4 had a siphon stenosis, and in 1 an ocular bruit was heard. In the same report there were 50 patients with a unilateral ICA occlusion and a contralateral angiographically normal ICA. Among the 50 occlusions, the contrast medium stopped in the siphon in 11 (cardiac embolism in 5; atherosclerotic thrombus or embolism in 2; 4 were undetermined). No ocular bruit but an ipsilateral cervical bruit in one patient and a bilateral cervical bruit in another patient were heard at the level of the common carotid bifurcation.[49] In 50 patients with tight stenoses or occlusions of the extracranial ICA, a unilateral ocular bruit contralateral to the side of ICA occlusion occurred in 9 of 10 patients; this occurred more often than an associated cervical bruit and was interpreted as a sign of augmentation flow.[284] In 18 patients with atherothrombotic ischemic cerebrovascular disease, 25 ocular bruits have been reported. Only 2 patients had a stenosis of the intracranial ICA as the main lesion.[39]

Some large surveys for arterial bruits in relation to cerebral ischemic accidents apparently did not include ocular auscultation, but it seems safe to conclude that the absence of an ocular bruit by no means rules out intracranial ICA lesions, and its presence by no means indicates intracranial ICA disease, inasmuch as many various pathologic conditions may give rise to ocular bruits.[191]

## CLINICAL SYNDROMES

The basic clinical features of extracranial carotid disease were described many years ago.[60,113–115,179,328] The characteristic clinical syndrome of internal carotid artery occlusion has long been known to include "premonitory fleeting symptoms including paresthesias, paralysis, monocular blindness, and aphasia."[113] Especially remarkable were the episodes of transient monocular blindness (TMB) described by patients with proven internal carotid artery occlusion. Interest in TMB, later stimulated by actual observations[118,308] of the retinal circulation during an attack, led to important ideas concerning the role of embolism in the production of transient ischemic attacks and stroke. As more clinical detail accumulated about TIAs, it became important to differentiate these spells from others of nonvascular origin. Even today, efforts continue in the difficult task of distinguishing among various types of spells that may have different pathogenesis and prognosis for stroke.

It was the prospect of therapy that prompted so much interest in carotid artery disease. Fisher[113–115] was mainly responsible for renewed interest in the clinical importance of carotid artery disease. In his early clinicopathologic studies, he described the prodromal transient neurologic events frequently preceding stroke, discussed possible stroke mechanisms, and even predicted the surgical treatment. Eastcott et al.[96] were the first to reconstruct successfully an extracranial internal carotid artery lesion. Thus occurred the beginning of the modern era in diagnosis and management of extracranial carotid artery disease.

### Transient Cerebral Ischemic Attacks

#### Definition

Transient ischemic attacks (TIAs) have been defined as a temporary, focal neurologic deficit presumably related to ischemia, lasting less than 24 hours.[145,172] The history of this time frame for a TIA seems to have arisen not so much from the documented time course of a typical attack, but more from uncertainty as to its cause. Because it has long been agreed that a focal deficit lasting longer than 24 hours would be expected to have a focus of ischemic infarction found at autopsy, the definition of a TIA as any spell lasting less than this time can be seen as a negative definition.

Where the subject has been studied using actual case material, the usual 24-hour criteria has been recognized to be excessive.[281] The typical carotid artery territory TIAs are brief, typically lasting only 7 to 10 minutes.[281] The brief spells have a better correlation with angiographic evidence of tight carotid artery stenosis.[281] However, the prognosis for subsequent stroke appears to be the same whether the spell is brief or long in duration.[227,296]

#### Natural History

The importance of carotid artery TIAs is highlighted when viewed from the perspective of carotid stroke. Patients who suffer carotid stroke from extracranial carotid artery occlusion disease have a known prior TIA incidence of 50 to 75 percent.[253,283,311] This contrasts sharply with the low incidence of TIAs (approximately 10 percent) in association with all types of stroke, and reinforces the strong relationship between these transient events and underlying atherothrombotic occlusive disease. The available data, both prospective and retrospective, indicate that the TIAs may be impressive warnings of stroke in some patients and their recognition provides the opportunity for therapeutic intervention.

Despite the large numbers of studies on TIAs, so many difference exist in definitions and methodology that all too many of them are disappointingly unhelpful. Some studies have emphasized incidence, while others describe prevalence. The TIAs have been documented by various methods, some by personal periodic examinations, others by search of clinical records, and even a questionnaire has been tried.[41,196,274,376,379,384] Few have focused on carotid artery territory TIAs alone, and even fewer have separated transient monocular blindness from transient hemispheral attacks. The available data show a wide spread of prevalence and incidence. The prevalence varies from 1.1

to 77/1,000 persons, the incidence rate from 2.2 to 8/1,000.[41,376,379] The stroke risk associated with TIAs is significant, although no well-designed, controlled, and randomized study has provided unequivocal information on the natural history of TIAs, nor is such a study likely to be done today. Past studies[1,14,15,117,134,135,223,235,272,277,327,403] have assessed the stroke risk to be between 2 and 50 percent, results so discrepant as to be useless in any individual case. These studies suffer from several limitations, including ambiguity of TIA definition, lumping together carotid and vertebral basilar TIAs, and, most importantly, no angiographic verification of underlying vascular disease. Despite the limitations of these early studies, the view has emerged that a considerable stroke risk attends TIAs, namely, in the range of 35 percent over 5 years, or 5 to 6 percent per year.[376] Many of the important questions relating TIAs to specific carotid artery lesion configurations, such as irregular plaque, ulcer, severe stenosis, or occlusion, remain unanswered despite all the effort that has gone into the subject thus far. At the least, the available evidence indicates that a serious stroke may follow TIA in a discouraging number of patients, but the factors contributing to the risks for individuals have remained elusive.

In view of the wide variation in reported stroke risk, it may be useful to describe some of the details in the studies that represent the extreme ends of the risk spectrum. Acheson and Hutchinson[1] reported the highest incidence of stroke following TIAs. Their 82 cases were confined to TIAs of less than 1 hour induration. After an average follow-up of 40 months, 42 (51 percent) developed a stroke, 12 died, 4 were totally disabled, and 7 were left with a moderate disability. An important aspect of this study is that the authors defined a stroke as "a clinical episode lasting more than 1 hour." Although they did not indicate how many patients had such a stroke, 19 patients made a complete recovery. This complete recovery in almost half their cases suggests many have had only a short-lived deficit. If so, the importance of this study as a predictor of major stroke following TIA may be exaggerated.

At the other end of the prognostic spectrum are three reports. The first study, by Pearce et al.,[277] reports a very low incidence of stroke: among 61 patients followed for an average of 45 months, only 1 (2 percent) suffered a complete stroke. In this study, the inclusion of a large number of patients with vertigo and vertebrobasilar TIAs, whose clinical outlook is thought to be more benign, may have accounted for the difference. In the second study, by Muuronen and Kaste,[267] a similarly low stroke rate (3.5 percent) was also documented among 228 untreated cases among 314 suffering from carotid artery territory TIA. The follow-up was carried over a mean period of 7.8 years. This group contained younger patients than is usually the case for TIA studies. In the third report, by Gärde et al.,[140] treatment with some form of anticoagulant or platelet inhibitor precluded natural history data. However, the course over an average of 20 months was followed for 241 cases with carotid TIAs, treated with either warfarin or aspirin. During this time only eight cases experienced cerebral infarction. This stroke rate of 3.1 percent is remarkably lower than any reported on any form of therapy. It is interesting that of the eight cases of stroke, four occurred in each treatment group, and two in each group had the stroke within a few weeks of the onset of treatment. Although all these studies are important, given their low incidence of stroke in cases with carotid territory TIAs, it may be equally important to note that, where the data are available, these cases did not have stenosis or occlusion of the symptomatic carotid artery, as best one can judge from the data.

Much of the variation in outcome data has been set aside now that the results of the North American Symptomatic Carotid Endarterectomy Trial (NASCET) have been published. The argument whether the outlook for TIA cases was too benign for endarterectomy to influence outcome favorably[93,180,193,267,303,322] has been put aside by the dramatic results of the studies for symptomatic patients: NASCET and the European Cooperative Study showed a clear advantage of surgery over medical (aspirin) therapy (see chapters on endarterectomy for further details). Neither trial tested surgery against anticoagulation and the positive findings were in those patients whose stenosis exceeded 70 percent. For NASCET, over a period of 18 months, of those symptomatic with TIA and found to have 70 to 90 percent stenosis, 7 percent of the 300 underwent surgery suffered stroke or death, mostly in the perioperative period, while 24 percent of the 295 on aspirin therapy had a stroke or died. This difference favoring surgery was highly significant ($P < 0.001$). The outcome and best management plan for those whose stenosis is in the 30 to 70 percent range remains unsettled. Judging from the data in the European trial, those whose stenosis is below 30 percent seem better managed with medical therapy. For patients with TIAs and over 70 percent stenosis, the effect of aspirin therapy alone was unimpressive.

## Transient Ischemic Attacks with Intracranial Internal Carotid Artery Disease

It can be expected that TIAs occur in atherosclerosis of the intracranial ICA as in extracranial ICA disease. However, precise data are lacking. One reason is that most studies of TIAs have not isolated those specifically due to intracranial ICA lesions, and the few which did so have not dealt with symptoms, only with duration or prevalence. The common association is the occurrence of TIAs with lesions elsewhere, and the common occurrence of tandem lesion renders it difficult to sort out those TIAs that could specifically result from intracranial ICA disease.

Harrison et al.[166] mentioned seven patients with stenosis ("any narrowing of the lumen") of the siphon in whom TIAs had lasted less than 1 hour; none of their 109 other patients had siphon stenosis. In the 66 patients of Marzewski et al.,[238] 24 had presented with TIAs (17 ICA territory, 25.7 percent). The onset of attacks before angiography had ranged from 3 years to 15 days with a median interval of 5 months. During follow-up, 8 patients (12.1 percent) had isolated TIAs (all ICA territory), and 6 of the 10 patients with stroke also experienced TIAs, all in the same territory as the stroke. Seven of the eight patients with isolated TIAs had ipsilateral intracranial ICA stenoses on their reference angiogram, but five had tandem stenoses. For this and other reasons, in only one of the eight patients was the intracranial ICA stenosis the only apparent cause of the ischemic episode. In the 58 patients of Craig et al.,[73] 16 (28 percent) presented with TIAs. During follow-up, eight patients suffered TIAs, of which 25 percent were appropriate to the lesion under study.

Since the ophthalmic artery arises from the intracranial ICA, it might be imagined that amaurosis fugax bears a special relationship to atherosclerosis of that stretch of the vessel. However, in reports of large series of cases no specific data about intracranial ICA atherosclerosis could be found.[3,80,236,262,281] Mungas and Baker[264] mentioned that among 107 patients 3 had an isolated intracranial stenosis of the carotid siphon and that a stenosis of the siphon was thought to be the source of an embolus in 5 of 36 patients studied with selective carotid artery angiography. Wilson et al.[381] reported that the siphon was abnormal in only 1 of 44 patients with branch-retinal-artery occlusion and in none of 18 with central retinal artery occlusion.

Very few specific cases have been recorded. Gerstenfeld[146] reported a 30-year-old man who suffered many attacks of amaurosis fugax of the right eye. White streaks were seen in the retinal arterioles. Angiography disclosed an ICA occlusion above the level of the ophthalmic artery. In addition, the ophthalmic artery had an unusually early origin from the ICA, since it arose from the infraclinoid part. It should be noted that a severe right frontal headache was mentioned, a very uncommon feature of amaurosis fugax, and in that young patient, atherosclerosis would appear unlikely. Dyll et al.[95] reported a patient with four attacks of amaurosis fugax and roughening and narrowing of the uncoiled carotid siphon proximal to the origin of the ophthalmic artery. David has reported a case of amaurosis fugax with siphon lesions and a possible embolic mechanism.[76]

Intracranial ICA atherosclerosis may of course be asymptomatic and angiography may be done for reasons that are not directly or certainly related. In 20 patients (30 percent) of Marzewski et al.[238] angiography had been done for asymptomatic carotid bruit in 13, encephalopathy in 2, dizziness in 2, seizures in 2, cranial nerve palsies in 1. Angiography was done in 11 (19 percent) of the patients of Craig et al.[73] for asymptomatic bruit (4 cases), stroke in other vascular territories (4 cases), confusional state due to metabolic encephalography (2 cases), and investigation prior to major vascular surgery (1 case).

## Transient Monocular Blindness

Transient monocular blindness, also known as amaurosis fugax, has been recognized as an important manifestation of carotid artery disease since early reports.[108] TMB may be considered a brief monocular visual obscuration described by patients as a "fog," "blur," "cloud," or "mist." A "shade" or "curtain" effect to the visual loss occurs in only a minority of cases, approximately 15 to 20 percent,[142,281] and is no more predictive of carotid artery disease than other variations of monocular visual loss. Several reports on TMB[3,114,264,281,308,363] have corroborated the brief duration of visual impairment, usually less than 15 minutes, rarely exceeding 30 minutes, with most patients affected only 1 to 5 minutes. Flashing lights, scintillations, colors, and fortification spectra rarely occur as a TIA manifestation and usually signify a migrainous event.[363] However, the presence of positive visual phenomena during TMB, in patients with 75 percent stenosis or greater, has been recorded by Goodwin et al.,[150] making differentiation from retinal migraine difficult, in some cases on clinical grounds alone.

The number of TMB attacks varies greatly from patient to patient before they seek medical attention. Patients may experience a few or as many as 100 attacks of TMB over a span of several days to a year or more.[281] Vision is usually fully restored following an attack, although in long-term followed-up studies of such patients,[236] a small number may sustain permanent visual loss from retinal infarction. TMB rarely occurs simultaneously with other neurologic deficits, and headache is not part of the disturbance. Hemisphere stroke is an infrequent sequel of TMB alone,[104,176,236] although careful studies of such cases occasionally reveal evidence of clinically inobvious cerebral embolism.[163] In most instances, clinically obvious stroke is preceded by one or more transient hemispheral attacks. TMB tends to precede the first transient hemispheral attack if a careful history can be documented.

### *Ophthalmoscopic Correlations*

Transient monocular blindness poses no end of diagnostic interpretation difficulties. The failure of the retinal arteries to show any abnormality during a period of transient monocular blindness has often been described. It has been speculated that the normal appearance of the retinal arteries may be a sign that the inferred embolic material or low flow state applies to the choroidal circulation that would not be visualized by the ophthalmoscope. However, experimental occlusion of the central retinal artery for up to 98 minutes[168] did not reveal itself by ophthalmoscopic change and no significant permanent neurologic damage was observed. Occlusion for 105 minutes or longer, however, produced irreversible damage, but even then no permanent injury was obvious in the retinal vascular bed. Only a transient leakage of fluorescein was observed 2.5 to 3 hours after the occlusion. These findings show that vessels that look normal by ophthalmoscope may be present even in a setting of complete retinal artery occlusion.[142]

### *Intravascular Material*

It is perhaps only whimsical speculation that Gowers[151] may have found intravascular material over a century ago in his report on embolic material in the vessels supplying the eye. In modern times, Hollenhorst, an ophthalmologist at the Mayo Clinic, is credited with the first description of cholesterol crystals (Hollenhorst plaques) in the retinal circulation.[175] His patients had all types of cerebrovascular symptoms, but he emphasized the association of the retinal material with systemic atherosclerosis and significant cardiovascular mortality, although he was uncertain about concomitant visual symptoms related to this particulate material.[142,175,291] In fact, in identifying a separate group of patients with TMB who did not have cholesterol plaques in their retinal circulation, he first documented that this embolic material was not necessarily associated with TMB. Clinical experience has corroborated Hollenhorst's observation that patients with TMB do not usually have cholesterol emboli in their retinal circulation during or between TMB attacks. The flat shape and small size of cholesterol emboli allow many to cause no interruption in blood flow.[142]

Reports[118,308] prompted by the rare opportunity to observe a patient during an attack of TMB have described white or grayish material passing through the retinal circulation, presumably platelet complexes, perhaps mixed with fibrin. This material is believed by many to be what is visualized by the ophthalmoscope in the rare instances of TMB studied during an attack. Although he has been credited with the first description of such material observed during an attack, Fisher[118] was careful not to make too great a claim as to how the material reached the vascular tree, and left open the possibility that it may have been embolic or generated by local events, such as sludging from inadequate perfusion. Gerstenfeld[146] found similar white bodies, but the disease was confined to the internal carotid artery above the origin of the ophthalmic artery. In other case reports[95] only pallor of the disc was found, even given a source for embolic material in the proximal internal carotid artery. McBrien and colleagues[242] succeeded in demonstrating a platelet origin to some of the embolic material seen in the retina in a 37-year-old man who suffered two episodes of blindness, the last one leaving him with a permanent nasal field defect. Platelet material was found in a superior nasal branch (apparently serving a portion of the visual field clinically unaffected). In the rare instances of calcium emboli to the retinal artery, opportunity was provided to document the visual loss associated with focal branch occlusions. Brockmeier et al.[43] described four patients whose accompanying visual loss corresponded to the location of the retinal embolus. Transient visual loss of the type attributed to retinal branch occlusion with platelet aggregates was not encountered. Brockmeier suggested that the small size of calcific emboli were sufficient to plug retinal arteries, but insufficient to precipitate clinical symptoms in the cerebrum. However, Beal et al.[22] documented several sites of cerebral infarction in a 69-year-old man who experienced numerous brief spells of numbness and weakness consistent with hemispheral transient cerebral ischemic attacks, indicating that some such particles can be large enough to precipitate symptoms. Cattle-trucking has also been seen in the vessels during some attacks.[142]

A rare case of transient vertical monocular hemianopsia was described,[388] the attacks attributed to an anomalous arteriolar pattern in that both the superior and inferior nasal quadrants were supplied by the same arterial branch. Microembolization to this common arteriolar trunk may have accounted for the six episodes of monocular vertical hemianopsia in a 3-day period.

An interesting variant of TMB has been reported by Furlan et al.,[139] in which exposure to bright light (often sunlight) precipitated transient unilateral visual loss in five patients with high-grade internal carotid artery stenosis or occlusion. All the patients also had typical, unprovoked TMB, reduced retinal artery pressure in the affected eye, and three patients also had hemispheric TIAs. Hemodynamic insufficiency of the retinal circulation was the probable mechanism leading to reduced photochemical resynthesis of visual pigments by the retinal rods and cones. Donnan et al.[87] recorded impaired visual evoked responses in four patients with similar symptoms. Recently, Wiebers et al.[378] extended these observations to include four patients with episodic bilateral visual blurring or dimming in response to bright light; all the patients had severe bilateral carotid occlusive disease. Apart from transient monocular blindness, persisting visual deficit from ocular infarction may also occur (see below).

## Transient Hemispheral Attacks

Symptoms reflecting a transient cerebral disturbance are common in carotid artery disease and have been called transient hemispheral attacks (THAs). Weakness and/or numbness of part or all of the contralateral body with or without a speech disturbance, depending on whether the dominant hemisphere is affected, are the general manifestations. It is an inherent problem in studying THAs that an accurate history may be difficult to obtain because the episodes are brief and frightening to the patient, not usually observed by another person, and may involve the right hemisphere making the patient's report unreliable. Nevertheless, the usual features of THAs have been characterized in several studies.[18,119,235,247,281]

The most common constellation of symptoms are motor and sensory dysfunction of the contralateral limbs, followed by pure motor dysfunction, then pure sensory dysfunction, and, lastly, isolated dysphasia.[281] The contralateral distal arm and hand is the body part that most consistently suffers in the attack and may be the only manifestation. The deficit presumably reflects ischemia to a portion of the motor cortex in the distal field of the carotid circulation, whether by means of embolism or perfusion failure.

THAs are typically brief in duration, less than 15 minutes, with the majority 1 to 10 minutes. In one study,[281] patients with THAs lasting 1 hour or more tended to have wide open carotid arteries with evidence of intracranial branch occlusion, suggesting that the THAs reflected a short-lived cerebral embolus.

Patients may have one or many THAs before coming to medical attention, a few have 20 or more.[281] Most patients have THAs over several weeks to a few months, while some patients may have a history spanning months to a year, but rarely longer.

An uncommon form of THA involves limb shaking, a manifestation identified in early reports on carotid TIAs[119] and in more recent reports.[17,112,310,339,394] Patients with major internal carotid artery occlusive disease (severe stenosis or occlusion) may experience recurrent, involuntary, irregular, wavering movements of the contralateral arm or leg. The movements are described as "shaking," "trembling," "twitching," "flap," or "wavering". Other more typical carotid TIAs are usually part of the overall picture, but limb shaking may be an initial manifestation, making distinction from focal epilepsy an important differential point. In the limited number of patients reported to date, it appears that endarterectomy may be beneficial. The mechanism underlying the shaking TIAs is presumed to be hemodynamic insufficiency, recently well documented in a single case reported by Tatemichi et al.[339] Using xenon-133 regional cerebral blood flow and transcranial ultrasonography with additional challenges of hypercapnia and hypotension, they showed perfusion insufficiency in the distal field of their patient with high-grade carotid stenosis and limb-shaking TIAs. Following endarterectomy, cerebral blood flow and blood velocities improved, and the TIAs ceased.

## Nonsimultaneous Transient Monocular Blindness and Transient Hemispheral Attacks

Patients with carotid territory TIAs, depending on when they come to medical attention, may have had TMB, THA, or both types of TIA, although rarely simultaneously. There may be a stronger correlation with severe extracranial carotid artery disease in patients with a history of separate episodes of eye and hemisphere TIAs, compared to either type of spell alone.[281]

## Angiographic Correlations with Transient Ischemic Attacks

### *Severe Stenosis or Occlusion*

There is a strong relationship between carotid territory TIAs (either TMB or THA) and extracranial carotid artery disease. Several prospective studies[105,177,185,281,294,349] have found an occurrence of significant carotid artery occlusive disease in 30 to 50 percent of patients with carotid artery territory TIAs. One prospective study[281] of patients with carotid artery territory TIAs found a bimodal distribution of angiographically documented extracranial carotid artery disease, either severe stenosis or occlusion, or a widely patent, nonobstructed artery supporting the view that symptoms do not occur with any degree of stenosis. This severe a stenosis is by no means a chance occurrence. It is prevalent in only 7 percent of an autopsy population asymptomatic for carotid disease,[128] and in less than 10 percent of patients with stroke due to another mechanism, such as hemorrhage.[253]

Lesser degrees of stenosis do not have the same high correlation with TIA. However, misestimation of the stenosis is common. A severe stenosis found at surgery may be misread on angiogram as a lesser degree of stenosis due to minor variations in lumen display or in the judgment of individuals[61,74] (Fig. 14-11). Oblique filming of the carotid bifurcation, in addition to the standard anterior-posterior and lateral views, will disclose irregular or ulcerative lesions not appreciated on the standard views.

### *Transient Ischemic Attack Type and Severe Stenosis or Occlusion*

The correlation between transient ischemic attack and severe stenosis in approximately 50 percent of patients applies equally well when the transient ischemic attack is transient monocular blindness or transient hemispheric attacks.

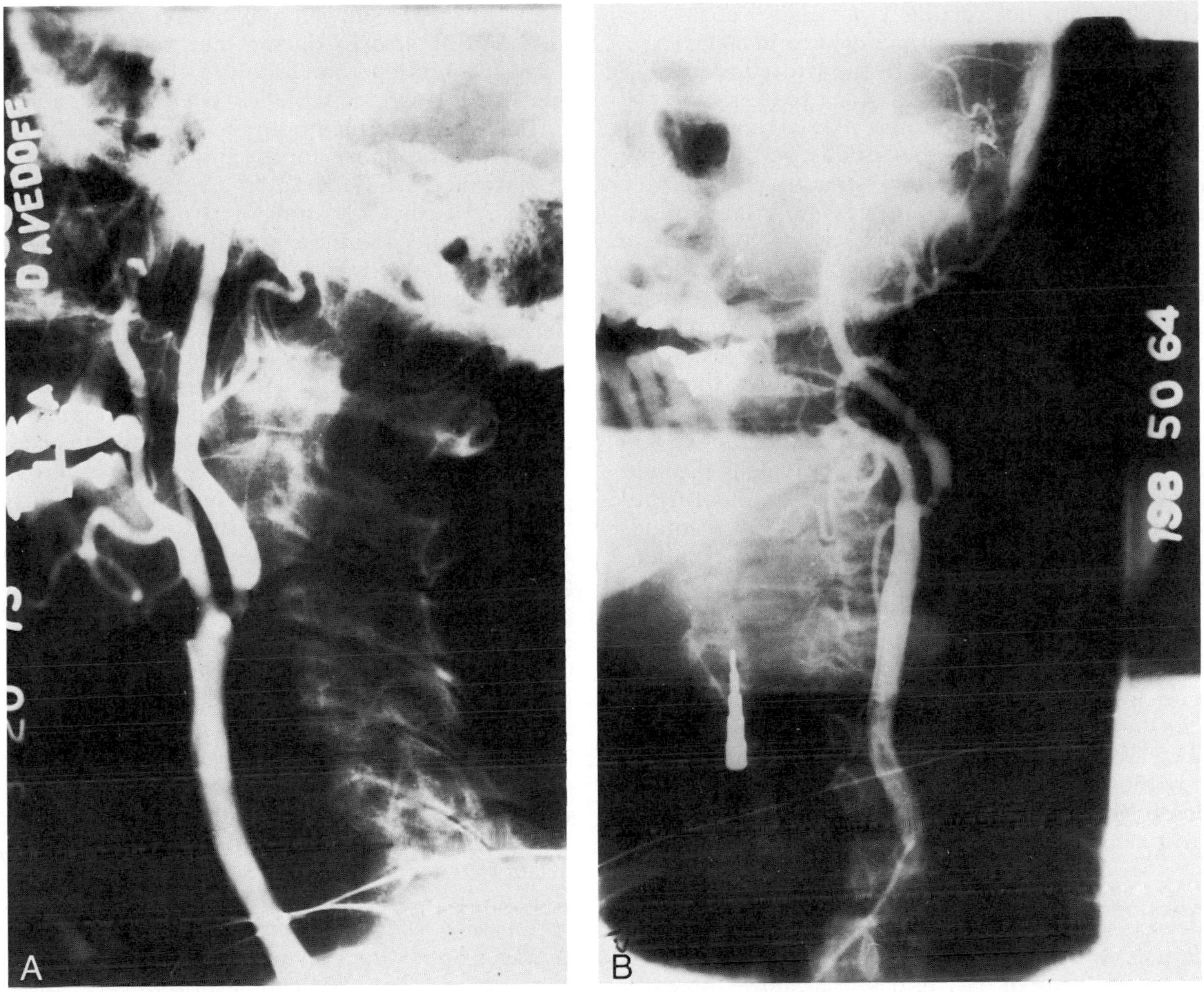


**Fig. 14-11.** (**A & B**) Two views of the same stenosis.

TMB poses a special problem in angiographic correlation. In a few studies, the correlations between the attacks, funduscopic findings, and angiography have been somewhat disappointing. Sandok et al.[314] found 43 patients with transient monocular blindness among 1,080 patients undergoing carotid angiography. In other studies there has been a poor correlation between the funduscopic findings and the angiographic findings. Of 112 patients, 53 were examined by funduscopy, and 24 showed retinal artery occlusion (intra-arterial plaques or some other evidence of retinal ischemia). Of these 53 patients, 20 had abnormal angiograms, but 24 of 29 with no retinal changes also had abnormal angiograms. No description of the clinical details of the TMB was given.

A handful of patients have been observed to show TMB associated with local stenosis of the ophthalmic artery independent of any disease in the carotid. Angiographic documentation of stenosis of the ophthalmic artery itself is extremely difficult to demonstrate. Weinberger et al.[369] documented a 50 percent stenosis near the origin of the ophthalmic artery in a patient with two episodes of transient monocular blindness. The details of the visual loss were not described. Their report was the first to correlate transient monocular blindness with ophthalmic artery stenosis. Gross et al.[156] had previously described local stenosis of the ophthalmic artery as a cause of a false positive pulse delay measured by oculoplethysmography, but they did not describe the visual symptoms in the 2 patients among 287 studied angiographically.

### *Transient Ischemic Attacks and Nonstenosing Carotid Lesions*

If TIAs are symptoms and not a unified diseased state, then the clinician's task is to correlate these transient deficits with appropriate carotid artery lesions. A migrainous event, dizziness, syncope, or seizure in a patient with a carotid lesion should not lead to the erroneous conclusion that the vascular lesion is the cause. That this important effort in clinical vascular correlation is not regularly pursued probably accounts for the excessive number of carotid endarterectomies performed each year in the United States.[375]

The problem arises from the idea that any form of carotid artery atheromatous plaque can harbor thrombus and serve as an embolic source causing TIAs. Plaque formation, either smooth, irregular, or even with ulceration seen on the angiogram, have all been implicated as "significant" lesions, although no obstruction to flow is present. The natural history of severe carotid artery stenosis in terms of its stroke risk has never been adequately settled and even fewer data are available on these other types of lesions. It still remains unsettled what to think about the presence of intraluminal thrombus removed at endarterectomy and not appreciated at angiography.[257,261] Many argue that intraplaque hemorrhage is the substrate for intraluminal thrombus when endothelialization has not occurred, and therefore even minor plaque formation should be removed if the patient has symptoms.[232] And if the minor lesions are important, their difficulty of being detected by angiography poses a major treatment dilemma.[103] The logical extension of these arguments leads to surgery for cases that are angiographically normal or show only minor plaque formation on the suspicion that significant stroke risk exists. Since carotid plaque formation is commonly seen angiographically in large numbers of patients, this may in part account for the excessive carotid artery surgery.

### *Plaques and Ulcerations*

Plaques and ulcerations have been recognized as potential sources of TIA and stroke since the early years of this century.[60] Early studies appeared to consider that TIAs could be attributable to any degree of stenosis[177,259,349] by means of microembolization. Evidence in support of this view arose from individual case reports, to which were later added whole series of cases.[34,77,101,190,200,246,260,389,401]

Compared with stenosis and occlusion, however, ulcerations are not a common finding in cases with TIAs. In a study of 95 consecutively angiogrammed cases with unilateral carotid territory TIAs, by Pessin et al.,[281] no correlation was found with ulcerations of the carotid artery; ulcerations were present in approximately 6 percent of cases and occurred with equal frequency ipsilateral and contralateral to the symptomatic side. In other studies,[104,105] although some degree of ulceration was found in 47 percent of cases suffering amaurosis fugax (transient monocular blindness) and 49 percent of cases with transient hemispheral attacks, fully 50 percent showed the expected ipsilateral tight stenosis or occlusion. In that study, no information was given as to the frequency of ulcers or stenosis in the nonsymptomatic artery. Finally, a retrospective study of 79 cases with 91 asymptomatic shallow ulcers or ulcerated plaques over a mean of 3 years showed only a 9 percent incidence of TIAs and no strokes during that period.[205] The published discussion that followed the paper was conducted by Moore, Machleder, Levin, Javid, and Eastcott, whose combined opinions supported the notion of a benign prognosis for asymptomatic patients with shallow ulcers and ulcerated plaques. Fisher and Ojemann's[131] pathologic study of carotid endarterectomy plaques found no important clinical correlation with ulcerations or cul-de-sacs (defined as rounded pouches of diverticuli protruding from the lumen into the plaque) in 90 patients with hemispheric TIAs, TMB, asymptomatic, or in a separate group of 51 patients with a persistent neurologic deficit. Of 30 cases of ulceration and 7 cul-de-sacs in the TIA patients, no definite examples of clinical embolic events occurred. This point is underscored by the observation that 9 ulcerations and 5 cul-de-sacs were found in 33 asymptomatic patients. Similarly, in 51 patients with a persistent neurologic deficit signifying infarction, only 10 had ulcerations or cul-de-sacs, and 6 of these were in association with a severe stenosis (residual lumen less than 1 mm). The remaining 4 patients, with widely patent lumens, had minor neurologic signs. However, the TIA and stroke risk for complex, deep ulcers is still a subject of dispute.[205,259]

Despite these findings, the mere demonstration of ulcer continues to be taken as a risk for stroke. Julien et al.[190] found 17 ulcerated atheromatous plaques among 231 carotid bifurcation specimens in surgery performed for TIA. Wood and Correll[389] found such changes in 54 percent of 160 cases, adding the observation that a few of the cases showed a small ulcer that was not evident on angiogram. All of their ulcers were found within cervical carotid bifurcation atheromas, and were especially common in the larger atheromas, measuring 3 to 4 mm in length. In most cases, only one microscopic area of ulceration was found. Their traced angiograms showed the ulcers were quite obvious and of fairly large size.

Despite the announced results of the North American Symptomatic Carotid Endarterectomy Trial and European Cooperative Study, debate continues on whether ulcers are important in stroke. They are often found in surgical specimens.[34,101,183,200] The smaller ulcers are difficult to demonstrate angiographically, and considerable interobserver variation exists in the diagnosis of ulceration.[103] As many as 40 percent are missed on routine angiogram, and many ulcers are found at operation in "smooth, benign-appearing plaques."[101] Ulceration may be an erroneous angiographic diagnosis for a lesion, actually due to subintimal hemorrhage into a shallow plaque,[101] a finding that may even resolve spontaneously.[201]

Nonobstructive but irregular and/or ulcerated lesions seen angiographically seem to have a benign natural history unless they are very large, and when large they are usually associated with advanced stenosis. Deep ulcer craters or severe irregularities on angiography are associated with an increased TIA and stroke risk, even in the absence of significant flow obstruction.[257,260] Mural lesions carry a higher stroke risk,[370] but none as high as obstructive lesions. Because of the known morbidity and mortality (3 percent) associated with carotid endarterectomy in the best series[188] and the uncertain stroke risk associated with these nonobstructive carotid lesions, we have adopted guidelines for "significant" carotid disease characterized by severe stenosis causing the residual lumen to be 2 mm or less as measured on the angiogram. Two millimeters has been selected as the criterion, based on the regular occurrence of clinical symptoms and the fact that hemodynamic mechanisms may operate at this level of stenosis.[42]

### Differential Diagnosis of Transient Ischemic Attacks

Many types of spells similar or even identical in part to TIAs have different pathogeneses and stroke prognosis.[92,119] The concept of TIA is based on an atherothrombotic mechanism, and this factor alone distinguishes them from other types of spells.

Seizures, migraine accompaniments, syncope, isolated dizziness, and transient memory disturbance are common disturbances that may be confused with TIAs. These spells, however, have no proven atheromatous basis and their treatments and outcomes differ significantly from TIAs. Even spells considered to meet the definition of TIAs may have an underlying vascular mechanism other than large-artery atherothrombotic disease. TIAs may be related to small, penetrating arterial disease that causes lacunar infarction.[253,281] They may occur as a flurry in the hours before stroke or as isolated events without stroke. The clinical features of lacunar TIAs may be indistinguishable from large-artery TIAs, yet diagnostic evaluation, treatment, and stroke risk are probably different. Also, rapidly fading cerebral embolism may give rise to a short-lived neurologic deficit consistent with the time criterion of TIA, but no atherothrombotic mechanism exists. In one study,[281] such TIAs of presumed embolic mechanism tended to be of longer duration, 1 hour or longer, than TIAs of carotid atheromatous cause.

All these variations should alert the clinician to the heterogeneous nature of TIAs. They are best viewed as symptoms, much like seizure and headache, and not as a homogeneous, pathogenic state. Further clarification of the underlying cerebrovascular mechanisms may help lead to more rational therapy and reliable prognostication.

### Reversible Ischemic Neurologic Deficit

The usefulness of the older concept of reversible ischemic neurologic deficit (RIND) has recently been questioned on the grounds that it has no prognostic value.[51,227] In fact, a slowly, but greater than 24-hour, clearing deficit probably reflects infarction, and many times the CT scan will corroborate this.[366]

Some carotid artery-related strokes begin and progress in a fashion that accumulation of neurologic deficit occurs over hours to a day or more giving rise to the term *progressive or evolving stroke.* Clearly the brain has suffered infarction in this situation, but the patient may have only a submaximal neurologic deficit for the arterial territory affected. For example, if a patient has only mild to moderate right arm and hand weakness, but face, leg, speech, and visual field functions are spared, then this will be considered a submaximal deficit for the territory involved, although infarction may be present even on CT scan. The mechanism responsible for this deficit might recur, leading to further disability unless treatment is offered. This approach, stressing submaximal deficit rather than whether or not the brain has suffered infarction, allows for the opportunity of treatment (surgical or medical) in the hope of preventing further disability.

## Ischemic Stroke from Carotid Artery Disease

### Ocular Infarction

The ipsilateral eye and brain are the usual sites of clinical symptoms in stroke affecting a given internal carotid artery territory. Although both the eye and the brain are susceptible, it is remarkable how infrequently the eye is affected by permanent deficit compared with the brain. Even rarer is the simultaneous occurrence of eye and brain infarction from hemodynamic carotid artery disease, called "optico-cerebral syndrome" by Bogousslavsky et al.[38] in 3 (0.5 percent) of 612 consecutive patients with carotid artery territory stroke. In our experience,[281] this syndrome is rare and gives too much emphasis to the notion that the eye and brain are involved at the same time in TIAs, a view that should be deemphasized, not resurrected.

The relationship between retinal infarction (eye stroke) and extracranial carotid artery disease is complicated. Since Marshall and Meadows'[236] study of the natural history of transient monocular blindness, it has been known that associated retinal infarction may occur in a small percentage of patients followed over the long run. The presumed mechanism is embolic occlusion of either a retinal branch or the central retinal artery. Considerable controversy, however, has centered on the relationship between the embolic material and associated carotid artery disease as a potential source. Cholesterol crystals discovered in the retinal circulation, a marker for systemic atherosclerosis known from Hollenhorst's original reports,[175,278] are often incidentally noted on routine ophthalmologic examination in asymptomatic patients.[45,282,318] Hollenhorst first documented that TMB was not usually associated with cholesterol emboli, an observation corroborated in clinical practice.

Even the role of cholesterol emboli in causing other types of permanent monocular visual loss is unclear. Some studies suggest a relationship to retinal branch occlusion with the carotid artery as the embolic source.[308,381] Other studies, however, identify a strong correlation between retinal infarct from branch occlusion and carotid artery occlusive disease, but the embolic material is usually platelet debris and not cholesterol. When permanent visual loss related to central retinal artery occlusion is included, a condition in which the embolic obstruction may not be visualized, cardiac embolic sources, albeit occult, as well as the carotid artery may be the underlying embolic mechanism. The simple and unitary idea that TMB and retinal stroke are all manifestations of one entity, with extracranial carotid artery disease giving rise to cholesterol emboli as the offending material, is probably incorrect. However, the possibility that moderate to severe carotid disease is similarly associated with different retinal embolic events has been raised by the finding of Pessin et al.[282] that in 39 patients with 42 instances of retinal cholesterol plaques, branch retinal artery occlusion, and central retinal artery occlusion, the incidence of carotid artery disease, 56 to 60 percent, was not different for the three groups.

### *Central Retinal Artery Occlusion*

Several large series of patients with central retinal artery occlusion, who had cerebral angiography, have documented ipsilateral carotid artery disease (ulcerative nonstenotic, stenosis without ulceration or irregularity, occlusion) consistent with an embolic source in 50 to 70 percent of cases.[89,282,323] Carotid artery territory TIAs, including transient monocular blindness, occurred in many patients before central retinal artery occlusion.

### *Ischemic Optic Neuropathy*

A host of ocular pathologies, encompassed by the term ischemic optic neuropathy, may attend chronic orbital ischemia as a result of extracranial carotid artery occlusive disease. Remarkably, it is an uncommon complication of carotid artery occlusive disease estimated to affect approximately 5 percent of patients in one of the early series.[198] Embolism may be the cause.[233] The ocular abnormalities include pupillary dilation with poor light reaction, neovascularization of the iris (rubeosis iridis), elevated intraocular pressure with secondary glaucoma, and proliferative retinopathy (Figs. 14-12 and 14-13) with microaneurysms, scattered flame-shaped hemorrhages, and prominent venous stasis.[121,169,198,233,399] Significant visual loss, sometimes ending in blindness with optic atrophy, makes this a serious condition. The presumed pathogenesis of reduced orbital blood flow has led to claims[102] that the chronic ocular ischemia changes may be reversible with extracranial-intracranial arterial grafting, but others[399] have not found this beneficial.

### *Unusual Syndromes*

A small series of cases have been described with symptoms and signs referable to the orbit in cases of

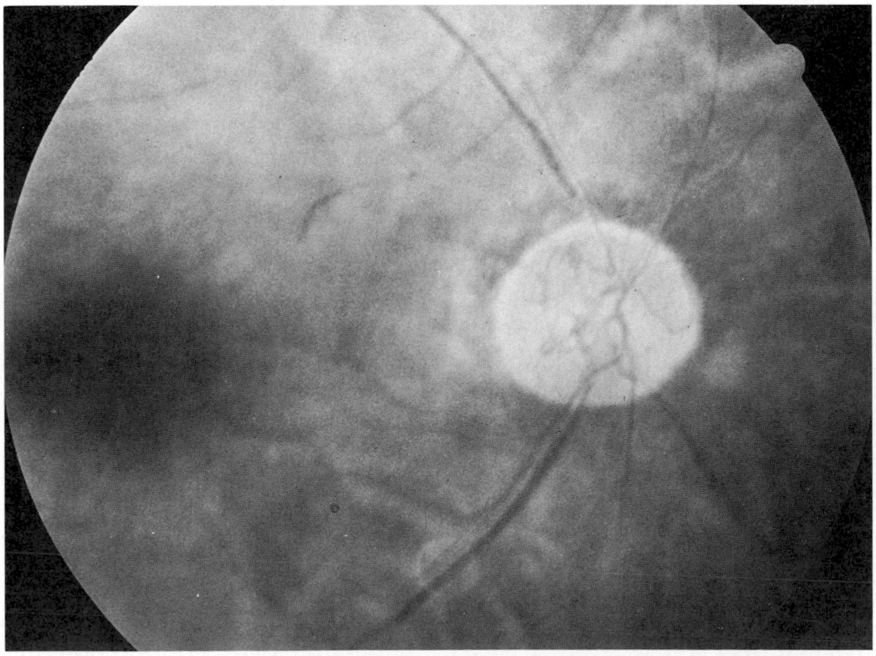

**Fig. 14-12.** Attenuated retinal vessels.

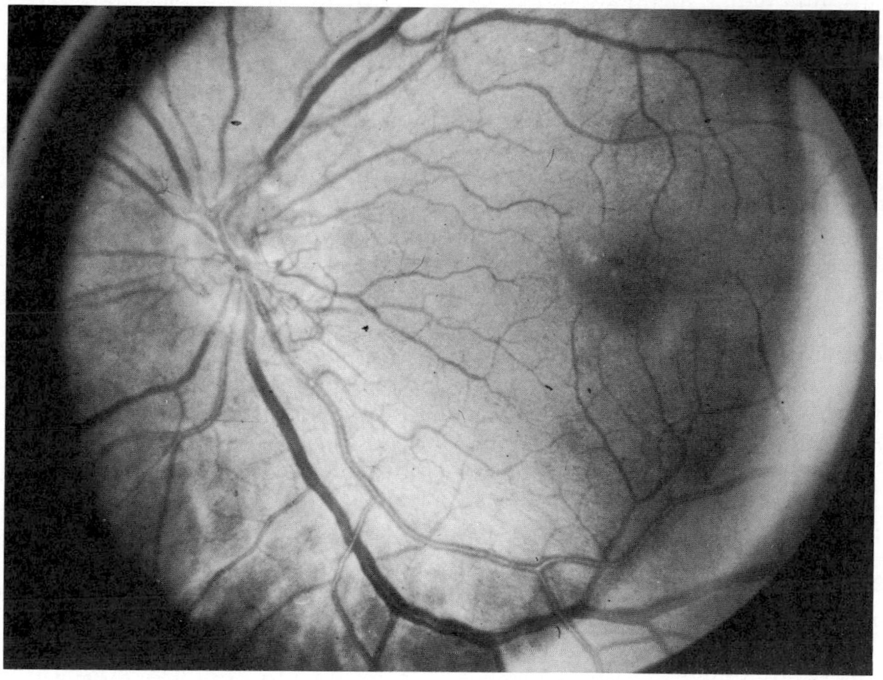

**Fig. 14-13.** Neovascular proliferation affecting the disc.

carotid artery disease. For some, a variant of migraine, Raeder's paratrigeminal syndrome, and the like have been described. Gelmers[144] described two cases with facial pain and ipsilateral oculosympathetic paresis, which he labeled as the "pericarotid syndrome." The angiogram demonstrated disease affecting the cervical portion of the internal carotid artery, to which Gelmers attributed the ocular disturbance.

## Cerebral Infarction

The number of instances of cerebral infarction in the territory of the internal carotid artery far exceed the instances in which the mechanism of the stroke is determined.[155] The difficulties in determining whether the internal carotid artery is occluded, severely stenosed, slightly stenosed, ulcerated, or merely the conduit for the embolic material remains a major obstacle to progress in the analysis of cases of stroke in the carotid territory. Yet this difficulty is brushed aside when the clinical syndromes of carotid artery disease are discussed in detail, as is apparent in the discussion that follows.

Following a variable number of TIAs, the completed stroke that results from severe stenosis or occlusion of the internal carotid artery reflects infarction from either distal flow failure[113] or embolization.[58,60] The latter mechanism is probably the most common, as it accounts for virtually two-thirds of strokes with internal carotid artery occlusion.[283] Distal insufficiency appears to account for the other third. Simultaneous infarction of the eye and brain[151] is rare.[35,281]

*Infarction with Distal Insufficiency*

The pathophysiologic basis for the concept of infarction with distal insufficiency has already been covered in detail (see above). The clinical syndromes from cerebral infarction in this distribution should be characterized by a prominent visual field defect, aphasia or hemi-inattention features (from dominant or nondominant hemisphere involvement, respectively), and variable degrees of contralateral sensorimotor deficit. The latter should affect the proximal more than the distal segments of the upper limb, reflecting the location of the infarct along the upper portions of the frontoparietal convexity.[250] Although the above constellation of symptoms is commonly found—bilaterally—in cases of cardiac arrest and hypotension with resulting bilateral distal field infarction, its unilateral occurrence from ICA atherothrombosis has only recently been documented by CT scan.[36]

In the study of symptoms with carotid artery occlusion by Pessin et al.[283] the clinical differences between two groups of patients were a higher frequency of preceding TIAs and less severe clinical deficits in those of nonembolic mechanism. These authors could not separate two groups of patients with clinically well-defined neurologic findings to assist in delineating a different topography of the infarcts.

From these considerations, it is apparent that a distal insufficiency mechanism of reduced cerebral flow, although a possible explanation for recurrent stereotypic TIAs,[92] has proved to be hard to document as the source of cerebral infarction from internal carotid artery disease, a situation in which distal embolism appears to account for the great majority of events. As a result, the neurologic examination findings in themselves have no distinctive elements to suggest extracranial ICA atherothrombosis as the cause of the stroke.

Numerous autopsy-documented studies have detailed the clinical picture in suprasylvian unilateral cerebral infarcts, even when the cause of the infarction has been unclear.[58,113,115,116,128,217,250,304,317] Many of these cases developed the infarct in relation to carotid occlusion, under which circumstances the main bulk of the endangered territory lay between the anterior and middle cerebral arteries, which caused the softening in the upper frontal lobe.

The most frequently reported effects have been unilateral infarction. The symptoms to be expected in such cases have received the descriptive attention of a number of authors.[113,115,220,222,278,283,299,304,332] Common symptoms have included weakness, paralysis, dyspraxia, numbness and tingling, and stereodysnomia in one or more fingers, hand, wrist or arm, and leg. The grasp reflex has been observed. Transient impaired ocular motility is often reported, but, when not referred to the meaning, the omission is unclear. Disturbances in higher cerebral function have included episodes of speechlessness, change in personality,[115,406] and dysgraphia of both the paretic and dyspraxic type.

A few well-known examples from the older literature will also indicate the long-standing recognition of the syndrome. Elder[107] described a 69-year-old messenger who developed stepwise attacks of right arm and leg paresis with slight dysarthria. Sensation was said to be normal, and he had no hemianopia. The left eye was frequently painful. A right grasp was noted. The progressing hemiplegia spared the face. His speech was intact, as were auditory comprehension and repetition. His writing was clumsy, large, and confined to his own name and few letters; copying was difficult. He named objects presented at sight easily. He was unable to read aloud, and could manage only a few letters with frequent repetitions. At autopsy white vessel and extensive infarction was observed extending from the upper frontal region to involve almost the entire lateral parietal and occipital regions.

Spatz's famous case[332] was a 43-year-old man whose problems began with attacks of headache and shimmering in the left eye. He later developed a weak right arm and disturbance of speech in which he often failed to find a word. A right homonymous hemianopia was observed. No tests of reading are reported. At autopsy, the suprasylvian territory of the left cerebral hemisphere from frontal through posterior parietal regions was involved with granular atrophy.

Attempts to clarify the clinical picture in a setting of carotid occlusion documented in life have been less striking, perhaps because such case material includes a mixture of examples of distal insufficiency, cerebral embolism, and anterograde extension of thrombus into the stem of the middle cerebral artery. In one of the first attempts at such a clinical study, 64 consecutively encountered cases of internal carotid artery occlusion among 5,000 angiograms performed over a 3-year period were reported by Pessin et al.[283] They found 22 cases whose clinical picture and radiologic findings suggested the stroke occurred through the mechanism of distal insufficiency.[283] No angiographic evidence of arterial branch occlusion was found. In this group of 22 cases, 16 had one or more prior TIAs, and the 13 who suffered a stroke showed only a modest deficit, mostly confined to weakness in the upper limb. Clinically, the cases attributed to hemodynamic cause conformed to the formula found by Pessin et al.,[283] with a milder deficit and better clinical outlook in such cases compared with those attributed to embolism.

Clinical syndromes of pure dementia have often been alluded to in the literature but have proved difficult to document. Claims of improvement in mental function after carotid endarterectomy have appeared from time to time. The most recent[184] is of interest for its attempt to focus on those cases presumed to be suffering from the "low flow" state. Using a battery of tests of memory and mental agility, the authors found a more dramatic change postoperatively in their 12 cases thought to have "low flow" state preoperatively than they did in the matched controls having no hemodynamically significant lesions.

Less attention has been accorded to bilateral infarcts. Perhaps because of the dramatic clinical picture, some of the literature of symptomatic bilateral cerebral infarction from bilateral carotid artery occlusion has emphasized the devastating nature of the clinical deficits. Cases of bilateral traumatic thrombosis of the carotid artery, although somewhat unusual, have been particularly striking: Petrov et al.[285] described a 30-year-old woman who developed bilateral traumatic carotid artery occlusions after an automobile accident and presented in coma. The coma deepened over a period of 24 hours and an autopsy appeared to involve virtually the entire territories of both internal carotid arteries, including not only the proximal fields as well as the distal but also the hypophysis.

Castaigne et al.[56] reported the case of a 51-year-old man with bilateral internal carotid artery occlusion, the distal end of the occlusion being below the ophthalmic artery on both sides. The patient survived for 2 years and died from cancer of the colon. Neuropathologic examination showed bilateral "watershed" lesions, more marked on the left hemisphere. On the left side the posterior cerebral artery as well as the anterior and middle cerebral arteries arose from the internal carotid artery. Microscopically, the pial arteries were patent, thin-walled, and stained pale pink with eosin. Clinically, the deep reflexes were brisk on both sides; there was a bilateral Babinski sign and *marche à petits pas*. The appearance and demeanor of the patient were quite remarkable. He had a masklike face with an impressive absence of mimicry. Day after day he lay for hours in his bed, motionless, head and eyes turned toward the left. At long intervals he winked and sighed or made a few clumsy movements with both hands. However, when encouraged he appeared well oriented in time and space. He could name objects and colors and recognized faces. He clumsily and slowly but correctly carried out spoken commands. There was no severe ideomotor apraxia. In Pierre Marie's three-paper test two out of three of the orders were correctly performed. However, as soon as the examination ended the patient reverted to his motionless state.

A few of the cases of bilateral infarction have presented less dramatic clinical syndromes. Romanul and Abramowicz[304] described a man (case 1) with left arm weakness, hyperreflexia, and impaired pin appreciation whose ability to understand newsprint, to draw, and to calculate were impaired. The patient showed bilateral carotid artery occlusion and bilateral lesions.

The predominance of high convexity infarction in carotid syndromes of distal insufficiency have yielded some distinctive syndromes. In a study of clinical features separating embolic from carotid artery thrombotic syndrome, Timsit et al.[346] found the carotid artery syndrome contained examples of fractional (different degrees of) weakness in the shoulder versus the hand, which was thought to reflect the upper convexity infarction from distal insufficiency. Examples of embolism more often showed comparable degrees of weakness of the hand and shoulder, consistent with the larger and lower convexity infarction. The probability of carotid artery disease increased over embolism when fractional arm weakness (shoulder different from hand) was present (odds ratio: 5.3; 95 percent confidence interval: 3.1 to 9.0). An example from the recent experience of the Salpêtrière hospital illustrates these points: A 56-year-old right-handed man awoke with a weakness of the right upper and lower limbs without any other symptoms. On neurologic examination 60 hours after onset, he was alert with a slight uneasiness for right finger movements without any other weakness. There was right-sided hyperesthesia for warm, cold, pinprick, touch, and joint position sense in the right shoulder extending to the upper third of the arm. Neurologic examination was otherwise unremarkable. CT scan showed an infarct in the upper prerolandic region on the left side (Fig. 14-14), and an angiogram showed 75 percent stenosis of the left internal carotid artery. Within several weeks the distal weakness had almost disappeared, but the sensory findings remained unchanged. Carotid endarterectomy was performed without complication.

Another unusual clinical variation of distal insufficiency in carotid occlusive disease, ipsilateral leg weakness, has been described in two separate reports.[62,395] Yanagahara et al.[395] reported 19 patients with episodic or progressive lower extremity weakness, contralateral to severe extracranial internal carotid artery occlusive disease (16 patients) or carotid siphon stenosis (3 patients). Cerebral blood measurements using xenon-133 in some of the patients, corroborated reduced hemispheric flow on the appropriate side localized to the borderzone in the frontoparietal to parietal areas corresponding to motor function of the lower extremity. Chimowitz et al.[62] described a 52-year-old man with separate transient episodes of left eye TMB, right hemiparesis and aphasia, and left leg weakness. The left leg weakness occurred on one occasion with simultaneous right arm weakness. When he developed a fixed deficit, his examination showed a right hemiparesis and expressive aphasia, left leg weakness, bilateral hyperreflexia, and Babinski signs. CT showed bilateral distal field infarcts involving the right frontoparietal, left frontal, and left parietal areas. Angiography showed an 80 percent stenosis of the left internal carotid artery and a 60 percent stenosis of the right internal carotid artery. Both anterior cerebral arteries filled from the left carotid artery circulation due to a presumably atretic right A1 segment, and the distal right anterior cerebral artery filled incompletely. Following left carotid endarterectomy the patient improved, and no further TIAs occurred in a 4-month follow-up. The

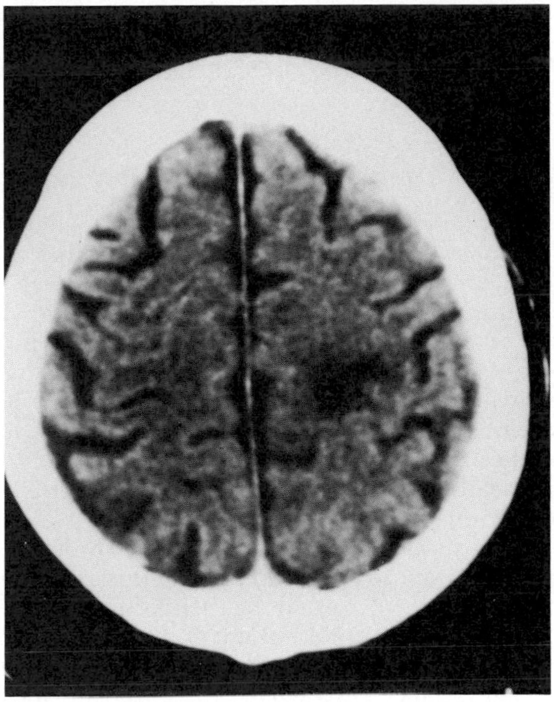

**Fig. 14-14.** High convexity infarct in a case of fractional weakness (see text).

case strongly suggests that distal insufficiency, bilaterally manifested because of an incomplete circle of Willis, accounted for the clinical signs.

*Intracranial Internal Carotid Artery Embolism*

Intracranial embolism was also found frequently in prior autopsy studies.[58,128,181,217] Embolism has also been the proposed mechanism in prior studies for some of the strokes that are delayed in onset following carotid artery occlusion.[19,58,75,128,133,352] This type of outlook is far more serious and seems to occur with far less warning.

The embolus may arise from several sources. Anterograde propagation of the thrombosis intracranially may result in a "tail" of thrombus that lies at the top of the internal carotid, the "tail" being available to be swept distally via retrograde flow through the ophthalmic and into the middle and anterior cerebral arteries above.[111,308] Lethal hemispheric stroke has been encountered in one patient 3 days after angiographically documented occlusion of the ipsilateral cerebral internal carotid artery. The autopsy evidence was consistent with embolism from the distal intracranial tail of the propagated carotid thrombus. An infarct this large has not previously been reported.[111] Embolization may also arise from the "stump" of the internal carotid artery that remains emanating from the bifurcation of the common carotid artery after internal carotid artery occlusion; the Venturi effect of blood passing up the common carotid artery to the external carotid artery may sweep material from the stump distally to reach the intracranial arteries.[19] Other sources have not yet been defined.

Embolism may be a frequent cause of stroke associated with carotid artery thrombosis. In the series reported by Pessin et al.[283] fully 25 of the 64 angiogrammed cases showed angiographic evidence of intracranial main stem or branch middle cerebral artery occlusion, while another 17 had angiographic findings consistent with or suggestive of earlier embolization. The clinical picture in these 43 cases contrasted sharply with the 22 who had no signs of embolism: less than half the cases (17 of 43) experienced prior TIA, and 12 suffered severe strokes, seven that were moderately severe, and only six that were mild. This difference in TIA frequency and stroke severity was the reverse pattern of the group whose symptoms were attributed to distal insufficiency.

This form of infarction has proved difficult to distinguish on clinical or radiographic grounds from embolism of cardiac source. At the present state of knowledge, there appears to be no essential difference between the type and severity of the syndromes caused by carotid artery or cardiac sources.[283,299] The subject of such syndromes is discussed in greater detail elsewhere in this volume.

*Anterograde Extension of Thrombus*

Pathologic studies of internal carotid artery thrombosis have documented anterograde extension of thrombus intracranially for varying distances. In a few cases, extension occurred across the circle of Willis into the stems of the anterior cerebral and middle cerebral arteries, yielding devastating cerebral infarction.[58,113,115,128,217]

One result of this form of extension may be the rare *telodiencephalic syndrome*.[316] The syndrome consists of contralateral brachiofacial hemiparesis occasionally accompanied by hemianopia and aphasia but mainly accompanied by ipsilateral hemihypohidrosis with an ipsilateral Horner syndrome. Schiffter and Reinhart[316] believe this syndrome is caused by an ischemic lesion of the crossed pathways descending from the cerebrum and the uncrossed hypothalamic-spinal sympathetic pathways. The syndrome was attributed to occlusion of the internal carotid artery and occasionally the middle cerebral artery.

## VASCULAR EXAMINATION

### Auscultation and Palpation

The clinical evaluation of cases of carotid territory stroke involve not only the neurologic examination but also the assessment of the extracranial vascular tree. The most reliable of these signs are a locally generated bruit and abnormalities in the pattern of facial pulses.

The bruit heard in roughly 70 to 80 percent of cases with severe stenosis[143,278] is most often found in front of the upper portion of the thyroid cartilage, which corresponds to the usual location of the carotid artery bifurcation.[284] Radiation of the bruit into the ocular region is usually a sign the carotid artery below is patent. Because intracranial vascular volume changes dramatically with intrathoracic pressure, great diminution in the bruit intensity with the Valsalva maneuver should be a sign of internal carotid artery stenosis. However, this sign has not proved very reliable.[209]

Palpation of the facial pulses is another bedside test that should be of considerable value in the diagnosis of carotid artery stenosis or occlusion. The collateral flow that develops in a setting of severe stenosis or occlusion of the internal carotid artery from branches of the external carotid through anastomoses in the orbit includes the distal orbital branches of the ophthalmic artery.[50] By palpation of these brow arteries, it is common to find an increase in the amplitude of the pulse in external carotid artery branches (facial, preauricular, temporal arteries) on the side of the internal carotid artery disease, resulting from increased collateral flow.[122] A more sensitive sign is the demonstration, by facial palpation, of reversal of flow in the frontal[50] or supratrochlear[8] arteries, which are a fairly reliable indicator of hemodynamically significant stenosis or occlusion of the internal carotid artery. However, the pulse is often feeble and the direction of flow is difficult to demonstrate by palpation alone. Any anxiety of precipitating a stroke by this manoeuver is unwarranted: the flow through these collateral channels are trivial compared with the greater volumes carried by the maxillary artery through the floor of the orbit, regions inaccessible to the examiner. This pattern of abnormal collateral flow can be determined more precisely by the use of directional Doppler testing. The demonstration of reversal of flow in frontal or supratrochlear arteries is strong evidence of ipsilateral internal carotid artery disease, ranging from residual lumens of 1.5 mm to complete occlusion.[8]

### Doppler Examination

The rapid development of Doppler technology for carotid artery disease has assumed so great a state as to have become the subject of a special chapter in this volume, to which the reader is referred: see Chapter 12.

### Angiography

Cerebral angiography has been the definitive evaluation for assessment of stenosis or occlusion of the extracranial internal carotid artery and detailed visualization of the intracranial circulation. Since our review in the first edition of this book, however, MR angiography[99,225] has emerged as the noninvasive competitor and even replacement for conventional angiography for, at least, initial screening. Other relatively inexpensive noninvasive methods, including B-mode and duplex Doppler imaging,[5,7,66,184,353,394] quantitative phonoangiography,[78,189,190] radionuclide imaging of the carotid artery lesion itself,[198] and digitized angiography,[104,127,220] continue to offer reliable and sensitive prescreening assessment prior to a more definitive evaluation with MR or conventional angiography. Early problems in MR angiography sensitivity in depicting severe stenosis or occlusion, compared to conventional angiography, have been resolved with so-called "black blood" techniques.[100] Definitive documentation of extracranial internal carotid artery disease may now be achieved with MR angiography, but details of the intracranial circulation, usually visualized with conventional intra-arterial angiography, are in the process of continued refinement.

Symptomatic stenoses leading to either TIAs or infarction are usually "tight," with residual lumens of 2 mm or less, a level of stenosis shown to be associated with hemodynamic changes.[10,42] Occluded cervical ICAs can have a number of angiographic patterns, some of which indicate a pathogenetic mechanism for the occlusion: a sharp-pointed, tapering stenosis of the ICA, distal to which there is a threadlike luminal filling that may open distally into a normal-sized lumen—the so-called "string sign"[132]—is a picture commonly seen in carotid artery dissection. In the atherosclerotic variety of ICA occlusion, on the other hand, several angiographic patterns have been recognized[280] (Fig. 14-15): sharp, pointed stump; amputation of the artery at its origin; rounded, blunt stump. The old notion that the first pattern indicates recent occlusion, and the other two are found in the chronic stage has not proved justified, as all three patterns were seen when arteriograms were performed within 6 days from stroke onset.[280]

Finally, the demonstration of the mechanism of stroke (embolic versus nonembolic) and the pattern of collateral circulation adds to the unique value of angiography in assisting the planning for definitive therapy of carotid artery atherosclerotic disease. Further discussion is found in the section on angiography in this chapter.

## PROGNOSIS FOR INTRACRANIAL INTERNAL CAROTID ARTERY

Two reports are available on the prognosis of intracranial ICA disease. In the 66 patients of Marzewski et al.,[238] the mean age at the time of angiography was 61.5 years, and follow-up averaged 3.9 years. Ten patients (15.2 percent) had a stroke (eight ICA territory), and the observed stroke rate for patients 35 years and older was 13 times the expected infarction rate for a normal population of a similar age and sex distribution. However, due to associated cerebral arterial lesions the intracranial ICA stenosis was the only apparent cause for only 2 of the 10 strokes. Half the patients died during follow-up. Eighteen deaths (54.6 percent of all deaths) were known to be cardiac-related. There were no known stroke deaths. The risk of stroke and death appeared to be increased when compared to that of ICA occlusion.[238] Craig et al.[73] followed, for a mean of 30 months (2 to 78 months), 58 patients whose mean age was 62.4 years. During follow-up 25 of the patients (43 percent) died: 44 percent of the deaths were cardiac-related and 36 percent stroke related. At the end of follow-up only 33 percent were alive and free from subsequent cerebral vascular events, and only 47 percent were functioning well: 17 patients (29 percent) had suffered a stroke, and 11 of these (65 percent) were appropriate to the intracranial ICA stenosis; there were 9 fatal strokes, 5 appropriate to the intracranial ICA stenosis. The asymptomatic patients had as poor a prognosis as the symptomatic ones, but women fared better than men, although the number of deaths was similar.[73]

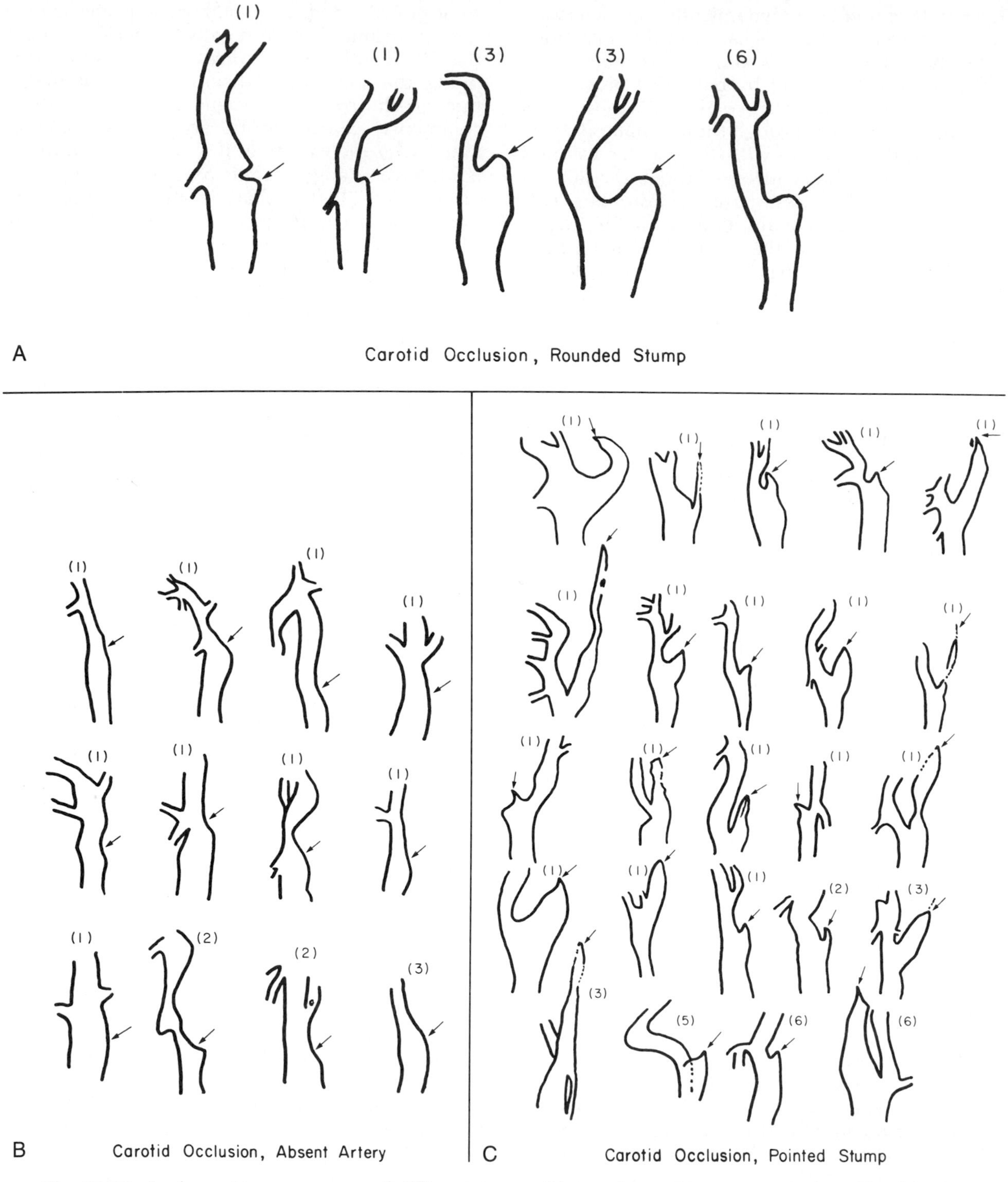


**Fig. 14-15.** Angiographic appearance of different types of internal carotid artery occlusion. Numbers in parentheses indicate days between stroke onset and angiogram.

## REFERENCES

1. Acheson J, Hutchinson EC: Observations on the natural history of transient cerebral ischemia. Lancet 2:871, 1964
2. Adams HP, Gross CE: Embolism distal to stenosis of the middle cerebral artery. Stroke 12:228, 1981
3. Adams HP, Jr, Putnam SF, Corbett JJ et al: Amaurosis fugax: the results of arteriography in 59 patients. Stroke 14:742, 1983
4. Adams RD, Fisher CM: Pathology of cerebral arterial occlusion. In Fields WS (ed): Houston Symposium on Pathogenesis and Treatment of Cerebrovascular Disease, CC Thomas, Springfield, IL, 1961
5. Adiga KR, Fresso SJ, Nayden J: Noninvasive methods in the diagnosis of extracranial carotid artery disease: a correlation with carotid arteriography in eighty patients. Angiology 35:331, 1984
6. Akelatis AJ: Symmetrical bilateral granular atrophy of the cerebral cortex of vascular origin: a clinico-pathologic study. Am J Psychiatry 99:447, 1942
7. Anderson DC, Loewenson R, Yock D et al: B-mode, real-time carotid ultrasonic imaging: correlation with angiography. Arch Neurol 40:484, 1983
8. Anderson JM, Stevens JC, Sundt TM et al: Ectopic internal carotid artery seen initially as middle ear tumor. JAMA 249:2228, 1983
9. Angeloni U, Bozzao L, Fantozzi L et al: Internal borderzone infarction following acute middle cerebral artery occlusion. Neurology (NY) 40.1196, 1990
10. Archie JP, Feldtman RW: Critical stenosis of the internal carotid artery. Surgery 89:67, 1981
11. The Asymptomatic Carotid Atherosclerosis Study Group: Study design for randomized prospective trial of carotid endarterectomy for asymptomatic atherosclerosis. Stroke 20:844, 1989
12. Awad I, Little JR, Modic MT et al: Intravenous digital subtraction angiography: an index of collateral cerebral blood flow in internal carotid artery occlusion. Stroke 13:469, 1982
13. Awad I, Modic M, Little JR et al: Focal parenchymal lesions in transient ischemic attacks: correlation of computed tomography and magnetic resonance imaging. Stroke 17:399, 1986
14. Baker RN, Broward JA, Fang HC et al: Anticoagulant therapy in cerebral infarction. Neurology (NY) 12:823, 1962
15. Baker RN, Ramseyer JG, Schwartz WS: Prognosis in patients with cerebral ischemic attacks. Neurology (NY) 18:1157, 1968
16. Banker BQ: Cerebral vascular disease in infancy and childhood. I. Occlusive vascular diseases. J Neuropathol Exp Neurol 20:127, 1961
17. Baquis GD, Pessin MS, Scott RM: Limb shaking—a carotid TIA. Submitted for publication
18. Barnett HJM: Delayed cerebral ischemic episodes distal to occlusion of major cerebral arteries. Neurology (NY) 28:769, 1978
19. Barnett HJM, Peerless SJ, Kaufmann JCE: The "stump" of internal carotid artery—a source for further cerebral embolic ischemia. Stroke 9:448, 1978
20. Baron JC, Bousser MG, Rey A et al: Reversal of focal "misery-perfusion syndrome" by extra-intracranial arterial bypass in hemodynamic cerebral ischemia. Stroke 12:454, 1981
21. Bauer RB, Boulos RS, Myer JS: Natural history and surgical treatment of occlusive cerebral vascular disease evaluated by serial angiography. AJR 104:1, 1968
22. Beal MF, Williams RS, Richardson EP, Fisher CM: Cerebral embolism as a cause of transient ischemic attacks and cerebral infarction. Neurology (NY) 31:860, 1981
23. Benditt EP, Benditt JM: Evidence for a monoclonal origin of atherosclerotic plaques. Proc Natl Acad Sci USA 70:1753, 1973
24. Benoit P, Destée A, Verier A et al: Sténose post-radiothérapique de l'artere carotide interne supraclinoïdiene: réseau de moyamoya. Rev Neurol 141:666, 1985
25. Bernasconi V, Cassinari V: Caratteristiche angiografische dei meningioma del tentorio. Radiol Med 43:1015, 1957
26. Berguer R, Hwang NHC: Critical arterial stenosis: a theoretical and experimental solution. Ann Surg 180:39, 1974
27. Bernstein NM, Norris JW: Benign outcome of carotid occlusion. Neurology (NY) 39:6, 1989
28. Berry RG, Alpers BJ: Occlusion of the carotid circulation: pathologic considerations. Neurology (Minneapolis) 7:223, 1957
29. Bickerstaff ER: Aetiology of acute hemiplegia in childhood. Br Med J 2:82, 1964
30. Björkesten G, Troupp H: Changes in the size of intra-cranial arterial aneurysms. J Neurosurg 19:583, 1962
31. Blackwood W: Pathological aspects of cerebral and spinal vascular disease. In Ross Russell RW (ed): Vascular Disease of the Central Nervous System. 2nd Ed. Churchill Livingstone, Edinburgh, 1983
32. Blackwood W, Hallpike JF, Kocen RS, Mair WGP: Atheromatous disease of the carotid arterial system and embolism from the heart in cerebral infarction: a morbid anatomical study. Brain 92:897, 1969
33. Bladin PF: A radiologic and pathologic study of embolism of the internal-middle cerebral arterial axis. Radiology 82:615, 1964
34. Blaisdell FW, Glickman M, Trunkey DD: Ulcerated atheroma of the carotid artery. Arch Surg 108:491, 1974
35. Bogousslavsky J, Regli F: Cerebral infarction with transient signs (CITS): do TIAs correspond to small deep infarcts in internal carotid artery occlusion? Stroke 15:536, 1984
36. Bogousslavsky J, Regli F: Borderzone infarctions distal to internal carotid artery occlusion: prognostic implications. Ann Neurol 20:346, 1986
37. Bogousslavsky J, Regli F, Hungerbühler J-P, Chrzanowski R: Transient ischemic attacks and

external carotid artery occlusion: a retrospective study of 23 patients with an occlusion of the internal carotid artery. Stroke 12:627, 1981
38. Bogousslavsky J, Regli F, Zografos L, Uske A: Optico-cerebral syndrome: simultaneous hemodynamic infarction of optic nerve and brain. Neurology (NY) 37:263, 1987
39. Bousser MG, Touboul P, Cabanis E et al.: The significance of ocular bruits in ischemic cerebrovascular disease. J Clin Neuro Ophthalmol 1:211, 1981
40. Boyd JD: Absence of the right common carotid artery. J Anat 68:551, 1934
41. Boysen G, Jensen G, Schnor P: Frequency of focal cerebral transient ischemic attacks during a 12-month period. Stroke 10:533, 1979
42. Brice JG, Dowsett DJ, Lowe RD: Haemodynamic effects of carotid artery stenosis. Br Med J 2:1363, 1964
43. Brockmeier LB, Adolph RJ, Gustin BW et al: Calcium emboli to the retinal artery in calcifics aortic stenosis. Am Heart J 101:32, 1981
44. Brown MF, Graham JM, Feliciano DV et al: Carotid artery injuries. Am J Surg 144:748, 1982
45. Bunt TJ: The clinical significance of the asymptomatic Hollenhorst plaque. J Vasc Surg 4:559, 1986
46. Burnbaum MD, Selhorst JB, Harbison JW, Brush JJ: Amaurosis fugax from disease of the external carotid artery. Arch Neurol 34:532, 1977
47. Busuttil RW, Baker DJ, Davidson RK, Machleder HI: Carotid artery stenosis—hemodynamic significance and clinical course. JAMA 245:1438, 1981
48. Byar D, Fiddian RV, Quereau M et al: The fallacy of applying the poisseulle equation to segmental arterial stenosis. Am Heart J 70:216, 1965
49. Callow AD: Recurrent stenosis after carotid endarterectomy. Arch Surg 117:1082, 1982
50. Caplan LR: The frontal artery sign—a bedside indicator of internal carotid occlusive disease. N Engl J Med 288:1008, 1973
51. Caplan LR: Are terms such as completed stroke or RIND of continued usefulness? Stroke 14:431, 1983
52. Caplan LR, Baker R: Extracranial occlusive vascular disease: does size matter? Stroke 11:63, 1980
53. Capron L: Athérosclérose: déscription et mécanismes. Rev Neurol (Paris) 139:167, 1983
54. Carpenter DA, Grubb RL Jr, Powers WJ: Borderzone hemodynamics in cerebrovascular disease. Neurology (NY) 40:1587, 1990
55. Carson SN, Demling RH, Esquivel CO: Aspirin failure in symptomatic atherosclerotic carotid artery disease. Surgery 90:1084, 1981
56. Castaigne P, Lhermitte F, Gautier JC: Obstruction bilateral des carotids internes. Presse Med 71:757, 1963
57. Castaigne P, Lhermitte F, Gautier JC: Rôle des lésions artérielles dans les accidents ischémiques cérébraux de l'athérosclérose. Rev Neurol (Paris) 113:1, 1965
58. Castaigne P, Lhermitte F, Gautier JC et al: Internal carotid artery occlusion: a study of 61 instances in 50 patients with post-mortem data. Brain 93:321, 1970
59. Cerebral Embolism Study Group: Immediate anticoagulation of embolic stroke. Stroke 14:668, 1983
60. Chiari H: Über das Verhalten der Teilungswinkels der Carotid communis bei der Endarteritis chronica deformans. Verh Dtsch Ges Pathol 9:326, 1905
61. Chikos PM, Fisher LD, Hirsch JH et al: Observer variability in evaluating extracranial cerotid artery stenosis. Stroke 14:885, 1983
62. Chimowitz MI, Lafranchise EF, Furlan AJ, Awad IA: Ipsilateral leg weakness associated with carotid stenosis. Stroke 21:1362, 1990
63. Cioffi FA, Meduri M, Tomasello F et al: Kinking and coiling of the internal carotid artery. J Neurosurg Sci 19:15, 1975
64. Coakham HB, Duchen LW, Scaravilli F: Moyamoya disease Clinical and pathological report of a case with associated myopathy. J Neurol Neurosurg Psychiatry 42:289, 1979
65. Cogan DG: Neurology of the Visual System. CC Thomas, Springfield, IL 1966
66. Comerota AJ, Cranley JJ, Cook SE: Real-time B-mode carotid imaging in diagnosis of cerebrovascular disease. Surgery 6:718, 1981
67. Cooperman M, Martin EW, Evans WE: Significance of asymptomatic carotid bruits. Arch Surg 113:1229, 1978
68. Correll JW, Quest DO, Carpenter DB: Nonatheromatous lesions of the extracranial cerebral arteries. p. 321. In Smith RR (ed): Stroke and the Extracranial Vessels. Raven Press, New York, 1984
69. Corrin LS, Sandok BA, Houser OW: Subsequent cerebral ischemic events in patients with carotid artery fibromuscular hyperplasia, abstracted. Stroke 12:120, 1981
70. Cote R, Barnett HJM, Taylor DW: Internal carotid occlusion: a prospective study. Stroke 14:898, 1983
71. Countee RW, Vijayanathan T, Wu SZ: External carotid occlusion as a cause of recurrent ischemia after carotid endarterectomy. Neurosurgery 11:518, 1982
72. Countee RW, Sapru HN, Vijayanathan T, Wu SZ: "Other syndromes" of the carotid bifurcation. p. 345. In Smith RR (ed): Stroke and the Extracranial Vessels. Raven Press, New York, 1984
73. Craig DR, Meguro K, Watridge C et al: Intracranial internal carotid artery stenosis. Stroke 13:825, 1982
74. Croft RJ, Ellam LD, Harrison MJG: Accuracy of carotid angiography in the assessment of atheroma of the internal carotid artery. Lancet 1:997, 1980
75. Dandy WE: Results following ligation of the internal carotid artery. Arch Surg 45:521, 1942
76. David NJ: Amaurosis fugax and after. In Glaser JS (ed): Neuroophthalmology. Vol. 9. CV Mosby, St. Louis, 1979

77. David NJ, Gordon KK, Friedberg SJ et al: Fatal atheromatous cerebral embolism associated with bright plaques in the retinal arterioles. Neurology (NY) 13:708, 1963
78. Davis DO, Rumbaugh CL, Gilson JM: Angiographic diagnosis of small-vessel cerebral emboli. Acta Radiol (Stockh) 9:264, 1969
79. Day AL, Rhoton AL, Quisling RG: Resolving siphon stenosis following endarterectomy. Stroke 11:278, 1980
80. DeBono DP, Warlow CP: Potential sources of emboli in patients with presumed transient cerebral or retinal ischemia. Lancet 1:343, 1981
81. Delal PM, Shah PM, Aiyar RR: Arteriographic study of cerebral embolism. Lancet 2:358, 1965
82. DeMarinis M, Fieschi C, Prencipe M et al: Circulating platelet aggregates: a chronic platelet activation in patients with transient ischaemic attacks. Ital J Neurol Sci 3:163, 1980
83. Denton IC, Gutmann L: Surgical treatment of symptomatic carotid stenosis and asymptomatic ipsilateral intra-cranial aneurysm. J Neurosurg 38:662, 1973
84. Dilenge D, Heon M: The internal carotid artery. p. 1202. In Newton TH, Potts DG (ed): Radiology of the Skull and Brain. Vol. 2, Book 2: Angiography. CV Mosby, St. Louis, 1974
85. Dixon S, Pais SO, Raviola C et al: Natural history of nonstenotic, symptomatic ulcerative lesions of the carotid artery: a further analysis. Arch Surg 117:1493, 1982
86. Djindjian R, Merland JJ: Super-Selective Arteriography of the External Carotid Artery. Springer-Verlag, Berlin, 1978
87. Donnan GA, Sharbrough FW, Whisnant JP: Carotid occlusive disease: effect of bright light on visual evoked responses. Arch Neurol 39:687, 1982
88. Doughtery JR, Jr, Levy DE, Weksler BB: Platelet activation in acute cerebral ischaemia. Lancet 1:821, 1977
89. Douglas DJ, Schuler JJ, Buchbinder D et al: The association of central retinal artery occlusion and extracranial carotid artery disease. Ann Surg 208:85, 1988
90. Ducos de Lahitte M, Marc-Vergnes JP, Rascol A et al: Intravenous angiography of the extracranial cerebral arteries. Radiology 137:705, 1980
91. Duncan GW, Gruber JO, Dewey CF et al: Evaluation of carotid stenosis by phonoangiography. N Engl J Med 293:1121, 1975
92. Duncan GW, Pessin MS, Mohr JP, Adams RD: Transient cerebral ischemic attacks. Adv Intern Med 21:1, 1976
93. Durward QJ, Ferguson GG, Barr HWK: The natural history of asymptomatic carotid bifurcation plaques. Stroke 13:459, 1982
94. Dyken ML, Doepker JF, Kiovsky R et al: Asymptomatic occlusion of an internal carotid artery in a hospital population: determined by directional Doppler ophthalmosonometry. Stroke 5:714, 1974
95. Dyll LM, Margolis M, David NJ: Amaurosis fugax: funduscopic and photographic observations during an attack. Neurology (Minneapolis) 16:136, 1966
96. Eastcott HG, Pickering GW, Rob CG: Reconstruction of internal carotid artery in a patient with intermittent attacks of hemiplegia. Lancet 2:994, 1954
97. Easton JD, Sherman DG: Stroke and mortality rate in carotid endarterectomy: 228 consecutive operations. Stroke 8:566, 1977
98. Easton JD, Sherman DG: Management of cerebral embolism of cardiac origin. Stroke 11:433, 1980
99. Edelman RR, Mantle HP, Atkinson DJ, Hoogewoud HM: MR angiography. Am J Radiol 154:937, 1990
100. Edelman RR, Mantle HP, Wallner B et al Extracranial carotid arteries: evaluation with "black blood" MR angiography. Radiology 177:45, 1990
101. Edwards JH, Kricheff II, Riles T, Imparato A: Angiographically undetected ulceration of the carotid bifurcation as a cause of embolic stroke. Radiology 132:369, 1979
102. Edwards MS, Chater NL, Stanley JA: Reversal of chronic occular ischemia by extracranial-intracranial arterial bypass: case report. Neurosurgery 7:480,1980
103. Eikelboom B, Riles TR, Mintzer F et al: Inaccuracy of angiography of the diagnosis of carotid ulceration. Stroke 14:882, 1983
104. Eisenberg RL, Mani RL: Clinical and arteriographic comparison of amaurosis fugax with hemispheric transient ischemic attacks. Stroke 9:254, 1978
105. Eisenberg RL, Nemzek WR, Moore WS, Mani RL: Relationship of transient ischemic attacks and angiographically demonstrable lesions of carotid artery. Stroke 8:483, 1977
106. Ekbom K, Greitz T: Carotid angiography in cluster headache. Acta Radiol [Diagn] (Stockh) 10:177, 1970
107. Elder W: The clinical varieties of visual aphasia (case 1). Edinb Med J 49:433, 1900
108. Elschnig A: Über den Einfluss des Verschlüsses der Arteria ophthalmica und der Carotis auf das Sehorgan. Graefes Arch Clin Exp Ophthalmol 39:151, 1893
109. Fields WS: The asymptomatic carotid bruit-operate or not. Stroke 9:269, 1978
110. Fields WS, Weibel J: Coincidental internal carotid stenosis and intra-cranial saccular aneurysm. Trans Am Neurol Assoc 95:237, 1970
111. Finklestein S, Kleinman GM, Cuneo R, Baringer JR: Delayed stroke following carotid occlusion. Neurology (Minneapolis) 30:84, 1980
112. Fisch BJ, Tatemichi TK, Prohovnik I et al: Transient ischemic attacks resembling simple partial motor seizures, abstracted. Neurology (NY), suppl 1. 38:264, 1988
113. Fisher CM: Occlusion of the internal carotid artery. Arch Neurol Psychiatry 69:346, 1951
114. Fisher CM: Transient monocular blindness associated with hemiplegia. Arch Ophthalmol 47:167, 1952
115. Fisher CM: Occlusion of the carotid arteries: fur-

ther experiences. Arch Neurol Psychiatry 72:187, 1954
116. Fisher CM: Cerebral thromboangiitis obliterans. Medicine (Baltimore) 36:169, 1957
117. Fisher CM: The use of anticoagulants in cerebral thrombosis. Neurology (NY) 8:311, 1958
118. Fisher CM: Observations of the fundus oculi in transient monocular blindness. Neurology (NY) 9:337, 1959
119. Fisher CM: Concerning recurrent transient cerebral ischemic attacks. Can Med Assoc J 86:1091, 1962
120. Fisher CM: Cranial bruit associated with occlusion of the internal carotid artery. Neurology (NY) 7:299, 1962
121. Fisher CM: Some neuro-ophthalmological observations. J Neurol Neurosurg Psychiatry 30:383, 1967
122. Fisher CM: Facial pulses in internal carotid artery occlusion. Neurology (NY) 20:476, 1970
123. Fisher CM: Cerebral ischemia-Less familiar types. Clin Neurosurg 18:267, 1971
124. Fisher CM: Clinical syndromes of cerebral thrombosis, hypertensive hemorrhage, and ruptured saccular aneurysm. Clin Neurosurg 22:117, 1975
125. Fisher CM: The natural history of carotid occlusion. p. 194. In Austin GM (ed): Microneurosurgical Anastomoses for Cerebral Ischemia. CC Thomas, Springfield, IL, 1976
126. Fisher CM: Discussion. In Moosy J, Reinmuth OM (eds): Cerebrovascular Diseases. Proceedings of the Twelfth Research Conference. Raven Press, New York, 1981
127. Fisher CM, Adams RD: Observations on brain embolism with special reference to the mechanism of hemorrhagic infarction. J Neuropathol Exp Neurol 10:92, 1951
128. Fisher CM, Gore I, Okabe N, White PD: Atherosclerosis of the carotid and vertebral arteries-extracranial and intracranial. J Neuropathol Exp Neurol 24:455, 1965
129. Fisher CM, Gore I, Okabe N, White PD: Calcification of the carotid siphon. Circulation 32:538, 1965
130. Fisher CM, Karnes WE: Local embolism. J Neuropathol Exp Neurol 24:174, 1965
131. Fisher CM, Ojemann RG: A clinico-pathologic study of carotid endarterectomy plaques. Rev Neurol (Paris) 142:573, 1986
132. Fisher CM, Ojemann RG, Roberson GH: Spontaneous dissection of cervico-cerebral arteries. Can J Neurol Sci 5:9, 1978
133. Fleming JFR, Petrie D: Traumatic thrombosis of the internal carotid artery with delayed hemiplegia. Can J Surg 11:166, 1968
134. Frank G: Comparison of anticoagulation and surgical treatments of TIA: a review and consolidation of recent natural history and treatment studies. Stroke 2:369, 1971
135. Friedman GD, Wilson WS, Mosier JM et al: Transient ischemic attacks in a community. JAMA 210:1428, 1969
136. Frisen L, Kjällman L, Lindberg B, Svendsen P: Detection of extracranial carotid stenosis by computed tomography. Lancet 1:1319, 1979
137. Furlan AJ, Little JR, Dohn DF: Arterial occlusion following anastomosis of the superficial temporal artery to middle cerebral artery. Stroke 11:91, 1980
138. Furlan AJ, Whisnant JP: Long-term prognosis after carotid artery occlusion. Neurology (Minneapolis) 30:986, 1980
139. Furlan AJ, Whisnant JP, Kearns TP: Unilateral visual loss in bright light: an unusual symptom of carotid artery occlusive disease. Arch Neurol 36:675, 1979
140. Gärde A, Samuelson K, Fahlgren H et al: Treatment after transient ischemic attacks: a comparison between anticoagulant drug and inhibition of platelet aggregation. Stroke 14:677, 1983
141. Gautier JC: L'angiopathie cérébrale moniliforme des toxicomanes: signification physiopathologique: role possible du spasme. Bull Acad Natl Med 172:87, 1988
142. Gautier JC: Clinical presentation and differential diagnosis of amaurosis fugax. In Bernstein EF (ed): Amaurosis Fugax. Springer-Verlag, New York, 1990
143. Gautier JC, Rosa A, Lhermitte F: Auscultation carotidienne: correlations chez 200 patients avec 332 angiographies. Rev Neurol (Paris) 131:175, 1975
144. Gelmers HJ: The pericarotid syndrome. Acta Neurochir (Wien) 57:37, 1981
145. Genton E, Barnett HJM, Fields WS et al: XIV. Cerebral ischemia: the role of thrombosis and of antithrombotic therapy. Joint Committee for Stroke Resources. Stroke 8:147, 1977
146. Gerstenfeld J: The fundus oculi in amaurosis fugax. Am J Ophthalmol 58:198, 1964
147. Gillilan LA: Anatomy of the blood supply to the brain and spinal cord: In NINCDS and NHLI: Cerebro-vascular Survey Report for Joint Council Subcommittee on Cerebrovascular Disease. Office of Scientific and Health Reports, Bethesda, MD, 1980
148. Glagov S: Mechanical stresses on vessels and the non-uniform distribution of atherosclerosis. Med Clin North Am 57:63, 1973
149. Goldberg HI, Grossman RI, Gomori JM et al: Cervical internal carotid artery dissecting hemorrhage: diagnosis using MR. Radiology 158:157, 1986
150. Goodwin JA, Gorelick PB, Helgason CM: Symptoms of amaurosis fugax in atherosclerotic carotid artery disease. Neurology (NY) 37:829, 1987
151. Gowers WR: On a case of simultaneous embolism of central retinal and middle cerebral arteries. Lancet 2:794, 1875
152. Grand W: Microsurgical anatomy of the proximal middle cerebral artery and the internal carotid artery bifurcation. Neurosurgery 7:151, 1980
153. Grillo P, Paterson RH: Occlusion of the carotid artery: prognosis (natural history) and the possibilities of surgical revascularization. Stroke 6:17, 1975
154. Grobe T: Diagnostik und Behandlungsmöglichkeiten extrakranieller Verschlussprozesse der

Arteria carotis. Fortschr Neurol Psychiatr 49:335, 1981
155. Gross CR, Kase CS, Mohr JP et al: Stroke in south Alabama: incidence and diagnostic features: a population-based study. Stroke 15:249, 1984
156. Gross W, Verta MJ, VanBellen B et al: Comparison of non-invasive diagnostic techniques in carotid artery occlusive disease. Surgery 82:271, 1977
157. Gunning AJ, Pickering GW, Robb-Smith AHT et al: Mural thrombosis of the internal carotid artery and subsequent embolism. Q J Med 33:155, 1964
158. Hammond JH, Eisinger RP: Carotid bruits in 1000 normal subjects. Arch Med 109:563, 1962
159. Handa J, Nakasu Y, Kidooka M: Transient cerebral ischemia evoked by yawning: an experience after superficial temporal artery-middle cerebral artery bypass operation. Surg Neurol 19:46, 1983
160. Hanson MR, Conomy JP, Hodgman JR: Brain events associated with mitral valve prolapse. Stroke 11:499, 1980
161. Harrington HJ, Mayman CI: Carotid body tumor associated with partial Horner's syndrome and facial pain ("Raeder's syndrome"). Arch Neurol 40:564, 1983
162. Harris FS, Rhoton AL: Anatomy of the cavernous sinus. J Neurosurg 45:169, 1976
163. Harrison MJG, Marshall J: Evidence of silent cerebral embolism in patients with amaurosis fugax. J Neurol Neurosurg Psychiatry 40:651, 1977
164. Harrison MJG, Marshall J: Does the geometry of the carotid bifurcation affect its predisposition to atheroma. Stroke 14:117, 1983
165. Harrison MJ, Marshall J: The variable clinical and CT findings after carotid occlusion: the role of collateral blood supply. J Neurol Neurosurg Psychiatry 51:269, 1988
166. Harrison MJG, Marshall J, Thomas DJ: Relevance of duration of transient ischemic attacks in carotid territory. Br Med J 2:1578, 1978
167. Hart RG, Easton DF: Dissections of cervical and cerebral arteries. Neurol Clin North Am 1:155, 1983
168. Hayreh SS, Weingeist TA: Experimental occulsion of the central artery of the retina. I. Ophthalmoscopic and fluorescein fundus angiographic studies. Br J Ophthalmol 64:896, 1980
169. Hedges TR: Ophthalmoscopic findings in internal carotid artery occlusions. Bull Johns Hopkins Hosp 111:89, 1962
170. Hennerici M, Rautenberg W: Stroke risk from symptomless extracranial arterial disease. Lancet 2:1180, 1982
171. Hertzer NR, Beven EG, Modic MT et al: Early patency of the carotid artery after endarterectomy: digital substraction angiography after 200 operations. Surgery 92:1049, 1982
172. Heyman A, Leviton A, Nefzger D et al: XI. Transient focal cerebral ichemia: epidemological and clinical aspects. Stroke 5:277, 1974
173. Heyman A, Wilkinson WE, Heyden S et al: Risk of stroke in asymptomatic persons with cervical arterial bruits. N Engl J Med 302:838, 1980
174. Hodge CJ Jr, Leeson M, Cacayorin E et al: Computed tomographic evaluation of extracranial carotid artery disease. Neurosurgery 21:167, 1987
175. Hollenhorst RW: Significance of bright plaques in the retinal arterioles. *JAMA* 178:23, 1961
176. Hooshmand H, Vines FS, Lee HM, Grindal A: Amaurosis fugax: diagnostic and therapeutic aspects. Stroke 5:643, 1974
177. Horenstein S, Hambrook G, Roat GW et al: Arteriographic correlates of transient ischemic attacks. Trans Am Neurol Assoc 97:132, 1972
178. Hu HH, Liao KK, Wong WJ et al: Ocular bruits in ischemic cerebrovascular disease. Stroke 19:1229, 1988
179. Hulqvist GT: Über Thrombose und Embolie der Arteria carotis und herbei vorkommende Gehirnveränderungen: eine pathologish-anatomische Studie. Fischer, Stockholm, 1942
180. Humphreys AW, Young JR, Santilli PH et al: Unoperated, asymptomatic significant carotid artery stenosis: a review of 182 instances. Surgery 80:695, 1976
181. Hutchinson EC, Yates PO: Carotico-vertebral stenosis. Lancet 1:2, 1957
182. Huvos AG, Leaming RH, Moore OS: Clinicopathologic study of the resected carotid artery. Am J Surg 126:570, 1973
183. Imparato AM, Riles TS, Gorstein F: The carotid bifurcation plaque: pathologic findings associated with cerebral ischemia. Stroke 10:238, 1979
184. Jacobs LA, Ganji S, Shirley JG et al: Cognitive improvement after extracranial reconstruction for the low flow-endangered brain. Surgery 93:683, 1983
185. Janeway R, Toole JF: Vascular anatomic status of patients with transient ischemic attacks. Trans Am Neurol Assoc 97:137, 1971
186. Javid H, Ostermiller WE, Jr, Hengesh JW et al: Natural history of carotid bifurcation atheroma. Surgery 67:80, 1970
187. Javid H, Ostermiller WE, Hengesh JW et al: Carotid endarterectomy for asymptomatic patients. Arch Surg 102:389, 1971
188. Jonas S, Hass WK: An approach to the maximum acceptable stroke complication rate after surgery for transient cerebral ischemia (TIA), abstracted. Stroke 10:104, 1979
189. Jorgensen L, Packham MA, Rowsell HC, Mustard JF: Deposition of formed elements of blood on the intima and signs of intimal injury in the aorta of rabbit, pig, and man. Lab Invest 27:341, 1972
190. Julian OC, Dye WS, Javid H: Ulcerative lesions of the carotid artery bifurcation. Arch Surg 86:803, 1963
191. Lancer SR, Guttierrez LF, Pillay VKG: Orbital bruits in patients on maintenance hemodialysis. Br Med J 1:481, 1975
192. Ley-Pozo J, Ringelstein EB: Noninvasive detection of occlusive disease of the carotid siphon and middle cerebral artery. Ann Neurol 28:640, 1990
193. Kagan A, Popper J, Rhoads GG et al: Epidemiologic studies on coronary artery disease and stroke in Japanese men living in Japan, Hawaii,

and California: prevalence of stroke. p. 267. In Scheinberg P (ed): Cerebrovascular Diseases. Raven Press, New York, 1976
194. Kapp JP, Smith RR: Spontaneous resolution of occlusive lesions on the carotid artery. J Neurosurg 56:73, 1982
195. Karis R: Asymptomatic carotid artery disease. (Letter to the Editors.) Stroke 14:443, 1983
196. Karp HR, Heyman A, Heyden S et al: Transient cerebral ischemia: prevalence and prognosis in a biracial community. JAMA 225:125, 1973
197. Kartchner MM, McRae LP: Noninvasive evaluation and management of the "asymptomatic" carotid bruit. Surgery 82:840, 1977
198. Kearns TP, Hollenhorst RW: Venous-stasis retinopathy of occlusive disease of the carotid artery. Mayo Clin Proc 38:304, 1963
199. Kirgis MD, Llewellyn RG, Peebles EMcG: Functional trifurcations of the internal carotid artery and its potential clinical significance. J Neurosurg 17:1062, 1960
200. Kishore PRS, Chase NE, Kricheff II: Carotid stenosis and intracranial emboli. Radiology 100:351, 1971
201. Kishore PRS, Dick AR: Spontaneous disappearance of carotid stenosis. Radiology 129:721, 1978
202. Kistler JP, Lees RS, Friedman J et al: The bruit of carotid stenosis vs radiated basal heart murmurs. Circulation 57:975, 1978
203. Kistler JP, Lees RS, Miller A et al: Correlation of spectral phonoangiography and carotid angiography with gross pathology in carotid stenosis. N Engl J Med 305:417, 1981
204. Krayenbühl H, Yasargil MG: Die zerebrale Angiographie. Thieme, Stuttgart, 1965
205. Kroener JM, Dorn PL, Shoor PM et al: Prognosis of asymptomatic ulcerating carotid lesions. Arch Surg 115:1387, 1980
206. Kusske JA, Kelly WA: Embolization and reduction of the "steal" syndrome in cerebral AVMs. J Neurosurg 40:313, 1974
207. Lasjaunias P, Moret J: The ascending pharyngeal artery: normal and pathological radioanatomy. Neuroradiology 11:77, 1976
208. Leblanc R, Yamamoto YL, Tyler JL et al: Borderzone ischemia. Ann Neurol 22:707, 1987
209. Lees RS, Kistler JP: Carotid phonoangiography. p. 187. In Bernstein E (ed): Noninvasive Diagnostic Techniques in Vascular Disease. CV Mosby, St. Louis, 1978
210. Lees RS, Lees AM, Strauss WH: External imaging of human atherosclerosis. J Nucl Med 24:154, 1983
211. Lennihan L, Kupsky WJ, Mohr JP et al: lack of association between carotid plaque hematoma and ipsilateral cerebral symptoms. Stroke 18:879, 1987
212. Levin SM, Sondheimer FK, Levin JM: The contralateral diseased but asymptomatic carotid artery: to operate or not?—an update. Am J Surg 140:203, 1980
213. Levine RL, Dobkin JA, Rozental JM et al: Blood flow reactivity to hypercapnia in strictly unilateral carotid disease: preliminary results. J Neurol Neurosurg Psychiatry 54:204, 1991
214. Levinson SA, Close MB, Ehrenfeld WK et al: Carotid artery of occlusive disease following external cervical irradiation. Arch Surg 107:395, 1973
215. Lhermitte F, Gautier JC: Sites of Cerebral Arterial Occlusions. In Williams D (ed): Modern Trends in Neurology 6. Butterworths, London, 1975
216. Lhermitte F, Gautier JC, Derouesne C: Anatomie et physiopathologie des sténoses carotidiennes. Rev Neurol (Paris) 115:641, 1966
217. Lhermitte F, Gautier JC, Derouesne C: Nature of occlusions of the middle cerebral artery. Neurology (Minneapolis) 20:82, 1970
218. Liapis CD, Satiani B, Florance CL et al: Motor speech malfunction following carotid endarterectomy. Surgery 89:56, 1981
219. Lie TA: Congenital Anomalies of the Carotid Arteries. Exerpta Medica Foundation, Amsterdam, 1968
220. Liebers M: Alzheimerische Krankheit bei schwerer Gehirnarteriosklerose. Z Ges Neurol Psychiatry 124:639, 1932
221. Liebeskind A, Chinichian A, Schechter MM: The moving embolus seen during serial cerebral angiography. Stroke 2:440, 1971
222. Lindenberg R, Spatz F: Über die Thromboendarteritis obliterans der Hirngefässe. Virchows Arch [A] 305:531, 1940
223. Link H, Lebram G, Johansson I, Radberg C: Prognosis in patients with infarction and TIA in carotid territory during and after anticoagulant therapy. Stroke 10:529, 1979
224. Lipchik EO, DeWeese JA, Schenk EA et al: Diaphragm-like obstructions of the human arterial tree. Radiology 113:43, 1974
225. Litt AW, Eidelman EM, Pinto RS et al: Diagnosis of carotid artery stenosis: comparison of 2DFT time-of-flight MR angiography with contrast angiography in 50 patients. Am J Radiol 156:149, 1991
226. Little JR, Shawhan B, Weinstein M: Pseudo-tandem stenosis of the internal carotid artery. Neurosurgery 7:574, 1980
227. Loeb C, Priano A, Albano C: Clinical features and long-term follow-up of patients with reversible ischemia attacks (RIA). Acta Neurol Scand 57:471, 1978
228. LoGerfo FW, Crawshaw HN, Nowak M et al: Effect of flow split on separation and stagnation in a model vascular bifurcation. Stroke 12:660, 1981
229. LoGerfo FW, Nowak MD, Quist WC et al: Flow studies in a model carotid bifurcation. Arteriosclerosis 1:235, 1981
230. Ludwig JW, Verhoeven LHJ, Engels PHC: Digital video subtraction angiography (DVSA) equipment: angiographic technique in comparison with conventional angiography in different vascular areas. Br J Radiol 55:545, 1982
231. Luessenhop AJ: Occlusive disease of carotid artery: observations on the prognosis and surgical treatment. J Neurosurg 16:705, 1959
232. Lusby RJ, Ferrell LD, Ehrenfeld WK et al: Carotid plaque hemorrhage: its role in production of cerebral ischemia. Arch Surg 117:1479, 1982

233. Magargal LE, Sanborn GE, Zimmerman A: Venous stasis retinopathy associated with embolic obstruction of the central retinal artery. J Clin Neuro Ophthalmol 2:113, 1982
234. Maitland CE, Black JL, Smith WA: Abducens nerve palsy due to spontaneous dissection of the internal carotid artery. Arch Neurol 40:448, 1983
235. Marshall J: The natural history of transient ischemic cerebrovascular attacks. Q J Med 33: 309, 1964
236. Marshall J, Meadows S: The natural history of amaurosis fugax. Brain 91:419, 1968
237. Martin GM, Sprague CA: Symposium on in vitro studies related to atherogenesis: life histories of hyperplastoid cell lines from aorta and skin. Exp Mol Pathol 18:125, 1973
238. Marzewski DJ, Furlan AJ, St. Louis P et al: Intracranial internal carotid artery stenosis: long-term prognosis. Stroke 13:821, 1982
239. Mathew NT, Abraham J, Taori GM et al: Internal carotid artery occlusion in cavernous sinus thrombosis. Arch Neurol 24:11, 1971
240. Mawad ME, Hilal SK, Michelsen WJ et al: Occlusive vascular disease associated with cerebral arteriovenous malformations. Radiology 153: 401, 1984
241. May AG, DeWeese JA, Rob CG: Hemodynamic effects of arterial stenosis. Surgery 53:513, 1963
242. McBrien DJ, Bradley RD, Ashton N: The nature of retinal emboli in stenosis of the internal carotid artery. Lancet 1:697, 1963
243. McCollum CH, Wheeler WG, Noon GP, DeBakey ME: Aneurysms of the extracranial artery. Am J Surg 137:196, 1979
244. McGill HG Jr, Strong JP: Natural history of human atherosclerotic lesions. p. 39. In Sandler M, Bourne GH (eds): Atherosclerosis and Its Origin. Academic Press, Orlando, FL, 1963
245. Merino MJ, Livolsi V: Malignant carotid body tumors. Cancer 47:1403, 1981
246. Meyer WW: Cholesterinkrystall embolie kleiner Organarterien und ihre Folgen. Virchows Arch [A] 314:616, 1947
247. Millikan CH: The pathogenesis of transient focal cerebral ischemia. Circulation 32:438, 1965
248. Millikan CH, Siekert RG, Shick RM: Studies in cerebrovascular diseases. V. The use of anticoagulant drugs in the treatment of intermittent insufficiency of the internal carotid arterial system. Mayo Clin Proc 30:578, 1955
249. Mitchell JRA, Schwartz CJ: Arterial Disease. Blackwell, Oxford, 1965
250. Mohr JP: Neurological complications of cardiac valvular disease and cardiac surgery including systemic hypotension. p. 143. In Vinken PJ, Bruyn GW (eds): Handbook of Clinical Neurology. Vol. 38: Klawans HL (ed): Neurological Manifestations of Systemic Diseases. North-Holland Publishing, Amsterdam, 1979
251. Mohr JP: Asymptomatic carotid artery disease. Stroke 13:431, 1982
252. Mohr JP: Discussion. In Reivich M, Hurtig H (ed), Cerebrovascular Diseases. Proceedings of the Thirteenth Research Conference. Raven Press, New York, 1983
253. Mohr JP, Caplan LR, Melski JW et al: The Harvard Cooperative Stroke Registry: a prospective registry. Neurology (NY) 28:754, 1978
254. Mokri B, Piepgras DG, Houser OW: Traumatic dissections of the extracranial internal carotid artery. J Neurosurg 68:189, 1988
255. Mokri B, Sundt TM, Houser OW: Spontaneous internal carotid artery dissection, hemicrania and Horner's syndrome. Arch Neurol 36:677, 1979
256. Moniz E, Lima A, deLacerda R: Hemiplegies par thrombose de la carotide interne. Presse Med 45:977, 1937
257. Moore WS, Boren C, Malone JM et al: Natural history of non-stenotic asymptomatic ulcerative lesions of the carotid artery. Arch Surg 113:1352, 1978
258. Moore WS, Boren C, Malone JM et al: Asymptomatic carotid stenosis: immediate and long-term results after prophylactic endarterectomy. Am J Surg 138:228, 1979
259. Moore WS, Hall AD: Ulcerated atheroma of the carotid artery: a major cause of transient cerebral ischemia. Am J Surg 116:237, 1968
260. Moore WS, Hall AD: Importance of emboli from carotid bifurcation in pathogenesis of cerebral ischemic attacks. Arch Surg 101:708, 1970
261. Moosy J: Cervical and cranial arteries: thrombosis, embolic and infarction. Stroke 14:120, 1983
262. Morax PV, Aron-Rosa D, Gautier JC: Symptomes et signes ophthalmologiques des stenoses et occlusions carotideinnes. Bull Soc Ophthalmol N Spec 1970
263. Morimoto T, Nitta K, Kazekawa K, Hashizume K: The anomaly of a non-bifurcating cervical carotid artery: case report. J Neurosurg 72:130, 1990
264. Mungas JE, Baker WH: Amaurosis fugax. Stroke 8:232, 1977
265. Murphy EA, Rowsell HC, Downie HG et al: Encrustation and atherosclerosis: the analogy between early in vivo lesions and deposits which occur in extracorporeal circulations. Can Med Assoc J 87:259, 1962
266. Mustard JF, Packham MA: Factors influencing platelet function: adhesion, release, and aggregation. Pharmacol Rev 22:97, 1970
267. Muuronen A, Kaste M: Outcome of 314 patients with transient ischemic attacks. Stroke 13:24, 1982
268. Norrving B, Nilsson B, Olsson J-E: Progression of carotid disease after endarterectomy: a Doppler ultrasound study. Ann Neurol 12:548, 1982
269. North American Symptomatic Carotid Endarterectomy Trial: Clinical alert: benefit of carotid endarterectomy for patients with high-grade stenmosis of the internal carotid artery. Stroke 22:816, 1991
270. O'Dwyer JA, Moscow N, Trevor R et al: Spontaneous dissection of the carotid artery. Radiology 137:379, 1980
271. Ojemann RG, Crowell RC, Roberson GH, Fisher CM: Surgical treatment of the extracranial carotid occlusive disease. Clin Neurosurg 22:214, 1975
272. Olsson JE, Muller R, Berneli S: Long term anti-

coagulant therapy for TIAs and minor strokes with minimum residuum. Stroke 7:444, 1976
273. Orr AE: A rare anomaly of the carotid arteries (internal and external). J Anat Physiol 41:51, 1906
274. Ostfeld AM, Shekelle RB, Klawans HL: Transient ischemic attacks and risk of stroke in an elderly poor population. Stroke 4:980, 1973
275. Parkinson D: A surgical approach to the cavernous portion of the carotid artery: anatomical studies and case report. J Neurosurg 23:474, 1965
276. Parkinson D, Shields CB: Persistent trigeminal artery: its relationship to the normal branches of the cavernous carotid. J Neurosurg 39:244, 1974
277. Pearce JMS, Gubbay SS, Walton JN: Long-term anticoagulant therapy in transient cerebral ischemic attacks. Lancet 1:6, 1965
278. Pentschew A: Die granuläre Atrophie der Grosshirnrinde. Arch Psychiatr Nervenkr 101:80, 1934
279. Perrone P, Candelise L, Scotti G et al: CT evaluation in patients with transient ischemic attack: correlation between clinical and angiographic findings. Eur Neurol 18:217, 1979
280. Pessin MS, Duncan GW, Davis KR et al: Angiographic appearance of carotid occlusion in acute stroke. Stroke 11:485, 1982
281. Pessin MS, Duncan GW, Mohr JP, Poskanzer DC: Clinical and angiographic features of carotid transient ischemic attacks. N Engl J Med 296:358, 1977
282. Pessin MS, Estol CJ, DeWitt LD et al: Retinal emboli and carotid disease, abstracted. Neurology (NY), suppl 1. 40:249, 1990
283. Pessin MS, Hinton RC, Davis KR et al: Mechanisms of acute carotid stroke. Ann Neurol 6:245, 1979
284. Pessin MS, Panis W, Prager RJ et al: Auscultation of cervical and ocular bruits in extracranial carotid occlusive disease: a clinical and angiographic study. Stroke 14:246, 1983
285. Petrov V, Waltregny A, Reznik M et al: Thrombose carotidienne bilaterale post-traumitique. Acta Neurol Belg 73:110, 1973
286. Picard L, Andre JM, Roland J et al: Moyamoya syndrome of the adult: transient forms. J Neuroradiol 1:69, 1974
287. Pode JCF: The monoclonal theory of atherosclerosis. Br J Clin Pract 32:219, 1978
288. Podore PC, DeWeese JA, May AG, Rob CG: Asymptomatic contralateral carotid artery stenosis: a five-year follow-up study following carotid endarterectomy. Surgery 88:748, 1980
289. Portnoy HD, Avellanosa A: Carotid aneurysm and contralateral carotid stenosis with successful surgical treatment of both lesions. J Neurosurg 32:476, 1970
290. Powers WJ, Press GA, Grubb RL et al: The effect of hemodynamically significant carotid artery disease on the hemodynamic status of the cerebral circulation. Ann Intern Med 106:27, 1987
291. Praffenbach DD, Hollenhorst RW: Morbidity and survivorship of patients with embolic cholesterol crystals in the ocular fundus. Am J Ophthalmol 75:66, 1973
292. Quisling RG, Friedman WA, Rhoton AL: High cervical dissection: spontaneous resolution. AJNR 1:463, 1980
293. Raichle M: Discussion. In Reivich M, Hurtig H (eds): Cerebrovascular Disorders. Proceedings of the Thirteenth Research Conference. Raven Press, New York, 1983
294. Ramirez-Lassepas M, Sandok BA, Burton RC: Clinical indicators of extracranial carotid artery disease in patients with transient symptoms. Stroke 4:537, 1973
295. Reed RL, Siekert RG, Merideth J: Rarity of transient focal cerebral ischemia in cardiac dysrhythmia. JAMA 223:893, 1973
296. Regli F: Die flüchtigen ischämischen zerebralen Attacken. Dtsch Med Wochenschr 96:526, 1971
297. Ricotta JJ, Ouriel K, Green RM, DeWeese JA: Use of computerized cerebral tomography in selection of patients for elective and urgent carotid endarterectomy. Ann Surg 202:783, 1985
298. Ring BA: Diagnosis of embolic occlusions of smaller branches of the intracerebral arteries. AJR 97:575, 1966
299. Ringelstein EB, Zeumer H, Angelou D: The pathogenesis of strokes from internal carotid artery occlusion. Stroke 14:867, 1983
300. Robb CG: Discussion of paper by JE Thompson, RD Patman, and CM Talkington: Asymptomatic carotid bruit: long-term outcome of patients having endarterectomy compared with unoperated controls. Ann Surg 188:316, 1978
301. Roberts AB, Strauss HW, Lees RS et al: Low density lipoproteins concentrate in damaged arterial wall, abstracted. Circulation, suppl 3. 62:97, 1980
302. Roederer GO, Langlois YE, Chan AT et al: Is siphon disease important in predicting the outcome of carotid endarterectomy?, abstraced. Stroke 14:8, 1983
303. Roederer GO, Langlois YE, Jager KA et al: The natural history of carotid arterial disease in asymptomatic patients with cervical bruits. Stroke 15:605, 1984
304. Romanul FCA, Abramowicz A: Changes in brain and pial vessels in arterial borderzones. Arch Neurol 11:40, 1964
305. Ropper AH, Wechsler LR, Wilson LS: Carotid bruit and the risk of stroke in elective surgery. N Engl J Med 307:1388, 1982
306. Ross R, Glomset JA: Atherosclerosis and the arterial smooth muscle cell. Science 180:1332, 1973
307. Ross R, Glomset J, Kariya B, Harker L: A platelet-dependent serum factor that stimulates the proliferation of arterial smooth muscle cells in vitro. Proc Natl Acad Sci USA 71:1207, 1974
308. Ross Russell RW: Observations on the retinal blood vessels in monocular blindness. Lancet 2:1422, 1961
309. Ross Russell RW: Atheromatous retinal embolism. Lancet 2:1354, 1963
310. Ross Russell RW, Page NGR: Critical perfusion of brain and retina. Brain 106:419, 1983

311. Russo LS: Carotid system transient ischemic attacks: clinical, racial, and angiographic correlations. Stroke 12:470, 1981
312. Sacquegna T, DeCarolis P, Pazzaglia P et al: The clinical course and prognosis of carotid artery occlusion. J Neurol Neurosurg Psychiatry 45:1037, 1982
313. Samuel KC: Atherosclerosis and occlusion of the internal carotid artery. J Pathol 71:391, 1956
314. Sandok BA, Tratmann JC, Ramirez-Lassepas M et al: Clinical angiographic correlations in amaurosis fugax. Am J Ophthalmol 78:137, 1974
315. Santamore WP, Bove AA, Carey RA: Hemodynamics of a stenosis in a complaint [sic] artery. Cardiology 69:1, 1982
316. Schiffter R, Reinhart K: The telodiencephalic ischemic syndrome. J Neurol 222:265, 1980
317. Schneider M: Durchblutung and Sauerstoffversorgung des Gehirns. Verh Dtsch Ges Herz Kreislauforsch 19:3, 1953
318. Schneider PA, Rossman ME, Bernstein EF et al: Noninvasive assessment of cerebral collateral blood supply through the ophthalmic artery. Stroke 22:31, 1991
319. Schuler JJ, Falnigan DP, Lim LT et al: The effect of carotid siphon stenosis on stroke rate, death, and relief of symptoms following elective carotid endarterectomy. Surgery 92:1058, 1982
320. Schwarcz TH, Eton D, Ellenby MI et al: Hollenhorst plaques: retinal manifestations and the role of carotid endarterectomy. J Vasc Surg 11:635, 1990
321. Scott SN, Sethi GK, Bridgman AH: Perioperative stroke during carotid endarterectomy: the value of intra-operative angiography. J Cardiovasc Surg (Torino) 23:353, 1982
322. Shah AB, Coull BM, Howieson J et al: Does natural history of transient ischemic attacks (TIAs) justify surgery? (Letter to the Editor.) Stroke 14:828, 1983
323. Sheng FC, Quinones-Baldrich W, Machleder HI et al: Relationship of extracranial carotid occlusive disease and central retinal artery occlusion. Am J Surg 152:175, 1986
324. Shillito J, Jr: Carotid arteritis: a cause of hemiplegia in childhood. J Neurosurg 31:540, 1964
325. Shipley RE, Gregg DE: The effect of external constriction of a blood vessel on blood flow. Am J Physiol 141:389, 1944
326. Shoumaker RD, Avant WS, Cohen GH: Coincidental multiple asymptomatic intra-cranial aneurysms and symptomatic carotid stenosis. Stroke 7:504, 1976
327. Siekert RG, Whisnant JP, Millikan CH: Surgical and anticoagulant therapy of occlusive cerebrovascular disease. Ann Intern Med 58:637, 1963
328. Sindermann F: Krankheitsbild und Kollateralkreislauf bei einseitigem und doppleseitigem Carotisverschluss. J Neurol Sci 5:9, 1967
329. Sipponen JT, Kaste M, Sepponen RE et al: Nuclear magnetic resonance imaging in reversible cerebral ischaemia. Lancet 1:294, 1983
330. Sobel J, Espinas OE, Friedman SA: Carotid artery obstructions following LSD capsule ingestion. Arch Int Med 127:290, 1971
331. Spallone A: Occlusion of the internal carotid artery by intracranial tumors. Surg Neurol 15:51, 1981
332. Spatz A: Uber die Beteiligung des Gehirns bei v. Winiwarter-Buergerische Krankheit. Dtsch Z Nervenheilk 136:86, 1935
333. Stanton PE, McClusky DA, Lamis PA: Hemodynamic assessment and surgical correction of kinking of the internal carotid artery. Surgery 84:793, 1978
334. Stehbens WE: The role of lipid in the pathogenesis of atherosclerosis. Lancet 1:724, 1975
335. Stemerman MB: Haemostasis, thrombosis and atherogenesis. Atheroscler Rev 6:105, 1979
336. Stringer WL, Kelly DL: Traumatic dissection of the extracranial internal carotid artery. Neurosurgery 6:123, 1980
337. Sundt TM Jr, Sandok BA, Whisnant JP: Carotid endarterectomy: complications and preoperative assessment of risk. Mayo Clin Proc 50:301, 1975
338. Suzuki J, Kodama N: Moyamoya disease—a review. Stroke 14:104, 1983
339. Tatemichi TK, Chamorro A, Petty GW et al: Hemodynamic role of ophthalmic artery collateral in internal carotid artery occlusion. Neurology 40:461, 1990
340. Tatemichi TK, Young WL, Prohovnik I et al: Perfusion insufficiency in limb shaking transient ischemic attacks. Stroke 21:341, 1990
341. Taveras JM, Wood EH: Diagnostic Neuroradiology. 2nd Ed. Vol. 2, Sect. 4: Vascular Diseases. p. 850. Williams & Wilkins, Baltimore, 1976
342. Thiele BL, Young JV, Chikos PM et al: Correlation of arteriographic findings and symptoms in cerebrovascular disease. Neurology (NY) 30:1041, 1980
343. Thompson JE: Operative mortality following carotid endarterectomy. (Letter to the Editor.) Stroke 14:115, 1983
344. Thompson JE, Patman RD, Persson AV: Management of asymptomatic carotid bruits. Am Surg 42:77, 1977
345. Thompson JE, Patman RD, Talkington CM: Asymptomatic carotid bruit: long-term outcome of patients having endarterectomy compared with unoperated controls. Ann Surg 188:308, 1978
346. Timsit SG, Sacco RL, Mohr JP et al: Early clinical differentiation of atherosclerotic and cardioembolic infarction: the Stroke Data Bank (SDB). First European Stroke Conference, Düsseldorf, 1990
347. Tolosa E: Periarteritic lesions of the carotid siphon with the clinical features of a carotid infraclinoidal aneurysm. J Neurol Neurosurg Psychiatry 17:300, 1954
348. Tomsak RL, Hanson M, Gutman SA: Carotid artery disease and central retinal artery occlusion. Cleve Clin Q 46:7, 1979
349. Toole JF, Janeway R, Choi K et al: Transient ischemic attacks due to atherosclerosis: a prospective study of 160 patients. Arch Neurol 32:5, 1975

350. Toole JF, Patel AN: Cerebrovascular Disorders. 2nd Ed. McGraw-Hill, New York, 1964
351. Torvik A: The pathogenesis of watershed infarcts in the brain. Stroke 15:221, 1984
352. Torvik A, Jörgensen L: Thrombotic and embolic occlusion of the carotid arteries in an autopsy series. 1. Prevalence, location and associated diseases. J Neurol Sci 1:24, 1964
353. Torvik A, Jörgensen L: Thrombotic and embolic occlusion of the carotid arteries in an autopsy series. 2. Cerebral lesions and clinical course. J Neurol Sci 3:410, 1966
354. Torvik A, Jörgensen L: Ischemic cerebrovascular disease in an autopsy series. 1. Prevalence, location and predisposing factors in verified thrombo-embolic occlusion and their significance in the pathogenesis of cerebral infarction. J Neurol Sci 3:490, 1966
355. Torvik A, Jorgensen L: Ischemic cerebrovascular disease in an autopsy series. 2. Prevalence, location; pathogenesis and clinical course of cerebral infarcts. J Neurol Sci 9:285, 1969
356. Toyama H, Takeshita G, Takeuchi A et al: SPECT measurement of cerebral hemodynamics in transient ischemic attack patients evaluation of pathogenesis and detection of misery perfusion. Kaku Igaku 26:1487, 1989
357. Treiman RL, Foran RF, Shore EH, Levin PM: Carotid bruit. Arch Surg 106:803, 1973
358. Turnbill I: Agenesis of the internal carotid artery. Neurology (NY) 12:588, 1962
359. Van der Eecken HM: Anastomoses Between the Leptomeningeal Arteries of the Brain. CC Thomas, Springfield, IL, 1959
360. Vorstrup S, Hemmingsen R, Henriksen L et al: Regional cerebral blood flow in patients with transient ischemic attacks studied by xenon-133 inhalation and emission tomography. Stroke 14:903, 1983
361. Wade JG, Larson CP, Hickey RR et al: Effect of carotid endarterectomy on carotid chemoreceptor and baroreceptor functions in man. N Engl J Med 282:823, 1970
362. Wade JPH, Wong W, Barnett HJM, Vandervoort P: Bilateral occlusion of the internal carotid arteries: presenting symptoms in 74 patients and a prospective study of 34 medically treated patients. Brain 110:667, 1987
363. Wagener HP: Amaurosis fugax: a specific type of transient loss of vision. Ill Med J p. 21, Jan 1957
364. Waller FT, Simons RL, Kerber C et al: Trigeminal artery and micro-emboli to the brain stem: report of two cases. J Neurosurg 46:104, 1977
365. Walsh PN, Pareti FI, Corbett JJ: Platelet coagulant activation and serum lipids in transient cerebral ischemia. N Engl J Med 295:854, 1976
366. Waxman SG, Toole JF: Temporal profile resembling TIA in the setting of cerebral infarction. Stroke 14:435, 1983
367. Weaver RG Jr, Howard G, McKinney WM et al: Comparison of Doppler ultrasonography with arteriography of the carotid bifurcation. Stroke 4:402, 1980
368. Weibel J, Fields WS: Tortuosity, coiling, and kinking of the internal carotid artery: etiology and radiographic anatomy. Neurology (NY) 15:7, 1965
369. Weinberger J, Bender AN, Yang WC: Amaurosis fugax associated with ophthalmic artery stenosis: clinical simulation of carotid atery disease. Stroke 11:290, 1980
370. Weinberger J, Robbins A: Neurologic symptoms associated with non-obstructive plaque at carotid bifurcation analysis by real-time B-mode ultrasonography. Arch Neurol 40:489, 1983
371. Weisman AD: Cavernous sinus thrombophlebitis: report of a case with multiple cerebral infarcts and necrosis of the pituitary body. N Engl J Med 231:118, 1944
372. Welling RE, Taha A, Goel T et al: Extracranial carotid artery aneurysms. Surgery 93:319, 1983
373. Wesolowski SA, Fries CC, Sabini AM, Sawyer PN: The significance of turbulance in hemic systems and in the distribution of the atherosclerotic lesions. Surgery 57:155, 1965
374. Whisnant JP: Multiple particles injected may all go to the same cerebral artery branch. Stroke 13:720, 1982
375. Whisnant JP: The role of the neurologist in the decline of stroke. Ann Neurol 14:1, 1983
376. Whisnant JP, Matsumoto N, Elveback LR: The efffect of anticoagulant therapy on the prognosis of patients with transient cerebral ischemic attacks in a cummunity: Rochester, Minnesota, 1955 through 1969. Mayo Clin Proc 48:844, 1973
377. Whisnant JP, Matsumoto N, Elveback LR: Transient cerebral ischemic attacks in a community. Mayo Clinic Proc 48:194, 1973
378. Wiebers DO, Swanson JW, Cascino TL, Whisnant JP: Bilateral loss of vision in bright light. Stroke 20:554, 1989
379. Wilkinson WE, Heyman A, Burch JG et al: Use of a self-administered questionnaire for detection of transient cerebral ischemic attacks. Survey of elderly persons living in retirement facilities. Ann Neurol 6:40, 1979
380. Wilkinson IMS, Ross Russell RW: Arteries of the head and neck in giant cell arteritis. Arch Neurol 27:378, 1972
381. Wilson LA, Warlow CP, Ross Russell RW: Cardiovascular disease in patients with retinal arterial occlusion. Lancet 1:292, 1979
382. Wodarz R: Watershed infarctions and computed tomography: a topographical study in cases with stenosis or occlusion of the carotid artery. Neuroradiology 19:245, 1980
383. Wodarz R, Ratzka M, Grosse D: Der Grenzzoneninfarkt als besondere Infarktkonstellation bei Karotisinsuffizienz. Fortschr Geb Rontgenstr Nuklearmed Erganzungsband 134:128, 1981
384. Wolf PA, Dawber TR, Colton T et al: Transient cerebral ischemic attacks and risk of stroke: the Framingham study. CVD Epidemiol Newslett 22:52, 1977
385. Wolf PA, Kannel WB, Sorlie P, McNamara P: Asymptomatic carotid bruit and the risk of stroke. JAMA 245:1442, 1981
386. Wolinsky H: Mesenchymal response of the blood

vessel wall: a potential avenue for understanding and treating atherosclerosis. Circ Res 32:543, 1973
387. Wolpert SM, Stein BM: Catheter embolization of arteriovenous malformations as an aid to surgical excision. Neuroradiology 10:73, 1975
388. Wolpow ER, Lupton RG: Transient vertical monocular hemianopsia with anomalous retinal artery branching. Stroke 12:691, 1981
389. Wood EH, Correll JW: Atheromatous ulceration in major neck vessels as a cause of cerebral embolism. Acta Radiol [Diag] (Stockh) 9:520, 1969
390. Wood CPL, Smith BR, McKinney CL, Toole JF: Non-invasive detection of boundary layer separation in the normal carotid artery bifurcation. Stroke 13:120, 1982
391. Woods BT, Strewler GJ: Hemiparesis occurring six hours after intravenous heroin injection. Neurology (NY) 22:863, 1972
392. Wylie EJ, Ehrenfeld WK: Extracranial Occlusive Cerebral Vascular Disease-Diagnosis and Management. WB Saunders, Philadelphia, 1970
393. Yamauchi H, Fukuyama H, Kimura J et al: Hemodynamics in internal carotid artery occlusion examined by positron emission tomography. Stroke 21:1400, 1990
394. Yanagihara T, Klass DW: Rhythmic involuntary movement as a manifestation of transient ischemic attacks. Trans Am Neurol Assoc 106:46, 1981
395. Yanagihara T, Sundt TM, Jr, Piepgras DG: Weakness of the lower extremity in carotid occlusive disease. Arch Neurol 45:297, 1988
396. Yates PO, Hutchinson EC: Cerebral Infarction: The Role of the Extracranial Cerebral Arteries. Special report series N 300. HM Stationery Office, London, 1961
397. Young B, Meacham WF, Allen JH: Documented enlargement and rupture of a small arterial sacculation. J Neurosurg 34:814, 1971
398. Young DF, Cholvin NR, Kirkeeide RL, Roth AC: Hemodynamics of arterial stenoses at elevated flow rates. Circ Res 41:99, 1977
399. Young LHY, Appen RE: Ischemic oculopathy: a manifestation of carotid artery disease. Arch Neurol 38:358, 1981
400. Zarins CK, Giddens DP, Balasubramanian K et al: Carotid plaques localized in regions of low flow velocity and shear stress. Circulation 64:44, 1981
401. Zatz LM, Iannone AM, Eckman PB, Hecker SP: Observations concerning intracerebral vascular occlusion. Neurology (NY) 15:390, 1965
402. Ziegler DK: Carotid lesions-to operate or not to operate? Stroke 14:824, 1983
403. Ziegler DK, Hassanein RS: Prognosis in patients with transient ischemic attacks. Stroke 4:666, 1973
404. Ziegler RE, Bandyk DF, Thiele BL, Strandness DE: Carotid artery stenosis following endarterectomy. Arch Surg 117:1408, 1982
405. Zülch KJ: Predilection of cerebral atherosclerotic stenosis: a morphologic and radiologic demonstration. In Zülch KJ, Kaufman W, Hossmann FA, Hossmann V (eds): Brain and Heart Infarct II. Springer-Verlag, Berlin, 1979
406. Zülch KJ, Kleihues P: Neuropathology of Cerebral Infarction. Thule International Symposium. p. 57. Nordiska, Stockholm, 1957
407. Zwiebel WJ, Crummy AB: Sources of error in Doppler diagnosis of carotid occlusive disease. Am J Neuroradiol 2:231, 1981

# 15
# ANTERIOR CEREBRAL ARTERY DISEASE

John C.M. Brust

## ETIOLOGY

Infarction in the territory of one or both anterior cerebral arteries (ACAs) is frequently secondary to vasospasm following rupture of saccular aneurysms of the ACA or the anterior communicating artery (ACoA). When such patients are excluded, ACA infarcts have been reported to represent 0.6 to 3 percent of acute ischemic strokes.[28,103,157] As with middle cerebral artery territory infarcts, those involving the ACA are more often associated with internal carotid artery (ICA) atherosclerosis than with primary stenosis or thrombosis of the ACA itself.[264] In a clinical series of 27 patients, 17 (63 percent) had probable emboli from the ICA or the heart; other causes were isolated proximal ACA occlusion, paraneoplastic disseminated intravascular coagulation, ICA dissection with embolic occlusion of the opposite ACA, acute ethanol intoxication, and hypertensive occlusion of a small penetrating ACA branch. Six patients with no obvious cause were over 50 years of age and five of these had risk factors for atherosclerotic stroke.[28] In an autopsy series of 55 patients with ACA infarcts 10 had probable cardiac emboli and only 5 had atherosclerosis primarily involving the ACA itself.[55] ACA territory infarction has resulted from vessel compression during transfalcial herniation.[269] Dissecting aneurysm of the ACA has followed minor head trauma.[8] One patient had transient ischemic attacks and fibromuscular dysplasia of both pericallosal arteries.[291] Another, with sickle cell trait, had bilateral ACA infarction during acute ethanol intoxication and withdrawal.[311] Another had bilateral ACA infarction from intracranial extension of Wegener's granulomatosis.[276]

Symptoms and signs including weakness, sensory loss, and behavioral disturbance vary widely among patients with ACA infarcts. To understand this variety one must be familiar with relevant anatomy.

## ANATOMY

The ACA can be divided into a proximal or A1 segment, from its origin as the medial component of the internal carotid bifurcation to its junction with the (ACoA), and a distal or postcommunicating artery segment[69,167,247,248,305] (Fig. 15-1). The distal segment has been variably subdivided by different authors,[17,19,64,95,167,176,187,204,218,219,247,261,275,299,305,346] for example, into an A2 segment beginning at the ACoA and passing in front of the lamina terminalis as far as the junction of the rostrom and genu of the corpus callosum, an A3 segment passing around the genu of the corpus callosum, an A4 segment above the corpus callosum to just beyond the coronal suture, and an A5 segment to the artery's termination.[95] The A2 and A3 segments have together been referred to as the ascending segment, and the A4 and A5 segments as the horizontal segment.[248]

The A1 segment passes over the optic chiasm (in 70 percent of cases) or optic nerve (30 percent), varying in length from 7.2 to 18 mm (average 12.7 mm).[247] Its diameter ranges from 0.9 to 4.0 mm (average 2.6 mm), and is greater than 1.5 mm in 90 percent of brains. In 74 percent both A1 segments are larger than the ACoA, the diameter of which ranges from 0.2 to 3.4 mm (average 1.5 mm).[247]

The ACAs pass over the corpus callosum side by side in only a minority of cases, and so the ACoA is most

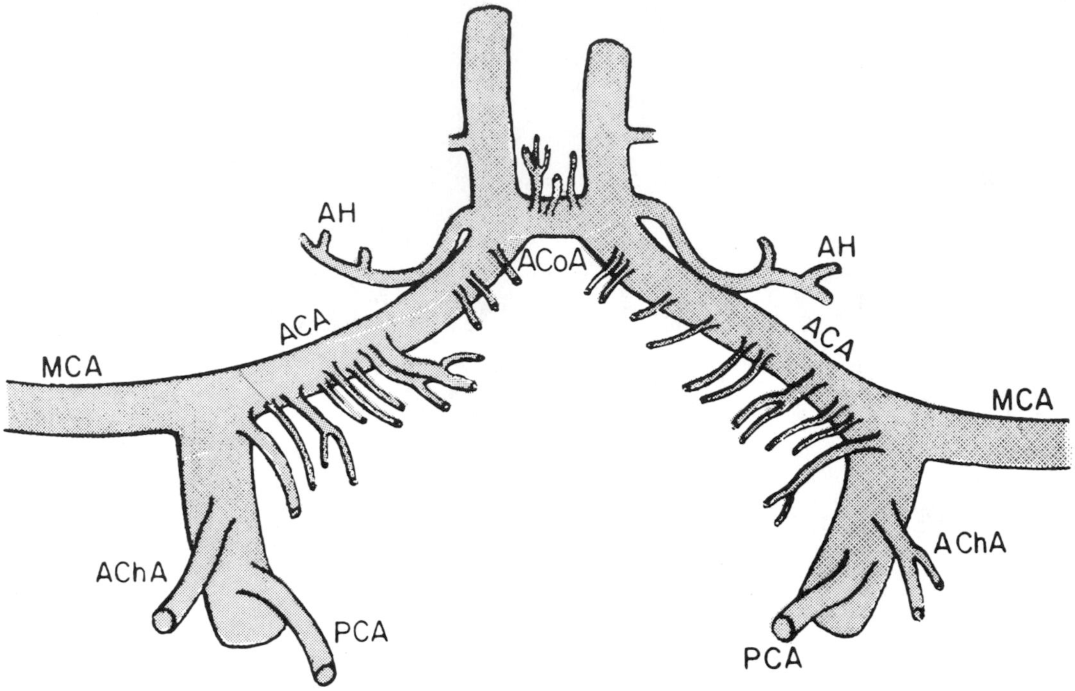


**Fig. 15-1.** Diagram of the dorsal surface of the anterior circle of Willis, showing branches from the A1 segment of the anterior cerebal artery and from the anterior communicating artery. PCA, posterior communicating artery; AChA, anterior choroidal artery; MCA, middle cerebral artery; ACA, anterior cerebral artery; AH, Heubner's artery; ACoA, anterior communicating artery. (From Dunker and Harris,[86] with permission.)

often directed obliquely or even anteroposteriorly; thus it is often best seen angiographically on oblique projections.[247]

The recurrent artery of Heubner[137] arises either at the level of the ACoA or just proximal or distal to it;[324] in different series it arose most often from the A1 segment,[234] from the A2 segment,[247] or at the level of the ACoA.[86,123,124] Usually the largest branch of the A1 or proximal A2 segments, Heubner's artery doubles back on the ACA for a variable distance and then, either as a single trunk or with as many as 12 branches, penetrates the anterior perforated substance above the internal carotid artery bifurcation or lateral to it in the sylvian fissure; some branches enter the olfactory sulcus, the gyrus rectus, or more lateral inferior frontal areas.[2,247] Heubner's artery, of obvious importance to the neurosurgeon,[92,118,134] most consistently supplies the head of the caudate, the anterior inferior part of the internal capsule's anterior limb, the anterior globus pallidus, and parts of the uncinate fasciculus, olfactory regions, and anterior putamen and hypothalamus.[2,5,64,86,117,234,247,324,353]

In addition to Heubner's artery the A1 and A2 segments give off smaller "basal perforating branches," up to 15 from each A1[86,247] and up to 10 from each A2.[116,247,248,305] One of these, called the *short central artery,* is considered more consistent than others, in some people supplying part of the caudate nucleus and anterior limb of the internal capsule.[49,286] Other proximal branches penetrate the anterior perforated substance and the optic tract and supply, variably, paraolfactory structures, the medial anterior commissure, globus pallidus, caudate, and putamen, and the anterior limb of the internal capsule; these vessels also frequently supply the genu and contiguous posterior limb of the internal capsule, part of the anterior nucleus of the thalamus, and most of the anterior hypothalamus.[86] More distal A1 penetrating branches are smaller and supply the optic nerve, chiasm, and tract,[77,86] gyrus rectus and inferior frontal lobe, anterior perforated substance, and suprachiasmatic area.[247] Additional supply to the anterior inferior striatum and anterior hypothalamus comes from A2 segment branches, which can arise either separately or from a larger common trunk (the precallosal artery).[248] Similar penetrating branches from ACoA, up to 13 in number,[65,86] supply the suprachiasmatic and paraolfactory areas, dorsal optic chiasm, anterior perforated substance, inferior frontal lobe, septum pellucidum, columns of the fornix, corpus callosum, septal region, and anterior hypothalamus and cingulum.[65,77,86,247]

Vascular anastomoses are less functional in the diencephalon and basal ganglia than elsewhere in the cerebral hemispheres, and the territories supplied by these ACA penetrating "end-zone" arteries are no exception. Capillary anastomoses, which are difficult to demonstrate by standard perfusion techniques, exceed arterial.[1,4,19,63,86,290,334]

The distal ACAs, deep in the interhemispheric fissure, are the only example of major cerebral arteries running side by side, although, as noted, one (usually the left) is often posterior to the other, and crossover of branches to the opposite hemisphere means that occlusion of either artery can cause contralateral or bilateral infarction.[248] Beyond the lamina terminalis the main trunk of the ACA, the pericallosal artery, runs above the corpus callosum in the pericallosal cistern (or, less often, over the cingulate gyrus or in the cingulate sulcus[17]), passes around the splenium of the corpus callosum, and terminates in the choroid plexus of the third ventricle; its posterior extent depends on the anterior extent of the posterior cerebral artery (PCA).[188,248] Except most posteriorly, the pericallosal artery lies below the free edge of the falx cerebri and can therefore shift across the midline.

The pericallosal artery has been variably defined as beginning at the ACoA[299,305] or at the point where the ACA gives off the callosomarginal artery; however, the latter is absent in 18 to 60 percent of brains.[219,248,261] The callosomarginal artery has been defined as that branch of the ACA traveling in or near the cingulate sulcus and giving off at least two major cortical branches.[219] It originates from just beyond the ACoA to the genu of the corpus callosum, most often from the A3 segment,[248] and can be of the same diameter, larger, or smaller than the pericallosal artery.[167,248] Any or all of the callosomarginal's usual branches can arise from the pericallosal artery;[248] these branches supply the inferior frontal lobe (including the gyrus rectus, the orbital part of the superior frontal gyrus, the medial part of the orbital gyri, and the olfactory bulb and tract), the medial surface of the hemisphere (including the cingulate gyrus, the superior frontal gyrus, the paracentral lobule, and the precuneus), and the superior 2 cm of the lateral convexity (including the superior frontal, precentral, central, and postcentral gyri), anastomosing there with branches of the middle cerebral artery (MCA).[17] (These "border zones" of shared arterial territory are of clinical importance: in a radionuclide study of 365 consecutive stroke patients, infarction in the "watershed" between the ACA and the MCA occurred in 5 percent of patients, compared with 28 percent in the MCA territory and 1 percent in the ACA territory.[31,347,350]) The band of lateral convexity supplied by the ACA is wider anteriorly than posteriorly and may extend into the middle frontal gyrus.

Although variable in number and in whether they arise directly from the pericallosal artery or from its callosomarginal branch, eight major cortical branches of the distal ACA can usually be defined.[248] The orbitofrontal artery arises from the A2 segment except, infrequently, when it shares a common trunk with the frontopolar artery[248] or arises just proximal to the ACoA.[247] Running forward in the floor of the anterior fossa as far as the planum sphenoidale, it supplies the gyrus rectus, olfactory bulb and tract, and the orbital surface of the frontal lobe. The frontopolar artery arises from the A2 segment (or, infrequently, from the callosomarginal artery), passes to the frontal pole along the medial hemispheric surface, and supplies parts of the medial and lateral surfaces of the frontal pole.

The anterior, middle, and posterior frontal arteries arise separately from the A2, A3, or A4 segments of the pericallosal artery or from the callosomarginal artery; infrequently they arise from a common stem.[248,261] They supply the anterior, middle, and posterior parts of the superior frontal gyrus and the cingulate gyrus. The paracentral artery, arising from A4 or the callosomarginal artery, supplies premotor, motor, and sensory areas of the paracentral lobule.

The superior parietal artery, arising anterior to the splenium of the corpus callosum from A4, A5, or the callosomarginal artery, passes through the marginal limb of the cingulate sulcus and supplies the superior part of the precuneus. The inferior parietal artery, subdivided by some into the precuneal and parieto-occipital arteries,[17,64] is the most frequently absent cortical branch of the ACA (36 percent of brains in one series[248]); it arises from the A5 segment (or rarely from the callosomarginal artery) just above the splenium of the corpus callosum and supplies the posterior inferior part of the precuneus and portions of the cuneus.

The rostrum, genu, body, and splenium of the corpus callosum are supplied by "short callosal arteries," pericallosal artery branches that pass through the callosum to supply, additionally, the septum pellucidum, anterior pillars of the fornix, and anterior commissure.[17,248] Posteriorly the pericallosal artery extends around the splenium of the corpus callosum (the "posterior pericallosal artery"[305]) and then passes forward, ending on the inferior surface of the splenium[173] or extending all the way to the foramen of Monro.[305]

## ANOMALIES AND SPECIES DIFFERENCES

The anatomy of the anterior circle of Willis is so varied among otherwise normal people that it is sometimes difficult to define when a variation should be called an anomaly. Especially common are hypoplastic A1 segments, from mildly narrow to nonfunctionally threadlike, with both distal ACAs filling from the larger A1.[7,92,253,324,358] In one study 7 percent of brains had a stringlike A1 segment and 6 percent had a hypoplastic ACoA.[260] In another study 22 percent of brains had A1-segment hypoplasia, severe in 8 percent, and in 82 percent associated with additional anomalies of the ACA or the posterior cerebral, posterior communicating, or basilar arteries.[203] Such anomalies are associated with an increased frequency of saccular aneurysms.[163,304,335,358]

A smaller ACA often occurs on the same side as a smaller internal carotid artery,[180] and a hypoplastic A1 segment tends to be associated with an ACoA of larger than usual diameter.[247,325] Small A1 segments are several times more common among patients with symptomatic cerebrovascular disease than in the general population.[353] A young man with episodic vertigo, loss of consciousness, and left leg weakness had, on cerebral angiography, absent ACAs with the MCAs and one intracavernous carotid providing collaterals to the medial cerebral hemispheres.[168]

In 50 adult autopsy specimens, 60 percent had one ACoA, 30 percent had two, and 10 percent three;[247] other investigators[64,359] have also found doubling and tripling, and some[64,359] have found absence of ACoA. A1 segment duplication also occurs,[247] as well as a third or median ACA arising from ACoA ("arteria termatica"),[23,64,86] which sometimes is as large as the two other ACAs[64,86,305] and may be the major supplier to the posterior medial hemispheres.[23]

The recurrent artery of Heubner rarely arises from the internal carotid at its bifurcation, from the middle cerebral artery, or from the ACoA itself.[247] Absence or doubling has occurred.[2]

Another well-recognized anomaly is a supernumerary vessel arising from the internal carotid artery at the level of the ophthalmic artery, coursing below the optic nerve, ascending in front of the optic chiasm, and terminating on the ipsilateral ACA near the ACoA. The A1 segment may be normal, hypoplastic, or absent;[40,143,213,227,263] in one instance both ACAs were absent.[288] Such an anomaly, which may be bilateral,[21] is frequently associated with ACA saccular aneurysm[143,227,235,288,324] and with other anomalies, such as duplicated MCA,[215] median corpus callosum artery, distal moyamoya, aortic coarctation,[179] facial congenital defects, cerebral lipoma,[40] and absent internal carotid artery (with the remaining carotid artery giving off a branch that passes beneath the optic nerve and divides into two ACAs, the opposite MCA arising from the PCA).[331] The anomalous vessel itself can cause visual symptoms from compression of the optic nerve or chiasm.[32]

The infraoptic ACA has been considered a remnant of the embryonic primitive maxillary artery, present in 3- to 4-mm embryos as an internal carotid artery branch, and normally becoming a cavernous carotid branch, the inferior hypophyseal artery. (The ACA normally arises from the primitive olfactory artery, eventually becoming the dominant vessel.[32,40,143,236])

Other reported anomalies include, in an autopsied infant, unilaterally absent proximal MCA, ACA, and anterior choroidal artery with much of the ipsilateral inferior frontal lobe supplied by branches from the opposite ACA and secondary porencephaly of the orbital frontal lobe.[306] Autopsy on a neurologically normal man revealed a plexiform anterior communicating system connected to the left internal carotid artery by an anomalous vessel arising from the internal carotid artery near the ophthalmic artery, a single distal ACA, marked right A1 segment hypoplasia, and right plexiform vessels in the area of Heubner's artery, plus other anomalies of the posterior circulation.[209] Such anomalies, rare in combination, are not unusual individually. For example, in a series of 1,250 consecutive autopsies, a plexiform anterior communicating system was found in 15 percent, hypoplastic ACAs in 4 percent, and fused distal ACAs in 4 percent; a plexiform Heubner's artery was much less common.[209] An ophthalmic artery arising from the ACA has also been reported.[130,173]

In a study of 381 brains distal ACA anomalies were present in 25 percent,[17] including pericallosal artery triplication, absence of ACA pairing, branches from one ACA to the opposite hemisphere, and bihemispheric branches[7,23,64,217,248,336,359] (Fig. 15-2). Triplicate ACAs with a variably developed midline accessory artery arising from the ACoA and supplying little, much, or most of either or both hemispheres have been observed in up to 22 percent of autopsies.[7,17,23,84,94,165,177,337,359] Also, a "long callosal artery" ("medial artery of the corpus callosum," "anterior middle cerebral artery") can arise from the pericallosal artery and pass parallel to it, giving off callosal perforating branches.[248,305] These anomalies, like a hypoplastic A1 segment, produce at angiography apparent bilateral ACA filling after unilateral carotid injection.[17,67,218,271,326] Bihemispheric ACAs, with either ACA taking over the supply of part or all of the opposite hemisphere, have been reported in up to 64 percent of brains.[17,217,248,337] (The high figure refers to a study in which any contralateral supply, however small, was included; brains in which most of both hemispheres are supplied by one of two ACAs are less common.[217,248])

In the fetus there is gradual embryonic transition from one to two ACAs.[84,182] An unpaired or azygous ACA, arising by proximal union of the ACAs without an ACoA, occurs in up to 5 percent of adult brains.[7,17,23,84,94,165,177,181,312,337,359] Sometimes the ACAs fuse for up to 3.9 cm with an absent ACoA.[168] Azygous ACAs are associated with a variety of other anomalies, including hydranencephaly, septum pellucidum defects, meningomyelocele, hydroencephalodysplasia, and vascular malformations[225] and, like other ACA anomalies, with an increased frequency of saccular aneurysm.[102,156] In holoprosencephaly (fusion of the frontal neocortex and absence of the interhemispheric fissure) an azygous ACA courses just beneath the inner table of the skull.[233]

As noted, ACA anomalies are associated with an increased frequency of saccular aneurysms, especially at the ACoA, but also on distal or anomalous

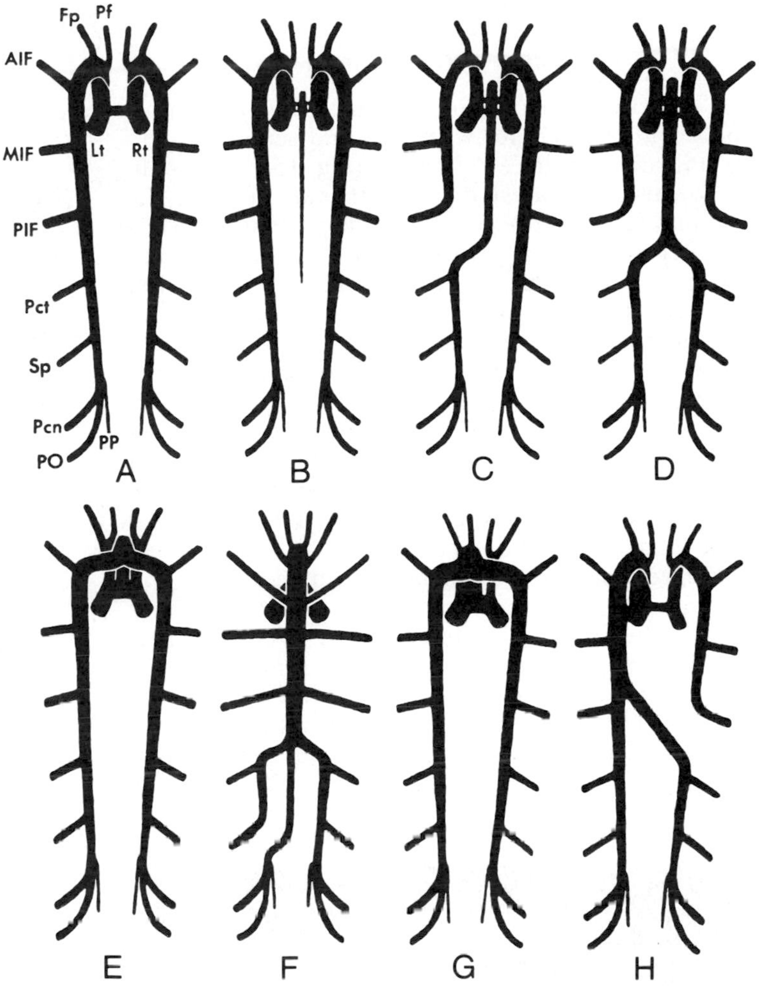


**Fig. 15-2.** Variations in the distal anterior cerebral artery including patterns without (*A*) and with (*B*) a medial artery of the corpus callosum, and variously developed accessory (*C,D,E*), unpaired (*F*), and bihemispheric lateral arteries (*G,H*). Pf, prefrontal (orbitofrontal); Fp, frontopolar; AIF, anterior internal frontal; MIF, middle internal frontal; PIF, posterior internal frontal; Pct, paracentral; Sp, superior parietal; Pcn, precuneal; PO, parieto-occipital; PP, posterior pericallostal. (From Baptista,[17] with permission.)

branches.[29,129,164,230,231,277,328] Of 206 patients with ACoA aneurysms 44 (21.4 percent) had ACA anomalies, especially a median artery of the corpus callosum and duplication of the ACoA.[231] Ruptured fusiform aneurysm of the ACA A1 segment has been reported.[228] Following subarachnoid hemorrhage a congenitally narrow A1 segment may be mistaken for vasospasm. Furthermore, proximal ACA ligation in patients with surgically unclippable ACoA aneurysms is not a valid option if one A1 segment fills both distal ACAs or if, in the absence of cross-compression, the aneurysms fills well from either side.[59,66,88,226,253,324]

A common anomaly, ACA fenestration has no clinical significance except when it is mistaken for an aneurysm angiographically.[144]

Species differences in the anatomy of the ACA (and other cerebral vessels) must be kept in mind in interpreting animal studies of cerebral ischemia and stroke. For example, birds, amphibians, and anteaters have paired arteries without an ACoA or other left–right anastomoses.[64] In most mammals both ACAs join to form a single pericallosal (azygous) artery, which may or may not bifurcate distally. There is no ACoA.[64] In subhuman primates several recurrent medial striate arteries (the equivalent of Heubner's artery in humans) supplying the anterior caudate, putamen, and globus pallidus have rich preparenchymal anastomoses with lateral lenticulostriate arteries from the MCA; the orbitofrontal artery, supplying most of the orbital surface of the frontal lobe, arises from the MCA and anastomoses with branches of the ACA; and extensive anastomoses exist between the ACA and the proximal MCA in the sylvian fissure.[48,117,154,216,348] In cats the presence of an ACoA has been both claimed[131,132] and denied.[153] The feline ACA supplies medial hemisphere cortex containing hindlimb motor representation,[321] but cerebral arterial occlusion tends to cause smaller and deeper infarcts than in higher primates. In rats the rostral caudatoputamen is supplied by penetrating ACA branches and a vessel running alongside the lateral olfactory tract, and this area accounts for 25 percent of strokes in stroke-prone spontaneously hypertensive rats.[259,369]

## SYMPTOMS AND SIGNS

### Weakness and Sensory Loss

ACA occlusion causes infarction of the paracentral lobule and, as a result, weakness and sensory loss in the contralateral leg[26,42,43,76,257,323] (Fig. 15-3). The deficit is usually greatest distally, in part because the proximal leg is represented on the primary sensorimotor cortex either superiorly on the medial hemisphere or on the high convexity with, therefore, richer collaterals from the MCA, and, in part, because proximal muscles have substantial representation in the ipsilateral hemisphere.[241] If infarction extends to the upper convexity, there may be proximal arm weakness, or, as is usual with cortical lesions, clumsiness or slowness out of proportion to actual loss of strength. Muscle tone is initially most often flaccid, becoming spastic over days or weeks; tendon reflexes at the outset may be decreased, normal, or increased. (This frequent early dissociation between tone and tendon reflexes has been attributed to loss of supraspinal influence upon different kinds of muscle spindle afferents, for example, phasic vs tonic.[41]) Babinski's sign may be present.

The sensory modalities most often affected are discriminative (two-point discrimination, localization, stereognosis) and proprioceptive (position sense). Pain and temperature sensation and gross touch are usually only mildly decreased; the patient can tell sharp from dull, but the pinprick does not feel as sharp or as "normal" as on the unaffected side. Vibratory loss is variable. Depending on the posterior ex-

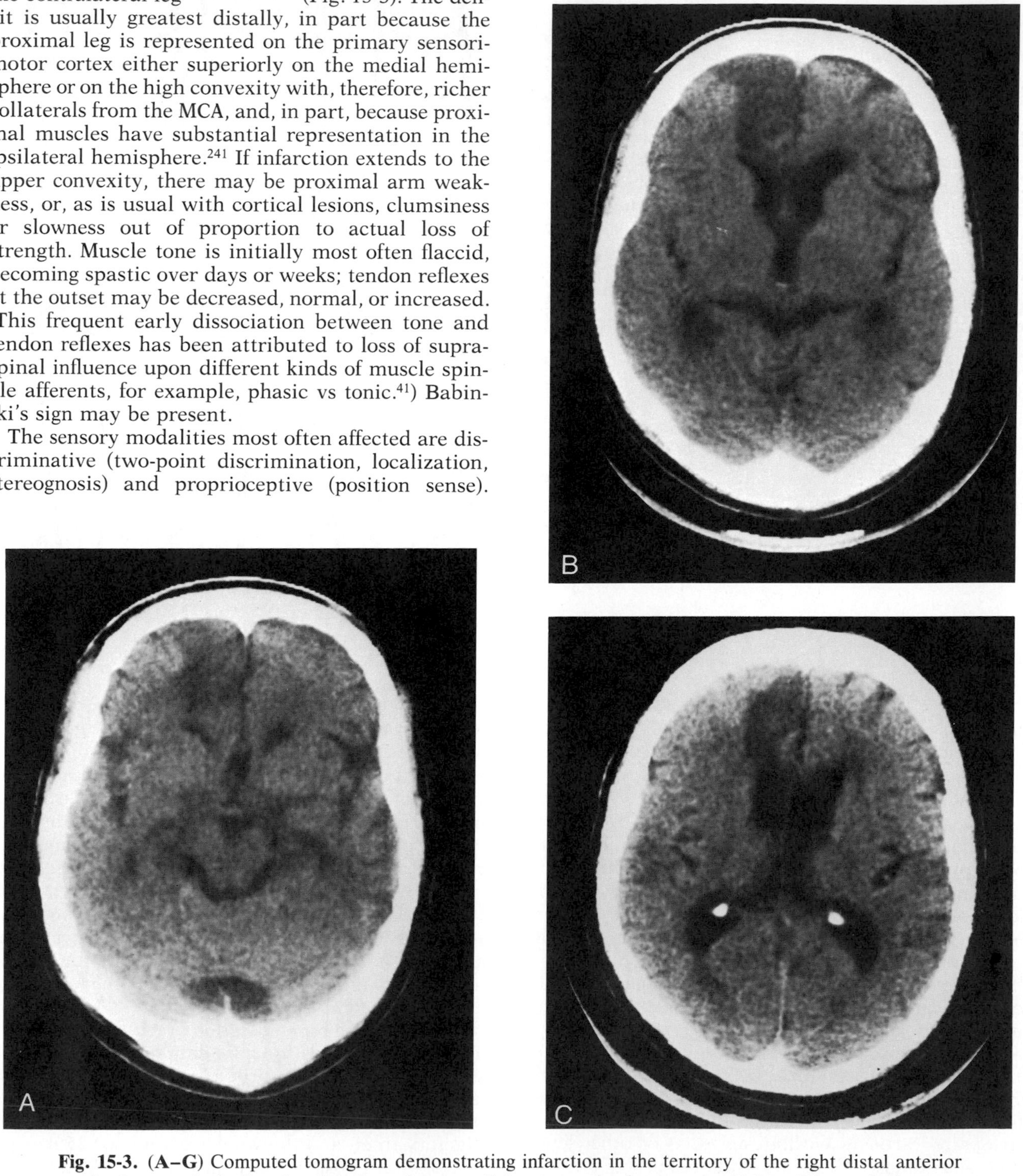


**Fig. 15-3.** (**A–G**) Computed tomogram demonstrating infarction in the territory of the right distal anterior cerebral artery, including the orbitofrontal and medial and superior frontoparietal lobes. Diencephalic structures supplied by proximal anterior cerebral artery penetrating branches are not involved. (*Figure continues.*)

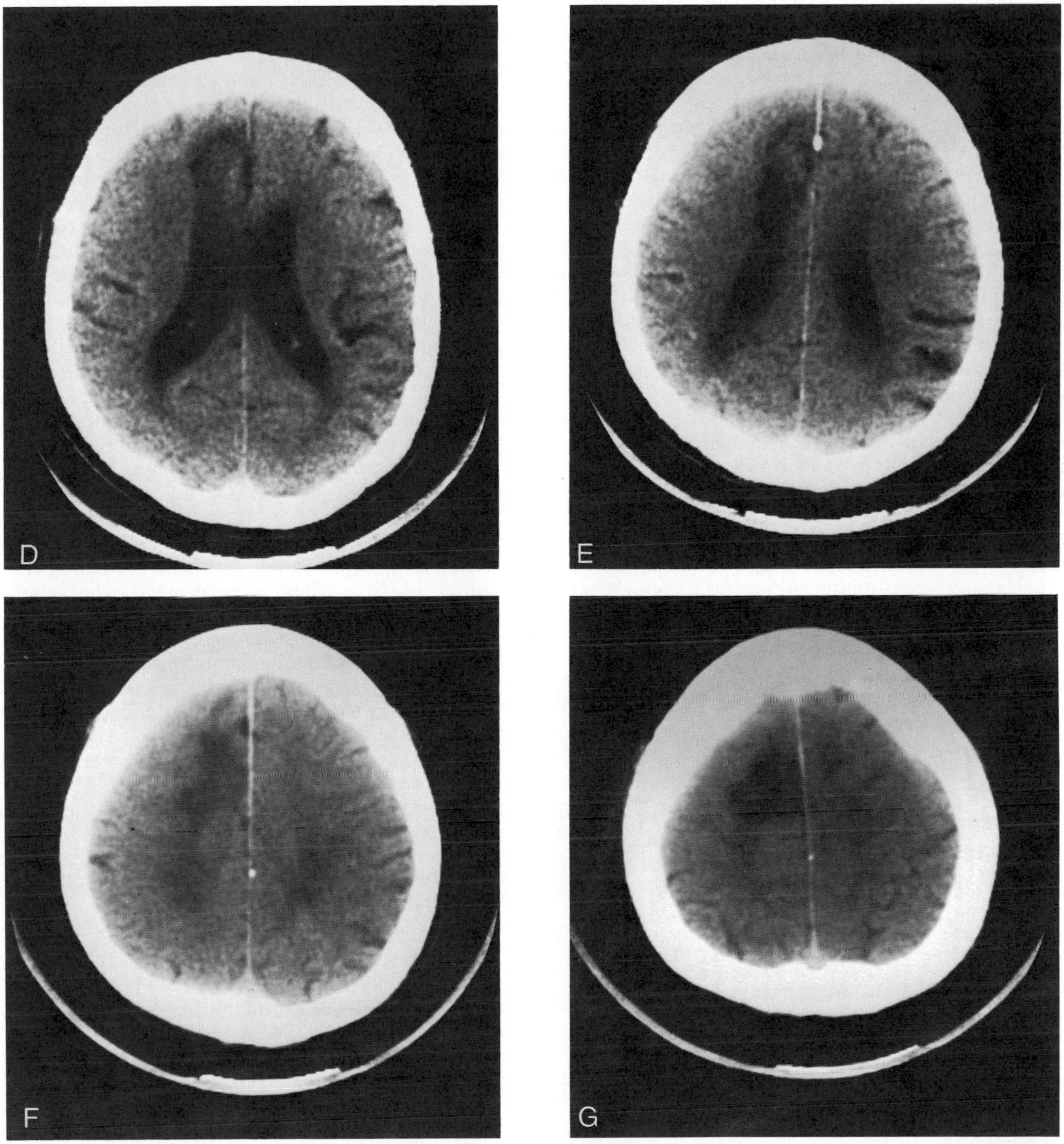


**Fig. 15-3** (*Continued*).

tent of the ACA and collaterals from the PCA, sensory loss may be mild or even absent in the presence of marked crural hemiparesis.[64] Sensation may be similarly spared when occlusion is not of the ACA or the pericallosal artery but of the paracentral branch.[64,194,195,357,360]

Acutely the head and eyes may be deviated toward the side of the lesion.[15,64,99] Forced grasping and groping of the contralateral hand, whether or not it is weak, follows damage to the posterior superior frontal gyrus.[64,186,281,289] Such forced grasping has been considered "a type of limb-kinetic apraxia," and "only one aspect of a total change in behavior, toward a compulsive exploration of the environment";[81] foot grasping[170] can cause the lower limb to seem "glued to the floor"[81] on attempted walking. Such patients also display sucking and biting,[81] "ansaugen" (a movement of lips and tongue toward stimulation of the skin near the lower lip),[281] bradykinesia (or an "absence of movement intension"[64,121,122]), catalepsy,[30] and "tonic innervation" ("amorphous movements of a pseudospontaneous character"[64]) on attempted voluntary action of the affected arm or leg.[121,122,170]

Pronounced weakness of the arm and face in the presence of ACA occlusion has been attributed to involvement of Heubner's artery and its supply to the anterior limb and genu of the internal capsule[64,257] (Fig. 15-4). If the circle of Willis is complete, such proximal thrombosis must extend as far as the ACoA to produce complete hemiplegia, or the contralateral ACA will take over the supply of both medial hemispheres and weakness will be limited to the face and arm. Paralysis of the right arm, paresis of the right face, and only slight weakness of the right leg occurred in a man who at autopsy had infarction of the left putamen, caudate, and anterior limb of the internal capsule, plus a "shrunken and occluded artery of Heubner."[64] (The leg weakness was attributed to additional softening in the territories of the ACA's middle and posterior internal frontal branches.) On the other hand, more recent anatomic studies have shown that Heubner's artery supplies only the most anterior striatum and anterior limb of the internal capsule and is, therefore, probably infrequently the responsible vessel when brachial or facial palsy accompanies ACA occlusion. More likely in such a situation is involvement of penetrating branches arising from the most proximal ACA and the internal carotid bifurcation which supply, in addition to the hypothalamus and the rostral thalamus, not only the genu but also the anterior part of the internal capsule's posterior limb.[86] Moreover, caudate infarction can cause contralateral limb bradykinesia, clumsiness, and loss of associated movements mistakenly interpreted as "weakness."[49] Dysarthria has followed unilateral infarction of either the left or right anterior limb of the internal capsule, and in one report dysarthria followed infarction apparently confined to the caudate nucleus.[49] Five patients with unilateral capsular genu infarction had contralateral facial and lingual weakness with dysarthria; three also had unilateral mastication-palatal-pharyngeal weakness, and one had unilateral vocal cord paresis; the only limb involvement was mild hand weakness in three.[27]

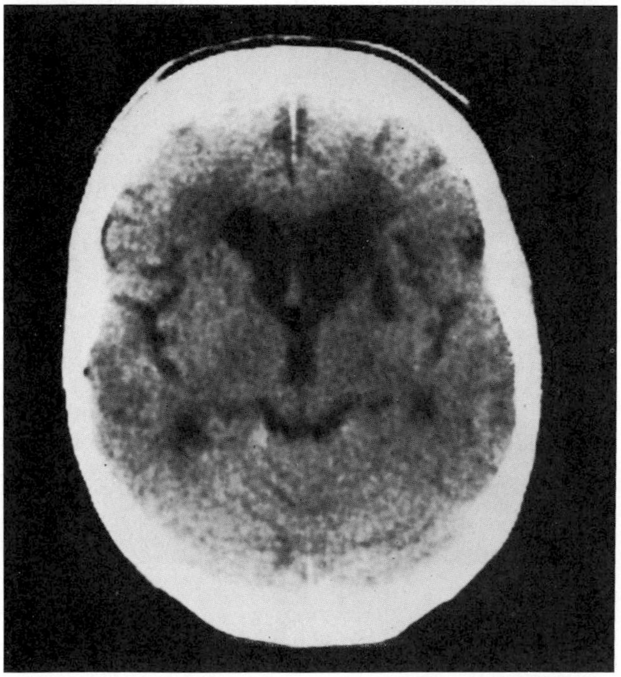

**Fig. 15-4.** Computed tomogram showing infarction in the territory of either the left artery of Heubner or another penetrating branch of the proximal anterior cerebral artery. Brain supplied by the distal anterior cerebral artery was radiographically normal, and at autopsy infarction was limited to the head of the caudate, the anterior part of the internal capsule's anterior limb, and the anterior putamen.

Infarction in the territories of both ACAs causes paraparesis, with or without sensory loss.[324] It is of course likeliest when there is a vascular anomaly, such as a hypoplastic A1 segment or an azygous distal ACA.[15,58,64,102,279,280] Particularly when symptoms are stutteringly progressive, spinal cord disease may be erroneously suspected.[17,202,248,333] Even if weakness is mild or absent there may be severe gait disturbance, with inability to initiate the first step with either foot, to lift either foot off the ground, or to turn to either side[214,332] ("slipping clutch syndrome"[81]). Grasp reflexes of the feet (or hands) are not present in all such patients, and although some can move their legs freely in the air (e.g., bicycling motions),[81] others cannot.[214] When severe, such medial prefrontal damage can produce a pronounced immobility of all four limbs, from bradykinesia to catatonic (perseverative) posturing with gegenhalten, sucking, and biting.[81]

The gait disability bears obvious resemblance to that found with hydrocephalus and with the "paraplegia in flexion" of degenerative disease that mainly affects the frontal lobes[36]; in these conditions the pathophysiology is not understood, and the possible roles of descending frontal and prefrontal fibers[96,365] or the globus pallidus[366] are uncertain. Pulsatile flow in the ACAs is decreased in infantile hydrocephalus,[138] and it has been suggested that secondary ACA ischemia may be the cause of lower extremity spasticity in hydrocephalic infants, as well as contributing to the gait disturbance of adult normal pressure hydrocephalus.[208]

## Callosal Disconnection Signs

In addition to either right or left leg weakness ACA occlusion can cause left apraxia, agraphia, and tactile anomia.[62,121,183,187,199,281,339,367] Early cases are difficult to interpret, however.[115,133] For example, the patient of Liepmann and Maas[187] had right hemiplegia, including his arm, and so it is uncertain if his agraphia and apraxia were truly unilateral. The patient of Goldstein[121] had left-sided weakness, greatest in the leg, with a pronounced left hand grasp reflex, adding another possible reason for left-sided motor difficulty.[35,81] Agraphia, apraxia, and tactile anomia have occurred, however, in otherwise normal left limbs of patients with ACA occlusion, right leg weakness, and normal right arms.[114,199,278,339]

Following surgical occlusion of the left ACA, a patient of Geschwind and Kaplan[115] had right hemiparesis worse in the leg, a marked grasp reflex in the right hand, and mild right proprioceptive loss. He also had left-handed agraphia, writing incorrectly and paragraphically both spontaneously and to dictation, and could not do written calculations with his left hand. He could not name objects, letters, or numbers placed in his left hand out of vision, but he could identify them afterward with his left hand by pointing to them or demonstrating their use. Using either hand he could not correctly select from a group of objects placed out of sight in the other hand. Finally, he had difficulty performing verbal commands with his left hand (e.g., draw a square, point to the examiner, show how to brush teeth). Despite the grasp reflex his right hand could write normally, and his left hand could slavishly copy writing. Either hand could imitate the examiner's movements or manipulate objects. Following the lead of earlier authors,[187] Geschwind and Kaplan attributed their patient's findings to anterior callosal destruction, with disconnection of the right hemisphere from the left, or, more specifically, of the right sensorimotor cortex from the left language areas. (Earlier writers who claimed that callosal lesions could cause left astereognosis[113,121] were undoubtedly observing tactile anomia rather than true agnosia, although a patient who could identify objects but not letters placed in the left hand is less easily explained.[330]) Preservation of the posterior corpus callosum was manifested by Geschwind and Kaplan's patient's ability to read words presented to either visual field. Retained ability to perform tasks requiring both hands, such as threading a needle, suggested that the two hemispheres could cooperate like two individuals on such visually guided activities.

A left-handed patient[223] had a stroke with weakness of the right leg but not the right arm, plus loss of ability to write with his right but not his left hand; if he is presumed to have had right cerebral language dominance, callosal disconnection might explain his agraphic right hand. Another patient, considered to have "pure agraphia," may represent a similar example of ACA occlusion.[251]

Some patients with presumed ACA occlusion and anterior callosal damage have had difficulty not only in performing verbal commands with the left hand but also in imitating the examiner and using actual objects.[30,113,186,198] Inaccessibility of verbal information to the right sensorimotor cortex would not explain this type of apraxia, and it has been suggested that in right-handers engrams for skilled movements ("space–time" or "visuokinesthetic" engrams[352]) reside in the left hemisphere and that callosal apraxia with impaired imitation and object use is the result of disconnection between these motor engrams and the right hemisphere.[119,352] In support of such a view is the observation, in a left-hander, that dominance for language and dominance for skilled motor acts appeared to be in different hemispheres.[133] That some patients with ACA occlusion have impaired imitation and object use and some do not has been explained by the hypothesis that "verbal motor programs" may be transmitted to the right hemisphere across the genu of the corpus callosum, whereas visuokinesthetic engrams may be transmitted across the body.[352]

Not all patients with ACA occlusion and left-sided apraxia perform well on bimanual tasks,[113,119,352] and sometimes the hands actually seem to be fighting one another (the "alien hand sign"[119,210]). It has been claimed[119] and denied[352] that extracallosal medial hemispheric damage is responsible for this phenomenon.

Occlusion of an ACA that extends around the splenium of the corpus callosum can produce pure alexia in the left visual field or other visual anomic or agnostic problems.[248,352]

A problem in interpreting these patients is the degree to which they differ from those who have undergone surgical callosectomy. Left-sided apraxia to verbal commands occurs acutely following complete section of the corpus callosum and anterior commissure, usually with preserved ability to carry out the act in imitation of the examiner.[104,106] Right-sided movements, when governed by the right hemisphere (e.g., drawing an object seen only in the left visual field), are also impaired.[24] Such deficits tend to improve over days, however,[106] unless severe extracallosal brain damage is present.[104] Lasting deficit after callosal and commissural section is most likely to affect homolateral control of fingers (e.g., moving the left fingers to identify areas corresponding to regions stimulated on the right fingers, or mimicking with the left hand postures shown pictorially to the right visual field). When there is left hemispheric damage early in life, the minor hemisphere can comprehend spoken or written names of familiar objects,[105,110,301,302] but except in the setting of prolonged stimulus exposure[372] or in rare instances of unusual plasticity in speech organization[111,293] it usually cannot comprehend verbs or action nouns.[108–110] Such lack of comprehension accounts for the callosectomized patient's inability to follow verbal commands with either hand when the information is given to the minor hemisphere. Recovery of all but the most distal and subtle apraxia when commands are given to the language hemisphere is explained by each hemisphere's control over homolateral as well as contralateral limbs.

A patient with anterior callosal hemorrhage and bilateral ACA vasospasm had alexia in the left hemifield, anomia for objects held in the left hand, and left-handed agraphia and apraxia (including imitation and object use). She also had bilateral "pseudoneglect": visual or tactile line bisection produced left hemineglect with the right hand in left hemispace and right hemineglect with left hand in right hemispace. The explanation offered was disconnection of "the hemisphere important for directing attention intention into the contralateral hemispace" from "the hemisphere important for controlling sensory motor processing of limb."[135] By contrast, left hemispatial neglect "confined to right-hand and verbal responses" occurred in a patient with infarction of the posterior genu and whole trunk of the corpus callosum plus the left medial frontal and temporo-occipital lobes.[155] These findings were considered consistent with the hypothesis that "the left hemisphere is only concerned with attending to the contralateral hemispace," whereas "the right hemisphere is specialized for attending to both sides of space." It was further observed, consistent with previous reports, that hemineglect does not seem to occur with lesions restricted to the corpus callosum but requires additional destruction (e.g., medial frontal lobe) that block transmission through extracallosal commissures.[120,294]

In a right-handed callosectomized patient with unusually rich right hemispheric verbal comprehension, there was no left-sided apraxia to verbal information presented to the right hemisphere.[109] This finding argues against the notion of motor engrams residing solely in one hemisphere, language-dominant or not.[113,136,160–162,273,342,344] In other callosectomized patients visual nonverbal stimulation has also produced normally coordinated contralateral motor acts.[344]

Consistent with the view that extracallosal damage is probably crucial to the appearance of "anterior callosal disconnection syndrome" following ACA occlusion[106] is the finding that left tactile anomia, apraxia for verbal commands, and agraphia did not occur in two patients who underwent section of the anterior commissure and only the anterior two-thirds of the corpus callosum. These patients, moreover, performed a variety of nonverbal cross-integration tasks, matching visual or tactile stimuli directed separately to each hemisphere.[125] Conversely, selective sectioning of the splenium, sparing the genu and body, did produce verbal deficits for left visual field and tactile stimuli,[207,330] as well as for tactile-motor tasks requiring interhemispheric integration.[342,344] It appears that "the anterior commissure and the rostral callosum do not transfer either lateralized visual images that elicit motor activity or the specific motor program needed to carry out the appropriate movement."[344] An isolated 3-cm midcallosal section impairs interhemispheric transfer of tactile data but not of information obtained visually.[148] Section of the most posterior 1.5 cm of the callosum disrupts naming of visual stimuli in the left visual field,[107,145,207,309] and an additional 1.5 cm section further impairs sensorimotor integration and tactile naming.[70,344] What information gets transferred across the rostral callosum, that part most often damaged following ACA occlusion, is unclear; it has been suggested that the anterior callosum transfers information after processing it into higher-order abstraction.[292,344] (Following posterior callosal section, interhemispheric transfer of sensory information from the right hemisphere is lost, but transfer of semantic information is still possible; after complete section, neither sensory nor semantic information can be transferred.[292])

## Akinetic Mutism (Abulia)

Coma probably can follow bilateral proximal ACA occlusion, but when aneurysm surgery[238] or vasospasm after subarachnoid hemorrhage[314] is the cause, interpretation is difficult. Dandy[74] believed that left ACA occlusion (i.e., surgical ligation) caused permanent coma and this view was promulgated by Poppen,[254] who, however, considered hypotension during surgery to be a critical factor. Subsequent authors have perpetuated the idea that coma can follow unilateral ACA occlusion.[17,57] However, Dandy's attribution of coma to striatal damage was soon discredited,[222,322] and it is now recognized that coma requires either bihemispheric or ascending reticular activating system lesions.[252] Probably those patients in whom coma seemed to follow ACA occlusion either had, as a result of one of the several vascular anomalies described above, brain damage not restricted to one hemisphere, or were akinetic, mute, and more alert than they seemed.

Akinetic mutism is "a state of limited responsiveness to the environment in the absence of gross alteration of sensory-motor mechanisms operating at a more peripheral level."[284] Neither paralysis nor coma accounts for the symptoms. Patients may open their eyes and seem alert, and brief movement, speech, or even agitation may follow powerful stimuli, but patients are otherwise "indifferent, detached, frozen, and apathetic."[284] The term akinetic mutism was used by Cairns[46] to describe such a state in association with a tumor of the third ventricle. With such lesions there is often ophthalmoparesis and fluctuating or continuous somnolence.[37,53,54,91,101,178,184]

Akinetic mutism also occurs with lesions of the anteromedial frontal lobes, including infarction.[45,100,127,238] Ophthalmoparesis (except for early gaze preference) is then not present, and the patient, whose open eyes may follow objects, is more obviously alert than with mesencephalic or thalamic lesions; there may be brief, monosyllabic, but appropriate responses to questions. Striking dissociation occurs between spontaneous verbal communication, which is often totally absent, and solicited communication, which is often retained though restricted.[45] The term *abulia* refers to a continuum of such abnormalities, from mild to severe, having in common decreased spontaneous movement and speech, latency in responding to verbal and other stimuli, and impersistence in responses and tasks.[97,233] While verbal responses are "late, terse, incomplete, and emotionally flat," patients sufficiently prodded sometimes reveal a cognitive capacity much more normal than expected.[49] When the patient is literally akinetic and mute, however, the condition must be differentiated from true stupor or coma, the locked-in state, extrapyramidal akinesia, catatonia, hysteria, and persistent vegetative state.

Abulia has followed bilateral cingulate gyrus lesions. A woman developed a sudden headache and then "lay staring at the ceiling, not asking for water or food, and never speaking spontaneously." She was incontinent of urine, ate and drank when food or water were brought, comprehended spoken speech, answered questions monosyllabically, and did not display any emotional reaction. There were right-sided hyperreflexia and bilateral Babinski signs. At autopsy there was embolic hemorrhagic infarction of both cingulate gyri and the corpus callosum.[224] A clinically and pathologically similar patient showed Babinski signs but no hypertonus, and there were "no visible reactions to pain."[18] Inability to walk despite normal strength has been specifically mentioned in other reports.[9] On the other hand, unilateral cingulate infarction in two patients was followed by seizures in one and personality change in another, with no reduction in motor activity.[9] Akinetic mutism occurred in one patient with presumed unilateral cingulate (and pontine) damage, but autopsy findings were incomplete.[295] A patient with hemorrhage into his right medial frontal lobe had marked bradykinesia of his left limbs, improving when they were placed in his right hemispace. The disturbance was considered "motor neglect" ("a failure of the intentional systems that lead to preparation and activation of movement"), possibly secondary to supplementary motor area damage.[211]

Cingulectomy in monkeys caused reduction of motor activity and "loss of social conscience"; the animals treated their fellows as inanimate objects not to be feared.[348] Monkeys in which the medial temporal lobes were removed and with Klüver-Bucy syndrome (quietness, no fear, and increased curiosity with compulsive nosing and smelling of all objects) had gradual clearing of symptoms, which, however, returned following bilateral cingulectomy.[158] In cingulectomized cats, motor signs suggested catatonia.[158] Human surgical cingulate ablation for psychiatric disturbance is difficult to interpret, since the amount of cingulate removed is usually small,[327,354] and the importance of cingulothalamic disconnection in frontal lobotomy has never been defined.[9,80]

The full syndrome of akinetic mutism or abulia has thus not been produced in animals by experimental cingulectomy or in humans by surgical cingulectomy, and even bilateral ACA ligation in humans has on occasion failed to cause the syndrome.[100,254] In an autopsy report of eight patients with akinetic mutism and bilateral cingulate destruction, there was no difference in the clinical picture whether or not additional lesions existed in the medial orbital cortex or septal region.[9] Most reports, however, have emphasized additional lesions or diffuse compressive cerebral injury,[45,100,252] and electroencephalograms (EEGs) usually show bilateral cerebral slowing.[100,252] An angiographic study of patients with subarachnoid hemorrhage showed correlation of unilateral or bilateral ACA vasospasm with akinetic mutism, but it was unclear if brain damage was limited to one hemisphere in the patients with unilateral vasospasm.[98]

Abulia has also followed unilateral or bilateral caudate infarction (most likely from occlusion of the recurrent artery of Heubner). In one series of unilateral caudate infarction, it was the most prominent feature in 10 of 17 patients (6 left, 4 right).[49] In four patients the lesions (by CT) were restricted to the caudate; in others the anterior limb of the internal capsule was involved. Three abulic patients had alternating restlessness and hyperactivity, and in four others hyperactivity was present without abulia. In another report it was proposed that abulia resulted from damage to the dorsolateral caudate (which connects to the dorsolateral frontal lobe) and disinhibition from damage to the ventromedial caudate (which connects to orbitofrontal areas).[212]

Acutely following surgical partial section of the anterior corpus callosum there is often akinetic mutism that tends to recover over days.[300,310] Positron emission tomography studies in baboons have shown that the procedure causes transient depression of cortical metabolism in widespread areas of both frontal lobes ("diaschisis").[368]

## Language Disturbance

Unilateral ACA occlusion can produce language disturbance, but whether it is aphasic is uncertain.[112] Details are often lacking in case reports.[324] In some patients "reduction of spontaneous verbal expression"[47] or muteness, often in association with more global psychomotor bradykinesia,[47,73] seems to be a manifestation of abulia; in such patients comprehension of spoken speech may be untestable.[166] Some reports have described truly impaired speech comprehension,[206] word-finding difficulty, alexia,[187] and phonemic or verbal paraphasias on spontaneous speech, reading aloud,[206,338] or writing.[206] Others, however, have emphasized the absence of paraphasias,[6,73,185,270] or considered the difficulty "partly defects of an aphasic order and partly those of a dysarthria."[64] A number of reports have described impaired spontaneous speech with normal repetition and, sometimes, echolalia (transcortical aphasia),[6,14,72,159,166,270,338] and in one instance echolalia and palilalia occurred without other evidence of aphasia.[15] A man with transcortical motor aphasia, although lacking echolalia or echopraxia, could not refrain from completing the sentences of others.[270] Some patients have had transcortical aphasia (or, as Luria calls it, "dynamic aphasia"[196,198]) with a strikingly greater impairment of list naming than naming to confrontation,[6] or particularly impaired speech initiative, as in attempts to narrate stories or describe complex pictures.[270]

In one report a patient with transcortical mixed aphasia had infarction of both the medial frontal and the medial parietal lobes, whereas two other patients with transcortical motor aphasia had infarction of only the medial frontal lobe.[268] One patient following a large left ACA infarct had transcortical motor aphasia and mirror writing.[26] Another, right-handed, had left-handed mirror writing following infarction of the right medial frontal cortex sparing the corpus callosum, leading the authors to conjecture that the supplementary motor area (SMA) is "responsible for nonmirror transformation of motor programs originating in the left hemisphere prior to execution by the primary motor area in the right hemisphere."[51] A woman with aphasia that included impaired comprehension, repetition, reading, and writing had medial frontal infarction plus an old infarct over the rolandic convexity.[255] In some patients speech disturbance was transient, whereas paucity of other movements, including writing, persisted.[206]

Reports of severely impaired language after pathologically documented ACA occlusion have involved left-sided lesions[26] with one exception,[44] a right-handed woman with left hemiparesis, diffuse bradykinesia, speech limited to short replies to questions, and a tendency to echolalia; naming and comprehension of spoken or written language seemed impaired, but were difficult to test. At autopsy there was infarction in the territory of the right ACA, including the head of the caudate, the anterior limb of the internal capsule, the anterior putamen, the anterior cingulate and superior frontal gyri, and the entire SMA (Fig. 15-5). Several reports exist of language disturbance after bilateral ACA occlusion,[139,166,205] and one, with neither postmortem examination nor disclosure of the patient's handedness, of occlusion of the right ACA.[47]

Most investigators, whether or not they consider these abnormalities to be truly aphasic, attribute them to damage to the SMA[112,142,245,246,355] on the medial surface of the frontal lobe, anterior to the paracentral lobule, and between the cingulate and superior frontal gyri (i.e., the medial hemispheric part of Brodmann's area 6). Of 10 right-handed patients with left ACA territory infarcts, four had transcortical motor aphasia, and in each the SMA was involved. Three other patients with sparing of the SMA but involvement of the cingulate had only "alterations of verbal memory."[25] In monkeys, stimulation of this area

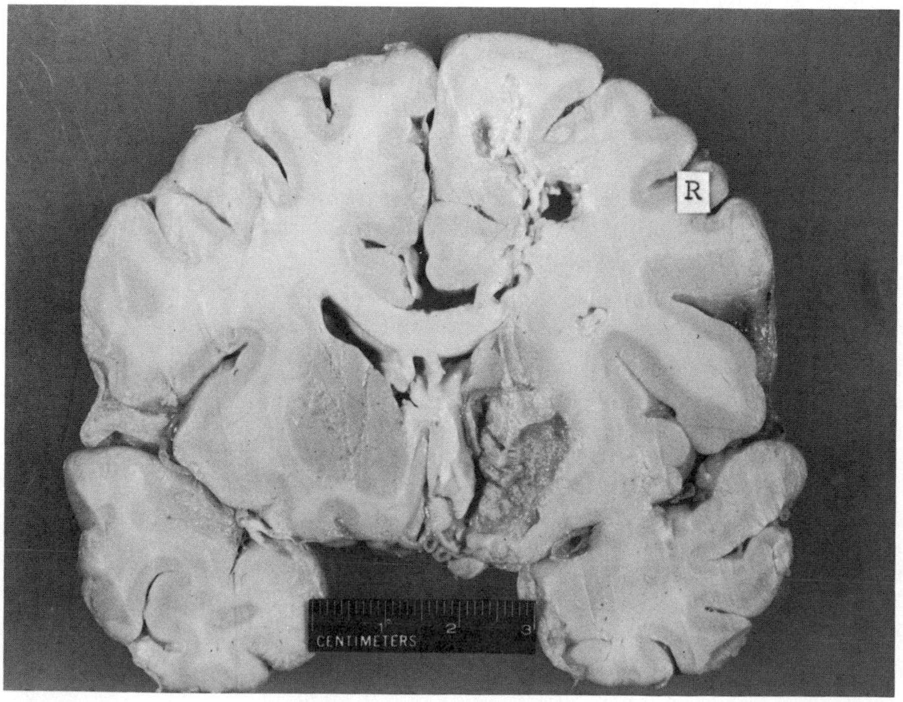


**Fig. 15-5.** Autopsy specimen showing a coronal section of the anterior frontal and temporal lobes. There is infarction in the territories of both the proximal and distal right anterior cerebral artery. Affected areas include the caudate, putamen, internal capsule's anterior limb, cingulate gyrus, and supplementary motor area. (From Brust et al.,[44] with permission.)

causes arm and leg movements and head turning,[220] and there seems to be rostral–caudal forelimb–hindlimb somatotopy.[39,200,296,318,319,361,364] Unilateral ablation of SMA in monkeys produces a deficit in tasks of bimanual coordination.[38] In humans SMA stimulation induces bodily postures (e.g., turning of head and eyes toward a contralaterally uplifted arm) or repetitive movements (e.g., stepping or hand-waving).[246] Such responses are often bilateral and can occur after ablation of area 4 (the primary motor cortex). SMA stimulation can also cause speech and movement arrest or vocalization.

Whereas stimulation of the face region of area 4 causes vocalization of continuous vowel sounds,[239,242] SMA stimulation on either hemisphere[241] produces intermittently repeated words, syllables, or meaningless combinations of syllables[246] ("saccadic vocalization"[355]). The repeated word might be a palilalia of what was being said at the onset of stimulation. Rhythmic mouth and jaw movements sometimes accompany the vacalization. Speech arrest, hesitation, or slowing also occur, sometimes with mouth movements suggesting attempted speech or with arrest of other voluntary movement. Speech comprehension is usually preserved, but anomia and paraphasias have occurred.[241]

Such symptoms, with or without other motor, sensory, or autonomic phenomena, may be the manifestation of seizures caused by structural lesions affecting the SMA, especially meningiomas[3,13,34,51,52,90,128,146,249,315,355] Although experimental stimulation of either the right or left SMA can cause speech arrest or repetition, seizures causing altered speech have only rarely occurred in dextrals with lesions of the right SMA.[33,50] Both stimulation and seizure phenomena raise the questions of whether true aphasia is occurring and which brain structures are in fact responsible.

Destructive lesions, including infarction, are similarly problematic. Medial hemispheric structural lesions such as neoplasm,[13,61,68,72,89,90,128,201,273] vascular malformation,[198,249] subdural empyema,[175] surgical ablation,[128,171,244,282] and trauma[197] not only can directly affect more regions than the SMA, but can also produce distant effects from edema or brain distortion. SMA excision for the treatment of epilepsy has led to language disturbance, but interpretation of such cases has varied. One group found that excision of the language hemisphere's SMA back to area 4 caused muteness, whereas excision of the language hemisphere's anterior SMA or the non-language hemisphere's entire SMA produced "no specific deficit."[243] Others found, after excision of either SMA, more lasting speech disturbances, which, however, seemed nonaphasic and secondary to bradykinesia.[171] Transcortical motor aphasia followed excision of the left SMA.[282] Bilateral ideomotor apraxia without aphasia affected two patients with ACA infarction involving both the left SMA and the corpus callosum.[351]

The SMA receives afferents from the ipsilateral primary and secondary somatosensory cortex and has reciprocal connections with the ipsilateral area 4, posterior parietal cortex, upper convexity premotor cortex (area 6), several thalamic nuclei, and, across the corpus callosum, the contralateral SMA and convexity area 6.[149–151,355] It has been suggested, therefore, that the SMA is "an area of sensory convergence."[39] Efferents project bilaterally to the cingulate gyrus and striatum,[73,83,148,169] ipsilaterally to the red nucleus, pontine nuclei, and dorsal column nuclei,[39] and contralaterally to area 4 and the midconvexity "premotor" region (area 8).[73] There are also SMA neurons that project to the spinal cord.[22,200,221] Regional cerebral blood flow (rCBF) increases in the SMA during automatic speech and during repetitive finger movement but not during isometric hand muscle contraction.[140,141,172,174,272] CBF also increases in the SMA during planning of sequential movements.[232,265,266] (By contrast, area 4's CBF increases only during execution of such movements.[265]) In monkeys, medullary pyramidal section did not affect movements produced by SMA stimulation,[363] increased discharge of SMA neurons preceded stereotyped learned motor tasks of either the ipsilateral or contralateral extremities, and SMA neurons fired in response to sensory signals "only when the signal called for a motor response."[319] Neurons in the SMA are, however, less responsive to peripheral stimuli than those in area 4,[39,361] suggesting that part of the SMA's function may be "to 'gate' or suppress the afferent influences on area 4"[360] (perhaps accounting for the transient contralateral grasp reflex frequently seen after SMA ablation[90,241,246,258,297,329,361]). Such suppression would convert area 4's activity from a closed loop to an open loop mode,[356,361] consistent with the further notion that the SMA develops "a preparatory state" for impending movement[319,320] or that it elaborates "programs for motor subroutines necessary in skilled voluntary motion,"[267] including, with its "sequences of fast isolated muscular contraction," human speech.[265] ACA occlusion and SMA damage may therefore affect "an elementary part of language, very primitive, and lacking . . . symbols and intellectual features";[249] the resulting disturbance would not be, strictly speaking, aphasic.

The oft-cited case of Bonhoeffer[30] may represent ACA occlusion causing language disturbance by a different mechanism. This patient developed right hemiplegia, with the leg weaker than the arm, plus reduction of speech to one or two words, relatively preserved comprehension of spoken speech, alexia, agraphia, and apraxia (difficulty following commands, imitating, and handling objects), that was greater on the left than right. Abnormalities at autopsy included infarction of the posterior left middle and superior frontal gyri, the anterior four-fifths of the corpus callosum, the anterior limb of the left internal capsule, and a small part of the left posterior inferior parietal lobule. Bonhoeffer[30] (and Geschwind,[113] reviewing the case) explained the left apraxia as resulting from the callosal lesion and the aphasia from the combined callosal and capsular lesions, which in effect isolated Broca's area; the posterior parietal lesion probably contributed to the alexia, agraphia, and right apraxia. Neither author discussed the possible contribution of SMA destruction to the language disturbance, which, theoretically, could have occurred without it.

## Other Mental Abnormalities

Besides abulia, apraxia, and language impairment, patients with ACA occlusion can have a variety of other emotional or intellectual disturbances, usually attributed to involvement of structures supplied by branches of the proximal ACA (A1 segment or ACoA).[34,134,287] Anxiety, fear, insomnia, talkativeness, or agitation have occurred with or without weakness, bradykinesia, or grasp and suck reflexes.[9,15,34,64] A young woman, awakening from coma after ACoA aneurysm rupture, had severe withdrawal with unprovoked agitation and screaming; at autopsy there was bilateral infarction of the orbital gyri, gyri recti, septal nuclei, cingulate gyri, hippocampal formations, and right amygdala.[93] Damage to hypothalamic or other limbic structures has also been considered responsible for these symptoms,[86] which, when they predominate, can suggest "nonstructural" neurotic or psychotic illness.[17,57] In any event, the notion that apathy and poor motivation predictably follow dorsolateral frontal lesions, whereas orbitofrontal damage causes disinhibited behavior, appears to be an oversimplification.[126,308]

Confusion, disorientation, and memory loss, sometimes severe, also occur.[9,76,85,139,153,192,193,238,248,256,283,324] Retrograde and anterograde amnesia following ACoA aneurysm rupture may be subtle or severe,[71,147,237,307,340] with variable denial or confabulation.[79,197,316,343,371] In one report a patient with bilateral infarction of both medial frontal lobes as well as the right inferior temporal lobe and pole had severely impaired recognition of previously presented words or pictures yet could spontaneously recall them.[78] In another report five patients with lesions restricted to basal forebrain structures (sparing the hippocampi and temporal lobes) were able to recall particular stimuli (e.g., someone's name or face) but could not bring such differently learned components together as an integrated memory.[71] Structures implicated in these amnestic syndromes have included the hypothalamus, medial forebrain bundle, septum, nucleus of Meynert, nucleus accumbens, and fornix, with possible secondary dysfunction of medial temporal regions.[71,250,362]

Visuospatial disturbance with difficulty dressing, drawing, or copying or with left hemineglect has followed infarction of the caudate and anterior limb of the internal capsule. Depression has been associated with left caudate lesions.[303]

## Incontinence and Other Autonomic Changes

Urinary (and less often fecal) incontinence can occur with either unilateral or bilateral ACA occlusion.[17,50,64,353] Involvement of the paracentral lobule (presuming homuncular representation of motor and sensory components of micturation) has been offered as an explanation,[20,60,248] even though paracentral stimulation produced only contralateral sensation in the penis without motor response.[240] Damage to the superiormedial frontal lobe, especially the midportion of the superior frontal gyrus, the cingulate, and the white matter in-between, is a more likely cause, since such damage (e.g., from frontal leukotomy) causes transient or permanent disturbance of urination and defecation, including urgency and incontinence.[10,11,36,262]

Cardiorespiratory alterations are frequent following stroke, whether or not limbic structures are specifically damaged.[191,341] Such changes following ACA occlusion are therefore open to interpretation, but it is not unreasonable to incriminate damage to the hypothalamus, cingulate gyrus, or other limbis areas. Fever not always related to infection, tachycardia, and unexpected death have followed human cingulate infarction.[9,18,238] Human and animal cingulate stimulation can produce altered respirations, bradycardia, temporary respiratory or cardiac arrest, hyper- or hypotension, pupillary dilatation, and piloerection.[9,18,87,152,285,298,349] Diabetes insipidus, perhaps from anterior hypothalamic infarction, has occurred after surgical occlusion of a proximal ACA for ACoA aneurysm.[59,134] Gastrointestinal bleeding following ACoA aneurysm rupture has also been blamed on hypothalamic damage.[317]

## Periventricular Leukomalacia of Infancy

Brains of infants dying within hours or months of birth may have necrotic foci along the lateral ventricles,[16] considered by some to be infarcts at border zones between the territories of the anterior, middle, and posterior cerebral arteries.[16,190,345] Others[82] have stressed that the periventricular areas are more properly called end zones, and are not in anastomatic areas but rather within a few millimeters of the ventricular wall "between the terminal distributions of ventriculopetal and ventriculofugal branches of small arteries that penetrate deeply into the brain,"[82] including those from the ACA passing through the cingulate gyrus.[313] Such lesions usually spare the cerebral cortex, for the fetus has rich meningeal anastomoses between pial vessels, and the newborn has a relatively higher metabolic rate in white matter.[75,82] Hypotensive newborn dogs develop decreased white matter blood flow and lesions resembling periventricular leukomalacia.[370] Infants with periventricular leukomalacia and no apparent perinatal asphyxia have shown poorly developed ventriculofugal branches at autopsy.[12,313] Affected infants display lethargy, hypotonia, difficulty feeding, and seizures; survivors are usually mentally retarded with spastic quadriparesis.

Because cerebral autoregulation is impaired in neonates with asphyxia, periventricular hemorrhage in the newborn may be the result of capillary dilatation and rupture in these same deep end zones.[345]

## REFERENCES


1. Abbie AA: The morphology of the fore-brain arteries, with especial reference to the evolution of the basal ganglia. J Anat 68:433, 1934
2. Ahmed DS, Ahmed RH: The recurrent branch of the anterior cerebral artery. Anat Rec 157:699, 1967
3. Alajouanine T, Castaigne P, Sabouraud O, Contamin F: Palilalie paroxystique et vocalisations itératives au cours de crises épileptiques par lesion intéressant l'aire motrice supplémentaire. Rev Neurol 101:685, 1959
4. Alexander L: The vascular supply of the striopallidum. Res Publ Assoc Res Nerv Ment Dis 21:77, 1942
5. Alexander MP, Freedman M: Amnesia after anterior communicating artery aneurysm rupture. Neurology (NY), suppl 2. 33:104, 1983
6. Alexander MP, Schmitt MA: The aphasia syndrome of stroke in the left anterior cerebral artery territory. Arch Neurol 37:97, 1980
7. Alpers BJ, Berry RG, Paddison RM: Anatomical studies of the circle of Willis in normal brain. Arch Neurol Psychiatry 81:409, 1959
8. Amagasa M, Sato S, Otabe K: Posttraumatic dissecting aneurysm of the anterior cerebral artery: case report. Neurosurgery 23:221, 1988
9. Amyes EW, Nielsen JM: Clinicopathologic study of vascular lesions of the anterior cingulate region. Bull Los Angeles Neurol Soc 20:112, 1955
10. Andrew J, Nathan PW: Lesions of the anterior frontal lobes and disturbances of micturition and defecation. Brain 87:233, 1964
11. Andrew J, Nathan PW: The cerebral control of micturition. Proc R Soc Med 58:553, 1965
12. Armstrong D, Norman MG: Periventricular leukomalacia in neonates: complications and sequelae. Arch Dis Child 49:367, 1974
13. Arseni C, Botez MI: Speech disturbances caused by tumours of the supplementary motor area. Acta Psychiatr Scand 36:279, 1961
14. Atkinson MS: Transcortical motor aphasia associated with left frontal lobe infarction. Trans Am Neurol Assoc 96:136, 1971
15. Baldy R: Les Syndromes de l'Artère Cérébrale Antérieure. Jouve, Paris, 1927
16. Banker BQ, Larroche JC: Periventricular leukomalacia of infancy: a form of neonatal anoxic encephalopathy. Arch Neurol 7:386, 1962
17. Baptista AG: Studies on the arteries of the brain. II. The anterior cerebral artery: some anatomic features and their clinical implications. Neurology (NY) 13:825, 1963
18. Barris RW, Schuman HR: Bilateral anterior cingulate gyrus lesions. Syndrome of the anterior cingulate gyri. Neurology NY 3:44, 1953
19. Beevor CE: The cerebral arterial supply. Brain 30:403, 1907
20. Berman SA, Hayman LA, Hinck VC: Correlation of CT cerebral vascular territories with function. 1. Anterior cerebral artery. AJR 135:253, 1980
21. Besson G, Leguyader J, Mimassi N et al: Anomalie rare du polygone de Willis: trajet sous-optique des deux artères cérébales antérieures: aneurysme associé de la bifurcation du tronc basilaire. Neurochirurgie 26:71, 1980
22. Biber MP, Kneisley LW, LaVail JH: Cortical neurons projecting to the cervical and lumbar enlargements of the spinal cord in young and adult rhesus monkeys. Exp Neurol 59:492, 1978
23. Blackburn IW: Anomalies of the encephalic arteries among the insane. J Comp Neurol Psychol 17:493, 1907
24. Bogen JE, Gazzaniga MS: Cerebral commissurotomy in man: minor hemisphere dominance for certain visuospacial functions. J Neurosurg 23:394, 1965
25. Bogousslavsky J, Regli F: Infarctus du territoire de l'artere cerebrale anterieure gauche. 1. Correlations clinico-tomodensitometriques. Rev Neurol 143:21, 1987
26. Bogousslavsky J, Assal G, Regli F: Infarctus du territoire de l'artere cérébrale anterieure gauche. 2. Troubles du langage. Rev Neurol 143:121, 1987
27. Bogousslavsky J, Regli F: Capsular genu syndrome. Neurology (NY) 40:1499, 1990
28. Bogousslavsky J, Regli F: Anterior cerebral artery territory infarction in the Lausanne Stroke Registry: clinical and etiological patterns. Arch Neurol 47:144, 1990
29. Bollar A, Martinez R, Gelabert M, Garcia A: Anomalous origin of anterior cerebral artery associated with aneurysm—embryological considerations. Neuroradiology 30:86, 1988
30. Bonhoeffer K: Klischer u. anatomischer Befund zur Lehre von der Apraxie und der motorischen Sprachbahn. Monatsschr Psychiatr Neurol 35:113, 1914
31. Booker J, Morris N, Huang C-Y: Cerebral radionuclide scintigraphy in the stroke syndrome. Med J Aust 1:625, 1978
32. Bosma NJ: Infra-optic course of anterior cerebral artery and low bifurcation of internal carotid artery. Acta Neurochir 38:305, 1977
33. Botez MI, Wertheim N: Expressive aphasia and amusia following right frontal lesions in a right-handed man. Brain 82:186, 1959
34. Boudouresques J, Bonnal J: Les troubles psychiques des tumeurs frontales. Rev Prat 7:1375, 1957
35. Bouman L, Grunbaum AA: Über motorische Momente der Agraphie. Monatsschr Psychiatr Neurol 77:223, 1930

36. Bradley WE, Timm GW, Scott FB: Innervation of the detrusor muscle and urethra. p. 3. In Lapides J (ed): Symposium on Neurogenic Bladder, The Urologic Clinics of North America. WB Saunders, Philadelphia, 1974
37. Brage D, Morea R, Copello AR: Syndrome nécrotique tegmento-thalamic avec mutisme akinétique. Rev Neurol 104:126, 1961
38. Brinkman C: Lesions in supplementary motor area interfere with a monkey's performance of a bimanual coordination task. Neurosci Lett 27:267, 1981
39. Brinkman C, Porter R: Supplementary motor area in the monkey: activity of neurons during performance of a learned motor task. J Neurophysiol 42:681, 1979
40. Brismar J, Ackerman R, Roberson G: Anomaly of anterior cerebral artery: a case report and embryologic considerations. Acta Radiol [Diagn] (Stockh) 18:154, 1977
41. Brodal A: Neurological Anatomy in Relation to Clinical Medicine. 3rd Ed. Oxford University Press, New York, 1981
42. Brust, JCM: Stroke: diagnostic, anatomical, and physiological considerations. p. 667. In Kandel ER, Schwartz JH (ed): Principles of Neuralscience. Elsevier/North-Holland, New York, 1981
43. Brust JCM: Cerebral infarction. p. 162. In Rowland LP (ed): Merritt's Textbook of Neurology. 7th Ed. Lea and Febiger, Philadelphia, 1984
44. Brust JCM, Plank C, Burke A et al: Language disorder in a right-hander after occlusion of the right anterior cerebral artery. Neurology (NY) 32:492, 1982
45. Buge A, Escourelle R, Rancurel G: "Mutisme akinétique" et ramollissement bilingulaire: trois observations anatomo-clinique. Rev Neurol 131:121, 1975
46. Cairns H, Oldfield RC, Pennybacker JB: Akinetic mutism with an epidermoid cyst of III ventricle. Brain 64:273, 1941
47. Cambier J, Dehen H: Les syndromes de l'artère cérébrale antérieure. Rev Med Toulouse [Suppl]:277, 1973
48. Campbell JB, Forster FM: The anterior cerebral artery in the macaque monkey (*Macaca mulatta*). J Nerv Ment Dis 99:229, 1944
49. Caplan LR, Schmahmann JD, Kase CS et al: Caudate infarcts. Arch Neurol 47:133, 1990
50. Caplan LR, Zervas NT: Speech arrest in a dextral with a right mesial frontal astrocytoma. Arch Neurol 35:252, 1978
51. Carrieri G: Sindrome da sofferenza dell'area supplementaria motoria sinistra nel corso di un meningioma parasaggitale. Riv Patol Nerv Ment 84:29, 1963
52. Castaigne P: Vocalisations itératives et crises palilaliques dans les lésions prérolandiques de la face interne du lobe frontal. Neurologia 9:39, 1964
53. Castaigne P, Buge A, Cambier J et al: Démence thalamique d'origine vasculaire par ramollissement bilateral, limité au territoire du pedicule retromammilaire. Rev Neurol 114:89, 1966
54. Castaigne P, Buge A, Escourelle R, Masson M: Ramollissement pedonculaire median, tegmento-thalamique avec ophthalmoplegie et hypersomnie. (Étude anatomo-clinique.) Rev Neurol 106:357, 1962
55. Castaigne P, Lhermitte F, Escourelle R et al: Etude anatomopathologique de 74 infarcts de l'artère cérébrale anterieure (55 observations). Rev Med Toulouse, suppl. 339, 1975
56. Chan J-L, Ross ED: Left-handed mirror writing following right anterior cerebral artery infarction: evidence for non-mirror transformation of motor programs by right supplementary motor area. Neurology (NY) 38:59, 1988
57. Chavany JA, Messimy R, Pertuiset B, Hagenmuller D: Les fonctions du territoire cortical de l'artère cérébrale antérieure: parentés séméiologiques des syndromes vasculaires traumatiques et tumoraux. Nouv Presse Med 63:512, 1955
58. Chimowitz MI, Lafranchise EF, Furlan AJ, Awad IA: Ipsilateral leg weakness with carotid stenosis. Stroke 9:1362, 1990
59. Choudhury AR: Proximal occlusion of the dominant anterior cerebral artery for anterior communicating aneurysms. J Neurosurg 45:484, 1976
60. Chusid JG: Correlative Neuroanatomy and Functional Neurology. 16th Ed. Lange Medical, Los Altos, CA, 1976
61. Chusid JG, de Gutiérrez-Mahoney CG, Margules-Lavergne MP: Speech disturbances in association with parasaggital frontal lesions. J Neurosurg 11:193, 1954
62. Claude H, Loyez M: Etude anatomique d'un cas d'apraxie avec hémiplégie droite et cécité verbale. Encéphale 8:289, 1913
63. Cobb S: The cerebral circulation. 13. The question of "end-arteries" of the brain and the mechanism of infarction. Arch Neurol Psychiatry 25:273, 1931
64. Critchley M: The anterior cerebral artery and its syndromes. Brain 53:120, 1930
65. Crowell RM, Morawetz RB: The anterior communicating artery has significant branches. Stroke 8:272, 1977
66. Cuatico W: The phenomenon of ipsilateral innervation: one case report. J Neurosurg Sci 23:81, 1979
67. Curry RW, Culbreth GC: The normal cerebral angiogram. AJR 65:345, 1951
68. Cushing H, Eisenhardt L: Meningiomas: Their Classification, Regional Behavior, Life History, and Surgical End Results. Charles C Thomas, Springfield, IL, 1938
69. Czochra M, Kozniewska H, Muszynski A, Trojanowski T: Surgical treatment of aneurysms of the anterior communicating artery using Yasargil's approach. Neurol Neurochir Pol 13:71, 1979
70. Damasio AR, Chui HC, Corbett J, Kassel N: Posterior callosal section in a non-epileptic patient. J Neurol Neurosurg Psychiatry 43:351, 1980
71. Damasio AR, Graff-Radford NR, Eslinger PJ et al: Amnesia following basal forebrain lesions. Arch Neurol 42:263, 1985
72. Damasio AR, Kassel NF: Transcortical motor

aphasia in relation to lesions of the supplementary motor area. Neurology (NY) 28:396, 1978
73. Damasio AR, Van Hoesen GW: Structure and function of the supplementary motor area. Neurology (NY) 30:359, 1980
74. Dandy WE: Surgery of the brain. p. 51. In Lewis D (ed): Practice of Surgery, Vol. 12. WF Prior, Hagerstown, MD, 1932
75. Davison AN, Dobbing J: Applied Neurochemistry. FA Davis, Philadelphia, 1968
76. Davison C, Goodhart SP, Needles W: Cerebral localization in cerebrovascular disease. Res Publ Assoc Res Nerv Ment Dis 13:435, 1934
77. Dawson BH: The blood vessels of the human optic chiasma and their relation to those of the hypophysis and thalamus. Brain 81:207, 1958
78. Delbecq-Derouesné J, Beauvois MF, Shallice T: Preserved recall versus impaired recognition: a Case Study. Brain 113:1045, 1990
79. DeLuca J, Cicerone KD: Cognitive impairments following anterior communicating artery aneurysm. J Clin Exp Neuropsychol 11:47, 1989
80. Denny-Brown D: The frontal lobes and their function. p. 13. In Feiling A (ed): Modern Trends in Neurology. Hoeber, New York, 1951
81. Denny-Brown D: The nature of apraxia. J Nerv Ment Dis 126:9, 1958
82. De Reuck J, Chatta AS, Richardson EP: Pathogenesis and evolution of periventricular leukomalacia in infancy. Arch Neurol 27:229, 1972
83. De Vito JL, Smith OA: Projections from the mesial frontal cortex (supplementary motor area) to the cerebral hemispheres and brain stem of the *Macaca mulatta*. J Comp Neurol 11:261, 1959
84. De Vriese B: Sur la signification morphologique des artères cérébrales. Arch Biol 21:357, 1904/05
85. Dimitri V, Victoria M: Síndrome de la arteria cerebral anterior. Rev Neurol Buenos Aires 1:81, 1936
86. Dunker RO, Harris AB: Surgical anatomy of the proximal anterior cerebral artery. J Neurosurg 44:359, 1976
87. Dunsmore RH, Lennox MA: Stimulation and strychninization of supracallosal anterior cingulate gyrus. J Neurophysiol 13:207, 1950
88. Durity F, Logue V: The effect of proximal anterior cerebral occlusion on anterior communicating artery aneurysms. Post-operative radiological survey of 43 cases. J Neurosurg 35:16, 1971
89. Elsberg CA: The parasagittal meningeal fibroblastomas. Bull Neurol Inst NY 1:389, 1931
90. Erickson TC, Woolsey CN: Observations on the supplementary motor area of man. Trans Am Neurol Assoc 76:50, 1951
91. Facon E, Steriade M, Werthein N: Hypersomnie prolongée engendrée par des lesions bilaterales du système activateur médial: le syndrome thrombotique de la bifurcation du tronc basilaire. Rev Neurol 98:117, 1958
92. Falconer MA: The surgical treatment of bleeding intracranial aneurysms. J Neurol Neurosurg Psychiatry 14:153, 1951
93. Faris AA: Limbic system infarction. J Neuropathol Exp Neurol 26:174, 1967
94. Fawcett E, Blachford JV: The circle of Willis: an examination of 700 specimens. J Anat Physiol 40:63a, 1905/06
95. Fischer E: Die Lageabweichungen der vorderen Hirnarterie im Gefässbild. Zentralbl Neurochir 3:300, 1938
96. Fisher CM: Hydrocephalus as a cause of disturbances of gait in the elderly. Neurology (NY) 32:1358, 1982
97. Fisher CM: Abulia minor versus agitated behavior. Clin Neurosurg 31:9, 1983
98. Fisher CM, Kistler JP, David JM: Relation of cerebral vasospasm to subarachnoid hemorrhage by computerized tomographic scanning. Neurosurgery 6:1, 1980
99. Foix C, Hillemand P: Les syndromes de l'artère cérébrale antérieure. Encéphale 20:209, 1925
100. Freeman FR: Akinetic mutism and bilateral anterior cerebral artery occlusion. J Neurol Neurosurg Psychiatry 34:693, 1971
101. French JD: Brain lesions associated with prolonged unconsciousness. Arch Neurol Psychiatry 68:727, 1952
102. Fujimoto K, Waga S, Kojima T, Shimosaka S: Aneurysm of distal anterior cerebral artery associated with azygous anterior cerebral artery. Acta Neurochir 59:79, 1981
103. Gacs G, Fox AJ, Barnett HJM, Vinuela F: Occurrence and mechanism of occlusion of the anterior cerebral artery. Stroke 14:952, 1983
104. Gazzaniga MS, Bogen JE, Sperry RW: Some functional effects of sectioning the cerebral commissures in man. Proc Natl Acad Sci 48:1765, 1962
105. Gazzaniga MS, Bogen JE, Sperry RW: Observations on visual perception after disconnection of the cerebral hemispheres in man. Brain 88:221, 1965
106. Gazzaniga MS, Bogen JE, Sperry RW: Dyspraxia following division of the cerebral commissures. Arch Neurol 16:606, 1967
107. Gazzaniga MS, Freedman H: Observations on visual processes after posterior callosal section. Neurology (NY) 23:1126, 1973
108. Gazzaniga MS, Hillyard SA: Language and speech capacity of the right hemisphere. Neuropsychologia 9:273, 1971
109. Gazzaniga MS, LeDoux JE, Wilson DH: Language, praxis, and the right hemisphere: clues to some mechanisms of consciousness. Neurology (NY) 27:1144, 1977
110. Gazzaniga MS, Sperry RW: Language after section of the cerebral commissures. Brain 90:131, 1967
111. Gazzaniga MS, Volpe BT, Smylie CS et al: Plasticity in speech organization following commissurotomy. Brain 102:805, 1979
112. Gelmers HJ: Non-paralytic motor disturbances and speech disorders: the role of the supplementary motor area. J Neurol Neurosurg Psychiatry 46:1052, 1983
113. Geschwind N: Disconnection syndromes in animals and man. Brain 88:237, 1965
114. Geschwind N: The apraxias: neural mechanisms of disorders of learned movement. Am Sci 63:188, 1975
115. Geschwind N, Kaplan E: A human cerebral dis-

connection syndrome: a preliminary report. Neurology (NY) 12:675, 1962
116. Ghika JA, Bogousslavsky J, Regli F: Deep perforators from the carotid system: template of the vascular territories. Arch Neurol 47:1097, 1990
117. Gillilan LA: The arterial and venous blood supplies to the forebrain (including the internal capsule) of primates. Neurology (NY) 18:653, 1968
118. Gillingham FJ: The management of ruptured intracranial aneurysms. Ann R Coll Surg Engl 23:89, 1958
119. Goldberg G, Mayer NH, Toglia JU: Medial frontal cortex infarction and the alien hand sign. Arch Neurol 38:683, 1981
120. Goldenberg G: Neglect in a patient with partial callosal disconnection. Neuropsychologia 24:397, 1986
121. Goldstein K: Zur Lehre von der motorischen Apraxie. J Psychol Neurol 11:169, 270, 1908
122. Goldstein K: Der makroskopiesche Befund in meinem Fall v. linksseiter motorischen Apraxie. Zentralbl Neurol 28:898, 1909
123. Gomes F, Dujouny M, Umansky F et al: Microsurgical anatomy of the recurrent artery of Heubner. J Neurosurg 60:130, 1984
124. Gorczyca W, Mohr G: Microvascular anatomy of Heubner's recurrent artery. Neurol Res 9:254, 1987
125. Gordon HW, Bogen JE, Sperry RW: Absence of deconnection syndrome in two patients with partial section of the neocommissures. Brain 94:327, 1971
126. Grafman J, Vance SC, Weingartner H et al: The effects of lateralized frontal lesions on mood regulation. Brain 109:1127, 1986
127. Gugliotta MA, Silvestri R, DeDomenico P, Galatioto S: Spontaneous bilateral anterior cerebral artery occlusion resulting in akinetic mutism: a case report. Acta Neurol (Napoli) 11:252, 1989
128. Guidetti B: Désordres de la parole associés à des lésions de la surface interhémisphérique frontale postérieure. Rev Neurol 97:121, 1957
129. Hanakita J, Nagayasu S, Nishi S, Suzuki T: An aneurysm of the distal anterior cerebral artery with a remarkably anomalous configuration. No Shinkei Geka 16:781, 1988
130. Hassler W, Zentner J, Voigt K: Abnormal origin of the ophthalmic artery from the anterior cerebral artery: neuroradiological and intraoperative findings. Neuroradiology 31:85, 1989
131. Hayakawa T, Waltz AG: Immediate effects of cerebral ischemia. Evolution and resolution of neurological deficits after experimental occlusion of one middle cerebral artery in conscious cats. Stroke 6:321, 1975
132. Hayakawa T, Waltz AG: On the importance of the anterior cerebral artery. Stroke 7:523, 1976
133. Hecaen H, Gimeno-Alava A: L'apraxie idéomotrice unilatérale gauche. Rev Neurol 102:648, 1960
134. Hegenholtz H, Morley TP: The results of proximal anterior cerebral artery occlusion for anterior communicating aneurysms. J Neurosurg 37:65, 1972
135. Heilman KM, Bowers D, Watson RT: Pseudoneglect in a patient with partial callosal disconnection. Brain 107:519, 1984
136. Heilman KM, Coyle JM, Gonyea EF, Geschwind N: Apraxia and agraphia in a left-hander. Brain 96:21, 1973
137. Heubner O: Zur Topographie der Ernährungsgebiete der einzelnen Hirnarterien. Zentralbl Med Wissenschaften 10:817, 1872
138. Hill A, Volpe J: Decrease in pulsatile flow in the anterior cerebral arteries in infantile hydrocephalus. Pediatrics 69:4, 1982
139. Hyland HH: Thrombosis of intracranial arteries: report of three cases involving, respectively, the anterior cerebral, basilar and internal carotid arteries. Arch Neurol Psychiatry 30:342, 1933
140. Ingvar DH, Philipson L, Torlof P, Ardo A: The average rCBF pattern of resting consciousness studied with a new colour display system. Acta Neurol Scand, suppl 64. 56:252, 1977
141. Ingvar DH, Schwartz MS: Blood flow patterns induced in the dominant hemisphere by speech and reading. Brain 97:273, 1974
142. Iragui VJ: Ataxic hemiparesis associated with transcortical motor aphasia. Eur Neurol 30:162, 1990
143. Isherwood I, Dutton J: Unusual anomaly of anterior cerebral artery. Acta Radiol [Diagn] (Stockh) 9:345, 1969
144. Ito J, Washiyama K, Kim CH, Ibuchi Y: Fenestration of the anterior cerebral artery. Neuroradiology 21:277, 1981
145. Iwata M, Sugishita M, Toyokura Y et al: Etude sur le syndrome de disconnection visuo-lingual après le transéction du splenium du corps calleux. J Neurol Sci 23:421, 1974
146. Jackson JH: Localized convulsions from tumour of the brain. Brain 5:364, 1882
147. Janowsky JS, Shimamura AP, Kritchevsky M, Squire LR: Cognitive impairment following frontal lobe damage and its relevance to human amnesia. Behav Neurosci 103:548, 1989
148. Jeeves MA, Simpson DA, Geffen G: Functional consequences of the transcollosal removal of intraventricular tumours. J Neurol Neurosurg Psychiatry 42:134, 1979
149. Jones EG, Coulter JD, Burton H, Porter R: Cells of origin and terminal distribution of corticostriatal fibers arising in the sensory-motor cortex of monkeys. J Comp Neurol 173:53, 1977
150. Jones EG, Coulter JD, Hendry SHC: Intracortical connectivity of architectonic fields in the somatic sensory, motor, and parietal cortex of monkeys. J Comp Neurol 181:291, 1978
151. Jones EG, Powell TPS: Connections of the somatic sensory cortex of the rhesus monkey. I. Ipsilateral cortical connections. Brain 92:477, 1969
152. Kaada BR, Pribram K, Epstein JA: Respiratory and vascular responses in monkeys from temporal pole, insular, orbital surface, and cingulate gyrus. J Neurophysiol 12:347, 1949
153. Kamijyo Y, Garcia JH: Carotid arterial supply of

the feline brain: applications to the study of regional cerebral ischemia. Stroke 6:361, 1975
154. Kaplan HA: Vascular supply of the base of the brain. p. 138. In Fields WS (ed): Pathogenesis and Treatment of Parkinsonism. Charles C Thomas, Springfield, IL, 1958
155. Kashiwagi A, Kashiwagi T, Nishikawa T et al: Hemispacial neglect in a patient with callosal infarction. Brain 113:1005, 1990.
156. Katz RS, Horoupian DS, Zingesser L: Aneurysm of azygous anterior cerebral artery: a case report. J Neurosurg 48:804, 1978
157. Kazui S, Sawada T, Kuriyama Y et al: A clinical study of patients with cerebral infarction localized in the territory of anterior cerebral artery. Jpn J Stroke 9:317, 1987
158. Kennard M: The cingulate gyrus in relation to consciousness. J Nerv Ment Dis 121:34, 1955
159. Kertesz A, Lesk D, McCabe P, Isotope localization of infarcts in aphasia. Arch Neurol 34:590, 1977
160. Kimura D: Neuromotor mechanisms in the evolution of human communication. p. 197. In Steklin HD, Raleigh MJ (eds): Neurobiology of Social Communication in Primates. Academic Press, San Diego, CA, 1979
161. Kimura D, Archibald Y: Motor functions of the left hemisphere. Brain 97:337, 1974
162. Kimura D, Archibald Y: Acquisition of a motor skill after left hemisphere damage. Brain 100:527, 1977
163. Kirgis HD, Fisher WL, Llewellyn RC, Peebles EM: Aneurysms of the anterior communicating artery and gross anomalies of the circle of Willis. J Neurosurg 25:73, 1966
164. Klein SI, Gahbauer H, Goodrich I: Bilateral anomalous anterior cerebral artery and infraoptic aneurysm. AJNR 8:1142, 1987
165. Kleiss E: Die verschiedenen Formen des circulus arteriosus cerebralis Willisi. Anat Anz 92:216, 1942
166. Kornyey E: Aphasie transcorticale et écholalie: le problème de l'initiative de la parole. Rev Neurol 131:347, 1975
167. Krayenbuhl HA, Yasargil MS: Cerebral Angiography. 2nd Ed. Lippincott, Philadelphia, 1968
168. Kruyt RC: Aplasia of the anterior cerebral arteries: angiographic study of a case. Neurochirurgia 14:172, 1971
169. Kunzle H: Bilateral projections from precentral motor cortex to the putamen and other parts of the basal ganglia: an autoradiographic study in *Macaca fascicularis*. Brain Res 88:195, 1975
170. Landau WM, Clare MH: Pathophysiology of the tonic innervation phenomenon of the foot. Arch Neurol 15:252, 1966
171. Laplane D, Talairach J, Meininger J et al: Clinical consequences of corticectomies involving the supplementary motor area in man. J Neurol Sci 34:301, 1977
172. Larson B, Skinhoj E, Larsen NA: Variations in regional cortical blood flow in the right and left hemispheres during automatic speech. Brain 101:193, 1978
173. Lasjaunias P, Vignaud J, Clay C: Radioanatomie de la vascularisation artérielle de l'orbite, à l'éxception du tronc de l'artère ophtalmique. Ann Radiol 18:181, 1975
174. Lassen NA, Roland PE, Larsen B et al: Mapping of human cerebral functions: a study of the regional cerebral blood flow pattern during rest, its reproducibility and the activation seen during basic sensory and motor functions. Acta Neurol Scand, supp 64. 56:262, 1977
175. Lazorthes G, Anduze-Acher H, Coll J: Empyème sous-dural intérhemisphérique (considerations sur les centres inhibiteurs de la face interne des hémisphères). Rev Otoneuroophtalmol 26:149, 1954
176. Lazorthes G, Bastide G, Gomes FA: Les variations du trajet de la carotide interne d'après une étude artériographe. Arch Anat Pathol 9:129, 1961
177. Lazorthes G, Gaubert J, Poulhes J: La distribution centrale et corticale de l'artère cérébrale antérieure: étude anatomique et incidences neuro-chirurgicales. Neurochirurgie 2:237, 1956
178. Lechi A, Marchi G: Nécrose méso-diencephalique au cours d'une méningo-encephalite subaiguë: observation anatomoclinique. Acta Neurol Belg 67:475, 1967
179. Lehmann G, Vincentelli F, Ebagosti A: Anomalies rares du polygone de Willis: le trajet infraoptique des artères cérébrales antérieures. Neurochirurgie 26:243, 1980
180. Lehrer HZ: Relative calibre of the cervical internal carotid artery. Normal variation with the circle of Willis. Brain 91:339, 1968
181. LeMay M, Gooding CA: The clinical significance of the azygous anterior cerebral artery (ACA). AJR 98:602, 1966
182. Lesem WW: The comparative anatomy of the anterior cerebral artery. Postgrad Med 20:445, 1905
183. Levin HS, Goldstein FC, Ghostine SY et al: Hemispheric disconnection syndrome persisting after anterior cerebral artery aneurysm rupture. Neurosurgery 21:831, 1987
184. Lhermitte F, Gautier JC, Marteau R, Chain F: Troubles de la conscience et mutisme akinetique: étude anatomoclinique d'un ramollissement paramedian bilateral du pedoncule cérébral et du thalamus. Rev Neurol 109:115, 1963
185. Lhermitte J, Schiff P: Le phénomène de la préhension forcée, expression d'un ramollissement complet de la première circonvolution frontale. Rev Neurol 35:175, 1928
186. Lhermitte J, Schiff P, Curtois A: Le phénomène de la préhension forcée, expression d'un ramollissement complet de la première convolution frontale. Rev Neurol 15:1218, 1907
187. Liepmann H, Maas O: Fall von linksseitiger Agraphie und Apraxie bei rechtsseitiger Lähmung. J Psychol Neurol 10:214, 1907
188. Zeal AA, Rhoton AL: Microsurgical anatomy of the posterior cerebral artery. J Neurosurg 48:534, 1978
189. Lin J, Kirsheff I: Normal anterior cerebral artery complex, p. 1319. In Newton TH, Potts DG

(eds): Radiology of the Skull and Brain. Vol. 2, Book 2. CV Mosby, St. Louis, 1974

190. Lindenberg R: Patterns of CNS vulnerability in acute hypoxemia including anesthesia accidents. p. 189. In Shade JP, McMenemey WH (eds): Selective Vulnerability of the Brain in Hypoxemia. FA Davis, Philadelphia, 1963
191. Lloyd T Jr: Effect of stroke on lung function and the pulmonary circulation. p. 371. In Price TR, Nelson E (eds): Cerebrovascular Diseases. Proceedings of the Eleventh Research Conference. Raven Press, New York, 1979
192. Löhr W: Erkrankungen des Hirngefässe in arteriographischer Darstellung. Arch Klin Chir 186:298, 1936
193. Löhr W, Jacobi W: Gefässkrankheiten des Gehirns in arteriographischer Darstellung. Arch Klin Chir 177:510, 1933
194. Long E: Contributions à l'étude des fonctions de la zone motrice du cerveau. Rev Neurol 15:1218, 1907
195. Long E: Monoplegia crurale, par lésion du lobule paracentrale. Nouv Icon Salpetr 21:37, 1908
196. Luria AR: Traumatic Aphasia. Mouton, The Hague, 1970
197. Luria AR: Disturbances of memory and consciousness after rupture of an aneurysm of the anterior communicating artery. p. 255. In Luria AR (ed): The Neuropsychology of Memory. Wiley, New York, 1976
198. Luria AR, Tsvetkova LS: Towards the mechanism of "dynamic aphasia." Acta Neurol Belg 67:1045, 1967
199. Maas O: Ein Fall von linksseitiger Apraxie und Agraphie. Zentralbl Neurol 26:789, 1907
200. Macpherson JM, Marangoz C, Miles TS, Wiesendanger M: Microstimulation of the supplementary motor area (SMA) in the awake monkey. Exp Brain Res 45: 410, 1982
201. Magnan. On simple aphasia, and aphasia with incoherence. Brain 2:112, 1879/1880
202. Marie P, Foix C: Paraplégie en flexion d'origine cérébrale par nécrose sous épendymaire progressive. Rev Neurol 27:1, 1920
203. Marinkovic S, Kovacevic M, Milisavljevic M: Hypoplasia of the proximal segment of the anterior cerebral artery. Anat Anz 168:145, 1989
204. Marino R: The anterior cerebral artery. I. Anatomo-radiological study of its cortical territories. Surg Neurol 5:81, 1976
205. Masdeu JC: Language disturbance after mesial frontal infarction. Neurology (NY), suppl 2. 33:243, 1983
206. Masdeu JC, Schoene WC, Funkenstein H: Aphasia following infarction of the left supplementary motor area: a clinical pathological study. Neurology (NY) 28:1220, 1978
207. Maspes PE: Le syndrome expérimental chez l'homme de la section du splenium du corps calleus. Alexie visuelle pure hémianopique. Rev Neurol 80:100, 1948
208. Mathew NT, Hartmann A, Meyer JS et al: The importance of "CSF pressure-regulated cerebral blood flow dysregulation" in the pathogenesis of normal pressure hydrocephalus. p. 145. In Lundberg N, Panton V, Brock M (eds): Intracranial Pressure Two: Proceedings. Springer-Verlag, New York, 1975
209. McCormick WF: A unique anomaly of the intracranial arteries of man. Neurology (NY) 10:77, 1969
210. McNabb AW, Carroll WM, Mastaglia FL: "Alien hand" and loss of bimanual coordination after dominant anterior cerebral artery territory infarction. J Neurol Neurosurg Psychiatry 51:218, 1988
211. Meador KJ, Watson RT, Bowers D, Heilman KM: Hypometria with hemispacial and limb motor neglect. Brain 109:293, 1986
212. Mendez MF, Adams NL, Lewandowski KS: Neurobehavioral changes associated with caudate lesions. Neurology (NY) 39:349, 1989
213. Mercier P, Velvt S, Fournier D et al: A rare embryologic variation: carotid-anterior cerebral artery anastomosis or infraoptic course of the anterior cerebral artery. Surg Radiol Anat 11:73, 1989
214. Meyer JS, Barron DW: Apraxia of gait: a clinicophysiological study. Brain 83:261, 1960
215. Milenkovic Z: Anastomosis between internal carotid artery and anterior cerebral artery with other anomalies of the circle of Willis in a fetal brain. J Neurosurg 55:701, 1981
216. Molinari GF, Moseley JI, Laurent JP: Segmental middle cerebral artery occlusion in primates: an experimental method requiring minimal surgery and anesthesia. Stroke 5:334, 1974
217. Moniz E: Die Cerebral Arteriographie und Phlebographie. Springer-Verlag, Berlin, 1940
218. Morris AA, Peck CM: Roentgenographic study of variation in normal anterior cerebral artery. One hundred cases studied in the lateral plane. AJR 74:818, 1955
219. Moscow N, Michotey P, Salamon G: Anatomy of the cortical branches of the anterior cerebral artery, p. 1411. In Newton TH, Potts DG (eds): Radiology of the Skull and Brain. Vol. 2, Book 2. CV Mosby, St. Louis, 1974
220. Munk H: Über die Functionen der Grosshirnrinde: Gesammelte Mitteilungen aus den Jahren 1877–80, mit Einleitung und Anmerkungen. Hirschwald, Berlin, 1881
221. Murray EA, Coulter JD: Organization of corticospinal neurons in the monkey. J Comp Neurol 195:339, 1981
222. Myers R: Dandy's striatal theory of "the center of consciousness." Surgical evidence and logical analysis indicating its improbability. Arch Neurol Psychiatry 65:659, 1951
223. Nielsen JM: Agnosia, Apraxia, Aphasia. 2nd Ed. Hoeber, New York, 1946
224. Nielsen JM, Jacobs LL: Bilateral lesions of the anterior cingulate gyri. Bull Los Angeles Neurol Soc 16:231, 1951
225. Niizuma H, Kwak R, Uchida K, Susuki J: Aneurysms of the azygos anterior cerebral artery. Surg Neurol 15:225, 1980

226. Nornes H, Wikeby P: Cerebral arterial blood flow and aneurysm surgery. 1. Local arterial flow dynamics. J Neurosurg 47:810, 1977
227. Nutic S, Dilence D: Carotid-anterior cerebral artery anastomosis: case report. J Neurosurg 44:378, 1976
228. Oba M, Suzuki M, Onuma T: Two cases of ruptured fusiform aneurysm of the proximal anterior cerebral artery (A1 segment). No Shinkei Geka 17:365, 1989
229. Odake G: Carotid-anterior cerebral artery anastomosis with aneurysm: case report and review of the literature. Neurosurgery (NY) 23:654, 1988
230. Ogasawara H, Inagawa T, Yamamoto M, Kamiya K: Aneurysm in a fenestrated anterior cerebral artery—case report. Neurol Med Chir 28:575, 1988
231. Ogawa A, Suzuki M, Sakurai Y, Yashimoto T: Vascular anomalies associated with aneurysms of the anterior communicating artery: microsurgical observations. J Neurosurg 72:706, 1990
232. Orgogozo JM, Larsen B: Activation of the supplementary motor area during voluntary movement in man suggests it works as a supramotor area. Science 206:847, 1979
233. Osaka K, Matsumoto S: Holoprosencephaly in neurosurgical practice. J Neurosurg 48:787, 1978
234. Ostrowski AZ, Webster JE, Gurdjian ES: The proximal anterior cerebral artery: an anatomic study. Arch Neurol 3:661, 1960
235. Padget DH: The circle of Willis. Its embryology and anatomy. p. 67. In Dandy WE (ed): Intracranial Arterial Aneurysms. Comstock, Ithaca, NY, 1945
236. Padget DH: The development of the cranial arteries in the human embryo. Contrib Embryol 32:205, 1948
237. Parkin AJ, Leng NRC, Stanhope N, Smith AP: Memory impairment following ruptured aneurysm of the anterior communicating artery. Brain Cognition 7:231, 1988
238. Patricolo A, Chiappetta F, Esposito S, Gazzeri G: Complicanze ipotalamiche nel trattamento chirurgio degli aneurismi della communicante anteriore. Minerva Neurochir 15:146, 1971
239. Penfield W: The cerebral cortex in man. I. The cerebral cortex and consciousness. Arch Neurol Psychiatry 40:417, 1938
240. Penfield W, Boldrey E: Somatic motor and sensory representation in cerebral cortex of man as studied by electrical stimulation. Brain 60:384, 1937
241. Penfield W, Jasper H: Epilepsy and the Functional Anatomy of the Human Brain. Little-Brown, Boston, 1954
242. Penfield W, Rasmussen T: Vocalization and arrest of speech. Arch Neurol Psychiatry 61:21, 1949
243. Penfield W, Rasmussen T: The Cerebral Cortex of Man: A Clinical Study of Localization of Function. Macmillan, New York, 1950
244. Penfield W, Roberts L: Speech and Brain Mechanisms. Princeton University Press, Princeton, NJ, 1959
245. Penfield W, Welch K: The supplementary motor area, in the cerebral cortex of man. Trans Am Neurol Assoc 74:179, 1949
246. Penfield W, Welch K: The supplementary motor area of the cerebral cortex: a clinical and experimental study. Arch Neurol Psychiatry 66:289, 1951
247. Perlmutter D, Rhoton AL: Microsurgical anatomy of the anterior cerebral–anterior communicating–recurrent artery complex. J Neurosurg 45:259, 1976
248. Perlmutter D, Rhoton AL: Microsurgical anatomy of the distal anterior cerebral artery. J Neurosurg 49:204, 1978
249. Petit-Dutaillis D, Guiot G, Messimy R, Bourdillon C: À propos d'une aphémie par atteinte de la zone motrice supplémentaire de Penfield, au cours de l'évolution d'un aneurisme artério-veineux: guérison de l'aphémie par l'ablation de la lesion. Rev Neurol 90:95, 1954
250. Phillips S, Sangalang V, Sterns G: Basal forebrain infarction: a clinicopathologic correlation. Arch Neurol 44:1134, 1987
251. Pitres A: Considerations sur l'agraphie. Rev Med 4:855, 1884
252. Plum P, Posner J: The Diagnosis of Stupor and Coma. 3rd Ed. FA Davis, Philadelphia, 1980
253. Pool JL: Aneurysms of the anterior communicating artery. Bifrontal craniotomy and routine use of temporary clips. J Neurosurg 18:98, 1961
254. Poppen JL: Ligation of the left anterior cerebral artery: its hazards and means of avoidance of its complications. Arch Neurol Psychiatry 41:495, 1939
255. Racy A, Jannotta FS, Lehner LH: Aphasia resulting from occlusion of the left anterior cerebral artery: report of a case with an old infarct in the left rolandic region. Arch Neurol 36:221, 1979
256. Reichert T: Die Arteriographie der Hirngefässe. JF Lehmann, Berlin, 1943
257. Reivich M: Embryology, anatomy, and pathophysiology of the cerebral circulation. p. 749. In Goldensohn ES, Appel SH (eds): Scientific Approaches to Clinical Neurology. Lea and Febiger, Philadelphia, 1977
258. Richter CP, Hines M: Experimental production of the grasp reflex in adult monkeys by lesions of the frontal lobes. Am J Physiol 101:87, 1932
259. Rieke GK, Bowers DE, Penn P: Vascular supply pattern to rat caudatoputamen and globus pallidus: scanning electronmicroscopic study of vascular endocasts of stroke-prone vessels. Stroke 12:840, 1981
260. Riggs HE, Rupp C: Variation in form of circle of Willis. Arch Neurol 8:8, 1963
261. Ring BA, Waddington MM: Roentgenographic anatomy of the pericallosal arteries. AJR 104:109, 1968
262. Risso M, Poeck K, Creutzfeld O, Pilleri G: Katamnestische Untersuchungen nach frontaler Leukotomie. I. Klinische Beobachtungen. II.

Anatomischklinische Korrelationen. Bibl Psychiatr Neurol 116:1, 1962
263. Robinson LR: An unusual human anterior cerebral artery. J Anat 93:131, 1959
264. Rodda RA: The arterial patterns associated with internal carotid disease and cerebral infarcts. Stroke 17:69, 1986
265. Roland PE, Larsen B, Lassen NA, Skinhoj E: Supplementary motor areas in organization of voluntary movements in man. J Neurophysiol 43:118, 1980
266. Roland PE, Meyer E, Shibasaki T et al: Regional cerebral blood flow changes in cortex and basal ganglia during voluntary movements in normal human volunteers. J Neurophysiol 48:467, 1982
267. Roland PE, Skinhoj E, Lassen NA, Larsen B: Different cortical areas in man in organization of voluntary movements in extrapersonal space. J Neurophysiol 43:137, 1980
268. Ross ED: Left medial parietal lobe and receptive language functions: mixed transcortical aphasia after left anterior cerebral artery infarction. Neurology (NY) 30:144, 1980
269. Rothfus WE, Goldberg AL, Tabas JH, Deeb ZL: Callosomarginal infarction secondary to transfalcial herniation. AJNR 8:1073, 1987
270. Rubens AB: Aphasia with infarction in the territory of the anterior cerebral artery. Cortex 11:239, 1975
271. Ruggiero G: Factors influencing the filling of the anterior cerebral artery in angiography. Acta Radiol 37:87, 1952
272. Ryding E, Bradvik B, Ingvar DH: Changes of regional cerebral blood flow measured simultaneously in the right and left hemisphere during automatic speech and humming. Brain 110:1345, 1987
273. Sabouraud O, Pecker J: Suspension de langage non aphasique après intervention sur la region interhémisphérique. Rev Otoneuroophtalmol 1:42, 1960
274. Saita I, Shigeno T, Aritake K et al: Vasospasm assessed by angiography and computerized tomography. J Neurosurg 51:466, 1979
275. Salamon G, Huang YP: Radiologic Anatomy of the Brain. Springer-Verlag, Berlin, 1976
276. Satoh J, Miyasaka N, Yamada T et al: Extensive cerebral infarction due to involvement of both anterior cerebral arteries by Wegener's granulomatosis. Ann Rheum Dis 47:606, 1988
277. Schick RM, Rumbaugh CL: Saccular aneurysm of the azygous anterior cerebral artery. AJNR suppl. 10:S73, 1989
278. Schott B, Michel F, Michel D, Dumas R: Apraxie idéomotrice unilatérale gauche avec main gauche anomique: syndrome de déconnection calleuse? Rev Neurol 120:359, 1969
279. Schuster P: Zwangsgreifen u. Nachgreifen, zweipost-hemisplegische Bewegungsstörungen. Z Ges Neurol Psychiatr 83:586, 1923
280. Schuster P: Autoptische Befunde bei Zwangsgreifen u. Nachgreifen. Z Ges Neurol Psychiatr 108:751, 1927
281. Schuster P, Pinéas M: Weitere Beobachtungen über Zwangsgreifen u. Nachgreifen u. deren Bezeihungen zu ahnlichen Bewegungsstorungen. Dtsch Z Nervenheilkd 91:16, 1926
282. Schwab O: Über vorübergehende aphasische Störungen nach Rindenexzision aus dem linken Stirnhirn bei Epileptikern. Dtsch Z Nervenheilkd 94:177, 1926
283. Scott M: Ligation of an anterior cerebral artery for aneurysms of the anterior communicating artery complex. J Neurosurg 38:481, 1973
284. Segarra JM: Cerebral vascular disease and behavior. I. The syndrome of the mesencephalic artery (basilar artery bifurcation). Arch Neurol 22:408, 1970
285. Segundo JP, Naquet R, Buser P: Cortical stimulation in monkeys. J Neurophysiol 18:236, 1955
286. Selman J, Dujovny M, Vasquez M et al: Microanatomical basis for lenticulostriate surgery. In Microsurgery for Cerebral Ischemia. Proceedings of the Ninth International Symposium. Springer-Verlag, Vienna, 1990
287. Sengupta RP: Direct surgery of anterior communicating aneurysms and its effect on intellect and personality. J Neurol Neurosurg Psychiatry 38:406, 1975
288. Senter HJ, Miller DJ: Interoptic course of the anterior cerebral artery associated with anterior cerebral artery aneurysm: case report. J Neurosurg 56:302, 1982
289. Seyffarth H, Denny-Brown D: The grasp reflex and the instinctive grasp reaction. Brain 71:9, 1948
290. Shellshear JC: The basal arteries of the forebrain and their functional significance. J Anat 55:27, 1920
291. Shimauchi M, Kaji Y, Goya T, Kinoshita K: A case report of fibromuscular dysplasia presenting symptoms like moyamoya disease: "string of beads" appearance of the pericallosal artery. No Shinkei Geta 17:981, 1989
292. Sidtsi JJ, Volpe BT, Holtzman JD et al: Cognitive interaction after staged callosal section: evidence for transfer of semantic activation. Science 212:344, 1981
293. Sidtis JJ, Volpe BT, Wilson DH et al: Variability in right hemisphere language function after callosal section: evidence for a continuum of generative capacity. J Neurosci 1:323, 1981
294. Sine RD, Soufi A, Shah M: Callosal syndrome: implications for understanding the neuropsychology of stroke. Arch Phys Med Rehab 65:606, 1984
295. Skultety FM: Clinical and experimental aspects of akinetic mutism: report of a case. Arch Neurol 19:1, 1968
296. Smith AM: The activity of supplementary motor area neurons during a maintained precision grip. Brain Res 172:315, 1979
297. Smith AM, Bourbonnais D, Blanchette G: Interaction between forced grasping and learned precision grip after ablation of the supplementary motor area. Brain Res 222:395, 1981
298. Smith WK: The functional significance of the rostral cingular cortex as revealed by its responses to electrical excitation. J Neurophysiol 8:241, 1945

299. Snyckers FD, Drake CG: Aneurysms of the distal anterior cerebral artery: a report on 24 verified cases. S Afr Med J 47:1787, 1973
300. Spencer SS: Corpus callosum section and other disconnection procedures for medically intractable epilepsy. Epilepsia, suppl 2. 29:S85, 1988
301. Sperry RW, Gazzaniga MS: Language following surgical disconnection of the hemispheres. In Millikan CH (ed): Brain Mechanisms Underlying Speech and Language. Grune & Stratton, New York, 1966
302. Sperry RW, Gazzaniga MS, Bogen JE: Interhemispheric relationships: the neocortical commissures; syndromes of hemispheric disconnection. p. 273. In Vinken PJ, Bruyn GW (eds): Handbook of Clinical Neurology. Vol. 4. North-Holland Publishing, Amsterdam, 1966
303. Starkstein SE, Robinson RG, Berthier ML et al: Differential mood changes following basal ganglia vs thalamic lesions. Arch Neurol 45:725, 1988
304. Stebbens WE: Aneurysms and anatomic variation of cerebral arteries. Arch Pathol 75:45, 1963
305. Stephens RB, Stilwell DL: Arteries and Veins of the Human Brain. Charles C Thomas, Springfield, IL, 1969
306. Stewart RM, Williams RS, Luhl P, Schoenen J: Ventral porencephaly: a cerebral defect associated with multiple congenital anomalies. Acta Neuropathol 42:231, 1978
307. Stuss DT, Alexander MP, Lieberman A, Levine H: An extraordinary form of confabulation. Neurology (NY) 28:1166, 1978
308. Stuss DT, Benson DF: Neuropsychological studies of the frontal lobes. Psychol Bull 95:3, 1984
309. Sugishita M, Iwata M, Toyokura Y et al: Reading ideograms and phonograms in Japanese patients after partial comcissurotomy. Neuropsychologia 16:417, 1978
310. Sussman NM, Gur RC, Gur RE, O'Connor MJ: Mutism as a consequence of callosectomy. J Neurosurg 59:514, 1983
311. Swanson TH, Zinkel JL, Peterson PL: Bilateral anterior cerebral artery occlusion in an alcohol abuser with sickle cell trait. Henry Ford Hosp Med J 35:67, 1987
312. Szdzuy D, Lehmann R, Nickel B: Common trunk of the anterior cerebral arteries. Neuroradiology 4:51, 1972
313. Takashima S, Tanaka K: Development of cerebrovascular architecture and its relationship to periventricular leukomalacia. Arch Neurol 35:11, 1978
314. Takeuchi K, Hara M, Yokata H et al: Factors influencing the development of moyamoya phenomenon. Acta Neurochir 59:79, 1981
315. Talairach J, Bancaud J: The supplementary motor area in man. Int J Neurol 5:330, 1966
316. Talland GA, Sweet WH, Ballantine HT: Amnestic syndrome with anterior communicating artery aneurysm. J Nerv Ment Dis 145:179, 1967
317. Tanaka S, Mori T, Ohara H et al: Gastrointestinal bleeding in cases of ruptured cerebral aneurysms. Acta Neurochir 48:223, 1979
318. Tanji J, Kurata K: Neuronal activity in the cortical supplementary motor area related with distal and proximal forelimb movements. Neurosci Lett 12:201, 1979
319. Tanji J, Kurata K: Comparison of movement-related activity in two cortical motor areas of primates. J Neurophysiol 48:633, 1982
320. Tanji J, Taniguchi K, Saga T: Supplementary motor area: neuronal responses to motor instructions. J Neurophysiol 43:60, 1980
321. Thompson FJ, Campbell ML: Arterial supply of the feline motor cortex. Stroke 12:233, 1981
322. Thompson GN: Cerebral area essential to consciousness. Bull Los Angeles Neurol Soc 16:311, 1951
323. Tichy F: The syndromes of the cerebral arteries. Arch Pathol 48:475, 1949
324. Tindall GT: The treatment of anterior communicating aneurysms by proximal anterior cerebral artery ligation. Clin Neurosurg 21:134, 1974
325. Tindall GT, Kapp J, Odom GL, Robinson SC: A combined technique for treating certain aneurysms of the anterior communicating artery. J Neurosurg 33:41, 1970
326. Tonnis W, Brandt P, Walter W: The roentgenological diagnosis of tumors of the corpus callosum: with a contribution to the normal roentgenological anatomy of the anterior cerebral artery. J Neurosurg 17:183, 1966
327. Tow PM, Whitty CWM: Personality changes after operations on the cingulate gyrus in man. J Neurol Neurosurg Psychiatry 16:189, 1953
328. Tracy PT: Unusual intracarotid anastomosis associated with anterior communicating artery aneurysm: case report. J Neurosurg 67:765, 1987
329. Travis AM: Neurological deficiencies following supplementary motor area lesions in *Macaca mulatta.* Brain 78:155, 1955
330. Trescher JH, Ford FR: Colloid cyst of the third ventricle. Arch Neurol Psychiatry 37:959, 1937
331. Turnbull I: Agenesis of the internal carotid artery. Neurology (NY) 12:588, 1962
332. Ueno E: Clinical and physiological study of apraxia of gait and frozen gait. Rinsho Shinkeigaku 29:275, 1989
333. Van Bogaert L, Ley R: Contribution à la connaissance de la paraplegie en flexion, type Babinski, d'origine cérébrale. J Neurol Psychiatry 26:547, 1926
334. Van den Bergh R, Vander Eecken H: Anatomy and embryology of cerebral circulation. Prog Brain Res 30:1, 1968
335. VanderArk GD, Kempe LC: Classification of anterior communicating aneurysms as a basis for surgical approach. J Neurosurg 32:300, 1970
336. Van der Eecken HM: Anastomosis Between the Leptomeningeal Arteries of the Brain. Their Morphological, Pathological and Clinical Significance. Charles C Thomas, Springfield, IL, 1959
337. Vander Eecken H: Discussion of "collateral circulation of the brain." Neurology (NY) 11:16, 1961
338. Van Stockert TR: Aphasia sine aphasia. Brain Lang 1:277, 1974
339. Van Vleuten CF: Linksseitige motorische Apraxie. Z Psychiatr 64:203, 1907

340. Vilkki J: Amnestic syndromes after surgery of anterior communicating artery aneurysms. Cortex 21:431, 1985
341. Vincent GM: Cardiac electrophysiologic abnormalities in the stroke syndrome. p. 365. In Price TR, Nelson E (eds): Cerebrovascular Diseases. Proceedings of the Eleventh Research Conference. Raven Press, New York, 1979
342. Volpe BT: Observation of motor control in patients with partial and complete callosal section: implications for current theories of apraxia. In Reeves A (ed): Epilepsy and the Corpus Callosum. Plenum Press, New York, 1983
343. Volpe BT, Hirst W: Amnesia following rupture and repair of an anterior communicating artery aneurysm. J Neurol Neurosurg Psychiatry 46:704, 1983
344. Volpe BT, Sidtis JJ, Holzman JD et al: Cortical mechanisms involved in praxis; observations following partial and complete section of the corpus callosum in man. Neurology (NY) 32:645, 1982
345. Volpe JJ: Cerebral blood flow in the newborn infant: relations to hypoxic–ischemic brain injury and periventricular hemorrhage. J Pediatr 94:170, 1979
346. Waddington MM: Atlas of Cerebral Angiography with Anatomic Correlation. Little, Brown, Boston, 1974
347. Waltz AG, Sundt TM: The microvascular and microcirculation of the cerebral cortex after arterial occlusion. Brain 90:681, 1967
348. Ward AA: The anterior cingular gyrus and personality. Res Publ Assoc Nerv Ment Dis 27:438, 1948
349. Ward AA: The cingular gyrus: area 24. J Neurophysiol 11:13, 1948
350. Watanabe O, Bremer AM, West CR: Experimental regional cerebral ischemia in the middle cerebral artery territory in primates. 1. Angioanatomy and description of an experimental model with selective embolization of the internal carotid artery bifurcation. Stroke 8:61, 1977
351. Watson RT, Fleet S, Gonzolez-Rothi L, Heilman KM: Apraxia and the supplementary motor area. Arch Neurol 43:787, 1986
352. Watson RT, Heilman KM: Callosal apraxia. Brain 106:391, 1983
353. Webster JE, Gurdjian ES, Lindner DW, Hardy WG: Proximal occlusion of the anterior cerebral artery. Arch Neurol 2:19, 1960
354. Whitty CWM, Duffield JE, Tow PM, Cairns H: Anterior cingulectomy in the treatment of mental disease. Lancet 1:475, 1952
355. Wiesendanger M: Organization of secondary motor areas of cerebral cortex. p. 1121. In Brookhart JM, Mountcastle VB, Brooks VB, Geiger SR (eds): Handbook of Physiology, Section 1: The Nervous System, Volume II: Motor Control, Part 2. American Physiological Society, Bethesda, MD, 1981
356. Wiesendanger M, Ruegg DG, Lucier GE: Why transcortical reflexes? Can J Neurol Sci 2:295, 1975
357. Wilson G. Crucal monoplegia. Arch Neurol Psychiatr 10:699, 1923
358. Wilson G, Riggs HE, Rupp C: The pathologic anatomy of ruptured cerebral aneurysms. J Neurosurg 11:128, 1954
359. Windle BCA: On the arteries forming the circle of Willis. J Anat Physiol 22:289, 1888
360. Winkelman NW: Two brains showing the lesions producing cerebral monoplegia. Arch Neurol Psychiatr 12:241, 1924
361. Wise SP, Tanji J: Supplementary and pre-central motor cortex: contrast in responsiveness to peripheral input in the hindlimb area of the unanesthetized monkey. J Comp Neurol 195:433, 1981
362. Wolfe N, Linn R, Babikian VL et al: Frontal systems impairment following multiple lacunar infarcts. Arch Neurol 47:129, 1990
363. Woolsey CN: Cortical motor map of *Macaca mulatta* after chronic section of the medullary pyramid. p. 19. In Zulch KJ, Creutzfeldt O, Galbraith GC (eds): Springer-Verlag, Berlin, 1975
364. Woolsey CN, Settlage PH, Meyer DR et al: Patterns of localization in precentral and "supplementary" motor areas. Res Publ Assoc Res Nerv Ment Dis 30:238, 1952
365. Yakovlov PI: Paraplegias of hydrocephalics (clinical note and interpretation). Am J Ment Defic 51:561, 1947
366. Yakovlev PI: Paraplegia in flexion of cerebral origin. J Neuropathol Exp Neurol 13:267, 1954
367. Yamadori A, Osumi Y, Ikeda H, Kanazawa Y: Left unilateral agraphia and tactile anomia: disturbances after occlusion of the anterior cerebral artery. Arch Neurol 37:88, 1980
368. Yamaguchi T, Kunimoto M, Pappata S et al: Effects of anterior corpus callosum section on cortical glucose utilization in baboons: a sequential positron emission tomography study. Brain 113:937, 1990
369. Yamori Y, Horie R, Akiguchi I et al: Pathogenic mechanisms and prevention of stroke in stroke-prone spontaneously hypertensive rats. Prog Brain Res 47:219, 1977
370. Young RSK, Hernandez MJ, Yagel SK: Selective reduction of blood flow to white matter during hypotension in newborn dogs: a possible mechanism of periventricular leukomalacia. Ann Neurol 12:445, 1982
371. Youngjohn JR, Altman IM, Van Doren J: Amnesia following anterior communicating aneurysm surgery. J Clin Exp Neuropsychol 11:61, 1989
372. Zaidel E: Unilateral auditory language comprehension on the Token Test following cerebral commissurotomy and hemispherectomy. Neuropsychologia 15:1, 1977

# 16
# MIDDLE CEREBRAL ARTERY DISEASE

J.P. Mohr
J.C. Gautier
Daniel B. Hier

## ANATOMY

The middle cerebral artery (MCA) is the artery most commonly affected in stroke syndromes. It is the largest of the major branches of the internal carotid artery, frequently as much as twice as large as the anterior cerebral artery. Studies of the anatomy of the MCA have been reported repeatedly over the past century,[1,2,40,146,163,360,410] some of the more recent utilizing angiography as well as dissections,[188,282,401] others using the dissecting microscope to pursue the fine details of vascular anatomy of the MCA stem.[197]

The MCA supplies most of the convex surface of the brain. Only the frontal pole, the superior posterior rim, and the extreme posterior rim of the convex surface are supplied by other cerebral arteries.[6] Within the brain, it supplies almost all of the basal ganglia and capsules, including the extreme capsule, claustrum, putamen, upper parts of the globus pallidus, parts of the substantia innominata of Reichert, posterior portion of the head and all of the body of the caudate nucleus, and all but the very lowest portions of the anterior and posterior limbs of the internal capsule. The thalamus is supplied almost entirely by the posterior cerebral artery, but a few cases have been reported in which an infarct arising in the thalamus produced slight ischemia in the adjacent internal capsule.[340]

The internal capsule has a complex arterial supply:[15] the inferior part of the anterior limb is supplied by the branch of the anterior cerebral artery known as Heubner's artery, although the MCA supplies even this territory in one-third of cases; the corona radiata and most of the anterior and posterior limbs are fed by the MCA; the lowest portion of the posterior limb is supplied by the anterior choroidal artery, which usually arises from the internal carotid artery.

### Classification

The anatomy of the MCA tree has been classified by two major criteria, one based on the branching of the artery itself, the other based on the relationship between the vessel and the anatomic landmarks of the cerebral surface.

#### Stem, Divisions, and Branches

The traditional terminology analogizes the vessel as a tree with a trunk and branches (Fig. 16-1). This scheme has proved useful in pathology, since emboli tend to arrest at bifurcations, while atheromatous lesions occur most often at bifurcations and curves. Because this classification is still commonly used clinically, it will be used throughout this chapter.

The MCA regularly begins as a single trunk or stem. The length of the stem varies from 18 to 26 mm. Its diameter at the site of origin is roughly 3 mm. Actual measurements range from 2.5 to 4.9 mm,[401] averaging 3 mm.[188,197]

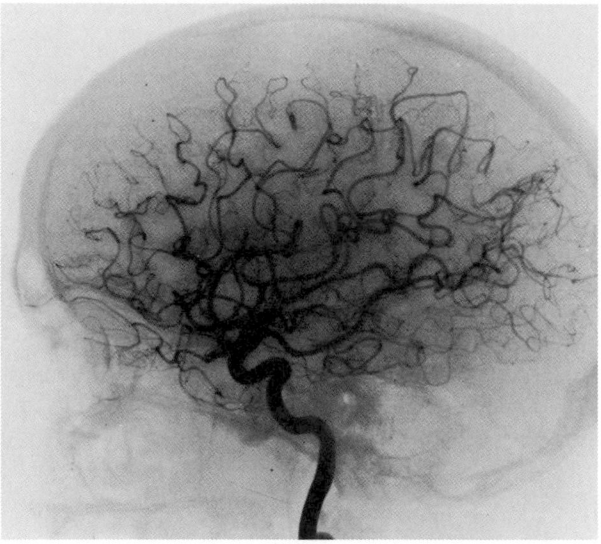

**Fig. 16-1.** Lateral view of middle cerebral artery anatomy.

The stem is generally considered to give rise to the lenticulostriate branches, those small arteries that take their name because they penetrate into the brain to supply the lentiform nucleus (putamen and pallidum) and caudate of the basal ganglia, and also supply the internal capsule.[185] (The claustrum and extreme capsule are supplied by vessels from the surface penetrating through the insula.[312]) Between 5 and 17 lenticulostriates arise from a given MCA.[197] A few of the smaller lenticulostriates may arise from the distal internal carotid artery, but the larger penetrating vessels do not do so.[197] No clear correlations exist between the length of the MCA stem and the pattern or number of the lenticulostriates. Nor does the pattern on one side predict that on the other.[197] Usually, the lenticulostriates arising more medially on the MCA stem are the smaller vessels, while the larger are more lateral. Three patterns of origin of the lenticulostriates from the MCA have been described.[197] In the most common variant (49 percent), one or more of the larger lenticulostriates arise just beyond the major bifurcation. In the next most common permutation (39 percent), all of the larger lenticulostriates arise from the stem just proximal to its bifurcation. In the least commonly encountered pattern, some of the larger penetrators arise from the medial portion of the stem. One important anatomic feature they all share is their lack of anastomoses between themselves and only rare anastomotic links to the cerebral surface vessels (see Chapter 26 on moyamoya disease). They are, with rare exceptions, physiologically endarteries.

The cerebral surface, claustrum and extreme capsule, and hemispheral cortex and white matter are supplied by those MCA branches that form beyond the lenticulostriates, usually 12 in number. They arise from the MCA stem in a variety of patterns, by far the most common pattern (78 percent[188] of cases) being two large divisions whose composition varies considerably. Less often (12 percent[188] of cases), the 12 branches arise from three major trunks (trifurcation pattern). The least differentiated and least common (10 percent of cases[188]) is the continuation of the stem with no major divisions, each of the surface branches arising in turn from the common trunk until the primary vessel has given off 11 of the usual 12 branches, after which it terminates as the angular artery.

In the bifurcation patterns, the superior division always contains the orbitofrontal and prefrontal; the inferior division always contains the temporal polar, anterior temporal, and middle temporal. The distribution of the remaining branches in a given division vary widely. The central (rolandic) branch is almost always in the upper division, while the posterior temporal is almost always in the lower. In like manner, the anterior parietal is usually in the upper division, while the temporo-occipital is usually in the lower. The posterior parietal and angular branches, which arise in the middle of this fanlike array of vessels, have an almost equal chance of being in either division.

In the trifurcation pattern, the orbitofrontal, prefrontal, and precentral division supplying the frontal lobe are regularly represented in the upper division. The middle division is made up of the central (rolandic) branch, the anterior parietal branch, and the angular branch. Less often the precentral branch is a member of this trunk on the frontal side, while in a few other instances the temporo-occipital and superior temporal branches are added on the inferior side. The inferior division regularly contains the temporal polar, anterior and middle temporal branches, to which the posterior temporal and temporo-occipital are less often added.

Although the frequency with which a given branch occurs in a given division may vary, the branches provide fairly reliable supply to certain brain regions and do not appear to cross one another. No branch arising from the upper division irrigates the brain which would be expected to be supplied from a branch of the lower division or vice versa. Within their band or wedge of the convexity, remarkable variations have been found in the exact position over gyri and sulci by individual branches.

The brain regions differ in the number and size of the vessels ramifying over their surface. The smallest and the shortest branches supply the frontal lobe.[91,188] Only 27 percent of the orbital frontal branches are as large as 1 mm.[188] The largest artery is usually the artery of the central (rolandic) sulcus. The more posterior regions of the brain are supplied by fewer arteries, which are larger in size, give off fewer major branches, and have the longest course from the circle of Willis to their termination in a borderzone (Fig. 16-2). The temporo-occipital artery is 1 mm in size in

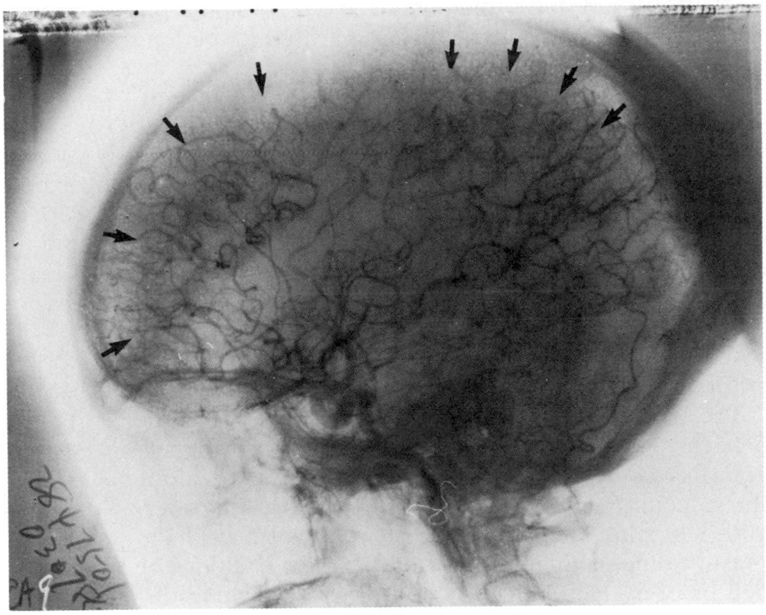

**Fig. 16-2.** Anatomy of the borderzone anastomoses (individual anastomoses shown by arrows).

90 percent of cases and over 1.5 mm in size in up to 63 percent of cases.[188] This large size and ease of being followed on the surface for long distances made this branch preferred by surgeons when the extracranial-intracranial anastomosis operation was in its heyday. The three vessels with the longest course on the cortical surface are the angular, postparietal and temporo-occipital arteries.[91,188] Intraluminal diameters greater than a millimeter had been encountered in up to 86 percent of angular arteries, 68 percent of temporo-occipital arteries, 52 percent of posterior parietal arteries, but only 14 percent of central sulcus arteries.[441]

## Arterial Segments in Relation to Anatomic Landmarks

Another method of classifying the branches of the MCA is based on the relationship of the artery to the major landmarks on the brain, especially the sylvian fissure, the operculum, and the convex surface. This scheme has found its greatest use in angiographic descriptions of the MCA and its branches.[153,271] By this scheme, the MCA is divided into four major segments (Fig. 16-3). The first, or M1, segment occupies the space from the origin of the MCA to the limen insulae. The second, or M2, segment encompasses the portions of the MCA that overlie the insula. The M3 segments are those portions that curve along the surface of the operculum, and the fourth or M4 describe those portions of the branches of the MCA over the convex surface of the brain.

Gibo et al.[186] found the *M1 or sphenoidal segment* composed of two components. The first was the undivided MCA stem from which the lenticulostriate branches arose; it occupied the majority of the length of this segment. The second consisted of the short segments from the bifurcation of the MCA into its major divisions to their entry into the sylvian fissure.

The *M2 or insular* segment gives rise to most of the cerebral surface branches. Most of them develop over the anterior portion of the insula.[186] Branches supplying the frontal and central regions of the convexity ascend sharply upward over the course of the insula,

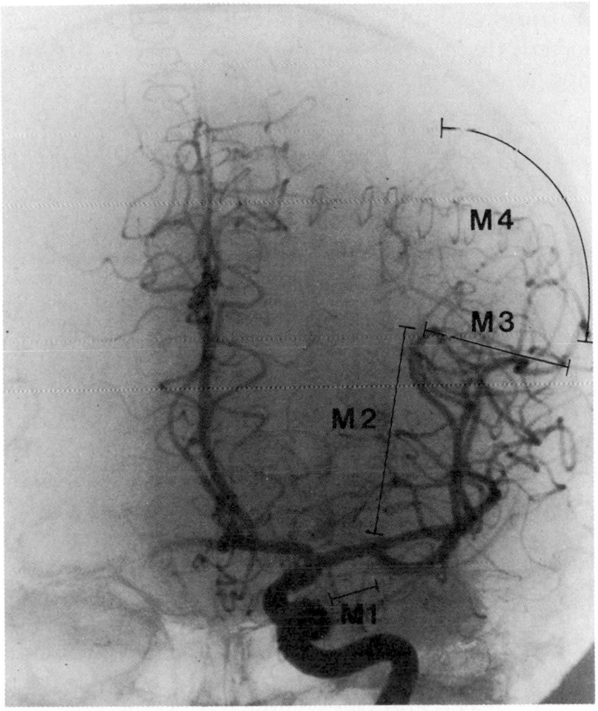


**Fig. 16-3.** Classification of the middle cerebral artery by segments.

while those supplying the posterior temporal and parietal regions course more or less parallel to the long axis of the insula.

The MCA branches that constitute the *M3 or opercular segment* follow the curve of the operculum back over the surface of the insula. Some of these branches reverse course over as much as 180 degrees,[282] especially those ascending over the frontal and central operculum to gain access to the frontal half of the cerebral convexity. Those passing over the parietal and temporal operculum make less striking reversals of direction, some turning only a few degrees before reaching the convex surface of the temporal and parietal regions.

The *M4 or cortical segments* are those portions of the branches of the MCA after they emerge from the sylvian fissure beyond the operculum and course along the sulci and gyri of the cerebral convexity. Considerable variation in their path is found from brain to brain. Some of them follow a path mainly along the depths of a given sulcus, while others pass long distances over the surface of a gyrus.

### Anomalies

A few anomalies have been described, but all types together appear to occur in no more than 3 percent of cases.[188,243,427] Some dispute even the occurrence of the anomalies.[197] Duplication of the MCA is the more common of the anomalies.[432,437] The duplicated vessel usually arises from the internal carotid artery, and supplies the same regions that would otherwise have been supplied by the original MCA. In the few cases reported, the regions supplied have mainly been the temporal pole and anterior and middle temporal areas. An accessory MCA has also been described.[243,427] It arises from the anterior cerebral, usually supplying frontal polar areas.

### Borderzone Anastomoses

For each cerebral surface branch of the major cerebral arteries, the terminal twigs end in a narrow network of vessels that form the borderzone (see Fig 16-2) between the major arterial territories.[9,77,231,388] Within the borderzone, anastomoses form end-to-end, end-to-side, and side-to-side in remarkable permutations.[266] Although such channels exist, the actual size of the anastomosis at any given point is usually quite small, on the order of 300 to 400 $\mu$m.[335] More often, the available anastomotic vessels are 200 to 400 $\mu$m, too small to provide adequate collateral to an endangered arterial territory. Only occasionally are the borderzone anastomoses larger than 500 $\mu$m. There are wide individual variations in the anastomotic artery-to-artery network. Direct, end-to-end anastomoses as large as 1 mm are rare. While these tiny vessels scarcely seem of the size that could sustain collateral flow, it has proved remarkable how useful, but unpredictable, a role they play in limiting the size of a given infarct. The dynamics of their dilation in response to occlusions of proximal arteries are still poorly understood.

Anastomoses between continguous branches of the MCA are either scanty or quite small, and play little or no useful role in collateralizing occlusion of adjacent branches, when compared to the value of end-to-end anastomoses via the borderzones.[40,434,435]

### Histology

The MCA contains the same intima, media, and adventitia as other arteries, but the relative thickness of these component parts differ from peripheral arteries of comparable size. The differences begin even within the intracranial internal carotid artery, which changes toward the histologic character of the MCA in such a way that the two blend in a smooth continuum.[418] Compared to extracranial vessels of comparable size, the MCA has a more narrow adventitia with little elastic tissue and little perivascular supporting structures; the media is also thinner, with some 20 circular muscle layers.[27,418,425] The internal elastic lamina is thicker[465] and finely fenestrated. The intima, although somewhat thin, seems essentially the same as that of comparable sized vessels elsewhere.[418] No evidence of vasa vasorum has been demonstrated to date.[95,418,463]

The implications for pathology of these differences from extracranial vessels is still unclear. The thinner adventitia of intracranial vessels may be a sign of the lower exposure to stretch and trauma compared with the environment in which the extracranial vessels live.[316] As for the elastic tissue, its concentration in the internal elastic lamina, instead of being scattered through the vessel, may make intracranial arteries more prone to dampen pulse waves.[465] Whatever their differences from extracranial arteries, intracranial vessels are susceptible to the same atherosclerosis, embolization, inflammation, and other diseases as are extracranial vessels. Whether their less frequent involvement by atherosclerosis is for reasons of histology alone is unsettled, as is whether the comparative rigidity of the MCA makes it less compliant in cases of embolization.

## PATHOLOGY

### Embolism

Although atherosclerosis is a major cause of disease of the extracranial carotid and intracranial basilar arteries, embolism is by far the more common cause of occlusion for the major cerebral arteries beyond the circle of Willis. As a cause of stroke, it accounts for between 15 and 30 percent of cases,[199,272,343] most of which occur in the territory of the MCA.

## Particle Size and Composition

To arrest in the stem of the MCA, the embolic mass must be at least a few millimeters in diameter. Rigid materials, such as shotgun pellets[251] (described first by Leceve and Lhermitte in 1920), catheter tips, and the like, may be this large. Some materials seem too small to be regular candidates, especially calcific plaques.[420,425] Calcific plaques large enough to occlude the stem occur in unusual circumstances, such as direct-puncture carotid arteriography[111,116] and perhaps from carotid atheroma itself. Most of the embolic material is elements of thrombus. These complexes, alone or mixed with bacteria, are a frequent cause of embolism of the middle cerebral stem,[166] the largest-diameter vessel in the middle cerebral artery system. This material seems remarkably compressible,[303] and may alter its length and width remarkably as it passes through the system. The important issue of how large an embolic particle may arise from angiographically inobvious carotid ulceration unfortunately remains unresolved.[147,239]

## Distribution

Although emboli have access to the entire cerebral arterial tree, their distribution is decidedly nonrandom. The two sides of the brain are equally affected, but the MCA is the most commonly embolized.[169,343] Beyond the stem, flow seems equally directed to the two divisions. In the upper division, the four posterior branches are arranged in series, providing an orderly set of opportunities for emboli to lodge.[60,169,343] The orbital frontal branch is rarely embolized, possibly because it is acutely angulated away from the main direction of flow. The lower division passes unbranched across the insula until it reaches the superior temporal plane where it gives off its three main branches within the space of a centimeter or less. As a result, embolization into lower division often results in the simultaneous occlusion of more than one, or even all, of the branches of the division.

## Persistence

It is common to find autopsy evidence of infarction with no occlusion at the site. In the 17 cases attributed to embolism in the series reported by Fisher and Pearlman,[161] an embolus at the site of the infarct was not always found. Yet in these cases, a source was available in the heart, and no evidence was found for atheromatous stenosis of the branch involved. In other studies of acute ischemic stroke clinically diagnosed as embolism, branch occlusions were found in the first 24 hours in over 75 percent of cases.[343] When the angiogram was delayed beyond 48 hours in cases with the same clinical features, the intracranial branches were widely patent.[126,343] Although it is inferred that the more friable materials will disperse rapidly, no reliable means have been developed thus far to predict which embolic occlusions will persist and which will disappear.[151] Transcranial Doppler studies have documented a few instances in which the occlusion has become recanalized within 40 minutes,[339] but it remains unknown with what frequency and how quickly emboli are dissipated past their point of initial lodgement. From the scant data available, persistence of embolic occlusion seems to be the exception rather than the rule, yet some branches originally affected may be found occluded well beyond 48 hours, while in others the occlusion has disappeared.[151] Persistence of the occlusion seems to carry a worse functional prognosis.[343] When persistent, the material has proved difficult to differentiate from in-situ thrombus at autopsy.

## Collateral

Unless adequately collateralized, embolic occlusion of the MCA stem yields a gigantic infarct affecting both the superficial and deep territory of supply. Where collateral flow is readily available, the resultant infarct may be remarkably circumscribed, sometimes confined to little more than those branches of the lenticulostriates caught by the occluding embolus.[16,333] There is little knowledge of what allows collateral flow to be so generous and readily available in some cases and so trivial in others, depending on the variations in the congenitally determined vascular pattern.

## Etiology

For this discussion, it is worthwhile to separate embolism to the stem from that to the branches of the MCA. It has been known since the time of Chiari[92] that embolic occlusion affecting the distal intracranial internal carotid may also affect the MCA *stem* across the circle of Willis. But particles large enough to lodge in the MCA stem alone are less easily documented. A literature survey was undertaken in an effort to document examples of the variety of settings in which an embolus occluded the MCA stem. Examples for each of the following was found documented by autopsy or angiogram: "paradoxical" embolus from a leg vein source,[166] atrial fibrillation,[241] mitral valve prolapse,[62] marantic embolus,[268] fragmented thrombus complexes from a nonobstructing internal carotid artery plaque,[116] shotgun pellet,[251] metal fragment from a penetrating neck wound,[252] traumatic dissection of the internal carotid artery,[231,232,296] internal carotid artery occlusion of various causes,[375] and automobile accident with angiographically normal ipsilateral internal carotid.[231,297]

Embolism to the *surface branches* involves additional considerations. Although it is a commonplace observation that occlusion of one or more branches of the MCA may occur from almost any source of embolism, it is not easy to find autopsy or angiographic evidence in support of such claims.[88,117] In a similar literature survey, the following etiologies were uncovered with an appropriate angiographic finding or autopsy proof: calcific material from the ipsilateral internal carotid artery;[92] spontaneous dissection of the internal carotid artery from fibromuscular hyperplasia,[386] traumatic internal carotid artery dissection,[423] mucin and emulsified fat from breast metastasis[120] endocaritis due to *Candida*,[189] mitral valve prolapse,[32] cardiac myxoma,[472] arterial wall fragments after resuscitation,[200] giant fusiform MCA aneurysm,[24,96] marantic embolus,[268] and internal carotid artery occlusion from various causes.[31,32,90,336] Recent work has also made clear the importance of transcardiac emboli via a patient cardiac foramen ovale.

## Clinical Syndromes

The disastrous effects of poorly or uncollateralized occlusion of the MCA are so familiar that only those with limited infarction warrant mention (Fig. 16-4). Collateral this effective seems to be rare.[1]

A variety of temporal profiles occur in embolism to *branches* of the MCA. In some instances, the deficits are only transient even with angiographic evidence of persisting occlusion or brain image evidence of focal infarction, which confounds traditional clinical definitions of transient ischemic attack (TIA).[375] Aberrant embolism in the days of Silastic pellet therapy for arteriovenous malformations (AVMs) was a well-recognized risk,[467] usually occurring near the end of the embolization procedure when conditions initially favoring the entry of the pellets directly into the AVM vessels changed as the fistula became clogged with pellets.[274,467] In Kusske and Kelly's series of 10 cases,[274] two showed focal ischemia, one involving the ipsilateral retina lasting 5 days, another involving the contralateral MCA with "transient" dysesthesia of the left hand. Wolpert and Stein[466] described six cases in which aberrant embolization occurred. One case had two beads into an angular branch of the MCA and experienced 15 minutes of contralateral arm numbness—a complaint not entirely predicted by classical clinicopathologic correlation—and also showed immediate distal retrograde collateralization. The pellet remained in place. Single beads occluded parietal branches of the MCA in two others and an ascending frontal in a third, none of whom experienced any deficits; in all cases, immediate collaterals occurred retrograde into the embolized branch.

Emboli initially occluding the MCA stem, and then later migrating to the convexity branches, may leave lesions in the deep and superficial territories as *discontinuous multifocal infarction.* The lack of collaterals to the lenticulostriates make this territory especially vulnerable to ischemia. The distally placed embolic fragment in a cortical branch is usually considerably smaller than the mass of which it was a part which initially blocked the MCA stem. The clinical picture may be predominantly that of the deep infarction affecting the penetrating vessels of the MCA stem.

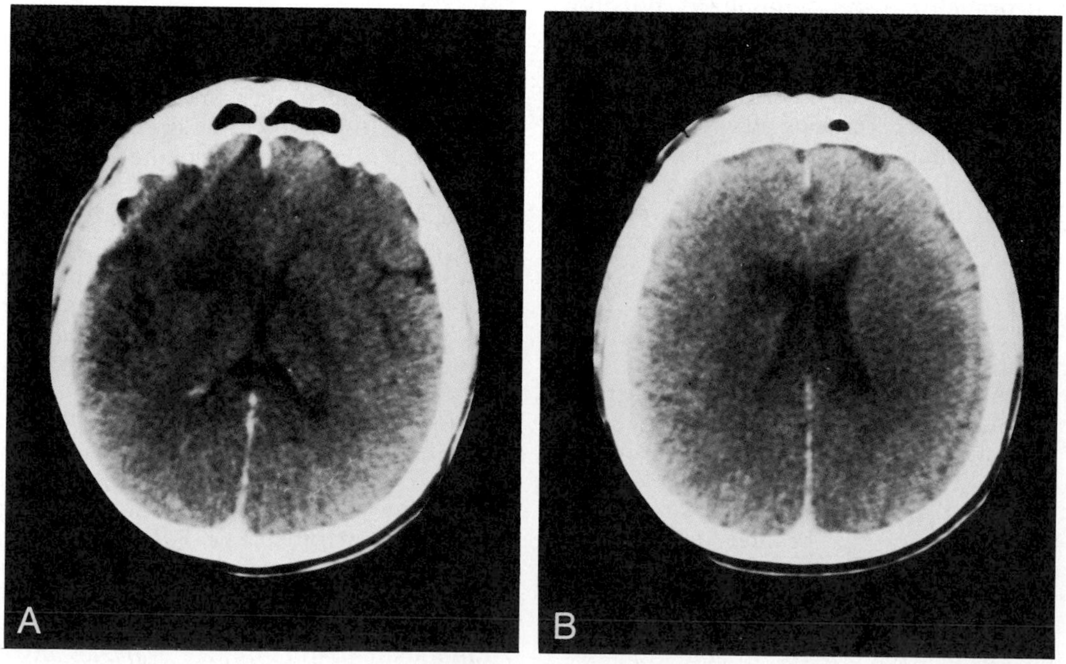


**Fig. 16-4. (A & B)** Computed tomography scan of a deep infarct, which was the only effect of an occlusion of the stem of the middle cerebral artery. Angiogram showed full collateral of the surface branches from the adjacent anterior and posterior cerebral arteries.

A spectacular shrinking deficit (given the initials SSS by Minematsu et al.[331]) in presentations can occur when the embolus occludes the internal carotid artery, causing a profound full hemisphere syndrome, after which it passes up the internal carotid artery to its final resting place in, say, the angular branch of the MCA, leaving only a mild aphasia after a few days or a week. Especially characteristic of this type of migratory embolism is a syndrome of fading hemiparesis with persisting Wernicke's aphasia: the embolus presumably lodges initially at the stem of the MCA, occluding the penetrating lenticulostriate branches long enough to produce scattered foci of infarction through the basal ganglia and internal capsule, the involvement of the latter producing the hemiparesis. Distal migration of the embolus then occurs, usually finally occluding the lower division of the MCA at the superior temporal plane and beyond, yielding the Wernicke's aphasia. Two separate foci of infarction occur, but both result from the same embolic event (Fig. 16-5).

Non-sudden or fluctuating onset occurs in 5 to 6 percent of documented embolic strokes, the syndrome often requiring 36 hours or so to evolve.[161,343] A clinical diagnosis of multiple transient ischemic attack is often entertained.

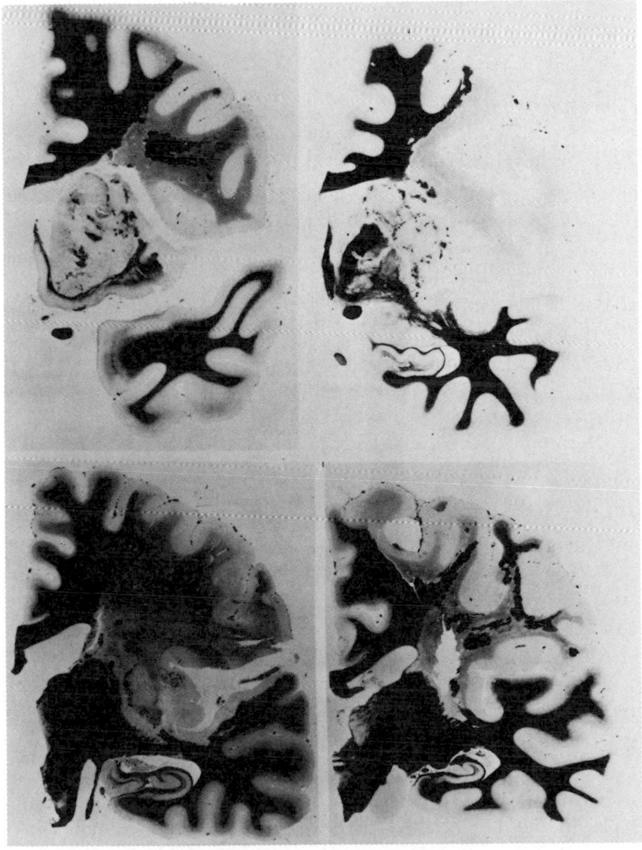

**Fig. 16-5.** Deep and superficial infarction from the same embolic occlusion. (Myelin stain of celloidin section.) (Reprinted from Friedlich et al.,[166] with permission.)

## Atherosclerosis

In current times primary atherosclerotic occlusive thrombosis is recognized as a decidedly uncommon cause of symptomatic disease of the MCA.[20] Yet, for years, most instances of MCA ischemia were casually attributed to thrombosis of the MCA. As long ago as 1951, Fisher[154] noted that "in case after case neuropathological examination failed to confirm the clinical impression of disease of the middle cerebral artery." In the past 40 years, studies have repeatedly demonstrated that this impression was correct. None of the 178 autopsied cases collected by Fisher et al.[160] to determine the distribution of atherosclerosis in the carotid or vertebrobasilar system showed thrombotic occlusion of an intracranial cerebral artery in the carotid system, including the MCA. Blackwood et al.[59] searched back through the records at the National Hospital, and found great difficulty uncovering many convincing examples of thrombosis of the MCA, attesting to its rarity. Likewise, in a clinical and autopsy study of 122 cases of infarction in the territory of the MCA, Lhermitte et al.[298] diagnosed atherosclerosis in 8 of 94 cases on clinical and angiographic grounds, while in a companion series studied by autopsy, only 2 (1 occlusion, 1 stenosis) were attributed to atherosclerosis. Resurveying the scene almost 20 years after his initial observation, Fisher[156] diagnosed atherosclerotic thrombosis in only 7 percent of 68 cases of MCA occlusion by clinical, angiographic, or pathologic criteria.

These findings lend support to the diagnosis of embolism for angiographically documented occlusions of the MCA and its branches, unless shown to be otherwise at autopsy. Angiographically demonstrated middle cerebral stenosis found a normal internal carotid artery suggests recanalizing embolism. Except for rare instances, the angiographic appearance of occlusion of the MCA or its branches does not permit a reliable separation between embolism and primary thrombosis. Admittedly, when lysis and disappearance of the initial occlusion occurs the usual cause is embolism,[126,231,241] but the hazards of angiography discourage repeat studies. In those cases with persisting occlusion, the diagnostic problem remains unsettled, defeating the diagnostic efforts of even the best clinicians.[87]

## Thrombotic Occlusion

Autopsy studies indicate that thrombotic occlusion accounts for only 2 percent of cases of ischemic events in the MCA territory.[295,298] In life, thrombotic occlusion of the MCA is indistinguishable from that caused by embolism. When repeat angiography shows the lesion has resolved, a diagnosis of embolism can be inferred, but persisting occlusion does nothing to clarify the etiology.

Although the distinction between thrombus and embolus on clinical grounds is difficult, the syndrome of occlusion is worthy of mention in its own right. Asymptomatic occlusion of the MCA stem must be rare, if it occurs at all.[101,156,201,280] Lascelles and Burroughs[279] found 18 of their 22 cases had major neurologic deficits and only 4 underwent satisfactory clinical improvement. Fisher[156] found no such cases among the 40 with occlusion of the MCA stem from his experience at the Massachusetts General Hospital. Almost all of the cases had a syndrome featuring hemiplegia or hemiparesis. He uncovered 23 cases, in only 5 did the stroke begin with no prodrome. In 3 patients the stroke developed in a stepwise fashion, requiring several days to reach the peak. Fully 15 had previous TIAs, in many instances multiple, and over periods as long as a year.

## Stenosis

Stenosis, that familiar problem in the extracranial carotid, is uncommon anywhere in the MCA, and when found is almost always in the stem (Fig. 16-6). Thus far, no reliable means have been developed to determine what the lesion represents when seen the first time. Atheroma not fully developed, recent embolus undergoing recanalization, the stenosis of moyamoya, dissection, postradiation effects, and other etiologies, including infection are all possibilities. Examples of atherosclerosis confined to the MCA stem are difficult to find, and the information is somewhat scanty and the clinical course has been surprisingly mild. Five of the nine cases reported by Lascelles and Burroughs[279] made almost a complete recovery. Kawase et al.[251] described only examples of TIA. Hinton et al.[228] reported 17 cases, only 3 of whom were left with focal neurologic deficits, although all were treated with Coumadin. Minor deficit characterized 8 of the 13 described by Feldmeyer et al.[150] A progressive course was described in five, evolving over 12 hours or more. The leisurely mode of onset even led to a clinical diagnosis of tumor in three instances. Day[119] mentioned TIAs alone or with mild stroke in 12 of the 18 cases of stenosis. The experience of Corston et al.[101] was less fortunate: 14 of their 21 cases presented with stroke; yet even in this series only 3 patients had a severe disability, and 7 patients presented with TIA alone.

Remarkably enough, only a small literature exists regarding the *clinical syndromes* of stenosis. Judging from the handful of studies available, stenosis can cause lenticulostriate or hemispheral syndromes by at least three mechanisms. Local lacunar-type syndromes affecting the lenticulostriate branches may occur if they become trapped in the atheroma affecting the MCA itself. Ischemic events in the hemisphere

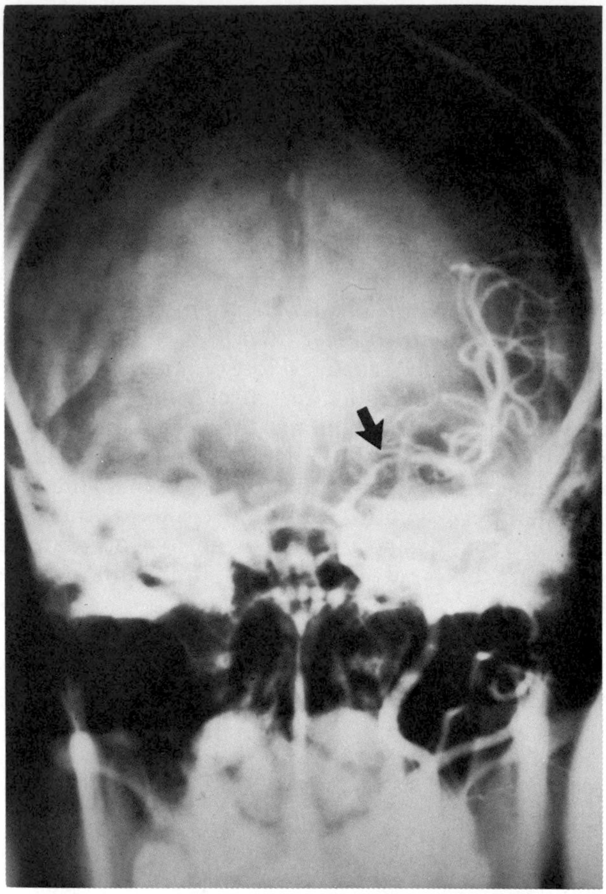

**Fig. 16-6.** Angiogram showing middle cerebral artery stem stenosis.

distal to the stenosis may occur because of hemodynamic insufficiency[229] or by embolism.[4] Kawase et al.[251] found four examples of capsular low density on CT scans ipsilateral to angiographically documented stenosis of the M1 segment of the MCA in 52 Japanese patients with TIAs affecting the carotid territory. They attributed the clinical syndrome and CT abnormality to the MCS stem stenosis. However, in one, the stenosis was so far distal in the stem that it was beyond the usual point of departure of even the lateral lenticulostriates, but in two of the others the stenosis lay at the origin of the stem and the last lay in its midportion.

Several of the cases (cases 2, 3, 4) reported by Hinton et al.[228] had similar syndromes, limited to pure motor weakness. In each instance, however, there was considerable shift of the borderzone seen angiographically, with anterior cerebral branches collateralizing the MCA. The pure motor character of the attacks and the obvious borderzone shift posed a problem in interpretation of the mechanism involved. Corston et al.[101] may have had similar experiences, as three of their cases were described with severe hemiplegia, but details on the remainder of the clinical syndrome in these cases was not provided. Shift of the borderzone was encountered in some of these cases. Other examples of lacunar syndromes in a setting of MCA stem stenosis may be found scattered through the literature.[18,335]

Hemispheral hemodynamic insufficiency was suggested by the clinical syndromes of 13 of the 16 cases reported by Hinton et al.[228] Their TIAs or minor permanent deficit was accompanied by mutism, dysarthria, or numbness. In each case, obvious shift had occurred in the borderzone, with striking collateral into the MCA territory. Even given the occurrence of ischemic stroke, the syndromes were quite mild. Less encouraging results were reported by Corston et al.[101] who described nine with some disturbance in higher cerebral function, one with no accompanying hemiparesis. In only one was shift of the borderzone described. These cases leave no doubt that some are left with a severe disability.

Some reports suggest there may be untoward effects attributed to surgical intervention. Extracranial-intracranial (EC/IC) bypass surgery, a procedure which at first sight could appear to be a rational step in therapy, has been reported in a few disheartening instances followed by symptomatic occlusion. Furlan et al.[167] described a symptomatic case (case 2) with angiographically documented advancing MCA stem stenosis. He had developed aphasia and right hemiparesis, which cleared within a few days leaving only mild right hemiparesis. Six days postoperatively, an angiogram demonstrated occlusion of the supraclinoid portion of the left internal carotid artery with good filling of the MCA territory through the anastamosis. Immediately after the angiogram, he developed "fluent dysphasia with jargon speech and numerous paraphasia errors. There was increased right arm weakness." A computed tomography (CT) scan showed no evidence of recent infarction. He returned to his posteroperative state and was discharged uneventfully. Gumerlock et al.[200] found that two of the seven cases of MCA stem stenosis had progressed to occlusion within days of successful EC/IC. One case presented with a 10-minute episode of aphasia; his postoperative course was described as "stormy" and within 4 days he had "increased speech deficit and generalized weakness, which improved slowly." The other case had two episodes of right-sided weakness with dysphasia. Posteroperatively, she "demonstrated intermittent right hemiparesis, hyper-reflexia, and Babinski signs." The deficits are not easily explained in any of these three, but some of the features seem reminiscent of the pre-EC/IC deficit. Perhaps the collateral through the bypass was sufficient to permit stagnation at the MCA stem, yet insufficient to keep the hemisphere continually perfused. In any case, none of these three had a syndrome obviously of the lenticulostriate or lacunar type, suggesting the occlusion did not trigger a large deep infarct.

Turning back to the issue faced by the angiographic demonstration of MCA stem stenosis, it is a disappointment that there are no distinctive angiographic criteria that permit the separation of recanalizing embolus from stenosis due to atherosclerosis on the basis of a single angiogram.[241] This difficulty nags at every study of the course of angiographic stenosis, since each group of cases contains an unknown subset of emboli.[101] The angiographic abnormality has been found at various points along the course of the stem, from its origin all the way to the bifurcation.[228]

## Dissection

Dissection confined to the MCA is quite rare. It is described here, since it seems to pursue a somewhat different course from dissection affecting other vessels. Over three dozen cases have been reported. A host of settings for dissection are recognized: trauma,[238] strenuous physical exertion,[466] surgery,[52] fibromuscular hyperplasia,[230] atherosclerosis,[14] mucoid degeneration of the media,[238] moyamoya disease,[471] split or frayed internal elastic lamina,[143] congenital defect of the media,[471] syphilis,[433] and even migraine.[14,414] The disorder has been most often reported in younger patients, many of them children. The usual site affected is a short section of the stem, although the disorder may spread into adjacent branches;[245] one remarkable case showed a continuous dissection involving the distal intracranial carotid, middle, and anterior cerebral arteries.

When a precipitating factor, such as trauma, has been documented, symptoms developed at that time or where delayed for minutes,[245] hours,[470] or up to 4 days.[139] Once the clinical syndrome was set in motion, events proceed rapidly, but in a few cases the decline was over a day or more. Since the dissections occur most often in the stem of the MCA, severe clinical deficits usually occur.

As the literature consists of the autopsied cases, the expected fate of cases diagnosed in life is poorly understood. Distinguishing dissection from other causes of stenosis or occlusion of the MCA stem has proved too difficult a diagnosis to be made with confidence.

## Other Diseases

The MCA, like other vessels, may fall victim to arteritis, fibromuscular hyperplasia, altered coagulation states, delayed effects of radiation,[250] and the like. From the available literature, there do not appear to be enough features of such involvement in the MCA to warrant separate consideration.

# CLINICAL SYNDROMES OF MIDDLE CEREBRAL ARTERY TERRITORY INFARCTION

## General Aspects

The major syndromes of MCA disease described by Foix and Levy[163] in their classical article have been repeated over and over in textbooks. In such accounts, the description of the syndrome from each trunk and branch is usually based on the assumption that the entire territory at risk is involved and that a description of the deficit at its maximum will suffice. However, it has been recognized for some time that the effects of an arterial occlusion are determined by the collateral flow via borderzone vessels shared with the anterior or posterior cerebral arteries. Effective collateral may rescue the endangered territory, resulting in the striking reduction in the symptoms and signs. Recent work with CT, positron emission tomography (PET), and now magnetic resonance (MR) scanning is demonstrating a wide spectrum of deficits, both acute and chronic, that are occasioned by a given arterial occlusion.

## Standard Syndromes

The main principles of clinical correlation found in textbook accounts[344,346,389] are briefly reviewed here as a backdrop for some of the details that follow. Uncollateralized occlusion of the *main trunk* of the MCA artery causes softening of the basal ganglia and internal capsule within the substance of the hemisphere and a large portion of the cerebral surface and subcortical white matter. The large infarct produces contralateral hemiplegia, deviation of the head and eyes toward the side of the infarct, hemianesthesia, and hemianopia. Major disturbances also occur in behavior: global aphasia occurs when the hemisphere dominant for speech and language is involved, while impaired awareness of the stroke is expected when the nondominant hemisphere is affected. When the infarct is large, the hemianopia may be due to involvement of the visual radiations deep in the brain. More often, the hemianopia is part of a syndrome of hemineglect for the opposite side of space, and is accompanied by failure to turn toward the side of the hemiplegia in response to sounds from that side, a problem separate from the head and eye deviation toward the side of the infarct.

When the occlusion is confined to the *upper division*, the initial deficit mimics that from occlusion of the main trunk: contralateral hemiparesis and hemisensory syndromes are the rule, accompanied by hemineglect for the opposite side of space, aphasia when the dominant hemisphere is involved, or by impaired awareness of the deficit when the opposite hemisphere is affected. However, the hemiparesis usually affects the face and arm more than the leg, a picture opposite from that in anterior cerebral artery disease. Because the occlusions usually affect the anterior branches of the upper division, the aphasia from dominant hemisphere infarction is usually of the motor (Broca) type, while the disturbance in behavior from nondominant hemisphere infarction may be mild.

In the *lower division* syndromes, hemiparesis does not usually occur, head and eye deviation are rarely encountered, and even disorders of sensation are infrequent. When the infarct affects the dominant hemisphere, pure aphasia (Wernicke type) is the rule, while the in nondominant hemisphere infarction, the behavior disturbances may appear in relative isolation. Hemianopia may be a prominent sign.

In cases where the involvement is limited to the territory of a small *penetrating artery* branch of the main stem, a small, deep infarct (lacune) occurs, affecting part or all of the internal capsule, producing a syndrome of pure hemiparesis, unaccompanied by sensory, visual, language, or behavior disturbances (See Chapter 20 on lacunes).

Enough exceptions occur that the foregoing can only be accepted as a guide, subject to modification from individual case experience. Analysis of individual cases has also yielded enough to indicate that the cerebral response to infarction expressed in the clinical picture is more than the effects of ischemia, edemia, and collateral blood flow.

In the formulations presented throughout this chapter, efforts have been made to confine the presentation to the case material representing the effects of ischemia in the MCA territory. Those studied by autopsy are given the closest consideration, followed by those documented by CT scan, angiogram, and magnetic resonance imaging (MRI). Although sorely tempted, we have made every effort to avoid analysis based only on textbook descriptions, clinical essays, or case material drawn from other etiologies. In pursuit of this policy some cases of interest from other etiologies have necessarily been neglected, but in the end it is hoped the findings reflect the syndromes of ischemia as opposed to other etiologies. Not the least of the points made is the thin support for many of the classical tenets of clinical correlation in neurology.

# DEFICITS FROM INFARCTION OR EITHER HEMISPHERE

## Loss of Consciousness

Transient loss of consciousness seems uncommon in all forms of ischemic stroke. It occurs only rarely in cases of MCA territory infarction. As an initial sign, it occurs in only 8.4 percent of carotid artery ischemic strokes,[73] a frequency slightly higher than the 5.7 percent in vertebrobasilar territory strokes. In half of the

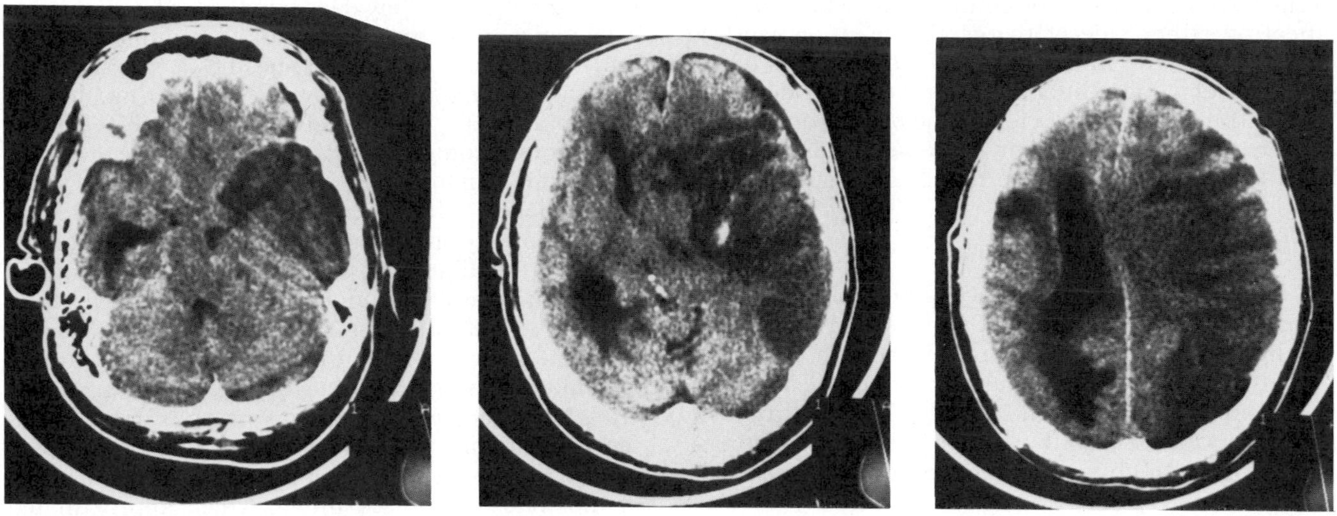

A B C

**Fig. 16-7.** Axial computed tomography scans showing infarction of the entire middle cerebral territory. (**A**) From the level of the temporal pole; (**B**) through the basal ganglia; (**C**) to the upper convexity, with coma and fatal midline shift.

cases, the loss is attributable to seizure. The mechanism is unclear in the others. Diaschisis[440] might be considered as a possible explanation,[73] assuming it to be secondary to sudden embolization of the stem of the carotid artery with temporary global ischemia.

Delayed loss of consciousness is more common. Following hemispheral infarcts ranging in size from the entire MCA territory to that limited to the frontotemporal region, delays from 36 hours to 4 and 5 days may occur in cases with loss of consciousness.[385] The decline in consciousness is usually part of a larger clinical picture of impending cerebral herniation, and not from an injury to a specific brain region in the MCA territory controlling consciousness (Fig. 16-7).

## Hemiplegia and Hemiparesis

The terms hemiplegia and hemiparesis have been used too loosely to permit a clear correlation between the formula and severity of weakness and a given site of infarction. Weakness of some degree and formula has been encountered most often in infarcts of the branches of the upper division, but is not regularly reported in infarcts affecting the territory of the lower division.

A disappointingly small number of cases correlate the hemiparesis formula and autopsy findings. Many authors have reviewed large numbers of cases, but not usually in pursuit of the formulas of hemiparesis. Henschen's[222] review of the published autopsy literature on higher cerebral function was typical of most authors: the occurrence of hemiparesis on a case by case basis was mentioned only in passing, and details of the syndrome were rarely given. The literature contains many surprising instances of apparent amelioration of motor deficit following infarction affecting the MCA territory on either side. Since the improvement of the motor deficit was not the main focus of most of the studies, it is difficult to know how seriously to take the findings into account. A discouraging point is that some of the earlier publications devoted to the clinical correlations of MCA occlusions lack credibility. For example, the effort by Davison et al.[118] contains several actual case descriptions, one of which is a photograph of a hemorrhage in a case described as an infarct. Among the recent larger series of cases, the basis for the diagnosis of MCA territory infarction varies considerably. For example, branch occlusions documented angiographically were the most common finding in 9 of the 38 cases reported by Barnett et al.[31]

After several attempts, we abandoned efforts to assemble the expected syndromes from large review articles and concentrated, instead, on detailed individual case reports found among the huge mass of published material on MCA territory infarcts. The result has been a necessarily haphazard collection of material, which may prove little better than the rough collections attempted by our many predecessors, but which is all that appears to be available, as reflected in the following material.

Middle cerebral artery stem occlusions affecting either side of the brain presumably produce the same basic motor deficit and can be described under the same heading. The pilot phase of the NINCDS Stroke Data Bank project,[345] involving some 488 cases of stroke confined to a cerebral hemisphere, showed no difference in the occurrence or the formula of the weakness from stroke of comparable source or size affecting either side of the cerebrum. More work is needed on this point, since some components of the motor deficit may differ according to the side of the stroke: De Renzi et al.[130] found the occurrence of conjugate eye deviation from right hemisphere stroke greatly to exceed that from the left hemisphere.

## Hemiplegia

The most reliable occurrence of hemiplegia follows complete occlusion of the MCA at its stem. The effect of the occlusion may produce infarction involving both the deep and superficial territory of the MCA, the deep only, or the superficial only. The syndrome of hemiplegia is essentially similar in all three settings, but varies enough to warrant separate description.

### *Hemiplegia From Deep and Superficial Infarction*

Foix and Levy[163] described in some detail the hemiplegia from deep and superficial infarction. The typical picture includes dense contralateral hemiplegia, hemianesthesia, homonymous hemianopia, and conjugate gaze deviation to the contralateral side. The severity of the syndrome increases when the occlusion approaches the MCA stem.[29,163,278,390,399] Huge infarctions affecting the territory of the MCA territory artery have been documented with a variety of autopsy studies,[5,51,358,384] but the syndrome descriptions echo the same findings as Foix and Levy, with a few embellishments. Among the cases that pursue a fatal course within days, contralateral hemiplegia is the rule, usually accompanied by hemianesthesia and hemianopia.[177] Kookier et al.[267] described an example of sudden complete hemiplegia with decerebration associated with angiographic occlusion of the MCA and delayed emptying. Hemorrhagic softening, affecting of the entire right cerebral hemisphere, was found on autopsy 3 days later.

Cases of MCA artery territory infarction, with brain swelling massive enough to promote hemicraniectomy, serve to indicate the expected course of hemiplegia in the most extensive strokes. Deterioration with massive brain edema may occur in these cases within periods as early as 36 hours, but often is more evident by the 4th day. After the reversal of the incipient herniation, the persistent neurologic deficit is usually severe hemiplegia. The syndrome among survivors without hemicraniectomy seems similar. For example, complete hemiplegia occurred in the five cases of MCA stem occlusion reported by Irino et al.,[239] all of whom were said to survive with severe neurologic deficits. Our experience includes an example of occlusion of the MCA stem from foreign body embolism documented by angiogram and CT scan.[251] This previously healthy man suffered a shotgun wound to the chest without neurologic complications but experienced a pellet embolus during resuscitation for cardiac arrest a few days later. His postarrest neurologic deficit featured a complete hemiplegia, with tonic eye deviation, hemihypesthesia, hemianopia, and stupor. Angiogram showed the pellet had lodged proximal to the lenticulostriate territories. The CT scan showed complete infarction of both the deep and superficial territories of the MCA.

The deficit after hemispherectomy in cases of chronic infarction gives a separate insight into motor functions mediated by the contralateral hemisphere and brain stem. Obrador[362] reported hemispherectomy on 10 patients ranging in age from 3 to 29 years, and noted in particular that 3 patients showed only slight facial paresis. Another 7 patients had only moderate lower facial paresis, and 4 patients were able to move facial muscles on each side easily. This degree of control of the lower face contrasted with the formula of the weakness of the limbs, which approximated that predicted by the principles attributed to Broadbent.[78] The distal functions of the limbs were very much impaired. Complete paralysis of the movements of the hand and fingers was seen in 6 patients and the foot was completely paralyzed in 9 patients. By contrast, the upper limbs moved well at the shoulder and elbow in 7 cases and motility of the muscles of the hip and knee was fairly well preserved, enough for walking in all cases.

### *Hemiplegia With Deep Infarction*

Several different syndromes occur when hemiplegia with deep infarction occurs. Foix and Levy[163] described two varieties of hemiplegia in the condition they characterize as deep infarction of the sylvian artery. The motor deficit was the same in right and left hemisphere infarcts. In the first type massive hemiplegia occurred, which had the same appearances that they found when the infarct involved both the superficial and the deep territories. Initial hemiplegia gave way to marked contracture. The authors observed no instances of involuntary movements, choreoathetosis, parkinsonism, or disturbances in balance. A second type was described with a more marked hemiplegia in the leg than in the arm, rendering the patient unable to walk. Contracture in this syndrome was more frequent in the leg and often was associated with a permanent flaccid hemiplegia. The prognosis for recovery was poor, but the outlook for life appeared to be good.

Few cases are to be found in the literature. Some[67] focused on a different problem, and the description of the motor abnormalities was limited to terms such as hemiparesis or hemiplegia. Two described the deficits in some detail. One of the cases described by Fisher and Curry[159] as "pure motor hemiplegia" seems to have been a large, deep infarct, presumably of an embolic mechanism. Hanaway et al.[201] encountered an elderly woman with complete hemiplegia with some degree of movement of the face, whose autopsy within

2 days of onset showed a larger hemorrhagic infarct affecting the entire lenticulostriate territory of the right MCA. Some of the hemorrhagic component may have been due to therapy with urokinase. Healton et al.[207] described an autopsy-documented case with a large, deep, hemorrhagic infarct affecting the head of a caudate nucleus, putmamen, and the anterior limb, genu, and superior aspect of the posterior limit of the internal capsule and extreme capsule. Contralateral supranuclear facial weakness, deviation of the tongue, paralysis of the arm and leg, hyperreflexia and extensor plantar reflex were described. Death occurred 10 days after onset.

Several reports have appeared in which lesion topography was documented by CT scan. Under the title of "giant lacunes," Rascol et al.[381] have described a small series of cases with capsuloputaminocaudate infarction. These infarcts spread over both the anterior and posterior limb of the capsule and involve the adjacent striatum. Their large size far exceeded that typical for lacunes, which prompts their inclusion in this discussion. The clinical presentation featured a profound hemiplegia, but, remarkably enough, incomplete syndromes of hemiparesis were also encountered. In a few instances, the course of the hemiparesis was surprisingly mild. Adams et al.[3] described two patients with large deep infarcts seen on CT scan, associated with arterial occlusion of the first segment of the MCA with no visualization of the lenticuloustriate branches. Retrograde filling collateralized the hemisphere surface branches. Severe hemiparesis was present, including the face. In the first case, no accompanying disturbances were documented in sensation, vision, or language, from an infarct that involved the head of the caudate nucleus, the anterior limit of the internal capsule, and the putamen. In the second patient, flaccid hemiplegia involving the face was associated with mild hypesthesia with normal visual fields and a mild language disturbance. In this instance the CT revealed low density involving the head of the caudate nucleus and the anterior limit of the internal capsule and putamen. The clinical course was not further described. Santamaria et al.[401] reported eight cases with large, deep infarcts seen on CT that they attributed to cerebral embolism. Five patients suffered complete hemiplegia, but only one patient had it as a pure syndrome. Complete recovery of the hemiplegia occurred in two patients, recovery was slight in two, and no improvement occurred in the last two. The only adult described by Demierre and Prondot[128] suffered sudden hemiplegia contralateral to a stroke with a CT scan appearance of hypodensity with central hyperdensity affecting the right lenticulocapsulocaudate region. Partial regression of the hemiplegia occurred over 4 days. By 4 weeks, dystonic disorders had developed. Grimes et al.[197] described three cases studied by CT scan who showed initial hemiparesis or hemiplegia from infarcts affecting the head of the caudate and the putamen, presumably also affecting the capsule to some degree. In all three, the initial deficit regressed to mild weakness within 3 months.

Our collection includes an elderly woman with a deep infarct whose CT scan showed a high-density lesion outlining the striatum and capsule, interpreted as a hemorrhagic infarct in the lenticulostriate territories (Fig. 16-8). Her clinical presentation featured a complete hemiplegia affecting the face and limbs, involving both the proximal and distal portions of the upper and lower extremities to equal degree. The deficit improved slightly over the following month only in the hip and foot; the face, shoulder, and hand remained completely paralyzed for the 6-week period she was under clinical observation.

More recent reports describing the syndromes of striatocapsular infarction have emphasized the difficulty in separating the syndrome of large, deep infarction from superficial cortical infarction on clinical grounds alone, and have cited numerous instances of dysphasia, dyspraxia, and hemineglect among the prominent clinical features.[142,448]

Other case reports have focused on the disturbances in language, and little detailed description of the hemiparesis is available. The subcortical, nonhemorrhagic lesions affected the basal ganglia and capsule, and were large enough to be beyond the usual size expected in lacunes.[30,110,365]

### *Hemiplegia From Surface Infarction*

Finally, there are the syndromes of hemiplegia from surface infarction. The syndrome of hemiplegia from infarction of the entire surface territory of the MCA is

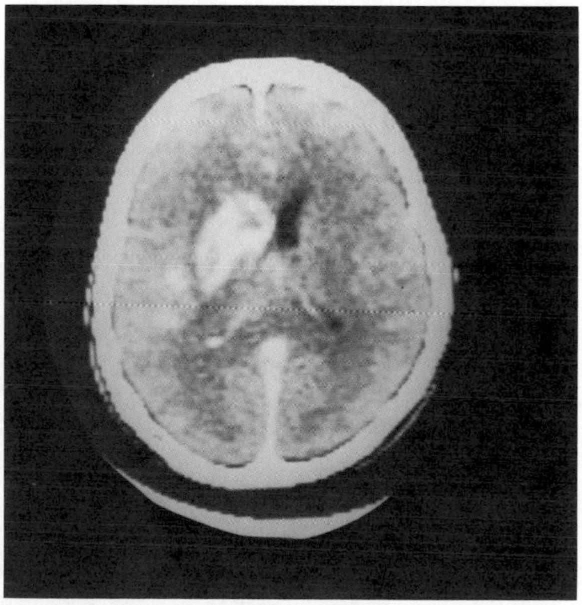

**Fig. 16-8.** Large deep infarction of the middle cerebral artery lenticulostraite territories shown by computed tomography scan.

essentially identical to that found when the deep territory is also affected. Few are to be found in the literature and the clinical deficits in those few are described only in part. A case of surface infarction among those in our collection was a 35-year-old man who suffered a subarachnoid hemorrhage without focal deficit, and underwent surgical repair of an aneurysm located at the bifurcation of the MCA. Aneurysmal rupture during the operation necessitated the placement of a clip across the MCA stem just distal to the territory of the lenticulostriate. From the time he awoke postoperatively, he was affected by a dense aphasia, contralateral hemiplegia, and hemisensory syndrome. Reexamination 2 years later showed complete lower facial plegia, deviation of the tongue, his fingers and hand lacked any voluntary movements, and the arm hung by his side with slight flexion at the elbow. The leg supported the body for walking, but the immobile toes and ankle required support by a brace. A few months later he committed suicide. At autopsy the entire MCA surface territory was found infarcted, with complete sparing of the territory supplied by the lenticulostriates (Fig. 16-9).

Some examples surface infarcts confined to the cortical surface of the insula and operculum have been described.[83] The cases have infarcts confined to the region of the insula and upper and lower banks of the operculum. The syndrome was described as a hemiplegia with faciobrachial predominance, which soon fades to a facioplegia with mild, predominantly distal, paresis of the arm.

Hemiplegia seems rather uncommon from individual branch occlusions.[163] In most cases, hemiparesis occurs, or the syndrome of paralysis is incomplete, confined to one or more body part(s). The most reliable deficit is encountered among those suffering occlusion of the ascending frontal branch. Glew[187] described an example of embolic occlusion of the back branches of the upper division: the patient suffered sudden onset of complete hemiplegia, lethargy, and mumbling of unintelligible sounds. Except for slight movement of the right ankle, the right side was immobile and flaccid, with paralysis of the face and no movement of the tongue. The CT scan showed a large low density in the back branches of the upper division. At autopsy, evidence was found of embolic infarction in the rolandic and ascending parietal regions of the MCA territory.

The clinical course of an initial hemiplegia has been described in disappointingly few cases. A survey of this case material interestingly indicates that some remarkable improvement may occur, but usually only in cases with branch occlusion. Barnett et al.[32] described a case of sylvian branch occlusion, with contralateral hemiplegia, who underwent substantial recovery in 1 week. Two years later, only minimal right-sided weakness was found on examination. A second case[32] had total hemiplegia with aphasia that remitted within a period of 1 week.

## Syndromes of Partial Hemiparesis

The most commonly encountered formula of hemiparesis seems to be one with equivalent weakness of the hand, shoulder, foot, and hip. This formula occurred in 71.2 percent of cases of the 488 unilateral hemisphere strokes studied during the pilot phase of the NINCDS Stroke Data Bank project.[345] Yet a few

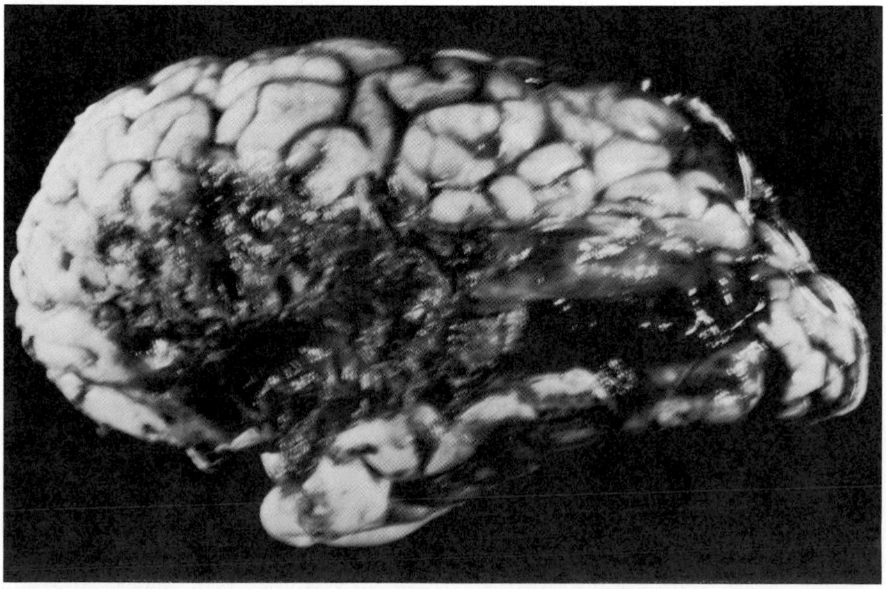

**Fig. 16-9.** Complete infarction of the surface territory of the middle cerebral artery following occlusion of the stem by an aneurysm clip.

other formulas of hemiparesis are also well known. Among them are the classical syndromes of distal predominance to the hemiparesis (Broadbent principle[78]), faciobrachial paresis, and monoplegia.

### *Hemiparesis With Distal Predominance*

The formula of hemiparesis with distal predominance, attributed to Broadbent,[78] has been widely accepted as typical of MCA territory infarction. The weakness affects the lower face, the fingers and the forearm, and the toes and lower leg, with relative sparing of the forehead, shoulder and upper arm, hip and thigh, and neck and trunk. This lower facial and distal predominance of hemiparesis has been taken to represent the density of the homocular representation over the hemispheral surface.[376,377] Although its occurrence is said to typify ischemic stroke involving the MCA territory, it seems to be a rather uncommon sign. Among the 488 cases with unilateral weakness affecting the cerebrum, studied in the pilot phase of the NINCDS Stroke Data Bank project, this formula was encountered in only 23.5 percent of cases.[345] Further, it occurred with approximately the same frequency whether the infarct was confined to a single lobe or was as large as several lobes, and whether the area involved was frontal, parietal, temporal, or opercular. As expected, hemiparesis of any kind did not occur in infarcts of the occipital region.

### *Faciobrachial Paresis*

Almost as common as distal predominance is the syndrome of faciobrachial paresis. In an angiographic study of MCA occlusion done in the days before CT scanning and with no autopsy data, Lascelles and Burrows[279] found that the lower face was affected in 51 of 59 MCA infarcts, and among those who could be assessed, the deficit was greater in the upper than in the lower limb. In cases with involvement of the insula and operculum,[10,83] the weakness of the face and oropharynx may be profound: in addition to the expected lower facial plegia, the upper face may fail to wrinkle for some days or weeks. Obvious weaknesses are present in the muscles of the jaw. Movements of the tongue and oropharynx show impaired swallowing, and occasionally impaired vocalization. These lower face and oral pharyngeal disturbances may persist long after the forehead movement has been restored. The initial appearance at times is similar to that of Bell's palsy, but the upper deviation of the eyes, typical of peripheral facial palsy (Bell's phenomenon), is usually not present even in the earliest stages. The involvement of the upper extremity is usually more obvious in the impaired movement of the fingers and hand. One such autopsied case was studied in life by our group (Fig. 16-10). On the day of the stroke, the patient showed a dense right supranuclear facioplegia, flaccid paralysis of the arm and hand, and

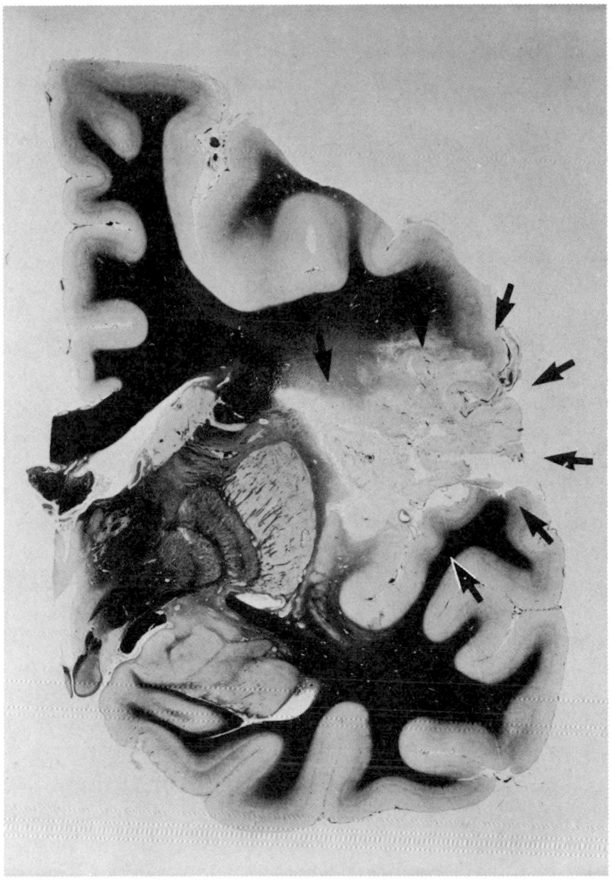

**Fig. 16-10.** Coronal view of insular and upper opercular infarction from embolism to the upper division of the middle cerebral artery (Myelin stain of celloidin section).

moderate paresis of the leg, with rare small spontaneous movements of the foot. By the 3rd day the arm could be elevated from the bed, but no movement of the fingers or forearm was found. By the next day she was able to produce a slight pressure on attempted handshake, but the face remained plegic. At 2 weeks the hand was able to produce a moderate grip, the arm could be elevated easily, and the leg supported the patient for standing in a few short steps. Other facial paralysis had improved to the point of moderate paresis and moderate weakness. By the end of the 3rd week, although she showed an obvious extensor plantar response, the weakness of the shoulder and hip were further improved, and a moderate grip with movements of the fingers was observed. The central facial weakness was present at rest and during voluntary movements, but smiling was symmetrical, the gag was intact, and the tongue moved freely. At 2 months the deep tendon reflexes had become roughly symmetrical. No further improvements were noted in the limbs, and the face showed a moderate paresis, which was more obvious than the weakness in the arm and leg. By the end of the 2nd month, the patient had reached a static condition with regard to the hemiparesis, but she made no further improvements until her death 14 months later. The autopsy revealed an infarct that destroyed the insula and adjacent banks of the operculum, but which spared the internal capsule, centrum semiovale, and cerebral surface above the operculum.

A faciobrachial predominance of the hemiparesis may occur in cases of small surface infarcts of the anterior rolandic and opercular area. One of our autopsied cases[333] of inferior frontal infarction had severe right central facial weakness with only moderate right hemiparesis (Fig. 16-11, case 1). Within a week the face and hand remained plegic, the arm strength improved to the point of being able to lift the arm off the bed, the leg had full power, and the eyes moved freely. Within 1 month the face and hand remained unchanged, but the arm moved freely, and she walked easily. By 5 months the face and fingers remained unchanged, but the wrist now was capable of making moderate movements and the arm and leg remained essentially free of trouble. Another case (Fig. 16-11, case 2), with more extensive spread of the infarct up the rolandic cortex, had a severe right facial and distal arm paralysis, including the hand, which persisted unchanged for 90 days before death.

A patient whose focal inferior frontal infarct was documented by angiogram and CT scan was struck mute while talking but did not lose balance. Examination within an hour revealed dense right lower facial plegia during attempts to talk, grimace, or smile, preserved wrinkling of the forehead, deviation of the tongue to the right, slight weakness of the grip, barely detectable weakness of the shoulder, but full movement of the trunk and leg. The right plantar response was extensor. Within 3 weeks the tongue moved freely, and the face showed only slight weakness, but the weakness of the hand persisted. By 3 months, the facial asymmetry was barely detectable under any conditions, and the grip was improved but still noticeably weak.

Another similar case indicates that the deficit may follow a similar course when the infarct affects the right hemisphere. Over a 2-hour period, in stuttering fashion, this 54-year-old man developed dysarthria and left facial plegia, with mild weakness of the grip, but retained full movement of the shoulder, trunk, and leg. Angiogram revealed occlusion of the MCA at the origin of the upper division, with collateral flow retrograde from the anterior cerebral territory to the point of the occlusion and a normal CT scan. The focal deficit persisted for over a week unchanged, then faded steadily within weeks to a barely detectable lower facial weakness on forced grimace.

Faciobrachial paresis may even occur as an isolated sign. One of our patients had a mild faciobrachial paresis of sudden onset unaccompanied by other findings, which was correlated with a contrast-enhancing CT scan and branch occlusion on angiogram. Even the possibility of facial weakness as an isolated sign has also been mentioned.[124]

## Monoplegias

Monoplegia is a circumscribed disturbance that is described in standard texts on the subject,[438] but is not easily found in the literature. Von Monakow[438] made reference to the possibility of an isolated brachial plegia arising from a lesion confined to the middle of the second frontal gyrus, provided that the lesion is acute and does not extend too deep into the white matter ("wenn sie akut einsetzt und nicht zu tief in das subcorticale Mark übergrieft . . . ")[438] Dejerine and Regnard[125] found a case with weakness

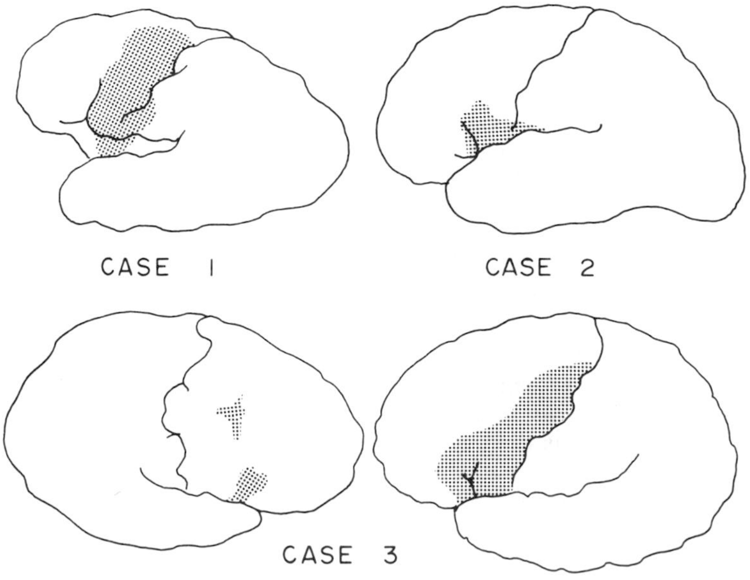


**Fig. 16-11.** Three examples of embolic infarction of the Broca area and surrounding cerebrum. (From Mohr,[332] with permission.)

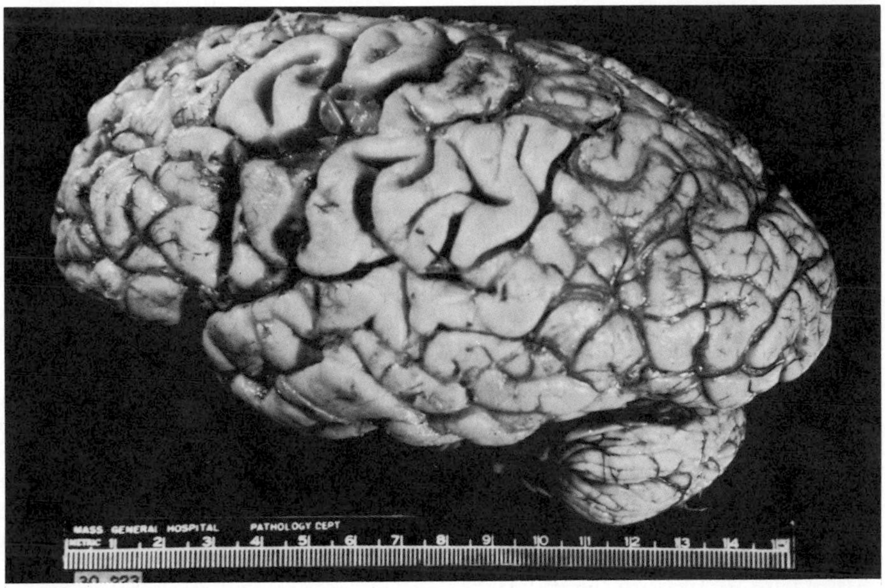


**Fig. 16-12.** Small upper rolandic infarction. (Courtesy of J.M.C. Pearce.) The pia-arachnoid has been stripped away to show the infarct.

limited to the muscles of the thenar, hypothenar, and interosseous muscles; no confirmation of the presumed vascular nature of the lesion was mentioned. Garcin[174] described a monoparesis with weakness predominating in the flexor movements mimicking a median nerve palsy; the locus of the lesion was inferred in the absence of autopsy data.

The only case of focal upper rolandic infarction that we encountered, with autopsy documentation (Fig. 16-12), was an elderly woman whose examination within hours of onset revealed normal power in the upper extremity, including the hands and fingers, sparing the limb entirely. The only clinical signs were slight right facial weakness with initial mutism. She was followed for months, during which time the initial deficit improved, but no disturbance of limb power occurred at any time.

Isolated brachial monoplegia has been described often as a clinical sign in carotid artery territory transient ischemic attacks. It has also been encountered as a transient syndrome in abberant emboli during pellet embolization in the treatment of arteriovenous malformations, regardless of the middle cerebral branch embolized. These findings are of great interest, but must be interpreted with caution, since the setting (an angiogram suite with the patient under a drape) does not lend itself to detailed evaluation of the leg and axial structures during the frantic period when the physicians are striving to reverse the acute deficit.

The data from the pilot phase of the NINCDS Stroke Data Bank project contained a mere 31 cases of monoplegia involving the arm among the 488 patients with cerebral stroke.[345] Yet even this small number showed a significant correlation with a single lobe infarct than with one involving multiple lobes ($P > 0.002$). Although monoplegia seems to be uncommon, it has some value as a sign of circumscribed infarction. Of interest, monoplegia was encountered in infarcts involving the frontal, temporal, or parietal lobe.

## Infarcts Without Hemiparesis

Infarction confined to the *lower division* of the middle cerebral artery is not expected to produce hemiparesis in any form, since the site of the infarct lies so far posterior to the rolandic sulcus. This point also seems to apply to the *postRolandic branches of the upper division* as well. Occlusion of the ascending parietal branch is uncommonly reported, but the few cases documented have been remarkably free of focal motor deficit.[138] The pilot phase of the NINCDS Stroke Data Bank[345] documented a handful of instances of hemiparesis following *opercular infarction.* Several notable cases exist with autopsy correlation in which weakness did not occur in either the face or the limbs at any time during an acute infarct affecting the inferior frontal region, the anterior operculum.[76] Reports of infarction confined to the *orbital frontal branch* of the upper division are exceedingly rare. Waddington and Ring[439] described a 62-year-old man with a grasp reflex, inappropriate laughing "witzelsucht," inappropriate advances toward his employees, and poor business judgment. His only motor deficit was the grasp reflex and contralateral extensive planar response. The case was studied by angiogram only. Rare reports of occlusion may be a result of the low frequency of embolism into this particular branch.

## Contraversive Eye and Head Deviation

Deviation of the head and eyes following unilateral lesion was first described clinically by Prevost[380] in 1868. The basic clinicopathologic correlations seem to have been so well accepted that reference to actual clinical cases in review articles has become rather uncommon.[42,56,372] Remarkably little recent documentation has been made of the lesions responsible for the deviation, and even less of the setting in which the deviation either persists or is transient. Most of the authorities writing on the subject seem to infer that the deviation of the eyes represents disruption of the frontal eye fields in and around area 8$\alpha$ located in the premotor region of the superior frontal lobe.[56,57,115,233,372,405] Given this long-standing assertion, it is remarkable how many cases with deviation of the head or eyes have lesions more centrally located in the middle cerebral artery territory, near the operculum or insula, and how few had actually been reported with eye deviation from a superior frontal central infarction.[345]

## Types of Deviation

De Renzi et al.[130] encountered three types of deviations in their 120 patients with occular motility disorders. In the first group, the head and eyes were in the midline and moved spontaneously to either side in response to stimulus, but eye movements were less complete to the side of space served by the damaged hemisphere. In a certain group the head and eyes were found completely to one side with absent spontaneous movements to the contralateral side, and only fleeting voluntary deviation of the eyes into the side of space served by the damaged hemisphere. In the most severely affected group the head and or eyes were completely deviated away from the side of space served by the damaged hemisphere and failed to turn in response to verbal or sensory stimuli, with no spontaneous or voluntary movements observed to the midline or beyond.

In the study by De Renzi et al.[130] hemi-inattention or neglect of the contralateral side of space usually accompanied those with head and eye deviation.

## Eye Deviation and Infarct Topography

Eye deviation is the expected finding after massive infarction of the *entire* middle cerebral artery territory. Lascelle and Burrows[279] noted conjugate deviation in a few of their patients with angiographically documented occlusion of the middle cerebral artery, all of whom died. It seems to have been taken as a sign of major cerebral infarction. In the *upper division* syndromes encountered in studies of Broca aphasia, we[334] uncovered 10 autopsy cases from the Massachusetts General files, all of whom experienced head and eye deviation to the site of the lesion, persisting for days and clearing within a week. There is less evidence bearing on the occurrence of eye deviation in opercular infarcts. One of our own cases showed head and eye deviation as part of the acute clinical syndrome occasioned by a left insula and opercular infarction. The infarct spared the suprasylvian hemispheral surface centrum semiovale capsular and basal ganglia structures. The deviation was reversed by passive head rotation. By the 5th day, occular motility was normal.

Ocular deviation in cases with *deep infarction* has attracted special interest. Two cases have been described. Hanaway et al.[201] found their elderly woman, with a large hemorrhagic infarct involving the entire territory of the lenticulostriates on the right side, had deviation of the eyes to the right. The eyes could not be fully moved to the left. She died within 2 days. Healton et al.[207] studied a 75-year-old woman whose autopsy showed a large hemorrhagic infarct involving the striatum. The infarct was smeared across the anterior limb, genu, and superior aspect of the posterior limb of the internal capsule. The patient's head and even the trunk remained deviated to the side of the infarct through the 10 days of life after the stroke, despite an alert state and interaction with the examiner sufficient to test language and praxis.

De Renzi et al.[130] found a higher frequency of occular motor deviation in *right* hemisphere infarcts compared with left. Patients with sensory motor stroke, and presumably larger lesions, suffered occular deviation in nearly half the cases with less difference between the right and left hemisphere group than in the posterior lesions where the right hemisphere lesion experience deviation in 61 percent compared to 13 of those on the left. The frequency of occular deviation in frontal lesions was extremely lower on both sides on the order of 5 to 6 percent. The authors point out the variance of these findings with the traditionally accepted rules of localization for eye movement disturbances. Experience in the NINCDS Stroke Data Bank may bear on this point.[345] Among the 531 cases of hemispheral stroke diagnosed by clinical or radiologic criteria, 86 cases (16 percent) had supratentorial-type conjugate ocular deviation. The occurrence of ocular deviation was significantly correlated with the larger infarcts, but among the infarcts confined to single lobes, those involving the right side were more frequently associated with ocular deviation. A frontal predominance over parietal infarcts was not found, and a parietal location was not the explanation for the effect of the right-sided stroke. The prevalence of frontal or parietal lobe location did not differ significantly among single-lobe infarcts. Ocular deviation occurred from infarction as low on the surface as the operculum. Gaze deviation of less than 5 days duration did not correlate with lesion side, size, site, cause, or positive initial CT scan. However, the larger lesions predominated among the nine cases whose ocular deviation persisted beyond 20 days.

## Duration of the Deviation and Severity of Infarct

In the study of De Renzi et al.[130] the severity of the initial ocular motility deficit seemed greater in right hemisphere cases than in left for the first 6 to 9 days, but at the end of 2 and 3 weeks most of the cases showed only mild or no disturbance. Contralateral hemineglect often outlasted the disturbance in occular motility in the cases studied by De Renzi et al.[130] Cases of infarct affecting the *operculum and insula* show what has been labeled pseudo-ophthalmoplegic for the first few days of the stroke.[83] Conjugate deviation of the head and eyes lasts for several days and then disappear. The lesion causing this condition is far away from area 8$\alpha$ and is considered a reliable feature of infarcts of the insula and operculum.

The duration of ocular deviation following *branch occlusion* in the upper division is less well documented. One of our cases[333] had head and eyes deviated to the left for a period of several weeks. In that case, the branch occlusion affected the anterior ascending branch of the middle cerebral as high as the borderzone with the anterior cerebral artery.

## Infarction With No Eye Movement Disturbances

One case of De Renzi et al.[130] showed a cortical subcortical lesion (a frontal hematoma) on the left, involving the areas of the rolandic fissure, who was completely free of any gaze disturbance.

The few cases with focal infarction confined to the superior frontal region, near area 8$\alpha$ have been a disappointment to the thesis that this region is vital for ocular motility.

# Sensory Disturbances

Because most of the attention has been paid to the more obvious deficits in language and motor function, surprisingly little is described regarding the sensory disturbances, outside the usual claims in the textbooks. The presence of a disturbance in sensation carries an important indication of a large lesion when it accompanies hemiparesis: in the pilot data from the NINCDS Stroke Data Bank project, this correlation was highly significant for infarcts greater than a single lobe in size ($P < 0.001$).[280]

## Hemispherectomies

Because the sensory disturbance from hemispheral disease may improve with time, it is worth emphasizing that the anatomic substrate may not be the surviving portions of the damaged hemisphere. The data from hemispherectomy cases[362] permit assessment of the sensory disturbance expected under extreme conditions of tissue removal. Studies have shown relative preservation of sensory function on the face. Blunted sensation to several modalities was found the more distally the test were performed in the arm. Complete astereognosia was common in his patients. Vibration and position sense were heavily effected. Of interest, no patients showed definite alteration of the body scheme.

## Pure Sensory Deficits

Focal sensory deficits have been described in detail in only a handful of cases with autopsy correlation, most of whom were described because they seemed to show an unusual variant of the expected deficit. One syndrome described has shown a pseudoradicular pattern of sensory loss[124] with impaired joint position sense, stereognosis, graphesthesia, and two-point discrimination. In the few cases studied, the hand is the most severely affected, but two cases have been described with both hand and foot disturbance. Hemianesthesia has also been described in a few other cases.[162,300,439] The persistence of the deficit outlasts the complaints of sensory disturbances.

## Hemisensory Deficits and Lesion Topography

Foix et al.[162] are credited with the demonstration that an infarct affecting the anterior parietal region may produce a profound hemisensory loss—pseudothalamic syndrome with little or no accompanying hemiparesis. Their patient had a large anterior parietal infarct, which was so deep it created almost a cleft in the hemisphere to the ventricular wall. Lhermitte et al.[295] had a similar patient studied by CT scan. Few other cases have been described. Derouesen et al.[138] reported a 50-year-old man with sudden numbness of the left thumb and index and middle fingers, which felt like they were frozen or asleep. Normal power was found on examination, but the patient dropped small objects held in the hand. The next day he experienced numbness in the distal foot and clumsiness in putting on the slipper. On examination, fine movements of the fingers and toes were inaccurately detected, and severe impairments were noted in graphesthesia, two-point discrimination, and stereoagnosis, although light touch, heat and cold, vibration, and pinprick were normally appreciated. No other disturbances were noted. A hypodense cortical and subcortical lesion was found on CT scan 17 days after the onset consistent with an infarction affecting the parietal region. The symptoms disappeared in 3 weeks, but the sensory deficit persisted unchanged on reexamination 2 months later. Paillard and colleagues[367] described a case of left middle cerebral artery lower division occlusion with a large infarct including the posterior parietal region and part of the superior parietal lobule. Very little motor deficit was noted deep tendon reflexes were symmetrical. However, a right hemianesthesia persisted for several years. The disturbance affected the right cheek and gums manifested by frequent failure of the patient to notice food had gone to the right side of the mouth. The hand was so anesthetic that she experienced cuts and burns without noticing them. The foot was anesthetic enough that several times the patient stumbled climbing stairs. Specific testing of the hand disclosed no joint position sense to point discrimination or ability to report pressure. However, the occurrence of touch was discriminable both as to direction and general speed whether fast or slow and the patient proved capable of discriminating the gross size of an object large or small and was capable of rough location of points of touch along the surface of the limb.

## Correlations With Motor Deficits

The correlation of the sensory disturbance with motor disturbance is infrequently reported. A few unusual cases exist that suggest a sensory disturbance may effect an area far smaller than that of the accompanying motor disturbance. Gacs et al.[168] described a 50-year-old woman, with a large low-density area in the right frontal region, whose clinical deficit included a dense left hemiplegia, including the face, with left hemianopia. The sensory disturbance was described only as diminution and pinpricking vibration in the left arm.

# Visual Field Disturbances

## Hemianopia

Standard textbook accounts of middle cerebral artery territory infarction regularly refer to hemianopia accompanying hemiparesis, hemisensory disturbance, and alterations in behavior.[344,346] But little clarification is given to the value of this sign as an index of infarct site and size, and even less to the pathoanatomic correlate. There is little doubt hemianopia accompanies the huge infarcts.[163,179,241,251] Traditionally, the hemianopia was ascribed to involvement of the visual radiation, even though the middle cerebral artery supplies only the upper half of the radiation.[330]

For less global infarcts, hemianopia has been described with infarcts involving the frontal region,[168] some as low as the sylvian fissure.[333] Yet hemianopia has been absent in some instances of focal infarction, even when impaired opticokinetic nystagmus was found. It is difficult to sustain the notion that edema involving the visual radiations explains hemianopia when the infarct is far away from these structures. Instead, it seems more likely that the hemianopia as described is actually a disturbance in hemispatial responding, which is part of a hemineglect syndrome.[449] In such cases, other faulty responses to spatial stimuli are noted, such as the patient suffering a left hemispheral infarction turning toward the left in response to a voice from the right, when also showing failure to blink to threat stimulus from the right side. The subject requires further investigation.

## Quadrantanopia

Parietal infarction deep enough to affect the fibers of the upper half of the visual radiation is presumably responsible for the infrequently described inferior quadrantanopsia of middle cerebral artery territory infarction (Fig. 16-13). Bounds et al.[70] described a 45-year-old woman who experienced left inferior quadrantanopsia 8 days after aortocoronary bypass surgery, attributed to embolism of the middle cerebral artery. Clinical worsening occurred 5 days later with hemiplegia, coma, and death from herniation. The autopsy report showed softening of most of the right hemisphere, and a specific focus of infarction correlating the earlier quadrantanopsia was not described. Remarkably enough, it is difficult to find the clinical setting in which lower quadrantanopia is found; it is even more difficult to determine if the quadrantanopia indicates a deep cleft of infarction reaching the visual radiation, or may occur in a more superficial infarct.

## Impaired Opticokinetic Nystagmus

The test for opticokinetic nystagmus is assumed to detect disorders of the gaze mechanism mild enough that conjugate ocular is not present at rest. Considering the number of patients tested for opticokinetic nystagmus (OKN), it is remarkable that there is still considerable controversy over the usual locus of the lesion, the pathways injured, and even the nature of the disturbance. The early view[174,416] was that OKN

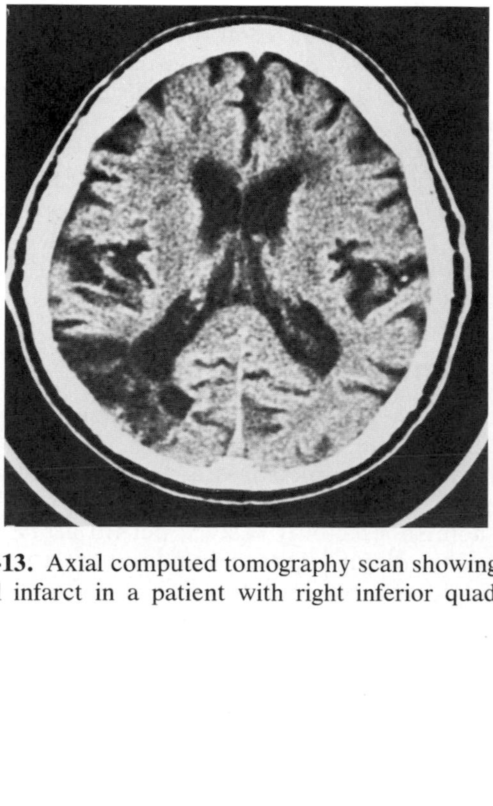

**Fig. 16-13.** Axial computed tomography scan showing a left parietal infarct in a patient with right inferior quadrantanopia.

was a reflex activity of the cerebral cortex, the slow component initiated from the occipital region, the fast corrective phase from the frontal, the OKN response blunted by lesions at any point in the pathway. However, the higher prevalence of abnormal OKN in parietal lesions supported another view[104,416]: the slow component from the occipital region passed directly to the brain stem through a pathway adjacent to the visual radiations, organized in ipsilateral pathways. Still another line of work[176] argued that the pathway runs deep through the parietal region to the frontal lobe, crosses the posterior limb of the corpus callosum, and controls fast-phase components generated in the opposite frontal lobe. More recently, arguments have been put forward for separate mechanisms controlling foveal pursuit and full-field pursuit.[28] These studies showed the main disturbance to be in the slow component when targets were moved into vision from the side of space served by the damaged hemisphere.

The actual documented sites vary considerably, not all in the parietal lobe, and hemianopia need not occur. Impaired opticokinetic nystagmus has been encountered in a small high rolandic infarct whose visual fields were intact (see Fig. 16-12). One of my (JPM) autopsied cases,[333] with superficial infarction confined to the inferior frontal region showed a brisk response by blinking from visual threat to the right side, but had absent opticokinetic nystagmus for targets moving from right to left on initial examination (see Fig. 16-10). And the patient reported by Baloh et al.[28] had a large infarct apparently involving the posterior cerebral artery territory, accompanied by right hemianopia, alexia but no language disturbance. To date, the author has encountered large numbers of cases with abnormal opticokinetic nystagmus testing when the resting eye position has been normal, but thus far no cases whose opticokinetic nystagmus testing has been normal in the face of tonic conjugate deviation of the eyes from a hemispheral infarct.

## Neglect

The term neglect is taken to indicate disturbances shown by patients in responding to stimuli from the right side of space, including opticokinetic nystamus, turning to the left in response to auditory stimuli from the right, or faulty reading aloud or naming of objects in the right side of space.

### Neglect From Frontal Lesion

It has long been appreciated that a parietal lesion, infarct or hemorrhage, even other etiologies, may be associated with impaired response to stimuli from the opposite side of space, whether from visual, auditory, or even somatosensory source.[12,100] These deficits are thought to reflect impaired input from sensory to motor regions. But a similar disturbance occurs from frontal lesions as well[114,217,257] whether cortical or subcortical.[419] Using PET scanning, Deuel and Collins[139] found widespread metabolic suppression in the basal ganglia and thalamus after a unilateral frontal lesion with little evidence of cortical hypometabolism beyond the immediate confines of the lesion. Their findings suggested that part of the syndrome may result from impaired activation of subcortical structures involved in planning motor movements. In the human, the signs of neglect from frontal lesions are remarkably transient, usually fading within a week in all but the largest infarcts. This subject is discussed more fully in the section on right hemisphere disease; the following discussion applies mainly to left hemisphere cases.

### Motor Neglect

Motor neglect, said to be characterized by underutilization of one side without defects in strength reflex sensibility, was described by Laplane and Degos.[278] Of the 20 cases reported, 1 was an ischemic type located only by radionuclide scan in a prerolandic area manifested by abnormal placement, lack of withdrawal of pain, reduced amplitude of movements, and visual hemineglect of the opposite side of space. This condition has a long history in clinical neurology. Under most circumstances of clinical examination, the patient with this syndrome appears to have a hemiparesis, yet with special efforts on examination normal strength and dexterity can be demonstrated. Usual features included a lack of spontaneous placing reaction such as failure to place the hand in the lap or on the arm of a chair when sitting, letting it instead drag down beside the body; delayed or insufficient assumption of correct postures, resulting in heavy falls to the affected side with no attempts to minimize the effect of the fall by reaching out or correcting the balance; impaired automatic withdrawal reaction to pain; excursions of the limb necessary to achieve a movement such as touching the nose, the patient instead leaning the head forward to compensate for failure to bring the finger far enough up. This disturbance may occur in the absence of sensory disturbance or demonstrable hemiparesis. An autopsy case with this similar disturbance was described by Hartmann,[205] secondary to an infarct affecting the second frontal gyrus of the right frontal lobe.

Animal studies have demonstrated a similar transitory disturbance observed after selective research high over the prefrontal region in the monkey.[449]

### Neglect for Verbal Material

Leicester et al.[286] described a form of visual neglect in which the occurrence and frequency of errors were determined by the verbal content of the test materials. Required to select from an array of choices displayed directly in front of the patient, errors were seen with those materials that the patient found the most difficult to name or write; in such instances, responses were made less frequently to choices on the right-hand side of the display. When the test materials were easily named by the patient, little or no evidence of neglect for the right side of space was noted. This form of neglect, which is commonly encountered in testing patients with aphasia, was shown not to be obligatory, but highly dependent on the verbal material being in the test itself. It was not explained by defective spatial responding nor by defective sensory function, and occurred from left-sided lesions, not right-sided ones.

## Movement Disorders

Temporary or permanent movement disorders, including hemichorea, atheosis, or dystonias are uncommon sequelae of middle cerebral artery territory infarcts. In a few cases the infarct has affected the lenticulostriate territories. The most common cause among these cases appear to be lacunes, but a few have been associated with relatively large, deep infarcts consistent with occlusion of the middle cerebral stem or embolism into many branches of the lenticulostriate territories.

Despite a large literature on the subject in children, few reports have appeared on adults. Only one has been described with chorea: a 68-year-old woman, reported by Austreglio and Borges-Forte,[25] developed immediate torsion spasms with choreiform movements from what was presumed to have been a stroke affecting the head of the caudate nucleus, putamen, and pallidum.

Dystonia has been the subject of the other reports. The one adult described in the series reported by Demierre and Prondot[128] was a 17-year-old with left hemiplegia, which improved slightly within 4 weeks, by which time signs of dystonia had appeared. The fingers, wrist, and left elbow extended on walking, the left arm showed retropulsion-abduction with elevation of the shoulders, and the lower limb was held in external rotation. No specific involuntary movements were observed. A large hypodensity affecting the putamen, anterior capsule, and caudate was seen on CT scan. Grimes et al.[197] encountered two cases of stroke in adulthood documented by CT scan. The first, a 32-year-old woman, suffered dense hemiplegia and "cortical" sensory loss from a large deep infarct affecting the caudate and putamen, which regressed considerably by 5 months. A month later, she began to experience involuntary abduction and extension of the affected fingers with ulnar deviation of the wrist; the arm flexed behind the back as she walked; she had coarse tremor of the outstretched hand. The deficit progressed for 2 months then stabilized. Medical therapy was ineffective. The second case, a 50-year-old man, pursued a similar course with the addition of orofacial dyskinesia and dystonia developed in the fingers and arm, with flexion of the limb behind the back during walking. The syndrome worsened for 3 months before stabilizing, unaffected by medical therapy.

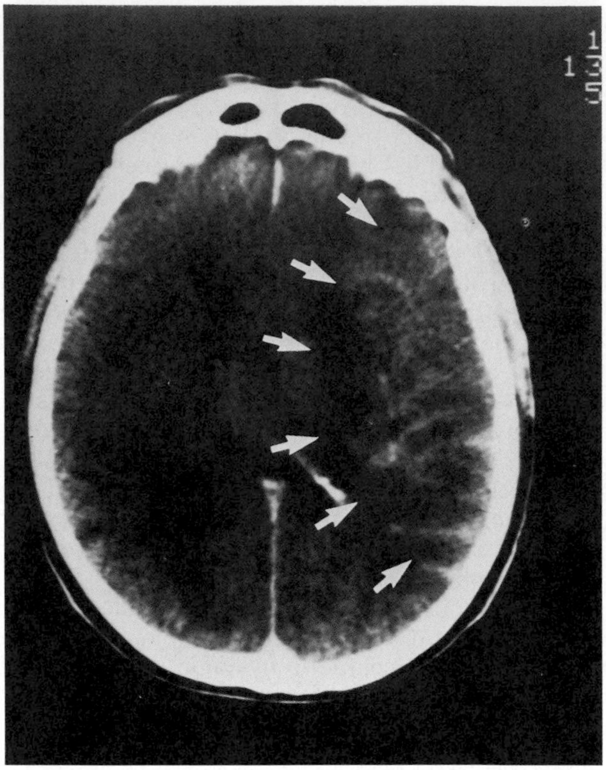

**Fig. 16-14.** Non-contrast enhanced CT scan showing hemorrhagic infarction of the entire middle cerebral artery territory. Hemihyperhydrosis and distal arm edema was part of the clinical picture.

## Autonomic Disturbances

Excess of sweating contralateral to a middle cerebral artery territory infarction is encountered only rarely. In the small series of cases reported, all cases had major syndromes of hemiparesis, hemisensory, hemianopia, and altered behavior states to indicate a large lesion affecting both the superficial and deep territory of the middle cerebral artery.[273] Sweating in these few cases affected the face, neck, axilla, and upper trunk contralateral to the infarct and faded to normal within days.

Appenzeller[17] published an autopsy case described clinically as showing hyperhidrosis on the contralateral side of the body. No further details were mentioned, including none regarding the extent of the other clinical deficits. The published photographs show a site of small hemorrhagic infarction in the upper bank of the insula and adjacent orbital surface of the operculum.

Contralateral rubbery edema of the affected hands and feet may occur from large middle cerebral artery territory infarction (Fig. 16-14). The syndrome usually becomes evident within a few hours and persists for up to 2 weeks. The exact anatomic correlates are unknown.

## SYNDROMES REFERABLE TO LEFT HEMISPHERE INFARCTION

### Aphasia

The cerebrum irrigated by the left middle cerebral artery is of prime importance in language function. The sylvian fissure of the hemisphere dominant for speech and language is the region most likely to show symptoms of dysphasia following a focal brain lesion. Over 95 percent of right-handed people and even the majority of left-handed people have dominance for speech and language in the left hemisphere. Right hemisphere dominance for speech and language in a right-handed person is distinctly uncommon.

Many of the traditional clinicopathologic correlations of brain and language function have undergone some revisions in recent years. Among them has been the demonstration of smaller, focal brain lesions that were once thought to produce the major syndromes of aphasia, which are now known to cause only transient or minor abnormalities in production or comprehension of speech sounds and shapes. Much larger lesions are necessary to produce major disruptions in language function.[34] Recent work has also made it apparent the vital speech and language role played by the deeper role structures, especially the thalamus.

### Global or Total Aphasia

Few studies have indicated the different types of aphasia expected in a setting of acute stroke. Brust et al.[80] studied 850 patients admitted to Harlem Hospital, noting that 177 (21 percent) had acute aphasia. In 57 patients (32 percent) the speech disturbance was characterized by fluent aphasia, while in 120 (68 percent) of the cases it was of the nonfluent type. A significant correlation ($P < 0.01$) was found between the occurrence of nonfluency and a poor prognosis for mortality. While within both the fluent and nonfluent a greater mortality was associated with the occurrence of hemiparesis or a visual field disturbance. Presumably the occurrence of the nonfluent type of aphasia was a reflection of larger lesions. CT scanning was not performed in this series of cases. A similar poor outlook for aphasia with acute stroke was noted in Marquardson[313] in his study of 769 acute stroke patients. Aphasia occurred in acute state in 133 (33 percent) of these cases. The author noted that hemiplegia was less likely to improve if accompanied by aphasia and aphasia had a better outlook when unaccompanied by hemiplegia.

*Clinical Features*

Occlusion of the trunk of the middle cerebral artery or the upper division produces a global disruption of language function. Its effect puts out of action virtually all of the brain regions responsible for language. The initial disturbance is so profound that it goes by the term *total aphasia.* Within weeks or months, comprehension improves, especially for nongrammatical forms, and the casual observer may be impressed that the patients speaking and writing are more disturbed than are listening and reading. This emphasis on dysphasia more in speaking and writing is known as Broca's aphasia or major motor aphasia.

*Lesion Size in Total Aphasia*

With the advent of CT scanning, a volumetric measure of the lesion became possible, permitting an inquiry into the issue not only of the usual lesion size associated with the syndrome, but also the minimal and maximal dimensions. Large lesions have been documented in several CT scan studies.[254,322] In the most recent report, Naeser[353] documented the lesion volume in two groups of cases, those labeled as "mixed" aphasia, a term that broadly encompasses the clinical picture of total aphasia, and those labeled as "global" aphasia.

The sites of the lesion in seven cases of "mixed" aphasia has proved heterogeneous, usually reflecting a large infarct affecting the sylvian region and beyond, but in a few instances the Broca area or Wernicke area proper were not mapped in the CT-scanned lesion. The lesion size in these cases was approximately 3.9 cm × 3.9 cm on the slices showing a lesion, and such a lesion was usually seen on five slices. The lesion volume in five cases of "global" aphasia was considerably larger, on the order of 5.8 cm × 5.8 cm in the slices showing a lesion. The lesion was usually seen in five slices. Like the mixed aphasia cases, the site of the minimal lesion lay in the sylvian region, and the major contribution to the larger volume was its centrifugal spread into the adjacent frontal, parietal, and temporal regions.

A few specific clinical examples should serve to indicate the main features of these cases. A 35-year-old man who underwent ligation of the middle cerebral artery stem just distal to the lenticulostriate branches remained globally aphasic for the remaining 3 years of life. Examined at 2 years, he interacted with the examiner and responded properly on tests that did not obviously require the use of language. Single examples represent in his consistent failure include his ability to select a picture of a cow on hearing the sound "moo" when presented with eight animal pictures; his ability to point to a picture of a dog when shown a picture of another dog; his ability to point to pots boiling on the stove in the background when a picture showing an elderly lady telling stories to children; his ability to point to his home state when shown a map of the United States. Tests of this type were carried out for many trials demonstrating his ability to see, hear, point, and respond to the elements of his stimulus when no spoken or written commands were involved from the examiner. Yet he obeyed no spoken or printed commands of even such single words as the printed word "smile." He vocalized only poorly understandable syllables and did not repeat aloud. He made only crude marks on a page using his left hand to guide a pen. He was easily dismayed by failure, flushing and bursting into tears when the examiner shook his head after a faulty response. Autopsy over a year later showed complete infarction of the entire hemispheral territory of the middle cerebral arteries, sparing only the basal ganglia and capsule supplied by the lenticulostriate territories (see Fig. 16-9).

## Motor Aphasia

For almost 100 years a syndrome has been recognized in which the ability to communicate by speaking or writing seems far more impaired than the comprehension of words heard or words seen.[79] Although Boulliaud[69] deserves credit for popularizing the notion that a lesion of both frontal lobes disrupts the power of spoken speech, his son-in-law's friend Paul Broca has received most of the credit for the documentation that a left-sided sylvian infarct more reliably causes the syndrome. In the years since Broca's description of his two patients who appeared to him to have lost their memory for how to speak, considerable controversy has persisted concerning the locus of the minimal lesion to precipitate the major syndrome and the effects of a lesion confined to the third frontal convolution, which Broca took to be the site of the lesion causing the syndrome that bears his name.

### *Major Motor Aphasia*

In its usual form, major motor aphasia develops as a late sign in the course of the major cerebral infarct. The responsible infarct encompasses at least the insula and usually the adjacent frontoparietal operculum, roughly approximating the large sylvian infarct encountered in Broca's original description (Fig. 16-15). In such patients, there is a sharp contrast between the hesitant, agrammatic speech and the relatively better comprehension evident in conversational tests, so long as the examiner keeps the sentences and questions simple.

In the initial period following the acute infarct, the distinction between speech and language production and comprehension is not obvious. The later state of Broca's aphasia is usually buried in a deficit so profound that the term *total aphasia* is used.[13,124,217,267,333,334,341,456] With the passage of a few months, however, the syndrome of Broca's aphasia begins to emerge from the total aphasia. Whether the motor aphasia that emerges is a disturbance confined to speaking and writing or contains a global disturbance in the brains capacity to deal with grammatical functions has remained the subject of dispute. The difficulties authors have had over the years settling this point is reflected in the variety of terms used in attempts to substitute for the eponym in Broca's aphasia: expressive dysphasia,[460] efferent motor dysphasia,[310] motor dysphasia,[192] and verbal dysphasia.[207] Most authors echo the impression of Liepmann[303] that in such cases the symptoms of motor aphasia predominate; the limited capacity at spoken expression conceals the deeper language disturbances that persist but are less obvious.

The *speech disturbance* is evident to a similar degree whether the utterances are produced in spontaneous conversation, during efforts to repeat aloud, or to read aloud. The spoken responses are hesitant, demonstrating impaired skilled interaction (dyspraxia) between the settings of the oropharynx and the respiratory elements that permit smooth vocalization.[11] In the production of individual words, the transitions from sound to sound are accomplished with difficulty,[308] an effect of the speech dyspraxia that conveys an impression of stuttering. The effect is especially obvious when polysyllabic words are spoken. The disturbance also impairs the usual clustering of words to

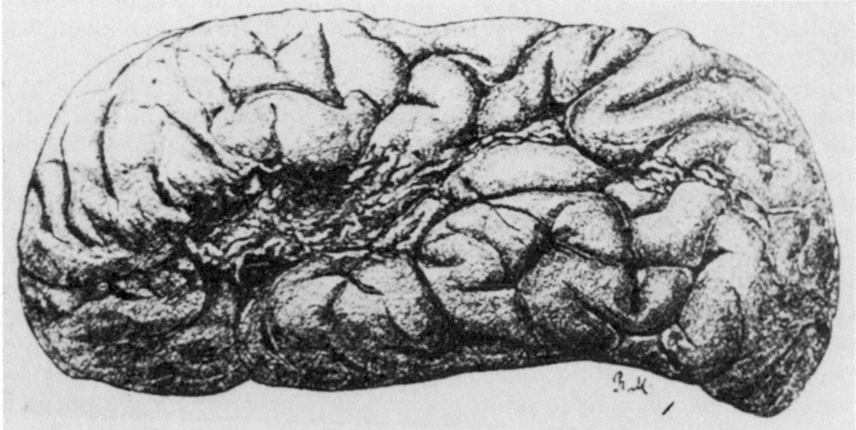

**Fig. 16-15.** One of Broca's original cases.

form phrases, and interferes with the normal melodic intonation that serves to indicate differences between exclamations, questions, and declarative statements. There is a high correlation between the degree of buccolingual dyspraxia and speech loss in patients with Broca's aphasia.[136] Apart from these signs of *speech dyspraxia*, the structure of the spoken phrases may be grammatically simplified, consisting largely of single words, which function as predicative elements; these responses strike the listener as having the laconic style of a telegram. In more severe cases, the responses consist of single nouns or verbs. These are so condensed that the disorder is not merely one of simplified speaking, but indicates impaired use of grammatical skills. These grossly condensed utterances are labeled as *agrammatism*. In some, the utterances have been limited to a single word or phrase[43,355] characterized as *verbal stereotypes*, a clinical sign carrying a discouraging prognosis for improvement.

Because of its common usage, mention must be made of *nonfluency*,[266] a term is use widely to capture the essence of the complex disturbance in spoken speech and language in these cases. The inherent ambiguities in the term has limited its value, since it is not clear if the user means the hesitancy, the dysmelodic flow of sounds, or the condensed grammar. Each of the elements alone may reflect lesions other than those responsible for motor aphasia. However, the term as defined recently apparently now encompasses all the elements together: "effortful, dysmelodic speech, often with impaired articulation and impoverishment of grammatical form."[266] As often defined, the persistence of nonfluency correlates well with lesion size. Among the group of infarcts studied by Knopman et al.,[266] 10 of the 17 with persisting nonfluency had lesions whose CT size measured greater than 100 $cm^3$, 6 were larger than 25 $cm^3$, and only 1 was smaller. Among the cases with smaller lesions, the surface component lay in the inferior rolandic region with a sizeable subcortical component, presumably a combination of cortical surface infarct and deep infarction affecting the lenticulostriate territories.

Other features of the language deficit are important elements of the syndrome. Numerous authors have commented on the difficulties such patients have in responding to spoken or written material that features small grammatical words such as "the," "are," "then," and so on, or involves spelling.[334] The disturbances observed extend beyond the acts of speaking or writing into comprehension of the material itself. Silent reading comprehension, which requires no overt vocalization, is usually only a little disturbed, unless the material to be read contains a particularly high density of such grammatical words. When it does, the comprehension may be strikingly abnormal. This condition has been termed *deep dyslexia*, and has been described as a third form of dyslexia.[43] Similar disturbances can be documented in tests that require the patient to point to visual displays containing single letters or grammatical words in response to hearing the names of the letters. Some have even shown faulty selection of a single letter among a visually presented display of letters when the test stimulus was a printed word whose pronounced sound (homophone) is identical to that of a given letter (i.e., "eye" to "i").[342] These examples indicate of the global disturbances in language that occur and persist in patients with the major syndrome of Broca's aphasia.

The *clinicopathologic correlation* has been better understood in recent years. Major motor or Broca's aphasia is not a syndrome expected from Broca's area infarction. It usually reflects a major infarction involving most of the territory supply of the upper division of the left middle cerebral artery. Accompanying disturbances in motor, sensory, and visual function usually make the diagnosis easy. The usually large size of the sylvian infarct sets the stage for contralateral hemiplegia.[234] At times, however, the main weight of the lesion may fall on the sylvian region alone, which may produce a surprisingly slight hemiparesis considering the major effect on language function[360] (Fig. 16-16). In these cases, the hemiparesis may be limited to the face and hand. Ideomotor dyspraxia of the unaffected left upper extremity is the rule as is bilateral buccofacial dyspraxia, which has been reported in 90 percent of patients.[136,182,184] Contralateral hemineglect is the rule in the acute stage.

Autopsy documentation of the major syndrome of Broca's aphasia comes largely from the older literature. In our[334] review, the 19 autopsy cases found with a syndrome described as Broca's aphasia passed beyond the period of 10 months; all were examined for major sylvian lesions or insular opercular lesions at the least. The two notable exceptions were both cases reported by Broca in which he mistakenly attributed the responsible lesions as limited to the third frontal convolution, even though he described the large sylvian opercular infarct that was actually found at autopsy (see Fig. 16-15). Similarly, 15 of 39 cases uncovered during a search of the records at the Massachusetts General Hospital for a 10-year period documented large sylvian infarcts.[333] Two cases reported, based on CT scans by the same author,[334] showed enormous lesions affecting the sylvian region and adjacent operculum and frontoparietal regions of the left hemisphere. In all of these cases, hemiplegia was present on onset, none were able to stand for a week after onset, and all walked in the chronic state with a circumducted gait carrying a spastic arm and a densely paretic lower face. Head and eye deviation was present for several days after onset and hemianopia was documented initially and persisted for several days.

Large aphasic populations have been studied using CT scan,[29,258,341,355,364] but not thus far with MR scanning. The CT scan lesions with persistent Broca's aphasia have largely been opercular and insular. The

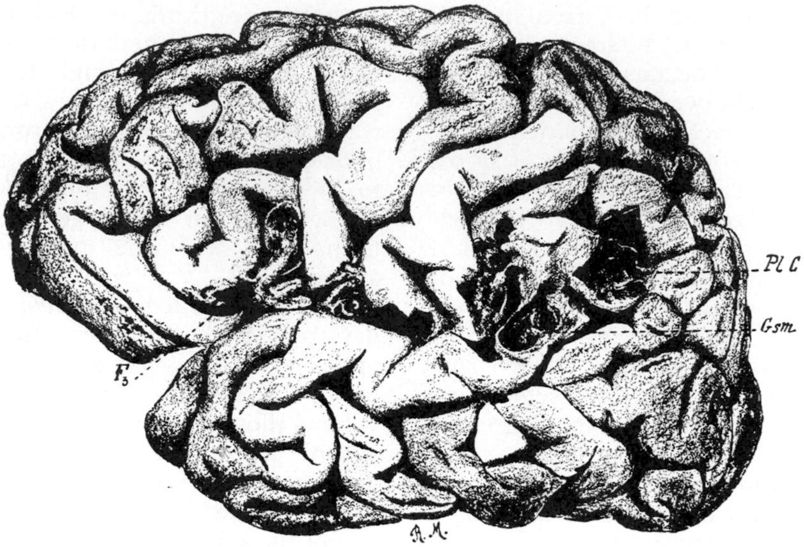


**Fig. 16-16.** Lithograph of an example of infarction limited to the "sylvian lip." (From Moutier,[350] with permission.)

lesion location and volume in Naeser's[353] four cases studied by CT scan showed a frontosylvian location, sparing the temporal lobe, with lesions on the order of 3.1 cm × 3.1 cm in CT slices where the lesion was present. The most recent such study,[267] focusing on the issue of nonfluency, showed the larger sylvian lesions associated with persistent nonfluency. Among the cases with the smaller lesions, destruction of the region taken to represent Broca's area was not necessary for persistent nonfluency, but was associated with transient deficits. No details of the remainder of the neurologic deficit was presented in this study. Although rare, a large lesion of the right hemisphere may precipitate the syndrome in a right-handed person.[228]

A few notable exceptions to the usual clinical picture accompanying Broca's aphasia may occur when the lesion is confined to the insula and adjacent operculum. Moutier's case,[350] Chissadon, acutely suffered a hemiplegia, but in the chronic state had only the slightest motor deficit. A remarkably circumscribed infarct was found along the lip of the upper bank of the sylvian fissure, which may have sufficed to interfere with language function and not with sensory motor function. A few cases of this type have been described under Benson's term, the *sylvian lip syndrome.* One of Broca's cases was also described as having no detectable motor disturbance, but was examined several years after the onset of his original deficit.

The issue of the smallest lesion that is sufficient to produce the persisting syndrome of Broca's aphasia remains unresolved. To date no known case of an infarct confined to the Broca area alone has produced a lasting, severe Broca's aphasia.[292]

### *Minor Motor Aphasia*

Focal infarcts affecting the operculum produce a very different form of disturbance. Infarcts confined to Broca's area are not the expected cause of the syndrome of Broca's aphasia. The syndrome has been described repeatedly in recent years.[289,315,333,334] In the acute stages, complete mutism with ideomotor and buccofacial dyspraxis is commonly encountered. Auditory and visual comprehension for language is virtually intact, and some of the individuals are capable of writing properly with the unaffected left hand. Improvement from the initial mutism begins within hours or at the least days and, rarely, weeks later. Any language deficit evident in speaking and writing is extremely transitory and often disappears before it can be tested in full detail. The accompanying buccolinguofacial and ideomotor limb dyspraxia likewise disappear quickly. The dyspraxia appears to contribute to most of the disturbances in speaking. The oral cavity positions closely approximate those desired to generate given sounds, but the slightly inaccuracies strike the listener's ears as mispronounciations. The dyspractic disturbance in respiration interferes with the smooth flow of sounds and transition from syllable to syllable in running speech. The disorder is not a result of weakness of the muscle serving articulation.

The initial mutism is usually accompanied by contralateral hemiparesis, but limitation of the weakness to the lower face and hand is not uncommon. Head and eye deviation have been documented but not often.[333] A few cases of Broca's area infarction have presented with no hint of motor paresis.[76] The most recent such reported case[315] became mute over a period of 20 minutes after initially experiencing 5 minutes of numbness affecting the right side of his face and arm, and difficulty repeating aloud. The neurologic examination revealed a mild orofacial dyspraxia but no weakness, and sensation and visual fields were normal. The disturbance in speaking faded to normal within 9 days. The CT scan at day 14 showed a low density with abnormal enhancement over the foot of the inferior frontal gyrus and inferior aspect of the second frontal gyrus. The operculum and insula were not involved.

In the six autopsied cases personally studied, three of whom were reported[333] (see Fig. 16-11), the initial right-sided motor deficit and ideomotor dyspraxia with initial mutism and language deficit gave way to emerging spoken speech that showed scant evidence of agrammatism. A larger series based on CT scan[341] showed similar findings, only one of which showed any evidence of grammatical condensation and simplified sentence structure at any time. When the speech and language production has been described as "nonfluency,"[267] a similarly transient disturbance has been seen in the smaller lesions found by CT scan.

The rate in extent of improvement vary considerably.[23] Some patients appear normal in all but the most complex language tasks within days.[341,423] Others become fluent after a few months and appear abnormal only to those most familiar with their daily routines (Fig. 16-17).

The *clinicopathologic correlation* has proved remarkably reproducible in the reported cases. There appear to be few exceptions to the rule that a Broca's area infarction does not precipitate either the acute or the chronic forms of Broca aphasia.[334,341] The exceptions to this rule appear infrequent enough to warrant special comment. Van Gehuchten[435] described a 60-year-old man with total sudden loss of speech accompanied by paresis of the right upper limb with a small amount of facial involvement. The paresis diminished progressively, but the speech disturbance persisted unchanged until death 1 year later. Van Gehuchten[435] described the clinical picture as "pure motor aphasia with agraphia with no word blindness or deafness." The patient was incapable of speaking. He uttered only a few sounds and sometimes a word or two. However, he could express himself adequately by gestures, wrote some letters or ordinary words from dictation, but was unable to write spontaneously or dictation under more demanding circumstances. Autopsy revealed an infarct affecting the inferior half of the middle frontal gyrus from the top to the bottom of what was described as Broca's area. The accompanying photograph disclosed the infarct, but did not indicate the involvement or sparing of the insula, nor whether the lesion extended deep into the brain. Kleist[264] considered that the rare instances of a persistent and severe deficit associated with a Broca's area infarction to be explained by an extension of the infarct extend deep into the hemisphere to disrupt the white matter fibers that serve as projection and association pathways for Broca's area. Foix[161a] earlier made a similar inference by referring to infarcts effecting the deeper branches of the middle cerebral artery. Goldstein[191] made similar suggestions, but failed to specify the vascular territory involved in these larger lesions.

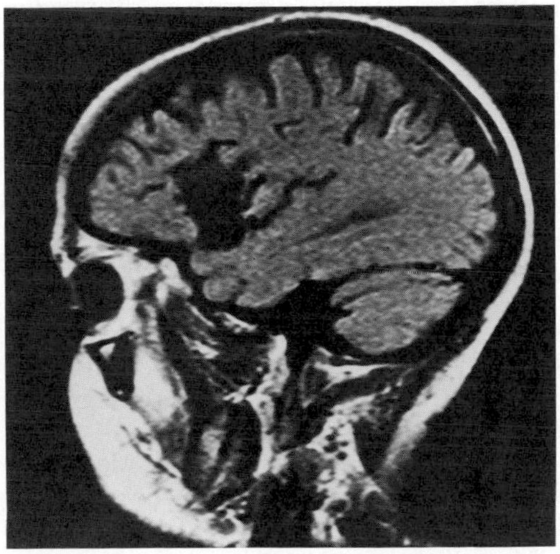

**Fig. 16-17.** Sagittal T1-weighted magnetic resonance, showing left inferior frontal infarction.

## Speech Disturbances With Lower Rolandic Infarction

The role of the lower rolandic cortex in the motor aphasias has not received wide attention. Few cases have been reported since the days of Moutier,[350] whose studies suggested that infarcts in this region did not cause motor aphasia. Niessl and von Mayendorf[360] described a case of infarction involving the rolandic operculum that spread to the supramarginal and angular gyri, including the first, second, and third temporal gyri, but which spared Broca's region. A disorder of speech articulation occurred in the absence of signs suggesting motor aphasia. A similar disturbance was suggested by Kleist[264] by the term *aphasic dysarthria*.

Three autopsied cases have appeared in the literature. Tonkonogy and Goodglass[427] described a 63-year-old man with moderate right central facial paresis, deviation of the tongue to the right, and slight right hemiparesis predominantly in the right arm with normal sensory function and visual fields. The speech was slow and dysprosodic, involving both stuttering and poor control of pitch. Articulations were deformed to the point of approximating literal paraphasias. Very slight disturbance in word-finding was present. Dysprosody and articulatory disturbances remained, and moderate brachial facial dyspraxia was present. Comprehension for reading and writing were practically intact. By 3 weeks the speech function had recovered fully, or almost, with just mild dysprosody, and the right hand had only slight weakness. Autopsy showed an infarct affecting the lower cortex of the rolandic sulcus of superficial size approximately 1.0 × 1.5 cm linked to an infarct in the anterior limb of the internal capsule. Lacours and Lhermitte[274] described a case whose infarct was limited to the rolandic operculum, lacking any disturbance in language but suffering the syndrome of "phonetic disintegration." Levine and Sweet[292] added a third case of rolandic infarction involving most of the precentral gyrus. The patient was only able to vocalize grunting or moaning sounds for the 10 days she was testable before death. Autopsy disclosed a highly focal hemorrhage involving the midportion of the precentral gyrus, sparing the frontal region in Broca's area.

The overlap of this syndrome with cases producing predominantly literal peraphasias has been noted by Luria[309] under the term *afferent motor aphasia*, attributed to faulty sensory feedback from a postrolandic lesion, leading to inaccurate anatomic settings of the oropharynx, with resultant mispronounciations.

The concern to settle the role of the lower rolandic region is not merely an exercise in trivia. Levine and Sweet[292] have updated the long-overlooked thesis of the role of the precentral gyrus lesion in the occurrence of the major syndrome of Broca's aphasia. As early as 1926, Niessl von Mayendorf[360] noted the invariable association of precentral gyrus lesions in the larger infarcts that set the stage for motor aphasia. Trojanowski et al.[429] encountered a case of persisting Broca's aphasia, with infarction limited to the cortex and subcortical white matter of the precentral gyrus, sparing the deeper structures and largely sparing the adjacent third frontal convolution. For the present, initial mutism must be considered an expected sign in lower rolandic infarcts, and its occurrence can be taken as a sign against an alternative diagnosis of a deep, lacunary-type infarct in a case presenting of isolated hemiparesis. Should more cases of inferior frontal-lower rolandic infarction be documented with persisting Broca's aphasia, the current clinical point that such cases mean a larger lesion would lose much of its force.

## Speech Disturbances From Deep Infarcts

Two forms of speech disorder have occurred: the first type, infarcts affecting the motor outflow of both sides, have produced mutism as part of a syndrome of paralysis of both sides of the face, oropharynx, and tongue; the second, and more interesting, type involves a single deep infarct, which has produced enough disturbance in speech and language described as an aphasic disorder by the observer. Bonhoeffer's classic case,[67] unable to speak anything more than a few poorly formed vowels, had a large, deep infarct of the type described as a "giant lacune."[382] However, given its large size and the second infarct in the cortical surface territory of the anterior cerebral, it seems more likely the cause was embolism to the stem of the middle cerebral artery. The infarct spread from the corner of the lateral ventricle through the caudate and internal capsule, even reaching the external capsule. The speech deficit was formulated as a double disconnection from Broca's area: the giant lacune prevented innervation of the bulbar apparatus from ipsilateral pathways, while the anterior cerebral territory infarct cut off transcallosal projections.

Severe dysarthria and rare paraphasias with little disturbance in comprehension, resulting from a single large, deep infarct, was also reported by Kleist[264] in the case of Bühlmeir. As best we can make out from the combination of the text and pictures, the infarct involved both limbs of the internal capsule, the putamen and caudate, and much of the corona radiata and centrum semiovale, of the size also usually associated with occlusion of the stem of the middle cerebral artery. No mention was made of the vascular pathology. The syndrome was formulated as a disruption of both efferent pathways from Broca's area from the single large lesion: one pathway to the bulbar apparatus ipsilaterally was destroyed by the capsular component of the lesion, the other transcallosal pathway through the centrum semiovale destroyed by another part of the lesion.

Fisher[157] described a case of "modified PMH with 'motor aphasia' " due to a large infarct involving the genu and anterior limb of the internal capsule and adjacent white matter of the corona radiata. Speech initially was dysarthric, progressed later to mispronounciation of words, then to a state of utterance of single-syllable unintelligible sounds, and ended as mutism. Comprehension was reportedly intact. Santamaria et al.[401] encountered the last among their series of eight cases with "expressive dysphasia." The language disorder was characterized by "nonfluent conversational speech, naming and reading difficulties, dysgraphia and normal auditory comprehension." The disorder had disappeared a year later. Marie[311] also presented a case—due to a putaminal hemorrhage—with "anarthria" but no aphasic symptoms.

Other cases of mutism with more circumscribed lacunes have been due to bilateral capsular infarction. One of Fisher's cases was documented by microscopic vascular pathology.[156] His case became mute with the second infarct, which involved the left internal capsule. The left capsular lacune was 4 × 4 × 5 mm and lay at the genu. A case in my[337] south Alabama collection was similar, with an earlier infarct in the posterior limb of the right internal capsule and a more recent infarct affecting the left internal capsule at the genu. This last infarct was so small as to be barely visible on CT scan, yet it yielded virtual anarthria, severe dysphonia, and dysphagia, but only a mild right arm weakness. None of the purely lacunar cases appear to qualify for the term aphasia, if the term is taken to imply a disturbance in language function independent of impaired articulation.

Imprecise definitions prevent any comparison of these terms with the classic syndrome of *subcortical motor aphasia.* Of interest, unusual syndromes of dysphasia have been described from deep infarcts, but, to date, the neuropathologic nature of the lesions remains unclarified. The six cases reported by Damasio et al.[110] were diagnosed by CT scan; there were no angiographic and no autopsy data. A similar database underlies the seven cases of ischemic mechanism reported by Naeser et al.,[354] at least three of which had accompanying surface infarcts. These uncertainties aside, the CT abnormalities encountered in the wholly deep lesion cases were predominantly in the anterior limb of the internal capsule, putamen, and caudate, and all were among the larger size consistent with the "giant lacunes" of the type 1 of Rascol et al.[381] Clinically, remarkable dysprosody, at times accompanied by dysarthria, little or no dyspraxia of limbs on either side, and a mixture of deficits in syntactic and semantic functions not typical of any of the classical syndromes of dysphasia.[110,248,356,448] Other studies showing impaired frontal reactivity in studies of cerebral blood flow suggest the disorder may be explained by damage to thalamofrontal pathways, the diminished verbal behavior being a part of a syndrome of abulia.[105,276]

## Sensory Aphasia

The vast majority of cases labeled Wernicke's aphasia are associated with occlusion of the lower division and its branches. The cause of the occlusion is usually embolism. Because the lower division gives off its branches over an extremely short distance, occlusion at its origin may give rise to several distinct variants in the size and topography of the infarction. Although little effort has been made in pursuit of the point in the literature on aphasia, there is a rough degree of correlation between the extent of the language deficit and its intensity as a function of the lesion size, which will be reflected in the section that follows.

### *Major Sensory Aphasia*

When the embolus blocks all the branches with no retrograde collateral from the posterior cerebral, a large infarct occurs, which encompasses the whole posterior temporal, inferior parietal, and lateral temporo-occipital regions (Fig. 16-18). Infarcts of such huge size generate a profound deficit in language function, often described by the eponym *Wernicke's aphasia.*

In contrast to motor aphasia, patients with sensory aphasia show little or no disturbance in the ability to vocalize, make smooth transitions between syllables, assemble utterances in the form of phrases, and achieve an intonation of their utterances that sound like questions, replies, and declarative statements, regardless of the severity of the language disturbance reflected in the content of their speech.[13]

In the acute stage of the major infarcts, the disturbance in language content reflected in such gross paraphasias in spontaneous speech that the utterances often contain no understandable words, a condition known as *jargon paraphasia.* The specific words expected to be uttered—the target words—are often distorted in their phonetic structure (literal paraphasia) both in vowels and consonants, or substituted by other words in the same class (verbal paraphasias), occasionally distorted by the addition of unwonted suffixes—less often prefixes—at times even omitted, and often contaminated by the recurrence (perseverations) of previously uttered words or word fragments. The effects on language behavior are almost the reverse of the insular-opercular syndromes: speech is filled with small grammatical words but missing the key words—the predicative elements—that contain the essence of the message. The extent of the language disturbance is often revealed only in prolonged conversation. The casual or hurried examiner may find the patient speaks easily, engages in simple conversational exchanges, and even appears to be making an effort at communication. Because the utterances often flow in a manner suggesting attempts at declarative statements, questions, or explanations, and are accompanied by gestures of the face and limbs, the patients seem to be making efforts to communicate. Yet attempts to engage the patient in testing often fail to yield much evidence the patient has understood the task and is attempting to respond. When the patient does not respond properly, the examiner is faced with the difficulty deciding whether the fault lies in comprehension, praxis, or failure of the examiner to make clear to the patient what is required.

The writing is usually disturbed in a manner similar to spoken speech. The cursive script is usually legible, since there is no hemiparesis, but the content varies considerably. Instances have been reported with writing far superior to oral naming.[223] Because quantitative comparison between written and spoken responses are not the rule for most analyses of cases of Wernicke's aphasia, it remains uncertain whether these observations are the exceptions or common.

The disturbance in comprehension of language in spoken and written form has long been assumed to be of the same type as that reflected in the spoken and written speech, which would reflect the essentially unitary nature of the disorder.[194] Although the brain lesion interferes with auditory comprehension, it has been difficult to demonstrate the presumed disturbance in phonemic processing.[419] Instead of a disturbance in elemental phonemic precessing,[175] the problem seems to lie at the level of determining the

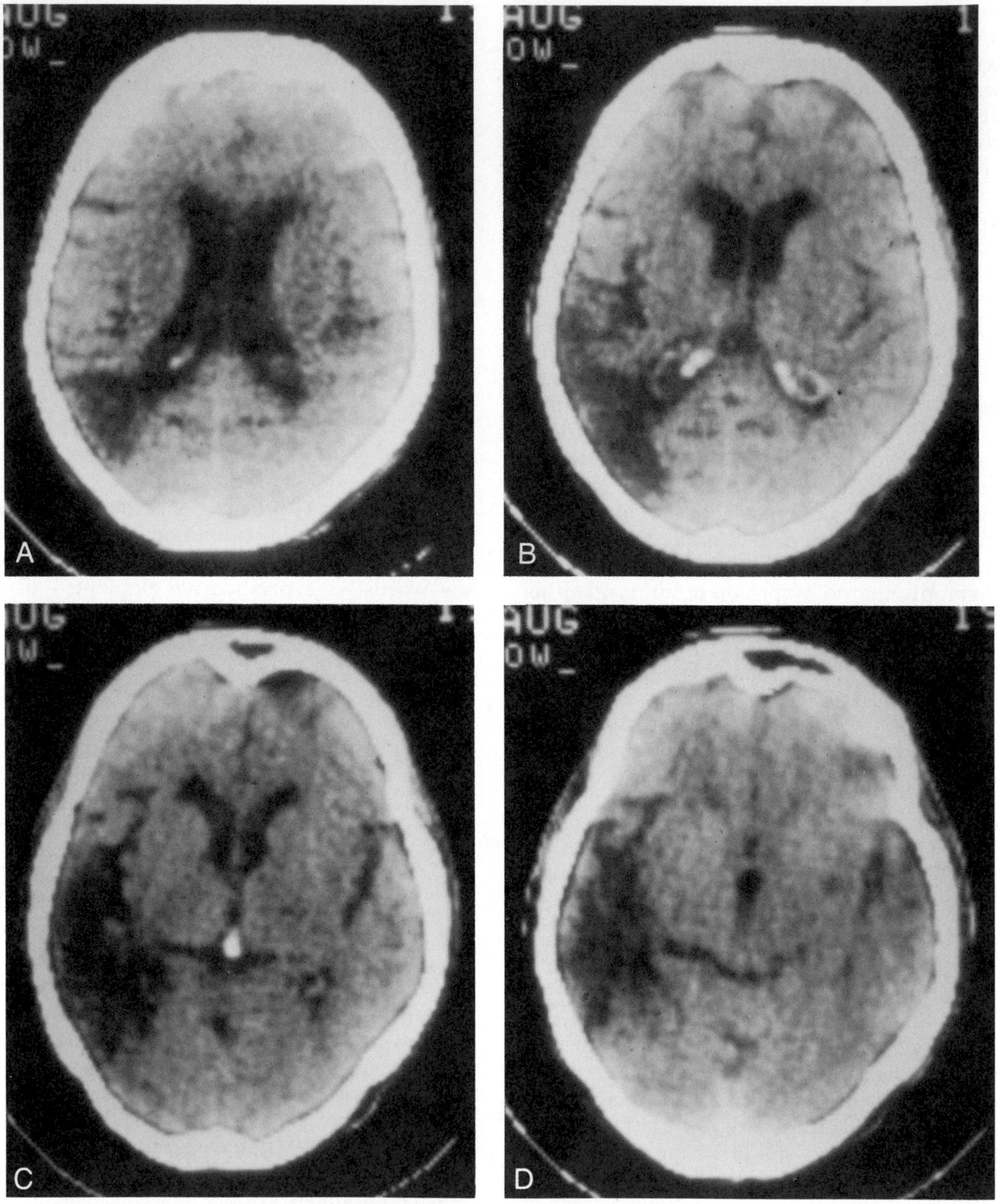


**Fig. 16-18. (A–D)** Computed tomography evidence of large infarct involving the lower division of the middle cerebral artery in a right-handed woman; no aphasia.

linguistic significance of the adequately discriminated auditory stimuli.[61] It has likewise proved difficult to determine the extent to which disturbances in reading comprehension parallels that of auditory comprehension. A few patients with rather larger lesions have shown a relative superiority of reading for comprehension compared with auditory comprehension.[223]

The *clinicopathologic correlation* has shown a rather large lesion. The cerebral infarction responsible for the major syndrome affects the lower division of the middle cerebral artery. Characteristically, the embolic material arrests at the first bifurcation of the lower division, which occurs at the superior temporal plane adjacent to Heschl's transverse gyrus. Uncollateralized occlusion of one or more branches of the lower division can produce an infarct so deep that it creates a schizencephalic cleft, reaching from the surface all the way through the white matter to the ventricular wall. Collateral retrograde into the lower division from the posterior cerebral artery territory may reduce the perimeter of the infarct, in some cases to a fairly small zone just beyond the point of the occlusion.

In most of the recent literature, the full syndrome of Wernicke's aphasia has been correlated mainly with the larger posterior hemispheral lesions.[354,355,428] In the four cases clinically diagnosed as Wernicke's aphasia in Naeser's study,[353] the lesions were relatively large, on the order of 2.5 to 31 × 3.1 cm on the slices showing low-density lesions, and the findings were seen on 3 slices around the level of Wernicke's area.

Although the lesion seems to be large in cases labeled clinically as Wernicke's aphasia, there is little known about the correlation of the lesion site and size and the features of the syndrome. We have encountered over 40 such cases of large infarction over the past 10 years. In this group of cases with large lesions, some degree of correlation seems to exist between lesion size and the performance on special language studies comparing the spoken and written response to auditory and visual presentation of words, pictures, and sounds: cases suffering the large lesions were no better at language response to words, sounds or pictures of the same items, that is, the disturbance was equally severe for words heard as for words seen, for sounds heard as for pictures seen. Other patients with smaller lesions have shown more limited disturbance in either auditory or visual comprehension, but not both to the same degree.[223] We believe that patients with protracted and exaggerated spontaneous speaking (logorrhea) have been those with the larger infarcts, and that those with the smaller infarcts rarely show this sign, a point that could be studied in more detail.

It has recently been recognized that some of the patients with a fairly large lesion across the lower division did not show a clinical picture of Wernicke's aphasia at all, but, instead, showed one suggestive of the syndrome of conduction aphasia.[47,113,397] In these cases the comprehension is so satisfactory that the main finding is the difficulty in repeating aloud. The implications are discussed in detail below.

A few cases have been reported in which no detectable initial deficit in language occurred, or at the most only it was slight and transient,[66,265,319] despite an infarct affecting the posterior superior temporal region large enough to have been expected to produce Wernicke's aphasia. We had a similar case, an elderly right-handed lady whose cerebral embolus occurred while walking in her garden in the company of her internist son. She was immediately tested and found able to read aloud and write correctly, to repeat and converse normally, but experienced signs of a right hemianopia. Examination within days also failed to disclose and language disturbance (see Fig. 16-18). Cases of this sort serve to indicate the limitations of our present understanding of language organization in the brain.

### *Minor Sensory Aphasia and Variants*

When the embolus occluding at the origin of the lower division is collateralized retrogradely from the branches of the posterior cerebral artery, some reduction in total infarct size occurs, the infarction zone shrinking backward toward the site of occlusion. How often such cases occur is only recently being appreciated with the widespread use of CT scanning. Prior to CT scanning, the mere angiographic demonstration of an occluded lower division at its origin left the physician unable to be certain how large an infarction was present distal to the occlusion. Less is known about the spectrum of syndromes that occur. However, these cases provide an opportunity to determine how small a lesion is sufficient to precipitate the full syndrome of Wernicke's aphasia.

At issue is the vital question of the precise location and size of Wernicke's area. The thorough review by Bogen and Bogen[64] has amply demonstrated that scarcely anyone agrees. Over the years, the region attributed to the Wernicke area seems to have shrunk steadily from Wernicke's original notion that it was the posterior end of the sylvian fissure and adjacent parietotemporooccipital region. From an initially large zone, actually encompassing much of the lower division as suggested by 19th century authors, the area critical for the syndrome is considered by more recent authorities to be smaller and smaller, shrinking most recently to the small size of the posterior superior temporal plane in Geschwind's diagrams.[182] This tendency to focus attention on this smaller zone may arise, in part, from the currently popular means of mapping a lesion by CT scan in several cases, then seeking the site where the lesions overlap.[255] The approach has the advantage of targeting the focal lesion site common to all the cases. Since the site common to all cases is the posterior superior temporal plane, it would be easy to assume this site represents the critical zone. But this site may simply be an artifact of the diagrammatic method, since it is along the posterior superior temporal plane that the lower division bifurcates, and where most of the embolic infarcts begin. If so, this location may merely be the essential focus of the infarct, not the site of the lesion producing Wernicke's aphasia. The precise relationship needs to be established by cases whose lesion is confined to this small site.

Cases of Wernicke's aphasia with a lesion *confined to the superior temporal plane* appear remarkably rare. A 20-year effort at three large hospital-based populations by the author and colleagues has failed to reveal any examples. No less an authority than Charles Foix,[161a] writing on vascular causes of Wernicke's aphasia in 1928, admitted he had seen none. In 1939, Nielsen[359] found 12 cases in the literature with Wernicke's aphasia, whose deficit included reading disturbances with lesions that spared the angular gyrus. These were the same cases Benson and Geschwind later used to support their claim that severe alexia (part of the full Wernicke aphasia syndrome) can arise from a lesion confined to the superior temporal plane.[46] Yet of these 12 cases, three had been reported by the original authors (and also so noted previously by Henschen[222] in his long review) to have had no alexia. Six others had large posterior sylvian lesions of which the superior temporal plane portion was merely a part. Two by detailed description appear to have been old residual subcortical hematomas, a lesion argueably much larger when initially symptomatic than later at autopsy.

In more recent times, Luria[308] considered the superior temporal plane to be the Wernicke area, but his case materials were of traumatic origin from World War II, a notoriously inadequate source material for precise localization. More recently, Kertesz and Benson[255] reported four autopsied cases with lesions involving the superior temporal plane. But the lesions in these cases also spread into the insula and supramarginal gyri, even into the angular gyri. Naeser[353] described lesion larger than the superior temporal plane in a study of four cases documented by CT scan.

In our literature search, only three superior temporal plane lesions have been found with Wernicke's aphasia among 89 published cases with autopsy correlation. Two are subject to criticisms that minimize their utility, while the third is described too briefly to permit much analysis. The first, Gilbert Ballet's case,[222] was actually reported as an example of pure word deafness, a more restricted syndrome. Examined in March 1900 shortly after the stroke, he had pure word deafness, paraphasic speech both spontaneously and on repeating aloud, word blindness, and agraphia. At autopsy in October 1901, 19 months later, the description of the findings fits that of a residue of an old subcortical (so-called slit) hemorrhage, which one can presume was larger at the time of the evaluation of the original clinical deficit. In any case, it is certainly not a isolated lesion of the superior temporal plane.

The second, Souques' case,[222] was followed for 14 years clinically. The deficit faded from an initial picture of Wernicke's aphasia to almost normal within 2 years. Unfortunately, the patient was illiterate before the stroke occurred, so reading and writing were not tested. At autopsy, he appeared to have had an old hematoma, a lesion presumably large enough in the acute stage to have caused the full syndrome of Wernicke's aphasia.

The third case was Kleist's case,[264] Papp, who was said to have sensory aphasia for 2 months, until another stroke altered the clinical picture. No details of reading tests were described. The lesion was, however, confined to the temporal plane.

Henschen,[222] in a review of the literature up to the mid-1920s, concluded that a superior temporal plane lesion does not cause the full picture of Wernicke's aphasia (i.e., both "pure word deafness" and "alexia"). He based this opinion on review of 35 cases with temporal lobe lesions, 20 of whom had "pure word deafness." In none was alexia present. Earlier, Bastian[37] had found alexia and sensory (Wernicke) aphasia in only 5 of 16 temporal lobe cases, and in most of these the lesion was large. Recent studies add no qualitatively new cases: the study of Nazaer et al.[354] contained cases with medium to large lesions, while that of Mazzocchi and Vignolo[318] reported only one case with a smallish lesion, which the authors described as an exception to the other cases in that "anomias were in the foreground."

These data provide little support for the view that a superior temporal plane lesion alone makes the full syndrome of Wernicke's aphasia. The infarction needed to precipitate the full syndrome in the reported cases has been much larger, well beyond the confines of the superior temporal plane.

There is no lack of superior temporal plane cases, but simply a lack of such cases showing the full syndrome of Wernicke's aphasia. Many of the cases with an infarct limited to less than the whole lower division territory lesion appear to have been labeled as "conduction aphasia," "pure word deafness," or "alexia with agraphia."

## Pure Word Deafness

Over 40 cases of pure word deafness described with CT or autopsy correlation are reported. According to the classical formulations, the only deficit should be auditory; spontaneous speech should be normal as should reading comprehension and writing. Eight well-known cases exist with a unilateral lesion confined to the superior temporal plane in the dominant hemisphere. In seven, paraphasic speaking was prominent, a clinical picture not permitted in formulation of "pure word deafness," which, by definition, should be free of a disturbance in speaking. In many, the elements of paraphasic speech later cleared.

Schuster and Taterka's[405] case has been repeatedly cited, but is a disappointment: in addition to the word deafness, in the acute phase the patient had paraphasia for well over a month; more disappointing, when examined at 7 months, no tests of reading were performed. Finally, autopsy revealed the residue of an old slit hemorrhage, scarcely the stuff of precise correlation. Although this case is famous, the early phase of the illness makes it difficult to maintain the "purity" of syndrome of "pure word deafness." In Nielsen's case,[359] Sult, a left superior temporal plane lesion was shown, which was said to be associated with pure word deafness, but there are few satisfying details in the clinical text.

Many of the cases with bilateral lesion also experienced paraphasic speaking with poor comprehension during the acute phase of the stroke. In the famous case reported by Pick,[377] bilateral lesions, including a large left temporal plane lesion, left the patient paraphasic for 4 years. The deficit was only slight when she was examined by the author 10 years later. The most recent case described as pure word deafness[113] had only a few paraphasic errors in spoken speech and in tests indicating comprehension of printed words. He suffered bilateral temporal lobe infarction, documented by CT scan, which the authors inferred had affected the primary auditory cortex. The largest lesion was on the right side.

From the foregoing, it must be concluded that examples of the syndrome of pure word deafness occur only rarely. There is not even much current evidence that unilateral infarcts of the left temporal lobe create a state of impaired auditory discrimination.[13] Instead, temporal lobe infarcts of small size or parenchymatous hemorrhages seem usually to set the stage for a transient form of Wernicke's aphasia whose major clinical feature is a disturbance in auditory comprehension. The spontaneous speech contains many paraphasic errors, especially in the acute stages, enough that the listener may make a preliminary diagnosis of Wernicke's aphasia. When taxed in tasks of reading aloud or for comprehension, the patients make enough errors that the notion of a pure disorder in auditory comprehension is not easily maintained.

### *Cortical Deafness*

The issue of cortical deafness is another matter. At least one autopsied case exists who was well-studied clinically with deafness occasioned by an infarct confined to Heschel's transverse gyrus.[281] This case supports Henschen's claim[222] that such an event can occur. Examples are rare enough that the unilateral lesion is difficult to predict on clinical grounds alone. Bilateral infarcts affecting the temporal plane are a well-recognized course of deafness, although only a few reports have appeared. The 24-year-old man reported by Khurana et al.[260] was a typical example: after the second cerebral embolus, he became completely deaf to all sounds, speech and nonspeech in character, and could not be startled by loud noise. The brain stem auditory evoked studies showed normal waveforms through wave V. The patient's spontaneous speech contained the expected paraphasias, which were of the phonetic type; communication was achieved by writing, and occasional paragraphic errors were observed. The bilateral superior temporal plane infarcts were rather circumscribed.

### *Alexia With Agraphia*

The syndrome of alexia with agraphia has proved remarkably difficult to encounter in actual case descriptions in the literature. Henschen[222] found five "pure" cases among the more than 250 cases with dyslexia and dysgraphia as part of a larger clinical syndrome, noting that the paraphasia in speaking was a frequent accompaniment of the syndrome.

Its general characteristics have been repeatedly described by a number of authorities[46] as a disturbance in reading comprehension and in the morphology and language content of writing that far exceeds the disturbance in auditory comprehension or in spontaneous speech. The original case of Dejerine's[122,123] suffered a lateral parietal infarct which penetrated as far as the ventricular wall. The disturbance in writing and reading was all out of proportion to the modest dysphasia in conversation, but Dejerine did not see the patient in the acute phase. Touche[428] described a similar case, whose remarkably focal cerebral infarct involved the right posterolateral parietal region in a left-handed man; his case also showed mild paraphasia in spoken speech, but not to the degree as the disturbance in reading and writing.

Among the many accounts, mention is usually made[47] that "almost all patients suffering alexia with agraphia have some degree of aphasia which ranges from a minimal degree of word-finding difficulty to a more marked sensory aphasia with paraphasia and comprehension disturbance." This observation raises the possibility the syndrome may be another variant of Wernicke's aphasia. DeMassary[127] suggested that Dejerine himself considered this form of alexia as a form of the syndrome of sensory aphasia, which is more evident when the patient is seen in the early phase of the stroke. We studied such a case for many years who eventually came to autopsy, showing a large lesion affecting much of the posterior left hemisphere (Fig. 16-19). His deficit began as sensory aphasia, affecting all forms of language and all conditions of testing.[412,413] As time passed, the spoken response to auditory language stimuli improved, but that of written response to any tests and response to printed words remained impaired, a disturbance that could be classified grossly as dyslexia with dysgraphia.

The clinical problem posed by the syndrome is not whether it exists but whether it is only a transient acute disorder, or occurs mainly in the chronic state of an initially more severe Wernicke's aphasia. The anatomy of the lesion requires a circumscribed infarction beyond the superior temporal plane. Embolism is the only reliable source of such an infarct, apart from a focal form of vasculitis. In the unusual case in which the posterior cerebral artery takes its origin from the carotid, the main weight of the distal infarction could fall on the parieto-occipital lobe, as happened in our case,[413] but such an event would be most unusual. The available clinical data do not permit the determina-

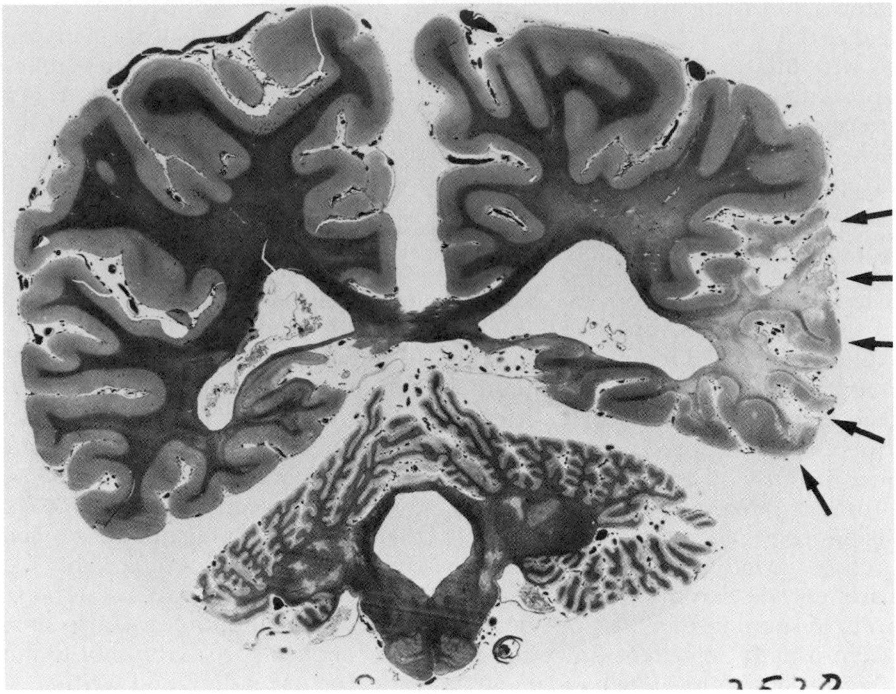

**Fig. 16-19.** Coronal section from posterior half of brain in a case with Wernicke's aphasia, which evolved over years toward a syndrome of dyslexia with dysgraphia.

tion of how acutely this syndrome can occur. The cases in the literature suggest it is a late development from an earlier syndrome of more extensive deficits. The few cases of the syndrome from nonvascular causes do not bear on this problem and are beyond the scope of this book.

## Conduction Aphasia

Conduction aphasia occupies a special position in aphasiology, mainly because its occurrence is more a result of its having been predicted by theories of aphasia than for its isolated occurrence as a clinical entity. For Wernicke,[453–455] who first defined the syndrome, it was presumed to represent the interruption of fiber pathways connecting the sensory language zone of the posterior half of the brain with the Morot language zone in the frontal. For Goldstein,[191] the disorder represented disruption of a brain region located between the major sensory and motor centres, concerned with both functions simultaneously. As has been well documented by Levine and Calvanio,[293] its clinical features are not accounted for by either of the two major theories.

The name has become accepted in clinical circles to characterize those cases with poor repetition, especially for unfamiliar material, and far better auditory and visual comprehension of language than that evident in their spontaneous spoken and written efforts. That spontaneous speech is often contaminated by paraphasic utterances goes unemphasized. Although auditory and visual language comprehension is relatively preserved, neither is normal at any stage of the disorder.[13] The ease with which such disturbances are demonstrated disturbance has proved a major stumbling block to the satisfactory application of the label, conduction aphasia, when faced with such a patient at the bedside.

The disturbance in repeating aloud, on which great stress has been laid,[47,181] is not as useful a distinguishing point in the acute stage of the syndrome. In assessing the deficits in conversation, Burns and Canter[85] found a greater incidence of unwonted phonemes and intrusion of semantically related words among those classified as Wernicke's aphasia than among those with conduction aphasia, but careful testing was required to make this distinction. Patients with conduction aphasia are also said to have a greater tendency to efforts at self-correction[46] than are those with Wernicke's aphasia; in my own experience, this point has applied only to those cases of Wernicke's aphasia with the major syndrome. For ordinary clinical purposes, the distinctions between the errors patterns in speaking in cases with conduction aphasia and Wernicke's aphasia is not an easy one.

Because the site of the infarct lies behind the rolandic region, there is usually no contralateral hemiparesis. Disturbances in eye movements and visual fields are also minor or not present. Buccolinguofacial dyspraxia is a common accompaniment,[46] as is bimanual ideomotor dyspraxia. The dyspraxia of the latter state is different in the two limbs, the limb served by the infarcted hemisphere taking the form of a deafferentation,[138] while the other conforms more to the picture expected in ideomotor dyspraxia.[183]

The syndrome often proves surprisingly evanescent and initially is diagnosed as Wernicke-type aphasia, evolving later into the picture of conduction aphasia.[397] Demonstration of the deficit in the chronic state often requires testing with difficult words which the patient is to repeat aloud.

The *clinicopathologic correlation* is at odds with the theory. The most popular current thesis envisions the interruption of the arcuate fasciculus as the mechanism for the errors.[47,181,182] Presumably, the interruption prevents adequate control from the auditory system over the speech apparatus. Because this thesis hinges on a lesion interrupting the arcuate fasciculus, the expected brain disturbance would be mainly subcortical. The autopsy evidence in support of this thesis is surprisingly slight. The documented lesions[43] have all been superficial infarcts, whose penetration into the subcortical white matter has varied considerably. In some instances, the infarction was completely superficial; in only a few has it been profound enough to produce a cleft deep enough to reach the arculate fasiculus beyond doubt. Recent work by the Damasios[112,113] indicate that two projecting systems may exist, and follow pathways susceptible to injury in even superficial lesions. The cases used for their analysis were not "pure," however, since some degree of disturbance in auditory and reading comprehension was present, although no more than in the usual cases classified as conduction aphasia. Over 20 cases with CT or autopsy correlation are reported with this syndrome, and many show the lesion located in the same area usually attributed to Wernicke's aphasia. Naeser[353] found no difference in the lesion size per slice in cases with conduction or Wernicke's aphasia, but the mean percentage left hemispheral tissue damage was larger in the Wernicke cases than those with conduction aphasia ($P < 0.01$).

Another major thesis of the conduction aphasia considers the deficit to represent a disturbance in kinestetic feedback. Luria[308] coined the term *afferent motor aphasia* to characterize the behavior. He assumed the lesion to lie in the sylvian operculum posterior to the rolandic fissure, yielding a disturbance in pronounciation resulting from faulty anatomic oropharyngeal positionings. The words pronounced would contain sounds different from those intended. These errors, analogous to the typing errors of a novice typist, require considerable listener training for their detection, rather like the recognition of typing errors to those familiar with the typewriter keyboard. The novice listener may easily mistake them as language errors (paraphasias), and assume the speaker has a language disorder. Such an interpretation may be inacurrate, but it remains common medical practice to refer to errors of this type as literal paraphasias. The doubting examiner may well wonder how the patient's language comprehension can be so intact when his speech utterances are so distorted, in some cases to the point of meaningless jargon. This thesis assumes a surface lesion, such as would be expected from the embolic infarction that is almost invariably the responsible lesion. It matches with studies that suggest the major difficulty experienced by these patients in repeating aloud can be considered to represent a disturbance in *en*coding accompanied by a disturbance in short-term memory.[408] A recent patient with this syndrome showed CT scan evidence of an anterior parietal infarct.[300]

As a result of the more modern studies using CT scan, it has been recognized for some time that the syndrome may result from a lower division infarct, a point that should make further trouble for the thesis that Wernicke's aphasia results from superior temporal plane disease. Kleist[264] suggested that some form of mixed hemisphere dominance accounted for those with conduction aphasia instead of Wernicke's aphasia from an infarction of the superior temporal plane. For others, including myself, the disturbance has been considered merely a mild form of sensory aphasia.[306,421] Many such cases show some degree of decreased auditory comprehension when tested, but their ability to read aloud and for comprehension is so much superior that they do not easily qualify for the full syndrome of Wernicke's aphasia as traditionally defined. But they would easily be described as examples of the mild form of Wernicke's aphasia.

## Apraxia

Apraxias are acquired disorders of execution. They represent an inability to perform a previously learned skilled act that is unexplained by weakness, visual loss, incoordination, dementia, sensory loss, or aphasia. Liepmann[301,302] described apraxia as the "incapacity for purposive movement despite retained mobility." Apraxic patients are unable to perform skilled acts because the motor engrams (programs) that guide skilled acts have either been lost or cannot be accessed. Since these deficits in skilled movement are rarely complete, the term dyspraxia is often used. Apraxic deficits may affect movements of the body, face, or limbs. Liepmann proposed that the left hemisphere possessed the motor engrams necessary for skilled movements just as it possessed the linguistic engrams necessary for speech. Left hemisphere dominance for skilled motor activity has been postulated by Kimura and Archibald[261] as well. The overwhelming proportion of dextrals with motor apraxia have left hemisphere lesions.[210] Ajuriagurerra et al.[8] noted 47 cases of ideomotor apraxia and 11 cases of ideational apraxia among 206 left retrorolandic cases and

55 bilateral hemisphere cases. Motor apraxia was absent in their 151 right retrorolandic cases.

## Ideomotor Apraxia

The most common type of motor apraxia is ideomotor apraxia. Liepmann[303] believed that a dissociation occurred between the brain areas that contained the "ideas" for movements and the "motor" areas responsible for execution. As a result, skilled movements involving the limbs are not executed accurately. Ideomotor apraxia may be elicited by asking the patient to show how he would salute, wave goodbye, hammer a nail, saw wood, and so on. In the most severe cases, the action cannot be performed at all. In moderately severe cases the actions are vague and confused. In milder cases the actions are clumsy and lack precision. In general, the worst performance is elicited upon verbal command. Performance may improve on imitation, but still remains abnormal.[210] The best performance is elicited upon actual use of the object.[215] Ideomotor apraxia can take two forms: a bilateral ideomotor apraxia in which both extremities are affected and sympathetic apraxia (callosal apraxia) in which the apraxia is limited to the nondominant left arm. Although the left hemisphere is dominant in most dextrals for both language and skilled motor activity, apraxia does not depend upon the presence of dysphasia. Furthermore, although aphasia commonly accompanies ideomotor apraxia, there is no close relationship between either the severity or the type of aphasia.[34,135,283] Geschwind[182] has suggested cerebral disconnection between the language area and the premotor area in the frontal lobe as an explanation for ideomotor apraxia. Lesions in the vicinity of the left supramarginal gyrus with deep extension into the subjacent white matter could interrupt impulses originating in Wernicke's area that were directed toward the premotor area. Heilman[215] suggests an alternative explanation. He believes that the motor programs for skilled motor movements are stored in the left superior parietal lobe. Skilled motor activity depends upon the transmission of these programs to the premotor area in the left frontal lobe. Ideomotor apraxia may then arise from two different mechanisms:[216] direct destruction of motor programs in the left superior parietal lobe or destruction of the pathways from the left superior parietal lobe to the premotor area of the left frontal lobe (i.e., disconnection).

Typically, bilateral ideomotor apraxia is associated with retrorolandic lesions in the vicinity of the parietal lobe.[211,215] These lesions are usually superficial cortical infarcts in the distribution of the posterior division of the left middle cerebral artery. Although ideomotor apraxia is more common with superficial as opposed to deep lesions, larger deep lesions may produce ideomotor apraxia.[7] Ideomotor apraxia does not occur with smaller lacunar-type infarctions. Little is known about recovery from ideomotor apraxia.[215] However, recovery may be surprisingly rapid in certain cases. Anterior lesions have a better prognosis for recovery than posterior cases.[35]

## Ideational Apraxia

Ideational apraxia bears an uncertain relationship to ideomotor apraxia. Ideational apraxia is a disorder of the sequencing and planning of complex motor acts. It can be elicited by asking the patient to demonstrate complex motor tasks, such as lighting a cigarette or mailing a letter. Hecaen and Gimeno[214] reported 8 cases of ideational apraxia among 47 cases of ideomotor apraxia. Sittig[414] believed that ideational apraxia was only a severe form of ideomotor apraxia. Others believe that ideational apraxia is a distinct entity different from ideomotor apraxia.[133,282]

Ideational apraxia is generally observed after dominant hemisphere parietal lobe lesions. Associated findings may include a fluent aphasia (anomic, semantic, or Wernicke), constructional apraxia, and elements of Gerstmann syndrome. Dementia and confusion are noted in some cases. The localization is the same that might be expected to produce ideomotor apraxia. Bilateral parietal lesions are present in some cases,[8,134] but isolated right parietal lesions seem to produce ideational apraxia only in individuals with anomalous cerebral dominance.[379] Little is known about recovery from ideational apraxia.

## Limb-Kinetic Apraxia

Limb-kinetic apraxia (also innervatory apraxia or melokinetic apraxia) is manifested as a lack of rapidity, skill, and delicacy in the performance of learned motor movements.[210] Liepmann held that in limb-kinetic apraxia "the virtuosity which practice lends to movement is lost. Therefore the movements are . . . clumsy, without precision" (quoted by Kerstesz[253]). The patient is clumsy in the execution of common motor acts such as the manipulation of objects (eating utensils, combs, brushes, saws, hammers, playing cards, etc.). Limb-kinetic apraxia is unilateral and affects the limb contralateral to the cerebral lesion. It may be difficult to distinguish between limb-kinetic apraxia and paresis in some cases.[210] Commonly associated neurologic signs include ataxia, choreoathetosis, grasping, spasticity, weakness, and dystonic posturing. However, the clumsiness in using objects is out of proportion to these other deficits. The perseverative and conceptual disturbances that characterize ideational apraxia are not prominent. Patients with limb-kinetic apraxia perform poorly to command or imitation. Performance may improve slightly with use of the object, but patients often act as if they were somewhat unfamiliar with the use of the object.

Limb-kinetic apraxia may occur after injury to either the right or left premotor cortex or subjacent white matter.[359] Slight weakness is usually present, suggesting that injury to the pyramidal pathways is an essential feature of limb-kinetic apraxia. However, injury limited solely to the pyramidal pathways does not produce limb-kinetic apraxia. Patients with pure motor hemiplegia due to lacunar infarction in the internal capsule do not manifest limb-kinetic apraxia. Thus the elicitation of this sign is a useful indicator that surface cortex or subjacent white matter has been injured. The diagnosis of limb-kinetic apraxia is rarely made, reflecting the doubts of some as to its validity as an apraxic entity discrete from either pyramidal weakness or ideomotor apraxia.[210,253]

### Callosal Apraxia

Callosal apraxia (sympathetic apraxia) represents a restricted form of ideomotor apraxia in which the apraxia is limited to the nondominant arm. Liepmann and Maas[304] first described a patient with a right hemiplegia who was unable to perform skilled movements with his nonparetic left arm. Similar patients have been described by Geschwind and Kaplan[184] and by Watson and Heilman.[445]

Critical to the syndrome is disruption of the anterior portions of the corpus callosum. Infarction of the medial or anterior left frontal lobe with Broca's aphasia and right hemiplegia is often present, but these elements are not critical to the genesis of the apraxia. The apraxia is unilateral and limited to the nondominant arm. If the right arm is not paretic it can be demonstrated to be free of apraxia. The apraxia of the left arm is similar to the bilateral apraxia that characterizes ideomotor apraxia. Two somewhat similar hypotheses have been offered to explain callosal apraxia. Geschwind[182] has suggested that callosal apraxia is due to a disconnection of the right premotor region from the speech area in the left temporal lobe. Verbal instructions are unable to traverse the anterior corpus callosum and reach the right premotor cortex. Hence, the left arm is deprived of verbal instructions to guide its motor activity. The patient of Geschwind and Kaplan[184] was able to perform skilled movements with his left arm on imitation but not on verbal command. However, this has not been the general experience.[215] Thus, this hypothesis does not explain why patients with callosal apraxia continue apraxic upon use of an object or on imitation of the examiner. Heilman[215] suggests that the left arm is apraxic because it is disconnected from the motor engram centers in the left hemisphere.

The lesion producing callosal apraxia may be a rare isolated lesion of the corpus callosum. More commonly the crossing callosal fibers are disrupted in the mesial left hemisphere by either a left anterior cerebral artery territory infarction or an infarction in the distribution of the anterior division of the left middle cerebral artery. These anterior division left middle cerebral artery territory infarctions are associated with right hemiplegia and Broca's aphasia. Injury to the corpus callosum rather than injury to the left supplementary motor cortex is critical to the syndrome.[195]

### Oral-Buccal-Lingual Apraxia

Orofacial or oral-buccal-lingual apraxia is the inability to perform skilled movements with the oral and facial musculature on command. John Hughlings-Jackson[236] had noted that some patients are unable to protrude their tongue on command. In addition these patients may be unable to pucker their lips, cough, lick their lips, puff up their cheeks, or whistle on verbal command. These same acts may be performed well spontaneously. De Renzi et al.[136] found oral apraxia in 90 percent of Broca's aphasics and 33 percent of conduction aphasics. Oral apraxia is unusual in cases of anomic or Wernicke's aphasia. Although oral apraxia is common in global aphasia, testing for oral apraxia may be difficult due to comprehension disturbances. Hecaen and Angelergues[213] have emphasized that oral-buccal-lingual apraxia is not synonymous with Broca's aphasia, as some Broca's aphasics will not be dyspraxic and some subjects with oral-buccal-lingual apraxia will not be aphasic. Oral-buccal-lingual apraxia generally results from an inferior frontal lesion in the premotor cortex adjacent to the face area on the motor strip. Most lesions are cortical and superficial.[426] Occasionally, oral buccal-lingual apraxia may occur after larger deep lesions.[7]

## SYNDROMES OF RIGHT HEMISPHERAL INFARCTION

A wide variety of behavior abnormalities may follow stroke in the right middle cerebral artery territory. These deficits are governed in general by several unifying observations:

1. Despite some rudimentary capacity to comprehend language, language plays no important role in the activities subserved by the right hemisphere.
2. The commitment of cerebral cortex to a specific higher cortical function within the right hemisphere is less precise than in the left hemisphere. While higher cortical functions in the left hemisphere appear to be governed by identifiable "centers" of function, higher cortical functions of the right hemisphere appear to be governed by far-flung "networks."
3. The right hemisphere is dominant for certain aspects of attention[327] including directed attention, focused attention, and vigilance. This specialization for attention may be reflected in a variety of right hemisphere deficits such as neglect, extinction, and impersistence.

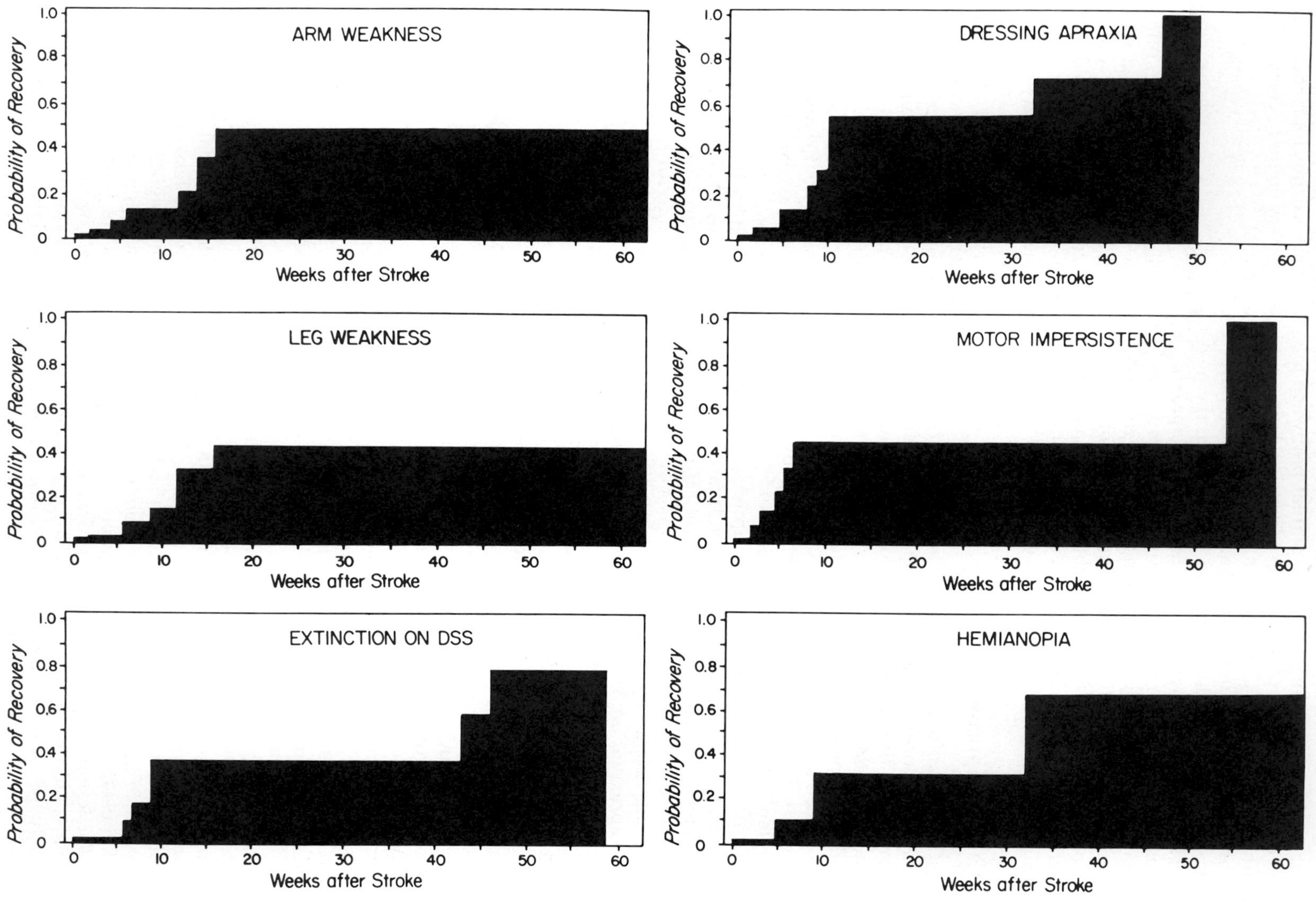
ARM WEAKNESS
DRESSING APRAXIA
LEG WEAKNESS
MOTOR IMPERSISTENCE
EXTINCTION ON DSS
HEMIANOPIA
Probability of Recovery
Weeks after Stroke

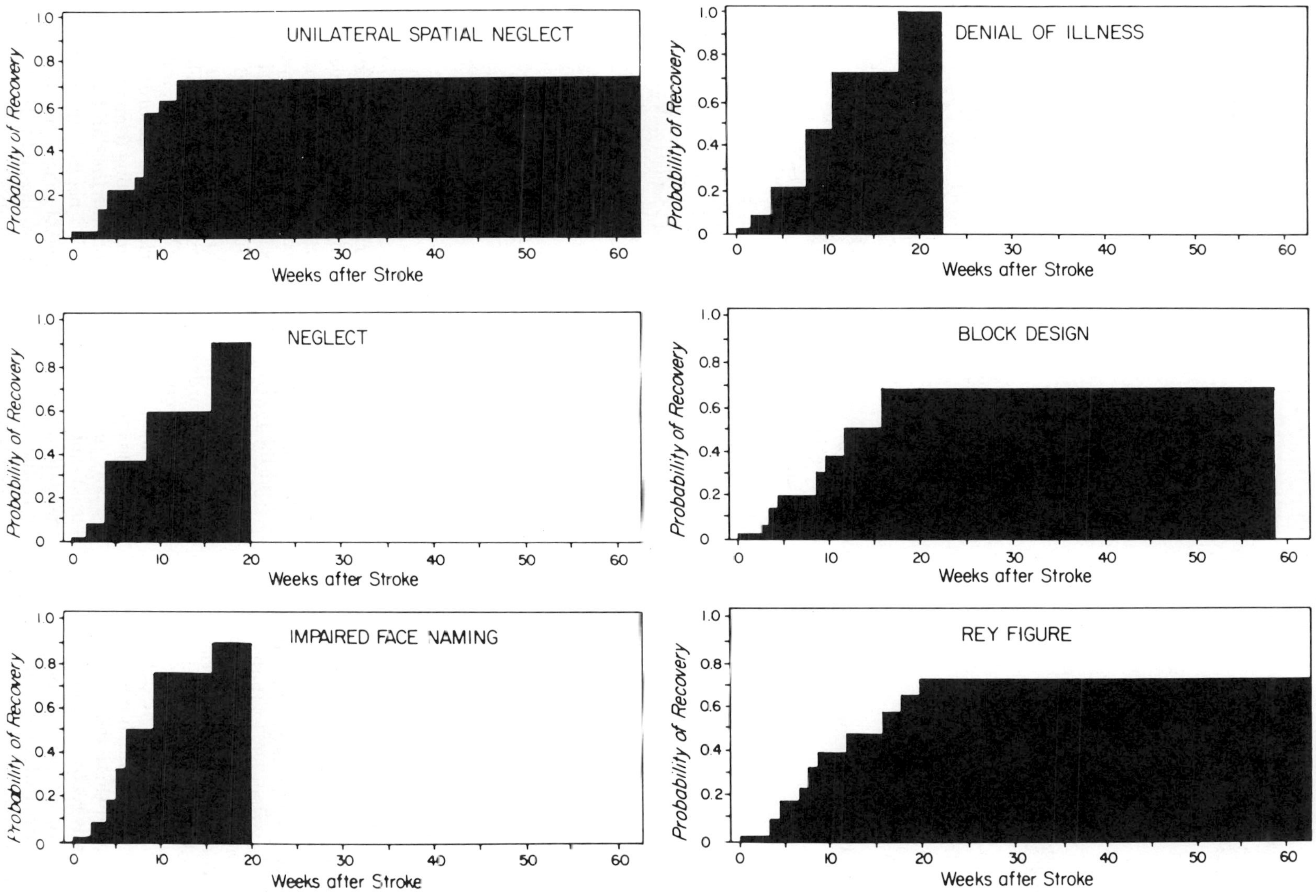


**Fig. 16-20.** The course of deficits in nondominant hemisphere infarction. (From Hier et al.,[226] with permission.)

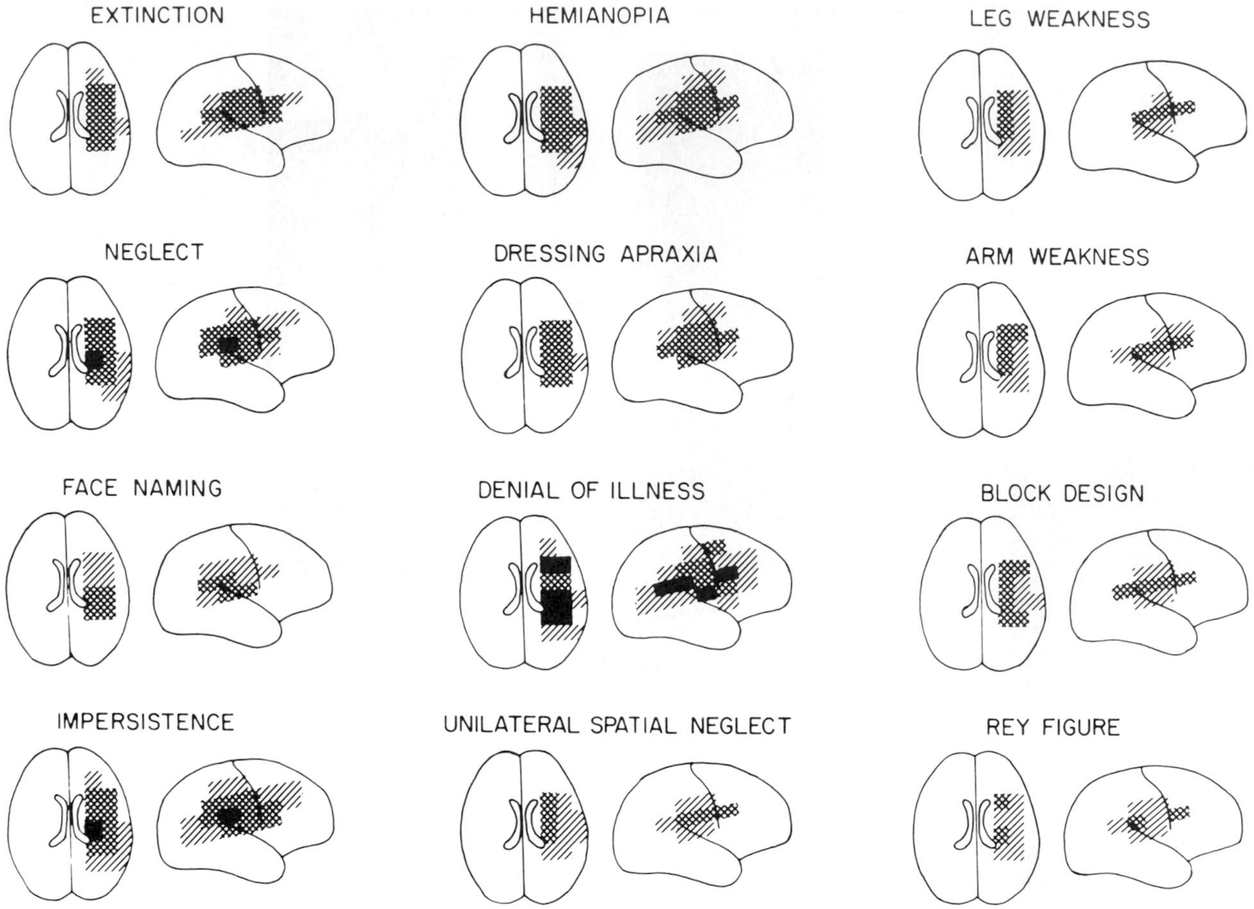


**Fig. 16-21.** Topography of infarction documented by computed tomography scan for cases with nondominant hemisphere deficits. (From Hier et al.,[226] with permission.)

4. Many spatial and quasi-spatial operations are performed by the right hemisphere. This specialization for spatial operations may be reflected in such right hemisphere deficits as prosopagnosia, topographic disorientation, constructional apraxia, and dressing apraxia.
5. Confabulatory behaviors are more common after right hemisphere injury than left.[181] Both reduplicative paramnesia and anosognosia may be considered forms of confabulation occurring after right hemisphere stroke.

Patients without the many neurologic deficits from right hemispheral infarction do much better in rehabilitation than patients with these deficits. Although some patients show a steady recovery from these deficits (Fig. 16-20), others are left with persistent and disabling behavioral abnormalities that include constructional and dressing apraxia, left neglect, and motor impersistence. The size of the lesion, rather than its exact location, is a better prodictor of behavioral deficits after right hemisphere damage (Fig. 16-21).

## Neglect and Extinction

Extinction and neglect are two forms of hemi-inattention that may occur after right hemisphere stroke. Extinction implies that a "stimulus is not perceived only when a second stimulus is presented simultaneously—usually but not necessarily on the opposite side of the body."[406] Unilateral spatial neglect (USN) is a restricted syndrome in which patients fail to copy one side (usually the left) of a figure, failure to read one side of words or sentences, and bisect lines far to the right of center. The term neglect implies a more flagrant syndrome characterized by a failure of the patient to attend to new stimuli coming from one side (usually the left). Neglect is often trimodal (auditory, visual, and tactile). In left-sided neglect, the patient may fail to explore the left side of space; the eyes and body may be turned tonically to the right. Neglect is characterized by "a lack of responsivity to stimuli on one side of the body, in the absence of any sensory or motor deficit severe enough to account for the imperception."[406]

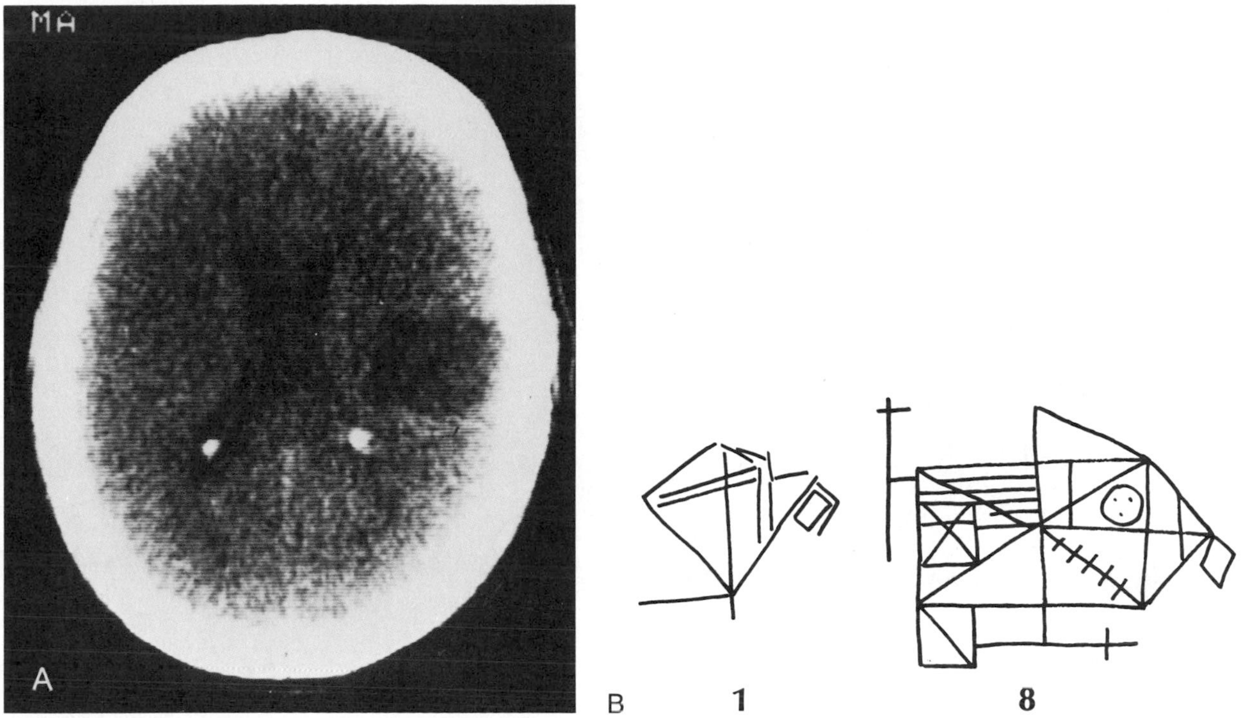


**Fig. 16-22.** (**A**) Computed tomography scan of small right middle cerebral artery territory infarct and (**B**) drawings done at 1 and 8 weeks after stroke.

Battersby et al.[38] found unilateral spatial neglect in 29 percent of their right-brain damaged patients and 12 percent of their left-brain damaged patients. Most subjects with USN had lesions involving either the parieto-occipital or temporo-occipital regions. Using a line-bisection test, Schenkenberg et al.[402] found USN to be more common after right than left brain damage. The mechanism underlying USN is uncertain. Neither hemianopia, oculomotor disorders, nor dementia can account for the phenomenon. Heilman and Valenstein[219] suggest that hemispatial hypokinesia due to hypoarousal explains USN on drawing tasks.

Related to the syndrome of USN is more gross ignorance of the neglect. These patients behave as if they have completely lost the left side of space and the left side of his body. They may ignore visitors on the left side or fail to attend to sounds coming from the left. Marked left neglect tends to occur in conjunction with other markers of severe right hemisphere damage, including anosognosia and motor impersistence. In contrast, USN may occur with smaller right hemisphere strokes which usually have a good prognosis (Fig. 16-22).

Neglect has been traditionally attributed to injury in the vicinity of the right parietal lobe. However, neglect may follow injury to the right frontal lobe, right cingulum, right lenticular nucleus, or right thalamus.[65] Since injury to a variety of cortical and subcortical structures produces left neglect, a cortical network in the right hemisphere underlying directed attention has been proposed.[220,221,327,438] Mesulam[327] posited a network model for attention that includes a reticular element (providing arousal and vigilance), a parietal element (providing sensory and spatial mapping), a frontal element (providing the motor programs for exploration), and a limbic element prosopagnosia, constructional apraxia, and left-sided neglect. Anosognosia is more likely to be associated with severe as opposed to mild hemiparesis.[225] Willanger et al.[460] also noted an association between anosognosia and severity of hemiparesis. Nonetheless, Bisiach et al.[54] have shown that anosognosia for either hemianopia or hemiparesis can be dissociated from elementary neurologic deficits or neglect. Babinski[26] noted that the anosognosia often resolves quickly. Hier et al.[225] found that in all 15 cases of acute right hemisphere stroke followed longitudinally, all recovered from anosognosia within 22 weeks.

The lesion producing anosognosia is usually large. Hier et al.[225] found that the responsible lesion is often extended beyond the parietal lobe to the frontal and temporal lobes (Fig. 16-23). Extension of the lesion to the deep white matter and basal ganglia was frequent. It is probably incorrect to call anosognosia a "right parietal" phenomenon, since many of the lesions are massive and involve much of the right middle cerebral territory (both deep and superficial struc-

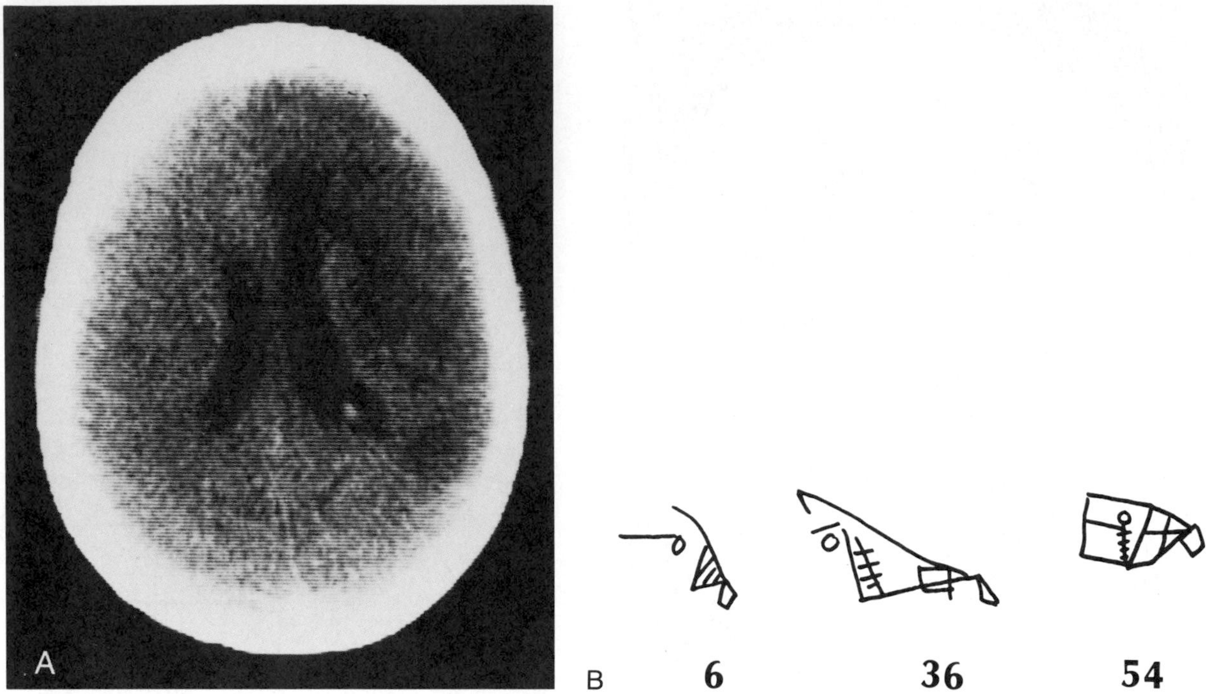


**Fig. 16-23.** (**A**) Computed tomography scan of large right middle cerebral artery territory infarct and (**B**) drawings done at 6, 36, and 54 weeks after stroke.

tures). Involvement of the occipital lobe does not appear to be essential to development of anosognosia. On occasion smaller deep lesions (often basal ganglionic hemorrhages) may produce anosognosia, presumably by undercutting and isolating the cortex of the right hemisphere.

Neither sensory loss, confusion, nor dementia can adequately account for anosognosia. Gerstmann[180] has viewed anosognosia as a disorder of a hypothetical "body image." Although he believed that this body image was "mapped" in the left parietal lobe, input from the right parietal lobe was essential in updating the left parietal lobe as to the condition of the left side of the body. Injury to the right parietal lobe, or to connecting pathways between right and left parietal lobes could lead to anosognosia. Geschwind[182] suggested anosognosia may be due to a disconnection syndrome that prevents sensory impressions from reaching the central language zone in the left hemisphere. Another explanation for anosognosia is that structures essential for the recognition of hemiplegia or other body defects are localized to the right hemisphere. Injury to the right hemisphere could produce an agnosia for illness by disrupting structures essential for the recognition of illness. Finally, anosognosia may be viewed as a variation of "neglect" or "inattention" in that the patient with anosognosia fails to "attend" to his hemiplegia.

## Impersistence

In 1956 Fisher[155] described 10 patients with left hemiplegia who were unable to persist at a variety of willed acts including eye closure, breath holding, conjugate gaze deviation, tongue protrusion, and hand gripping. Fisher introduced the "new term impersistence" to describe "this failure to persist in a motor act." He noted that "mental impairment of some degree was always present" and that impersistence was "encountered almost exclusively in association with left hemiplegia. . . ." Many of the patients had accompanying left neglect, constructional apraxia, and anosognosia. Joynt et al.[245] tested for impersistence in 48 left hemisphere-damaged patients and 34 right hemisphere-damaged patients. Impersistence was found in 26 percent of the patients with right hemisphere damage and 19 percent of the patients with left hemisphere damage. Joynt et al.[245] found impersistence to be more common in patients with mental impairment, especially visuospatial deficits. However, Levin[287] could not demonstrate an increased incidence of impersistence after right as compared to left hemisphere damage. Ben-Vishay et al.[50] found a correlation between impersistence and visuomotor and visuospatial deficits. In addition, impersistence proved to bode poorly for rehabilitation efforts. More recent studies confirm a right hemisphere localization for motor impersistence.[259] Hier et al.[225] found impersistence in 46 percent of 41 subjects with acute right hemisphere strokes. Impersistence correlated with a variety of other deficits, including severity of hemiparesis, prosopagnosia, dressing apraxia, constructional apraxia, left neglect, and anosognosia. Motor impersistence occurred only after the largest lesions. Injury generally extended to the frontal, parietal, temporal, and deep structures. No specific locus of injury for "impersistence" was found within the right hemisphere. Rather, impersistence reflected diffuse and widespread dysfunction. Hier et al.[225] found recovery from motor impersistence to be quite indolent.

The mechanism underlying impersistence is unknown. Motor impersistence may reflect a depletion of vigilance or sustained attention following widespread injury to the right hemisphere. The anatomic locus of those structures involved in sustained attention and vigilance is unknown. Widespread networks in the right hemisphere may underlie focused attention.

### Dressing Apraxia

"Apraxia for dressing" was described in 1941 by Brain.[74] Dressing apraxia refers to confusions in the orientation of clothing during dressing. As McFie et al.[320] commented these "difficulties appeared to be due to confusions regarding top and bottom, back and front, and right and left with reference to the garments." Roth[395] noted the close association between constructional apraxia and dressing apraxia. Dressing apraxia occurs almost exclusively with lesions of the right hemisphere. Although constructional apraxia occurs with either right or left hemisphere lesions, the constructional apraxia that occurs with left hemisphere lesions is rarely associated with dressing apraxia. After right hemisphere damage, stroke large enough to produce both dressing apraxia and constructional apraxia are larger than those strokes producing only constructional apraxia. Unilateral spatial neglect contributes to difficulties in dressing as well. Dressing apraxia should not be diagnosed in the presence of disabling hemiplegia that interferes with dressing.

### Loss of Topographic Memory and Disorientation for Place

Loss of topographic memory is the inability of some patients to find their way in familiar surroundings, to recognize familiar surroundings, and to learn new routes in unfamiliar surroundings. Loss of topographic memory is somewhat different from disorientation to place, which refers to patients who are confused as to their current location.[158] Critchley[104] described several patients who were constantly getting lost in familiar surroundings. Many of his subjects had biparietal injury. A few had lesions limited to the posterior right hemisphere. Critchley described one patient with a right middle cerebral artery territory infarction who "will often pass his home without knowing that it is his, and will wander around for many minutes trying to decide where he does live. . . ." In milder cases, patients recognize surroundings as familiar, in more severe cases even very familiar surroundings may seem strange. Critichley described another patient with a right middle cerebral artery occlusion who could not recognize "the countryside he should have known so well. His home and surroundings are no longer familiar. . . ." Loss of topographic memory is uncommon. Hecaen[208] reported 40 cases of loss of topographic memory, 29 with right hemisphere lesions and 3 with bilateral lesions. Many patients have bilateral parietal lesions, although some have unilateral right parietal lesions.[22] Landis et al.[277] described 16 patients with loss of topographic familiarity, all had right medial temporoparietal lesions. The mechanism underlying loss of topographic memory is uncertain. The failure to recognize familiar surroundings suggests an agnostic defect similar to that underlying prosopagnosia. The inability to follow familiar routes and the inability to orient oneself in space suggests a failure to create an internal spatial representation of the external world. Ross[390] has suggested that visual-modality specific memory defects may underlie both loss of topographic memory deficits and prosopagnosia.

### Disorders of Spatial Localization

The right hemisphere plays a special role in the spatial localization of stimuli. This effect has been demonstrated for both visual and auditory stimuli. With regard to determination of spatial orientation of objects in space, the severest deficits have been noted after posterior right hemisphere damage.[132,325] Short-term spatial memory (a skill analogous to the auditory short-term memory task of digit span) is a dominant function of the posterior right hemisphere.[131] Auditory localization of sounds in space also depends upon an intact posterior right hemisphere.[54]

### Confusion and Delirium

Acute confusion and delirium are states characterized by impaired orientation, diminished attention, and aberrant perception. Alertness is usually well maintained, clarity and speed of thinking are diminished, and memories are poorly formed. Inattentiveness, poor concentration, and alerting to irrelevant stimuli are present. There is overlap between confusional and delirious states with delirium considered by some to be a subset of a confusion. Delirium is characterized by disturbed perception with terrifying hallucinations, vivid dreams, fantasies, insomnia, and overactivity. Acute confusional states have been reported after right middle cerebral artery infarctions.[404] Mesulam and colleagues[328] reported three cases of sudden onset of acute confusion accompanied by retropulsion, unsteady gait, incontinence, difficulty in using common objects, and lack of concern for the illness. Mental agitation evolved into a state of irritable sluggishness, inattention, and memory disorder. Mullaley et al.[351,352] reported acute confusion in 13 patients with right parietal lobe lesions and 4 with right temporal lobe lesions. Levine and Finklestein[293] added eight patients with a behavioral disorder characterized by hallucinations, delusions, agitation, and confusion remotely related (1 month to 11 years) to right temporoparietal stroke or trauma. Dunne et al.[145] found that 19 (3 percent) of 661 stroke patients presented as delirium, confusion, dementia, or psychosis. Nearly all had right hemisphere lesions. Elementary neurologic findings were either absent or subtle. In 41 patients with right middle cerebral territory infarctions, Mori and Yamadori[349] found acute confusion in 25 and acute delirium in 6. Caplan et al.[89] found posterior right temporal lesions more likely to produce acute confusion than posterior right parietal lesions. The propensity of temporal lesions to produce confusional states may be explained by the proximity of these lesions to the underlying limbic system. Confusional states that follow brain infarction may result from one of two processes: disrupted modulation of affective responses in the limbic system or disruption of right hemisphere networks subserving attention.

## Confabulation and Reduplicative Paramnesia

Confabulation is the unintentional production of inappropriate and fabricated information. Confabulation is often associated with a failure to inhibit incorrect responses, poor error awareness, and poor self-correction abilities. Impaired memory, poor motivation, and anosognosia are often present. Since many of these associated behaviors are characteristics of frontal lobe pathology, confabulation is often linked to frontal lobe damage. Although impaired memory is often associated with confabulation, the two behaviors vary independently in severity.[45,326] Reduplication is a special form of confabulation. It appears to reflect an attempt of the brain-injured patient to fuse experiences from two disparate periods in his life. In instances of reduplication for place, the patient holds an inaccurate belief that two versions of a geographic location exist. The patient wrongly believes that he is residing in a second version of a familiar setting. The hospitalized patient may persist in a belief that he is at home or at another hospital despite repeated attempts to orient him to his current location. Luria[309(p.168)] describes several patients with right hemisphere lesions and reduplication for place. He says he "shall never forget a group of patients with deep lesions . . . of the right hemisphere. . . . They firmly believed that at one and the same time they were in Moscow and also in another town. They suggested that they had left Moscow and gone to the other town. They suggested that they were still in Moscow where an operation had been performed on their brain. Yet they found nothing contradictory about these conclusions." Environmental reduplication occurs most commonly after right frontoparietal lobe injury. Reduplication of person (a false belief that two versions of an individual exist) may also occur after right hemisphere injury. Like reduplication of place, reduplication of person is a restricted form of confabulation.

## Constructional Apraxia

In 1934 Kleist[264] described constructional apraxia as "a disturbance which appears in formative activities (arranging, building, drawing) and in which a spatial part of the task is missed, although there is no apraxia of single movements." Kleist's definition entails the key aspects of constructional apraxia: patients fail at tasks that require the manipulation of objects in space. A variety of tests have been utilized to identify constructional apraxia, including the copying of block designs, the copying of simple and complex figures, puzzle constructions, mental rotations, and three-dimensional model building. Constructional apraxia is synonymous with other terms, including apractognosia, constructional disability, and visuospatial agnosia. Constructional apraxia occurs after injury to either cerebral hemisphere.[19] Among 67 patients with constructional apraxia, Piercy et al.[378] reported 42 with right-sided lesions and 25 with left-sided lesions. Arrigoni and De Renzi[21] found constructional apraxia to be more prevalent in right-brain damaged than left-brain damaged subjects. Most lesions are in the vicinity of the parietal lobe.[398] The nature of constructional apraxia differs according to the hemisphere injured. Although unilateral spatial neglect is prominent after right hemisphere lesions, it is absent with left hemisphere lesions. Patients with left-sided lesions improve their drawings when aided by visual cues, whereas patients with right-sided lesions do not. Warrington et al.[443] suggested that the constructional apraxia that follows right-hemisphere damage is a visuospatial disorder whereas the constructional apraxia that follows left hemisphere damage is an executive disorder. The drawings of left hemisphere damaged patients are oversimplified with reduced detail, whereas left unilateral neglect characterizes the drawings of right hemisphere damaged patients. However, Gainotti et al.[173] were not able to distinguish right-sided from left-sided constructional. Based upon this work and the work of Heilman et al.,[217] Ross and Mesulam[394] proposed that the right hemisphere was dominant for the modulation of affective language, and that this modulation was organized in a fashion analogous to left hemisphere organization for propositional language.

In a subsequent study, Ross[391] provided additional confirmatory evidence of the functional-anatomic organization of the affective components of language in the right hemisphere. By utilizing a bedside examination strategy, analogous to a routine aphasia examination, combined with CT scan mappings, he observed that the organization of affective language in the right hemisphere mirrored that of propositional language in the left hemisphere. The resulting disturbances of affective modulation were coined the aprosodias. In analogy with the aphasias, Ross[391,393] proposed the existence of motor, sensory, global, conduction, and transcortical aprosodias. In motor aprosody, the patient is unable to utilize prosody to inject affect in his speech nor is he able to repeat the affect-laden prosody of others. Yet he can comprehend the affect conveyed by the prosody of other speakers. The patient with sensory aprosody shows poor comprehension of affective prosody and cannot repeat affective prosody, but has normal spontaneous affective prosody in his own speech. Global aprosody is reflected in apraxics according to drawing errors. Hecaen and Albert[210] suggest that "constructional apraxia may result from a breakdown in different underlying neuropsychological mechanisms, depending on the hemisphere damaged." Critchley[104] sees constructional apraxia as "an executive defect within a visuospatial domain." Constructional apraxia may also be viewed as a spatial agnosia, that is a defect in the comprehension of spatial relationships.[383] Similarly, Whitty and Newcombe[459] argued that "the nature of the visual spatial difficulty appears to be of an agnostic rather than simple perceptual type. The term constructional apraxia is not entirely satisfactory."

## Allesthesia

Allesthesia (also allochiria) is the referral of a sensory stimulus (visual, tactile, or auditory) from one side of the body to the other.[240,242] Allesthesia is most often seen in the setting of right hemisphere damage with left-sided neglect. When the left side is touched, the sensation may be experienced by the patient on the right side. Allesthesia may also occur in the setting of spinal cord injury or conversion hysteria.

## Amusia

Amusia (loss of musical ability secondary to brain disease) has been an elusive deficit to study.[48] Brust[81] concluded that no simple relationship exists between the location of a lesion and extent of musical disability. Case reports of expressive amusia after right hemisphere lesions are numerous. These patients are unable to sing or whistle but have preserved language function and melody recognition. Receptive amusia may also occur with right hemisphere lesions. Because of its complexity, the neural basis of music remains obscure. Amusia as an isolated phenomena may occur after right hemisphere lesions of varying location, size, and etiology.

## Aprosody and Affective Agnosia

Monrad-Krohn[348] defined prosody as the musical quality of speech which is produced by "variations in pitch, rhythm, and stress of pronunciation. . . ." After right hemisphere damage, some patients are unable to intone affect into their speech. This deficit is known as aprosody. Heilman and colleagues[217] noted that right temporoparietal lesions caused defects in the comprehension of affective speech and termed this disorder affective agnosia. Tucker and colleagues[430] observed that right temporoparietal lesions caused both affective comprehension deficits and deficits in evoking emotional intonation on a speech repetition task. Ross and Mesulam[392] described a loss of spontaneous affective behavior in patients with right frontal opercular lesions and thought these patients could experience emotions inwardly and could comprehend the affective behaviors of others. It is characterized by defective spontaneous affective prosody, impaired repetition of affective prosody, and impaired comprehension of affective prosody. Transcortical aprosody is characterized by preserved repetition of affective prosody, whereas conduction aprosody is characterized by defective repetition of affective prosody.

## REFERENCES

1. Abbie AA: The morphology of the forebrain arteries with especial reference to the evolution of the basal ganglia. J Anat 68:432, 1934
2. Abbie AA: The vascular supply of the internal capsule. Med J Aust 1934
3. Adams HP, Demasio HC, Putman SF, Demasio AR: Middle cerebral artery occlusion as a cause of isolated subcortical infarction. Stroke, 1983
4. Adams HP, Gross CE: Embolism distal to stenosis of the middle cerebral artery. Stroke 12:228, 1981
5. Adams JH, Graham DI: Twelve case of fatal cerebral infarction due to arterial occlusion in the absence of atheromatous stenosis or embolism. J Neurol Surg Psychiatr 30:4379, 1957
6. Adams RD, Victor M: Principles of Neurology. McGraw-Hill, New York, 1984
7. Agostini E, Coletti A, Orlando G, Tredici G: Apraxia in deep cerebral lesions. J Neurol Neurosurg Psychiatry 46:804, 1983
8. Ajuriaguerra J, Hecaen H, Angelergues R: Les apraxies: varietes clinique et lateralisation lesionelle. Rev Neurol (Paris) 102:494, 1960
9. Akelatis AJ: Symmetrical bilateral granular atrophy of the cerebral cortex of vascular origin: a

clinico-pathologic study. Am J Psychiatry 99:447, 1942
10. Alajouanine T, Boudin G, Pertuiset B, Pepin B: Le syndrome operculaire unilateral avec atteinte contralaterale du territoire des V,VII,IX, XI,XXIIème nerfs craniens. Rev Neurol (Paris) 101:167, 1959
11. Alajouanine T, Obredane A, Durand M: Le Syndrome de Desintegration Phonetique dans l'Aphasie. Masson, Paris, 1939
12. Albert ML: A simple test for neglect. Neurology (NY) 23:658, 1973
13. Albert ML, Goodglass H, Helm NA et al: Clinical Aspects of Dysphasia. Springer-Verlag, New York, 1981
14. Alexander CB, Burger PC, Gore JA: Dissecting aneurysms of the basilar artery in 2 patients. Stroke 10:294, 1979
15. Alexander L: The vascular supply of the striatopallidum. Res Pub Assoc Nerv Ment Dis 21:77, 1941
16. Amyes EW, Nielsen JM: Clinicopathologic study of vascular lesions of the anterior cingulate region. Bull Los Angeles Neurol Soc 20:112, 1955
17. Appenzeller O: The Autonomic Nervous System. North-Holland Publishing, Amsterdam, 1970
18. Araki G: Small infarctions of the basal ganglia with special reference to transient ischemic attacks. Recent Adv Gerontol 469:161, 1978
19. Arena R, Gainotti G: Constructional apraxia and visuoperceptive disabilities in relation to laterality of cerebral lesions. Cortex 14:463, 1978
20. Aring CD, Merritt HH: Differential diagnosis between cerebral hemorrhage and cerebral thrombosis. Arch Intern Med 56:435, 1935
21. Arrigoni G, De Renzi E: Constructional apraxia and hemispheric locus of lesion. Cortex 1:170, 1964
22. Assal G: Regression des troubles de la reconnaissance des physionomies et de la memoire topographique. Rev Neurol (Paris) 121:184, 1969
23. Atkins R: Case of sudden and complete aphasia and partial right hemiplegia, lesion of Broca's convolution, with a small haemorrhage in substance of corpus callosum. J Ment Sci 22:406, 1876
24. Auld AW, Shafey S: Transient ischemic attacks not produced by extracranial vascular disease: a plea for early and complete angiographic evaluation. South Med J 69:722, 1976
25. Austregesilo A, Borges-Forte A: Sur un cas de hemischorée avec lésion du noyau caude. Rev Neurol (Paris) 67:477, 1937
26. Babinski J: Anosognosie. Rev Neurol (Paris) 31:365, 1918
27. Baker AB: Structure of the small cerebral arteries and their changes with age. Am J Pathol 13:453, 1937
28. Baloh RW, Yee RD, Honrubia V: Optokinetic nystagmus and parietal lobe lesions. Ann Neurol 7:269, 1980
29. Barat M, Constant P, Mazaux JM, Caille JM, Arne L: Correlations anatomo-cliniques dans l'apasie: apport de la tomodensitomatrie. Rev Neurol (Paris) 134:611, 1978
30. Barat M, Mazaux JM, Bioulac B et al: Troubles due langage de type aphasique et lesions putamino-caudees. Rev Neurol (Paris) 137:343, 1981
31. Barnett HJM, Boughner DR, Taylor DW et al: Further evidence relating mitral valve prolapse to cerebral ischemic events. N Engl J Med 302:139, 1980
32. Barnett HJM, Jones MW, Boughner DR, Kostuk WJ: Cerebral ischemic events associated with prolapsing mitral valve. Arch Neurol 33:777, 1976
33. Barnett HJM, Peerless SJ, Kaufmann JCE: "Stump" of internal carotid artery: a source for further cerebral embolic ischemia. Stroke 9:448, 1978
34. Basso A, Capitani E, Luzzatti C, Spinnler H: Intelligence and left hemisphere disease: the role of aphasia, apraxia and size of lesion. Brain 104:721, 1981
35. Basso A, Luzzatti C, Spinnler H: Is ideomotor apraxia the outcome of damage to well-defined regions of the left hemisphere? J Neurol Neurosurg Psychiat 43:118, 1980
36. Basso A, Taborelli A, Vignolo A: Dissociated disorders of speaking and writing in aphasia. J Neurol Neurosurg Psychiat 41:556, 1978
37. Bastian HC: Some problems in connection with aphasia and other speech defects. Lancet 1:933, 1005, 1131, 1187, 1897
38. Battersby WS, Bender MB, Pollack M: Unilateral spatial agnosia (inattention) in patients with cerebral lesions. Brain 79:68, 1956
39. Beal MF, Williams RS, Richardson EP, Fisher CM: Cerebral embolism as a cause of transient ischemic attacks and cerebral infarction. Neurology (NY) 31:860, 1981
40. Beevor CE: On the distribution of the different arteries supplying the human brain. Phil Trans R Soc Ser B, CCI, 1908
41. Bender MB: Extinction and other patterns of sensory interaction. Adv Neurol 18:117, 1977
42. Bender MB: Brain control of conjugate horizontal and vertical eye movements: a survey of the structural and functional correlates. Brain 103:23, 1980
43. Benson DF: Aphasia, Alexia and Agraphia. Churchill Livingstone, New York, 1979
44. Benson DF, Barton M: Constructional disability. Cortex 6:19, 1970
45. Benson DF, Gardner H, Meadows JC: Reduplicative amnesia. Neurology (NY) 26:147, 1976
46. Benson DF, Geschwind N: The aphasias and related disorder. In Baker AB, Baker LH (eds): Clinical Neurology. Vol 1. Harper & Row, Hagerstown, 1976
47. Benson DF, Sheremata WA, Bouchard R et al: Conduction aphasia. Arch Neurol 28:339, 1973
48. Benton AL: The amusias. In Critchley M, Henson RA (eds): Music and the Brain. Heinemann, London, 1977
49. Benton AL, Van Allen MW: Facial recognition in patients with cerebral disease. Cortex 4:344, 1968
50. Ben-Yishay Y, Diller L, Gerstman L et al.: The

relationship between impersistence, intellectual function and outcome of rehabilitation in patients with left hemiplegia. Neurology (NY) 18:852, 1968
51. Berry RG, Alpers GJ: Occlusion of the carotid circulation: pathological consideration. Neurology (NY) 7:233, 1957
52. Bigelow NH: Intracranial dissecting aneurysms: an analysis of their significance. Arch Pathol 60:271, 1955
53. Birch HG, Belmont I, Karp E: Delayed information processing and extinction following cerebral damage. Brain 90:113, 1967
54. Bisiach E, Cornacchia L, Sterzi R, Vallar G: Disorder perceived auditory lateralization after lesions of the hemisphere. Brain 107:37, 1984
55. Bisiasch E, Luzzatti C: Unilateral neglect of representational space. Cortex 14:129, 1978
56. Bizzi E: Discharge of frontal eye field neurons during eye movements in unanesthetized monkeys. Science 157:1588, 1967
57. Bizzi E: Discharge of frontal eye field neurons during saccadic and following eye movements in unanesthetized monkeys. Exp Brain Res 6:69, 1968
58. Black FW, Strub RL: Constructional apraxia in patients with discrete missile wounds of the brain. Cortex 12:212, 1976
59. Blackwood W, Bratty P, Mair WGP: p. 146. In Jakob H (ed): Observations on Occlusive Vascular Disease of the Brain. Vol 3. Thieme, Stuttgart, 1963
60. Bladin PF: A radiologic and pathologic study of embolism of the internal carotid-middle cerebral arterial axis. Radiology 82:614, 1964
61. Blumstein SE, Baker E, Goodglass H: Phonological factors in auditory comprehension in aphasia. Neuropsychologia 15:19, 1977
62. Bluschke V, Hennerici M, Scharf RE et al: Mitralklappenprolaps-Syndrom und Thrombozytenaktivität bei jungen Patienten mit zerebralen Ischämien. Dsch Med Wochenschr 107:410, 1982
63. Bodamer J: Die Prosop-Agnosie. Arch Psychiatr Nervenkr 179:6, 1947
64. Bogen JE, Bogen GM: Wernicke's region—where is it? Ann NY Acad Sci 280:834, 1976
65. Bogousslavsky J, Miklossy J, Regli F et al: Subcortical neglect: neuropsychological, and neuropathological correlations with anterior chor artery territory infarction. Ann Neurol 23:448, 1988
66. Boller F: Destruction of Wernicke's area without language disturbance: a fresh look at crossed aphasia. Neuropsychologia 11:243, 1973
67. Bonhoeffer K: Klinischer und anatomischer Befund zur Lehre von der Apraxie und der "Motorischen Sprachbahn." Monatsschr Psychiatr Neurol 35:113, 1914
68. Botez MI, Wertheim N: Expressive aphasia and amusia following right frontal lesion in a right-handed man. Brain 82:186, 1959
69. Boulliaud J: Recherches cliniques propres a demonstrer que la perte de la parole correspond a la lesion des lobules anterieurs du cerveau, et a confirmer l'opinion de M. Gall sur le siege de l'organe du langage articule. Arch Gen Med 8:25, 1825
70. Bounds JV, Sandok BA, Barnhorst DA: Fatal cerebral embolism following aorto-coronary bypass graft surgery. Stroke 7:611, 1976
71. Bourneville: Atherome generalise: obliterations multiples (aphasie; sphacele du pied, etc.). Prog Med 2:278, 1874
72. Bourneville: Atherome generalise: obliterations multiples (aphasie; sphacele du pied, etc.). Prog Med 2:296, 1874
73. Bousser MG, Dubois B, Castaigne P: Perts de connaissance breves au cours des accident ischemiques cerebraux. Ann Med Interne 132:300, 1981
74. Brain WR: Visual disorientation with special reference to the lesions of the right hemisphere. Brain 64:244, 1941
75. Brain WR: Speech Disorders. Butterworths, London, 1962
76. Bramwell B: A remarkable case of aphasia. Brain 21:343, 1898
77. Brierley JB, Adams JH, Connor RCR, Triep CS: The effects of systemic hypotension upon the human brain. Brain 89:235, 1966
78. Broadbent WH: On the cerebral mechanism of speech and thought. Trans R Med Chiar Soc (London) 55:145, 1872
79. Broca P: Remarques sur le siege de la faculte du language articule, suivies d'une observation d'aphemie (pere de la parole). Bull Soc Anatom Paris 6:330, 1861
80. Brown JW: Aphasia, Apraxia, and Agnosia. CC Thomas, Springfield, Ill, 1972
81. Brust JCM: Music and language. Brain 103:367, 1980
82. Brust JCM, Shafer SQ, Richter RW, Bruun B: Aphasia in acute stroke. Stroke 7:167, 1976
83. Bruyn GW, Gathier JC: The operculum syndrome. p. 776. In Vinken PJ, Bruyn GW (eds): Handbook of Clinical Neurology. Vol 2. North-Holland Publishing, Amsterdam, 1976
84. Buck R, Duffy RJ: Nonverbal communication of affect in brain-damaged patients. Cortex 16:331, 1980
85. Burns MS, Cantor CJ: Phonemic behavior of aphasic patients with posterior cerebral languages. Brain Lang 4:492, 1977
86. Campbell DC, Oxbury JM: Recovery from unilateral visuo-spatial neglect. Cortex 12:303, 1976
87. Caplan LR: A 62-year-old Haitian woman with strokes, renal disease and abdominal pain. N Engl J Med 315:567, 1986
88. Caplan LR, Hier DB, D'Cruz I: Cerebral embolism in the Michael Reese Stroke Registry. Stroke 14:30, 1983
89. Caplan LR, Kelly M, Kase CS et al: Infarcts of the inferior d of the right middle cerebral artery: mirror image of Wernicke's aphasia. Neurology (NY) 36:1015, 1986
90. Castaigne P, Lhermitte F, Gautier J-C et al: Internal carotid artery occlusion: a study of 61 instances in 50 patients with post-mortem data. Brain 93:231, 1970

91. Chater N, Spetzler R, Tonnemachar K et al: Microvascular bypass surgery. I. Anatomical studies. J Neurosurg 44:712, 1976
92. Chiari H: Über das Verhalten des Teilungswinkels der Carotis communis bei der Endarteritis chronic deformans. Verh Dtsch Ges Pathol 9:326, 1905
93. Chouppe: Ramollissement superficiel du cerveau interessant surtout la troisieme circonvolution frontale gauche, sans aphasie. Bull Soc Anatom Paris 45:365, 1870
94. Cicone M, Wapner W, Gardner H: Sensitivity to emotional expressions and situations in organic patients. Cortex 16:145, 1980
95. Clower BR, Sullivan DM, Smith RR: Intracranial vessels lack vasa vasorum. J Neurosurg 61:44, 1984
96. Cohen MM, Hemalatha CP, D'Addario RT, Goldman HW: Embolism from a fusiform middle cerebral artery aneurysm. Stroke 11:58, 1980
97. Cohn R, Neumann MA, Wood DH: Prosopagnosia: a clinicopathological study. Ann Neurol 1:177, 1977
98. Cole MF, Cole M: Pierre Marie's Papers on Speech Disorders. Hafner, New York, 1971.
99. Columbo A, DeRenzi E, Faglioni P: The occurrence of visual neglect in patients with unilateral cerebral disease. Cortex 12:221, 1976
100. Cords R: Optisch-motorisches Feld und optisch-motorishe Bahn. Albrecht von Graefes Arch Ophthalmol 117:58, 1926
101. Corston RN, Kendall BE, Marshall J: Prognosis in middle cerebral artery stenosis. Stroke 15:237, 1984
102. Coslett HB, Brashear HR, Heilman KM: Pure word deafness after bilateral primary auditory cortex infarcts. Neurology (Cleveland) 34:347, 1984
103. Costa LD, Vaughan G Jr, Horwitz M et al: Patterns of behavioral deficit associated with visual spatial neglect. Cortex 5:242, 1969
104. Critchley M: The Parietal Lobes. Hafner Press, New York, 1953
105. Croisile B, Henry E, Trillet M, Aimard G: Loss of motivation for speaking with bilateral lacunes in the anterior limb of the internal capsule. Clin Neurol Neurosurg 91:3257, 1989
106. Cutting J: Study of anosognosia. J Neurol Neurosurg Psychiatry 41:548, 1978
107. Daffner KR, Ahern GL, Weintraub S, Mesulam MM: Dissociation neglect behavior following sequential strokes in the hemisphere. Ann Neurol 28:97, 1990
108. Damasio AR, Damasio H: Musical faculty and cerebral dominance. In Critchley M, Henson RA (eds): Music and the Brain. CC Thomas, Springfield, IL, 1977
109. Damasio A, Damasio H, Chang Chi H: Neglect following damage to frontal lobe or basal ganglia. Neuropsychologia 18:123, 1980
110. Damasio AR, Damasio H, Rizzo M et al: Aphasia with non hemorrhagic lesions of the basal ganglia and the internal capsule. Arch Neurol 39:15, 1982
111. Damasio AR, Damasio H, Van Hoesen GW: Prosopagnosia: anatomic basis and behavioral mechanisms. Neurology (NY) 32:331, 1982
112. Damasio H, Damasio AR: The anatomic basis of conduction aphasia. Brain 103:337, 1980
113. Damasio H, Damasio AR: Localization of lesions in conduction aphasia. p. 231. In Kertesz A (ed): Localization in Neuropsychology Academic Press, New York, 1983
114. Damasio H, Damasio AR, Hamsher K, Varney N: CT scan correlates of aphasia and allied disorders. Neurology (Minneapolis) 29:572, 1979
115. Daroff RB, Hoyt WF: Supranuclear disorders of occular control system in man: Clinical, anatomical and physiological correlates. p. 175. In Bach-Y-Rita P, Collins CC et al (eds): The Control of Eye Movements. Academic Press, New York, 1971
116. David NJ, Gordon KK, Friedberg SJ et al: Fatal atheromatous cerebral embolism associated with bright plaques in the retinal arterioles. Neurology (NY) 13:708, 1963
117. Davis DO, Rumbaugh CL, Gilson JM: Angiographic diagnosis of small-vessel cerebral emboli. Acta Radiol (Stockh) 9:264, 1969
118. Davison C, Goodhart SP, Needles W: Cerebral localization and cerebral vascular disease. Arch Neurol Psychiatry 30:749, 1933
119. Day AL: Anatomy of the extracranial vessels. p. 9. In Smith RR (ed): Stroke and the Extracranial Vessels. Raven Press, New York, 1984
120. Deck JHN, Lee MA: Mucin embolism to cerebral arteritis: a fatal complication of carcinoma of the breast. J Can Sci Neurol 5:327, 1978
121. Dee HL: Visuoconstructive and visuoperceptive deficits in patients with unilateral cerebral lesions. Neuropsychologia 8:305, 1970
122. Dejerine J: Sur un cas de cecite verbale avec agraphie, suivi d'autopsie. Mem Soc Biol 3:197, 1891
123. Dejerine J: Des differentes varietes de cecite verbale. Mem Soc Biol 1:30, 1892
124. Dejerine J: Semeiologie de Affections du Systeme Nerveux. Masson, Paris, 1914
125. Dejerine J, Regnard M: Monoplegie brachiale gauche limitée aux muscles des éminences thénar, hypothénar et aux intérosseux: astereognosie, épilepsie jacksonianne. Rev Neurol 1:285, 1912
126. Delal PM, Shah PM, Aiyar RR: Arteriographic study of cerebral embolism. Lancet 2:358, 1965
127. DeMassary J: L'alexie. Encephale 27:134, 1934
128. Demierre B, Prondot P: Dystonia caused by putamino-capsulo-caudate vascular lesions. J Neurol Neurosurg Psychiatry 46:404, 1983
129. Denes G, Semenza C, Stoppa E et al: Unilateral spatial neglect and recovery from hemiplegia: a follow-up study. Brain 105:543, 1982
130. DeRenzi E, Colombo A, Faglioni P, Gilbertoni N: Conjugate gaze paresis in stroke patients with unilateral damage. Arch Neurol 39:42, 1982
131. DeRenzi E, Faglioni P, Previdi P: Spatial memory and hemispheric locus of lesion. Cortex 13:424, 1977
132. DeRenzi E, Faglioni P, Scotti G: Judgement of

spatial orientation in patients with focal brain damage. J Neurol Neurosurg Psychiatry 34:489, 1971
133. DeRenzi E, Faglioni P, Sorgato P: Modality-specific and supramodal mechanisms of apraxia. Brain 105:301, 1982
134. DeRenzi E, Lucchelli F: Ideational apraxia. Brain 198:1173, 1988
135. DeRenzi E, Motti F, Nichelli P: Imitating gestures: a quantitative approach to ideomotor apraxia. Arch Neurol 37:6, 1980
136. DeRenzi E, Pieczuro A, Vignola L: Oral apraxia and aphasia. Cortex 2:50, 1966
137. DeRenzi E, Pieczuro A, Vignolo L: Ideational apraxia: a quantitative study. Neuropsychologia 6:41, 1968
138. Derouesen C, Mas JL, Bolgert AF, Castaigne P: Pure sensory stroke caused by a small cortical infarct in the middle cerebral artery territory. Stroke 15:660, 1984
139. Deuel RK, Collins RC: The functional anatomy of frontal lobe neglect in the monkey: behavioral and quantitative 2-deoxyglucose studies. Ann Neurol 15:521, 1984
140. Dimond S: Depletion of awareness and double-simultaneous stimulation in split-brain man. Cortex 14:604, 1978
141. Dimond SJ: Performance by split-brain humans on lateralized vigilance tasks. Cortex 15:43, 1979
142. Donnan GA, Bladin PF, Berkovic SF et al: The stroke syndrome of striatocapsular infarction. Brain 114:51, 1991
143. Dratz HM, Woodhall B: Traumatic dissecting aneurysm of left internal carotid, anterior cerebral and middle cerebral arteries. J Neuropathol Exp Neurol 6:286, 1947
144. Duman S, Stephans JW: Post-traumatic middle cerebral artery occlusion. Neurology (NY) 13:613, 1963
145. Dunne JW, Leedman PJ, Edis RH: Inobvious stroke: a ca delirium and dementia. Aust NZ J Med 16:771, 1986
146. Duret H: Recherches anatomiques dur la circulation de l'encephale. Arch Physiol Norm Pathol 1:919, 1874
147. Edwards JH, Kricheff II, Riles T, Imparato A: Angiographically undetected ulceration of the carotid bifurcation as a cause of embolic stroke. Radiology 132:369, 1979
148. Ellenberg L, Sperry RW: Capacity for holding sustained attention following commissurotomy. Cortex 15:421, 1979
149. Fairfax AJ, Lambert CD, Leatham A: Systemic embolism in chronic sinoatrial disorder. N Engl J Med 275:190, 1976
150. Feldmeyer JJ, Merendaz C, Regli F: Stenoses symptomatiques de l'artère cérébrale moyenne. Rev Neurol (Paris) 139:725, 1983
151. Fieschi C, Argentino C, Lenzi GL et al: Clinical and instrumental evaluation of patients with ischemic stroke within the first six hours. J Neurol Sci 91:311, 1989
152. Finklestein S, Kleinman GM, Cuneo R, Baringer JR: Delayed stroke following carotid occlusion. Neurology (NY) 30:84, 1980
153. Fischer E: Die Lageabweichungen der vordern Hirnarterie im Gefaessbild. Zentralbl Neurochir 3:300, 1938
154. Fisher CM: Occlusion of the internal carotid artery. Arch Neurol Psychiatry 69:346, 1951
155. Fisher CM: Left hemiplegia and motor impersistence. J Nerv Ment Dis 123:201, 1956
156. Fisher CM: Cerebral ischemia-less familiar types. Clin Neurosurg 18:267, 1971
157. Fisher CM: Capsular infarcts. Arch Neurol 36:65, 1979
158. Fisher CM: Topographic disorientation. Arch Neurol 19:33, 1982
159. Fisher CM, Curry HB: Pure motor hemiplegia of vascular origin. Arch Neurol 13:30, 1965
160. Fisher CM, Gore I, Okabe N, White PD: Atherosclerosis of the carotid and vertebral arteries-extracranial and intracranial. J Neuropathol Exp Neurol 24:455, 1965
161. Fisher CM, Pearlman A: The non-sudden onset of cerebral embolism. Neurology (Minneapolis) 17:1025, 1967
161a. Foix C: Aphasies. p. 135. In Roger GH, Widal F, Teissier PJ (eds): Nouveau Triete de Medecine. Vol. 19. Masson, Paris, 1928
162. Foix C, Chavany J-A, Levy M: Syndrome pseudo-thalamique d'origine parietale: lesion de l'artere du sillon interparietal (Pa P1 P2 antereurs, petit territoire insulo-capsulaire). Rev Neurol (Paris) 35:68, 1927
163. Foix C, Levy M: Les ramollissement sylviens. Rev Neurol (Paris) 11:51, 1927
164. Fox JC, Holmes G: Optic nystagmus and its value in the localization of cerebral lesions. Brain 49:333, 1926
165. Fredericks JAM: Disorders of body schema. p. 209. In Vinken PJ, Bruyn GW (eds): Handbook of Clinical Neurology. Vol. 4. North-Holland Publishing, Amsterdam, 1969
166. Friedlich AL, Castleman B, Mohr JP: Case records of the Massachusetts General Hospital. N Engl J Med 278:1109, 1968
167. Furlan AJ, Little JR, Dohn DF: Arterial occlusion following anastamoses of the superficial temporal artery to middle cerebral artery. Stroke 11:91, 1980
168. Gacs G, Fox AJ, Barnett HJM, Vinuela F: CT visualization of intracranial arterial thromboembolism. Stroke 14:756, 1983
169. Gacs G, Merei F, Bodosi M: Balloon catheter as a model of cerebral emboli in humans. Stroke 13:39, 1982
170. Gainotti G: Emotional behavior and hemispheric side of lesion. Cortex 8:41, 1972
171. Gainotti G, Caltagirone C, Micelli G: Poor performance of right brain-damaged patients on Raven's coloured matrices. Neuropsychologia 15:675, 1977
172. Gainotti G, Messerli G, Tissot R: Qualitative analysis of unilateral spatial neglect in relation to laterality of cerebral lesion. J Neurol Neurosurg Psychiatry 35:545, 1972
173. Gainotti G, Tiacci C: The relationships between disorders of visual perception and unilateral spatial neglect. Neuropsychologia 9:451, 1971

174. Garcin R: Paralysie dissociee du median d'origine corticale (sur le caractere durement familial de certains accidents vasculaires cerebraux). Medecine (Baltimore) 137, 1932
175. Gardner H, Albert ML, Weintraub S: Comprehending a word: the influence of speed and reduncy on auditory comprehension in aphasia. Cortex 11:155, 1975
176. Gay AJ, Newman NM, Keltner JL: Eye Movement Disorders. Mosby, St. Louis, 1974
177. Gazengel JGL: Etude de 276 emboles cerebrales d'origine cardiaque. p. 123. Thèse Faculté de Médecine de Paris. Editions AGEMP, Paris, 1966
178. Gazzaniga M: Pure word deafness: a case history. Cortex 9:183, 1973
179. Gazzaniga M, Bogen J, Sperry R: Dyspraxia following division of the cerebral commissures. Arch Neurol 16:606, 1967
180. Gerstmann J: Problem of imperception of disease and of impaired body territories with organic lesions. Arch Neurol Psychiatry 48:890, 1942
181. Geschwind N: Disconnection syndromes in animals and man. Brain (Parts 1 & 2) 88:237, 1965
182. Geschwind N: Problems in the anatomical understanding of the aphasias. In Benton AL (ed): Contributions to Clinical Neuropsychology. Aldin, Chicago, 1969
183. Geschwind N: The Apraxias: neural mechanisms of disorders of learned movement. Am Sci 63:188, 1975
184. Geschwind N, Kaplan E: A human disconnection syndrome. Neurology (NY) 12:675, 1962
185. Ghika JA, Bogousslavsky J, Regli F: Deep perforators from the carotid system: template of the vascular territories. Arch Neurol 47:1097, 1990
186. Gibo H, Carver CP, Rhoton AL et al: Microsurgical anatomy of the middle cerebral artery. J Neurosurg 54:151, 1981
187. Glew RH: Case records of the Massachusetts General Hospital. N Engl J Med 301:36, 1979
188. Gleysteen JJ, Silver D: Paradoxical arterial embolism: collective review. Am Surg 36:47, 1970
189. Gloning I, Gloning K, Quatember R: A case of "prosopagnosia" with necropsy findings. Neuropsychologia 8:199, 1970
190. Goldstein K: Die Transkortikal Aphasien. G. Fischer, Jena, 1917
191. Goldstein K: Language and Language Disturbances. Grune & Stratton, New York, 1948
192. Goodglass H, Kaplan E: Disturbance of gesture and pantomime in aphasia. Brain 86:703, 1963
193. Goodglass H, Kaplan E: The Assessment of Aphasia and Related Disorders. Lea & Febiger, Philadelphia, 1972
194. Gordon HW, Bogen JE: Hemispheric lateralization of singing after intracarotid sodium amylobarbitone. J Neurol Neurosurg Psychiatry 37:727, 1974
195. Graff-Radford NR, Welsh K, Godersky J: Callosal apraxia. Neurology (NY) 37:100, 1987
196. Grand W: Microsurgical anatomy of the proximal middle cerebral artery and the internal carotid artery bifurcation. Neurosurgery 7:151, 1980
197. Grimes JD, Hassan MN, Quarrington AM, d'Alton J: Delayed-onset post hemiplegic dystonia: CT demonstration of basal ganglia pathology. Neurology (NY) 32:1033, 1982
198. Gross CR, Kase CS, Mohr JP et al: Stroke in south Alabama: incidence and diagnostic features—a population-based study. Stroke 15:249, 1984
199. Gulkin TA, Asbury AK: Fragment of great-vessel wall causing cerebral embolism. N Engl J Med 277:751, 1967
200. Gumerlock MK, Ono H, Neuwelt EA: Can a patent extracranial-intracranial bypass provoke the conversion of an intracranial arterial stenosis to a symptomatic occlusion? Neurosurgery 12:391, 1983
201. Hanaway J, Torack R, Fletcher AP, Landau WM: Intracranial bleeding associated with urokinace therapy for acute ischemic hemispheral stroke. Stroke 7:143, 1976
202. Harris LJ: Sex differences in spatial ability: possible environmental, genetic, and neurological factors. p. 405. In Kinsbourne M (ed): Asymmetrical Function of the Brain. Cambridge University Press, Cambridge, 1978
203. Harrison MJG, Hampton JR: Neurologic presentation of bacterial endocarditis. Br Med J 2:148, 1967
204. Harrison MJG, Marshall J: Evidence of silent cerebral embolism in patients with amaurosis fugax. J Neurol Neurosurg Psychiatry 40:651, 1977
205. Hartmann F: Beitrage zur Apraxielehre. Monatsschr Psychiatr Neurol 21:97, 1907
206. Head H: Aphasia and Kindred Disorders of Speech. Cambridge University Press, London, 1926
207. Healton EB, Navarro C, Bressman S, Brust JCM: Subcortical neglect. Neurol (NY) 32:776, 1982
208. Hecaen H: Clinical symptomatology in right and left hemisphere lesions. p. 215. In Mountcastle V (ed): Interhemispheric Relations and Cerebral Dominance. Johns Hopkins University Press, Baltimore, 1962
209. Hecaen H, de Ajuriaguerra J: L'Apraxie de l'habillage: Ses rapports avec la planotopokinesie et les troubles de la somatognosie. Encephale 35:113, 1942
210. Hecaen H, Albert ML: Human Neuropsychology. John Wiley, New York, 1978. p. 982
211. Hecaen H, Angelergues R: Etude anatomoclinique de 280 lesions retrorolandiques unilaterales des hemispheres cerebraux. Encephale 6:533, 1961
212. Hecaen H, Angelergues R: Agnosia for faces. Arch Neurol 7:92, 1962
213. Hecaen H, Angelergues R: Localization of symptoms in aphasia. In Dereuck A.V.S., O'Connor M (eds): Disorders of Language, Little, Brown, Boston, 1978
214. Heilbronner K: Die aphasischen, apraktischen und agnostichen Störungen. In Lewandowsky M (ed): Handbuch der Neurologie. Vol. 1. Springer-Verlag, Berlin, 1910
215. Heilman KM: Apraxia. In Heilman K, Valen-

stein E (eds): Clinical Neuropsychology. Oxford University Press, New York, 1979
216. Heilman KM, Rothi LJ, Valenstein E: Two forms of ideomotor apraxia, Neurology (NY) 32:342, 1982
217. Heilman KM, Scholes R, Watson RT: Auditory affective agnosia: disturbed comprehension of affective speech. J Neurol Neurosurg Psychiat 38:69, 1975
218. Heilman K, Valenstein E: Frontal lobe neglect in man. Neurology (Minneapolis) 22:660, 1972
219. Heilman KM, Valenstein E: Mechanisms underlying hemispatial neglect. Ann Neurol 5:166, 1979
220. Heilman KM, Van Den Abell T: Right hemispheric dominance for mediating cerebral activation. Neuropsychologia 17:315, 1979
221. Heilman KM, Van Den Abell T: Right hemisphere dominance for attention: the mechanism underlying hemispheric asymmetries of inattention (neglect). Neurology (NY) 30:327, 1980
222. Henschen SE: Klinische und Anatomische Beitrage zur Pathologie des Gehirns. Nordiska, Stockholm, 1920
223. Hier DB, Kaplan J: Verbal comprehension deficits after right hemisphere damage. Appl Psycholinguistics 2:279, 1980
224. Hier DB, Mohr JP: Incongruous oral and written naming: evidence for a subdivision of the syndrome of Wernicke's aphasia. Brain Lang 4:115, 1977
225. Hier DB, Mondlock J, Caplan LR: Behavioral abnormalities after right hemisphere stroke. Neurology (NY) 33:337, 1983
226. Hier DB, Mondlock J, Caplan LR: Recovery of behavioral abnormalities after right hemisphere stroke. Neurology (NY) 33:345, 1983
227. Hindson DA, Westmoreland DE, Carroll WA, Bodmer BA: Persistent Broca's aphasia after right cerebral infarction in a right-hander. Neurology (Cleveland) 34:387, 1984
228. Hinton RC, Mohr JP, Ackerman RA et al: Symptomatic middle cerebral artery stenosis. Ann Neurol 5:152, 1979
229. Hirsch CS, Roessmann U: Arterial dysplasia with ruptured basilar artery aneurysm: report of a case. Hum Pathol 6:749, 1975
230. Hollin SA, Silverstein A: Transient occlusion of the middle cerebral artery. JAMA 194:243, 1965
231. Hollin SA, Sukoff MH, Silverstein A, Gross SW: Post-traumatic middle cerebral artery occlusion. J Neurosurg 25:526, 1966
232. Holmes G: The cerebral integration of the ocular movements. Br Med J 2:108, 1938
233. Horenstein S, Chamberlin Q, Conomy J: Infarction of the fusiform and calcarine regions: agitated delirium and hemianopsia. Trans Am Neurol Assoc 92:85, 1967
234. Howes D, Boller F: Simple reaction time: evidence for focal impairment from lesions of the right hemisphere. Brain 98:317, 1975
235. Howes D, Geschwind N: Quantitative studies of aphasic language. in Disorders of Communication Proceedings. Assoc Res Nerv Ment Dis. William & Wilkins, Baltimore, 1964
236. Hughlings-Jackson J: On affections of speech from the brain. Brain 38:106, 1915
237. Hyland HH: Thrombosis of intracranial arteries. Arch Neurol Psychiatry 30:342, 1933
238. Imparato AM, Riles TS, Gorstein F: The carotid bifurcation plaque: pathologic findings associated with cerebral ischemia. Stroke 10:238, 1979
239. Irino T, Tandea M, Minami T: Angiographic manifestations in postrecanalized cerebral infarction. Neurology (NY) 27:471, 1977
240. Jacobs L: Visual allesthesia. Neurology (NY) 30:105, 1980
241. Jain KK: Some observations on the anatomy of the middle cerebral artery. Can J Surg 7:134, 1964
242. Joanette Y, Brouchon M: Visual allesthesia in manual pointing: some evidence for a sensorimotor cerebral organization. Brain Cognition 3:152, 1984
243. Johnson AC, Graves VB, Pfaff JP, Jr: Dissecting aneurysm of intracranial arteries. Surg Neurol 7:49, 1977
244. Joynt RJ, Zimmerman G, Khalifett R: Cerebral emboli from cardiac tumors. Arch Neurol 12:84, 1965
245. Joynt RL, Benton AL, Fogel ML: Behavioral and pathological correlates of motor impersistence. Neurology (NY) 12:876, 1964
246. Kanshepolsky J: A cortical auditory disorder: clinical, audiologic and pathologic aspects. Neurology (NY) 23:699, 1973
247. Kaplan J, Hier DB: Visuospatial deficits after right hemisphere sroke. J Occup Ther 36:314, 1982
248. Kase CS, Troncoso JF, Court JE et al: Global spatial disorientation. J Neurol Sci 34:267, 1977
249. Kase CS, White L, Vinson L, Eichelberger P: Shotgun Pellet Embolus to the middle cerebral artery. Neurology (NY) 31:458, 1981
250. Katoh M, Kamiyama H, Abe H et al: Complete occlusion of right middle cerebral artery by radiation therapy after removal of pituitary adenoma: case report. No Shinkei Geka 18:855, 1990
251. Kawase T, Mizukami M, Tazawa T, Araki G: The significance of lenticulostriate arteries in transient ischemic attack—neuroradiological and regional cerebral blood flow studies. Brain Nerve 31:1033, 1979
252. Kerbler S, Schober PH, Steiner H: Traumatische Embolisierung der Arteria cerebri media. Z Kinderchir. 45:301, 1990
253. Kertesz A: Aphasia and Associated Disorders: Taxonomy, Localization and Recovery. Grune & Stratton, New York, 1979
254. Kertesz A: Localization of lesions in Wernicke's aphasia. Page 209-230 In Kertesz A (ed): Localization in Neuropsychology. Academic Press, New York, 1983
255. Kertesz A, Benson DF: Neologistic jargon: a clinical pathologic study. Cortex 6:362, 1970
256. Kertesz A, Dobrowolski S: Right hemisphere deficits, lesion size and location. J Clin Neuropsychol 3:283, 1981
257. Kertesz A, Harlock W, Coates R: Computer to-

mographic localization, lesion size and prognosis in aphasia and nonverbal impairment. Brain Lang 8:34, 1979
258. Kertesz A, Lesk D, McCabe P: Isotope localization of infarcts in aphasia. Arch Neurol 34:590, 1977
259. Kertesz A, Nicholson I, Cancelliere A, Kassa K: Motor impersistence: a right-hemisphere syndrome. Neurology (NY) 35:662, 1985
260. Khurana RK, O'Donnell PP, Suter CM, Inayatullah M: Bilateral deafness of vascular origin. Stroke 12:521, 1981
261. Kimura D, Archibald Y: Motor functions of the left hemisphere. Brain 97:337, 1974
262. Klein R: The problem of agnosia in the light of a case of pure word deafness. J Ment Sci 102:112, 1956
263. Kleist K: Gehirnpathologische and Lokalisatorische Ergebnisse uber Horstorungen: Gerauschtaubheiten und Amusie. Monatsschr Psychiatr Neurol 66:853, 1928
264. Kleist K: Gehirnpathologie. Barth: Leipsig, 1934
265. Klosovskii
266. Knopman DS, Selnes OA, Niccum N et al: A longitudinal study of speech fluency in aphasia: CT correlates of recovery and persistent nonfluency. Neurology (Cleveland) 33:1170, 1983
267. Kooiker JC, MacLean JM, Sumi SM: Cerebral embolism, marantic endocarditis, and cancer. Arch Neurol 33:260, 1976
268. Kostuk WJ, Baughner DR, Barnett HJM, Silver MD: Strokes: a complication of mitral valve prolapse? Lancet 2:131, 1977
269. Kotila M, Niemi ML, Laaksonen R: Four-year prognosis stroke patients with visuospatial inattention. Scand Rehabil Med 18:177, 1986
270. Krayenbuehl HA, Yasargil MG: Cerebral Angiography. 2nd Ed. Butterworths, London, 1968
271. Kunitz S, Gross CR, Heyman A et al: The pilot stroke data bank: definition, design, data. Stroke 15:740, 1984
272. Kusske JA, Kelly WA: Embolization and reduction of the "steal" syndrome in cerebral AVMs. J Neurosurg 40:313, 1974
273. Labar DR, Mohr JP, Nichols FT, Tatemichi TK: Unilateral hyperhidrosis after cerebral infarction. Neurology (NY) 38:1679, 1988
274. LaCours AR, Lhermitte F: The "pure form" of the phonetic disintegration syndrome (pure anathria): anatomical-clinical report of a historical case. Brain Lang 3:88, 1976
275. Lafon R, Gross C, Betoulieres P et al: Mise en evidence angiographic d'anastomoses distales entre arteres cerebrales. J Radiol Electrol 37:960, 1956
276. Laitinen LV: Loss of motivation for speaking with bilateral lacunes in the anterior limb of the internal capsule. Clin Neurol Neurosurg Psychiatry 92:1778, 1990
277. Landis T, Cummings JL, Benson DF, Palmer EP: Loss of topographic familiarity: an environmental agnosia. Arch Neurol 43:132, 1986
278. Laplane D, Degos JD: Motor neglect. J Neurol Neurosurg Psychiatr 46:152, 1983
279. Lascelles RG, Burrows EH: Occlusion of the middle cerebral artery. Brain 88:85, 1966
280. Lawson IR: Visual-spatial neglect in lesions of the right cerebral hemisphere: a study in recovery. Neurology (NY) 12:23, 1962
281. Lazorthes G, Gouaze A, Salomon G: Vascularisation et Circulation de l'Encephale. Masson, Paris, 1976
282. Lehmkuhl G, Poeck K: A disturbance in the conceptual organization of actions in patients with ideational apraxia. Cortex 17:153, 1981
283. Lehmkuhl G, Poeck K, Willmes K: Ideomotor apraxia and aphasia: an examination of types and manifestations of apraxic symptoms. Neuropsychologia 21:199, 1983
284. Leicester J: Central deafness and subcortical motor aphasia. Brain Lang 10:224, 1980
285. Leicester J, Sidman M, Stoddard LT, Mohr JP: Some determinants of visual neglect. J Neurol Neurosurg Psychiatry 32:580, 1969
286. Leicester J, Sidman M, Stoddard LT, Mohr JP: The nature of aphasic responses. Neuropsychologia 9:141, 1971
287. Levin HS: Motor impersistence and proprioceptive feedback in patients with unilateral cerebral disease. Neurology (NY) 23:833, 1973
288. Levine DN: Prosopagnosia and visual object agnosia: a behavioral study. Brain Lang 5:341, 1978
289. Levine DN, Calvanio R: Conduction aphasia. p. 79. In Kirshner HS, Freemon FR (eds): The Neurology of Aphasia. Swets & Zeitlinger, Lisse, 1982
290. Levine DN, Mohr JP: Language after bilateral cerebral infarctions: role of the minor hemisphere and speech. Neurology (NY) 29:927, 1979
291. Levine DN, Sweet E: The neuropathologic basis of Broca's aphasia and its implications for the cerebral control of speech. in Arbib M, Kaplan D, Marshall J (eds): Neural Models of Language Processes. Academic Press, New York, 1982
292. Levine DN, Sweet E: Localization in lesions in Broca's motor aphasia. p. 185. In: Kertesz A (ed): Localization in Neurophyschology. Academic Press, New York, 1983
293. Levine RA, Finkelstein S: Delayed psychosis after right temporoparietal stroke or trauma: relation to epilepsy. Neurology (NY) 32:267, 1982
294. Lhermitte F: Unusual anatomy in fluent jargon aphasia. Cortex 9:436, 1973
295. Lhermitte F, Desi M, Signoret JL, Deloche G: Aphasie kinesthetique associée à un syndrome pseudothalamique. Rev Neurol (Paris) 136:675, 1980
296. Lhermitte F, Gautier JC, Derouesne C, Guiraud B: Anatomie et physiopathologie des stenoses carotidiennes. Rev Neurol (Paris) 115:641, 1966
297. Lhermitte F, Gautier JC, Derouesne C, Guiraud B: Ischemic accidents in the middle cerebral artery territory (a study of the causes in 122 cases). Arch Neurol 19:248, 1968
298. Lhermitte F, Gautier JC, Derouesne C: Nature of occlusions of the middle cerebral artery. Neurology (Minneapolis) 20:82, 1970

299. Lhermitte J, Trelles JO: Sur l'apraxie pure constructive. Encephale 28:413, 1933
300. Liebeskind A, Chinichian A, Schechter MM: The moving embolus seen during serial cerebral angiography. Stroke 2:440, 1971
301. Liepmann H: Aufsätze aus den Apraxiegebeit. Karger, Berlin, 1908
302. Liepmann H: Diseases of the brain. p. 467. In Barr CW (ed): Curschmann's Textbook of Nervous Diseases. Vol. 1. Blakiston, Philadelphia, 1915
303. Liepmann H: The syndrome of apraxia (motor asymboly) based on a case of unilateral apraxia. (Translated by W.H.O. Bohne K. Liepmann and D.A. Rottenberg from Monatsschr Psychiatr Neurol 8:15, 1900.) In Rottenberg DA, Hochberg FH (eds): Neurological Classics in Modern Translation. Hafner Press, New York, 1977
304. Liepmann H, Maas O: Fall von linksseitiger Agraphie und Apraxie bei rechtsseitiger Lähmung. Z Psychologie Neurolog 10:214, 1907
305. Liepmann H, Papenheim M: Über einen Fall von sogenannter Leitungsaphasie mit anatomischen Befund. Z Gesamt Neurol Psychiatr 27:1, 1914
306. Liepmann H, Storch E: Ein Fall von Reiner Sprachtaubheit. Psychiatr Abhandlung von Wernicke. Haft 7/8, 1898
307. Luria AR: Higher Cortical Functions in Man. Basic Books, New York, 1966
308. Luria AR: Human Brain and Psychological Processes. Harper, New York, 1966
309. Luria AR: The Working Brain. Basic Books, New York, 1976
310. Malone DR, Morris HH, Kay MC et al: Prosopagnosia: a double dissociation between the recognition of familiar and unfamiliar faces. J Neurol Neurosurg Psychiatry 45:820, 1982
311. Marie P: Revision de la question de l'aphasie: la troisieme circonvolution frontale gauche ne joue aucun role special dans la fonction du langage. Sem Med 26:241, 1906
312. Marinkovic R, Markovic L: The role of the middle cerebral artery in the vascularization of the claustrum. Med Pregl 43:361, 1990
313. Marquardson J: The natural history of acute cerebral vascular disease: a retrospective study of 769 patients. Acta Neurol Scand [Suppl] 45:38, 1969
314. Masdeu JC, O'Hara RJ: Motor aphasia unaccompanied by faciobrachial weakness. Neurology (Cleveland) 33:519, 1983
315. Maksimow AA, Bloom W: A Textbook of Histology. 4th Ed. Saunders, Philadelphia, 1942
316. Mazziotta JC, Phelps ME, Carson RE et al.: Tomographic mapping of human cerebral metabolism: auditory stimulation. Neurology (NY) 32:921, 1982
317. Mazzocchi F, Vignolo LA: Computer assisted tomography in neuropsychological research: a simple procedure for lesion mapping. Cortex 14:136, 1978
318. Mazzochi F, Vignolo LA: Localisation of lesions in aphasia: clinical-CT scan correlations in stroke patients. Cortex 15:627, 1979
319. Mazzuchi A, Marchini C, Budai R et al: A case of receptive amusia with prominent timbre perception defect. J Neurol Neurosurg Psychiatry 445:644, 1982
320. McFie J, Piercy MF, Zangwill OL: Visual spatial agnosia associated with lesions of the right cerebral hemisphere. Brain 73:167, 1950
321. McFie J, Zangwill OL: Visual-constructive disabilities associated with lesions of the left cerebral hemisphere. Brain 83:243, 1960
322. Meadows JC: The anatomical basis of prosopagnosia. J Neurol Neurosurg Psychiatry 37:489, 1974
323. Medina JL, Chokroverty S, Rubino FA: Syndrome of agitated delirium and visual impairment: a manifestation of temporo-occipital infarction. J Neurol Neurosurg Psychiatry 40:861, 1977
324. Medina JL, Rubino FA, Ross E: Agitated delirium caused by infarctions of the hippocampal formation and fusiform and lingual gyri. Neurology (NY), 24:1181, 1974
325. Meerwaldt JD, Van Harskamp F: Spatial orientation in right-hemisphere infarction. J Neurol Neurosurg Psychiatry 45:586, 1982
326. Mercer B, Wapner W, Gardner H, Benson DF: A study of confabulation. Arch Neurol 34:429, 1977
327. Mesulam M-M: A cortical network for directed attention and unilateral neglect. Ann Neurol 10:309, 1981
328. Mesulam M-M, Waxman SG, Geschwind N et al: Acute confusional states with right middle cerebral artery infarctions. J Neurol Neurosurg Psychiatry 39:84, 1976
329. Miller NR: Walsh and Hoyt's Clinical Neuro-Ophthalmology. 4th Ed. Williams & Wilkins, Baltimore, 1983
330. Milner B: Laterality effects in audition. In Mountcastle V (ed): Interhemispheric Relations and Cerebral Dominance. Johns Hopkins Press, Baltimore, 1962
331. Minematsu K, Yamaguchi T, Omae T: Spectacular shrinking deficit: rapid recovery from a full hemispheral syndrome by migration of an embolus. Neurology (NY) (Suppl.) 41:329, 1991
332. Mohr JP: Rapid amelioration of motor aphasia. Arch Neurol 28:77, 1973
333. Mohr JP: Broca's area and Broca's aphasia. p. 201. In Whitaker H (ed): Studies in Neurolinguistics. Academic Press, New York, 1976
334. Mohr JP: Neurological complications of cardiac valvular disease and cardiac surgery including systemic hypotension. Ch 7 in Klawans HL (Ed) Neurological Manifestations of Systemic Diseases, vol 38 of Vinken PJ, Bruyn GW (Eds): *Handbook of Clinical Neurology,* New York: North-Holland, 1979, P. 143.
335. Mohr JP: The vascular basis of Wernicke aphasia. Trans Am Neurol Assoc 105:133, 1980
336. Mohr JP: Lacunar infarctions. p. 201. In Barnett HJM (ed): Neurological Clinics of North America. Saunders, Philadelphia, 1983
337. Mohr JP: Differential diagnosis of stroke. In

Rowland LP (ed): Merritt's Textbook of Neurology. 7th Ed. Lea & Febiger, Philadelphia, 1984
338. Mohr JP, Caplan LR, Melski JW et al: The Harvard cooperative stroke registry: a prospective registry. Neurology (NY) 28:754, 1978
339. Mohr JP, Duterte DI, Oliveira VR et al: Recanalization of acute middle cerebral artery occlusion. Neurology 38:215, 1988
340. Mohr JP, Hier DB, Krishner HS: Modality bias in Wernicke's aphasia. Neurology (NY) 4:395, 1978
341. Mohr JP, Kase CS, Adams RD: Cerebral vascular disorders. p. 2028. In Petersdorf RG et al (eds): Harrison's Principles of Internal Medicine. 10th Ed. McGraw-Hill, New York, 1983
342. Mohr JP, Kase CS, Meckler RJ, Fisher CM: Sensorimotor stroke due to thalamocapsular ischemia. Arch Neurol 34:739, 1977
343. Mohr JP, Pessin MS, Finkelstein S et al: Broca aphasia: pathologic and clinical aspects. Neurology (NY) 28:311, 1978
344. Mohr JP, Rubinstein LV, Kase CS et al: Gaze palsy in hemispheral stroke: the NINCDS Stroke Data Bank. Presented at the annual meeting, American Academy of Neurology, Boston, 12 April 1984
345. Mohr JP, Rubinstein LV, Kase CS et al: Hemiparesis profiles in stroke: the NINCDS Stroke Data Bank. Presented at the annual meeting, American Neurologial Association, Baltimore, 8 October 1984
346. Mohr JP, Sidman M, Stoddard LT et al: Evolution of the deficit in total aphasia. Neurology (NY) 23:1302, 1973
347. Monrad-Krohn GH: Dysprosody or altered "melody of speech." Brain 70:405, 1947
348. Monrad-Krohn GH: The prosodic quality of speech disorders. Acta Psychiatr Neurol Scand 22:255, 1947
349. Mori E, Yamadori A: Acute confusional state and acute agitated delirium: occurrence after infarction in the middle cerebral artery territory. Arch Neurol 4:1139, 1987
350. Moutier F: *L'aphasie de Broca.* Thèse Medicine. Paris, 1908
351. Mullally W, Huff K, Ronthal M et al: Frequency of acute confusional states with lesions of the right hemisphere. Ann Neurol 12:113, 1982
352. Mullally W, Huff K, Ronthal M et al: Chronic confusional state with right middle cerebral artery occlusion. Neurology (NY) 32:96, 1982
353. Naeser MA: CT scan lesion size and lesion locus in cortical and subcortical aphasias. p. 63. In Kertesz A (ed): Localization in Neuropsychology. Academic Press, New York, 1983
354. Naezer MA, Alexander MP, Helm-Estabrooks N et al: Aphasia with predominantly subcortical lesion sites. Arch Neurol 39:2, 1982
355. Naezer MA, Hayward RW: Lesion localization in aphasia with cranial computerized tomography and The Boston Diagnostic Aphasia Examination. Neurology (NY) 28:545, 1978
356. Neufield HN, Cadman NL, Miller AW, Edwards JE: Embolism from marantic endocarditis as a manifestation of occult carcinoma. Proc Mayo Clin 35:292, 1960
357. Ng LKY, Nimmannitya J: Massive cerebral infarction with severe brain swelling: a clinical pathologic study. Stroke 1:158, 1970
358. Nielsen JM: The unsolved problems in aphasia. Bull Los Angeles Neurol Soc 162, 1939
359. Nielsen JM: Agnosia, Apraxia, Aphasia. Hoeber, New York, 1946
360. Niessl von Mayendorf E: Über die sognannter brocasche Windung und ihre angebliche Bedeutung für den motorischen Spracht. Monatsschr Psychiatr Neurol 61:129, 1926
361. Niessl von Mayendorf E: Vom lokalisation problem der articulierte Sprache. Barth, Leipsig, 1930
362. Obrador S: Nervous integration after hemispherectomy in man. p. 133. Schaltenbrand G, Woolsey CN: Cerebral localization and organization. University of Wisconsin Press, Madison, 1964
363. Obredane A: *L'aphasie et l'elaboration de la pensee explicite.* Presses Universitaires de France, Paris, 1951
364. Ojemann GA: Brain organization for language from the prospective of electrical stimulation mapping. The Behavioral and Brain Sciences 6:189, 1983
365. Ojemann RG, Crowell RC, Roberson GH, Fisher CM: Surgical treatment of the extracranial carotid occlusive disease. Clin Neurosurg 22:214, 1975
366. Oxbury JM, Campbell DC, Oxbury SM: Unilateral spatial neglect and impairments of spatial analysis and visual perception. Brain 97:551, 1974
367. Paillard J, Michel F, Stelmach G: Localization without content: a tactile analogue of "blind sight." Arch Neurol 40:548, 1983
368. Pallis CA: Impaired indentification for faces and places with agnosia for colours. J Neurol Neurosurg Psychiatry 18:218, 1955
369. Paterson A, Zangwill OL: A case of topographic disorientation associated with a unilateral cerebral lesion. Brain 68:188, 1945
370. Pearce J, Miller E: Clinical Aspects of Dementia. p. 41. Ballière Tindall, London, 1973
371. Pederson RA, Troost BT: Abnormalities of gaze in cerebrovascular disease. Stroke 12:251, 1981
372. Penfield W, Rasmussen T: The Cerebral Cortex of Man. Macmillan, New York, 1952
373. Pessin MS, Duncan GW, Mohr JP, Poskanzer DC: Clinical and angiographic features of carotid transient ischemic attacks. N Engl J Med 296:358, 1977
374. Pessin MS, Hinton RC, Davis KR et al: Mechanisms of acute carotid stroke. Ann Neurol 6:245, 1979
375. Phillips CG: Some thoughts on the organization of the motor cortex. In Eccles JC (ed): The Brain and Conscious Experience. Springer-Verlag, New York, 1966
376. Phillips CG: Changing concepts of the precentral motor area. In Eccles JC (ed): Brain and Con-

scious Experience. Springer-Verlag, New York, 1966
377. Pick A: Studien uber Motorische Apraxie und ihre Mahestehende Erscheinungen. Deuticke, Liepzig, 1905
378. Piercy M, Hecaen H, de Ajuriaguerra J: Constructional apraxia associated with unilateral cerebral lesions: left and right cases compared. Brain 83:225, 1960
379. Poeck P, Lehmkuhl G: Ideatory apraxia in a left-handed patient with right-sided brain lesion. Cortex 16:273, 1980
380. Prevost JL: De la Déviation Conjuguée des Yeux et de la Rotation de la Tête. Thèse, Paris, 1896
381. Rascol A, Clanet M, Manelfe C: Pure motor hemiplegia: CT study of 30 cases. Stroke 13:11, 1982
382. Rasmussen TH, Penfield W: Movement of the head and eyes from stimulation of human frontal cortex. p. 346. In: *The Frontal Lobes.* Vol 27. Williams & Wilkins, Baltimore, 1947
383. Ratcliff G: Spatial thought, mental rotation and the right cerebral hemisphere. Neuropsychologia 17:49, 1979
384. Rengachary SS, Batnitzky S, Morantz RA et al: Hemicraniectomy for acute mass of cerebral infarction. Neurosurgery 8:321, 1981
385. Ringel SP, Harrison SH, Norenberg MD, Austin JH: Fibromuscular dysplasia: multiple "spontaneous" dissecting aneurysms of the major cervical arteries. Ann Neurol 1:301, 1977
386. Ruesen RJ, Daly DD: Auditory cortex disconnection associated with thalamic tumor. Neurology (NY) 24:555, 1974
387. Romanul FCA, Abramowicz A: Changes in brain and pial vessels in arterial borderzones. Arch Neurol 11:40, 1964
388. Rondot P: Syndromes of central motor disorder. p. 169. In Vinken PJ, Bruyn GW (eds): Handbook of Clinical Neurology. Vol 1. Disturbances of Nervous Function. North-Holland Publishing, Amsterdam, 1969
389. Rosegay H, Welch KJ: Peripheral collateral circulation between cerebral arteries. J Neurosurgery 11:363, 1954
390. Ross ED: Sensory-specific and fractional disorders of recent memory in man: isolated loss of visual recent memory. Arch Neurol 37:193, 1980
391. Ross ED: The aprosodias. Arch Neurol 38:561, 1981
392. Ross ED: Right hemisphere's role in language, affecting behavior and emotion. *Trends in Neurosciences* 7:342, 1984
393. Ross ED, Harney JH, deLacoste-Utamsing et al: How the brain integrates affective and propositional language into a unified behavioral function. Arch Neurol 38:745, 1981
394. Ross ED, Mesulam M-M: Dominant language functions of the right hemisphere. Arch Neurol 36:144, 1979
395. Roth M: Disorders of body image caused by lesions of the right parietal lobe. Brain 72:89, 1949
396. Rothi LJ, McFarling D, Heilman KM: Conduction aphasia, syntaxic alexia, and the anatomy of syntactic comprehension. Arch Neurol 39:272, 1982
397. Rovira M, Jacas R, Lay A: The collateral circulation in thrombosis of the internal carotid and its branches. Acta Radiol (Stockh) 50:101, 1958
398. Ruessman K, Sondag HG, Beneicke U: On the cerebral localization of constructional apraxia. Int J Neurosci 42:59, 1991
399. Ruff RL, Volpe BT: Environmental reduplication associated with right frontal and parietal lobe injury. J Neurol Neurosurg Psychiatry 44:382, 1981
400. Salamon G, Huang YP: Radiologic Anatomy of the Brain. Springer-Verlag, New York, 1976
401. Santamaria J, Graus F, Rubio F et al: Cerebral infarction of the basal ganglia due to embolism from the heart. Stroke 14:911, 1983
402. Schenkenberg T, Bradford DC, Ajax ET: Line bisection and unilateral visual neglect in patients with neurological impairment. Neurology (NY) 30:509, 1980
403. Schiller PH, True SD, Conway JL: Effects of frontal eye field and superior colliculus ablations on eye movements. Science 206:590, 1979
404. Schmidley JW, Messing RO: Agitated confusional states patients with right hemisphere infarctions. Stroke 19:883, 1988
405. Schuster P, Taterka H: Beitrag zur Anatomie und Klinik der reinen Wourttaubheit. Z Neurol Psychiatr 105:494, 1926
406. Schwartz AS, Marchok PL, Kreinick CJ et al: The asymmetric lateralization of tactile extinction in patients with unilteral cerebral dysfunction. Brain 102:669, 1979
407. Shallice T, Warrington EK: The possible role of selective attention in acquired dyslexia. Neuropsychologia 15:31, 1977
408. Shaw CM, Foltz EL: Traumatic dissecting aneurysm of middle cerebral artery and carotid-cavernous fistula with massive intracerebral hemorrhage: case report. J Neurosurg 28:475, 1968
409. Shellshear JC: The basal arteries of the forebrain and their functional significance. J Anat 55:35, 1920
410. Shellshear JC: A contribution to our knowledge of the arterial supply of the cerebral cortex in man. Brain 50:236, 1927
411. Sidman M: The behavioral analysis of aphasia. J Psychiatr Res 8:413, 1971
412. Sidman M, Stoddard LT, Mohr JP, Leicester J: Behavioral studies of aphasia: methods of investigations and analysis. Neuropsychologia 9:119, 1971
413. Sinclair W Jr: Dissecting aneurysm of the middle cerebral artery associated with migraine syndrome. Am J Pathol 29:1083, 1953
414. Sittig O: Über Apraxie. Karger, Berlin, 1931
415. Smith JL: Optokinetic Nystagmus. CC Thomas, Springfield, IL, 1963
416. Starr A: The pathology of sensory aphasia. Brain 12:82, 1889
417. Stehbens WE: Focal intimal proliferation in the cerebral arteries. Am J Pathol 36:289, 1960
418. Stein S, Volpe B: Classical "parietal" neglect

syndrome after subcortical right frontal lobe infarction. Neurology (Cleveland) 33:797, 1983
419. Steiner TJ, Rail DL, Rose FC: Cholesterol crystal embolization in rat brain—a model for atherosclerotic cerebral infarction. Stroke 11:184, 1980
420. Stengel E, Lodge Patch IC: Central aphasia associated with parietal symptoms. Brain 78:401, 1955
421. Stenvers HW: Ueber die klinische Bedeutung des optischen Nystagmus für die zerebrale Diagnostik. Schweiz Arch Neurol Psychiatr 14:279, 1925
422. Stringer WL, Kelly DL: Traumatic dissection of the extracranial internal carotid artery. Neurosurgery 6:123, 1980
423. Strong KC: A study of the structure of the media of the distrubting arteries by the method of microdissection. Anat Rec 72:151, 1938
424. Sunderland A, Wade DT, Langton Hewer R: The natural history of visual neglect after stroke: indications from two of assessment. Int Disabil Stud 9:55, 1987
425. Teal JS, Rumbaugh CL, Bergeron RT et al: Anomalies of the middle cerebral artery: accessory artery, duplication, and early bifurcation. AJNR 118:567, 1973
426. Tognola G, Vignola LA: Brain lesions associated with oral apraxia in stroke patients: a clinico-neuroradiological investigation with the CT scan. Neuropsychologia 18:257, 1980
427. Tonkonogy J, Goodglass H: Language function, foot of the third frontal gyrus, and rolandic operculum. Arch Neurol 38:486, 1981
428. Touche: Contribution a l'etude anatomo-clinique des aphasies. Arch Gen Med 6:326, 1901
429. Trojanowski JQ, Green RC, Levine DN: Crossed aphasia in a dextral: a clinical pathological study. Neurology (NY) 30:709, 1980
430. Tucker DM, Watson RT, Heilman KM: Discrimination and evocation of affectively intoned speech in patients with right parietal disease. Neurology (NY) 27:947, 1977
431. Turnbull HM: Alterations in arterial structures, and their relation to syphilis. Q J Med 8:201, 1915
432. Umansky F, Dujovny M, Ausman JI, Diaz FG, Mirchandani HG: Anomalies and variations of the middle cerebral artery: a microanatomical study. Neurosurgery 22:1023, 1988
433. van der Eecken HM: Anastomoses Between the Leptomeningeal Arteries of the Brain. CC Thomas, Springfield, IL, 1959
434. van der Eeken HM, Adams RD: The anatomy and functional significance of the meningeal arterial anastamoses of the human brain. J Neuropathol Exp Neurol 12:132, 1953
435. Van Gehuchten P: *The Scientific Work of Arthur Van Gehuchten*. p. 60. Francqui Fondation, Louvain, 1974
436. Vighetto A, Aimard G, Confavreux C et al: Une observation anatamo-clinique de fabulation (ou délire) topographique. Cortex 16:501, 1980
437. Vincentelli F, Caruso G, Andriamamonji C et al: Modalities of origin of the middle cerebral artery: incidence on the arrangement of the perforating branches. J Neurosurg Sci 34:7, 1990
438. von Monakow K: Die Lokalisation im Grosshirn und der Abbau der Funktion durch Kortikale Herde. Begman, Wiesbaden, 1914
439. Waddington MM: Intraluminal diameter of middle cerebral branches for microanastomosis. Neurol Res 1:65, 1979
440. Waddington M, Ring BA: Syndromes of occlusion of middle cerebral artery branches, angiographic and clinical correlation. Brain 91:685, 1968
441. Walsh KW: Neuropsychology. p. 1197. Churchill Livingstone, Edinburgh, 1978
442. Warrington EK, James M: An experimental investigation of facial recognition in patients with unilateral cerebral lesions. Cortex 3:317, 1967
443. Warrington EK, James M, Kinsbourne M: Drawing disability in relation to laterality of cerebral lesion. Brain 89:53, 1966
444. Watson RT, Heilman KM: Thalamic neglect. Neurology (NY) 29:690, 1979
445. Watson RT, Heilman KM: Callosal apraxia. Brain 106:391, 1983
446. Watson RT, Heilman KM, King FA: Neglect after cingulectomy. Neurology (NY) 23:1003, 1973
447. Watson RT, Valenstein E, Heilman KM: Thalamic neglect: possible role of the medial thalamus and nucleus reticularis in behavior. Arch Neurol 38:501, 1981
448. Weiller C, Ringelstein EB, Reiche W, Thron A, Buell U: The large striatocapsular infarct: a clinical and pathophysiological entity. Arch Neurol 47:1085, 1990
449. Weinstein EA, Kahn RL: The syndrome of anosognosia. Arch Neurol Psychiatr 64:772, 1950
450. Weintraub S, Mesulam M-M, Kramer L: Disturbances in prosody. Arch Neurol 38:742, 1981
451. Weisenberg T, McBride K: Aphasia: A Clinical and Psychological Study. Hafner, New York, 1935
452. Welch K, Stuteville P: Experimental production of unilateral neglect in monkeys. Brain 81:341, 1958
453. Wernicke C: Lehrbuch der Gehirnkranheiten. Th. Fischer, Kassel, 1881
454. Wernicke C: Der Aphasische Symptomencomplex. Breslau, 1874, reprinted in gesammelte Aufsatze, Fischer, Berlin, 1893
455. Wernicke C: The symptom-complex of aphasia. In Church A (ed): Modern Clinical Medical Disease of the Nervous System. Appleton, New York, 1908
456. Wertheim N: Disturbances of the musical functions. In Halpern L (ed): Problems of Dynamic Neurology. Port Press, Jerusalem, 1963
457. Wertheim N: The amusias. p. 195. In Vinken PJ, Bruyn GW (eds): Handbook of Clinical Neurology. Vol. 4. North-Holland, Amsterdam, 1969
458. Wertheim N, Botez MI: Plan d'investigation des fuctions musicales. Encephale 3:246, 1959
459. Whitty CWM, Newcombe F: Disabilities associated with lesions in the posterior parietal region

of the non-dominant hemisphere. Neuropsychologia 3:175, 1965
460. Willanger R, Danielsen VT, Ankerhus J: Denial and neglect of hemiparesis in right-sided apoplectic lesions. Acta Neurol Scand 64:310, 1981
461. Willanger R, Danielsen UT, Ankerhus J: Visual neglect of right-sided apoplectic lesions. Acta Neurol Scand 64:327, 1981
462. Winternitz MC, Thomas RM, LeCompte PM: The Biology of Arteriosclerosis. CC Thomas, Springfield, IL, 1938
463. Wolf PA, Dawber TR, Thomas HE, Kannel WB: Epidemiologic assessment of chronic atrial fibrillation and risk of stroke: the Framingham Study. Neurology (Minneapolis) 28:973, 1978
464. Wolff HG: The cerebral blood vessels—anatomical principles. In: The Circulation of the Brain and Spinal Cord. Ass Res Nerv Men Dis 18:39, 1938
465. Wolman L: Cerebral dissecting anerysms. Brain 82:276, 1959
466. Wolpert SM, Stein BM: Catheter embolization of intracranial arteriovenous malformations as an aid to surgical excision. Neuroradiology 10:73, 1975
467. Wood EH, Correll JW: Atheromatous ulceration in major neck vessels as a cause of cerebral embolism. Acta Radiol [Diag] 9:520, 1969
468. Wyllie J: The Disorders of Speech. p. 340. Oliver & Boyd, Edinburgh, 1894
469. Yamashita M, Tanaka K, Matsuo T et al: Cerebral dissecting aneurysms in patients with moyamoya disease. J Neurosurg 58:120, 1983
470. Yonas H, Agamanolis D, Takaoka Y et al: Dissecting intracranial aneurysms. Surg Neurol 8:407, 1977
471. Yufe R, Karpati G, Carpenter S: Cardiac myxoma: a diagnostic challenge for the neurologist. Neurology 26:1060, 1976
472. Zatz LM, Iannone AM, Eckman PB, Hecker SP: Observations concerning intracerebral vascular occlusion. Neurology (NY) 15:390, 1965

# 17 POSTERIOR CEREBRAL ARTERY DISEASE

J.P. Mohr
Michael S. Pessin

## ANATOMY

### General Features

The posterior cerebral artery usually arises from a terminal bifurcation of the basilar artery. In its initial course across and around the peduncle, it gives off the small thalamoperforant branches that penetrate and supply the midbrain, and through it supplies the thalamus and adjacent lateral geniculate body. During this course it gives rise to the medial and lateral posterior choroidal arteries that supply the posterior portion of the thalamus and the choroid plexus. It courses downward and backward around the brain stem in the ambient cistern, immediately below the tentorium cerebelli just above, and slightly lateral to the superior cerebellar artery. Beyond the brain stem, it curves upward and medially in the quadrigeminal cistern. By crossing the free medial edge of the tentorium, it reaches the medial surface of the occipital lobe near the anterosuperior border of the lingual gyrus just below the splenium of the corpus callosum. As it reaches the surface, it usually divides into two major divisions. The anterior division gives rise to the two inferior temporal arteries, the anterior and the posterior. The posterior division yields three major branches in sequence: the first bifurcation gives rise to the occipitotemporal artery and the calcarine artery; the calcarine artery gives rise to the occipitoparietal artery. The anterior and posterior inferior temporal artery and the occipitotemporal artery supply the orbital surface of the temporal and orbital lobes. Their terminal branches anastamose with the middle cerebral artery via a borderzone network that runs roughly along the margin of the hemisphere where the orbital surfaces become the convex surface. The calcarine artery supplies the calcarine cortex and medial surfaces of the occipital lobe as far distally as the occipital pole, anatomosing with terminal branches of the middle cerebral artery. The branches of the occipitoparietal artery supply the precuneus, and, along a borderzone network, and terminal vessels anastomose with branches of the anterior cerebral artery.

In approximately 70 percent of cases, both the posterior cerebral arteries arise from the basilar artery. In the remainder, one or, rarely, both arise from the internal carotid artery, fed by a large posterior communicating artery.

### Brain Stem and Thalamic Territory

The posterior cerebral artery branches that supply the midbrain and adjacent thalamus are considered[77] to follow the general plan of the arteries of the brain stem, in which the vessels are divided into three major groups: paramedian penetrating, short circumferential, and long circumferential arteries.[1] The *thalamoperforant* arteries are the midbrain equivalent of the paramedian penetrating branches encountered lower in the brain stem, and of the lenticulostriate arteries of the anterior circle of Willis. The thalamoperforant arteries, measuring between 200 and 400 μm in size, arise from the posterior communicating artery and the proximal portions of the posterior cerebral artery, the most constant being those arising from the posterior cerebral artery.[121] They are divided into three groups: the first two, the premamillary and the postmamillary, which follow an upward curvilinear course into the anterior nuclei of the thalamus, and a third group, which pursues a horizontal course and supplies the cerebral peduncle.[121]

The arteries making up the midbrain-thalamic equivalent of the short circumferential group arise from the posterior cerebral artery as it winds around the stem. Measuring from 320 to 800 μm in diameter and numbering between 8 and 10 branches, these *thalamogeniculate, posterior thalamic,* and *pulvinarian* branches curve upward into the posterior portions of the thalamus, supplying the posterolateral nuclei and the pulvinar. One to three thalamogeniculate branches have been found in individual brains.[97]

The medial and lateral posterior choroidal arteries[49] are the equivalent of the long circumferential group of the lower brain stem. Both arise from the posterior cerebral artery in the circummesencephalic course. The *posterolateral choroidal artery* arises first. It follows the curve of the pulvinar, which it supplies only superficially,[102] irrigates the optic tract and the lateral geniculate body,[102] and then enters the choroidal fissure to supply the choroid plexus of the lateral ventricle. In the terminal branches, it anastomoses with the anterior choroidal artery. The *posteromedial choroidal artery* arises a few millimeters behind the posterolateral, passing first over the medial and lateral geniculate bodies (Fig. 17-1). This double-humped course gives the vessel the appearance of a 3 on the angiogram.[121] After entering the choroidal fissure, it supplies the choroid plexus of the 3rd ventricle, and its terminal branches supply the anterior nucleus of the thalamus. The last branch of the arteries supplying the deep territory is the posterior pericallosal or splenial artery.[121]

Ghika and colleagues[53] have recently mapped the deep perforators from the carotid system, and they found that the thalamotuberal artery may rarely take its origin from the middle cerebral artery instead of its more common origination from the posterior communicating artery.

## Cortical Territory

Although the cortical branches of the posterior cerebral artery are well known, there has been considerable disagreement as to their names. Salamon and Huang[121] label the three major orbital temporal branches the inferior temporal and occipitotemporal arteries, while the vessel supplying the calcarine region is known as the calcarine artery. Kaul et al.[69] refer to the former group as the anterior, middle, and posterior temporal arteries. The term parieto-occipital artery describes the branches that supply the calcarine cortex, cuneus, and precuneus (Fig. 17-2). Whatever their names, three vessels usually supply the entire orbital surface of the temporal and occipital lobes. The anterior inferior temporal and the posterior inferior temporal may arise from a single trunk,

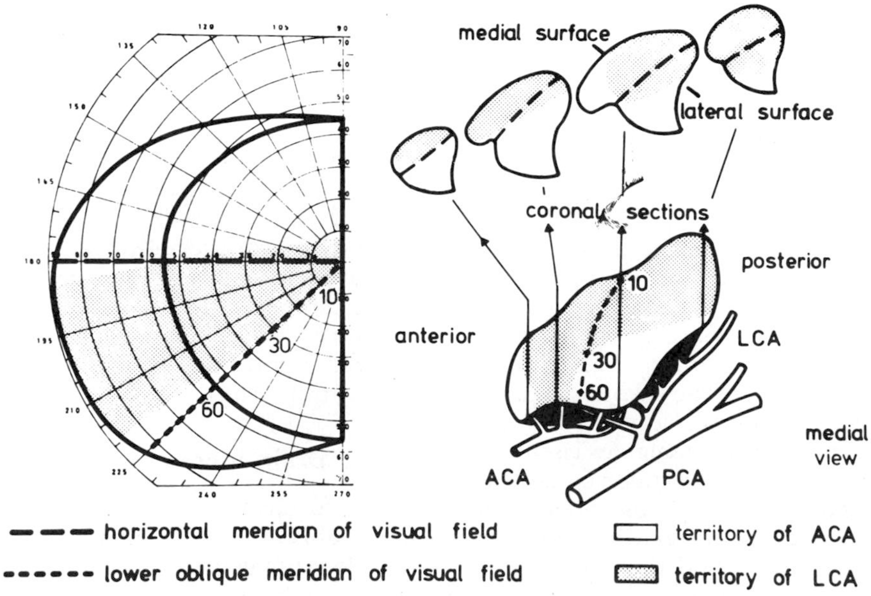


**Fig. 17-1.** Arterial supply to the lateral geniculate body. (From Frisen et al.,[47] with permission.)

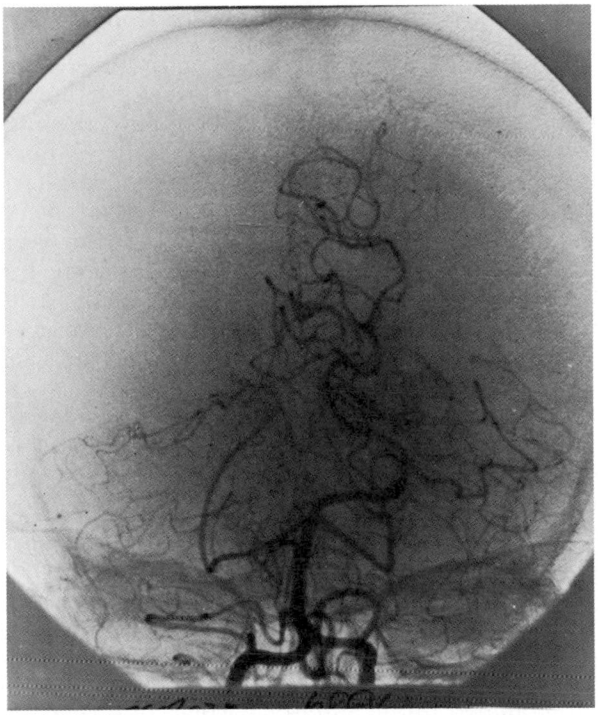

**Fig. 17-2.** Anteroposterior view of the posterior cerebral artery territory showing the cerebral surface branches that supply the inferior surface branches that supply the inferior surface of the temporal lobe and the mesial occipital region.

separate from the occipitotemporal, or the three may arise from a common trunk. The two anterior arteries supply the entire under- (orbital) surface of the temporal lobe. The undersurface of the occipital lobe, including the posterior portion of the fusiform and lingual gyri, are supplied by the occipitotemporal branch.

The calcarine artery may be single or double.[69] Although it has been claimed to be the exclusive supply to the visual cortex in the calcarine fissure,[124] the striate area may at times be supplied in part by the occipitotemporal or occipitoparietal arteries.[132] The termination of the supply of the calcarine artery and its branches is far posterior along the occipital pole.[88] The supply commonly passes around the edge of the occipital pole and as far forward as 1 cm on the convex surface of the hemisphere, where anastomoses are formed with terminal branches of the middle cerebral artery.

### Collaterals

The posterior cerebral artery has abundant collaterals with the middle and anterior cerebral arteries.[9] The collaterals occur in the borderzone, a narrow (usually 1-mm) strip separating two major arterial territories. Within this zone, anastamoses between end arteries occur freely in a variety of forms: end to end, side to side, and end to side. The actual size of the anastomosing vessels vary considerably, but the majority are on the order of 300 to 600 $\mu$m, only rarely as large as 1 cm. As a result, although a potential collateral exists at any point along a borderzone, it is all but impossible to anticipate that a given terminal branch will receive the immediate flow through the borderzone it may need to prevent infarction when its territory is suddenly compromised.

The anastomoses with the anterior cerebral artery usually takes place along a narrow borderzone of vessels between the precuneus and the parieto-occipital fissure, from the isthmus of the gyrus fornicati inferiorly to the margin of the central sulcus superiorly. Some three to four branches enter the borderzone.

With the middle cerebral artery, anastomoses occur from the orbital surface of the anterior tip of the temporal lobe inferiolaterally along the margin of the hemisphere as far back as the occipital pole. Between five and eight such branches can be traced into the borderzones in most hemispheres.

## PATHOGENESIS

### Frequency of Occlusion

Occlusion affecting the posterior cerebral artery or its branches is uncommon compared to involvement of the middle cerebral artery. Among 329 cases of infarction reported by Kleihues and Hizawa,[72] the posterior cerebral artery was affected in 35 cases. Castaigne et al.[23] found 22 posterior cerebral arteries occluded in their series of 44 autopsied cases of vertebrobasilar territory occlusions; in only 8 was the posterior cerebral artery occlusion unaccompanied by occlusions in the more proximal vessels.

Bilateral involvement is rather common, occurring in 25 percent of the cases reported by Kleihues and Hizawa.[72]

### Topography of Infarcts

Infarction of the entire deep and superficial territory of the posterior cerebral artery bilaterally must be quite rare. In their 7-year study of infarction documented by computed tomography (CT) scan, Kinkel and coworkers[71] found six examples, only one of which was bilateral (Table 17-1). However, posterior cerebral artery territory infarction was an uncommon diagnosis: only 54 occurred among the 1,050 infarcts (5 percent). The 6 cases, among only 54 eligible, were fully 11 percent of the total posterior cerebral artery territory infarcts. Pessin et al.[111] found several varieties of infarcts in their series of 35 cases, depending on the mechanism; embolism was the most common (10 cases). Infarction of individual branches, alone or

**TABLE 17-1. Regional Distribution of Infarcts**

| Infarction | Number |
|---|---|
| PCA | 6 |
| CA | 7 |
| PTA | 7 |
| ATA | 1 |
| POA | 2 |
| PTA + ATA | 7 |
| CA + POA | 6 |
| CA + PTA | 10 |
| CA + PTA + ATA | 11 |
| CA + PTA + POA | 1 |
| CA + PTA + POA + PPA | 2 |

*Abbreviations*: PCA, posterior cerebral artery; CA, calcarine artery; PTA, posterior temporal artery; ATA, anterior temporal artery; POA, parieto-occipital artery; PPA, posterior pericallosal artery.
(Adapted from Kinkel et al.,[71] with permission.)

in combination, is more common. Among the surface branches, the calcarine artery is the most commonly affected.[71] The least commonly affected is the anterior temporal artery, and clinical details in such cases are lacking.

Reports vary as to the frequency of cortical and deep infarction: 6 of 38 were diagnosed by Goto et al.,[55] but only 2 of 56 by Kinkel and colleagues.[71]

## Occlusion from Embolization

Embolic material may reach the posterior cerebral artery via the vertebral or basilar arteries or from the internal carotid artery (ICA). Uncommonly, the initial presentation of extracranial carotid occlusive disease may be a hemianopia from embolism to the posterior cerebral artery (PCA) through a fetal origin of the PCA from the ICA.[110] A cardiac source for embolism seems rare compared with embolic material arising from plaques in the vertebral arteries or the basilar artery itself: Castaigne et al.[23] found 10 atherosclerotic emboli, but only 1 from cardiac cause in their autopsied series.

Emboli up the posterior circulation are often arrested at the top of the basilar artery,[19] where they may produce bilateral posterior cerebral artery occlusions, fragment into branches bilaterally, or arrest in one posterior cerebral artery at any point along its course (Fig. 17-3). Common sites of arrest are the stem of the posterior cerebral artery, where it winds around the brain stem, at the origin of the cortical surface branches, or along the course of the branches serving the occipital lobe. Although embolic occlusions confined to the anterior cortical branches serving the undersurface of the temporal lobe are theoretically possible, we found no cases in the literature in our preparation for this chapter.

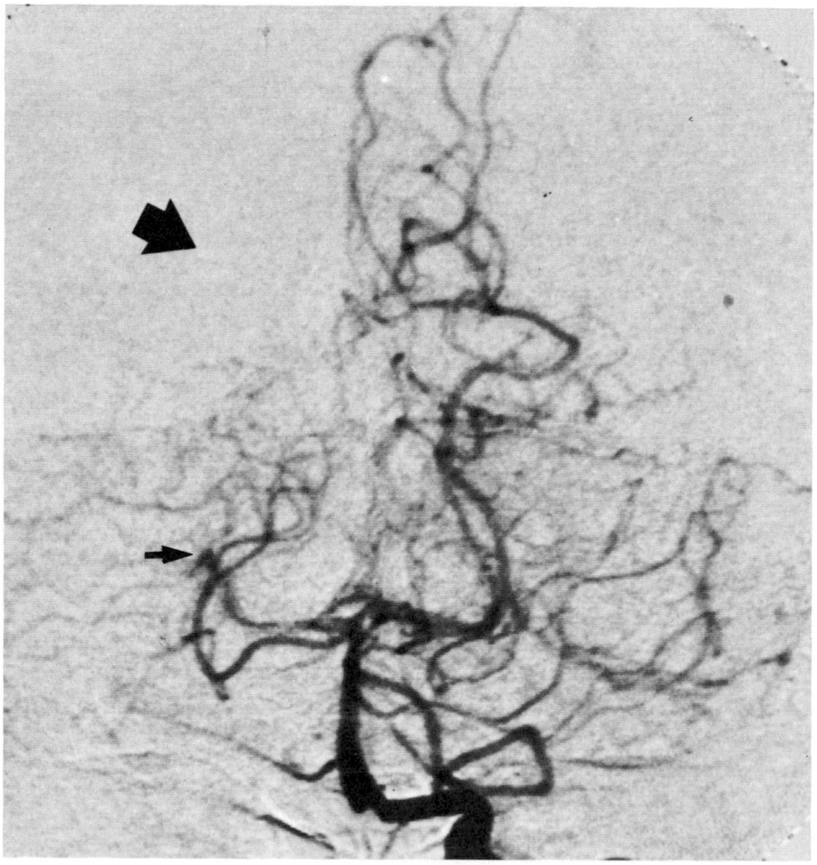

**Fig. 17-3.** Anteroposterior view of a selective left vertebral angiogram. There is occlusion of the ambient segment of the right posterior cerebral artery (*small arrow*). There is no opacification of the terminal branches of this artery (*large arrow*).

Embolic occlusions often produce incomplete infarction of the territory distal to the occluded site. Subcortical infarction, often inobvious on gross inspection of the brain, seems a common finding, and has been the common finding in many of the case reports.[12,35,79,102,114,147] Complete infarction affecting the gray matter and subcortical white matter to the depths of the ventricular wall are rather uncommon findings.[17] Patchy infarction is often encountered.[114]

## Occlusion from Thrombosis

Atheromatous thrombosis of the posterior cerebral artery seems rather uncommon. Occlusion in a setting of preexisting atheromatous stenosis were encountered in only 2 of 22 cases studied by Castaigne et al.[23] In this series, the occlusion was almost always embolic, although the source of the embolus was usually an atherosclerotic lesion more proximally situated in the basilar or vertebral arteries.

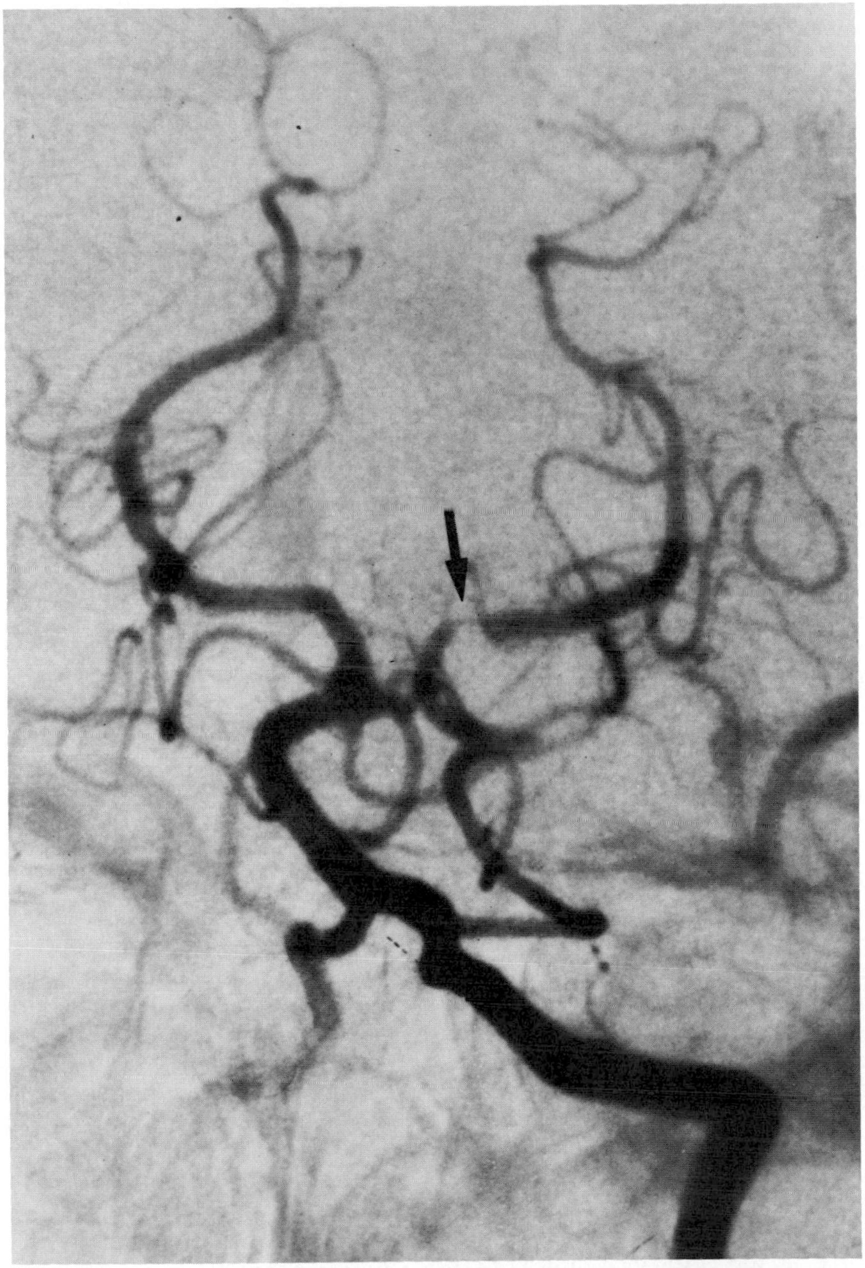

**Fig. 17-4.** Anteroposterior view of a selective left vertebral angiogram with simultaneous compression of the left carotid artery. There is a high-grade stenosis (*arrow*) in the proximal left posterior cerebral artery just distal to its junction with the left posterior communicating artery. Compression of left carotid artery eliminated the possibility of flow artifact created by nonopacified blood from the anterior circulation. (From Pessin,[109] with permission.)

The atheroma usually affects the posterior cerebral artery as it winds around the brain stem,[109] at approximately the same sites where embolic material is arrested. (Fig. 17-4). Thrombus atop preexisting stenosis is rare.[23] No clinical features specifically distinguish thrombosis from embolic syndromes where the occlusion is in the proximal posterior cerebral artery stem.

Occlusion may also occur from anterograde extension of thrombus from an occlusion of the upper basilar artery occlusion or even from the internal carotid if the posterior communicating artery is patent.[23,74] This mechanism may account for as many as half the instances of bilateral posterior cerebral artery occlusion.

Reference is often made[93,118,137] to the possibility that the occipital lobes may suffer ischemia as a "distal field" effect from occlusion of the vertebral arteries bilaterally or the basilar artery itself. Evidence to support this notion is more circumstantial than readily available, as most of the autopsy material suggests that embolism is the cause.[23]

Few studies have been made of stenosis of the posterior cerebral artery stem. Pessin et al.[109] found six examples in a 7-year period. From this slender database they found five had had transient ischemic attacks (TIAs) as the major presenting complaint, while two had homonymous visual field deficits. The TIAs were predominantly visual disturbances in the contralateral half-field, or sensory complaints in the form of paresthesiae involving the arm and hand, occasionally the face and leg. Three patients had visual and sensory spells together. During a period of follow-up, ranging from 4 months to 4 years, no patient had a new stroke in the PCA territory, and only one continued to have TIAs.

## SYNDROMES OF INFARCTION

### Infarction Affecting the Brain Stem and Thalamus

Brain stem infarction attributable to occlusion of the posterior cerebral artery arises incidental to a large occlusion affecting the top of the basilar artery, from local stenosis or thrombus confined to the stem of the posterior cerebral artery, or from an isolated occlusion of the many penetrating branches of the posterior cerebral artery itself.

#### Bilateral Infarcts Affecting the Midbrain and Thalamus

Occlusions affecting the top of the basilar artery are discussed in detail in Chapter 18. In this section, the discussion will be confined to those syndromes in which the posterior cerebral artery is affected as part of the basilar artery occlusion.

Among the 28 cases of paramedian midbrain and thalamic infarction, Castaigne et al.[22] described 4 cases from pathologically proven occlusion of the posterior cerebral artery. Two cases showed an extension of an occlusion of the upper portion of the basilar artery or the portion of the posterior cerebral artery between the basilar artery and the junction with the posterior communicating artery. Atherosclerotic thrombus explained one, and cardiac embolism explained two, but no satisfactory explanation was found for the other. In all four cases the infarct affected the red nucleus and the intralamellar, parafascicular, central, and median nuclei of the thalamus. The clinical picture was dominated by profound deficits in all four cases: obtundation, stupor or coma, disturbance in memory, hemiplegia, varying degrees of hemihypesthesia, and isolated instances of hemianopia or partial 3rd cranial nerve paresis.

Sieben et al.[128] described two patients with unilateral thalamopeduncular infarction from occlusion of the posterior cerebral stem between the basilar artery and the junction of the posterior communicating artery: hemiparesis occurred in both cases; somnolence, Horner syndrome, and hemianopia occurred in one, and 3rd cranial nerve paresis with dysarthria in the other.

The literature is also scanty for cases documented only by angiogram or CT scan.[144] Gacs[48] described a 60-year-old man with atrial fibrillation, who presented with a right 3rd cranial nerve palsy, left hemiparesis, left-sided loss of pain sensation, and left upper quadrant field defect. The CT scan showed a low-density area affecting the posterior cerebral artery territory with enhancement in the right occipital lobe, medial temporal lobe, and thalamus, corresponding to the distribution of the right posterior cerebral artery. The motor function improved, but the partial 3rd cranial nerve paresis, diminished pain sensation, and upper quadrant field deficit did not change. CT scan showed a high-density area on noncontrast, which was considered to reflect occlusion of the posterior cerebral artery stem.

From the limited literature available, it is apparent that occlusion of the posterior cerebral artery stem between the basilar artery and the junction of the posterior communicating artery is sufficient to precipitate a hemiparesis from peduncular infarct, ocular motility disorder from deeper infarction of the midbrain, and complex disturbances in consciousness, memory, and even language for those whose infarct penetrates deeper into medial thalamic structures. In some cases, hypersexuality and changes in appetite occur as well.

#### Unilateral Occlusion of the Posterior Cerebral Artery Stem

A few instances have been reported to unilateral occlusion of the posterior cerebral artery stem, which caused syndromes mimicking those of middle cerebral artery territory infarction. Chambers et al.,[26] Hommel et al.,[66] and Caplan et al.[20] described a total of 17 patients with occlusion of the proximal posterior cerebral artery. The clinical syndrome, affecting the midbrain, mimicked many of the elements of middle cerebral artery occlusion, including contralateral hemiparesis, homonymous hemianopia, hemispatial neglect, and sensory loss or sensory inattention. For all of the eight patients whose infarction involved the dominant hemisphere, aphasia was present as well. CT scan was needed for accurate diagnosis, suggesting the specific clinical features did not distinguish the syndromes clearly.

## Sensory Syndromes

### Hypesthesia

Hypesthesia or anesthesia might be an expected consequence of posterior cerebral artery occlusion near the stem, since the vascular supply to the ventral tier nuclei of the thalamus are in the territory of its penetrating branches.[129] Most of the literature on this subject is discussed in more detail in this book in Chapter 20 on lacunes, in the section on pure sensory stroke. The subject of sensory loss has received only passing mention in most of the reviews, but has been described in detail in few case reports. Remarks such as sensorimotor deficit, hypesthesia, even "considerable anesthesia"[147] are commonly encountered, but not given further elaboration. Rarely, the syndrome may be mentioned as having begun in one part or been confined to one body part.[104] One of Wyllie's patients, with a large autopsy-documented dominant hemisphere occipital infarction but no lesions described in the thalamus (by gross inspection), complained that ". . .the whole right side of the body [felt] cold and heavy . . . the difference of sensation in the two sides being so marked he felt as if a plumb line down the middle of the head and trunk had divided him into two halves".[147]

Among the individual posterior cerebral artery territory branches, the supply to the ventral tier nuclei of the thalamus comes most regularly from the thalamogeniculate branch of the posteromedial choroidal artery (Fig. 17-5). On its course to the thalamus, it passes through the lateral geniculate nucleus. Cases of occlusion of this artery appear to be uncommon. Frisen et al.[47] speculated that its occlusion could produce not only a hemianopia from involvement of the lateral geniculate body, but also hemiparesis and hemihypesthesia from involvement of the ventral tier nuclei of the thalamus, although they did not report such a syndrome in their two patients. The only case we have studied had normal motor function and no abnormality of sensation.[102]

### Dejerine-Roussy Syndrome

Occlusion of the thalamogeniculate branch of the posteromedial choroidal artery was the source of the thalamic pain syndrome of Dejerine and Roussy,[36]

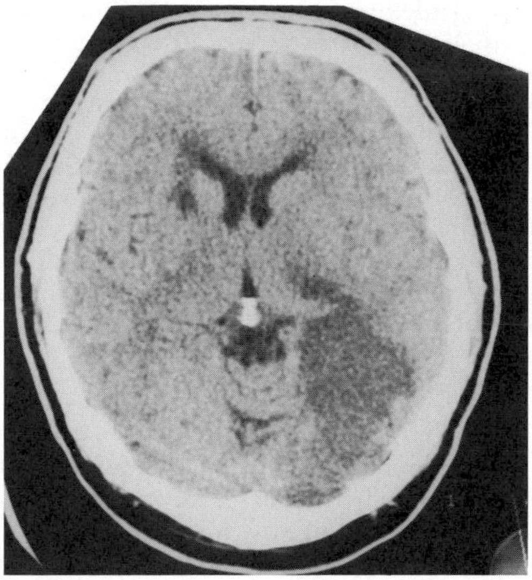

**Fig. 17-5.** Deep thalamic and occipital infarction from occlusion of the posterior cerebral artery in a patient with severe sensory loss and dense hemianopia.

who reviewed the literature up to 1906, and concluded that the occlusion of this artery produced a syndrome of rapidly improving hemiparesis with choreic movements and ataxia, persisting hypesthesia, and severe paroxysmal pain in the hypesthestic side. Their pathologic correlation has been reconfirmed by others over the years[36] and, rarely, by CT scan. The only case we uncovered in preparation for this chapter was reported by Hayman and colleagues,[60] whose clinical details were limited to the remark that the "patient had Dejerine-Roussy (thalamic) syndrome of altered sensation."

The sensory disturbance in these cases has many features. There is usually some degree of hypesthesia, although, rarely, sensation may eventually be normal. Dysesthesia, a feeling of excessive heaviness, and a disagreeable sensation of coldness are common. Either at the onset or after a period up to several months, the unusual pain syndrome may appear. This hyperpathia may be spontaneous or precipitated by stimuli, constant or paroxysmal, temporary or permanent. The pain varies from tingling and aching to intense unbearable discomfort. The site stimulated often feels normal at first, but after a brief delay the pain begins and spreads over larger areas, at times increasing steadily in intensity, usually far outlasting the duration of the original stimulus. Once established, such cases may become permanent.

More often, the disorders occur in partial form. Complaints of dysesthesia, such as tingling, receive frequent mention.[35] The patient described by Caplan and Hedley-Whyte[21] had totally anesthetic right limbs, but when pinched firmly, they experienced a "weak tingling sensation." Geschwind and Fusillo[52] detailed the clinical features of a patient with right hemianopia, alexia, color anomia, and transient memory disturbance experienced from a large left posterior cerebral artery territory infarction. He experienced ". . .vague pains over the right side of the body, especially the thorax, which were diffuse and difficult to characterize. They were increased by repetitive sensory stimulation. [They] were repeatedly complained of, [but] they never became agonizing." The serial section autopsy study showed an infarct in the ventral posteriolateral nucleus of the thalamus.

No treatment has been devised. L-Dopa has been recommended.

## Visual Fields

The lower portions of the visual radiations, throughout their entire course, lie in the territory of the posterior cerebral artery. Most of the upper portion is supplied by branches of the middle cerebral artery, especially the angular and posterior temporal branches. Disruption of the pathway may occur from infarction involving the lateral geniculate body, the radiations along their course in the temporal lobe, and at the calcarine cortex itself.

### Bilateral Infarction

The best described bilateral infarction are the visual field disturbances from infarction involving the calcarine cortex in one or both territories of the posterior cerebral artery.

#### *Complete Infarction*

Complete destruction of the entire territory of supply of the cerebral branches of the posterior cerebral artery bilaterally has been reported infrequently, and only occasionally have the clinical effects been reviewed in detail.[45,72,133,137]

The remarkable patient studied by Brindley and Janota[17] typifies the striking syndrome in massive infarction. Virtually complete infarction of the territories of both posterior cerebral arteries was found at autopsy. Severe stenosis (described as "pinhole") was present in both posterior cerebral stems. The infarcts extended bilaterally along the entire undersurface of the temporal and occipital lobes. In the inferior temporal region, the hippocampus, parahippocampal gyri, and inferior temporal gyri were destroyed. The medial surface of the occipital lobes were affected, including both fusiform gyri, lingual gyri and cunei, and banks of each calcarine cortex; the infarction affected the posterior portions of the corpus callosum the pillars of the fornix, and extended as high as the parieto-occipital fissure. Of interest, each occipital pole was spared. Throughout the remainder of her life after the stroke, the patient remained blind. She had no response to opticokinetic nystagmus and no visual evoked potentials. She was unable to distinguish steady darkness from steady light, nor could she detect a light moving in front of her. However, she consistently distinguished sudden darkening of a lighted room and sudden lighting of a darkened room.

Electrophysiologic studies of a similar case[25] revealed preservation of visual evoked potentials to pattern stimulation, despite a complete lack of vision when tested by clinical methods: the patient was unable to detect the occurrence of a strong light flashed directly at the face, nor when moving in a vertical, horizontal, or diagonal direction. She vigorously denied visual loss and claimed an ability to see well. In contrast to the patient described above, this patient could not distinguish sudden darkening from sudden lighting in a room. CT scan showed a huge bilateral posterior cerebral artery territory infarction. More often, the visual evoked responses have been attenuated or absent.[105]

Examples in the literature[14] and our own experience suggest these huge infarcts can be expected to be associated with severe amnesic states, amnesic aphasia, amnesic color dysnomia, topographic disorientation, and implicit unawareness of the extent of the deficit and perhaps even its existence. This last point suggests that the preservation or lack of awareness of the visual loss is of little value in differentiating middle from posterior cerebral artery territory infarction.[19]

#### *Incomplete Infarction*

Incomplete bilateral posterior cerebral artery territory infarction produces a remarkable variety of syndromes. Such cases have been the basis for the understanding of the projections of the visual fields on the calcarine cortex: the upper radiations in the upper banks, the lower radiations in the lower banks, and the macula at the pole end. Some cases have begun as complete blindness only to evolve within hours or days to less striking deficits.[93] Of interest, during the time of complete blindness, the patient commonly volunteers no complaints and is unaware of the deficit. Description of a few of the autopsied cases suffice to indicate an extremely sharp correlation between the visual fields and the surviving calcarine cortex. In a series of 25 patients recently described,[15] detection of movement of objects in visual space was sufficient for localization, but no discrimination of size or shape was noted. Tests were done in the blind areas, arguing for some extracalcarine vision.

Superficial infarction may involve almost the whole of the calcarine cortex, but if it spares the occipital pole and the subcortical visual radiations, visual function for complex activities such as reading may be spared even if only a tiny portion of the central field remains.[45,95,118,137] Holmes[65] described a case with a narrow wedge of preserved vision extending from the fixation points upward on either side of the vertical meridian, its apex at the fixation point and its base at the periphery. Serial sections of the autopsy specimen showed total calcarine infarction except for a small region, nearly symmetrical bilaterally, extending along the inferior lip of the striate cortex from the anterior end to the pole.

Bilateral altitudinal hemianopia is an expected consequence of incomplete occipital infarction, but has been reported in detail in few cases. The loss of vision is presumed to be from infarction, but whether from embolism or otherwise has not been established. The onset in several cases has been preceded by hallucinations of lights, prismatic or geometric forms, and other phenomena suggestive of migrainous scintillations. After the hemianopias have been developed, associated visual disturbances have included color dysnomias, difficulties with visual form discrimination, spatial disorientation, and disordered visual search behavior of the type encountered in the Balint syndrome. However, others have had little such disturbance[114] and one of our patients, a construction foreman, was annoyed most by his inferior altitudinal hemianopia because it prevented his easy scanning of blueprints and his difficulty reaching for his floor-mounted gearshift in his pickup truck while driving. Only a handful of autopsy-documented cases have been published, all suffering from inferior altitudinal hemianopia.[64,114,137] In each case, however, the superior quadrants were slightly affected as well. Autopsy studies showed foci of infarction scattered through the calcarine cortex with varying degrees of subcortical involvement. The visual field disturbances seemed more homogeneous than was indicated by the discontinuous foci of infarction. Two remarkably homogeneous cases of altitudinal hemianopia were reported documented by CT scan,[105] one with superior, the other with inferior visual field defects. Neither case showed a visual field defect that crossed the horizontal meridian as did those documented by autopsy. No angiographic data were provided.

For most of the cases of cortical blindness with bilateral infarction, the deficits are described as persisting and unchanging. However, scattered reports and our own experience indicate that some cases of bilateral cortical blindness may undergo considerable remission of the deficit. Presumably, the infarction is incomplete, and the acute syndrome is misleading in its failure to predict the subsequent improvement. Although Bergman[14] addressed the issue of remission in 12 examples of cortical blindness, in only 1 of the 5 due to infarction was any improvement noted. Vision recurred within a month but was confined to the macular region, suggesting sparing of the radiations and the occipital pole. The description of the autopsy specimen does not settle this point.

Clinical events that herald cortical blindness are not often reported. A scattering of cases began with a unilateral hemianopia, which was followed by cortical blindness. Bogousslavsky et al.[16] followed 58 patients, with unilateral infarction in the superficial area supplied by the posterior cerebral artery, for a period of up to 39 months; 13 of these cases experienced cortical blindness associated with a delayed contralateral occipital infarction. The authors noted that the lack of visual field improvement most accurately predicted a high risk of cortical blindness.

## Unilateral Infarction

### *Temporal Crescent Sparing Infarction*

Preservation of the temporal crescent has been described in a few instances of unilateral infarction with sparing of the anterior end of the inferior lip of the calcarine cortex.[13]

### *Macular Sparing Infarction*

Macular sparing is frequently encountered in unilateral (and also in bilateral) infarction of the posterior cerebral artery territory. The most common explanation is that the collateral flow available from the middle cerebral artery territory spares the pole. For macular vision to remain, the infarct must remain superficial enough to spare the visual radiations; when they are involved, anatomic integrity of the occipital pole does not suffice to preserve central vision.[17] Infarcts limited to the middle fields of supply of the posterior cerebral artery involve the anterior portions of the calcarine cortex and lingual gyrus.[9,69,72] The most frequent finding in such instances is a homonymous hemianopia, with the most consistent deficit in the area adjacent to the horizontal meridian.[69] The regions covered by the infarct may have an extremely sharp correlation with the visual field in the chronic state: the autopsy of a well-known pathologist, whose visual field deficit showed a small upper quadrantanopia occupying 10 degrees of the vertical and 20 degrees of the horizontal meridian, showed an extremely circumscribed infarct involving the inferior lip of the calcarine fissure almost at the occipital pole; the infarct spread anteriolaterally in a broader brand, undercutting the lingual gyrus but sparing the radiation.[114]

### *Infarction in Individual Branches*

Infarction in the territory of individual branches of the posterior cerebral artery, other than the calcarine artery, has not been found to have a reliable correlation between the severity and type of visual field deficit.[69] CT correlations, by contrast, have been more reliable.[89]

### *Infarction in Visual Radiations*

Infarctions confined to the visual radiations have been reported rarely. In contrast to middle cerebral artery territory disease, infarctions of the posterior cerebral artery territory have often been reported in which the subcortical component was more evident than was the infarction involving the cortical surface.[12,102,137] However, in most instances, the damage found subcortically affected the white matter of the lingual or fusiform gyrus, often sparing the visual radiations, which pass deeper, adjacent to the ventricular wall. Infarcts in this deep territory are rare unless they are the result of a full-thickness infarct, one which forms a schizencephalic cleft extending from the pial surface of the cortex all the way to the ependyma of the ventricle.

### *Lateral Geniculate Body Infarcts*

Lateral geniculate infarcts make up but a small fraction of the literature[47,98,102] (Fig. 7-6). The anterior choroidal artery supplies the anterior hilum and the anterior and lateral aspects of the nucleus. The posterior choroidal artery supplies the remainder, including the crown. The two sources of supply do not anastamose before or in the nucleus; they appear to be end-arteries, with no collaterals. The visual field is represented in three parts in the nucleus: the anteromedial, which subserves inferior quadrant vision; the crown, which serves macular vision; and the lateral, which serves upper quadrantic vision. The only pathologically documented infarcts produced a *congruous*, complete upper quadrantanopsia involving the macula, with a few degrees of involvement of the upper portion of the lower quadrant.[85,102] Upper and lower homonymous sectoranopia has been reported following ligation of the anterior choroidal artery, but was documented only by CT scanning.[46,47] Although such attention to detail might seem excessive, the occlusion of the posterior choroidal artery may yield a rather unusual syndrome: The artery supplies the lateral geniculate body, the fornix, the dorsomedial nucleus, and the posterior pulvinar. Infarction of these structures might cause hemianopia, hemidysesthesia, and disturbance of memory, all from an occlusion very difficult to visualize by angiography and almost as difficult to document by the best CT scanners.

### *Clinical Course*

The clinical course of unilateral partial or complete hemianopia has received little attention. It has been assumed that, like bilateral large infarctions, visual field deficit from unilateral infarctions should also be permanent. However, a few remarkable cases raise the possibility that the initial visual field deficit may undergo gradual shrinkage and the size of the infarct at autopsy may exceed that predicted by the final, shrunken visual field deficit. The pathologist referred to above[114] initially experienced a large visual field deficit which later "cleared up." It was not better characterized historically. As late as 1 year after the

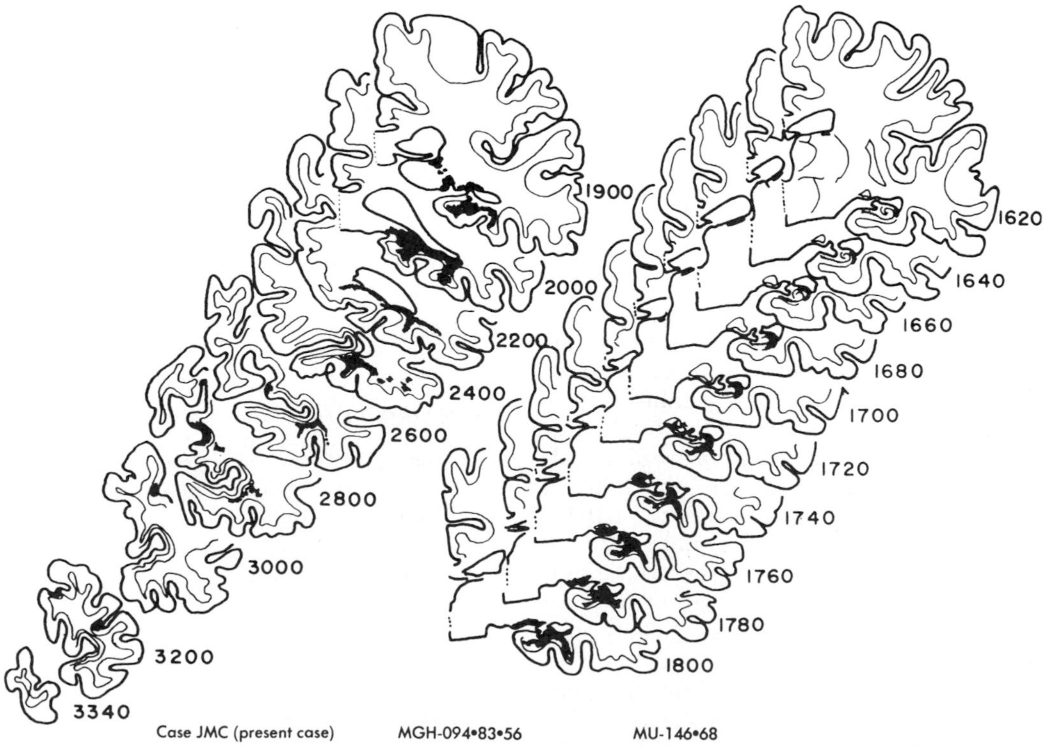


**Fig. 17-6.** Traced serial sections of a posterior cerebral artery territory infarct with involvement of the lateral geniculate body, hippocampus, and subcortical portions of the calcarine region. (From Mohr et al.,[102] with permission.)

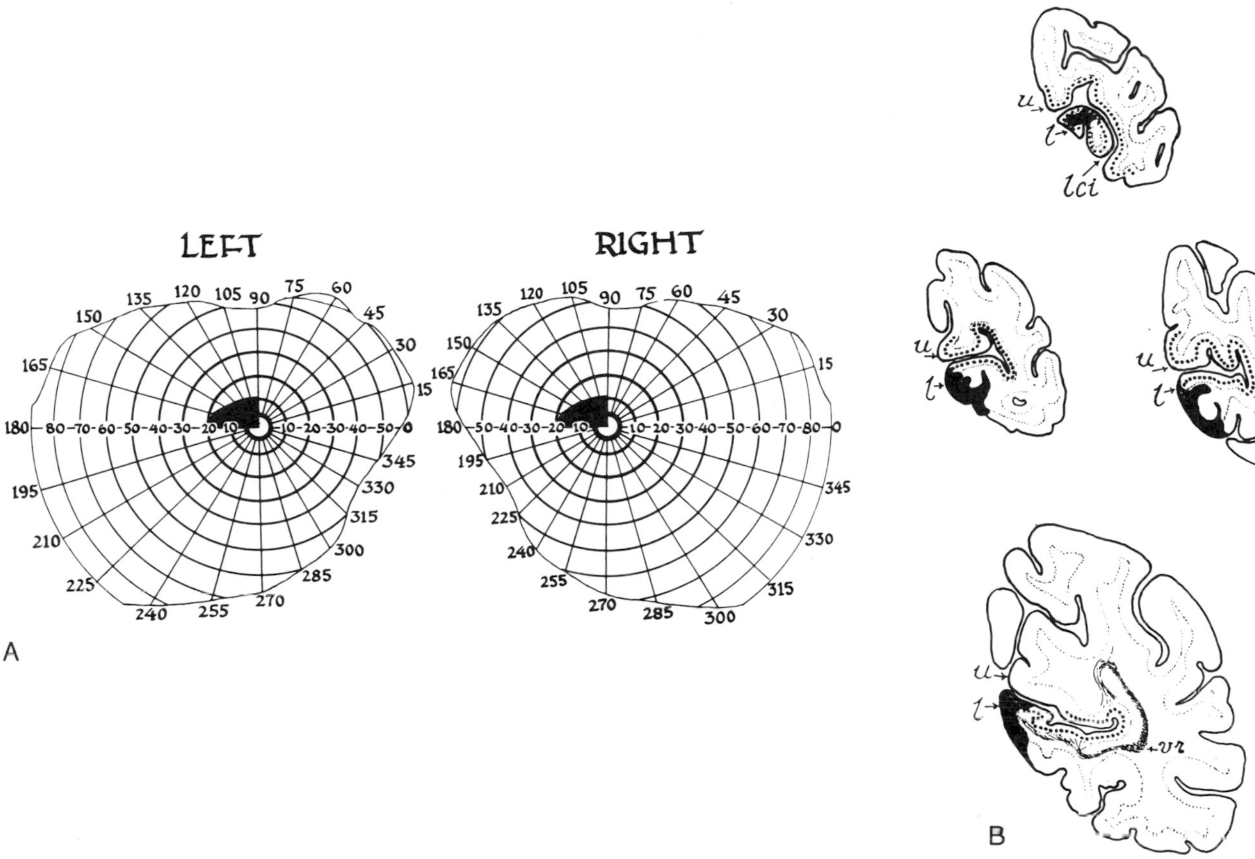


**Fig. 17-7. (A & B).** Case Mallory. The visual field years after the stroke showed a circumscribed upper quadrantanopia. (From Polyak,[114] with permission.)

onset, he was examined by an ophthalmologist who described a large hemianopic scotoma in the left upper fields "too far from the macula to cause him any disturbances in microscopic work." Twenty-four years later his formal visual fields were plotted by a tangent screen and showed only a dense but highly circumscribed upper quadrananopsia confined to the macular region some 20 degrees in the horizontal and 10 degrees in the vertical plane (Fig. 17-7). At autopsy, the only site of infarction affecting the calcarine cortex was a small wedge of the lower bank near the pole. However, a larger area of infarction had undermined much of the lingual gyrus and adjacent inferior bank of the calcarine cortex, within which the cellular elements were much reduced in number (Fig. 17-7). The findings were interpreted[114] as indicating that the surviving cells sufficed to permit the initial visual field deficit to undergo functional resolution.

## Klüver-Bucy Syndrome

The Klüver-Bucy syndrome is described here because its cause is usually bilateral lesions. In the tiny number of cases reported from infarction, the lesions have been very large, affecting most of the undersurface of the temporal lobes,[28,67,81,83,126] including the fusiform and lingual gyri, hippocampal gyri, and the medial hippocampal structures. In addition to the fearless exploration of environment, the syndromes precipitated by these infarctions frequently include a prominent state of exaggerated motor activity: restlessness, agitation, delirium, crying out, and unwonted excessive reaction to visual, auditory, or cutaneous stimuli may be the most striking features noted in the acute phase.[92] Within hours to days, these states usually subside.

## Visual Agnosia

Extensive bilateral occipital infarction is the usual cause of visual agnosia, a rare disorder. The majority of the few cases described occurred in a setting of cardiac arrest. Even fewer have been described from bilateral posterior cerebral artery territory infarction.

A great deal of effort has been made to assert[84,120] or deny[8,10,61] such syndromes exist. Those opposed to the notion argue the deficits are a combination of a "primary" visual field deficit, a secondary perceptual disorder, and some degree of dementia. Those in support of the notion[3,12,93,120] admit few cases have been fully described, but in those the strict criteria have been met: intact primary visual function and no language disturbance. Two forms are said to exist: an apperceptive form, caused by "interference with the processing of primary visual sensory data,[120] and an associative form, "caused by disorders affecting associative cortex where visual percepts wee matched with previously processed sensory data for recognition."[120]

The small number of cases of vascular cause show essentially the same syndrome. There are important but seemingly minor differences in the formulas of the deficits. Because no standard method of examining these rare cases has yet been developed, it remains uncertain how many of the differences reflect variations in the syndrome from minor differences in lesion site and size, and how many represent nothing more than differences in the approach to testing the individual patients.

### Bilateral Posterior Cerebral Artery Territory Infarction

The case reported by Rubens and Benson[120] was later the subject of an autopsy report.[12] The visual agnosia was accompanied by right hemianopia, dyslexia with preserved ability to write, color "agnosia," "impaired verbal learning," and prosopagnosia. The visual agnosia was demonstrated by the patient's ability to produce approximate drawn copies of the picture stimuli he was unable to name or point to after hearing the item named by the examiner. By comparison, he was able to name the same object immediately by palpation or when its characteristic sound was heard. At autopsy, the let posterior cerebral was found firmly occluded from its junction with the posterior communicating artery to its first temporal branch. On cut section, a predominantly subcortical infarct was found that undermined the left parahippocampal gyrus, undermined the entire lingual gyrus, and reached the surface at its distal end. A smaller subcortical infarct undermined most of the right lingual gyrus.

The authors speculated that the combination of lesions prevented visual stimuli discriminated by the right hemisphere from arousing associations in the left, analogous to the alexia and color associative defect also found.

A similar case of the "associative" type was reported by Albert et al.,[3] with later autopsy,[5] whose deficit was somewhat more circumscribed. Although able to read aloud, describe pictures, copy by drawing, and match words heard to pictures seen, he had difficulty naming pictures shown to him. He was initially blind, but regained some sight within 2 days. By day 8, he showed a right upper quadrantic field defect. The lesion was documented by radionuclide scan with increased uptake in both occipital regions. In a later publication[5] gross cut sections were reported. On the right side, an infarct was found over the entire parahippocampal and lingual gyrus; on the left, a similar infarct affected the parahippocampal gyrus and another affected part of the lingual and fusiform gyri. A small infarct was found in the left pulvinar.

One patient, reported by Cambier et al.,[18] had bilateral infarctions, quite large on the right, but the infarct affecting the left side was confined to the fusiform gyrus. Hemianopia was confined to the left side. He had alexia without agraphia, but no "agnosia for colors."

Another variant of the bidirectional disconnection was described in a case studied only by CT scan.[7] Although objects could be matched at sight with one another, naming was deficient and so was the praxic gesture characteristically associated with the use of the object. The authors added the term *visual apraxia* to the list.

### Unilateral Left Posterior Cerebral Artery Territory Infarction

We have not found any autopsy cases showing unilateral left posterior cerebral artery territory infarction, but one case documented by CT scan has been reported, which showed a large hemorrhagic infarction. The syndrome featured a right homonymous hemianopia, right visual spatial hemineglect, difficulty naming visual stimuli, and alexia with spared writing.[113] The patient proved able to copy by drawing; when presented with a picture of an object, he could select the exact picture among six choices or even another pictured item having some functional relationship to the original picture, that is, another view of the same object. Yet he showed great difficulty showing the use of an object pictured and had difficulty grouping objects together by their functional class. The authors noted that the deficits were not explainable as a bidirectional disconnection, but indicated a disorder in the appreciation of the significance or functional value of the stimulus, as might be implied by the original use of the term visual agnosia.

The authors expressed the opinion that these disturbances would not be encountered in right hemispheral infarcts.

## Prosopagnosia

The intriguing syndrome of prosopagnosia may be but a component of the larger problem currently labeled as visual agnosia. Prosopagnosia is said to be present when the sufferer fails to name other individuals at sight. In the published literature on the subject, recently reviewed by Damasio et al.,[32] this special deficit has been found always associated with unilateral or bilateral visual field defects, dyslexia or color dysnomia is usually also present, and in a few instances, more striking disturbances of visual neglect or the Balint syndrome are present. However, the patient reported by Cambier et al.,[18] with a large right occipital infarct and a small one on the left limited to the fusiform gyrus, had no trouble with colors. These authors argued for a bilateral mesial occipital lesion in such cases, affecting the inferior visual radiations, and not necessarily caused by large infarcts. They marshaled evidence against the traditional claims[12] that prosopagnosia was a sign of right hemisphere dysfunction.[146] Their findings also indicated that the larger of the bilateral lesions could be on the left, not the right, side. The condition does not appear to be confined to difficulty with faces, as many other classes of visual stimuli may be similarly affected. The syndrome does not seem to occur in isolation.

The case of Landis et al.[75] was of importance because the woman patient died in the acute phase (after 10 days) and was found to have a large unilateral right occipitotemporal infarct, arguing that unilateral involvement is sufficient for the syndrome to occur.

## Palinopsia

Like prosopagnosia, palinopsia has been regarded as a bit of a curiosity, not commonly a result of vascular disease. The syndrome is usually encountered in a visual field that is impaired but not entirely blind.[11] Many authors have grouped together the two variants and their frequently associated experiences:[90] in one form, there is a persistence of some or all of a visual image immediately after it has disappeared from the environment; in the other form, the image reappears only some time later, and persists for varying periods of time. This last group is quite striking, as the delay between the disappearance of the original stimulus and its reappearance may be within hours or days, and the image may persist into the following day. A peculiar feature of the palinopic images is their tendency to be incorporated in the appropriate position into visual stimuli in the present environment, such as a cigar and beard appearing on the faces of the all the people at a party. Frank hallucinations, and illusions of visual movement are common accompaniments of both types.[29]

A small literature exists on cases of vascular cause, however. Meadows and Munro[99] described three cases of palinopsia, one of whom was autopsied. The autopsied patient experienced a severe headache lasting but a few hours, then suffered palinopic images beginning the next day and recurring for the remaining 7 days of her life, unaccompanied by any other obvious complaints. A congruous, left upper quadrantanopsia was documented. The autopsy showed a predominantly subcortical infarct undermining the right lingual and fusiform gyri, which had the appearance of at least several months of age.

Michel and Troost[96] studied three patients by CT scan only, whose palinopic images also occurred in the affected visual field following presumed unilateral occipital infarction. Two affected the right, but one was left-sided. The lesions were all large.

Whether the palinopic effect represents a form of seizure remains unknown, although it is still common practice to treat such patients with anticonvulsants.

## Micropsia

Micropsia is an unusual complaint, in which objects appear smaller than expected, is infrequently reported, and rarely described with posterior cerebral artery territory infarction. The example from Yamada et al.[148] was a 63-year-old man whose complaint occurred suddenly, was associated with an acute amnesic state, as expected from large posterior cerebral artery territory infarction, but his visual field disturbance was limited to a right upper quadrantanopsia. CT scan and MR showed an infarct of the left occipital lobe and hippocampus. All the clinical features improved within a month, save for the persistence of the quadrantanopsia.

## Topographic Disorientation

The infrequently described syndrome of topographical disorientation features a striking inability of patients to find their way around.[59] In most instances, there has been infarction in the right hemisphere and left hemianopia, occasionally a disorder in recognition of faces, and other signs of involvement of the nondominant hemisphere. Yet, rarely, the syndrome may occur in isolation: in one case we studied, there was no other disturbance discovered despite intense testing: while suffering a spatial disorientation so severe that he could not find the bathroom in the apartment he had lived in for more than 40 years, he successfully conducted a high-level law practice, with no errors in language, memory, or judgment noted by any of his many colleagues.

## Disorders of Reading

Ischemic lesions in the territory of the posterior cerebral artery produce a variety of disorders labeled as alexia or dyslexia. These syndromes have proved of interest for the opportunity they provide to test mechanisms of cerebral function as well as for the different forms of disturbance encountered. Several distinctive disorders have been encountered. At the present time, all of them are casually classified as alexia or dyslexia. Yet the nature of the disorder and the extent of the lesions that underlie them differ enough that they each deserve a different descriptive term. Unfortunately, no such terms have yet come into common use.

## Pure Alexia

Major infarction in the posterior cerebral artery territory of the hemisphere dominant for speech and language may precipitate the striking disorder of pure or absolute alexia, usually the left hemisphere, but reported in the right in some instances.[112] The lexical stimuli are treated as though they are the text of an unfamiliar language. The patient usually rejects truly novel lexical stimuli, such as the alphabet of a foreign language sharing no characters in common (like Arabic compared with English), but does not separate among languages sharing the same characters as his own (e.g., English and Italian). It makes little difference whether the letters and words are presented in typed, printed, or handwritten form; even the patient's own handwriting is not read successfully. Some words ordinarily presented in a distinctive form (i.e., the script form in which the word, Coca-Cola, appears in advertisements) may be read aloud easily, but the meaning of the words is derived from the unique shape of the stimuli, not from the letters themselves. This point may be demonstrated by presenting other letters in the same general configuration. Of interest are the occasional instances in which the letters can be named when the hand is passively traced over the shapes, a pont that indicates the patient's problem is with the visual forms. Spelling aloud and naming words heard in spelled form is usually spared. In some of the cases, single letters may be read aloud and for comprehension. Characteristically, when presented with lexical stimuli, the patient names them with little hesitation and often displays little awareness his responses are well off the mark. For example, Wyllie's case III[147] (Fig. 17-8) named the word "Dugald" as a series of single letters "k-a-n-i-o-i", and similarly responded to the digit set "123456" as "i-r-e-i-u-e", and even named the mathematical symbols "+ × =" as "n-e-a." Musical notes and digits are classifiable separate from letters, but the items themselves do not convey meaning. The best-known example of this effect was described by Dejerine in his report of the first patient with absolute alexia:[37] the patient was an accomplished musician, but after his stroke he lost the power to read musical scores, although he retained the ability to play and sing from memory.

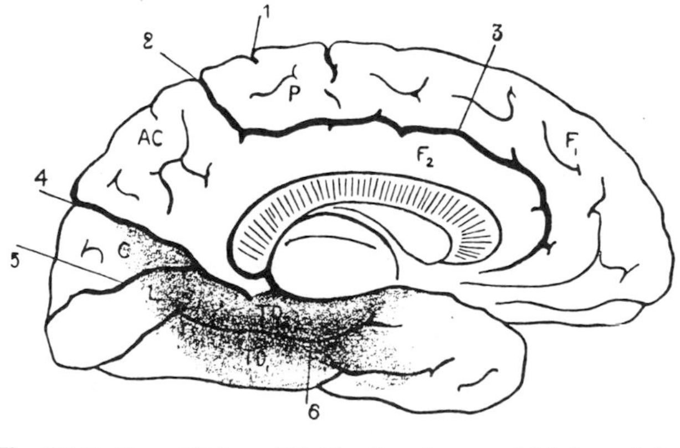


**Fig. 17-8.** Case III from Wyllie showing mesial left occipital infarction that produced absolute atexia. (From Wyllie,[147] with permission.)

This clinical picture has been described in several striking cases and is often accompanied by many other disorders.[39] In some, the alexia has been accompanied by a dense right homonymous hemianopia, and has been accompanied by color dysnomia, amnesic aphasia, and memory disturbance indicative of a major left posterior cerebral artery territory infarction.[21,34,52] In other cases, the deficits accompanying the alexia have been less spectacular.[34] Color dysnomia, in particular, occurs with the larger lesions[34,68,102] and may be absent in some cases[142] (see Fig. 17-6).

The *neuropathology* of this condition has been subject to many interpretations,[44,52,57,102,140] recently reviewed in detail.[34] In Dejerine's frequently discussed case,[35] the lesion, an old infarct, had damaged the inferior edge of the posterior portion of the corpus callosum, the cortex of the cuneus and adjacent calcarine region, and penetrated completely through the underlying white matter to the wall of the ventricle. Although Dejerine's case is commonly interpreted as having hemianopia, the right visual field function was intact enough that Landolt's[76] original examination demonstrated only a hemiachromatopsia (see the section on color in this chapter); the patient had full, if dim, vision in the right visual field to white targets. Dejerine emphasized that the subcortical component of the infarct served to disrupt the projections to the angular gyrus (which he held as the site where the lexical information gained access to the language zone) from both the ipsilateral calcarine cortex and the opposite side, this latter pathway via the corpus callosum. Dejerine made little mention of the callosal lesion, nor did Vialet[140] in a thorough review of the case. In both instances, emphasis was placed on the deep paraventricular lesion. Damasio and Damasio[34] resurrected these observations, drew attention to the likelihood that the inferior fibers of the forceps major, which cross in the inferior portion of the corpus callosum and terminate in the inferior visual association cortices, were the fibers of relevance for the conveyance of lexical information from the right to the left hemisphere. The anatomic course of these fibers places them in the position to be caught in a deep infarct, which penetrates to the wall of the ventricle. In his original publication, Dejerine did not specify whether he believed this information was conveyed from the right hemisphere via transcallosal pathways directly to the language zone without interruption, or by an indirect route through the left calcarine region. The lesion shown in his often-reproduced diagram can be interpreted either way, but is placed laterally enough to emphasize his original point that it served to interrupt the pathway from both calcarine regions. The point is not trivial: should the indirect path be the route, the occurrence of absolute alexia would necessitate a hemianopia; should the direct route apply, hemianopia from calcarine infarction could occur without alexia if the fibers crossing the callosum are spared (Fig. 17-9).

The widely quoted modern cases[21,31,52] do not bear on this point, since the infarcts were so extensive that the entire left calcarine pathway was destroyed. Both of Wyllie's cases[147] showed a major infarction in the proximal calcarine and lingual gyrus regions, which spread sufficiently deep to destroy the entire visual radiations, functionally nullifying the intact calcarine cortex farther back toward the occipital pole.

*Incomplete right hemianopia,* with macular sparing, is commonly encountered without disorders of reading, but such cases should come as no surprise, as the pathway is still intact through the macular zone of the calcarine cortex. Vialet[140] demonstrated that *complete right hemianopia* from a calcarine lesion could occur without alexia, provided the deep paraventricular regions are spared. Foix and Hillemand[44] called attention to a role for posterior portion of the corpus callosum by documenting a similar case. Stommel and colleagues[135] described a case of alexia without agraphia with spleniogeniculate infarction. In some of the cases with incomplete hemianopia[80] the disorder of reading has taken the form of slowed and incomplete responses to the stimuli, with particular difficulties in discriminating the right-hand portions of the words (see below).

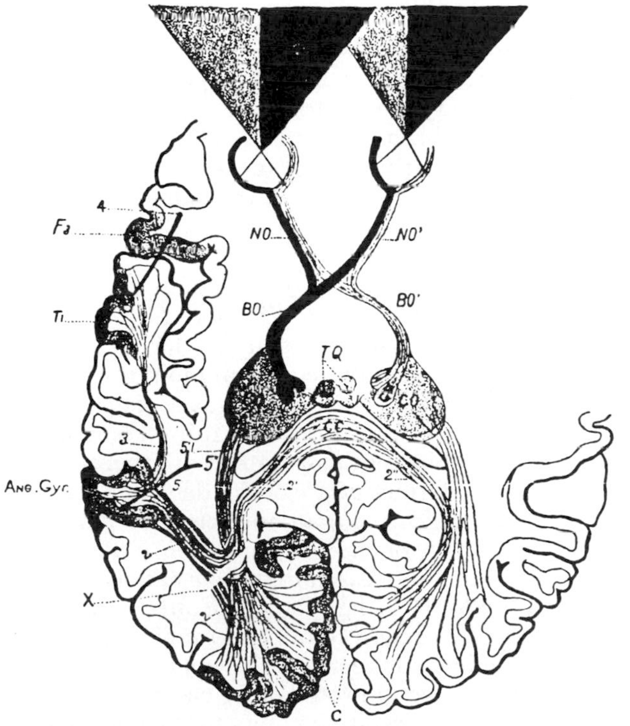


**Fig. 17-9.** Diagram of the possible site (X) of interruption of the visual pathways linking the calcarine cortices (C) with the angular gyrus (Ang. Gyr.). (Adapted from Dejerine and Vialet,[37] with permission.)

Orgogozo et al.[104] and Damasio and Damasio[34] have described instances of alexia in the presence of a *right upper quadrantanopsia.* The locus of the infarction was documented by CT scan. The authors argued for the original notion of Dejerine and Vialet that the lesion interrupted the deep paraventricular pathways. The patient described by Orgogozo et al.[104] was able to read small and large letters without hesitation, but reading words was described as laborious, slow, proceeding from letter to letter to arrive at the syllables, finally the word, but with numerous errors. The reading of long words was impossible. Certain common words such as "good morning" were read as a whole ("globalment"). This patient's deficit seems to strain the notions of pure alexia, arguing instead for some degree of disordered visual discrimination. Patient 3 of Damasio and Damasio[34] was described as having "pure alexia"; no clinical details were given.

A small literature documents that alexia may occur in the *absence* of any evidence of right hemianopia. The first description of the syndrome was made without autopsy data:[108] a 20-year-old woman, walking in the street, suddenly noticed she could not read the letters on a sign nor the names of the subway stations. Her alexia was described as complete for all variety of reading tasks, including musical notes. The handful of autopsied cases, the first of which was described by Greenblatt,[57] have been from tumors, arteriovenous malformations, and the like, but not from infarction.[58]

## Hemidyslexia

Hemidyslexia, which was described by Wilbrand[145] as a macular hemianopic disturbance of reading (*makulär-hemianopische Lesestörung*), has received little attention in the literature.[80] In our experience, it is a frequent accompaniment of a homonymous hemianopia contralateral to infarction, affecting the posterior cerebral artery territory of the hemisphere dominant for speech and language. In some instances, the hemianopia is limited to the macular region, as demonstrated by Polyak's case, Harry Kraft.[114] It may even occur without hemianopia.[24]

For most patients so afflicted, the syndrome occurs from left-sided infarction and presents as misreading of the right-hand end of longer words. The errors occur whether the task is reading aloud or for comprehension, whether the words are printed or written, large or small, isolated or embedded in text, so long as the words are lengthy, on the order of four letters or more. They occur less often when the right-hand end of the word is easily predicted by the left-hand end, that is, words such as "eight." The errors are present more often when the right-hand end has many possibilities not predicted by the left-hand end, that is, "predator." The term hemidyslexia is not quite accurate, as the errors do not occur beginning at the midpoint of the stimulus, but, instead, only at some point beyond the midline of the word.

The hemianopia that accompanies hemidyslexia is usually incomplete. Most often it takes the form of upper quadrantanopsia with or without macular sparing, a sign that the lower bank of the calcarine cortex has suffered infarction. At times, colors seem dimmer in the affected field.

The quadrantanopsia with sparing of the other quadrant or the macula indicates the infarct was not large enough to destroy the underlying visual radiations. The limited infarction appears to spare the pathways involved in conveying the lexical information decoded by the right calcarine cortex; it is inferred that this information concerning the left-hand side of the lexical stimulus does not pass through the left calcarine surface gray matter on its way to whatever brain regions derive the language value of the stimulus.

Hemidyslexia is often part of a complex syndrome of impaired response to complex visual stimuli, which has been explored in detail only rarely, the most elegantly by Levine and Calvanio.[80]

Hemidyslexia for stimuli from the left side of space occurs following section of the corpus callosum, but has not been reported in ischemic vascular disease thus far. A small branch of the posterior cerebral artery supplies the posterior corpus callosum. Its occlusion could possibly precipitate such a syndrome.

## Dyschromatopsia, Color and Color-Name Disconnection, and Color Dysnomia

### Dyschromatopsia

Some degree of faulty color discrimination may occur with dysfunction at any level along the visual pathway.[56,125] The lateral geniculate body is considered to play a role in color discrimination,[78] but deficits in color discrimination would be expected to occur only when the lesion is bilateral. However, when infarction is the cause of dyschromatopsia, it usually lies in the occipital lobe inferior to the calcarine cortex in the lingual gyrus.

This type of disturbance has been described in numerous instances of unilateral lingual gyrus involvement, either with full-thickness infarction or with subcortical infarction that undermined the gyrus.[31,35,37,76,94,149] The lesion may be unilateral on either side[76,114,116] or bilateral.[79,107] This correlation has also been established by CT scan studies.[33,73]

Color blindness from cerebral disease shows impaired performance on tests of color discrimination, for example, Ishihara plates. In typical cases, the colors in the affected field are described as gray, pale, or washed-out in the involved field(s). At times, a given color is misnamed for another having similar hue or brightness. This last finding is of little clinical value, since it also occurs in patients whose performance on the Ishihara plates is intact (see below). Recall is normal for the color-name characteristically associated with a given object (e.g., green with grass). A degree of improvement over time has been reported, even though an upper quadrantanopsia might remain.[3,73] Prosopagnosia and spatial and topographic disorientation have been reported as associated findings in a few cases with right posterior cerebral artery territory infarction.[27] Dyslexia often accompanies right hemidyschromatopsia.

One among these cases[35,37,76] was explained by subsequent reviewers as a disconnection syndrome.[51] Unfortunately, few of the reports described the exact means of testing for color, often omitting such details as whether the testing was done unilaterally or bilaterally, whether the patient was asked to name the color or simply point to it when named, or whether the patient simply had the visual fields tested with different color stimuli. As a result, the literature remains rather disappointing concerning the clinical points that differentiate between hemidyschromatopsia for the field contralateral to an infarct and a "disconnection" between two sides of the brain.

### Color and Color-Name Disconnection

The term color and color-name disconnection was designed to describe a bidirectional impairment in relating a color to its name in the absence of deficits in color discrimination. The term *color agnosia* has also been used. The absence of deficits in color discrimination are revealed by the normal performance on tests such as the Ishihara color plates. The bidirectional impairment in relating a color to its name is shown by errors in naming colors at sight and in matching color names heard or color names seen to color choices, or vice versa.

It is to this type of case that Geschwind and Fusillo[52] have applied the term *disconnection syndrome* to stress the point that the lesion may have separated the adequately discriminated visual input in the right hemisphere from access to the language region of the left hemisphere. As a result, visual stimuli would presumably be unable to be associated with their names, causing alexia (letters and words), defective naming of colors, and defective matching of color names to colors. In support of the disconnection notion, Geschwind and Fusillo stressed that their patient "would answer at random"[52] when shown an object and asked whether it was a certain color. This random quality of color naming has not been a feature of other reported cases, however, even in some other cases with a bidirectional failure in relating colors to their names.[120]

The infarct in the best-known case[52] was in the distribution of the left posterior cerebral artery, destroying most of the gray and deep white matter of the medial occipital lobe, including the visual radiations, inferior longitudinal fasciculus, and the crossing fibers through the splenium of the corpus callosum in the tapetum. A subsequent case[120] showed more circumscribed subcortical infarction[12] underlining the left lingual gyrus. Another case used by these authors in support of their thesis[35,37,84] appears to have had right hemidyschromatopsia; it is not clear from the details of the clinical case report that a disturbance as thoroughly documented as that by Geschwind and Fusillo[52] was present.

Unfortunately, for most of the other reported cases whose deficits might represent the bidirectional disconnection, precise documentation of a disconnection state was lacking.[62,106,117,122,130,131,134,139] In only a few cases was complete testing done for color discrimination, impaired color naming, and impaired matching of colors with color names.[52,82,84] Clinically, these cases also showed a right homonymous hemianopia and dyslexia.

## Color Dysnomia

Color dysnomia, often considered synonymous with the bidirectional disconnection syndromes, appears to be the more common of the acquired cerebral disturbances involving response to color stimuli. Its existence provides another indication that I (JPM) have had experience with some unusual examples of color dysnomia.[102]

In the initial days after onset, our patient (see Fig. 17-6) showed errors both in naming colors and in selecting the correct color from among an array of color choices when a color name was dictated aloud to him. However, within several days, he became able to select a color from among several choices when its name was shown to him or dictated to him. He also was easily able to recall the name of a color commonly associated with given items and items commonly associated with given a color. Yet he persisted in having difficulties in naming a color shown to him and in selecting its name among several choices. His naming errors were not random nor of the confabulatory type. He often named a given color using the name of another color close to it on the spectrum of hue or brightness, such as green for blue, yellow for orange. The errors were mild enough to be overlooked on casual testing and might have been attributed to dim light in less rigorous test settings. Casual explanations such as these probably account for the infrequency with which the dysnomia is reported in cases with an infarct in a similar locale. When sought in such cases, the deficit is often easily demonstrated. The infarct is often quite modest, and may be confined to the subcortical structures of the lingual gyrus.

The syndrome of color dysnomia is also of interest, since it may be present without a dyslexia, that is, with preserved reading. Although the two deficits frequently coexist, color dysnomia and alexia do not reflect a common mechanism for their occurrence; rather, they show that spatially proximate regions of the cerebrum serving different functions are susceptible to simultaneous involvement by the same lesion if it is large enough.[115]

It usually persists for many months and may be permanent.

## Amnesic Color Dysnomia

Amnesic color dysnomia, an almost vanishingly rare syndrome, refers to a disturbance in the recall of the names of the colors that are characteristic of a given object, that is, green for grass, and vice versa. Tests of color discrimination and cross-matching of color with color names are said to be performed well.[54] No definite neuropathologic basis for these disorders has been established.

## Unusual Variants

Other types of disturbances in response to colors occur in cerebral disease.[30] However, none of them have as yet been related to a focal lesion. The delineation of most of them requires the examiner to depend on the patient's subjective description of the altered appearance of color and of its relationship to the environment. The syndromes include illusory spread of color.

# Transcortical Sensory Aphasia

An unusual disturbance in language function, transcortical sensory aphasia suffers both from lack of autopsy correlation and disagreements concerning its clinical features. Whether to place this syndrome among the consequences of posterior cerebral artery territory infarction is subject to argument, but it is discussed here because of the high frequency of accompanying heminaopia, visual object agnosia, and medial occipital low density seen on CT scan.

Kertesz et al.[70] are the latest group to try and define satisfactorily. Using CT scan and the results of the Western Aphasia Battery tests, 15 patients were collected for study. In 12 patients the lesion was diagnosed by isotope brain scan, in 6 by CT scan. This manner of documentation probably reflects the very low incidence of the disorder and the long span of time over which the 15 cases were accumulated. A contralateral hemianopia occurred in 12, one of whom had only an inferior quadrantanopsia. Some form of sensory loss was present in 11 patients. Only five had any degree of weakness, in four of whom it was described as "slight." In five cases the disturbed higher cerebral function was accompanied by "visual agnosia." An unusual disturbance in speech and language was described by the authors[70] as fluent and circumlocutory speech, whose content was mainly semantic jargon.

The lesion locations were equally unusual, as practically all of the cases seem to show massive involvement of the posterior half of the brain, spreading from the occipital pole forward on both the medial and lateral surfaces, and in many the abnormality reached far forward along the mesial occipital lobe, well within the territory of the posterior cerebral artery. The authors suggested the sites of infarction were "in the posterior cerebral artery territory or in the watershed area . . . between posterior cerebral and middle cerebral arteries. . . ."[70]

The mechanism of the infarctions is unclear. It is possible that this syndrome may be the result of an internal carotid artery occlusion with distal field infarction affecting the parieto-occipital region in the unusual instances where the posterior cerebral artery is a branch of the internal carotid artery. For embolism to achieve this result would require some remarkable anatomy. At least one of their cases was an arteriovenous malformation, a lesion suitable for such an unusual location, crossing as it does between two major arterial territories. Little more is currently known of this interesting syndrome, and it awaits further study.

## Amnesic Aphasia

Amnesic aphasia is characterized by a failure to recall the names of people as well as many other individual nouns when the stimuli were presented in visual or auditory form. Commonly, the expected response fails to occur, the patient often falling silent or hesitating as if the name is about to be produced momentarily ("tip of the tongue" phenomenon). When the name fails to appear, it is rare for a neologism or other substitutive error to be produced. Instead, attributes of the item are described, indicating the patient's familiarity with the item in question. The failures in naming are often associated with circumlocutions, lame excuses for failure, and a general acceptance of the correct name when offered.[54]

Although classically considered a sign of deep temporal lobe involvement,[54] amnesic aphasia has occasionally been reported, often incidentally,[62,147] in cases showing infarction in the territory of the dominant posterior cerebral artery. The exact pathologic correlation for such deficits remains unclear, as does the issue of whether memory deficit and amnesic aphasia are functionally related or simply result from a lesion simultaneously involving physically proximate regions of the cerebrum serving separate functions.[116]

## Memory Deficits

Posterior cerebral artery territory infarction may have a profound effect on memory function. Both embolism and thrombus have been found responsible.[137] The occlusions have usually been found proximally in the posterior cerebral artery in the stem and precortical portion. Amnesic disorders have also been reported from occlusion of thalamoperforants, but in these cases the possibility of simultaneous infarction of structures supplied by larger posterior cerebral artery branches is not ruled out.

Based on the available literature, the occurrence of an amnesic state is no guide to whether the infarct is of thrombotic or embolic origin.

## Bilateral Infarction

The literature contains numerous examples of bilateral posterior cerebral artery territory infarction of varying size described at autopsy[138] or by CT scan.[113] In these bilateral cases, the infarcts frequently are found spread along most of the undersurface of the cerebrum, involving the hippocampus, lingual and fusiform gyri, some as far posteriorly as the cuneus,[17] while others have been extensive enough to include the fornices and fimbria of the hippocampus.[141] The hippocampus seems to be the most commonly affected of these various structures in amnesic cases. A single case report with infarction confined to the region of the hippocampus lacked most of the essential clinical details needed to determine the clinical features of isolated hippocampal infarction.[38] In case reports where it is described, the memory disorder itself seems to have the characteristics found in surgical removals of the hippocampus bilaterally.

A large literature has accumulated indicating bilateral hippocampal involvement as a necessary condition for amnesia to occur and to persist.[101] A single surgical case suggests that a bilateral disruption of the fornix may achieve the same effect,[136] but no long-term follow-up was reported on this patient. In another similar case,[99] later examination revealed improvement in the memory deficit. Other cases showed no such effects occur.[2,36,42] The exact role of fornix section in the occurrence and persistence of recent memory deficits has been difficult to determine, since instances of isolated bilateral fornix interruption are rare.[63] In a literature search, we did not find any cases of isolated infarction.

The rare case with bilateral posterior cerebral artery territory infarction with unilateral hippocampal or limbic infarction exists to confound efforts to settle the role of the bilateral lesion in memory disorder. Benson et al.[12] described a 47-year-old physician with right hemianopia, alexia, visual agnosia, color agnosia, prosopagnosia, and "impaired verbal learning." This disturbance was manifested by an "inability to learn the names of ward personnel, considerable difficulty in learning the Babcock sentence, and ability to remember only one or two of four unrelated words after five minutes." He was noted to have made some improvements in the first few months after onset but remained disabled. Although bilateral fusiform gyrus and posterior callosal infarcts were found, the hippocampal infarct was confined to the left side. The autopsy findings were described only on cut section.

## Unilateral Infarcts

Few cases have been reported of memory loss with a unilateral nonvascular lesion,[41,50,103,136] and only a handful from autopsy-documented infarction. Geschwind and Fusillo[52] described a man with thrombosis of the left posterior cerebral artery whose infarct was detailed in serial sections. On admission, he was able to recall his name, stated his age incorrectly and was unable to recall his address. He failed to recall any of four objects after 1 minute. In addition, prominent deficits were encountered in reading aloud and in naming colors and simple objects. Severe disturbances in topographic orientation and topography were also noted. No further description was given concerning his memory disorder, but when he was seen 7 weeks after onset, the recent memory deficits were said to have "cleared completely." The topographic disorientation "cleared to normal in the next few weeks." He died 15 months after the stroke occurred. On serial sections, the left hippocampus was infarcted and the left fornix had undergone complete degeneration.

Our own case[102] (Fig. 17-11) showed a severe memory disorder from onset, which persisted unchanged until his death on day 82. On initial examination within 12 hours of onset, this patient also stated his name, failed to recall his exact age, and was unable to state his address nor where he had been the evening of his stroke. He repeatedly asked many questions, such as "Where is my wife?," accepted the examiner's answer, and within seconds asked the question again. When his wife arrived hours after onset and mentioned her brother by name, he asked "Ed who?." He repeatedly attempted to learn the examiner's name, often wrote it on a pad, and when the examiner reappeared, failed to recall the name, and failed to consult his notepad. Weeks after discharge, when returning to the laboratory for reexamination, he regularly introduced himself to the staff whom he had met on every previous occasion, and only rarely walked spontaneously in the correct direction toward the examining room. He showed a retrograde and anterograde amnesia for the events surrounding his admission, faulty retention of verbal material, impaired retention of a form discrimination test, and an amnesic dysnomia. Whether his deficit would have persisted over a longer period remains an open question. The pathologic findings indicated only unilateral infarction of the left hippocampus, with secondary degeneration of the left fornix and the precommissural bed nuclei of the septum.

Escourolle and Gray[43] reported an important autopsied case with memory disturbance whose infarct affected the left occipital and temporal lobe with atrophy of the fimbria of the hippocampus, the fornix, and the anterior nucleus of the thalamus. An amnesic state from occlusion of the left anterior choroidal artery was recently reported by Amarenco et al.[6] the first such report.

## Clinical Features of the Memory Deficit

Where details were provided, the cases reported on the clinical features of memory deficit have shown profound disturbances in memory, especially for recent events when tested by conversational methods. The characteristics of the memory impairment and the performance on special laboratory tests are essentially identical to those reported[127] on bilateral medial temporal regions that include the hippocampus[123] and from unilateral temporal lobe removals.[41,100,119,143] An acute confusional state in left posterior cerebral artery territory infarction has also been described.[40]

## Associated Symptoms and Signs

An isolated amnesic state has yet to be reported from infarction in the posterior cerebral artery territory. To date, such cases have produced other deficits accompanying the amnesic state.

## REFERENCES


1. Abbie AA: The blood supply of the visual pathways. Med J Aust 2:199, 1938
2. Akelaitis AJ: Study of language functions unilaterally following section of the corpus callosum. J Neuropathol Exp Neurol 2:226, 1943
3. Albert ML, Reches A, Silverberg R: Associative visual agnosia with alexia. Neurology (NY) 25:322, 1975
4. Albert NL, Reches A, Silverberg R: Hemianopic colour blindness. J Neurol Neurosurg Psychiatry 38:546, 1975
5. Albert NL, Soffer D, Silverberg R, Reches A: The anatomic basis of visual agnosia. Neurology (NY) 29:876, 1979
6. Amarenco P, Cohen P, Roullet E et al: Syndrome amnésique lors d'un infarctus du térritoire de l'artère choroidienne antérieure gauche. Rev Neurol (Paris) 144:36, 1988
7. Assal G, Regli F: Syndrome de disconnexion visuo-verbale et visuo-gestuelle. Rev Neurol (Paris) 136:365, 1980
8. Bay E: Agnose und Funktionswandel: Eine hirnpathologische Studie. Springer-Verlag, Berlin, 1950
9. Beevor CE: On the distribution of the different arteries supplying the human brain. Phil Trans R Soc Ser B 200:1, 1909
10. Bender MB, Feldman M: The so-called visual agnosias. *Brain* 95:173, 1972
11. Bender MB, Feldman M, Sobin AJ: Palinopsia. Brain 91:321, 1968
12. Benson DF, Segarra J, Albert ML: Visula agnosia—prosopagnosia. Arch Neurol 30:307, 1974

13. Benton S, Levy I, Swash M: Vision in the temporal crescent in occipital infarction. Brain 103:83, 1980
14. Bergman PS: Cerebral blindness. Arch Psychiatr Neurol 78:568, 1957
15. Blythe IM, Kennard C, Ruddock KH: Residual vision in patients with retrogeniculate lesions of the visual pathways. Brain 110:887, 1987
16. Bogousslavsky J, Regli F, van Melle G: Unilateral occipital infarction: evaluating the risks of developing bilateral loss of vision. J Neurol Neurosurg Psychiatry 46:78, 1983
17. Brindley GS, Janota I: Observations on cortical blindness and on vascular lesions that cause loss of recent memory. J Neurol Neurosurg Psychiatry 38:459, 1975
18. Cambier J, Masson M, Elghozi D et al: Agnosie visuelle sans hemianopsie droite chez un sujet droitier. Rev Neurol (Paris) 136:727, 1980
19. Caplan LR: "Top of the basilar" syndrome. Neurology (NY) 30:72, 1980
20. Caplan LR, DeWitt LD, Pessin MS et al: Lateral thalamic infarcts. Arch Neurol 45:959, 1988
21. Caplan LR, Hedley-Whyte T: Cuing and memory dysfunction in alexia without agraphia—a case report. Brain 97:251, 1974
22. Castaigne P, Lhermitte F, Buge A et al: Paramedian thalamic and midbrain infarcts: clinical and neuropathological study. Ann Neurol 10:127, 1981
23. Castaigne P, Lhermitte F, Gautier JC et al: Arterial occlusions in the vertebro-basilar system—a study of forty-four patients with post-mortem data. Brain 96:133, 1973
24. Castro-Caldas A, Salgado V: Right hemifield alexia without hemianopsia. Arch Neurol 41:84, 1984
25. Celesia GG, Archer CR, Kuriowa Y: Visual function of the extrageniculo-calcarine system in man. Arch Neurol 37:704, 1980
26. Chambers BR, Brooder RJ, Donnan GA: Proximal posterior cerebral artery occlusion simulating middle cerebral artery occlusion. Neurology (NY) 41:385, 1991
27. Cogan DG: Visuospatial dysgnosia. Am J Ophthalmol 88:361, 1979
28. Conomy JP, Laureno R, Massarweh W: Transient behavioral syndrome associated with reversible vascular lesions of the fusiform-calcarine region in humans. Abstracted. Ann Neurol 12:83, 1982
29. Critchley M: Types of visual preseveration: "palinopsia" and "illusory visual spread." Brain 74:267, 1951
30. Critchley M: Acquired disturbances of color perception of central origin. Brain 88:711, 1965
31. Cumming WJK, Hurwitz LJ, Perl NT: A study of a patient who had alexia without agraphia. J Neurol Neurosurg Psychiatry 33:34, 1970
32. Damasio A, Damasio H, Van Hoesen GW: Prosopagnosia: anatomic basis and behavioral mechanisms. Neurology (NY) 323:331, 1982
33. Damasio A, Yamada T, Damasio H: Central achromatopsia: Behavioral and anatomic and physiologic aspects. Neurology (NY) 30:1064, 1980
34. Damasio AR, Damasio H: The anatomic basis of pure alexia. Neurology (NY) (Cleveland) 33:1573, 1983
35. Dejerine J: Differentes varietes de cecite verbale. C R Soc Biol Paris 4:61, 1892
36. Dejerine J, Roussy G: La syndrome thalamique. Rev Neurol (Paris) 14:521, 1906
37. Dejerine J, Vialet N: La localisation anatomique de la cécite verbale pure. C R Soc Biol Paris 5:790, 1893
38. DeJong RN, Itabashi HH, Olson JR: Memory loss due to hippocampal lesions. Arch Neurol 20:339, 1969
39. De Renzi E, Zambolin A, Crisi G: The pattern of neuropsychological impairment associated with left posterior cerebral artery infarcts. Brain 110:1099, 1987
40. Devinsky O, Bear D, Volpe BT: Confusional states following posterior cerebral artery infarction. Arch Neurol 45:160, 1988
41. Dimsdale H, Logue V, Piercy M: A case of persisting impairment of recent memory following right temporal lobectomy. Neuropsychologia 1:287, 1964
42. Dott NM: The Hypothalamus. Oliver & Boyd, London, 1938
43. Escourolle R, Gray F: Las accidents vasculaires du systeme limbique. p. 195. In Proceedings of the Seventh International Congress of Neuropathology. Excerpta Medica, Amsterdam, 1975
44. Foix C, Hillemand P: Contribution à l'étude des ramollisemments protuberantiels. Rev Neurol (Paris) 43:287, 1925
45. Förster O: Über Rindenblindheit. Graefes Arch Ophthalmol 36:94, 1890
46. Frisen L: Quadruple sectoranopia and sectorial optic atrophy: a syndrome of the distal anterior choroidal artery. J Neurol Neurosurg Psychiatry 42:590, 1979
47. Frisen L, Holmegaard L, Rosencrantz M: Sectorial optic atrophy and homonymous horizontal sectoranopia: a lateral choroidal artery syndrome? J Neurol Neurosurg Psychiatry 41:374, 1978
48. Gacs G, Fox AJ, Barnett HJM, Vinuela F: CT visualization of intracranial arterial thromboembolism. Stroke 14:756, 1983
49. Galloway JR, Greitz T: The medial and lateral choroidal arteries An anatomic and roentgenographic study. Acta Radiol [Diagn] (Stockh) 53:353, 1960
50. Garcia-Bengochea F, De La Torre O, Esquivel O et al: The section of the fornix in the surgical treatment of certain epilepsies. Trans Am Neurol Assoc 176:1954, 1959
51. Geschwind N: Disconnexion syndromes in animals and man. Brain 88:237, 1965
52. Geschwind N, Fusillo M: Color-naming defects in association with alexia. Arch Neurol 15:137, 1966
53. Ghika JA, Bogousslavsky J, Regli F: Deep perforators from the carotid system: template of the vascular territories. Arch Neurol 47:1097, 1990
54. Goldstein K: Language and Language Disturbances. New York Grune & Stratton, New York, 1948

55. Goto K, Takagawa K, Uemura K et al: Posterior cerebral artery occlusion: clinical computed tomographic and angiographic correlation. Radiology 132:357, 1979
56. Green GJ, Lessell S: Acquired cerebral dyschromatopsia. Arch Ophthalmol 95:121, 1977
57. Greenblatt SH: Alexia without agraphia or hemianopsia. Brain 96:307, 1973
58. Greenblatt SH: Subangular alexia without agraphia or hemianopia. Brain Lang 3:229, 1976
59. Habib M, Sirigu A: Pure topographical disorientation: a definition and anatomical basis. Cortex 23:73, 1987
60. Hayman LA, Berman SA, Hinck VC: Correlation of CT cerebral vascular territories with function. II. Posterior cerebral artery. AJNR 2:219, 1981
61. Head H: Aphasia: An historical review. Brain 43:340, 1920
62. Heidenhain A: Beitrag zur Kenntnis der Seelenblindheit. Monatsschr Psychiatr Neurol 66:61, 1927
63. Heilman KN, Sypert GW: Korsakoff's syndrome resulting from bilateral fornix lesions. Neurology (NY) 27:490, 1977
64. Heller-Bettinger I, Kepes JJ, Preskorn SH et al: Bilateral altitudinal anopia caused by infarction of the calcarine cortex. Neurology (NY) 26:1176 1976
65. Holmes G: Selected Papers of Sir Gordon Holmes p. 195. London, 1956
66. Hommel M, Besson G, Pollak P et al: Hemiplegia in posterior cerebral artery occlusion. Neurology (NY) 40:1496, 1990
67. Horenstein S, Chamberlin W, Conomy J: Infarction of the fusiform and calcarine regions: agitated delirium and hemianopia. Trans Am Neurol Assoc 92:85, 1967
68. Johansson T, Fahlgren H: Alexia without agraphia: lateral and medial infarction of the occipital lobe. Neurology (NY) 29:390, 1979
69. Kaul SN, DuBoulay GH, Kendall BE, Ross Russell RW: Relationship between visual field defects and arterial occlusion in the posterior cerebral circulation. J Neurol Neurosurg Psychiatry 37:1033, 1974
70. Kertesz A, Sheppard A, MacKenzie R: Localization in transcortical sensory aphasia. Arch Neurol 39:475, 1982
71. Kinkel WR, Newman RP, Jacobs L: Posterior cerebral artery branch occlusions: CT and anatomic considerations. p. 117. In Berguer R, Bauer RB (eds): Vertebrobasilar Arterial Occlusive Disease: Medical and Surgical Management. Raven Press, New York, 1984
72. Kleihues P, Hizawa K: Die Infarkte der A. Cerebri posterior. Arch Psychiatr Z Ges Neurol 208:263, 1966
73. Kolmel HW: Pure homonymous hemiachromatopsia. Findings with neuro-ophthalmologic examination and imaging procedures. Eur Arch Psychiatr Neurol Sci 237:237, 1988
74. Kubik CS, Adams RD: Occlusion of the basilar artery: a clinical and pathological study. Brain 69:73, 1946
75. Landis T, Regard M, Bliestle A, Kleihues P: Prosopagnosia and agnosia for noncanonical views: an autopsied case. Brain 111:1287, 1988
76. Landolt E: De la cécite verbale. p. 418. In: Nederlansch Tijdschrift voor geneeskunde Feestbundel oan Franciscus Corneilius Donders op den 27 Mei 1888. F Van Rossen, Amsterdam, 1888
77. Lazorthes G, Salamon G: Etude anatomique et radio-anatomique de la vascularisation arterielle du thalamus. Ann radiol 14:905, 1971
78. LeGros Clark WE: The laminar pattern of the lateral geniculate nucleus considered in relation to color vision. Docum Ophthalmol 3:57, 1949
79. Lenz G: Zwei Sektionsfalle doppelseitigen zentraler Farbenhemianopsie. Z Ges Neurol Psychiatr 71:135, 1921
80. Levine DN, Calvanio R: A study of the visual defect in verbal alexia-simultanagnosia. Brain 101:65, 1978
81. Levine DN, Finklestein S: Delayed psychosis after right temporoparietal stroke or trauma: relation to epilepsy. Neurology (NY) 32:267, 1982
82. Lewandowsky M: Über Abspaltung des Farbensinnes. Monatsschr Psychiatr Neurol 23:488, 1908
83. Lilly R, Cummings JL, Benson DF, Frankel M: The human Klüver-Bucy syndrome. Neurology (Cleveland) 33:1141, 1983
84. Lissauer H: Ein Fall von Seelenblindheit nebst einem Beitrage zur Theorie derselben. Arch Psychiatr Nervenkr 21:222, 1890
85. Mackenzie I, Meighan S, Pollock EN: On the projection of the retinal quadrants on the lateral geniculate bodies and the relationship of the quadrants to the optic radiations. Trans Ophthalmol Soc UK 53:142, 1933
86. Manfredi M, Curccu G: Thalamic pain revisited. p. 73. In Loeb C (ed): Studies in Cerebrovascular Disease Masson Italia Editori, Milan, 1981
87. Margolis MT, Newton TH, Hoyt WF: Cortical branches of the posterior cerebral artery anatomic-radiologic correlation. Neuroradiology 2:127 1971
88. Margolis MT, Smith CG, Richardson WF: The course and distribution of the arteries supplying the visual (striate) cortex. Am J Ophthalmol 61:1391, 1966
89. McAuley DL, Ross Russell RW: Correlation of CAT scan and visual field defects in vascular lesions of the posterior visual pathways. J Neurol Neurosurg Psychiatry 42:298, 1979
90. Meadows JC, Munro SS: Palinopsia. J Neurol Neurosurg Psychiatry 40:5, 1977
91. Medina JL, Chokroverty S, Rubino FA: Syndrome of agitated delirium and visual impairment: a manifestation of medial temporooccipital infarction. J Neurol Neurosurg Psychiatry 40:861, 1977
92. Medina JL, Rubino FA, Ross E: Agitated delirium caused by infarctions of the hippocampal formation and fusiform and lingual gyri: a case report. Neurology (NY) 24:1181, 1974
93. Melamed E, Abraham FA, Lavy S: Cortical blindness as a manifestation of basilar artery occlusion. Eur Neurol 11:22, 1974

94. Merle P: Aphasie et hemiachromatopsie. Rev Neurol (Paris) 21:1129, 1908
95. Meyer O: Ein- und doppleseitige homonyme Hemianopsia mit Orientirungsstörungen. Monatsschr Psychiatr Neurol 8:440, 1900
96. Michel EM, Troost BT: Palinopsia: cerebral localization with computed tomography. Neurology (NY) 30:887, 1980
97. Milisavljevic MM, Marinkovic SV, Gibo H, Puskas LF: The thalamogeniculate perforators of the posterior cerebral artery: the microsurgical anatomy. Neurosurgery 28:523, 1991
98. Miller NR: Walsh and Hoyt's Clinical Neuro-Ophthalmology. 4th Ed. Vol. 1. Williams & Wilkins, Baltimore, 1982
99. Milner B: Discussion of Sweet WH et al: loss of recent memory following section of fornix. Trans Am Neurol Assoc 84:78, 1959
100. Milner B: Laterality effects in audition. p. 177. In VB Mountcastle (ed): *Interhemispheric Relations and Cerebral Dominance.* Johns Hopkins University Press, Baltimore, 1962
101. Milner B: Amnesia following operations on the temporal lobes. p. 109. In Whitty CMW, Zangwill OL (ed): Amnesia. Butterworth, London, 1966.
102. Mohr JP, Leicester J, Stoddard LT, Sidman M: Right hemianopia with memory and colors in circumscribed left posterior cerebral artery territory infarction. Neurology (NY) 21:1104, 1971
103. Ojemann GA, Blick KI, Ward AA: Improvement and disturbance of short-term verbal memory during human ventrolateral thalamic stimulation. Trans Am Neurol Assoc 94:72, 1969
104. Orgogozo JM, Pere JJ, Strube E: Alexie sans agraphie "agnose" des colours et atteinte de l'hemichamp visuel droite: un syndrome de l'artère cérébrale posterieure. Sem Hop 55:1389, 1979
105. Newman RP, Kinkel WR, Jacobs L: Altitudinal hemianopia caused by occipital infarctions. Arch Neurol 41:413, 1984
106. Pallis CA: Impaired identification of faces and places with agnosia for colors. J Neurol Neurosurg Psychiatry 18:218, 1955
107. Pearlman AL, Birch J, Meadows JC: Cerebral color blindness: and acquired defect in hue discrimination. Ann Neurol 5:253, 1979
108. Peron N, Gutner V: Alexie pure sans hemianopsie. Rev Neurol (Paris) 76:81, 1944
109. Pessin MS, Kwan ES, DeWitt LD et al: Posterior cerebral artery stenosis. Ann Neurol 21:85, 1987
110. Pessin MS, Kwan ES, Scott RM, Hedges TR: Occipital infarction with hemianopsia from carotid occlusive disease. Stroke 20:409, 1989
111. Pessin MS, Lathi ES, Cohen MB et al: Clinical features and mechanism of occipital infarction. Ann Neurol 21:290, 1987
112. Pillon B, Bakchine S, Lhermitte F: Alexia without agraphia in a left handed patient with a right occipital lesion. Arch Neurol 44:1257, 1987
113. Pillon B, Signoret J-L, Lhermitte F: Agnosie visuelle associative: role de l'hémisphere gauche dans la perception visuelle. Rev Neurol (Paris) 137:831, 1981
114. Polyak S: The Vertebrate Visual System. University of Chicago Press, Chicago, 1957
115. Pötzl O: Die zweite Gruppe der optischen Agnosien. p. 80. In Aschaffenburg G (ed): Handbuch der Psychiatrie. Die Aphasielehre: I. Optischeagnostischen Storungen. Franz Deuticke, Wien, 1928
116. Pötzl O: Über einige zentrale Probleme des Farbensehens. Wien Klin Wochenschr 61:706, 1949
117. Reinhard C: Zur Frage der Hirnlocalisation mit besonderen Berücksichtigung der cerebralen Sehstörungen. Arch Psychiatr Nervenkr 18:240, 1887
118. Riley HA, Yaskin JC, Riggs ME, Torney AS: Bilateral blindness due to lesions in both occipital lobes. NY J Med 43:1619, 1943
119. Ross ED: Sensory-specific and fractional disorders of recent memory in man. I. Isolated loss of visual recent memory. Arch Neurol 37:193, 1980
120. Rubens AB, Benson DF: Associative visual agnosia. Arch Neurol 24:305, 1971
121. Salamon G, Huang YP: Radiologic Anatomy of the Brain. Springer-Verlag, Berlin 1976
122. Schober H: Erworbene Farbenblindheit nach Schadeltrauma. Graefe Arch Ophthalmol 148:93, 1948
123. Scoville W, Milner B: Loss of recent memory after bilateral hippocampal lesions. J Neurol Neurosurg Psychiatry 20:11, 1957
124. Shellshear JL: A contribution to our knowledge of the arterial supply of the cerebral cortex in man. Brain 50:236, 1927
125. Sheppard JJ: *Human Color Perception.* p. 98. Elsevier, New York, 1968
126. Shraberg D, Weisberg L: The Klüver-Bucy syndrome in man. J Nerv Ment Dis 166:130, 1978
127. Sidman M, Stoddard LT, Mohr JP: Some additional quantitative observations of immediate memory in a patient with bilateral hippocampal lesions. Neuropsychologia 6:245, 1968
128. Sidman M, Stoddard LT, Mohr JP, Leicester J: Behavioral studies of aphasia: methods of investigation and analysis. Neuropsychologia 9:119, 1971
129. Sieben G, De Reuck J, Eecken HV: Thrombosis of the mesencephalic artery: a clinico-pathological study of two cases and its correlation with the arterial vascularization. Acta Neurolog Belg 77:151, 1977
130. Siemerling: Ein Fall sogenannter Seelenblindheit nebst anderweitigen cerebralen Symptomen. Arch Psychiatr Nervenkr 21:284, 1889
131. Sittig O: Störungen in Verhalten gegenuber Farben bei Aphasischen. Monatsschr Psychiatr Neurol 49:63, 1921
132. Smith CG, Richardson WFG: The course and distribution of the arteries supplying the visual striate cortex. Am J Ophthalmol 61:1391, 1966
133. Spector RH, Glaser JS, David NJ, Vining DQ: Occipital lobe infarctions: perimetry and computed tomography. Neurology (NY) 31:1198, 1981

134. Stengel E: The syndrome of visual alexia with color agnosia. Br J Psychiatry 94:46, 1948
135. Stommel EW, Friedman RJ, Reeves AG: Alexia without agraphia associated with spleniogeniculate infarction. Neurology (NY) 41:587, 1991
136. Sweet WH, Talland GA, Ervin FR: Loss of recent memory following section of fornix. Trans Am Neurol Assoc 84:76, 1959
137. Symonds C, Mackenzie I: Bilateral loss of vision from cerebral infarction. Brain 80:415, 1957
138. Trillet M, Fischer C, Serclerat D, Schott B: Le syndrome amnésique des ischémies cérébrales postériores. Cortex 16:421, 1980
139. Urechia CI, Cremene V, Popescu P: Hemianopsie avec chromoagnosie. Rev Neurol (Paris) 80:70, 1948
140. Vialet N: Las Centres Cerebraux de la Vision el l'Appareil Nerveux Visuel Intra-cerebral. Faculte de Medecine de Paris, Paris, 1893
141. Victor M, Angevine JB, Mancall EL: Memory loss with lesions of the hippocampal formation. Arch Neurol 5:244, 1961
142. Vincent FM, Sadowsky CH, Saunders RL, Reeves AG: Alexia without agraphia hemianopia or color-naming defect: a disconnection syndrome. Neurology (NY) 27:689, 1977
143. Walker AE: Recent memory impairment in unilateral temporal lesions. Arch Neurol Psychiatry 78:543, 1957
144. Waterston JA, Stark RJ, Gilligan BS: Paramedian thalamic and midbrain infarction: the "mesencephalothalamic syndrome." Clin Exp Neurol 24:45, 1987
145. Wilbrand H: Über die makulär-hemianopische Lesestörung und die v Monakowsche Projektion der Makula auf die Sehspäre. Klin Monatsbl Augenh 45:1, 1907
146. Whiteley AM, Warrington EK: Prosopagnosia: a clinical psychological and anatomical study of three patients. J Neurol Neurosurg Psychiatry 40:395, 1977
147. Wyllie J: The Disorders of Speech. p. 340. Oliver & Boyd, Edinburgh, 1894
148. Yamada A, Miki H, Nishioka M: A case of posterior cerebral artery territory infarction with micropsia as the chief complaint. Rinshoshinkeigaku 30:894, 1990
149. Ziehl-Lübeck: Über einem Fall von Alexia and Farbenhemiagnosie. Verh Ges Dtsch Natur Aertze 67:184, 1895

# 18

# *VERTEBROBASILAR OCCLUSIVE DISEASE*

Louis R. Caplan
Michael S. Pessin
J.P. Mohr

Clinicians of the nineteenth century described in detail the clinical and pathologic findings in patients with softening or hemorrhage limited to portions of the brain stem. Interest lay primarily in defining the anatomy and function of the various brain stem nuclei and tracts. The nature and location of the responsible vascular lesion and the mechanism of the parenchymatous damage were given little attention because they were at that time of no practical concern.

In the early years of the twentieth century, attention turned to the pathology and anatomy of the intracranial vessels. Although isolated cases[227,294] of basilar artery occlusion, usually attributed to syphilitic endarteritis, had been described in the later nineteenth century, in 1911 Marburg[309] first reviewed the topic of brain stem infarction and described clinical examples of basilar territory syndromes. In 1932 Pines and Gilinsky[384] published a detailed report that included serial sections of the brain stem in a patient with thrombosis of the rostral basilar artery. Meanwhile Stopford[443,444] in England and Foix and colleagues[71,190,194] in France had defined the anatomy of the branches of the basilar artery and described syndromes caused by paramedian and lateral ischemia. By 1934 Lhermitte and Trelles[295] showed that arteriosclerosis (as well as syphilis) affected the cerebral vessels and led to softening, and that the basilar artery and its branches were especially vulnerable to atheroma formation.

In 1946 Kubik and Adams[281] published a meticulous analysis of 18 cases studied clinically and at postmortem of patients with occlusion of the basilar artery. They emphasized the severity of the disorder and believed it was diagnosable during life. In their series, the onset was usually abrupt, and death invariably ensued from extensive brain stem infarction. The possibility of patients occasionally surviving was also entertained, and clinical details of four living patients suspected of having basilar artery occlusion were included. This landmark report brought the subject of basilar artery occlusion to the full attention of the neurologic community. With the advent of arteriography, and careful pathologic studies of the entire vascular tree, the 1950s saw an awakening of interest in the extracranial vessels. Fisher[153] showed that severe atherosclerotic occlusive vascular disease within the internal carotid artery in the neck was a common cause of hemispheral softening. Hutchinson and Yates[251] carefully dissected the cervical vertebral arteries and demonstrated that severe occlusive disease also occurs frequently in these vessels. Meyer and colleagues[328] corroborated arteriographically the frequency of occlusive disease in the basilar and nuchal vertebral arteries during life. In his monograph on carotid artery disease, Fisher[151] emphasized that warning spells, transient ischemic attacks, frequently occurred prior to cerebral hemisphere infarctions. Others called these attacks "carotid insufficiency."

As the clinical findings associated with posterior circulation infarction became more widely recognized, Williams and Wilson,[491,492] Denny-Brown,[114] Fang and Palmer,[139] Millikan and Siekert,[331] and others called attention to transient episodes of dysfunction within the posterior circulation territory.[495] The term *vertebrobasilar insufficiency* was born, and interest in the 1960s shifted away from the pathology and clinical symptoms to an attempt to understand the pathophysiology of these vascular lesions. Microembolization, intermittent obstruction of the vertebral arteries by bony osteophytes, and clotting and viscosity factors within the blood were identified as important factors. Intense physiologic studies of Denny-Brown[115] added emphasis to the nature and capability of the collateral circulation with its dependence on systemic factors such as blood pressure, blood volume, cardiac output, body position and activity, and pharmacologic agents.

During the 1970s and 1980s, emphasis had shifted from diagnosis to treatment. As a result of a number of uncontrolled observations,[332,333] enthusiasm for the use of warfarin anticoagulation grew in the 1960s. In a review in 1969 Browne and Poskanzer[57] stated, "If anticoagulation has value, it may be more useful in the patient with vertebrobasilar disease, with its high morbidity, than in other forms of cerebral vascular thrombosis." More recently, aspirin and other agents that affect platelet agglutination, such as dipyridamole and sulfinpyrazone, have been used in an attempt to modify coagulation factors in patients with posterior circulation disease. Surgically created shunts from occipital artery to long circumferential cerebellar artery branches of the vertebral and basilar arteries and to the posterior cerebral artery[20,271,450] have been devised to increase circulation to the brain stem and posterior cerebral hemispheral regions. Vertebral[253] and carotid endarterectomy[319] and bypass and transluminal dilatation of the basilar artery[449] involve more direct surgical correction of occlusive disease in the posterior circulation.

Advances in interventional neuroradiology now make it possible to introduce catheters and therapeutic agents into the vertebral artery and the larger intracranial arteries within the posterior circulation. Intravenous and intra-arterial thrombolytic agents such as streptokinase and recombinant tissue plasminogen activator (rtPA) have been infused to lyse clots in patients with vertebral artery and basilar artery[145,213,379,505,506] thromboses.

During the 1980s there were also dramatic improvements in diagnostic technology. Brain imaging became possible in the 1970s after the introduction of computed tomography (CT). CT proved useful for posterior circulation hemorrhages but was less helpful in occlusive disease, since the brain stem was difficult to image by CT. Magnetic resonance imaging (MRI), introduced in the 1980s, permitted far superior imaging of brain stem and cerebellar infarcts.[39,275,431] Axial, sagittal, and coronal sections allow localization of brain stem lesions in rostrocaudal, tegmentobasal, and medial-lateral directions. Flow voids on MRI give information about anuerysms and occlusions in the plane of the section. Technology for study of the posterior circulation arteries has also improved greatly. Duplex scanning, color-coded Doppler imaging, and continuous-wave Doppler sonography allow detection of lesions in the extracranial vertebral arteries,[2,41,132,231,297,464,468,476] and transcranial Doppler ultrasound has improved detection of intracranial lesions.[75,232,464,476] Magnetic resonance angiography has promise in allowing safe imaging of the vertebrobasilar vessels without risk to patients.[124,128,129] Echocardiography, cardiac imaging, and sophisticated rhythm monitoring now also allow detection of cardiac sources of embolism to the posterior circulation.[84] Angiography using standard arterial catheterization and dye opacification has also become safer with improvements in catheters, dyes, filming, and experienced personnel. Clearly, physicians practicing in the 1990s have much greater capabilities for defining the brain and vascular lesions in patients with vertebrobasilar arterial occlusive disease than was possible a decade ago.

The physicians of the nineteenth and early twentieth centuries had virtually no therapy that could influence the course of serious cerebrovascular disease. In the 1990s, we have a variety of potent treatments. Even more important, we have sophisticated technology. But despite the advances, many basic questions remain: How does disease within the vessels produce transient ischemic attacks[4] or stroke, and why in some cases with severe occlusive disease do many regions escape damage? Why do clinical signs fluctuate? Which patients do we treat? When? With what? For how long?

Posterior circulation disease is not a homogeneous entity. Many patients are severely disabled or die, while others suffer only transient or minor disability. The prognosis varies and is dependent on multiple factors, including (1) the nature, locus, and severity of the vascular lesions, (2) the presence of coexisting vascular lesions elsewhere, (3) hemodynamic, circulatory, and coagulation factors, and (4) the congenital constitution of the individual vascular bed. Somehow the studies of the preceding generations have not provided enough specific details regarding the pathophysiology and diagnosis of posterior circulation disease to allow the present-day clinician to be eclectic and precise in choosing optimal treatment for the individual patient. We need to know more about the less frequent causes of posterior circulation vascular disease such as fibromuscular hyperplasia, temporal arteritis, and arterial dissection. Within the large entity of vertebrobasilar occlusive disease, we need to delineate recognizable subdivisions that share a common clinical course and prognosis. Treatment could then be studied within somewhat homogeneous subdivisions, rather than being used indiscriminately against an amalgam of heterogeneous lesions that we list under the loose classification of vertebrobasilar disease.

This chapter begins by summarizing the important anatomic relations and variations within the posterior circulation. The pathology of the diseases that affect the extracranial and intracranial vasculature of the posterior circulation are then reviewed, emphasizing the frequency and locale of lesions. Pathophysiologic mechanisms are discussed briefly, since our knowledge of the relative importance of individual mechanisms is scanty. Clinical findings are then subdivided into groups of patients with known documented vascular lesions in the various vessels within the posterior circulation, and then findings are organized into clinical presentations that reflect the kinds of problems the clinician encounters. Finally, diagnostic techniques and treatment are reviewed briefly, even though the value of individual treatment for each problem is almost entirely speculative at present.

## ANATOMY

The vertebrobasilar arterial system has several unique features. For a period in the embryologic life of the fetus, most of the blood to the hindbrain structures comes from the carotid circulation. Because of its paired systems and the many changes that it undergoes during fetal development, the vertebrobasilar system has a high incidence of variations, anomalies, and persistent fetal vessels. It is one of the only regions in the body where two large arteries merge into a single larger trunk. The posterior circulation also supplies the anterior spinal artery, which usually forms from smaller arterial branches of each vertebral artery. In addition, because the vertebral arteries course through and around many bony structures and ligaments and are fixed in a part of their course, they are especially vulnerable to traumatic injury.

Traditionally, the vertebral artery is divided into segments[279,440,458] (Fig. 18-1). In the first segment, the artery courses directly cephalad from its origin as the first branch of the subclavian artery to enter the costotransverse foramen of C6 or C5. The second segment is entirely within the transverse foramina from C6 to C2. The third segment is very tortuous: the vertebral artery emerges from the transverse foramen of C2 and courses posteriorly and laterally toward the costotransverse foramen of the atlas. It circles the posterior arch of C1 and passes between the atlas and occiput within the suboccipital triangle. During its course, the third segment of the vertebral artery is covered by muscles and nerves and is pressed against bone while

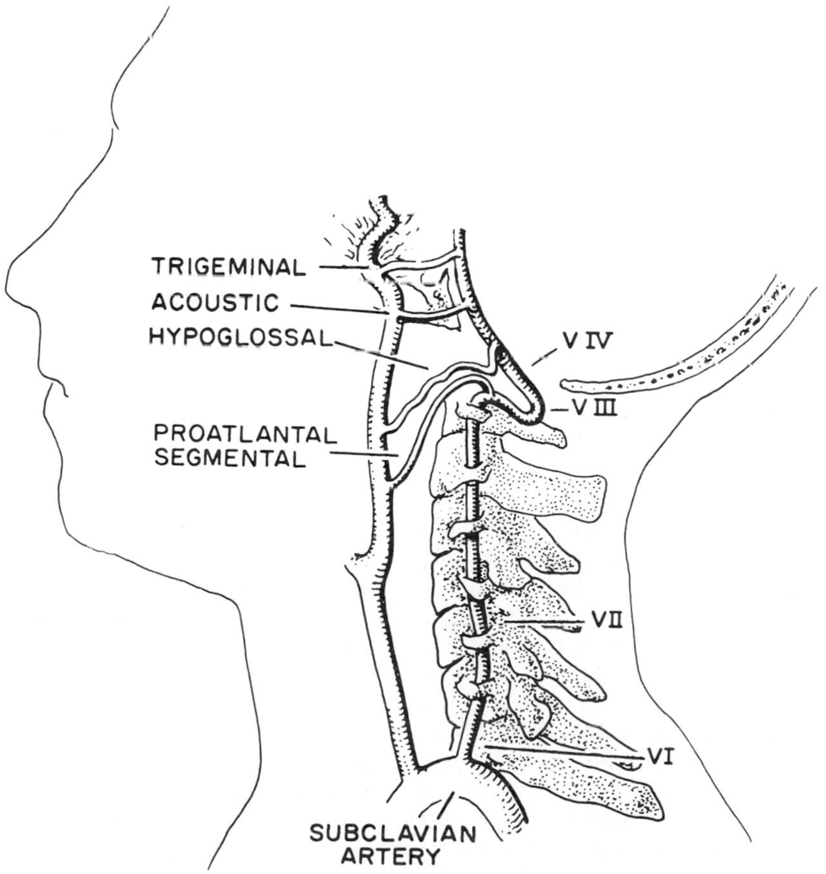


**Fig. 18-1.** Vertebral artery segments and persisting primitive anastomotic connections with the carotid arterial tree (VI to VIV denote vertebral artery segments 1 to 4).

being covered by the atlanto-occipital membrane. The fourth segment of the vertebral artery is its intracranial portion after the vessel pierces the dura mater to enter the foramen magnum. As the vertebral artery pierces the dura, its adventitial and medial coats are less thick, and there is a gross reduction in elastic fibers in its media and external elastic lamina.[489] Usually at the level of the pontomedullary junction, the two vertebral arteries merge to form the basilar artery. The junction is sometimes higher, in which case the vertebral artery supplies the mid- and lower pons; occasionally there is a low origin of the basilar artery. The basilar artery becomes somewhat smaller as it travels distally, and frequently it curves slightly in the direction away from the larger vertebral artery. It divides near the pontomesencephalic junction to form the two posterior cerebral arteries.

Variations are relatively common. In approximately 8 percent of humans, the left vertebral artery originates directly from the aortic arch and not the subclavian artery (in which case the left vertebral artery would not fill from a left brachial injection). Rarely, the right vertebral artery arises as a separate branch from the innominate artery and not from the subclavian artery. The posterior inferior cerebellar artery (PICA) is usually the largest branch of the vertebral artery and arises from its intradural segment approximately 1.5 cm from the origin of the basilar artery. The PICA most often arises from the vertebral artery an average of 8.6 mm above the foramen magnum, but occasionally may originate from the vertebral artery as low as 24 mm below the foramen magnum.[300] Occasionally, the PICA arises extracranially and courses cephalad within the spinal canal.[140] The vertebral artery may terminate in the PICA, in which case the distal segment (which usually communicates with the basilar artery) is hypoplastic or nonexistent, and the vertebral artery is small compared to the contralateral side.[211] The vertebral arteries are frequently asymmetric (in 45 percent of people the left is larger, in 21 percent the right is larger, and in 24 percent the arteries are of equal size). The posterior spinal arteries may arise from the PICA rather than from their usual vertebral artery origin.[198] The PICA and anterior inferior cerebellar artery (AICA) are often reciprocally related in size; for example, a large PICA may supply most of the inferior surface of the cerebellum, while the AICA on the same side is quite small and has little cerebellar supply. In the case of a large AICA, the PICA is frequently small. The lateral medulla is usually fed primarily from the PICA as it courses around the medulla, but in many cases the major blood supply is from direct lateral medullary branches of the vertebral artery. The distal PICA usually bifurcates into a medial trunk that supplies the vermis and adjacent hemisphere and a lateral trunk supplying the cortical surface of the tonsil and cerebellar hemisphere. The cerebellum is supplied by the long circumferential vessels; the PICA encircles the medulla and supplies the suboccipital surface, whereas the AICA encircles the pons and relates to the rostrosal surface of the cerebellum, while the superior cerebellar artery (SCA) supplies the tentorial surface after encircling the midbrain.

The major branches of the basilar artery are generally uniform, the most common variation being that the internal auditory artery, usually an AICA branch, may arise directly from the basilar artery. The SCAs are occasionally duplicated or arise from the posterior cerebral artery. Even more uniform are the smaller penetrating branches of the vertebral and basilar arteries.[89,183,189] There are three groups of arterial penetrators (Fig. 18-2): (1) median arteries, which usually take a slightly caudal course and then penetrate the brain stem and supply the paramedian basal and tegmental regions; (2) short lateral circumferential arteries, which give rise to branches that penetrate the brain stem and supply the intermediate tegmental and basal regions; and (3) long lateral circumferential arteries, which course around the brain stem and supply the lateral basal and tegmental regions. Stephens and Stilwell,[440] using elegant injection techniques, have shown that there are many lateral circumferential vessels that arise from the vertebral and basilar arteries directly, as well as from the long cerebellar vessels. In the medulla and midbrain there are also posterior branches, which arise from the long lateral circumferential cerebellar vessels (SCA, PICA, and AICA) to course in a horizontal and dorsoventral direction to supply the lateral tegmentum (Fig. 18-2). Penetrating vessels are usually less than 100 $\mu$m in diameter, their size being roughly proportional to their length.[202] The medial penetrating vessels arise from the anterior spinal, vertebral, basilar, AICA, and posterior cerebral arteries; lateral penetrators frequently enter the brain stem along the laterally emerging nerve roots. The medial tegmental region has a prominent rich collateral supply, making it more resistant to ischemia than the base or lateral tegmentum.

The distal basilar segments are also the source of occasional variations. During early fetal life, the internal carotid artery supplies the posterior hemispheres and brain stem via the posterior communicating arteries. In one-third of humans, this primitive vascular pattern persists (variously called the basilar communicating artery or mesencephalic artery), and the connecting segment from the basilar artery to the posterior cerebral artery remains vestigial.[201,202,456] In these cases, the posterior cerebral artery may fill from carotid injection, and not after vertebral artery opacification. In 2 percent of humans, this primitive circulatory pattern is bilateral; even more rarely the basilar artery may be hypoplastic in its distal segment and end in the SCAs.[456] Penetrating branches from the distal basilar communicating artery and su-

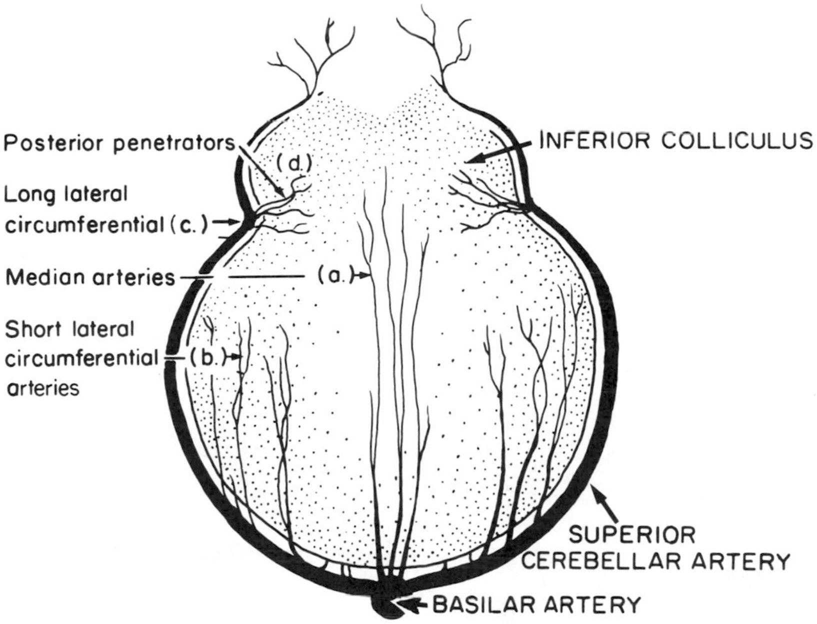


**Fig. 18-2.** Rostral pons with the usual arterial distribution. (**a**) Median penetrating arteries. (**b**) Short lateral circumferential arteries. (**c**) Long lateral circumferential artery. (**d**) Posterior penetrating arteries.

perior cerebellar and proximal posterior cerebral arteries pass through the posterior perforating substance and supply the paramedian midbrain and diencephalon.

The paramedian mesencephalic arteries arise from the proximal portion of the basilar communicating artery to supply the cerebral peduncle and red nucleus.[246] The lateral midbrain is supplied by peduncular perforating branches arising from the proximal portion of the posterior cerebral arteries.[246] There are usually two separate paramedian thalamoperforating arteries:[69,2098,248,374,458,475] (1) the polar artery (also called the tuberothalamic artery) and the preliminary pedicles;[88,188,208] (2) the thalamic-subthalamic arteries (also called paramedian thalamic[374] deep interpeduncular profunda,[208] and the thalamoperforating pedicle.[88,190] The polar artery arises from the posterior communicating artery and supplies the anterolateral thalamus, including the mamillothalamic tract, the paraventricular region and a part of the reticular nucleus.[46,69,208] The lateral portions of the thalamus are supplied by a series of thalamogeniculate arteries,[90,440] often called the thalamogeniculate pedicle, and not a large vessel as was formerly believed (Fig. 18-3). The thalamogeniculate pedicle arises from the ambient segment of the posterior cerebral arteries and penetrates into the thalamus between the geniculate bodies.[77] These arteries supply the posterolateral and posteromedial ventral somatosensory nuclei, part of ventralis lateralis, part of the centromedian nucleus, and the rostrolateral portion of the pulvinar. The posterior choroidal arteries arise from the posterior cerebral arteries more laterally and supply portions of the medial nuclei, the habenular nucleus, and the rostromedial pulvinar.

Occasionally, primitive connections from the internal carotid artery to the posterior circulation vessels persist into adult life.[295,440,458] The most common persisting anastomotic channel is the trigeminal artery, which remains in 0.1 to 0.2 percent of adults.[296] The trigeminal artery arises from the internal carotid artery as it enters the cavernus sinus proximal to the carotid siphon, and penetrates the sella turcica or the dura near the clivus to join the basilar artery between the AICA and SCA branches. Frequently, the vertebral arteries and proximal basilar artery are small or hypoplastic, as is true in many patients with other persistent anastomoses. Persistence of the hypoglossal artery is the next most common variant.[274,296,385] This vessel originates from the internal carotid artery in the neck, usually between C1 and C3, and courses posteriorly to enter the hypoglossal canal, from which it joins the lower basilar artery.[385] A persistent otic artery is a rarer anomaly; this vessel leaves the internal carotid artery within the petrous bone and enters the posterior fossa with the 7th and 8th cranial nerves at the internal acoustic meatus, later to join the mid-basilar artery. The rarest fetal communicating channels are the persistent proatlantal intersegmental arteries, which originate from the nuchal internal or external carotid artery at C2 to C3 and join the horizontal (third) segment of the vertebral artery suboccipitally.[359] Isolated reports have documented communications between the common or proximal

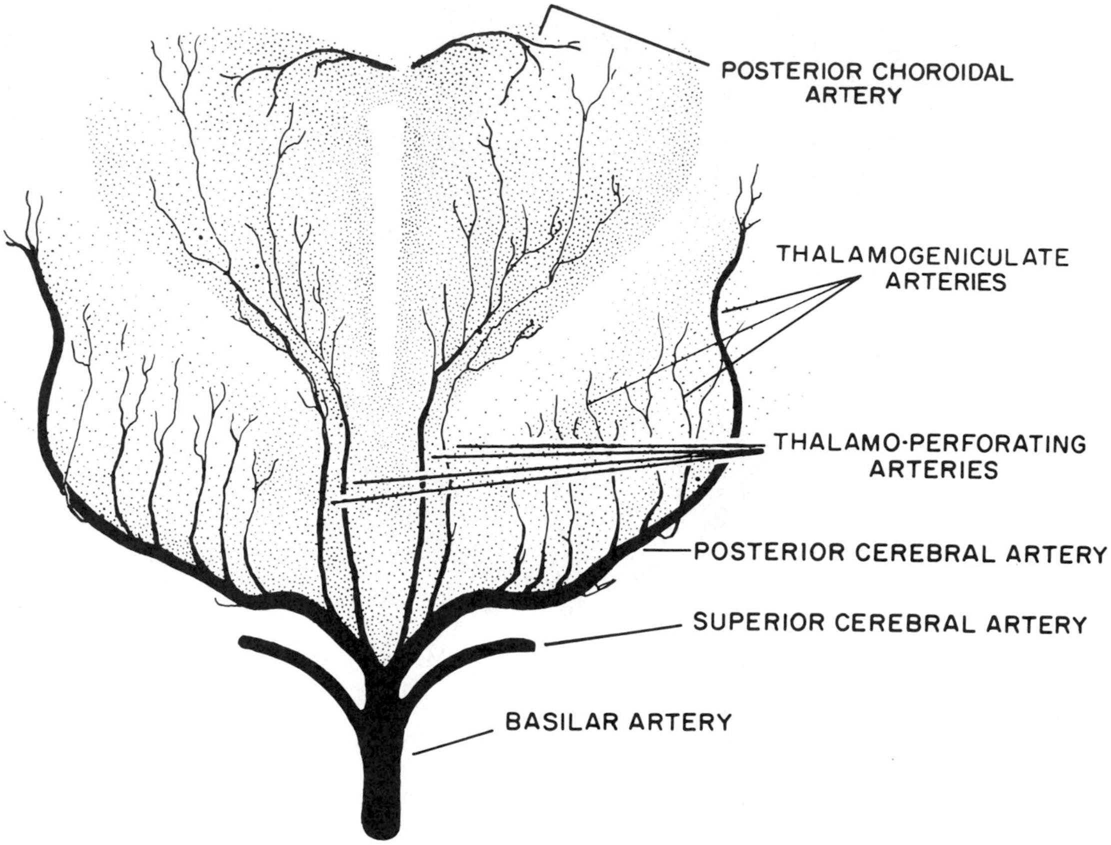


**Fig. 18-3.** Thalamus with the usual arterial distribution. Note the multiple thalamogeniculate arteries.

internal carotid artery and the lower vertebral arteries.[363]

## PATHOLOGY

### Atherosclerosis

Atherosclerosis is by far the most common vascular condition responsible for posterior circulation ischemia. Fatty streaks, fibrous plaques, calcified lesions, and complicated lesions (fibrous plaques upon which hemorrhage, ulceration, or thrombosis has developed) have all been frequently identified within the larger vessels of the vertebrobasilar system and do not differ qualitatively from atherosclerosis of other vessels.[16,54,63,98,127,143,416] Ulceration in plaques is less frequent in the posterior circulation.[184,416] However, when ulceration occurs, it usually involves the subclavian artery at the origin of the vertebral artery or in the most proximal portion of the vertebral artery.[373,416] As in the anterior circulation, thrombosis may occur in the absence of severe preexisting atherosclerosis of the vessel wall.[398]

The most common site of atherosclerotic stenosis is at the origin of the vertebral arteries.[181,251,345,416,484] Plaque forms and may assume a ringlike extension from the subclavian artery to encircle the vertebral artery orifice.[181] The left and right vertebral arteries are approximately equally affected by atherosclerosis, but there is some indication that when the two vessels are unequal in diameter, the smaller vessel is more frequently occluded.[73,416] The intracranial vertebral artery, after it pierces the dura, is another frequent site of occlusive disease.[91,181,345] Aside from these sites, fibrous plaques and fatty streaks are distributed along the vertebral artery without any single site of predilection.[91,181,251,345] Often in the second segment of the vertebral artery, during its course through the transverse foramina, a ladderlike arrangement of fibrous plaques, seemingly related to the anatomy of the adjacent cervical spine structures, is found.[345] When thrombosis occurs within the extracranial vertebral artery, the clot usually develops at a site of atherosclerotic stenosis and seldom forms a long anterograde or retrograde extension.[91,181] In contrast, a thrombus within the extracranial internal carotid artery often extends the length of the vessel up to the first branch, the ophthalmic artery. The limited length of the vertebral artery thrombus may be related to this vessel's more extensive branching and the possibility that extensive collateral channels keep blood circulating above and below the clot.[147] Thrombus formed within the intracranial vertebral artery, however, frequently extends into the proximal basilar artery.[91]

Within the basilar artery, fatty sudanophilic plaques are more prevalent on the ventral surface,[98] and stenosis or occlusion is frequent in the proximal 2 cm of the vessel. In the series of Castaigne et al.[87,89] there were six occlusions of the lower third of the basilar artery, five in the middle third, and three in the distal third. In a review of reported cases of basilar artery occlusion, the middle segment of the artery was most often involved, followed in frequency by involvement of the proximal and then the distal third of the artery.[379] In 14 percent of cases the entire length of the artery was occluded.[379] Atherostenosis of the distal portion of the basilar artery may be more common in blacks.[80] Clots within the basilar artery also tend to have limited propagation;[88] frequently they extend only to the orifice of the next long circumferential cerebellar artery (AICA or SCA). The proximal posterior cerebral arteries are also sites of atherosclerotic lesions, but lesions occur less frequently there than in the middle cerebral artery.[24,345] Embolic material is most often found within the distal basilar tributaries, especially the posterior cerebral artery branches; less often, an embolus lodges in the more proximal vertebral or basilar arteries, especially at sites of luminal encroachment by preexisting atherosclerotic lesions.[84,88,281] In a series of 30 pathologically verified posterior cerebral artery occlusions studied by Castaigne et al.,[88] 15 were artery to artery emboli arising as atheromatous debris or clot originating in the more proximal vertebral or basilar artery. One posterior cerebral artery was occluded by an embolus of cardiac origin, and eight occlusions represented extensions of clot from the basilar artery into a posterior cerebral artery. Only three patients had in situ development of thrombosis of the posterior cerebral artery.[88]

Atherosclerotic stenosis of the extracranial internal carotid artery occurs approximately twice as often as stenosis of the extracranial vertebral artery,[181,184,345,416] but often both vessels are severely compromised.[250] However, the location and severity of occlusive disease in these two vessels are extremely variable and unpredictable; for example, 60 percent of patients studied by Castaigne et al.,[88] who had occlusions within the vertebrobasilar system, had no serious occlusive disease within the anterior circulation. Angiographic studies[32,328,439,473] have corroborated that the origin of the vertebral artery, the intradural vertebral artery,[466] the basilar artery,[328] and the subclavian artery proximal to the vertebral artery origin are the most common sites of occlusive disease.

The frequency of atherosclerotic lesions in the subclavian and proximal vertebral arteries is different in men and women and in persons of different racial backgrounds.[80,146,207] Patients with atheromatous lesions at the origins of the vertebral arteries share epidemiologic and demographic features with those who have lesions at the carotid artery bifurcation in the neck.[80,251] There is a strong association of vertebral and carotid artery lesions with coronary and peripheral vascular occlusive disease, smoking, hypertension, and hypercholesterolemia.[80] Men predominate over women.[80] Whites have a relatively higher incidence of severe extracranial occlusive disease, while blacks and persons of Japanese and Chinese ancestry have a preponderance of intracranial occlusive disease, especially of medium-sized branches (PICA, AICA, SCA, PCA).[80,144,207,273,395] Blacks, Japanese, Chinese, and women with predominantly intracranial branch disease have a high incidence of hypertension, but a relatively low frequency of coronary and peripheral vascular occlusive disease and hypercholesterolemia. Occlusive lesions of the intracranial vertebral artery and the basilar artery have less clear sex and racial preponderance.[207]

Atherosclerosis may also compromise the branches of the vertebral and basilar arteries.[70] The larger branches (PICA, AICA, anterior spinal artery, and SCAs) are surprisingly infrequently affected by atherosclerosis; most infarctions in the vascular territories of these vessels are due to narrowing of the parent vessel that blocks or diminishes blood flow into these major tributaries. The smaller penetrating branches (approximately 0.5 mm in diameter) are vulnerable to occlusive disease. Fisher and Caplan[179] fund four such small "basilar branch occlusions" in serial section (Fig. 18-4). Two branches were blocked as they traversed the intramural portion of the parent basilar artery, one by a foamy macrophage plaque causing blockage of the orifice of the branch. In the other two vessels, a "junctional plaque" extended from the parent basilar artery into the proximal branch and occluded the branch lumen. Microatheroma, usually consisting of foamy, fatty macrophage plaques, are frequently seen within the proximal portions of small branches in hypertensive patients. In diabetic patients without documented hypertension, infarction in regions of the pons and diencephalon supplied by paramedian penetrating branches are found three or four times more commonly than in nondiabetics.[375] The morphology of the presumed branch disease in these patients has not been studied but could represent similar microatheroma;[70] Figure 18-4 depicts mechanisms of branch occlusion.

## Lipohyalinosis

The pathology of smaller penetrating arteries (less than 200 $\mu$m) within the brain stem parenchyma is qualitatively quite different from atherosclerosis of larger vessels.[63,156,159,168,171] The smaller vessels become occluded by a distinctive process that Fisher has called "lipohyalinosis,"[156,159] which can lead to disorganization and disruption of the lumen of the vessel.

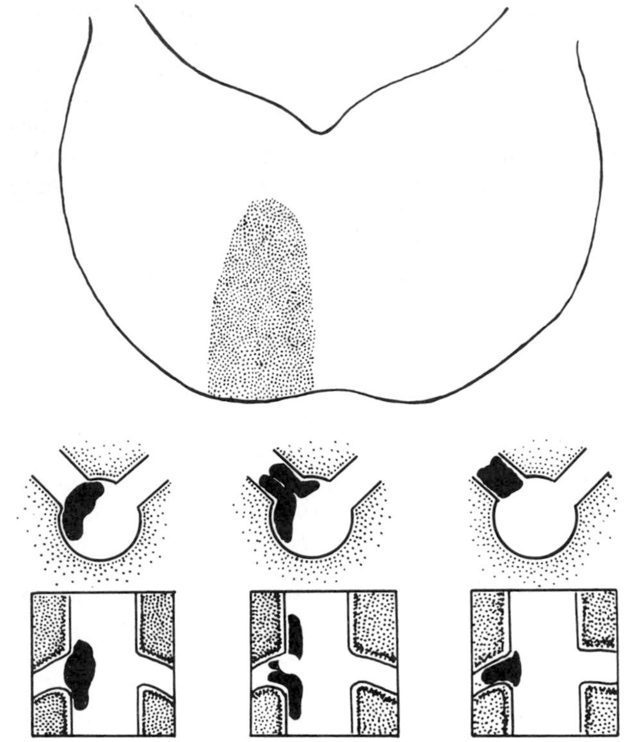

**Fig. 18-4.** Diagrammatic representation of types of branch occlusion. Luminal plaque blocking the orifice of a branch, junctional plaque spreading into a branch, and clot in the proximal part of a branch.

In this process, a hyaline material, which readily takes up stains used for fat, accumulates subintimally. The wall of the vessel is weakened and aneurysmal dilatations occur. At times red blood cells are extravasated through the disintegrating wall.

Lipohyalinosis leads to functional occlusion of the vessel by a subintimal process that obliterates the lumen and leads to ischemia distal to the lesion. Because the ischemic lesions are generally small and somewhat round, the term lacune (hole) has been applied. In addition, the same vascular process can lead to a break in the vessel wall and parenchymatous hemorrhage.[167] Most patients with lipohyalinosis and lacunar infarctions are or have been hypertensive, although lipohyalinosis is not limited to patients with hypertension.[25] The incidence of lipohyalinosis increases with the age of the patient. Aging itself is associated with adventitial and medial fibrosis in smaller blood vessels, but is not correlated with atheroma of larger vessels.

## Aneurysms

Saccular aneurysms are usually discovered during evaluation of subarachnoid hemorrhage. Occasionally these aneurysms block the orifice of tributary vessels or a clot within the aneurysm embolizes distally; either mechanism leads to an ischemic stroke.[30] Saccular aneurysms are not common in the posterior circulation, but did account for 3.6 percent (64 of 1,769) of the aneurysms analyzed in the large series of Bull.[59] The most common site within the posterior circulation for saccular aneurysms is the basilar apex (60 percent); the vertebral-PICA junction (20 percent) and the basilar-SCA junction (11 percent) are also common sites, and occasionally aneurysms involve the junction of the vertebral and basilar arteries (3 percent).[59,365,458] Other sites are quite rare. Aneurysms of the basilar apex may grow quite large,[18] splaying the cerebral peduncles (Fig. 18-5); when these apex aneurysms leak, blood in the interpeduncular fossa may lead to spasm and infarction in the territory of vessels within the posterior perforated substance, producing a complex clinical picture of rostral brain stem ischemia.

Despite their frequency, it is unusual for basilar apex aneurysms to present as an isolated third nerve palsy. Barnes and Ferrario[27] studied 30 patients with posterior circulation aneurysms; all had the clinical features of subarachnoid hemorrhage, and none had a third nerve palsy. Only 4 percent of aneurysms causing a third nerve palsy arise from the vertebrobasilar system.[27] A single patient with a large aneurysm at the junction of the basilar and left posterior cerebral arteries had paroxysmal hypertension closely simulating a pheochromocytoma;[133] blood pressure normalized after clipping of the aneurysm. Partially thrombosed giant basilar aneurysms are seen on CT scan as calcified, partially enhancing lesions, often near the cerebellopontine angle (Fig. 18-6).[352]

Fusiform (dolichoectatic) aneurysms are tortuous, elongated, ectatic variations of the normal arterial anatomy[503] (see Fig. 18-6). Once viewed as uncommon, fusiform aneurysms are now increasingly identified by CT scanning where they appear as dilated enhancing channels crossing the cerebellopontine angle. Fusiform aneurysms of the vertebrobasilar vessels produce symptoms by either compression and traction on posterior fossa structures[347,377] or by ischemia[241] from obstruction of blood flow related to atherostenosis of the vertebrobasilar arteries, local embolism from in situ thrombus within the aneurysm, and by compromising the orifice of tributary vessels.[108,116,131] Headache, located in the occipital-nuchal area, is a common accompaniment. Cranial nerve compression and traction may result in neuropathies, usually affecting the 7th and 8th cranial nerves, resulting in hemifacial spasm, tinnitus, deafness, and occasionally vertigo.[269,365,370] Glossopharyngeal and trigeminallike pain,[269] hiccoughs, and hypoglossal paralysis also result from cranial nerve traction by the aneurysms. Large basilar artery aneurysms may also compress the basis points or cerebral peduncle, may cause hydrocephalus,[131] or may present as cerebellopontine angle masses.[392,398] Verte-

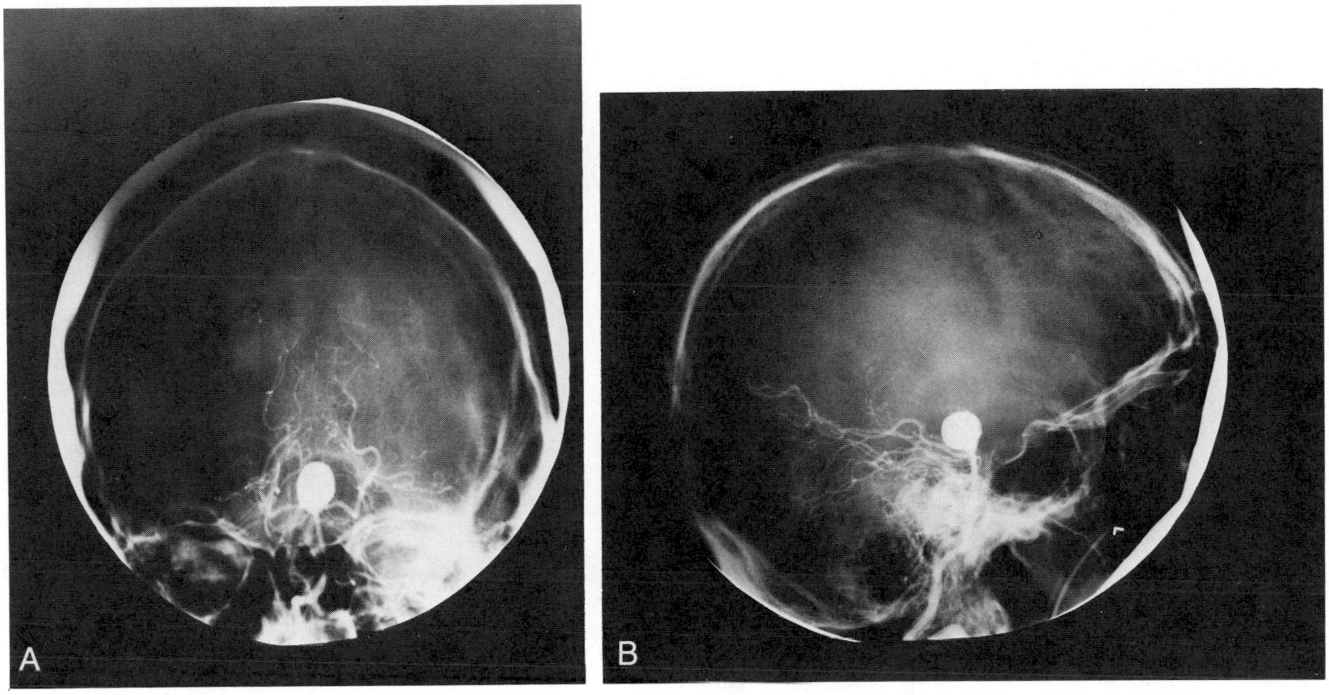


**Fig. 18-5.** Basilar apex aneurysm. (**A**) Anteroposterior view. (**B**) Lateral view.

bral artery (VA) aneurysms may compress the medulla[312] or upper brain stem.[131]

The pathogenesis of these aneurysms involves congenital and degenerative factors, occasionally genetic influences. Several reports have documented underlying structural arterial defects, including connective tissue replacement and deficient elastin,[369] fibrous dysplasia and degeneration of internal elastic lamina,[240] and fibrous and collagen replacement of the media. In adults, atherosclerotic changes in the vessels may interact with congenital structural defects to result in fusiform aneurysm formation. Recently, a genetic deficiency in $\alpha$-glucosidase was found in three teenage brothers with fusiform basilar aneurysms, two of whom had ruptures of the aneurysms, and the third had cerebellar infarction.[307] In some patients with structural defects, the arterial abnormalities are widespread, affecting other vessels.[301,357] Fusiform aneurysms therefore appear to represent a heterogeneous mixture of vascular etiologies. Atherosclerosis may be a prominent factor in many adult patients, and other arteriopathies play a role in some patients, especially children.

Dolichoectatic vertebral and basilar artery aneurysms are also readily imaged by MRI. The heterogeneity of echo densities and morphology of flow voids usually allows detection of thrombus within the aneurysms. MR angiography accurately detects the vast majority of sizable saccular and fusiform aneurysms.[126,129,130] Angiography or metrizamide CT cisternography can confirm the diagnosis but are not usually needed if high quality plain and contrast-enhanced CT or MRI have been performed with special attention to the posterior fossa[113] or if MR angiography is available.

## Spondylosis

In 1960 Sheehan et al.[424] popularized the idea that compression of the vertebral artery by osteophytes was a common cause of vertebrobasilar insufficiency. Spondylitic osteophytes project from the vertebral joints adjacent to the transverse foramina through which the vertebral arteries course. In cadavers, extreme neck turning can cut off vertebral artery flow. When Tatlow and Bammer[462] injected dye into cadavers, turning of the neck revealed minor compression of the vertebral artery in the region of C5 to C6 osteophytes. In 26 patients studied clinically and by brachial angiography,[424] the vertebral arteries were very tortuous with many sigmoid curves, and frequently the lateral concavities of the curves were opposite an intervertebral space. "Stenosis" was frequent but occlusion rare at the point of maximal concavity.[424] The most frequent loci of disease were at the C5 to C6 and C4 to C5 interspaces. However, only two patients developed symptoms on neck turning (dizziness, blurred vision, and confusion, and in only two other patients (not the symptomatic patients) was angiographically measured stenosis worsened by turning. In 6 of the 26 patients, the only symptom was drop attacks, dubiously attributable to vascular disease. Several cogent arguments militate against the argument that spondylosis is a frequent cause of symptomatic vascular compression.

1. In postmortem studies, though slight ridging or streaks are frequently seen in the midcervical area,[345] this region is infrequently a site of severe stenosis or occlusion;[88,181,416] in large radiographic series, severe lateral displacement by osteophytes is rare (2 of 203 cases of Radner[391]).
2. The majority of reported patients with intermittent posterior circulation ischemia and spondylosis have coexistent atherosclerosis,[220,424] and some degree of spondylosis is ubiquitous in patients over the age of 40.
3. In some patients, spondylosis itself may cause

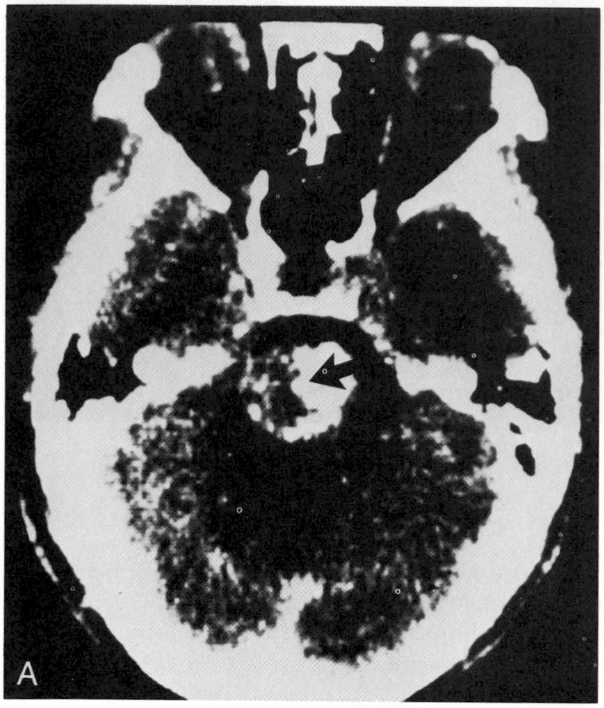

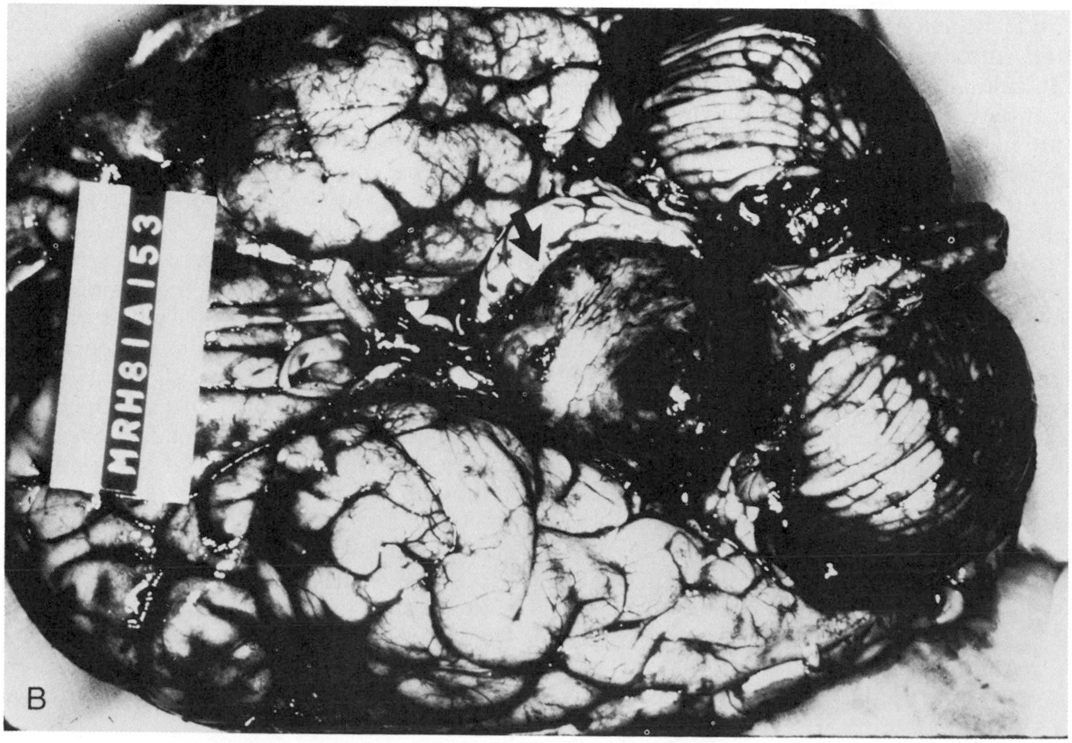

**Fig. 18-6.** (**A**) Computed tomography enhancement of a large circular lesion partially opacified by contrast. (**B**) Necropsy of a partially thrombosed giant basilar aneurysm.

transient rostral spinal cord signs, for example, drop spells.

In other supposed examples of "spondylosis-vascular disease," the only symptom is vertigo upon neck motion, a common phenomenon in the elderly and one frequently produced by labyrinthine and other nonvascular mechanisms.[161,460] Blood normally flows in the vertebral arteries under arterial pressure; neither cadaver studies nor dye injection in patients accurately depicts the real pressure relationships in each vertebral artery in life. Although turning or sudden motion may further compromise kinks or smaller atherosclerotic vessels and can lead to vascular occlusion or dissection, it is unlikely that the mechanism involves spondylosis. Until a clearer relationship between spondylosis and vascular disease can be demonstrated, surgery upon spondylitic lesions should not be performed for the sole purpose of treating "vertebrobasilar insufficiency."

## Neck Rotation or Trauma

Though earlier reports have described individual case histories of posterior circulation infarction that occurred after neck manipulation, only recently has the mechanism been further elucidated. In 1947 Pratt-Thomas and Berger[389] provided an account of two previously healthy individuals, a 32-year-old man and a 35-year-old woman, who became unconscious during chiropractic manipulation and died in less than 24 hours without regaining consciousness. Occlusion of the basilar artery, left AICA, and right PICA with brain stem and bilateral cerebellar hemisphere softenings were found in one patient, and occlusion of the right vertebral and basilar arteries and left PICA in the other. Since this original report, over 50 additional patients have been described in whom posterior circulation stroke followed neck rotation or injury.[192,219,234,280,293,351,401,402,425,499,502] The majority of cases occur after chiropractic manipulation, but manipulation of the neck by a patient's wife,[192] neck turning while driving a car, wrestling,[402] and practicing archery and yoga[219] have also been implicated. Most of the patients have been young (average 37 years)[426] and have had no evidence of preexisting vascular disease, cervical fractures, or dislocations.

In the majority of patients the syndrome is unilateral, and ischemia is limited to the lateral medulla or pons and the ipsilateral cerebellum.[126,219,293,351,402,425] Arteriography in the patients with predominantly unilateral findings has documented narrowing or occlusion of the vertebral artery in its third segment, usually in the region of C2 or C1 before the vessel penetrates the dura. In one patient the occlusive process was in the intracranial vertebral artery;[128] in a single patient with neck trauma and paraplegia the vertebral artery was occluded at C6.[440] Only one patient[293] had a lesion at the level of the vertebral artery origin, but this patient, who suffered an acute traumatic injury, was studied 7 weeks after the initial injury, a period that would allow retrograde extension of clot. Pseudoaneurysm formation has been seen in five patients, also at the C2 to C1 region. Unilateral lesions tend to develop at the time of neck rotation and often (14 out of 21 cases) do not progress.[280] Only 1 of these 21 patients died of the unilateral stroke. Cerebellar softening with subsequent edema and increased posterior fossa pressure may occur and require surgical decompression.[371]

When there are initial findings indicative of bilateral brain stem lesions, the course is often progressive (9 of 13 cases) and fatal (6 of 13 cases). In approximately one-third of patients symptoms appear at the time of neck rotation or injury, in one-third symptoms develop minutes or days later, and in one-third symptoms progress after the onset.[425] Autopsy usually confirms extensive brain stem and cerebellar infarctions and thrombosis in the basilar or vertebral arteries. In one patient, the right vertebral artery was perforated with disruption of the media and internal elastic membrane, and hemorrhage surrounded the vertebral artery and vein;[425] in one other patient (an 8-year-old boy who fell from a tree) a true traumatic aneurysm of the right vertebral artery ruptured, leading to death from subarachnoid hemorrhage.[371] In some patients, the radiographic appearance of pseudoaneurysm suggests dissection of the vertebral artery, but this has not often been verified by postmortem examination.

Especially susceptible to injury during neck rotation is the third segment of the vertebral artery, which lies in relation to the atlas, axis, and atlanto-occipital membrane. Injury to the intima activates clotting mechanisms and leads to the formation of thrombus in the vertebral artery, usually at the C2 to C1 region. Thrombus may propagate distally or embolize to more rostral portions of the basilar arterial tree. Filling defects in the distal vascular bed are occasionally verified angiographically.[85,425] In unusual instances the vertebral artery may be perforated, or a dissection may be initiated at the injured segment. Anticoagulation has been occasionally used in an attempt to stop clot propagation and embolization.[425] The variability of the natural course and the scarcity of treated patients make it impossible at present to estimate the utility of anticoagulation in this group of patients.

## Dissection

Dissection of the vertebral and basilar arteries has been increasingly recognized in recent years following the clinical and angiographic descriptions of internal carotid artery (ICA) dissection.[185] In the posterior circulation, the artery most involved in dissection is the extracranial VA, usually well above the origin from the subclavian, and below the intradural intracranial penetration of the vessel. The initial reports of dissection of the extracranial VA were in patients who had chiropractic or other neck manipulations,[126,192,197,203,249,280] but "spontaneous" or dissection related to trivial trauma has also been recognized. Recently, several studies of patients with extracranial VA dissection have been described.[9,85,91,192,313,343] The most common symptom is pain in the head or neck. Usually the pain is in the posterior neck with radiation to the occiput, and sometimes to the shoulder. In some patients, headache and neck pain may be the only complaints. Ischemic symptoms and signs may develop at the same time as the pain or after a delay of hours to a few days. The brain stem regions most susceptible to ischemia from extracranial VA dissection are the lateral medulla and cerebellum.[87] The clinical features usually correspond to a partial lateral medullary syndrome. Vertigo and isolated face dysesthesia are common symptoms. Visual blurring, diplopia and oscillopsia also occur. Ipsilateral cerebellar dysfunction and gait ataxia occur frequently. A Horner's syndrome is usually present. If isolated cerebellar infarction occurs, then dizziness, and ataxia predominate. Unilateral symptomatic VA dissection may be associated with asymptomatic dissection of the other VA or even the ICA.

Intracranial VA dissections are less common compared to extracranial VA dissection. Two major clinical presentations have been described; SAH, and brainstem infarction.[74] Less commonly, the dissection may act as a mass lesion compressing posterior fossa structures.[74] SAH as a complication of intracranial VA dissection reflects, in part, the differences in vessel morphology of intracranial and extracranial arteries. The intracranial arteries have a thinner media and adventitial layers, and only an internal elastic lamina, while extracranial arteries have thicker media and adventitia and an external as well as an internal elastic lamina. If an intracranial dissection involves the media and spreads to the outer layers then rupture and subarachnoid hemorrhage may occur. When the dissection occurs in the media and subintimal layers, then obstruction to blood flow from a narrowing of the lumen, or local embolism may lead to brainstem infarction. When SAH is present, it is not different from SAH due to saccular aneurysm rupture. Headache, often chronic, is common in all presentations of intracranial VA dissection. Acute headaches associated with prodromal leaks have been suspected. As with subarachnoid hemorrhage (SAH) from saccular aneurysms, the outcome is poor. When brain stem infarction occurs, it is usually severe and often fatal. Initial unilateral signs frequently become bilateral with coma and quadriparesis. Deficits limited to the lateral medulla, as in extracranial VA dissection, are unusual when the dissection involves the intracranial VA. Dissecting aneurysms of the intracranial VA may present as mass lesions without SAH or stroke. Headache, neck pain, and progressive lower cranial nerve compressive signs have been the hallmark.[8,78,109]

Dissection of the basilar artery and its major branches is very uncommon compared to VA dissection. Most descriptions are isolated case reports diagnosed at postmortem.[6,134,185,400,480] The commonest clinical presentation is sudden coma with no history of preceding events. Major brain stem infarction correlates with the clinical findings. Subarachnoid hemorrhage as the initial presentation of basilar dissection has also been documented. At least one report described dissection beginning in the right intracranial VA and extending into the basilar artery.[133] Watson[480] described a 32-year-old man who developed headache, confusion, blindness, and "pontine" dysfunction. The spinal fluid contained no blood. At postmortem examination there was a dissection of the basilar artery between the media and internal elastic lamina, which had narrowed the basilar lumen to a small slit. Unusual "loose" connective tissue was identified in the media and may have contributed to the dissection. Wolman[496] described a similar case: a 33-year-old man suddenly became comatose and died of brain stem and cerebellar infarction. The basilar artery dissection had begun at the distal end and spread into the posterior and superior cerebellar arteries. The lumen of the basilar artery was occluded by compression from the large clot within the vessel wall. A congenital defect in the media of the involved segment of the basilar artery may have predisposed this patient to the dissection. Alexander et al.[6] also reported two patients with basilar dissection. One had a month-long chronic course characterized by altered mental state and paraparesis; the basilar dissection had enlarged the vessel, producing considerable mass effect. The other patient, with long-standing migraine, developed sudden brain stem infarction secondary to dissection of the basilar artery. In none of these cases of basilar dissection were premonitory symptoms noted. However, Escourolle and colleagues[135] described a patient with a positive serologic test for syphilis who developed severe headache and episodes of left hemiplegia prior to a fixed quadriplegic deficit. Postmortem examination revealed a dissection beginning in the right intracranial vertebral artery extending up the basilar artery to the superior cerebellar artery.

The principal features that were thought to distinguish carotid artery dissection from atherosclerotic occlusion are (1) local neck or jaw pain, (2) migrainous spells of scintillation, (3) relatively rapid onset with multiple spells ("carotid allegro"), and (4) Horner syndrome.[185] We have seen several patients in whom vertebral artery occlusion was heralded by severe headache, local posterior occipital and nuchal discomfort, and caudal brain stem dysfunction. In some of these cases, angiography has shown a vertebral artery occlusion, but the extent of the vascular lesion could not be clarified angiographically, and so the presence of dissection could not be verified. Some authors have proposed that migraine may predispose to dissection by producing edema of the media of vessels.[480,501] Are we failing to diagnose most examples of vertebral artery dissection? Is dissection a more common cause of posterior circulation stroke than is presently appreciated?

## Fibromuscular Dysplasia

Fibromuscular dysplasia (FMD) is characterized by hyperplasia of the intima and media of arteries with adventitial sclerosis and breakdown of normal elastic tissue. Thickened septa and ridges protrude into the lumen. At postmortem, basilar occlusion with brain stem infarction was documented; the basilar artery was severely ectatic and atherosclerotic with focal variations in wall thickness an aneurysm formation. Frens et al.[195] and Osborn and Anderson[361] reported patients with homonomous hemianopia and posterior cerebral artery FMD. Cephalic FMD is strongly associated with accompanying intracranial aneurysm.[195,218,325] Six patients in Osborne and Anderson's report presented with SAH from aneurysm rupture. In the Mayo Clinic series reported by Corrin et al.[99] there were 10 of 79 patients with FMD and aneurysm, some with SAH. In a collection of 109 patients with cervical FMD there were 23 intracranial aneurysms, So et al.[436] reported 7 patients with Berry aneurysms in their series of 32 patients with FMD, 5 patients with SAH. A relationship between cephalic FMD and dissection has also been noted. In a dramatic example, Ringel et al.[400] reported dissecting aneurysms in all four major extracranial arteries in one patient with FMD. The angiographic changes of pseudoaneurysm formation seen in FMD are also commonly described in dissection of cervical vessels.[185] The abnormalities of the media and elastic lamina in patients with FMD may predispose to dissection more often than is presently recognized. The mechanisms of ischemia distal to lesions of FMD are unclear, as are the need for and the types of treatment.

## Temporal Arteritis

Headache and visual loss, the most common clinical manifestations of temporal arteritis, are caused by giant cell granulomatous disease of the ophthalmic branches to the optic nerve and central retinal arteries and the superficial temporal and occipital artery branches of the external carotid artery. Larger vessels are frequently also involved and occasionally lead to symptoms that dominate the clinical picture. Hamrin[217] examined the major branches of the aortic arch in patients with temporal arteritis and found 10 of 10 had segmental involvement of the subclavian arteries. Klein et al.[276] described symptoms related to ischemic involvement of the upper extremities (subclavian artery and its branches) in 20 of 248 patients with temporal arteritis. The subclavian steal syndrome also has been reported as a result of subclavian artery occlusion in temporal arteritis.[388] Vertebral artery involvement also has been documented in temporal arteritis.[206] The changes invariably affect the vertebral artery before it pierces the dura matter, and usually there is an abrupt transition to normal, 5 mm within the dura. Just inside the dura, the normal vertebral artery undergoes a decrease in its medial and adventitial coats and thereafter has fewer elastic fibers in the media and external elastic lamina.[490] Similarly, the internal carotid artery is affected in its petrous and intracavernous portions just before the artery becomes intradural. Vertebral artery arteritis can produce brain stem infarction.[490] The most frequently described intracranial vessel pathology in temporal arteritis is thrombus formation without local arteritis; this is probably due to embolization[206] from the extracranial arteritic occlusive disease. Rarely, smaller intracranial vessels, including posterior circulation branches, may demonstrate granulomatous arteritis.[206] The related clinical findings are headache, cerebrospinal fluid pleocytosis, and multifocal cranial nerve and parenchymatous dysfunction, usually without a clear history of strokes.[91,206]

## Other Pathology

Less common diseases affecting vascular structures of the posterior fossa will be mentioned only briefly because of their rarity and the lack of data on their special features within the posterior circulation.

*Fibrous bands* crossing the proximal vertebral artery before it enters the transverse foramina may constrict the vessel when the neck is turned.[308]

*Sickle cell disease* is associated with occlusion of small and larger vessels;[497] the larger vessels frequently show extensive intimal proliferation of fibrodysplasia, possibly related to abnormal flow mechanisms.[323] Stroke often occurs during a sickle cell crisis and is heralded by seizures. Few data are available concerning the findings related to posterior circulation occlusion in this group of patients; pseudobulbar signs are more common than bulbar paralysis.

*Fungal and tuberculous meningitis* commonly produces changes within vessels, most often in branches of the middle cerebral artery and in arteries that traverse the interpeduncular fossa to penetrate the rostral brain stem. The exudate somehow produces a reaction in the media of these vessels usually referred to as "Huebner's arteritis." Sudden stupor may be due to infarctions of the brain stem, often with 3rd cranial nerve palsies and bilateral pyramidal tract dysfunction. Headache, fever, cranial nerve palsies, and confusion dominate the clinical picture, and examination of the cerebrospinal fluid usually confirms the diagnosis.

*Young women on oral contraceptives* may suffer occlusion of the extracranial vertebral artery, and for unclear reasons basilar artery occlusion occasionally occurs in the first 2 decades of life.

*Syphilis* can also produce an arteritis and can be associated with brain stem infarcts, usually in branch distribution.

*Systemic lupus erythematosus* and *granulomatous angiitis* do affect cerebral blood vessels, but a stroke-like picture is rarely found.

*Homocystinuria, Marfan syndrome, Ehlers-Danlos syndrome, pseudoxanthoma elasticum, polyarteritis no-*

*dosa*, *Kohlmeyer-Degos disease*, and *Fabry's disease* are associated with ischemic strokes, but little is known of the incidence and site of involvement in the vertebrobasilar system in these diseases.

*Takayasu's pulseless disease* often involves the subclavian and vertebral artery orifices as well as the aorta.[256,306] Occasionally, the intracranial arteries also show intensive inflammation typical of Takayasu's arteritis.[342] Brain stem lesions are especially common in Behçet's syndrome.[318]

*Behçet's disease* was described by a Turk and seems common in the Middle East. Clinical findings include aphthous stomatitis and genital ulcers, uveitis, cells in the spinal fluid and multifocal neurologic signs.[236,420] The neurologic symptoms often relate to the brain stem and develop quickly or gradually. CT usually shows a low-density abnormality in the brain stem, cerebellum, or cerebral white matter which enhances acutely.[236] Mass effect may be seen. With time, enhancement is lost, and the patient stabilizes or improves. Angiography usually does not show arterial occlusions, but dural sinus occlusions are common. At necropsy inflammatory lesions are seen with perivascular lymphocytic cuffing around capillaries and venules, especially in the brain stem.[236]

## PATHOPHYSIOLOGY

Many factors determine whether or not an ischemic tissue becomes infarcted. Blockage of the lumina of blood vessels by atheroma, clot, or swollen vessel wall, embolization of intraluminal material distally, and activation of clotting factors with propagation of clot all act to increase luminal obstruction and diminish blood flow to a given region. However, concomitantly, reduction of flow to a region leads to accumulation of metabolites, especially lactate, and an increase in collateral circulation. Fibrinolysis and other enzymatic processes act to lyse and solidify the local clot. Embolic fragments pass through the vascular bed, allowing resumption of flow. In addition, systemic factors such as blood pressure cardiac output, blood viscosity, red blood cell count, and pulmonary function all affect the rheology and oxygen-carrying capacity of the blood reaching a given ischemic region. The sum of these factors determines survival of a given ischemic zone. The process can be viewed schematically (Table 18-1) as the summation of vectors, those tending to increase ischemia and those promoting additional blood flow to reduce the ischemic deficit. Within the posterior circulation, there are multiple collateral channels for augmenting flow. Reduction of flow through a vertebral artery can often be compensated for by collaterals from the opposite vertebral artery, the thyrocervical trunk, and occipital artery branches of the external carotid artery, which direct flow toward the nuchal vertebral artery. Intracranially, the long circumferential cerebellar arteries (AICA, PICA, and SCA) form an active collateral system. For example, in a lesion blocking flow in the proximal basilar artery, blood can course from the vertebral artery to the PICA and into hemispheral branches of the AICA and back to the basilar artery beyond the region of blockage. Similarly, blood may pass from the SCA to AICA or PICA branches. The internal carotid artery may serve as a major source of collateral circulation, with blood flowing via the posterior communicating artery to the posterior cerebral and superior cerebellar arteries, the latter supplying collaterals to the lower brain stem through the cerebellar hemispheral branches. Collateral circulation is especially rich in the brain stem tegmentum, making this region more resistent to ischemia.

**TABLE 18-1. Pathophysiology Tenuous Equilibrium After Occlusion of an Artery**

| Factors Promoting Deficit | Factors Defending Against Deficit |
|---|---|
| Blood flow to lesion diminished by stenosis of occlusion | Collateral circulation and autoregulation |
| Embolization from plaque or clot | Passing of emboli |
| Activation of clotting factors | Thrombolysis (?) |

The time course of development and progression of symptoms is well correlated with prognosis and gives information about the sum of pathophysiologic vectors operative in the individual patient. Symptoms develop in one of the following temporal patterns: (1) transient ischemic attacks (TIAs), either as an isolated finding or preceding a stroke; (2) sudden-onset deficits which are maximal at onset; (3) fluctuating clinical deficits punctuated by improvements and deteriorations; and (4) gradually progressive stroke. In a series of personally observed cases of vertebral or basilar occlusion,[65,81] the temporal course was analyzed. The majority of patients had TIAs. These often were multiple and variegated and increased in frequency as the stroke approached. In these patients, the stroke often was noticed on arising. Symptoms and signs of brain stem, cerebellar, and posterior cerebral territory ischemia then fluctuated for a period of 2 to 3 weeks and stabilized thereafter. During this 2- to 3-week period, clinical fluctuations were quite sensitive to blood pressure and postural changes.[65,83] Simply sitting up or raising the head of the bed to eat could cause temporary aggravation of a deficit, which was quickly relieved by lowering the head. The presence of preceding TIAs indicates some chronicity to the occlusive process, allowing more time for collateral circulation to develop. Improvement in function indicates that collateral circulation has developed or the occlusive process is less operant (e.g., lysis of embolic clot). Perhaps for these reasons patients with TIAs and a fluctuating course have a better prognosis. Other patients had sudden-onset deficits sometimes heralded by TIAs or progressive accumulation of deficit without significant temporary improvement in function. Sudden-onset deficits are usually embolic. Prognosis depends on the length of time the embolus blocks the vessel and clot lysis or passage. Steady progression of symptoms without stabilization or improvement indicates poor formation of collaterals and has a bad prognosis.

Few reports have considered the temporal course. Jones et al.[259] analyzed the course of 37 patients with vertebrobasilar territory infarction: 12 had at least one preceding TIA, and in 30 patients the onset of stroke was precipitous. Fluctuations commonly occurred during the first week but were unusual thereafter. Progressive deterioration in function was common (16 of 37 cases), usually reached its maximum within the first 4 days, and had a bad prognosis. Similarly, Patrick et al.[367] reviewed 39 patients with vertebrobasilar territory infarction and commented on the instability of the early clinical course but rarity of late (over 3 weeks) progression. In neither series was there frequent corroboration of the nature and locus of the vascular lesion during life.

Transient ischemic attacks are caused by either diminished blood flow (with temporarily insufficient collateral circulation) or embolization of clot or plaque material. In our experience, frequently recurring brief TIAs (machine-gunlike flurries) usually indicate a severe proximal stenosis or occlusion, whereas occasional but longer-lasting spells are more likely embolic. The fixed deficit is often noticed in the morning, having accumulated at night during a time of more sluggish flow. Once the vertebral or basilar artery is occluded, propagation of clot, embolization, and diminished blood flow may result. The critical period for development of neurologic deficit is at the time of occlusion and during the next few weeks. During this time collateral circulation is developing and the clot becomes adherent to the vascular wall and is thereafter more resistent to embolization. Denny-Brown[114] emphasized a contributory role of systemic factors in compounding the clinical deficit and called these fluctuations "reversible hemodynamic crises." These factors seem most operant in the first 2 weeks after vascular occlusion and were less clinically important thereafter. Sundt and Piepgras[447] also emphasized the importance of postural changes on flow during the early critical period. Naritomi et al.[353] showed that reduction in regional blood flow to the posterior circulation, as measured by xenon inhalation, rarely persisted 3 weeks after transient ischemic symptoms, but that defective autoregulation (i.e., change in flow after induced postural hypotension) was more widespread and long-lasting after "vertebrobasilar insufficiency" than after carotid attacks. Careful scrutiny of blood pressure, maintenance of blood volume and optimal oxygenation, and careful surveillance of patients when they assume sitting or upright postures is very important during the first few weeks after a vertebrobasilar territory stroke, because collateral circulation is still developing. This is especially true in occlusive disease of larger vessels (vertebral or basilar artery), but extension of deficit after reduced blood pressure may also occur in basilar branch occlusion.[178]

Embolic occlusion is considered by some to be unusual in patients with vertebral basilar infarction; however, Castaigne et al.[88] have documented the frequency of emboli within the posterior cerebral arteries, and syndromes related to the rostral basilar artery are likely to be more frequently embolic.[67] In several previously reported cases distal embolic lesions arose from an occluded vertebral artery. Artery to artery emboli do occur within the posterior circulation, but their frequency has not been documented. Emboli probably account for the sudden-onset deficits.

A recent report reviews prior documentation of intra-arterial emboli within the posterior circulation.[84] The most frequent donor sites are the vertebral artery origin (either recent thrombosis or ulcerated plaque[373]), and the intracranial vertebral artery. Among a series of 67 patients with brain stem and cerebellar ischemia, 9 (13 percent) had intra-arterial embolism as the mechanism of stroke.[84] Among these 9 patients, the donor site was the proximal extracranial vertebral artery in 5, distal extracranial vertebral artery dissection in 3, and a thrombus within the intracranial vertebral artery in 1. Emboli went to the intracranial vertebral artery-PICA in 3, the basilar artery in 3, and the distal basilar artery-superior cerebellar artery region in another 3.[84]

Generally, progressive neurologic deficits usually imply propagation of clot or failure of collateral circulation to compensate for the reduced flow. If a larger vessel is involved, this usually implies a poor prognosis.[65,265] Another cause of worsening of symptoms within the posterior circulation is infarction of the cerebellum with progressive swelling and pressure on the brain stem and ventricular pathways.[289] This problem is serious and has high mortality, but it is amenable to surgical decompression. Progression of deficit can also occur within the territory of a basilar branch, but this usually occurs over a shorter period of hours to 1 week, and the deficit is limited to the territory supplied by the single branch or its previously occluded neighboring branches.[170]

Worsening can also be caused by alterations in cardiovascular and respiratory function resulting from ischemic brain stem dysfunction. Lability of blood pressure and blood flow can result from lesions of the medulla and pons.[272] Reis[393] has also documented the importance of the fastigial nucleus of the cerebellum in altering cerebral blood flow. Stimulation of regions within the brain stem tegmentum can alter heart rate and rhythm.[28,299] Khurana[272] described persistent tachycardia, orthostatic hypotension without cardiac acceleration, episodic bradycardia and even cardiorespiratory arrest in four patients with bilateral pontomedullary lesions. Even unilateral lesions can be accompanied by tachycardia and lability of blood pressure. Bogousslavsky et al.[43] reported two patients studied clinically and at necropsy with severe hypoventilation related to unilateral lateral tegmental pontomedullary infarcts. Intermittent apnea, especially during sleep, and failure to respond during $CO_2$ retention were prominent features, and each patient died of the complications of respiratory failure.

Activation of clotting factors, polycythemia, or thrombocytosis can exaggerate occlusive disease and in some situations may alone be responsible for sluggish posterior circulation flow and clinical attacks. One patient with an elevated hemoglobin and platelet count and increased platelet agglutination developed frequent spells of vertebrobasilar ischemia and claudication of the legs; no lesion could be seen angiographically and the spells disappeared after aspirin therapy. This experience prompts the suggestion that a hematologic survey be part of the evaluation of all patients with transient or persisting ischemic symptoms. In the individual patient, the anatomic location of the lesion producing the neurologic signs and the time course of development of the deficit help the physician predict the affected vessel, the nature of the pathologic process in the vessel, and the adequacy of collateral circulation. Laboratory investigations, especially angiography, confirm the location of the responsible vascular lesion, give additional information concerning previous pathology or maldevelopment in other extracranial and intracranial vessels, and help define the source and adequacy of collateral circulation.

## CLINICAL FINDINGS IN PATIENTS WITH VASCULAR LESIONS AT VARIOUS LOCATIONS

### Subclavian and Innominate Artery Occlusive Disease and the "Subclavian Steal"

In 1961 Reivich and colleagues[394] reported their observations of two patients with transient ischemic attacks referable to the posterior circulation. Each patient had diminished pulse and blood pressure in the left arm. Attacks were precipitated by exercise in one patient and by change of head posture in the other. Angiography in each case revealed stenosis of the subclavian artery proximal to the origin of the left vertebral artery. In one case the left internal carotid artery was also occluded. Blood flowed from the normal right vertebral artery into the cranium and then down the left vertebral artery in a retrograde fashion and filled the distal left subclavian artery. In the laboratory, these investigators occluded the left subclavian artery of dogs and measured blood flow in the other great vessels. In this artificially induced situation they documented a compensatory increase in flow through the right vertebral artery and a reversal of flow in the left vertebral artery. Fisher,[154] in an accompanying editorial in the same edition of the *New England Journal of Medicine,* coined the term *subclavian steal,* referring to the siphoning of blood away from its proper cranial destination toward the ischemic arm.

Within the next few years angiography in similar groups of patients documented reversal of flow in the vertebral artery due to subclavian artery occlusive disease. These reports[105,149,238,358,366,426] showed that the phenomenon was not rare. The reaction to these reports was immediate and widespread. Coming at a time of rapid growth in the use of angiography and surgical interest in cerebral vascular disease, lesions of the subclavian artery were avidly sought and surgically repaired. More importantly, the concept of blood flowing from one vessel to rescue a more distant circulation gave rise to the concept that the cerebrovascular bed was an open net in which decreased input at any point of entry could conceivably lead to decreased flow in any distant site. To determine "ischemia at a distance," clinicians would fully opacify the entire vascular bed, including the aortic arch and the four major extracranial vessels. Any obstructive lesion, even if it did not directly supply the ischemic region, would then be surgically repaired.

In the two decades since the original report, a clearer definition of the clinical findings and further reflections on the place of surgery in the treatment of subclavian steal has been worked out. Patients with subsequently verified subclavian steal may present with one of several types of symptoms: (1) headache, (2) intermittent episodes of cerebral ischemia, or (3) claudication or pain in the ischemic arm. However, many patients have no symptoms referable to the subclavian lesion. They are discovered only when angiographic or noninvasive evaluation of pulse or blood pressure changes in the arm, peripheral vascular disease in the legs, or abnormalities in the carotid circulation reveal the subclavian lesion. In a recent study of 324 patients with subclavian steal detected by noninvasive techniques, 116 of the 155 patients (74 percent) who had a unilateral isolated subclavian steal and no severe carotid artery disease had no neurologic symptoms.[230]

Headache is common and is usually located in the mastoid, occiput, or neck. The major symptom of the first patient of Reivich et al.[394] was recurrent throbbing pain in the left mastoid area, which radiated to the left parietal and occipital regions. The headache may be more generalized and may be isolated or accompany symptoms of cerebral ischemia. The headache may be precipitated by exercise. Surprisingly, symptoms of severe ischemia in the involved arm are rare. Patients may complain of fatigue, claudication on exercise, paresthesia, sensitivity to cold, and sensations of heaviness or coolness in the arm. These are often exercise related. The usual slow development of the occlusive lesion and the richness of collateral supply tend to make the upper extremity ischemia a relatively minor problem unless the patient exercises the arm frequently, as would be the case in a golfer or baseball pitcher.

Athletes, especially baseball pitchers, seem to have an increased incidence of subclavian artery occlusive disease, or at least the sufferers are brought more frequently to public attention.[148,150,445] Sudden downward arm motions can cause angulation of the artery over the first rib or a cervical rib where the subclavian artery courses over the flat surface of the first rib on its way out of the thorax. Pitchers and cricket bowlers may subject the subclavian arteries of their throwing arms to chance trauma with subsequent thrombosis. Fatigue, arm pain, loss of pitching velocity and accuracy, and lack of stamina in the throwing arm results. In the large series of Hennerici et al.,[230] one-third of patients reported pain, numbness, or fatigue in the arm, but only 15 of 324 patients (4.8 percent) had objective signs of severe brachial ischemia or embolism.

Cerebral symptoms are common but usually transient, lasting seconds to minutes but often recurring over a period of months or even years.[358,426] In many patients, subclavian stenosis is caused by severe atherosclerotic disease; coexistent significant atherosclerotic lesions in the carotid artery and other extracranial and intracranial vessels are quite common and might even be considered the rule rather than the exception. This fact often makes the origin of transient ischemic cerebral symptoms difficult to discover. For example, the second case of Reivich et al.[394] had a transient episode of aphasia and right-hand paresis. Evaluation revealed complete occlusion of the left internal carotid artery, which at surgery contained fresh clot, as well as a subclavian steal. Of the nine patients with subclavian steal, reported by North et al.,[358] only three had permanent deficits; each patient with a lasting deficit had hemiparesis, and all had significant internal carotid artery occlusive disease (two bilateral and one unilateral). In all other series, the incidence of associated vascular lesions is high.[230] In the series of Hennerici et al.[230] lateralized hemispheric symptoms of cerebral ischemia were about twice as frequent in patients with unilateral subclavian steal and associated carotid disease as in those without carotid lesions. Hemispheric brain symptoms occurred more often (29 patients, 66 percent) in patients with severe carotid artery stenosis than in those with less severe obstruction (18 patients, 32 percent). The arm may show more cyanosis when held above heart level. A bruit may be heard in the supraclavicular region and radiate into the axilla or along the posterior neck to the mastoid region. Sometimes one can distinguish the subclavian or vertebral origin of a bruit by pumping the blood pressure cuff above systolic pressure. This maneuver decreases distal subclavian flow but may increase cephalad flow in the vertebral artery, because blood goes into the proximal branches rather than the arm. In disease of the proximal subclavian artery, the bruit usually decreases because of less flow through the stenotic segment and less retrograde vertebral flow; in stenosis of the vertebral artery, the bruit is usually augmented. Focal neurologic deficits caused by subclavian-vertebral siphonage are rare and are usually explained by coexistent carotid artery disease, which should be sought on examination.

The most common etiology of subclavian occlusive disease is atherosclerosis, although congenital lesions such as preductal coarctation of the aorta with patent ductus arteriosis,[109] atresia of the left subclavian artery,[199] and a pseudocoarctation of the aorta with kinked left subclavian artery[302] occasionally produce the syndrome. Sometimes subclavian steal follows surgical manipulation of the subclavian artery, as in the Blalock-Taussig procedure for tetralogy of Fallot, in which the subclavian artery is anastamosed to the pulmonary artery. Traumatic injury, embolism, and arteritis (temporal arteritis and Takayasu's arteritis) may also cause subclavian steal. In the large series of North et al.[358] the left subclavian artery was affected alone in 33 instances, whereas the right subclavian or innominate artery was affected in 13 cases, and 13 cases were bilateral.

The frequency with which the arteries are affected varies. The left subclavian artery is involved approximately three times more frequently than the right innominate or subclavian arteries. Among 155 patients with a unilateral subclavian steal in one series, 111 (71 percent) were left-sided, and 29 percent occurred on Raynaud's phenomenon. In the subclavian artery, occlusive disease does not always cause retrograde vertebral flow. Of 20 cases of subclavian artery stenosis evaluated by Berguer et al.,[36] only one-half had evidence of reversed vertebral artery flow. There are many other possible collateral channels to augment distal subclavian flow, including the inferior and external thyroid, internal mammary, intercostal, and ascending cervical arteries.[26] At times, the vertebral artery ipsilateral to the subclavian artery stenosis originates from the aortic arch, ends distally in the PICA, or is tiny or occluded, and so is unavailable as a source of collateral supply.[140]

The anatomy of the right side of the aortic arch differs from that of the left. The innominate artery is larger and usually rises higher in the supraclavicular fossa than its left counterpart. The right subclavian artery has a more intimate relationship with the right common carotid artery. Clot in the right axillary or subclavian artery may propagate into the innominate artery and extend or embolize to the carotid system. Though this phenomenon is rare, most of the patients have been young and have presented a striking clinical picture. Symonds[454] described two patients with diminished arterial pulsation in the right arm, probably due to a cervical rib in which sudden left hemiplegia developed. Yates and Guest[502] reported a patient with progressive pain and weakness in the right arm who had an ununited fracture of the right clavicle.

This patient suddenly experienced visual loss, went into a coma, had left hemiplegia, and subsequently died. The right subclavian artery at postmortem was displaced by the fractured bone and occluded. Clot extended into the innominate artery and had embolized to the basilar artery bifurcation. Hoobler[247] reported a similar patient with a cervical rib, weak right arm pulses, and sudden left hemiparesis. Damage to the subclavian artery may be caused by cervical ribs, trauma, or the use of crutches. Clot or aneurysm forms at the site of compression and leads to symptoms of ischemia or Raynaud's phenomenon in the arm; the clot will embolize, on the right, into the distal carotid or vertebral arterial tree. Though a similar lesion could occur on the left, it would only involve the left vertebral artery and might be difficult to recognize.

Stenosis or occlusion of the innominate artery is less common than is subclavian artery disease. Brewster and colleagues[51] collected 71 patients operated on in one hospital for innominate artery lesions during a 20-year period. In this series, 36 patients had atherosclerotic occlusive disease involving the origin of the innominate artery from the aortic arch or the heart.

Diagnosis of subclavian steal in the early series was usually confirmed by angiography, which is best done by selective transfemoral or transaxillary catheterization of the normal vertebral artery with delayed films to show retrograde flow down the contralateral vertebral artery toward the subclavian artery. Furthermore, the internal carotid and intracranial circulation can also be visualized during the procedure. Arch angiography provides suboptimal detail of the involved vessels and poor visualization of the intracranial vessels. In addition, more dye is required for arch angiography, and complications are more frequent. Digital subtraction angiography, using intravenous dye installation, has also been used to show the subclavian-vertebral artery anatomy in the neck.[284,481] However, the complication rate is relatively high and often opacification and imaging is suboptimal and not diagnostic. Arterial injection using computerized subtraction technology is much more effective and is relatively safe. Magnetic resonance angiography may in the future allow accurate imaging without the need for invasive dye injections.[124,128,129]

Now noninvasive testing accurately documents severe innominate and subclavian artery occlusive disease with a high degree of reliability.[231,232,476] Ekestrom and colleagues[132] used serial measurements to test subclavian flow and detect reversed vertebral artery flow; these techniques included forearm blood flow measurement by oscillography, venous occlusive plethysmography of the arm, Doppler ultrasound with the patient in a sitting position, and directional flow recorded in the vertebral artery below the transverse process of the atlas. Liljequist et al.[297] demonstrated that directional Doppler ultrasound analysis of flow in the vertebral artery located just below the transverse process of the atlas reliably detected the presence of retrograde vertebral artery blood flow in angiographically verified patients with subclavian steal. Berguer and colleagues[36] measured the relative velocity of pulsed-wave propagation in the two arms and concluded that a delay in propagation was well correlated with angiographically verified reversal of vertebral artery flow in the innominate and subclavian arteries by angiographic correlation. All 21 patients with Doppler-detected innominate stenosis and all 66 patients with subclavian steal had angiography that agreed with the noninvasive findings. Combining the patients with subclavian and vertebral artery extracranial disease, 92 percent of these that had lesions by Doppler had angiographic agreement. However, provocative tests such as decreasing peripheral resistance in the upper arm could cause temporary basilar artery flow reversal. Transcranial Doppler (TCD) also documents flow changes in the intracranial vertebral artery.[79,476] A variety of surgical procedures have been devised to treat subclavian artery occlusive disease.

Endarterectomy of the subclavian lesion usually requires a thoracotomy. Cervical or thoracic prosthetic or venous bypass grafts or ligation of the ipsilateral vertebral artery are other techniques which have been used.[26] Vertebral ligation can cause thrombosis of the vertebral artery with later propagation of clot into the cranium or distal embolization.[194,248] The question is not whether surgery can be done to remedy vertebral artery siphonage, but whether it should be done in a particular patient. In deciding this question, three points should be kept in mind: (1) Subclavian steal is a relatively benign phenomenon. Though transient spells are common, brain stem infarction is rare. Cerebellar infarction has been observed, but only after hypotension. In other words, there is usually "more smoke than fire." (2) Coexistent serious extracranial and intracranial vascular disease is the rule! It is easy to be seduced by the intriguing collateral pathways and the clearly demonstrable physical signs of subclavian disease and miss the more important, more relevant vascular lesion in the individual patient. (3) Subclavian or innominate surgery is somewhat more complex and is associated with more morbidity than other extracranial vascular surgery if a thoracotomy is needed. Patients who could tolerate a local neck procedure such as carotid endarterectomy or venous bypass grafting may not be able to survive a thoracotomy satisfactorily. Unfortunately, the open net theory of cerebral circulation has given license for surgical repair of an angiographic stenosis whether or not it is directly related to the symptomatology.

## Extracranial Vertebral Artery Occlusive Disease

The extracranial vertebral artery is a frequent site of atheromatous disease[181,254,345,416] and also exhibits an unusually high incidence of congenital variability (asymmetry, small size, residual embryologic anastomosis, and termination in the PICA). Atherostenosis at the vertebral artery origin is more common in men than in women[80,207] and is often associated with carotid artery occlusive disease.[252] Whites have a higher frequency of vertebral origin disease than blacks or persons of Chinese or Japanese ancestry.[80,207] At times, the proximal vertebral artery lesions represent extension of plaque material from the parent subclavian artery.

Despite the high incidence of disease, serious brain stem or posterior circulation strokes have only rarely been caused by occlusive disease limited to an extracranial vertebral artery. During the nineteenth century Alexander[5] treated epilepsy with apparent impunity by placing a ligature on the vertebral artery; he ligated one or both vertebral arteries low in the neck in 21 young epileptics, at times tying both vessels at one operation. Surgeons have ligated the vertebral artery as a treatment of subclavian steal, eliminating the siphonage through this vessel. Fisher[166] reported in detail five patients in whom bilateral occlusions of the proximal vertebral system could be demonstrated angiographically. All patients had transient episodes, but in only one was there a persisting neurologic deficit, and that patient also had an occlusion of the internal carotid artery at the siphon on the appropriate side to explain the findings. Extensive collateral circulation may develop, especially if the vertebral artery occlusion occurs gradually. The occipital branch of the external carotid artery is a prominent source of collateral supply, often filling the deep muscular branches of the vertebral artery near the atlas.[166,399] The ascending cervical and transverse cervical branches of the thyrocervical trunk originating from the subclavian artery may also fill the vertebral artery in its midcervical course. Compensatory flow from the contralateral vertebral artery and retrograde flow down the basilar artery from the carotid-posterior communicating system is also frequently visualized. The most common transient symptoms are dizziness, faint feelings, blurred vision, and imbalance. Fisher[166] has argued that occlusion of the proximal vertebral artery, like subclavian steal, is usually a benign syndrome rarely accompanied by serious brain stem infarction.

In the past, proximal vertebral artery lesions were said not to ulcerate.[345] However, a recent report by Pelouze[373] documents the finding of an ulcerated vertebral artery plaque as a source of intra-arterial embolism to the intracranial posterior circulation. The patient was a 79-year-old man who had many attacks during a period of months characterized by vertigo, falling, and diplopia. Angiography showed an irregular stenosing lesion at the origin of the left vertebral artery, and a B-mode scan of the region suggested the presence of an ulcerated plaque. Two of my cases[81] document that embolism may occasionally arise from a previously occluded extracranial vertebral artery. A 58-year-old man had two isolated episodes of brain stem dysfunction, separated by a month, one probably pontine and the other thalamic. Angiography revealed opacification of the left vertebral artery only through muscular branches of the thyrocervical trunk. The right vertebral artery and intracranial vessels were normal. Spells ceased after anticoagulant therapy. A 38-year-old man suddenly developed headache and quadraparesis some days after a stormy airplane ride.[65] Angiography revealed nonfilling of the right nuchal vertebral artery and a midbasilar artery occlusion. After anticoagulation therapy there were no further episodes during the next 3 years. A 34-year-old man had persistent left posterior neck pain and headache for 4 days, then developed a right pontine infarct.[378] Angiography showed a left VA occlusion at the C2 level and an intraluminal filling defect (embolus) in the distal basilar artery and proximal superior cerebellar artery. He was anticoagulated for 6 months. Repeat angiography showed an unchanged left VA occlusion, but the distal basilar artery was now normal. George and Laurian[198] described two patients with VA occlusive disease and suspected basilar embolism. Koroshetz and Ropper[278] studied local embolism of the posterior circulation and found the suspected embolic source in either the extracranial (5 patients), intracranial (3 patients), or both VA segments (3 patients), in 11 patients undergoing angiography. Castaigne et al.[88] observed three cases in which emboli had arisen from a tight stenosis of the proximal vertebral artery. The frequency of embolism arising in vertebral artery occlusive disease or plaques is not known. If a comparable situation in the carotid artery is examined, emboli arising from a fresh occlusion usually occur soon after the occlusion and are rare later. Traumatic occlusions within the nuchal vertebral artery are clearly not as benign (see previous section on pathology). Chiropractic and other manipulation and closed head and neck trauma often cause damage to the third segment of the vertebral artery just before it pierces the dura. Tears, dissection, and thrombosis develop acutely and may give rise to extension of the clot intracranially or to distal clot embolization. The sudden occurrence of the pathology hampers development of adequate collateral circulation. Furthermore, rapidly developing thrombi are usually less adherent to the vascular wall and are closer to the intradural vertebral artery than in the situation of slowly developing atherosclerotic occlusion of the proximal vertebral arteries. In most examples of traumatic injury, the peril of brain stem infarction occurs at the time or soon after the injury. Late occurrences are rarely seen, if ever.

Occasionally, vertebral artery aneurysms in the neck can serve as a donor site for intra-arterial emboli. Maruyama et al.[311] reported the case of a 40-year-old man who had numerous attacks of double vision, sensory abnormalities, and alternating hemiparesis. Angiography performed after he had developed a fixed quadrantanopia showed a large (nearly $3 \times 3$ cm) aneurysm near the origin of the left vertebral artery. Platelet scintigraphy, using radionuclide-labeled platelets, showed a well-defined focus of activity within the aneurysm. After aspirin, repeat scintigraphy showed no activity in the lesion, but spells persisted. At surgery, a brown thrombus was found firmly attached to the wall of the aneurysm. We recently consulted on an adolescent boy who had been rendered quadriplegic due to a traumatic neck injury and a cervical vertebral fracture with displacement. During the first week, he suddenly went blind and became agitated and later somnolent. Investigation showed that one vertebral artery was occluded at the site of the injury, and an intra-arterial embolus had traveled to the rostral basilar artery. We are aware of no prospectively collected series of patients with serious cervical spine injuries who have had systematic studies of the frequency of important accompanying injury to the infraspinous segment of the vertebral arteries. In a series of 24 patients with pontine infarcts and a "locked-in" state, 5 of the 10 patients had neck injuries and delayed onset of brain stem signs. Four patients had cervical fractures, two of whom had documented occlusions of the VA in the neck.[267] Noninvasive ultrasound testing of the vertebral arteries should be capable of determining patency of the arteries above the site of bony trauma.

There are few systematic studies of the incidence of symptoms and signs and prognosis in untreated patients with occlusive disease of the proximal vertebral arteries. Labauge et al.[282] reported 100 personally collected cases of vertebral artery occlusion but included lesions at various sites along the extracranial and intracranial vertebral artery. Headache and "cerebellovestibular" symptoms were common. Many patients presented because they were already symptomatic. Moufarrij and colleagues[349,350] performed a prospective study on patients with angiographically detected vertebral artery stenosis. Most lesions (93 percent) were located at the vertebral artery origin and brain stem strokes were rare at presentation or during follow-up. They followed 89 patients with 75 percent stenosis of at least one vertebral artery origin for an average of 4.6 years. None developed definite vertebrobasilar TIAs; 19 had nonlocalizing spells, among whom 9 had a stroke. Only two patients had brain stem infarcts and each also had basilar artery stenosis. Hennerici and colleagues[229] studied a large group of patients who had no neurovascular symptoms but had severe atherosclerosis of the large peripheral arteries, the aorta or the coronary arteries. In 426 patients, both continuous-wave Doppler insonation and angiograms of the vertebral arteries were available; 183 patients (43 percent) had significant disease of the vertebral or subclavian arteries, indicating that asymptomatic vertebral artery disease is quite common. Doppler insonation of the vertebral artery origin is quite accurate when performed by experienced sonographers in detecting reduced anterograde flow.[229,476] Insonation at the distal extracranial vertebral artery can detect distal alteration in flow.[79,231,476] In the study of Hennerici et al.,[229] the accuracy of continuous-wave Doppler in detecting angiographically confirmed vertebral artery lesions was excellent. Among the 183 patients with lesions, the Doppler results did not agree with angiography in only 8 percent. Considering the total series, 183 patients with lesions and 243 controls without lesions, the accuracy was 90.1 percent. More recently, duplex scanning has been used to image the proximal vertebral artery region.[2,41,468] The technique that combines B-mode ultrasound with Doppler has been shown to accurately detect severe disease from the vertebral artery origin to the C3 to C4 level.[468] Color-coded Doppler imaging of the nuchal vertebral artery is also quite accurate and useful diagnostically.[469]

Intravenous digital subtraction angiography (DSA) can also be helpful. Among 111 patients who had venous DSA in one study, 90 percent had vertebral artery images considered to be of diagnostic quality.[237] Magnetic resonance angiography may become the diagnostic method of choice because of its capability of noninvasively providing longitudinal images of the arteries, but to date the accuracy of detecting proximal vertebral artery lesions is unknown.[124,128,129] At times, films of the vertebral artery origin taken during standard angiography by arch injection are difficult to interpret because of kinking of the vertebral artery origin. The origin is often behind the opacified subclavian artery and difficult to see on standard projections.

Surgical reconstruction of proximal vertebral artery occlusive lesions is most often performed by bypassing the occlusive disease.[35,130,252–254,288,396,407,438] Connections are most often created with the carotid arterial system. The operations can be performed safely by surgeons experienced with the procedure with very low morbidity and mortality. At times, the bypass procedure is performed at the time of carotid endarterectomy.[288] Endarterectomy can also be performed but has been sparingly reported.[375,465] More recently, interventional radiologists have begun to perform angioplasty using catheter techniques, but results are not yet available from series of patients so treated. Fear of distal intracranial embolization after plaque dilatation has made most neurologists and neurosurgeons wary of the technique until technology is available to trap distally moving emboli at the time of angioplasty. The indication for surgery and/or angioplasty are not clear, since collateral circulation is usually restored naturally and the risk of severe brain stem infarction without treatment is low.[349,350]

Theoretically, agents that affect platelet function could prevent fibrin-platelet nidi from forming plaques or stenotic lesions. Heparin given during the first week after a recent vertebral artery occlusion might prevent propagation and embolization of clot while the thrombus organizes and becomes adherent to the vascular wall. Coumadin could theoretically prevent occlusion or embolization in patients with preocclusive stenosis of the proximal vertebral artery. Unfortunately, none of the treatments in use has been systematically studied in trials. Trials would be difficult to perform because the low incidence of adverse events of the lesions would necessitate a very large number of study patients.

## Intracranial Vertebral Artery Occlusive Disease

Occlusive disease of the intracranial portion of the vertebral artery is much more serious than extracranial disease and is commonly associated with infarction of posterior circulation structures. When the one vertebral artery that is responsible for supplying the lion's share of the blood flow (the contralateral vertebral artery being tiny, previously occluded, severely narrowed, or ending in the PICA) is occluded, the resulting syndrome is indistinguishable from occlusion of the basilar artery. In fact, Fisher[163] has used the term *basilarization* of the vertebral artery to describe the situation of dependence on one vertebral artery for maintenance of the posterior circulation. In addition, clot formed within the distal vertebral artery may propagate into the proximal basilar artery, again producing a syndrome indistinguishable from basilar occlusion.

In the more usual situation of bilaterally competent vertebral arteries, occlusion of a single vertebral artery usually is associated with one of several clinical pictures: (1) lateral medullary infarction, (2) cerebellar infarction, (3) ischemia of the ipsilateral hemimedulla and pons, (4) embolic occlusion in vessels of the distal basilar arterial tree, the embolus originating from the vertebral artery clot, or (5) transient spells without infarction. Because these syndromes are common, quite distinct, and clinically important, they are considered separately and in detail.

### Lateral Medullary Infarction

In 1895 Wallenberg[479] reasoned from the clinical findings in a single case and what he knew of brain stem anatomy and physiology that the responsible lesion should be in the lateral medulla.[488] Furthermore, Wallenberg injected the vessels of seven other autopsied human brains in order to define the arterial supply to the lateral medulla and concluded that the posterior inferior cerebellar artery should be occluded in patients with infarcts in the lateral medulla. In fact, postmortem examination of the single case studied clinically did verify infarction of the cerebellum and medulla and occlusion of the PICA. However, when Fisher et al.[183] examined the pattern of vascular occlusion in 17 of their own cases of lateral medullary infarction, in only 2 cases was the occlusive lesion solely within the PICA. In 13 cases the vertebral artery was occluded, and in 1 case severely stenosed. In 20 earlier reports in which the responsible vascular lesion had been documented, 15 had vertebral artery occlusion; only 4 had occlusion within the PICA itself. In about half the cases the thrombus in the vertebral artery extended to block the PICA orifice.

Among the patients studied at necropsy, 14 were thought to have atherostenotic thrombotic occlusions and 3 were thought to represent embolic occlusions. Two patients with embolism had cardiac sources in the form of congenital heart disease and bacterial endocarditis; the other patient with presumed embolism had multiple scattered brain infarcts and no occlusion of the vertebral artery or PICA at necropsy, suggesting an embolism that fragmented and passed. Fisher and colleagues[183] also reviewed prior reports of embolism causing lateral medullary infarcts. The first reported case was described by Hallopeau and was a patient, studied at necropsy by Charcot, who was thought to have a distal vertebral artery embolus that arose from ulcerated atheromatous plaques in the aorta. A patient of Breuer and Marbury had a cardiac mural thrombus and nonadherent gray embolic clot in the intracranial vertebral artery leading to a lateral medullary infarct.[84,183] A patient studied by Richter had a PICA embolus from a bicuspid aortic valve, and Wintler's patient with the lateral medullary syndrome had rheumatic heart disease and an atrial thrombus but patent arteries (presumably indicating a migrant clot) leading to the medullary infarct. Escourolle and colleagues[135] found 14 vertebral artery occlusions and 3 occlusions of the PICA among 23 examples of lateral medullary infarction. When the infarctions were located in the dorsal medulla the occlusion was more likely to be in the stem of the PICA (4 of 5 patients). Although Foix and colleagues[191] had postulated that the syndrome was caused by occlusion of "the artery of the lateral sulcus of the medulla," this has not been observed by others.[183] In fact, in the original case of Foix et al.[191] the suspected blockage was a plaque in the wall of the basilar artery supposedly obstructing the mouth of this lateral sulcal artery. Thus their evidence for incriminating this vessel was quite tenuous. The occlusive lesion within the vertebral artery is most commonly thrombosis engrafted upon preexisting arteriosclerosis.

The infarct usually involves a wedge of the medulla extending medially from the lateral edge (Fig. 18-7). It usually involves a portion of the olive ventrally, and in some cases extends dorsally, to involve the restiform body. Currier et al.[102] divided the pattern of infarction into ventral, superficial, and dorsal lesions, indicating that the extent of infarction was quite variable. When the dorsal medulla is infarcted, the lesion is almost always accompanied by cerebellar infarction.[226] Since the lesion extends dorsally to the olive, the older terminology referred to the lesion as the "retro-olivary" syndrome.[423] The zone of infarction usually extends 7 to 10 mm in a rostrocaudal dimension, occurring most commonly in the middle part of the olive but frequently extending into its upper or lower third.[183] In 9 of 24 lateral medullary infarcts studied by Hauw and colleagues,[226] the lesion extended to the pontomedullary junction. As with

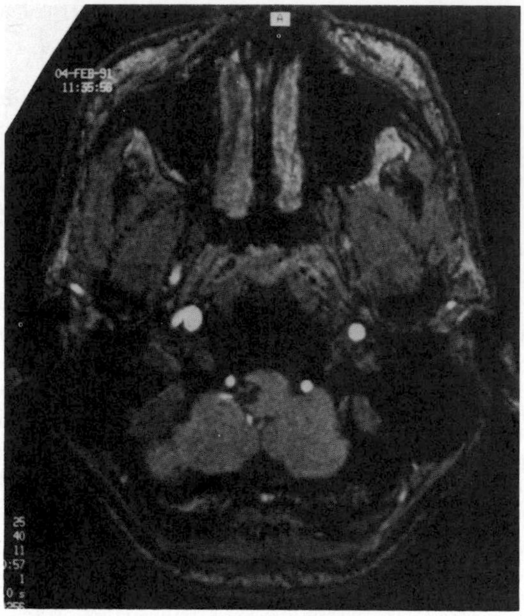

**Fig. 18-7.** T1-weighted magnetic resonance showing lateral medullary infarct sparing the cerebellum.

thrombosis elsewhere, transient attacks frequently precede the stroke by days or weeks, more rarely months, and are noted in about half the patients with lateral medullary infarction.

### *Symptoms*

The symptoms are explained by the distinctive anatomy of the lesion (Fig. 18-8).

**Vertigo.** The most common symptom is dizziness or vertigo, often accompanied by staggering and double vision. Difficulty in focusing and numbness of the face are other common components of the transient attacks. Headache, especially in the occipital region, may accompany other symptoms or may occur alone. The deficit may develop suddenly, but more commonly it progresses gradually or stepwise over 24 to 48 hours. Fluctuations or stepwise deterioration frequently characterizes the first week after the stroke onset, but is less common thereafter, and is distinctly unusual after 2 weeks.

**Headache.** Moderate or severe headache is common in lateral medullary infarction and is related to involvement of the descending spinal tract of the 5th cranial nerve and its nucleus, or to vascular distension produced by the occlusive process within the vertebral artery. In 1836 Bright[53] called attention to posterior headache in vascular disease. He described a "gentleman past the meridian of life" who had apoplectic attacks and complained, "I feel completely knocked up and have much pain in the back of the head, like a rheumatic pain, generally at the same spot the right side of the back part of the head." Bright commented, "This pain would itself chiefly direct our suspicions to disease of the vertebral arteries." Steady or, less commonly, pulsatile headache is located most often in the occipital region and is unilateral in about half of cases.[163] Aching headache is usually centered just below the external occipital protuberance and extends into the suboccipital and nuchal regions, usually nearer the midline than the ear. Frequently it extends into the frontal region, and occasionally the headache may be dull and only frontal in location.

**Facial Pain.** Facial pain is more diagnostic and is a cardinal feature of the syndrome. Of 39 patients studied in one large series,[102] 27 had persisting (18 patients) or transient face pain ipsilateral to the lesion. Sharp, single stabs or jolts of pain are felt in the eye or face. Occasionally, these may occur in flurries like a machine gun. Sticking, burning, stinging, tingling, or numbness are other commonly used descriptive terms. The eye is the most commonly affected region, but the pain may be limited to the ear or isolated spots on the forehead or cheeks. Pain frequently affects the entire face, including the lips and inside the mouth, but is rarely if ever limited to the mandibular division of the trigeminal nerve. Unpleasant facial sensations, when present, usually appear at the very onset of the stroke and are often the first symptom perceived by the patient. The coexistent contralateral hemianalgesia of the body is seldom mentioned, but is usually evident to the patient only after pain or temperature testing. The striking contrast between the spontaneous sudden facial pain due to involvement, presumably, of the nucleus of the descending tract of the 5th cranial nerve and the lack of perception of the hemianalgesia related to ischemia of the spinothalamic tract has led Fisher[169] to postulate that dysfunction of sensory neurons (either within the dorsal root ganglia or buried within the central nervous system, as in the nucleus of the tract of the 5th cranial nerve or in its main sensory nucleus) produces spontaneous pain, but lesions of white matter or nerves do not generally evoke pain as an early finding. Occasionally burning facial pain, likened by one patient to having salt and pepper thrown on the face, may be seen transiently in tegmental ischemia other than in a lateral medullary location.[79] The presence of facial pain or dysesthetic feelings may not be mentioned spontaneously by the patient because of their bizarre or unusual nature. Since these are so diagnostic of brain stem involvement, their presence should be diligently sought when the patient is questioned.

**Feelings of Disequilibrium.** Vertigo or other feelings of disequilibrium are nearly always present. Though frank whirling or rotational turning may be described, feelings of swaying, falling, feeling "seasick" or "being off balance" are the most common terms

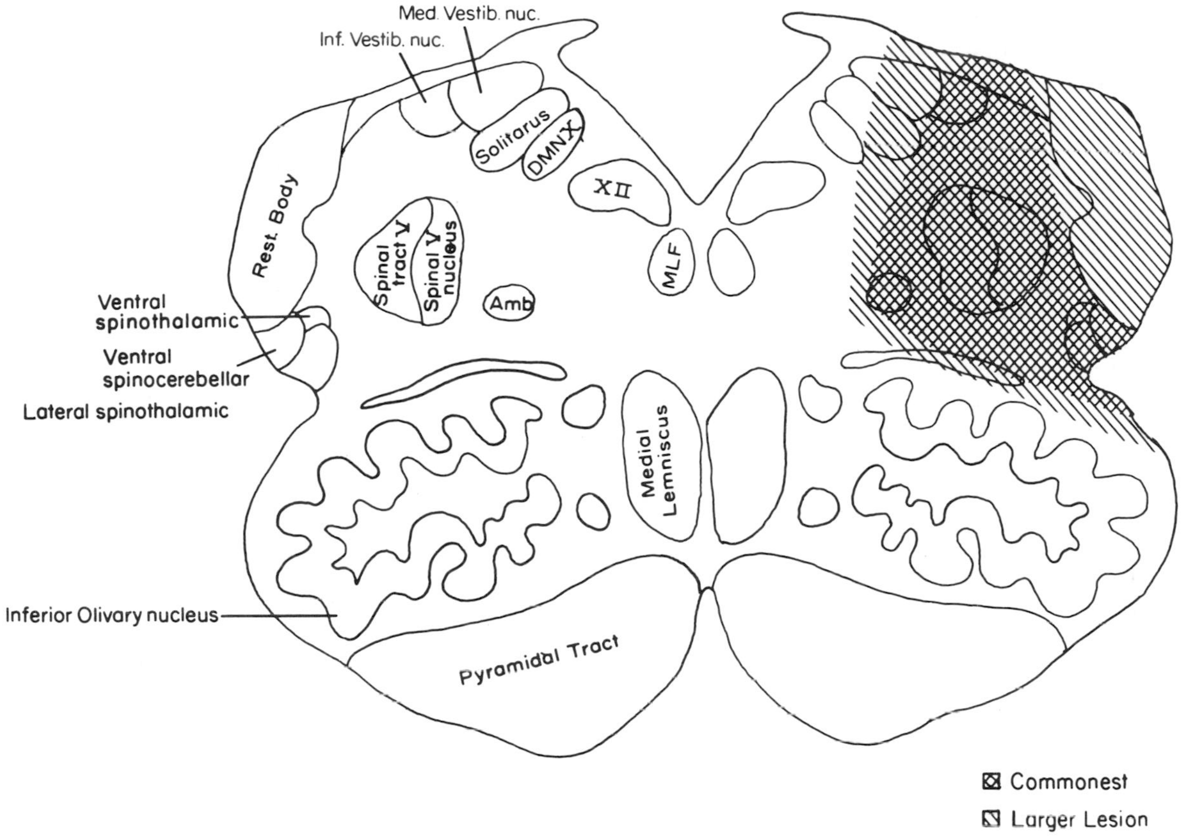


**Fig. 18-8.** Lateral medullary infarction. The most common involvement and largest extent of the lesion are designated by checkerboard markings as described in the key. (Based on figure in Currier et al.,[102] with permission.)

used. These perceptions are probably due to involvement of the vestibular nuclei or their connections. Alteration of vision is another frequent complaint and may even be described as diplopia (18 of 39 cases)[102] or, less commonly, as the illusion of objects oscillating or moving. The visual deficit is not monocular, and decreased visual acuity, visual field defects, or extraocular muscle palsies are not found to explain the visual symptoms. In the patient complaining or altered vision, the most common neuro-ophthalmologic finding is nystagmus; the visual complaints are probably due to sudden alteration in the vestibulo-ocular system. Occasionally patients with lateral medullary infarction complain of tilting of the visual world with a 90- to 180-degree inversion of the visual images.[135] Even with persisting nystagmus, the patient's visual symptoms are usually transient, indicating the nervous system's compensatory ability to adapt to chronic nystagmus and vestibular dysfunction.

**Nausea and Vomiting.** Nausea and vomiting are also common symptoms (18 of 35 patients in the series of Peterman and Siekert[381] and 27 of 39 patients in the series of Currier et al.[102]) and are due to vestibular dysfunction or to involvement of the dorsal tegmentum—"the vomiting centers" of Borison and Wang[48] in the floor of the 4th ventricle. Since the nucleus ambiguus is near "the vomiting centers," some authors[102] have argued that because signs of 9th and 10th cranial nerve dysfunction frequently occur in patients with vomiting, the floor of the 4th ventricle is incriminated as the site of origin of the vomiting. We have not seen a patient with nausea and vomiting without accompanying dizziness or nystagmus, and we wonder if vomiting is simply a reflection of disease of the vestibular nuclei and their connections.

**Ataxia.** Ataxia is the rule rather than the exception. Virtually no patient with documented lateral medullary infarction walks normally, and all patients complain of altered gait. Walking is usually characterized by veering to the side, leaning, or stumbling. The patient is also aware of the ipsilateral cerebellar dysfunction and describes the arm as clumsy, unreliable, or weak.

**Hiccups.** Hiccups (19 of 74 patients in the series of Currier et al.[102]) are a frequent complaint, usually developing some time after the onset. In most patients with hiccups, the lateral medullary infarct is typically complete and is usually not ventral or superficial. The origin of the hiccups is uncertain but could relate to dysfunction of "respiratory centers" or to involvement of 10th cranial nerve fibers.[102,304] Difficulty in swallowing is common (55 of 74 patients in the series of Currier et al.[102] and Peterman and Siekert[381]). Food or secretions may have unusually free influx into the air passages, a phenomenon unusual in patients with peripheral 9th and 10th cranial nerve involvement at the jugular foramen. Disturbances of the coordination of epiglottic closure and palatal and pharyngeal function may be more likely with a central lesion of the nucleus ambiguus. Food gets stuck in the piriform recess of the pharynx adjacent to the larynx; patients attempt to extricate the material by an unusual coughlike maneuver. This crowinglike cough is characteristic, and its presence in a stroke patient is virtually diagnostic of lateral medullary infarction. Hoarseness is also frequent, but may be absent in the ventral or more superficial lesions. Some patients with involvement of the spinothalamic tract mention numbness, burning, or perverted sensations in the contralateral limbs or trunk, but these most commonly occur later in the course, sometimes weeks or months after the stroke.[437] Ipsilateral stuffy nose, altered taste, and dysarthria are less common.

### *Signs*

The signs accompanying lateral medullary infarction have been extensively reviewed by others.[102,183,304,324,381,437] A review of the seven main signs follows.

**Diminished Sensation in the Ipsilateral Face.** Involvement of the descending tract of the 5th cranial nerve and its nucleus usually produces decreased pain and temperature sensation of the ipsilateral face. Almost invariably, the corneal reflex is lost or severely reduced. The forehead and rest of the ophthalmic division are more analgesic than the lower face. Pain and cold sensitivity are generally affected equally. At times, although single pinpricks feel less sharp and less discrete, there may be a dysesthetic quality, with spread and persistence of the perceived stimulus. When the ipsilateral face is severely analgesic, the lower border does not usually conform to the limits of the peripheral mandibular division of the 5th cranial nerve but can be portrayed as a gentle curve sloping downward and medially from the tragus to the mandible where the facial artery lies.[381] Touch may also be diminished[437] in the analgesic face. The facial sensory defect usually clears more quickly than that on the contralateral body, although usually the loss of corneal reflex persists.[437]

**Diminished Pain and Temperature Sensation on the Contralateral Body.** Ischemia of the lateral spinothalamic tract is responsible for diminished pain and temperature sensation on the contralateral body. As previously noted, patients infrequently report the contralateral hemianalgesia, but some described a "numbness" or cold feeling. The sensory loss may affect the entire hemicorpus, but often the cervical region is spared. At onset, a level of pain and temperature sensation may be delimited either near the nipple line or on the trunk or abdomen, in which case the arm frequently has normal sensibility. Pain and temperature should always be checked in the lower extremity; some examiners will retire their pin in order to abbreviate the examination when pain has been perceived normally in the arm. The fibers within the spinothalamic tract are laminated, with the sacral fibers most lateral and the arm more medial. The arm and upper neck and trunk are spared in more superficial lesions. When the lesion extends far medially, it may even involve the quintothalamic fibers, which have already crossed to joint the medial border of the spinothalamic tract, producing a complete contralateral hemianalgesia including the contralateral face. In patients with bilateral facial analgesia, the pin feels different on the two sides of the face, the loss being more severe ipsilaterally. Without very careful testing, the contralateral face could be passed as "normal" unless the pin sensibility here is compared to the normal ipsilateral arm or trunk. With time, the hemianalgesia frequently improves and a level may become apparent over the trunk.[314] Less often the analgesia clears both rostrally and caudally, leaving a band of altered sensibility on the trunk.[304] Although at onset the loss of pain and temperature sensibility tends to be homogeneous over affected areas, greater degrees of sensibility appear later, leaving patches of perverted sensation. The analgesia usually extends to the midline at onset, but the paramedian region of the body often clears more in the front than in the back.[437]

At times, the loss to pain and temperature can be entirely crossed, occurring in the face, arm, trunk, and leg contralateral to the infarct. The lesions that cause this "unilateral" pattern of sensory loss are located more medially and involve the crossing fibers in the ventral trigeminal thalamic tract and the fibers in the crossed lateral spinothalamic tract. At times, the discomfort is severe and is comparable to "thalamic pain," with which it probably shares a common mechanism. Rubbing of the involved part, the pressure of tight clothing, or excessive heat or cold may aggravate the discomfort. When pain makes a delayed appearance on the contralateral body, it generally persists and is relatively resistant to pharmacologic treatments.[437]

**Horner Syndrome.** Sympathetic nervous system fibers course through the lateral reticular substance and are involved in most cases of lateral medullary infarction (25 of 35 patients in the series of Pierrot-Deseilligny et al.[382]) resulting in the Horner syndrome ipsilaterally. Usually the Horner syndrome is incomplete; ptosis is the most common element and leads to drooping of the upper eyelid and some elevation of the lower lid, narrowing the palpebral fissure. Miosis is also very common, the pupil usually retaining its reactivity to light. Anhydrosis is the least common element of the Horner syndrome in lateral medullary infarction.

**Ataxia.** Gait and limb ataxia are very important signs of lateral stem infarction and are due to ischemia of the restiform body, or the spinocerebellar tract which will later join the restiform body, or to infarction of the inferior cerebellum, which is also supplied by the PICA. The gait ataxia seen in the lateral medullary syndrome is different from that seen with the vermal degeneration of alcoholism. Leaning, veering, falling, or toppling to the side when the patient is placed in an erect or sitting position is characteristic of medullary infarction and can be contrasted to the wide-based gait with truncal titubation of vermal lesions. The ipsilateral limbs are often called "weak" by the patient, but on examination striking rebound and finger to nose ataxia are found. The most sensitive test to elicit the cerebellar limb abnormality is to have the patient quickly lift or drop his arms and brake them suddenly: the affected limb will overshoot. When the cerebellum is infarcted, a posterior fossa pressure cone can develop and may lead to a fatal outcome unless medical or surgical decompression is instituted. The presence of cerebellar infarction thus alters the management and prognosis. How can one clinically distinguish involvement of the cerebellum from involvement of the inferior cerebellar components? No study has definitely settled this point. Head tilt, decreased alertness, prominent occipital headache, and a tendency to hold the head stiffly, resisting passive or active movement, probably indicate involvement of the cerebellum itself. A radiolucent region within the cerebellum on CT scan is also very helpful. We encountered two patients with extensive cerebellar softening accompanying lateral medullary infarction, in whom the initial CT scan, taken within the first 48 hours of stroke, appeared normal. Days later, when the patients worsened clinically, a large region of radiolucency in the cerebellum appeared on their CT scans. One of the patients recovered after surgical decompression and the other patient succumbed. (The serial CT scans of one of these patients is shown in Fig. 18-9.) Therefore a normal CT scan at the onset of a stroke does not eliminate the possibility of a serious cerebellar infarct. The ataxia of the usual patient with lateral medullary infarction has a tendency to clear remarkably, leaving only minor clumsiness. It is usually safe to reassure the patients that they will be back on their feet within 3 to 6 months.

**Nystagmus.** The vestibular nuclei and their connections are affected in the lateral tegmentum and very frequently lead to nystagmus. The nystagmus is horizontal and frequently rotatory;[102,183] the quick component of the rotation usually moves the upper border of the iris toward the side of the lesion.[102] Vertical nystagmus is seldom if ever seen with ischemic lesions in the lateral medulla.[183] The eyes frequently drift away

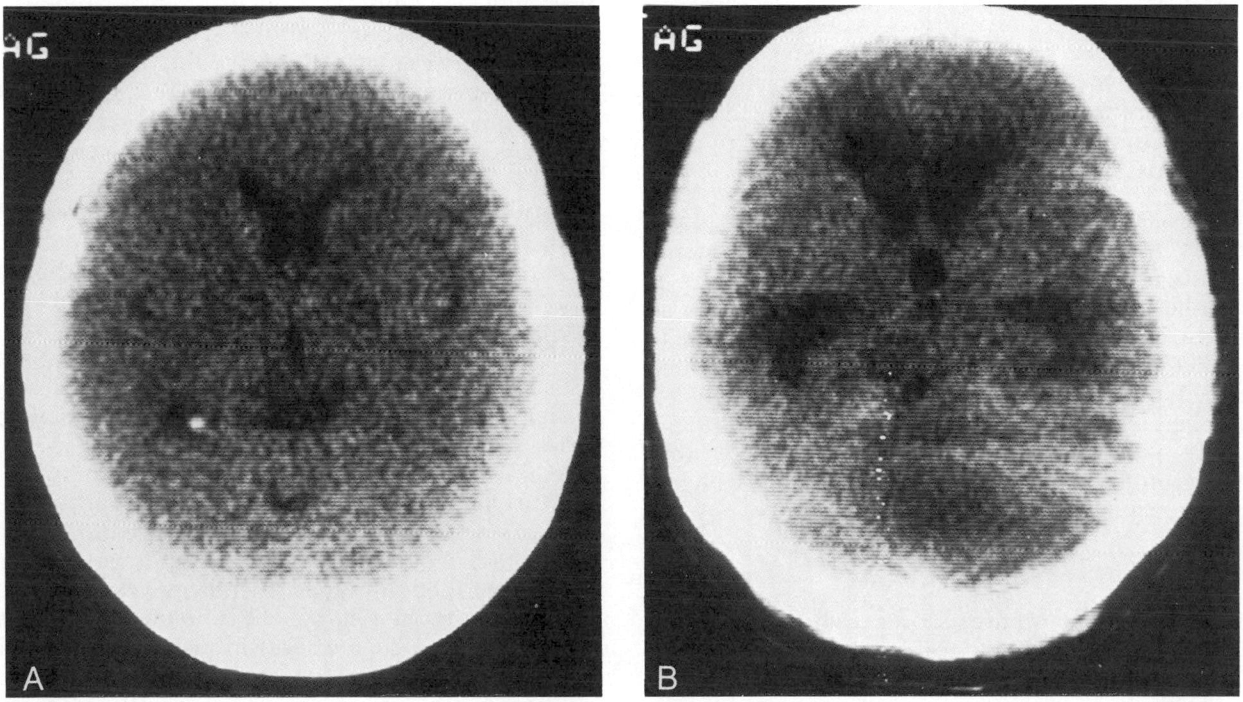


**Fig. 18-9.** Cerebellar infarct computed tomography scans. (**A**) Day 1: no definite lesion seen. (**B**) Day 3: large right cerebellar hypodense lesion, nonvisualization of the 4th ventricle, and hydrocephalus.

from the side of the lesion; small-amplitude, quick nystagmus is present on voluntary gaze to the contralateral side, and coarser, larger-amplitude, but slower nystagmus is present on ipsilateral gaze. In some cases, this pattern is reversed, with coarser horizontal nystagmus to the opposite side. The directional preponderance of nystagmus probably depends on the rostrocaudal location of the lesion.[344] The nystagmus may be torsional as it was in three patients reported by Morrow and Sharp.[344] These patients had skew deviation with hypotropia on the side of the infarct. The torsional nystagmus beats away from the lesion side in all patients but in one the nystagmus changed direction as the eyes drifted about a neutral position of torsion: most often lateral gaze is characterized by hypermetric saccades to the side of the lesion and hypometric saccades to the opposite side.[136] At times the eyes are forcibly deviated to the side of the lesion, so-called lateropulsion.[40,277,329] Reflex and voluntary eye movements are full but at rest the eyes may be deviated far to the side closely mimicking conjugate eye deviation from a hemispheric lesion. Skewing and slight dysconjugacy (the abducting eye lagging on gaze to the ipsilateral side) may explain the patient's complaints of diplopia. Diplopia is relieved in some patients by tilting the head to the side of the lesion.[136]

**Paralysis of the Ipsilateral Vocal Cord and Weakness of the Ipsilateral Palate.** Involvement of the nucleus ambiguus is responsible for paralysis of the ipsilateral vocal cord and weakness of the ipsilateral palate. These signs are frequently absent in more superficial lesions that do not extend far medially. The patient's ability to swallow usually improves despite persistent documentation of pharyngeal and palatal weakness. Unexplained tachycardia has accompanied lateral medullary infarction and could be due to involvement of vagal fibers arising from the dorsal motor nucleus of the vagus.

**Slight Weakness of the Ipsilateral Face.** Although it is a common occurrence, a slight weakness of the ipsilateral face is difficult to explain, since the lesion is below the facial nucleus. Dejerine commented on an aberrant corticobulbar tract that coursed dorsal to the other corticospinal and corticobulbar fibers and looped a bit caudally before traveling rostrally toward the facial nucleus. Involvement of this bundle or, more likely, affection of descending extrapyramidal fibers might explain the facial weakness, which is generally transient and minor in degree.

### *Prognosis*

Contralateral hemiparesis or a Babinski sign are not components of the lateral medullary syndrome; their presence indicates a wider zone of ischemia and possibly a more serious prognosis. In the patient with a pure lateral medullary syndrome, the prognosis is usually quite good.[103] However, death may ensue from cerebellar infarction with development of a posterior fossa pressure cone. Some patients with lateral medullary infarction do die unexpectedly without an obvious explanation, that is, either cerebellar infarct or a more extensive occlusion or ischemia.[183]

Levin and Margolis[291] described a single patient with failure of automatic respiration (Ondine's curse) from a unilateral lateral medullary infarct. Others[118] have described altered automatic respiration in bilateral lateral medullary lesions, and one of us (LRC)[68] have examined two stroke patients with failure to initiate respirations: one had postmortem confirmation of a bilateral lateral medullary lesion, and the other patient had a lateral pontine infarct on one side and a lateral medullary infarct on the other. Khurana[272] described a patient with a fatal unilateral lateral medullary infarct with well-documented central hypoventilation, episodic hypotension and hypertension, and profound bradycardia. Bogousslavsky et al.[43] described in detail the clinical and autopsy findings in two patients with severe respiratory failure and unilateral lateral medullary infarcts that extended into the lower pons. The patient had a very severe central hypoventilation syndrome with loss of respiratory drive despite high $Paco_2$. Despite being fully conscious, no ventilatory response could be obtained at 62 mmHg $Paco_2$ during a $CO_2$ retention procedure similar to that used for assessment of brain death. Their second patient had periods of apnea during sleep consistent with Ondine's curse. Bogousslavsky and colleagues[43] posited that the hypoventilation was caused by involvement of the nucleus of the solitary tract, nucleus ambiguus, nucleus retroambiguus, nucleus reticularis parvocellularis, and nucleus reticularis gigantocellularis. Evidence that these structures are related to respiratory control and drive is cited. Might apneic periods, arrhythmia, and autonomic abnormalities[292] be more common than is usually recognized in patients with lateral medullary infarcts?

Patients with lateral medullary infarcts may worsen owing to extension of ischemia. Embolization of clot from the vertebral artery distally to the top of the basilar artery was observable on postmortem examination in 3 of 16 patients examined by Fisher et al.[183] Clot may also extend from the vertebral artery into the basilar artery, leading to more widespread ischemia. Embolization or clot extension occur early in the course (less than 7 days) and are very rare after 2 weeks. Prior compromise of the contralateral vertebral artery does affect the ultimate prognosis, but in patients with prior contralateral disease the early syndrome, in our experience, is usually not limited to the lateral medulla alone. Insufficient data are available to clarify the risk/benefit ratio of short-term heparin therapy (1 to 3 weeks) in preventing early clot extension or embolization. Surely long-term warfarin therapy is not indicated in patients with lateral medullary infarctions.

MRI often defines the location of lateral medullary

infarcts on transcranial images of the brain stem and is far superior to CT in sensitivity for detection of these lesions.[408]

## Cerebellar Infarction

Though cerebellar softening has long been recognized pathologically, the clinical picture and pathogenesis have only recently been clarified. In 1956 Fairburn and Oliver[138] and Lindgren[299] reported stuporous patients in whom diagnostic procedures (usually ventriculography) demonstrated hydrocephalus and posterior fossa mass lesions; the lesions were unexpectedly discovered to be large infarcts when surgically explored or studied at postmortem. In the 1960s McKissock et al.[317] and later Fisher and colleagues[186] described in detail the clinical findings of groups of patients with cerebellar hemorrhage. To the surprise of most of the neurologic community, the classic "cerebellar signs" described and analyzed by Holmes[244,245] in patients with bullet wounds of the cerebellum and well known in cerebellar system degenerations were not prominent; instead, the cardinal features were vomiting, inability to walk, and stupor. In 1970, prior to the widespread use of CT scanning, Lehrich et al.[289] described three patients whose clinical and radiographic features were compatible with cerebellar hemorrhage, but at surgical decompression the lesions were discovered to be infarctions. (These same patients were also seen by one of us (JPM), who can vouch for the difficulty Lehrich and his coworkers faced in attempting to make differential diagnosis.) Lehrich's group emphasized the difficulty in distinguishing hemorrhage from infarction but were able to do so in their fourth case by arteriography, which documented occlusive disease with retrograde filling of the basilar system after carotid injection.

Subsequent studies have clarified the underlying vascular cause[127,455] and CT findings.[414,417] Sypert and Alvord[455] analyzed the postmortem findings in 28 patients dying with large acute cerebellar infarcts. In all but two cases the infarct was in the posterior-inferior portion of the cerebellum (bilaterally in three). The most frequent vascular cause was occlusion of the vertebral artery (unilateral in 17 and bilateral in 1). Occlusion of the PICA was found in 10 cases. In addition, a separate group of four postmortem specimens harboring old, healed large cerebellar infarcts was also analyzed; in 18 cases the infarcts were in territory supplied by the PICA, and past occlusion of the vertebral artery was found in 11. Associated lateral-medullary infarction occurred in three cases.

Others[125,289] have confirmed the preponderance of PICA territory lesions. Emboli from valve prostheses or atrial fibrillation were responsible in two of three patients of Duncan et al.,[125] and six patients in Sypert and Alvord's series[455] had embolic occlusion of the vertebral artery (three due to recent myocardial infarction, three due to atrial fibrillation). Amarenco and colleagues[14] studied the distribution and underlying vascular lesions in 28 patients in whom PICA territory cerebellar infarcts were found at necropsy. All of their cases had a benign outcome and many of the infarcts were found incidentally at autopsy: 15 infarcts were limited to PICA territory of the cerebellum, while 13 had additional AICA or SCA territory infarction; 9 patients had cerebellar infarction limited to the medial branch, 5 of whom also had dorsal and lateral medullary infarcts. Infarction limited to the lateral territory of the PICA was never associated with lateral medullary infarction, corroborating the view that the lateral branch of the PICA does not supply the medulla.[10] Instead the lateral medulla is fed by short circumferential arteries arising from the vertebral artery directly. An arterial occlusion was found at necropsy in 20 of these 28 patients:[14] in 13 patients the occlusion involved the distal intracranial portion of the vertebral artery, in 6 patients the occlusion involved the PICA, and in 1 patient the occlusion was in the basilar artery which gave off the PICA. The vascular occlusion was judged to have been an in situ thrombosis engrafted on preexisting atherosclerotic stenosis in 12 of the 20 occlusions (60 percent). The occlusive lesion was considered embolic in 7 of the 20 thrombi (35 percent), and 1 lesion was due to a post-angiography dissecting vertebral artery aneurysm. Among the 8 patients without occlusion at necropsy, 6 had emboligenic cardiac lesions. In total then, the mechanism of infarction was probably embolic in 13 of the 28 cases (46 percent). Combining these series, the most common vascular lesion is occlusion of the intracranial vertebral artery (approximately two-thirds of patients); thrombotic and embolic occlusions are nearly equally represented.

Some of the variation may be accounted for by the anatomy. The origin and supply territory of the PICA is very variable. Most often the PICAs originate from each vertebral artery within 2 cm of the basilar artery origin. In about 7 percent of patients the vertebral artery "ends in PICA," and the distal intracranial vertebral segment is hypoplastic. A common trunk can sometimes supply both traditional PICA and AICA territories. The PICA divides into a medial branch that usually supplies a portion of the dorsal medulla and the vermis, uvula, nodulus, and tonsil, and sometimes the pyramid and clivus, and a lateral branch that supplies the posterior portion of the cerebellar hemisphere on the undersurface of the cerebellum and sometimes the cerebellar tonsil.

There are three different clinical patterns of signs and symptoms in patients with PICA territory cerebellar infarcts. There are: (1) infarction in the medial branch territory affecting mostly the vermis and vestibulocerebellum; (2) infarcts in the lateral cerebellar hemispheres in the supply of the lateral PICA branch; and (3) combined dorsal and lateral medullary and cerebellar infarction. When infarction includes both the medulla and cerebellum, the pathogenesis is either occlusion of the intracranial vertebral artery with compromise of both short circumferential lateral medullary branches and the PICA, or occlusion of the medial PICA branch supplying dorsal medulla and the vermis.[14] Combined lateral medullary-cerebellar infarction occurred in only 5 of the 28 patients in the Sypert and Alvord series, and 5 of the 28 patients in the Amarenco and colleagues series. Infarction in the vermis and territory of the medial PICA branch produces a predominantly vestibular syndrome. The flocculus, nodulus, and uvula all have important connections with the vestibular nuclei. Vertigo, often with spinning, is usually increased by head movement. There may be feelings of being pulled or propelled to the side of the lesion and the gait is usually ataxic. Initially, the eyes may be deviated to the side of the lesion.[382] Nystagmus is often prominent with larger amplitude oscillations to the side of the lesion. Foveal smooth pursuit and opticokinetic nystagmus is often abnormal in all directions of gaze. Recovery is usually good but dizziness may persist. Often these patients with medial infarcts have been misdiagnosed as having labyrinthine or peripheral vestibular disease, but pure vestibular presentations of cerebellar infarction are becoming more widely recognized.[13,125,212,410,413]

Small lateral cerebellar infarcts present with unilateral clumsiness and limb and gait ataxia. Promonitory transient spells of dizziness or vertigo, ataxia, or blurred vision sometimes precede the cerebellar softening, as is true of other syndromes related to vertebral artery occlusion. The most common symptom at onset is an inability to stand or walk or a sudden fall. Vomiting, dizziness, and dysarthria are also very common. In some cases the patient is found in a stuporous state and cannot clearly describe the onset and progression. In most cases, there is then a period of 6 to 12 hours of stable findings, but in fatal cases a progressive decline transpires between 12 hours and 6 days.[455] In some patients, there is a more progressive but subacute course in which days or weeks of headache and dizziness are followed by the gradual onset of ataxia and mental clouding, the course simulating a posterior fossa tumor.[299] The pupils are generally small but reactive, and the pupil ipilateral to the cerebellar lesion may be smaller. Dysarthria and gait ataxia are common findings, but limb dysmetria and ataxia are more variable and more often than not are absent or not testable. The key diagnostic findings involve the oculomotor system. The eyes may be conjugately deviated to the contralateral side with course nystagmus or a gaze paresis to the side of the infarct. The gaze defect is frequently dysconjugate, with more severe weakness of the abducting eye; at times, a frank ipsilateral 6th cranial nerve paralysis is found. In larger infarctions, there is drowsiness, confusion, and decreased spontaneity of activity and verbal communication. The occiput may be tilted to the side of the infarct, and frequently patients resist head movement, which leads to a "stiff neck" appearance. Lateralized motor or sensory findings are unusual, although bilateral hyperreflexia is frequent. At times the swollen cerebellum presses on nerve structures within the cerebellopontine angle, giving rise to a reduced ipsilateral corneal reflex and ipsilateral facial nerve paralysis. Papilledema has also been noted, albeit rarely.[455] Larger cerebellar infarcts (at least one-third of a cerebellar hemisphere) produce a progressive syndrome by gradually enlarging to produce mass effects. Once significant swelling develops, it seems as if a vicious cycle is begun in which edema becomes self-perpetuating. The swollen cerebellar hemisphere compresses the 4th ventricle, leading to hydrocephalus.[209] The lower brain stem tegmentum is compressed directly, and the cerebellar tonsils are forced into the foramen magnum, thus sealing the inferior outlet of the posterior fossa. In addition, "upward transtentorial herniation" can develop with distortion of the midbrain and cerebral aqueduct and buckling of the quadrigeminal plate.[101] Pressure on the midbrain or 3rd cranial nerve is responsible for the ipsilateral dilated pupil late in the course of cerebellar infarction.

If taken within the first 48 hours, CT scan may not visualize the area of cerebellar infarction (see Fig. 18-9A); however, in large infarcts, compression of the fourth ventricle and hydrocephalus are apparent and give a clue to the location of the lesion.[418] Newer generation CT scanners and MRI usually provide accurate images of the size and location of the infarcts. The posteroinferior surface is hypodense on CT. The hypodensity often has a crescentic shape with more superior extension posteriorly. The anterior petrosal surface is spared because of its supply from AICA. On T2-weighted sagittal images, the characteristic shape and pattern of PICA territory infarction is usually evident.[414] Edema may surround the infarcts and compression of the 4th ventricle and brain stem can also be seen.

Arteriography may corroborate hydrocephalus and posterior fossa mass effect and may also document the occlusive lesion, which is usually within the vertebral artery. When a patient with vertebral artery occlusion and cerebellar infarction becomes stuporous, the usual differential consideration is the swelling of a cerebellar infarct with pressure cone or extension of the thrombosis and infarction to involve the bilateral brain stem. Since the treatments of the two situations are so different, clarification is important prior to active treatment. Angiography and CT may help make the distinction. Removal of the swollen cerebellum decompresses the posterior fossa and can be life-saving.[125,138,235,289,418,498] Furthermore, the deficit after nearly total cerebellar hemispherectomy may be negligible. "Medical" decompression using mannitol, corticosteroids, or glycerol helps reduce the swelling while the patient is being prepared for surgery. In occasional cases, these agents might obviate the need for surgical decompression. Placement of a temporary or permanent ventricular shunt may also decompress the patient with hydrocephalus caused by a lesion impinging on the 4th ventricle.[418] Patients with smaller cerebellar infarcts recover nicely without aggressive therapy.

## Hemimedullary or Pontine Infarction (Elements of Medial and Lateral Ischemia)

The lateral medulla and inferior cerebellar hemispheres are the most frequent sites of infarction in patients with occlusion of a single vertebral artery intracranially. The ischemia may extend more rostrally to affect the inferolateral pons[123,183] (pyramidal tract; 5th, 6th, and 7th cranial nerves; and motor dysfunction of the 5th cranial nerve). Also, the infarction may extend to the medial medulla as well as the lateral tegmentum;[123,183] this presumably was the mechanism of hemiparesis or Babinski sign in the Babinski-Nageotte syndrome,[25] which includes elements of the lateral medullary syndrome with a crossed hemiparesis or Babinski signal. Transient hemiparesis also occurs in vertebral occlusion, presumably due to decreased flow in the medial medullary branch or more rostral brain stem ischemia.

The hemiparesis is usually crossed, that is, contralateral to the infarct and on the same side as the body and limb pain and temperature loss. The anatomic bases for the hemiparesis is infarction of the medullary pyramid,[368] a region supplied usually by the anterior spinal artery, which originates from the distal vertebral artery.[135] Occasionally, the hemiparesis is ipsilateral to the infarct and on the side of the cerebellar signs and contralateral to the pain loss.[121] The anatomic explanation is infarction of the pyramid more caudally in the lower medulla and rostral spinal cord after the pyramidal decussation. This results from ischemia in anterior spinal artery supply more distally. Theoretically, a cruciate hemiplegia (one arm and opposite leg) could occur, but we know of no such documented cases.

## Embolization of Clot from a Region of Vertebral Occlusion

Fisher and colleagues[183] documented distal embolization in three of their patients with vertebral occlusion and the lateral medullary syndrome. In one patient, embolic material blocked both superior cerebellar arteries, and in the other two patients branches of the posterior cerebral arteries were blocked. McCusker and colleagues[315] described a patient with a locked-in syndrome likely due to an embolus to the basilar artery arising from a previously occluded vertebral artery. Fisher and Karnes[182] noted 18 examples of local artery to artery embolism within the posterior circulation, 5 in relation to a unilateral vertebral artery occlusion. Castaigne et al.[88] also described examples of artery to artery emboli within the posterior circulation, and Caplan[65] reported a patient (case 5) with spells of transient dizziness, who developed a stroke when embolic material originating in a unilateral vertebral occlusion embolized to the superior cerebellar artery. George and Laurian[198] described two patients with unilateral vertebral artery stenosis and subsequent angiographically verified occlusion, who suffered embolism arising from the diseased vertebral arteries. George and Laurian found that 80 percent of patients with a lateral medullary or cerebellar infarct and 65 percent of patients with "basilar trunk" territory infarcts had greater than 50 percent stenosis of a vertebral artery, leading the authors to suspect that the stenotic vertebral artery was a common source of embolism.

Koroshetz and Ropper[278] systematically studied patients with PCA territory strokes who also had brain stem symptoms. Six patients had occlusive lesions of the intracranial VA (combined with extracranial lesions in three patients), which the authors considered had served as the donor site for intra-arterial emboli to the posterior cerebral artery. Pessin et al.[378] reported a patient with a major basilar artery territory infarct in whom angiography showed occlusion of one intracranial VA and an intraluminal filling defect embolus in the distal basilar artery. Among a series of 85 patients with recent basilar artery thrombi who underwent acute thrombolytic treatment, 16 had stenotic or occlusive lesions of the intracranial vertebral arteries that likely served as a source of artery to artery emboli to the basilar artery. Figure 18-10 de-

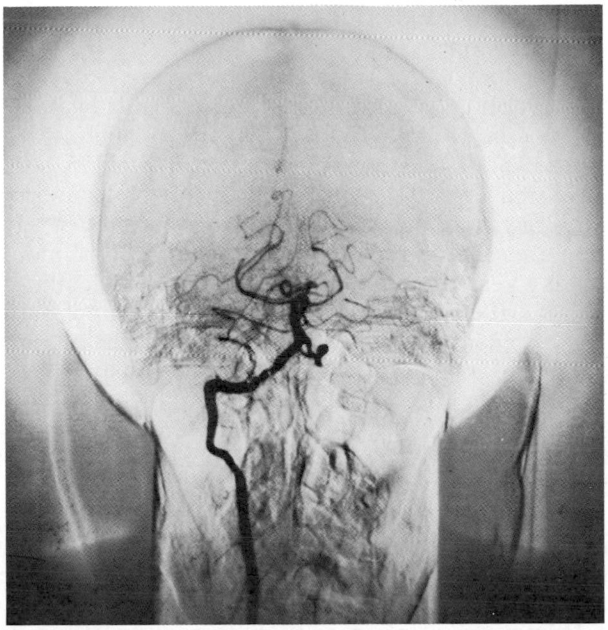

**Fig. 18-10.** Vertebral angiogram showing right vertebral artery intracranial occlusion. The top of the basilar artery and posterior cerebral arteries are not opacified, probably owing to embolus from the vertebral artery clot.

picts an example of vertebral artery intracranial occlusion with embolus to the distal basilar artery. In patients with distal basilar territory infarction, scant data are available concerning the incidence of coincidentally discovered vertebral occlusion that might have provided an embolic source. Within the anterior circulation, occlusion of the internal carotid artery is frequently heralded by a distal embolus.

## Transient Ischemic Attacks or No Deficit

As in the case of occlusive disease of other major vessels, some patients suffer an intracranial vertebral artery occlusion without permanent deficit. On some occasions, the occlusion may be totally silent or produce only occipital headache. The most common transient symptom is dizziness or vertigo. In a review of patients who subsequently developed a lateral medullary syndrome, dizziness accompanied other symptoms in 17 of 36 cases and was an unaccompanied symptom in 7 cases.[161] However, when vertigo was unaccompanied, if an infarct was to develop, it usually did so within 3 weeks. Chronic recurrent unaccompanied spells of vertigo (lasting longer than 6 weeks) are seldom if ever attributable to vertebral artery occlusion or other known vascular disease. Similarly, drop attacks (the patient, through awake, falls precipitously to the ground, but then arises without a deficit) are considered by some to be typical of vertebrobasilar occlusion. It is often forgotten that similar dropping may occur for a variety of heterogeneous nonvascular reasons; isolated drop spells in the absence of other symptoms of brain stem ischemia have seldom, in our experience, been due to vertebral artery occlusion.

Occlusion of the vertebral artery can be verified, angiographically, although attention must be paid to the specific radiologic features; the vertebral artery may be small, originate in an aberrant fashion, or end blindly in the PICA, producing a "physiologic occlusion" or, more simply, poor opacification.[461,464] Tatsumi and Shenkin[463] consider an irregular or "mouse-bitten" vertebral-artery termination and collateral filling of the basilar artery as reliable signs of pathologic occlusion. A smooth vertebral termination and faint basilar opacification are more consistent with "physiologic" nonfilling. Figure 18-11 depicts occlusion of the vertebral artery after the PICA branch, with filling of the superior cerebellar artery from PICA branches.

Transcranial Doppler (TCD) can now give accurate indications of stenotic and occlusive lesions in the intracranial VAs using insonation through a suboccipital foramen magnum window.[461,464] A recent study of TCD-angiographic correlation revealed excellent TCD results in patients with intracranial VA disease.[464] MR angiography also may allow accurate detection of these lesions, although looping of the vertebral artery may present technical problems for imaging. Surgeons are now beginning to operate on patients with lesions of the intracranial VA. Direct endarterectomy in this segment have been performed.[7,22,254] More often bypass procedures are constructed to supply the distal system, especially when there are bilateral occlusive intracranial VA lesions.[254] Angioplasty, using modern endovascular techniques is technically feasible, but as yet series of treated patients have not been reported.

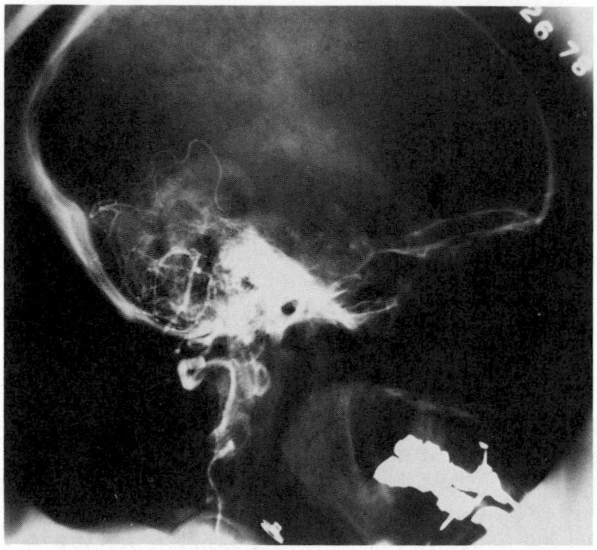

**Fig. 18-11.** Vertebral angiogram. The vertebral artery does not fill past the posterior inferior cerebellar artery branch, and superior cerebellar artery branches fill from the posterior inferior cerebellar artery.

## Bilateral Vertebral Artery Occlusion

Occlusion of the origins of the vertebral arteries even when bilateral, can be surprisingly well tolerated because of the potential plethora of available collateral vessels that may supply the more rostral cervical and intracranial vertebral arteries. Intracranial occlusion of both vertebral arteries, in contrast, is generally poorly tolerated by the patient and usually leads to severe cerebellar and brain stem infarction. Caplan[68] recently reviewed his experience with nine patients with bilateral distal vertebral artery occlusion. Most patients had known severe systemic vascular disease, especially hypertension, coronary artery disease, and diabetes mellitus. The neurologic deficit usually developed gradually. Four patients had discrete TIAs, and three had multiple TIAs. Six patients, including two with TIAs, had vague prodromal symptoms that included dizziness, blurred vision, ataxia, and headache; these warning symptoms did not have a discrete onset or end and so could not be easily classified as TIAs. The prodromal period was long and varied from 12 to 60 days (average 17.3 days) before the stroke. Only one of the nine patients developed a stroke without warnings. The fixed neurologic deficit usually began on awakening or while resting. All patients had prominent cerebellar dysfunction in the form of limb and gait ataxia. Limb weakness was severe in eight patients, six of whom became quadriplegic. Nystagmus, facial weakness, and bilateral miotic pupils were also common signs. Two patients had associated posterior cerebral artery hemispheral deficits, each a homonymous hemianopia accompanied by an amnestic defect in one. Fluctuation of the neurologic deficits was common early in the course, and some patients became suddenly worse when they sat or stood or when their blood pressure was lowered. All patients died. Only one patient survived for an extended period, and he was the only one in whom a successful surgical posterior circulation shunt had been created. He died 5 months after the surgery, but was quadriplegic and "locked in," and resided in a nursing home prior to his septic death. Anticoagulation was of no obvious benefit. In the six patients studied at postmortem, infarction decimated the medulla, pons, and cerebellar hemispheres, but tended to spare the upper pons and midbrain. Two patients had additional posterior cerebral artery territory infarcts.

Few examples of bilateral intracranial VA occlusion have been reported in clinical detail. Roski et al.[407] reviewed patients treated with occipital artery to PICA bypass and include six patients with bilateral intracranial vertebral artery occlusion. Three of these patients had only TIAs, one had a stroke, and two had both TIAs and stroke. Cerebellar, limb, and gait abnormalities were present in four patients, one had nystagmus, and one had a normal neurologic examination. After the shunt, two patients were considered normal or "asymptomatic," three were improved, and one was unchanged. None worsened later. These authors also treated five other patients with unilateral intracranial vertebral artery occlusion and contralateral severe vertebral artery stenosis with occipital artery to PICA shunts, intracranial vertebral artery occlusion who had many spells, often positional, of vertigo and alternating hemiparesis not responsive to heparin. An external carotid artery to posterior cerebral artery shunt was successful.

In contrast, Bogousslavsky et al.[42] followed 10 patients with bilateral intracranial VA occlusions and reported a more benign prognosis: 4 presented with TIAs only, 4 had nondevastating strokes, and only 2 had severe brain stem infarcts. During follow-up, no severe brain stem strokes occurred, and only one patient died of brain stem infarction. The onset of symptoms was more abrupt than in the series of Caplan.[68]

In patients with basilar artery occlusion the most severely damaged regions are the pontine bases bilaterally;[283] the lateral basis pontis, the tegmentum, and the cerebellum are relatively spared. The likely explanation for this distribution is found from analyzing the pattern of collateral circulation that develops when the basilar artery is occluded (Fig. 18-12). When the vertebral artery is patent, blood courses from the vertebral artery to the PICA and then to the cerebellar hemispheral AICA and superior cerebellar artery branches, ultimately nourishing the lateral brain stem and cerebellum. The pontine and midbrain tegmentum are supplied through the superior cerebellar artery.[38] In patients with bilateral vertebral artery occlusion, the PICA supply is usually compromised, leading to cerebellar infarction and poor collateral supply to the lower brain stem. Bilateral distal vertebral artery occlusion is rare. The full neurologic deficit in this condition develops over a longer period of time as compared to patients with basilar artery occlusion, branch disease, lacunes, or embolic infarction. The principal pathogenesis of posterior circulation ischemia in this condition is chronically reduced vertebrobasilar perfusion. Desmet and Brucher[117] described a patient with bilateral lateral medullary infarcts and reviewed the clinical and necropsy features of five other cases. Abnormal control of respiratory function may have led to death in these patients. All were considered asymptomatic or normal after surgical treatment. Of interest, 8 of these 12 patients had "orthostatic cerebral ischemia," that is, postural sensitivity of their neurologic signs. Hopkins et al.[248] also studied a single patient with recurrent rostral brain stem ischemia, often positional, who had bilateral intracranial vertebral artery occlusion. A superficial temporal artery to posterior cerebral artery shunt seemed to stop his ischemic attacks. Ausman and colleagues[21] describe a single patient with bilateral vertebral artery occlusion treated with a vertebral artery to PICA shunt using an interposed radial artery graft. This patient had intermittent left facial numbness, dysarthria, diplopia, limb and gait ataxia, and a lucent lesion on CT in the left brain stem and cerebellum. Aspirin and warfarin had not stopped the spells. After the surgical shunt, the patient had slight residual gait ataxia. Postural sensitivity was also a feature in this patient. Ausman et al.[19] described another patient with unilateral intracranial vertebral artery occlusion and contralateral vertebral artery stenosis, who had spells of diplopia, vertigo, and blindness nearly daily, which were not stopped by aspirin, dipyridamole, or heparin. An occipital artery to AICA anastomosis was performed with good results. Sundt et al.[450] described 14 patients treated with occipital to PICA bypass: 7 had bilateral vertebral artery occlusion, 3 had bilateral vertebral artery stenosis, and 3 had unilateral vertebral occlusion with contralateral stenosis. Cerebellar signs were prominent. In the patients with bilateral vertebral artery occlusion, four had an excellent result, two had good results, and one was improved. Sundt et al.[450] also emphasized that orthostatic ischemia was present in six of the seven patients with bilateral vertebral occlusion. Sundt and colleagues[450] later also described a single patient with bilateral anticoagulants, and the success of surgically

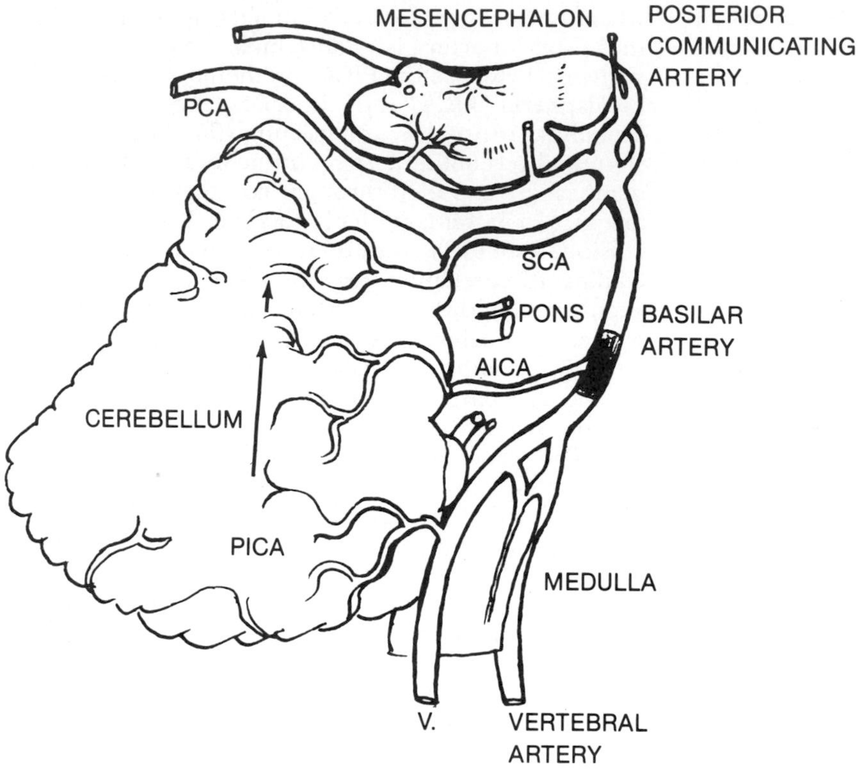


**Fig. 18-12.** Diagrammatic representation of oblique view of the base of the brain. The pattern of collaterals can be seen (*arrows*) when the basilar artery is segmentally occluded.

constructed artificial conduits to bring more blood flow to the posterior circulation provide strong evidence for a low-flow state.[19,21,407,448,450] As in unilateral vertebral artery occlusion, bilateral lateral medullary infarction can lead to sudden death, perhaps due to autonomic, cardiovascular, or respiratory mechanisms.

The prognosis of bilateral intracranial vertebral artery occlusion is variable. Some patients develop adequate collateral circulation and survive without major subsequent infarction.[42] In others, progressive ischemia develops, and the prognosis is grave.

## Basilar Branch Disease

This group is heterogeneous and includes all occlusive disease arising in small or larger branches of the vertebral or basilar arteries. Convenient subdivisions are (1) lacunar infarctions due to hypertensive disease, usually within the tiny penetrating parenchymatous vessels, (2) occlusion of small branches, such as median pontine or thalamogeniculate arteries, usually by miniature atheromatous plaques or junctional lesions,[170,179] and (3) stenosis or occlusion of larger circumferential branches, such as the PICA, AICA, and SCA by atherosclerosis.

### Lacunar Infarctions

Lacunes are the single most common lesion found in the brain stem at postmortem examination. These small deep infarcts are caused by disruption of vessels less than 200 μm in diameter by lipohyalinosis[159] or, less commonly, by blockage of arteries 0.1 to 1 mm in diameter by miniature atherosclerotic plaques. Precise clinicopathologic correlation has been infrequent, since the prognosis for recovery from the individual strokes is good, leaving less opportunity for pathologic confirmation. At postmortem, lacunes tend to be multiple, providing a dilemma as to which lacunes were responsible for which symptoms or signs. A lacunar infarct can vary from a tiny pinpoint hole to a larger cavitated lesion 1.5 cm in diameter. They are most common in the pons and thalamus, but do occur in the medulla and midbrain. In the medulla, pons, and midbrain they usually occupy the basal portion, especially medially, seldom extend far into the tegmentum, and are never limited solely to the tegmentum. Fisher's[176] intent in describing specific lacunar syndromes was to call attention to combinations of clinical findings that had an extremely high probability of being caused by lacunar infarctions; many lacunes, however, present a slight deficit impossible to distinguish from an incomplete stroke due to larger vessel disease or embolism. Several syndromes known to be caused by brain stem lacunes are reviewed in the following sections.

#### *Syndromes*

**Pure Motor Hemiplegia.** In this syndrome weakness of the face, arm, and leg is not accompanied by visual or sensory signs or deficits of higher cortical function. Of the nine original cases studied by Fisher,[158] three had lesions in the basis pontis. One of these patients also had a conjugate gaze paresis to the ipsilateral side, identifying the pontine locus of the stroke. Transient tegmental symptoms or signs (diplopia, dizziness, nystagmus, or internuclear ophthalmoplegia), prominent dysarthria, an ataxic quality to the movements of the hemiparetic side, and bilateral extensor plantar reflexes sometimes give a clue to the brain stem origin. To date, CT has not been effective in predictably verifying these lesions, although we have seen one patient with a past pure motor hemiparesis in whom months after the stroke a definite pontine lacune was seen on CT. A lacune in the medial medullary pyramid[243,368,406] or cerebral peduncle[242] also can produce a pure motor hemiparesis, usually with sparing of the face in medullary lesions.

**Dysarthria-Clumsy Hand Syndrome.** The cardinal features of this syndrome are moderate to severe dysarthria, corticobulbar weakness of the lower face and tongue, and slowness of fine movements of one hand. At times there is slight ataxia, hyperreflexia, or a Babinski sign on the side of the clumsy hand. The lesion is a small infarct in the dorsal basis pontis just below the medial lemniscus, which disrupts the corticobulbar fibers in this location.[160] The limb findings are due to dysfunction of extrapyramidal or pyramidal fibers within the basis pontis.

**Ataxic Hemiparesis.** This term describes a syndrome in which motor hemiparesis, usually of slight degree, occurs with incoordination of the cerebellar type.[171] Occasionally the pyramidal and cerebellar dysfunction is limited to the lower extremity; this variant is then called "homolateral ataxia and crural paresis."[180] The lesion responsible for ataxic hemiparesis is usually in the more rostral pons, interrupting crossing cerebellar fibers as well as the pyramidal fibers in the pontine base. We have also seen a patient with this syndrome whose postmortem lesion involved the brachium conjunctivum and cerebral peduncle at the midbrain level. Slight ataxia of the contralateral (normal) leg has been a clue to the pontine location of this syndrome. At times, horizontal or vertical nystagmus and dysarthria accompany the limb ataxia and hemiparesis.[171]

**Pure Sensory Stroke.** A lacune in the somatosensory nuclei of the thalamus and ventral posterolateral and ventral posteromedial nuclei produces sensory symptoms on the opposite side of the body and face without motor, cerebellar, or higher cortical function abnormalities.[157,175,176] Paresthesiae are usually characterized as tingling, prickling, or a sleepy, cold, hard, numb, or dead feeling. Usually at least two parts, face and arm or arm and leg, are involved.[175] The limbs are involved more than the face, but often the whole hemicorpus is affected, including the abdomen, chest, and face (including the eye, ear, and inside of the mouth). Cortical representation in the postcentral gyrus for the ear, eye, and trunk is quite small. Involvement of these structures usually means a lesion in a tract or a thalamic nucleus rather than in a parietal cortical lesion. When the hand is affected, usually all the digits are affected. The symptoms of sensory dysfunction usually far exceed the objective signs; in fact, objective parameters of sensory function may be completely normal. In one reported patient with a right lateral thalamic lacune, the sensory loss consisted only of proprioceptive loss with intact pain and temperature sensation.[411]

**Sensorimotor Stroke.** A lacune may involve both the thalamic sensory nuclei and the adjacent posterior limb of the internal capsule. This leads to a combination of hemiparesis, pyramidal signs, and hemisensory loss all on the contralateral side, unaccompanied by visual or intellectual dysfunction.[341] This syndrome is nearly impossible to differentiate from larger vessel ischemic disease or deep hemorrhage except by CT and angiography.

The tempo of lacunar infarctions in the posterior circulation has been similar to that of infarctions in a supratentorial location.[340] Transient ischemic attacks occur, but are less common than with larger vessel disease. The neurologic deficit usually develops over a period of hours to a few days and rarely evolves over more than 7 days. There is no accompanying headache. The patients generally remain alert. Hypertension, either in the past or present, is the nearly invariable requirement for the development of lacunes; the diagnosis should not be made in its absence. Other syndromes also occur, including pure dysarthria, toppling to the side whenever the erect position is attained, but an absence of symptoms and signs when the patient is examined supine or seated, and pure sensory stroke of just half the face and head. The pathologic basis for these lesions is unknown, but the ecology, tempo of onset, clinical course, and negative radiologic findings do suggest lacunar infarction as the most probable etiology.

## Occlusion of Penetrating Branch Arteries in Their Extraparenchymatous Course

Occlusion of medium-sized penetrating vessels is probably quite common, but the pathology within these vessels has only been verified in detail in three cases.[170,179] All of these patients were hypertensive and, in addition, two had known diabetes. Atheromatous branch disease is probably more common than is presently realized.[70] Diagnosis rests on a clinical syndrome limited to dysfunction in a unilateral branch and findings on CT or MRI of infarction in the territory of a single branch. The infarct may extend to the pontine basal surface, confirming that the occlusive process must have involved the branch before penetration of the parenchyma (Fig. 18-13). MR angiography or standard arterial opacification though catheters shows the patency of the parent basilar artery.

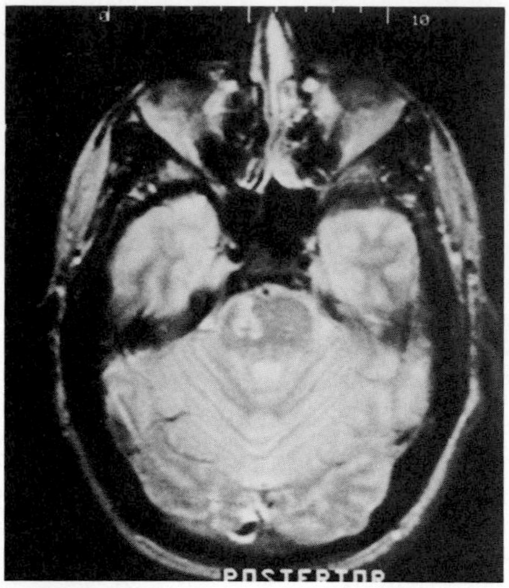


**Fig. 18-13.** T2-weighted magnetic resonance showing paramedian infarct, inferred as basilar branch occlusion.

### *Basilar Branch*

The two patients with unilateral basilar branch occlusion[179] had transient tegmental signs: ipsilateral small pupil in one patient, and lateral gaze palsy, internuclear ophthalmoplegia, and horizontal and vertical nystagmus in the other. The patient with bilateral branch occlusion,[70] was a hypertensive diabetic man who, 2 months previously, had a minor stroke characterized by right hemiparesis, dysarthria, and transient diplopia. This lesion was later traced to a bead of atheroma blocking a left pontine paramedian branch. He then developed dysarthria and a severe left hemiparesis. After his blood pressure was lowered precipitously and heparin was given, he became quadriplegic and lost all lateral gaze. Those caring for the patient (including the senior author) thought he had an occlusion of the main basilar artery with extensive pontine infarction. To everyone's surprise, the basilar artery was widely patent at postmortem and the vascular lesions were limited to two adjacent paramedian branches. There was an old infarct in the left pons and fresh infarctions superimposed in both the left and right paramedian zones of the pontine base. In this case, prior branch occlusion and rapid reduction in blood pressure led to a large zone of ischemia much wider than would be expected in disease of a single branch. The pathology of the branch lesions has been described in the section of this chapter dealing with pathology.

### *Thalamogeniculate Arteries*

A more common clinical syndrome is referable to the posterolateral thalamus in the distribution of one of the thalamogeniculate branches of the posterior cerebral arteries. The clinical findings were described by Dejerine and Roussy[110] in 1906 and include (1) paresthesia or numbness of the contralateral limbs and face, frequently without prominent objective loss, mimicking the situation in pure sensory stroke, (2) cerebellar-type dysmetria of the contralateral arm and leg, (3) dystonic posturing of the contralateral limbs, often with choreic or athetoid features, (4) contralateral transient hemiparesis, and (5) the delayed appearance of pain in the previously paresthetic side weeks or months after the stroke. Some patients also have slight dizziness, a smaller pupil ipsilateral to the lesion, slight horizontal nystagmus, and ipsilateral ptosis. The infarction involves the sensory nuclei (ventral posterior lateral and ventral posterior medial) and the ventral anterior and ventral lateral nuclei and their connection with the ansa lenticularis, brachium conjunctivum, and red nucleus. The posterior limb of the internal capsule can also be involved. This lesion commonly occurs in diabetics and has the same tempo as other examples of branch disease. A large lacunar infarction is sometimes visualized as a low attenuation zone in the lateral thalamus. The posterior cerebral artery has been patent when these patients were studied angiographically. To date, the elucidation of the vascular lesion underlying these infarcts is unknown, but it is presumed it is identical to that shown in other basilar branch cases.

### *Anterior Spinal Artery*

Another penetrating branch that is occasionally occluded is the anterior spinal artery. Each vertebral artery usually gives rise to a small paramedian anterior spinal branch, which join to form the anterior spinal artery. Unilateral occlusion of the anterior spinal branch can give rise to a paramedian medullary infarction involving the pyramid, medial lemniscus, and occasionally the hypoglossal nerve or nucleus. Though the supply of the anterior spinal branch is well known, and lesions are frequently postulated, documented occlusion of these vessels is extremely rare. Davison[106] reported one patient with infarction of the right pyramid and medial lemniscus who had severe paralysis of the left arm and leg, with tingling in those limbs. Dementia prevented careful sensory observations. Thrombosis of an anterior spinal artery branch and "partial" occlusion of the right vertebral artery were found at postmortem. Another patient had bilateral but asymmetric signs of damage to the medullary pyramid and medial lemniscus, with bilateral vibration and position sense loss and a unilateral brachiocrural hemiplegia with hyperreflexia and Babinski sign on the other side. Occlusion of the anterior spinal artery after its fusion was verified. Ropper et al.[406] described a medullary infarct in the distribution of the anterior spinal artery that had been associated with paralysis of the arm and leg and subjective tingling. Unfortunately, the responsible occlusive lesion could not be identified. Ho and Meyer[243] reviewed the clinical findings in 15 reported cases of medial medullary syndrome. Hypertension was common. Necropsy usually revealed lacunar infarctions affecting the pyramid and medial lemniscus; the responsible vascular lesions were usually not identified. In a postmortem analysis of medullary infarcts, 7 of 10 medial infarcts were due to occlusion of the distal intracranial vertebral artery blocking the anterior spinal artery branch.[135]

Embolic occlusion of the anterior spinal artery territory may be more common than is presently recognized. Kase et al.[264] described a 23-year-old woman with sudden onset of fibrocartilaginous disc material embolization to the anterior spinal artery branches of the vertebral arteries, causing bilateral medial medullary and rostral cord infarction. Of interest, despite the fact that the most rostral level of infarction was below the pontomedullary junction, the patient had bilateral facial weakness, vertical nystagmus, and ocular bobbing, in addition to a flaccid quadriplegia. Mitzutani and colleagues[336] also described foreign body emboli in each anterior spinal branch of the vertebral arteries; their patient had introduced foreign material into the circulation by intravenous injection of drugs designed for oral use. Nearly one-half of all reported examples of medial medullary infarction are bilateral;[243] usually the lesions occur simultaneously, but may rarely develop on separate occasions.[176,470] Emboli reaching a single anterior spinal artery may flow into the point of junction of both anterior spinal arteries, or emboli reaching the vertebral artery junction might preferentially pass into the anterior spinal artery orifices nearby.

## Occlusion of Large Circumferential Branches: Posterior Inferior, Anterior Inferior, and Superior Cerebellar Arteries

The most common mechanism of occlusion of the PICA, AICA, and SCA is by atheroma or clot in the parent vertebral or basilar arteries blocking the orifice of these branches. However, in some cases, atheroma or thrombosis is confined to these branches without major disease of the parent vessels.

### *Posterior Inferior Cerebellar Artery*

PICA occlusions occur and account for approximately 15 percent of examples of lateral medullary infarction. They do not differ clinically from occlusion of the vertebral artery or smaller lateral circumferential vessels, except for a much higher incidence of infarction of the cerebellum. These syndromes have been considered under vertebral artery occlusion.

### *Anterior Inferior Cerebellar Artery*

AICA occlusion has been documented even more infrequently than occlusion of the PICA. Atkinson[17] carefully studied by injection techniques the anatomy of the AICA. This vessel arises from the lateral aspect of the basilar artery at the junction of its lower and middle thirds, crosses the cerebellopontine angle and 8th cranial nerves, and gives off an internal auditory branch. The vessel then divides into a medial and lateral branch. The proximal stem of the AICA supplies the lateral pons, and the lateral branch supplies the brachium pontis and the caudal lateral pontine tegmentum. The AICA also supplies a variable part of the inferior cerebellum, depending upon its size in relationship to the ipsilateral PICA. The AICA also supplies the flocculus.[10]

AICA territory infarcts on CT usually involve the lateral pons and may extend laterally toward the cerebellopontine angle cistern.[414] Atkinson[17] described postmortem studies of seven patients in whom the AICA had been compromised during surgery for cerebellopontine angle tumors. Infarctions extended rostrocaudally from the lateral uppermost medulla (as low as a plane 3 mm above the olive) to as high as the midbrain at the lower limit of the red nucleus. The maximal area of infarction usually was at the midpontine level and extended from the lateral margin to near the midline. Unfortunately, most of the patients never awakened from surgery and so a clinical correlation could not be made. Some of the patients became acutely hypertensive, a phenomenon Atkinson related to ischemia of the central tegmental tract in the upper pons or midbrain because alterations of this region in animals can lead to blood pressure changes. So many other considerations applied to this group of surgical patients that this hypothesis must remain entirely speculative. Adams[3] reported a single patient with postmortem verification of occlusion of the AICA. A 48-year-old man became quite dizzy and noted tinnitus, nausea, and vomiting. The findings included the following: (1) right Horner syndrome, (2) right peripheral facial paralysis, (3) right ear deafness and decreased left auditory activity, (4) nystagmus greatest on left gaze, (5) loss of pain and temperature sensibility and to a lesser extent touch on the right face and decreased right corneal reflex, (6) cerebellar-type ataxia of the right arm and leg, and (7) decreased pain and temperature sense over the left neck and arm. As can be seen, the symptoms and signs are identical to those of lateral medullary infarction except for the involvement of the 7th and 8th cranial nerves instead of the 9th and 10th. The lesion involves the lateral and tegmental regions of the pons rostral to those affected by a comparable lateral medullary infarct.

Extensive cerebellar infarction is not as common with AICA occlusion. Adams[3] commented that infarction limited to the AICA territory had a more benign prognosis than involvement of the parent vessel. Goodhart and Davison[205] described one patient with AICA occlusion, but like other patients with this lesion, there were other extensive widespread areas of infarction throughout the neuraxis. Occlusion of the proximal AICA with compromise of its inconstant paramedian penetrating branches could theoretically cause a hemiplegia due to paramedian infarction.[56,376] Brouckaert et al.[56] found that 2 of 278 brains at necropsy harbored an infarct that they attributed to AICA ischemia. Their first patient had a pure motor hemiplegia with a patent AICA. The second patient had left Horner syndrome, decreased left corneal reflex, right hemiplegia, and right hemisensory loss due to a large paramedian pontine infarct. The basilar artery showed atherosclerosis with stenosis of the AICA origin by a plaque. A large combined paramedian and lateral pontine infarct could theoretically be caused by an isolated AICA occlusion, but we know of no published case proving this point. One of us (LRC) saw one patient who had a syndrome identical to that described by Adams.[3] This patient had a Novocain-like feeling in the ipsilateral face, ipsilateral deafness, diplopia, crossed sensory loss to pin and temperature, and ipsilateral cerebellar signs; angiography documented occlusion of the proximal AICA. Wallenberg,[479] who become famous for his description of lateral medullary infarction, also recorded the first verified case of AICA territory infarction,[17] but few cases have since been added.

In some patients, AICA territory infarction can be preceded by a syndrome of vertigo and tinnitus or unilateral deafness. Ischemia of the peripheral labyrinth or cochlear apparatus, or the 8th cranial nerve, is due to ischemia in the territory of the internal auditory artery, most often a branch of AICA. The offending vascular lesion in patients with AICA territory infarction has seldom been documented. When AICA territory cerebellar infarcts are accompanied by corticospinal tract infarction the vascular lesion usually involves the distal vertebral or basilar arteries.[13] In diabetics and others, microatheroma presumably involves the AICA origin, sometimes originating in a plaque in the main basilar artery.

### *Superior Cerebellar Artery*

SCA occlusion is of special interest. This artery is the most anatomically consistent of all the vertebral and basilar branches. It originates at the pontomesencephalic junction and circles the upper pons or midbrain, giving off medial and lateral branches.[221,500] In its course around the brain stem, short circumferential and penetrating vessels provide blood supply to the stem. Biemond[38] has attributed great importance to this vessel because of its extensive supply to the tegmentum of the midbrain and upper pons.

Occlusion of the SCA itself is unusual; most examples of SCA territory infarction are related to occlusion of the basilar apex, most often by emboli. In the index case described by Mills,[334] and later examined pathologically by Spiller, there was deafness, bilateral tremor, worse ipsilaterally, ipsilateral cerebellar ataxia, and contralateral loss of pain and temperature sensation. The superior aspect of the cerebellum and the midbrain tegmentum were infarcted. Davison and colleagues[107] described seven patients with involvement of the SCA, but there were detailed clinical notes for only one patient; a 51-year-old woman with subsequently proven lues developed right cerebellar signs, a left hemisensory loss, and a left gaze palsy. Luetic arteritis had led to occlusion of the SCA as well as extensive left middle cerebral artery territory infarction. The brain stem lesion involved the right brachium conjunctivum, right superior cerebellum, and the right lateral tegmentum of the rostral pons and midbrain. Freeman and Jaffe[193] described a single case in which the prominent clinical features were deafness, involuntary movements, and the Horner syndrome. However, this patient had subacute bacterial endocarditis with embolic occlusion that involved the midbrain and the thalamus bilaterally, and certainly was not an example of pure SCA occlusion. Luhan and Pollock[305] also described six cases, but, similarly, none was a verified example of isolated SCA occlusion (three were studied clinically, two had subacute bacterial endocarditis with multiple vascular lesions, and one had hemorrhage and no vascular occlusion). They considered ipsilateral cerebellar dysfunction and contralateral hemisensory loss of pain and temperature sensation as the cardinal features of SCA occlusion, and these were the criteria for choosing the clinical cases. Ipsilateral Horner syndrome, contralateral central facial weakness, and deafness, often contralateral, were also mentioned. These authors described involuntary ipsilateral adventitious movements or static tremor, but had no example of this among their own patients. Guillain et al.[210] described a single patient with necropsy-proven SCA territory infarction. Ipsilateral slow, involuntary movements of the arm, ipsilateral arm dysmetria, and contralateral loss of pain and temperature sensation were the principal findings. De Visser[119] studied a single patient with a necropsy-proven isolated SCA occlusion and an infarct in the right midbrain; clinical findings included a right third nerve palsy, ataxia, and a left hemiplegia.

Adams' review[3] of the findings in cases of SCA occlusion agrees with those of Luhan and Pollock,[305] Guillain et al.,[210] and Kase et al.[265] Because the lesion is above the spinal tract and the main sensory nucleus of the 5th cranial nerve, the ipsilateral facial pain and loss of facial sensitivity seen in the PICA and AICA territory lesions are not found; instead there is a contralateral hemisensory loss, usually affecting only pain and temperature sensation. In a more rostral lesion, loss of sensation could include touch and position sense because of involvement of the medial lemniscus after merger of the spinothalamic tract with proprioceptive fibers that course in the medial lemniscus in the pons. The mechanisms of the spontaneous abnormal ipsilateral arm movements and ipsilateral dysmetria are uncertain. Are these findings related to dysfunction of the superior aspect of the cerebellum or to lesion in the superior cerebellar peduncle? Since the decussation of the brachium conjunctivum usually falls within the boundaries of SCA supply, could the involuntary movements occasionally be contralateral or bilateral? Lateral tegmental hemorrhage within the same region is occasionally associated with bilateral dysmetria and delayed onset of a contralateral rest and action tremor despite the fact that the cerebellum is not involved.[78]

The "classic" clinical syndrome of SCA territory infarction is usually considered to include ipsilateral limb ataxia and the Horner syndrome, contralateral thermoanalgesia involving the face, arm, trunk, and leg, and a fourth cranial nerve palsy.[12,13] These patients all had ischemia in the brain stem supply of the SCA. A recent study by Amarenco and Hauw[12] shows a much wider range of clinical findings in patients with necropsy-proven SCA territory infarcts. These authors studied 33 patients with infarcts involving the SCA at necropsy. Isolated SCA territory infarction occurred in only 7 patients (21 percent), most of the remainder had infarction in other regions supplied by the distal basilar and posterior cerebral arteries. When the brain stem was spared the findings were limited to "cerebellar signs." At times, infarction was limited to medial branch territory (four patients) or lateral branch hemispheral supply (five patients). Infarcts restricted to the medial or lateral branches were accompanied by lateral pontine tegmental infarcts, as was also the case in the series by Kase et al.[265]

In the series of Amarenco and Hauw,[12] the predominant mechanism of SCA territory infarction was embolism either from a cardiac or proximal intra-arterial source. Amarenco and colleagues[13] also reviewed and summarized their experience at the Sâlpétrière hospital concerning the underlying arterial pathology and mechanisms in 88 patients with necropsy-studied cerebellar infarction. The extracranial and intracranial arteries were carefully dissected and examined in this group of patients.

The intracranial VA and basilar arteries were most often the seat of occlusion, but 12 patients had occlusions of the long circumferential cerebellar arteries (PICA, AICA, or SCA).[13] In 38 infarcts the artery leading to the infarct was patent, and 26 of the 38 patients (68 percent) had a cardiac source of embolism. In total, the authors considered that 35 percent of infarcts were caused by local atherosclerosis, 43 percent by cardiac origin emboli, and others by intra-arterial embolism from proximal sources.

A review of recorded cases in the literature and our own experience verifies the fact that documented examples of infarction due to occlusion of long circumferential branches (PICA, AICA, and SCA) are rather common. Infarction in paramedian branches due to lesions of small penetrating vessels is, in contrast, quite common. This experience runs exactly parallel to the situation in the anterior circulation. In the prearteriographic era the clinical diagnosis of middle cerebral artery and middle cerebral artery branch occlusion was routinely proposed. Careful clinical and radiologic and clinicopathologic study has led to the realization that occlusion of the anterior cerebral and middle cerebral arteries is unusual. More common are lacunae due to disease of penetrating vessels and ischemia related to disease of the larger, more proximal internal carotid artery. Ischemia in the carotid territory of superficial branch distribution is usually due to small emboli from the heart and proximal carotid artery, or to reduced distal flow secondary to proximal occlusion. Similarly, in the posterior circulation, lacunae and disease of larger vessels (vertebral and basilar arteries) are common; ischemia in the territory of lateral branch arteries is commonly related to emboli or disease of the parent vessels. The lateral circumferential cerebellar branches are the posterior circulation homologues of the middle cerebral artery in the anterior circulation. An exception to this might be the AICA; unilateral ischemia in the territory of this vessel alone is usually due to occlusion of the AICA, because basilar occlusion at this level produces more widespread findings. In contrast, PICA territory ischemia is more usually due to vertebral artery occlusion, and SCA territory ischemia is more often due to emboli or occlusive disease of the rostral basilar artery. Table 18-2 reviews the usual findings in long circumferential branch disease.

## Occlusion or Severe Stenosis of the Basilar Artery

Kubik and Adams,[281] in their landmark description of occlusion of the basilar artery, summarized the findings as follows:

> The onset is sudden and not preceded by tangible causal factors. The first symptom is usually headache, dizziness, confusion, or coma. Difficulty in speaking and unilateral paresthesiae occur in a large proportion of the cases. Common findings are pupillary abnormalities, disorders of ocular movement, facial palsy, hemiplegia and/or quadriplegia, and bilateral extensor plantar reflexes. Cranial nerve palsies and contralateral hemiplegia may be combined. . . . It is common for temporary improvement, lasting hours or days, to occur during the course of the illness. In the majority of cases death takes place in from two days to five weeks.

In an angiographic study Archer and Horenstein[15] also found severe deficits in 20 patients with angiographically confirmed basilar artery occlusion: 15 patients were stuporous or comatose and 2 were "locked in"; 15 patients died and the other 5 patients were left severely disabled. In contrast, Caplan[65] described four patients among six with verified basilar occlusion who survived the associated acute ischemic event with little (one patient) or no deficit (three patients).

**TABLE 18-2. Most Frequent Findings in Long Circumferential Branch Territory Infarcts**

| Artery | Anatomic Structure | Symptoms and Signs: Ipsilateral | Symptoms and Signs: Contralateral |
|---|---|---|---|
| PICA | Restiform body or cerebellum | Limb and gait ataxia | |
| | Vestibular nuclei | Dizziness and nystagmus | |
| | Descending tract and nucleus of V | Loss of facial pain and temperature sensation and corneal reflex | |
| | Spinothalamic tract | | Loss of pain and temperature sensation on the body |
| | Descending sympathetic system | Horner syndrome | |
| | Nucleus ambiguus | Hoarseness; dysphagia; paralysis of pharynx, palate, and vocal cord; hiccups | |
| | Solitary tract and nucleus | Loss of taste | |
| AICA | Brachium pontis or cerebellum | Limb and gait ataxia | |
| | Cranial nerve VII and nucleus | Facial paralysis | |
| | Cranial nerve VIII | Deafness | |
| | Spinothalamic tract | | Loss of pain and temperature sensation on the body |
| | Vestibular nuclei | Nystagmus and dizziness | |
| | Descending tract of cranial nerve V and sensory nucleus of cranial nerve V | Decreased pin and temperature sensation over the face and occasional decrease in touch | |
| | Descending sympathetic system | Horner syndrome | |
| SCA | Brachium conjunctivum or cerbellum | Limb and gait ataxia | Limb dysmetria (?) |
| | Descending sympathetic system | Horner syndrome | |
| | Dentate nucleus or brachium conjunctivum | Static tremor | |
| | Sensory lemniscus | Trochlear nerve palsy | Loss of pain and temperature sensation over the body and face, and loss of position sense in the limbs |
| | Lateral lemniscus | | Decreased hearing |

*Abbreviations*: PICA, posterior inferior cerebellar artery; AICA, anterior inferior cerebellar artery; SCA, superior cerebellar artery.

Others[16,152,331,346,387] have also noted examples of survival without crippling deficit after basilar artery occlusion, and, in fact, Kubik and Adams,[281] in their original paper, mention four patients with clinical findings identical to those with documented basilar occlusion who survived the stroke and were alive months later.

Basilar artery atheromatous disease has been recognized at the preocclusive stage of severe stenosis (Fig. 18-14). It is a relatively uncommon lesion compared to basilar artery occlusion. In the Joint Study of Extracranial Arterial Occlusion,[224] basilar artery stenosis was identified in 7.7 percent of 3,788 patients undergoing four-vessel angiography. In our own survey we identified nine patients with angiographically proven middle or distal segment basilar stenosis,[380] and in reviewing other angiographic and pathologic cases we found that occlusion affected all three basilar artery segments (proximal, middle, and distal) in relatively equal frequencies. TIAs were a common feature of the clinical presentation in patients with basilar artery stenosis, occurring in six of our nine cases. The TIAs usually preceded brain stem stroke, but in two patients they were the sole clinical manifestation. The TIA features included the brief duration of two or more of the following symptoms; dizziness, slurred speech, double vision, dysphagia, and unilateral or bilateral weakness. The TIAs occurred during a period of 1 day to 6 months before stroke. Stroke severity and infarct location varied, but the pons was a frequent locus of injury. The short-term prognosis was good; the majority of patients remained free of symptoms for periods of 1 month to 2 years, usually on anticoagulation or on antiplatelet treatment. Three patients died, one of the original stroke, another from a new basilar territory infarct, and one from unrelated causes.

It should now be quite obvious that there is no uniform syndrome or outcome applicable to all patients with basilar artery occlusion. Should this come as a surprise? The situation in the carotid artery is clearly comparable. Sometimes when the internal carotid artery is occluded, patients complain of amaurosis fugax followed by symptoms and signs of total ischemia of the anterior and middle cerebral artery branches of the internal carotid artery. Such patients are readily diagnosed. Other patients with internal carotid artery occlusion have transient or partial deficits, and diagnosis can only be made by laboratory confirmation, usually angiography. There is a wide spectrum of

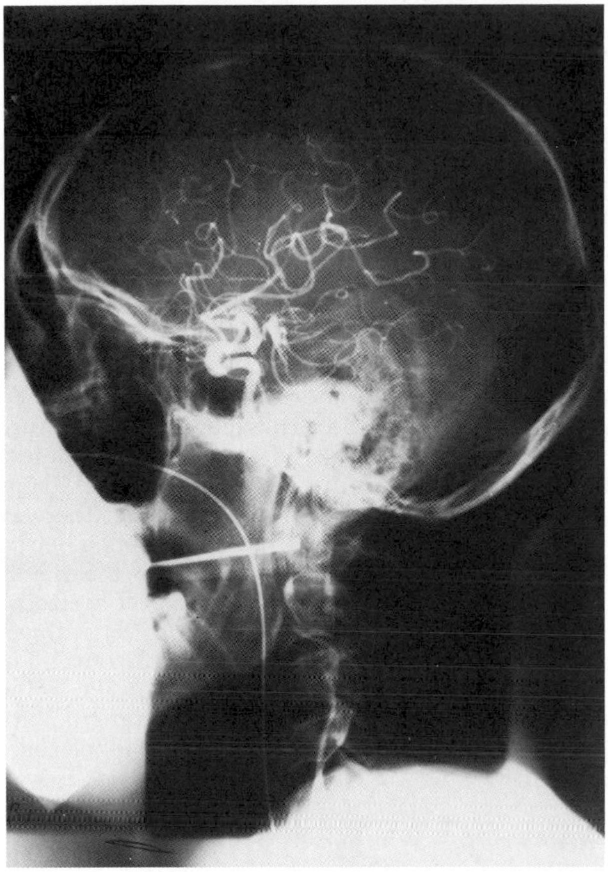

**Fig. 18-14.** Carotid arteriogram demonstrating retrograde filling of the basilar artery and the posterior cerebral and superior cerebellar arteries. Note the midbasilar occlusion.

symptomatology severity of signs, and outcome.[1] The situation in basilar artery occlusion is not very different. Since confirmation of basilar artery occlusion depends on angiography, at present, the frequency of this angiographic diagnosis will depend on the indications for angiography in a given institution. Archer and Horenstein[15] angiographically studied severely ill patients; Meyer and colleagues[328] excluded patients with severe brain stem infarction from angiography, but nevertheless identified two patients with unsuspected basilar artery occlusion. Prognosis depends upon the rate and extent of occlusion, presence of collateral circulation, systemic factors (see the section on pathophysiology), and possibly treatment.

Patients with documented severe stenotic lesions of the basilar artery or the intracranial vertebral arteries have a relatively poor prognosis for subsequent brain stem infarction or death.[350] In one series, the stroke rate for such patients was 17 times the expected rate for a matched normal population. Since there is no absolutely uniform syndrome of basilar artery occlusion, this discussion will describe common neurologic findings not previously commented on that occur with basilar artery occlusion, characterize the common patterns of infarction documented at postmortem, and discuss angiographic diagnosis and clinical tempo.

## Common Clinical Phenomena

### *Internuclear Ophthalmoplegia*

In the 1950s Cogan and colleagues[94,96,434] revised the nomenclature and described the usual findings of patients with internuclear ophthalmoplegia. Lutz had originally designated two types of internuclear ophthalmoplegia: "an anterior" type, in which the "internus" (i.e., medial rectus) is paralyzed for conjugate movements toward the side of the lesion but functions normally in convergence and the externus (i.e., lateral rectus) operates normally on lateral gaze, and a "posterior" type, in which both, internal recti function normally on convergence and lateral gaze movements but the "externus" on the side of the lesion is paralyzed for voluntary conjugate movements but can function on labyrinthine stimulation. Smith and Cogan[434] said that, Lutz's posterior internuclear ophthalmoplegia was merely a partial sixth cranial nerve palsy and these authors proposed a new designation, which is now in common usage. In their terminology, internuclear ophthalmoplegia always involved paralysis of the adducting eye; the posterior type, in their terminology, designates cases in which the medial rectus works normally during convergence, and the anterior type refers to absence of medial rectus function in either convergence or conjugate lateral gaze. In either type nystagmus of the abducting eye occurs, a phenomenon that had led others to designate internuclear ophthalmoplegia as "ataxic nystagmus,"[223] a term still in use in some regions. Furthermore, analysis of 58 cases (29 unilateral and 29 bilateral) led Smith and Cogan[434] to assert that bilateral internuclear ophthalmoplegia was "invariably indicative of multiple sclerosis" and unilateral internuclear ophthalmoplegia was most commonly vascular in etiology.

Christoff and colleagues,[93] among others, reviewed past examples of clinicopathologic correlation in patients with internuclear ophthalmoplegia and added three examples of their own; they implicated the ipsilateral medial longitudinal fasciculus (MLF) in the production of internuclear ophthalmoplegia. Damage to the right MLF would produce an absence of adduction of the right medial rectus on leftward gaze and abducting nystagmus of the left eye. Vertical nystagmus and skew deviation were frequent concomitant findings. More recently, Gonyea[204] described a number of patients with bilateral internuclear ophthalmoplegia due to vascular disease (only one had documented basilar artery occlusion) and reviewed past examples in the literature and, as a result, took exception to the dictum of Smith and Cogan[434] that bilateral involvement was invariably due to multiple sclerosis. In basilar artery occlusion with extensive pontine infarction, tegmental infarcts are frequently patchy and asymmetric so that unilateral internuclear ophthalmoplegia is more common than bilateral. Absence of associated convergence does not necessarily implicate the more rostral midbrain MLF, as Cogan[95,96] initially believed.

Though the eyes are generally conjugate at rest in patients with internuclear ophthalmoplegia, some patients have bilateral exotropia; this situation has been referred to as "wall-eyed bilateral internuclear ophthalmoplegia."[104] Outward deviation of the eyes has been used as evidence of medial rectus nuclear involvement, but Gonyea[204] and Cogan[95,96] emphasize that exotropia is to be anticipated with dysconjugate impairment of media rectus function at any level, including the MLF.

MRI studies of patients with internuclear ophthalmoplegia MLF and adjacent structures.[55] When intranuclear ophthalmoplegia was associated with loss of convergence or abnormality of abduction of the contralateral eye, the medial tegmental lesions were usually more extensive than when the only defect was an intranuclear ophthalmoplegia.

### *Conjugate Horizontal Gaze Palsy*

Fibers from the frontal eye fields affecting conjugate lateral gaze cross at or near the level of the abducens nucleus in the pons[100] and end in the reticular gray region in the neighborhood of the contralateral abducens nucleus. This region is usually referred to as the paramedian pontine reticular formation (PPRF), or by some as the pontine lateral gaze center. Damage to the abducens nucleus probably can produce an ipsilateral gaze palsy for all lateral eye movements, voluntary and reflex (caloric or vestibulo-ocular).[383]

MRI shows that in patients with a unilateral abduction weakness (6th cranial nerve palsy), the lesion invariably involves the intrapontine nerve fascicles and not the abducens nucleus.[54] Involvement of the PPRF leads to absence of voluntary lateral gaze to the side of the lesion with preservation of reflex movements.[383] The PPRF also mediates ipsilaterally directed saccades within the contralateral hemifield of movement. Bilateral lesions in the pontine tegmentum involving the abducens nucleus and PPRF produce paralysis of all horizontal eye movements, with sparing of vertical gaze, since this is mediated at a more rostral level. Halsey et al.[216] described a patient with subsequently documented basilar artery occlusion and infarction restricted to the basis pontis ventral to the PPRF who had an absence of voluntary lateral gaze. Voluntary vertical gaze was preserved and labyrinthine stimuli produced full conjugate lateral gaze except for absence of adduction of one eye (due to a more rostral MLF lesion). These authors postulate that the descending fibers for voluntary conjugate gaze travel with the corticobulbar and aberrant corticobulbar fibers in the base of the pons in the region of the medial lemniscus. The senior author saw one patient with pontine hemorrhage who was conscious but could not look voluntarily to either side; reflex lateral gaze could be readily evoked by the doll's eye maneuver. In unilateral lesions of the PPRF there is often some conjugate deviation of the eyes toward the contralateral size, but this is less than that usually found with supratentorial lesions.

MRI studies of patients with unilateral conjugate gaze palsy show lesions in the paramedian pons, including the abducens nucleus, the nucleus reticularis pontis oralis, and the lateral portion of the nucleus reticularis pontis caudate. These latter two structures are identified in animals as responsible for lateral gaze and contain burst neurons of the PPRF. In patients with bilateral horizontal gaze palsies there are usually bilateral medial pontine lesions, but some patients have unilateral lesions that include the pontine tegmental raphe.[54] Patients with bilateral horizontal gaze palsies often also have slowness of vertical gaze saccades or limitation of up gaze. Horizontal gaze palsies are common in patients with basilar artery occlusive disease. In one series of 85 patients with proven basilar artery occlusion, 22 had a horizontal gaze palsy.[146]

### *One-and-a-Half Syndrome*

Fisher[162] introduced the term one-and-a-half syndrome to refer to "a paralysis of eye movements in which one eye lies centrally and fails completely to move horizontally while the other eye lies in an abducted position and cannot be adducted past the midline." A unilateral pontine lesion involving the PPRF produces an ipsilateral conjugate gaze palsy and also affects the MLF on the same side, leading to paralysis of adduction of the ipsilateral eye on conjugate gaze to the opposite side.[162,383] If normal conjugate gaze to either side is rated 1, full horizontal gaze would score 2. Patients with combined PPRF and MLF lesions on one side only move a single eye in abduction to one side, therefore lacking one and one-half components of normal gaze. Others[422] have called this deficit *paralytic pontine exotropia* because of the deviation of the eye at rest.

### *"Ocular Bobbing"*

Fisher[155] introduced the term "ocular bobbing" to describe an unusual vertical movement of the eyes: "The eyeballs intermittently dip briskly downwards through an arc of a few millimeters and then return to the primary position in a kind of bobbing action." He felt that this was a sign of "advanced pontine disease" and of little diagnostic importance because "the site of the disease process is usually obvious from the other ocular abnormalities" and clinical findings.

Fisher described three examples of bobbing in pontine disease: two patients had pathologic documentation of basilar artery occlusion with extensive infarction of the pontine base and tegmentum; one had a pontine hemorrhage. In the patients with pointine lesions, voluntary and reflex horizontal gaze was lost. The eyes moved conjugately but the vertical excursion of the bob was only one-fourth to one-third of the normal full voluntary vertical movement. Downward movement was quicker than upward; between downward jerks the eyes rested quietly. Fisher also noted "atypical bobbing," either dysconjugate, as in one case of cerebellar hemorrhage, or unilateral. Unilateral bobbing occurred in a patient with a left 6th cranial nerve palsy and consisted of a downward bob of the left eye on attempted left lateral gaze. Nelson and Johnston[355] added four cases of bilateral ocular bobbing, all in patients with pontine hemorrhage, one of whom had a hemorrhage confined to the tegmentum and 4th ventricle.

The mechanism of bobbing in pontine lesions proposed by Fisher[155] and supported by Nelson and Johnston relates the bobbing to roving eye movements. In patients with coma due to bilateral supratentorial lesions, the eyes rove from side to side freely. In pontine lesions, since horizontal gaze is lost and vertical gaze preserved owing to sparing of the midbrain tegmentum, the vertical vector of gaze is accentuated so that the eyes bob down. In addition, caloric irrigation increases the bobbing, acting as an afferent stimulus to gaze. Similarly, a unilateral bob, when that eye is directed toward the direction of paralytic lateral gaze, could evoke a downward movement.

Yap and colleagues[501] described two clinical cases of ocular bobbing (one vascular and one probably demyelinative) in which the ocular bobbing occurred synchronously with palatal myoclonus and raised the possibility of an unusual "tremor" or movement disorder affecting brain stem structures as a mechanism of the bobbing. Bosch et al.[49] questioned the value of bobbing as a reliable sign of intrapontine disease; they presented a case of "typical ocular bobbing" (referring to bilateral conjugate downward movements) in a patient with a large cerebellar hemorrhage who had no extensive pontine lesion. However, that patient was in deep coma, had distortion of the pons, and a small unilateral Duret-type hemorrhage in the adjacent pontine tegmentum. Surely, distortion with physiologic disruption of pontine function was the basis of the bobbing, absent horizontal gaze, and decerebrate state.

Others have described bobbing in cerebellar hemorrhage[155,362] and cerebellar infarction.[451] Newman et al.[356] described a patient in coma after cranial gunshot wounds. The necrotic temporal lobe was removed, at which time the patient had no spontaneous or reflex oculocephalic eye movements. He became alert after surgery, and ocular bobbing appeared and was accentuated during voluntary eye movements, especially when the patient attempted to gaze into fields of remaining limitations of horizontal eye movements. We have also noted in patients with pontine lesions (hemorrhage or infarction) and preserved consciousness the tendency for bobbing to occur, bilaterally or unilaterally, on attempted voluntary gaze into a field of limited gaze. Newman and colleagues[356] raised the possibility that the vertical vectors could originate inferior to the lesion, for example, in the medulla or vestibular nuclei; they emphasized the possibility of recovery.

Ocular bobbing occurs in a variety of situations in which horizontal gaze is affected despite sparing of vertical gaze capabilities. It usually indicates pontine dysfunction due to an intrinsic pontine lesion or to external pressure, or to toxic or metabolic disruption of function.[165]

### *Other Neuro-ophthalmologic Signs*

**Ptosis.** Ptosis is frequent in patients with basilar occlusion and is usually attributed to involvement of the descending sympathetic fibers in the lateral pontine tegmentum. However, even with severe bilateral ptosis, the pupils may not be miotic.[162] "Pontine ptosis" is often more severe than the ptosis that usually accompanies peripheral Horner syndrome or Horner syndrome found in patients with lateral medullary syndrome. Pontine ptosis is often modified by involvement of the 7th cranial nerve or a hemiparesis.[62] In patients with hemiparesis, whether brain stem or supratentorial, ptosis is often more severe on the hemiparetic side. A peripheral type of facial weakness will diminish the ptosis by paralyzing the orbicularis oculi muscle, widening the palpebral fissure. If basilar artery occlusion produces infarction of a third nerve nucleus, complete bilateral ptosis is the rule.

**Pontine Pupils.** Pontine pupils are frequently pinpoint,[162] but reaction can be seen if a bright light and magnification are used.[386] When pontine and midbrain infarction coexist, the pupils are often at midposition but poorly reactive. Lesions in the midbrain alone, with sparing of the pons, produce fixed dilated pupils. Pupillary constriction is more severe with pontine infarction or hemorrhage than with peripheral Horner syndrome; some have postulated parasympathetic irritation as well as a destructive sympathetic process to explain the pinpoint pupils.

**Nystagmus.** Nystagmus is common in patients with basilar occlusion but varies, depending on the locus of infarction and the degree of paresis of eye movements. Vertical nystagmus is an important sign of pontine infarction; rhythmic vertical nystagmus does not occur with higher brain stem lesions, though other disorders of vertical gaze are hallmarks of mesencephalic and diencephalic damage.[386]

**Skew Deviation.** Skew deviation refers to an altered vertical position of the eyes, with one eye situated above the other and the vertical displacement remaining nearly constant in all planes of gaze. Skew is quite frequent in patients with brain stem infarction, especially when lesions are asymmetric. When associated with a unilateral internuclear ophthalmoplegia, the elevated eye is usually ipsilateral to the lesion.[435] Asymmetric lesions in the region of the vestibular nuclei, dorsolateral medulla, brachium pontis, cerebellum, and rostral midbrain all may produce skewing.

### *Palatal Myoclonus*

Palatal myoclonus is a rhythmic involuntary jerking movement of the soft palate and pharyngopalatine arch, often involving the diaphragm and laryngeal muscles.[457] It usually appears some time after the acute brain stem process, which is most often an infarction. The locus and nature of the responsible vascular lesion have not been analyzed, but the parenchymatous lesion involves the dentate nucleus of the cerebellum, the red nucleus, the inferior olivary nucleus, or their connections (the "Guillain-Mollaret triangle"). The dentate nucleus and contralateral inferior olive are somatotopically related. Fibers from the dentate nuclei travel in the superior cerebellar peduncle and decussate in the midbrain to the region of the contralateral red nucleus from which the central tegmental tract descends to the inferior olivary nucleus of the same side.[286] The pathologic lesion most often seen in patients with palatal myoclonus is hypertrophic degeneration of the inferior olive, often associated with a lesion of the ipsilateral central tegmental tract or the contralateral dentate nucleus. The olivary lesion includes enlarged neurons, loss of other neurons, and gliosis, usually with enlargement of the olive; these changes are thought to be transsynaptic and secondary to lesions of the neuronal system afferent to the inferior olivary nucleus.

The branchial movement may vary in rate (40 to 200/min).[457] The patient may complain of an audible clicking noise due to movement of the eustachian tube or may be aware of a shake in their voice. The noise can be heard by the examiner if a stethoscope is applied to the lateral neck. The movements of the pharynx can be readily seen and are often accompanied by a fluttering of the diaphragm, which is usually obvious by chest fluoroscopy. Palatal myoclonus has surprisingly little effect on swallowing.

### *Coma*

Unresponsiveness to external stimuli occurs in some patients with basilar artery occlusion. Chase et al.[90] analyzed 8 of their own cases (7 basilar occlusions, 1 pontine hemorrhage) and 12 prior reports in an attempt to correlate the state of consciousness and electroencephalographic changes with the necropsy findings. Bilateral damage to the medial pontine tegmentum was present in all of the comatose patients, whereas of the 11 patients with no more than unilateral tegmental damage, 8 were either alert or only "slightly obtunded." No patient with bilateral tegmental damage was fully alert. There was no reliable relation between the resting electroencephalogram and the size or localization of the lesions, but attempts to activate the electroencephalograph by voice or painful cutaneous stimuli were unsuccessful in the unresponsive patient. Lesions of the mesencephalic reticular formation can produce prolonged coma.[255,268,386] In animals, damage to the central tegmental region in the rostral pons, midbrain, and dorsal hypothalamus are associated with unresponsiveness.[386] Lesions below the trigeminal nerve entry zone of the pons usually do not interrupt alertness in the experimental animal.[386]

### *"Locked-In" Syndrome*

Kemper and Romanul[268] described a patient who, though paralyzed and speechless, could move his eyes horizontally and raise his eyebrows. At postmortem, there was extensive destruction of the pontine base and only slight encroachment on the ventral part of the pontine tegmentum unilaterally. They sought to differentiate this paralytic state from "akinetic mutism," a condition in which the patient could, under certain circumstances, speak and move. Plum and Posner[386] coined the term "locked-in syndrome" to describe a state in which severe paralysis prevents the usual means of gestural or vocal communication. Usually the patient can communicate by way of vertical eye movements or blinking and can demonstrate full comprehension of his plight and the environment. In some locked-in patients, oral automatisms in the form of chewing and sucking movements can be reflex-induced by oral and perioral stimulation, indicating loss of voluntary control over bulbar masticatory function.[31] These patients have been likened to M. Noirtier de Villefort in the *Count of Monte Cristo* by Dumas, who, while encased in armor, could not communicate except with his eyes.

The most common vascular lesion underlying the locked-in syndrome is basilar artery occlusion with extensive destruction of the pontine base. Vertical eye movements are usually spared. Midbrain lesions may also produce a locked-in state. In one such patient,[262] the lesions were confined to the ventral mesencephalon, and eye and lid movement was preserved. In another patient, studied only clinically, bilateral 3rd cranial nerve paralysis, mutism, and quadriplegia were present, but the patient could signal with one hand.[321] Caplan and Zervas[86] described two similar patients with presumed Duret hemorrhages who could communicate by hand signals despite bilateral 3rd cranial nerve paralysis and mutism. The necessary substrate for the locked-in syndrome is bilateral paralysis despite preserved consciousness.

*Paresis*

Some degree of paresis, either transient or persistent, accompanies nearly all cases of basilar artery occlusion. Fisher[178] emphasized that the initial motor weakness can be quite lateralized and referred to this phenomenon as the "herald hemiparesis" of basilar artery occlusion. Fisher[178] described five examples, in four of whom quadriparesis soon developed, and one exhibited jerking of the limbs contralateral to the hemiparesis. Though hemiparesis may occur, the spared side invariably demonstrates some slight paresis, hyperreflexia, and a Babinski sign.[283] It is of practical importance to clinically separate the paramedian penetrating branch lesions with hemiplegia from the more serious basilar artery occlusion with bilateral involvement. When basilar occlusion begins with a hemiplegia, the other limbs are generally affected within 24 hours. In one such case, which one of us (LRC) personally examined, with angiographically verified basilar artery occlusion, the patient was hemiplegic when first seen, but the contralateral limbs had episodic shivering movements; the next day he was quadriplegic. At times, the hemiplegia alternates from one side to another. Biemond[38] described a patient who intially developed a right hemiplegia; later, after the right limb weakness had cleared, she became dysarthric and had a left hemiplegia. Right hemiplegia, bilateral tongue and face weakness, and bilateral extensor plantar responses then developed. At postmortem examination, the left vertebral artery was occluded, and the clot had extended into the caudal basilar artery. Asymmetries probably depend on vertebral artery involvement, adequacy of collaterals on each side, and presence of distal emboli. In the 18 cases carefully studied by Kubik and Adams,[281] one side of the body was generally more affected than the other. Stupor often made precise motor examination difficult. Crossed motor paralysis, ipsilateral facial or conjugate gaze paralysis, and contralateral hemiparesis were found in 4 of the 18 cases of Kubik and Adams. Among the 85 cases of Ferbert et al.,[145] with angiographically proven basilar artery occlusion, at presentation 31 patients had tetraparesis, 15 had tetraplegia, and 21 had hemiparesis.

*Decerebrate Responses*

Decerebrate responses are frequent in patients with extensive infarction, though at times the inferior extremity flexes as the arms extended, a response correlated with lesions at the level of the vestibular nuclei.[386]

*Sensory Findings*

Sensory findings are quite variable and clearly depend on the locus of infarction. Stupor or altered capability of communication often makes determination of sensory abnormalities imprecise. Usually the motor dysfunction far outweighs the sensory signs. Perhaps this is explained by the predominantly medial location of infarction; the more lateral regions, which contain the spinothalamic tracts, and, more rostrally, the main somatosensory lemniscus are supplied by lateral circumferential collaterals and are relatively spared. In the Ferbert et al.[145] series, 11 of 85 patients were said to have a hemihypoesthesia. In our experience hemisensory signs usually indicate additional involvement of the medulla (vertebral artery) or spread of infarction to the thalamus or posterior cerebral artery territory. Occasional patients with basilar artery disease have bilateral severe, unusual pain sensations in the face. Some patients have likened the feeling to having salt and pepper thrown on their face.[79] This symptom could be due to involvement of crossing fibers crossing the midline from the spinal trigeminal nuclei to join the medial border of the spinothalamic tracts. Alternatively, the symptoms could be explained by involvement of the nucleus raphe magnus in the periaqueductal gray matter. This nucleus has serotonergic projections to the spinal tracts of the 5th cranial nerve and their nuclei.

*Ataxia*

Ataxia is frequently hidden by weakness and has been difficult to analyze, although the location of necropsy findings would predict its presence. Nystagmus is common in patients with tegmental ischemia, but may be overshadowed by nuclear, internuclear, or gaze paresis. Vertical nystagmus frequently accompanies internuclear ophthalmoplegia and pontine infarction. Dysarthria, dysphagia, and facile laughing and crying can be due to pseudobulbar paralysis and are present to some degree in most patients with moderate to severe limb paresis.

*Abnormalities of Respiration*

Abnormalities of respiration are also frequent, but their mechanism is difficult to determine because of the extensiveness of the infarction and presence of general medical factors (aspiration, fever, hypoventilation). Apneustic breathing with a hangup of the inspiratory phase and grossly regular breathing ("ataxic" respirations) occasionally occur terminally in patients with basilar artery occlusion and carry an ominous prognosis. Fisher[165] and Plum and Posner[386] have outlined other respiratory irregularities and discussed their clinicoanatomic significance. Silverstein[428,429] has outlined the frequency of symptoms and signs in 83 patients with infarction within the "distribution of the basilar artery."

## Patterns of Infarction

The regions of infarction in patients with confirmed basilar artery occlusion vary considerably, depending on the portion of the basilar artery occluded. At times the occlusion is quite limited and segmental, whereas in other patients thrombosis can affect multiple segments or even occlude the entire basilar artery and extend into the vertebral and posterior cerebral arteries.[87,283]

Kubik and Adams[281] studied 18 patients with basilar artery occlusion, including 6 examples of presumed embolic occlusion: 8 involved the rostral basilar artery, 5 the proximal third, 2 the middle third, and 3 the entire artery. In their material, the pattern of infarction and vascular occlusion are neatly diagrammed. In the patients with sparing of the rostral tip of the basilar artery, the infarcts were predominantly pontine, usually centering around the midpons. In these cases, the most lateral margins of the basis pontis were often spared and the basis pontis was affected to a far greater degree than the tegmentum. When the basilar tip was occluded, the lesions were predominantly in the midbrain, diencephalon, and rostral pons, and the tegmentum of the pons and midbrain were more often involved than in occlusion of the caudal basilar artery. In a third of the cases, the infarcts were symmetric, and in many cases the softenings were patchy. The cerebellum was also spared in most cases; the extensive brain stem softening was in striking contrast to the normal or minimally damaged cerebellum.

Silverstein[428] included 11 examples of verified basilar artery occlusion in his series; in 8 patients the lesion included the distal third, in 1 the proximal third, and in 2 the middle third. Silverstein remarked, "Embolism was not recorded clinically or pathologically in our series," but three cases had minimal atherosclerosis of the basilar artery, brain stem infarcts, and emboli in various viscera. The infarctions centered around the midpons (again predominantly in a paramedian distribution), were occasionally patchy, and were almost invariably "anemic" (75 cases), as opposed to hemorrhagic (8 cases).

Loeb and Meyer[303] reviewed and tabulated (Table 5 on p. 86 of ref. 303) past reports of basilar artery occlusion and the pattern of brain stem infarction. Pontine infarcts always favored median and paramedian zones, with relative sparing of the lateral margins. Biemond[38] noted the frequent tegmental sparing and sought to explain it by emphasizing that the tegmentum is mainly supplied by the SCA and its branches. The SCA is the most anatomically constant of the long circumferential branch vessels and often has a prominent anastomosis with the posterior cerebral artery. Biemond[38] followed small branches of the SCA and found that they form a "corona" around the cranial part of the pontine tegmentum and anastomosed with the SCA branches of the opposite side. When a lateral branch of the SCA was injected, the tegmentum was stained bilaterally, but when the basilar artery was injected from the vertebral artery, the basis pontis was deeply stained, while the tegmentum remained entirely clear. Biemond[38] also obtained little tegmental staining from injection of the AICA. According to the study of Kubik and Adams,[281] the tegmentum was involved most frequently when the occlusive lesions extended to the basilar tip, thus obstructing the SCA orifices. Our[81] own angiographic material in patients with basilar occlusion also demonstrates retrograde filling of the posterior cerebral and superior cerebellar arteries from carotid injection and the prominence of cerebellar artery anastomotic vessels that fill other lateral circumferential cerebellar artery branches. Tegmental involvement thus depends on the involvement of the distal basilar artery and the adequacy of collaterals. Collateral circulation through the PICA is poor when the vertebral artery and the basilar artery are both obstructed. Archer and Horenstein[15] wondered whether hypertension, by reducing the number and adequacy of collateral vessels, might considerably affect prognosis.

## Angiographic Diagnosis

Angiography by the standard Seldinger technique or intra-arterial digital subtraction angiography have been the principal methods of corroborating the clinical impression of basilar artery occlusive disease. Now MRI can often suggest occlusion by the absence of a signal void in the artery in various sliced.[39] Magnetic resonance angiography shows great future promise of allowing corroboration of basilar artery occlusion without invasive catheterization or dye injection.[128,129] Transcranial Doppler is probably accurate in lesions of the proximal basilar artery but to date has not been sensitive to lesions of the mid and distal basilar artery.[464] Diagnosis of basilar artery occlusion hinges upon demonstration of blocked cephalad flow (not simply poor filling or the vertebral artery ending in the PICA) and collateral filling of rostral structures. Carotid injection frequently leads to flow through the posterior communicating artery to the posterior cerebral artery, basilar tip, and superior cerebellar artery. Figure 18-14 is an example of such retrograde filling. Even in the presence of a tiny incompetent posterior communicating artery, the posterior cerebral arteries may be opacified via anastomosis between the posterior branches of the middle cerebral artery and the branches of the posterior cerebral artery, with subsequent filling of the distal basilar artery. In addition to the anastomosis between the vermian and hemispheric branches of the PICA, AICA, and SCA, there is also filling via the posterior meningeal branches of the vertebral artery and the meningohypophyseal branch of the internal carotid artery.[346] Angiographic definition of the disease in the basilar artery can help determine whether long-term warfarin anticoagulation therapy should be used in a patient with slight deficits. Angiography must be done if surgery to create shunts to increase posterior circulation flow is under consideration. The risk of angiography for posterior circulation disease has been surprisingly low in large centers with trained neuroradiologists and a large number of cases. The CT scan is helpful in documenting cerebellar infarction, but to date has been disappointing in defining acute brain stem softenings.

Magnetic resonance imaging has been a great advance in mapping and defining infarcts in the brain stem and cerebellum. The pattern of brain stem infarction, that is, unilateral or bilateral, tegmental or basal, medial or lateral, rostrocaudal level, can indicate whether the lesion involves the territory of the unilateral or bilateral intracranial vertebral arteries, the basilar artery, or single penetrating or circumferential branches. The pattern of cerebellar infarction, most readily seen on T2-weighted sagittal sections, also helps define the likely arterial territory and pathology.

## Clinical Tempo and Course

Information correlating the usual tempo of neurologic deficit acquisition and the location of vascular occlusion is very scanty. Many studies include patients chosen solely because of the availability of necropsy material,[281,428] a factor that eliminates the less severely affected patients. The clinical studies often lack angiographic or pathologic confirmation.[263,495] Angiographic studies frequently do not include detailed temporal profiles.[152] Larger series of patients with basilar artery occlusion antedated the widespread use of angiography. Caplan[65] analyzed the clinical course of surviving patients with basilar artery occlusion that have been verified angiographically, but the series was quite small (six cases). Transient ischemic attacks were quite frequent prior to the stroke (four of six cases). The last TIA occurred within 1 month of the stroke in all of these patients (within 1 week in three cases). The initial TIA preceded the stroke by a wide range (1 week to 1 year). After onset of a prolonged deficit, five of the six patients had either progression of the deficit over a 2- to 3-day period or fluctuations. Fluctuations occurred over a 2-week period and were sensitive to position in bed.[83] Two patients had sudden-onset deficits, one of which subsequently fluctuated for less than 2 weeks. Only one patient had a progressive course without stabilization or fluctuation over the first 3 days. In another clinical series, Jones et al.[259] noted that a temporal profile consisting of an unstable course characterized by progression or remission and relapses was common in patients with "vertebrobasilar system infarction" (54 percent) as compared to patients with carotid system disease (26 percent). In this series the neurologic deficit in patients with vertebrobasilar disease rarely progressed after 4 days, and most changes occurred within the first 48 hours. Declining consciousness was an ominous sign. Patrick and colleagues[367] also analyzed the temporal profile in their series of 39 cases of clinical vertebrobasilar infarction (7 with angiography). Sudden onset followed by stabilization (12 patients) and gradual onset with later progression (9 patients) were common patterns. Only two patients' deficits progressed after 24 hours: one over 48 hours and the other over 1 week. A total of 13 patients progressed after the original deficit had been stable for 24 hours or more; 8 progressed on day 2, 2 on day 3, and 1 each on days 4, 6, and 7. Again coma was a poor prognostic sign. These studies indicate that sudden-onset deficits are frequent, a point also emphasized by Kubik and Adams.[281]

Ferbert and colleagues[145] analyzed the early symptoms and course in their 85 patients with angiographically proven basilar artery occlusion. More than half had some premonitory symptoms usually in the 2 weeks before stroke onset. Vertigo and headache were especially common symptoms. Acute onset of stroke was noted in 31 patients, 11 of whom had TIAs or other prodromal symptoms. In 54 of the 85 patients (64 percent) the course was progressive with or without prodromal symptoms.

Sudden onset might point to an embolic mechanism (clot breaking loose from a more proximal arterial site within the intracranial vertebral or the lower basilar artery). Fluctuations and progressions are common, but are almost invariably documented only within the first 2 weeks after stroke onset, usually within the first 48 hours; few occur between 1 and 2 weeks. Gradual progression without improvement, especially if stupor develops, is a grave prognostic sign. This evidence, in my view, favors treatment prior to the stroke in those with TIAs and emphasizes treatment during the first 1 to 2 weeks after the stroke onset. Vigorous treatment after the deficit is stable, especially after 2 weeks, would not seem to be warranted in patients with basilar artery occlusion because late deficits are rare.

The recent introduction of thrombolytic treatment in patients with basilar artery occlusion has brought new therapeutic promise for treatment of a potentially devastating illness. After angiography has confirmed a basilar artery occlusion, patients have been treated with local infusion by catheter of streptokinase or urokinase[213,506] or recombinant tissue plasminogen activator (rtPA),[233] and with intravenously administered rtPA.[487] The optimum route of administration, optimal dose, and need for and dangers of the concurrent or postinfusion use of platelet antiaggregants, heparin, or warfarin have still to be defined. Endovascular techniques for treatment of basilar artery disease also has untested promise for the future.

## "Top of the Basilar" Occlusion

Occlusive lesions of the rostral tip of the basilar artery lead to bilateral infarction of midbrain, thalamus, and occipital and medial temporal lobes. In this area, in addition to the major tributary branches of the basilar apex, the superior cerebellar, posterior communicating, and posterior cerebral arteries, there are numerous smaller perforating midbrain arteries and vessels that course through the posterior perforating substance to feed the hypothalamus and paramedian diencephalic structures (Fig. 18-15). Atherosclerosis is generally most severe in the proximal basilar artery; as the basilar artery travels cephalad, there is less incidence of atherosclerotic stenosis, and the vessel gradually tapers in size. Occlusions of the basilar apex are generally embolic clots originating from the heart or proximal vertebrobasilar system.[67,88] The extent of infarction depends on the size of the clot, the length of time it obstructs the main basilar artery, its eventual destination in tributary vessels, and the adequacy of collateral circulation. At times, the ischemic damage is limited to one or both posterior cerebral artery hemispheric territories, and on other occasions the brunt of the damage is to the rostral brain stem structures.

At times, the syndrome of rostral basilar territory ischemia follows posterior circulation angiography, usually when the posterior circulation vessels are widely patent and have no important occlusive disease. Cortical blindness, agitated delirium, and an amnesic state are the cardinal features usually with accompanying headache. The symptoms and signs reverse within 24 hours, leaving a permanent amnesia for the period of the angiography and its sequelae. Mehler[320] studied 61 patients with ischemia in the rostral basilar artery territory: 14 patients (23 percent) had vascular stroke risk factors, prior episodes of vertebrobasilar ischemia, and presented with severe bilateral vessel, oculomotor, and behavioral abnormalities. Thrombosis engrafted upon atherostenosis and artery to artery emboli from the proximal system were common stroke mechanisms in this group; 47 patients had less severe syndromes that were often reversible. Cardiac embolism was more prominent in

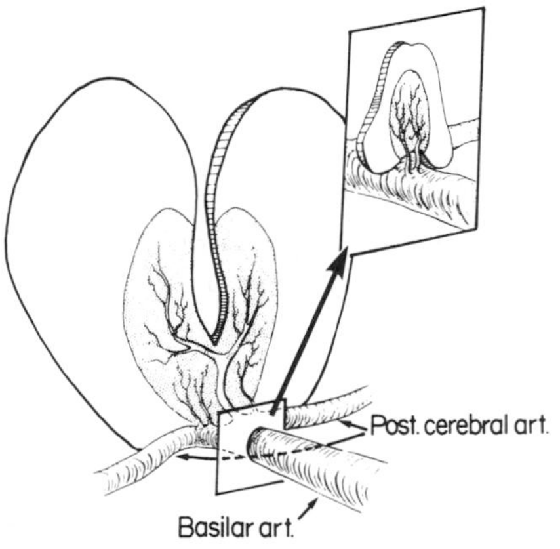


**Fig. 18-15.** Diagrammatic representations of blood supply from the distal basilar artery. Note the single midline vessel supplying the thalamus bilaterally. The area of infarction is shown in gray. *Insert:* Midbrain with shaded area of infarction.

this group. Among the total group of 61 patients, 28 (46 percent) were considered to have an embolic etiology—8 intra-arterial, 14 cardiac origin, and 6 unknown source. In situ thrombosis was believed to be responsible in 11 (18 percent), and 7 patients (11 percent) had symptoms after angiography, some of whom had documented transient contrast extravasation.

In the following section, we discuss just the findings in those patients with embolism or atherosclerotic occlusions of the basilar artery apex in whom ischemia involves multiple tributaries of the basilar artery. Similar findings, although of more limited extent, can occur in branch occlusions of these basilar apex branches, so they are also mentioned briefly.

## Major Clinical Syndromes

### Pupillary Abnormalities

When ischemia affects the medial midbrain tegmentum or medial diencephalon, pupillary reactivity is usually abnormal, because the afferent limb of the pupillary reflex arc is interrupted in its course from the optic tract of Edinger-Westphal nucleus. Midbrain pupils are frequently eccentric ("corectopia iridis") and may acutely shift position.[421,493] If the lesions only affects the Edinger-Westphal nucleus, the pupils will generally be fixed and dilated, but, if, in addition, rostral extension of the lesion occurs with resultant sympathetic paralysis, the deficit will include a midposition, fixed pupil. At times the pupil is oval,[174] a phenomenon that is usually transient and most often found in patients with supratentorial vascular catastrophes that lead to tentorial herniation. Occasionally a pupil will become oval in a patient with midbrain infarction when a 3rd cranial nerve paralysis is developing or recovering.[174] Thalamic infarcts are associated with small, poorly reactive pupils.

Among 61 patients with rostral basilar artery territory infarction Mehler[320] found that 18 (30 percent) had abnormal pupillary size, shape, or function. Six patients had discrepancies in pupillary reaction between accommodation and light stimuli. Despite abnormal light reactivity, 4 patients with dorsal midbrain infarcts had constriction on forced lid closure, normal dilatation with "psychosensory" stimuli, normal-sized pupils and normal dilation to drugs applied locally. Two other patients had normal pupillary light reactions but impaired response to convergence-accommodation.

### Oculomotor Dysfunction

Vertical gaze-vertical plane eye movements are voluntarily generated by bilaterally simultaneous activation of the frontal and parietal occipital conjugate "gaze centers." Vertical gaze pathways then converge on the periaqueductal region just beneath the collicular plate,[322,372,471] near the interstitial nucleus of Cajal and the posterior commissure. In this region in the monkey there is a cluster of neurons important in vertical gaze, which is situated among the fibers of the medial longitudinal fasciculus and is generally referred to as the "rostral interstitial nucleus of the MLF"[60] or the nucleus of the prerubral field.[471] Clinically there is often a disparity between paralysis of voluntary vertical gaze and vertical eye movements reflex-induced by vertical doll's eyes maneuver, bilateral simultaneous caloric stimulation, or Bell's phenomenon, although the anatomic basis for the disparity is not clear. Most commonly, up- and downgazes are affected together. Debate still centers around the question of the need for bilateral lesions, since unilateral stereotactically placed lesions[354] or unilateral vascular[435] and metastatic[18] lesions have on occasion produced upward gaze paralysis. In monkeys and humans, lesions of the pretectum in the posterior commissure region are necessary to produce paralysis of upward gaze.[92,364] Selective paralysis of downward gaze is much rarer; when it occurs, the lesions usually border the red nucleus and lie more ventral and caudal, producing paralysis of upward gaze.[214,257,471]

In one patient with selective downgaze palsy, the lesions were situated bilaterally in the dorsolateral periaqueductal gray, involving the crossing fibers of the commissure of the superior colliculus.[258] The eyes may rest down and are often skewed in asymmetric lesions of the mesodiencephalic junction.[67] Some patients with unilateral lesions of the paramedian midbrain and caudal diencephalon have abnormal control of head and eye posture in the roll plane.[215] Halmagyi and colleagues[215] reported four patients, and Mehler[320] reported two patients with "ocular tilt reactions." These patients all had a head tilt, conjugate eye torsion, and skewing with hypotropia all to the side ipsilateral or contralateral to the mesodiencephalic lesion. All patients with ocular tilt reactions also had vertical, predominantly upward gaze, palsies. Some patients with mesodiencephalic infarcts have had "vertical one-and-a-half" syndrome.[45,111,184] Deleu et al.[111] reported a patient in whom all downward saccadic and smooth pursuit eye movements were lost bilaterally, but only a monocular paresis of upgaze was present. The lesion on MRI was confined to the rostral interstitial nucleus of the medial longitudinal fasciculus bilaterally. The authors hypothesized that the lesion affected upgaze premotor fibers in the tracts from these nuclei before or after their decussation in the posterior commissure. Bogousslavsky and Regli[45] reported a patient with a unilateral mesodiencephalic lesion with bilateral upgaze palsy but only monocular paresis of downgaze. Unilateral lesions, by affecting crossing or commissural fibers, can produce bilateral defects in vertical gaze. Among Mehler's[320] series of 61 patients with "top of the basilar" territory infarction, 47 (77 percent) had some abnormality of vertical eye position or gaze.[322]

## Abnormalities of Convergence

Ocular convergence is probably controlled in the medial midbrain tegmentum, although there is considerable debate as to whether a formal nuclear structure, such as the nucleus of Perlia, subserves this function. One or both eyes may rest in, and convergence vectors are frequently evident on attempted upward gaze. Rhythmic "convergence nystagmus" may be elicited by following a downgoing opticokinetic target. Convergence vectors may also modify lateral gaze. Voluntary lateral movements of the lateral rectus are balanced against convergence vectors, thus limiting abduction and giving the superficial appearance of a 6th cranial nerve palsy (pseudosixth).[67] Lid abnormalities are also a frequent sign of rostral brain stem disease. Unilateral infarction of a 3rd cranial nerve nucleus can lead to complete bilateral ptosis.[62] Retraction of the upper lid, giving the eye a prominent stare (Collier's sign)[97] is also frequent in tectal lesions.

## Abnormalities of Alertness, Attention, and Behavior

The medial mesencephalon and diencephalon contain the most rostral portions of the reticular activating system. Infarcts in these regions frequently affect consciousness, sleep, and behavior. Facon and colleagues[137] and later Castaigne et al.[87] described patients with basilar apex occlusion in whom prolonged sleep and 3rd cranial nerve palsies were the most prominent features. Segarra[419] later outlined the distribution of the infarction that causes this syndrome, which he believed was due to occlusion of the perforating branches of the mesencephalic artery (the first portion of the posterior cerebral artery as it courses around the midbrain). These vessels have been studied by Foix and Hillemand,[188] Lazorthes,[287] Percheron,[374] and Castaigne and colleagues[88] and are called the paramedian mesencephalic arteries and the anterior and posterior thalamosubthalamic paramedian arteries. They form the most rostral group of vessels in the posterior perforated substance and supply the paramedian midbrain and diencephalon. There is some evidence that a single midline vessel may branch to supply both banks of the 3rd ventricle[88] (Fig. 18-16). Because the reticular gray is adjacent to the 3rd cranial nerve nuclei and the vertical gaze regions near the posterior commissure, somnolence is invariably associated with pupillary abnormalities, 3rd cranial nerve palsies, and defects of vertical gaze, although lateralized motor or sensory signs are often absent. A similar syndrome can occur after herniation, presumably due to extension pressure on these same vascular structures, caused by wedging of the

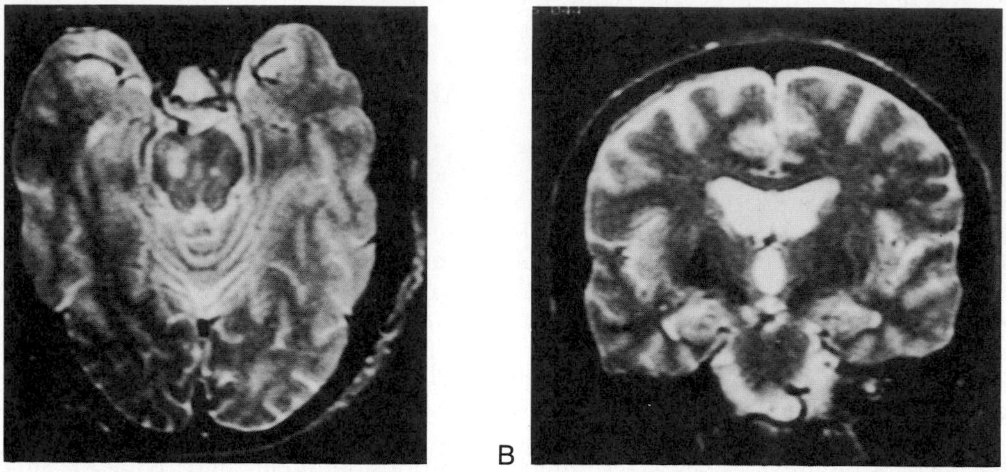

A B

**Fig. 18-16.** T2-weighted views of pontomesencephalic infarct. (**A**) Axial plane. (**B**) Coronal plane.

mamillary bodies into the interpeduncular fossa, a situation which causes either median brain stem infarction[298] or Duret hemorrhages.[86] Among our own patients, one with a large putaminal hemorrhage survived the acute stroke but was left with 3rd cranial nerve palsies and slept nearly continuously for 2 years at a nursing home. At postmortem an old slit cavity was found in the putamen and, in addition, butterfly distribution infarctions in the medial midbrain and thalamus developed, probably during the period of herniation. Of 28 patients with rostral brain stem infarcts studied by Castaigne and colleagues,[88] 15 had hypersomnia caused by paramedian tegmental lesions, usually bilateral.

## Hallucinations

Complaints of hallucination are also seen in cases of rostral brain stem infarction and have led to the term *peduncular hallucinosis.* All patients described with this phenomenon have had the hallucinations at twilight time or during the night and all have had a sleep disorder (nocturnal insomnia or daytime hypersomnolence).[67] The hallucinations are usually vivid and most commonly visual. Blood and red hair, horses and green serpents against a red background, and brightly plumed parrots are some examples. Occasionally auditory or tactile hallucinations are associated. Similar hallucinations also accompany sleep deprivation or drug intoxication and may relate to dysfunction of the reticular-activating system. In addition to hallucinations, impulsive reports, which have been called "extraordinary confabulation,"[446] are often made by patients with rostral brain stem infarcts. These consist of descriptions of behavior or present whereabouts that are totally unrealistic. The reports have no approximation to reality and are influenced by surrounding stimuli. For example, a 60-year-old woman was questioned while a newscast of a school incident was on an adjacent television set. She said that she was in school at a lunch bar ready to order English muffins, and if we did not get out of the way she would be late for her next seventh grade class. When asked why she was wearing a nightgown and seemed to be in a hospital bed, she said that she was too lazy that day to get fully dressed and simply came to school in her nightgown in bed. Similarly, others have incorporated into their replies reality items provided by the questioner. Many such patients "dream a lot" and they may be reporting their imaginings as reality.

In most patients with peduncular hallucinations, the lesions have been large, making it difficult to relate the abnormality to any particular anatomic structure. McKee et al.[316] reported a single patient with peduncular hallucinations who had very discrete small bilateral lesions in the medial portions of the substantia nigra pars reticulata. Their patient was a diabetic man with prior 3rd cranial nerve palsies that developed 2 years apart, each recovering within 2 months. After a seizure he reported visual hallucinations of animals and people with obscured faces walking across his field of vision. Often the visual hallucinations were preceded by the sensation of being touched on the shoulder or face. The lesions were limited entirely to the pars reticulata and may have affected adjacent fibers of the 3rd cranial nerve just medial to the infarcts, but tegmental structures were completely spared. The pars reticulata has connections with the pedunculopontine nucleus and show increased discharge during REM sleep.

## Hemiballism and Abnormal Movements

It has long been known that involuntary movements occur from deep upper brain stem lesions. In

1927 Martin[310] described a hypertensive man who suddenly developed violent movements of the right limbs associated with facial grimacing, dysarthria, agitation, and finally death. Necropsy revealed a small hemorrhage located in the left subthalamus in the region of the subthalamic nucleus (corpus Luysii). Martin[310] reviewed 12 earlier cases of "hemichorea" associated with lesions in this region that were verified at postmortem; 8 were small hemorrhages, 3 metastases, and 1 unspecified. Whittier[486] later reviewed the subject and attempted to differentiate ballism, that is, incessant violent flinging proximal movements, from other types of adventitious movements such as chorea. Lesions in 30 of the cases he reviewed involved the subthalamic region or "the connections of this region." The most common etiology was hemorrhage, but infarctions in this region were also described. Moersch and Kernohan[337] noted a single patient with hemiballism due to two small adjacent softenings in the subthalamic nucleus, but unfortunately did not comment on the offending vascular lesion. More recently, it has become clear from CT correlation that lesions in other sites, especially the striatum and thalamus,[265] can produce a movement disorder difficult to distinguish from that caused by lesions in the subthalamic nucleus. Infarction of the subthalamus can produce a severe movement disorder that is unilateral and characterized by nearly constant flinging and often rotatory proximal arm and leg movements on one side of the body. Frequently a hemiparesis precedes or follows the movement disorder, the movement disappearing as the limbs are paralyzed and returning when the paralysis clears. Unfortunately, the offending vascular lesion in the subthalamus, which is fed by branches of the posterior communicating, posterior choroidal, and posterior cerebral arteries,[337] has seldom if ever been characterized. One of us (LRC) has seen a patient in whom unilateral hemiballism was associated with stupor and eye signs typical of bilateral basilar apex brain stem infarction (no hemorrhage on CT), but unfortunately the vascular lesion was not verified.

Abnormal movements other than ballistic were present in 7 of 28 rostral brain stem infarcts studied by Castaigne and colleagues.[88] The movements were frequently delayed in onset and had a predilection for the face, arm, and thumb. Clonic, athetoid, and myoclonic movements were described in patients with bilateral paramedian thalamic infarcts that at times extended to the upper pole of the red nucleus and affected Meynert's tract and the decussation of the brachium conjunctivum. When emboli block the penetrating vessels of the basilar apex, limb paralysis is usually transient or absent. When the most proximal portion of the posterior cerebral is affected, a contralateral hemiplegia may occur, at times accompanied by a contralateral third nerve palsy.[249] Often, however, the clinical findings are dominated by unilateral or bilateral posterior cerebral artery territory hemispheral infarction.

## Midbrain Infarcts

Lipohyalinosis and atheromatous branch occlusions also occur frequently in arterial penetrating branches of the basilar artery apex and the adjacent basilar communicating, posterior communicating, and proximal posterior cerebral arteries. MRI is now able to identify infarcts limited to the territory of individual penetrating branches. However, the only pathologic studies of lesions in penetrating arteries have been Fisher's studies[157,172,175] of patients with pure sensory stroke due to lateral thalamic infarction.

Paramedian arteries originate from the proximal basilar communicating artery (also called the P1 segment of the posterior cerebral artery by some)[249,504] and supply the cerebral peduncles, medial portions of the substantia nigra, fascicles of the 3rd cranial nerve, and the red nuclei. Peduncular perforating arteries originate from the distal end of the basilar communicating arteries and the proximal portions (P2a) of the posterior cerebral arteries as they course around the cerebral peduncles.[249] These arteries supply the more lateral portions of the ventral midbrain, including the lateral portions of the cerebral peduncles and substantia nigra.

Infarctions in the territory of the paramedian penetrating mesencephalic arteries are probably responsible for some examples of Weber's syndrome (ipsilateral 3rd cranial nerve palsy and contralateral hemiplegia). Some diabetic 3rd cranial nerve palsies probably involve the parenchymatous portions of the 3rd cranial nerve before the fascicle exit from the midbrain. Pure motor hemiplegia could also result from infarction limited to the cerebral peduncle. In the case of peduncular hallucinosis related to bilateral infarcts in the substantia nigra pars reticulata cited earlier, infarction was probably due to bilateral small paramedian artery disease.[315] An organized occlusion with recanalization was identified in one small penetrating artery within the substantia nigra. Clinicopathologic correlations have not been reported in patients with penetrating mesencephalic infarcts.

## Thalamic Infarcts

There are four main groups of arteries that penetrate into the thalamus, arising from the region of the basilar artery bifurcation: two groups of thalamoperforating arteries, the polar (tuberothalamic) arteries and the thalamic-subthalamic (thalamoperforating) arteries, and the thalamogeniculate and the posterior choroidal arteries. To date, there have been no reports of infarction limited to posterior choroidal artery territory caused by branch disease, but reports of branch occlusion-related infarcts are known for the other arteries.

### *Polar Artery*

The polar artery (also called the anterior internal optic artery by Duret,[208] the premammillary pedicle by Foix and Hillemand,[187,188,208,374] and the tuberothalamic artery[69,208] usually arises from the middle portion of the posterior communicating artery to supply the anterolateral portion of the thalamus. In about a third of cases this artery is absent and the thalamic-subthalamic artery also supplies this territory. The polar artery supply includes the lateral portion of the anterior thalamic pole, but not the anterior nucleus. Portions of the ventral lateral, dorsomedial, and reticular nuclei are supplied as well as part of mammillothalamic tract.[46,69,208] Supply is said to be always unilateral by single branches.[46,69,208] Infarcts can result from penetrating branch disease or clipping of internal carotid artery or posterior communicating artery aneurysm.

Unilateral infarcts cause minor or negligible contralateral motor signs, for example, slight often transient hemiparesis, asymmetrical facial expression, slight asymmetry of arm swing and spontaneous or automatic use of the contralateral limbs. Sensory and oculomotor findings are generally absent.[46,69,208] Cognitive and behavioral abnormalities predominate. Initially, patients may appear confused and disoriented. Later, the predominant findings are lack of initiation and spontaneity, long latency in responding, and inability to persevere with protracted tasks. These deficits have been called abulia by Fisher.[177] They are identical to dysfunction found in patients with disease of the frontal lobes and caudate nuclei[82] and probably indicate loss of function of corticostriatothalamic projections from the anterior thalamic nuclei.[88]

Patients with left anterolateral thalamic infarcts also may have slight aphasic abnormalities with paraphasic errors and verbal perseverations but retain ability to repeat spoken language.[69] With right anterolateral thalamic infarction, constructional praxis and visual-spatial abnormalities may also be found.[46,69] Verbal memory is affected in left-sided lesions and visual memory in right-sided infarcts.[69,208] The abulia and cognitive and behavioral abnormalities are often transient and usually regress and substantially recover during the 3 to 6 months after the stroke. Although all reported cases to date are unilateral, one of the authors (LRC) is aware of several patients with MRI lesions restricted to the bilateral territories of the polar arteries who have persisting abulia and memory and cognitive and behavioral dysfunction. These cases raise the suspicion that unilateral polar artery branches could supply both sides, as is the case in the thalamic-subthalamic arteries. Polar territory infarcts are responsible for what has been referred to as acute "thalamic dementia."

### *Thalamic-Subthalamic Arteries*

The thalamic-subthalamic arteries (also called the deep interpeduncular profunda arteries, the paramedian thalamic arteries by Percheron, the posterior internal optic arteries by Duret, and the thalamoperforating pedicle by Foix and Hillemand.[187,188,208,374,459] These arteries arise from the basilar communicating artery segment of the posterior cerebral artery. The arterial pattern is quite heterogeneous. Single arteries to each side can arise, or bilateral branches may arise from a unilateral single artery, or arteries to both sides may arise from a pedicle.[69,88,322] These arteries may also supply territory usually supplied by the polar arteries. Medial thalamic infarcts in the territories of the thalamic-subthalamic arteries usually involve the subthalamus, the rostral interstitial nucleus of the medial longitudinal fasciculus, the nucleus parafascicularis, and the medial part of the centromedian nucleus.[69,208,459] Ischemia in the territory of these arteries can be caused by atheromatous branch disease, emboli to the basilar apex, or aneurysms at the basilar bifurcation.

Reported patients with unilateral paramedian left thalamic infarcts all have had upgaze pulses and loss of convergent eye movements.[44,208,343,478] Temporary downgaze paresis also may be present. The vertical gaze abnormality affects voluntary saccades, smooth pursuit, and vestibulo-ocular reflex motions.[69] Disorientation and severe amnesic deficits have also been noted.[44,208,343] Some patients have also had aphasic abnormalities characterized by occasional paraphasic errors and loss of naming abilities. A minor right hemiparesis characterized by decreased spontaneous and associated movements of the right limbs may be present.[44,208] One patient had decreased pain and touch sensation in the right face.[44,69] Insufficient examples of unilateral right-sided paramedian infarction limited to the territory of the thalamic-subthalamic artery are reported that might permit clinicopathologic correlation. Bilateral paramedian infarcts cause hypersomnolence, vertical gaze palsies predominantly of upgaze, loss of ocular convergence, and amnesic syndrome.[69,322,453,475] Elements of 3rd cranial nerve palsies may also be present. Patients with bilateral paramedian thalamic infarcts usually have persistent severe amnesia and vertical gaze palsies. The thalamogeniculate arteries arise as a pedicle or group of arteries from the ambient segment of the posterior cerebral artery. The pedicle usually consists of six to eight arteries that vary widely in diameter and penetrate into the ventral lateral thalamus between the geniculate bodies.[77,188,458] These arteries supply the somatosensory, the ventral posterolateral and posteromedial nuclei, the inferior and posterior portions of the ventral lateral nucleus, the lateral portion of the centromedial nucleus, and the rostrolateral portion of the pulvinar.[77] The thalamogeniculate arteries also, in most cases, probably also supply a portion of the posterior limb of the internal capsule, as can be seen from the lesions in the original cases of Dejerine and Roussy.[77,110]

### *Thalamogeniculate Arteries*

There are three somewhat distinct syndromes that result from infarction in the territorial supply of the thalamogeniculate arteries and their branches. These vessels are the posterior circulation counterpart of the lenticulostriate branches of the middle cerebral arteries. Lesions of small branches can produce infarction restricted to the somatosensory nuclei causing the clinical syndromes of pure sensory stroke or sensory loss limited to the face.[172,175] Occlusion of branches supplying the lateral thalamus and posterior limb of the internal capsule can give rise to a "sensorimotor" stroke in which the deficits are restricted to paresis, decreased pin and touch perception, and pyramidal signs without cognitive or behavioral abnormalities.[77,341] Larger lateral thalamic infarcts cause a syndrome originally described by Dejerine and Roussy,[110] which includes hemiataxia, hemichorea, transient hemiparesis, and hemisensory symptoms and signs.[77,112]

### *Choroidal Artery*

The anterior choroidal artery is also known to supply a small portion of the thalamus, but infarction restricted to the thalamus after occlusion of this artery has not been reported.[228] Lateral geniculate infarction can occur secondary to occlusive lesions of either the anterior or posterior choroidal arteries and produce characteristic visual field deficits. Posterior choroidal artery territory branch occlusion has not ben reported, but infarction of the lateral geniculate body after occlusion of lateral choroidal branches of the posterior cerebral artery has been described.[196,228] Undoubtedly, the advent of MRI and MR angiography will allow further recognition of penetrating artery disease at the basilar apex improving clinicopathologic correlation of vascular disease at this level.

## Low-Flow States with Resultant Borderzone Ischemia in the Posterior Circulation

Occlusion of a blood vessel, whether due to in-situ thrombosis or embolus, results in a region of infarction usually within the center of distribution of that vessel. Collateral circulation is apt to supply the more peripheral zones and thus limit the centrifugal extent of the infarct. When, however, flow is diffusely diminished, for example, during shock due to blood loss or cardiogenic hypotension, the distribution of ischemia more often straddles the borderzone regions between major blood vessels. Schneider labeled these borderzones as "distal fields" comparable to the far zones of an agricultural irrigation system.[507] Zülch and Behrend,[508] Romanul and Abramowicz,[403,404] Mohr,[338] and Brierley[52] have discussed the localization and pathophysiology of this phenomenon in clinical and experimental hypotension.

Few examples of necropsy-confirmed posterior circulation borderzone infarction have been reported. Romanul and Abramowicz[404] described a single patient, a 70-year-old woman, who never awakened from surgical hypotension. Extensive supratentorial and infratentorial boundary zone lesions were found. The posterior circulation lesion was a zone of infarction in the cerebellum at the junction of supply of the inferior cerebellar arteries (AICA and PICA) and the SCA; no brain stem lesion was mentioned. Hutchinson and Yates[251] described four patients with combined vertebral and carotid disease who developed infarction bilaterally in the cerebellum in or adjacent to territory usually supplied by the SCAs after systemic hypotension. We have also seen infarction in this junctional region of the cerebellum in patients with a past history of decreased cerebral blood flow. In the reported cases and our own observations, the dominant clinical features in severe cases was coma, and in milder forms visual agnosia and branchial weakness were due to the accompanying supratentorial lesions.

Brain stem lesions due to hypotension have been hypothesized but seldom documented. Romanul[403] identified the medial zone at the tegmentobasal junction of the midpons (the area damaged in central pontine myelinolysis) as a possible zone of vulnerability between medial penetrating branches and tegmental supply from the circumferential cerebellar vessels supplying the tegmentum, but did not refer to necropsy specimens supporting this idea. Jurgensen et al.[261] described a 44-year-old epileptic woman who was found hypotensive, hypothermic, and comatose after presumed multiple drug injection. At necropsy, there were bilateral, symmetric, round, hemorrhagic infarcts distributed in a columnar fashion in the lateral brain stem tegmentum extending the length of the lower pons and medulla. They were between the short lateral circumferential penetrators and the lateral edge. There were also bilateral hemorrhagic regions in the lateral putamen. Gilles[200] described isolated necrosis of brain stem nuclei in children after hypotension. The authors have seen two adult patients with a clinical picture following hypotension that closely mimicked pontine hemorrhage: small pupils, absent horizontal gaze, and deep coma. One of these patients had no gross lesion visible at postmortem, but extensive necrosis of brain stem nuclei was seen microscopically, especially in the pons. The other patient had no postmortem examination. Lance and Adams[285] described patients with hypotension who made fine or course muscular jerks, especially on conscious attempts at precise movement. They called this phenomenon intention and action myoclonus. Myoclonus was related to probable cerebellum system damage, but was not more precisely localized. Keane[266] wondered if the sustained upward gaze found in 15 patients who had suffered a cardiorespiratory arrest could be due to "symmetrical cerebellar hypoxic change" that was found at postmortem in the 6 autopsied patients. Downward nystagmus and severe truncal and extremity cerebellar dysfunction was also noted in several patients, leading Keane[266] to suggest a posterior circulation locus for the pathogenic mechanism. Hutchinson and Yates[251] and Romanul[403] also speculate that hypotension in patients with preexisting severe occlusive disease in the vertebral arteries may modify the usual locus of infarction. Hinshaw et al.,[239] in a radiographic analysis, described one patient with bilateral borderzone lesions in the cerebellum visible on CT scan who had critical stenosis of one vertebral artery while the other vertebral artery ended in the PICA. At this time data are insufficient either to specify the anatomic loci of vulnerability to hypotension in the posterior circulation or to characterize the associated clinical picture.

## Migraine

In 1961 Bickerstaff[37] reported a distinct symptom complex occurring in adolescent girls, consisting of repeated episodes of altered vision, vertigo, ataxia, dysarthria, and numbness and tingling of the limbs and sometimes face, followed by headache. The frequent family history of migraine and clearing of the ischemic symptoms by the time the headache began stamped the disorder as migrainous for Bickerstaff and he coined the descriptive term *basilar artery migraine.* Swanson and Vick[452] have corroborated the existence of this syndrome, noted its occasional onset in adult life, and described an occasional familial tendency.[64]

Though traditionally considered a disorder beginning in the first 2 to 3 decades of life, migraine occurring late in life is more frequent than is generally realized. Fisher[164] analyzed the nature of migraine accompaniments and compared their clinical features with a comparable group of patients in whom ischemia was due to verified atherosclerotic occlusive disease. Migrainous deficits developed over a period of 15 to 30 minutes. "Positive" phenomena (for example, scintillations or brightness in the visual sphere or tingling in the tactile sphere) were perceived first and gradually spread within each sensory modality; for example, scintillations traveled gradually across the visual field and paresthesiae spread from one digit to the next and slowly up the limbs. The "positive" phenomena left in their wake "negative" phenomena, for example, blackness or numbness. As positive and later negative phenomena spread within the sensory modality, the earliest affected regions would clear, and finally all symptoms related to that modality would return to normal before a second modality would be affected. Headache would usually, but not always, appear after the deficits had disappeared. Using these clinical criteria and the absence of appropriate angiographic atherosclerotic lesions that might explain the clinical phenomenon, Fisher[173] defined a group of patients who he believed had transient migrainous spells beginning after the age of 50. Our experience with such patients include those with (1) a clinical tempo matching that described by Fisher,[164] (2) multiple attacks in a variety of regions, (3) absence of angiographic disease or a source of cerebral emboli, and (4) response to commonly used prophylactic antimigraine agents such as propanalol, phenytoin, and methysergide. In many such patients, attacks are within the distribution of the posterior circulation.

The term basilar artery migraine is perhaps redundant, because it has long been known, but not understood, that migraine tends to involve the basilar artery and its branches. Visual scintillations are the most common accompaniments of migraine and are occipital (posterior cerebral artery) in origin. Examples of transient global amnesia are known in migraine,[76] and the pathologic anatomy and physiology of memory suggest a dominant posterior cerebral artery localization. Physiologic studies[430,432] using xenon-133 have documented oligemia as an early finding or subsequent to focal hyperemia. Blood flow changes are maximal in the occipitoparietal regions.[360] Also, angiographically performed during the prodromal phase of migraine has demonstrated filling of the posterior cerebral artery from carotid injection, which suggests low pressure in the basilar system. An example of adult basilar migraine might serve to illustrate this problem.

A 58-year-old physician had no past history of important headache or transient neurologic dysfunction. In January 1980, 5 minutes after intercourse, he noted dizziness and a wobbly, unsteady gait, which was followed by unclear vision and diplopia. An unpleasant "dysesthetic" feeling was then apparent in his right hand and spread to his right leg and trunk. He became unable to walk and vomited. The attack lasted 20 minutes and left no residue. Subsequently, he had more than 30 nearly identical attacks frequently beginning after intercourse or exertion. During some attacks, his wife noted outward deviation of one eye. Dysphagia, drooling of saliva, and hiccups occasionally accompanied the vertigo, ataxia, diplopia, and right dysesthesia, all of which were invariable features. A neurologist found an intranuclear ophthalmoplegia and gait ataxia during one attack and was examined during another attack. He was dysarthric. The right eye was deviated to the right and there was prominent horizontal nystagmus on left gaze. On right gaze he did not adduct the left eye but had abducting nystagmus of the outwardly deviated right eye (intranuclear ophthalmoplegia). Gait was grossly ataxic. Spells varied from 15 minutes to 24 hours. Headache was not experienced during or after any attack. Electroencephalography, CT scan with and without contrast, and vertebral angiography were all normal. Heparin, warfarin, aspirin, and dipyridamole was used sequentially to no avail. After the beginning of phenytoin therapy, there was a transient decrease in the frequency of the attacks, which had by now become very disabling. After methysergide therapy was begun in July 1980, the spells completely disappeared, except for some insignificant intermittent dysesthetic feeling in the physician's right hand. Methysergide therapy was stopped in December 1980, with no further recurrence of the episodes. The tempo of the symptoms, normality of the vertebrobasilar system angiographically, and response to methysergide strongly suggest a migrainous mechanism, that is, adult "basilar" migraine. Five years after his last attack, he first noted spells of typical migrainous scintillating scotomas that lasted 20 to 30 minutes without headache.

Some patients who have transient basilar artery territory deficits but normal angiography are, in fact, suffering migrainous spells. Is this more common than we now appreciate? Does physiologic alteration in vascular size with inefficient delivery of blood (spasm?) occur in patients who would not fall within the usually accepted nosology of migraine?[76]

Caplan[72] recently reviewed his experience with patients who had migraine, classical or common, and posterior circulation ischemic attacks and strokes, who had also had angiography. Nine patients were presented, including the case described above. Men and women of widely varying ages were included. The clinical patterns included patients with just TIAs, single strokes, single stroke followed by attacks, and multiple strokes. In some patients classic migraine developed only months or years later. CT and MRI confirmed infarctions in patients who had strokes with persistent neurologic deficits (7 of 9 patients).[72] Angiography showed basilar artery occlusions, severe diffuse narrowing of vertebrobasilar arteries (rather persistent in one patient), or normal posterior circulation vessels. The mechanism of infarction was not elucidated but clearly vasoconstriction, often protracted, and basilar artery occlusion did occur. Ischemia is presumably due to protracted vasoconstriction, or to vascular thrombosis precipitated by activation of platelet adhesion and agglutination and activation of the intrinsic and extrinsic coagulation pathways.

## CLINICAL PRESENTATIONS

The preceding section contains descriptions of the variety of clinical findings in patients with vascular lesions at known locations. Unfortunately, the patient usually does not come to the physician with an already known vascular lesion. Nevertheless, patient presentations can be grouped into different general classes of problems or recurrent themes. The task for the clinician is to gauge from the type of clinical problem the patient's prognosis and then to plan the evaluation and treatment accordingly. Assessment of the prognosis and likely natural course of the stroke will be most accurate when knowledge of the vascular lesion and location and state of the brain lesion is most inclusive and accurate. In some patients, the clinical signs will be clear enough to allow reliable prediction of the vascular lesion without arteriography; in others, the clinical syndrome could fit several vascular etiologies, and precise diagnosis will depend on further laboratory and radiographic investigations.

### Ischemia in the Distribution of a Penetrating Branch

Some patients presenting symptoms and signs will fit neatly into the typical distribution of a basilar branch.

A 71-year-old hypertensive woman during a few hours developed a right hemiparesis, tingling of the right hand, and diplopia on looking to the right. Examination confirmed a right hemiparesis, decreased position sense in the right hand, and a left internuclear ophthalmoplegia.

In this case the lesion must involve the left paramedian brain stem, including the left medial longitudinal fasciculus, medial lemniscus, and pyramidal tract in the basis pontis. When such a patient also has a history of hypertension, the deficit develops over a short period (hours to a week), and there have not been prior transient ischemic attacks that indicate a wider zone of ischemia (e.g., dizziness, bilateral limb weakness, or blindness), one can predict with a high degree of confidence that the responsible vascular lesion lies within a basilar branch. The likelihood of more widespread further ischemia during the acute stroke is small. Treatment might be limited to keeping cerebral perfusion pressure high during the acute stroke but subsequently controlling blood pressure more vigorously. Other more aggressive evaluation and treatment are not very likely to be of additional help. The important features that allow diagnosis of a branch lesion include the following:

1. Ecology (usually the patient is hypertensive or diabetic)
2. Rate of deficit acquisition (usually hours to days, often with smooth gradual progression)
3. Anatomic localization (lesion limited to the territory of a penetrating branch)
4. Absence of features common in large-vessel occlusion (e.g., headache, decreased alertness, and vomiting).

When the basilar artery is occluded, the earliest signs can resemble branch disease, but, within 48 hours, signs indicating involvement of the contralateral side of the brain stem are added. Computed tomography may help corroborate branch disease in a negative way by failing to delineate cerebellar or posterior cerebral artery territory infarctions.

MRI often is capable of confirming the infarct and showing that it is limited to the territory of a paramedian branch. MRI and MR angiography may help establish patency of the parent basilar artery.

### Ischemia of the Lower Brain Stem Bilaterally, Evolving Gradually or After Warnings

In patients whose signs and symptoms indicate bilateral dysfunction of the basis and/or tegmentum of the pons, the most common vascular lesion is basilar artery occlusion or severe stenosis.

> A 60-year-old diabetic man had 20 transient spells during a few months, which were varied and included vertigo, staggering, double vision, and on one occasion weak legs and slurred speech. On awakening, he was unable to lift his legs, and his arms were clumsy. He could not swallow and spoke in a slurred, low-volume voice. Examination confirmed a quadriparesis, worse on the right, and the only horizontal eye movement was abduction with nystagmus of the left eye. Though he improved transiently, leg weakness became more profound when his blood pressure was lowered.

In this patient, the findings indicate bilateral dysfunction of the pyramidal system in the basis pontis and extension into the left tegmentum to involve the left paramedian-pontine reticular formation and medial longitudinal fasciculus. Furthermore, the time course of symptoms is long (months) and the patient is sensitive to change in perfusion, both common features of large-vessel disease. The diagnosis of basilar artery occlusion is more likely if there have been transient nonstereotyped attacks of brain stem ischemia dating back weeks or months, especially if the attacks have been recurring more frequently in the period just before the stroke. Headache, decreased alertness, and a background that includes disease of other large vessels, such as coronary and peripheral limb arteries, support the likelihood of basilar artery occlusive disease. Separation of occlusion from severe stenosis may be warranted because the patient with a residual lumen probably has a higher long-term risk of further ischemia. In basilar artery occlusion the risk of severe infarction occurs at and shortly after the time of occlusion. Basilar branch occlusion, if extensive and bilateral, can occasionally mimic occlusive disease of the basilar artery. One of two strategies might be used: (1) employ maximal medical treatment, that is, nurse the patient in a head-down position, maintain systemic blood pressure, and begin therapeutic levels of intravenous heparin and delay arteriography, or (2) pursue immediate angiographic clarification to define the vascular lesion.

If MRI shows infarction that includes the cerebellum or structures outside the territories of the paramedian penetrators, then basilar artery occlusion can be reasonable inferred. If the patient treated with heparin without angiography improves to the level where long-term treatment might be considered, angiographic clarification could be pursued at the time a switch to warfarin is contemplated. Angiography, if normal, could indicate the likelihood of branch disease; if occlusive disease is corroborated, angiography should separate stenosis from occlusion. The risk of bleeding from the unnecessary use of warfarin outweighs the smaller risk of angiography.

Some patients with basilar artery occlusion (verified by angiographically documented obstruction, or inferred because of the distribution despite normal angiography) have cardiac origin or intra-arterial embolism to this site.[84] Especially when the onset of the disorder is sudden, or no thrombus is found at angiography, a search for a donor site for embolism should be made. In the case presented the multitude of transient prodromal attacks effectively excludes cardiogenic embolism as the cause.

### Lower Brain Stem Ischemia of Sudden Onset Not Limited to a Typical Branch

Sudden-onset lower brain stem ischemia is similar to gradually evolving ischemia of the lower brain stem discussed in the preceding section, except for the timing of deficit acquisition.

> A 50-year-old man suddenly developed tingling of the right arm and leg and could not walk. Examination revealed a slight quadriparesis that was worse on the left. Vertical nystagmus, slurred speech, and bilateral extensor plantar reflexes were also found, but sensory examination was normal. Within 24 hours, the deficit had cleared.

In this case the lack of prior warnings and absence of known coexistent vascular disease make the diagnosis less certain. Atherosclerosis with occlusion of the basilar artery and patchy ischemia, embolism to the basilar artery from the heart or great vessels, basilar migraine, or less common vascular disease, such as aneurysm or dissection, are all possible. In some cases, hemorrhages, either spontaneous or secondary to an arteriovenous malformation or telangiectasia, can produce a clinical picture that would fit into this general category. (Computed tomography is usually warranted to exclude hemorrhage and define regions of infarction.) Angiography is helpful in this group in order to plan appropriate therapy. A search for a cardiac origin for embolism is also important.[84]

## Rostral Brain Stem Ischemia

Especially when combined with ischemia in the territories of the posterior cerebral arteries, rostral brain stem ischemia usually indicates a basilar apex embolus.

A 47-year-old woman, while sitting on the toilet, suddenly pitched forward. Her daughter, a nurse, heard the fall and found her mother comatose. The eyes were each deviated laterally and the pupils were dilated. On arrival at the hospital, there was a bilateral 3rd cranial nerve palsy, weakness of the right limbs, and a right extensor plantar response.

In this example there are bilateral lesions in the midbrain (or 3rd cranial nerves) and dysfunction of the left cerebral peduncle. Initial evaluation should generally exclude rostral brain stem compression by a supratentorial space-taking lesion, such as intracerebral or subdural hemorrhage. Angiography or CT could exclude such a mass effect; angiography also might corroborate the basilar apex embolus, but is infrequently performed acutely. A source of embolization should be avidly sought, especially in the younger patient. The most common sources are the heart and proximal vessels (innominate, subclavian, or vertebral arteries). Transient preceding spells of headache or dizziness might point toward a vertebral artery source, possibly detectable by angiography. Treatment will depend on the site and nature of the source of embolus.

## Ischemia of the Cerebellum

Ischemia of the cerebellum is a life-threatening lesion that must be distinguished from other lesions because its management, possibly including surgical decompression, is so different.

A 59-year-old woman had three spells of transient whirling dizziness. On awakening she complained of diplopia and was unable to get to the bathroom because of staggering to the left. She vomited and had a left occipital headache. Examination revealed a sleepy woman with slow-course nystagmus on left gaze, decreased left corneal reflex, and a grossly ataxic gait with leaning to the left when she stood or sat. She held her head taut with the occiput to the left.

Headache, vomiting, gait ataxia, reduced alertness, and neck stiffness are symptoms and signs that suggest involvement of the cerebellum. In this case, prior warnings suggest an occlusive mechanism, usually occlusion of the vertebral artery. When onset is sudden, hemorrhage is difficult to distinguish clinically. The diagnosis of cerebellar infarction should also be considered in the patient with a lateral medullary syndrome who is sleepy, has severe headache, or resists head movement. Therapy with agents that might decrease intracranial pressure, for example, mannitol, corticosteroids, or glycerol, should be started immediately. Computed tomography will corroborate hemorrhage and may confirm infarction or pressure on the 4th ventricle. Remember that the early CT scan may miss a cerebellar infarct.

MRI may allow better delineation of the vascular territory of the infarction. T2-weighted sagittal sections are especially helpful in anatomic localization.[11,408] When the lesion is restricted to PICA territory, occlusion of the vertebral artery is likely, either by in situ thrombosis or embolism.[84] Superior cerebellar artery territory infarcts are predominantly embolic, especially when combined with thalamic and/or posterior cerebral artery territory infarction.[11,13,265]

The patient who continues to deteriorate despite administration of osmotic agents and steroids, surgical decompression may be lifesaving. In some cases, it may be difficult clinically to separate pressure signs produced by a swollen cerebellum from more extensive brain stem ischemia, in which case arteriography could better define the extent of the vascular lesion and collaterals.

## Ischemia in the Distribution of Lateral Circumferential Branches

When ischemia is limited to PICA, AICA, or SCA territory, occlusion of the main basilar artery is very uncommon.

A 70-year-old woman exhibited, over 2 days, dizziness, deafness in the left ear, left facial palsy, and ataxic gain. Examination revealed left Horner syndrome, decreased pain, and temperature sensation on the left face and right body, left limb ataxia, and nystagmus and corroborated palsy of the left 7th cranial nerve and left ear deafness.

Such a patient should be carefully observed for the development of a cerebellar pressure cone. In some cases, CT can confirm the limits of the infarction. In the case of a PICA territory lesion the underlying cause is usually occlusion of the vertebral artery. Occlusion of the AICA is usually due to occlusive disease within the branch. On occasion, an embolus may lodge in these lateral circumferential vascular territories; therefore a source for embolus should be sought. The yield of arteriography or prophylactic treatment is probably small in this group of patients, since they improve spontaneously and usually do not have a high risk of further brain stem ischemia.

## Recurrent Transient Ischemic Attacks Without a Fixed Deficit

Patients who have recurrent TIAs without a fixed deficit are the least homogeneous group, and perhaps the most difficult to decide on a course of action.

A 60-year-old woman had eight spells of vertigo, which were brief and, on one occasion, associated with diplopia and numbness about the left lip. Examination was normal.

Some recurrent transient episodes, especially vertigo and drop attacks, have nonvascular mechanisms. In this case, numbness of the face does suggest a central location. As in this patient, vertigo, dizziness, and diplopia or ataxia commonly point to a proximal lesion, such as subclavian steal or stenosis of the proximal or distal vertebral artery. When the lesion is in the basilar artery, paretic spells, sensory symptoms, and headache are more common, although these rules are not clear enough to allow confident distinction in the individual patient. Occasionally small-vessel lesions can give rise to TIAs, in which case these usually occur over a shorter period and are more frequently stereotyped. Many factors, for example, the general health of the patient, presence of hypertension or peptic ulcer, the variability, severity and frequency of attacks, and whether the pattern of attacks changes over time, will determine whether the clinician empirically tries aspirin, other platelet-agglutinating agents, or warfarin, or pursues more aggressive evaluation prior to treatment. In some circumstances the definition of the vascular lesion might lead to consideration of a surgical shunt.

In our opinion, such patients should all be studied by noninvasive ultrasound technology, studying both the extracranial vertebral and subclavian arteries and the intracranial vessels by transcranial Doppler, hematocrit, platelet count, and prothrombin; partial thromboplastin times should also be measured. MR angiography may also be helpful. When the etiology remains uncertain after these studies, or the preliminary studies indicate a region of severe stenosis or occlusion, angiography should be considered.

## Gradually Progressive Dysfunction of the Medulla and/or Cerebellum

In gradually progressive dysfunction of the medulla and/or cerebellum the lesions are usually maximal in the caudal stem and mimic brain tumor.

> A 60-year-old diabetic man complained of occipital and mastoid pain, and gradually, over a month, became more ataxic and immobile. Examination revealed striking left rotatory nystagmus, weakness of the right limbs, slurred speech, and left limb ataxia. Changing position made him cry out with dizziness and pain.

In this case, cerebellar and brain stem dysfunction evolved gradually but inexorably. A CT scan revealed pressure on the 4th ventricle and slight hydrocephalus. Steroids improved the headache. Transcranial Doppler showed no anterograde flow in either intracranial vertebral artery and retrograde flow down the basilar artery. Angiography confirmed occlusion of the intracranial left vertebral artery, a congenitally small or previously occluded right vertebral artery, and retrograde flow from the internal carotid artery

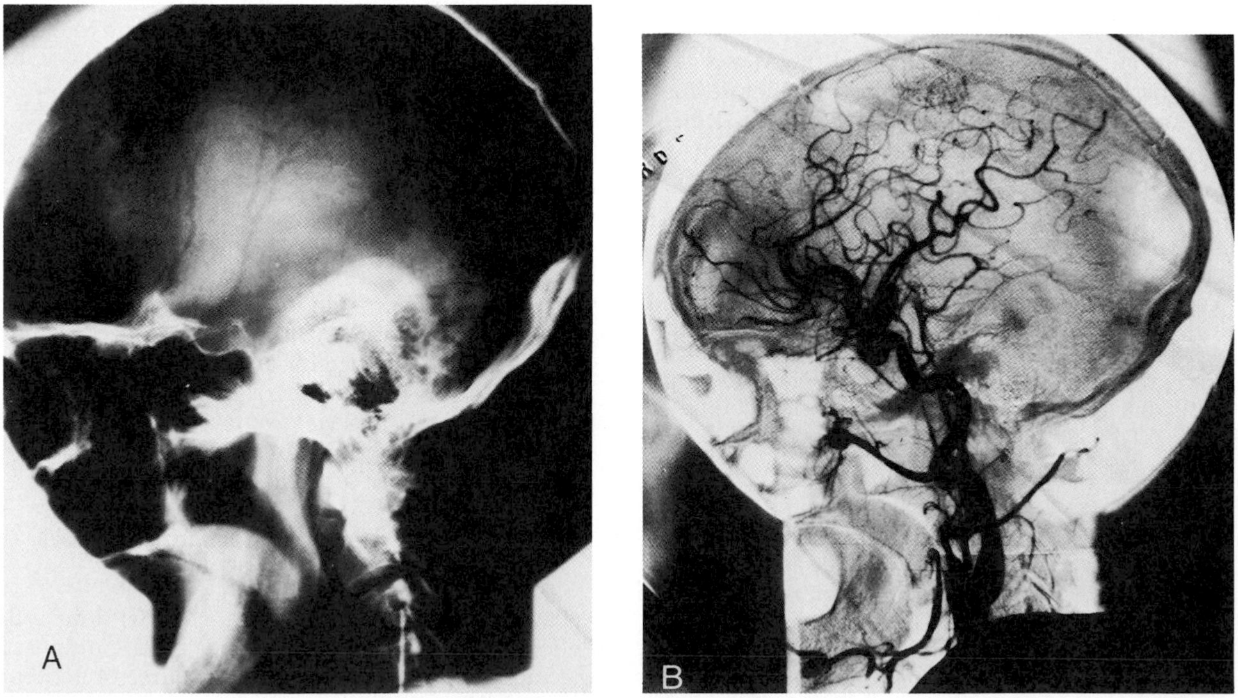


**Fig. 18-17.** (**A**) Cerebral angiography. The vertebral artery is opacified only very low in the neck, with a tapered ending. (**B**) Carotid angiography. There is retrograde filling of the basilar artery to near its origin. The right vertebral artery did not opacify from the subclavian artery or aortic arch.

down to the proximal basilar artery (Fig. 18-17). Progressive lower brain stem disease is usually due to bilateral vertebral artery disease. Occasionally a cerebellar infarction or hemorrhage can produce a slowly evolving course. This group of patients has a grim prognosis unless specific diagnosis and remedial treatment is initiated. An aggressive diagnostic and therapeutic strategy is warranted because of the poor outlook. If a large cerebellar infarct or hemorrhage is confirmed, surgical decompression is critical. If the mechanism is ischemia due to poor perfusion, a surgical shunt should be considered.

## DIAGNOSTIC TESTS

With the advent of high-quality magnetic resonance imaging, most regions of infarction can be diagnosed noninvasively, and less reliance is made on cerebral angiography, hitherto the principal diagnostic investigation in patients with vertebrobasilar occlusive disease. The use of the studies summarized below are cited widely throughout this chapter. Here attention will be paid briefly to general comments concerning the techniques themselves.

### Magnetic Resonance Imaging

The lack of signal from bone has given MR imaging a great advantage over CT for infarcts in the brain stem.[120,270] MR demonstrates signal abnormalities earlier than CT in the brain stem.[339] A long T2-weighted image has been preferred. In some studies, more MRI lesions were found than CT lesions: in 22 cases of TIA, among the 12 with negative CT scan, 5 were negative in MRI, 6 had a single MRI lesion, while in 10, with multiple MRI lesions, 5 had a negative CT, 4 showed a single CT abnormality, and only 1 had multiple abnormalities.[23] This study was done with modern equipment: a 1200 Picker CT scanner and 0.6 or 1.5 Tesla Technicare MRI. Similar observations on the sensitivity of MR have been made subsequently by others.[335,409] The imaging qualities have been good enough that it has been possible to find explanations for medial longitudinal fasciculus lesions not seen by CT.[24] Even cerebellar infarcts, usually imaged by CT, are better imaged by MR.[10]

Contrast enhancement using gadolinium-DTPA has been successful in demonstrating small infarcts of lacunar size[335] and has been useful in brain stem infarction.

In a few instances, it has been possible to identify stenosis of the basilar itself by performing the MR in the coronal or saggital plane.[39] The thickened walls of the dolicoectatic basilar has become a familiar sight as has the compression of the brain stem by the tortuous arteries, all of which are new findings clearly demonstrated by MR.[47]

### Computed Tomography

Newer generation CT scanners can reveal cerebellar, posterior cerebral hemisphere, and brain stem softenings.[339] In patients with only transient ischemic attacks in the posterior circulation, the scan is usually normal.[274] Cerebellar and pontine hemorrhages are almost always visible on CT; thus an early scan not demonstrating a dense lesion effectively excludes significant parenchymatous bleeding. Cerebellar infarcts scanned early, during the first 2 or 3 days, may be missed by CT. Brain stem softenings are also imperfectly imaged, although Hinshaw and colleagues[239] were able to delineate lucent regions among their patients with posterior circulation infarcts as follows: in the cerebellar territory of the posterior inferior cerebellar artery and in the lateral medulla in four patients, in the cerebellum and lateral pons in the territory of the anterior inferior cerebellar artery in four patients, and in the superior cerebellar artery territory in the cerebellum, midbrain, and pons in six other patients. Six patients had lucent lesions limited to the brain stem. In this study, most of the scans were performed after 5 days. Computed tomography is especially helpful in patients with cerebellar infarction. Even when a discrete region of cerebellar softening is not visible, the CT scan will visualize compression of the 4th ventricle, posterior fossa crowding with reduced cisternal size, and hydrocephalus; these may be useful clues to the diagnosis. In a CT study of 31 acute posterior fossa infarcts, 10 of 12 patients with fatal outcome showed complete obliteration of posterior fossa cisterns, small or absent 4th ventricles, and hydrocephalus.[472] At times, the basilar artery failed to opacify after the introduction of contrast. The principal uses of CT in posterior circulation disease are

1. To separate brain stem and cerebellar hemorrhage from occlusive disease
2. To establish cerebellar infarction and posterior fossa pressure
3. To determine the presence and distribution of distal basilar territory infarction (occipital and temporal lobe) in patients with symptoms of brain stem ischemia
4. To visualize basilar artery aneurysms

### Angiography

Opacification of the vertebral and basilar arteries and their major branches, either by venous[412] or arterial injection, and by digital[482] or cut-film techniques, is the only investigation that allows the clinician to determine the location, nature, and severity of occlusive disease within the posterior circulation. In 1960 Meyer et al.[328] reported the frequency of significant arterial lesions uncovered by arteriography in their patients with vertebrobasilar disease. Of 36 patients, 35 had significant lesions, most often in the basilar artery (11 cases) or in one or both vertebral arteries and the basilar artery (8 cases). Subsequent studies have documented the fact that arteriography can delineate the nature of vertebrobasilar occlusive lesions. The exact frequency of lesions varies with the indications for angiography and the criteria used to judge whether a given lesion is significant. In some series, the incidence of appropriate vertebrobasilar occlusive lesions is relatively low, for example, 41 percent.[466] Angiography of the posterior circulation has proved surprisingly safe. Torma and Fogelholm[467] described 7 serious complications in 249 vertebral angiograms (2.8 percent), all of which cleared within 72 hours. Weibel and Fields[481] had 9 percent total complications in 846 posterior circulation angiograms; all were slight or local and were not disabling. Pribram[390] cited only 2 serious complications in 357 vertebral artery studies (0.56 percent): 1 asymptomatic iatrogenic vertebral artery occlusion and 1 cerebellar syndrome. Lester and Klee[290] reported on complications of 337 percutaneous vertebral angiograms. There were only 7 cerebral complications: 5 (vertigo, increased migraine, and increased ischemic symptoms) cleared rapidly. Two patients died. One had a ruptured basilar aneurysm and the other basilar artery occlusion; each was deteriorating and desperately ill at the time of angiography. Faught et al.[141] reported 1 cerebral complication in 31 patients with vertebral basilar symptoms (3.2 percent). Field and colleagues[146] reported their experience with 1,000 brachial arteriograms; there was a total complication rate of 0.99 percent, 3.3 percent slight complications, and 0.60 percent serious. In their hands only 1 in 157 patients having a brachial arteriogram had a serious complication. Wishart[494] had 1 serious complication in 215 vertebral artery studies.

The advent of newer catheters and dyes, increasing numbers of studies performed by trained neuroradiologists, better filming techniques, and the likely widespread use of intravenous dye injection all promise to make posterior circulation arterial opacification even safer in the future. By allowing a more accurate diagnosis in uncertain cases, angiography should guide the clinician to a more rational choice of therapy.

## Doppler Examination of the Subclavian, Vertebral, and Basilar Arteries

The early attempts at estimating the presence of occlusive disease was by means of oscillographic measurement of forearm blood flow, venous occlusive plethysmography of the arm[33] and study of the relative velocity of propagation of pulse waves in the two arms[36] They served to detect subclavian occlusion and infer reversed flow in the vertebral supplying the distal subclavian.[297,485]

More recently, direct analysis of the velocity profiles in the vertebrobasilar using continuous-wave Doppler ultrasound techniques, which can detect flow and flow direction at the skull base (C2), and is capable of predicting vertebral artery stenosis or hypoplasia.[41,232]

The difficulty accessing the vertebral arteries in the neck has prevented extensive study of this vascular territory by duplex Doppler techniques, which entail the use of larger probes than those used for continuous-wave Doppler studies. The extracranial vertebrals gain access to the transverse processes at about C6, and course cephalad where they are accessible to Doppler insonation, where they cross the narrow spaces bridging the transverse processes. At the skull base, the sharp turns taken by the artery make it difficult to detect and follow a stable reflected signal from the blood flowing in the arteries. A further problem is that most of the arteriosclerosis is at the origin of the vertebral from the subclavian, which is located in a difficult place to insonate, behind the clavicle.[41,232]

Despite these limitations, duplex Doppler insonation of the accessible, small segments of the vertebral artery have allowed diagnosis of some instances of occlusion and reversal of flow. Color-flow Doppler imaging has made it easier to detect the signal between the transverse processes.[469] Even under the best of conditions, the quantitative assessments are more often frustrated by the considerable asymmetry in flow velocity and pulsatility in vertebral arteries due to asymmetric vessel diameters of both vertebrals and the many variations in the vertebra-basilar circulation.

Retrograde flow in one vertebral artery has proved a reliable sign of ipsilateral subclavian stenosis or occlusion causing retrograde vertebral artery flow. The discovery of no velocity or a high-resistance velocity profile on cephalad flow is also fairly reliable indicator of occlusion between the probe and the skull. Normal flow velocity, usually a sign the entire vessel is patent, may be found when the occlusion lies cephalad to the posterior inferior cerebellar artery, as flow into this branch often suffices to keep a normal velocity profile in the vertebral artery below the occlusion.[461]

Transcranial Doppler insonates the velocity profile of the intracranial vertebral and basilar arteries. The faint signal requires the operator to direct the Doppler beam almost exactly along the same axis as that of the artery. When the basilar curves dorsally over the pons, the signal is often lost to the probe placed at the base of the skull. Despite these limitations, transcranial Doppler has proved useful in estimating high-grade stenosis of the vertebral artery or basilar artery, and can often detect severe atheromatous stenosis that is typically located at the vertebrobasilar junction.[232]

Bidirectional flow in the basilar is also frequently detected when the subclavian steal is present.[477]

## Cerebral Blood Flow

Xenon-133 inhalation is a noninvasive method of quantifying regional cerebral blood flow in alert humans. Controversy has surrounded measurements in the vertebrobasilar territory.[122] Juge et al.[260] evaluated the validity of regional cerebral blood flow determinations in the brain stem and cerebellar region by studying contamination from surrounding extracerebral sources (nasopharynx, muscles, paranasal sinuses), establishing reproducibility, and comparing the results from xenon-133 inhalation with those derived from other normal human and animal studies. These investigators believe the xenon-133 inhalation values are reliable, reproducible, and indicative of cerebral blood flow to these regions. In addition, Meyer and colleagues,[326,327] among others,[225] have coupled the xenon-133 inhalation technique to CT imaging, making it possible to visualize regions of reduced blood flow and compare them with normal regions.

As with cerebral blood flow in the carotid territory, it is still unclear what use posterior circulation blood flow measurements have in the clinical evaluation of the patient. Without knowledge of the vascular lesion, blood flow measurements are difficult to interpret. For example, it would not be surprising to find reduced occipital and temporal lobe blood flow in a patient with basilar artery occlusion. Another individual with basilar occlusion might have sufficient collateral circulation to practically normalize cerebral blood flow; this patient's cerebral blood flow would be difficult to distinguish from a patient with a pontine lacune and a patent basilar artery. At present, for the clinician, cerebral blood flow data add to angiographic information but do not substitute for vascular opacification. Positron emission tomography scanning adds the capability of studying metabolism and blood flow, but to date has not been rigorously used to study posterior circulation occlusive disease.

## Nuclear Brain Scan

Technical factors have limited the capability of imaging the vertebral arteries by radionuclide angiography. Infarcts in the cerebellum and the temporal and occipital lobes may be seen on radionuclide scanning, but not usually well enough to help in differential diagnosis, and the anatomic detail is inferior to that obtained by CT. Small or early lesions are not well visualized by radionuclide techniques.

## Clinical Neurophysiology

### Electroencephalography

Approximately 70 percent of electroencephalograms (EEGs) in patients with vertebrobasilar disease are considered normal. Abnormalities are often slight or bilateral and include shifting focal slowing[90,474] and low-voltage fast activity. In a study of 20 patients with vascular lesions of the pons and caudal midbrain, 10 patients had normal EEGs; EEG abnormalities that were found had no relationship to the location or extent of the brain stem lesion or to the behavioral state of the patient.[90] The authors commented, "In the comatose patient, an EEG resembling that of the waking state is a pathognomonic sign of brain stem injury." Pontomesencephalic lesions are the cause of stupor in some patients with rhythmic alpha range activity not reactive to stimuli (alpha pattern coma). In one study, EEG slowing was well correlated with cerebral hemisphere infarction, but EEG abnormalities were quite variable in patients with vertebrobasilar disease.[85] The EEG has not usually yielded helpful diagnostic information.

### Brain Stem Auditory Evoked Responses

In several patients with "alpha coma," markedly abnormal brain stem auditory evoked responses supported the diagnosis of brain stem infarction.[222,442] Stern and colleagues[441] analyzed brain-stem auditory evoked responses in 35 patients with ischemic brain stem lesions. Abnormal responses predicted an unstable or poor outcome in pontomesencephalic lesions; in medullary infarcts the brain stem auditory evoked response was also frequently abnormal (7 of 11 cases) but was not helpful prognostically. Further clinicopathologic analysis is needed to define the role of auditory responses in the diagnosis and prognosis of posterior circulation ischemia.

## TREATMENT

Unfortunately not a single definitive study establishes the advantages or disadvantages of a given therapy for patients with well-defined occlusive vascular disease within the posterior circulation. Published studies are either small or not randomized or contain patients lumped together under the general term *vertebrobasilar insufficiency*, often without further definition of the severity and nature of the vascular lesion. Aspirin and other agents that affect platelet agglutination have been infrequently studied. The Canadian Cooperative Study[29] included 86 patients with vertebrobasilar TIAs and 49 patients with slight nonprogressive vertebrobasilar strokes. Of the 75 posterior circulation patients studied angiographically, 82 percent had significant appropriately situated lesions.[29] Aspirin reduced the risk of recurrent episodes, stroke, and death in men in both the vertebrobasilar and carotid groups, but not in women. Sulfinpyrazone had no definite effect. The American Aspirin Study[151] excluded patients with only vertebrobasilar attacks. A German study showed a slight statistically insignificant trend favoring a beneficial effect of aspirin in occlusive vertebrobasilar disease.[397]

Enthusiasm for the use of anticoagulants grew in the 1950s when this form of treatment was being evaluated for vascular disease of all varieties and locations. A number of reports from the Mayo Clinic cerebrovascular department[330,332,333,427,483] enthusiastically supported the use of anticoagulants for TIA and progressing stroke within the vertebrobasilar system. Millikan and colleagues[332] first reported 21 patients who had progressive vertebrobasilar symptoms and were given anticoagulants. Only 14 percent of these patients died, whereas during this same period 43 percent of 23 patients who were not treated with anticoagulation and had a similar clinical profile had died. All five patients with intermittent attacks in the vertebrobasilar system had clearing of the attacks. Whisnant[483] collected 140 patients with progressive symptoms due to vertebrobasilar occlusion who were treated with anticoagulants: 12 (8.5 percent) died, whereas 23 of 39 (58.9 percent) similar patients not on anticoagulants died. Patients in this study had ischemia that was assumed to be not restricted to a single arterial branch of the vertebral or basilar artery, and showed some signs of progressing deficit. The patients were not randomized, the study was retrospective, and most vascular lesions were not verified angiographically. Also, a high percentage of patients with intermittent spells of vertebrobasilar insufficiency had attacks cease after institution of anticoagulant therapy. Following these reports, it became customary in most centers to treat patients with vertebrobasilar ischemia with anticoagulants, though a true randomized study of anticoagulant treatment has not been performed. Other reports usually contain small numbers of nonrandomized patients. Fazekas et al.[142] described 26 patients of whom 10 had only vertebrobasilar TIAs and 16 had some clinical deficit; 14 were treated with anticoagulants for 6 to 50 months, and the remaining 12 were considered unsuitable for anticoagulant therapy because of "medical or personality disorders." All 26 patients improved; only 3 continued to have episodes (1 on anticoagulants, 2 not), but of decreased frequency. In a series of patients with vertebrobasilar disease seen by Bradshaw and McQuaid,[50] six were treated with anticoagulants. Of these, one with verified basilar occlusion died and five did well, although two had persistent attacks. Of 48 patients with vertebrobasilar disease not treated with anticoagulants, 38 did well.

The use of anticoagulants has been associated with dramatic cessation of attacks or improvement in a progressing vertebrobasilar deficit. Most experienced clinicians will verify their immediate effectiveness in some patients. Heparin and warfarin each have a role to play in patient management, but at present this opinion is conjectural and unproven. In our experience, patients with basilar artery stenosis and transient episodes have responded to warfarin and often have had recurrent spells after cessation of treatment; on the other hand, few patients with vertebral or basilar artery occlusion experience progressive symptoms during the weeks after their stroke, even without anticoagulants.[65] Perhaps these latter patients would better be treated with heparin for 4 weeks or less. Branch disease probably does not warrant use of heparin or warfarin.

The most promising new treatment of recent thromboembolic occlusions of the vertebral and basilar arteries is thrombolytic agents.[58,112,145,213,233,379,433,487,505,506] Hacke[213] and colleagues treated 65 consecutive patients with clinical signs of severe ischemia of the brain stem and thrombotic basilar artery occlusions shown angiographically: 43 were given local intra-arterial thrombolytic therapy (urokinase or streptokinase) and 22 were given anticoagulants or agents that alter platelet function. Recanalization was shown in 19 of the 43 patients treated with thrombolytic agents. All patients without recanalization died, but 14 of the 19 in whom the artery reopened survived, 10 with a good clinical outcome. Only 3 of 22 patients not treated with thrombolytic agents survived, all with moderately severe deficits. Local infusion by catheter of recombinant tissue plasminogen activator has also proven effective[233] but few patients have been reported. Systemic use of recombinant tissue plasminogen activator is also feasible and has been effective in a single case report.[487] del Zoppo[112,113] has recently reviewed the experience with thrombolytic agents in vertebrobasilar occlusive disease. Discussions at a meeting devoted to vertebrobasilar occlusive disease highlight our knowledge and lack of experience with thrombolytic agents in patients with posterior circulation disease.[34]

The utility of other medical regimens has not been studied in vertebrobasilar disease; for example, despite the widespread prescription of vasodilator agents such as papaverine for cerebrovascular disease, there are no well-designed studies that consider its effect on posterior circulation disease.[66] A wide range of surgical procedures has been performed. Vertebral artery reconstruction or bypass in the neck,[61,252,253,407] dilatation of vertebral artery stenosis by balloon[415] or transluminal angioplasty,[348] and intracranial vertebral artery endarterectomy[7] have been performed on occasion. Sundt and colleagues[449] have performed transluminal angioplasty on two reported patients with refractory ischemia due to tight basilar stenosis. These procedures can be effective, but to date the indications are uncertain and the operations are unwise in inexperienced hands. The open net theory of cerebrovascular disease has led many to perform carotid endarterectomy for patients with vertebrobasilar disease. When this procedure has been studied, the results were disappointing.[319]

Bypass grafts have been used to attempt to buoy up the flagging posterior circulation.[20,21,248,271,405,447,448] Donor vessels such as the occipital or superficial temporal arteries may be anastomosed to PICA, AICA, SCA, or even the posterior cerebral artery. The choice of recipient vessel depends on the site of occlusion; for example, with a lower basilar occlusion an anastomosis to the AICA is performed, whereas in vertebral occlusion a PICA recipient is chosen. An interposed venous or arterial graft is sometimes used.[22,450] It is also important to have blood from the donor vessel widely disseminated; a blocked recipient artery will not be of great help in restoring flow elsewhere in the posterior circulation. Surgical shunts can be created and in experienced hands usually remain patent. Greatest potential benefit of a shunt is in the patient with severe occlusive disease whose deficit is due to diminished flow and who has not responded to more conservative medical measures. Bilateral vertebral artery intracranial occlusion, basilar occlusion with progressing deficit, and continued TIAs due to severe basilar stenosis are all possible indications. Randomized controlled studies testing any form of posterior circulation surgery are wanting.

The advent of modern endovascular treatment capabilities and neuroradiologists and neurosurgeons trained and specialized in interventional radiographic techniques also opens up new potential treatments. To date, there is too little experience with the use of these techniques in occlusive posterior circulation disease, but undoubtedly their use will increase and be tested in the near future.

Diagnostic techniques are proliferating and we now have available potent medical and surgical therapies. It is hoped that the experience of the next decades will allow for more rational treatment of the complex, heterogeneous conditions that are included under the category of vertebrobasilar disease.

## REFERENCES


1. Ackerman E, Levinsohn M, Richards D et al: Basilar artery occlusion in a 10-year-old boy. *Ann Neurol* 11:204, 1977
2. Ackerstaff RG, Hoenefeld H, Slowikowski JM et al: Ultrasonic duplex scanning in atherosclerotic disease of the innominate, subclavian and vertebral arteries: a comparative study with angiography. Ultrasound Med Biol 10:409, 1984
3. Adams R: Occlusion of the anterior inferior cerebellar artery. Arch Neurol Psychiatry 49:765, 1983
4. Alajouanine T, Lhermitte F, Gautier J: Transient cerebral ischemia in atherosclerosis. Neurology (NY) 10:906, 1960
5. Alexander A: The treatment of epilepsy by ligature of the vertebral arteries. Brain 5:170, 1882
6. Alexander C, Burger P, Goree J: Dissecting aneurysms of the basilar artery. Stroke 10:294, 1979
7. Allen G, Cohen R, Preziosi T: Microsurgical endarterectomy of the intracranial vertebral artery for vertebrobasilar transient ischemic attacks. Neurosurgery 81:56, 1981
8. Alom J, Matias-Gurer J, Padeo L et al: Spontaneous dissection of intracranial vertebral artery: clinical recovery with conservative treatment. J Neurol Neurosurg Psychiatry 49:599, 1986
9. Alpert J, Gerson L, Hall R et al: Reversible angiopathy. Stroke 13:100, 1982
10. Amarenco P: Les infarctus du cervelet. Presse Med 18:909, 1991
11. Amarenco P, Hauw JJ: Anatomie des artères cérébelleuses. Rev Neurol 145:267, 1989
12. Amarenco P, Hauw JJ: Cerebellar infarction in the territory of the superior cerebellar artery. Neurology (NY) 40:1383, 1990
13. Amarenco P, Hauw JJ, Gautier JC: Arterial pathology in cerebellar infarction. Stroke 21:1299, 1990
14. Amarenco P, Hauw JJ, Henin D et al: Les infarctus du territoire de l'artère cérébelleuse postéro-inférieure: étude clinico-pathologique de 28 cas. Rev Neurol 145:277, 1989
15. Archer C, Horenstein S: Basilar artery occlusion: clinical and radiological correlation. Stroke 8:383, 1977
16. Asplund K, Wester P, Fodstad H et al: Long time survival after vertebral/basilar occlusion. Stroke 11:304, 1980
17. Atkinson WJ: The anterior inferior cerebellar artery. J Neurol Neurosurg Psychiatry 12:137, 1949
18. Auerbach S, De Piero T, Romanul F: Sylvian aqueduct syndrome caused by unilateral midbrain lesion. Ann Neurol 11:91, 1982
19. Ausman J, Diaz F, de los Reyes RA et al: Occipital artery to anterior inferior cerebellar artery anastamosis for vertebrobasilar junction stenosis. Surg Neurol 16:99, 1981
20. Ausman JI, Diaz FG, Pearce JE et al: Endarterectomy of the vertebral artery from C-2 to posterior inferior cerebellar artery intracranially. Surg Neurol 18:400, 1982
21. Ausman J, Nicoloff D, Chou S: Posterior fossa revascularization anastamosis of vertebral artery to PICA with interposed radial artery graft. Surg Neurol 9:281, 1978
22. Ausman J, Lee M, Chater N et al: Superficial artery to superior cerebellar artery anastomosis for distal basilar artery stenosis. Surg Neurol 12:277, 1979
23. Awad I, Modic M, Little JR et al: Focal parenchymal lesions in transient ischemic attacks: correlation of computed tomography and magnetic resonance imaging. Stroke 17:399, 1986
24. Awerbuch G, Brown M, Levin JR: Magnetic resonance imaging correlates of internuclear ophthalmoplegia. Int J Neurosci 52:39, 1990
25. Babinski J, Nageotte J: Hémiasynergie, latéropulsion et myosis bulbaires avec hémianesthésie et hemiplégie croisées. Rev Neurol 10:358, 1902
26. Baker R, Rosenbaum A, Caplan L: Subclavian steal syndrome. Contemp Surg 4:96, 1974
27. Barnes KL, Ferrario CM: Role of the central nervous system in cardiovascular regulation. In Furlan A (ed): The Heart and Stroke. Springer-Verlag, Heidelberg, 1987
28. Barnes M, Hunt B, Williams I: The role of verte-

bral angiography in the investigation of third nerve palsy. J Neurol Neurosurg Psychiatry 44:1153, 1981
29. Barnett HJ: The Canadian Cooperative Study of platelet suppressive drugs in transient cerebral ischemia. p. 221. In Price T, Nelson E (eds): Cerebrovascular Disease. Proceedings of the Eleventh Princeton Conference. Raven Press, New York, 1979
30. Barrows L, Kubik C, Richardson E: Aneurysms of the basilar and vertebral arteries: a clinicopathologic study. Trans Am Neurol Assoc 81:181, 1956
31. Bauer G, Prugger M, Rumpl E: Stimulus evoked oral automatisms in the locked-in syndrome. Arch Neurol 39:435, 1982
32. Bauer R, Sheehan S, Wechsler N et al: Arteriographic study of sites, incidence and treatment of arteriosclerotic cerebrovascular lesions. Neurology (NY) 12:698, 1962
33. Bergan J, MacDonald J: Recognition of cerebrovascular fibromuscular hyperplasia. Arch Surg 98:332, 1969
34. Berguer R, Caplan LR: Panel discussion: vertigo. p. 165. In: Vertebrobasilar Disease. Quality Medical Publications, St. Louis, 1991
35. Berguer R, Feldman AJ: Surgical reconstruction of the vertebral artery. Surgery 93:670, 1983
36. Berguer R, Higgins R, Nelson R: Non-invasive diagnosis of reversal of vertebral artery blood flow. N Engl J Med 302:1349, 1980
37. Bickerstaff E: Basilar artery migraine. Lancet 1:15, 1961
38. Biemond A: Thrombosis of the basilar artery and the vascularization of the brainstem. Brain 74: 300, 1951
39. Biller J, Yuh W, Mitchell GW: Early diagnosis of basilar artery occlusion using magnetic resonance imaging. Stroke 19:297, 1988
40. Bjewer K, Silkerskjold BP: Lateropulsion and imbalance in Wallenberg's syndrome. Acta Neurol Scand 44:91, 1968
41. Bluth EL, Merritt CR, Sullivan MA et al: Usefulness of duplex ultrasound in evaluating vertebral arteries. J Ultrasound Med 8:229, 1989
42. Bogousslavsky J, Gates PC, Fox AJ et al: Bilateral occlusion of vertebral artery. Neurology (NY) 36:1309, 1986
43. Bogousslavsky J, Khurana R, Deruaz JP et al: Respiratory failure and unilateral caudal brainstem infarction. Ann Neurol 28:668, 1990
44. Bogousslavsky J, Miklossy J, Deruaz JP et al: Unilateral left paramedian infarction of the thalamus and midbrain: a clinico-pathological study. J Neurol Neurosurg Psychiatry 49:686, 1986
45. Bogousslavsky J, Regli F: Upgaze palsy and monocular paresis of downgaze from ipsilateral thalamo-mesencephalic infarction: a vertical one-and-a-half syndrome. J Neurol 231:43, 1984
46. Bogousslavsky J, Regli F, Assal G: The syndrome of unilateral tuberothalamic artery territory infarction. Stroke 17:434, 1986
47. Bollensen E, Buzanoski JH, Prange HW: Brainstem compression by basilar artery anomalies as visualized by MRI. J Neurol 238:49, 1991
48. Borison H, Wang S: Physiology and pharmacology of vomiting. Pharmacol Rev 5:193, 1953
49. Bosch E, Kenlledy S, Aschenbrenner C: Ocular bobbing: the myth of its localizing valve. Neurology (NY) 25:949, 1975
50. Bradshaw P, McQuaid P: The syndrome of vertebrobasilar insufficiency. Q J Med 32:279, 1963
51. Brewster DC, Moncure AC, Darling C et al: Innominate artery lesions: problems encountered and lessons learned. J Vasc Surg 2:99, 1985
52. Brierley JB: The neuropathology of brain hypoxia. p. 243. In Critchley M, O'Leary J, Jennett B (eds): Scientific Foundations of Neurology. FA Davis, Philadelphia, 1972
53. Bright R: Cases illustrative of the effects produced when the arteries and brain are diseased. Guys Hosp Rep 1:9, 1836
54. Bronstein AM, Morris J, DuBoulay G et al: Abnormalities of horizontal gaze: clinical, oculographic and magnetic resonance imaging findings. I. Abducens palsy. J Neurol Neurosurg Psychiatry 53:194, 1990
55. Bronstein AM, Rudge P, Gresty MA et al: Abnormalities of horizontal gaze: clinical, oculographic and magnetic resonance imaging findings. II. Gaze palsy and internuclear ophthalmoplegia. J Neurol Neurosurg Psychiatry 53:200, 1990
56. Brouckaert L, Sieben G, De Reuck J et al: The syndrome of the anterior inferior cerebellar artery. Acta Neurol Belg 81:65, 1981
57. Browne T, Poskanzer D: Treatment of strokes. N Engl J Med 281:594, 1969
58. Bruckmann H, Ferbert A, del Zoppo G et al: The acute vertebrobasilar thrombosis: angiological-clinical comparison and therapeutic implications. Acta Radiol (Stockh), suppl. 369:38, 1986
59. Bull J: Contribution of radiology to the study of intracranial aneurysms. Br Med J 2:1701, 1962
60. Buttner-Ennever J, Buttner U, Cohen B et al: Vertical gaze paralysis and the rostral interstitial nucleus of the medial longitudinal fasciculus. Brain 105:125, 1982
61. Callow A: Surgical management of varying patterns of vertebral artery and subclavian artery insufficiency. N Engl J Med 270:546, 1964
62. Caplan L: Ptosis. J Neurol Neurosurg Psychiatry 37:1, 1974
63. Caplan LR: Lacunar infarction: a neglected concept. Geriatrics 3:71, 1976
64. Caplan L: A tale of two brothers. Headache 17:49, 1977
65. Caplan L: Occlusion of the vertebral or basilar artery. Stroke 10:277, 1979
66. Caplan L: Use of vasodilating drugs in cerebral symptomatology. p. 305. In Miller R, Greenblatt D (eds): Drug Therapy Reviews. Elsevier-North-Holland, Amsterdam, 1979
67. Caplan L: "Top of the basilar" syndrome: selected clinical aspects. Neurology (NY) 30:72, 1980
68. Caplan L: Bilateral distal vertebral artery occlusion. Neurology (NY) 33:552, 1983

69. Caplan LR: Vertebrobasilar system syndromes. p. 371. In Vinken PJ, Bruyn GW, Klawans HL (eds): Handbook of Clinical Neurology. North-Holland Publishing, Amsterdam, 1988
70. Caplan LR: Intracranial branch atheromatous disease: a neglected, understudied and underused concept. Neurology (NY) 39:1246, 1989
71. Caplan LR: Charles Foix—the first modern stroke neurologist. Stroke 21:348, 1990
72. Caplan LR: Migraine and vertebrobasilar ischemia. Neurology (NY) 41:55, 1991
73. Caplan L, Baker R: Extracranial occlusive disease: does size matter? Stroke 11:63, 1980
74. Caplan LR, Baquis G, Pessin MS et al: Dissection of the intracranial vertebral artery. Neurology (NY) 38:868, 1988
75. Caplan LR, Brass LM, DeWitt LD et al: Transcranial Doppler ultrasound: present status. Neurology (NY) 40:696, 1990
76. Caplan L, Chedru F, Lhermitte F et al: Transient global amnesia and migraine. Neurology (NY) 31:1167, 1981
77. Caplan LR, DeWitt LD, Pessin MS et al: Lateral thalamic infarcts. Arch Neurol 45:959, 1988
78. Caplan L, Goodwin J: Hypertensive lateral tegmental brainstem hemorrhage. Neurology (NY) 32:252, 1982
79. Caplan L, Gorelick P: Salt and pepper in the face pain in acute brainstem ischemia. Ann Neurol 13:344, 1983
80. Caplan LR, Gorelick PB, Hier DB: Race, sex and occlusive cerebrovascular disease: a review. Stroke 17:648, 1986
81. Caplan J, Rosenbaum A: Role of cerebral angiography in vertebrobasilar occlusive disease. J Neurol Neurosurg Psychiatry 38:601, 1975
82. Caplan LR, Schmahmann JD, Kase CS et al: Caudate infarcts. Arch Neurol 47:133, 1990
83. Caplan L, Sergay S: Positional cerebral ischemia. J Neurol Neurosurg Psychiatry 39:385, 1976
84. Caplan LR, Tettenborn B: Embolism in the Posterior Circulation in ·Vertebrobasilar Disease. p. 52. Quality Medical Publications St. Louis, 1991
85. Caplan L, Young RR: EEG findings in certain lacunar stroke syndromes. Neurology (NY) 22:403, 1972
86. Caplan L, Zervas N: Survival with permanent midbrain dysfunction after surgical treatment of traumatic subdural hematoma: the clinical picture of a Duret hemorrhage. Ann Neurol 1:587, 1977
87. Castaigne P, Buge A, Escourolle R et al: Ramollissement pédonculaire médiane, tégmentothalamique avec ophthalmoplégie et hypersomnie. Rev Neurol 106:357, 1962
88. Castaigne P, Lhermitte F, Buge A et al: Paramedian thalamic and midbrain infarcts: clinical and neuropathological study. Ann Neurol 10:127, 1981
89. Castaigne P, Lhermitte F, Gautier J et al: Arterial occlusions in the vertebral-basilar system. Brain 96:133, 1973
90. Chase T, Moretti L, Prensky A: Clinical and electroencephalographic manifestations of vascular lesions of the pons. Neurology (NY) 18:357, 1968
91. Chiras J, Marciano S, Vega Molina J et al: Spontaneous dissecting aneurysm of the extracranial vertebral artery (20 cases). Neuroradiology 27:327, 1985
92. Christoff N: A clinicopathological study of vertical eye movements. Arch Neurol 31:1, 1974
93. Christoff N, Anderson P, Nathanson M et al: Problems in anatomical analysis of lesions of the medial longitudinal fasciculus. Arch Neurol 2:293, 1960
94. Cogan DG: Supranuclear connections of the ocular motor system. p. 84. In Neurology of the Ocular Muscles. 2nd Ed. CC Thomas, Springfield, IL, 1956
95. Cogan D: Internuclear ophthalmoplegia, typical and atypical. Arch Ophthalmol 84:583, 1970
96. Cogan D, Kubik C, Smith WL: Unilateral interlluclear ophthalmoplegia. Arch Ophthalmol 44:783, 1950
97. Collier J: Nuclear ophthalmoplegia with especial reference to retraction of the lids and ptosis and to lesions of the posterior commissure. Brain 50:488, 1927
98. Cornhill J, Akins D, Hutson M et al: Localization of atherosclerotic lesions in the human basilar artery. Atherosclerosis 35:77, 1980
99. Corrin LS, Sandok BA, Houser W: Cerebral ischemic events in patients with carotid artery fibromuscular disease. Arch Neurol 38:616, 1981
100. Crosby E, Yoss R, Henderson J: The mammalian midbrain and isthmus regions. II. The fiber connections: D. The pattern for eye movement in the frontal eye fields and the discharge of specific portions of this field to and through midbrain levels. J Comp Neurol 97:357, 1952
101. Cuneo R, Caronna J, Pitts L et al: Upward transtentorial herniation. Arch Neurol 36:618, 1989
102. Currier R, Giles C, DeJong R: Some comments on Wallenberg's lateral medullary syndrome. Neurology (NY) 11:778, 1961
103. Currier R, Giles C, Westerberg M: The prognosis of some brainstem vascular syndromes. Neurology (NY) 8:664, 1958
104. Daroff R, Hoyt W: Supranuclear disorders of ocular control systems in man. p. 175. In Bach Y, Rita P, Collins C (eds): The Control of Eye Movements. Academic Press, Orlando, FL, 1977
105. Daves J, Treger A: Vertebral grand larceny. Circulation 29:911, 1964
106. Davison C: Syndrome of the anterior spinal artery of the medulla oblongata. J Neuropathol Exp Neurol 3:73, 1944
107. Davison C, Goodhart S, Savitsky N: The syndrome of the superior cerebellar artery and its branches. Arch Neurol Psychiatry 33:1143, 1935
108. DeBosscher J: Aneurysme de L'artère vertébrale gauche chez un homme 45 ans. Acta Neurol Psychiatr Belg 52:1, 1952
109. Deeb Z, Janetta P, Rosenbaum A et al: Tortuous vertebrobasilar arteries causing cranial nerve syndromes: screening by computed tomography. J Comput Assist Tomogr 3:774, 1965

110. Dejerine J, Roussy G: Le syndrome thalamique. Rev Neurol 14:521, 1906
111. Deleu D, Buisseret T, Ebinger G: Vertical one-and-a-half syndrome: supranuclear downgaze paralysis with monocular elevation palsy. Arch Neurol 46:1361, 1989
112. del Zoppo G: Fibrinolytic therapy. In Berguer R, Caplan LR (eds): Vertebrobasilar Arterial Disease. Quality Medical Publications, St. Louis, 1991
113. del Zoppo GJ, Zeumer H, Harker LA: Thrombolytic therapy in stroke: possibilities and hazards. Stroke 17:595, 1986
114. Denny-Brown D: Basilar artery syndromes. Bull N Engl Med Cent 15:53, 1953
115. Denny-Brown D: Recurrent cerebrovascular episodes. Arch Neurol 2:194, 1960
116. Denny-Brown D, Foley J: The syndrome of basilar aneurysm. Trans Am Neurol Assoc 77:30, 1952
117. Desmet Y, Brucher JM: L'infarctus bilatéral du territorie latéral du bulbe. Acta Neurol Belg 85:137, 1985
118. Deverereaux M, Keane J, Davis R: Automatic respiratory failure associated with infarction of the medulla: report of two cases with pathologic study of one. Arch Neurol 29:46, 1973
119. DeVisser B: Afferent limb of the human jaw reflex: electrophysiologic and anatomic study. Neurology (NY) 32:563, 1982
120. DeWitt LD, Buonanno FS, Kistler JP et al: Nuclear magnetic resonance imaging in evaluation of clinical stroke syndromes. Ann Neurol 16:535, 1984
121. Dhamoon SK, Igbal J, Collins GH: Ipsilateral hemiplegia and the Wallenberg syndrome. Arch Neurol 41:179, 1984
122. Drayer B, Gur D, Wolfson S et al: Regional blood flow in the posterior fossa: xenon enhanced CT scanning. Acta Neurol Scand, suppl 2. 60:218, 1979
123. Duffy P, Jacobs G: Clinical and pathologic findings in vertebral artery thrombosis. Neurology (NY) 8:862, 1958
124. Dumoulin CL, Hart HR: MR angiography. Radiology 161:717, 1986
125. Duncan G, Parker S, Fisher CM: Acute cerebellar infarction in the PICA territory. Arch Neurol 32:364, 1975
126. Easton JD, Sherman DG: Cervical manipulation and stroke. Stroke 8:594, 1977
127. Echiverri HC, Rubino FA, Gupta SR et al: Fusiform aneurysm of the vertebrobasilar arterial system. Stroke 20:1741, 1989
128. Edelman RR, Mattle HP, Atkinson DJ et al: MR angiography. AJR 154:937, 1990
129. Edelman RR, Mattle HP, O'Reilly GV et al: Magnetic resonance imaging of flow dynamics in the circle of Willis. Stroke 21:56, 1990
130. Edwards WH, Mulherin JL: The surgical reconstruction of the proximal subclavian and vertebral artery. In Berguer R, Bauer R (eds): Vertebrobasilar Arterial Occlusive Disease. Raven Press, New York, 1984
131. Ekbom K, Grietz T, Kugelberg E: Hydrocephalus due to ectasia of the basilar artery. J Neurol Sci 8:465, 1969
132. Ekestrom S, Eklund B, Liljequist L et al: Noninvasive methods in the evaluation of obliterative disease of the subclavian or innominate artery. Acta Med Scand 206:467, 1979
133. Emanuele M, Dorsch T, Scarff T et al: Basilar artery aneurysm simulating pheochromocytoma. Neurology (NY) 31:1560, 1981
134. Escourolle R, Gautier J, Rosa A et al: Aneurysme disséquant vertébrobasilaire. Rev Neurol 128:95, 1972
135. Escourolle R, Hauw J, Der Agopian P et al: Les infarctus bulbaires. J Neurol Sci 28:103, 1976
136. Estanol B, Lopez-Rios G: Neuro-otology of the lateral medullary infarct syndrome. Arch Neurol 39:176, 1982
137. Facon E, Steriade M, Werthein N: Hypersomnie prolongée engendrée par des lésions bilatérales du système activateur médial: le syndrome thrombotique de la bifurcation du tronc basilaire. Rev Neurol 98:117, 1958
138. Fairburn B, Oliver LC: Cerebellar softening: a surgical emergency. Br Med J 1:1335, 1956
139. Fang H, Palmer J: Vascular phenomena involving brainstem structures. Neurology (NY) 6:402, 1956
140. Fankhauser H, Kamano S, Hanamura T et al: Abnormal origin of the posterior inferior cerebellar artery. J Neurosurg 51:569, 1979
141. Faught E, Trader S, Hanna G: Cerebral complications of angiography for transient ischemia and stroke: prediction of risk. Neurology (NY) 29:4, 1979
142. Fazekas J, Alman R, Sullivan J: Vertebral-basilar insufficiency. Arch Neurol 8:215, 1963
143. Feigin I, Budzilovich G: The general pathology of cerebrovascular disease. p. 128. In Vinken P, Bruyn G (eds): Handbook of Clinical Neurology. Vol. 2. North-Holland Publishing, Amsterdam, 1972
144. Feldmann E, Daneault N, Kwan E et al: Chinese-white differences in the distribution of occlusive cerebrovascular disease. Neurology (NY) 40:1541, 1990.
145. Ferbert A, Bruckmann H, Drummen R: Clinical features of proven basilar artery occlusion. Stroke 21:1135, 1990
146. Field JR, Lee L, McBurney R: Complications of 1000 brachial arteriograms. J Neurosurg 36:324, 1972
147. Fields WS: Collateral circulation in cerebrovascular disease. p. 168. In Vinken P, Bruyn G (eds): Handbook of Clinical Neurology. Vol. 2. North-Holland Publishing, Amsterdam, 1972
148. Fields WS: Neurovascular syndromes of the neck and shoulders. Semin Neurol 1:301, 1981
149. Fields WS, Lemak N: Joint study of extracranial arterial occlusion. VII. Subclavian steal. JAMA 222:1139, 1972
150. Fields WS, Lemak NA, Ben-Menachem Y: Thoracic outlet syndrome: review and reference to a stroke in a major league pitcher. AJNR 7:73, 1986
151. Fields W, Lemak N, Frankowski R et al: Con-

trolled trial of aspirin in cerebral ischemia. Stroke 8:301, 1977
152. Fields W, Ratinov G, Weibel J et al: Survival following basilar artery occlusion. Arch Neurol 15:463, 1966
153. Fisher CM: Occlusion of the internal carotid artery. Arch Neurol Psychiatry 65:345, 1951
154. Fisher CM: A new vascular syndrome: "the subclavian steal." (Editorial.). N Engl J Med 265:912, 1961
155. Fisher CM: Ocular bobbing. Arch Neurol 11:543, 1964
156. Fisher CM: The vascular lesion in lacunae. Trans Am Neurol Assoc 90:243, 1965
157. Fisher CM: Pure sensory stroke involving face, arm, and leg. Neurology (NY) 15:76, 1965
158. Fisher CM: Pure motor hemiplegia of vascular origin. Arch Neurol 13:30, 1965
159. Fisher CM: The arterial lesions underlying lacunes. Acta Neuropathol 12:1, 1967
160. Fisher CM: A lacunar stroke: the dysarthria-clumsy hand syndrome. Neurology (NY) 17:614, 1967
161. Fisher CM: Vertigo in cerebrovascular disease. Arch Otolaryngol 85:529, 1967
162. Fisher C: Some neuro-ophthalmological observations. J Neurol Neurosurg Psychiatry 30:383, 1967
163. Fisher CM: Headache in cerebrovascular disease. p. 124. In Vinken P, Bruyn G (eds): Handbook of Clinical Neurology. Vol. 5. North-Holland Publishing, Amsterdam, 1968
164. Fisher CM: Migrainous accompaniments versus arteriosclerotic ischemia. Trans Am Neurol Assoc 93:211, 1968
165. Fisher CM: The neurological examination of the comatose patient. Acta Neurol Scand, suppl 36. 45:1, 1969
166. Fisher CM: Occlusion of the vertebral arteries. Arch Neurol 22:13, 1970
167. Fisher CM: Pathological observations in hypertensive cerebral hemorrhage. J Neuropathol Exp Neurol 30:536, 1971
168. Fisher CM: Cerebral ischemia: less familiar types. Clin Neurosurg 18:267, 1971
169. Fisher CM: Is pressure on nerves and roots a common cause of pain? Trans Am Neurol Assoc 97:282, 1972
170. Fisher CM: Bilateral occlusion of basilar artery branches. J Neurol Neurosurg Psychiatry 40:1182, 1977
171. Fisher CM: Ataxic hemiparesis: a pathologic study. Arch Neurol 35:126, 1978
172. Fisher CM: Thalamic pure sensory stroke: a pathologic study. Neurology (NY) 28:1141, 1978
173. Fisher CM: Transient migrainous accompaniments of late onset. Stroke 10:96, 1979
174. Fisher CM: Oval pupils. Arch Neurol 37:502, 1980
175. Fisher CM: Pure sensory stroke and allied conditions. Stroke 13:434, 1982
176. Fisher CM: Lacunar strokes and infarcts: a review. Neurology (NY) 32:871, 1982
177. Fisher CM: Abulia minor vs agitation behavior. Clinical Surgery. p. 9. In Clinical Surgery. Vol. 31. Williams & Wilkins, Baltimore, 1983.
178. Fisher CM: The "herald hemiparesis" of basilar artery occlusion. Arch Neurol 45:1301, 1988
179. Fisher CM, Caplan L: Basilar artery branch occlusion: a cause of pontine infarction. Neurology (NY) 21:900, 1971
180. Fisher CM, Cole M: Homolateral ataxia and crural paresis: a vascular syndrome. J Neurol Neurosurg Psychiatry 28:48, 1965
181. Fisher C, Gore I, Okabe N et al: Atherosclerosis of the carotid and vertebral arteries: extracranial and intracranial. J Neuropathol Exp Neurol 24:455, 1965
182. Fisher CM, Karnes WE: Local embolism. J Neuropathol Exp Neurol 24:174, 1965
183. Fisher CM, Karnes W, Kubik C: Lateral medullary infarction: the pattern of vascular occlusion. J Neuropathol Exp Neurol 20:323, 1961
184. Fisher CM, Ojemann RG: A clinico-pathologic study of carotid endarterectomy plaques. Rev Neurol (Paris) 142:573, 1986
185. Fisher CM, Ojemann R, Roberson G: Spontaneous dissection of cervico-cerebral arteries. J Can Sci Neurol 5:9, 1978
186. Fisher CM, Picard E, Polak A et al: Acute hypertensive cerebellar hemorrhage: diagnosis and surgical treatment. J Nerv Ment Dis 140:38, 1965
187. Foix C, Hillemand P: Irrigation du bulbe. CR Soc Biol Paris 42:33, 1924
188. Foix C, Hillemand P: Les artères de l'axe encéphalique jusqu'au diencéphale inclusivement. Rev Neurol 32:705, 1925
189. Foix C, Hillemand P: Irrigation de la protuberance. CR Soc Biol Paris 42:35, 1925
190. Foix C, Hillemand P: Contribution a l'étude des ramollissements protuberentiels. Rev Med 43:287, 1926
191. Foix C, Hillemand P, Schalit I: Sur le syndrome latéral du bulbe et l'irrigation du bulbe superieur: l'artère de la fosette latérale du bulbe, le syndrome de la cérébelleuse inferieure térritoire de ces artères. Rev Neurol 32:160, 1925
192. Ford F, Clark D: Thrombosis of the basilar artery with softenings in the cerebellum and brainstem due to manipulation of the neck. Bull Johns Hopkins Hosp 98:37, 1956
193. Freeman W, Jaffe D: Occlusion of the superior cerebellar artery. Arch Neurol Psychiatry 46:115, 1941
194. French LA, Haines GL: Unilateral vertebral artery ligation. J Neurosurg 7:156, 1950
195. Frens D, Petajan J, Anderson R et al: Fibromuscular dysplasia of the posterior cerebral artery: report of a case and review of the literature. Stroke 5:161, 1974
196. Frisen L, Holmegaard L, Rosencrantz M: Sectorial optic atrophy and homonymous horizontal sectoranopia: a lateral choroidal artery syndrome. J Neurol Neurosurg Psychiatry 41:374, 1978
197. Frumkin L, Baloh R: Wallenberg's syndrome following neck manipulation. Neurology 40:611, 1990

198. George B, Laurian C: Vertebro-basilar ischemia with thrombosis of the vertebral artery: report of two cases with embolism. J Neurol Neurosurg Psychiatry 45:91, 1982
199. Gerber N: Congenital atresia of the subclavian artery producing subclavian steal syndrome. Amer J Dis Child 113:709, 1967
200. Gilles F: Hypotensive brainstem necrosis. Arch Pathol 88:32, 1969
201. Gillilan L: The correlation of the blood supply to the human brainstem with brainstem lesions. J Neuropathol Exp Neurol 23:78, 1964
202. Gillilan L: Anatomy and embryology of the arterial system of the brainstem and cerebellum. p. 24. In Vinken P, Bruyn G (eds): Handbook of Clinical Neurology. Vol. 2. North-Holland Publishing, Amsterdam, 1972
203. Goldstein S: Dissecting hematoma of the cervical vertebral artery. J Neurosurg 56:451, 1982
204. Gonyea E: Bilateral internuclear ophthalmoplegia: association with occlusive cerebrovascular disease. Arch Neurol 31:168, 1974
205. Goodhart S, Davison C: Syndrome of the posterior inferior and anterior inferior cerebellar arteries and their branches. Arch Neurol Psychiatry 35:501, 1936
206. Goodwill J: Temporal arteritis. p. 313. In Vinken P, Bruyn G (eds): Handbook of Clinical Neurology. Vol. 39. North-Holland Publishing, Amsterdam, 1980
207. Gorelick PB, Caplan LR, Hier DB et al: Racial differences in the distribution of posterior circulation occlusive disease. Stroke 16:785, 1985
208. Graff-Radford NR, Damasio H, Yamada T et al: Non-haemorrhagic thalamic infarction. Brain 108:495, 1985
209. Greenberg J, Skubick D, Shenken H: Acute hydrocephalus in cerebellar infarct and hemorrhage. Neurology (NY) 29:409, 1979
210. Guillain G, Bertrand L, Peron N: Le syndrome de l'artère cérébelleuse supérieure. Rev Neurol 2:835, 1928
211. Guillard A: Pathologie ischémique cérébrale et anomalie de terminaison intracranienne de l'artère vertebrale. Sem Hop Paris 62:2755, 1986
212. Gulang RL, Ellington OB: Acute pure vertiginous disequilibrium in cerebellar infarction. Eur Neurol 16:11, 1977
213. Hacke W, Zeumer H, Ferbert A et al: Intra-arterial thrombolytic therapy improves outcome in patients with acute vertebrobasilar occlusive disease. Stroke 19:1216, 1988
214. Halmagyi G, Evans W, Hallinan J: Failure of downward gaze. Arch Neurol 35:22, 1978
215. Halmagyi MB, Brandt Th, Dieterich M et al: Tonic contraversive ocular tilt reaction due to unilateral mesodiencephalic lesion. Neurology (NY) 40:1503, 1990
216. Halsey J, Ceballos R, Crosby E: The supranuclear control of voluntary lateral gaze. Neurology (NY) 17:928, 1967
217. Hamrin B: Polymyalgia arteritica with morphological changes in the large arteries. Acta Med Scand, suppl. 533:4, 1972
218. Handa J, Kamijo Y, Handa H: Intracranial aneurysms associated with fibromuscular hyperplasia of the renal and internal carotid arteries. Br J Radiol 43:483, 1970
219. Hanus S, Homer T, Harter D: Vertebral artery occlusion complicating yoga exercises. Arch Neurol 34:547, 1977
220. Hardin C, Williamson W, Steegman T: Vertebral artery insufficiency produced by cervical osteoarthritic spurs. Neurology (NY) 10:855, 1960
221. Hardy D, Peace D, Rhoton A: Microsurgical anatomy of the superior cerebellar artery. Neurosurgery 6:10, 1980
222. Hari R, Sulkava R, Halti A: Brainstem auditory evoked responses and alpha-pattern coma. Ann Neurol 11:187, 1982
223. Harris W: Ataxic nystagmus: a pathognomonic sign in disseminated sclerosis. Br J Ophthalmol 28:40, 1944
224. Hass WK, Fields WS, North RR et al: Joint Study of Extracranial Arterial Occlusion. II. Arteriography, technique, sites, and complications. JAMA 203:159, 1986
225. Haughton V, Donegan J, Walsh P et al: Clinical cerebral blood flow measurements with inhaled xenon and CT. Am J Radiol 134:281, 1980
226. Hauw J, Der Agopian P, Trelles L et al: Les infarctus bulbaires. J Neurol Sci 28:83, 1976
227. Hayem G: Sur la thrombose par artérite du tronc basilaire comme cause de mort rapide. Arch Physiol Norm Pathol 1:270, 1868
228. Helgason C, Caplan LR, Goodwin J et al: Anterior choroidal artery territory infarction: case reports and review. Arch Neurol 3:681, 1986
229. Hennerici M, Aulich A, Sandmann W et al: Incidence of asymptomatic extracranial arterial disease. Stroke 12:750, 1981
230. Hennerici M, Klemm C, Rautenberg W: The subclavian steal phenomenon: a common vascular disorder with rare neurologic deficits. Neurology (NY) 38:669, 1988.
231. Hennerici M, Rautenberg W, Schwartz A: Transcranial Doppler ultrasound for the assessment of intracranial arterial flow velocity. II. Evaluation of intracranial arterial disease. Surg Neurol 27:523, 1987
232. Hennerici M, Rautenberg W, Sitzer G et al: Transcranial Doppler ultrasound for the assessment of intracranial arterial flow velocity. I. Examination of technique and normal values. Surg Neurol 27:439, 1987
233. Henze T, Boeer A, Tebbe U et al: Lysis of basilar artery occlusion with tissue plasminogen activator. Lancet 2:1391, 1987
234. Heros R: Cerebellar infarction resulting from traumatic occlusion of a vertebral artery. J Neurosurg 51:111, 1979
235. Heros R: Cerebellar hemorrhage and infarction. Stroke 13:106, 1982
236. Herskovitz S, Lipton RB, Lantos G: Neuro-Behçet's disease. Neurology (NY) 38:1714, 1988
237. Hesselink JR, Teresi L, Davis K et al: Intravenous digital subtraction angiography of arterio-

sclerotic vertebrobasilar disease. AJR 142:255, 1984
238. Heyman A, Young W, Dillon M et al: Cerebral ischemia caused by occlusive lesions of the subclavian or innominate arteries. Arch Neurol 10:581, 1964
239. Hinshaw D, Thompson J, Hasso A et al: Infarction of the brainstem and cerebellum: a correlation of computed tomography and angiography. Radiology 137:105, 1980
240. Hirsch CS, Roessmann U: Arterial dysplasia with ruptured basilar artery aneurysm: report of a case. Hum Pathol 6:749, 1975
241. Hirsh L, Gonzalez C: Fusiform basilar aneurysm simulating carotid transient ischemic attacks. Stroke 10:598, 1979
242. Ho K: Pure motor hemiplegia due to infarction of the cerebral peduncle. Arch Neurol 39:524, 1982
243. Ho K, Meyer K: The medial medullary syndrome. Arch Neurol 38:385, 1981
244. Holmes G: The symptoms of acute cerebellar injuries due to gunshot wounds. Brain 40:461, 1917
245. Holmes G: The Cloonian lectures on the clinical symptoms of cerebellar disease and their interpretations. Lancet 1:1177, 1922; 2:59, 1922
246. Hommel H, Besson G, Pollak P et al: Hemiplegia in posterior cerebral artery occlusion. Neurology (NY) 40:1496, 1990
247. Hoobler S: The syndrome of cervical rib with subclavian aterial thrombosis and hemiplegia due to cerebral embolism. N Engl J Med 226:942, 1942
248. Hopkins LN, Martin NA, Hadley MN et al: Vertebrobasilar insufficiency. II. Microsurgical treatment of intracranial vertebrobasilar disease. J Neurosurg 66:662, 1987
249. Houser OW, Baker H, Sandok B et al: Cephalic arterial fibromuscular dysplasia. Radiology 101:605, 1971
250. Hutchinson E, Yates P: The cervical portion of the vertebral artery: a clinic-pathological study. Brain 79:319, 1956
251. Hutchinson E, Yates P: Carotico-vertebral stenosis. Lancet 1:2, 1957
252. Imparato A: Vertebral artery reconstruction: a nineteen year experience. J Vasc Surg 2:626, 1985
253. Imparato A, Riles T, Kim G: Cervical vertebral artery angioplasty for brainstem ischemia. Surgery 90:842, 1981
254. Imparato A, Riles T, Kim G et al: Vertebral artery reconstruction. Stroke 12:125, 1981
255. Ingvar D, Sourander P: Destruction of the reticular core of the brainstem. Arch Neurol 23:1, 1970
256. Ishikawa K: Natural history and classification of occlusive thromboarteropathy (Takayasu' disease). Circulation 57:27, 1978
257. Jacobs L, Anderson P, Bender M: The lesion producing paralysis of downward but not upward gaze. Arch Neurol 28:319, 1973
258. Jacobs L, Heffner RR, Newman RP: Selective paralysis of downward gaze caused by bilateral lesions of the mesencephalic periaqueductal gray matter. Neurology (NY) 35:516, 1985
259. Jones HE, Millikan C, Sandok B: Temporal profile (clinical course) of acute vertebrobasilar system cerebral infarction. Stroke 11:173, 1980
260. Juge O, Meyer J, Sakai F et al: Critical appraisal of cerebral blood flow measured from brainstem and cerebellar regions after Xe-133 inhalations in humans. Stroke 10:428, 1979
261. Jurgensen J, Brennan R, Towfighi J: Brainstem arterial end-zone infarction following hypotension in man. Neurology (NY) 31:92, 1981
262. Karp J, Hurtig H: "Locked-in" state with bilateral midbrain infarcts. Arch Neurol 30:176, 1974
263. Kase C, Maulsby G, De Juan et al: Hemichoreahemiballism and lacunar infarction in the basal ganglia. Neurology (NY) 31:452, 1981
264. Kase C, Varakis J, Stafford J et al: Medial medullary infarction from fibrocartilogenous embolism to the anterior spinal artery. Stroke 14:413, 1983
265. Kase CS, White JL, Joslyn N et al: Cerebellar infarction in the superior cerebellar artery distribution. Neurology (NY) 35:705, 1985
266. Keane J: Sustained up gaze in coma. Ann Neurol 9:409, 1981
267. Keane JR: Locked-in-syndrome after head and neck trauma. Neurology (NY) 36:80, 1986
268. Kemper T, Romanul F: State resembling akinetic mutism in basilar artery occlusion. Neurology (NY) 17:74, 1967
269. Kerber C, Margolis M, Newton T: Tortuous vertebrobasilar system: a cause of cranial nerve signs. Neuroradiology 4:74, 1972
270. Kertesz A, Black SE, Nicholson L, Carr T: The sensitivity and specificity of MRI in stroke. Neurology (NY) 37:1580, 1987
271. Khodadad G, Singh R, Olinger C: Possible prevention of brainstem stroke by microvascular anastomosis in the vertebrobasilar system. Stroke 8:316, 1977
272. Khurana R: Autonomic dysfunction in pontomedullary stroke. Ann Neurol 12:86, 1982
273. Kieffer SA, Takeya Y, Resch JA et al: Racial differences in cerebrovascular disease: angiographic evaluation of Japanese and American populations. AJR 101:94, 1967
274. Kingsley D, Radue E, DuBoulay E: Evaluation of computed tomography in vascular lesions of the vertebrobasilar territory. J Neurol Neurosurg Psychiatry 43:193, 1980
275. Kistler JP, Buonnano FS, DeWitt LD et al: Vertebral-basilar posterior cerebral territory stroke: delineation by proton nuclear magnetic resonance imaging. Stroke 15:417, 1984
276. Klein R, Hunder G, Stanson A et al: Large artery involvement in giant cell (temporal) arteritis. Ann Intern Med 83:806, 1975
277. Kommerell G, Hoyt W: Lateropulsion of saccadic eye movements. Arch Neurol 28:313, 1973
278. Koroshetz WJ, Ropper AH: Artery-to-artery embolism causing stroke in the posterior circulation. Neurology (NY) 37:292, 1987

279. Krayenbuhl H, Yasargil M: Radiological anatomy and topography of the cerebral arteries. p. 65. In Vinken P, Bruyn G (eds): Handbook of Clinical Neurology. Vol. 2. North-Holland Publications, Amsterdam, 1972
280. Kreuger B, Okazaki H: Vertebral-basilar distribution infarction following chiropractic cervical manipulation. Mayo Clin Proc 55:322, 1980
281. Kubik C, Adams R: Occlusion of the basilar artery: a clinical and pathologic study. Brain 69:73, 1946
282. Labauge R, Boukobza M, Pages M et al: Occlusion de l'artère vertébrale. Rev Neurol 143:490, 1987
283. Labauge R, Pages M, Marty-Double C et al: Occlusion du tronc basilaire. Rev Neurol 137:545, 1981
284. Lahitte M, Marc-Vergnes J, Rascol A et al: Intravenous angiography of the extracranial arteries. Radiology 137:705, 1980
285. Lance J, Adams R: The syndrome of intention and action myoclonus as a sequel of hypoxic encephalopathy. Brain 86:111, 1963
286. Lapresle J, Ben Hamida M: The dentato-olivary pathway. Arch Neurol 22:135, 1970
287. Lazorthes G: Vascularisation et Circulation Cérébrales. Masson, Paris, 1961
288. Lee RE: Reconstruction of the proximal vertebral artery. In Berguer R, Caplan LR (eds): Vertebrobasilar Disease. Quality Medical Publications, St. Louis, 1991
289. Lehrich J, Winkler G, Ojemann R: Cerebellar infarction with brainstem compression: diagnosis and surgical treatment. Arch Neurol 22:490, 1970
290. Lester J, Klee A: Complications of 337 percutaneous vertebral angiographies. Acta Neurol Scand 41:301, 1965
291. Levin B, Margolis G: Acute failure of automatic respirations secondary to a unilateral brainstem infarct. Ann Neurol 1:583, 1977
292. Levine SR, Patel VM, Welch KMA et al: Are heart attacks really brain attacks? In Furlan A (ed): The Heart in Stroke. Springer-Verlag, Heidelberg, 1987
293. Levy R, Dugan T, Bernat J et al: Lateral medullary syndrome after neck injury. Neurology (NY) 30:788, 1980
294. Leyden E: Über die Thrombose der basilar Arterie. Z Klin Med 5:165, 1882
295. Lhermitte J, Trelles J: L'arteriosclérose du tronbasilaire et ses consequences anatomocliniques. Jahrb Psychiatr Neurol 51:91, 1934
296. Lie T: Congenital malformations of the carotid and vertebral arterial systems, including the persistent anastamoses. p. 289. In Vinken P, Bruyn G (eds): Handbook of Clinical Neurology. Vol. 12. North-Holland Publishing, Amsterdam, 1972
297. Liljequist L, Ekerstrom S, Nordhus O: Monitoring direction of vertebral artery blood flow by Doppler shift ultrasound in patients with suspected subclavian steal. Acta Chir Scand 147:421, 1981
298. Lindenberg R: Compression of brain arteries as pathogenetic factor for tissue necrosis and their areas of predilection. J Neuropathol Exp Neurol 14:223, 1955
299. Lindgren SO: Infarctions simulating brain tumors in the posterior fossa. J Neurosurg 13:575, 1956
300. Lister J, Rhoton A, Matsushima T et al: Microsurgical anatomy of the posterior inferior cerebellar artery. Neurosurgery 10:170, 1982
301. Little JR, St. Louis P, Weinstein M et al: Giant fusiform aneurysm of the cerebral arteries. Stroke 12:183, 1981
302. Lochaya S, Kaplan B, Shaffer AB: Pseudocoarctation of the aorta will bicuspid aortic valve and kinked left subclavian artery, a possible cause of subclavian steal. Am Heart J 73:369, 1967
303. Loeb C, Meyer JS: Strokes Due to Vertebro-basilar Disease. CC Thomas, Springfield, IL, 1965
304. Louis-Bar D: Sur le syndrome vasculaire de l'hemibulbe (Wallenberg). Monatsshr Psychiatr Neurol 112:53, 1946
305. Luhan J, Pollock S: Occlusion of the superior cerebellar artery. Neurology (NY) 3:77, 1953
306. Lupi-Herrera E, Sanchez-Torres G, Marcushamer J et al: Takayasu's arteritis: clinical study of 27 cases. Am Heart J 93:94, 1977
307. Makos MM, McComb RD, Hart MN et al: Alpha-glucosidase deficiency and basilar artery aneurysm: report of a sibship. Ann Neurol 22:629, 1987
308. Mapstone T, Spetzler R: Vertebrobasilar insufficiency secondary to vertebral artery occlusion from a fibrous band. J Neurosurg 56:581, 1982
309. Marburg O: Über die neuren Fortschritte in der topischen Diagnostic du Pons und Oblongata. Dtsch Z Nervenheilkd 41:41, 1911
310. Martin JP: Hemichorea resulting from a local lesion of the brain (the syndrome of the body of Luys). Brain 50:637, 1927
311. Maruyama M, Asai T, Kuriyama Y et al: Positive platelet scintigram of a vertebral aneurysm presenting thromboembolic transient ischemic attacks. Stroke 20:687, 1989
312. Maruyama K, Tanaka M, Ikeda S et al: A case report of quadriparesis due to compression of the medulla oblongata by the elongated left vertebral artery. Rinsho Shinkeigaku 29:108, 1989
313. Mas JL, Bousser MG, Hasboun D et al: Extracranial vertebral artery dissection: a review of 13 cases. Stroke 18:1037, 1987
314. Matsumoto S, Okuda B, Imai T et al: A sensory level on the trunk in lower lateral brainstem lesions. Neurology (NY) 38:1515, 1988
315. McCusker E, Rudick R, Honch G et al: Recovery from the locked-in syndrome. Arch Neurol 39:145, 1982
316. McKee AC, Levine DN, Kowall NW et al: Peduncular hallucinosis associated with isolated infarction of the substantia nigra pars reticulata. Ann Neurol 27:500, 1990
317. McKissock W, Richardson A, Walsh R: Spontaneous cerebellar hemorrhage: a study of 34 consecutive cases treated surgically. Brain 83:1, 1960
318. McMenemy WH, Lawrence BJ: Encephalo-

myelopathy in Behcet's syndrome. Lancet 2:353, 1957
319. McNamara J, Heyman A, Silver D et al: The value of carotid endarterectomy in treating transient cerebral ischemia of the posterior circulation. Neurology (NY) 27:682, 1977
320. Mehler MF: The neuro-ophthalmogic spectrum of the rostral basilar artery syndrome. Arch Neurol 45:966, 1988
321. Meienberg O, Mumenthaler M, Karbowski K: Quadriparesis and nuclear oculomotor palsy with total bilateral ptosis mimicking coma. Arch Neurol 36:708, 1979
322. Meissner I, Sapir S, Kokmen E et al: The paramedian diencephalic syndrome: a dynamic phenomenon. Stroke 18:380, 1987
323. Merkel K, Grinsberg P, Parker J et al: Cerebrovascular disease in sickle cell anemia: a clinical, pathological, and radiological correlation. Stroke 9:45, 1978
324. Merritt H, Finland M: Vascular lesions of the hindbrain (lateral medullary syndrome). Brain 53:290, 1930
325. Mettinger K: Fibromuscular dysplasia and the brain. II. Current concepts of the disease. Stroke 13:53, 1982
326. Meyer J, Hayman L, Amano T et al: Mapping local blood flow of human brain by CT scaning during stable xenon inhalation. Stroke 12:426, 1981
327. Meyer J, Hayman, Sakai F et al: High-resolution three-dimensional measurement of localized cerebral blood flow by CT scanning and stable xenon clearance: effect of cerebral infarction and ischemia. Trans Am Neurol Assoc 104:1, 1979
328. Meyer JS, Sheehan S, Bauer R: An arteriographic study of cerebrovascular disease in man: stenosis and occlusion of the vertebral basilar arterial system. Arch Neurol 2:27, 1960
329. Meyer K, Baloh R, Krohel G et al: Ocular lateropulsion: a sign of lateral medullary disease. Arch Ophthalmol 98:1614, 1980
330. Millikan C: Reassessment of anticoagulant therapy in various types of occlusive cerebrovascular disease. Stroke 2:201, 1971
331. Millikan C, Siekert R: Studies in cerebrovascular disease: the syndrome of intermittent insufficiency of the basilar arterial system. Proc Staff Meet Mayo Clin 30:61, 1955
332. Millikan C, Siekert R, Shick R: Studies in cerebrovascular disease: the use of anticoagulant drugs in the treatment of insufficiency or thrombosis within the basilar arterial system. Proc Staff Meet Mayo Clin 30:116, 1955
333. Millikan C, Siekert R, Whisnant J: Anticoagulant therapy in cerebrovascular disease: current status. JAMA 166:587, 1958
334. Mills CK: Hemianesthesia to pain and temperature and loss of emotional expression on the right side with ataxia of the upper limb on the left. J Nerv Ment Dis 35:331, 1908
335. Miyashita K, Naritomi H, Sawada T et al: Identification of recent lacunar lesions in cases of multiple small infarctions by magnetic resonance imaging. Stroke. 19:834, 1988
336. Mizutani T, Lewis R, Gonatas N: Medial medullary syndrome in a drug abuser. Arch Neurol 37:425, 1980
337. Moersch F, Kernohan J: Hemiballismus, a Clinicopathological study. Arch Neurol Psychiatry 41:365, 1939
338. Mohr JP: Neurological complications of cardiac valvular disease and cardiac surgery including systemic hypotension. p. 143. In Vinken P, Bruyn G (eds): Handbook of Clinical Neurology. Vol. 38. Noth-Holland Publications, Amsterdam, 1979
339. Mohr JP, Biller J, Hilal SK et al: MR vs CT Imaging in Acute Stroke. Proceedings of the Seventeenth International Conference on Stroke and the Cerebral Circulation. Phoenix, AZ, 1992
340. Mohr JP, Caplan L, Melski et al: Harvard Cooperative Stroke Registry: a prospective registry. Neurology (NY) 28:754, 1978
341. Mohr JP, Kase C, Meckler R et al: Sensomotor stroke due to thalmocapsular ischemia. Arch Neurol 34:739, 1977
342. Molnar P, Hegedus K: Direct involvement of intracerebral arteries in Takayasu's arteritis. Acta Neuropathol (Berl) 63:83, 1984
343. Mori E, Yamadori A, Mitani Y: Left thalamic infarction and disturbance of verbal memory: a clinicoanatomical study with a new method of computed tomographic stereotaxic lesion localization. Ann Neurol 20:671, 1986
344. Morrow MJ, Sharpe JA: Torsional nystagmus in the lateral medullary syndrome. Ann Neurol 24:390, 1988
345. Moosy J: Morphology, sites and epidemiology of cerebral atherosclerosis. Proc Assoc Res Nerv Ment Dis 51:1, 1966
346. Moscow N, Newton T: Angiographic implications in diagnosis and prognosis of basilar artery occlusion. Am J Radiol 119:597, 1973
347. Moseley I, Hollalld I: Ectasia of the basilar artery: the breadth of the clinical spectrum and the diagnostic value of computed tomography. Neuroradiology 18:83, 1979
348. Motarjeme A, Keifer J, Zuska A: Percutaneous transluminal angioplasty of the vertebral arteries. Radiology 139:715, 1981
349. Moufarrij NA, Little JR, Furlan AJ et al: Vertebral artery stenosis: long-term follow-up. Stroke 15:260, 1984
350. Moufarrij NA, Little JR, Furlan AJ et al: Basilar and distal vertebral artery stenosis: long-term follow-up. Stroke 17:938, 1986
351. Mueller S, Sahs A: Brainstem dysfunction related to cervical manipulation. Neurology (NY) 26:547, 1976
352. Naheedy M, Tyler H, Wolf M et al: Diagnosis of thrombotic giant basilar artery aneurysm on computed tomographic scan. Arch Neurol 39:64, 1982
353. Naritomi H, Sakai F, Meyer J: Pathogenesis of transient ischemic attacks within the vertebrobasilar arterial system. Arch Neurol 36:121, 1979
354. Nashold B, Seaber J: Defects of ocular mobility

after stereotactic midbrain lesions in man. Arch Ophthalmol 88:245, 1972
355. Nelson J, Johnston C: Ocular bobbing. Arch Neurol 22:348, 1970
356. Newman N, Gay A, Heilbrun M: Disconjugate ocular bobbing: its relation to midbrain, pontine and medullary function in a surviving patient. Neurology (NY) 21:633, 1971
357. Nishizaki T, Tamikl N, Takeda N: Dolichoectatic basilar artery: a review of 23 cases. Stroke 17:1277, 1986
358. North R, Fields W, DeBakey M et al: Brachial-basilar insufficiency syndrome. Neurology (NY) 12:810, 1962
359. Obayashi T, Furuse M: The proatlantal intersegmental artery. Arch Neurol 37:387, 1980
360. Olesen J, Larsen B, Lauritzen M: Focal hyperemia followed by spreading oligemia and impaired activation of CBF in classic migraine. Ann Neurol 9:344, 1981
361. Osborn A, Anderson R: Angiography spectrum of cervical and intracranial fibromuscular dysplasia. Stroke 8:617, 1977
362. Ott K, Kase C, Ojemann R et al: Cerebellar hemorrhage: diagnosis and treatment. Arch Neurol 31:160, 1974
363. Parkinson D, Reddy V, Ross R: Congenital anastomosis between the vertebral artery and internal carotid artery in the neck. J Neurosurg 51:697, 1979
364. Pasik P, Pasik T, Bender M: The pretectal syndrome in monkeys. I. Disturbance of gaze and body posture. Brain 92:521, 1969
365. Passerini A, Tagliabue G: Aneurysms of the vertebrobasilar system. Radiol Clin Biol 35:257, 1966
366. Patel A, Toole J: Subclavian steal syndrome: reversal of cephalic blood flow. Medicine (Baltimore) 44:289, 1965
367. Patrick B, Ramirez-Lassepas M, Snyder B: Temporal profile of vertebrobasilar territory infarction. Stroke 11:643, 1980
368. Paulson GW, Yates AJ, Paltan-Ortiz JD: Does infarction of the medullary pyramid lead to spasticity? Arch Neurol 43:93, 1986
369. Paulson G, Boesel C, Evans W: Fibromuscular displasia. Arch Neurol 35:287, 1978
370. Paulson G, Nashold B, Margolis G: Aneurysms of the vertebral artery. Neurology (NY) 9:590, 1959
371. Pawl G, Shaw C, Wray L: True traumatic aneurysms of the vertebral artery. J Neurosurg 53:101, 1980
372. Pedersen R, Troost BT: Abnormalities of gaze in cerebrovascular disease. Stroke 12:251, 1981
373. Pelouze GA: Plaque ulcerie de l'ostium de l'artère vertébrale. Rev Neurol 145:478, 1989
374. Percheron GMJ: Etude anatomique du thalamus de l'homme adulte et de sa vascularisation artérielle. Thesis, Paris, 1966
375. Peress N, Kane WC, Aronson SM: Central nenlous system findings in a tenth decade autopsy population. Prog Brain Res 40:473, 1973
376. Pernecsky A, Perneczky G, Tschabitscher M et al: The relationship between the caudolateral pontine syndrome and the anterior inferior cerebellar artery. Acta Neurochir 58:245, 1981
377. Pessin MS, Chimowitz MI, Levine SR et al: Stroke in patients with fusiform vertebrobasilar aneurysms. Neurology (NY) 39:16, 1989.
378. Pessin MS, Daneault N, Kwan E et al: Local embolism from vertebral artery occlusion. Stroke 19:112, 1988
379. Pessin MS, del Zoppo GJ, Estol C: Thrombolytic agents in the treatment of stroke. Clin Neuropharmacol 13:271, 1990
380. Pessin MS, Gorelick PB, Kwan ES et al: Basilar artery stenosis: middle and distal segments. Neurology (NY) 37:1742, 1987
381. Peterman A, Siekert R: The lateral medullary (Wallenberg) syndrome: clinical features and prognosis. Med Clin North Am 44:887, 1960
382. Pierrot-Deseilligny C, Amarenco P, Roullet E et al: Vermal infarct with pursuit eye movement disorders. J Neurol Neurosurg Psychiatry 53:519, 1990
383. Pierrot-Deserilligny C, Chain F, Serdaru M et al: The one and a half syndrome. Brain 104:665, 1981
384. Pines L, Gilinsky E: Über die Thrombose der Arteria basilaris und über die Vascularization der Brücke. Arch Psychiatr 26:380, 1932
385. Pinkerton J, Davidson K, Hibbard B: Primitive hypoglossal artery and carotid endarterectomy. Stroke 6:658, 1980
386. Plum F, Posner J: The Diagnosis of Stupor and Coma. 3rd Ed. FA Davis, Philadelphia, 1980
387. Pochaczevsky R, Uygur Z, Berman A: Basilar artery occlusion. J Can Assoc Radiol 22:261, 1971
388. Pollock M, Blennerhassett J, Clarke A: Giant cell arteritis and the subclavian steal syndrome. Neurology 23:653, 1973
389. Pratt-Thomas H, Berger K: Cerebellar and spinal injuries after chiropractic manipulation. JAMA 133:600, 1947
390. Pribram H: Complications of cerebral arteriography. p. 184. In Fields W, Sahs A (eds): Intracranial Aneurysms and Subarachnoid Hemorrhage. CC Thomas, Springfield, IL, 1965
391. Radner S: Vertebral angiography by catheterization. Acta Radiol [suppl] (Stockh) 87, 1951
392. Rao K, Woodlief C: Stimulation of cerebellopontine tumor by tortuous vertebrobasilar artery. Am J Roentgenol 132:602, 1979
393. Reis DJ, Iadecola C, Nakai M: Control of cerebral blood flow and metabolism by intrinsic neural systems in brain. p. 1. In Plum F, Pulsinelli W (eds): Cerebrovascular Diseases. Proceedings of the Fourteenth (Princeton) Conference. Raven Press, New York, 1985
394. Reivich M, Holling E, Roberts B et al: Reversal of blood flow through the vertebral artery and its effect on cerebral circulation. N Engl J Med 265:88, 1961
395. Resch JA, Okabe N, Loewenson RB et al: Patterns of vessel involvement in cerebral atherosclerosis: a comparative study between a Japanese and Minnesota population. J Atherosclerosis Res 9:239, 1969

396. Reul GJ, Cooley DA, Olson SK et al: Long-term results of direct vertebral artery operations. Surgery 96:854, 1984
397. Reuther R, Dorndorf W: Aspirin in patients with cerebral ischemia and normal angiograms or nonsurgical lesions: the results of a double-blind trial. p. 97. In Breddin K, Dorndorf W, Loew D et al (eds): Acetylsalicylic Acid in Cerebral Ischemia and Coronary Heart Disease. Schattauer, Stuttgart, 1978
398. Reznik M: Le ramollissement du tronc cérébral. Acta Neurol Belg 81:257, 1981
399. Richter R: Collaterals between the external carotid artery and the vertebral artery in cases of thrombosis of the internal carotid artery. Acta Radiol [Diagn] (Stockh) 40:108, 1953
400. Ringel S, Harrison S, Norenberg M et al: Fibromuscular dysplasia: multiple "spontaneous" dissecting aneurysms of the major cranial arteries. Ann Neurol 1:301, 1977
401. Robertson J: Neck manipulation as a cause of stroke. Stroke 12:1, 1981
402. Rogers L, Sweeney P: Stroke: a neurological complication of wrestling. Am J Sports Med 7:352, 1979
403. Romanul F: Examination of the brain and spinal cord. p. 131. In Tedeschi CG (ed): Neuropathology: Methods and Diagnosis. Little, Brown, Boston, 1970
404. Romanul F, Abramowicz A: Changes in brain and pial vessels in arterial boundary zones. Arch Neurol 11:40, 1964
405. Roon A, Ehrenfeld W, Cooke P et al: Vertebral artery reconstruction. Am J Surg 138:29, 1979
406. Ropper A, Fisher CM, Kleinman G: Pyramidal infarction in the medulla: a cause of pure motor hemiplegia sparing the face. Neurology (NY) 29:91, 1979
407. Roski R, Spetzler R, Hopkins L: Occipital artery to posterior inferior cerebellar artery bypass for vertebrobasilar ischemia. Neurosurgery 10:44, 1982
408. Ross MA, Biller J, Adams HP et al: Magnetic resonance imaging in Wallenberg's lateral medullary syndrome. Stroke 17:542, 1986
409. Rothrock JF, Lyden PD, Hesselink JR et al: Brain magnetic resonance imaging in the evaluation of lacunar stroke. Stroke 18:781, 1987.
410. Rubenstein RL, Norman D, Schindler R et al: Cerebellar infarction: a presentation of vertigo. Laryngoscope 90:505, 1980
411. Sacco RL, Bello JA, Traub R et al: Selective proprioceptive loss from a thalamic lacunar stroke. Stroke 18:1160, 1987
412. Sackett J, Strother C, Crummy A et al: Computerized fluoroscopic intravenous arteriography of the carotid arteries. Stroke 12:122, 1981
413. Samson M, Mihout B, Thiebot J et al: Forme benigne des infarctus cérébelleaux. Rev Neurol 137:373, 1981
414. Savoiardo M, Bracchi M, Passerini A et al: The vascular territories in the cerebellum and brainstem: CT and MR study. AJNR 8:199, 1987
415. Schutz H, Yeung H, Chiu M et al: Dilatation of vertebral artery stenosis. N Engl J Med 304:732, 1981
416. Schwartz C, Mitchell J: Atheroma of the carotid and vertebral arterial systems. Br Med J 2:1057, 1961
417. Scotti G, Spinnler H, Sterzi R et al: Cerebellar softening. Ann Neurol 8:133, 1980
418. Seelig J, Selhorst J, Young H et al: Ventriculostomy for hydrocephalus in cerebellar hemorrhage. Neurology (NY) 31:1537, 1981
419. Segarra J: Cerebral vascular disease and behavior. I. The syndrome of the mesencephalic artery (basilar artery bifurcation). Arch Neurol 22:408, 1970
420. Seldarogiu P, Yazici H, Ozdemir C et al: Neurologic involvement in Behcet's syndrome: a prospective study. Arch Neurol 46:265, 1989
421. Selhorst J, Hoyt W, Feinsod M et al: Midbrain corectopia. Arch Neurol 33:193, 1976
422. Sharpe J, Rosenberg M, Hoyt W et al: Paralytic pontine exotropia. Neurology (NY) 24:1076, 1974
423. Sheehan D, Smith G: A study of the anatomy of vertebral thrombosis. Lancet 2:614, 1937
424. Sheehan S, Bauer R, Meyer J: Vertebral artery compression in cervical spondylosis. Neurology (NY) 10:968, 1960
425. Sherman D, Hart R, Easton JD: Abrupt change in head position and cerebral infarction. Stroke 12:2, 1981
426. Siekert R, Millikan C, Whisnant J: Reversal of blood flow in the vertebral arteries. Ann Intern Med 61:64, 1964
427. Siekert RG, Whisnant JP, Millikan CH: Surgical and anticoagulation therapy of occlusive cerebrovascular disease. Ann Intern Med 58:637, 1963
428. Silverstein A: Acute infarctions of the brainstem in the distribution of the basilar artery. Conf Neurol 24:37, 1964
429. Silverstein A: Pontine infarction. p. 13. In Vinken P, Bruyn G (eds): Handbook of Clinical Neurology. Vol. 12. North-Holland Publishing, Amsterdam, 1972
430. Simard D: Cerebral vasomotor paralysis during migraine attack. Arch Neurol 29:207, 1973
431. Simmons Z, Biller J, Adams HP et al: Cerebellar infarction: comparison of computed tomography and magnetic resonance imaging. Ann Neurol 19:291, 1986
432. Skinhoj E: Hemodynamic studies within the brain during migraine. Arch Neurol 29:95, 1973
433. Sloan MA: Thrombolysis and stroke: past and future. Arch Neurol 44:748, 1987
434. Smith JL, Cogan D: Internuclear ophthalmoplegia. Arch Ophthalmol 61:687, 1959
435. Smith M, Laguna J: Upward gaze paralysis following unilateral pretectal infarction. Arch Neurol 38:127, 1981
436. So EL, Toole JF, Dalal P et al: Cephalic fibromuscular dysplasia in 32 patients: clinical findings and radiologic features. Arch Neurol 38:619, 1981
437. Soffin G, Feldman M, Bender M: Alterations of

sensory levels in vascular lesions of lateral medulla. Arch Neurol 18:178, 1968
438. Spetzler RF, Hadley MN, Martin NA et al: Vertebrobasilar insufficiency. I. Microsurgical treatment of extracranial vertebrobasilar disease. J Neurosurg 66:648, 1987
439. Stein B, McCormick W, Rodriques J et al: Incidence and significance of occlusive vascular disease of the extracranial arteries as documented by post-mortem angiography. Trans Am Neurol Assoc 86:60, 1961
440. Stephens R, Stilwell D: Arteries and Veins of the Human Brain. CC Thomas, Springfield, IL, 1969
441. Stern B, Krumholz A, Weiss H et al: Evaluation of brainstem stroke using brainstem auditory evoked responses. Stroke 13:705, 1981
442. Stockard J, Sharbrough F: Unique contributions of short latency auditory and somatosensory evoked potentials to neurologic diagnosis. p. 231. In Desmedt J (ed): Clinical Uses of Cerebral, Brainstem and Spinal Somatosensory Evoked Potentials. Karger, Basel, 1980
443. Stopford J: The arteries of the pons and medulla oblongata. I. J Anat Physiol 50:131, 1915
444. Stopford J: The arteries of the pons and medulla oblongata. II. J Anat Physiol 50:255, 1916
445. Strukel RJ, Garrick JG: Thoracic outlet compression in athletes: a report of four cases. Am J Sport Med 6:35, 1978
446. Stuss D, Alexander M, Lieberman A: An extraordinary form of confabulation. Neurology (NY) 28:1166, 1978
447. Sundt TM, Piepgras D: Occipital to posterior inferior cerebellar artery bypass surgery. J Neurosurg 49:916, 1978
448. Sundt T, Piepgras D, Houser O et al: Interposition saphenous vein grafts for advanced occlusive disease and large aneurysms in the posterior circulation. J Neurosurg 56:205, 1982
449. Sundt T, Smith H, Campbell J et al: Transluminal angioplasty for basilar artery stenosis. Mayo Clin Proc 55:673, 1980
450. Sundt T, Whisnant J, Piepgras D et al: Intracranial bypass grafts for vertebral basilar ischemia. Mayo Clin Proc 53:12, 1978
451. Susac J, Hoyt W, Daroff R et al: Clinical spectrum of ocular bobbing. J Neurol Neurosurg Psychiatry 33:771, 1970
452. Swanson J, Vick N: Basilar artery migraine. Neurology (NY) 28:782, 1978
453. Swanson R, Schmidley J: Amnestic syndrome and vertical gaze palsy: early detection of bilateral thalamic infarction by CT and MRI. Stroke 16:823, 1985
454. Symonds C: Two cases of thrombosis of subclavian artery with contralateral hemiplegia of sudden onset, probably embolic. Brain 50:259, 1927
455. Sypert G, Alvord E: Cerebellar infarction: a clinicopathological study. Arch Neurol 32:357, 1975
456. Szdzuy D, Lehman R: Hypoplastic distal part of the basilar artery. Neuroradiology 4:118, 1972
457. Tahmoush A, Brooks J, Keltner J: Palatal myoclonus associated with abnormal ocular and extremity movements. Arch Neurol 27:431, 1972
458. Takahashi S: Atlas of Vertebral Angiography. University Park Press, Baltimore, 1974
459. Takahashi S, Goto K, Fukasawa H et al: Computed tomography of cerebral infarction along the distribution of the basal perforating arteries. II. Thalamic arterial group. Radiology 155:119, 1985
460. Tandon P: Vertebrobasilar insufficiency secondary to cervical spondylosis: an overdiagnosed disease. J Indian Med Assoc 74:77, 1980
461. Tatemichi TK, Oropeza LA, Sacco RL et al: Doppler diagnosis of vertebral artery occlusion: role of runoff into the posterior inferior cerebellar artery. Ann Neurol 26:158, 1989.
462. Tatlow W, Bammer H: Syndrome of vertebral artery compression. Neurology (NY) 7:331, 1957
463. Tatsumi T, Shenkin H: Occlusion of the vertebral artery. J Neurol Neurosurg Psychiatry 28:235, 1965
464. Tettenborn B, Estol C, DeWitt LD et al: Accuracy of transcranial Doppler in the vertebrobasilar circulation. J Neurol 237:159, 1990
465. Thevenet A: Endarterectomy of the vertebral artery. In Berguer R, Caplan L (eds): Vertebrobasilar Arterial Occlusive Disease. Quality Medical Publications, St. Louis, 1991
466. Thompson JR, Simmons C, Hasso A et al: Occlusion of the intradural vertebrobasilar artery. Neuroradiology 14:219, 1978
467. Torma T, Fogelholm M: Complications of cerebral angiography with urograffin. Acta Neurol Scand 43:616, 1967
468. Touboul PJ, Bousser MG, LaPlane D et al: Duplex scanning of normal vertebral arteries. Stroke 17:97, 1986
469. Trattnig S, Hubsch P, Schuster H et al: Color-coded Doppler imaging of normal vertebral arteries. Stroke 21:1222, 1990
470. Trelles J, Trelles L, Urquraga C: Le ramollissemen médiane du bulbe. Rev Neurol 129:91, 1973
471. Trojanowski J, Wray S: Vertical gaze ophthlalmoplegia: selective paralysis of downgaze. Neurology (NY) 30:605, 1980
472. Tsai F, Teal J, Heishima G et al: Computed tomography in acute posterior fossa infarcts. Am J Neuroradiol 3:149, 1982
473. Ueda K, Toole J, McHenry L: Carotid and vertebrobasilar transient ischemia attacks: clinical and angiographic correlation. Neurology (NY) 29:1094, 1979
474. Van der Drift J: The EEG in cerebrovascular disease. p. 267. In Villken P, Bruyn G (eds): Handbook of Clinical Neurology. Vol. 2. North-Holland Publishing, Amsterdam, 1972
475. Von Cramm D, Hebel N, Schieri U: A contribution to the anatomical basis of thalamic amnesia. Brain 108:993, 1985
476. von Reutern GM, Budingen JH: Ultraschalldiagnostik der hirnversorgenden Arterien. Thieme, Stuttgart, 1989
477. von Reutern GM, Pourcelot L: Cardiac cycle-dependent alternating flow in vertebral arteries with subclavian artery stenoses. Stroke 9:229, 1978
478. Wall M, Slamovits T, Weisberg LA et al: Vertical

gaze ophthalmoplegia from infarction in the area of the posterior thalamo-subthalamic paramedian artery. Stroke 17:546, 1986
479. Wallenberg A: Acute bulbar affection. Arch Psychiatr Nervenheilkd 27:504, 1895
480. Watson AJ: Dissecting aneurysm of arteries other than the aorta. J Pathol Bacteriol 72:439, 1956
481. Weibel J, Fields W: Angiography of the posterior cervicocranial circulation. AJR 98:660, 1966
482. Weinstein M, Modie M, Little J et al: Digital subtraction angiography to evaluate carotid and intracranial arteriosclerotic disease. Stroke 12:123, 1981
483. Whisnant J: Discussion in cerebral vascular diseases. p. 156. In Millikan C, Siekert R, Whisnant J (eds): Transactions of the Third Princeton Conference on Cerebrovascular Disease. Grune & Stratton, Orlando, FL, 1961
484. Whisnant J, Martin M, Sayre G: Atherosclerotic stenosis of cervical arteries. Arch Neurol 5:429, 1961
485. White DN, Ketelaars EJ, Cledgett PR: Non-invasive techniques for the recording of vertebral artery flow and their limitations. Ultrasound Med Biol 6:315, 1980
486. Whittier J: Ballism and the subthalamic nucleus. Arch Neurol Psychiatry 58:672, 1947
487. Wildemann B, Hutschenreuter M, Krieger D et al: Infusion of recombinant tissue plasminogen activator for basilar artery occlusion. Stroke 21:1513, 1990
488. Wilkins R, Brody I: Wallenberg's syndrome. Arch Neurol 22:379, 1970
489. Wilkinson I: The vertebral artery. Arch Neurol 27:392, 1972
490. Wilkinson I, Russel R: Arteries of the head and neck in giant cell arteritis. Arch Neurol 27:378, 1972
491. Williams D: The syndromes of basilar insufficiency. p. 202. In Garland H (ed): Scientific Aspects of Neurology. Williams & Wilkins, Baltimore, 1961
492. Williams D, Wilson T: The diagnosis of the major and minor syndromes of basilar insufficiency. Brain 85:741, 1962
493. Wilson SAK: Ectopia pupillae in certain mesencephalic lesions. Brain 29:524, 1906
494. Wishart D: Complications in vertebral angiography as compared to nonvertebral cerebral angiography in 447 studies. Am J Roentgenol Radium Ther Nucl Med 113:527, 1971
495. Wolf J: The Classical Brainstem Syndromes. Thomas, Springfield, IL, 1971
496. Wolman L: Cerebral dissecting aneurysms. Brain 82:276, 1959
497. Wood D: Cerebrovascular complications of sickle cell anemia. Stroke 9:73, 1978
498. Woodhurst W: Cerebellar infarction: review of recent experience. Can J Neurol Sci 7:97, 1980
499. Woolsey R, Chang H: Fatal basilar artery occlusion following cervical spine injury. Paraplegia 17:280, 1979
500. Worster-Drought C, Allen I: Thrombosis of the superior cerebellar artery. Lancet 2:1137, 1929
501. Yap C, Mayo C, Barron K: "Ocular bobbing" in palatal myoclonus. Arch Neurol 18:304, 1968
502. Yates A, Guest D: Cerebral embolism due to an ununited fracture of the clavicle and subclavian thrombosis. Lancet 2:25, 1928
503. Yu Y, Moseley I, Pullicino P et al: The clinical pictures of ectasia of the intracerebral arteries. J Neurol Neurosurg Psychiatry 45:29, 1982
504. Zeal AA, Rhoton AL: Microsurgical anatomy of the posterior cerebral artery. J Neurosurg 48:534, 1978
505. Zeumer H: Vascular recanalyzing technique in interventional neuroradiology. J Neurol 231:287, 1985
506. Zeumer H, Hacke W, Ringlestein EB: Local intraarterial thrombolysis in vertebrobasilar thromboembolic dissease. Am J Neuroradiol 4:401, 1983
507. Zülch K: On circulatory disturbances in borderline zones of cerebral and spinal vessels. In Proceedings of the Second International Congress of Neurology. Excerpta Medica, London, 1955
508. Zülch KJ, Behrend R: The pathogenesis and topography of anoxia, hypoxia, and ischemia of the brain in man. p. 144. In Meyer J, Gastaut H (eds): Cerebral Anoxia and the EEG. CC Thomas, Springfield, IL, 1961

# 19
# *CEREBRAL VENOUS THROMBOSIS*

Marie-Germaine Bousser
Henry J.M. Barnett

In 1825, Ribes[101] described the clinical history of a 45-year-old man who died after a 6-month history of severe headache, epilepsy, and delirium. Postmortem examination showed thrombosis of the superior sagittal sinus, left lateral sinus, and of a cortical vein in the parietal region. This was probably the first detailed description of cerebral venous thrombosis (CVT) in man. Since then, numerous case reports and series have been published, most of them from autopsy material.[5,8,37,50,74,78,94,122,123] They had led to the classical description of a rare and severe disease characterized clinically by headache, papilledema, seizures, focal deficits, progressive coma, and death and pathologically by hemorrhagic infarction contraindicating the use of anticoagulants.

This early literature and the history of CVT have been extensively covered in two excellent French[50] and English[74] monographs. However, angiography[77,90,136] and, more recently, magnetic resonance imaging (MRI)[82,85,127] have made the intravitam diagnosis possible, and evidence has accumulated that many patients do not fall into this classical description.[3,6,13,26,51,52,65,81,89,103,113,131] This recent literature has convincingly shown that (1) CVT is far more common than previously assumed, (2) the spectrum of its clinical presentation is extremely wide, (3) its mode of onset is highly variable, and (4) its outcome is usually favorable either spontaneously or with heparin.[13,131]

Because of its frequently misleading presentation, its wide variety of causes, its unpredictable course, and certain treatment problems, CVT remains a challenge for the clinician.

## RELEVANT VENOUS ANATOMY

Blood from the brain is drained by cerebral veins, which empty into dural sinuses that are mostly drained by the internal jugular veins.[26,50,59,65,74,79]

### Dural Sinuses

The dural sinuses most commonly affected by thrombosis are the superior sagittal sinus, lateral sinuses, and cavernous sinuses (Figs. 19-1 and 19-2).

#### Superior Sagittal Sinus

The superior sagittal sinus (SSS) lies in the attached border of the falx cerebri. It starts at the foramen caecum and runs backward toward the occipital protuberance where it joins with the straight sinus (SS) and lateral sinuses (LS) to form the torcular herophili. Its anterior part is narrow, or sometimes absent, replaced by two superior cerebral veins that join behind the coronal suture.[74] This is why the anterior part of the sinus is often poorly visualized at angiography and its isolated lack of filling not sufficient to indicate thrombosis.[77,78]

The SSS receives superficial cerebral veins and drains the major part of the cortex. It also receives diploic veins connected to those of the scalp by emissary veins, which explains some cases of SSS thrombosis after cutaneous infections or contusions. SSS and other sinuses play a major role in cerebrospinal fluid (CSF) circulation because they contain most of

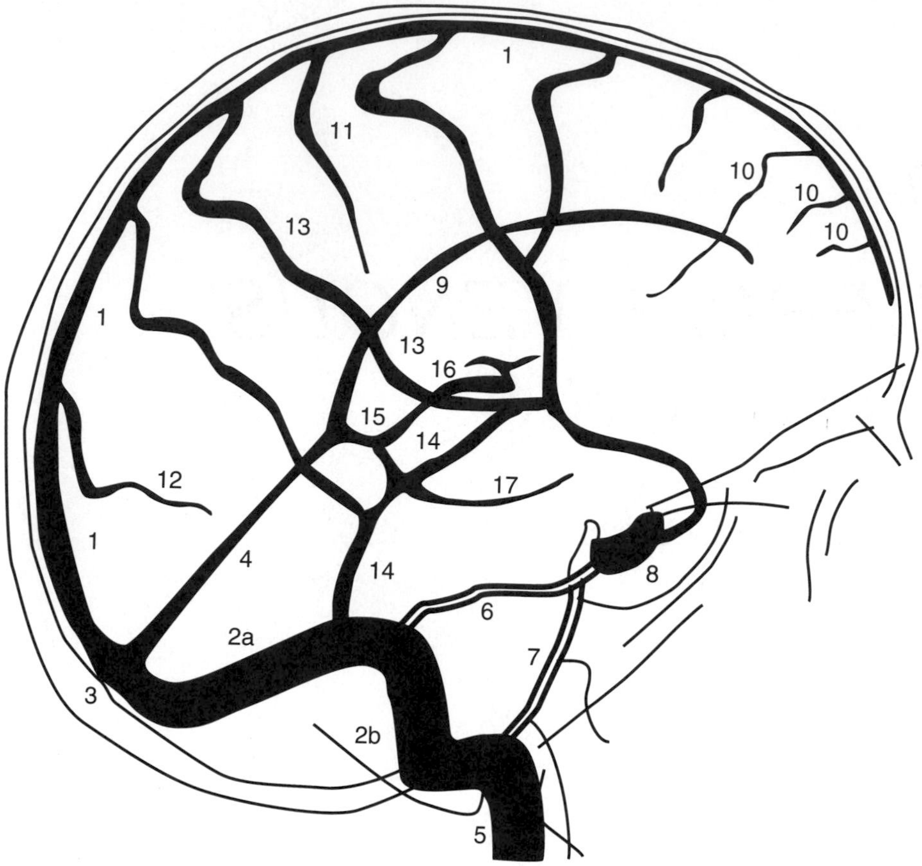


**Fig. 19-1.** Superficial and deep cerebral veins and dural sinuses: *1*, superior sagittal sinus; *2a*, transverse portion of lateral sinus; *2b*, sigmoid portion of; *3*, torcular herophili; *4*, straight sinus; *5*, internal jugular vein; *6*, superior petrosal sinus; *7*, inferior petrosal sinus; *8*, cavernous sinus; *9*, inferior sagittal sinus; *10*, frontal veins; *11*, parietal vein; *12*, occipital vein; *13*, Trolard's vein; *14*, Labbé's vein; *15*, great vein of Galen; *16*, internal cerebral vein; *17*, basal vein.

the arachnoid villi and granulations (pacchionian bodies) in which CSF absorption takes place. Thus there is a direct dependency of CSF pressure upon the intracranial venous pressure, accounting for the frequency of raised intracranial pressure in SSS or LS thrombosis.

## Lateral Sinuses

The lateral sinuses (LS) extend from the torcular herophili to the jugular bulbs and consist of two portions: the transverse portion, which lies in the attached border of the tentorium, and the sigmoid portion, which runs on the inner aspect of the mastoid process and is thereby susceptible to infectious thrombosis in patients with mastoiditis or otitis media. The LS drains blood from the cerebellum, brain stem, and posterior part of the cerebral hemispheres. They also receive some of the diploic veins and some small veins from the middle ear, still another possible source of septic thrombosis.

There are numerous LS anatomic variations that may be misinterpreted as sinus occlusion at angiography. In particular, the right LS, which is often a direct continuation of the SSS, is frequently larger than the left, which receives most of its supply from the straight sinus. In Hacker's study,[59] the transverse portions were not visualized on ipsilateral carotid angiograms in 14 percent of cases on the left side and in 3.3 percent on the right side, whereas sigmoid portions, which may be directly injected via cerebral veins, failed to fill in 4 percent of cases on the left side and were always demonstrated on the right. An isolated lack of filling of a left transverse sinus is thus more suggestive of hypoplasia than of thrombosis.

## Cavernous Sinuses

Cavernous sinuses consist of trabeculated cavities formed by the separation of the layers of the dura and are located on each side of the sella turcica, superolaterally to the sphenoid air sinuses. The oculomotor

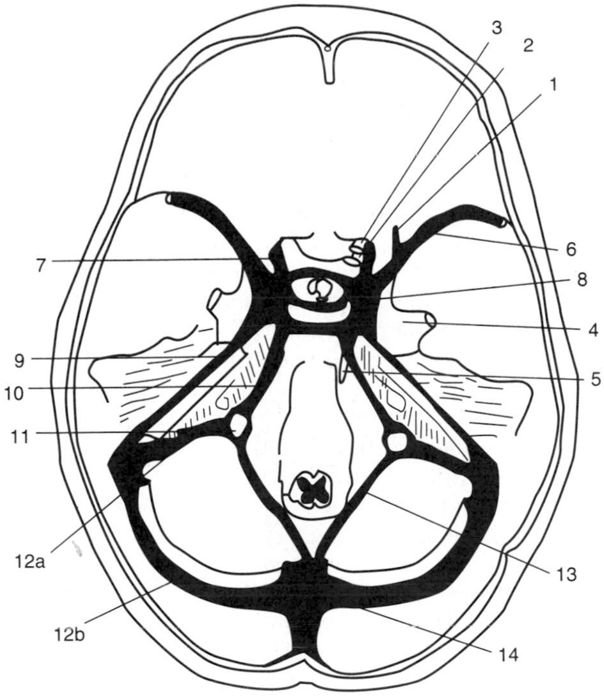


**Fig. 19-2.** Cavernous sinus and dural sinuses: *1*, trochlear cranial nerve; *2*, carotid artery; *3*, optic nerve; *4*, trigeminal nerve; *5*, oculomotor nerve; *6*, sphenoparietal sinus; *7*, ophthalmic vein; *8*, cavernous sinus; *9*, superior petrosal sinus; *10*, inferior petrosal sinus; *11*, internal jugular vein; *12a*, sigmoid portion of lateral sinus; *12b*, transverse portion of lateral sinus; *13*, posterior occipital sinus; *14*, torcular herophili.

and trochlear cranial nerves, along with the ophthalmic and maxillary branches of the trigeminal nerve, course along the lateral wall of the cavernous sinuses, whereas the abducens nerve and the carotid artery with its surrounding sympathetic plexus are located within the center of the sinus itself.

Cavernous sinuses drain the blood from the orbits through the ophthalmic veins and from the anterior part of the base of the brain by the sphenoparietal sinus and the middle cerebral veins. They empty into both the superior and inferior petrosal sinuses and ultimately into the internal jugular veins. Because of their situation, cavernous sinuses are often thrombosed in relation to infections of the face or sphenoid sinusitis, and, in contrast to other varieties of sinus thrombosis, infection is still the leading cause.[32,119]

Rarely injected on carotid angiograms, cavernous sinuses are now well visualized on computed tomography (CT) scans and MRI.

### Cerebral Veins

The three groups of veins that drain the blood supply from the brain are the superficial cerebral veins (or cortical veins), deep cerebral veins, and the veins of the posterior fossa (Fig. 19-1).

**Superficial Cerebral Veins.** Some of the superficial cerebral veins— the frontal, parietal, and occipital superior cerebral veins—drain the cortex ascendingly into the SSS, whereas others—mainly the middle cerebral veins—drain descendingly into the cavernous sinuses. These veins are linked by Trolard's great anastomotic vein, which connects the SSS to the middle cerebral veins, which are themselves connected to the LS by Labbé's vein. These cortical veins present some peculiarities[74] that are important for an understanding of some of the clinical features of CVT. They have thin walls, no muscle fibers, and no valves, thereby permitting both their dilatation and the reversal of the direction of blood flow when the sinus in which they drain is occluded. They are linked by numerous anastomoses, allowing the development of a collateral circulation (angiographically visible as "corkscrew" vessels), which probably explains the good prognosis of some CVT. The number and the location of cortical veins is inconstant, which makes the angiographic diagnosis of isolated cortical vein thrombosis extremely difficult and sometimes impossible. This anatomic variability, together with the possibility of flow reversal and of development of collateral circulation, accounts for the absence of well-delineated venous territories and consequently of well-defined clinical syndromes of cortical vein thrombosis.

**Deep Cerebral Veins.** Blood from the deep white matter of the cerebral hemispheres and from the basal ganglia is drained by internal cerebral and basal veins that join to form the great vein of Galen, which drains into the straight sinus. In constrast to the superficial veins, the deep system is constant and always visualized at angiography, so that its thrombosis is easily recognized.

**Veins of the Posterior Fossa.** The veins of the posterior fossa may be divided into three groups:[66,67] superior veins, draining into the galenic system, anterior veins, draining into the petrosal sinus, and posterior veins, draining into the torcular and neighboring straight and lateral sinuses. They are variable in course, and angiographic diagnosis of their occlusion is extremely difficult.

## PATHOLOGY

Pathologic findings have been extensively described in the past.[50,74,123] They vary, depending on the site of thrombosis and the interval between the onset of symptoms and death.

The *thrombus* itself is like other venous thrombi elsewhere in the body: when it is fresh, it is a red thrombus, rich in red blood cells and fibrin and poor in platelets; when it is old, it is replaced by fibrous tissue (Fig. 19-3), sometimes showing recanalization. Its formation is due to the usual pathogenetic factors: venous stasis, increased clotting tendency, changes in the vessel wall, and, less frequently, embolization. Its location and extension are variable. In autopsy series, extensive thrombosis of the SSS and tributary veins is the most frequent finding, but this pattern of involvement no longer reflects the real distribution of CVT (see the next section).

The consequences of CVT on the brain are again highly variable: massive brain edema can be the only consequence in thrombosis restricted to SSS,[74] whereas occlusion of cerebral veins usually leads to infarction. Venous infarcts affect the cortex and adjacent white matter and are often hemorrhagic, which explains the possibility of associated subarachnoid hemorrhage and subdural and intracerebral hematoma. The classical anatomic presentation is that of extensive bilateral hemorrhagic infarcts, located in the superior and internal part of both hemispheres, due to thrombosis of the SSS and its tributary cortical veins (Fig. 19-4).

## INCIDENCE

The true incidence of CVT is totally unknown because of the absence of epidemiologic study specifically devoted to this subject. In most autopsy series, the incidence was extremely low. Ehlers and Courville[37] found only 16 SSS thromboses in a series of 12,500 autopsies, and Barnett and Hyland[8] found only 39 noninfective CVT in 20 years. Kalbag and Woolf[74] indicated that CVT was the principal cause of death in only 21.7 persons per year in England and Wales between 1952 and 1961. By contrast, Towbin[128] found CVT in 9 percent of 182 consecutive autopsies, and Averback,[3] in a series of 7 cases, insists that primary CVT in young adults is an "under-recognized disease." The more recent publication of large clinical series[6,13,26,78,89,103,127] suggests that the true incidence is much higher than thought from autopsy series, possibly 10 times higher because of a current mortality rate of approximately 10 percent[13] or possibly less.[127] Three to four new cases are encountered each year in a neurology department in a general hospital.[13,89,127]

It has been suggested that the incidence of CVT is higher in females[41] and in the aged, reflecting the overall greater incidence of thromboembolic diseases in these categories. This was not confirmed in the majority of recent series, which showed that both sexes are equally affected, and all age groups, from the neonate to the very old, are concerned, with possibly a slight preponderance in young adults.[3,6,13,26,52,82,85,103,113,127]

## ETIOLOGY

A host of well-known conditions can cause or predispose to CVT (Table 19-1). They include all known surgical, gyneco-obstetric, and medical causes of deep-vein thrombosis as well as a number of local or

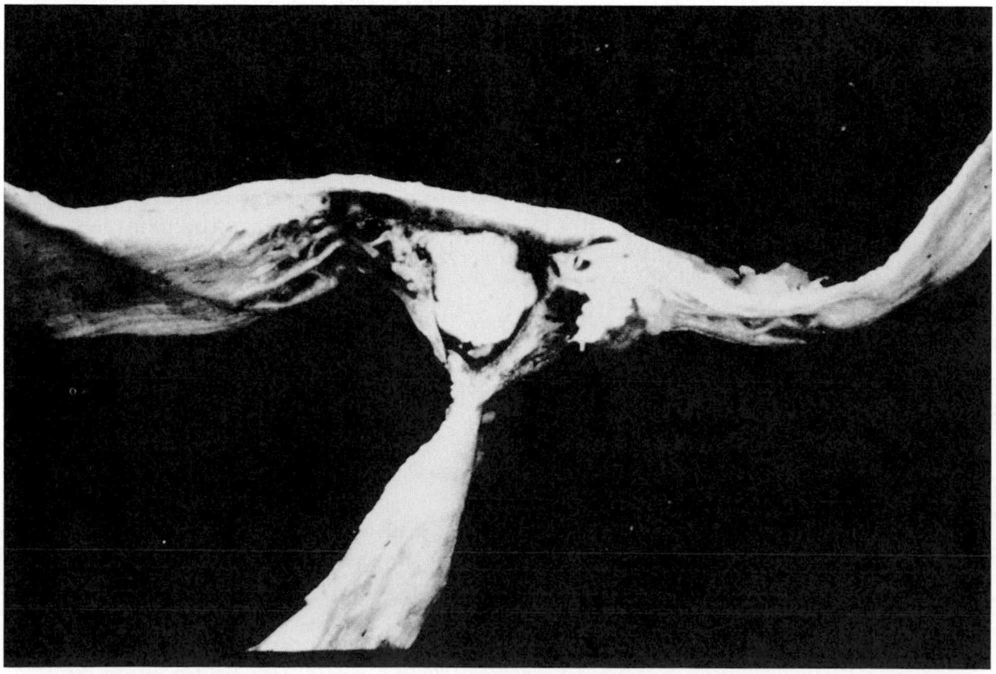

**Fig. 19-3.** Old superior sagittal sinus thrombosis.

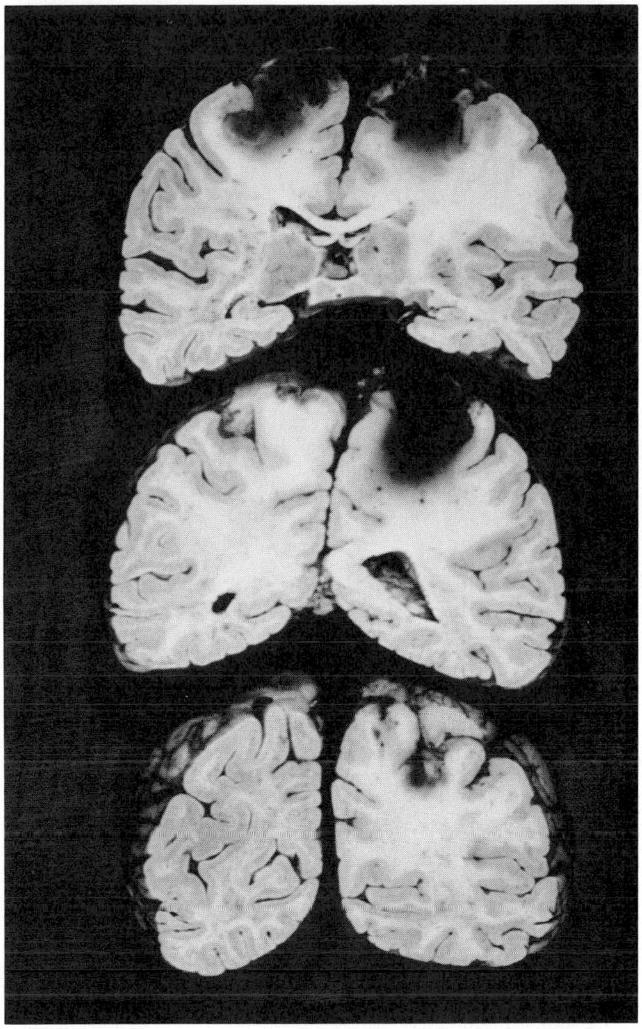

**Fig. 19-4.** Bilateral hemorrhagic infarcts in superior sagittal sinus thrombosis.

regional causes, either infective or noninfective, such as head trauma, brain tumors, and arterial infarcts. Although infection still constituted the major identifiable cause in a recent series[51] (27 out of 66), it is well established that the incidence of septic CVT has been greatly reduced in developed countries since the introduction of antibiotics.[32,36,119] In our own series of 38 cases published in 1985 there were only 4 septic cases,[13] and in our present series of 76 cases there are 8 septic cases (10.5 percent). Cavernous sinus thrombosis remains the most common form of septic thrombosis, usually following an infection of the middle third of the face due to *Staphylococcus aureus*. Other sites of infection include sphenoid or ethmoid sinusitis, dental abscess, and, less often, otitis media. In chronic forms, gram-negative rods and fungi such as *Aspergillus* species[110] are more commonly isolated.[32] Among general causes, parasitic infections such as trichinosis[42] and, more recently, HIV and CMV infections[87] have been added to the long list of infective conditions possibly leading to CVT.

In young women, CVT occurs more frequently during puerperium than during pregnancy[8,13,41,52,77,90] and remains very common in developing countries,[6] whereas in developed countries, the role of oral contraceptives (OC)[13,17,31,41,43,103] is more important. In our series of 76 cases, OC use was the only etiologic factor in 7 patients (9 percent). This had led us, as many others,[13,17,31,43,103] to stop OC and promptly look for CVT (now with MRI) in women presenting with any of the neurologic manifestations compatible with this condition. However, OC use was also found together with other conditions, such as systemic lupus or Behcet's disease, in 5 of our 76 patients, stressing the need for an extensive etiologic workup, even in young women taking OC.

Among the numerous noninfective medical causes of CVT, malignancies[3,4,26,44,63,86,96,113] and inflammatory diseases such as Behcet's disease[12,13] and connective tissue diseases[26,88,130] are the most frequent. Though rare, hereditary antithrombin III,[105] protein C,[126] and protein S[40] deficiencies should be systematically looked for in the absence of obvious cause because they indicate the need to conduct a family study and long-term treatment.

Despite the continuous description of new causes, the proportion of cases of unknown etiology remains in our recent series between 25[66] and 35 percent.[51,89,127] The search for a cause thus remains one of the most vexing problems in CVT. It necessitates an extensive initial workup and, when no cause is found, a long follow-up with repeated investigations. In some cases initially interpreted as idiopathic, a general disease can be discovered some months later.[13]

In neonates and children, the etiology of CVT is characterized by the frequency of regional infections (e.g., otitis and mastoiditis) neonatal asphyxia, severe dehydrations, and congenital heart diseases.[3,108] There are, however, also a number of idiopathic cases, 30 out of 80 in one old series.[3]

## CLINICAL ASPECTS

Cerebral venous thrombosis presents with a remarkably wide spectrum of symptoms and signs, as illustrated in our series of 76 patients (Table 19-2). Headache is in all series the most frequent (80 percent) and often the earliest sign.[6,13,26,50,51,74,78] However, the frequency of other symptoms differs from classical series: focal deficits (hemiparesis and hemisensory disturbances are found much more frequently than dysphasia or homonymous hemianopia) and seizures (partial, generalized, status epilepticus) were each present in approximately one-third of cases, whereas in most series they are found in 50 to 75 percent of cases.[6,26,50,51,74,78] The same applies to mental changes and disorders of consciousness, found in only one-fourth of our cases. By contrast, papilledema, present

**TABLE 19-1. Cerebral Venous Thrombosis: Recognized Causes or Predisposing Conditions**

| Cause | Local | General |
|---|---|---|
| Infective | Direct septic trauma[50,74]<br>Intracranial infection: abscess, empyema, meningitis[13,50,51,74,78]<br>Regional infections: otitis, tonsillitis, sinusitis, stomatitis, skin[13,26,50,51,74] | Bacterial: septicemia,[50,51,74,78], endocarditis,[50,51,74,78] typhoid,[50] tuberculosis[94]<br>Viral: measles,[74] hepatitis,[94] encephalitis,[74] (herpes, HIV), CMV[87]<br>Parasitic: malaria,[26] trichinosis[42]<br>Fungal: aspergillosis[110] |
| Noninfective | Head injury (open or closed, with or without fracture)[8,13,26,74,75,127]<br>Neurosurgical operation[50,74,94]<br>Cerebral infarcts and hemorrhages[8,74]<br>Tumors (meningioma, metastasis, glomus tumor)[50,74,85]<br>Porencephaly, arachnoid cysts[13,26,50]<br>Infusions into the internal jugular vein[118] | Surgical: any surgery with or without deep vein thrombosis[8,26]<br>Gyneco-obstetric<br>Pregnancy and puerperium[6,8,13,41,52,77]<br>Oral contraceptives (estrogens,[13,41,103] progestogens[17,31,43])<br>Medical<br>Cardiac: congenital heart disease,[26] cardiac insufficiency,[8,74,78,94] pacemaker[53]<br>Malignancies: any visceral carcinoma,[8,63,113] lymphoma,[4,86] leukemia,[26,86] carcinoid,[96] L-asparaginase therapy[44]<br>RBC disorders: polycythemia,[8] posthemorrhagic anemia,[51] sickle cell disease,[45] paroxysmal nocturnal hemoglobinuria[129]<br>Thrombocytemia (primary or secondary)[91]<br>Coagulation disorders: antithrombin III,[105] protein C[126] and protein S deficiencies,[40] circulating anticoagulants,[80] disseminated intravascular coagulation,[115] heparin- or heparinoid-induced thrombocytopenia[72]<br>Severe dehydration of any cause[50,51,74]<br>Digestive: cirrhosis,[26,50] Crohn's disease,[16] ulcerative colitis[78,137]<br>Connective tissue: systemic lupus,[130] temporal arteritis,[26] Wegener's granulomatosis[88]<br>Venous thromboembolic disease, Hughes-Stovin syndrome[69]<br>Others: Behçet's disease,[12,13] sarcoidosis,[22] nephrotic syndrome,[9,51] neonatal asphyxia,[51] parenteral injections,[39] androgen therapy[112] |
| Idiopathic | | |

**TABLE 19-2. 76 Patients with Cerebral Venous Thrombosis: Main Neurological Signs and Symptoms**

| | |
|---|---|
| Headache | 61 (80%) |
| Papilledema | 38 (50%) |
| Motor of sensory deficit | 27 (35%) |
| Seizures | 22 (29%) |
| Drowsiness, mental changes, confusion or coma | 18 (27%) |
| Dysphasia | 5 ( 6%) |
| Multiple cranial nerve palsies | 3 ( 4%) |
| Cerebellar incoordination | 2 ( 3%) |
| Nystagmus | 2 ( 3%) |
| Hearing loss | 2 ( 3%) |
| Bilateral or alternating cortical signs | 3 ( 4%) |

in 50 percent of our cases was more frequent than in previous series: 12,[51] 34,[6] and 43 percent.[127] It should also be noted that the classical picture of SSS thrombosis with its bilateral or alternating deficits and/or seizures[50,74] was encountered in only 4 percent of our patients. Although there might be a selection bias in our series because of an important referral from ophthalmologists, the main reason for this changing pattern of clinical presentation of CVT is most probably the possibility of early diagnosis now offered by modern neuroimaging techniques.

The mode of onset of symptoms is also highly variable: in our series of 76 patients, it was acute (less than 48 hours) in 22 patients (29 percent), of whom 20 had focal signs; it was subacute (more than 48 hours but less than 30 days) in 24 (32 percent), of whom 15 had focal signs, and it was chronic (more than 30 days) in 30 (39 percent), of whom 20 had focal signs.

With such a wide spectrum of neurologic signs and modes of onset, the clinical presentation of CVT is extremely variable. It can be separated into the following four groups: those with isolated intracranial hypertension, those with focal cerebral signs, those with the cavernous sinus syndrome, and those with unusual presentations.

**Isolated Intracranial Hypertension.** Isolated intracranial hypertension with headache papilledema and sixth nerve palsy, mimicking benign intracranial hypertension (pseudotumor cerebri), is the most homogeneous pattern, accounting for 38 percent of our 76 patients. There is no characteristic site or nature to the headache, which is usually diffuse, and sometimes associated with vomiting. It can evolve over days, months,[13] or even years.[7] Despite the fact that SSS and LS thrombosis have long been recognized as one of the leading causes of benign intracranial hypertension,[10,47,58,124] this syndrome has, in numerous reports,[28,117] been diagnosed purely on clinical, CSF, and CT findings. Since CVT can mimic all the features of benign intracranial hypertension,[13,34,127,135] normal four-vessel angiography or normal MRI should be added to the classical diagnostic criteria of this syndrome.[27,56]

**Focal Cerebral Signs.** The second group, characterized by the presence of focal signs, is the largest, accounting for roughly 75 percent of published cases, but it is a heterogeneous one depending upon the mode of onset of focal signs, their nature (deficits, seizures, or both), and their possible association with altered consciousness. Acute cases (21 percent in our series) simulate an arterial stroke, but the presence of seizures and the absence of a well-defined arterial syndrome should alert the clinician to the possibility of CVT, particularly if the patient steadily deteriorates. Chronic cases (16 percent) simulate tumors, whereas subacute cases (17 percent) mimic encephalitis or abscess, particularly in patients with fever, increased ESR, and CSF pleocytosis. Focal signs can be even more misleading when they present like transient ischemic attacks[13] or migrainelike phenomena.[92]

**Cavernous Sinus Syndrome.** Cavernous sinus thrombosis has a distinctive clinical picture,[26,29,32,50,51,81,119] which includes, in the classical acute cases, chemosis, proptosis, and painful ophthalmoplegia, initially unilateral but frequently becoming bilateral. Dramatic complications can occur, such as extension to other sinuses[115] and stenosis (with a mycotic aneurysm in one case) of the intracavernous portion of the internal carotid arteries.[29] However, cavernous sinus thrombosis is not always acute but can also take a more indolent form (either spontaneously or because of the masking effect of an inadequate antibiotic regimen), with an isolated abducens nerve palsy and only mild chemosis and proptosis, leading to great diagnostic difficulties.[32]

**Unusual Presentations.** The grouping of signs of CVT into the foregoing three main patterns does not account for every case. Some rare cases initially present with isolated intracranial hypertension and later develop focal neurologic signs.[7,13,45] Some patients may initially present with isolated headache, which can, for instance, be mistaken for a postdural puncture headache after delivery,[68] or with isolated grand mal seizures mimicking eclampsia and sometimes associated with it.[139] Psychiatric disturbances (irritability, lack of interest, anxiety, depression) are sometimes the prevailing symptoms,[104] as was recently shown in four cases during pregnancy and puerperium.[104] Other cases present with headache of sudden onset, neck stiffness, and CT scan or lumbar puncture evidence of subarachnoid hemorrhage simulating a ruptured intracranial aneurysm.[13] Finally, CVT may be so insidious that it is only discovered at postmortem, particularly in elderly patients dying of congestive heart failure.[8] It can even be totally asymptomatic, as recently shown in a patient given a routine CT scan after mastoidectomy, which showed a left LS thrombosis.[55]

It is clear from the above description that the clinical presentation of CVT is extremely variable and often misleading. One must therefore routinely make the appropriate investigations to reach the diagnosis.

## TOPOGRAPHIC DIAGNOSIS

The location of venous thrombosis in our 76 patients is indicated in Table 19-3. It shows that SSS (70 percent) and LS (72 percent) are the sinuses most frequently involved but rarely in isolation (25 percent). In other cases, thrombosis involved several sinuses (33 percent) or sinuses and cerebral veins (41 percent). In one case there was an isolated thrombosis of the deep venous system. This relative frequency slightly differs from the literature where SSS thrombosis ranks first and LS thrombosis second. The third commonest location in published data is cavernous sinus. Thrombosis of the galenic system is rare, with some 50 reported cases. Only a few cases have been described of petrosal sinus,[50] isolated cortical,[49] or cerebellar vein[13] thrombosis, but these conditions might be underdiagnosed because of the extreme difficulty in arriving at the diagnosis.

The frequent association of sinus and cerebral vein thrombosis explains the lack of well-defined topo-

**TABLE 19-3. Site of Venous Occlusion at Angiography in 76 Patients with Cerebral Venous Thrombosis**

| Location | Frequency |
|---|---|
| Superior sagittal sinus | 53 (70%) |
| Lateral sinuses | 55 (72%) |
| Right: 18 (24%) | |
| Left: 24 (31.5%) | |
| Both: 13 (17%) | |
| Straight sinus | 10 (13%) |
| Cavernous sinus | 2 (3%) |
| Cerebral veins | 29 (38%) |
| Superficial: 26 (34%) | |
| Deep: 3 (4%) | |
| Cerebellar veins | 3 (4%) |
| One sinus only | 19 (25%) |
| Superior sagittal sinus: 7 (9%) | |
| Lateral sinus: 11 (14%) | |
| Straight sinus: 1 (1%) | |
| Deep veins only | 1 (1%) |
| Isolated cortical veins | 0 |
| More than one sinus (superior sagittal sinus + lateral sinus + straight sinus) | 25 (33%) |
| Sinuses + cerebral or cerebellar veins | 31 (41%) |

graphic clinical syndromes, similar to those described in arterial occlusions, except for cavernous sinus thrombosis. Thus SSS thrombosis can present with any of the above-described patterns, and this also applies to LS thrombosis, although isolated intracranial hypertension is probably even more frequent, and, among focal signs, dysphasia is not unusual.[13] Thrombosis of the petrosal sinuses was described in the old literature[50,122] and was characterized mainly by a fifth nerve palsy for the superior sinus and by a sixth nerve palsy for the inferior one. As already stressed, angiographic diagnosis of isolated cortical vein thrombosis is extremely difficult,[49] but there are old reports of anatomic or surgical cases in patients presenting with an acute or rapid onset of focal deficits, seizures, or both.[25,35,50] The classical picture of deep cerebral venous thrombosis is that of an acute coma with signs of decerebration or extrapyramidal hypertonia leading to death in a few days or resolving, but with marked sequelae such as akinetic mutism, dementia, bilateral athetoid movements, vertical gaze palsy, and dystonia.[11,37,50,73,138] Recent reports have illustrated benign forms presenting mainly with confusion.[13,38,61,93] The few reported cases of cerebellar vein thrombosis are mainly anatomic,[94] but we reported a patient presenting with a 3-month history of cranial nerve palsies, cerebellar incoordination, and papilledema simulating a posterior fossa tumor,[13] and a somewhat similar case has been recently published.[102]

MRI studies should help to improve clinicoradiologic correlations and assist in defining the clinical patterns of the involvement of various sinuses and cerebral veins. At present, topographic diagnosis does not seem important for the management of thrombosis; the crucial step is to recognize CVT itself.

## INVESTIGATIONS

### Computed Tomography Scan

Computed tomography (CT) scan with and without contrast injection is the first neuroimaging examination to carry out when CVT is clinically suspected, both to rule out other conditions and to try to confirm CVT. CT findings have been described in detail in numerous reports[1,14,16,18,20,24,48,55,76,97,99,109,111,114,134] and are now well established.

**Direct Signs of Cerebral Venous Thrombosis.** Three abnormalities are considered as direct signs of CVT: the cord sign, the dense triangle, and the empty delta or empty triangle sign.

The *cord sign*, visible on unenhanced CT scans, represents the visualization of a thrombosed cortical vein;[20,48,99] it is extremely rare and its diagnostic value is debated.[24]

The *dense triangle* also reflects spontaneous SSS opacification by freshly congealed blood[18,97] (Fig. 19-5A); it is thus a very early sign, again extremely rare, present in less than 1 out of 50 cases. It is difficult to assess, particularly in other sinuses (lateral and straight sinus), which can be spontaneously hyperdense in normal children[95] or in patients with hemoconcentration.

The *empty delta sign*, described by Buonanno and associates,[20] appears after contrast injection and reflects the opacification of collateral veins in the SSS wall, contrasting with the noninjection of the clot inside the sinus (Fig. 19-5B). It is the most frequent direct sign, present in approximately 30 percent of published cases.[1,18,99,134] However, it is absent when thrombosis does not affect the posterior third of SSS or when the CT scan is performed in the first 5 days after the onset of symptoms or more than 2 months later.[111] Its sensitivity and specificity are increased with some technical refinements such as orthogonal sectioning, different window and level settings, and multiplanar reformations.[48,55,99,109,114] These reasons probably explain why the empty delta sign is found only in 10 to 20 percent of CT scans performed routinely to rule out other conditions in patients suspected of having CVT.[13,24] Furthermore, it is not pathognomonic, since the early division of the SSS can be responsible for a false delta sign.[95]

**Indirect and Nonspecific Signs of Cerebral Venous Thrombosis.** Indirect and nonspecific abnormalities are more frequent.

Intense contrast enhancement of the falx and tentorium[18,20,99] is present in some 20 percent of cases[24]

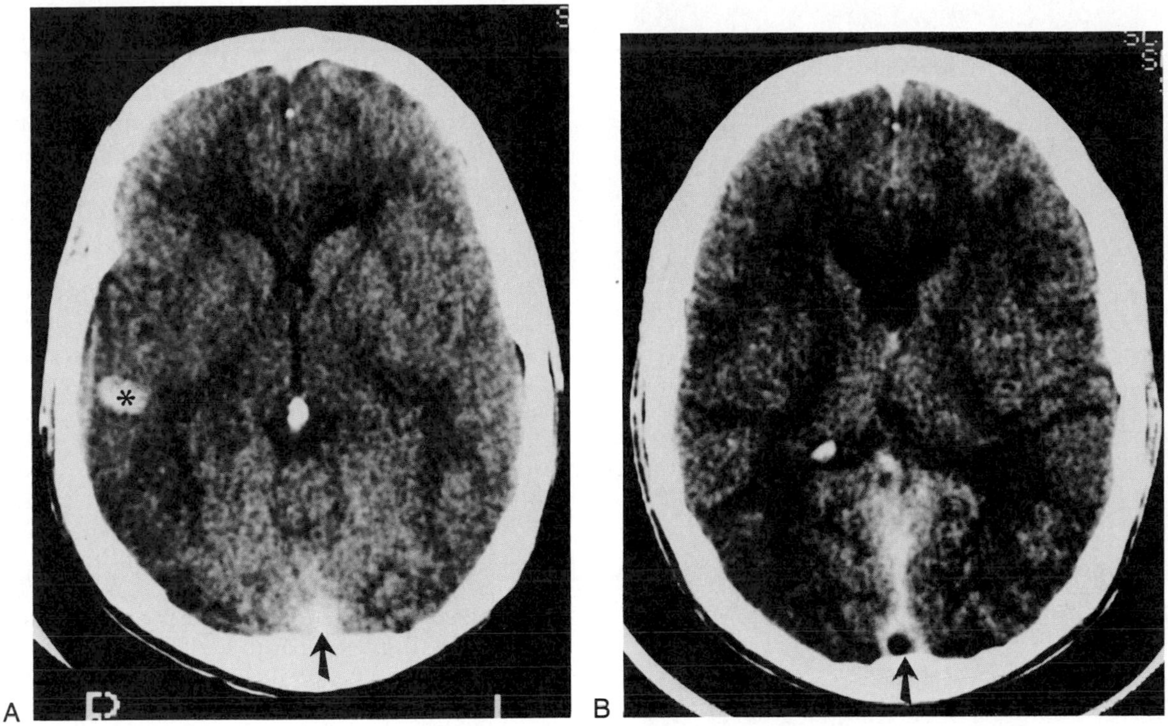

**Fig. 19-5.** (**A**) Unenhanced CT scan: dense triangle in a recent superior sagittal sinus thrombosis (*arrow*) with a small cortical hemorrhage (*star*). (**B**) Enhanced CT scan in the same patient 10 days later: empty delta sign (*arrow*).

(Fig. 19-6). It is easily recognized in the tentorium but can be difficult to assess in the falx, particularly in aged patients. It indicates venous stasis or hyperemia of the dura mater. Tentorial enhancement is usually thought to suggest straight sinus thrombosis,[99] but it is not rare in SSS thrombosis.[13,24]

A common finding is the presence of small ventricles resulting from cerebral swelling and at times accompanied by diffuse low density suggestive of edema.[13,20,24,76,99] Though reported in 20 to 50 percent of cases, it is not a useful sign because it is totally nonspecific and is frequently difficult to differentiate from normal brain, particularly in the young. In some cases the cerebral swelling can be confirmed by the later increase in size of ventricles that were initially small.[76] However, the opposite finding, that is, enlarged ventricles, is a possibility and therefore does not exclude the diagnosis.[13]

Usually described by pathologists as hemorrhagic, venous infarcts on CT scan present with a spontaneous hyperdensity in 10 to 50 percent of cases.[13,18,24,61,99] Two main features are encountered: large subcortical, often multifocal, hematomas[24,41] and petechial hemorrhages within large hypodensities[24] (Fig. 19-7). Nonhemorrhagic venous infarcts are frequent and protean in appearance:[24,99] focal hypodensity with gyral enhancement, areas of hypodensity without enhancement, and isolated gyral enhancement (Fig. 19-8). Hemorrhagic or nonhemorrhagic infarcts can be unilateral[13,18,24] or bilateral,[20,24,99] single[20,24] or multiple.[24,99] They are seen superficially in the hemispheres in SSS thrombosis and within the basal ganglia in deep venous system thrombosis.

**Normal Scan.** In 10 to 20 percent of cases, the CT scan is normal in patients with proven CVT, more frequently so in patients presenting with isolated intracranial hypertension than in those with focal signs.[24,99]

**Postcontrast Computed Tomography.** The CT scan can also be useful in demonstrating cavernous sinus thrombosis,[29,30] showing on postcontrast CT as multiple irregular filling defects with bulging cavernous sinuses and enlarged orbital veins.[30] The presence of air, seen on coronal sections, has been reported in a case of septic thrombosis.[29]

**Summary.** The place of CT scan in the diagnostic strategy of CVT is of crucial importance because CT scan rules out other conditions such as arterial stroke, abscess, tumors, and subarachnoid hemorrhage. It should be employed at the earliest clinical suspicion

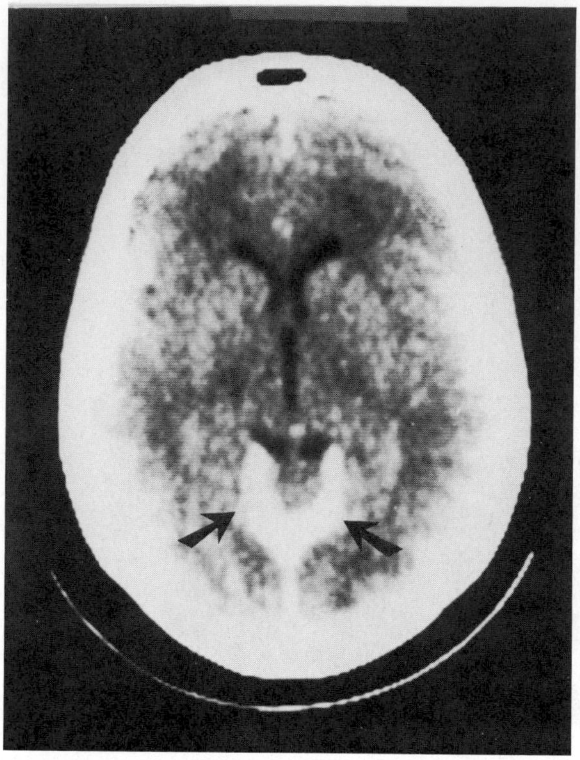

**Fig. 19-6.** Enhanced CT scan. Intense tentorial enhancement in a patient with thrombosis of the superior sagittal sinus and both lateral sinuses.

of CVT and performed at first without contrast, and, in the absence of hemorrhagic infarct, with contrast. Nevertheless, since most CT findings are nonspecific, and because the CT scan may occasionally be normal, angiographic and MRI confirmation should be obtained in all cases lacking CT pathognomonic changes.[13,127]

## Angiography

Angiography has been the key procedure in the diagnosis of CVT for many years and still remains the method of reference for evaluation of new methods. It requires a perfect technique: four-vessel angiography (conventional or digitalized intra-arterial) with visualization of the entire venous phase on at least two projections (frontal and lateral) and, if possible, three, oblique views being the best to entirely visualize the SSS.[2,13,77,90,133,136]

The partial or complete lack of filling of veins or sinuses is the best angiographic sign of CVT. Easily recognized when it affects the posterior part or the entire SSS (Fig. 19-9), both LS (Fig. 19-10), or the deep venous system (Fig. 19-11), it may be more difficult to interpret in other locations, such as the anterior third of the SSS or the left LS where it can be confused with hypoplasia.[59] For occlusion of the anterior part of the SSS to be established, it is necessary to have either involvement of another sinus or unequivocal indirect signs of CVT, such as delayed emptying and dilated

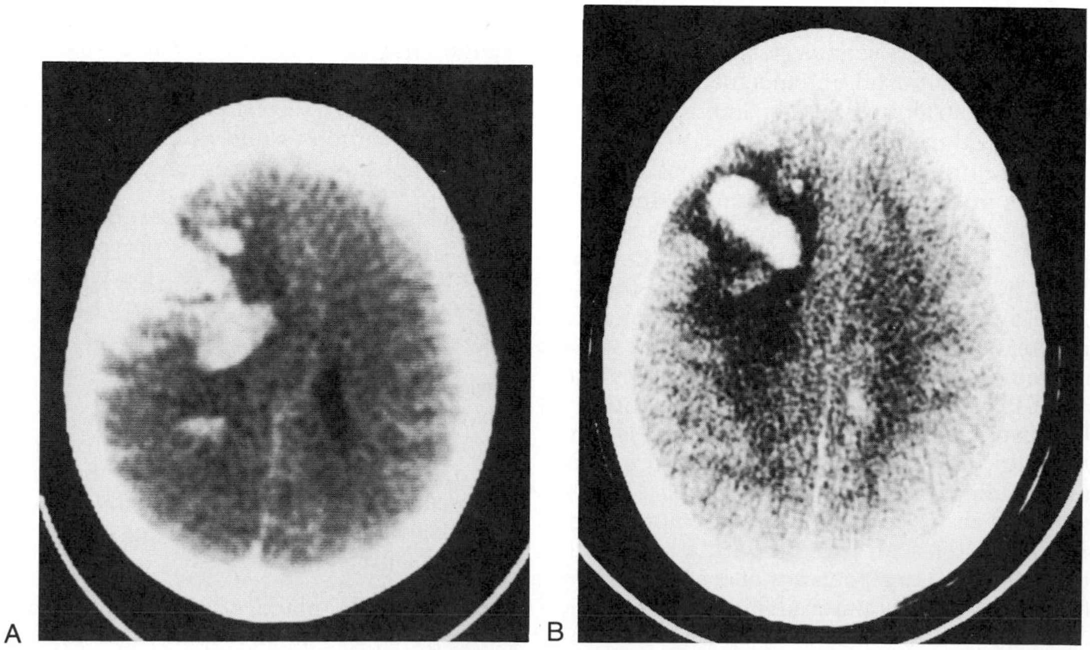


**Fig. 19-7.** Unenhanced CT scans in two patients with superior sagittal sinus thrombosis. (**A**) Spontaneous hyperdensity with severe mass effect suggestive of an hemorrhagic infarct. (**B**) Bilateral hemorragic infarct.

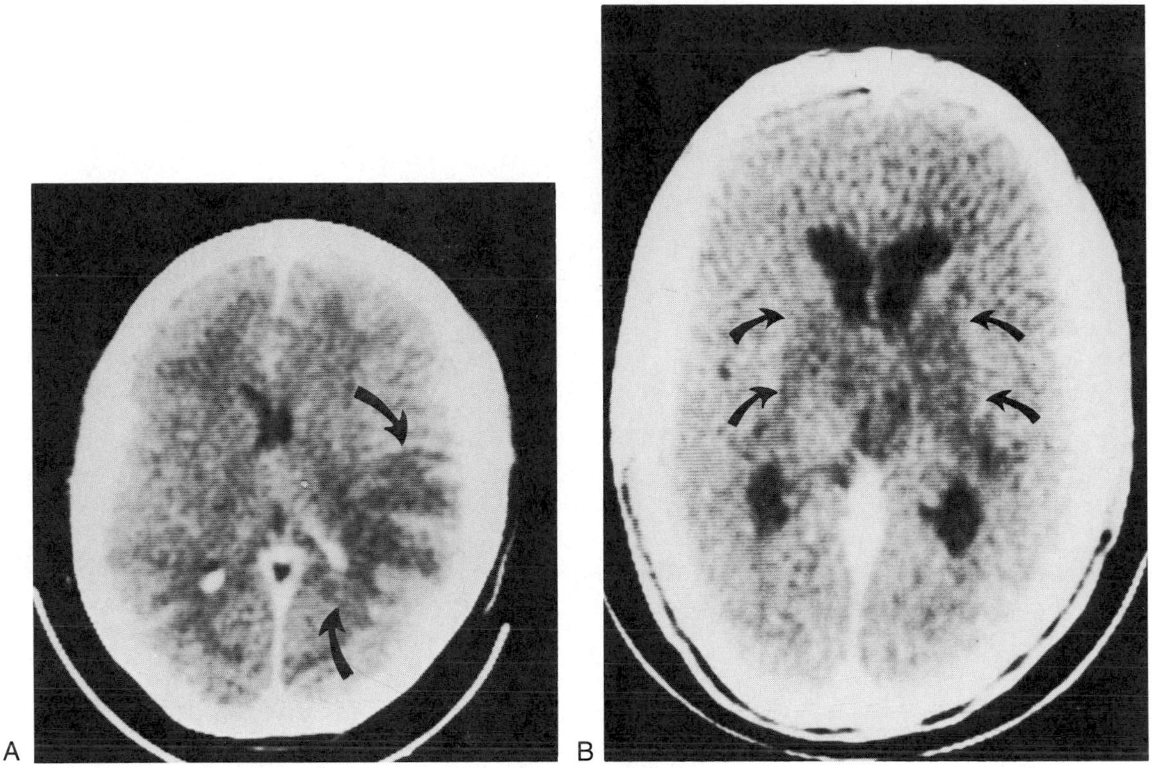

**Fig. 19-8.** Enhanced CT scans. (**A**) Large area of corticosubcortical hypodensity with mass effect on the lateral ventricle in a patient with superior sagittal sinus thrombosis (*curved arrows*). (**B**) Bilateral basal ganglia hypodensity (*curved arrows*) in a patient with deep cerebral vein thrombosis.

collateral veins. For LS thrombosis the main argument is the absence of filling of the totality of the sinus or of its sigmoid portion, which is in contrast to the presence of the sinus groove and normality of the jugular foramen on plain x-rays of the skull.[19] However, in some cases such signs are lacking, and MRI is required to differentiate between thrombosis and hypoplasia (Fig. 19-12).

The absence of a cortical vein is difficult and sometimes impossible to detect except when the vein is partly visualized but stops suddenly and is surrounded by dilated collateral veins (Fig. 19-9).

Other angiographic findings include delayed emptying and collateral venous pathways. Delayed emptying is found in 50 percent of cases[13,77,90] and explains why in old conventional angiography, the venous phase was frequently not visualized, and therefore CVT not diagnosed. Films taken up to 12 seconds after the injection of contrast were needed.[77] The development of collateral venous pathways is also found in approximately half the cases and almost invariably indicates SSS thrombosis. Dilated and tortuous cortical collateral veins with a corkscrew appearance are much more frequent Fig. 19-9) than transcerebral or intradural collaterals.[13,77,90,133,136] An important mass effect is extremely rare and has only been reported in a few cases.[13,133]

## Magnetic Resonance Imaging

MRI offers major advantages for the evaluation of patients suspected of having CVT because of its sensitivity to blood flow, its ability to visualize the thrombus itself, and its noninvasiveness. A variety of MR findings has been described, mainly related to the evolution of thrombosis.[34,61,82,106,116,127] At a very early stage, there is an absence of flow void and the occluded vessel appears isointense on T1-weighted image (WI) and hypointense on T2-WI. A few days later, the absence of flow void persists, but the thrombus becomes hyperintense, initially on T1-WI and then on T2-WI[82] (Fig. 19-13). In large vessels these changes start in the periphery and proceed toward the center. They represent the aging of the thrombus with biochemical conversion of oxyhemoglobin to methemoglobin, rather than extension of thrombosis.

Late changes (approximately 2 weeks after onset) can reveal the beginning of vascular recanalization with the resumption of flow void in the previously thrombosed vessel. MRI can thus not only reveal ve-

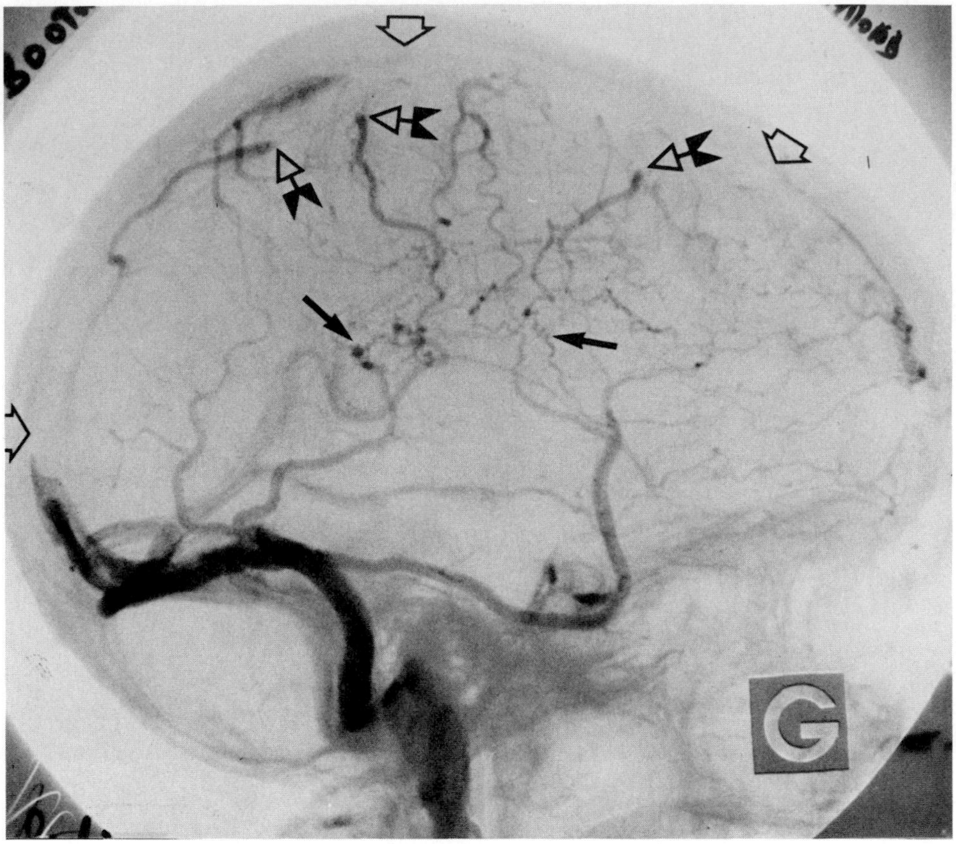

**Fig. 19-9.** Left carotid angiogram. Total superior sagittal sinus occlusion (*white arrows*) with occlusion of frontoparietal veins (*tailed arrows*) and anastomotic cortical veins with a corkscrew appearance (*straight arrows*).

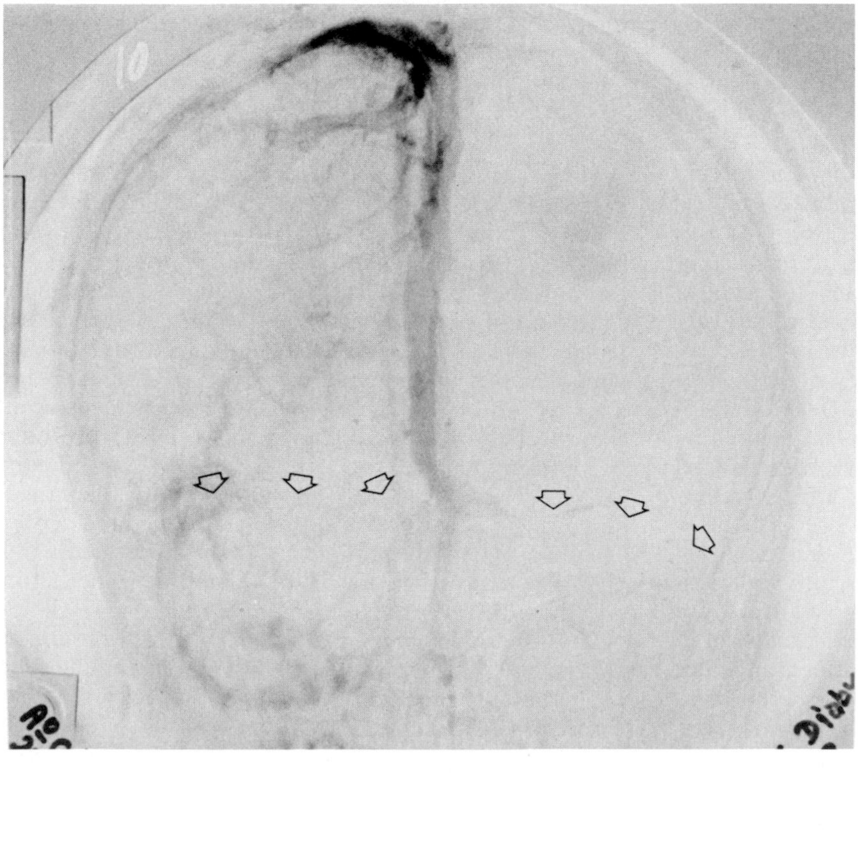

**Fig. 19-10.** Right carotid angiogram. Lack of filling of both lateral sinuses (*white arrows*). (From Bousser et al.,[13] with permission.)

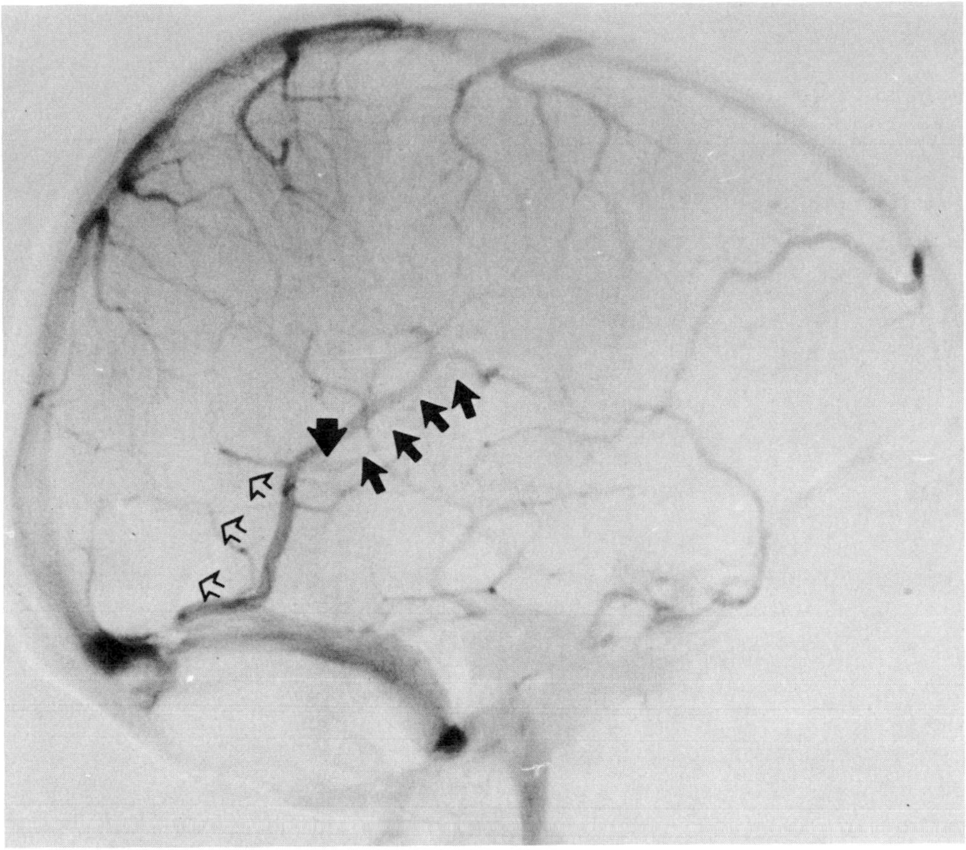

**Fig. 19-11.** Right carotid angiogram. Poor filling of internal cerebral vein (*thin black arrows*), vein of Galen (*wide arrow*), and lack of filling of straight sinus (*white arrows*). (From Bousser et al.,[13] with permission.)

nous thrombosis but also the natural history of the thrombotic process (Fig. 19-13). MRI diagnosis is particularly easy in SSS thrombosis,[34,82,116,127] but convincing images have also been obtained in cases of thrombosis involving the LS,[34,85,116] straight sinus[6,116] (Fig. 19-14), internal cerebral veins and great vein of Galen,[61,82] cavernous sinus,[106] and cortical veins.[106]

Besides its ability to detect thrombosis, MRI also offers the advantage of sometimes showing parenchymal lesions not visible on CT scan and demonstrating an underlying cause such as an adjacent tumor or an unsuspected mastoiditis.[85]

In some cases, however, interpretation of MRI images is not so easy because of false negative and false positive images.[71,85,125,127] With a high field unit, the very early decreased signal of thrombosis observed on T2-WI may be confused with patency. It may then be necessary to repeat the MR examination a few days later or to image the patient again at intermediate field strength. An increased signal mimicking thrombosis can be artifactually created by slowly flowing blood. Repositioning the patient, repeating the sequence in a different plane, using at least two sequences, and sometimes obtaining specialized acquisitions are helpful in eliminating these artifacts.[82,125] Another disadvantage of MRI techniques used so far has been that the venous system is not seen coherently, as it is in angiography, but is viewed on different slices, which limits its feasibility as a first-choice routine examination. Three-dimensional MR flow imaging (3D-MRFI) has overcome this shortcoming and convincing images of SSS thrombosis have been published.[132] This new technique offers theoretical advantages over angiography: it allows reconstruction from different angles of views, it is noninvasive and does not require contrast injection, and it can be coupled with spin echo imaging, simultaneously showing the vessels and the parenchymal lesions.[132] It is, however, too early for 3D-MRFI to replace angiography, although MRI is at present the method of choice for the diagnosis and follow-up of CVT, angiography being required only in difficult or doubtful cases.

## Other Neurologic Investigations

Other investigations were most useful and necessary in the pre-CT scan era. Constantly found in SSS thrombosis with extension to cortical veins, EEG

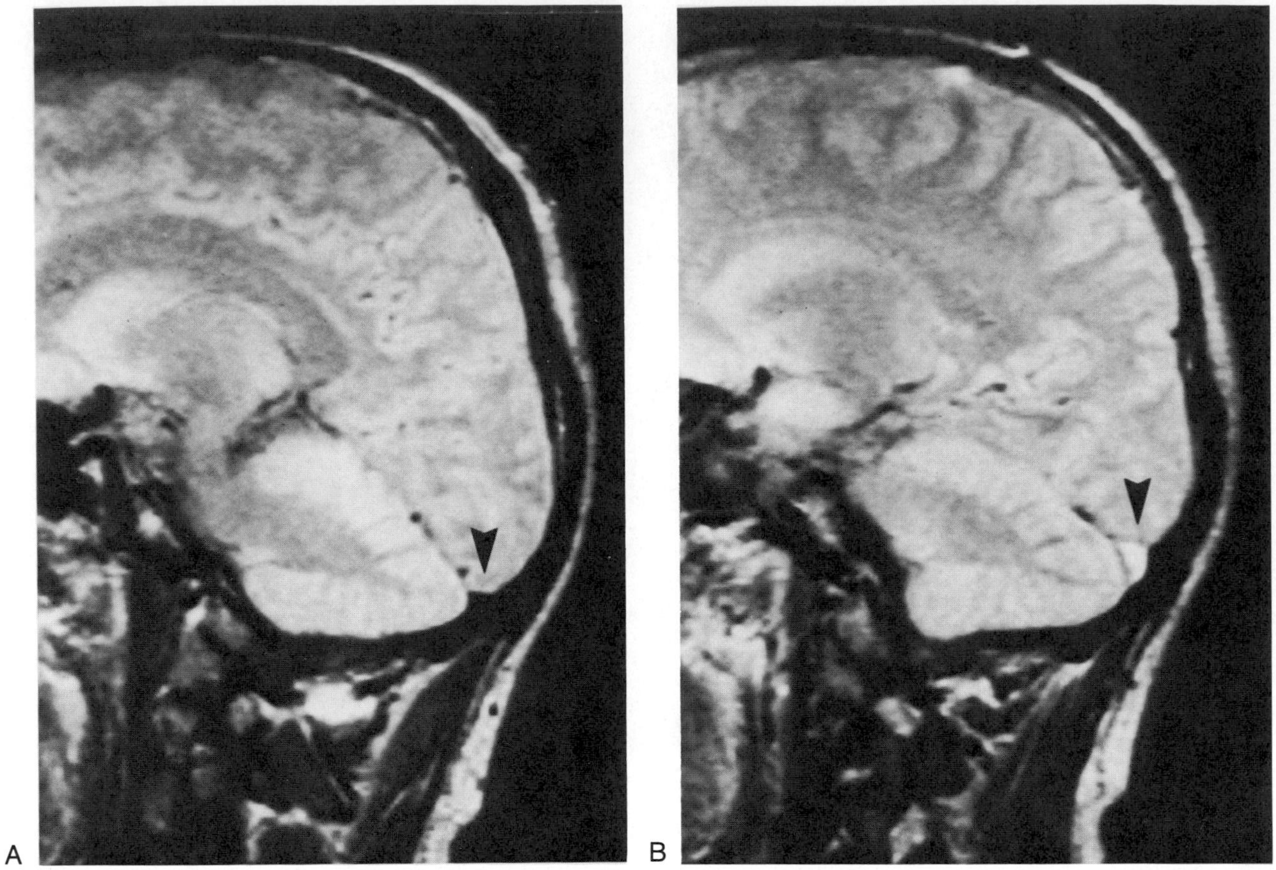


**Fig. 19-12.** MRI T2-WI. (**A**) Lateral sinus hypoplasia (*arrowhead*). (**B**) Lateral sinus thrombosis (*arrowhead*).

changes occur in roughly 75 percent of cases.[13,21,70] They are, however, nonspecific: the most common pattern is a severe generalized slowing more marked on one side with frequent superimposed epileptic activity. In some patients with focal symptoms, there is a generalized slowing, indicating a more diffuse lesion than clinically suspected.

**Isotope Brain Scanning.** Isotope brain scanning with $^{99m}Tc$ has been shown to be a useful tool in the diagnosis of SSS and LS occlusion.[7,54] However, some false negatives have been reported, probably due to the visualization of an intense collateral circulation in the sinus walls. A case has been published of SSS thrombosis demonstrated by indium-111 platelet scintigraphy.[15] Early scintigraphy showed a focal increase in activity at each end of the thrombus, while later examination showed diffuse increase in activity in the sinus. Over the 2 following weeks platelet uptake declined markedly, thus giving information about the natural history of thrombosis. However, this technique is of no use in an emergency, since images are taken at 24 and 48 hours after injection, and its interest is supplanted by that of MRI.

**Cerebrospinal Fluid Examination.** CSF examination is still a useful diagnostic tool because it is very rarely (10 percent) entirely normal in composition or in pressure.[4,13,26,50,74,78] Abnormalities in composition include raised protein content and the presence of red blood cells in two-thirds of cases[13] and pleocytosis in one-third. On rare occasions the amount of blood in the CSF is sufficiently extensive to suggest a subarachnoid hemorrhage due to aneurysm rupture. Mainly found when focal signs are present, pleocytosis and the presence of red blood cells also occur in patients presenting with "benign intracranial hypertension," suggesting that the presence of these abnormalities should point toward sinus thrombosis as the possible cause of this syndrome.[13] CSF examination is crucial to rule out meningitis, which is extremely difficult to exclude on clinical grounds only in patients with symptoms of CVT, of which it is sometimes the underlying cause. Although in the current CT scan and MRI era CSF study has become obsolete in most cases of nonseptic CVT presenting with focal signs, it remains of the utmost importance in patients with isolated intracranial hypertension, to rule out meningitis, to measure CSF pressure, and to remove CSF when vision is threatened.

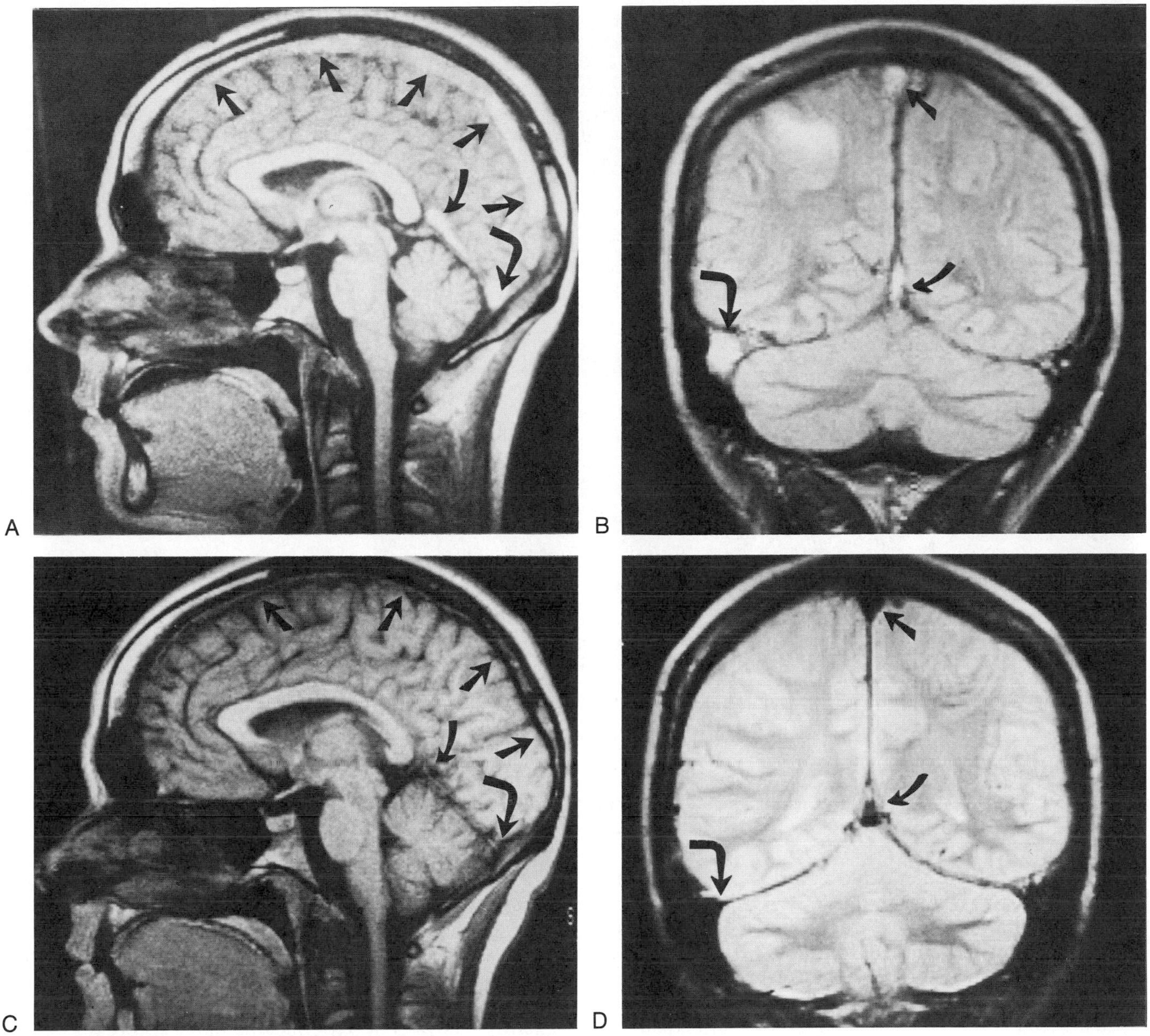


**Fig. 19-13.** MRI T1-WI. (**A & B**) Hypersignal indicating superior sagittal sinus (*straight arrows*), lateral sinus (*angle arrows*), and straight sinus (*curved arrows*) thrombosis. (**C & D**) Same patient 3 months later. Normal flow void in previously thrombosed sinuses.

## General Investigations

Once having established the presence of CVT, investigations should be directed toward demonstrating the underlying etiology. Because of the multiplicity of etiologies, this is a long and difficult task whenever the cause is not clinically evident. The presence of fever, of increased erythrocyte sedimentation rate, or of raised polymorphonuclear white blood cell count points to infective, inflammatory, or malignant causes. However, even with such underlying diseases, these abnormalities are sometimes lacking and, by contrast, they are occasionally found in idiopathic cases.[13] Their presence is particularly useful to point to CVT in patients presenting with benign intracranial hypertension.

Detailed coagulation studies have only rarely been performed in series of CVT, and their results have been conflicting. Some have found a "hypercoagulability state,"[31,98] that is, an increase in platelet adhesiveness and aggregability[6,31] and a decrease in fibrinolytic activity,[6] but this was during pregnancy

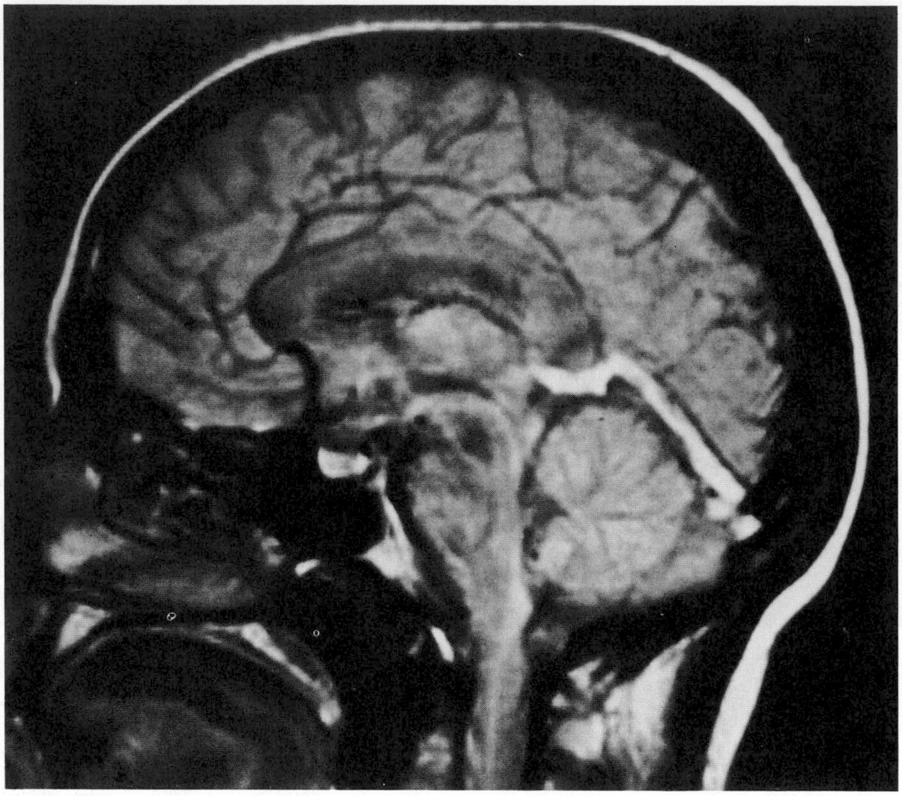

**Fig. 19-14.** MRI T2-WI (first echo) (TR 2,000 TE 40) hypersignal indicating great vein of Galen and straight sinus thrombosis.

and puerperium or in women taking oral contraceptives. Others did not confirm these results[41] or found that the only abnormality was an increased platelet aggregation with the lowest dose of epinephrine.[13] On the whole, detailed hemostasis studies are not recommended routinely for all patients with CVT. These investigations are necessary in all apparently "idiopathic cases" and for patients with a personal or familial history of recurrent venous thrombosis in order to detect possible causative conditions.[40,72,80,91,105,115,126].

## OUTCOME

Before the introduction of angiography, CVT was mainly diagnosed at autopsy and therefore was thought to be most often lethal.[50,74,94] In early angiographic series, mortality still ranked between 30 and 50 percent,[70,78] but later it was between 25 and 30 percent, further dropping to 10 to 15 percent in the most recent series[13,29,127,134] and to 6.5 percent in our series of 76 patients. This favorable outcome is one of the reasons for the low prevalence of CVT in autopsy studies.

Factors classically considered of bad prognosis are the rate of evolution of thrombosis,[74] the presence of coma,[78] the age of patients with a high mortality rate in infancy and in the aged,[74] the presence of focal symptoms pointing to an involvement of cerebral veins,[13,50,74] and the presence of a hemorrhagic infarct and of an empty delta sign on CT scan.[134] The topography of cerebral veins involved is also an important prognostic factor, deep cerebral vein thrombosis and cerebellar vein thrombosis carrying a much higher risk than cortical vein thrombosis.[11,32,28,50,78] The single most important prognostic factor is probably the underlying cause. In our series of 76 patients, the 5 deaths occurred in patients who had a severe underlying cause, such as subdural empyema, brain abscess, or end-stage systemic lupus. CVT, which complicates paroxysmal nocturnal hemoglobinuria, also seems to carry a higher risk.[129] Septic CVT remains a severe disease with a mortality rate of 30 percent in cavernous sinus thrombosis and 78 percent in SSS thrombosis.[36]

It has long been recognized that, if survival occurs in CVT, the prognosis for recovery of function is much better than in arterial thrombosis;[13,64,83,121,123] a minority (15 to 25 percent) of patients are left with sequelae such as optic atrophy or focal deficits.[13,26,127,134]

It is thus apparent that, though less severe than classically thought, the natural history and prognosis of CVT are highly variable. There are acute cases that can have a fulminating course leading to death in a few days, whereas others recover rapidly and completely, and still others are left with sequelae. There are chronic cases that worsen progressively, leading to sequelae, whereas others recover spontaneously. There are extremely benign forms limited to TIA or headache or epilepsy, which are probably still underrecognized. On the whole, isolated sinus thrombosis carries a good prognosis, provided intracranial hypertension is controlled; however, sinus thrombosis can, at any moment, extend to cerebral veins, and then possibly lead to death or sequelae, though only in a minority of cases.

Very little is known about the long-term outcome of patients with CVT.[13,64] A few reports suggest that LS thrombosis can later induce arteriovenous malformations affecting the transverse sinus.[64] Residual epilepsy and recurrences of CVT (2 out of 26 in our study)[13] seem uncommon, but this would have to be documented by long-term prospective studies.

## TREATMENT

The variability in the natural history of an uncommon disease explains the fact that treatment is still controversial. It is based on a combination of symptomatic medications (anticonvulsants, antibiotics, methods to reduce intracranial pressure) on a case by case basis and on antithrombotic treatments.

**Anticonvulsants.** As far as anticonvulsant treatment is concerned, some investigators favor its systematic use,[74] whereas the majority, including ourselves, restrict it to patients who present seizures.[13] The question of the duration of treatment remains open: in our series, it was progressively discontinued 2 years after CVT, but only in patients with normal EEG and CT scan who had neither recurrent seizures nor neurologic sequelae.[13]

**Antibiotics.** In septic CVT, all agree on the use of a wide-spectrum combination of antibiotics such as a penicillinase-resistant penicillin, together with a last generation cephalosporin and metronidazole (or chloramphenicol), as a reasonable initial regimen. This treatment may be subsequently modified pending culture results and should be given over a period of at least 2 weeks.[32,36,41,66,67,119,128]

**Methods to Reduce Intracranial Pressure.** Opinions are more divergent on reducing intracranial pressure and diverse approaches have been used: steroids,[13,26,52,103,127] mannitol,[13,26,45,103,127] acetazolamide,[13,26,45,103] daily lumbar punctures,[13,26,45] ventricular cerebrospinal fluid drainage,[45,62] lumbar peritoneal shunting,[13,40,104] barbiturate-induced coma,[45,55,62] LS venous bypass,[114] or even craniectomy.[100,103] In our series of 76 patients, only 2 required shunting procedures: in all others, the combination of antiedema agents, acetazolamide, and repeated lumbar punctures was sufficient to control raised intracranial pressure. We do not advise steroids. We particularly favor repeated lumbar punctures in patients with isolated intracranial hypertension with threatened vision. As long as vision does not deteriorate and consciousness remains normal, such a conservative approach seems reasonable in a condition where spontaneous recovery is the rule[6,13,26,68,85,89,103,106,127] and generally avoids the use of more drastic methods. Patients on anticoagulants do not receive lumbar puncture therapy because of the risk of subarachnoid, subdural or extradural hemorrhage.

**Anthrombotic Treatments.** The treatment of the thrombotic process is still controversial.

*Surgical thrombectomy* has been performed in some patients,[41,100] but an overwhelming majority of clinicians are against direct surgery, which might be harmful on a swollen and sometimes hemorrhagic brain.[26,33,78,103] Surgery may be mandatory in patients with an associated brain abscess and no improvement despite a wide-spectrum combination of antibiotics.[13]

The use of *anticoagulants* has long remained controversial because of the risk of further bleeding into an already hemorrhagic infarct, and such a complication has been well documented.[8,17,31,52] However, the risk of increasing intracranial hemorrhage has probably been overestimated in the past, and an increasing number of observations favor the use of heparin. First, there are a number of well-documented cases in which a dramatic improvement occurred 24 hours after the initiation of heparin in patients who had previously been steadily deteriorating,[13,23,43,57,122] and some of these patients worsened when high-dose heparin was changed to low-dose or oral anticoagulants, and they improved quickly after full-dose heparin therapy was resumed.[43,127] Second, heparin has been used in many patients since the pioneer observations of Martin and Sheenan[84] and Stansfield[120] without deleterious effect.[23,26,43,57,60,78,81,101,103,127] In our previous series of 23 heparin-treated patients, there was no death, and a complete recovery was observed in 19 patients. This being a retrospective study, no conclusion could be drawn on the efficacy of heparin, but it did indicate that, at least in this group, heparin was not harmful. Finally, the benefit of heparin has been demonstrated in the only randomized trial so far performed in CVT:[131] high-dose intravenous heparin was compared to placebo in patients with angiographically proved CVT. The study had to be stopped after the first 20 patients because of a statistically significant difference in favor of heparin ($P < 0.05$). After 3 months, all 10 heparin-treated patients had either completely recovered or were left with a slight neurologic deficit, whereas in the control group, 4 patients died or had severe sequelae.

There is good evidence that heparin has a beneficial effect in patients with CVT, but there is still disagreement on the best indications. All would agree that heparin is indicated in patients with coexistent pelvic or deep leg vein thrombosis and pulmonary embolism, or in conditions with an increased thrombotic tendency such as antithrombin III, protein C or S deficiencies, or presence of lupus anticoagulant. By contrast, heparin is usually contraindicated in CVT caused by paroxysmal nocturnal hemoglobinuria because of frequent thrombocytopenia.[129] When there is no formal indication of contraindication due to underlying or associated conditions, the use of anticoagulants is still controversial in a disease that recovers spontaneously in a majority of cases but also, though exceptionally, leads to fatal hemorrhage in some patients. For the majority, high-dose heparin is now the drug of choice in CVT, provided there is no hemorrhagic infarction on CT scan.[51,60,89,103] However, there are several reports of patients with hemorrhagic infarcts who did improve on anticoagulants,[13,55] and in the German randomized study,[131] heparin was found to be beneficial even in such patients.[131] Our attitude is, at present, to anticoagulate all patients with demonstrated CVT, with or without hemorrhagic infarcts, provided there is no general contraindication to the use of heparin. Low molecular weight heparin might prove as effective as conventional heparin, but experience is still limited.[46] The duration of anticoagulant treatment is not standardized. By analogy with deep-vein thrombosis, we have been using heparin for the first few days and oral anticoagulants for the next 2 to 3 months except when there is a known thrombotic tendency, in which case treatment is prolonged as necessary. We now tend to adapt the duration of treatment to the evolution of thrombosis as assessed by MRI, but it is too early yet to widely recommend this attitude.

The use of *fibrinolytics* is even more controversial. Fibrinolytics were found by some[52,103] to be dangerous because of bleeding into the infarct and by others to be beneficial by preventing extension of thrombosis and promoting recanalization.[57,133] Urokinase infusion has recently been performed locally inside the SSS, but this information appears in a single case report, which remains anecdotal.[107] There is at present no scientific reason to treat CVT patients with fibrinolytics (even tPA) rather than with heparin, but there is possibly a case for a randomized trial to compare these two treatment regimens.

## ACKNOWLEDGMENTS

We wish to thank most warmly Drs. Chiras, Dormont, Hauw, Mas, Meder, and Tehindrazanarivelo for providing us some of the figures and Mrs. Jocelyne Ruffie for her technical assistance.

## REFERENCES

1. Anderson SC, Shah CP, Murtagh FR: Congested deep subcortical veins as a sign of dural venous thrombosis: MR and CT correlations. J Comput Assist Tomogr 11:1059, 1987
2. Askenasy HM, Kosary IZ, Braham J: Thrombosis of the longitudinal sinus: diagnosis by carotid angiography. Neurology (NY) 12:288, 1962
3. Averback P: Primary cerebral venous thrombosis in young adults: the diverse manifestations of an underrecognized disease. Ann Neurol 3:81, 1978
4. Azzarelli B, Itani AL, Catanzaro PT: Cerebral phlebothrombosis: a complication of lymphoma. Arch Neurol 37:126, 1980
5. Bailey OT, Hass GM: Dural sinus thrombosis in early life, clinical manifestations and extent of brain injury in acute sinus thrombosis. J Pediat 11:755, 1937
6. Bansal BC, Gupta RR, Prakash C: Stroke during pregnancy and puerperium in young females below the age of 40 years as a result of cerebral venous/sinus thrombosis. Jpn Heart J 21:171, 1980
7. Barnes BD, Winestock DP: Dynamic radionuclide scanning in the diagnosis of thrombosis of the superior sagittal sinus thrombosis. Neurology (NY) 27:656, 1977
8. Barnett HJM, Hyland HH: Noninfective intracranial venous thrombosis. Brain 76:36, 1953
9. Barthelemy M, Bousser MG, Jacobs C: Thrombose veineuse cérébrale au cours d'un syndrome néphrotique. Nouv Presse Med 9:367, 1980
10. Boddie HG, Banna M, Bradley MG: "Benign" intracranial hypertension: a survey of the clinical and radiological features and long-term prognosis. Brain 97:313, 1974
11. Bots GAM: Thrombosis of the galenic system veins in the adult. Acta Neuropathol 17:227, 1971
12. Bousser MG, Bletry O, Launay M et al: Thrombose veineuse cérébrale au cours de la maladie de Behçet: à propos de deux cas. Rev Neurol (Paris) 136:753, 1980
13. Bousser MG, Chiras J, Sauron B et al: Cerebral venous thrombosis: a review of 38 cases. Stroke 16:199, 1985
14. Brant-Zawadzki M, Chang GY, McCarty GE: Computed tomography in dural sinus thrombosis. Arch Neurol 39:446, 1982
15. Bridgers SL, Strauss E, Smith EO et al: Demonstration of superior sagittal sinus thrombosis by indium-111 platelet scintigraphy. Arch Neurol 43:1079, 1986
16. Brismar J: Computed tomography in superior sagittal sinus thrombosis. Acta Radiol [Diagn] (Stockh) 21:321, 1980
17. Buchanan DS, Brazinsky JH: Dural sinus and cerebral venous thrombosis: incidence in young women receiving oral contraceptives. Arch Neurol 22:440, 1970
18. Buonanno FS, Moody DM, Ball RM: CT scan findings in cerebral sinovenous occlusion. Neurology (NY) 12:288, 1982
19. Buonanno FS, Moody DM, Ball MR et al: Radionuclide sinography: diagnosis of lateral sinus thrombosis by dynamic and static brain imaging. Radiology 130:207, 1979
20. Buonanno F, Moody DM, Ball MR, Laster DW:

Computed cranial tomographic findings in cerebral sino-venous occlusion. J Comput Assist Tomogr 2:281, 1978
21. Burkhardt S, Regli F: EEG Veränderungen bei 27 Fällen von zerebraler Thrombophlébitis. Schweiz Arch Neurol Neurochir Psychiatr 94:1, 1964
22. Byrne JV, Lawton CA: Meningeal sarcoïdosis causing intracranial hypertension secondary to dural sinus thrombosis. Br J Radiol 56:755, 1983
23. Castaigne P, Laplane D, Bousser MG: Superior sagittal sinus thrombosis. Arch Neurol 34:788, 1977
24. Chiras J, Bousser MG, Meder JF et al: CT in cerebral thrombophlebitis. Neuroradiology 27:145, 1985
25. Claude H: La phlébite des veines cérébrales. Rev Med 31:761, 1911
26. Coquillat G, Warter JM: Thromboses veineuses cérébrales: rapport de neurologie présenté au congrès de psychiatrie et de neurologie de langue française. Vol. 1. Masson, Paris, 1976
27. Corbett JJ: Problems in the diagnosis and treatment of pseudo-tumor cerebri. Can J Neurol Sci 10:221, 1983
28. Corbett JJ, Mehta MP: Cerebrospinal fluid pressure in normal obese subjects and patients with pseudotumor cerebri. Neurology (NY) 33:1386, 1983
29. Curnes JT, Creasy JL, Whaley RL, Scatliff JH: Air in the cavernous sinus thrombosis (Letter to the Editor.) AJNR 8:176, 1987
30. Deslegte RGM, Kaiser MC, Vanderbaan S, Smit L: Computed tomographic diagnosis of septic sinus thrombosis and their complications. Neuroradiology 30:160, 1988
31. Dindar F, Platts ME: Intracranial venous thrombosis complicating oral contraception. Can Med Assoc J 111:545, 1974
32. Dinubile MJ: Septic thrombosis of the cavernous sinuses: neurological review. Arch Neurol 45:567, 1988
33. DiRocco C, Lanelli A, Leone G et al: Heparin-urokinase treatment in a septic dural sinus thrombosis. Arch Neurol 38:431, 1981
34. Donohoe CD, Waldman SD, Resor LD: Magnetic resonance imaging in cerebral venous thrombosis, a case report. Headache 27:155, 1987
35. Dowman CE: Thrombosis of the rolandic vein. Arch Neurol Psychiatr 15:110, 1926
36. Editorial: Infections of the dural venous sinuses. Lancet 1:201, 1987
37. Ehlers H, Courville CB: Thrombosis of internal cerebral veins in infancy and childhood: review of literature and report of five cases. J Pediatr 8:600, 1936
38. Eick JJ, Miller KD, Bell KA, Tutton RH: Computed tomography of deep cerebral venous thrombosis in children. Radiology 140:399, 1981
39. Eikmeier G, Kuhlmann R, Gastpar M: Thrombosis of cerebral veins following intravenous application of clomipramine. J Neurol Neurosurg Psychiatry 52:1461, 1989
40. Engesser L, Broekmans AW, Briet E et al: Hereditary protein S deficiency: clinical manifestations. Ann Intern Med 106:31, 1987
41. Estanol B, Rodriguez A, Conte G et al: Intracranial venous thrombosis in young women. Stroke 10:680, 1979
42. Evans RW, Patten BM: Trichinosis associated with superior sagittal sinus thrombosis. Ann Neurol 11:216, 1982
43. Fairburn B: Intracranial venous thrombosis complicating oral contraception: treatment by anticoagulant drugs. Br Med J 2:647, 1973
44. Feinberg WM, Swenson MR: Cerebrovascular complications of L-asparaginase therapy. Neurology (NY) 38:127, 1988
45. Feldenzer JA, Bueche MJ, Venes JL, Gebarski SS: Superior sagittal sinus thrombosis with infarction in sickle cell trait. Stroke 18:656, 1987
46. Fevrier MJ, Nguyen JP, Brugieres P, Goujon C: Thrombophlébite du sinus longitudinal supérieur au stade chirurgical: a propos d'un cas: intérêt de l'héparine de bas poids moléculaire. Neurochirurgie 33:490, 1987
47. Foley J: Benign forms of intracranial hypertension; "toxic" and "otitic" hydrocephalus. Brain 78:1, 1955
48. Ford K, Sarwar M: Computed tomography of dural sinus thrombosis. Am J Neuroradiol 2:539, 1981
49. Gabrielsen TO, Seeger JF, Knake JE, Stilwill EW: Radiology of cerebral vein occlusion without dural sinus occlusion. Radiology 140:403, 1981
50. Garcin R, Pestel M: Thrombophlébites cérébrales. Masson, Paris, 1949
51. Gates PC: Cerebral venous thrombosis: a retrospective review. Aust NZ J Med 16:766, 1986
52. Gettelfinger DM, Kokmen E: Superior sagittal sinus thrombosis. Arch Neurol 34:2, 1977
53. Girard DE, Reuler JB, Mayer BS et al: Cerebral venous sinus thrombosis due to indwelling transvenous pacemaker catheter. Arch Neurol 37:113, 1980
54. Go RT, Chiu CL, Neuman LA: Diagnosis of superior sagittal sinus thrombosis by
55. Goldberg AL, Rosenbaum AE, Wang H et al: Computed tomography of dural sinus thrombosis. J Comput Assist Tomogr 10:16, 1986
56. Greer M: Management of benign intra-cranial hypertension (pseudo-tumor cerebri). Clin Neurosurg 15:161, 1967
57. Greitz T, Link H: Aseptic thrombosis of intracranial sinuses. Radiol Clin Biol 35:111, 1966
58. Guidetti B, Giuffre B, Gambacorta D: Follow up study of 100 cases of pseudo-tumor cerebri. Acta Neurochir 18:259, 1968
59. Hacker H: Normal supratentorial veins and dural sinuses. In Newton TH, Potts DG (eds): Radiology of the Skull and Brain. Angiography. CV Mosby, St. Louis, 1974
60. Halpern JP, Morris JGL, Driscoll GL: Anticoagulants and cerebral venous thrombosis. Aust NZ J Med 14:643, 1984
61. Hanigan WC, Rossi LJ, McLean JM, Wright RM: MRI of cerebral vein thrombosis in infancy: a case report. Neurology (NY) 36:1354, 1986
62. Hanley DF, Feldman E, Borel CO et al: Treatment of sagittal sinus thrombosis associated

with cerebral hemorrhage and intracranial hypertension. Stroke 19:903, 1988
63. Hickey WF, Garnick MB, Henderson JC, Dawson DM: Primary cerebral venous thrombosis in patients with cancer—a rarely diagnosed paraneoplastic syndrome. Am J Med 73:740, 1982
64. Houser OW, Campbell JK, Campbell RJ, Sundt TM: Arteriovenous malformation affecting the transverse dural venous sinus: an acquired lesion. Mayo Clin Proc 54:651, 1979
65. Huang YP, Wolf B: Veins of the white matter of the cerebral hemispheres (the medullary veins): diagnostic importance in carotid angiography. AJR 92:739, 1964
66. Huang YP, Wolf BS: Veins of posterior fossa-superior or galenic draining group. AJR 95:808, 1965
67. Huang YP, Wolf BS, Antin SP, Okudera T: The veins of the posterior fossa-anterior or petrosal draining group. AJR 104:36, 1968
68. Hubbert CH: Dural puncture headache suspected, cortical vein thrombosis diagnosed. (Letter to the Editor.) Anesth Analg 66:285, 1986
69. Hughes JP, Stovin PG: Segmental pulmonary artery aneurysms with peripheral venous thrombosis. Br J Dis Chest 53:19, 1959
70. Huhn A: Die thrombosen der intrakraniellen Venen und Sinus. Klinische und pathologisch-anatomische Untersuchungen. Thromb Haemost, suppl. 18: 1965
71. Hulcelle PJ, Dooms GC, Mathurin P, Cornelis G: MRI assessment of unsuspected dural sinus thrombosis. Neuroradiology 31:217, 1989
72. Jacquin V, Salama J, Leroux G, Delaporte P: Thromboses veineuses cérébrales et des membres supérieurs associées à une thrombopénie, induites par le polysulfate de pentosane. Ann Med Interne (Paris) 139:194, 1988
73. Johnsen S, Greenwood R, Fischman MA: Internal cerebral vein thrombosis. Arch Neurol 28:205, 1973
74. Kalbag RM, Woolf AL: Cerebral venous thrombosis. Vol. 1. University Press, London, 1967
75. Kinal ME: Traumatic thrombosis of dural venous sinuses in closed head injuries. J Neurosurg 27:142, 1967
76. Kingsley DPE, Kendall BE, Moseley LF: Superior sagittal sinus thrombosis, an evaluation of the changes demonstrated on computed tomography. J Neurol Neurosurg Psychiatry 41:1065, 1978
77. Krayenbuhl H: Cerebral venous thrombosis: the diagnostic value of cerebral angiography. Schweiz Arch Neurol Neurochir Psychiatr 74:261, 1954
78. Krayenbuhl H: Cerebral venous and sinus thrombosis. Clin Neurosurg 14:1, 1967
79. Lazorthes G, Gouazé A, Salamon G: Vascularisation et circulation de l'encéphale. Vol. 1. Masson, Paris, 1976
80. Levine SR, Kieran S, Puzio K et al: Cerebral venous thrombosis with lupus anticoagulants: report of 2 cases. Stroke 18:801, 1987
81. Levine SR, Twyman RE, Gilman S: The role of anticoagulation in cavernous sinus thrombosis. Neurology (NY) 38:517, 1988
82. Macchi PJ, Grossman RI, Gomori JM et al: High field MR imaging of cerebral venous thrombosis. J Comput Assist Tomogr 10:10, 1986
83. Martin JP: Venous thrombosis in the central nervous system. Proc R Soc Med 37:383, 1944
84. Martin JP, Sheenan HL: Primary thrombosis of cerebral veins (following childbirth). Br Med J 1:349, 1941
85. McMurdo SK, Brant-Zawadzki M, Bradley WG et al: Dural sinus thrombosis study using intermediate field strength MR imaging. Radiology 161:83, 1986
86. Meininger V, James JM, Rio B, Zittoun R: Occlusions des sinus veineux de la dure-mère au cours des hémopathies. Rev Neurol (Paris) 141:228, 1985
87. Meyohas MC, Roullet E: Cerebral venous thrombosis and dual primary infection with human immuno-deficiency virus and cytomegalovirus. J Neurol Neurosurg Psychiatry 52:1010, 1989
88. Mickle JP, McLennan JE, Lidden CW: Cortical vein thrombosis in Wegener's granulomatosis. J Neurosurg 46:248, 1977
89. Milandre L, Gueriot C, Girard N et al: Les thromboses veineuses cérébrales de l'adulte. Ann Med Interne (Paris) 139:544, 1988
90. Montrieul B, Janny P: Contribution à l'étude angiographique des thromboses veineuses cérébrales. Neurochirurgie 8:175, 1962
91. Murphy MF, Clarke CRA, Brearley RL: Superior sagittal sinus thrombosis and essential thrombocythaemia. Br Med J 287:1344, 1983
92. Newman DS, Levine SR, Curtis VL, Welch KMA: Migraine-like visual phenomena associated with cerebral venous thrombosis. Headache 29:82, 1989
93. Nishimura RN, Stepanek D, Howieson J, Hammerstad J: Internal cerebral vein thrombosis: a case report. Arch Neurol 39:439, 1982
94. Noetzel H, Jerusalem F: Die Hirnvenen und Sinusthrombosen. Monogr Gesamtgeb Psychiatr 106:1, 1965
95. Osborn AG, Anderson RE, Wing SD: The false falx sign. Radiology 134:421, 1980
96. Patchell RA, Posner JB: Neurologic complications of carcinoid. Neurology (NY) 36:745, 1986
97. Patronas NJ, Duda EE, Mirfakhraee M, Wollmann RL: Superior sagittal sinus thrombosis diagnosed by computed tomography. Surg Neurol 15:11, 1981
98. Poltera AA: The pathology of intracranial venous thrombosis in oral contraception. J Pathol 106:209, 1972
99. Rao KCVG, Knipp HC, Wagner EJ: CT findings in cerebral sinus and venous thrombosis. Radiology 140:391, 1981
100. Ray BS, Dunbar HS: Thrombosis of dural venous sinuses as cause of "pseudotumor cerebri." Ann Surg 134:376, 1951
101. Ribes MF: Des recherches faites sur la phlébite. Revue Médicale Française et Etrangère et Journal de Clinique de l'Hôtel-Dieu et de la Charité de Paris 3:5, 1825
102. Rousseaux M, Lesoin F, Barbaste P, Jomin M: Infarctus cérébelleux pseudotumoral d'origine veineuse. Rev Neurol (Paris) 144:209, 1988

103. Rousseaux P, Bernard MH, Scherpereel B, Guyot JF: Thrombose des sinus veineux intra-crâniens (à propos de 22 cas). Neurochirurgie 24:197, 1978
104. Ruel M, Montfort JC, Pinta P: Symptomatologie trompeuse des thrombophlébites cérébrales au cours de la grossesse et du post-partum. Nouv Presse Med 15:1367, 1986
105. Sauron B, Chiras J, Chain G, Castaigne P: Thrombophlébite cérébelleuse chez un homme porteur d'un déficit familial en antithrombine III. Rev Neurol (Paris) 138:685, 1982
106. Savino PJ, Grossman RI, Schatz NJ et al: High field magnetic resonance imaging in the diagnosis of cavernous sinus thrombosis. Arch Neurol 43:1081, 1986
107. Scott JA, Pascuzzi RM, Hall PV, Becker GJ: Treatment of dural sinus thrombosis with local urokinase infusion. J Neurosurg 68:284, 1988
108. Scotti LN, Goldman RL, Hardman DR, Heinz ER: Venous thrombosis in infants and children. Radiology 1121:393, 1974
109. Segall HD, Ahmadi J, McComb JG et al: Computed tomographic observations pertinent to intracranial venous thrombotic and occlusive disease in childhood. Radiology 143:441, 1982
110. Sekhar LN, Dujovny M, Rao GR: Carotid cavernous sinus thrombosis caused by *Aspergillus fumigatus*. J Neurosurg 52:120, 1980
111. Shinohara Y, Yosmitoshi M, Yoshii F: Appearance and disappearance of empty delta sign in superior sagittal sinus thrombosis. Stroke 17:1282, 1986
112. Shiozawa Z, Yamada H, Mabuchi C et al: Superior sagittal sinus thrombosis associated with androgen therapy for hypoplastic anaemia. Ann Neurol 12:578, 1982
113. Sigsbee B, Deck MDF, Posner JB: Nonmetastatic superior sagittal sinus thrombosis complicating systemic cancer. Neurology (NY) 29:139, 1979
114. Sindou M, Mercier P, Brunon J et al: Hypertension intra-crânienne "bénigne" par thrombose des deux sinus latéraux traitée par pontage veineux. Nouv Presse Med 9:439, 1980
115. Smith WDF, Sinar J, Carey M: Sagittal sinus thrombosis and occult malignancy. J Neurol Neurosurg Psychiatry 46:187, 1983
116. Snyder TC, Sachdev HS: MR imaging of cerebral dural sinus thrombosis. J Comput Assist Tomogr 10:889, 1986
117. Sorensen PS, Hammer M, Gjerris F: Cerebrospinal fluid vasopressin in benign intracranial hypertension. Neurology (NY) 32:1255, 1982
118. Souter RG, Mitchell A: Spreading venous cortical thrombosis due to infusion of hyperosmolar solution into the internal jugular vein. Br Med J 285:935, 1982
119. Southwick FS, Richardson EP Jr, Swartz MN: Septic thrombosis of the dural venous sinuses. Medicine (Baltimore) 65:82, 1986
120. Stansfield FR: Puerperal cerebral thrombophlebitis treated by heparin. Br Med J 1:436, 1942
121. Swanson HS, Fincher EF: Experience involving superior longitudinal sinus and rolandic veins. Neurology (NY) 4:801, 1954
122. Symonds CP: Hydrocephalic and focal cerebral symptoms in relation to thrombophlebitis of the dural sinuses and cerebral veins. Brain 60:531, 1937
123. Symonds CP: Cerebral thrombophlebitis. Br Med J 2:348, 1940
124. Symonds C: Otitic hydrocephalus. Neurology (NY) 6:681, 1956
125. Sze G, Simmons B, Krol G et al: Dural sinus thrombosis: verification with spin echo techniques. AJNR 9:679, 1988
126. Tarras S, Gadia C, Mester L et al: Homozygous protein C deficiency in a newborn: clinicopathologic correlation. Arch Neurol 45:214, 1988
127. Thron A, Wessel K, Linden D et al: Superior sagittal sinus thrombosis: neuroradiological evaluation and clinical findings. J Neurol 233:283, 1986
128. Towbin A: The syndrome of latent cerebral venous thrombosis: its frequency and relation to age and congestive heart failure. Stroke 4:419, 1973
129. Van Vleymen B, de Haenne I, van Hoof A, Pattyn G: Cerebral venous thrombosis in paroxysmal nocturnal haemoglobinuria. Acta Neurol Belg 87:80, 1987
130. Vidailhet M, Piette JC, Wechsler B et al: Cerebral venous thrombosis in systemic lupus erythematosus: report of 6 cases and review. Stroke 21:1226, 1990
131. Einhäupl KM, Villringer A, Meister W: Heparin treatment in sinus venous trombosis. Lancet 358:597, 1971.
132. Villringer A, Seiderer M, Bauer WM et al: Diagnosis of superior sagittal sinus thrombosis by three-dimensional magnetic resonance flow imaging. Lancet 1:1086, 1989
133. Vines FS, Davis DO: Clinical radiological correlation in cerebral venous occlusive disease. Radiology 98:9, 1971
134. Virapongse C, Cazenave C, Quisling R et al: The empty delta sign: frequency and significance in 76 cases of dural sinus thrombosis. Radiology 162:779, 1987
135. Williams RS, Richardson EP Jr: A 10-year-old boy with papilledema after treatment for otitis externa and tonsillitis. N Engl J Med 318:1322, 1988
136. Yasargil MG, Damur M: Thrombosis of the cerebral veins and dural sinuses. In Newton TH, Potts DG (eds): Radiology of the Skull and Brain. Angiography. CV Mosby, St. Louis, 1974
137. Yezrby MS, Bailey GM: Superior sagittal sinus thrombosis 10 years after surgery for ulcerative colitis. Stroke 11:294, 1980
138. Yoshii N, Seiki Y, Samejima H et al: Occlusion of the deep cerebral veins. Neuroradiology 16:287, 1978
139. Younker D, Jones MM, Adenwala J et al: Maternal cortical vein thrombosis and the obstetric anesthesiologist. Anesth Analg 65:1007, 1986

# 20
# *LACUNES*

J.P. Mohr

*Lacune* was a term coined to describe the small cavity remaining in the brain tissue, which developed after the necrotic tissue of a deep infarct had been removed. The process is no different from any other brain infarct except that the more common one affecting the convexity leave a depression or dent in the brain, while those confined to the depths must leave a hole, that is, a lacune.

Interest in these lesions arose from their unusual vascular pathology and their rather pure clinical pictures. Little trouble was encountered in separating them from postmortem gas bubble artifacts at autopsy. In later years, with improving brain images, some problems have been encountered in trying to determine if the small lesion is an infarct, the late product of a small hemorrhage, or merely an enlarged Virchow-Robin space, but even these problems occur infrequently. In the early years of study, they seemed best explained by a special arteriopathy encountered in hypertension,[35] although other etiologies, including embolism, were also found at autopsy. At first, the clinical syndromes seemed relatively pure, since they occurred mainly in the motor pathways or in the thalamus, producing pure motor or pure sensory stroke. Clinical recognition of a small infarct was initially considered important, since the hypertensive arteriopathy that affected the vessel feeding a lacune was too small to be seen on angiography, and too little of the brain substance was affected by infarction to disturb the electroencephalogram. Because the arteriopathy was the same as that in hypertensive parenchymatous hemorrhage, anticoagulation was considered too risky to warrant casual use. All told, the recognition of lacunar syndromes in the days before useful brain imaging was both challenging clinically and relevant therapeutically.

The initial concept of lacunes as a set of clinical syndromes with pathologic criteria was soon diluted by new findings. While none of the findings have fundamentally altered the basic concepts, so many exceptions to the basic concepts have appeared that some have challenged the utility of the concepts entirely. Numerous studies have claimed that the syndromes may have causes other than hypertensive arteriopathy.[35,47,55,102,119] Although the individual reports often contained one or more clinical elements that deviated from the original syndrome, the effect was to blunt the impact of a causal relation of the syndromes to hypertension. With the introduction of high-quality brain imaging, it was not long before a wider range of locations of small, deep infarcts were found, together with an expansion of the syndromes associated with such lesions, now including the brain stem, parts of the thalamus, other nuclei in the basal ganglia, corona radiata, centrum semiovale, and even some straddling the thalamus and internal capsule and expanding the concept to include syndromes overlapping with those caused by Binswanger's disease.[35,87,98,117,120,138] The earlier insistence on autopsy studies has largely been lost under the weight of publications based entirely on computed tomography (CT) or magnetic resonance (MR) findings. In recent years, it has been the exception, not the rule, to find a case report with autopsy correlation. Lamentably, the term lacune has passed into common use to refer to any small, deep lesion. Many authors at least attempt to show its cause is ischemic, but for some no such caution has been exercised, including the introduction of the notion that they may come from small hemorrhages.

## HISTORICAL ASPECTS

Pierre Marie[89] used lacune as his descriptive term for 50 cases of capsular infarction. He formulated a syndrome featuring sudden onset of incomplete hemiplegia, unaccompanied by persisting sensory loss, homonymous hemianopia, or permanent aphasia. Considerable improvement in the paralysis occurred within hours to days, but complete recovery was unusual. Walking was disturbed in a special fashion, the patients taking small steps described as "marche à petits pas de Déjerine." In modern times this latter state has been attributed to patients with many foci of lacunar infarction, the so-called *lacunar state.* Marie emphasized a capsular location for the syndrome. Ferrand[33] later claimed that the same syndrome occurred whether the lesion was capsular or pontine in location. Over 20 years later, Foix and Levy[51] reiterated these principles, adding the claim that a deep lesion produced a hemiparesis without visual or sensory disturbance, and also adding the formulation that the hemiparesis equally affected arm and leg. In another publication, Foix and Hillemand[50] described the effects of a pontine infarction as a "simple" hemiplegia affecting arm more than leg, with an associated mild dysarthria. From the 1930s to the 1960s, only passing reference to a capsular lesion producing a pure hemiplegia can be found in most standard textbooks of neurology.[3,141]

Lacunes began their modern comeback almost entirely through the efforts of C. M. Fisher. Largely alone, in a few instances accompanied by or in support of younger colleagues, he described pure motor hemiplegia,[48] pure sensory stroke,[35] homolateral ataxia and crural paresis,[47] dysarthria-clumsy hand syndrome,[36] sensorimotor stroke,[99] basilar branch syndromes,[46] and the vascular pathology underlying lacunes.[37] The position was so thoroughly developed that it triggered companion studies, many corroborating[69,92,99] and others enlarging upon the clinical entities,[131] vascular pathology, and clinicoradiologic correlations.[26,110,139] Other studies attacked the basic principles,[17,117,120,138] some arguing for other etiologies, including embolism,[96] some recommending the concepts be abandoned altogether.[81] Yet the high frequency of publications worldwide[137] indicates the subject has become firmly established among the syndromes of stroke. In some countries, notably China, the high frequency of deep infarcts has even been proposed to have a racial or ethnic basis.[22,67]

## DEFINITIONS

As a term based on neuropathologic findings, lacune refers to a small, deep infarct attributable to a primary arterial disease that involves a penetrating branch of a large cerebral artery (Fig. 20-1). It should not be used to describe lesions of nonvascular origin. Nor does it apply to deep infarction that is simply part of a larger stroke that affects the cerebral surface in continuity or separately, such as occurs in embolism affecting the middle cerebral artery. Nor is it applicable to describe deep infarction from disease involving the stems of the large cerebral arteries, such as the middle or anterior cerebral, which affects the penetrating branches.

The low frequency of autopsy studies has forced modification of the definitions to include, small, deep lesions found by brain imaging, whether CT or MR scanning. Numerous attempts at definitions have been made, but the most widely used is the attempt to separate between a small, deep infarct, the residue of a small hemorrhage and dilated Virchow-Robin spaces. For those inclined to use numbers, these are types I, II, and III lacunes, respectively.

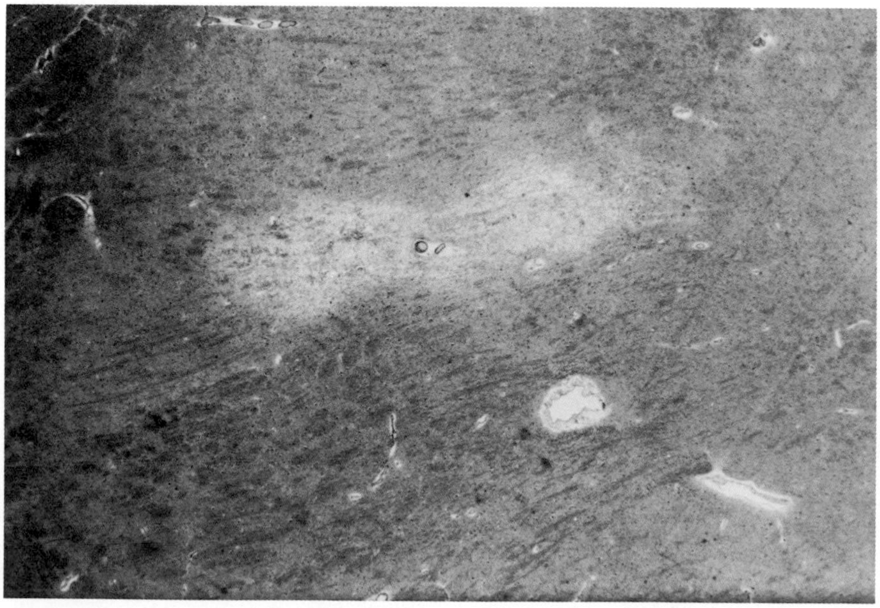

**Fig. 20-1.** Microscopic pathology of a lacune.

In an attempt to keep the presentation orderly, emphasis will be placed on the autopsy-based material, followed by those studies based only on brain imaging, and finally on clinical studies only.

## PATHOANATOMY

### Size

The majority of autopsy-documented lacunar infarcts are small, ranging from 0.2 to 15 $mm^3$ in size.[43] Their size varies according to the territory supplied by the occluded vessel feeding the infarct. In general, these vessels are 100 to 400 μm[41] in size, and serve territories varying from little more than a cylinder the size of the vessel itself to wedges as large as 15 mm on a side. While the smallest infarcts are unresolved by CT scanners, and occasionally even escape detection at autopsy,[110] the largest, the so-called superlacunes, are as large as 15 $mm^3$.[43] They are seen as obvious abnormalities at several levels in the CT scan. Thus far, few of these superlacunes have been examined at autopsy, and some that have been examined had no detailed search of the underlying vascular pathology. Embolism into the stem of the middle cerebral artery, which occlusion of several of the lenticulostriates, are possible causes of such infarcts, which do not deserve the name lacune, except for their location in the depths of the brain.

### Locations of Lacunes

Lacunes predominate in the basal ganglia, especially the putamen, the thalamus, and the white matter of the internal capsule and pons, and they occur occasionally in the white matter of the cerebral gyri. They are rare in the gray matter of the cerebral surface, in the corpus callosum, visual radiations, centrum semiovale of the cerebral hemispheres, medulla, or spinal cord.[35] In general, the larger the series, the more widespread have been the lesions.[25] In the largest autopsy series thus far reported, 169 among 2,859 patients, 81 percent of the lacunes seem to have been asymptomatic in life, arguing that many of those seen nowadays in brain imaging are of uncertain clinical significance.

Attempts to include the centrum semiovale and white matter of the temporal lobes in the regions subject to lacunes involves a challenge (thus far not justified by available data) to an important principle long thought important in the production of lacunes: the lack of gradual stepdown in vascular size between the major cerebral artery trunks and the penetrating vessels involved in lacunes. The medullary arteries of the white matter arise from the cortical branches and not directly from the large trunks. If their disease is the same as those of the lenticulostriates and thalamoperforants, it awaits such demonstration.

### Vascular Territories Involved

Most lacunes occur in the territories of the lenticulostriate branches of the anterior and middle cerebral arteries, the thalamoperforant branches of the posterior cerebral arteries, and the paramedian branches on the basilar artery. Their occurrence is rare in the territories of the cerebral surface branches.

The lenticulostriates arise from the circle of Willis and the stems of the anterior and middle cerebral arteries to supply the putamen, caudate nucleus, and internal capsule. They are comprised of two main groups, those more medial, whose lumen is 100 to 200 μm, and those more lateral whose diameters are 200 to 400 μm.[43] The thalamoperforants arise from the posterior half of the circle of Willis and the stems of the posterior cerebral arteries to supply the midbrain and thalamus. Their size varies from 100 to 400 μm. The paramedian branches of the basilar mainly supply the pons. Few branches have been measured, but sizes ranging from 40 μm to as large as 500 μm have been observed.[37,63] These arteries share in common both a tendency to arise directly from much larger arteries and an unbranching end-artery anatomy. The penetrators are all below 500 μm in size, and arise directly from the larger 6- to 8-mm internal carotid or basilar artery. Their small size and their point of origin rather proximal in the arterial network are thought to expose these vessels to forces that scarcely reach other similar sized arteries in the cerebral cortex.[53] These latter are apparently protected by a gradual stepdown in size from the 8-mm internal carotid to 3- to 4-mm middle cerebral to 1- to 2-mm surface branches from which the intracortical vessels whose diameters are less than 500 μm arise. Perhaps this difference explains the low frequency of lacunes in the cerebral surface vessels.[10,16]

The lack of collateral for the penetrators results in an infarct that spreads distally from the point of occlusion through the entire territory of the vessel affected. The exact volume of tissue supplied by each penetrator varies enormously.[37] Some arteries supply little more than the territory the same diameter as the artery,[43] while others arborize widely and supply a territory shaped like a wedge or cone.[37] The smaller the artery involved, the smaller the lacune. For example, most capsular infarcts arise from arteries 200 to 400 μm in size and produce infarcts 2 to 3 $mm^3$ or smaller.[43] These small infarcts require 1.5 Tesla MR imaging to be found regularly, are frequently missed by CT scaning, and are easily overlooked at autopsy.[110]

The arterial occlusion usually occurs in the first half of the course of the penetrating vessel, a location that ensures most lacunes will be quite small. These sites are not usually detected by angiography because the course of the individual vessels is difficult to plot to show one is missing. However, disease involving the stem of the cerebral artery from which the penetrator

**TABLE 20-1. Distribution of Lacunar Lesions Among Penetrating Arteries**

| | Lacunar Syndrome (%) | | | | |
|---|---|---|---|---|---|
| Location | PMH ($N$ = 181) | SMS ($N$ = 63) | AH ($N$ = 33) | PSS ($N$ = 21) | DCH ($N$ = 18) |
| Basal ganglia | 22 | 19 | 8 | 0 | 0 |
| Thalamus | 2 | 9 | 0 | 67 | 0 |
| Anterior limb of internal capsule | 15 | 6 | 15 | 33 | 11 |
| Genu | 8 | 7 | 15 | 0 | 0 |
| Posterior limb of internal capsule | 26 | 31 | 23 | 0 | 11 |
| Corona radiata | 20 | 22 | 31 | 0 | 28 |
| Pons | 1 | 0 | 0 | 0 | 0 |
| Cerebellum | 0 | 0 | 0 | 0 | 11 |
| Other | 6 | 6 | 8 | 0 | 39 |

*Abbreviations*: PMH, pure motor hemiparesis; SMS, sensorimotor syndrome; AH, ataxic hemiparesis; PSS, pure sensory syndrome; DCH, dysarthria-clumsy hand syndrome.
(From Chamorro et al.,[15] with permission.)

arises, or from one of the small number of large penetrators, a bigger infarction results. Occlusions at the ostium of a penetrator where it departs from the parent major cerebral artery may yield a swath of infarction some 15 mm$^3$. These so-called superlacunes[43] are large enough to produce a striking abnormality at several levels on the CT scan. In most instances, however, superlacunes result from occlusions of larger vessels and are not a sign of primary arteriopathy of the penetrating vessels (Table 20-1).

## Arteriopathies Underlying Lacunes

### Microatheroma

Several distinct but related arteriopathies cause lacunes. Microatheroma is believed to be the most common mechanism of arterial stenosis underlying lacunes.[38,40,43] The artery is usually involved in the first half of its course. Microatheroma stenosing or occluding a penetrating artery was found in 6 of 11 capsular infarcts in the only published pathologic study on the cause of capsular infarcts.[43] It was the cause of the only published case of thalamic lacune.[41] The histologic characteristics of the microatheroma are identical with those affecting the larger arteries.

These tiny foci of atheromatous deposits are commonly encountered in chronic hypertension. In the usual nonhypertensive case, atheroma appears mostly in the extracranial internal carotid and basilar arteries, but only rarely in the stems of the major cerebral arteries.[42] In hypertension, however, the lesions are not only more advanced for the patient's age, but they are spread more distally in the arterial system, at times involving even some of the cerebral surface arteries. In advanced hypertensive patients, miniature foci of typical atherosclerotic plaques are found even in arteries as small as 100 to 400 $\mu$m in diameter, resulting in a stenosis or occlusion that sets the stage for a lacune.

### Lipohyalinosis and Fibrinoid Necrosis

Other arterial disorders seem less common. *Lipohyalinosis,* formerly considered the most frequent cause of lacunes, affects penetrating arteries in a segmental fashion in chronic hypertension.[53] It was the cause attributed to 40 of 50 lacunes studied in serial section by Fisher in four cases of stroke.[38] It seems to occur most often in the smaller penetrating arteries, these below 200 $\mu$m in diameter, and accounts for many of the smaller lacunes, especially those that are clinically asymptomatic. Lipohyalinosis has been thought to be an intermediate stage between the fibrinoid necrosis of severe hypertension and the microatheroma associated with more long-standing hypertension.[16,38,63]

*Fibrinoid necrosis* is a related condition found in arterioles and capillaries of the brain, retina, and kidneys in a setting of extremely high blood pressure.[62] It appears histopathologically as a brightly eosinophilic, finely granular, or homogeneous deposit involving the connective tissue of blood vessels. The mechanism is believed to involve disordered cerebrovascular autoregulation[29,128] with a necrotizing consequence.[12] This thesis envisions that the thickened arterial walls are unable to constrict, resulting in a resetting of cerebrovascular autoregulation at higher blood pressure levels. Continued high pressure produces increased capillary hydrostatic pressure and capillary damage. The overdistension[55,64] of these small arteries occurs in segmental fashion,[54] leading to vascular necrosis,[10–12] which allows red blood cells, plasma, and protein ultrafiltrates into the stretched segments of the wall.[54]

That other vessels are spared such injury is not easily explained. However, the arteriole and capillary necrosis encountered in severe hypertension does not occur in renal arteries protected from hypertension distal to an experimental arterial clamp or to renal arterial stenosis. Larger vessels seem able to absorb enough in the subintima and in their thicker muscularis to resist such change, while the tiny cerebral cortical arteries of a size similar to the deep branches of the circle of Willis are protected by their more distal location.[12,16,55]

Fibrinoid necrosis shares some of the same histochemical, electron-microscopic,[56,143] and immunofluorescent[103] characteristics with lipohyalinosis,[32] another cause of lacunes. Both occur in the brain[37,43] in a setting of hypertension, and both occur in a segmental location along the course of the arteries.[37] The two conditions have also been labeled as hyalinosis, hyaline fatty change, hyaline arterionecrosis, angionecrosis, fibrinoid arteritis, plasmatic vascular destruction, atherosclerosis of small arteries, and segmental arterial disorganization. Although often considered identical,[37,43] the segmental fibrinoid necrosis and lipohyalinosis differ histochemically, in that fibrinoid necrosis is said to stain strongly for PTAH, whereas lipohyalinosis does not.[16] Lipohyalinosis[37] is found most commonly in a setting of chronic, nonmalignant hypertension,[63] whereas fibrinoid necrosis is said to be found only with extreme blood pressure elevations,[16,62] such as occurs in hypertensive encephalopathy[16] and eclampsia.

## Charcot-Bouchard Aneurysm

A long-standing, albeit little noted controversy, concerns whether lipohyalinosis or microatheroma is the precursor, the result, or is even related to another commonly encountered arteriopathy in chronic hypertensives, Charcot-Bouchard aneurysm.[18,37,39,119] The controversy also involves the questions whether the Charcot-Bouchard arteriopathy represents a true aneurysm formation or merely a dissection into the wall of a microatheroma; whether both lipohyalinosis and Charcot-Bouchard aneurysm deserve consideration as pathologic processes separate from microatheroma of the penetrating arteries; and whether these lesions are simply variants along a spectrum of vascular effects of hypertension. The available evidence suggests that lipohyalinosis is more significant than Charcot-Bouchard aneurysm in the development of lacunes.[37,39] No recent evidence has appeared to support an earlier suggestion that lipohyalinosis is the end stage of an earlier Charcot-Bouchard aneurysm.[119]

## Other Causes

*Microembolism* has been inferred in a few serially sectioned lacunes shown to have normal arteries leading to the infarct.[43] *Macroembolism* is considered elsewhere, but one such case (case 10) is to be found among Fisher and Curry's original descriptions of pure motor stroke[48] (Fig. 20-2). Even *polycythemia* has been thought to be a cause of lacunes,[104] the small vessels being obstructed by the sludged blood. *Dissection* of a tiny artery may occur in the process leading to Charcot-Bouchard aneurysm.[44] Recent attempts have been made[136] to relate severe extracranial carotid artery stenosis to deep infarcts on a *hemodynamic basis,* the lacunar infarct imaged on brain scan. Although the presumed mechanism has been via perfusion failure in the symptomatic deep territory, the lack of autopsy data leave unsettled whether such infarction is from embolism in carotid artery disease or from associated severe stenosis of a penetrating artery. Varying forms of *arteritis* may also occur, especially due to chronic meningitis (so-called Heubner's arteritis)[78,93] in chronic neurosyphilis, any severe granulomatous meningitis, and chronic fibrosing meningitis. Arteritis may have been a major cause of

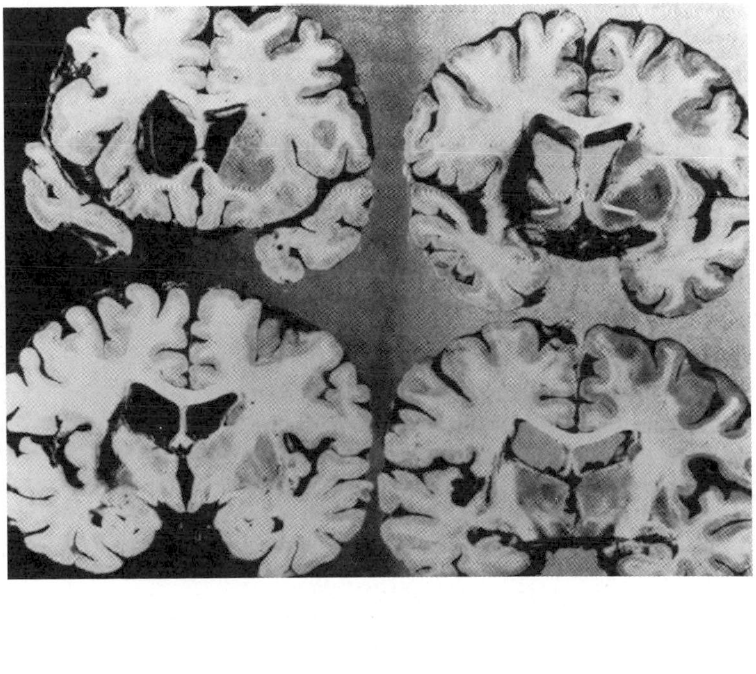

**Fig. 20-2.** Large, deep infarct reported in the original series of pure motor stroke.

small, deep infarcts[65] when chronic neurosyphilis was in its heyday. However, two major works[21,93] on the subject contain no specific cases, although the authors opined that "they undoubtedly occur."[93] This opinion was not shared by Pentschew[105] who expressed doubts whether "syphilitic endarteritis" was actually of syphilitic origin.

## GENERAL CLINICAL FEATURES

Lacunar infarctions share many risk factors, leading among them hypertension and diabetes mellitus. These two common accompaniments of lacunar disease have been present to comparable degrees in three clinical series exceeding 100 patients collected over the last 20 years: 75 percent and 29 percent, respectively, of lacunar cases diagnosed in the Harvard Cooperative Stroke Registry,[62] in 74 percent and 27 percent of cases in the south Alabama population study,[41] in 72 percent and 28 percent of the Barcelona series reported by Arboix and colleagues,[6] in which only 26 percent had cardiac disease. A high frequency (93 percent) of hypertension or left ventricular hypertrophy was found by Reimer et al.,[112] while no clear correlation between blood pressure or hypertension was found in some of the smaller series.[84,90] The largest currently reported autopsy-based study was of 2,859 patients by Tuszynski et al.,[134] who found lacunar infarctions in 169 patients (6 percent). Hypertension was present in 64 percent, diabetes in 34 percent, smoking in 46 percent, while there were no known risk factors for cerebrovascular disease in 18 percent. A correlation was found between high hematocrit and hypertension in the patients with lacunar syndromes in a population-based study.[83] In the Stroke Data Bank project 337 (27 percent) of the 1,273 patients diagnosed as infarction had a typical lacunar syndrome. In this large cohort, no striking differences were found among the risk factors for each of the lacunar subtypes but differences were found between lacunar syndrome stroke as a group and other types of infarcts. Lacunar syndrome strokes shared similar risk factors with large-vessel infarction except for fewer transient ischemic attacks (TIAs) (13 percent vs 40 percent) and prior stroke (19 percent vs 39 percent). Compared with cardioembolism, they had more hypertension (75 percent vs 60 percent) and diabetes (26 percent vs 17 percent) and less cardiac disease (24 percent vs 77 percent).[15]

Atrial fibrillation, one of the hallmarks of embolism, has a low frequency of small, deep infarcts. In a series of patients with atrial fibrillation versus a control series, neither group known to have symptomatic stroke, Kempster et al.[74] found all infarcts with atrial fibrillation peripheral and consistent with embolism. In the control group, three of asymptomatic infarcts were lacunes.

Prior transient ischemic attacks occur within approximately 20 percent of cases, a frequency intermediate between embolism (5 percent) and large artery atherostenosis (50 percent). No correlation has yet been documented between the type of lacune, severity of the clinical deficit, prognosis, and the occurrence of transient ischemic attacks.

Compared with the sudden onset more typical of infarction in other territories, a leisurely mode of onset has occurred in many lacunar strokes, delayed over enough time that opportunity often exists to determine the effects of intervention. In contrast to major atheromatous or embolic stroke, where a gradual onset is encountered in less than 5 percent of cases, as many as 30 percent of lacunes develop over a period up to 36 hours.[41,43,69,70] During this time a mild weakness may evolve to total paralysis, usually by intensifying the initial deficit, but occasionally by spreading into limbs not affected initially.[41] This smooth onset occurs with equal frequency in all types of lacunar syndromes. Sudden onset occurs in only 40 percent of cases.[70] The rate of evolution of the stroke appears not to predict the severity of the eventual defect, but this matter has not yet received much detailed study.

Lacunes typically present with highly focal symptoms described below, but a few nonfocal symptoms have been reported in clinical series of patients with the typical motor or sensory syndromes. Lability of mood was once taken as a sign of multiple lacunes. This sign occurs in 26 percent of cases with an equal frequency in single or multiple lacunes visible on CT scan.[25] It may simply be that multiple lacunes are present pathologically but are too small to be seen on CT scan. To date, neither headache, lightheadedness, hiccough, or asterixis occur in a predictable manner with a high frequency, nor have they been correlated with the presence of a CT scan abnormality, or with the size or location of the lacunes shown on CT scan. None appear to predict the clinical outcome.

## CLINICAL SYNDROMES OF LACUNES

### Lacunar State

For many years, lacunar state was what most clinicians understood was meant by the term lacunes. It was part of the original description by Marie.[89] His syndrome included a progressive decline in neurologic function punctuated by a few episodes of mild hemiparesis, followed by the appearance of dysarthria, imbalance, incontinence, pseudobulbar signs, and a short-step gait (described as *marche à petits pas*). It was easy to envision that the small infarcts, widely scattered throughout the deep white matter, might accumulate gradually, each individual infarct all but inobvious, but the cumulative effect devastating. Despite a few voices expressing disagreement, matters have remained thus over the years since.

Whether because of the effects of antihypertensive treatment, the lacunar state is a rarity in modern times. One reason might be that the syndrome had been due to other causes. Fisher[44] has pointed out that symptomatic occult hydrocephalus may have been the more common cause, and that Marie's own published cases show such findings. He further noted that most lacunar infarcts are symptomatic and that the number of infarcts are small compared with the greatly deteriorated state of the patients. Earnest et al.[28] and Koto et al.[77] have observed a correlation between lacunar infarcts and hydrocephalus, suggesting the former may arise from the pressure on the white matter.

## Pure Motor Stroke

Pure motor stroke syndrome undoubtedly occurs the most frequently of any of the forms, accounting for between one-half and two-thirds of cases, depending on the series.[6,100,112,135] It was the first lacunar syndrome recognized clinically,[48,89] and its features have been the most thoroughly explored.

### Clinicoanatomic Correlations

Pure motor stroke (PMS) has been reported from autopsied cases with focal infarction involving the corona radiata,[25] internal capsule,[43,48] pons,[46] and the medullary pyramid[48,85] (Fig. 20-3). The most frequent correlations have been with capsular locations. Of the two ends of the capsule, the greatest number have been reported from the posterior limb. The *posterior limb capsular lacunes*[111] usually involve the pallidum and posterior limb of the capsule, which are supplied by the lenticulostriate branches of the middle cerebral artery. The vessels occluded vary in size from small medially placed penetrators to the larger lateral lenticulostriates. The infarcts range from the genu to the back of the posterior limb. It is in this group that most of the data referable to the classical views of a homonculus in the internal capsule is to be found. Lesions in this region, especially those affecting the corona radiata, have also produced the syndrome of ataxic hemiparesis.

*Anterior limb capsular lacunes*[111] constitute a smaller number of cases and are smaller sized infarcts, which may affect the caudate in addition to the anterior limb of the capsule. Some of them are in the territory of supply of anterior cerebral artery, including the largest of the penetrating vessels, the recurrent artery of Heubner. Syndromes of hemiparesis are only one of the many permutations of anterior capsular infarcts,[111,140] which also includes ataxic hemiparesis[72] and some unusual speech and language disorders.[20,101]

Compared to the small number of cases with autopsy correlation, a steadily enlarging group of cases of PMS have been documented by CT scan alone. In the NINCDS Pilot Stroke Data Bank project,[100] fully 45 of the 100 cases of lacune were diagnosed by CT scan, most often instances of pure motor stroke. The pathology in such cases is rarely defined.

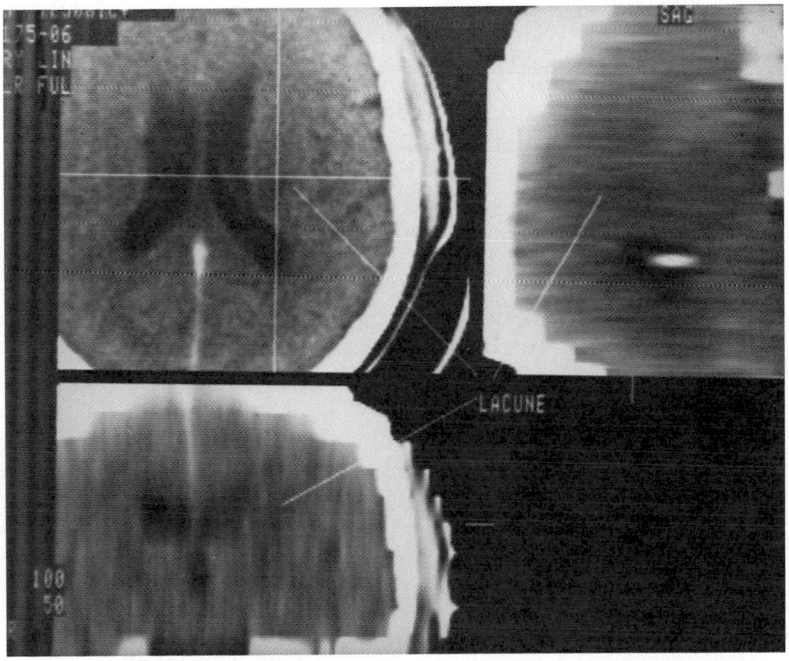


**Fig. 20-3.** Lacune affecting the corona radiata.

## Other Causes of Pure Motor Syndromes

Nonlacunar pure motor syndromes have also been described, indicating that the clinical picture alone is not invariably due to deep infarction. Less than a year passed after Marie's description of lacunes when protests against the syndromes were lodged. Abadie[1] contrasted the great frequency with which a capsular lesion was diagnosed clinically against the rarity with which such a lesion was found without other complaints that accompanied the hemiparesis. His objection set the stage for the many others down through the years.

After Fisher and Curry's report[48] of pure motor stroke, several articles appeared challenging the lacunar origin by detailing a similar syndrome due to a variety of other causes, ranging among nocardial abscess of the motor cortex,[138] ischemia-edema postcraniotomy for postoperative bleeding,[71] internal carotid artery occlusion in the neck,[2] and cerebral cortical surface infarction. Lesions rostral to the capsule have been described in cases studied only by CT scan,[139] and the syndrome has also been encountered with both deep and superficial low-density lesions on CT inferred to be from infarction.[110] Three such cases have even been reported from hemorrhage.[111,132]

The clinical picture itself has also come in for criticism. Richter et al.[113] studied all cases of stroke that occurred in a single hospital and found that pure motor stroke occurred rarely, was not more prevalent among hypertensive patients and did not usually have a good clinical outlook.

Yet even the most careful studies exploring the limits of the syndrome and its etiologies have found a remarkably high percentage of cases whose clinical and radiologic picture conformed to the original syndrome described by Fisher and Curry.[48] Pullicino et al.[110] studied 297 consecutive cases whose CT scan showed one or more foci of low density and found among them 42 single, small, deep lesions. Hypertension was more prevalent in this group than in the 122 cases with large lesions; 9 of the 42 (21 percent) had a pure motor deficit, in contrast to only three of 122 (2 percent) with large lesions, a highly significant difference ($P < 0.0005$). Further, in another 13 cases with isolated deep lesions, either the clinical deficit could not be related to the lesion or there was no clinical deficit at all, a point consistent with the observation that deep infarcts may spare the capsule.

## Clinical Features

PMS is most easily diagnosed when the stroke equally affects the face, arm and leg on the same side, sparing sensation, vision, language, and behavior.[48] The complete syndrome is somewhat uncommon, however. As a clinical rule, so long as the syndromes is purely motor, a diagnosis of PMS applies when the affected side involves one part more than the other, and a few cases have been described in which the face is essentially spared.[115] The term pure motor stroke was used initially to draw attention to the lack of the expected accompanying sensory, visual, or behavior disturbances, especially considering the severity of the weakness. In this sense only is it pure.

PMS has been described in both capsular and pontine locations, producing an essentially identical clinical picture as first suggested by Ferrand.[33] Some reports[37,48] suggested that the capsular infarct case might have an associated conjugate eye movement disturbance that would follow the "hemispheral" pattern, that is, deviation of the eyes toward the side of the lesion, while those involving the pons would have the opposite, so-called "wrong-way" eyes. However, this finding occurs too infrequently to serve a useful function.[98]

Despite earlier opinions by Ferrand[33] and by Foix and Levy,[51] it has become clear that pure motor stroke may be associated with considerable variations among the syndromes involving face, arm, and leg. Fisher and Curry[48] found the arm severely affected in all 50 cases of pure motor stroke, but the lower the lesion occurred in the neuraxis, the less the face was involved.

In cases where the lacune affects the internal capsule and corona radiata, a considerable variety of motor deficits have been encountered, both in severity and formula. Despite the many CT correlations with capsular lesions, only a handful of cases exist with a capsular infarct whose syndrome was fully studied in life. Among this small group, remarkable variations exist. The most compact lesion with a hemiplegia was an autopsied case with an infarct confined to the third quarter of the posterior limb of the internal capsule.[30] This location corresponds to the approximate pathway of the motor fibers as inferred from whole-brain anatomic dissections.[117] The clinical deficit had persisted for years, equally affecting face, arm, and leg. Yet in another autopsied case involving the same site in the posterior limb of the internal capsule, the deficit was less severe. Spastic hemiparesis, which developed over many hours and lasted for the remaining 9 months of life, paralyzing the tongue, palate, face, arm and hand, but the leg was only slightly affected.[62] In still another case, ischemia involving the posterior quarter of the internal capsule was associated with a hemiparesis that only slightly affected the face.[99]

Most of the recent studies have been documented by CT scan. Donnan et al.[26] found a hemiplegia involving face, arm, and leg in equivalent fashion in all 36 cases of infarction involving the capsule, but 22 other cases in the same series had incomplete syndromes, the most common being paresis of the arm and leg, sparing the face. The inferred lacune in these latter cases occurred more often in the fibers of the corona radiata, or at extreme ends of the capsule. One lacune with pure facial weakness was located at the genu, while another with pure leg weakness lay at the extreme posterior end of the capsule. Rascol et al.[111] also found a spectrum of syndromes of hemiparesis, which varied at one end from equal involvement of face, arm, and leg to partial syndromes faciobrachial weakness in a few cases purely crural;[111] similar incomplete formulas of hemiparesis occurred in the smaller capsulopallidal cases, and also in the anterior capsulocaudate infarcts. In the NINCDS Pilot Stroke Data Bank project[100] and in the population-based study of stroke in south Alabama,[59] lacunes located more posteriorly in the capsule produced a deficit greater in the leg than in the arm, but several varieties were encountered, including some whose arm was worse than leg. Lesions affecting the anterior limb and genu have also been a source of syndromes of partial hemiparesis, in a few cases featuring greater weakness of the face than the leg.[26] For those studied in the Stroke Data Bank, lesions seen in the corona radiata were associated with a hemiparesis, which took highly variable, forms while those lower in the capsule produced a wide variety of syndromes (Fig. 20-4).[15] Taken together, the CT-scan correlations with the syndromes of hemiparesis showed only slight support for the classical view of a homunculus in the internal capsule with face, arm, and leg displayed in an anteroposterior distribution.

When these findings are taken together, it is no longer possible to infer the exact site and size of the lesion in the motor pathway based on the clinical formulation based on the older dogma[23] that the motor fibers occupy a certain functionally reliable position in the posterior limb of the internal capsule. The case material only vaguely supports the traditional impression of a homunculus whose face is forward, and whose leg is located posteriorly. These findings suggest even more careful attention to the clinical details in future cases might permit a clearer understanding of the variability and reliability of the pathways that make up the capsule.[5,23,120] At the least, the findings thus far indicate partial syndromes of hemiparesis are common manifestations of lacunar infarction affecting the internal capsule and adjacent territory.

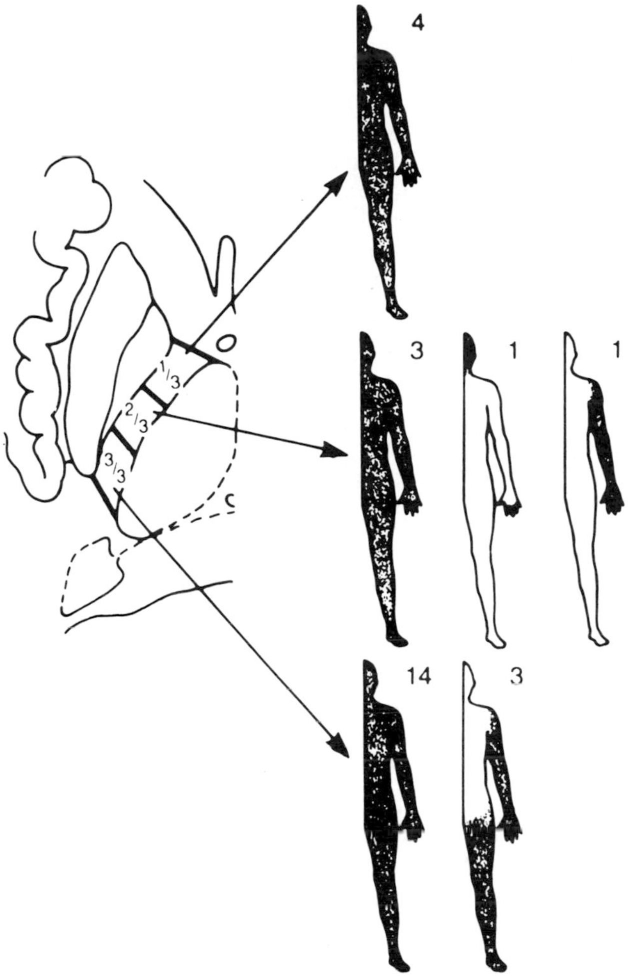


**Fig. 20-4.** Hemiparesis formulas for capsular lesions of the anterior, middle, and posterior thirds of the posterior limb of the internal capsule. (From Chamorro et al.,[15] with permission.)

## Associated Complaints

Although the main elements of the PMH syndromes are motor, other complaints are not rare, especially sensory disturbances, which occur initially in as many as 42 percent of cases.[26] These complaints usually present as numbness, heaviness, and loss of feeling. Only scant abnormalities are found on clinical examination. Given their vague, they are all too easily brushed aside or ignored. However, complaints of undue coldness, at times confined to the distal arm, are less easily ignored, and in a few cases personally observed, they have lasted for years.[98] The anatomic pathology of these complaints is not resolved. These sensory complaints are thought to reflect slight involvement of the projections to the sensory cortex from occlusion of the larger lateral striate vessels, although few such cases have actually been documented by autopsy.

No disturbance in visual field function has been described from such infarcts. Dysphasia, dyspraxia, and other disturbances of higher cerebral function have rarely been described.

## Clinical Course

Improvement is the result in a high percentage of cases. It is usually more rapid than that following cerebral surface infarction with a similar initial motor deficit.[110] The syndromes of partial hemiparesis show the best prognosis, as do those with the smaller infarct size on CT scan, but cases of complete plegia with virtual total recovery has been encountered. Rascol et al.[111] found that all of their cases regained the ability to walk. Fully 19 of their 30 cases experienced a favorable outcome, while another 6 were left with functional incapacity of the upper extremity. Of the 42 cases documented in the pilot phase of the NINCDS Stroke Data Bank,[100] 35 improved to a functionally useful level within a few months. The improvement occurred regularly in the cases whose initial syndrome was incomplete. Unfortunately, among the seven cases initially paralyzed, only two made much improvement in the first few months, and both of them improved almost to normal.

## Ataxic Hemiparesis

The syndrome of ataxic hemiparesis[42] has both cerebellar and pyramidal elements. It was initially described as homolateral ataxia with crural paresis,[47] its most familiar form. The original authors speculated that the lesion might lie either in the anterior limb of the internal capsule or in the adjacent corona radiata. However, the first autopsied cases showed a pontine lesion of the small size typical of lacunar infarction.[42]

Since these early observations, numerous case reports have shown a low-density CT lesion lying in the corona radiata[68] or in the posterior limb of the internal capsule.[25,42,70,122,140] These lesions have not been in the same site in each case and have been encountered as far forward as the head of the caudate and as far posterior as the posterior limb of the internal capsule.[25] As the lesion in all of these cases have been documented by CT scan alone, their exact correlation with the syndrome has been called into question somewhat by Kistler's disturbing case.[75] This patient had a CT scan showing a corona radiata lesion, while a nuclear magnetic resonance scan revealed a recent pontine lesion which better explained the deficit. The pontine lesion was not seen by CT scan due to the difficulty averaging the bone densities adjacent to the brain stem. Since this effect prevents all but the largest pontine infarcts from being seen by CT scan, other cases may have had a similar second lesion as well. Although the syndrome is best known from infarction, it has also been reported from tumor,[8] although not in as pure a form.

The clinical features have been rather similar from case to case. The usual form presents as a mild to moderate weakness of the leg, especially the ankle, with little or no weakness of the upper limb and face, accompanied by an ataxia of the arm and leg on the same side. In a few cases,[68,70] a mild and transient hemisensory deficit may initially accompany the motor findings. The syndrome commonly develops only gradually, requiring from hours[68] to a day or more to reach its peak. A few instances of a chronic state exist, but some degree of improvement within days or months is usual. In some cases, the syndrome changes, with the hemiparesis clearing off, leaving the ataxia.[68]

Only limited success has been met with efforts[47,68] to separate hemispheral from brain stem location: the latter have a slightly higher frequency of dysarthria and trigeminal weakness. In most instances, however, no distinctive features separate the cases of capsular or radiation origin from those involving the pons. The extent of weakness accompanying the ataxia is no guide to the location. In both the capsular and pontine cases, weakness may involve more structures than the leg, at times affecting the face and arm almost to the same degree. In all cases, the degree of ataxia is more striking than the weakness, and exceeds that attributable to weakness alone.

## Dysarthria-Clumsy Hand Syndrome

The dysarthria-clumsy hand syndrome has the advantage of emphasizing the distinctive elements of the stroke: in patients presenting with the syndrome, the dysarthria and the ataxia of the upper limb appear to be more prominent components of the overall clinical deficit than is usually expected. But they do not occur in isolation. The syndrome usually also includes facial weakness, which at times may be profound, dysphagia, some degree of weakness of the hand, and even of the leg. The reflexes on the affected side are usually exaggerated, and the plantar response is extensor. The clinical picture usually develops suddenly. The cases with autopsy correlation have shown no sensory deficit. In one case, the facial weakness was accompanied by impaired strength in opening of the jaw.[123] In the case from pontine hemorrhage, several features occurred, which differed from those reported with infarction: vomiting and lethargy occurred at onset; balance was impaired enough that the patient was unable to stand; and the facial weakness was mild. It was only after a week that the persisting deficit was reduced to dysarthria and a clumsy hand.

Some authors have equated the syndrome with ataxic hemiparesis,[134] while the originator has come to the view that it is a variant.[44] The best recognized association has been with lacunes of the anterior limb of the internal capsule.[36] Other sites have been reported less often: Spertell and Ransom[129] described a case with a low-density lesion near the genu; and two of Fisher's anterior capsular infarcts had combinations of mild ataxia and dysarthria. In a few other cases, the lesion has been in the basis pontis. The syndrome has also been reported from hemorrhage of the pons.[133]

The outlook for functional recovery is good.

## Movement Disorders

Several types of movement disorders have been described with small, deep infarcts. Although the exact vascular occlusion has not been demonstrated in many of these cases, the small size of the infarct and its occurrence in territories fed by small penetrating arteries justifies considering these disorders among the lacunar syndromes. The disorder may appear as the only sign of the infarct or develop later, after an initial syndrome, different in character, has resolved.

## Hemichorea-Hemiballismus

The form of movement disorder known as hemichorea or hemiballismus, is the most frequently documented. The infarcts found in different parts of the striatum have been of lacunar size[55,91] including those in the head of the caudate nucleus and adjacent corona radiata,[125] the subthalamic nucleus,[92,94] and the thalamus.[4,69,91] The onset is typically abrupt and usually unaccompanied by other complaints. The chorea usually involves the forearm, hand, and fingers. In one case, it was accompanied by hemiparesis, which faded within 3 months while the chorea persisted unchanged.[125] In some cases, it has been delayed by some weeks or months after the initial occurrence of hemiparesis. One patient familiar to the author, whose putaminal lesion was documented only by CT scan,[73] suffered choreic movements of the distal parts of the arm and leg, which interfered with normal activity and prevented easy walking for over 4 weeks. In this case the chorea improved only to relapse a few weeks later. Rare ballistic movements were superimposed. The examination revealed normal strength, sensation, and reflexes.

Treatment with haliperidol is a common approach, but has not been uniformly effective.[125] Doses as high as 5 mg tid have been required to suppress the chorea.[73]

## Dystonia

Two types of dystonia have been described. *Action-induced rhythmic dystonia* has been documented by an autopsy study. In the case reported,[131] the syndrome began as a sensorimotor stroke. Both these deficits improved within a month. By 3 months, the movement disorder began in the left leg, which had been the most severely affected part in the initial stroke. The disorder spread to involve his entire left side. The fingers of the affected hand became flexed into the palm, leaving only the thumb free. When examined 4 years later, the hand was unchanged, but strength was otherwise normal. Voluntary movements of any parts of the body, including even eye closure, precipitated rhythmic dystonic extension and rotation of the left arm and leg, sparing the trunk, and subsided a few seconds after the voluntary movements ceased. Clonazepam and 5-hydroxytryptophan were successful in suppressing the involuntary movement disorder. At autopsy, an infarct 5 × 1 × 2 mm was found straddling the ventral posterolateral nucleus and the adjacent posterior limb of the internal capsule.

The other type is a *focal dystonia*. One case has been described whose CT scan showed a low density in the right lenticular nucleus.[121] Like the cases of hemichorea and hemiballism, the deficit appeared abruptly, unaccompanied by weakness or sensory disturbances. Only the distal end of the upper extremity was affected. Although described as dystonic, the disorder featured changing postures: "The movements were slow and caused the patient's fingers to assume unusual positions. Activity exacerbated the movements. . . . The left hand and forearm showed involuntary movements that produced an unusual posture, with hyperpronation and flexion at the wrist, extension of the fingers, and opposition of the thumb." Haloperidol, 1 mg tid, relieved much of the movement and posture disorder. Attempts to remove the medication over 8 months later produced relapse, requiring reinstitution of therapy to suppress the disorder.

## Pure Sensory Stroke

Pure sensory stroke is assumed to be due to infarction of the sensory pathway of the brain stem, thalamus, or thalamocortical projections. Few autopsy-documented cases have been reported, and the syndrome was not noted in one large autopsy-based series.[134] In this small group, the most common location has been in the thalamus,[34,41,99] mostly in the ventral posterior tier nuclei, the main sensory relay nuclei to the cerebrum.[34] The only autopsied case with pure sensory stroke from a lesion outside the thalamus[58] was a small hemorrhage that involved the corona radiata of the posterior limb of the internal capsule.

CT scan has been the basis of the other sites associated with pure sensory stroke. One case inferred due to a lacune because of its small size, affected the centrum semiovale, presumably with involvement of the thalamocortical projection area.[117] Caution is necessary in this interpretation, as lacunes in the centrum semiovale are distinctly uncommon in series based on autopsy data.[25,35] Involvement of subthalamic brain stem pathways has not yet been reported to be associated with pure sensory stroke.

The observations on the arterial disease is confined to two cases. In one, a microatheroma was found narrowing the lumen of a small artery to the posterior thalamus,[37] which led to a lacunar infarct. Whether the lacune was symptomatic was unmentioned. In the other, a pure sensory syndrome was described clinically.[41] The 54-year-old patient was recovering from a right-sided pure motor hemiplegia, when a feeling of "pins and needles" developed in the left lower lip, left side of the mouth, and the fingers of the left hand; the sole of the left foot tingled, and felt numb, dull and swollen many hours later. No sensory deficit was evident on examination. Unpleasant paresthesias affected the left side of the face and the left foot. CT scan was normal on the 4th day. At autopsy 6 months later, a lacune 2 × 2 × 3.7 mm was found in the right ventral posterior nucleus, fed by four tiny arteries that arose from a single artery destroyed by lipohyalinosis.

The lacunes in both of the reported autopsied cases have been quite small. If they are typical, it is easy to understand why many thalamic lacunes have thus far escaped detection by CT scan and require the higher-grade images provided by MRI (Fig. 20-5). Larger lesions may be seen by both techniques (Fig. 20-6).

## Complete Hemisensory Syndromes

Typically, the disturbance in sensation extends over the entire side of the body, involving face, proximal well as distal limbs, and axial structures including the scalp, neck, trunk, and genitalia right to the midline, even splitting the two sides of the nose, tongue, penis, and anus.[34,99] This remarkable midline split, especially when the trunk or abdomen is involved, may be unique to thalamic or thalamocortical pathway lesions. This type of hemisensory syndrome affected one case with a thalamic infarction measuring 4 × 4 × 2 mm.

The earliest reported patient with a complete hemisensory syndrome[144] referred to a "plumb-bob" having been dropped down the exact center of the body. In this case, the responsible thalamic infarct was not reported: the main interest to the author was the associated disturbances in higher cerebral function from the remainder of the large left posterior cerebral artery territory infarction. This complaint of total hemisensory loss has also been part of the syndrome in the small number of cases with the syndrome of sensorimotor stroke.

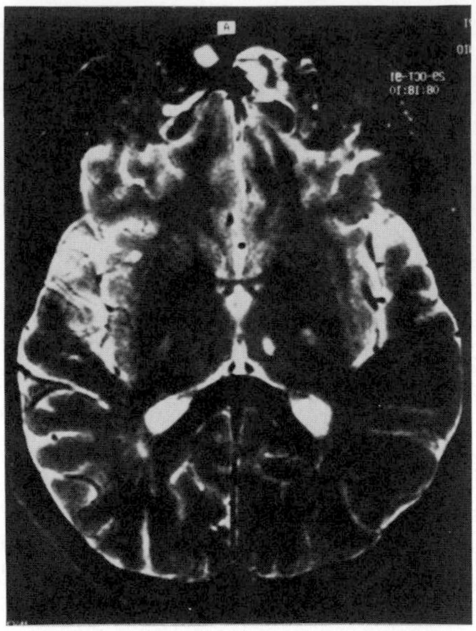

**Fig. 20-5.** Magnetic resonance imaging showing small thalamic lacune.

## Incomplete Hemisensory Syndromes

Variants in the topography of pure sensory stroke have been reported that involve less than the entire side of the body. One case, reported with autopsy correlation (case 9 in Fisher's original collection of pure sensory stroke)[34] suffered only transient ischemic attacks affecting the right fingers, and at another time the right upper and lower lips, right side of the tongue, and the two medial toes of the right foot. At autopsy, a lacune 7 mm in diameter affected the left

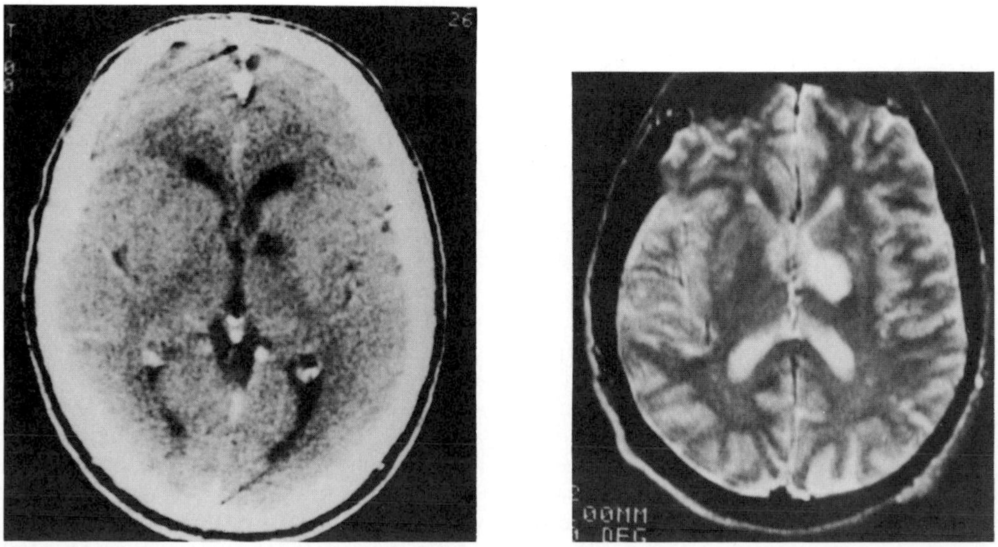

**Fig. 20-6.** Anterior thalamic infarct seen by (**A**) computed tomography and (**B**) magnetic resonance scans on the same patient.

ventral posterior nucleus. The complaints in other cases, without autopsy documentation, have involved the face, arm, and leg; head, cheek, lips, and hand; face, fingers, and foot; shoulder tip and lower jaw; distal forearm alone; fingers alone; and leg alone.[34] How many permutations exist is a subject of some interest, since it might serve to determine the organization of a sensory homonculus in the ventral tier nuclei.

Lapresle and Haguenau[82] found partial sensory syndromes involving the face, the arms, the leg, the oral cavity, the peribuccal area and forearm, and the peribuccal area and radial edge of forearm, all from focal thalamic softenings of lacunar size. Fisher's case 9 suffered only transient ischemic attacks affecting the right fingers, and at another time the right upper and lower lips, right side of the tongue and the two medial toes of the right foot.[41] A lacune 7 mm in diameter affecting the left ventral posterior nucleus was found at autopsy. Another case, a 54-year-old patient recovering from a right pure motor hemiplegia, developed a feeling of "pins and needles" in the left lower lip, left side of the mouth, and the fingers of the left hand; the sole of the left foot tingled, and felt numb, dull, and swollen many hours later. No sensory deficit was evident on examination. Unpleasant paresthesias affected the left side of the face and the left foot. CT scan was normal on the 4th day. At autopsy 6 months later, a 2 × 2 × 3 mm lacune was found in the right ventral posterior thalamus. The complaints in other cases, without autopsy documentation, have involved the face, arm, and leg; head, cheek, lips, and hand; face, fingers, and foot; shoulder tip and lower jaw; distal forearm alone; fingers alone; and leg alone. The full array of permutations has been subject to considerable study recently.[45]

Electrophysiologic studies have found a well-organized topographic arrangement of the ventroposterolateral nucleus of the thalamus in animals, which have been confirmed in man by single-unit studies of thalamic neurons The location and size of the receptive field have been mapped, showing a high number of cells concentrated on perioral and digital sensation and only a few for the forearm and upper arm.[86] The organization of the cells is in the sagittal plane with cutaneous and deep stimuli aligned toward one another. The failure of the clinical syndromes from infarction to reflect this type of organization may find its explanation in the vascular anatomy. The small vessels, individually occluded, may cause an infarct that cuts across the functional anatomic fields of somatosensory projections, causing clusters of symptoms and signs from lesions that are at variance with the normal organization.

## Nature of the Sensory Complaints

The patients complain of striking alterations in spontaneous sensations.[34,97] The parts feel stretched, hot, sunburned, "pins sticking," larger, smaller, heavier. Contacts or the skin from eyeglasses, bedclothes, rings, watches, and sheets feel heavier on the affected side and may transiently aggravate the sensory disturbance. The stimulus seems to persist a few seconds after its removal. In the cases with severe disturbances, the occurrence of a stimulus is better reported than its exact location.

The *Dejerine-Roussy syndrome*[24] is an uncommon accompaniment of lacunar infarction of the thalamus, although dysesthetic accompaniments are common in pure sensory stroke, as outlined above. The full Dejerine-Roussy syndrome was originally described as the effect of occlusion of the thalamogeniculate branch of the posterior cerebral artery, with infarction of the ventral posterolateral and ventral posteromedial nuclei, largely sparing the remaining nuclei of the thalamus. Cases documented only by CT scanning have shown a lesion small enough to qualify for a clinical diagnosis of lacunar infarction.[88] Here, suffice to say the initial deficit usually includes a hemiparesis and hemisensory syndrome. The pain, which is an inconstant feature in cases with such infarcts, may begin at the onset of the syndrome or appear only later. Delays up to several months are common. They are intermittent or constant, appear spontaneously or at other times are provoked by contact with the affected parts. They are usually accompanied by many other disturbances in sensation, including tingling, feelings of excessive weight, and feelings of cold, although a few cases exist in which the sensory function is normal to clinical testing. The special disturbance known as *hyperpathia* is particularly characteristic but not common: following a sensory stimulus, a disagreeable response occurs that is usually delayed in onset, may spread over a large area, persists after removal of the stimulus, and may even increase in intensity over several seconds. The syndrome may outlast other features of the original stroke syndrome and even become permanent. No reliable treatment has been devised but amitriptyline has been used.

## Associated Disturbances

Disturbances in motor function, language, and vision might be expected in a setting of thalamic infarction, but have thus far been unreported, save for a single example of sensorimotor stroke due to thalamic lacune[100] (see below). Given the anatomy of the thalamus and its widely varying projections to the cerebrum, such syndromes should be encountered, but have thus far eluded the most careful efforts of vascular neurologists in diagnosis.

## Clinical Course

Improvement appears to be the rule, often to normal within weeks.[45,108] The topography of the shrinking deficit may be rather unusual. Improvement in the trunk with persistence in the distal extremities, common in hemispheral disease, is only occasionally encountered. In one case, the deficit shrank to a vertical band from the axilla down the lateral trunk to the thigh,[69] a finding encountered by the author in several cases studied in south Alabama.

### Sensorimotor Stroke

Three autopsied cases of sensorimotor stroke[82,99,131] have been reported to date, only one published under the title "sensorimotor stroke."[99] Such cases, although rare, are important, since they attest to the occurrence of a combined motor and sensory deficit from a small, deep infarct. Their vascular anatomy also helps clarify the vascular supply to the thalamus and adjacent internal capsule. The rarity of these cases should set aside any casual assumptions that small, deep infarcts cause most instances of sensorimotor stroke.

The first case report I found was published by Garcin and Lapresle[52] as part of a review of sensory disorders from thalamic infarction. The patient was a 65-year-old woman who suddenly developed left hemiparesis and a combination of hypesthesia and dysesthesia in the left peribuccal area and forearm. At autopsy, a small infarct was found straddling the intersection of the ventral posterior lateral and medial nucleus of the right thalamus. Involvement of the internal capsule was not mentioned.

Our patient[99] was a 61-year-old man. The sensory component preceded the motor by several hours. The syndrome evolved smoothly and steadily over approximately a day then stabilized for many days before beginning to improve. The sensory component involved the entire half of the body, including the neck, ear, and genitalia. The sensory and motor deficits each followed a temporal course and clinical profile typical of pure sensory stroke and pure motor stroke, respectively. Neither deficit faded completely with time, but both underwent considerable improvement. The hemihypalgesia shrank to a vertical band from the axilla down the lateral trunk to the thigh. At autopsy, a well developed lacune 4 × 4 × 2 mm was present in the ventral lateral nucleus of the thalamus, while the adjacent internal capsule showed a slight degree of pallor (Fig. 20-7). Efforts to track down the vascular supply to the infarct by means of serial sections were frustrated by the prior gross horizontal section made prior to embedding. The small artery found in the infarct was tracked downward toward its expected source from the posterior cerebral artery. Instead of gradually enlarging, the vessel gradually became smaller and vanished, leaving the authors to infer its origin was from above the infarct. Efforts to trace the artery upward also proved futile when the serial sections crossed the plane of the original gross section. Here the discontinuity was too great to permit matching of sections to map the course of the artery.

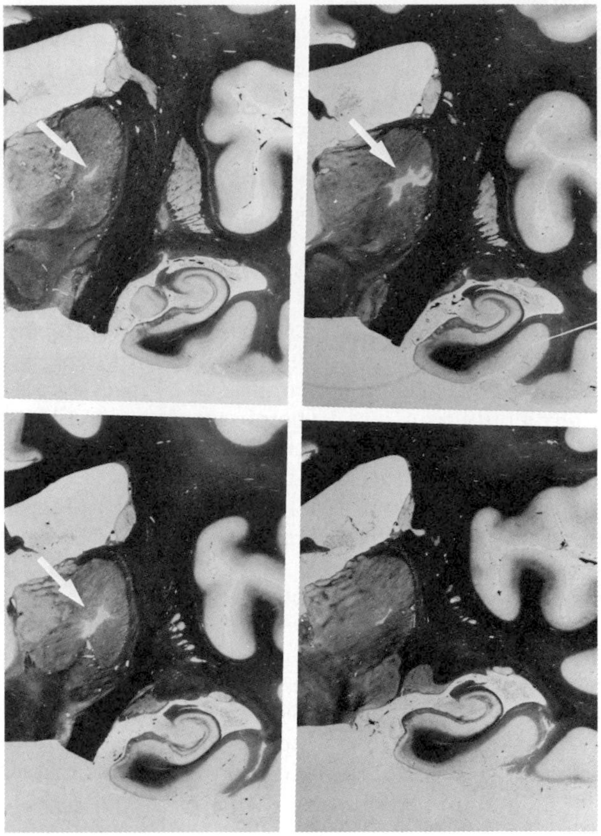

**Fig. 20-7.** Myelin stain of celloidin section in a case of sensorimotor stroke.

The third case attracted more interest to the observers by his action-induced rhythmic dystonia than by the sensorimotor stroke.[131] The stroke occurred when the patient was age 61, a known diabetic for 4 years. He fell suddenly, with left leg weakness. On examination, he was found to have a left hemiparesis "with loss of all sensory modalities." He improved within a week and was able to walk with support within a month. Involuntary movements began in the left leg by the 4th month. When examined by the authors 4 years after the stroke, he had slight lower facial weakness, slightly exaggerated left sided reflexes but normal strength and sensation. Autopsy revealed an infarct 3 × 3 × 10 mm involving the ventral posterolateral nucleus of the right thalamus and adjacent internal capsule. No mention was made of the arterial anatomy of the lesion.

The neurovascular issues raised by the case are also of importance. Before such cases were documented, it was believed that the vascular supply to the internal capsule was wholly separate from that to the thalamus. The lenticulostriate branches of the middle cerebral presumably supplied the capsule,[108] while the thalamus was presumed to receive its supply from the perforating branches of the posterior cerebral artery. The extreme posterior nuclei of the thalamus received a few branches from the choroidal arteries.[106] Yet three cases now exist showing that a single infarct may involve both the thalamus and the adjacent internal capsule. These cases suffice to overturn earlier claims and reopen the issues of the boundary line between the middle and posterior cerebral artery territories.

At least 13 clinical examples of sensorimotor stroke have been documented by CT scan.[26,61,100,140] In these cases, the lesions have been fairly large. Donnan et al.[26] described one extending from the left putamen to the corona radiata, not obviously involving the thalamus. We encountered two other examples in south Alabama. The first case began as an incomplete pure motor stroke to which the hemisensory component was added within hours. This pattern was the reverse of our autopsy-documented case of sensorimotor stroke. In Weisberg's series,[140] eight cases were described with "weakness and sensory disturbance and were found to have a hemiparesis and a decreased appreciation of pinprick, light-touch, vibration, and position sense involving the face, arm, and leg."[140] Large caudatoputaminal infarcts were seen on CT scan. It is presumed that these CT-documented cases affected the thalamocortical projections. However, apart from the cases reported by Groothius et al.,[58] no autopsy-documented material has appeared to clarify the course followed by the thalamocortical fibers.

## Speech and Language Disorders

### Mutism, Aphonia, and Anarthria

Bilateral capsular lacunar infarction has been a cause of mutism in the absence of any disturbance in language or praxis. One of Fisher's cases, documented by microscopic vascular pathology,[13] had no difficulty with speech on his first infarct, but became mute with the second infarct, involving the left internal capsule. The left capsular lacune was 4 × 4 × 5 mm and lay at the genu. Marie[90] had earlier reported a case of unilateral stroke with "anarthria" but no aphasic symptoms, but the cause of the small, deep lesion was a putaminal hemorrhage.

In subsequent years, several such cases have been reported with the lesion documented by brain imaging. None of these bilateral capsular infarct cases have had aphasia apart from the disturbance in articulation. Our collection includes a case of an infarct affecting the posterior limb of the right internal capsule followed by an infarct affecting the left internal capsule at the genu.[100] This last infarct was so small as to be barely visible on CT scan, yet it yielded virtual anarthria, severe dysphonia, and dysphagia, but only a mild right arm weakness. Three others have been reported, each with bilateral capsular infarcts, involving the genu or anterior limb of the capsule.[19,81,134]

### Disorders of Language

There still remains considerable doubt whether aphasic disturbances per se occur at all from lacunes. At least one case[44] indicates they may do so. In most instances, the cause is not the primary arteriopathy, but embolism into the stem of the middle cerebral artery with involvement of many lenticulostriates together. Fisher's is the only autopsy-verified case to date reported with a language disorder from an infarct involving the territory of a lenticulostriate. The syndrome included a modified pure motor hemiparesis with "motor aphasia." It was attributed to a large infarct involving the genu and anterior limb of the internal capsule and adjacent white matter of the corona radiata. Speech initially was dysarthric, progressed later to mispronounciation of words, then to a state of utterance of single-syllable unintelligible sounds, and ended as mutism (Fig. 20-8). Comprehension was reportedly intact. The accompanying weakness severely affected the right side of the face and moderately involved the right hand. This case is important not because of the large size of the infarct, but because the underlying lesion was a thrombosis of a lenticulostriate artery.

One case reported by CT scan only has also been associated with a small lesion.[124] It was but one among eight large, deep infarcts attributed to cardiac embolism, and presented with an "expressive dysphasia." The disturbance was characterized by "nonfluent conversational speech, naming and reading difficulties, dysgraphia and normal auditory comprehension." The case is of especial interest, given the small size of the lesion demonstrated on the CT scan, since a lacunar cause is in the differential diagnosis.

That unilateral, large, deep infarcts may disrupt language function to some degree has never been the subject of serious dispute. Several well-known cases attest to the correlation. Yet save for the case noted above, in each the infarct has been quite large, of the "superlacune" category, well beyond the usual limits of the infarcts caused by primary disease of the penetrating arteries. Although described in more detail in this volume, the subject is touched on here to settle this point of the larger size of the infarcts.

Two famous cases are on record with large infarction documented by autopsy. Bonhoeffer's classic case[9] was associated with a large, deep lesion of type 1 of Rascol et al.,[111] involving the caudate nucleus, internal capsule, and putamen as far laterally as the external capsule. He was unable to speak anything more than a few poorly formed vowels. The cause of the lesion was undetermined, but its large size suggested occlusion of the middle cerebral artery stem. An embolic mechanism was suggested by the second infarct, of fairly large size, affecting almost the entire anterior cerebral artery territory. Kleist[76] reported a case with an infarct of similar size and location (case

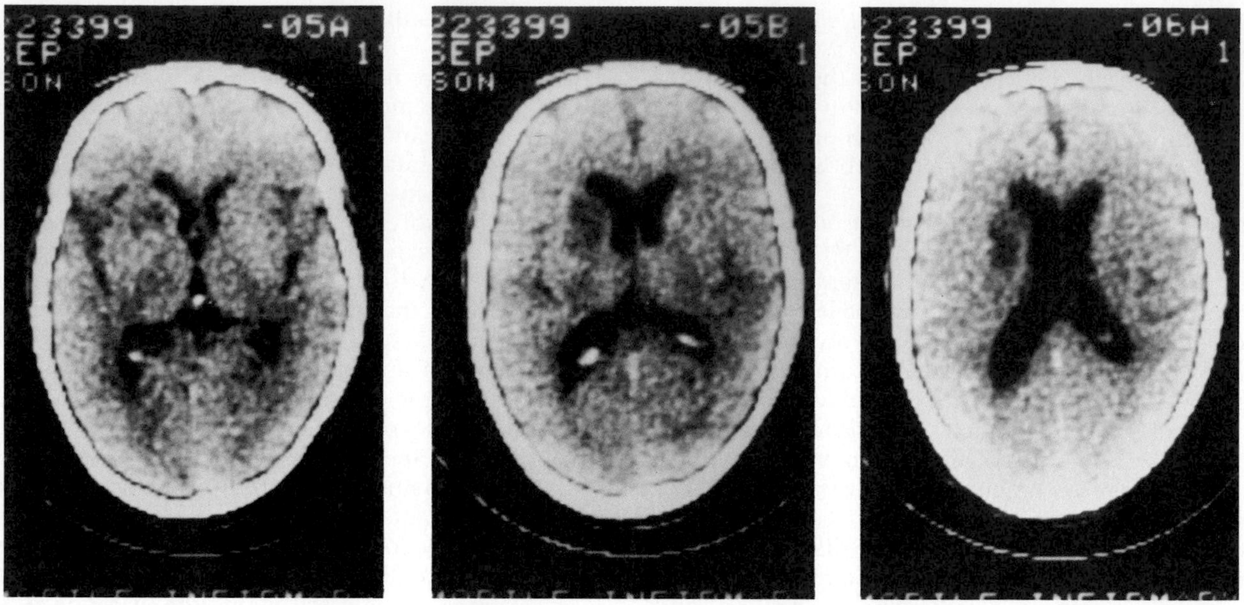

**Fig. 20-8.** Large anterior capsular infarct with dysnomia.

Bühlmeir) featuring severe dysarthria, rare paraphasias, and only slight disturbance in comprehension. No mention was made of the vascular pathology.

Thirteen other cases to date have been reported by CT scan, all of which showed large, deep infarcts.[20,101,124] In Naeser's series,[101] at least three had accompanying surface infarcts. That an accompanying surface infarct, inobvious on CT scan, might be the cause, keeps the value of the reports based entirely on CT scan well below those with autopsy documentation. These cases have been characterized by dysprosody, at times accompanied by dysarthria, and a mixture of deficits in syntactic and semantic functions not typical of any of the classical syndromes of dysphasia.

## Other Disorders of Higher Cerebral Function

A single instance of pure motor stroke with "confusion" has been recently referred to with a 1.2-cm lacune affecting the anterior limb and the anterior portion of the posterior limb of the right internal capsule.[43] The behavior disorder was characterized as "acute onset of confusion and impairment of attention and memory." Recent studies using brain imaging to document the lesion have found a few instances of deep infarction, usually affecting the genu or anterior limb of the internal capsule with greatly reduced level of activity. In a study comparing 11 patients with multiple lacunes against 11 controls, Wolfe et al.[143] found lacunar patients showed some neuropsychological signs of frontal system disturbance, although only 27 percent met clinical criteria for a diagnosis of dementia. The disturbances were described as shifting mental set, response inhibition, and executive function [and such patients] were more often rated apathetic on a behavior-rating scale.

Some insight into the underlying mechanisms was provided by the study of one patient by Satomi et al.,[126] who performed a single photon emission computed tomogram (SPECT) study with [$^{123}$I]iodoamphetamine, which showed decreased vasoreactivity predominantly to the frontal lobes. Tatemichi et al. studied a right-handed man whose infarct was limited to the genu of the capsule in the left hemisphere; they suggested that the impaired SPECT reactivity could be from interruption of thalamofrontal projections passing below the genu, producing a syndrome of frontal lobe dysfunction without direct lesion to the frontal lobe.

The literature continues to document disorders of language, memory, orientation, and activity following infarction of the paramedian thalamic nuclei. Save for two reports,[14,109] CT scanning has been the basis for the lesion localization. In many of these cases, including some of the autopsied material of Castaigne et al.,[14] embolism to the top of the basilar, to the posterior cerebral artery stem, or thrombosis of the basilar may have been the cause, not vascular disease of the lacunar type. Given the origin of these cases, the CT scan might not reveal all of the foci of infarction, making the correlation with CT findings a bit unreliable.[60,95,127,135] In the few cases with autopsy, the arterial disease has been rather unusual. In the case reported by Poirer et al.,[109] a picture of thalamic dementia was encountered. Autopsy showed many small, deep infarcts of lacunar size. The authors formed the impression the lesion was an angiitis hitherto undefined. Among those documented only by CT scan, a hypertensive patient, a normal angiogram, several spells typical of transient ischemic attacks before the final stroke, and then the emergence of a CT positive low density lesion have been documented in a few instances, which seems consistent with the course expected from lacunar disease. The patient reported by Michel et al.[95] is such an example, described by the authors as a thalamic lacune. The initial deficit included right hemiparesis with agitation, disorientation, and language disturbances. The language disorder was of the expressive type, with reduction in language, slowness in response, and some verbal paraphasias. Verbal memory was greatly disturbed and was the subject of a special investigation. The presence of the hemiparesis might mean the scope of the lesion exceeded that seen on CT scan, but this issue was not settled.

A single case with dysphasia with a small thalamic infarction documented by CT scan has been reported.[57] The size of the infarct was large enough to include the ventral anterior and rostral ventral lateral nucleus, which might be too large for an infarct from primary disease of the thalamoperforant vessels. No cause for the infarct was found. In the other cases in the literature, the infarcts were bilateral or large enough to make it unlikely they were due to primary arteriopathy of the penetrating vessels. These cases are detailed elsewhere in this volume. The last word has not been written on the syndromes of deep infarction with disturbances in speech and language.

## LABORATORY STUDIES

### Computed Tomography Scan

Technical limitations of the most modern CT scanners prevent the resolution of most lacunes smaller than 2 mm in the internal capsule and almost all of those in the thalamus and brain stem[110,139] due to obscuring artifact from the small size of the lesion.[139] For the lacunar syndromes in the Stroke Data Bank, a lesion was found in 39 percent on the first CT scan, most lesions located in the posterior limb of the internal capsule and corona radiata.[15] Repeat CT scan increased the yield to 35 percent. Brain stem lesions were not often visualized. The mean infarct volume in this cohort was greater in pure motor and sensorimotor stroke syndromes than in ataxic hemiparesis, dysarthria-clumsy hand, and pure sensory stroke syndrome. In those pure motor stroke patients with posterior capsule infarction, there was a correlation between lesion size and hemiparesis severity save for the small number of cases whose infarct involved the lowest portion of the capsule, supplied by the anterior choroidal artery, where severe deficits occurred without regard for the lesion size.

Magnetic resonance (MR) scanners may have a higher yield, as inferred from the experience of Kistler et al.[75] and by our recent experience at the New York Neurological Institute. To date, none of the cases whose lesion was seen by MR scan has had autopsy correlation. Autopsy correlations with CT scanners indicate the CT overestimates lacunar size by as much as 100 percent.[26] The yield on scans within 2 days of the stroke is very low, but by 10 days over 50 percent of the lacunes that eventually show on CT scan can be detected.[26,100,110,139,140] The high yield in the study by Rascol et al.[111] may have been an artifact of selection, but fully 29 of 30 cases of hemiparesis were documented by CT scan. The population-based study in south Alabama described 13 percent of strokes due to lacunes, of which 40 percent were documented by fourth generation CT scan.[59]

### Magnetic Resonance Scan

Magnetic resonance imaging, barely in use when the first edition of this book appeared, has greatly changed the frequency with which small infarcts are now being demonstrated. Although CT scanning is still the most common technique in use, MR imaging has now surpassed it in sensitivity for detection of lacunes.[7,66]

In their study of 227 patients with lacunar infarcts, Arboix et al.[6] found CT positive in 100 patients (44 percent), while MR was positive in 35 of 45 (78 percent). Magnetic resonance imaging was significantly better ($P < 0.001$) than computed tomography for imaging lacunes, especially those located in either the pons ($P < 0.005$) or the internal capsule ($P < 0.001$). Hommel et al.[66] used MR for 100 patients hospitalized with a lacunar infarct syndrome and also found MR more sensitive. MR imaging detected at least 1 lacune appropriate to the symptoms in 89 patients who had 135 lacunes found by imaging. These investigators found MR imaging more effective when it was performed a few days after the stroke. The superiority of MR over CT for detection of small lesions now seems generally accepted.

### Angiography

Similar technical limitations apply to arteriography. Since the artery affected is usually on the range of 100 to 500 $\mu$m conventional angiography does not often demonstrate abnormalities.[39] However, in the case of giant lacunes, stenosis of the middle cerebral artery stem, or occasionally one of the larger lateral lenticulostriates, may be documented.[111] Insufficient cases have been studied to determine how often the angiogram in classical lacunar syndromes will show major extracranial or intracranial atheroma (Fig. 20-9) and what prognostic interaction exists between such findings and the lacunar syndromes.[5]

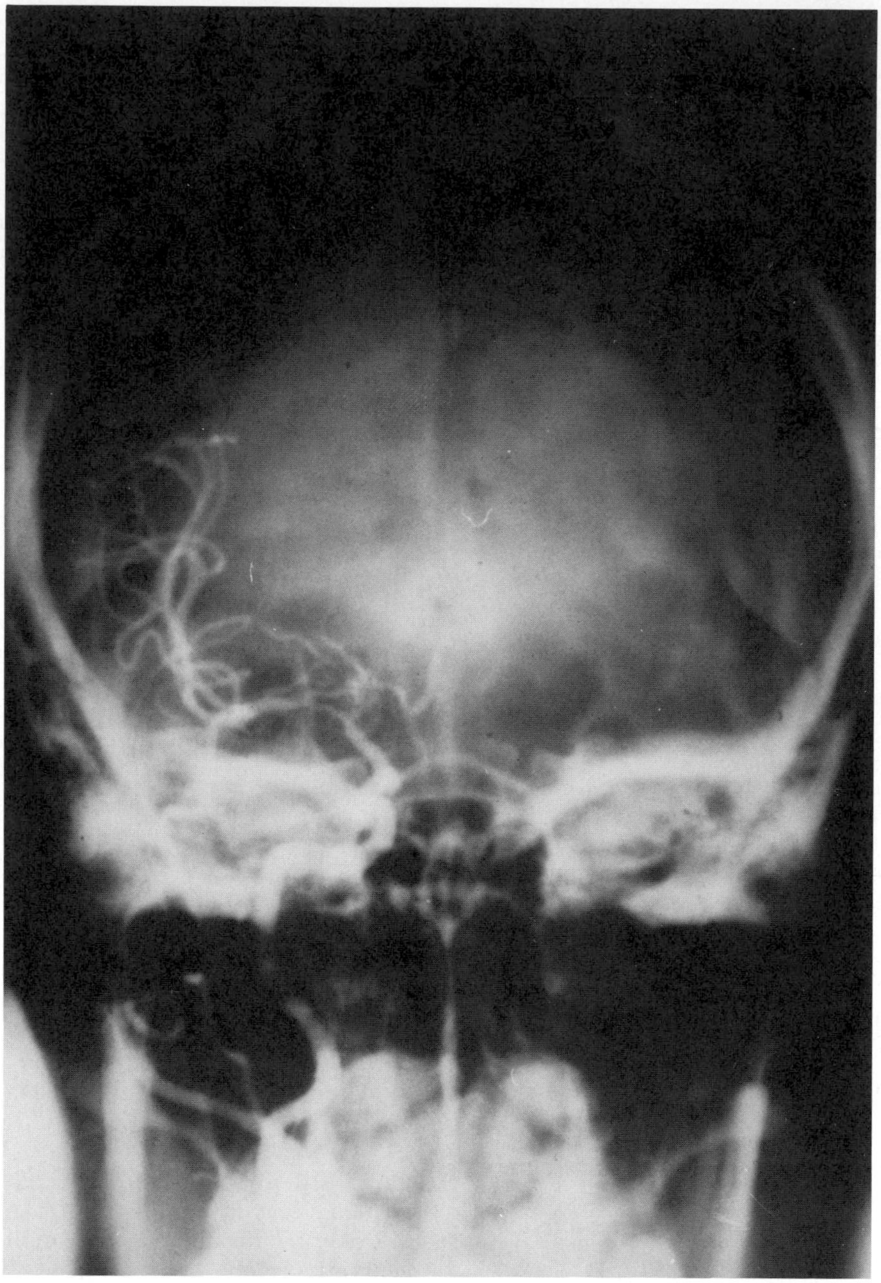

**Fig. 20-9.** Angiographic evidence of middle cerebral artery stem stenosis in patient with dysnomia. (The computed tomography scan of this patient is shown in Fig. 20-8.)

## Electroencephalogram

The small size prevents most individual lacunes from disrupting enough of the general brain function to produce changes in the conventional electroencephalogram.[13] In the recent study of the subject in the Pilot Stroke Data Bank, no significant electroencephalogram abnormalities were encountered, even in cases with a positive CT scan.[100] EEG abnormalities were so infrequent in their 56 lacunar patients that Falcone et al.[31] considered the normal EEG a helpful sign, suggesting lacune.

## Evoked Cerebral Responses

A few studies of the somatosensory response have shown alterations in the waveform, suggesting a subclinical sensory impairment in clinically pure motor strokes. Efforts to find an abnormality in the sensory evoked potential were disappointing in a series studied by our group[114]; only those with a large CT lesion and an accompanying motor deficit showed such abnormalities. Other even larger series also failed to show the usefulness of evoked potentials, save for those with the largest lesions and sensorimotor deficits.[79] As a test for brain-image-negative lacunes, the evoked potential seems thus far to have little use.

## REFERENCES


1. Abadie JL: Les localisations functionelles de la capsule interne. Thesis. Bordeaux, 1900
2. Aleksie SN, George AE: Pure motor hemiplegia with occlusion of the extracranial carotid artery. J Neurol Sci 19:331, 1973
3. Alpers BJ: Clinical Neurology. FA Davis, Philadelphia, 1958
4. Antin SP, Prockop LD, Cohen SM: Transient hemiballism. Neurology (Minneapolis) 17:1068, 1967
5. Araki G: Small infarctions of the basal ganglia with special reference to transient ischemic attacks. Recent Adv Gerontol 469:161, 1978
6. Arboix A, Marti-Vilalta JL, Garcia JH: Clinical study of 227 patients with lacunar infarcts. Stroke 21:842, 1990
7. Awad IA, Johnson PC, Spetzler RF, Hodak JA: Incidental subcortical lesions identified on magnetic resonance imaging in the elderly. II. Postmortem pathological correlations. Stroke 17:1090, 1986
8. Bendheim PE, Berg BO: Ataxic hemiparesis from a midbrain mass. Ann Neurol 9:405, 1981
9. Bonhoeffer K: Klinischer und anatomischer Befund zur Lehre von der Apraxie und der "motorischen Sprachbahn." Monatschr Psychiatr Neurol 35:113, 1914
10. Byrom FG: The pathogenesis of hypertensive encephalopathy and its relation to the malignant phase of hypertension. Lancet 2:201, 1954
11. Byrom FB: The Hypertensive Vascular Crisis. Grune & Stratton, New York, 1969
12. Byrom FB, Dodson LF: The causation of acute arterial necrosis in hypertensive disease. J Pathol Bacteriol 60:357, 1948
13. Caplan LR, Young RR: EEG findings in certain lacunar stroke syndromes. Neurology (NY) 22:403, 1972
14. Castaigne P, Lhermitte F, Buge A et al: Paramedian thalamic and midbrain infarcts: clinical and neuropathologic study. Ann Neurol 10:127, 1981
15. Chamorro AM, Sacco RL, Mohr JP et al: Lacunar infarction: clinical-CT correlations in the Stroke Data Bank. Stroke 22:175, 1991
16. Chester EM, Agamanolis DP, Banker Q, Victor M: Hypertensive encephalopathy: a clinicopathologic study of 20 cases. Neurology (NY) 28:928, 1978
17. Chokroverty S, Rubino FA, Haller C: Pure motor hemiplegia due to pyramidal infarction. Arch Neurol 2:647, 1975
18. Cole FM, Yates PO: Psuedo-aneurysms in relationship to massive cerebral haemorrhage. J Neurol Neurosurg Psychiatry 30, 1967
19. Croisile B, Henry E, Trillet M, Aimard G: Loss of motivation for speaking with bilateral lacunes in the anterior limb of the internal capsule. Clin Neurol Neurosurg 91:325, 1989
20. Damasio AR, Damasio H, Rizzo M et al: Aphasia with nonhemorrhagic lesions of the basal ganglia and internal capsule. Arch Neurol 39:15, 1982
21. Dattner B, Thomas EW, Wexler G: The Management of Neurosyphilis. Grune & Stratton, New York, 1944
22. Davis LE, Xie JG, Zou AH et al: Deep cerebral infarcts in the People's Republic of China. Stroke 21:394, 1990
23. Dejerine J, Dejerine Klumpke H: Anatomie des Centres Nerveux. Vol. 2. p. 128. Rueff, Paris, 1901
24. Dejerine J, Roussy G: La syndrome thalamique. Rev Neurol (Paris) 14:521, 1906
25. De Rueck J, van der Eecken H: The topography of infarcts in the lacunar state. p. 162. In Meyer JS, Lechner H, Reivich M (eds): Cerebral Vascular Disease. Seventh International Conference. Thieme, New York, 1976
26. Donnan GA, Tress BM, Bladin PF: A prospective study of lacunar infarction using computerized tomography. Neurology (NY) 32:49, 1982
27. Dustin P, Jr: Arteriolar hyalinosis. Int Rev Exp Pathol 1:73, 1962
28. Earnest MP, Fahn S, Karp JH, Rowland LP: Normal pressure hydrocephalus and hypertensive cerebrovascular disease. Arch Neurol 31:262, 1974
29. Ekstrom Jodal B, Haggendal E, Linder LE et al: Cerebral blood flow autoregulation at high arterial pressures and different levels of carbon dioxide tension in dogs. Eur Neurol 6:6, 1972
30. Englander RN, Netsky MG, Adelman LS: Location of human pyramidal tract in the internal capsule: anatomic evidence. Neurology (NY) 25:823, 1975
31. Falcone N, Fensore C, Lanzetti A et al: Clinical considerations and EEG-CT correlations in lacunar infarcts. Riv Neurol 56:396, 1986
32. Feigin I, Prose P: Hypertensive fibrinoid arteritis of the brain and gross cerebral hemorrhage: a form of "hyalinosis." Arch Neurol 1:98, 1959
33. Ferrand J: Essai sur L'hemiplegie des vieillards, les lacunes de desintergrations cerebrale. Thesis. Rousset, Paris, 1902.
34. Fisher CM: Pure sensory stroke involving face, arm and leg. Neurology (NY) (Minneapolis), 15:76, 1965
35. Fisher CM: Lacunes: small deep cerebral infarcts. Neurology (Minneapolis) 15:774, 1965
36. Fisher CM: A lacunar stroke: the dysarthria clumsy hand syndrome. Neurology (Minneapolis) 17:614, 1967
37. Fisher CM: Some neuroophthalmologic observations. J Neurol Neurosurg Psychiatry 30:383, 1967
38. Fisher CM: The arterial lesions underlying lacunes. Acta Neuropathol (Berl) 12:1, 1969
39. Fisher CM: Cerebral ischemia less familiar types. Clin Neurosurg 18:267, 1971
40. Fisher CM: Bilateral occlusion of basilar artery branches. J Neurol Neurosurg Psychiatry 40:1182, 1977
41. Fisher CM: Thalamic pure sensory stroke: a pathologic study. Neurology (NY) 28:1141, 1978

42. Fisher CM: Ataxic hemiparesis. Arch Neurol 35:126, 1978
43. Fisher CM: Capsular infarcts. Arch Neurol 36:65, 1979
44. Fisher CM: Lacunar strokes and infarcts: a review. Neurology (NY) 32:871, 1982
45. Fisher CM: Pure sensory stroke and allied conditions. Stroke 13:434, 1982
46. Fisher CM, Caplan LR: Bailar artery branch occlusion: a cause of pontine infarction. Neurology (Minneapolis) 21:900, 1971
47. Fisher CM, Cole M: Homolateral ataxia and crural paresis: a vascular syndrome. J Neurol Neurosurg Psychiatry 28:48, 1965
48. Fisher CM, Curry HB: Pure motor hemiplegia of vascular origin. Arch Neurol 13:30, 1965
49. Fisher CM, Gore I, Okabe N, White PD: Atherosclerosis of the carotid and vertebral arteries: extracranial and intracranial. J Neuropathol Exp Neurol 24:455, 1965
50. Foix C, Hillemand P: Contribution a l'etude des ramollissements protruberantiels, Rev Med 43:287, 1926
51. Foix C, Levy M: Les ramollissements sylviens. Rev Neurol 11:1, 1927
52. Garcin R, Lapresle J: Syndrome sensitif de type thalamique et atopographie cheiro orale par lesion localisee du thalamus. Rev Neurol 90:124, 1954
53. Gautier JC: Cerebral ischemia in hypertension. p. 181. In Russell R (ed): Cerebral Arterial Disease. Churchill Livingston, London, 1978
54. Giese J: The pathogenesis of hypertensive vascular disease. Dan Med Bull 14:259, 1967
55. Goldblatt D, Markesbery W, Reeves AG: Recurrent hemichorea following striatal lesions. Arch Neurol 31:51, 1974
56. Goldblatt H: Studies on experimental hypertension. VII. The production of the malignant phase of hypertension. J Exp Med 67:809, 1938
57. Gorelick PB, Caplan LR: Racial differences in the distribution of anterior circulation occlusive disease. Neurology (NY) 34:54, 1984
58. Groothius DR, Duncan GW, Fisher CM: The human thalamocortical sensory path in the internal capsule: evidence from a capsular hemorrhage causing a pure sensory stroke. Ann Neurol 2:328, 1977
59. Gross CR, Kase CS, Mohr JP, Cunningham SC: Stroke in south Alabama: incidence and diagnostic features. Stroke 15:249, 1984
60. Guberman A, Stuss D: The syndrome of bilateral paramedian thalamic infarction. Neurology (Cleveland) 33:540, 1983
61. Gursahani RD, Khadilkar SV, Surya N, Singhal BS: Capsular involvement and sensorimotor stroke with posterior cerebral artery territory infarction. J Assoc Physicians India 38:939, 1990
62. Hanaway J, Young RR: Localization of the pyramidal tract in the internal capsule of man. J Neurol Sci 34:63, 1977
63. Heptinstall RH: Pathology of the Kidney. 2nd Ed. Vol. 1. p. 121. Little, Brown, Boston, 1974
64. Hill GS: Studies on the pathogenesis of hypertensive vascular disease: effect of high pressure intraarterial injections in rats. Circ Res 27:657, 1970
65. Ho KL: Pure motor hemiplegia due to infarction of the cerebral peduncle. Arch Neurol 39:524, 1982
66. Hommel M, Besson G, Le Bas JF et al: Prospective study of lacunar infarction using magnetic resonance imaging. Stroke 21:546, 1990
67. Huang CY, Chan FL, Yu YL et al: Cerebrovascular disease in Hong Kong Chinese. Stroke 21:230, 1990
68. Huang CY, Lui FS: Ataxic hemiparesis: localization and clinical features. Stroke 15:363, 1984
69. Hyland HH, Forman DM: Prognosis in hemiballismus. Neurology (Minneapolis) 7:381, 1957
70. Ichikawa K, Tsutsumishita A, Fujioka A: Capsular ataxic hemiparesis: a case report. Arch Neurol 39:585, 1982
71. Igapashi S, Mori K, Ishijima Y: Pure motor hemiplegia after recraniotomy for postoperative bleeding. Arch Jpn Chir 41:32, 1965
72. Iragui VJ, McCutchen CB: Capsular ataxic hemiparesis. Arch Neurol 39:528, 1982
73. Kase CS, Maulsby GO, deJuan E, Mohr JP: Hemichorea hemiballism and lacunar infarction in the basal ganglia. Neurology (NY) 31:454, 1981
74. Kempster PA, Gerraty RP, Gates PC: Asymptomatic cerebral infarction in patients with chronic atrial fibrillation. Stroke 19:955, 1988
75. Kistler JP, Buonanno FS, DeWitt LD et al: Vertebra, basilar posterior cerebral territory stroke delineation by proton nuclear magnetic resonance imaging. Stroke 15:417, 1984
76. Kleist K: *Gehirnpathologie.* p. 930. Barth, Leipzig, 1934
77. Koto A, Rosenberg G, Zingesser LH et al: Syndrome of normal pressure hydrocephalus: possible relation to hypertensive and arteriosclerotic vasculopathy. J Neurol Neurosurg Psychiatry 40:73, 1977
78. Kribs M, Kleihues J: The recurrent artery of Heubner. p. 40. In Zulch KJ (ed): Cerebral Circulation and Stroke. Springer-Verlag, New York, 1971
79. Labar DR, Petty GW, Emerson RG et al: Abnormal somatosensory evoked potentials in patients with motor deficits due to lacunar strokes. EEG Clin Neurophysiol 67:74, 1987
80. Laitinen LV: Loss of motivation for speaking with bilateral lacunes in the anterior limb of the internal capsule. Clin Neurol Neurosurg 92;177, 1990
81. Landau WM: Clinical neuromythology VI. Au clair de lacune: holy, wholly, holey logic. Neurology (NY) 39:725, 1989
82. Lapresle J, Haguenau S: Anatomico clinical correlation in focal thalamic lesions. Z Neurol 205:29, 1973
83. LaRue L, Alter M, Lai SM et al: Acute stroke, hematocrit, and blood pressure. Stroke 18:565, 1987
84. Lazzarino LG, Nicolai A, Poldelmengo P et al: Risk factors in lacunar strokes: a retrospective study of 52 patients. Acta Neurol (Napoli) 11:265, 1989

85. Leestma JE, Noronha A: Pure motor hemiplegia, medullary pyramid lesion, and olivary hypertrophy. Arch Neurol 39:877, 1976
86. Lenz FA, Dostrovsky JO, Tasker RR et al: Single unit analysis of the human ventral thalamic nuclear group: somatosensory responses. J Neurophysiol 59:299, 1988
87. Loeb C: The lacunar syndromes. Eur Neurol 29:2, 1989
88. Manfredi M, Cruccu G: Thalamic pain revisited. p. 73. In Loeb C (ed): Studies in Cerebrovascular Disease. Masson, Milano, 1981
89. Marie P: Des foyers lacunaire de desintegration et de differents autres etats cavitaires du cerveau. Rev Med 21:281, 1901
90. Marie P: A case of transitory anarthria by lesion of the lenticular zone. Bull Mem Soc Med 23:1291, 1906. Translated in Cole MF, Cole M: Pierre Marie's Papers on Speech Disorders. p. 135. Hafner, New York, 1971
91. Martin JP: Hemichorea (hemiballismus) without lesions in the corpus Luysii. Brain 80:1, 1957
92. Melamed E, Korn Lubetzki I, Reches A et al: Hemiballismus: detection of focal hemorrhage in subthalamic nucleus by CT scan. Ann Neurol 4:582, 1978
93. Merritt HH, Adams RD, Solomon HC: Neurosyphilis. New York: Oxford, 1946
94. Meyers R: Ballismus. p. 476. In Vinken PJ, Bruyn GW (eds): Handbook of Clinical Neurology. Vol. 6. North-Holland Publishing, Amsterdam, 1968
95. Michel D, Laurent B, Foyatier N et al: Infarctus thalamique paramedian gauche. Rev Neurol (Paris) 138:6, 1982
96. Millikan C, Futrell N: The fallacy of the lacune hypothesis. Stroke 21:1251, 1990
97. Mohr JP: Lacunes. Neurol Clin North Am 1:201, 1983
98. Mohr JP, Caplan LR, Melski JW et al: The Harvard Cooperative Stroke Registry. Neurology (NY) 28:754, 1978
99. Mohr JP, Kase CS, Meckler RJ, Fisher CM: Sensorimotor stroke. Arch Neurol 34:739, 1977
100. Mohr JP, Kase CS, Wolf PA et al: Lacunes in the NINCDS Pilot Stroke Data Bank, abstracted. Ann Neurol 12:84, 1982
101. Naeser MA, Alexander MP, Helm Estabrooks N et al: Aphasia with predominantly subcortical lesion sites. Arch Neurol 39:2, 1982
102. Nelson RF, Pullicino P, Kendall BE, Marshall J: Computed tomography on patients presenting with lacunar syndromes. Stroke 11:256, 1980
103. Paronetto F: Immunocytochemical observations on the vascular necrosis and renal glomerular lesions of malignant nephrosclerosis. Am J Pathol 46:901, 1965
104. Pearce JMS, Chandrasekera CP, Ladusans EJ: Lacunar infarcts in polycythemia with raised packer cell volumes. Br Med J 287:935, 1983
105. Pentschew A: Gibt es eine Endarteritis luica der kleinen Hirnrindengefässe (Nissl Alzheimer)? Nervenartz 8:393, 1935
106. Percheron SMJ: Les arteries du thalamus humain. Rev Neurol 132:297, 1976
107. Perman GP, Racey A: Homolateral ataxic and crural paresis: case report. Neurology (NY) 30:1013, 1980
108. Plets C, DeReuck J, Vander Ecken H et al: The vascularization of the human thalamus. Acta Neurol Belg 70:685, 1970
109. Poirer J, Barbizet J, Gaston A, Meyrignac C: Demence thalamique. Rev Neurol (Paris) 139:5, 1983
110. Pullicino P, Nelson RF, Kendall BE, Marshall J: Small deep infarcts diagnosed on computed tomography. Neurology (NY) 30:1090, 1980
111. Rascol A, Clanet M, Manelfe C et al: Pure motor hemiplegia: CT study of 30 cases. Stroke 13:11, 1982
112. Reimers J, de Wytt C, Seneviratne B: Lacunar infarction: a 12-month study. Clin Exp Neurol 24:28, 1987
113. Richter RW, Brust JCM, Bruun B, Shafer SQ: Frequency and course of pure motor hemiparesis: a clinical study. Stroke 8:58, 1977
114. Robinson RK, Richey ET, Kase CS, Mohr JP: Somatosensory evoked potentials in pure sensory stroke and allied conditions, abstracted. Neurology (NY) 34:231, 1984
115. Ropper AH, Fisher CM, Kleinman GM: Pyramidal infarction in the medulla: a cause of pure motor hemiplegia sparing the face. Neurology (NY) 29:91, 1979
116. Rosenberg EF: The brain is malignant hypertension: a clinicopathological study. Arch Intern Med 65:545, 1940
117. Rosenberg NL, Koller R: Computerized tomography and pure sensory stroke. Neurology (NY) 31:217, 1981
118. Ross ED: Localization of the pyramidal tract in the internal capsule by whole brain dissection. Neurology (NY) 30:59, 1980
119. Ross Russell RW: Observations on intracerebral aneurysms. Brain 86:425, 1963
120. Rottenberg DA, Talman W, Chernik NL: Location of pyramidal tract questioned. Neurology (Minneapolis) 26:291, 1976
121. Russo LS: Focal dystonia and lacunar infarction of the basal ganglia. Neurology (NY) 40:61, 1983
122. Sage JI: Ataxic hemiparesis from lesions of the corona radiata. Arch Neurol 40:449, 1983
123. Sakai T, Murakami S, Ito K: Ataxic hemiparesis with trigeminal weakness. Neurology (NY) 31:635, 1981
124. Santamaria J, Graus F, Rubio F et al: Cerebral infarction of the basal ganglia due to embolism from the heart. Stroke 14:911, 1983
125. Saris S: Chorea caused by caudate infarction. Arch Neurol 40:590, 1983
126. Satomi K, Terashima Y, Goto K et al: Capsular pseudobulbar mutism in a patient of lacunar state. Rinsho Shinkeigaku 30:299, 1990
127. Schott B, Maugiere F, Laurent B et al: L'amnesie thalamique. Rev Neurol (Paris) 136:117, 1980
128. Skinhoj E, Strandgard S: Pathogenesis of hypertensive encephalopathy. Lancet 1:461, 1973
129. Spertell RB, Ransom BR: Dysarthria clumsy hand syndrome produced by capsular infarct. Ann Neurol 6:268, 1979
130. Strandgard S, Olesen J, Skinhoj E et al: Auto-

regulation of brain circulation in severe arterial hypertension. Br Med J 1:507, 1973
131. Sunohara N, Mukoyama M, Mano Y, Satoyoshi E: Action induced rhythmic dystonia: an autopsy case. Neurology (Cleveland) 34:321, 1984
132. Tapia JF, Kase CS, Sawyer RH, Mohr JP: Hypertensive putaminal hemorrhage presenting as pure motor hemiparesis. Stroke 14:505, 1983
133. Tuhrim S, Yang WC, Rubinowitz H, Weinberger J: Primary pontine hemorrhage and the dysarthria clumsy hand syndrome. Neurology (NY) 31:635, 1982
134. Tuszynski MH, Petito CK, Levy DE: Risk factors and clinical manifestations of pathologically verified lacunar infarctions. Stroke 20:990, 1989
135. Wallesch CW, Kornhuber HH, Kunz T, Brunner RJ: Neuropsychological deficits associated with small unilateral thalamic lesions. Brain 106:141, 1983
136. Waterston JA, Brown MM, Butler P, Swash M: Small deep cerebral infarcts associated with occlusive internal carotid artery disease: a hemodynamic phenomenon? Arch Neurol 47:953, 1990
137. Wei, Gang zhi: Lacunar infarction of the brain: report of 8 cases. Chin J Intern Med 22:473, 1983
138. Weintraub MI, Glaser GH: Norcardial brain abscess and pure motor hemiplegia. NY J Med 70:2717, 1970
139. Weisberg LA: Computed tomography and pure motor hemiparesis. Neurology (NY) 29:490, 1979
140. Weisberg LA: Lacunar infarcts. Arch Neurol 39:37, 1982
141. Weschler IS: Textbook of Clinical Neurology. WB Saunders, Philadelphia, 1943
142. Wiener J, Spiro D, Lattes RG: The cellular pathology of experimental hypertension. II. Arteriolar hyalinosis and fibrinoid change. Am J Pathol 47:457, 1965
143. Wolfe N, Linn R, Babikian VL et al: Frontal systems impairment following multiple lacunar infarcts. Arch Neurol 47:129, 1990
144. Wyllie J: The Disorders of Speech. p. 340. Oilver & Boyd, Edinburgh, 344, 1894

# 21
# *INTRACEREBRAL HEMORRHAGE*

Carlos S. Kase
J.P. Mohr
Louis R. Caplan

## EPIDEMIOLOGY

Intracerebral hemorrhage (ICH) occurs as a result of bleeding from an arterial source directly into the brain substance. Although its relative frequency in patients with stroke is subject to geographic and racial variations, figures between 5 and 10 percent are most commonly quoted.[173,207,262,291] In a consecutive series of 938 stroke patients entered into the NINCDS Stroke Data Bank, primary ICH accounted for 10.7 percent of the cases.[172] Similar figures were obtained in population studies from Denmark (10.4 percent),[133] Holland (9 percent),[138] the midwestern United States (10 percent), and southern Alabama (8 percent).[125] The incidence of ICH increases with advancing age,[69,262] a feature that applies to all types of stroke, both ischemic and hemorrhagic. The incidence rates are relatively constant in predominantly white populations, with rates between 7 and 11 cases per 100,000[28,70,272,265] (Table 21-1). The figures were higher in a United States population (southern Alabama) with a mixture of whites and blacks, since the former had an incidence rate of 12/100,000, whereas in blacks the rate was 32/100,000.[125] Some series from Oriental countries, such as that from Shibata, Japan,[284] report a severalfold increase (61/100,000 population) in incidence rates of ICH. Along with these differing incidence rates from various geographic locations, a general trend toward declining rates of ICH has been detected in recent decades, starting with the initial observation in Göteborg, Sweden,[9] subsequently confirmed in the U.S. population of Rochester, Minnesota.[107,108] From analysis of data encompassing a 32-year period (1945 to 1976), Furlan et al.[107] showed a significant decrease in incidence between the first and second parts of this period: 13.3/100,000 for 1945 to 1960, 6.7/100,000 for 1961 to 1976. These figures correlated with a similar decline in the frequency and severity of hypertension in the population studied. A similarly declining trend in the incidence of ICH has been reported from Hisayama, Japan,[297] where it was also related to a decrease in the frequency of hypertension.

The role of *hypertension* as a leading risk factor is well established, and its frequency has been estimated between 72 percent[207] and 81 percent.[107] The causative role of hypertension is supported by the high incidence of left ventricular hypertrophy in autopsy cases of ICH,[25,216,279] and the significantly higher admission blood pressure readings in ICH patients compared with those with other forms of stroke.[226] The autopsy study of McCormick and Rosenfield[194] has challenged the view that hypertension represents the main causative factor in ICH. Their series included a large number of cases of ICH due to blood dyscrasias, vascular malformations, and tumors, and hypertension was regarded as the sole basis for the bleeding in only 25 percent of the total. This discrepancy with most reported series of ICH may reflect in part a referral pattern bias, as well as more stringent criteria in establishing a causal relationship between hypertension and ICH. However, recently reported clinical series[27,265] have also questioned the validity of the concept of ICH as a condition most commonly

**TABLE 21-1. Incidence of Intracerebral Hemorrhage in Studies From Various Geographic Locations**

| Location | Ref. | Incidence of Intracerebral Hemorrhage: No. of Cases | Rate[a] |
|---|---|---|---|
| Rochester, Minnesota | 71 | 81 | 7 |
| Framingham, Massachusetts | 262 | 58 | 10 |
| Southern Alabama | 125 | 13 | 12 |
| Cincinnati, Ohio | 206 | 154 | 11 |
| Giessen, Germany | 265 | 100 | 11 |
| Shibata, Japan | 284 | 97 | 61 |

[a] Per 100,000 population.

related to hypertension: Brott et al.[28] found a history of hypertension in only 45 percent of 154 patients, a figure that rose to a modest 56 percent when electrocardiographic or chest radiographic evidence of cardiomegaly were added as criteria for the diagnosis of hypertension. Similarly, Schütz et al.[265] labeled only 59 percent of their ICH cases as due to hypertension. These data suggest that a sizable proportion of ICH cases are due to nonhypertensive mechanisms.

In addition to advancing age, hypertension, and race, a number of other risk factors have been recently evaluated, including cigarette smoking, alcohol consumption, and serum cholesterol levels. Abbott et al.[1] showed an increased risk of intracranial hemorrhage (both ICH and subarachnoid hemorrhage) in cigarette-smoking Hawaiian men of Japanese ancestry, and Donahue et al.[67] documented an increased risk of ICH in relation to alcohol ingestion, an effect that operated independently from hypertension, cigarette smoking, and low serum cholesterol levels. The latter, defined as serum cholesterol below 160 mg/dl, has been shown to be associated with an increased risk of ICH in Japanese men,[284] as well as in Hawaiian men of Japanese origin.[298] Other risk factors have been suggested in some studies, but have not been confirmed in others. Liver cirrhosis was highly represented (15.5 percent) in the autopsy series of Boudouresques et al.,[23] but its significance could not be assessed, since no comparison was available with a control autopsy series of the general population. This factor is regarded as of no significance by most epidemiologic studies[2] and autopsy series of ICH.[216,279] The occasional association of ICH to liver cirrhosis has been linked to thrombocytopenia and other abnormalities in coagulation.[195]

## PATHOLOGIC FEATURES AND PATHOGENESIS

Spontaneous ICH occurs predominantly in the deep portions of the cerebral hemispheres. Its most common location is the putamen; this site accounts for 35 to 50 percent of the cases.[87,107,159,172,207,318] The second site of preference varies in different series; in some it is the subcortical white matter,[107,159,207,216] in others the cerebellum,[141] with frequencies of 30 and 16 percent, respectively. The thalamus follows with a uniform frequency of 10 to 15 percent.[86,106,107,159,172,207,308,318] Pontine hemorrhage accounts for 5 to 12 percent of ICH cases.[86,107,159,172,207] The distribution figures for our series of 100 unselected cases of ICH are shown in Table 21-2.

The hemorrhages of putaminal, thalamic, and pontine location occur in the vascular distribution of small, perforating intracerebral arteries, the lenticulostriate, thalamoperforating, and basilar paramedian groups, respectively. Cerebellar hemorrhage occurs in the area of the dentate nucleus,[64,101] which is supplied by small branches of both the superior and the anterior-inferior cerebellar arteries.[37,64] Thus most ICHs originate from the rupture of small, deep arteries,[95] of diameters between 50 and 200 μm. These same arteries are recognized to be those occluded in cases of lacunar infarcts,[94] a form of stroke correlated with chronic hypertension.[91] Thus it is apparent that these various groups of small arteries, located in well-defined anatomic areas, become the target of chronic hypertension, and the result can be either occlusion or rupture, leading to lacunar infarcts or ICH, respectively.

### Vascular Rupture

The actual mechanism of vascular rupture leading to ICH has been the subject of considerable interest, and several detailed pathologic studies[50,52,255,322] have addressed this point. Because hypertension is one of its main causative factors,[53] arterial changes associated with it have been commonly implicated in its pathogenesis. Since Charcot and Bouchard[40] described "miliary aneurysms" in brain specimens from hypertensive ICH cases, these lesions have been the subject of extensive interest. Initially, they were thought to represent true dilatations of the arterial wall,[101] and their preferential location deep in the hemispheres lent support to their pathogenic role. However, with the use of a more precise histologic

**TABLE 21-2. Distribution by Site of 100 Cases of Intracerebral Hemorrhage at the University of South Alabama Medical Center**

| Type | No. of Cases |
|---|---|
| Putaminal | 34 |
| Lobar | 24 |
| Thalamic | 20 |
| Cerebellar | 7 |
| Pontine | 6 |
| Miscellaneous | |
| Caudate | 5 |
| Putaminothalamic | 4 |

technique, Ellis[78] was able to show that miliary aneurysms represented "false aneurysms," and were actually made of blood collected outside the vessel wall, as "masses of blood" surrounded by either "remains of the vessel wall" or fibrin. His view of the pathogenesis of ICH implied a primary intimal lesion, with or without secondary involvement of the media and adventitia, the former often leading to passage of blood into the vessel wall, with formation of a dissecting aneurysm. Either form of vascular abnormality (dissecting aneurysm or simple "weakening" of the vessel wall by the primary intimal lesion extending into the media and adventitia) would then be responsible for rupture and hemorrhage. Over the following years, miliary aneurysms in the brain of hypertensives were shown by the use of thick frozen sections[121] and x-ray imaging of brain specimens injected with radiopaque media.[257] Green's study[121] showed three such lesions, two of which were associated with a fresh hemorrhage in the pons and frontal lobe. His view was that these lesions were mainly related to atherosclerosis and that they "may be responsible for some cases of cerebral hemorrhage." However, the definitive work that established the relationship between hypertension and miliary aneurysms was performed by Ross Russell,[257] with the use of postmortem angiography combined with routine histologic study of brain specimens. He found miliary aneurysms in 15 of 16 brains of hypertensive patients and in 10 of 38 normotensive patients. They were mostly found in the basal ganglia, internal capsule, and thalamus, and less commonly in the centrum semiovale and cortical gray matter. He regarded these lesions as most likely acquired, strongly related to hypertension, and, possibly, causally related to ICH. He rejected the notion that they may be a consequence rather than a cause of ICH, as they were present in brains of hypertensives without ICH. This study was followed by a series of observations reported by Cole and Yates[50–52] in a systematic analysis of 100 brains from hypertensive patients and an equal number of brains from normotensive persons. Miliary aneurysms were found in 46 percent of hypertensives, but only in 7 percent of normotensives; furthermore, they occurred in 85 percent of the cases of hypertensives with massive ICH, and in all those with small "slit" hemorrhages, which suggested that small hemorrhages probably result from microaneurysmal "leaks."[50] However, these authors did not establish a relationship between microaneurysms and bleeding sites, thereby failing to prove these "leaks" had a causal role in ICH. In 1971, Fisher[95] reported the study of two brains containing three ICHs, one pontine and two putaminal, by serial sections of blocks of tissue containing the hemorrhage. In both putaminal hemorrhages the primary arterial bleeding sites were identified along with multiple sites of secondary bleeding. The latter were thought to result from mechanical disruption and tearing of smaller vessels at the periphery of the enlarging hematoma. In the pontine case only the secondary bleeding sites were recognized. No instances of microaneurysm formation were found in immediate relationship to the hematomas, whereas "lipohyalinosis" was a frequent abnormality of the walls of small arteries harboring the bleeding sites. Miliary aneurysms were identified in both hemorrhages, although not in relation to the bleeding points. Fisher regarded them as an unlikely source of major hemorrhage, but rather as the end result of old small sites of arterial rupture ("the end stage of a limited extravasation"). Following this study, Fisher[97] reported in 1972 a detail of the types of microaneurysms found in brains of hypertensives. He described "saccular," "lipohyalinotic," and "fusiform" varieties of microaneurysms, and suggested that the lipohyalinotic form may be the process underlying ICH (as well as lacunar infarcts). He regarded the saccular and fusiform varieties as less likely to be important factors in the pathogenesis of ICH. On the basis of these two studies,[95,97] Fisher concluded that hypertensive ICH most likely results from rupture of one or two lipohyalinotic arteries, followed by secondary arterial ruptures at the periphery of the enlarging hematoma in a cascade or "avalanche" fashion.

## Active Bleeding

Irrespective of the precise mechanism of arterial rupture, the period of active bleeding in ICH is commonly believed to last a fraction of an hour, which generally implies that the active bleeding has ceased by the time the patient arrives at the hospital.[226] Even in those patients in whom clinical deterioration is observed after admission, it is generally attributed to brain edema rather than continuing bleeding.[89,207] This point was studied by Herbstein and Schaumburg,[137] using injection of $^{51}$Cr-labeled erythrocytes in patients with ICH. Labeled erythrocytes were injected 2 to 5 hours after the onset of ICH, and radioactive counting was performed in the cerebral hematoma at postmortem examination in 11 cases. No significant local radioactivity was detected in any of the hematomas, indicating that bleeding had stopped by the time of injection and no further bleeding had occurred. These results suggested that ICH is commonly a monophasic event lasting 2 hours or less, and the authors indicated that maneuvers aimed at a "reduction in blood flow into the involved hemisphere" are not expected to benefit these patients. Although these temporal relations generally correspond to the course observed clinically in ICH, occasional exceptions occur,[3,162] and progressive clinical deterioration after admission can be correlated with CT documentation of continued enlargement of the hematoma. The following case illustrates this point.

A 56-year-old hypertensive man awoke with a mild headache on the morning of admission, and on attempting to stand up he noticed weakness of the left limbs. Relatives noticed that his speech had become dysarthric. On admission 1 hour later, blood pressure was 300/150, he was awake, alert, answered questions appropriately with moderately dysarthric speech, and could carry out commands without delay. Motor examination showed a left hemiparesis predominating in the arm and face, with a Babinski sign on that side. He had hypalgesia on the left limbs, trunk, and face, but localization of stimuli was adequate. On cranial nerve testing, he had a dense left homonymous hemianopia. Extraocular movements were full on command, but the eyes deviated conjugately to the right at rest. Pupils were irregular from old cataract surgery, but reacted sluggishly to light.

A computed tomography (CT) scan performed at 11 a.m. showed a moderate-sized hemorrhage originating at the lateral-posterior angle of the right putamen, with mild mass effect (Fig. 21-1). During the following hours his blood pressure remained markedly elevated, and intermittent use of nitroprusside was required. Blood pressures as high as 250/135 were recorded during the 8 hours following admission. After that time, he was lethargic and minimally responsive to verbal commands. Complete flaccid paralysis of the left limbs was present, along with marked hypesthesia to pinprick. He was partially unaware of the left hemiplegia, and the right gaze preference was unchanged. A repeat CT scan 24 hours after admission showed massive enlargement of the right putaminal hematoma, to two to three times the initial size, with marked mass effect (Fig. 21-2).

The laboratory evaluation revealed no abnormalities in coagulation parameters, and results of liver function tests were within normal limits. His hospital course was characterized by no significant improvement in his neurologic deficits, and on the 23rd hospital day, he suddenly became dyspneic and shortly thereafter had a respiratory arrest, from which he could not be resuscitated.

Pathologic examination showed moderate cardiomegaly, but no acute cardiorespiratory lesions (pulmonary embolus, myocardial infarction) to account for his sudden death. Sections of the brain disclosed a large right putaminocapsular hemorrhage (Fig. 21-3), that matched the size and configuration of the hematoma on the second CT scan (Fig. 21-2). Microscopic examination failed to disclose a vascular malformation as the cause of the hemorrhage, regarded on clinical and pathologic grounds as hypertensive in nature.

The foregoing case illustrates the point that, on occasion, hypertensive ICHs can continue to enlarge for hours after onset, in the absence of conditions known to lead to a more protracted course, such as anticoagulation[86,157,208] or vascular malformations.[250] This problem has been studied recently in a systematic manner. Broderick et al.[27] evaluated eight patients with ICH by CT within 2½ hours from onset, and again several hours later (within 12 hours from onset in seven patients), documenting a substantial increase in hematoma size (mean percentage increase: 107 percent). This increase in the volume of the hemorrhage was accompanied by clinical deterioration in six of the eight patients, all of whom had a greater than 40 percent increase in hematoma volume. In five of them the clinical deterioration occurred with blood pressure measurements of 195 mmHg or greater. The authors suggested that a prolongation of active bleeding for several hours (up to 5 or 6) from onset may not be uncommon as a mechanism of early clinical deterioration in ICH. Similarly, Fehr and Anderson[84] reviewed 56 cases of hypertensive ICH in the basal ganglia and thalamus, and documented enlargement of the hematoma by CT in 4 (7 percent); in 2 of them the increase in hematoma size was documented within 24 hours from onset, in the other 2 on days 5 and 6. Three of these patients had neurologic deterioration: in two who deteriorated within 24 hours, it occurred in the

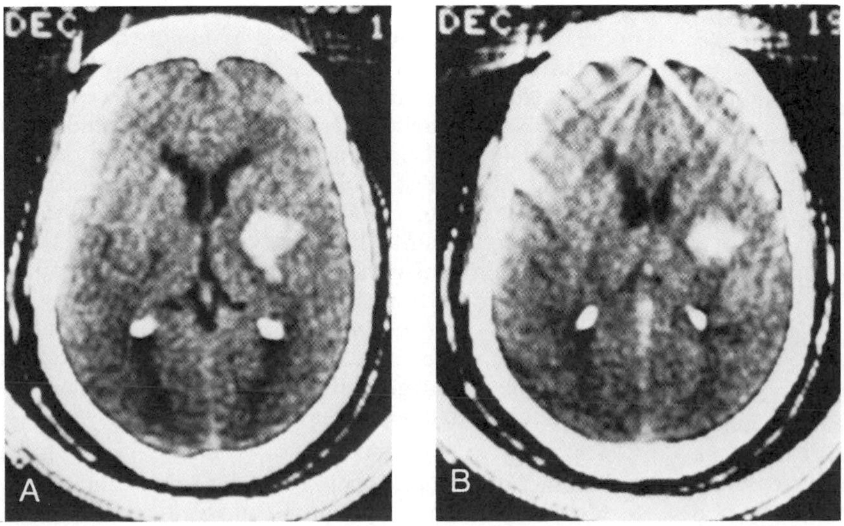

**Fig. 21-1.** (**A**) Moderate-sized right putaminal hemorrhage impinging upon the posterior limb of the internal capsule, with minimal effacement of the frontal horn of the right lateral ventricle. (**B**) Higher computed tomography section shows well-defined putaminal hemorrhage partially extending into the posterior limb of the internal capsule.

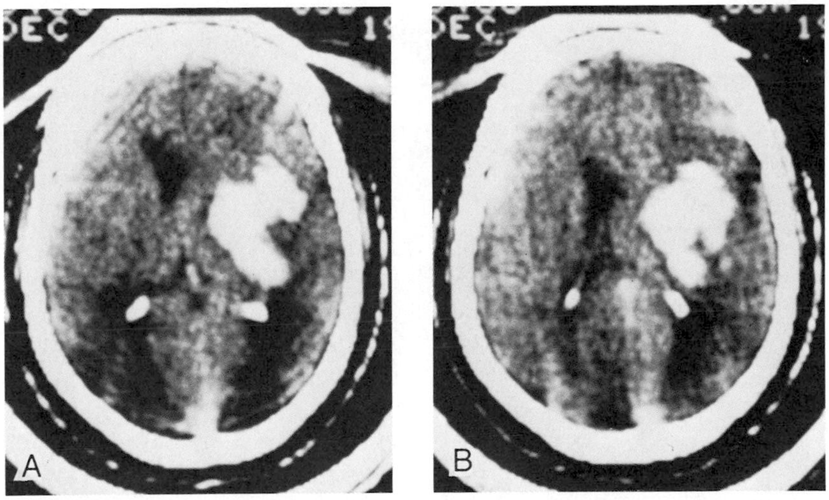

**Fig. 21-2.** (**A**) Marked enlargement of the putaminal hemorrhage, extending laterally and medially, with effacement of the frontal horn of the right lateral ventricle, midline shift, and extension into the ventricular system. (**B**) Higher level of section showing large putaminal hemorrhage.

setting of poorly controlled hypertension, whereas the others had adequate blood pressure control; one of the latter two patients was a chronic alcoholic, leading the authors to suggest that this may be a risk factor for delayed progression of ICH.

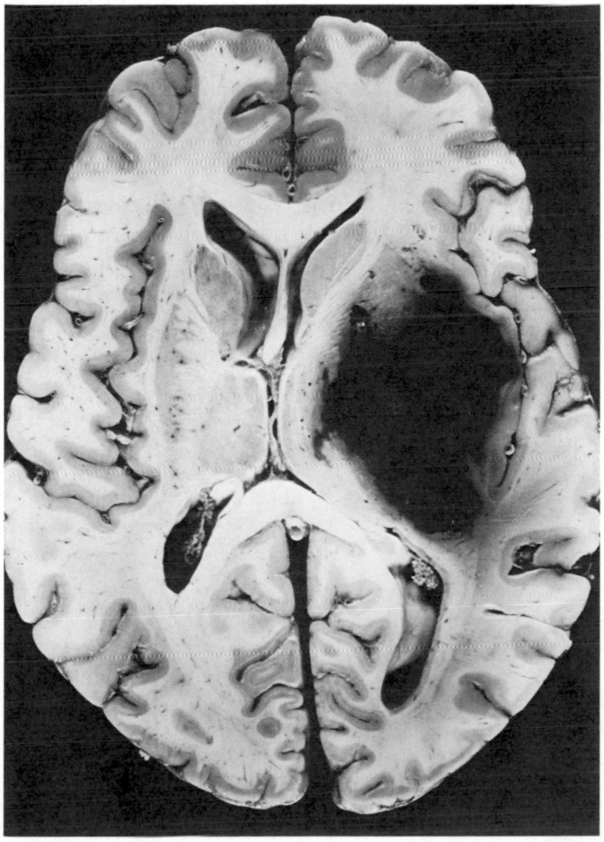

**Fig. 21-3.** Pathologic specimen of right-sided hemorrhage, involving the posterior half of the putamen, globus pallidus, posterior limb of the internal capsule, and claustral area. Effacement of the ipsilateral lateral ventricle, and midline shift occurred.

## Gross Pathologic Anatomy

The gross pathologic anatomy of ICH includes a number of features peculiar to the various locations of the hematomas. The common putaminal variety originates at the posterior angle of this nucleus, and spreads in a concentric fashion, but extends more in the anteroposterior than the transverse diameter.[86] This results in an ovoid mass of maximal anteroposterior diameter collected in the putamen and the structures located laterally to it, the external capsule and claustrum. As a result, the insular cortex is pushed laterally, whereas the internal capsule is either displaced medially or directly involved by the hematoma (Fig. 21-4). The fairly constant origin of this form of ICH in the lateral-posterior aspect of the putamen corresponds to the most common bleeding site being from a lateral branch of the striate arteries.[86] These laterally placed middle cerebral artery perforating branches have lumens between 200 and 400 μm wide on their entry to the brain,[257] and they supply the putamen, internal capsule, and the head of the caudate nucleus. From its initial putaminal-claustral location, a sufficiently large hematoma may extend to other structures in the vicinities: medially into the internal capsule and lateral ventricle, superiorly into the corona radiata, and inferiorly laterally into the white matter of the temporal lobe (Fig. 21-5). These variations in the pattern of extension result in clinical variants of putaminal hemorrhage. The extension of the hemorrhage from its site of origin can follow several patterns, the most common being dissection along the course of adjacent white matter fibers. The common medial extension of the hematoma results in communication with the lateral ventricle, through a process of slow leakage of blood rather than as direct communication between active bleeding site and ventricular system.[86] Direct communication of the hematoma with the ventricular system, at times with associated hydrocephalus, is more likely to result from bleeding at sites adjacent to the ventricular space,

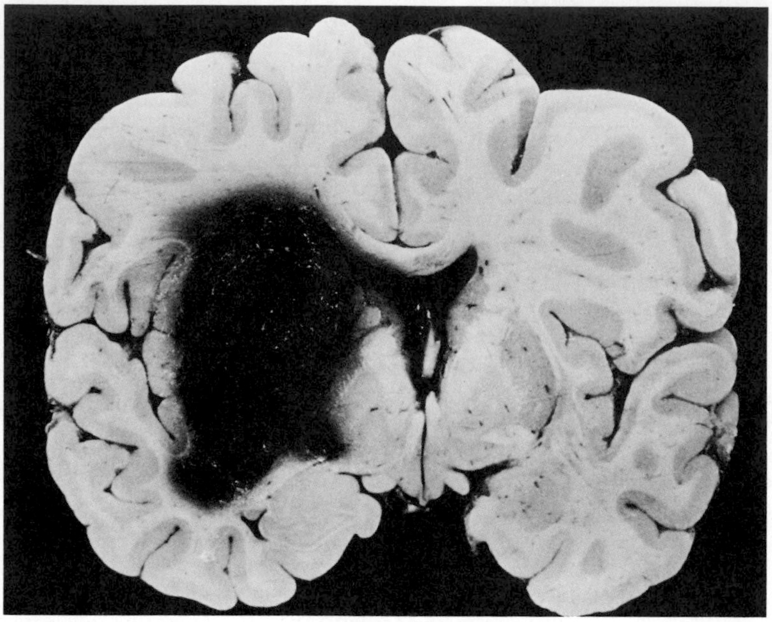

**Fig. 21-4.** Massive right putaminal hemorrhage, originating from the lateral aspect of this nucleus, extending as a large ovoid mass into the subcortical region of the insula. Midline shift, and extension of the hemorrhage into the frontal horn of the lateral ventricle are also present.

such as the thalamus[142] or the head of the caudate nucleus.[280] A putaminal hematoma that directly extends into the ventricle is usually of large size, and is then associated with high mortality.[142]

A variant of striatal hematomas is that occurring in the head of the caudate nucleus. Although the bleeding source is thought to be the same as in putaminal hemorrhage (the lateral group of striate arteries), this form of ICH is uncommon.[280] The recognized low frequency of this type of striatal hemorrhage in hypertensive patients leads the clinician to a search for a different underlying cause, such as an arteriovenous malformation (AVM) or aneurysm. This wide variation in the incidence of two types of striatal bleeding (putaminal and caudate) from the same arterial source is unexplained, and may reflect a higher frequency of arterial rupture at the more proximal segments of these arteries. This, in turn, may correlate with a higher frequency of "lipohyalinosis" or "microatheroma" at the more proximal segments of these vessels, as shown by Fisher[98] in serial studies of the underlying vascular lesions in cases of capsular infarcts. As it has been implied that the same basic vascular abnormality ("lipohyalinosis," "microatheroma") may be the basis for both lacunar infarcts and ICH in hypertensive patients,[86] the predominantly proximal location of these lesions could explain the very low frequency of caudate hemorrhage,

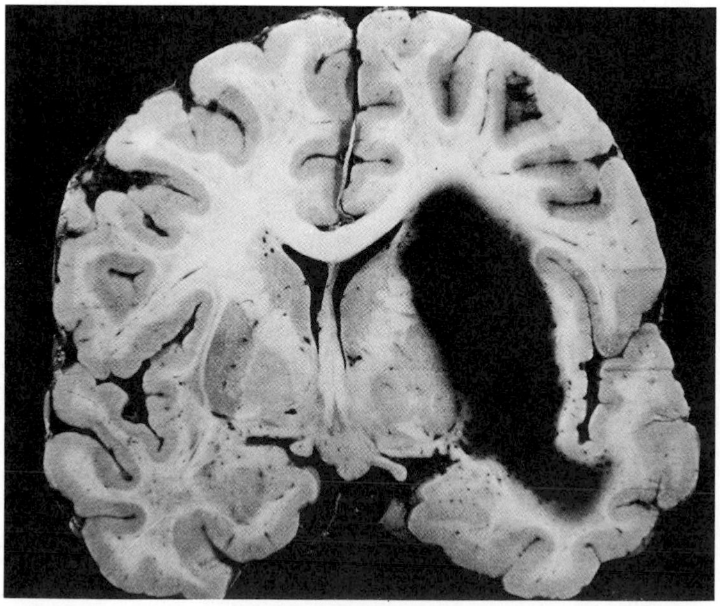

**Fig. 21-5.** Large left putaminal–capsular hemorrhage, with tracking into the white matter of the temporal lobe.

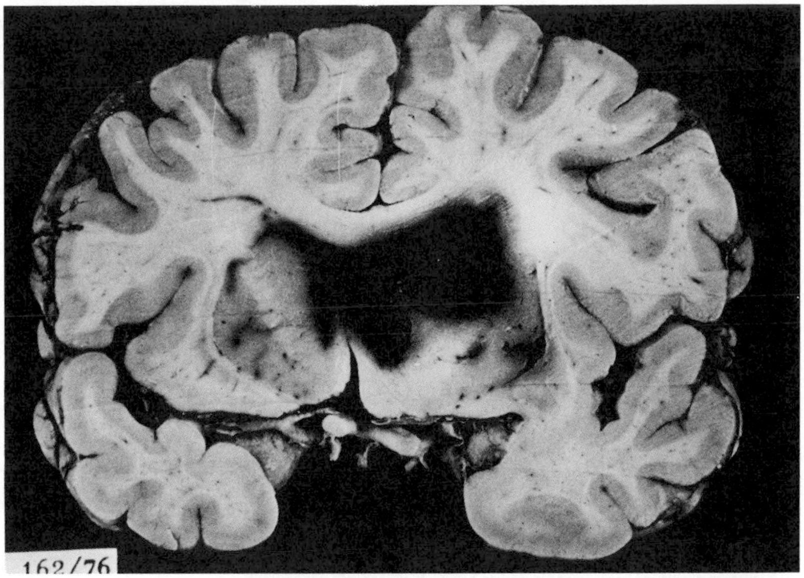

**Fig. 21-6.** Hemorrhage originating from the head of the left caudate nucleus, with involvement of the anterior limb of the internal capsule, and direct ventricular extension with formation of a ventricular cast.

originating from the distal ends of these lateral striate branches. Caudate hemorrhage occurs most commonly in the head of this nucleus (Fig. 21-6), and ventricular entry is an early event; this component sometimes exceeds by many times the size of the parenchymal hematoma.[280] Involvement of the anterior limb of the internal capsule is the rule.

Thalamic hemorrhages involve most or all of this nucleus, and their extension is mostly in the transverse direction, into the third ventricle medially and the posterior limb of the internal capsule laterally (Fig. 21-7). As commonly as the hemorrhage extends transversely, it produces pressure effect or directly extends inferiorly into the tectum and tegmentum of the midbrain. Moderate-sized and large thalamic hematomas will often extend superiorly into the corona radiata and parietal white matter, following the orientation of their fibers.

White matter ("lobar") hematomas collect along the fiber bundles of the cerebral lobes, most commonly at the parietal and occipital levels[107,159,226,253] (Fig. 21-8). Blood usually collects between the cortex and underlying white matter, separating them and often extending along the white matter pathways. Because of this tendency to collect in orientations roughly parallel to the overlying cortex, these are also known as "slit" hemorrhages.[322] By virtue of their sites of origin, these hematomas are close to the corti-

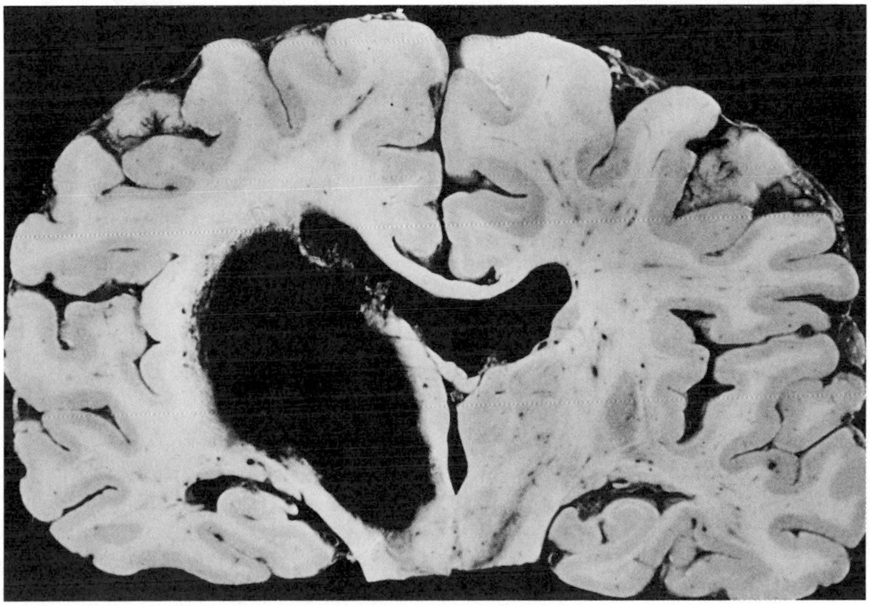

**Fig. 21-7.** Right thalamic hemorrhage, involving most of this nucleus, with extension into the corona radiata, as well as inferiorly into the subthalamic area, with compression of the dorsal midbrain.

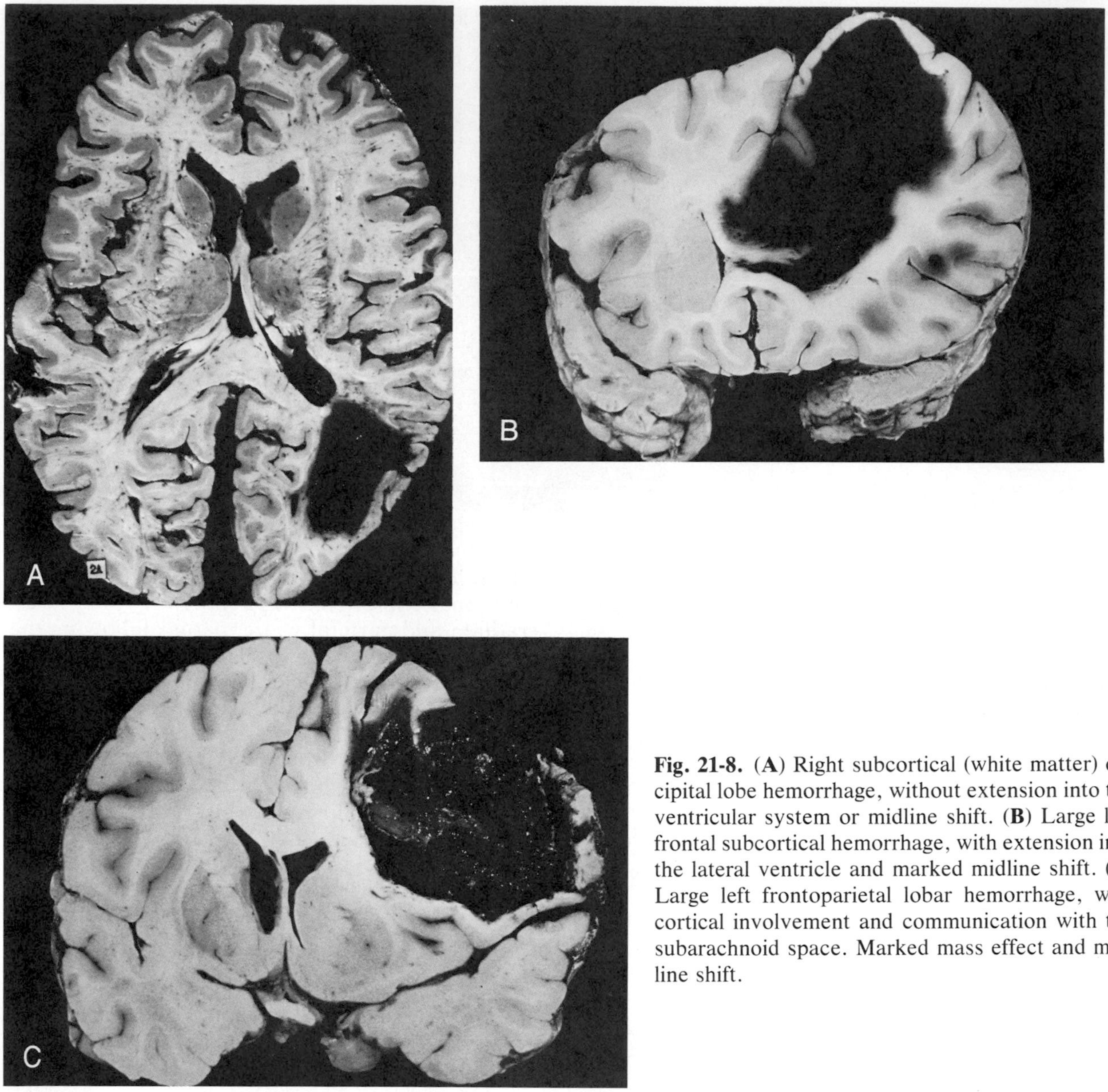


**Fig. 21-8.** (**A**) Right subcortical (white matter) occipital lobe hemorrhage, without extension into the ventricular system or midline shift. (**B**) Large left frontal subcortical hemorrhage, with extension into the lateral ventricle and marked midline shift. (**C**) Large left frontoparietal lobar hemorrhage, with cortical involvement and communication with the subarachnoid space. Marked mass effect and midline shift.

cal surface, at a distance from the ventricular system and midline structures and, usually, not in direct contact with deep hemispheric structures (internal capsule, basal ganglia).

Cerebellar hemorrhage usually occurs on one hemisphere, and it originates in the area of the dentate nucleus.[64,101] From here it extends into the hemispheric white matter, as well as the cavity of the 4th ventricle. The adjacent brain stem (pontine tegmentum) is rarely involved directly by the hematoma, but is often compressed by it, at times with resultant pontine necrosis. A variant of cerebellar hemorrhage, the midline hematoma originating from the cerebellar vermis is virtually always in direct communication with the 4th ventricle through its roof, and frequently extends into the pontine tegmentum bilaterally. The bleeding artery in this variety usually corresponds to distal branches of the superior cerebellar artery. These two forms of cerebellar hemorrhage have distinct clinical and prognostic differences.

In pontine hemorrhage, the bleeding sites correspond to small paramedian basilar perforating branches.[95] This produces a medially placed hematoma, which extends symmetrically to involve the basis pontis bilaterally, with variable degrees of tegmental extension (Fig. 21-9). Tracking of the hematoma into the middle cerebellar peduncle is rarely seen. A partial unilateral variety of pontine hematoma, predominantly tegmental in location, is being recognized clinically and documented by CT

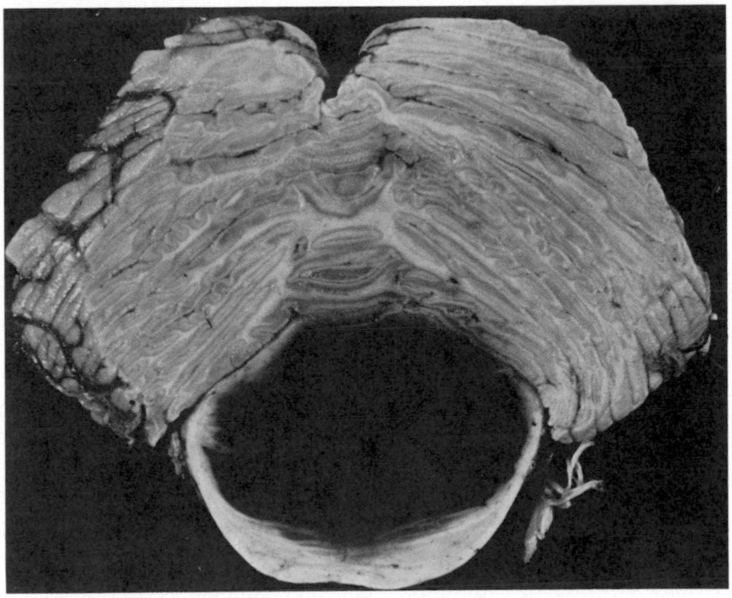

**Fig. 21-9.** Massive midline basal pontine hemorrhage, with destruction of basis and tegmentum bilaterally.

scan.[34,154] These hypertensive hemorrhages result from rupture of distal tegmental segments of long circumferential branches of the basilar artery.[34] The hematomas usually communicate with the 4th ventricle, and they extend laterally and ventrally into the tegmentum and upper part of the basis pontis on one side.

The ICH of hypertensive patients is classically a one-time event: in a group of 101 patients with ICH entered into the NINCDS Stroke Data Bank,[172] history of a prior hemorrhage was documented in only one instance. On the other hand, long-term follow-up studies in patients with ICH have failed to document instances of recurrent bleeding,[68] which clearly differentiate these cases from those due to aneurysms and AVMs, in which rebleeding is a prominent feature. Occasionally, however, multiple simultaneous ICHs can be documented.[141,315] In a series of 600 consecutive cases of ICH diagnosed by CT scan, Weisberg[315] found 12 instances (2 percent) of multiple hematomas. These double lesions were probably simultaneous (because of equal CT attenuation values) in 11 instances, and they occurred in the same intracranial compartment (supratentorial or infratentorial) in all instances but 1, in which a thalamic and cerebellar hematoma coexisted. The incidence of hypertension was unusually low (2 of 12 patients) in his series, suggesting that cases of multiple spontaneous ICHs may be frequently due to other causative factors. Similarly, Hickey et al.[141] have reported two instances of double ICHs in nonhypertensive patients, in whom pathologic brain examination failed to provide the mechanism for the hemorrhages. These reports suggest that the rare occurrence of multiple, nontraumatic ICHs in patients without known pathologic processes predisposing to multiple hemorrhagic brain lesions (cerebral amyloid angiopathy, metastases, venous sinus occlusion, leukemia or other blood dyscrasias) may reflect a different (still undetermined) pathologic process underlying these hemorrhages.

## Histopathologic Studies

The studies on the histopathology of ICH have been mostly concerned with pathogenic issues. However, the main features on the microscopic anatomy of ICH and its changes with time are well documented. The initial arterial rupture leads to local accumulation of blood, which in part destroys the parenchyma locally, displaces nervous structures in the vicinities, and dissects at some distance from the initial focus. The bleeding sites are at times difficult to locate, and serial sections are necessary to show them.[95] The bleeding sites appear as round collections of platelets admixed with and surrounded by concentric lamellae of fibrin, the so-called "bleeding globes"[192] or "fibrin globes."[95] These "fibrin" or "bleeding globes" at the primary and secondary sites are histologically identical, except for the larger size of the former.[95] The bulk of the hematoma is formed by a compact mass of red blood cells, and the bleeding sites are characteristically found at its periphery. Once the bleeding has stopped and the hematoma has become clotted, the microscopic characteristics remain unaltered for many days, until the first signs of a reparative process are observed, about 3 weeks from the onset.[4] A rim of hemosiderin-laden macrophages appears at this time, marking the beginning of a process of clot removal that proceeds slowly from the periphery into the center of the hematoma. While this process is occurring at its periphery, the center of the hematoma undergoes changes that transform it, by gross inspection,

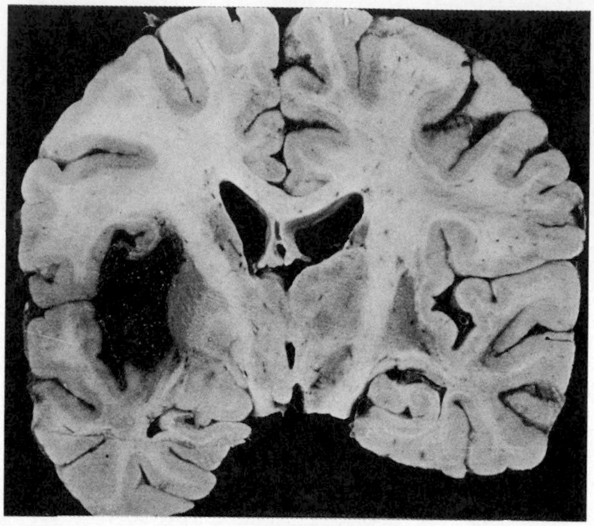

**Fig. 21-10.** A 2-month-old right putaminal–insular hemorrhage, with partial cavitation, good demarcation from the adjacent parenchyma, and lack of signs of mass effect.

into a soft, spongy mass of brick-red altered blood (Fig. 21-10). After many months of slowly progressing phagocytosis, the residual of the hematoma is confined to a flat collapsed cavity lined by reddish-orange discoloration resulting from the accumulation of hemosiderin-laden macrophages.[279] Astrocytic proliferation in the neighboring parenchyma extends for variable distances from the residual cavity.

## Nonhypertensive Causes of Intracerebral Hemorrhage

There are a number of instances in which ICH occurs in the absence of hypertension. These nonhypertensive mechanisms of ICH are (1) small vascular malformations, (2) sympathomimetic drugs, (3) cerebral amyloid angiopathy, (4) brain tumors, (5) anticoagulants, (6) fibrinolytic agents, and (7) vasculitis.

### Small Vascular Malformations

Small vascular malformations, also referred to as "angiomas," are frequently implicated in cases of ICH, especially in those of lobar location. The study of Margolis et al.[187] first called attention to these lesions when they reported four cases of fatal ICH in young patients, in whom pathologic examination disclosed small vascular malformations, one of which was arteriovenous, two venous, and one probably cavernous. Two other cases with incidentally found (not associated with ICH) malformations were added: a cavernous angioma and a so-called "telangiectasis." These authors stressed the need to consider these lesions in cases of nonhypertensive ICH, especially in the young. Since then, several authors have shared this point of view.[55,86,171,260] Fisher[86] recorded 17 such lesions in his series of ICH, and stressed that the hemorrhages they produce are less massive or slower to develop than most hypertensive ones. Russell and coworkers[55,260] reported 21 examples of ICH due to small vascular malformations, 20 of which were arteriovenous, and only 1 a cavernous angioma.[260] The 20 arteriovenous lesions were located in the cerebral convexity (10 cases), deep portions of the hemispheres (4 cases), and cerebellum (6 cases).[55] Because of their small size and the difficulties in diagnosing them in life, the term "cryptic" was proposed for these malformations.[55] These authors pointed out that lesions likely to bleed were arteriovenous, whereas cavernous angiomas, although not infrequently found in routine examination of brain specimens (Fig. 21-11), rarely are a source of bleeding. The latter are most commonly found in the cerebral subcortical white matter, basal ganglia, and pons.[261] Subsequently, more instances of association of ICH with small vascular malformations were recorded,[16,171,250] some occurring on a familial basis.[19,48]

In the series of 18 cases of Becker et al.,[16] the hemorrhages were predominantly lobar, reflecting the usually cortical location of the malformations. These authors found a mean age of 23 years in their series, and documented a 2.5:1 female:male ratio, similar to the sex distribution of 42 cases previously reported in the literature. Recent data have added further to the notion that small vascular malformations need to be considered in the differential diagnosis of ICH in the young: in a study of patients between 15 and 45 years of age with nontraumatic ICH, Toffol et al.[294] documented ruptured AVM as the most common mechanism, amounting to 38 percent of the 55 patients in whom a cause for the ICH could be determined.

Cavernous angiomas are thought to have a generally lower bleeding potential than the arteriovenous variety. However, they occasionally lead to progressive, subacute deficits that result from protracted bleeding or recurrent small hemorrhages, as documented by Roberson et al.[250] in a young normotensive woman who died from a pontomedullary hemorrhage secondary to a pathologically verified cavernous angioma. Recent data suggest that bleeding from cavernous angiomas may be more common than previously recognized: Weber et al.[311] documented intracranial hemorrhage in 3 of 34 (9 percent) cases of cavernous angioma, in 2 of them with meningocerebral hemorrhage, the other case with purely subarachnoid hemorrhage (SAH). Simard et al.[275] reviewed 138 cases of cavernous angiomas, 40 (29 percent) of which produced acute intracranial bleeding, in a recurrent pattern in 7 of them. Furthermore, with the current availability of magnetic resonance imaging (MRI), it has become apparent that cavernous angiomas, sometimes even incidentally found, frequently show signal characteristics that reflect extravasation of blood into the adjacent brain parenchyma.[324] Because of the above reports, it now seems well established that

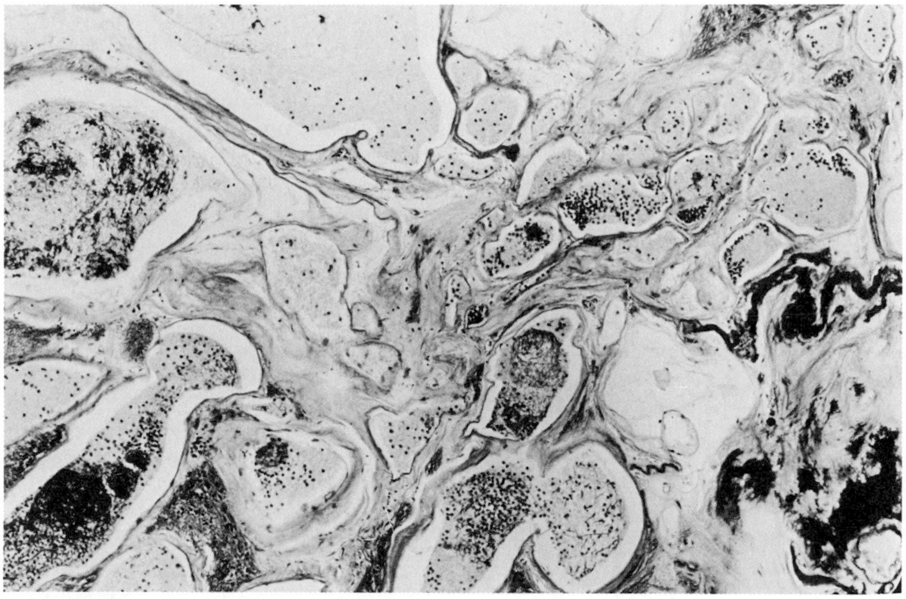

**Fig. 21-11.** Incidentally found cavernous angioma in the subcortical white matter of the left frontal lobe, showing widely separated vascular channels with primitive walls, without intervening brain parenchyma. Areas of calcification are shown in the right lower corner. (Hematoxylin and eosin; × 48.)

small vascular malformations, both arteriovenous and cavernous, are likely to bleed, and may be responsible for cases of nonhypertensive ICH. The frequency of this occurrence is difficult to establish, but one figure is available from the autopsy study of Russell,[260] in which 21 cases were obtained from a total of 461 cases of ICH, a frequency of 4.5 percent.

## Sympathomimetic Drugs

ICH related to the use of *amphetamines* has been documented in several publications.[61,71,134,182] The preparation most commonly implicated has been intravenous methamphetamine,[61] but cases related to intranasal[134] or oral[71] use of this drug and amphetamine have also been reported. Another sympathomimetic drug, *pseudoephedrine,* has been associated with yet another reported instance of ICH.[182] These patients have developed the ICHs usually within minutes (20 to 40) to a few hours (4 to 6) after the use of the drug, frequently representing an established pattern of drug abuse for months prior to the ICH, while at times ICH has followed their first-time use.[71] An association with transiently elevated blood pressure has been noticed in about 50 percent of the cases, and the majority of the hematomas have been located in the "lobar" subcortical white matter.[134,182] Their pathogenesis has been related to either transient drug-related elevation in blood pressure[71] or to an arteritislike vascular change histologically similar to periarteritis nodosa.[47] The latter is considered to be either a direct "toxic" effect of the drug on cerebral blood vessels, or a hypersensitivity reaction to the drug or its vehicle. The cerebral "arteritis" related to use of these drugs is characterized angiographically by "beading" (multiple areas of focal arterial stenosis or constriction) of medium-size and large intracranial arteries,[134,182,188,259,325] an effect that has been shown to be reversible, following use of steroids and discontinuation of drug abuse.[325] However, it is likely that these reversible vascular changes do not correspond to a true vasculitis but rather to a nonspecific phenomenon of multifocal spasm related to the effects of the sympathomimetic drug on the vessel wall. In isolated instances, intravenous use of methamphetamine precipitated an ICH from a sylvian-region AVM,[183] and oral use of dextroamphetamine was associated with SAH in the presence of a small middle cerebral artery aneurysm.[192] Most other reports of amphetamine-related ICH and SAH have failed to document preexisting vascular malformations or mycotic aneurysms.

Other sympathomimetic agents have been recently related to episodes of ICH. *Phenylpropanolamine* (PPA), which is contained in more than 70 "over-the-counter" nasal decongestants and appetite supressants,[214] has been associated with at least 20 reported instances of ICH and SAH. Most affected patients have been young (median age in the 30s), women more often than men, and generally lacking other risk factors for intracranial hemorrhage.[152] The hemorrhages have occurred within short periods of time from PPA ingestion, the majority between 1 and 8 hours.[11,18,81,152,165,282] The ICHs were most commonly of lobar location, and about two-thirds of the cases that underwent angiography showed widespread "beading" of intracranial arteries (Fig. 21-12), without doc-

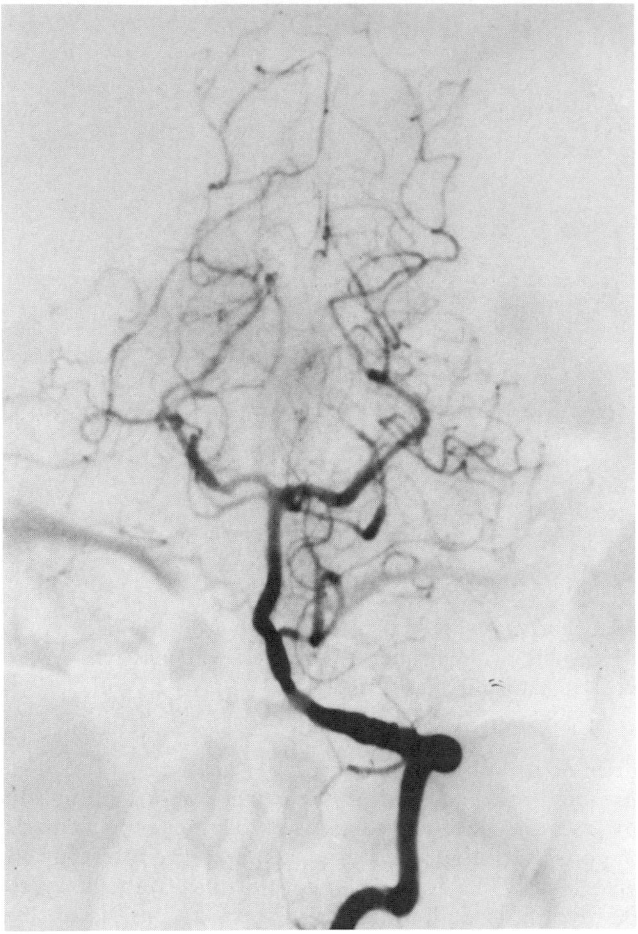

**Fig. 21-12.** Multifocal areas of arterial constriction and dilatation ("beading") in the vertebrobasilar system following an episode of severe headache and transient hypertension (200/110), shortly after the ingestion of a PPA-containing nasal decongestant. (From Kase et al.,[152] with permission.)

umentation of other vascular lesions responsible for bleeding, such as AVM or aneurysm. Histologic examination of blood vessels from biopsy material has been nondiagnostic except for one instance of documentation of changes consistent with vasculitis.[113] The pathogenesis of these PPA-related hemorrhages is obscure. Although rare patients have been previously hypertensive, about 50 percent of the reported cases have had transient hypertension at presentation with ICH.[152] This suggests that a possible mechanism of vascular rupture is drug-induced transient hypertension associated with multifocal arterial changes due to vasospasm or, less commonly, vasculitis.

*Cocaine* is being increasingly reported as a cause of cerebral hemorrhage in young individuals, especially in its precipitate form known as "crack." Instances of ICH and SAH have occurred within minutes to 1 hour from use of "crack" cocaine.[178] The ICHs are either lobar or deep ganglionic, occasionally with multiple hemorrhages in both locations.[122] The mechanism of these ICHs is unclear, although they are in many respects similar to those related to amphetamine and PPA use, the angiographic "beading" that characterizes the latter two is relatively uncommon in cocaine-related ICHs, which, in turn, have shown a higher association with AVMs or aneurysms as the bleeding mechanism.[178] This suggests that the hypertensive response that frequently follows cocaine use may act in some instances as a precipitant of ICH in preexisting vascular malformations.

## Cerebral Amyloid Angiopathy

Cerebral amyloid angiopathy (CAA) or "congophilic" angiopathy represents a unique form of cerebral angiopathy characterized by amyloid deposits in the media and adventitia of medium-sized and small cortical and leptomeningeal arteries.[111,148,186,227,245,301] The condition is not associated with systemic vascular amyloidosis and its most common form of clinical presentation is ICH. CAA virtually always occurs sporadically, but it has been described as a familial condition with autosomal dominant transmission in Iceland[126] and in the Netherlands,[310] where the instances of ICH have occurred at an early age (in the 3rd and 4th decades in the Icelandic cases,[126] in the 5th and 6th decades in the Dutch cases[310]). This angiopathy characteristically affects elderly individuals, its incidence in autopsy series rising steeply with age: 8 percent in the 7th decade,[290] 23 to 42.8 percent in the 8th decade, 37 to 46.4 percent in the 9th decade, and 57 to 58 percent in persons older than 90.[109,302] The condition has rarely been reported before age 55.[151] CAA is associated with a progressive senile dementia in about 30 percent of the cases,[111] and histopathologic features of Alzheimer's disease (neuritic plaques and neurofibrillary degeneration) are documented in about 30 percent of the cases. Hypertension has been infrequently associated with ICH in patients with CAA: only 2 of 9 cases with large ICHs were hypertensive in the series of Okazaki et al.,[227] 3 of 7 in the Wagle et al. report,[305] 3 of 11 in the series of Gilbert and Vinters,[109] 2 of 11 in the series of Gilles et al.,[111] and 2 of 17 in the series of Vonsattel et al.[303]

The Congo red-positive amyloid deposits occur in the media and adventitia of small and medium-sized cortical and leptomeningeal arteries, which also show characteristic birefringence under polarized light (Fig. 21-13). Under the electron microscope, these lesions contain typical nonramified amyloid fibrils, 90 to 110 Å diameter,[111,245] that are identical to those found in systemic amyloidosis and in the central cores of the neuritic plaques of Alzheimer's disease.[228] The amyloid deposits in the arterial wall frequently lead to stenosis of the arterial lumen, as well as thickening of the basement membrane, fragmentation of the internal elastic lamina, and loss of endothelial cells.[228,245] An association with fibrinoid necrosis of

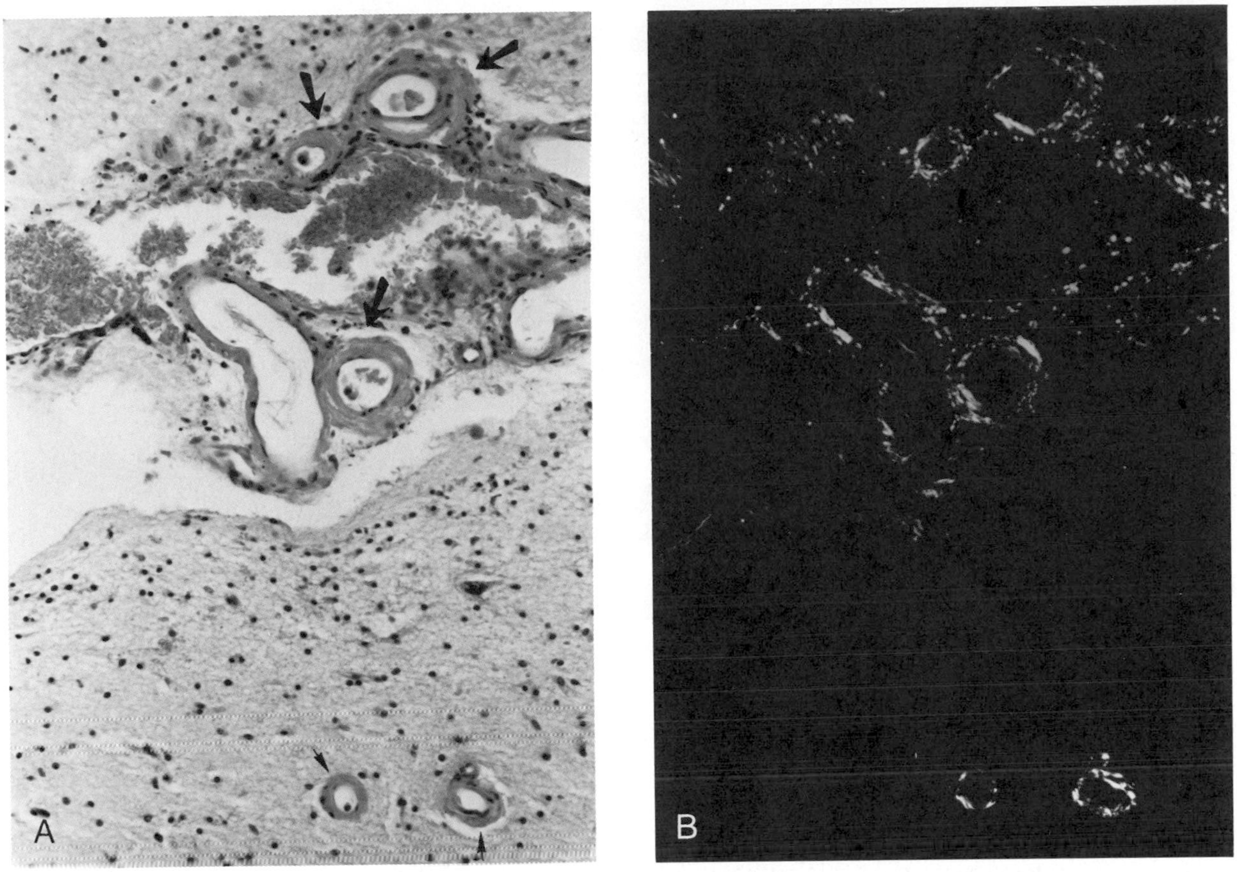


**Fig. 21-13.** (**A**) Arteries in leptomeninges (*large arrows*) and upper cortical layers (*small arrows*) with amyloid deposits in the vessel wall. (Congo red, × 48.) (**B**) Same field as in Fig. A under polarized light showing birefringence of amyloid deposits in the vessel wall. (Congo red, × 48.) (Histologic materials used for this figure were kindly provided by Dr. Jean-Paul Vonsattel, Neuropathology Laboratory, Massachusetts General Hospital, Boston, Massachusetts.)

affected vessels has been occasionally documented,[148,149,185,227,245] followed rarely by microaneurysm formation.[277] Recently, Vonsattel et al.[303] reported the results of a comparative histologic study of brains with CAA with and without ICH. They found that the features most consistently associated with the occurrence of ICH were a severe degree of vascular amyloid deposit and the coexistence of fibrinoid necrosis, with or without microaneurysm formation.

Cerebral infarcts and, especially, hemorrhages are the common consequences of CAA, both of which occur in superficial locations, since the angiopathy typically spares the deep white matter and basal ganglionic areas.[109,111,148,186,227,245] As a result, most instances of ICH have occurred as subcortical, "lobar" hemorrhages,[85,109,234,245,296,305] more often affecting the occipital and parietal lobes, where the angiopathy tends to predominate.[109,227,290] However, examples affecting the frontal subcortical white matter are not uncommon (Fig. 21-14), and Vinters and Gilbert[302] found ICH occurring more often in the frontal and frontoparietal areas than in the occipital or parietal lobes. An additional characteristic of these ICHs has been the tendency to recur over periods of months to years,[85,111,245,296] occasionally occurring simultaneously.[111,234]

In conclusion, CAA appears to be an important causative factor for ICHs in normotensive, elderly, and at times demented individuals, in particular in the event of subcortical (lobar) hemorrhage, at times in a recurrent pattern. The actual contribution of this factor in ICH in general will need to be determined by systematic search for this form of angiopathy in autopsy studies of ICH, as well as biopsy material obtained from the walls of surgically drained hematomas.

## Intracranial Tumors

Intracranial tumors are a well-recognized but uncommon cause of ICH. Underlying tumors have accounted for 1 to 2 percent of ICH cases in autopsy series,[216] while figures of 6 to 10 percent have been

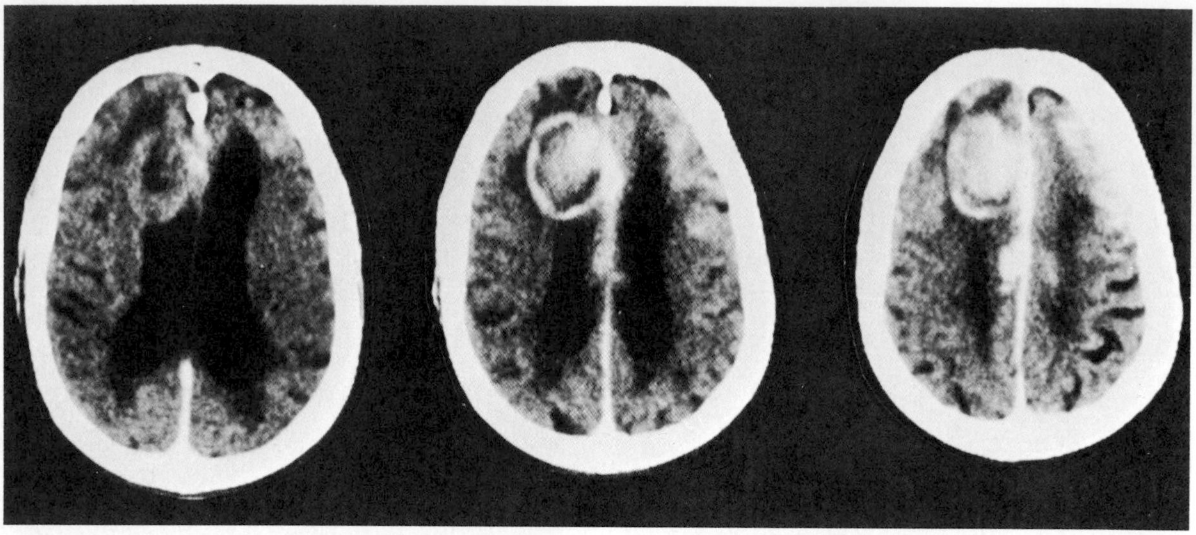

**Fig. 21-14.** Right subcortical frontal hematoma, of 10 to 12 days' duration, with postcontrast "ring" enhancement. Biopsy specimen of surgically drained hematoma demonstrated widespread amyloid deposits in cortical and leptomeningeal arteries.

found in clinical-radiologic series.[179,266] The great majority of the underlying neoplasms have been malignant, either primary or metastatic, and rarely meningiomas[206] or oligodendrogliomas[179] have presented with ICH. An example of a generally benign tumor with relatively high tendency to bleed is pituitary adenoma, which was associated with bleeding in over 15 percent of the cases in one large series of brain tumors.[306] Among the primary malignant brain tumors causing ICH, glioblastoma multiforme predominates,[179] while the metastatic ones have corresponded to melanoma, choriocarcinoma, renal-cell, and bronchogenic carcinoma.[110,128,184,266,300] The frequency of hemorrhagic metastases was estimated at 60 percent for germ-cell tumors, 40 percent for melanoma, and 9 percent for bronchogenic carcinoma.[120] The bleeding tendency in neoplasms is thought to be directly related to the richness of their vascular components, and their pathologic, neoplastic character.[328] In the case of metastatic choriocarcinoma these features are enhanced by the normal biologic tendency of trophoblastic tissue to invade the walls of blood vessels.[128,271] The location of the hemorrhage relates to some extent to the type of neoplasm involved: those occurring into glioblastoma multiforme are frequently deep into the hemispheres, basal ganglia, or corpus callosum,[179] whereas metastatic ones occur more often into the subcortical white matter[110] (Fig. 21-15) since metastatic nodules frequently deposit at the gray–white matter junction[261] (Fig. 21-16). In approximately one-half of the reported instances of ICH within intracerebral tumors, this event corresponded

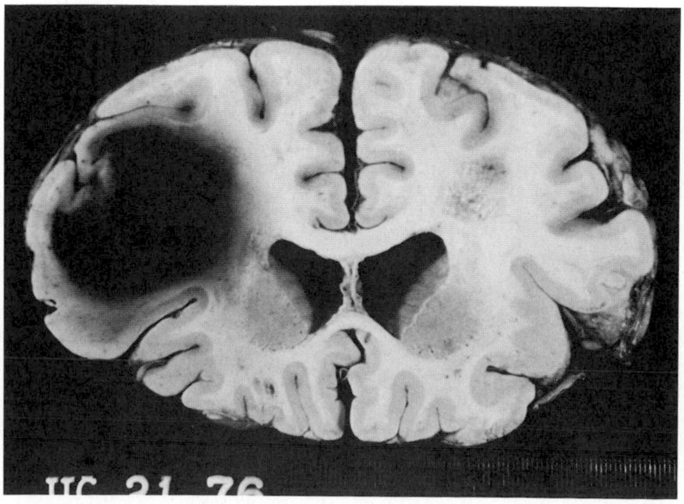

**Fig. 21-15.** Large hemorrhage into a metastatic lesion (from bronchogenic carcinoma) in the right frontal subcortical white matter. A second, nonhemorrhagic, metastasis is present in the white matter of the left frontal lobe.

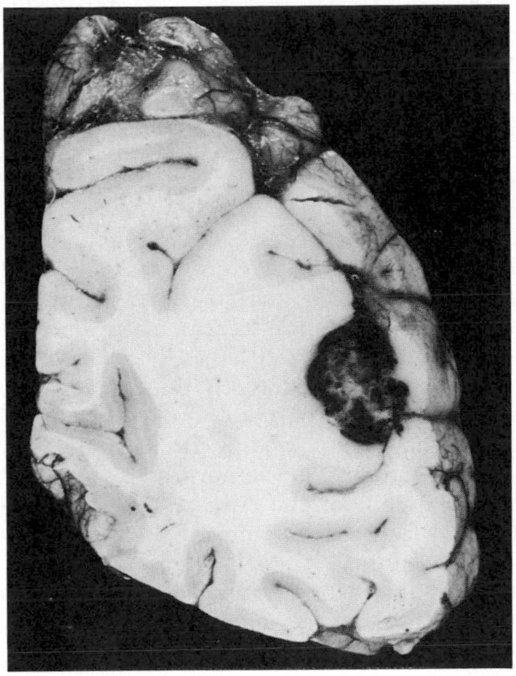

**Fig. 21-16.** Small hemorrhagic metastasis from melanoma in the gray–white matter junction of the right occipital lobe.

to the first clinical manifestation of the neoplasm. The radiologic diagnosis by CT can be established easily in instances of multiple metastatic lesions,[110] but cases of ICH into single tumors can be more difficult to diagnose. They need to be suspected with the finding of large areas of low-density edema surrounding the hematoma, or in the presence of an area of postcontrast enhancement at the periphery of the hematoma, frequently forming a "ring" pattern on initial presentation with ICH.[110,179] Since "ring" enhancement is not expected on presentation of spontaneous, hypertensive ICH,[139,314,326] its presence should strongly suggest the possibility of an underlying, previously asymptomatic primary or metastatic brain tumor. Other features suspicious of ICH into a brain tumor include[151] (1) finding of papilledema at presentation with acute ICH; (2) atypical location of the ICH, in sites such as the corpus callosum, which is rarely the site of "spontaneous" ICH and is commonly involved by malignant gliomas; (3) a "ringlike" high-density corresponding to blood around a low-density center, resulting from bleeding by tumor vessels at the junction of tumor and adjacent brain parenchyma. These clinical and radiologic features should prompt a search for a primary or metastatic brain tumor, with MRI and cerebral angiography. If the results of these tests are inconclusive, biopsy of the hematoma cavity should be considered to establish the diagnosis of an underlying brain tumor, since the therapeutic options and prognosis are radically different in comparison with nontumoral ICH.

## Anticoagulants

Chronic oral anticoagulation with warfarin probably represents an independent risk factor for ICH. In our consecutive series of 100 cases of ICH observed over a 3-year period, warfarin anticoagulation was a factor in 9 percent of the cases.[157] In the autopsy series of 500 cases of intracranial hemorrhage reported by Boudouresques et al.,[23] anticoagulation was implicated in 11 percent of the ICH cases. Rådberg et al.[244] documented an anticoagulant-related mechanism in 14 percent of 200 consecutive patients with ICH, excluding cases due to trauma, ruptured aneurysm, or concomitant brain tumor. Furthermore, anticoagulation follows hypertension as a causative factor in series of cerebellar[232] and lobar[253] locations. Its importance in ICH of other more common locations (putaminal, thalamic) is unknown, as most of the large series reported[142,308] have excluded from analysis cases due to oral anticoagulation or blood dyscrasias. On the other hand, chronic oral anticoagulation has been shown to increase by 8 to 11 times the risk of ICH in comparison with patients of similar age not receiving anticoagulants.[103,317,321] However, the true importance of oral anticoagulants as a risk factor separate from hypertension is unknown: 87 percent of the patients on anticoagulants were also hypertensive in the series of Boudouresques et al.,[23] 4 of 6 patients reported by Wells and Urrea,[316] 10 of 24 patients (42 percent) in our series,[157] and 80 percent of those reported by Wintzen et al.[321] were known to be previously hypertensive. Figures on the incidence of ICH in patients on oral anticoagulants have rarely been reported.[21,54,102,145] The study of Bjerkelund[21] indicated an incidence of ICH of 3.3 percent (4 of 119 cases) in patients receiving warfarin for myocardial infarction, and 3 of the 4 cases had documented hypertension. However, other large series[54,145] have failed to document a relationship between hypertension and bleeding during anticoagulant therapy.

Other characteristics of these hemorrhages include the tendency to occur in the absence of signs of systemic bleeding, lack of relationship of ICH with preceding cerebral infarction, frequent leisurely progression of the focal neurologic deficits, at times over periods as long as 48 or 72 hours, and high mortality (55 to 65 percent) related to hematoma sizes that are, in general, larger than the hypertensive varieties.[103,157,244]

Other features related to ICH on anticoagulants have shown different results in various series. These include (1) *duration of anticoagulation prior to ICH onset:* in two series, the majority of ICHs (70 percent,[157] 54 percent[244]) occurred during the first year after treatment onset, while in others[103] only one-third occurred over that period of time, the other two-thirds being scattered between 2 and 18 years from treatment onset; (2) *relationship between intensity of anticoagulant effect and ICH risk:* several studies[13,157,276] have suggested an increased rate of ICH with excessively prolonged prothrombin time, but others[103] found only a slight excess of ICH in overtreated patients as compared with those in the recommended therapeutic range of prothrombin time prolongation; (3) *location of ICH:* an unexpectedly high frequency of cerebellar location was found in two studies,[157,244] whereas others[103,321] found no differences in location between anticoagulated and nonanticoagulated patients.

The actual mechanism of ICH in anticoagulated patients is unknown, in part due to the lack of adequate pathologic studies with serial histologic sections aimed at identifying the type of bleeding vessel and the histopathologic abnormality at the bleeding site. Such studies should determine whether anticoagulant-related ICHs have a different microscopic pathology from "spontaneous" ICH, in terms of the type of affected vessel, as well as the eventual presence of local vascular pathology (microaneurysm, fibrinoid necrosis, lipohyalinosis, CAA) at the rupture site as a possible substrate for this complication of warfarin anticoagulation.

The occurrence of ICH during intravenous *heparin* anticoagulation represents a different situation, since this complication generally occurs in the setting of a preceding acute cerebral infarction (as ICH is extremely uncommon in patients receiving intravenous heparin for noncerebrovascular indications, such as deep vein thrombosis and myocardial infarction[69,131]). Thus, a recent cerebral infarction with local ischemic blood vessels is a likely site for the occurrence of secondary ICH, especially in embolic infarcts, that tend to become hemorrhagic as part of their natural history.[99] ICH in this setting occurs within 24 to 48 hours from onset of heparin treatment, and excessive prolongation of the activated partial thromboplastin time (aPTT) is frequently present.[10] In addition to excessive prolongation of aPTT, other risk factors for ICH in the setting of intravenous heparin therapy for acute cerebral infarction include infarcts of large size and uncontrolled hypertension (blood pressure [BP] above 180/100).[39] This has led to the recommendations of limiting the immediate use in intravenous heparin anticoagulation in acute nonseptic cerebral infarction to those cases with subtotal infarcts in a given vascular territory, without uncontrolled hypertension (i.e., BP below 180/100), and while maintaining close adherence to a prolongation of the aPTT within the recommended "therapeutic" range (one and one-half times the control value).

## Fibrinolytic Agents

Fibrinolytic agents, including streptokinase, urokinase, and tissue-type plasminogen activator (tPA) are increasingly being used in the treatment of coronary and arterial and venous thrombosis in the limbs and pulmonary circulation. The ability of these agents to produce clot lysis and a relatively low degree of systemic hypofibrinogenemia makes them ideal choices for the treatment of acute thrombosis. However, the major complication, although relatively infrequent, continues to be hemorrhage, in particular ICH. ICH has been reported in 0.4 to 1.3 percent of patients with acute myocardial infarction (MI) treated with the single-chain tPA "alteplase."[289] The clinical and CT features of ICHs related to coronary thrombolysis with tPA have been recently reviewed.[117,155,156,224] The hemorrhages tend to occur early after onset of tPA treatment: in one study 40 percent of them started during the infusion, and another 25 percent occurred within 24 hours from onset of treatment.[117] In 70 to 90 percent of the cases, the hemorrhages are lobar, with virtually no examples of deep ganglionic hemorrhages (Fig. 21-17). In about 30 percent of the cases the hemorrhages are multiple,[155] and their mortality is high (44 to 66 percent).[117,155,156,224]

The mechanism of bleeding in this setting is unknown. On several occasions[155,156,224] patients have had excessively prolonged aPTTs at the time of onset of intracranial hemorrhage as a result of the use of intravenous heparin (aimed at preventing reocclusion of reperfused coronary arteries). Other factors suggested as significant in increasing the risk of ICH after the use of tPA in acute MI have included old age (over 65 years), history of hypertension, and pre-tPA use of aspirin,[224] but they were not found to be significantly different in comparison with the nonbleeders in a recent study.[156] A possible role for local cerebral vascular pathology has been considered, since examples of pretreatment head trauma[156] and concomitant CAA[236] have been recently documented in association with ICH after use of tPA. Other coagulation defects related to this treatment, such as hypofibrinogenemia and thrombocytopenia, have not been found to correlate with this complication.

## Vasculitis

The cerebral vasculitides generally result in arterial occlusion and cerebral infarction, and only rarely are they responsible for ICH. Most of these unusual examples of ICH secondary to cerebral arteritis have been secondary to *granulomatous angiitis of the nervous system* (GANS).[168] This primary cerebral vasculitis occurs in the absence of systemic involvement, and histologically it is characterized by mononuclear inflammatory exudates with giant cells in the media and adventitia of small and medium-sized arteries and veins. This is occasionally associated with the formation of microaneurysms. The cerebral disease evolves with chronic headache, progressive cognitive decline, seizures, and recurrent episodes of cerebral infarction.[212] Due to its primary cerebral location, systemic features such as malaise, fever, weight loss, arthralgias, myalgias, anemia, and elevated sedimenta-

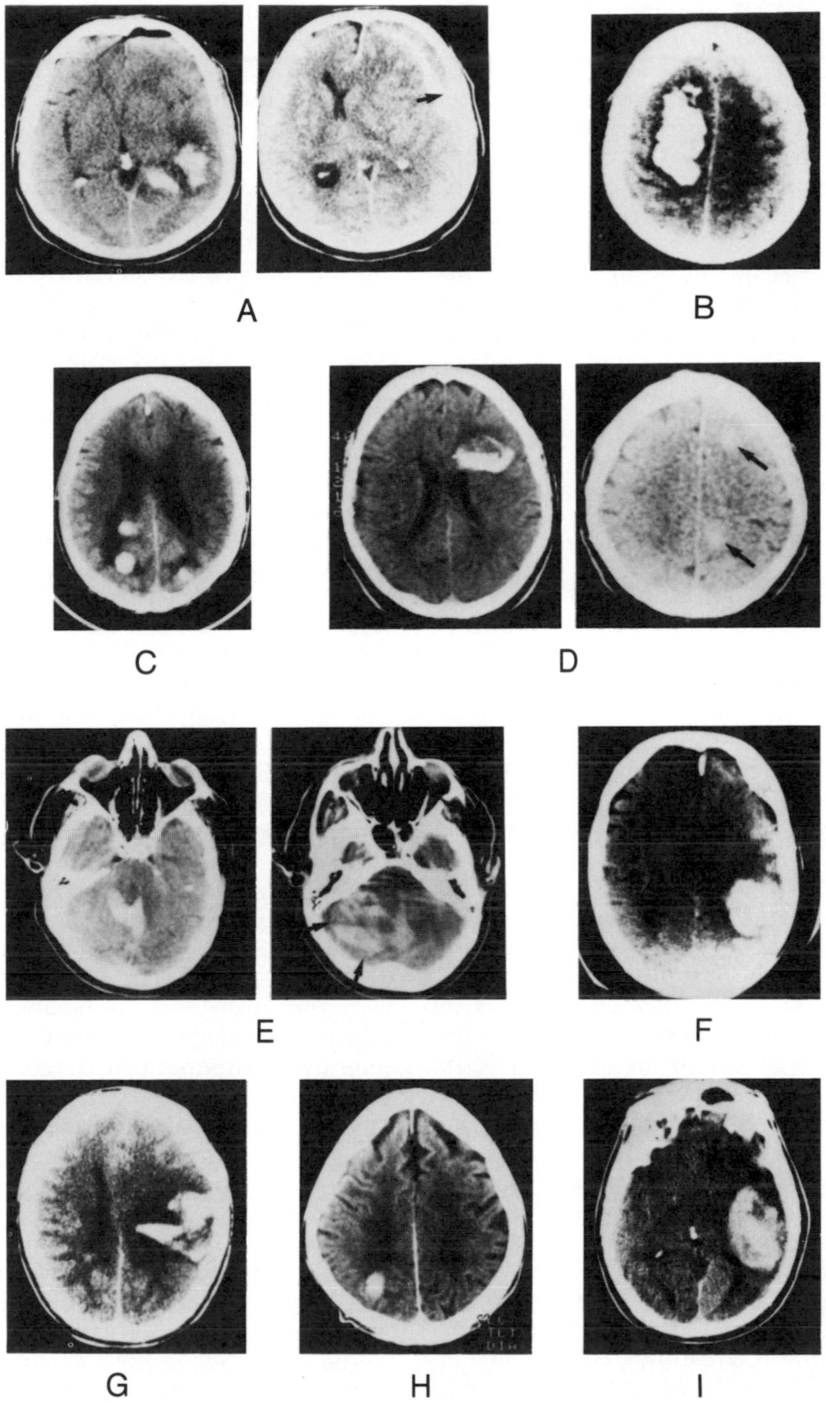


**Fig. 21-17.** Location of intracranial hemorrhage in nine patients treated with tPA for acute myocardial infarction. (**A**) Left temporal lobar hematoma (left panel), and chronic and acute subdural hematoma (*arrow*) (right panel). (**B**) Right parasagittal frontoparietal lobar hemorrhage. (**C**) Bilateral multiple occipital lobar hematomas. (**D**) Left frontal and occipital hematomas (*arrows*). (**E**) Right cerebellar hemorrhage (*arrows*) (right panel), with extension to the vermis and 4th ventricle (left panel). (**F**) Left posterior temporal lobar hematoma. (**G**) Left frontoparietal lobar hematoma with ventricular extension. (**H**) Small right posterior parietal parasagittal hematoma. (**I**) Left temporoparietal lobar hemorrhage. (From Kase et al.,[156] with permission.)

tion rate are absent.[132,212] The diagnosis is favored by lymphocytic CSF pleocytosis with elevated protein, and angiography may show a "beading" pattern in multiple medium and small-sized intracranial arteries. The instances of ICH reported in patients with GANS have occurred in the setting of progressive encephalopathy or myelopathy,[49,63] although occasionally ICH has been the first manifestation of the condition.[20] The hemorrhages have had a predominant lobar location, and in rare instances histologic examination of cerebral vessels has shown the association of GANS with CAA,[243,270] suggesting that either vascular lesion could have been responsible for the episode of ICH.

## BRAIN IMAGING

### Computed Tomography Scan

Computed tomography (CT) has had an impact on several aspects of the diagnosis of ICH. This noninvasive test allows not only a precise localization of the hemorrhage and its effects (midline shift, surrounding edema, ventricular extension),[166,267,326] but also provides rapid diagnosis of small or clinically atypical hemorrhages that in the past either were misdiagnosed as infarcts or required extensive invasive diagnostic efforts. This impact is reflected in several modern series of ICH that show lower mortality figures than in the past,[142,258,314,318] a difference largely due to the CT diagnosis of small (usually nonfatal) hemorrhages that were not usually detected in pre-CT series. The widespread use of this technique has also resulted in an apparent increase in the incidence of ICH in some areas, where the rise in hospital admissions for ICH has paralleled an increase in the use of CT.[258] In addition, the use of contrast infusion in CT in ICH offers the possibility of diagnosing an underlying cause in nonhypertensive or atypically located hematomas. An AVM can be suspected when post-contrast scans show the characteristic serpentiginous pattern of enlarged arteries and/or veins, seen in as many as two-thirds of the cases.[164] However, delayed scans may be necessary for the diagnosis of an underlying AVM in ICH, since the lesion can be missed in the acute phase, presumably as a result of its compression by the adjacent clot.[253] Finally, bleeding into an unsuspected tumor can be detected with CT scan by the presence of post-contrast enhancement in the area of the ICH,[110] a change not expected in the acute stages of primary ICH.[139]

The characteristic CT aspect of ICH is an area of increased attenuation in the parenchyma, with absorption values in the range of 40 to 90 Hounsfield units.[267] This high attenuation value of hematomas is mainly due to the hemoglobin protein (globin) contained in the extravasated blood.[221] This raises the possibility that ICH in anemic patients may not show as an area of increased CT attenuation, but rather as an isodense or hypodense area.[221] One such instance has been reported by Kasdon et al.,[150] in a severely anemic patient (hematocrit of 20 percent) with a surgically and pathologically proven cerebellar hematoma with an attenuation value of 17 Hounsfield units. In another instance, Jacome[147] reported two recurrent isodense cerebellar hematomas in a patient with a small AVM of the cerebellum. The reason for the lack of the characteristic CT hyperdensity was not found.

The acute hematoma is commonly surrounded by a thin halo of low absorption in the adjacent parenchyma, representing edema.[220] After 7 to 10 days, the high attenuation values of the hematoma start to decrease, always from the periphery into the center.[139,220] Depending on its size, the whole hematoma will become isodense, in 2 to 3 weeks if small, in 2 months if large,[220] and 2 to 4 months later the result will be an area of decreased density indicative of cavity formation.[30] The reduction in size and attenuation values in ICH has been shown to occur at a rate of 0.65 mm and 1.4 Hounsfield units per day, respectively.[66] The mass effect lags behind these two variables in its rate of resolution,[139] starting to decline after an average of 16.7 days after ictus.[66] This finding reflects the fact that the early signs of CT resolution (judged by reduction in size and attenuation values) merely represent changes in the physical properties of the extravasated blood, rather than actual reduction in hematoma size. In addition to these changes, resolving hematomas frequently show the appearance of "ring enhancement" after contrast infusion[139,326] (Fig. 21-18). This change can appear between 1 and 6 weeks from the onset,[314,326] can be abolished by administration of steroids,[318] and often disappears after 2 to 6 months.[326] This pattern is recognized as part of the natural CT course of ICH, and needs to be differentiated from the similar change observed in cerebral abscess.[326] The mechanism of production of "ring enhancement" in ICH is unclear. It has been suggested that it is due to hypervascularity at the periphery of the resolving hematoma[326] and/or disruption of the blood-brain barrier at this level, akin to that observed in cerebral infarction,[65] in which post-contrast enhancement occurs regularly.

The final stage in the CT evolution of an ICH represents the complete absorption of the necrotic and hemorrhagic tissue, leaving a residual cavity often ovoid or slitlike in shape (Fig. 21-19). This stage is reached after periods between 8 and 10 weeks from the initial hemorrhage. At times, the residual cavity from old ICH can be indistinguishable from that of old cerebral infarction.

A difficult differential diagnosis involves the differentiation between ICH and hemorrhagic infarction. The latter is a pathologic process of primary embolic ischemic necrosis with secondary aggregation of microspheres of red blood cells spread throughout the

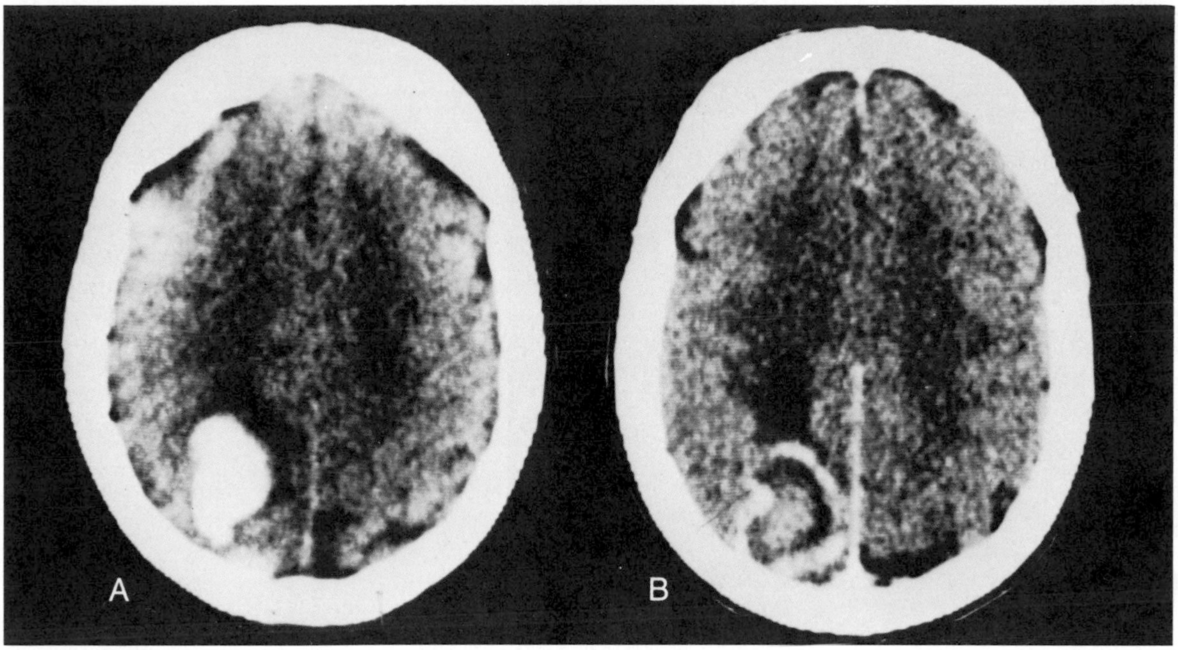


**Fig. 21-18.** (**A**) Right occipital hematoma shown on day 1 as a well-circumscribed homogeneous high-density lesion. (**B**) Repeat computed tomography scan 3 weeks later shows marked reduction in the size and density of the central high-density component, with a well-developed "ring" following intravenous contrast infusion.

area of infarction[99] (Fig. 21-20). This aggregation of petechiae into the infarcted area results in a change of the gross pathologic aspect of the infarct from pale to hemorrhagic. In instances of sparse accumulation of petechiae, their number may not be sufficient to change the attenuation values in the area of infarction by CT, and the lesion will be indistinguishable from a pale, nonhemorrhagic infarction.[59] On the other hand, a densely confluent aggregation of petechiae can result in a homogeneously high-density CT lesion, that may not be possible to differentiate from a primary ICH.[59,143] These high-density CT lesions corresponding to densely hemorrhagic infarctions usually show some degree of post-contrast enhancement. In

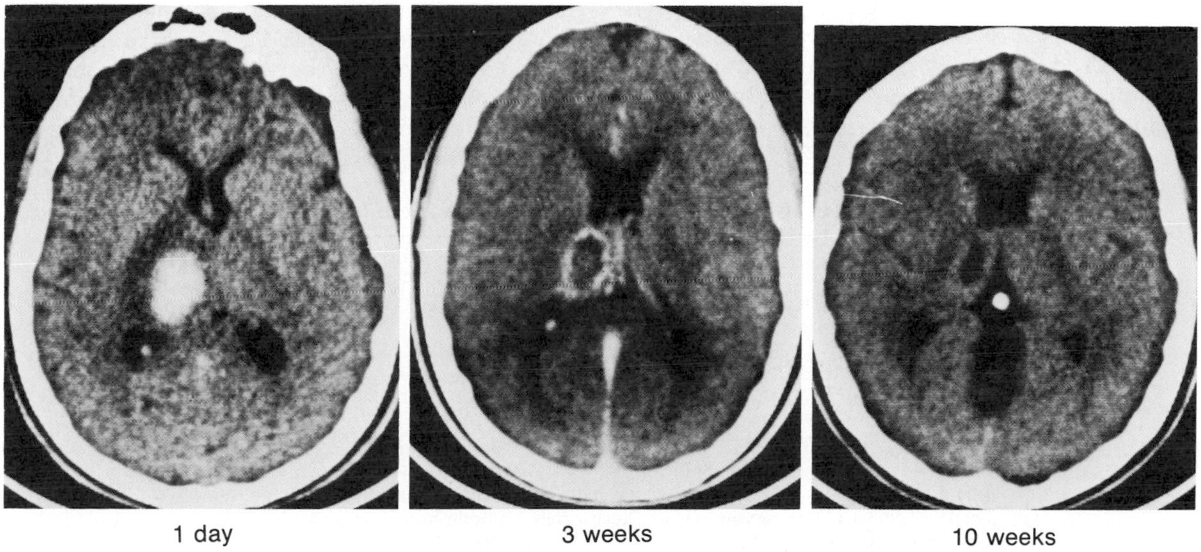


**Fig. 21-19.** Right thalamic hemorrhage shown in three stages of evolution, from the initial homogeneous high-density lesion (*left*), through an intermediate stage of "ring" enhancement following contrast infusion (*center*), into the chronic stage of cavity formation (*right*).

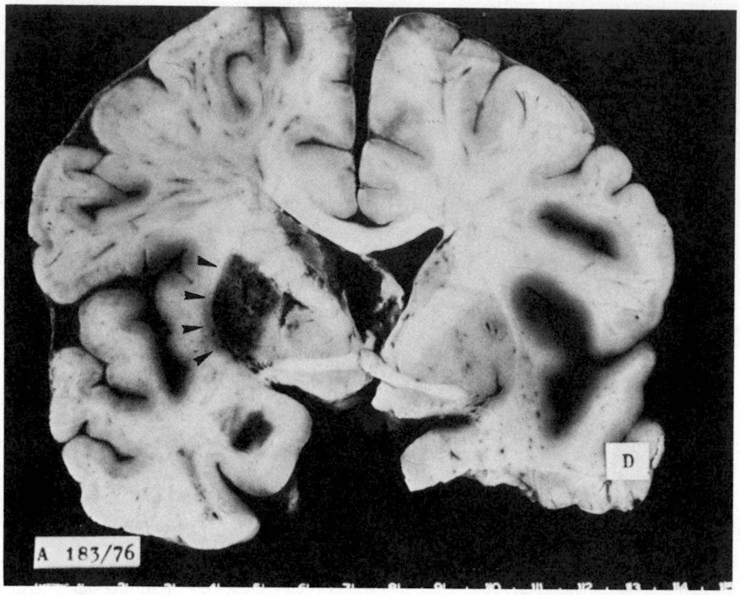


**Fig. 21-20.** Hemorrhagic infarction at the level of the left putamen, shown as an irregularly hemorrhagic area (*arrowheads*), without mass effect.

instances when it is difficult to separate densely hemorrhagic infarctions from ICHs, a combination of clinical, CT, and angiographic features usually allow for their differentiation (Table 21-3). The clinical differences stem from the fact that hemorrhagic infarction almost always results from arterial occlusion by an embolic mechanism, whereas ICH is a classic "mass lesion" associated with increased intracranial pressure (ICP). The differential criteria on CT include the morphology of the high-attenuation lesion (mottled or "spotted" in hemorrhagic infarction (Fig. 21-21), dense in ICH), presence or absence of mass effect, topography (subcortical vs corticosubcortical), distribution within or beyond arterial territories, pattern of post-contrast enhancement ("gyral" vs "ring"), and presence or absence of blood in the ventricular system. These CT criteria can be further enhanced by angiographic data, showing intracranial branch occlusions in embolic hemorrhagic infarction, and avascular mass effect in ICH. Among these criteria, those that categorically point to ICH are mass effect and presence of intraventricular blood. Features suggestive of hemorrhagic infarction are areas of high density in the brain parenchyma that follow strict anatomic patterns of arterial distribution, in addition to lack of mass effect.

## Magnetic Resonance Imaging

Magnetic resonance imaging (MRI) has become invaluable in the diagnosis of ICH. This technique not only separates hemorrhage from cerebral infarct, but also provides accurate information on the evolution of intracerebral hematoma, to a more precise degree than that obtained with CT scanning. The ability of MRI to distinguish between acute, subacute, and chronic hematomas is based primarily on its detection of the various chemical changes undergone by

**TABLE 21-3. Hematoma versus Hemorrhagic Infarction**

| | Distinguishing Features | |
|---|---|---|
| | Intracerebral Hematoma | Embolic Hemorrhagic Infarction |
| Clinical | | |
| Onset | Sudden → progression | Maximal from onset |
| ↑ ICP | Prominent | Absent |
| Embolic source | No | Yes |
| CT scan | | |
| High attenuation | Dense, homogeneous | Spotted, mottled |
| Mass effect | Prominent | Absent or mild |
| Location | Subcortical white matter | Cortex > subcortical white matter |
| Distribution | Beyond arterial territories | Along branch distribution |
| Late enhancement | "Ring" | "Gyral" |
| Ventricular blood | Yes | No |
| Angiogram | Mass effect (avascular) | Branch occlusion |

*Abbreviations:* ICP, intracranial pressure; CT, computed tomography.

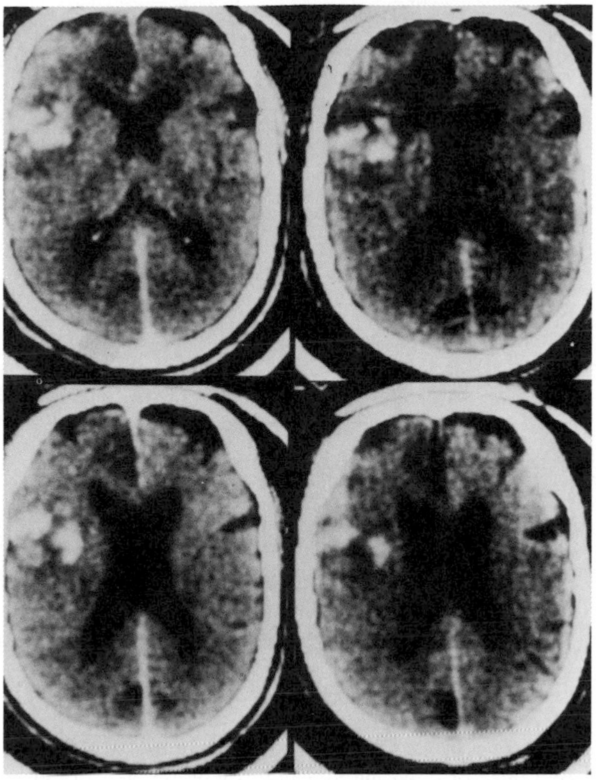

**Fig. 21-21.** Computed tomography aspect of hemorrhagic infarction, shown as irregular mottled areas of high density superimposed in a background of low density corresponding to ischemic infarction.

the hemoglobin molecule within the substance of the hemorrhage. In addition, the associated features of mass effect and perilesional edema can be further correlated with the hemoglobin changes to provide a precise picture of the evolution of ICH. Furthermore, the use of different MRI sequences, including the T1-weighted, T2-weighted, proton density, and gradient-echo (GE) images, provides a predictable change in signal intensity within the mass of the hemorrhage, in correlation with the specific time-dependent biochemical changes in the hemoglobin molecule, adding further precision to the estimated age of an intracerebral hematoma. These changes in the MRI characteristics of ICH have been recently summarized by Williams et al.[320] (Table 21-4).

In the *acute* stage of ICH, which is considered to be between onset and 1 week from onset, the mass of the hemorrhage is rich in oxygen-saturated hemoglobin (oxyhemoglobin). However, within short periods (hours from onset), oxygen is released from the hemoglobin molecule, and the mass of the hematoma increases its contents of deoxyhemoglobin, which is the predominant biochemical form of hemoglobin during the acute phase of ICH. Gomori et al.[116] have postulated that at this early stage of the evolution of a hematoma, its central portion is made of mostly intact red blood cells that contain high concentrations of intracellular deoxyhemoglobin. The change from oxyhemoglobin to deoxyhemoglobin takes place in the central portions of the hemorrhage and then proceeds gradually toward its periphery, thus resulting in a typical aspect on T2-weighted images of a hypointense central area, frequently surrounded by a rim of high signal change, the latter corresponding to surrounding edema[116] (Fig. 21-22). This central hypointensity on T2-weighted images correlates well with the hyperintensity of acute hematomas on CT scan.[116] The aspect of the acute hematoma on T1-weighted images is less characteristic, since it can be either hypointense or isointense, in comparison with the adjacent gray matter.[116]

The MRI characteristics of hyperacute ICH, within minutes of onset, are unknown in clinical cases because of the obvious limitations in scanning at such an early stage of bleeding. In experimental animals, Weingarten et al.[312] showed that T1- and T2-weighted sequences can fail to detect small ICHs in the hyperacute stage, whereas the use of GE sequences consistently documented the hemorrhages as hypointense

**TABLE 21-4. Appearance of Stages of a Hematoma on Magnetic Resonance Imaging**

| | Hematoma Center | | Hematoma Periphery | | Rim of Adjacent Brain | | Nearby White Matter | |
|---|---|---|---|---|---|---|---|---|
| Stage | SI T1 | SI T2 | SI T1 | SI T2 | SI T1 | SI T2 | SI T1 | SI T2 |
| Acute (1 day-week) | — or ↓ | ↓ ↓ (IC DHgb) | — | — | — | — | — | ↑ ↑ (Edema) |
| Early subacute (1–2 weeks) | — or ↓ | ↓ | ↑ ↑ (IC MHgb) | ↓ (IC MHgb) | — | — or ↓ | — | ↑ |
| Late subacute (2–4 weeks) | ↑ ↑ (EC MHgb) | ↑ ↑ (EC MHgb) | ↑ ↑ (EC MHgb) | ↑ ↑ (EC MHgb) | — | ↓ | — | ↑ |
| Early chronic (1–6 months) | ↑ | ↑ | ↑ | ↑ | — | ↓ ↓ (Hemosiderin) | — | — |
| Late chronic (>6 months) | — | ↓ | — | ↓ | — | ↓ ↓ (Hemosiderin) | — | — |

*Abbreviations and symbols:* SI T1, signal intensity T1-weighted image; SI T2, signal intensity T2-weighted image; —, normal signal intensity; ↓, decreased signal intensity; ↑, increased signal intensity; IC, intracellular; EC, extracellular; DHgb, deoxyhemoglobin; MHgb, methemoglobin.

(From Williams et al.,[320] with permission.)

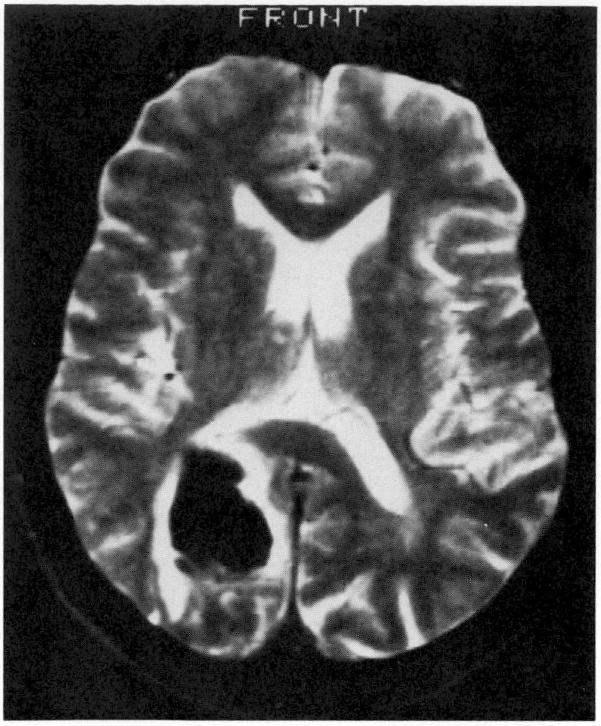


**Fig. 21-22.** Spin-echo sequence, T2-weighted (TR = 3,000 ms, TE = 90 ms) of right occipital hematoma with hypointense center and hyperintense halo of surrounding edema. (Courtesy of Dr. Jared K. Thomas, Department of Neuroradiology, Boston University Medical Center, Boston, MA.)

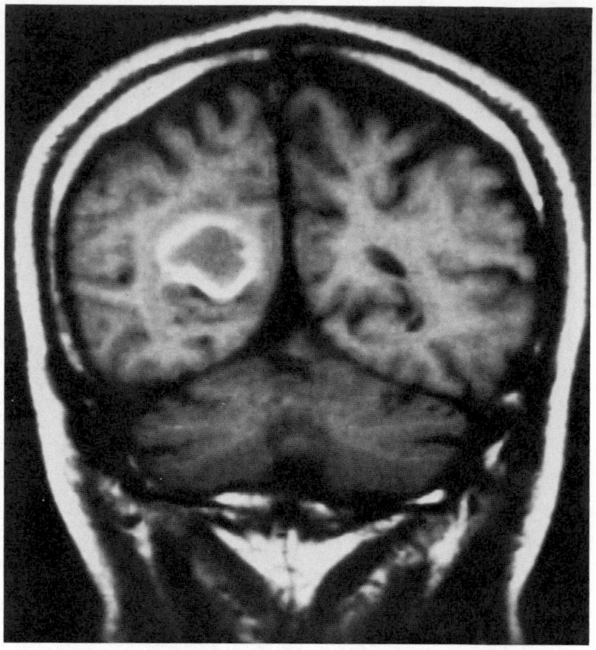

**Fig. 21-23.** Spin-echo sequence, T1-weighted (TR = 600 ms, TE = 15 ms) of right medial occipital hematoma with central isointense core, surrounded by hyperintense halo. (Courtesy of Dr. Jared K. Thomas, Department of Neuroradiology, Boston University Medical Center, Boston, MA.)

areas at this early stage. In the clinical setting, the high sensitivity of GE sequences for the detection of ICH of any age was recently supported by Zyed et al.,[329] who documented hypointense GE signal in 45 of 46 cases studied.

In the *subacute* stage of ICH, which encompasses the period between 1 and 4 weeks from onset, the main biochemical change is the progressive transformation of deoxyhemoglobin into methemoglobin. This change tends to occur first at the periphery of the hematoma, and it then gradually progresses centrally. As a result, the presence of methemoglobin produces a characteristic high signal change in T1-weighted images at the periphery of the hematoma, a change that subsequently involves the body of the hematoma further as the biochemical change progresses centrally[116] (Fig. 21-23). At this stage, T2-weighted images are typically hypointense, whereas in the later stages of the subacute phase of the hematoma the T2-weighted images become progressively more hyperintense, thus both T1 and T2 sequences having the same signal characteristic at the late subacute stages.

The *chronic* stage of intracerebral hematoma includes the period beyond 1 month from onset, at which time the hemoglobin molecule is progressively changing into hemosiderin, located primarily inside macrophages. This biochemical change correlates with marked hypointensity on T2-weighted images[116] (Fig. 21-24). The hypointensity will be more diffuse the more chronic the hematoma, whereas in the early phases of the chronic stage there may be a residual hyperintense center due to the presence of methemoglobin that has not yet changed into hemosiderin. The changes on T1-weighted images are basically the same as those described for the T2-weighted sequences. In a recent study of experimental ICH in rats, Thulborn et al.[287] reported the finding of ferritin, as well as hemosiderin, as the predominant iron-storage substances in chronic hematomas. These authors suggested that both compounds are responsible for the MRI changes observed at the late stage of evolution of intracerebral hematomas.

Although these MRI features of ICH are generally accurate, one has to be aware of a certain variability in the characteristics of the hematomas, in particular in their subacute and chronic stages. This relates primarily to the fact that the changes in the hemoglobin molecule take place gradually, and at times there may be mixture of the various components; for instance, residual methemoglobin may persist in the chronic stage, making the signal characteristics deviate partially from the schematic sequence depicted in Table 21-4.

In addition to its ability to determine the approximate age of the hematoma, MRI has the additional

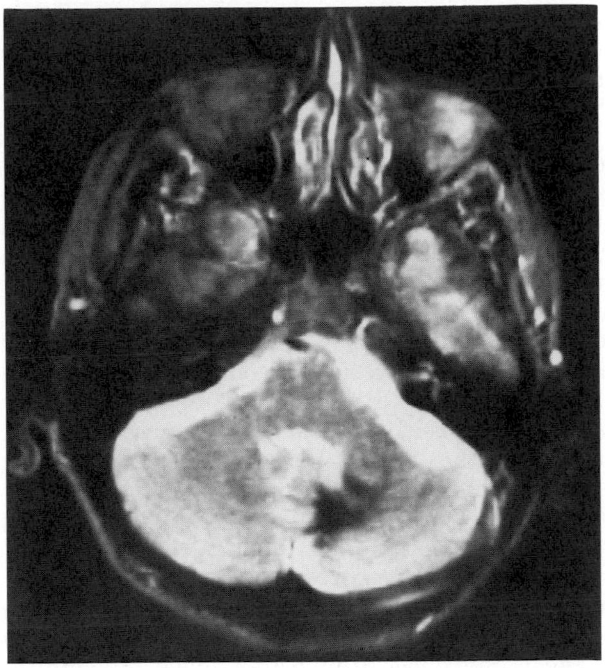

**Fig. 21-24.** Spin-echo sequence, T2-weighted (TR = 2,500 ms, TE = 90 ms) of old left cerebellar hemorrhage showing diffuse hypointensity, with no surrounding edema. (Courtesy of Dr. Jared K. Thomas, Department of Neuroradiology, Boston University Medical Center, Boston, MA.)

advantage of suggesting at times the mechanism of a nonhypertensive form of ICH. Among these are included (1) the demonstration of an adjacent vascular malformation (AVM or cavernous angioma) in the vicinities of an intracerebral hematoma, the vascular malformation being suggested by the presence of either a serpentiginous "flow void" or a round, at times calcified, vascular structure; and (2) the documentation of an underlying brain tumor, either primary or metastatic, adjacent to an acute ICH.

## GENERAL CLINICAL AND LABORATORY FEATURES

The different forms of ICH share a number of clinical features, that result from the progressive accumulation of a mass of blood in the parenchyma. These features include mode of onset, as well as clinical manifestations reflecting increased ICP. ICH occurs characteristically during activity,[95,101] and onset during sleep is extremely rare.[89] It occurred in only one instance in Fisher's series,[89] and in only 3 percent of ICH cases included in the NINCDS Stroke Data Bank.[172] The type of onset was studied in 70 cases of ICH prospectively included in the Harvard Cooperative Stroke Registry,[207] and was found to be one of gradual and smooth progression in two-thirds of the cases, the deficit being maximal from the onset in the remainder. No cases showed a regressive course in the acute phase, which supports the clinical dictum that a definite improvement in the early hours of a stroke syndrome rules out ICH.[226] Along with a gradual onset over periods of 5 to 30 minutes, patients with ICH frequently show some degree of decreased alertness at the time of admission, as a consequence of increased ICP. The frequency and severity of this sign vary to some extent according to the location of the hemorrhage, but when all forms are considered, it is present in at least 60 percent of the cases,[142,207] in two-thirds of them to a level of coma.[207,318] Coma has been correlated with ventricular extension of the hemorrhage,[68,89,318] large size of the hematoma,[68,142] and poor vital prognosis.[68,142,242,292,318]

Clinical features of ICH associated with increased ICP are headache and vomiting. Although they also vary widely in their frequency, depending on the location of the hemorrhage, their overall importance at the onset of ICH is limited.[207] Of 54 patients alert enough to report the symptom, only 36 percent reported headache in the series of Mohr et al.[207] Aring's[6] series disclosed a frequency of headache of 23 percent. The reporting of vomiting at onset follows similar frequencies, of 44 percent[207] and 22 percent[6] in these two series. These findings stress the important clinical point that absence of headache or vomiting does not rule out ICH. On the other hand, when present, these signs suggest ICH (or SAH) as the most likely diagnosis, since occlusive strokes show them in less than 10 percent of cases.[207]

Seizures at the onset of ICH are uncommon. They have been reported at rates as low as 7 percent,[207] 11 percent,[107] and 14 percent[6] when all forms of ICH are considered together. In some specific groups, frequencies go from zero[142,232,253] to as high as 32 percent in the lobar variety.[159] Their low general frequency is similar to that of occlusive stroke,[6,207] especially embolism,[207] and thus does not serve as a useful diagnostic feature.

In the general physical examination, a virtually constant abnormality is hypertension, found in as many as 91 percent of the cases in some series.[207] The high frequency of elevated blood pressure on admission in all forms of ICH correlates with other physical signs indicative of hypertension, such as left ventricular hypertrophy[2] and hypertensive retinopathy.[89] The examination of the ocular fundi in a case of suspected ICH serves the dual purpose of detecting signs of hypertensive retinopathy and allowing careful search for subhyaloid hemorrhages. These represent blood collections in the preretinal space, and their presence is virtually diagnostic of SAH,[226] since they rarely occur in primary ICH.[226,232,253] Although an occasional case of massive primary ICH will show this sign,[307] its presence has a high correlation with ruptured aneurysm as the cause of the intracranial hemorrhage. The findings on neurologic examination permit the differentiation of the different topographic varieties of ICH (see below).

The most reliable general laboratory examination for the diagnosis of ICH is examination of the cerebrospinal fluid (CSF). Communication of the hematoma with the ventricular space accounts for the presence of bloody or xanthochromic CSF in 70 to 90 percent of cases.[6,89,107,207,217,232,318] A somewhat lower frequency of bloody CSF (63 percent) has been reported in hematomas of lobar location,[253] probably reflecting the less frequent communication with the ventricular system[159] due to the subcortical location of the hematoma. The small percentages of cases with clear CSF in all series of ICH reflect hematomas of smaller size that do not reach the ventricular system, despite being at times located close to it. Furthermore, on account of their smaller size, the clinical presentation may not be clearly indicative of an ICH, as signs of increased ICP may be inconspicuous, making the differential diagnosis with ischemic stroke difficult. It is in this particular group of strokes that CT scan has had its most dramatic impact.

In addition to simple inspection of the CSF for bloody or xanthochromic aspect, spectrophotometric CSF analysis can disclose blood products in virtually 100 percent of cases.[167] However, this technique is not used routinely, as the widely available anatomic means of diagnosis (CT and MRI) has made CSF examination less crucial in establishing the presence of an ICH. The microscopic examination shows red blood cells in variable concentrations, sometimes as low as $100/mm^3$, more often[89] between several thousand and $1,000,000\ mm^3$. A second useful piece of information to be obtained from lumbar puncture is CSF pressure, which directly correlates with hematoma size, which in turn relates to prognosis.[68,142,159] The value of CSF examination in the diagnosis of ICH is still high, but this test is now less widely used as the availability of CT and MRI examination increases. Moreover, the uncommon but well-recognized precipitation of uncal or tonsilar herniation by lumbar puncture in supratentorial ICH[86,226,241] has contributed to the trend to defer the use of this test whenever CT scan examination is readily available.

The value of angiography in the evaluation of ICH cases has similarly declined since the introduction of CT and MR scanning. Most commonly, it shows the nonspecific signs of mass effect at the site of the hematoma,[286] and, occasionally, extravasation of contrast medium has been detected.[170,203] The study of Mizukami et al.[204] correlated the angiographic pattern of displacement of the lenticulostriate arteries with functional prognosis in putaminal hemorrhage. The obvious advantages of CT and MRI in disclosing most of the anatomic features of ICH has rendered angiography a procedure now used only in selected instances. Its main role at present is in the evaluation of nonhypertensive forms of ICH, multiple ICHs, or those located in "atypical" sites (hemispheral white matter, head of caudate nucleus), to look for possibilities of AVM, aneurysm, or tumor as the cause of the hemorrhage. Even this role is steadily diminishing with improvement in noninvasive brain imaging.

Recent studies have separated the clinical features and outcome of hematomas affecting the cerebral lobes from those involving deep structures (Table 21-5).[190] They have often been lumped together for the purpose of clinical trials, but some evidence suggests they should be considered separately. Headache at onset was an important finding in patients with lobar hemorrhage, but was not related to history of hypertension, size of the lesion, or outcome. This may be explained by local distension, distortion, or stretching of pain-sensitive intracranial superficial structures as responsible for the greater frequency of severe headache. Hypertension was less common in lobar than in deep hemorrhage. Seizures, which occur more often in lobar hemorrhage, were not associated with a higher early mortality or worsening. When a motor deficit was absent on admission neurologic examination, lobar hemorrhage was far more often the diagnosis than was deep hemorrhage, probably because many lobar hematomas affect the brain in areas other than the motor pathways, while deep hemorrhages rarely spare these pathways. The superficial location of lobar hematomas resulted in a greater frequency of visual field deficits. Otherwise, the neurologic examination does not readily differentiate the two groups. Hematoma size is usually smaller for deep hemorrhages than for lobar, making size alone a difficult measure for hemorrhages in general. The proximity of the ventricular system to the site of deep hemorrhage probably accounts for the greater fre-

**TABLE 21-5. Comparison of Lobar versus Deep Hemorrhages**

| | Lobar Hemorrhage | | | Deep Hemorrhage | | |
|---|---|---|---|---|---|---|
| CT Variables | Total | Coma | % | Total | Coma | % |
| Volume <15 ml | 14 | 3 | 21.4 | 48 | 8 | 16.7 |
| IVH | | | | | | |
| Yes | 1 | 1 | 100 | 21 | 7 | 33.3 |
| No | 13 | 2 | 15.4 | 27 | 1 | 3.7 |
| Volume 15–50 ml | 23 | 8 | 34.8 | 37 | 14 | 37.8 |
| IVH | | | | | | |
| Yes | 4 | 3 | 75.0 | 23 | 12 | 52.2 |
| No | 19 | 5 | 26.3 | 14 | 2 | 14.3 |
| Volume >50 ml | 28 | 15 | 53.6 | 22 | 18 | 81.8 |
| IVH | | | | | | |
| Yes | 11 | 9 | 81.8 | 14 | 12 | 85.7 |
| No | 17 | 6 | 35.3 | 8 | 6 | 75.0 |
| All volumes | 65 | 26 | 40.0 | 107 | 40 | 37.4 |
| IVH | | | | | | |
| Yes | 16 | 13 | 81.3 | 58 | 31 | 53.5 |
| No | 49 | 13 | 26.5 | 49 | 9 | 18.4 |

*Abbreviations:* CT, computed tomography; IVH, intraventricular hemorrhage.

(Modified from Massarro et al.,[190] with permission.)

quency of ventricular extension in this group of patients. A relationship between hematoma volume and intraventricular extension of the hemorrhage exists for lobar hemorrhage, but not the same as for deep hemorrhages, where even small hematomas present with a high frequency of intraventricular hemorrhage (IVH). Although clinical outcome correlates with hematoma volume, the different relationship between intraventricular extension and hematoma size in lobar versus deep hemorrhage may help explain why these two groups have a similar prognosis in spite of larger mean hematoma volume for those with lobar hemorrhage.

The design of future clinical trials for supratentorial ICH may need to account for these complex interrelationships with volume, brain displacement, and coma scores, particularly when treatment is aimed at evacuating or reducing the hematoma volume.

## SUPRATENTORIAL INTRACEREBRAL HEMORRHAGE

The majority of cases of intracerebral hemorrhage occur in the supratentorial compartment, mostly involving the deep structures of the cerebral hemispheres, the basal ganglia, and the thalamus.[68,87,107,159,207,225,318] In addition, a significant number of hemispheral ICH cases occur at the level of the subcortical white matter of the cerebral lobes, the so-called "lobar" hemorrhages.[159,253] These various forms of ICH have distinctive features in terms of clinical presentation, CT aspects, course, and therapy.

### Putaminal Hemorrhage

Putaminal hemorrhage is the most common form of ICH and has several clinical subtypes determined by the size and pattern of extension of the hematoma. Each of these variables independently determines the prognosis. Overall, a mortality of 37 percent is expected,[142] a figure that is far lower than those quoted in the pre-CT literature,[199] which did not include the undiagnosed smaller cases.[68]

The "classical" presentation putaminal hemorrhage described the massive hemorrhages, with rapidly evolving unilateral weakness accompanied by sensory, visual, and behavioral abnormalities. Headache is common, as is vomiting, within a few hours from the onset.[207] Although the onset is abrupt, there is typically a gradual evolution of both the focal deficit and the level of consciousness in the following minutes or hours.[89,226] A deficit maximal from the onset is uncommon. Whether sudden or gradual in evolution, moderate or large hematomas are invariably accompanied by a decreased level of alertness correlated with hematoma size. Once the syndrome is well developed, neurologic examination shows a dense flaccid hemiplegia with a hemisensory syndrome and homonymous hemianopia, with global aphasia in dominant hemisphere hematomas, or hemi-inattention in nondominant lesions.[89,226] A conjugate horizontal gaze palsy, with the eyes conjugately deviated toward the side of the lesion, is usually found, which can be reversed momentarily by doll's head maneuver or ice-water caloric testing.[241] The pupillary size and reactivity are normal unless uncal herniation has occurred, in which case signs of an ipsilateral 3rd cranial nerve palsy will be present.[89] These abnormalities in oculomotor function have a poor prognosis.[142] Total unilateral motor deficit, coma, and clinical progression following admission, all correlate with large hematoma size and poor functional and vital prognosis, as does ventricular extension of the hematoma by CT scan.[142] In all probability, the increased mortality reflects the large size of the hematoma required to dissect a course from the laterally placed original site of bleeding into the paramedian ventricular wall, rather than any primary independent effects of blood entering the ventricular system.[280] Further support of this point is the occurrence of ventricular extension in other varieties of ICH, such as caudate ICH,[280] which has an excellent vital prognosis (see below).

The patient whose CT scan is shown in Figure 21-25 illustrates many of these points. A healthy man, aged 60, collapsed at work and vomited while being transported to the hospital. On arrival, showing left hemiplegia and conjugate ocular deviation to the right, he was initially conversant, but sank into a state of lethargy over an hour, and spontaneous speech was no longer present. He was minimally responsive to painful stimuli only, and, if unstimulated, he would fall into moderately deep sleep. The right limbs withdrew

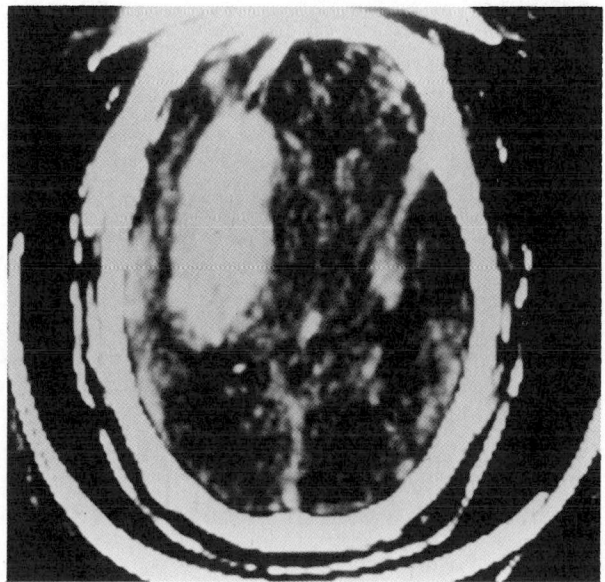

**Fig. 21-25.** Massive right putaminal hemorrhage with marked midline shift and ventricular extension.

appropriately to pain, but similar stimuli on the left limbs only produced stereotypic movements of shoulder adduction. At times, he moved the right limbs in a nonpurposeful way during periods of agitation, but the left limbs were densely plegic. A CT scan revealed a massive right putaminal hemorrhage with marked shift of midline structures and extension of the hemorrhage into the ventricular system (Fig. 21-25). He was treated with antihypertensive medications and supportive measures until his death 12 hours after admission. Postmortem examination revealed a massive recent right putaminal hemorrhage, in addition to a small recent hemorrhage originating from the posterior corner of the contralateral putamen (Fig. 21-26).

The presence of two hypertensive putaminal hemorrhages, one recent and one old, has been described several times in pathologic material,[95,106,195,216,291] but the occurrence of simultaneous fresh bilateral putaminal hemorrhages is distinctly uncommon: it was observed in only 2 of 86 cases in Fisher's series,[87] and in none of 42 hypertensive ICH cases from McCormick and Schochet's series.[195] Multiple ICHs are rare unless due to bleeding diathesis associated with thrombocytopenia,[87,272] metastatic tumor,[110] or cerebral amyloid angiopathy.[111]

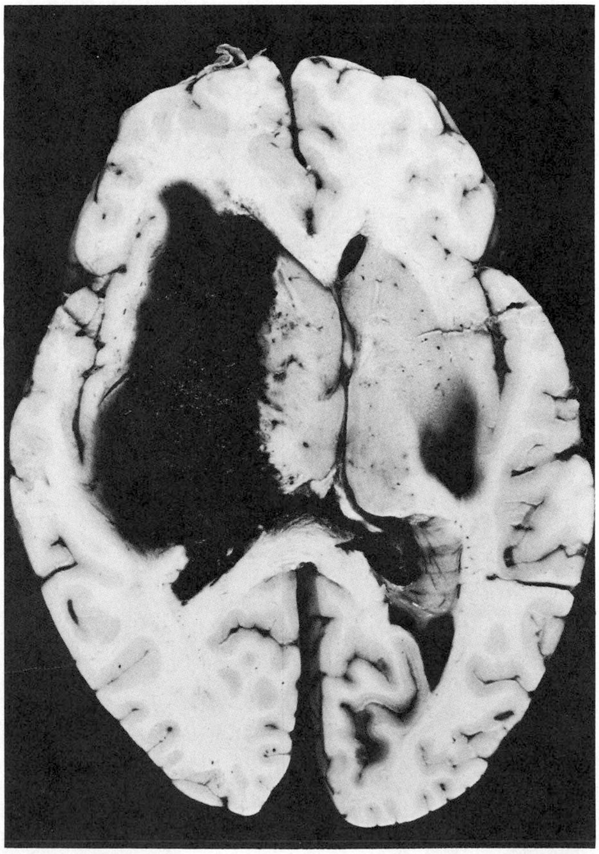

**Fig. 21-26.** Postmortem specimen showing extensive right putaminal hemorrhage (left side of picture) with ventricular extension. Incidental finding of small hemorrhage on the posterior corner of the contralateral (left) putamen.

## Syndromes of Smaller Hematomas

Although many variants of putaminal hemorrhage are recognized, few are well known clinically. Most of the tiny putaminal hemorrhages in pathologic material have occurred along with large hematomas that have dominated the clinical picture.[95] The smallest examples reported by Hier et al.[142] (Cases 1 through 6), showed motor deficits in a level of hemiparesis rather than hemiplegia, contralateral hemisensory deficits, and normal extraocular movements; five of six had full visual fields, and five of six were alert. They all survived and left the hospital with a mild functional disability. Rarely, syndromes of pure hemiparesis have been described from a small putaminal hemorrhage.[223,285] Their rarity suggests that a putaminal hemorrhage large enough to compress or destroy the adjacent internal capsule wall is expected to involve the sensory capsular or paracapsular pathways, leading to a combined sensorimotor syndrome.

Signs of good functional and vital prognosis in putaminal hemorrhage include partial motor deficit, alert mental status, normal extraocular movements and full visual fields.[142] Mizukami and colleagues, who analyzed the prognosis for recovery in relationship to angiographic[204] and CT[205] findings, found their angiographic data correlated the pattern of displacement of the lenticulostriate arteries in the anteroposterior views; pattern of medial displacement of the distal branches of these arteries was a poor prognostic sign, as it indicated medial extension of the hematoma into the posterior limb of the internal capsule, frequently transecting it. The preservation of the normal configuration of these arteries was associated with a better functional prognosis. From CT scan, the main prognostic feature was the upward extension of the hematoma: cases with hematomas restricted to a CT level corresponding to the posterior limb of the internal capsule had in general better functional prognosis than those in whom the hematoma was also visible on higher cuts.[205]

Hemichorea-hemiballismus, usually described from lacunes,[153] has been reported with CT-documented hemorrhage,[181] which showed the lesion in the subthalamic nucleus, and a case of bilateral ballism with CT-proven hemorrhagic lesions in the basal ganglia[308] disclosed lesions compatible with hemorrhagic infarction rather than primary ICH.

Partial capsular involvement by a small adjacent putaminal hematoma could result in a sensorimotor deficit, with marked dissociation between upper and lower limb involvement, but instances of upper or lower limb monoparesis or monoplegia have thus far not been documented in putaminal hemorrhage,[89] probably on account of the closely packed arrangement of corticospinal fibers in the internal capsule,[79,130,256] which make selective fiber involvement by a lesion of expanding character difficult to achieve.

Between the extreme varieties of putaminal hemorrhage lies the common type of medium-sized putaminal hematoma. This intermediate variety is characterized by moderate to severe sensorimotor deficit, with minimal or no involvement of oculomotor, visual, or language functions, and is at times associated with remarkably rapid and complete recovery of function. These cases with good prognosis usually compress but do not destroy the internal capsule, by remaining confined to the putaminoclaustral area, without extending medially into the ventricular system.[142] The case documented by Figure 21-27 illustrates these points. This previously healthy 52-year-old man awoke able to get out of bed and walk unassisted, at that time moving the left arm less than normal with the left side of his face "drooping." He had no headache, was able to eat, and had no vomiting. Examination shortly thereafter found a mild proximal paresis of the left arm and leg, the sensory examination was intact for touch and pin, joint position sense and vibration, and he showed a mild left-sided extinction for double simultaneous tactile stimulation of the limbs, trunk, and face. His eyes were conjugately deviated to the right, and attempts at voluntary left gaze would only produce about 1 to 2 mm deviation across the midline to the left, but horizontal gaze was conjugate and full in both directions on testing of ocular pursuit.

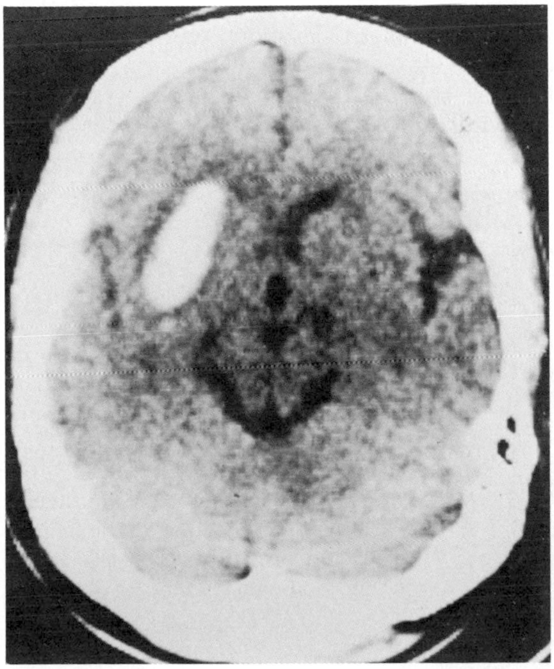

**Fig. 21-27.** Moderate-sized right putaminal hemorrhage with mild effacement of the frontal horn of the lateral ventricle.

## Patterns of Extension from the Putamen

Extension laterally or superiorly from the putamen greatly increases the severity of the syndrome, even when the hematoma remains small. Lateral extension into the dominant frontotemporal white matter leads to aphasia,[5] and the nondominant parietal lobe produces hemi-inattention and neglect.[226,299] Of interest concerning the aphasia theory, lateral extension into the arcuate fasciculus is thought to be the cause of "conduction" aphasia,[17] yet such extension, common in putaminal hemorrhage,[5,226] has not caused this syndrome, global aphasia,[142,210] or relatively nonspecific aphasias with fluent, poorly articulated speech, prominent paraphasias, and relatively spared repetition[5] being the rule.

When a putaminal hematoma expands vertically, it collects along the white fiber tracts of the corona radiata and centrum semiovale. This extension into the nondominant frontal and parietal lobes results in prominent inattention and neglect syndromes,[142] which at times may acquire more relevance than the sensorimotor deficit.

## Caudate Hemorrhage

This variety of ICH called caudate hemorrhage has been rarely reported in the literature, since it is usually included with putaminal hemorrhage as an example of "basal ganglia" hematoma.[106,260] Caudate hemorrhage represents approximately 5 to 7 percent of cases of ICH[280] (see Table 21-2), a frequency similar to that of cerebellar hemorrhage.[101,232] Most cases in the literature have been isolated instances reported because of unusual etiologic factors such as eclampsia[4] or vascular malformations of arteriovenous[16,38] or cavernous type.[193] However, as in all varieties of ICH, its most common etiology has been arterial hypertension.[280] The bleeding vessels correspond to deep penetrating branches of the anterior and middle cerebral arteries, vessels of diameter similar to those that supply the putamen and thalamus.[281] Due to its paraventricular location, the caudate also receives blood supply from ependymal arteries that flow outward from the ventricular surface into the parenchyma. These arteries originate beneath the ependymal surface as terminal branches of the anterior choroidal artery, posterior choroidal artery, and striatal rami of the middle cerebral artery.[29]

A number of reported cases of spontaneous hemorrhage in the caudate nucleus has delineated a relatively consistent clinical picture[14,31,100,280] (Table 21-6). The onset has generally been abrupt, with headache and vomiting commonly followed by variable degrees of decreased level of consciousness. Seizures at onset have been rarely reported,[16] and were not encountered in the series of 12 patients reported by Stein et al.[280] Consistent findings in the physical examination have included neck stiffness and various types of be-

**TABLE 21-6. Clinical Picture in Five Cases of Caudate Nucleus Hemorrhage**

| | Patients | | | | |
|---|---|---|---|---|---|
| | 1 | 2 | 3 | 4 | 5 |
| History | | | | | |
| Age | 67 | 56 | 48 | 20 | 50 |
| Hypertension | − | + | + | + | − |
| Symptoms | | | | | |
| Headache | ? | Yes | Yes | Yes | Yes |
| Nausea/vomiting | No | Yes | Yes | Yes | Yes |
| Seizures | No | No | No | No | No |
| Loss of consciousness | − | − | − | − | − |
| Findings on physical exam | | | | | |
| Obtundation | | + | | | |
| Lethargy | + | | + | + | + |
| Abulia | + | − | − | − | + |
| Weakness | Yes | No | Yes | Yes | Yes |
| Plantars (L-R) | ↓ ↓ | ↓ ↓ | ↑ ↑ | ↓ ↑ | ↓ ↓ |
| Sensory deficit | − | − | − | − | + |
| Extraocular movements | Full | Full | Paresis, horizontal and vertical | Full | Paresis, vertical |
| Neck stiffness | + | + | + | + | + |
| Computed tomography scan | | | | | |
| Ventricular extension | (+) | (+) | (+) | (+) | (+) |
| Hydrocephalus | (−) | (+) | (+) | (+) | (+) |
| Arteriogram | Not done | Normal | Incidental aneurysm | Not done | Normal |

havioral abnormalities, the latter most often in the form of disorientation and confusion, occasionally accompanied by a prominent short-term memory defect.[43,280] All these features tend to be temporary.[280] The clinical picture is similar to that of subarachnoid hemorrhage from ruptured aneurysm.

In approximately 50 percent of the cases the common clinical features are accompanied by others, most often taking the form of transient gaze paresis and contralateral hemiparesis, a rare case showing elements of an ipsilateral Horner syndrome.[280] The abnormalities described in gaze mechanisms have most often been horizontal gaze palsies with conjugate deviation or preference toward the side of the hemorrhage, with full correction by oculocephalic maneuvers. Less commonly, vertical gaze palsy has been described, either combined with a horizontal gaze palsy or, more commonly, as an isolated phenomenon. Occasionally, the motor deficit is accompanied by a transient hemisensory syndrome. In those instances in which hemiparesis is a feature, the weakness tends to be slight (never to a degree of hemiplegia) and transient, resolving within days from the onset.[14,100,280]

The case shown in Figure 21-28 is typical of the minor syndromes. This 48-year-old diabetic and hy-

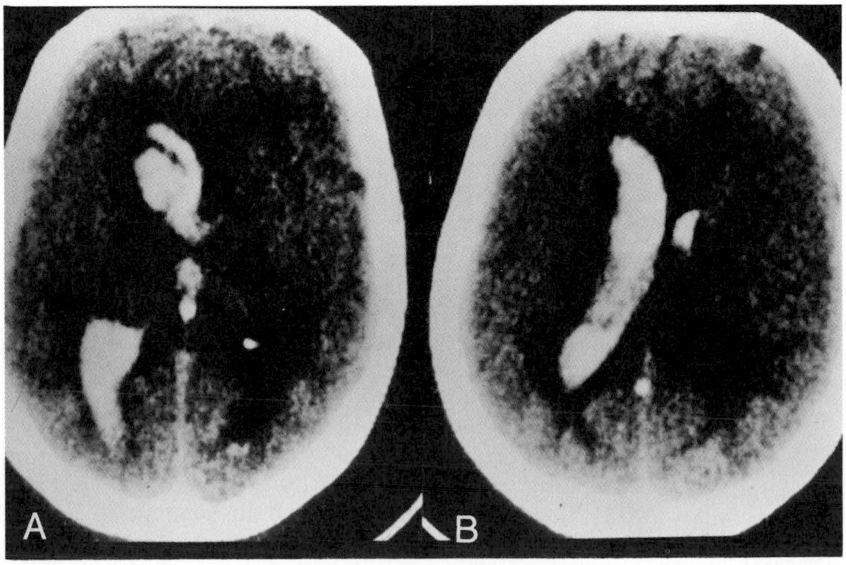


**Fig. 21-28.** (**A**) Hemorrhage originating in the head of the right caudate nucleus with extension into the anterior limb of the internal capsule and into the ipsilateral ventricle and third ventricle. (**B**) Extensive amount of intraventricular blood in the body of the lateral ventricles, primarily on the right side, associated with moderate hydrocephalus.

pertensive female had sudden severe headache and collapsed to the ground, regaining consciousness within 5 to 10 minutes, somnolent but able to talk with dysarthric speech. She vomited repeatedly. On initial examination she was lethargic, with paralysis of the left arm and weakness of the leg, the eyes conjugate and in midposition. There was no horizontal or vertical deviation to the doll's eyes maneuver or ice-water stimulation. The pupils were 3 mm, minimally reactive to light. She showed no facial motility to pain. A CT scan revealed a right intracerebral hematoma at the level of the head of the caudate nucleus and anterior limb of the internal capsule, with ventricular extension and massive amounts of blood into the 3rd and 4th ventricles and accompanying hydrocephalus. She improved remarkably within 12 hours and could answer to questions with full sentences, and follow verbal commands. Over the following days she was able to deviate the eyes to the right voluntarily, lacking only about 1 mm of full excursion, but they could not cross the midline to the left. Over a period of 24 hours, she became alert, was able to answer questions appropriately, and had slight left arm weakness, but now had full and conjugate eye movements.

In typical cases, CT scan shows a hematoma located in the area of the head of the caudate nucleus. Ventricular extension into the frontal horn of the ipsilateral ventricle is an invariable feature.[280] In approximately 75 percent of cases, mild to moderate hydrocephalus of the body and temporal horns of the lateral ventricles has been present.

In general, hemorrhages present a picture of a subarachnoid hemorrhage; those of medium and large size are frequently accompanied by transient gaze palsies and hemiparesis, and those featuring an ipsilateral Horner syndrome have a more inferior and lateral extension of the hemorrhage. Occasionally, the hematomas extend from the region of the head of the caudate nucleus into the anterior portions of the thalamus (Fig. 21-29). In two such isolated instances,[43,280] the clinical syndrome has featured a prominent but transient short-term memory defect. Prior to the introduction of CT scan, these cases of caudate ICH with consistent extension into the ventricular system may have been diagnosed as cases of "subarachnoid hemorrhage with negative arteriography," or even as cases of so-called "primary intraventricular hemorrhage."[29] The latter is probably a very rare condition,[225] in most instances reflecting a lack of documentation of the parenchymal or meningeal (in cases of ruptured aneurysm) site of origin of the bleed, rather than a hemorrhage truly confined to the ventricular space. Such an occurrence has not been documented in our institution in a consecutive series of over 250 cases of intracranial hemorrhage observed over a 6-year period.

Caudate hemorrhage can be separated from putaminal and thalamic hemorrhage clinically and radiographically. Headache, nausea, vomiting, and stiff neck regularly accompany caudate hemorrhage,[280] but are less common manifestations in putaminal hemorrhage.[142] Disorders of language are regular features of putaminal and thalamic hemorrhage in the dominant hemisphere,[142,211,308] whereas hemorrhages that remain confined to the caudate nucleus have not been associated with aphasia.[280] Furthermore, caudate hemorrhages in the nondominant hemisphere do not show the behavioral abnormalities of hemi-inattention and anosognosia associated with thalamic[32,264,309] and putaminal[142] hemorrhages in that hemisphere. Caudate hemorrhage needs also to be distinguished from anterior communicating artery aneurysms that bleed into the brain parenchyma. In primary caudate hemorrhage there is no accumulation of blood in the interhemispheric fissure, and the majority of the blood is located in the lateral ventricle adjacent to the involved caudate nucleus. In addition, extension of the hemorrhage into the basal frontal region, a feature invariably seen when hemorrhage into the parenchyma results from ruptured anterior communicating aneurysm, is rarely present in caudate ICH.[280]

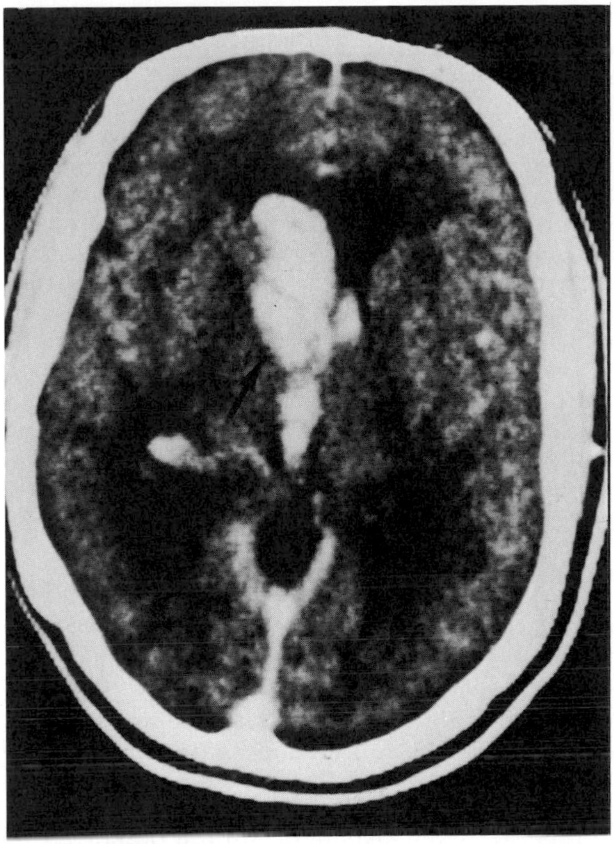

**Fig. 21-29.** Hemorrhage originating from the head of the left caudate nucleus with extension into the anterior-dorsal aspect of the thalamus (*arrow*), lateral ventricle, and third ventricle.

The outcome in caudate hemorrhage is usually benign, and the majority of patients recover fully, without permanent neurologic sequelae.[280] The accompanying hydrocephalus characteristically tends to disappear as the hemorrhage resolves, and ventriculoperitoneal shunting for persistent hydrocephalus has been rarely required.[280] This generally benign outcome in caudate ICH occurs despite the almost constant ventricular extension of the hemorrhage, stressing the fact that the latter in itself is not necessarily a bad prognostic sign in hemorrhages originating in the vicinities of the ventricular system, such as in caudate and thalamic ICH. The documented poor prognostic value of this feature in putaminal ICH[68,142] reflects the required large size of a laterally originated putaminal hematoma to be able to extend enough medially to open into the ventricular system.

## Thalamic Hemorrhage

The thalamic form of ICH represents from 10 to 15 percent of parenchymatous hemorrhage.[87,106,107,159,172,207,308,318] Its clinical and pathologic characteristics are well recognized, and the spectrum of clinical variations reflects the size and pattern of extension of the hematoma. The mass originates in the thalamus and, if it enlarges, extends laterally (into the internal capsule), medially (into the 3rd ventricle), or inferiorly (into the subthalamus and dorsal midbrain).[226] Even upward extension into the parietal white matter can occur in the larger cases (see Case 5).

The characteristic clinical picture has several distinctive features. These are shown in Table 21-7, which includes a total of 41 patients from the two largest series reported.[12,308] A typical mode of presentation features a rapid onset of unilateral sensorimotor deficit, frequent occurrence of vomiting (about half of the cases), but a low frequency of headache (less than one-third of the cases). Infrequently noted[12,83,86,226] is the more abrupt onset than in putaminal hemorrhage.[112,247,309] In some the onset was as coma.[83,308] In our studies,[158] only a third had the gradual progression that characterizes two-thirds of ICHs in general[207] and 70 percent of putaminal bleeds.[142] A slowly progressive initial course with headache preceding the focal deficits is distinctly uncommon,[226] and only 4 of 13 patients in the series of Walshe et al.[308] evolved with symptoms for 1 to 2 hours before developing hemiparesis. Few present initially with unilateral sensory symptoms (numbness) preceding the onset of hemiparesis and stupor.[83,304,308]

The physical findings (Table 21-7) include hemiparesis or hemiplegia in 100 percent of the cases,[12,83,308] virtually all of them with an associated severe hemisensory syndrome. The latter usually occurs as a decrease or loss of all sensory modalities over the contralateral limbs, face, and trunk,[226] but small hematomas have affected superficial sensation in a partial distribution in some cases.[308] The motor deficit is severe and equal in upper and lower limbs, but at times the lower limb has been relatively less affected.[308] The severity and distribution of the motor and sensory symptoms are similar to those of putaminal hemorrhage, therefore not serving as useful differential points. A homonymous hemianopia is an uncommon finding, and tends to be transient,[86,89] probably reflecting the location of the lateral geniculate body below and lateral to the bleed. This sign would be expected in large bleeds with extrathalamic extension, but those, in addition, affect consciousness severely, precluding the detection of the visual field defect.

**TABLE 21-7. Clinical Features of Thalamic Hemorrhage**

| | Walshe et al.[308] ($N$ = 18) | Barraquer-Bordas et al.[12] ($N$ = 23) |
|---|---|---|
| History | | |
| Age (mean) | 64 | 68 |
| Headache | 22% | 30% |
| Vomiting | 77% | 48% |
| Physical findings | | |
| Level of consciousness | | |
| Alert | 6% | 21% |
| Drowsy | 33% | 40% |
| Stuporous | 33% | 18% |
| Comatose | 28% | 21% |
| Hemiplegia–hemiparesis | 100% | 100% |
| Hemisensory deficit | 100% | 100% |
| Homonymous hemianopia | — | 18% |
| Aphasia | 4/7[a] | 4 |
| Mutism | 1 | 1 |
| Anosognosia | 2/3[a] | 2 |
| Upward gaze palsy | 94% | 35% |
| Horizontal ocular deviation | | |
| Toward side of lesion | 6 | 3 |
| Opposite side of lesion | 3 | 6 |
| Pupillary abnormalities | | |
| Miosis | 100% | 70% |
| Loss light reflex | 62% | 13% |
| Mortality | 50% | 39% |

[a] Number of patients with deficit/number of patients tested.

The landmark in the clinical presentation of thalamic hemorrhage is in the oculomotor findings. The most characteristic combination is one of upward gaze palsy with miotic unreactive pupils[12,83,86,89,308] elements of Parinaud syndrome, caused by the enlarging mass exerting effects on the upper midbrain. The upward gaze palsy determines the ocular position at rest of conjugate downward deviation, sometimes associated with convergence, as if the eyes were "peering at the tip of the nose."[86] In addition, convergence paralysis, nystagmus retractorius on attempted upward gaze, and skew deviation are frequently present.[86,89,226] Other less common oculomotor abnormalities reported in thalamic hemorrhage include downward gaze palsy;[86,89] anisocoria with ipsilateral miosis, sometimes associated with palpebral ptosis;[89] transient opsoclonus;[161] ipsilateral[12,308] or contralateral[12,160,308] horizontal ocular deviation.

Figure 21-30 illustrates an example of thalamic hemorrhage. This previously healthy 58-year-old male was found unresponsive with signs of vomitus and urinary and fecal incontinence. On admission examination his blood pressure was 180/100, and he was comatose. He promptly showed decerebrate posturing on the right and decorticate posturing occurred on the left in response to painful stimuli. The eyes showed no skew at rest and were engaged in regular roving horizontal movements. The doll's head maneuver in the vertical plane produced only full conjugate depression, whereas upward movements were limited only to 2 mm on the right and 1 mm on the left eye. Pupils were 2 mm, unreactive to bright light. He expired 8 days after the onset. A CT scan on admission showed a left thalamic hemorrhage with extension into the 3rd ventricle, both lateral ventricles, aqueduct and 4th ventricle, with moderate hydrocephalus (Fig. 21-30A). There was significant upward extension into the left parietal white matter with midline shift (Fig. 21-30B).

The classical combination of upward gaze palsy with miotic unreactive pupils has high diagnostic value, and it is due to compressive or destructive effects of the thalamic hematoma on the underlying midbrain tectum.[12,86,89,308] The precise anatomic structures involved in these oculomotor abnormalities have been delineated by experimental studies in monkeys[62,233] and a number of observations in humans.[45,46,219] The experimental observations of Pasik et al.[233] established that involvement of the posterior commissure and the "nucleus interstitialis of the posterior commissure" was consistently associated with upward gaze palsy. Areas that were not essential for the development of the gaze palsy included the superior colliculi, nuclei of Cajal and Darkschewitsch, and the medial thalamus. The observations of Christoff et al.[45,46] in human clinicopathologic material concluded that most lesions producing upward gaze palsy required bilateral or midline involvement of the midbrain tectum, particularly when loss of pupillary light reflex coexisted.[46] However, Denny-Brown and Fischer[62] performed unilateral midbrain tegmental lesions in monkeys, which resulted in upward gaze palsy, skew deviation (with the ipsilateral eye in a higher position than the contralateral eye), and head tilt. In addition, after unilateral stereotactic lesions of the dorsolateral midbrain tegmentum performed in humans for the treatment of pain syndromes, Nashold and Seaber[219] recorded symmetric upward gaze palsy in 13 of 16 subjects. In 10 subjects, downward gaze was impaired as well, but never without upward gaze palsy. Of the 16 patients, 15 had miotic nonreactive pupils, 11 had convergence paralysis, and 10 showed skew deviation, two-thirds with the ipsilateral eye in a lower position. In summary, virtually all the oculomotor findings observed in thalamic hemorrhage have been described after unilateral tegmental midbrain lesions in humans. This supports the view that the oculomotor findings in this condition are due

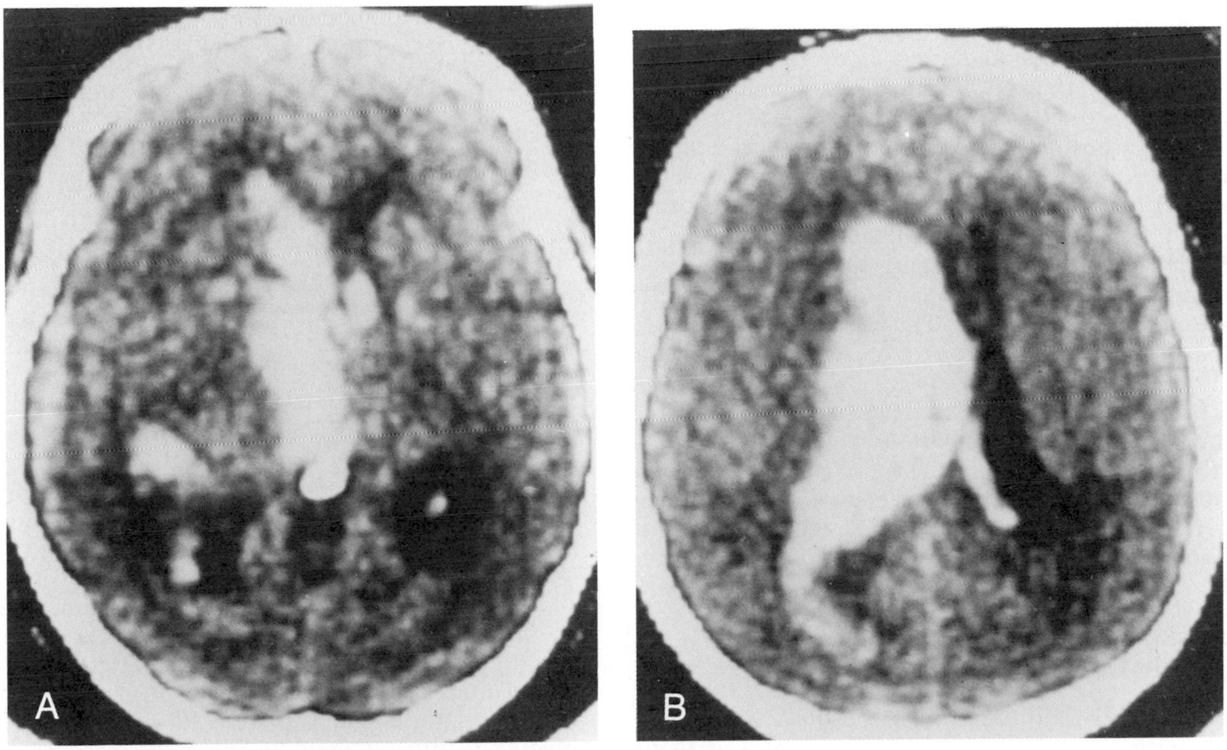


**Fig. 21-30.** (**A**) Left thalamic hemorrhage extending into the third and lateral ventricles. (**B**) Upward extension of the hemorrhage into the lateral ventricles and parietal white matter, with midline shift to the right.

to compression or extension of the hemorrhage into the midbrain tegmentum. However, other observations[112,247,304] suggest that CSF hypertension and hydrocephalus associated with the bleed may play an additional role in the production of the oculomotor findings, as ventricular shunting has been shown to reverse these manifestations. In conclusion, a compressive effect upon the tegmental-tectal portion of the midbrain, either directly by unilateral compression by the hematoma or indirectly through hydrocephalus, results in the classical oculomotor and pupillary abnormalities of thalamic hemorrhage.

Although these oculomotor abnormalities occur frequently, they are not invariably present, as shown in Table 21-7. This table indicates that some cases of thalamic hemorrhage will occur as a sensorimotor deficit (present in virtually 100 percent of the cases), without the diagnostic oculomotor features. In those instances the differential diagnosis with putaminal hemorrhage may be difficult. However, a number of clinical manifestations may be present and thus suggest the diagnosis. These findings include contralateral eye deviation, aphasia in the dominant hemisphere, neglect in the nondominant, and unusual sensory syndromes.

## Contralateral Conjugate Eye Deviation

In some instances, thalamic hemorrhage cases may show horizontal eye deviation, with or without the characteristic downward deviation at rest. This horizontal eye deviation is more commonly ipsilateral (toward the side of the lesion),[308] as is routinely observed in putaminal hemorrhage, but a contralateral conjugate deviation (toward the side of the hemiplegia) occasionally occurs.[12,308] This eye deviation occurs in the direction opposite that expected in a supratentorial lesion, thus being labeled the "wrong-way" eye deviation.[92] Although this peculiar sign has been recorded in an instance of unilateral subarachnoid-sylvian hemorrhage with frontal and insular extension,[238] most reported cases have occurred in association with thalamic hemorrhage.[92,160] The mechanism of the sign is obscure. Postdecussation involvement of horizontal oculomotor pathways by dissection of the hematoma into the ipsilateral brain stem has been suggested, but pathologic studies have failed to confirm it.[92,160,238] Furthermore, this ocular deviation usually behaves as a supratentorial gaze palsy, as oculocephalic and ice-water caloric testing produces full excursion in both horizontal directions.[160,238,241]

## Aphasia in Dominant Hemisphere Thalamic Hemorrhage

Occasionally, left thalamic bleeds have been associated with a peculiar form of language disturbance.[5,12,89,308] Its relatively low reported frequency is probably due to the fact that its detection is restricted to cases of small dominant hemisphere bleeds, as large ones are likely to be accompanied by stupor or coma.[247] A detailed analysis of three cases by Mohr et al.[211] stressed the main features of this syndrome: fluctuating performance in language function from an almost normal one to a profusely paraphasic fluent speech akin to a delirium. The almost "uncontrollable" character of the paraphasias, in conjunction with intact repetition, led the authors to postulate the removal by the thalamic lesion of a controlling influence of that structure over the intact cerebral surface speech areas. Similar clinical observations were reported by Reynolds et al.[247] These authors commented on the frequency of aphasic abnormalities after left stereotactic thalamotomy, and suggested that the language disorders following acute thalamic lesions may to some extent be mediated by disturbances in attention and recent memory. The study of Alexander and LoVerme[5] included nine cases of aphasia in left thalamic hematomas, and the speech profile was a fluent, relatively well-articulated speech with poor naming, relatively good repetition, and prominent paraphasias. These authors commented on the lack of distinctive features in aphasias from putaminal and thalamic hemorrhage. They also suggested a prominent role for memory and attention deficits in the production of the language disturbances.

## Neglect in Nondominant Thalamic Hemorrhage

Syndromes of hemineglect are classically associated with destructive lesions of the nondominant parietal lobe.[56] Other areas, such as the frontal lobe,[135] have rarely given rise to a similar set of symptoms. Among ICHs, the putaminal location can be associated with this syndrome.[142] This occurrence in thalamic hemorrhage is rare: Walshe et al.[308] and Barraquer-Bordas et al.[12] each described two patients with anosognosia from right thalamic hemorrhage. Watson and Heilman[309] described hemineglect in three cases of right thalamic hemorrhage. These patients exhibited prominent anosognosia and hemispatial agnosia, and Cases 1 and 2 showed limb akinesia, manifested as lack of spontaneous movements of the left limbs despite mild objective weakness. These patients, in particular Cases 1 and 2, had relatively small thalamic hemorrhages that disrupted sensation only partially in Case 1 and affected motor function partially, to a level of weakness only, in Cases 1 and 2. Case 3 had a larger bleed associated with arm paralysis, marked leg weakness, absent sensation, bilateral Babinski signs, and drowsiness, while the other two patients were alert and cooperative. These cases illustrated a neglect syndrome similar to that observed in nondominant cortical surface disease, from documented medium-size and small right thalamic hematomas.

## Unusual Sensory Syndromes

Unusual sensory syndromes are infrequently encountered. The best recognized is the thalamic pain syndrome of Dejerine and Roussy,[60] which is usually regarded as a feature of thalamic infarction in the distribution of the perforating branches of the posterior cerebral artery.[237,319] The profoundly distressing dysesthesias and spontaneous pain characteristically arise with a latency of days to weeks from the onset.[60] Its occurrence after thalamic hemorrhage is probably rare: the 8-month follow-up information in the nine survivors from the series of Walshe et al.[308] did not mention this sequela. However, Alexander and LoVerme[5] commented on the presence of a central pain syndrome in six of their nine patients with thalamic hemorrhage. The relative rarity of this syndrome in the setting of hemorrhage has suggested that partial thalamic lesions of a precise lateral-posterior location are necessary to produce it.[319] This is in agreement with the finding of this syndrome in two of four cases of CT-documented lacunar infarcts of the posterolateral thalamus reported by Robinson et al.[251] This sensory syndrome is an uncommon feature of the usually more massive thalamic destruction due to hematoma. However, the diagrams of the three original cases of Dejerine and Roussy[60] show old posterolateral thalamic lesions extending laterally well beyond the thalamic boundaries, into the posterior limb of the internal capsule and slightly into the caudal putamen. As the latter areas are outside the territory of supply of the posterior cerebral perforating branches,[179] it is conceivable that they may have represented old bleeds rather than infarcts, as the lesions seem to have straddled across two neighboring vascular territories. We have observed classical examples of the syndrome following both infarcts[251] and hemorrhages[158] affecting the thalamus.

A second unusual sensory syndrome is a form of "pure sensory stroke," classically associated with small (lacunar) thalamic infarcts,[90] which thus far has not been described in hemorrhage confined to the thalamus. The only instance of a small hemorrhage in that area detected by CT scan occurred in the subthalamic region, and the clinical presentation was hemiballismus.[198] In another single report, Groothuis et al.[124] documented in a patient with a "pure sensory stroke" a small hemorrhage in the posterior limb of the internal capsule rather than in the thalamus. It is conceivable, however, that a small thalamic bleed will eventually be documented in the setting of "pure sensory stroke."

The CT aspects of thalamic hemorrhage are shown in Table 21-8. Of interest are the high frequency of ventricular extension (reflecting the location of the bleed immediately adjacent to the 3rd ventricle), and the resulting high frequency (about 25 percent)[12,308] of hydrocephalus. As already mentioned, the latter may allow a successful therapeutic intervention in thalamic hemorrhage.[112,247,304] In addition, the CT information on the size of the hematoma has useful prognostic significance: hematomas larger than 3.3 cm were uniformly fatal in two series,[12,308] and all cases with hematomas smaller than 2.7 cm survived in the report of Walshe et al.[308] Piepgras and Rieger[239] described two cases in their series who survived with hematomas of more than 4.0 cm diameter. In addition to the diameter or volume of the hemorrhage, the level of consciousness on admission and the presence of hydrocephalus have a strong relationship to outcome, whereas the age of the patient, side of the hematoma, ventricular extension, and midline shift have shown no prognostic significance.[174,239] The mortality figures in thalamic hemorrhage (Table 21-7) have been slightly higher than in putaminal hemorrhage[109,221] in some series, comparable in others.[12] In summary, the CT information in thalamic hemorrhage does not only have value in diagnosis, but also gives useful prognostic information and suggests the need for some forms of early surgical intervention.

**TABLE 21-8. Computed Tomography Aspects of Thalamic Hemorrhage**

| | Walshe et al.[308] ($N$ = 18) | Barraquer-Bordas et al.[12] ($N$ = 23) |
|---|---|---|
| Side of hematoma | | |
| Right/left | 8/10 | 17/6 |
| Size of hematoma | | |
| Below 3.3 cm | 11 | — |
| Above 3.3 cm | 7 | — |
| Ventricular extension | 66% | 50% |
| Hydrocephalus | 27% | 21% |

## White Matter (Lobar) Hemorrhage

The scattered location of lobar ICHs made it difficult to describe them as a clinical entity, but the use of imaging has led to increasing publications lumping the locations together as lobar. The main clinical features were defined only in the last decade,[159,253] and reliable criteria for a choice of therapy are still not available.[189]

### Anatomy

The pathologic anatomy is well known. They occur in the subcortical white matter of the cerebral lobes, usually extending longitudinally in a plane parallel to the overlying cortex, hence their label as "slit" hemorrhages as mentioned in Greenfield.[323] As they attain larger sizes, their shape changes into the more common oval or round one. They occur in all cerebral lobes, but have a predilection for the parietal, temporal, and occipital lobes[107,159,253] (Table 21-9). This predilection for the posterior half of the brain in lobar ICH is unexplained, and is probably not a reflection of differences in relative lobe size, as the ratio of 3:1 be-

**TABLE 21-9. Location of Lobar Intracerebral Hematomas**

| Location | Number | |
|---|---|---|
| Frontal | 4 | |
| Parietal | 3 | 18 (82%) |
| Temporoparietal | 8 | |
| Parieto-occipital | 2 | |
| Parietotemporo-occipital | 1 | |
| Parietofrontal | 2 | |
| Occipital | 2 | |
| Total | 22 | |

(From Kase et al.,[159] with permission.)

tween parietotemporo-occipital and frontal hematomas[159] is larger than the anatomic volumetric ratio of 2:1[10] or 3:2[18] between these two areas. A possible explanation for this finding is the preponderance of intracerebral microaneurysms for the parieto-occipital area found by Cole and Yates.[51] These authors found that the junction of cortical gray and white matter contained about 30 percent of the microaneurysms, and the diagrams included in their paper show a significantly higher concentration of these lesions on the parieto-occipital areas, and proportionately smaller numbers of them in the frontal and temporal poles. Although the causal relationship between microaneurysms and ICH has not been established,[95] these anatomic correlations in lobar ICH lend some support to it.

## Etiology

The etiologic factors in lobar ICH may be somewhat different than those of other forms of ICH, in particular with regard to a less significant role of arterial hypertension.[159,194,216,253,314] Ropper and Davis[253] reported chronic hypertension in only 31 percent of their cases of lobar ICH, and in our series[159] only 50 percent of the cases had elevated blood pressure on admission, half of whom had documented high blood pressure anteceding the bleed. In Weisberg's[314] series only 33 percent of the cases with lobar ICH were hypertensive, whereas this factor was present in 81 percent of the deep ("ganglionic-thalamic") group of ICH. Hence, etiologic factors other than hypertension are relevant in lobar ICH: AVMs, which occur in frequencies between 7 and 14 percent, tumors in 7 to 9 percent, and blood dyscrasias or anticoagulation responsible for 5 to 20 percent[50,89,106] of the bleeds, leaving a large group (22 percent in our series[159]) in whom the mechanism for the ICH remains unknown. This raises the possibility that this variety of ICH may have some etiologic factors that are more common than in other forms of ICH. One such etiologic factor may be "cerebral amyloid angiopathy," which is being increasingly recognized as the substrate of recurrent, sometimes multiple ICH in elderly nonhypertensive individuals.[85,109,111,234,245,296,305] These hemorrhages have a strong tendency to occur in the lobar subcortical white matter,[85,109,234,296,305] since the classical anatomic location of the amyloid-infiltrated arteries is in the superficial layers of the cortex and leptomeninges, being absent in the deep gray nuclei.[109,111,227] In addition, the arteries affected by the amyloid deposits are more commonly found on the posterior portions of the hemispheres (parietal and occipital areas),[109,227,290] which are the sites in which lobar ICH classically occurs.[107,159,253] These facts suggest that lobar ICH in the elderly may be related to this etiologic factor, which, on the other hand, does not play a significant role in other forms of ICH.

## Clinical Features

The clinical manifestations of lobar ICH have been analyzed recently,[159,253] and a number of differences with other types of ICH have been noted (Table 21-10). The circumstances at onset are depicted in Table 21-9, comparing series of lobar ICH[159,192] with those considering all forms of ICH together.[6,207] The distinguishing features of lobar ICH by frequency of single findings are less arterial hypertension, less coma on admission, more headaches, more seizures. The higher frequency of headache at onset may reflect the higher number of patients who are awake and can give a history in lobar ICH. Ropper and Davis[253] described the headaches in and around the ipsilateral eye in occipital hematomas, around the ear in temporal bleeds, bilateral anteriorly in frontal hemorrhage, and anterior temporal ("temple") in location in parietal lobe hematomas. The low incidence of coma on admission in lobar ICH is probably related to the peripheral location of the hematoma, at a distance from midline structures.[253] The two series of lobar ICH[159,253] cited coma on admission at 0.3 percent and 17 percent, respectively. The lower figure is from a large referral center where deeply comatose patients are less likely to be referred on account of their being poor therapeutic candidates. Our figure of 18 percent of coma on admission in an unselected population of

**TABLE 21-10. Clinical Manifestations at Onset of Lobar ICH vs. All Forms of ICH**

| | All Forms ICH (%) | | Lobar ICH (%) | |
|---|---|---|---|---|
| | Mohr et al.[153] | Aring[6] | Ropper and Davis[253] | Kase et al.[159] |
| Hypertension | | | | |
| By history | 72 | — | 31 | 36 |
| On admission | 91 | — | 46 | 45 |
| Headache | 36 | 23 | 46 | 68 |
| Vomiting | 44 | 22 | 61 | 45 |
| Seizures | 7 | 14 | 0 | 23 |
| Coma | 42 | 51 | 0.3 | 18 |

*Abbreviation:* ICH, intracerebral hemorrhage.
(From Kase et al.,[159] with permission.)

ICH cases probably reflects more accurately the true frequency of coma in this condition.

Seizures in our series of lobar ICH[159] was significantly higher than in other forms of ICH. Only the series of Ropper and Davis[253] show no seizures, a finding difficult to explain. The seizure type in our group of patients was most commonly generalized, but on several occasions they occurred as focal status epilepticus. The mechanism of seizures in lobar hematomas may reflect the location of the bleed in the gray matter-white matter interface, creating a situation similar to the surgical isolation of cortex by subcortical injury that results in sustained paroxysmal activity from the isolated cortex.[77]

The scan shown in Figure 21-31 is typical of lobar hemorrhage on CT. The patient, a 45-year-old diabetic and hypertensive woman, "collapsed to the ground" and had focal motor convulsions involving the left face and arm, shortly after which she vomited. Valium and intravenous Dilantin were required to control the focal seizure activity. In the postictal period she was stuporous, barely able to follow commands, unable to answer questions. The left limbs were paralyzed and flaccid, and response to pain was minimal and nonpurposeful on the left side. A CT scan revealed a fresh hematoma in the midportion of the right temporal lobe, in a subcortical position (Fig. 21-31). No mass effect or ventricular extension were present. Within a day after she was seizure-free she was alert and oriented, with the left limbs mildly paretic. By day 4, she had regained full strength the left leg, the arm was slightly weak distally, and no facial asymmetry was present.

The neurologic deficits on lobar ICHs depend on the location and size of the hematoma. A number of features in the neurologic examination have been documented[253]: sudden hemiparesis, worse in the arm, with retained ability to walk, in frontal hematoma; combined sensory and motor deficits, the former predominating, and visual field defects in parietal bleeds; fluent paraphasic speech with poor comprehension and relatively spared repetition in left temporal lobe hematomas; homonymous hemianopia, occasionally accompanied by mild sensory changes (extinction to double simultaneous stimulation), in occipital lobe hemorrhages. In our group of 24 patients,[159] hemiparesis and visual field defects were the most common abnormality, found in 60 percent and 30 percent of those patients who were not comatose on admission, respectively. Those cases in whom both signs coexisted represented larger and more anteriorly placed hematomas, whereas those with hemianopia and no hemiparesis were located posteriorly. From these data, the clinical picture of the patient with a lobar parieto-occipital hematoma emerges as one of sudden onset of headache, sometimes associated with vomiting, not uncommonly associated with seizure activity, with state of consciousness in the alert or obtunded level, associated with mild contralateral hemiparesis and visual field defect. The specific deficits in speech and spatial function will be added when the bleeds are of dominant frontotemporal or nondominant parietal location, respectively, mimicking those of infarction.[209,218]

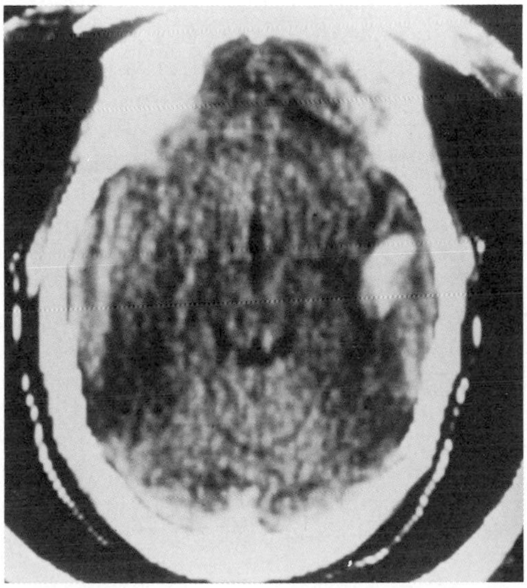

**Fig. 21-31.** Small subcortical white matter hematoma in the right temporal lobe without mass effect or ventricular extension.

## Prognosis

The prognosis in lobar hematomas is usually less grave than in other forms of ICH. The mortality figures reported have been 11.5 percent,[253] 14 percent,[249] 20 percent,[314] and 29 percent,[159] all below the mortality rates of each of the other varieties of ICH. A low frequency of 6 percent has been reported in an autopsy series,[106] whereas in clinical series they represent between 10 and 32 percent of the cases.[159,253,314] In addition, the functional outcome for survivors is said to be generally good, and Richardson[249] reported full recovery in more than half the survivors in his series, the other half being partially disabled. In the group of 17 survivors in our series,[159] 4 died within 6 months from discharge, 1 of whom had probably a recurrent ICH (in the setting of polycythemia vera), the other 3 from unrelated causes. Two patients were lost to follow-up. The functional outcome in the other 11 patients showed complete recovery in 3, mild disability in 5, and moderate disability in 3. These small figures indicate a trend toward a generally less severe degree of disability in survivors from lobar ICH as compared with other supratentorial sites of ICH.

## Computed Tomography Aspects

The CT aspects of lobar ICH have not been carefully analyzed in the literature. Ropper and Davis[253] provided two-dimensional measurements of their 26 he-

**TABLE 21-11. Computed Tomography Aspects and Outcome of Lobar Intracerebral Hematomas**

| Hematoma Size | Number of Cases | Midline Shift | Ventricular Extension | Outcome/Operated |
|---|---|---|---|---|
| Small (<20 cc) | 5 | 1 | 0 | 5 improved/0 |
| Moderate (20–40 cc) | 7 | 6 | 1 | 6 improved/3<br>1 died/0 |
| Massive (>40 cc) | 10 | 10 | 7 | 4 improved/2<br>6 died/1 |
| Total | 22 | 17 | 8 | |

(From Kase et al.,[159] with permission.)

matomas, and commented on their tendency to enlarge mostly in the transverse and anteroposterior planes of the CT section. In Weisberg's[314] series of 45 cases of lobar ICH, 10 were found to have intraventricular extension, a factor that did not affect the mortality rates in his group. The CT aspects of our 22 cases[159] are shown in Table 21-11. The volume of the hematoma fell into three main groups, which, in turn, correlated with the presence of mass effect. Ventricular extension was a factor that correlated with location (proximity to ventricular system) rather than size of the hematoma. The outcome was in part a function of hematoma size, as no patient with a hematoma larger than 60 $cm^3$ survived, whereas all those with small hematomas (less than 20 $cm^3$) survived. In the group of intermediate size hematoma, 75 percent survived, and the functional level was in general poorer than in the group with small hematomas. These figures, in addition, provide some indication of the possible role of surgical drainage as a therapeutic option in lobar ICH. In some series of lobar ICH it has been stated that surgery offers no advantage over medical therapy,[196,253] whereas in our uncontrolled study[159] a trend toward improved outcome following surgery was suggested. This option for lobar hematomas is further encouraged by the superficial location of the bleed that makes it more easily accessible.[57] This form of therapy is particularly indicated in patients with medium-size or large hematomas who show signs of progressive neurologic deterioration following diagnosis.[159,225]

## HEMORRHAGE AFFECTING THE BRAIN STEM AND CEREBELLUM

### Cerebellar Hemorrhage

Early morphologists were aware of apoplectic hemorrhage into the cerebellum and reported single instances in the early nineteenth century. In 1875 Carion[36] described seven examples of cerebellar hemorrhage in a doctoral thesis and noted some of the major clinical features. Childs[42] reported the first American patient in 1858, a 19-year-old who became ill while shaking her head to amuse a child. Starr[277] analyzed American necropsy cases up to 1906, and Guillain et al.[127] reviewed the major clinical features of cerebellar hemorrhage in 1923. In 1932, Michael[201] reported 10 of his own patients and provided a literature review. He divided patients according to their clinical course, that is, fulminating, grave, or benign. Headache, vertigo, and asthenia developed quickly and he suggested that "antemortem localization is practically impossible in these cases," an opinion shared by McKissock and colleagues[197] in 1960, who described 34 instances of cerebellar hemorrhage, among which were 6 angiomas and 2 aneurysms. The authors commented, "The neurological signs presented by these patients were in the main singularly unhelpful. Localizing signs could not be elicited in those patients who were unconscious except most of them had constricted and non-reactive pupils and periodic respirations. The signs of cerebellar dysfunction were present in less than half."[197]

In a landmark paper in 1959, Fisher and colleagues[101] responded to this challenge in their analysis of the clinical features. Especially important in diagnosis were the inability to walk, gaze palsy without hemiplegia, and the absence of unilateral limb paresis. They found surgical decompression could be lifesaving, occasionally even in patients in deep coma prior to surgery. More important, patients who had been treated surgically were often able to return to active lives without the overwhelming disability often retained by survivors of basal ganglionic hemorrhage. Although these diagnostic formulations were initially subject to dispute, CT scanning has made the detection of smaller cerebellar hematomas possible[180,215] and has essentially confirmed them and the clinical spectrum of the disease.

Cerebellar hemorrhage appears with a frequency variously quoted as between 5 and 15 percent.[33,64,87,104,146,246,248] The average frequency is about 10 percent, approximating the relative percentage of weight of the cerebellum in reference to the entire brain. Although this represents a relatively low frequency, the importance of establishing this diagnosis resides in its good prognosis after prompt surgical treatment.[24,87,232] Cerebellar hemorrhage usually occurs in one of the hemispheres, usually originating in the region of the dentate nucleus, probably from distal branches of the superior cerebellar artery[101] or occasionally the posterior-inferior cerebellar artery

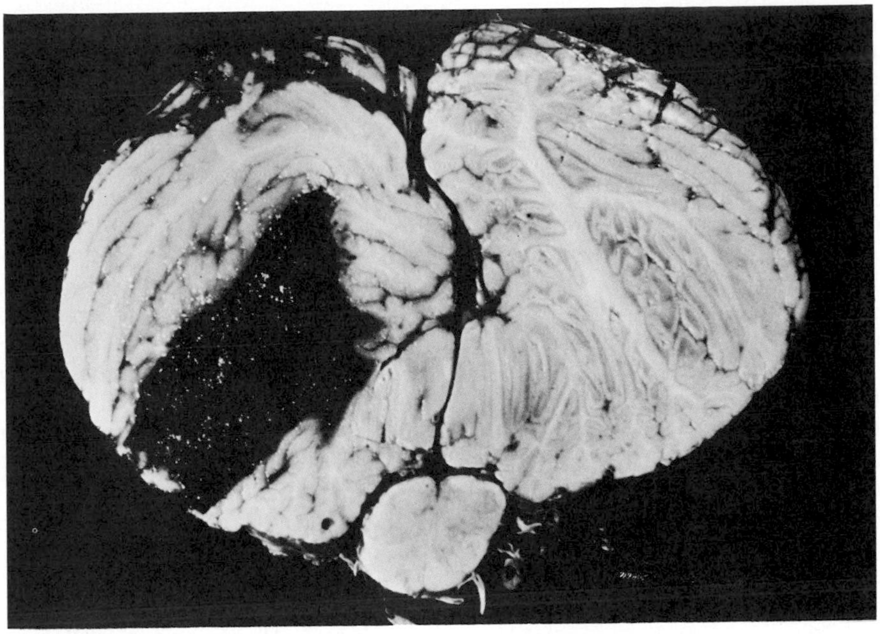

**Fig. 21-32.** Large dentate area cerebellar hemorrhage.

(PICA).[104] In the series of Fisher et al.,[101] the left hemisphere was affected twice as often as the right. McKissock et al.[197] also commented on a left cerebellar predominance. Most other series do not report hemorrhage laterality.

The hematoma collects around the dentate and spreads into the hemispheral white matter (Fig. 21-32), frequently extending into the cavity of the 4th ventricle as well. The adjacent brain stem (pontine tegmentum) is rarely involved directly by the hematoma, but is often compressed by it, at times resulting in pontine necrosis. The midline variant of cerebellar hemorrhage originates from the vermis, and represents only about 5 percent of the cases.[101] It virtually always directly communicates with the 4th ventricle through its roof, and frequently extends into the pontine tegmentum bilaterally (Fig. 21-33). The bleeding vessel in this variety usually corresponds to distal branches of the PICA. These two forms of cerebellar hemorrhage have distinctive clinical and prognostic features (Fig. 21-34).

Etiologic factors have a similar distribution to other forms of intracerebral hemorrhage, arterial hy-

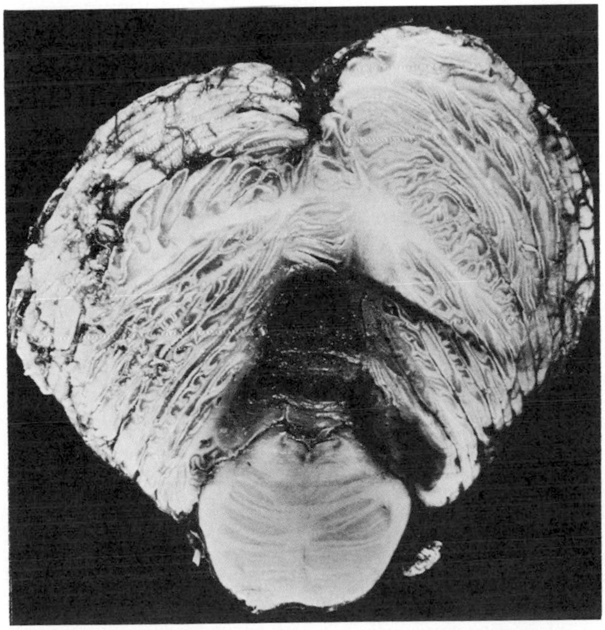

**Fig. 21-33.** Vermian cerebellar hemorrhage with pressure on the pontine tegmentum.

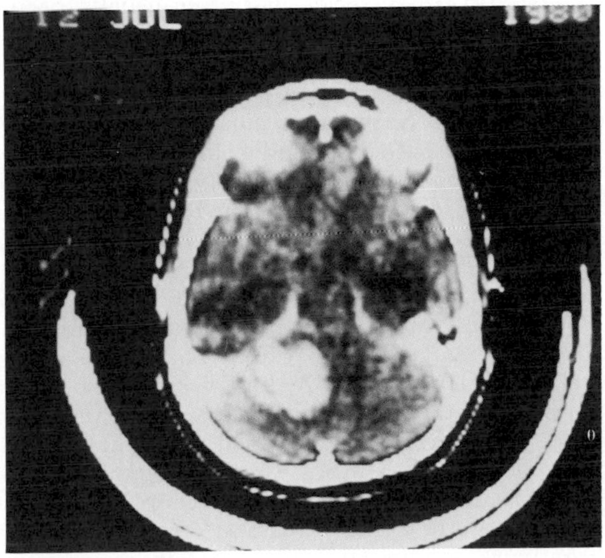

**Fig. 21-34.** Computed tomography of large cerebellar hemorrhage, left dentate region.

pertension being the leading cause.[101,232] Arteriovenous malformations are said to be frequent in the cerebellum;[197,246] they accounted for 5 of 15 cerebellar hematomas in the autopsy series of McCormick and Rosenfield.[194] In other series[232] a lower frequency of arteriovenous malformations has been reported (4 percent), a rate similar to that in other sites of intracerebral hemorrhage.[253] Anticoagulation is an important etiologic factor in cerebellar hemorrhage, and was the second most frequent cause reported by Ott et al.[232] Among 24 cases of intracerebral hemorrhage in patients on oral anticoagulants,[157] 9 hematomas occurred in the cerebellum. Three of these were of the less common vermian or midline variety. Although these small numbers do not allow definitive conclusions, anticoagulant-related intracerebral hemorrhages may show a relative predilection for the cerebellum. Fisher[101] commented on a relative female preponderance in his series: 13:8; but in other series the female:male ratios were 26:30,[232] 6:6,[64] 1:9,[201] 5:14,[222] and 17:17.[197]

Symptoms usually develop during the working day while the patient is active. Occasionally a single prodromal episode of dizziness or facial numbness may precede the hemorrhage. The most constant symptom is *an inability to stand or walk*. In many patients this has been dramatic. One man leaned against a fence while painting and could not right himself; another bumped downstairs on his bottom in order to call for help. Crawling or propelling oneself prone on the floor in order the get to the bathroom to vomit have been mentioned. Rare patients maintain their ability to walk a few steps, but scarcely any patient with a sizable hemorrhage (more than 2 cm) walks into the emergency ward or office. Vomiting is also very frequent and was present in 42 of 44 patients in the series of Ott et al.,[232] and 12 of 12 patients[24] and 14 of 18 patients[101] in other series. *Vomiting* usually occurs soon after the onset in cerebellar and subarachnoid hemorrhage but often develops later, following other symptoms, in patients with putaminal hemorrhage. *Dizziness* is also common, occurring in 24 of 44 patients,[232] 8 of 21 patients,[88] and 4 of 12 patients.[24] More often the feeling is one of insecurity, a "drunken feeling," or wavering rather than true rotational vertigo. *Headache* is also very common and occurred in 32 of 44 patients,[232] 10 of 21 patients,[101] and 12 of 12 patients.[64] Most often the pain is occipital, but occasionally it can occur on the side of the head or frontally. At times the headache is abrupt and excruciating, closely mimicking subarachnoid hemorrhage. In other patients the pain can be primarily in the neck or shoulder. An early case described by Thyne[288] developed severe neck stiffness resembling meningitis. Dysarthria, tinnitus, and hiccups occur, but are less frequent. Loss of consciousness at onset is distinctly unusual,[93,232] and by the time the patient reaches hospital only one-third are obtunded.[232] Most patients gradually worsen over a period of 1 to 3 hours, as in other forms of intracerebral hemorrhage.[33,35,207]

The physical findings are classically those of a combination of a unilateral cerebellar deficit with variable signs of ipsilateral tegmental pontine involvement. These are detailed in Table 21-12, from an analysis of 38 noncomatose patients from the series of Ott et al.[232] Appendicular and gait ataxia occurred in 65 percent and 78 percent of the cases, respectively, among the patients who were alert enough to cooperate for cerebellar function testing. Other patients lean to the side when placed upright. On the side of the hemorrhage there usually is overshoot or inability to brake the limb quickly. This sign is more common than finger-to-nose or -to-object ataxia. Signs of involvement of the ipsilateral pontine tegmentum include peripheral facial palsy, ipsilateral horizontal gaze palsy, 6th cranial nerve palsy, depressed corneal reflex, and miosis. In some patients the hemorrhage presses laterally in the area of the cerebellopontine angle, producing peripheral facial palsy, deafness, and diminished corneal response.

From analysis of the relative frequency of signs in noncomatose patients, a characteristic triad of appendicular ataxia, ipsilateral gaze palsy, and peripheral facial palsy was suggested,[232] since at least two of the three signs were present in 73 percent of those patients tested for all three signs. Skew ocular deviation is also common.[104] Additional findings useful in differential diagnosis are hemiplegia and subhyaloid hemorrhages, both being uncommon enough in cerebellar hemorrhage that their presence essentially rules out the diagnosis.[232] The frequency of unilateral limb weakness in cerebellar hemorrhage has been a matter

**TABLE 21-12. Neurologic Findings in Cerebellar Hemorrhage for Noncomatose Patients**

| Neurologic Finding | Number | % |
|---|---|---|
| Appendicular ataxia | 17/26 | 65 |
| Trunkal ataxia | 11/17 | 65 |
| Gait ataxia | 11/14 | 78 |
| Dysarthria | 20/32 | 62 |
| Gaze palsy | 20/37 | 54 |
| Cranial nerve findings | | |
| Peripheral facial palsy | 22/36 | 61 |
| Nystagmus | 18/35 | 51 |
| Miosis | 11/37 | 30 |
| Decreased corneal reflex | 10/33 | 30 |
| Abducens palsy | 10/36 | 28 |
| Gag reflex loss | 6/30 | 20 |
| Skew deviation | 4/33 | 12 |
| Trochlear palsy | 0/36 | — |
| Hemiparesis | 4/35 | 11 |
| Extensor plantar response | 23/36 | 64 |
| Respiratory irregularity | 6/28 | 21 |
| Nuchal rigidity | 14/35 | 40 |
| Subhyaloid hemorrhage | 0/34 | — |

(From Ott et al.,[232] with permission.)

of controversy. In the series of Fisher et al.[101] hemiplegia was observed only in the setting of a prior stroke, and similar findings were recorded by Ott et al.[232] However, in two autopsy series[24,246] hemiplegia was reported in 50 percent and 20 percent of the cases, respectively, and Richardson[248] noted contralateral hemiplegia in more than 50 percent of the cases in his clinical series. Although in some instances reports of ipsilateral hemiplegia may have corresponded to decreased mobility of grossly ataxic limbs or decreased spontaneous movement, a contralateral hemiplegia cannot be explained on those bases, and one has to assume involvement of the corticospinal tract in the ipsilateral basis pontis.

Other findings on neurologic examination add little specific diagnostic data: the pupils are commonly small and reactive to light, dysarthria is present in two-thirds of the cases, and the respiratory rhythm is usually unaffected.[232] Unilateral involuntary eye closure has been occasionally observed,[92,200] the involved eye usually being contralateral to the hematoma. This sign has been interpreted as eye closure for avoidance of diplopia, but this is probably not always the case, as it occurs in the absence of diplopia, in both infratentorial and supratentorial strokes.[92] Other less common oculomotor abnormalities, such as ocular bobbing, have occasionally been reported in cerebellar hemorrhage,[22,88,232] but with a lower frequency than in pontine hemorrhage or infarction. Some patients have a head tilt. Neck stiffness and unwillingness to move the head or neck either actively or passively probably signify increased pressure in the posterior fossa. Along with these focal manifestations on neurologic examination, patients with cerebellar hemorrhage may present with variable degrees of decreased alertness. Of the 56 cases reported by Ott et al.,[232] 14 (25 percent) were alert, 22 (40 percent) drowsy, 5 (9 percent) stuporous, and 15 (26 percent) comatose. That two-thirds of the patients are responsive (alert or drowsy) on admission justifies the intensive efforts at diagnosing this condition early, as the surgical prognosis is largely dependent on the preoperative level of consciousness. In one of our cases, the patient was unable to stand or walk, and sank into a lethargic state within 2 hours of onset, the eyes conjugately deviated with a partial 6th cranial nerve palsy. CT scan showed a 3-cm, round cerebellar hematoma in the left hemisphere, without intraventricular extension (Fig. 21-35). After evacuation of the hematoma, the patient was discharged 16 days after admission, walking with assistance because of moderate left-sided ataxia, but extraocular movements were normal. By 1 month she was further improved, and 2 months later she had resumed full activity, including sports.

The clinical course in cerebellar hemorrhage is notoriously unpredictable: patients who are alert or drowsy on admission can deteriorate suddenly to coma and death without warning,[101,232] while others in a similar clinical status have an uneventful course with complete recovery of function. Of those patients who were not comatose on admission, only 25 percent had a smooth, uneventful recovery in the series of Ott et al.,[232] whereas 80 percent deteriorated to coma, one-fourth of them within 3 hours from the onset (Fig. 21-36). A similar frequency was observed in the series of Fisher et al.,[101] where only 2 of 18 patients had a benign course, the other 16 deteriorating to coma at variable intervals, mostly within a few hours after onset. Although most cases deteriorate early in the

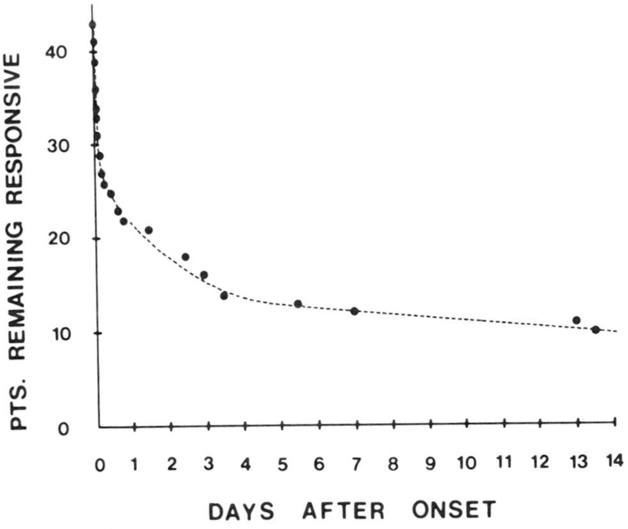


**Fig. 21-35.** Coma in patients with cerebellar hemorrhage as a function of time after onset. (From Ott et al.,[232] with permission.)

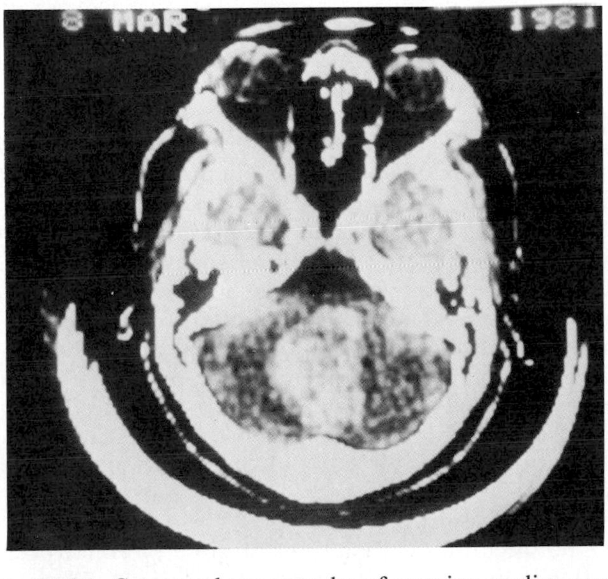


**Fig. 21-36.** Computed tomography of massive median cerebellar hemorrhage, vermian.

course, occasional patients have shown fatal decompensations at a later stage, even a month later, although they were stable in the interim.[26] Since prediction of the clinical course cannot be made based on clinical parameters on admission, the recommendation followed that surgical evacuation of the hematoma should be undertaken whenever the diagnosis is made within 48 hours from the onset.[232] The need for prompt diagnosis and emergency surgery had its justification in the documented poor surgical outcome with worsening preoperative mental status, the surgical mortality being 17 percent for responsive and 75 percent for unresponsive patients.[232] These figures have proven generally accurate, despite occasional reports of good surgical results in comatose patients.[323]

Because of the marked tendency toward clinical deterioration without warning signs, several authors[24,101,232] advised against the use of time-consuming angiographic diagnostic procedures, and advocated surgery on the basis of a clinical diagnosis of cerebellar hemorrhage. This approach was considered too risky by some,[254] arguing that the reliability of the clinical diagnosis of cerebellar hemorrhage is not high enough to justify exploratory posterior fossa craniotomy. The clinical dilemma between surgery based on clinical data alone and the risk of deterioration while performing procedures has fortunately been avoided by the use of CT scanning, the most valuable investigation in patients with suspected cerebellar hematoma. The use of CT scan in cerebellar hemorrhage has permitted the recognition of many different aspects of these lesions, some of which are useful early predictors of clinical course.[123,180,215] Little et al.[180] reported two groups of patients with cerebellar hemorrhage: one group had abrupt onset, a more severely depressed level of consciousness, and a tendency toward progressive deterioration, while the other group had a more benign, stable course. The first group required surgical treatment, whereas the second group did well on a medical program. CT scans of the first group showed hematomas of 3 cm or more in diameter, obstructive hydrocephalus, and ventricular extension of the hemorrhage, whereas these features were absent in the second group of patients, all of whom had hematomas of less than 3 cm in diameter. These observations and others[136] have identified a group of cerebellar hemorrhages with benign course, and accurate predictions may be possible by the combined analysis of clinical and CT data at the time of onset. Especially important is careful monitoring of the status of the patient. The development of obtundation and extensor plantar responses is ominous and is virtually always followed by a fatal outcome without surgery. Heros[140] has outlined the course of the progression.

The uncommon variety of midline (vermian) cerebellar hematoma still represents a serious diagnostic challenge, and its outcome is generally poor. Its frequency in autopsy series has been 6 percent of all cerebellar hemorrhages.[64] Our experience has documented syndromes featuring relatively acute onset of coma, ophthalmoplegia, and respiratory abnormalities, with variable degrees of bilateral limb weakness. Early extension of the vermian hematoma into the midline pontine tegmentum is probably responsible for the abrupt onset of coma and bilateral oculomotor signs, which can mimic a picture of barbiturate intoxication. This variant of cerebellar hematoma carries a poor prognosis, similar to that of primary pontine hemorrhage. At times, a relatively small hematoma in this location results in fatal brain stem compression (Fig. 21-34). A small vermian hematoma is illustrated in Figure 21-37 in a patient with uremia and hypertension.

## Midbrain Hemorrhage

Spontaneous, nontraumatic mesencephalic hemorrhage is rare. In most instances the hemorrhage dissects down from the thalamus or putamen, or is part of a lesion originating in the cerebellum or pons, or arises from blood dyscrasias or arteriovenous malformations. From frequency data alone, this subject could be placed at the end of the chapter but is placed here, ahead of the more common problem of pontine hemorrhage, to conform to an orderly anatomic description of brain stem hemorrhage.

Mesencephalic arteriovenous malformations are known to occur, and generally produce a stepwise but progressive deterioration. Ataxia and ophthalmoplegia (especially 3rd cranial nerve paralysis and paralysis of upward gaze) are common. Aqueductal or 3rd ventricular blockage or distention often leads to hydrocephalus. Bleeding diathesis can lead to isolated midbrain hemorrhage as is seen in Figure 21-38 from an elderly leukemic woman who developed a 3rd cra-

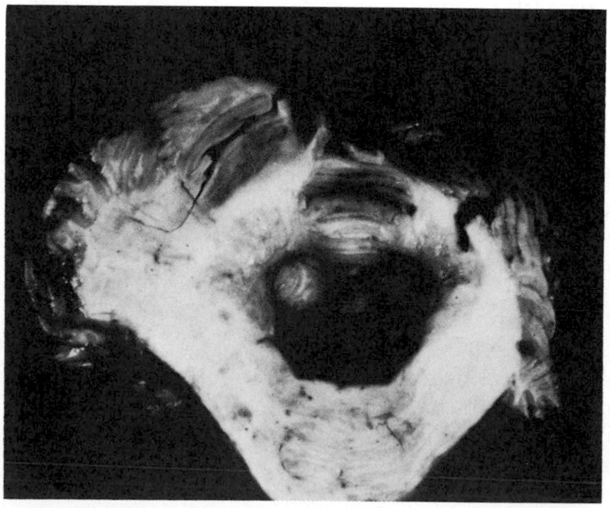

**Fig. 21-37.** Vermian cerebellar hemorrhage with dissection into the 4th ventricle in a hypertensive uremic patient.

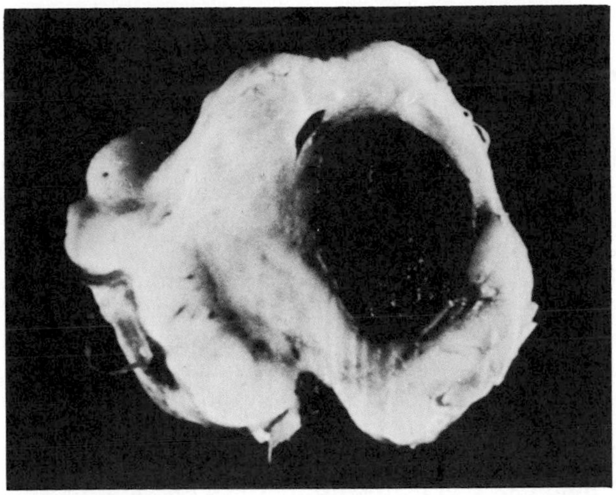

**Fig. 21-38.** Midbrain hemorrhage in patient with bleeding diathesis.

nial nerve palsy and contralateral intention tremor shortly before death. Hypertensive primary mesencephalic hemorrhage is very rare but does occur. One might predict that the hemorrhage would be in the tegmentum in the territory supplied by branches of the superior cerebellar arteries, as in the hypertensive patients of Roig et al.,[252] Durward et al.,[76] and Morel-Maroger et al.[213] The details of these cases follow.

Durward and colleagues[76] described two patients with mesencephalic hematomas. Their first patient was a 71-year-old hypertensive man (blood pressure 230/130) who suddenly could not stand nor open his eyes. Signs included bilateral 3rd cranial nerve paralysis, bulbar weakness, and extensor plantar responses. CT scan revealed a 1-cm hematoma in the ventral tegmentum of the midbrain with rupture into the 3rd ventricle. He developed obstructive hydrocephalus, treated by a ventriculoperitoneal shunt, and survived with bilateral 3rd cranial nerve palsies and poor balance with a tendency to fall backward. Arteriography was normal. Although there was no pathologic confirmation, this case may represent a primary hypertensive mesencephalic tegmental hematoma. The second patient was a normotensive young man who developed Weber syndrome (crossed 3rd cranial nerve palsy and hemiparesis) after a week of prodromal headache. The CT scan showed a right midbrain hematoma. After further deterioration the hematoma was surgically decompressed, and microscopic examination of the wall of the hematoma revealed an arteriovenous malformation. This patient survived but was grossly ataxic.

Morel-Maroger and colleagues[213] also describe a patient with midbrain hemorrhage caused by hypertension. A 71-year-old patient treated for hypertension for 5 years suddenly lost consciousness and awakened confused and dizzy. He had a diffuse headache and vomited. Findings included a right 3rd cranial nerve palsy, left hemiparesis, and a cerebellar-type ataxia of the right limbs. Blood pressure was 290/110. CT scan documented a 12 × 16 mm hematoma in the right superior cerebellar peduncle. The patient recovered after antihypertensive therapy without surgical intervention.

Roig et al.[252] also described two patients with hypertensive mesencephalic hematomas detected by CT scan. In one patient there was an ipsilateral 3rd cranial nerve paralysis, and contralateral hemihypesthesia and limb ataxia. The hyperdense lesion was high in the right mesencephalic tegmentum near the midline, probably draining into the 3rd ventricle. Vertebral angiography was normal. A second patient had a right 3rd cranial nerve palsy and left hemiparesis. The lesion was high in the right side of the midbrain. Both patients survived.

Humphreys[144] reported a 10-year-old boy who suddenly developed a right hemiparesis and confusion. Neuro-ophthalmologic findings were not given in detail. CT scan showed a large hematoma in the basis pedunculi extending into the interpeduncular fossa. The lesion was drained surgically and contained nuclear debris. The nature of the lesion is unknown, but it was likely a hemorrhage into an arteriovenous malformation or a benign tumor.

LaTorre et al.[175] described a 38-year-old woman who, after complaining of headache and intermittent diplopia for 2 years, vomited and developed bilateral 6th cranial nerve palsies and paralysis of upward gaze. The spinal fluid was bloody, and ventriculography visualized a beaded aqueduct and hydrocephalus. Exploration of the midbrain revealed an arteriovenous malformation of the quadrigeminal plate with blood clot embedded in the sylvian aqueduct.

Scoville and Poppen[268] also reported a single patient, a 44-year-old woman, who developed an ataxic right hemiparesis in stepwise fashion during 1½ years. Vomiting, bilateral 3rd cranial nerve paralysis, stupor, and pinpoint pupils suddenly supervened. A blood clot was drained from the left cerebral peduncle, and she awakened. Normal blood pressure and coagulation studies and the gradual onset favored an AVM in this patient.

## Pontine Hemorrhage

Pontine hemorrhage was recognized as a postmortem finding by morphologists early in the nineteenth century. As early as 1812, Cheyn[41] cited an example of pontine hemorrhage, as did Serres and Burdach several years later. Gowers,[119] in his 1893 textbook, included a picture of a typical large pontine hemorrhage (Fig. 21-39). By the early years of the twentieth century, the usual findings of pontine hemorrhage were recognized.[119]

In 1903, Danaby described the syndrome as follows:

1. Headache, malaise, vomiting
2. Sudden and profound coma

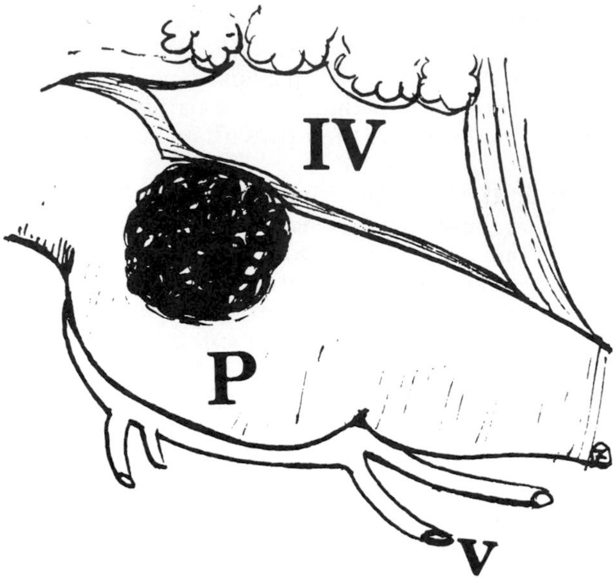


**Fig. 21-39.** Artist's rendition of illustration of pontine hemorrhage in Gowers' textbook. (From Gowers,[119] with permission.)

3. Twitching of the face and limbs or both
4. Miosis and convergent strabismus or conjugate deviation away from the side of the lesion
5. Slow irregular breathing
6. Irregular pulse
7. Dysphagia
8. Paralysis of limbs or crossed paralysis and exaggerated reflexes
9. Gradual rise of temperature, sometimes to high point
10. Death inside of 24 hours

The works of Oppenheim,[231] in 1905, who reviewed the literature and Attwater,[8] in 1911, who analyzed 77 examples of pontine hemorrhage found at necropsy, led to the separation of primary hemorrhage from those secondary to sudden increases in intracranial pressure. Attwater[8] postulated that some pontine hemorrhages could be due to "an increase in intracranial tension produced by the rapid entry of blood into the closed cranial cavity." Duret[75] elaborated these ideas several years later in a monograph, having previousy described some details of the blood supply of the brain stem.[72–74]

In the second half of the twentieth century, clinicians extended the observations, invariably focusing on patients with large pontine hemorrhages found at autopsy. Steegmann[278] described 17 patients, noting that death was usually not instantaneous, no patients dying in less than 22 hours. Pinpoint pupils were very common. All patients had bulbar paralysis, and most had some irregular limb movements. He attributed the "shaking of the limbs, twisting all over and trembling" to abnormal motor phenomena and did not believe, as had earlier authors, that the movements represented true epileptiform convulsions. He also emphasized the frequency of respiratory abnormalities. Five of his 17 patients had respiratory "failure," four had slow labored breathing, and some patients had shallow gasping and increased or irregular respirations. Epstein[80] reviewed a 33-year experience and found 7 patients with pontine hemorrhage among 74 autopsied intracerebral hemorrhages (9.1 percent). Most patients had severe hypertension before the hemorrhage. Fang and Foley[82] and later Dinsdale[64] reviewed the necropsies at Boston City Hospital and found 511 intracerebral hemorrhages among 19,093 autopsies, of which 30 were pontine (6 percent). Two-thirds of the patients were comatose when first seen, 13 percent vomited, and 78 percent were dead within 48 hours. One patient who survived for 23 days had a small hemorrhage in the right pontine tegmentum. All the remainder had massive hemorrhage, usually in the midpons at the junction of the basis pontis and tegmentum, that frequently spread rostrally into the midbrain; the hemorrhages almost never spread caudally to the medulla but frequently ruptured into the 4th ventricle.

In 1971 Fisher,[95] using serial sections from a patient with a massive fatal pontine hemorrhage, identified numerous small vessels with "fibrin globes," which he thought were related to the vascular rupture causing the hemorrhage: "From the gaping end of each of these torn vessels there protruded a large mass of platelets partially encircled by thin concentric layers of fibrin." He suggested the primary hemorrhage led to pressure on surrounding vessels which subsequent ruptured these vessels, causing a cascade or avalanche effect producing gradual enlargement of the hematoma. Ross Russell[257] had demonstrated large asymptomatic fusiform enlargements on the penetrating vessels of the pons in patients with "atherosclerosis" and hypertensive vascular disease. Cole and Yates,[50] Rosenblum,[255] Fisher,[95] and Caplan[33] all explained bleeding in hypertensive patients as leakage from tiny penetrating vessels damaged by lipohyalinosis and containing small microaneurysms. Kornyey[169] reported a patient whose pontine hemorrhage occurred under clinical observation: The slow march of signs was similar to the pattern of development seen in ganglionic and thalamic hemorrhages, and he provided evidence to support Fisher's postulation of the slowly evolving avalanche. Kornyey's patient was a 39-year-old man referred for admission because of malignant hypertension. While his admission history was being taken, he complained of numb hands, weakness, and dizziness. The blood pressure was 245/170. He became restless and apprehensive and complained that he could not hear and had difficulty swallowing and breathing. He developed a bilateral 6th cranial nerve palsy and dilated pupils, and his corneal reflexes disappeared. Spech became "bulbar," he was deaf, and he could not move his left leg.

Within 15 minutes he was comatose; the pupils were small, and the eyes were converged. There was bilateral bulbar palsy, stiff limbs with exaggerated reflexes, and extensor plantar responses. Two hours after the onset he died. A large hemorrhage in the tegmentum of the pons, with some spread into the right basis pontis was found at necropsy.[169] In other patients observed during the onset of pontine hemorrhage, development of the deficit usually evolved gradually over minutes (1 to 30 minutes), and was not as instantaneous as is aneurysmal subarachnoid hemorrhage.

In the pons, the largest penetrating arteries enter the pons medially, arise perpendicular to the basilar artery, and course from the base to the tegmentum. Other small penetrating arteries originate from the short and long circumferential vessels and enter more laterally, also coursing from base to tegmentum. Some arteries enter the tegmentum laterally and course horizontally across it.[34] Since vessels in all of these sites are potentially susceptible to hypertensive damage and lipohyalinosis, they could theoretically also be sites for pontine bleeding. Silverstein[273,274] reviewed the pathologic material from the Philadelphia General Hospital and corroborated that these loci (Fig. 21-40) were the usual regions of pontine hemorrhage. Of 50 cases, 28 were massive central hemorrhages presumably arising from large paramedian penetrators; 11 were more lateralized, usually spreading from base to tegmentum; and 11 had a tegmental location, 4 remaining unilateral and 7 involving the tegmentum bilaterally. Not until the late 1970s when CT became available, was it possible to accurately diagnose smaller nonfatal pontine hemorrhages and to positively separate them from pontine infarction during life. The clinical correlation of the various loci of hemorrhage predicted from anatomic studies and found by Silverstein was now possible. However, the clinicopathologic correlation of these smaller lateral basal and tegmental hemorrhages is still evolving.

## Large Paramedian Pontine Hemorrhage

Massive pontine hemorrhage results from rupture of parenchymal midpontine branches originating from the basilar artery. The bleeding vessel is thought to be a paramedian perforator in its distal portion,[64] causing initial hematoma formation at the junction of tegmentum and basis pontis,[64,274] from which the mass grows into its final round or oval shape and replaces most of both subdivisions of the pons (Fig. 21-41). The lesion usually begins in the middle of the pons and extends along the longitudinal axis of the brain stem into the lower midbrain. The hematoma may track into the middle cerebellar peduncles but usually does not extend caudally beyond the pontomedullary junction.[64] In the process of rapid hematoma expansion, destruction of tegmental and ventral pontine structures results, with the classical combination of signs caused by involvement of cranial nerve nuclei, long tracts, autonomic centers, and structures responsible for maintenance of consciousness. Large pontine hematomas also regularly rupture into the 4th ventricle.[64,273,274]

The "classic" form of pontine hemorrhage, bilateral and massive, is almost exclusively of hypertensive origin. Other etiologies such as "cryptic vascular malformation" account for 10 percent or less of the cases in

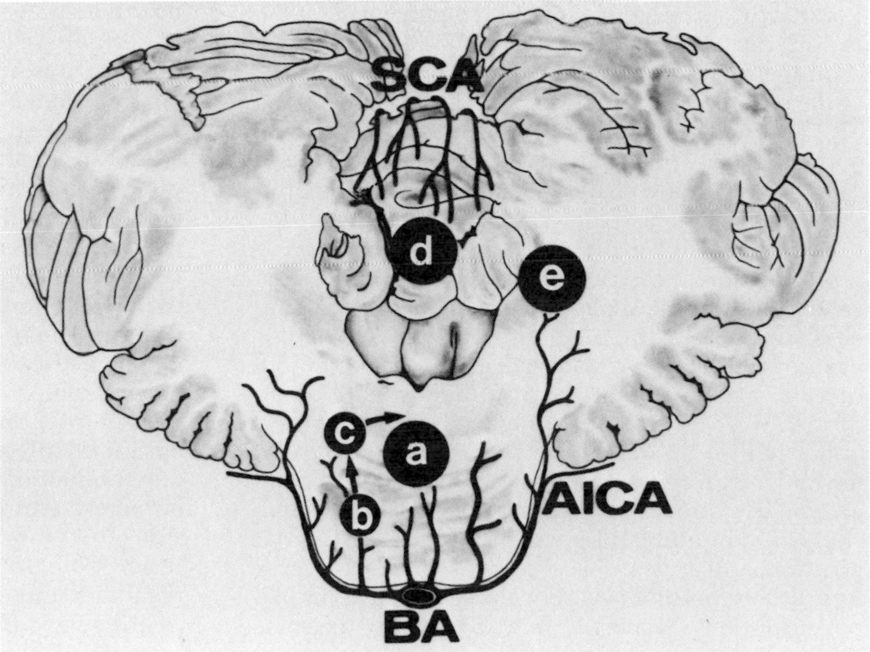


**Fig. 21-40.** Schematic representation of common loci of hypertensive pontine and cerebellar hemorrhages: (**A**) Massive, paramedian pontine, (**B**) Basal pontine. (**C**) Lateral tegmental pontine. (**D**) Cerebellar vermian. (**E**) Cerebellar hemispheral.

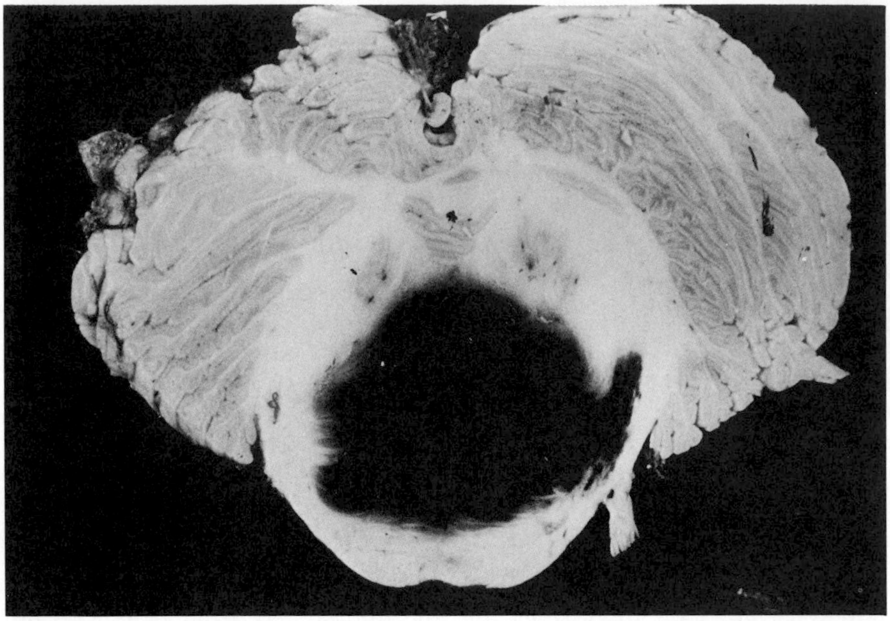

**Fig. 21-41.** Massive pontine hemorrhage with dissection into brachium pontis and 4th ventricle.

most series.[64,274] Russell[260] regarded pontine hemorrhage as a form of intracerebral hemorrhage most likely to occur in patients with malignant hypertension or hypertension associated with chronic nephropathy. Clinical presentation is characteristically one of rapid development of coma (80 percent of cases) without warning signs. Dana[58] recognized that some patients were conscious when first examined: in three different series, 4 of 19 (22 percent),[82] 10 of 30 (33.3 percent), and 5 of 50 (10 percent)[273,274] patients were alert when initially seen. By 48 hours, approximately 80 percent were dead.[64,82] In some patients (30 percent) a complaint of severe occipital headache preceded by minutes the catastrophic onset of coma.[229,273] Vomiting was noted in 4 of 30 (13 percent)[64] and 4 of 19 (22 percent)[82] patients, and occasionally was a prominent early symptom. The frequency of seizures at the onset, estimated as high as 22 percent,[273] probably represents a combination of true convulsive phenomena in rare instances, along with episodes of spasmodic decerebrate posturing, and even the sometimes violent shivering associated with autonomic dysfunction and rapidly evolving hyperthermia. Some patients will present prior to the development of coma with focal pontine signs, such as facial or limb numbness, deafness, diplopia, bilateral leg weakness, or progressive hemiparesis. Physical examination often reveals an abnormal respiratory rhythm or apnea.[64,274,278] Steegmann[278] analyzed these respiratory abnormalities in detail and reported a variety of abnormal respiratory patterns, including "inspiratory gasps of apneustic respiration," Cheyne-Stokes rhythm, slow and labored respirations, "gasping" respiration, and apnea. Two-thirds of his 17 cases exhibited either apnea or severely abnormal patterns of hypoventilation. Hyperthermia frequently coexisted, with temperatures above 39°C in more than 80 percent of the cases,[229] in one-fourth of whom it reached levels of 42 to 43°C,[273] usually in the preterminal stages. Neurologic examination findings characteristically result from involvement of cranial nerve nuclei and long tracts: quadriplegia with decerebrate posturing, bilateral Babinski signs, absent corneal reflexes, pinpoint miotic pupils, and various forms of ophthalmoplegia.[34,229,278]

The oculomotor findings include the following. *(1) Miotic pinpoint pupils:* These are usually about 1 mm in diameter. They react to light if a strong light source is used, a tiny constriction detected with a magnifying lens.[92,93] Hare noted that pontine hemorrhage could be confused/with opium poisoning.[278] The pupillary abnormality probably results from bilateral interruption of descending sympathetic pupillodilator fibers.[92,93] Since in Kornyey's patient pupillary dilatation preceded miosis,[169] it is possible that early stimulation of these fibers could lead to transient pupillary dilatation. *(2) Absent horizontal eye movements:* Their absence by reflex testing with the doll's head maneuver or ice-water caloric stimulation reflects bilateral injury of the paramedian pontine reticular formation. This sign occurs in partial forms or variants such as the "one-and-a-half syndrome,"[92] which is also referred to as "paralytic pontine exotropia,"[269] which represents a combination of unilateral horizontal gaze palsy plus ipsilateral internuclear ophthalmoplegia, resulting in one immobile eye with only abduction preserved in the contralateral one. It is more commonly seen in the smaller unilateral lesions from infarcts,[92,269] partial hematomas,[15,154,240] arteriovenous malformations[269] or tumors,[269] which result in unilateral involvement of the paramedian pontine reticular formation and the dorsally located ipsilateral medial longitudinal fasciculus. In one of our patients with a hematoma limited to the basis pontis, there was no voluntary horizontal gaze, but reflex movements were preserved. This situation has been described by Halsey et al.[129] and reflects damage to supranuclear fibers traveling with corticobulbar fibers in the pontine basis before they reach the tegmental paramedian pontine reticular formation. *(3) Ocular bobbing:* Described by Fisher,[88] the term denotes brisk movements of conjugate ocular depression, followed within seconds by a slower return to midposition. It occurs most commonly from a pontine lesion, either hemorrhage or infarction, although it has also been described in cerebellar hemorrhage.[88,140,232,283] Typically, it affects both eyes simultaneously and is accompanied by bilateral paralysis of horizontal gaze.[88] Atypical varieties include unilateral or markedly asymmetric forms, and those occurring when horizontal eye movements are still present.[88,283] The latter form is less strictly localizing to pontine disease, as it can be seen in cerebellar hemorrhage, subarachnoid hemorrhage, and even in comas of nonvascular etiologies.[88]

Weakness of pontine and bulbar musculature is invariable in the larger median hemorrhages but is difficult to assess, since patients with bilateral tegmental damage are always comatose. Puffing of the cheeks with expiration, diminished eyelid tone, and pooling of secretions in the oropharynx are commonly elicited signs. Deafness, dysarthria, dizziness, and facial numbness occasionally precede the development of coma. Facial weakness is often asymmetric and may be associated with a crossed hemiplegia at the time the patients are first seen.[118]

Limb motor abnormalities are also always present in large tegmental-basal hemorrhages, usually quadriplegia with stiffness of all limbs. "Hemiplegia" was noted in 4 of 15 tegmental-basal hemorrhages by Goto et al.,[118] but was present in only 3 of 28 of Silverstein's bilateral hemorrhages.[273,274] The motor abnormality is usually bilateral with minor asymmetries. Asymmetries in decerebrate posturing, rflexes, or clonus are commonly detected. Tremor, shivering, restless limb movements, and dystonic postures have been common in our own experience; patients may suddenly stiffen, giving the false impression of convulsive phenomena. Shivering occurs as the patient is worsening and can be indicative of failing motor function. Decerebrate posturing was noted in 12 of 15 of the patients of Goto et al.[118] Surprisingly, only 2 of 28 of Silverstein's series of large bilateral pontine hematomas were reported to have decerebrate rigidity,[273,274] but 13 had flaccid quadriplegia and 10 "generalized flaccidity," the frequent bilaterality of the motor dysfunction.

Massive pontine hemorrhages are always fatal, though death does not come instantaneously. Steegmann[278] noted no deaths among 17 patients in less than 2 hours. Death usually occurs between 24 and 48 hours.[64,82,274,278] Survival for 2 to 10 days is not unusual and depends on the vigor of nursing and supportive care and the presence of complicating respiratory or urinary sepsis. Some patients with medium size hemorrhages survive.[235] On rare occasions a patient has survived the surgical removal of a pontine and a 4th ventricular clot,[15,230] usually due to bleeding from a pontine AVM. Since the development of the lesion is so rapid, it is unlikey that surgical treatment could be provided early enough in the larger hemorrhages to be helpful. No other medical or surgical therapy seems likely to help these grave lesions.

## Unilateral Basal or Basotegmental Hemorrhages

Unilateral basal or basotegmental hemorrhages are less common than the large paramedian lesions already discussed. In his autopsy-based series, Silverstein described 11 (22 percent) of such lesions in his report;[274] 3 were limited to the base and 8 were basotegmental. The larger lesions ruptured into the 4th ventricle. Reports based on CT scan have shown more restricted syndromes,[215,327] increasing the range of causes of a pure motor syndrome.[313] Gobernado et al.[114] described a hypertensive woman with the gradual development over a 3-day period of a pure motor hemiplegia affecting the right arm and leg, sparing the face. CT scan defined a small hematoma limited to the base of the left pons. Another patient with a small hematoma confined to the right basis pontis had an "ataxic hemiparesis" of his left limbs.[263] Small unilateral hematomas limited to the base present with syndromes indistinguishable from lacunar infarction in the same region. Tuhrim et al.[293] reported a patient with dysarthria, limb ataxia and extensor plantar response due to a small basal pontine hematoma; though the authors labeled this case as a "dysarthria-clumsy hand syndrome" it more closly resembles "ataxic hemiparesis."[96]

Bleeding originating from a pontine penetrating artery may start in the basis pontis, but also frequently dissects dorsally into the tegmentum. Whn the lesion spreads to the tegmentum, an ipsilateral facial palsy and conjugate gaze or 6th cranial nerve palsy to the ipsilateral side often accompany the contralateral hemiplegia.[105] Larger unilateral lesions may rupture into the 4th ventricle after spreading within the tegmentum (Fig. 21-42). In Silverstein's series[274] these larger unilateral basal tegmental lesions usually lead to hemiplegia, coma, and death.

## Lateral Tegmental Brain Stem Hematomas

Lateral tegmental brain stem hematomas usually originate from vessels penetrating into the brain stem from long circumferential vessels. They enter the tegmentum laterally and course medially. Small hematomas remain confined to the lateral tegmentum, while larger lesions spread across to the opposite side

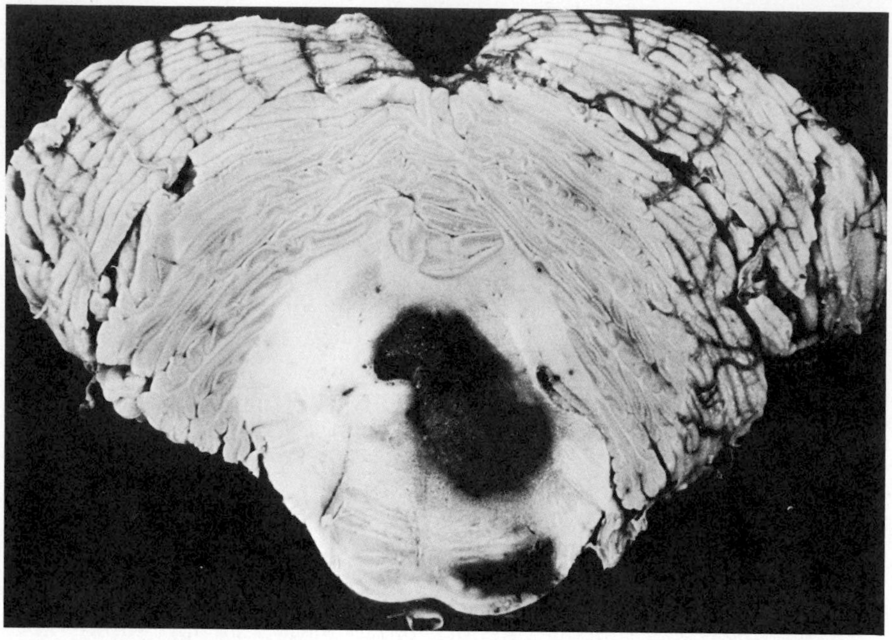

**Fig. 21-42.** Unilateral basotegmental pontine hemorrhage with rupture into 4th ventricle.

and can destroy the entire tegmentum. Neurologic examination reveals a predominantly unilateral tegmental lesion with variable degrees of basilar involvement.[34,154] Oculomotor abnormalities, especially the "one-and-a-half syndrome," horizontal gaze palsy, internuclear ophthalmoplegia, partial involvement of vertical eye movements, and ocular bobbing have been described.[34,105,154,215,235,295] The tegmental location of the spinothalamic tract makes sensory symptoms common. Ataxia, either unilateral or bilateral also may accompany the oculomotor signs.[34,154] Action tremor has developed as the transient hemiparesis improves, possibly explained by involvement of the red nucleus or its connections.[34] Facial numbness, ipsilateral miosis, and hemiparesis also have been noted.[34,154] Two patients[154] developed Cheyne-Stokes respirations, one of the "short-cycle" type,[93,241] the other of the classic variety. Table 21-13 reviews reported examples of tegmental pontine hematomas.

**TABLE 21-13. Tegmental Pontine Hemorrhages**

| Author | EOMs | Motor | Sensory | Other CN | Cerebellar |
|---|---|---|---|---|---|
| *CT Diagnosis* | | | | | |
| Caplan, Goodwin[34] | No vertical, R gaze, R 6th, bilat INO | L ↑ toe | L ↓ pin | R 7th, dysarthria, ptosis | Ataxia R > L |
| Caplan, Goodwin[34] | "1½" vertical nystagmus | L hemip, ↑ ↑ toes | L ↓ pin | R 7th, 8th, ptosis, dysarthria | Ataxia L > R |
| Müller et al.[215] | R INO | L hemip, ↑ ↑ toes | L ↓ pin | R 5th, 7th | — |
| Kase et al.[154] | "1½" No ↑ gaze, | R hemip | R ↓ pin & JPS | Dysarthria, L 7th | Ataxia L |
| Kase et al.[154] | L INO & 6th, R 4th, bobbing | R hemip | R ↓ pin | Dysphagia, L 7th | Ataxia R & L |
| *Autopsy Cases* | | | | | |
| Caplan, Goodwin[34] | "1½", bobbing, OD ↓ & inward | L hemip, Babinski | L ↓ pin | Dysarthria | Ataxia R > L |
| Tyler, Johnson[295] | No horizontal or ↑ gaze, bobbing, skew | L hemip, ↑ ↑ toes | L ↓ pin | R 5th, 7th, dysarthria, dysphagia, ptosis | R tremor |
| Dinsdale[64] | R gaze palsy | L hemip | L ↓ pin | R 7th, 8th | — |
| Silverstein[274] | R gaze palsy | L hemip, ↑ ↑ toes | L ↓ pin | R 7th, ptosis, dysphagia | — |
| Pierrott-Deseilligny et al.[240] | "1½" | L hemip, ↑ ↑ toes | L hemis | R 7th, 5th, 8th | Ataxia R arm |

*Abbreviations and symbols:* CT, computed tomography; INO, internuclear ophthalmoplegia; ↑ upward, ↓ decreased; 1½, the "one-and-a-half" syndrome; hemip, hemiparesis; JPS, joint position sense; hemis, hemisensory syndrome; CN, cranial nerve; R, right; L, left.

A small hypertensive hemorrhage could be confined to the paramedian pontine tegmentum, arising from a vessel penetrating from the dorsal region or from rupture of the distal portion of a paramedian vessel penetrating from the base. One of our cases reprsents the benign form of pontine hemorrhage: This 47-year-old normotensive female had a left horizontal gaze palsy on admission for asthma. She was severely dyspneic, but oriented, with clear speech. Motor strength, coordination, and sensation were normal and plantar responses flexor. She had a marked left lateral gaze palsy, with only 1 mm of conjugate excursion beyond the midline. Both medial recti adducted about 3 mm, an excursion larger than the 1 mm observed in right eye on left lateral gaze. Right lateral and vertical gaze were full. She reported no diplopia, and no palpebral ptosis was present. Pupils were 3 mm, reactive to light and near vision. The following morning the oculomotor findings were unchanged, but a left peripheral facial palsy had developed, along with inconsistent hypesthesia on the lower third of the face on the left. A CT scan disclosed a small hematoma in the midline pontine tegmentum (Fig. 21-43), which in its uppermost extension appeared immediately ventral to the floor of the 4th ventricle (Fig. 21-43). Her condition did not progress further her coordination improved by day 6. A repeat CT scan 2 weeks after admission showed resolution of the midline pontine hematoma, but incomplete "ring-enhancement" was detected after contrast infusion (Fig. 21-43). By discharge on day 18, the gaze palsy had improved.

We examined two patients with tegmental pontine hemorrhage and Lawrence and Lightfoote[176] studied a patient with a pontine arteriovenous malformation; all three patients showed vertical pendular ocular oscillations with dizziness and vertical oscillopsia

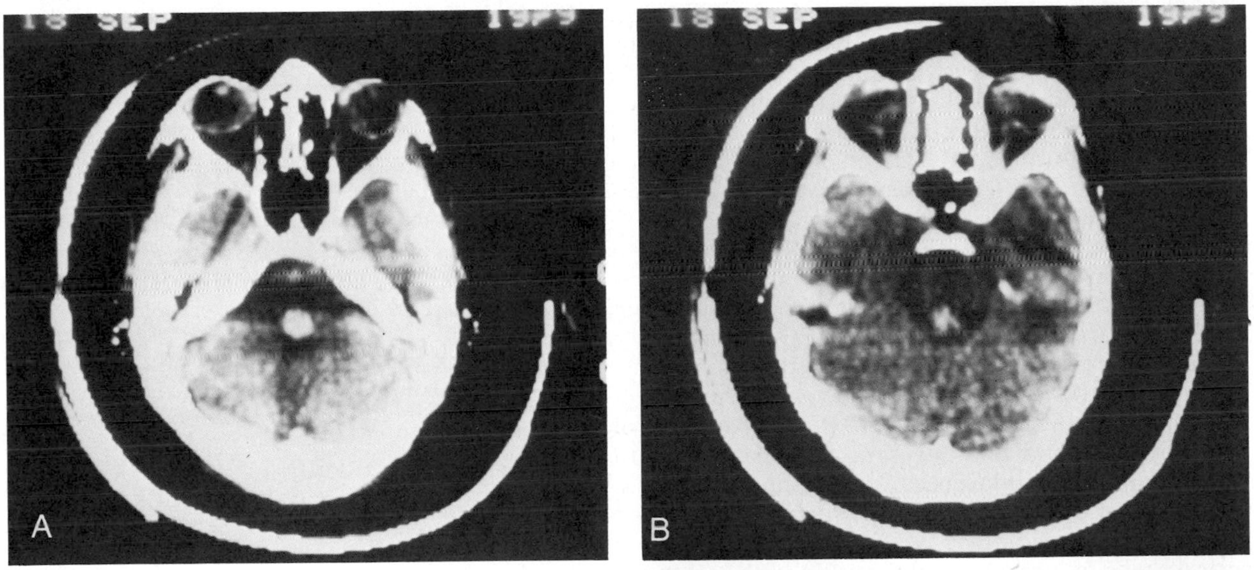


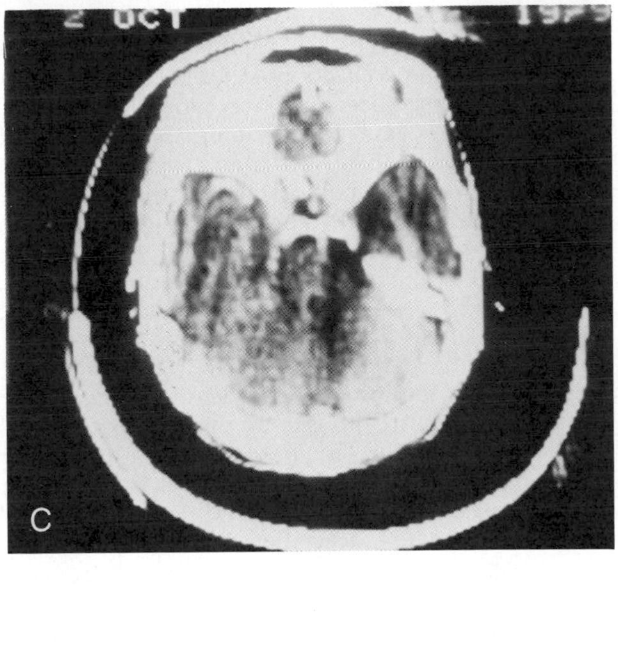


**Fig. 21-43.** Computed tomography of tegmental pontine hematoma. (**A**) Midline hematoma. (**B**) Uppermost extent just ventral to the floor of the 4th ventricle. (**C**) Repeat computed tomography 2 weeks later showing contrast "ring" enhancement of lesion.

weeks after the hemorrhage. Delayed pain in the contralateral limbs, as in the "thalamic pain syndrome," began during recovery from a unilateral tegmental hemorrhage in an additional patient.

## Medullary Hemorrhage

Hemorrhage into the medulla oblongata is even more rare than hemorrhage into the midbrain. We are still unable to find a single, well-studied patient with primary hypertensive medullary hemorrhage who did not have contiguous associated pontine hemorrhage. However, cavernous angioma and arteriovenous malformations have caused hemorrhage in the medulla.

Arseni and Stanciu[7] described a 40-year-old woman with dizziness, vomiting, and headache with diplopia and right limb paresthesiae. She suddenly became somnolent and ataxic with a stiff neck, left hemiparesis, diminished pin and temperature sensation on the left side of the face, left limb ataxia, nystagmus, dysphonia, and dysphagia. Surgical exploration found a hematoma on the floor of the 4th ventricle laterally. After drainage of the clot the patient was said to do well. Kempe[163] described a similar patient who developed a lateral medullary hematoma. A 25-year-old woman noted diminished hearing on the left and then suddenly became ill with headache, vomiting, vertigo, and hiccups. She was ataxic and fell to the left. Findings included left nystagmus, diminished pain and temperature sensation on the left side of the face, and left facial weakness; the left ear was deaf and unreactive to caloric stimuli. After PEG documented a defect in the rhomboid fossa of the 4th ventricle, exploration revealed a clot bulging through the floor of the 4th ventricle medial to the restiform body. Both of these patients had findings similar to patients with lateral medullary infarcts, and each had a stepwise course. Arteriography was not performed and CT and MRI were not available. We suspect the underlying process was a cavernous angioma in both instances. In another patient[241] the explanation was arteriovenous malformation: At age 37, this woman developed weakness and decreased position sense in her left limbs. Right vocal cord and hypoglossal paralysis developed at age 60, and 2 years later she became gradually and then abruptly worse and was hypertensive. Necropsy revealed a hemorrhage in the medial medullary tegmentum with spread into the dorsal medulla and right lateral medulla.

Mastaglia et al.,[191] reported two instances of medullary hemorrhage with quite different clinical features. An 87-year-old hypertensive woman was found unconscious with a right gaze palsy, right facial weakness, and left hemiplegia. The hemorrhage was largest in the lateral pons and descended into the medullary pyramid. This case seems to have been a pontine basal-tegmental hemorrhage with unusual caudal dissection, but it did not differ from the clinical picture already described in unilateral pontine hemorrhage. The other patient was hypertensive and had been taking warfarin anticoagulation. She developed an unusual clinical picture with markedly decreased postural sensation and incoordination of her left limbs, diminished left arm reflexes, numbness over the right eye, and subjective numbness of the right limbs. Autopsy revealed a hemorrhage into the rostral spinal cord with dissection rostrally into the left medullary pyramid. The most likely etiologic factor in this patient was anticoagulation, perhaps compounded by increased arterial pressure.

There is one well-documented case of medullary hemorrhage due to hypertension, but it is not certain whether the hemorrhage arose in the medulla or in the caudal pontine tegmentum and dissected into the medulla.[213] A 56-year-old, previously hypertensive man developed difficulty swallowing, and examination revealed paralysis of the left side of the face, soft palate, vocal cord, and tongue. A left Horner syndrome, deafness in the left ear, and paresthesiae of the right limbs were also found. CT scan showed a left medullary tegmental hematoma, but the signs of deafness and facial palsy might indicate some pontine involvement.

## REFERENCES

1. Abbott RD, Yin Y, Reed DH, Yano K: Risk of stroke in male cigarette smokers. N Engl J Med 315:717, 1986
2. Abu-Zeid HAH, Choi NW, Maini KK et al: Relative role of factors associated with cerebral infarction and cerebral hemorrhage. Stroke 8:106, 1977
3. Adams RD: Pathology of cerebral vascular disease. p. 23. In Wright IS, Millikan CH (eds): Cerebral Vascular Disease: Second Conference. Grune & Stratton, New York, 1958
4. Adams RD, Sidman RL: Introduction to Neuropathology. p. 176. McGraw-Hill, New York, 1968
5. Alexander MP, LoVerme SR: Aphasia after left hemispheric intracerebral hemorrhage. Neurology (NY) 30:1193, 1980
6. Aring CD: Differential diagnosis of cerebrovascular stroke. Arch Intern Med 113:195, 1964
7. Arseni C, Stanciu M: Primary hematomas of the brain stem. Acta Neurochir 28:323, 1973
8. Attwater H: Pontine hemorrhage. Guys Hosp Rep 65:339, 1911
9. Aurell M, Head B: Cerebral hemorrhage in a population after a decade of active anti-hypertensive treatment. Acta Med Scand 176:377, 1964
10. Babikian VL, Kase CS, Pessin MS et al: Intracerebral hemorrhage in stroke patients anticoagulated with heparin. Stroke 20:1500, 1989
11. Barinagarrementeria F, Méndez A, Vega F: Hemorragia cerebral asociada al uso de fenilpropanolamina. Neurologia 5:292, 1990
12. Barraquer-Bordas L, Illa I, Escartin A et al: Tha-

lamic hemorrhage: a study of 23 patients with a diagnosis by computed tomography. Stroke 12:524, 1981
13. Barron KD, Fergusson G: Intracranial hemorrhage as a complication of anticoagulant therapy. Neurology (NY) 9:447, 1959
14. Beck DW, Menezes AH: Intracerebral hemorrhage in a patient with eclampsia. JAMA 246:1442, 1981
15. Becker DH, Silverberg GD: Successful evacuation of an acute pontine hematoma. Surg Neurol 10:263, 1978
16. Becker DH, Townsend JJ, Kramer RA, Newton TH: Occult cerebrovascular malformations: a series of 18 histologically verified cases with negative angiography. Brain 70:530, 1979
17. Benson DF, Sheremata WA, Bouchard R et al: Conduction aphasia: a clinicopathological study. Arch Neurol 28:339, 1973
18. Bernstein E, Diskant BM: Phenylpropanolamine: a potentially hazardous drug. Ann Emerg Med 11:311, 1982
19. Bicknell JM, Carlow TJ, Kornfeld M et al: Familial cavernous angiomas. Arch Neurol 35:746, 1978
20. Biller J, Loftus CM, Moore SA et al: Isolated central nervous system angiitis first presenting as spontaneous intracranial hemorrhage. Neurosurgery 20:310, 1987
21. Bjerkelund CJ: The effect of long-term treatment with dicumarol in myocardial infarction. Acta Med Scand, suppl. 158:1, 1957
22. Bosch EP, Kennedy SS, Aschenbrener CA: Ocular bobbing: the myth of its localizing value. Neurology (NY) 25:949, 1975
23. Boudouresques G, Hauw JJ, Meininger V et al: Etude neuropathologique des hemorrhagies intracraniennes de l'adulte. Rev Neurol 135:197, 1979
24. Brennan RW, Bergland RM: Acute cerebellar hemorrhage: analysis of clinical findings and outcome in 12 cases. Neurology (NY) 27:527, 1977
25. Brewer DB, Fawcett FJ, Horsfield GI: A necropsy series of non-traumatic cerebral haemorrhages and softenings, with particular reference to heart weight. J Pathol Bact 96:311, 1968
26. Brillman J: Acute hydrocephalus and death one month after non-surgical treatment for acute cerebellar hemorrhage. J Neurosurg 50:374, 1979
27. Broderick JP, Brott TG, Tomsick T et al: Ultra-early evaluation of intracerebral hemorrhage. J Neurosurg 72:195, 1990
28. Brott T, Thalinger K, Hertzberg V: Hypertension as a risk factor for spontaneous intracerebral hemorrhage. Stroke 17:1078, 1986
29. Butler AB, Partian RA, Netsky MG: Primary intraventricular hemorrhage: a mild and remediable form. Neurology (NY) 22:675, 1972
30. Butler JF, Cancilla PA, Cornell SH: Computerized axial tomography of intracerebral hematoma: a clinical and neuropathological study. Arch Neurol 33:206, 1976
31. Cambier J, Elghozi D, Strube E: Hemorrhagie de la tete de du noyau caude gauche. Rev Neurol (Paris) 135:763, 1979
32. Cambier J, Elghozi D, Strube E: Trois observations de lesions vasculaires du thalamus droit avec syndrome de l'hemisphere mineur: discussion du concept de negligence thalamique. Rev Neurol (Paris) 136:105, 1980
33. Caplan LR: Intracerebral hemorrhage. p. 185. In Tyler HR, Dawson DM (eds): Current Neurology. Vol II. Houghton Mifflin, Boston, 1979
34. Caplan LR, Goodwin JA: Lateral tegmental brainstem hemorrhages. Neurology (NY) 32:252, 1982
35. Caplan LR, Mohr JP: Intracerebral hemorrhage: an update. Geriatrics 33:42, 1978
36. Carion F: Contribution à l'étude symptomatique et diagnostique de l'hemorrhagie cerebelleuse. Adrien Delhaye, Paris, 1875
37. Carpenter MB: Human Neuroanatomy. p. 23. 7th Ed. Williams & Wilkins, Baltimore, 1976
38. Carton CA, Hickey WC: Arteriovenous malformation of the head of the caudate: report of a case of total removal. J Neurosurg 12:414, 1955
39. Cerebral Embolism Study Group: Immediate anticoagulation of embolic stroke: brain hemorrhage and management options. Stroke 15:779, 1984
40. Charcot JM, Bouchard C: Nouvelles recherches sur la pathogénie de l'hemorragie cerebrale. Arch Physiol Norm Pathol 1:110, 1868
41. Cheyn J: Cases of apoplexy and lethargy with observations upon the comatose diseases. Thomas Underwood, London, 1812
42. Childs T: A case of apoplexy of the cerebellum. Am Med Month (NY) 9.1, 1858
43. Choi D, Sudansky L, Schachter S et al: Medial thalamic hemorrhage with amnesia. Arch Neurol 40:611, 1983
44. Chokroverty S, Rubino FA, Haller C: Pure motor hemiplegia due to pyramidal infarction. Arch Neurol 32:647, 1975
45. Christoff N: A clinicopathologic study of vertical eye movements. Arch Neurol 31:1, 1974
46. Christoff N, Anderson PJ, Bender MB: A clinicopathologic study of associated vertical eye movements. Trans Am Neurol Assoc 87:184, 1962
47. Citron BP, Halpern M, McCarron M et al: Necrotizing angiitis associated with drug abuse. N Engl J Med 283:1003, 1970
48. Clark JV: Familial occurrence of cavernous angiomata of the brain. J Neurol Neurosurg Psychiatry 33:871, 1970
49. Clifford-Jones RE, Love S, Gurusinghe N: Granulomatous angiitis of the central nervous system: a case with recurrent intracerebral hemorrhage. J Neurol Neurosurg Psychiatry 48:1054, 1985
50. Cole FM, Yates PO: Intracranial microaneurysms and small cerebrovascular lesions. Brain 90:759, 1967
51. Cole FM, Yates PO: The occurrence and significance of intracerebral microaneurysms. J Pathol Bact 93:393, 1967
52. Cole FM, Yates PO: Pseudo-aneurysms in rela-

tionship to massive cerebral hemorrhage. J Neurol Neurosurg Psychiatry 30:61, 1967
53. Cole FM, Yates PO: Comparative incidence of cerebrovascular lesions in normotensive and hypertensive patients. Neurology (NY) 18:255, 1968
54. Coon WW, Willis PW: Hemorrhagic complications of anticoagulant therapy. Arch Intern Med 133:386, 1974
55. Crawford JV, Russell DS: Cryptic arteriovenous and venous hamartomas of the brain. J Neurol Neurosurg Psychiatry 19:1, 1956
56. Critchley M: The Parietal Lobes. p. 326. Hafner, New York, 1966
57. Crowell RM, Ojemann RG: Surgery for brain hemorrhage. p. 233. In Moossy J, Reinmuth OM (eds): Cerebrovascular Diseases. Twelfth Research Conference. Raven Press, New York, 1981
58. Dana C: Acute bulbar paralysis due to hemorrhage and softening of the pons and medulla. Med Rec 64:361, 1903
59. Davis KR, Ackerman RH, Kistler JP, Mohr JP: Computed tomography of cerebral infarction: hemorrhagic, contrast enhancement, and time of appearance. Comput Tomogr 1:71, 1977
60. Dejerine J, Roussy G: Le syndrome thalamique. Rev Neurol (Paris) 12:521, 1906
61. Delaney P, Estes M: Intracranial hemorrhage with amphetamine abuse. Neurology (NY) 30:1125, 1980
62. Denny-Brown D, Fischer EG: Physiological aspects of visual perception. II. The subcortical visual direction of behavior. Arch Neurol 33:228, 1976
63. De Reuck J, Crevits L, Sieben G, DeCoster W: Granulomatous angiitis of the nervous system: a clinicopathological study of one case. J Neurol 227:49, 1982
64. Dinsdale HB: Spontaneous hemorrhage in the posterior fossa: a study of primary cerebellar and pontine hemorrhage with observations on the pathogenesis. Arch Neurol 10:200, 1964
65. Dolinskas CA, Bilaniuk LT, Zimmerman RA et al: Computed tomography of intracerebral hematomas. II. Radionuclide and transmission CT studies of the perihematoma region. AJR 129:689, 1977
66. Dolinskas CA, Bilaniuk LT, Zimmerman RA, Kuhl DE: Computed tomography of intracerebral hematomas. I. Transmission CT observations on hematoma resolution. Am J Roentgenol 129:681, 1977
67. Donahue RP, Abbott RD, Reed DM, Yanko K: Alcohol and hemorrhagic stroke: the Honolulu Heart Program. JAMA 255:2311, 1986
68. Douglas MA, Haerer AF: Long-term prognosis of hypertensive intracerebral hemorrhage. Stroke 13:488, 1982
69. Drapkin A, Merskey C: Anticoagulant therapy after acute myocardial infarction: relation of therapeutic benefit to patient's age, sex, and severity of infarction. JAMA 222:541, 1972
70. Drury I, Whisnant JP, Garraway WM: Primary intracerebral hemorrhage: impact of CT on incidence. Neurology (NY) 34:653, 1984
71. D'Souza T, Shraberg D: Intracranial hemorrhage associated with amphetamine use. (Letter.) Neurology (NY) 31:922, 1981
72. Duret H: Études experimentales et cliniques sur les traumatisms cérébraux. Adrien Delhaye, Paris, 1873
73. Duret H: Sur la distribution des artères nourricières du bulbe rachidien. Arch Physiol Norm Pathol 5:97, 1873
74. Duret H: Recherches anatomiques sur la circulation de l'encéphale. Arch Physiol Norm Pathol 6, 1:60, 919, 1874
75. Duret H: Traumatismes cranio-cérébraux. Librairie Felix Alcan, Paris, 1919
76. Durward QJ, Barnett HJM, Barr HWK: Presentation and management of mesencephalic hematoma. J Neurosurg 56:123, 1982
77. Echlin FA, Arnett V, Zoll J: Paroxysmal high voltage discharges from isolated and partially isolated human and animal cerebral cortex. EEG Clin Neurophysiol 4:147, 1952
78. Ellis AG: The pathogenesis of spontaneous cerebral hemorrhage. Proc Pathol Soc (Philadelphia) 12:197, 1909
79. Englander RN, Netsky MG, Adelman LS: Location of human pyramidal tract in the internal capsule: anatomic evidence. Neurology (Minneapolis) 25:823, 1975
80. Epstein AW: Primary massive pontine hemorrhage. J Neuropathol Exp Neurol 10:426, 1951
81. Fallis RJ, Fisher M: Cerebral vasculitis and hemorrhage associated with phenylpropanolamine. Neurology (NY) 35:405, 1985
82. Fang HCM, Foley JM: Hypertensive hemorrhages of the pons and cerebellum. Arch Neurol Psychiatry 72:638, 1954
83. Fazio C, Sacco G, Bugiani O: The thalamic hemorrhage: an anatomo-clinical study. Eur Neurol 9:30, 1973
84. Fehr MA, Anderson DC: Incidence of progression or rebleeding in hypertensive intracerebral hemorrhage. J Stroke Cerebrovasc Dis 1:111, 1991
85. Finelli PF, Kessimian N, Bernstein PW: Cerebral amyloid angiopathy manifesting as recurrent intracerebral hemorrhage. Arch Neurol 41:330, 1984
86. Fisher CM: The pathologic and clinical aspects of thalamic hemorrhage. Trans Am Neurol Assoc 84:56, 1959
87. Fisher CM: The pathology and pathogenesis of intracerebral hemorrhage. p. 295. In Fields WS (ed): Pathogenesis and Treatment of Cerebrovascular Disease. CC Thomas, Springfield, IL, 1961
88. Fisher CM: Ocular bobbing. Arch Neurol 11:543, 1964
89. Fisher CM: Clinical syndromes in cerebral hemorrhage. p. 318. In Fields WS (ed): Pathogenesis and Treatment of Cerebrovascular Disease. CC Thomas, Springfield, IL, 1961
90. Fisher CM: Pure sensory stroke involving face, arm and leg. Neurology (Minneapolis) 15:76, 1965
91. Fisher CM: Lacunes: Small, deep cerebral infarcts. Neurology (Minneapolis) 15:774, 1965
92. Fisher CM: Some neuro-ophthalmological obser-

vations. J Neurol Neurosurg Psychiatry 30:383, 1967
93. Fisher CM: The neurological examination of the comatose patient. Acta Neurol Scand, suppl. 45:1, 44, 1969
94. Fisher CM: The arterial lesions underlying lacunes. Acta Neuropathol 12:1, 1969
95. Fisher CM: Pathological obsrvations in hypertensive cerebral hemorrhage. J Neuropathol Exp Neurol 30:536, 1971
96. Fisher CM: Cerebral ischemia—less familiar types. Clin Neurosurg 18:267, 1971
97. Fisher CM: Cerebral miliary aneurysms in hypertension. Am J Pathol 66:313, 1972
98. Fisher CM: Capsular infarcts. Arch Neurol 36:65, 1979
99. Fisher CM, Adams RD: Observations on brain embolism with special reference to the mechanism of hemorrhagic infarction. J Neuropathol Exp Neurol 10:92, 1951
100. Fisher CM, Curry HB: Pure motor hemiplegia of vascular origin. Arch Neurol 13:30, 1965
101. Fisher CM, Picard EH, Polak A et al: Acute hypertensive cerebellar hemorrhage: diagnosis and surgical treatment. J Nerv Ment Dis 140:38, 1965
102. Forfar JC: A 7-year analysis of haemorrhage in patients on long-term anticoagulant treatment. Br Heart J 42:128, 1979
103. Franke CL, deJonge J, van Swieten JC et al: Intracerebral hematomas during anticoagulant treatment. Stroke 21:726, 1990
104. Freeman RE, Onofrio BM, Okazaki H, Dinapoli RP: Spontaneous intracerebellar hemorhage. Neurology (NY) 23:84, 1973
105. Freeman W, Ammerman HH, Stanley M: Syndromes of the pontile tegmentum, Foville's syndrome: report of 3 cases. Arch Neurol Psychiatry 50:462, 1943
106. Freytag E: Fatal hypertensive intracerebral haematomas: a survey of the pathological anatomy of 393 cases. J Neurol Neurosurg Psychiatry 31:616, 1968
107. Furlan AJ, Whisnant JP, Elveback LR: The decreasing incidence of primary intracerebral hemorrhage: a population study. Ann Neurol 5:367, 1979
108. Garraway WM, Whisnant JP, Drury I: The continuing decline in the incidence of stroke. Mayo Clin Proc 58:520, 1983
109. Gilbert JJ, Vinters HV: Cerebral amyloid angiopathy: incidence and complications in the aging brain. I. Cerebral hemorrhage. Stroke 14:915, 1983
110. Gildersleve N, Koo AH, McDonald CJ: Metastatic tumor presenting as intracerebral hemorrhage. Radiology 124:109, 1977
111. Gilles C, Brucher JM, Khoubesserian P, Vanderhaeghn JJ: Cerebral amyloid angiopathy as a cause of multiple intracerebral hemorrhages. Neurology (NY) 34:730, 1984
112. Gilner LI, Avin B: A reversible ocular manifestation of thalamic hemorrhage: a case report. Arch Neurol 34:715, 1977
113. Glick R, Hoying J, Cerullo L, Perlman S: Phenylpropanolamine: an over-the-counter drug causing central nervous system vasculitis and intracerebral hemorrhage. Neurosurgery (NY) 20:969, 1987
114. Gobernado JM, Fernandez de Molina AR, Gimeno A: Pure motor hemiplegia due to hemorrhage in the lower pons. Arch Neurol 37:393, 1980
115. Goldblatt D, Markesberry W, Reeves AG: Recurrent hemichorea following striatal lesions. Arch Neurol 31:51, 1974
116. Gomori JM, Grossman RI, Goldberg HI et al: Intracranial hematomas: imaging by high-field MR. Radiology 157:87, 1985
117. Gore JM, Sloan M, Price TR et al: Intracerebral hemorrhage, cerebral infarction, and subdural hematoma after acute myocardial infarction and thrombolytic therapy in the Thrombolysis in Myocardial Infarction Study: Thrombolysis in myocardial infarction, phase II, pilot and clinical data. Circulation 83:448, 1991
118. Goto N, Kaneko M, Hosaka Y, Koga H: Primary pontine hemorrhage: clinicopathologic correlations. Stroke 11:84, 1980
119. Gowers WR: A Manual of Diseases of the Nervous System. 2nd Ed. Vol. II. p. 395. JA Churchill, London, 1893
120. Graus F, Rogers LR, Posner JB: Cerebrovascular complications in patients with cancer. Medicine 64:16, 1985
121. Green FHK: Miliary aneurysms in the brain. J Pathol Bact 33:71, 1930
122. Green RM, Kelly KM, Gabrielsen T et al: Multiple intracranial hemorrhages after smoking "crack" cocaine. Stroke 21:957, 1990
123. Greenberg J, Skubick D, Shenkin H: Acute hydrocephalus in cerebellar infarct and hemorrhage. Neurology (NY) 29:409, 1979
124. Groothuis DR, Duncan GW, Fisher CM: The human thalamocortical sensory path in the internal capsule: evidence from a small capsular hemorrhage causing pure sensory stroke. Ann Neurol 2:328, 1977
125. Gross CR, Kase CS, Mohr JP et al: Stroke in south Alabama: incidence and diagnostic features—a population based study. Stroke 15:249, 1984
126. Gudmundsson G, Hallgrimsson J, Jonasson TA, Bjarnason O: Hereditary cerebral haemorrhage with amyloidosis. Brain 95:387, 1972
127. Guillain G, Alajouanine T, Marquezy R: Hemorrhagie cerebelleuse avec spasms toniques et attitude de rigidité des membres inferieures. Bull Mem Soc Med Hop Paris 47:1120, 1923
128. Gurwitt LJ, Long JM, Clark RE: Cerebral metastatic choriocarcinoma: a postpartum cause of "stroke." Obstet Gynecol 45:583, 1975
129. Halsey JH, Ceballos R, Crosby EC: The supranuclear control of voluntary lateral gaze. Neurology (NY) 17:928, 1967
130. Hanaway J, Young RR: Localization of the pyramidal tract in the internal capsule of man. J Neurol Sci 34:63, 1977
131. Handley AJ, Emerson PA, Fleming PR: Heparin in the prevention of deep vein thrombosis

after myocardial infarction. Br Med J 2:436, 1972
132. Hankey GJ: Isolated angiitis/angiopathy of the central nervous system. Cerebrovasc Dis 1:2, 1991
133. Hansen BS, Marquardsen J: Incidence of stroke in Frederiksberg, Denmark. Stroke 8:663, 1977
134. Harrington H, Heller HA, Dawson D et al: Intracerebral hemorrhage and oral amphetamine. Arch Neurol 40:503, 1983
135. Heilman JM, Valenstein E: Frontal lobe neglect in man. Neurology (Minneapolis) 22:660, 1972
136. Heiman TD, Satya-Murti S: Benign cerebellar hemorrhages. Ann Neurol 3:366, 1978
137. Herbstein DJ, Schaumburg HH: Hypertensive intracerebral hematoma: an investigation of the initial hemorrhage and rebleeding using chromium Cr 51-labeled erythrocytes. Arch Neurol 30:412, 1974
138. Herman B, Schulte BPM, van Luijk JH et al: Epidemiology of stroke in Tilburg, The Netherlands: the population-based stroke incidence register. 1. Introduction and preliminary results. Stroke 11:162, 1980
139. Herold S, von Kumer R, Jaeger CH: Follow-up of spontaneous intracerebral haemorrhage by computed tomography. J Neurol 228:267, 1982
140. Heros RC: Cerebellar hemorrhage and infarction. Stroke 13:106, 1982
141. Hickey WF, King RB, Wang A-M, Samuels MA: Multiple simultaneous intracerebral hematomas: clinical, radiologic, and pathologic findings in two patients. Arch Neurol 40:519, 1983
142. Hier DB, Davis KR, Richardson EP, Mohr JP: Hypertensive putaminal hemorrhage. Ann Neurol 1:152, 1977
143. Houser OW, Campbell JK: Computed tomography in cerebrovascular disease: influences of morphology, topography, clinical factors, and temporal profile. p. 181. In Moossy J, Reinmuth OM (eds): Cerebrovascular Diseases. Proceedings of the Twelfth Research Conference. Raven Press, New York, 1981
144. Humphreys RP: Computerized tomographic definition of mesencephalic hematoma with evacuation through pedunculotomy. J Neurosurg 49:749, 1978
145. Husted S, Andreasen F: Problems encountered in long-term treatment with anticoagulants. Acta Med Scand 200:379, 1976
146. Hyland HH, Levy D: Spontaneous cerebellar hemorrhage. Can Med Assoc J 71:315, 1954
147. Jacome DE: Isodense cerebellar hematoma. Neurology (Cleveland) 33:1201, 1983
148. Jellinger K: Cerebrovascular amyloidosis with cerebral hemorrhage. J Neurol 214:195, 1977
149. Jellinger K: Cerebral hemorrhage in amyloid angiopathy. (Letter.) Ann Neurol 1:604, 1977
150. Kasdon DL, Scott RM, Adelman LS, Wolpert SM: Cerebellar hemorrhage with decreased absorption values on computed tomography: a case report. Neuroradiology 13:265, 1977
151. Kase CS: Intracerebral hemorrhage: non-hypertensive causes. Stroke 17:590, 1986
152. Kase CS, Foster TE, Reed JE et al: Intracerebral hemorrhage and phenylpropanolamine use. Neurology (NY) 37:399, 1987
153. Kase CS, Maulsby GO, deJaun E, Mohr JP: Hemichorea-hemiballism and lacunar infarction in the basal ganglia. Neurology (NY) 31:452, 1981
154. Kase CS, Maulsby GO, Mohr JP: Partial pontine hematomas. Neurology (NY) 30:652, 1980
155. Kase CS, O'Neal AM, Fisher M et al: Intracranial hemorrhage after use of tissue plasminogen activator for coronary thrombolysis. Ann Intern Med 112:17, 1990
156. Kase CS, Pessin MS, Zivin JA et al: Intracranial hemorrhage following coronary thrombolysis with tissue plasminogen activator. Am J Med 92:384, 1992
157. Kase CS, Robinson RK, Stein RW et al: Anticoagulant-related intracerebral hemorrhage. Neurology (NY) 35:943, 1985
158. Kase CS, White JL, Mohr JP: Intracerebral hemorrhage: clinical and CT observations in 100 consecutive cases. (In preparation).
159. Kase CS, Williams JP, Wyatt DA, Mohr JP: Lobar intracerebral hematomas: clinical and CT analysis of 22 cases. Neurology (NY) 32:1146, 1982
160. Keane JR: Contralateral gaze deviation with supratentorial hemorrhage: three pathologically verified cases. Arch Neurol 32:119, 1975
161. Keane JR: Transient opsoclonus with thalamic hemorrhage. Arch Neurol 37:423, 1980
162. Kelley RE, Berger JR, Scheinberg P, Stokes N: Active bleeding in hypertensive intracerebral hemorrhage: computed tomography. Neurology (NY) 32:852, 1982
163. Kempe LG: Burgical removal of an intramedullary hematoma simulating Wallenberg's syndrome. J Neurol Neurosurg Psychiatry 27:78, 1964
164. Kendall BE, Claveria LE: Vascular conditions. p. 161. In du Boulay GH, Moseley IF (eds): Computerized Axial Tomography in Clinical Practice. Springer-Verlag, Berlin, 1977
165. Kikta DG, Devereaux MX, Chandar K: Intracranial hemorrhages due to phenylpropanolamine. Stroke 16:510, 1985
166. Kistler JP, Hochberg FH, Brooks BR et al: Computerized axial tomography: clinicopathologic correlation. Neurology (NY) 25:201, 1975
167. Kjellin KG, Soderstrom CE: Cerebral haemorrhages with atypical clinical patterns: a study of cerebral hematomas using CSF spectrophotometry and computerized transverse axial tomography ("EMI scanning"). J Neurol Sci 25:211, 1975
168. Kolodny EH, Rebeiz JJ, Caviness VS, Richardson EP: Granulomatous angiitis of the central nervous system. Arch Neurol 19:510, 1968
169. Kornyey S: Rapidly fatal pontile hemorrhage: clinical and anatomic report. Arch Neurol Psychiatry 41:793, 1939
170. Kowada M, Yamaguchi K, Matsuoka S, Ito Z: Extravasation of angiographic contrast material in hypertensive intracerebral hemorrhage. J Neurosurg 36:471, 1972

171. Krayenbuhl H, Siebenmann R: Small vascular malformations as a cause of primary intracerebral hemorrhage. J Neurosurg 22:7, 1965
172. Kunitz SC, Gross CR, Heyman A et al: The Pilot Stroke Data Bank: definition, design and data. Stroke 15:740, 1984
173. Kurtzke JF: Epidemiology of Cerebrovascular Disease. Springer-Verlag, Berlin, 1969
174. Kwak R, Kadoya S, Suzuki T: Factors affecting the prognosis in thalamic hemorrhage. Stroke 14:493, 1983
175. LaTorre E, Delitala A, Sorano V: Hematoma of the quadrigeminal plate. J Neurosurg 49:610, 1978
176. Lawrence WH, Lightfoote WE: Continuous vertical pendular eye movements after brainstem hemorrhage. Neurology (NY) 25:896, 1975
177. Leestma JE, Noronha A: Pure motor hemiplegia, medullary pyramid lesion, and olivary hypertrophy. J Neurol Neurosurg Psychiatry 39:877, 1976
178. Levine SR, Brust JCM, Futrell N et al: Cerebrovascul complications of the use of the "crack" form of alkaloid cocaine. N Engl J Med 323:699, 1990
179. Little JR, Dial B, Bellanger G, Carpenter S: Brain hemorrhage from intracranial tumor. Stroke 10:283, 1979
180. Little JR, Tubman DE, Ethier R: Cerebellar hemorrhage in adults: diagnosis by computerized tomography. J Neurosurg 48:575, 1978
181. Loder J, Baard WC: Paraballism caused by bilateral hemorrhagic infarction in basal ganglia. Neurology (NY) 31:484, 1981
182. Loizou LA, Hamilton JG, Tsementzis SA: Intracranial hemorrhage in association with pseudoephedrine overdose. J Neurol Neurosurg Psychiatry 45:471, 1982
183. Lukes SA: Intracerebral hemorrhage from an arteriovenous malformation after amphetamine injection. Arch Neurol 40:60, 1983
184. Mandybur TI: Intracranial hemorrhage caused by metastatic tumors. Neurology (NY) 27:650, 1977
185. Mandybur TI: Cerebral amyloid angiopathy: possible relationship to rheumatoid vasculitis. Neurology (NY) 29:1336, 1979
186. Mandybur TI, Bates SRD: Fatal massive intracerebral hemorrhage complicating cerebral amyloid angiopathy. Arch Neurol 35:246, 1978
187. Margolis G, Odom GL, Woodhall B, Bloor BM: The role of small angiomatous malformations in the production of intracerebral hematomas. J Neurosurg 8:S64, 1951
188. Margolis MT, Newton TH: Methaamphetamine ("speed") arteritis. Neuroradiology 2:179, 1971
189. Masdeu JC, Rubino FA: Management of lobar intracerebral hemorrhage, medical or surgical. Neurology (Cleveland) 34:381, 1984
190. Massaro AR, Sacco RL, Mohr JP et al: Clinical discriminators separate lobar and subcortical hemorrhage: the Stroke Data Bank. Neurology (NY) 41:1881, 1991
191. Mastaglia FL, Edis B, Kakulas BA: Medullary hemorrhage: a report of two cases. J Neurol Neurosurg Psychiatry 32:221, 1969
192. Matick H, Anderson D, Brumlik J: Cerebral vasculitis associated with oral amphetamine overdose. Arch Neurol 40:253, 1983
193. McConnell TH, Leonard JS: Microangiomatous malformations with intraventricular hemorrhage. Neurology (NY) 17:618, 1967
194. McCormick WF, Rosenfield DB: Massive brain hemorrhage: a review of 144 cases and an examination of their causes. Stroke 4:946, 1973
195. McCormick WF, Schochet SS: Atlas of Cerebrovascular Disease. p. 328. WB Saunders, Philadelphia, 1976
196. McKissok W, Richardson A, Taylor J: Primary intracerebral hemorrhage: a controlled trial of surgical and conservative treatment in 180 unselected cases. Lancet 2:221, 1961
197. McKissock W, Richardson A, Walsh L: Spontaneous cerebellar hemorrhage: a study of 34 consecutive cases treated surgically. Brain 83:1, 1960
198. Melamed E, Korn-Lubetzki I, Reches A, Siew F: Hemiballismus: detection of focal hemorrhage in subthalamic nucleus by CT scan. Ann Neurol 4:582, 1978
199. Merritt HH: A Textbook of Neurology. p. 160. 6th Ed. Lea & Febiger, Philadelphia, 1979
200. Messert B, Leppik IE, Sato Y: Diplopia and involuntary eye closure in spontaneous cerebellar hemorrhage. Stroke 7:305, 1976
201. Michael JC: Cerebellar apoplexy. Am J Med Sci 183:687, 1932
202. Mitchell N, Angrist A: Spontaneous cerebellar hemorrhage: report of 15 cases. Am J Pathol 18:235, 1942
203. Mizukami M, Araki G, Mihara H et al: Arteriographically visualized extravasation in hypertensive intracerebral hemorrhage: report of seven cases. Stroke 3:527, 1972
204. Mizukami M, Araki G, Mihara H: Angiographic sign of good prognosis for hemiplegia in hypertensive intracerebral hemorrhage. Neurology (NY) 24:120, 1974
205. Mizukami M, Nishijima M, Kin H: Computed tomographic findings of good prognosis for hemiplegia in hypertensive putaminal hemorrhage. Stroke 12:648, 1981
206. Modesti LM, Binet EF, Collins GH: Meningiomas causing spontaneous intracranial hematomas. J Neurosurg 45:437, 1976
207. Mohr JP, Caplan LR, Melski JW et al: The Harvard Cooperative Stroke Registry: a prospective registry. Neurology (NY) 28:754, 1978
208. Mohr JP, Kase CS, Adams RD: Cerebrovascular Disorders. p. 2028. In Petersdorf RG et al: Harrison's Principles of Internal Medicine. 10th Ed. McGraw-Hill, New York, 1983
209. Mohr JP, Pessin MS, Finkelstein S et al: Broca aphasia: pathologic and clinical aspects. Neurology (Minneapolis) 28:311, 1978
210. Mohr JP, Sidman M: Aphasia: behavioral aspects. p. 279. In Reiser MF (ed): American Handbook of Psychiatry. Basic Books, New York, 1975

211. Mohr JP, Watters WC, Duncan GW: Thalamic hemorrhage and aphasia. Brain Lang 2:3, 1975
212. Moore PM, Cupps TR: Neurological complications of vasculitis. Ann Neurol 14:155, 1983
213. Morel-Maroger A, Metzger J, Bories J et al: Les hematomes benins du tronc cérébral chez les hypertendus artériels. Rev Neurol (Paris) 138:437, 1982
214. Mueller SM: Phenylpropanolamine: a non-prescription drug with potentially fatal side effects. (Letter.) N Engl J Med 308:653, 1983
215. Müller HR, Wüthrich R, Wiggli U et al: The contribution of computerized axial tomography to the diagnosis of cerebellar and pontine hematomas. Stroke 6:467, 1975
216. Mutlu N, Berry RG, Alpers BJ: Massive cerebral hemorrhage: clinical and pathological correlations. Arch Neurol 8:74, 1963
217. Myoung CL, Heany LM, Jacobson RL, Klassen AC: Cerebrospinal fluid in cerebral hemorrhage and infarction. Stroke 6:638, 1975
218. Naeser MA, Hayward RW: The resolving stroke and aphasia: a case study with computerized tomography. Arch Neurol 36:233, 1979
219. Nashold BS, Seaber JH: Defects of ocular motility after stereotactic midbrain lesions in man. Arch Ophthalmol 88:245, 1972
220. New PFJ: Computed tomography in the diagnosis of hemorrhagic stroke. p. 145. In Thompson RA, Green JR (eds): Advances in Neurology. Raven Press, New York, 1977
221. New PFJ, Aronow S: Attenuation measurements of whole blood and blood fractions in computed tomography. Radiology 121:635, 1976
222. Norris JW, Eisen AA, Branch CL: Problems in cerebellar hemorrhage and infarction. Neurology (NY) 19:1043, 1969
223. Obeso JA, Marti-Masso JF, Carrera N, Astudillo W: Pure motor quadriplegia secondary to bilateral capsular hematomas. Arch Neurol 37:248, 1980
224. O'Connor CM, Aldrich H, Massey EW et al: Intracranial hemorrhage after thrombolytic therapy for acute myocardial infarction: clinical characteristics and in-hospital outcome, abstract ed. J Am Coll Cardiol 15:213A, 1990
225. Ojemann RG, Heros RC: Spontaneous brain hemorrhage. Stroke 14:468, 1983
226. Ojemann RG, Mohr JP: Hypertensive brain hemorrhage. Clin Neurosurg 23:220, 1976
227. Okazaki H, Reagan TJ, Campbell RJ: Clinicopathologic studies of primary cerebral amyloid angiopathy. Mayo Clin Proc 54:22, 1979
228. Okoye MI, Watanabe I: Ultrastructural features of cerebral amyloid angiopathy. Hum Pathol 13:1127, 1982
229. Okudera T, Uemura K, Nakajima K et al: Primary pontine hemorrhage: correlations of pathologic features with postmortem microangiographic and vertebral angiography studies. Mt Sinai J Med 45:305, 1978
230. O'Laoire SA, Crockard HA, Thomas DGT, Gordon DS: Brain-stem hematoma. J Neurosurg 56:222, 1982
231. Oppenheim H: Trattato della Malattie Nervose. Vol II. S.E.I., Milano, 1905
232. Ott KH, Kase CS, Ojemann RG, Mohr JP: Cerebellar hemorrhage: diagnosis and treatment. Arch Neurol 31:160, 1974
233. Pasik P, Pasik T, Bender MB: The pretectal syndrome in monkeys. I. Disturbances of gaze and body posture. Brain 92:521, 1969
234. Patel DV, Hier DB, Thomas CM, Hemmati M: Intracerebral hemorrhage secondary to cerebral amyloid angiopathy. Radiology 151:397, 1984
235. Payne HA, Maravilla KR, Levistone A et al: Recovery from primary pontine hemorrhage. Ann Neurol 4:557, 1978
236. Pendlebury WW, Iole ED, Tracy RP, Dill BA: Intracerebral hemorrhage related to cerebral amyloid angiopathy and t-PA treatment. Ann Neurol 29:210, 1991
237. Percheron SMJ: Les artères du thalamus humain. Rev Neurol (Paris) 132:297, 1976
238. Pessin MS, Adelman LS, Prager RJ et al: "Wrong-way eyes" in supratentorial hemorrhage. Ann Neurol 9:79, 1981
239. Piepgras U, Rieger P: Thalamic bleeding: diagnosis, course and prognosis. Neuroradiology 22:85, 1981
240. Pierrott-Deseilligny C, Chain F, Serdaru M et al: The "one-and-a-half" syndrome: electro-oculographic analysis of five cases with deductions about the physiological mechanisms of lateral gaze. Brain 104:665, 1981
241. Plum F, Posner JB: The Diagnosis of Stupor and Coma. 3rd Ed. FA Davis, Philadelphia, 1980
242. Portenoy RK, Lipton RB, Berger AR et al: Intracerebral hemorrhage: a model for the prediction of outcome. J Neurol Neurosurg Psychiatry 50:976, 1987
243. Probst A, Ulrich J: Amyloid angiopathy combined with granulomatous angiitis of the central nervous system: report on two patients. Clin Neuropathol 4:250, 1985
244. Rådberg JA, Olsson JE, Radberg CT: Prognostic parameteres in spontaneous intracranial hematomas with special reference to anticoagulant treatment. Stroke 22:571, 1991
245. Regli F, Vonsattel J-P, Perentes E, Assal G: L'Angiopathie amyloïde cérébrale: une maladie cerebro-vasculaire peu connue—etude d'une observation anatomo-clinique. Rev Neurol (Paris) 137:181, 1981
246. Rey-Bellet J: Cerebellar hemorrhage: a clinicopatholo ic study. Neurology 10:217, 1960
247. Reynolds AF, Harris AB, Ojemann GA, Turner PT: Aphasia and left thalamic hemorrhage. J Neurosurg 48:570, 1978
248. Richardson AE: Spontaneous cerebellar hemorrhage. p. 54. In Vinken PJ, Bruyn GW (eds): Handbook of Clinical Neurology. Vol. 12. North-Holland Publishing, Amsterdam, 1972
249. Richardson A: Spontaneous intracerebral and cerebellar hemorrhage. p. 210. In Russell RWR (ed): Cerebral Arterial Disease. Churchill-Livingstone, New York, 1976
250. Roberson GH, Kase CS, Wolpow ER: Telangiectases and cavernous angiomas of the brainstem:

"cryptic" vascular malformations. Neuroradiology 8:83, 1974
251. Robinson RK, Richey ET, Kase CS, Mohr JP: Somatosensory evoked potentials in pure sensory stroke and allied conditions. abstract ed. Neurology, suppl 1. 34:231, 1984
252. Roig C, Carvajal A, Illa I et al: Hemorragies mesencaphaliques isolées. Rev Neurol (Paris) 138:53, 1982
253. Ropper AH, Davis KR: Lobar cerebral hemorrhages: acute clinical syndromes in 26 cases. Ann Neurol 8:141, 1980
254. Rosenberg GA, Kaufman DM: Cerebellar hemorrhage: reliability of clinical evaluation. Stroke 7:332, 1976
255. Rosenblum WI: Miliary aneurysms and "fibrinoid" degeneration of cerebral blood vessels. Hum Pathol 8:133, 1977
256. Ross ED: Localization of the pyramidal tract in the internal capsule by whole brain dissection. Neurology (NY) 30:59, 1980
257. Ross Russell RW: Observations on intracerebral aneurysms. Brain 86:425, 1963
258. Rowe CC, Donnan GA, Bladin PF: Intracerebral haemorrhage: incidence and use of computed tomography. Br Med J 297:1177, 1988
259. Rumbaugh CL, Bergeron RT, Fang HCH, McCormick R: Cerebral angiographic changes in the drug abuse patient. Radiology 101:335, 1971
260. Russell DS: The pathology of spontaneous intracranial haemorrhage. Proc Soc Med 47:689, 1954
261. Russell DS, Rubinstein LJ: Pathology of Tumours of the Nervous System. 4th Ed. Williams & Wilkins, Baltimore, 1977
262. Sacco RL, Wolf PA, Bharucha NE et al: Subarachnoid and intracerebral hemorrhage: natural history, prognosis, and precursive factors in the Framingham Study. Neurology (NY) 34:847, 1984
263. Schnapper RA: Pontine hemorrhage presenting as ataxic hemiparesis. Stroke 13:518, 1982
264. Schott B, Laurent B, Mauguiere F, Chazot G: Negligence motrice par hematome thalamique droit. Rev Neurol (Paris) 137:447, 1981
265. Schütz H, Bodeker R-H, Damian M et al: Age-related spontaneous intracerebral hematoma in a German community. Stroke 21:1412, 1990
266. Scott M: Spontaneous intracerebral hematoma caused by cerebral neoplasms: report of eight verified cases. J Neurosurg 42:338, 1975
267. Scott WR, New PFJ, Davis KR, Schnur JA: Computerized axial tomography of intracerebral and intraventricular hemorrhage. Radiology 112:73, 1974
268. Scoville WB, Poppen JL: Intrapenduncular hemorrhage of the brain. Arch Neurol Psychiatry 61:688, 1949
269. Sharpe JA, Rosenberg MA, Hoyt WF, Daroff RB: Paralytic pontine exotropia: a sign of acute unilateral pontine gaze palsy and internuclear ophthalmoplegia. Neurology (NY) 24:1076, 1974
270. Shintaku M, Osawa K, Toki J et al: A case of granulomatous angiitis of the central nervous system associated with amyloid angiopathy. Acta Neuropathol 70:340, 1986
271. Shuangshoti S, Panyathanya R, Wichienkur P: Intracranial metastases from unsuspected choriocarcinoma: onset suggestive of cerebrovascular disease. Neurology (NY) 24:649, 1974
272. Silverstein A: Intracranial hemorrhage in patients with bleeding tendencies. Neurology (NY) 11:310, 1961
273. Silverstein A: Primary pontile hemorrhage. Conf Neurol 29:33, 1967
274. Silverstein A: Primary pontine hemorrhage. p. 37. In Vinken PJ, Bruyn GW (eds): Handbook of Clinical Neurology. Vol. 12, Part II. North-Holland Publishing, Amsterdam, 1972
275. Simard JM, Garcia-Bengochea F, Ballinger WE et al: Cavernous angioma: a review of 126 collected and 12 new clinical cases. Neurosurgery 18:162, 1986
276. Snyder M, Renaudin J: Intracranial hemorrhage associated with anticoagulation therapy. Surg Neurol 7:31, 1977
277. Starr M: Cerebellar apoplexy. Med Rec 69:743, 1906
278. Steegmann AT: Primary pontile hemorrhage. J Nerv Ment Dis 114:35, 1951
279. Stehbens WE: Pathology of the cerebral blood vessels. CV Mosby, St. Louis, 1972
280. Stein RW, Kase CS, Hier DB et al: Caudate hemorrhage. Neurology (NY) 34:1549, 1984
281. Stephen R, Stillwell D: Arteries and veins of the human brain. Springfield, IL, CC Thomas, 1969
282. Stoessl AJ, Young GB, Feasby TE: Intracerebral haemorrhage and angiographic beading following ingestion of catecholaminergics. Stroke 16:734, 1985
283. Susaç JO, Hoyt WF, Daroff RB, Lawrence W: Clinical spectrum of ocular bobbing. J Neurol Neurosurg Psychiatry 33:771, 1970
284. Tanaka H, Ueda Y, Date C et al: Incidence of stroke in Shibata, Japan, 1976–1978. Stroke 12:460, 1981
285. Tapia JF, Kase CS, Sawyer RH, Mohr JP: Hypertensive putaminal hemorrhage presenting as pure motor hemiparesis. Stroke 14:505, 1983
286. Taveras JM, Wood EH: Diagnostic Neuroradiology. 2nd Ed. Vol. 2. p. 1018. Williams & Wilkins, Baltimore, 1976
287. Thulborn KR, Sorensen AG, Kowall NW et al: The role of ferritin and hemosiderin in the MR appearance of cerebral hemorrhage: a histopathologic biochemical study in rats. AJNR 11:291, 1990
288. Thyne W: A case of cerebellar hemorrhage presenting with well marked opisthotonus and Kernig sign. Lancet 79(1):397, 1901
289. TIMI Study Group: Comparison of invasive and conservative strategies after treatment with intravenous tissue plasminogen activator in acute myocardial infarction: results of the Thrombolysis in Myocardial Infarction (TIMI) phase II trial. N Engl J Med 320:618, 1989
290. Tomonaga M: Cerebral amyloid angiopathy in the elderly. J Am Geriatr Soc 29:151, 1981
291. Toole JF, Patel AN: Cerebrovascular Disorders. 2nd Ed. p. 335. McGraw-Hill, New York, 1967

292. Tuhrim S, Dambrosia JM, Price TR et al: Prediction of intracerebral hemorrhage survival. Ann Neurol 24:258, 1988
293. Tuhrim S, Yang WC, Rubinowitz H, Weinberger J: Primary pontine hemorrhage and the dysarthriaclumsy hand syndrome. Neurology (NY) 32:1027, 1982
294. Toffol GJ, Biller J, Adams HP: Nontraumatic intracerebral hemorrhage in young adults. Arch Neurol 44:483, 1987
295. Tyler HR, Johnson PC: Case records of the Massachusetts General Hospital 36–1972. N Engl J Med 287:506, 1972
296. Tyler KL, Poletti CE, Heros RC: Cerebral amyloid angiopathy with multiple intracerebral hemorrhages. J Neurosurg 57:286, 1982
297. Ueda K, Omae T, Hirota Y et al: Decreasing trend in incidence and mortality from stroke in Hisayama residents, Japan. Stroke 12:154, 1981
298. Ueshima H, Iida M, Shimamoto T et al: Multivariate analysis of risk factors for stroke: eight-year follow-up of farming villages in Akita, Japan. Prevent Med 9:722, 1980
299. Valenstein E, Heilman KM: Unilateral hypokinesia and motor extinction. Neurology (NY) 31:445, 1981
300. Vaughan HG, Howard RG: Intracranial hemorrhage due to metastatic chorionepithelioma. Neurology (NY) 12:771, 1962
301. Vinters HV: Cerebral amyloid angiopathy: a critical review. Stroke 18:311, 1987
302. Vinters HV, Gilbert JJ: Cerebral amyloid angiopathy: incidence and complications in the aging brain. II. The distribution of amyloid vascular changes. Stroke 14:924, 1983
303. Vonsattel JPG, Myers RH, Hedley-Whyte ET et al: Cerebral amyloid angiopathy without and with cerebral hemorrhages: a comparative histological study. Ann Neurol 30:637, 1991
304. Waga S, Okada M, Yamamoto Y: Reversibility of Parinaud syndrome in thalamic hemorrhage. Neurology (NY) 29:407, 1979
305. Wagle WA, Smith TW, Weiner M: Intracerebral hemorrhage caused by cerebral amyloid angiopathy: radiographic pathologic correlation. AJNR 5:171, 1984
306. Wakai S, Yamakawa K, Manaka S, Takakura K: Spontaneous intracranial hemorrhage caused by brain tumors: its incidence and clinical significance. Neurosurgery 10:437, 1982
307. Walsh FB, Hoyt WK: Clinical Neuro-ophthalmology. 3rd Ed. p. 1786. Williams & Wilkins, Baltimore, 1969
308. Walshe TM, Davis KR, Fisher CM: Thalamic hemorrhage: a computed tomographic-clinical correlation. Neurology (NY) 27:217, 1977
309. Watson RT, Heilman KM: Thalamic neglect. Neurology (NY) 29:690, 1979
310. Wattendorff AR, Bots GTAM, Went LN, Endtz LJ: Familial cerebral amyloid angiopathy presenting as recurrent cerebral haemorrhage. J Neurol Sci 55:121, 1982
311. Weber M, Vespignani H, Bracard S et al: Les angiomes caverneux intracérébraux. Rev Neurol 145:429, 1989
312. Weingarten K, Zimmerman RD, Deo-Narine V et al: MR imaging of acute intracranial hemorrhage: findings on sequential spin-echo and gradient-echo images in a dog model. AJNR 12:457, 1991
313. Weintraub MI, Glaser GH: Nocardial brain abscess and pure motor hemiplegia. NY State J Med 70:2717, 1970
314. Weisberg LA: Computerized tomography in intracranial hemorrhage. Arch Neurol 36:422, 1979
315. Weisberg L: Multiple spontaneous intracerebral hematomas: clinical and computed tomographic correlations. Neurology (NY) 31:897, 1981
316. Wells CE, Urrea D: Cerebrovascular accidents in patients receiving anticoagulant drugs. Arch Neurol 3:553, 1960
317. Whisnant JP, Cartlidge NEF, Elveback LR: Carotid and vertebral-basilar transient ischemic attacks: effect of anticoagulants, hypertension, and cardiac disorders on survival and stroke occurrence in a population study. Ann Neurol 3:107, 1978
318. Wiggins WS, Moody DM, Toole JF et al: Clinical and computerized tomographic study of hypertensive intracerebral hemorrhage. Arch Neurol 35:832, 1978
319. Wilkins RH, Brody IA: The thalamic syndrome (Neurological Classics 18). Arch Neurol 20:559, 1969
320. Williams KD, Drayer BP, Bird CR: Magnetic resonance imaging in the diagnosis of intracerebral hematoma. Barrow Neurological Institute, Phoenix, 5:16, 1989
321. Wintzen AR, de Jonge H, Loeliger EA, Bots GTAM: The risk of intracerebral hemorrhage during oral anticoagulant treatment: a population study. Ann Neurol 16:553, 1984
322. Yates PO: Vascular disease of the central nervous system. p. 86. In Blackwood W, Corsellis JAN (eds): Greenfield's Neuropathology. Year Book Medical Publishers, Chicago, 1977
323. Yoshida 5, Sasaki M, Oka H et al: Acute hypertensive cerebellar hemorrhage with signs of lower brainstem compression. Surg Neurol 10:79, 1978
324. Young IR, Bydder GM, Hall AS et al: NMR imaging in the diagnosis and management of intracranial angiomas. AJNR 4:837, 1983
325. Yu YJ, Cooper DR, Wellenstein DE, Block B: Cerebral angiitis and intracerebral hemorrhage associated with methamphetamine abuse. J Neurosurg 58:109, 1983
326. Zimmerman RD, Leeds NE, Naidich TP: Ring blush associated with intracerebral hematoma. Radiology 122:707, 1977
327. Zuccarello M, Iavicoli R, Pardatscher K et al: Primary brain stem hematomas, diagnosis and treatment. Acta Neurochir 54:45, 1980
328. Zülch KJ: Neuropathology of intracranial haemorrhage. Progr Brain Res 30:151, 1968
329. Zyed A, Hayman LA, Bryan RN: MR imaging of intracerebral blood: diversity in the temporal pattern at 0.5 and 1.0 T. AJNR 12:469, 1991

# 22
# *INTRACRANIAL ANEURYSMS*

J.P. Mohr
J. Philip Kistler
M.E. Fink

## EPIDEMIOLOGY

Rupture of an intracranial saccular aneurysm is the most common cause of subarachnoid hemorrhage, far exceeding that of ruptures of other forms of aneurysms, mycotic or myxomatous, or from other anomalies or tumors, including arteriovenous malformations. Estimates based on the Cooperative Study data[194] indicate that roughly 80 percent of nontraumatic subarachnoid hemorrhage is a result of aneurysmal rupture. Apart from subarachnoid hemorrhage, aneurysmal rupture can also affect the brain substance, the ventricular system, or the subdural space.[19,82,137,145,159,178,201,210]

In the United States, the peak age for aneurysm rupture is between 55 and 60 years of age.[196] In children and adolescents intracranial aneurysms remain uncommon, even rare, whether revealed by angiogram or postmortem examination. In this group bleeding from an arteriovenous malformation is the more common cause. Beyond the age of 20, hemorrhage is more likely to be the result of aneurysmal rupture (Fig. 22-1).

Autopsy studies estimate that as much as 5 percent of the population may harbor aneurysms.[37,42,103,227,243] Clinically, the frequency of ruptured aneurysms has ranged from as low as 3.9 per 100,000 per year[172], a median value of 11 per 100,000 per year[179] to as high as 17.5[165] to 19.4 per 100,000 per year.[71] Of all strokes entered in the Harvard Cooperative Stroke Registry between 1972 and 1976, subarachnoid hemorrhage from ruptured saccular aneurysm accounted for 6 percent.[146] In 1981 the Cooperative Study[194] estimated the incidence in the United States at 26,000 cases per year, a higher figure than the 20,000 figure cited by Sypert[235] in 1978, who estimated that 400,000 adults in the United States harbor unruptured aneurysms, and that every year 5 percent of these people undergo a major neurologic catastrophe.

Of the risk factors associated with subarachnoid hemorrhage, pregnancy seems to increase the risk, with aneurysms predominating over arteriovenous malformations.[105,189] Intracranial aneurysmal rupture is often cited as a factor in 12 to 25 percent of maternal deaths, but has been reported in one series as contributing to 80 percent of maternal mortality.[89]

The true prevalence of intracranial aneurysms remains difficult to ascertain. No agreement has been reached about the size at which an arterial defect should be designated an aneurysm. McCormick and Acosta-Rua[136] demonstrated that manual perfusion of unruptured aneurysms with saline under a pressure of 70 mmHg caused the size to increase by 30 to 60

The work of JPM was supported in part by a gift from the Horace W. Goldsmith Foundation; the work of JPK was supported in part by the Eliot B. Shoolman Fund, and by Vera and J.W. Gilliland.

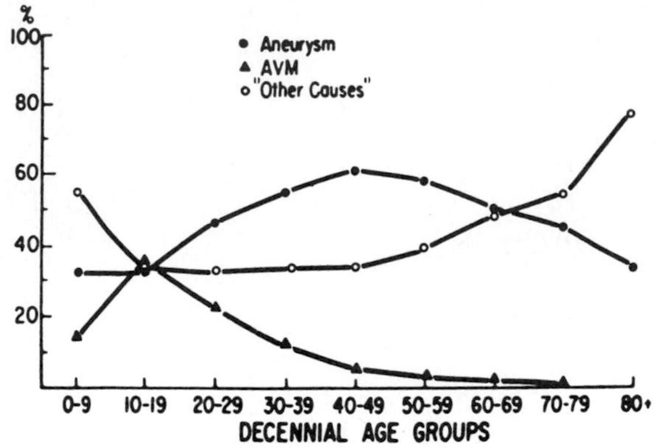


**Fig. 22-1.** Relative probability of major causes of subarachnoid hemorrhage in each decade of life. AVM, arteriovenous malformation. (From Sahs et al.,[196] with permission.)

percent, a finding that indicates that many smaller aneurysms may be overlooked at autopsy. If aneurysms as small as 2 mm are considered, 17 percent of routine autopsies reveal an unruptured intracranial aneurysm.[92] If only those lesions larger than 3 mm are included, the incidence in autopsy series will still be less than 4 percent.[221]

There seems to be a constancy of the incidence of aneurysmal rupture.[253] Although the incidence of other forms of stroke and generalized cardiovascular disease appears to be declining, subarachnoid hemorrhage is apparently not following this pattern.[159]

The fatality rate in aneurysmal rupture remains high. Better classification by severity grade on admission and timing of surgery may be reducing these rates to near 23 percent overall in some studies,[165,177] with mortality rates as low as 3 to 5 percent for those in good clinical condition who are operated on later.[110] Since many of the studies of subarachnoid hemorrhage are from referral institutions, such favorable fatality rates could reflect a referral bias and provide false reassurance regarding the expected course of this disease without effective and prompt treatment. In the 1980 population study of south Alabama, Mohr and Kase[146] found an incidence of death above 50 percent, much of it early in the course (Fig. 22-2), when those diagnosed within 24 hours of rupture were also included. In some locations rates have been as high as 68 percent.[129] Between 45 percent[179] and 49 percent[71] have been reported to die within the first 3 months. Those entering a hospital with a giant aneurysm or with a neurologic deficit have a particularly bad outcome.[56]

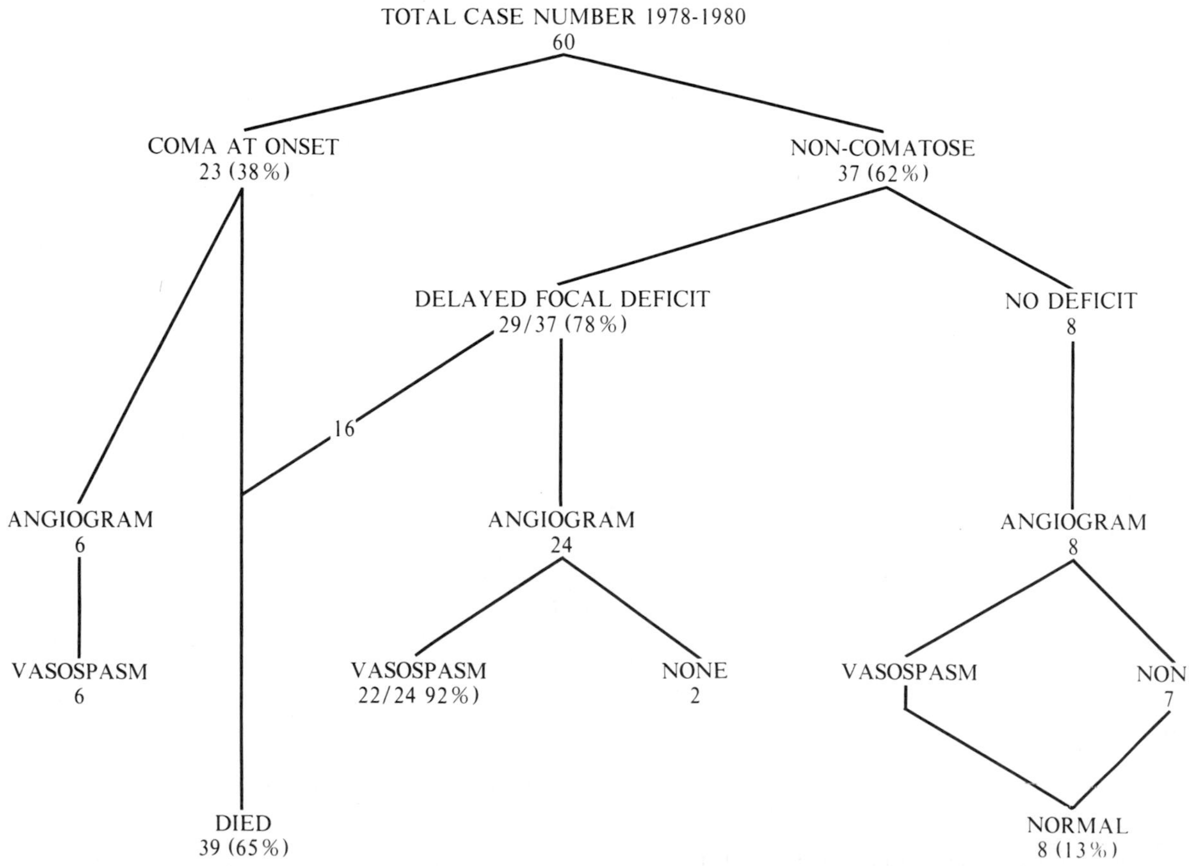


**Fig. 22-2.** Course of acute subarachnoid hemorrhage in a population study. (From Mohr and Kase,[146] with permission.)

Beyond the issue of case fatality is disability. For more than half the survivors, disability is major, and fully 64 percent of those patients well enough to be discharged home after neurosurgical obliteration of the aneurysm never achieve the quality of life they enjoyed before the rupture.[192]

## ANATOMY AND HISTOPATHOLOGY

Cerebral aneurysms are classified as saccular, mycotic, traumatic, dissecting, neoplastic, and arteriosclerotic. It is generally believed that the pathogenesis of the saccular aneurysm—often called congenital aneurysms—differs from that of the arteriosclerotic aneurysm. While this distinction is controversial, we will use the term *saccular aneurysm* to include all arterial outpouchings of an unknown origin that are not associated with inflammation or tumor, and will reserve the term *arteriosclerotic aneurysm* for the unusual, tortuous, dolichoectatic aneurysm that is associated with severe, widespread, atheromatous vascular disease.

### Saccular Aneurysms

Saccular aneurysms occur at the bifurcations of the large arteries at the base of the brain and rupture into the subarachnoid space of the basal cisterns (Fig. 22-3). By contrast, mycotic aneurysms usually occur at distal branch points of the convexity or brain stem arteries and rupture into the subarachnoid space or surrounding cerebral or cerebellar hemisphere. The most common sites for saccular aneurysms to occur are in the basal arteries. Approximately 85 percent occur in the anterior circulation,[166,167] the usual sites being the junction of the anterior communicating artery with the anterior cerebral artery and the junction of the posterior communicating artery with the internal carotid artery and the bifurcation of the middle cerebral artery. The posterior fossa sites are the top of the basilar artery, the junction of the basilar artery and the superior cerebellar artery or the anterior inferior cerebellar artery, or the junction of the vertebral artery and the posterior inferior cerebellar artery.[102] From 12 to 31 percent of aneurysms are multiple,[198] particularly in mirror locations (9 to 19 percent).[210]

The pathogenesis of cerebral aneurysms remains controversial,[35] but can be condensed to three major views: (1) aneurysms are thought to arise from congenital defects in the muscular layer of the cerebral arteries[37,72,243]; (2) degenerative changes within the vessel wall eventually result in damage to the internal elastic membrane, creating a local weakness that allows formation of an aneurysm[80,221,222,225]; (3) aneurysms are never a result of developmental deficiencies or degenerative changes alone, but are always due to the combined effects of these two processes.[30,201]

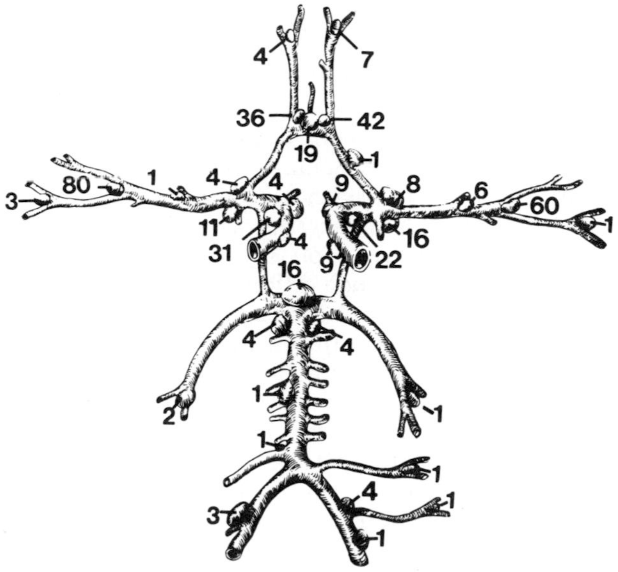


**Fig. 22-3.** A drawing of the arteries at the base of the brain showing the location of 429 saccular aneurysms in 316 consecutive patients with aneurysms on an autopsy service. Approximately 90 percent of the aneurysms occur on the anterior cerebral circulation. Aneurysms are slightly more common on the right side of the intracranial vessels than on the left for reasons that are not apparent. (From McCormick,[135] with permission.)

Because the majority of cerebral aneurysms arise at points of arterial branching, many studies have been directed at this region. Aneurysms typically grow out from a base on the arterial wall, forming a neck with a dome on top.[207] The thickness and length of this neck and the size of the dome show great variation, making microsurgical obliteration an individual matter. An internal elastic lamina is not found at the origin of the neck. The normal vascular media of thin and smooth muscle cells are replaced by collagenous connective tissue. At the site of rupture, most often thought to be the dome, the wall may be thinner than 0.3 mm. In one of the rare reported cases where the site of rupture was documented by microscopic serial section,[70] the site of rupture was actually at the base, not at the dome. A small fibrin-filled gap, measuring 0.5 × 0.14 mm, marked the site of rupture. Although small, it allowed enough blood to escape into the subarachnoid space to engulf the middle cerebral artery stem and the A1 segment of the anterior cerebral artery. This rupture site was on the neck proximal to the usual site of clip placement.

The issue of defects in the media still excites controversy.[207] Small gaps in the musculature of the media at the points of bifurcation of the cerebral vessels of the circle of Willis were first reported by Forbus[73] in 1930, who postulated that these defects were an important factor in the development of noninflammatory aneurysms. In 1940 Glynn[81] found these "medial defects" in 80 percent of the bifurcations of cerebral arteries in both aneurysmal and control cases. After observing that vessels with an intact internal elastic membrane tolerated pressures in excess of 600 mmHg without deformity, he concluded that degeneration of the elastic layer was crucial to the genesis of cerebral aneurysms. Glynn suggested that the greater frequency with which aneurysms occur in the arteries of the circle of Willis was probably due to a difference in the elastic tissue. Of such differences the most readily detected is one of position: in the cerebral vessels the elastic tissue is concentrated in the internal elastic lamina. By virtue of its position it was probably more susceptible to injury and degeneration than if it were more widely distributed through the media and adventitia as in other vessels.

In 1963 Stehbens[222] reported studies differentiating the congenital medial defects described by Forbus[73] from those lesions that develop later, apparently on a degenerative basis: funnel-shaped dilatations, areas of thinning, and small outpouchings that probably signify the first stages of aneurysmal formation were described at vessel forks. Severe histologic degenerative changes and fragmentation of the internal elastic lamina were apparent at these points of thinning and evagination, and were thought to be the result of hemodynamic stress. He supported the hypothesis that aneurysms result from acquired degenerative processes. In 1975, in an electron-microscopic examination of five cerebral aneurysms, three preaneurysmal lesions, and three arteriovenous malformations, Stehbens[225] observed that these vascular lesions were remarkably similar to one another and also to the degenerative changes he had previously described in experimental arteriovenous malformations. Since aneurysmal dilatation and degenerative changes can be induced hemodynamically, Stehbens[223,224] reasoned that hemodynamic stress plays a major role in the development of cerebral aneurysms. Hydrodynamic studies, using both rigid and elastic models, have also demonstrated that the greatest point of stress in the vasculature occurs at the forks of arterial branches.[72,92]

Hereditary factors may also play a role, especially a familial occurrence, which suggests genetic factors in the development of these defects.[2,18,25,85] Infundibular widening at the origin of the posterior cerebral artery was documented in 8 of 11 members of one family, 5 of whom also developed frank saccular aneurysms.[59] Aneurysms have been reported at the same site in twins.[29,63,64,85,163] Intracranial aneurysms are also commonly associated with certain congenital malformations such as polycystic kidneys,[49] arteriovenous malformations,[14,184,230] moya-moya disease,[152] coarctation of the aorta,[190] Ehlers-Danlos syndrome,[16,84,193] fibromuscular hyperplasia,[21,258] and possibly other connective tissue diseases.[139,176] Certain arterial anomalies of the circle of Willis are also more frequently found in patients harboring aneurysms. The most commonly encountered anomaly is hypoplasia of one or both proximal anterior cerebral arteries in association with an anterior cerebral aneurysm. Of these various associations, only those for polycystic kidney disease, coarctation of the aorta, and fibromuscular hyperplasia are known to be statistically significant. However, since each of these disorders may present with early onset of hypertension, there is reason to question whether the pathogenesis for the increased occurrence of cerebral aneurysms is a function of hereditary or congenital factors or hypertensive degeneration.

The role of systemic arterial hypertension in the genesis of intracranial aneurysms or in their subsequent rupture has not been clearly established. While many authors[27,55,57,58,129] have favored a role for hypertension, others disagree. McCormick and Schmalotieg[138] have argued otherwise in their study of 250 patients with aneurysms—150 patients with rupture and 100 with unruptured saccular aneurysms studied by autopsy. Andrews and Spiegel[16] found that hypertension was not significantly more prevalent in the aneurysm population than in the age-matched general population, except for females under 55 years of age. They noted that hypertension appears to be associated with an increased frequency of multiple aneurysms.

## Arteriosclerotic Aneurysms

Arteriosclerotic—so-called dolichoectatic—aneurysms occur most frequently along the basilar artery, but are also found in the internal carotid, middle cerebral, and anterior cerebral arteries.[77] The affected artery is tortuous, widened, and elongated, and cause symptoms from compression, embolic phenomenon, or the obstruction of cerebrospinal fluid (CSF) pathways. They rarely present with subarachnoid hemorrhage. Arteriosclerosis and hypertension are unquestionably of paramount importance in the etiology of these aneurysms, as they occur almost entirely in patients who have widespread arteriosclerotic disease.

## Mycotic Aneurysms

Mycotic aneurysms typically are located in the distal cerebral circulation as might be expected from their microembolic origin (Fig. 22-4). Mycotic cerebral aneurysms may be caused by extension of infection from emboli lodged in the arterial lumen, bacterial embolism of the vasa vasorum, or a combination of these two factors.[147,212] Once established, the infective process leads to septic degeneration of the elastic lamina and muscular coats of the vessel wall, with resultant rupture and subarachnoid hemorrhage.

Mycotic aneurysms constitute approximately 5 percent of all cerebral aneurysms, primarily as a complication of subacute bacterial endocarditis (SBE), obvious clinically or occult, and from natural or artificial

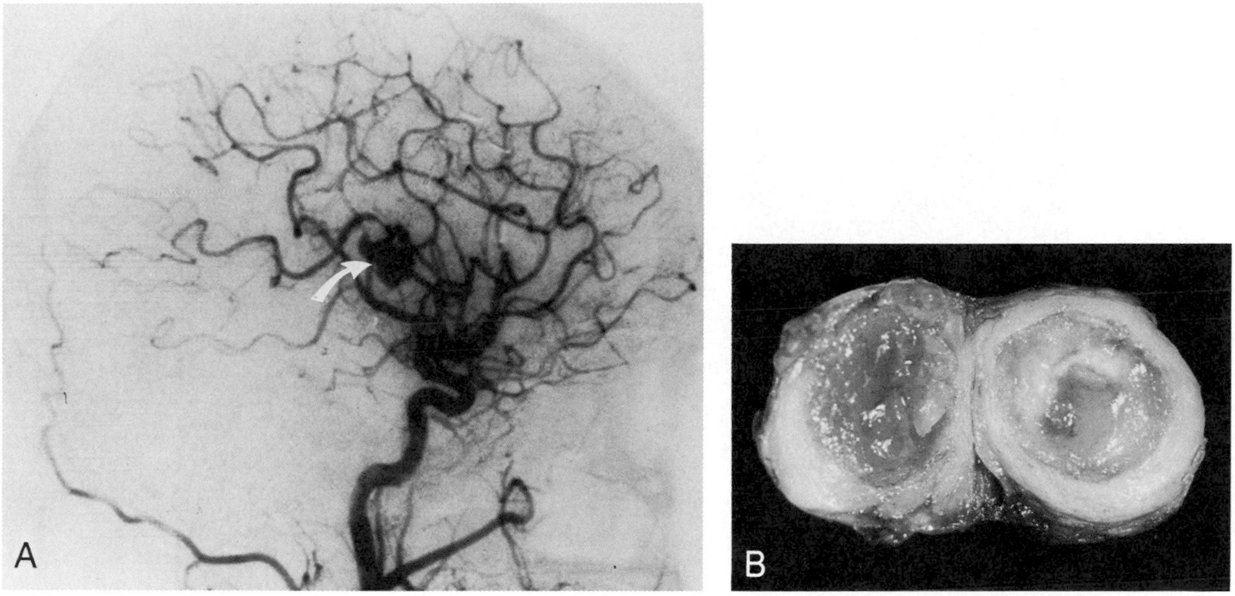


**Fig. 22-4.** (**A** & **B**). Angiographic and gross pathologic appearance of mycotic middle cerebral artery aneurysms in a middle-aged male who presented with signs and symptoms of subacute bacterial endocarditis, including dyspnea, fever, chills, and Grade V/VI holosystolic murmur.

valve surfaces.[122] Some 15 to 20 percent of all mycotic aneurysms are in the brain, ranking only below the aorta and its major abdominal and peripheral branches.[217] For patients with bacterial endocarditis, about 17 percent have been reported to have symptoms of cerebral embolization,[36,91,121] and mycotic cerebral aneurysms are demonstrated in approximately 4 percent.[149,151]

Angiography has been recommended for all patients with embolic symptoms to identify aneurysms prior to the occurrence of subarachnoid hemorrhage, but this policy has never been widely adopted. Those who harbor an aneurysm can be treated with high doses of the appropriate antibiotic, and the aneurysm followed with repeat angiograms. If the aneurysm thromboses, no further treatment is necessary. However, if it enlarges, it should be clipped.[151]

## Dissecting Aneurysms

Dissecting intracranial aneurysms were once believed to be quite rare and are included here only because of the name, aneurysm. Prior to 1960 there was a total of only 10 pathologically verified cases in the world's literature. In recent years, there has been a great increase in the number of case reports. Primary intracranial dissections have been documented most often in young persons with little or no evidence of atherosclerotic disease and with identified trauma, such as a cuff on the head or other injuries, major or minor.[86,247,259] When recognized clinically, the course has been calamitous. No satisfactory criteria have been developed for antemortem diagnosis, which requires a high level of suspicion. Antecedent headache seems common.[204] The consistent occurrence of headache, often focal and severe, correlates with documented patterns of intracranial pain referral when the intracranial vessels are stimulated during operative procedures performed under local anesthesia[181] or temporarily occluded by balloon catheters.[160]

These lesions have been separated into two groups.[259] The more common presents as a stroke without subarachnoid hemorrhage and has a dissection between the elastica and media. It is ascribed to defects in the internal elastic lamina and can result from trauma. Therapy for these patients is usually directed toward the management of the expectant cerebral edema and prevention of medical complications. The second type is more unusual, only six cases having been described in the literature. Here, dissection occurs between the media and adventitia, presumably as the result of rupture of a vasa vasorum. These cases occur more commonly in the vertebrobasilar system, usually without a history of trauma. If adequate collateral circulation exists, the dissection can be treated by proximal ligation or a trapping procedure.[210] If the collaterals are inadequate, they can be established first with a bypass procedure before the trapping.[219,220]

## Traumatic Aneurysms

True traumatic intracranial aneurysms are rare. Aneurysms of the meningeal vessels and false aneurysms have also been reported as a complication of major head trauma. When trauma produces disrup-

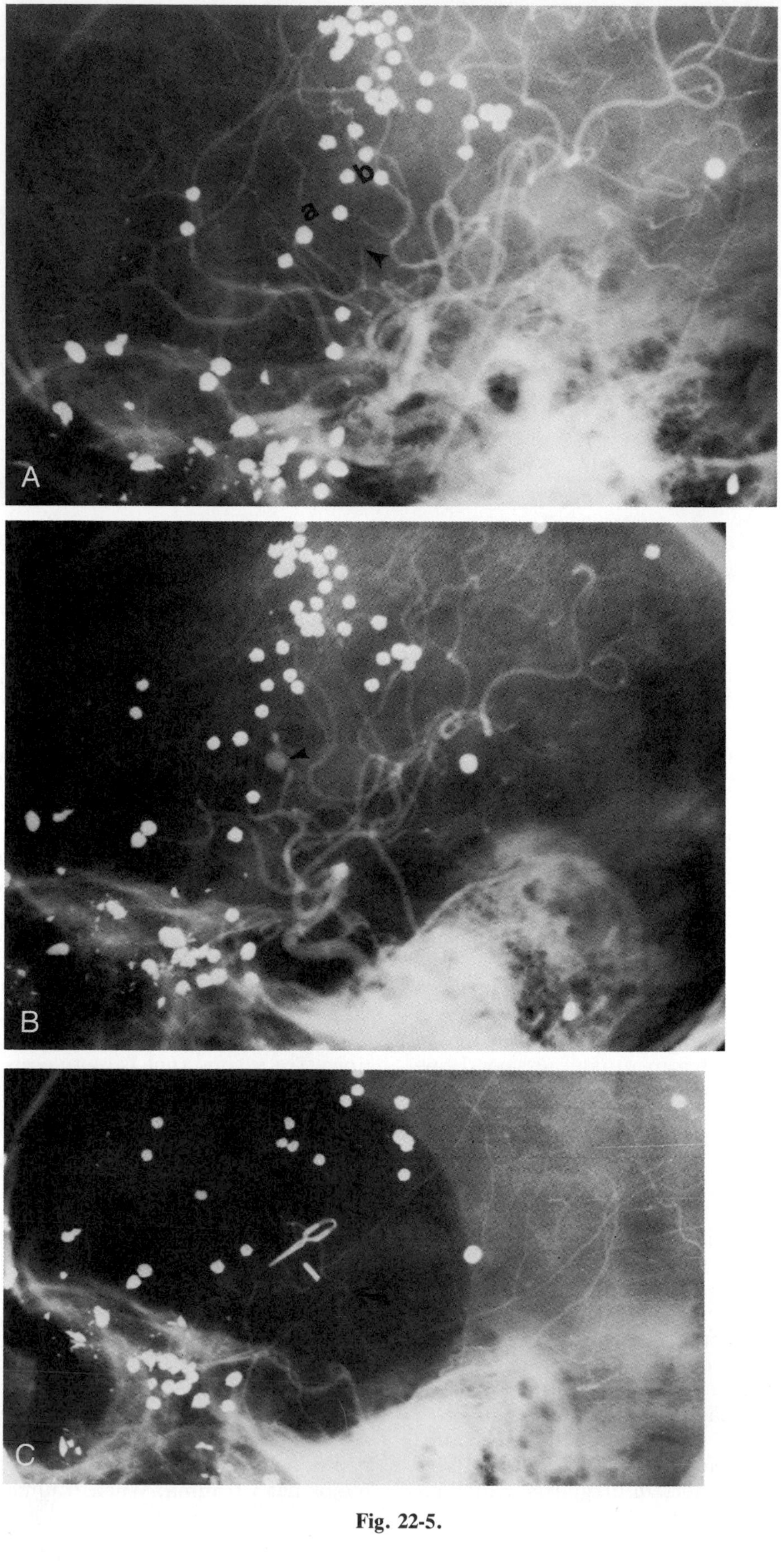


**Fig. 22-5.**

tion of an artery, a hematoma forms around it, producing a false aneurysm. When, however, only the internal elastic lamina is damaged, the intima may herniate through this defect, producing a true aneurysm. Mixed types may also occur. Traumatic intracranial aneurysms occur most commonly on the internal carotid artery, the middle cerebral artery in relation to bony fractures and penetrating trauma, and the anterior cerebral artery in relation to the falx. Rupture resulting in death occurs in 50 percent of the reported cases, suggesting that operative management, when clinically feasible, is the therapy of choice[23,219] (Fig. 22-5).

### Neoplastic Aneurysms

Emboli from an atrial myxoma may lodge in cerebral arteries, invade the arterial wall, and lead to the formation of a neoplastic aneurysm. Cardiac myxomas are benign intracavitary tumors, constituting about 50 percent of primary cardiac tumors. Approximately 75 percent of these tumors arise in the left atrium. Systemic emboli have been reported in up to 45 percent of patients with this tumor type, and about half of these are cerebral. Angiographic abnormalities include irregular filling defects in major and minor cerebral artery branches, fusiform and saccular aneurysms, and occlusion of vessels[156] (Fig. 22-6). Tumor emboli apparently remain viable, and can penetrate the endothelium at the site of lodgment, grow subintimally, and eventually infiltrate and destroy the arterial wall.[156]

### Multiple and Incidental Aneurysms

Unruptured multiple aneurysms may occur in up to 13 percent of cases.[64,198] The incidental aneurysms are at risk of rupture. This risk seems to be in the range of 1 to 3 percent per year for each year of survival.[95,258] While it would appear that aneurysms under 5 mm in diameter are at lower risk for subsequent rupture,[62,127,136] it is not possible to separate, angiographically or clinically, those lesions that will remain stable from those that will continue to grow or rupture spontaneously, with devastating consequences to the patient.[8,62]

The operative risks for the elective surgical management of unruptured aneurysms are extremely favorable. Usually there is no mortality and little operative morbidity.

### Giant Aneurysms

Here, the term "giant aneurysm" is used for lesions exceeding 25 mm in greatest diameter. This coincides with the largest size (Group 5) in the Cooperative Study.[127] In the literature, lesions of this size make up about 5 percent of all intracranial aneurysms, and are unusual in that the majority (approximately 80 percent) present with symptoms of mass effect or embolic phenomenon rather than subarachnoid hemorrhage.[150] Giant aneurysms often have such a wide neck and/or become so large that obliteration of the sac becomes impossible (Fig. 22-7). Furthermore, in some cases, calcifications and partial thrombosis make mobilization of these aneurysms extremely hazardous. Despite advances in anesthesia and the development of microsurgical techniques, the risk of dealing directly with giant intracranial aneurysms remains high.[169] The surgical management of these aneurysms presents special problems that are discussed at length elsewhere in the volume.

## NATURAL HISTORY

### Unruptured Aneurysms

There is relatively little information available to determine the possibility of an asymptomatic aneurysm rupturing in the future. Data from a small number of patients in the Cooperative Study,[127] and more recently from 65 patients with unruptured aneurysm from the Mayo Clinic,[228] suggest that aneurysmal size is the only important variable associated with subsequent rupture. In the 65 patients with unruptured aneurysms followed at the Mayo Clinic, 8 of 29 aneurysms greater than 1 cm in size ruptured, while none of 44 aneurysms less than 1 cm in size ruptured over a mean follow-up interval of 98.5 months. Some have advised microsurgical obliteration of asymptomatic aneurysms larger than 7 mm.[167]

**Fig. 22-5.** A 20-year-old patient was hospitalized after sustaining a close-range shotgun blast to the left side of the face. **(A)** Left common carotid artery angiogram demonstrated spasm (*arrowhead*) at the location where an aneurysm was later demonstrated to arise. The two vessels irrigated by that branch of the middle cerebral artery are labeled *a* and *b*. **(B)** Repeat common carotid artery angiogram 5 days after the initial study reveals an aneurysm (*arrowhead*). **(C)** A left external carotid artery angiogram 2 weeks after clipping of the traumatic aneurysm. Obliteration of the aneurysm. Obliteration of the aneurysm necessitated occlusion of the parent vessel. Therefore, the superficial temporal artery (*large arrow*) was anastomosed to a distal cortical segment of the occluded artery to ensure adequate arterial flow. The site of anastomosis (*long arrow*) and perfusion of middle cerebral artery vessels *a* and *b* via the bypass are demonstrated. (From Spetzler and Owen,[219] with permission.)

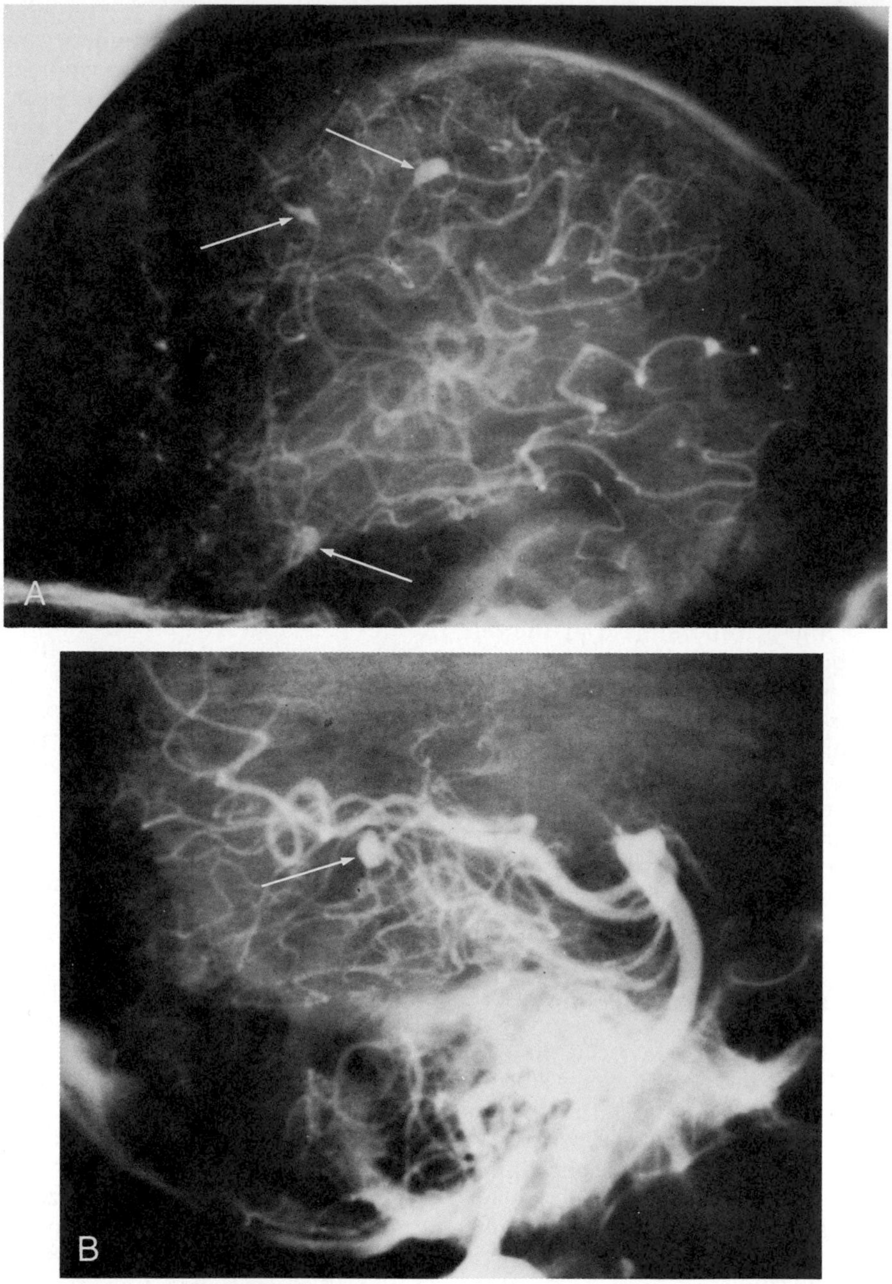


**Fig. 22-6.** (**A**) Internal carotid artery and (**B**) posterior cerebral artery angiograms demonstrating multiple neoplastic aneurysms in a 30-year-old female who presented with a history of transient cerebral ischemic events. Echocardiogram demonstrated a large atrial myxoma, which was surgically removed.

## Subarachnoid Hemorrhage

Many retrospective studies have been conducted in an effort to elucidate the natural history of subarachnoid hemorrhage.[76] Such attempts to assemble a representative series have been plagued by the difficulty evaluating those undergoing no treatment because of selection criteria, and by the lack of statistical data on the many patients who die as a result of subarachnoid hemorrhage without ever reaching a hospital. Including both these points makes higher fatality rates in any series.

The Cooperative Study[127] indicated the mortality rate during the first week after subarachnoid hemorrhage could be as high as 27 percent. Reevaluation of risks by grades has shown a striking spectrum of outlook. Locksley[127] defined three patient groups: (1) a high-risk group of 9 percent of the population, whose

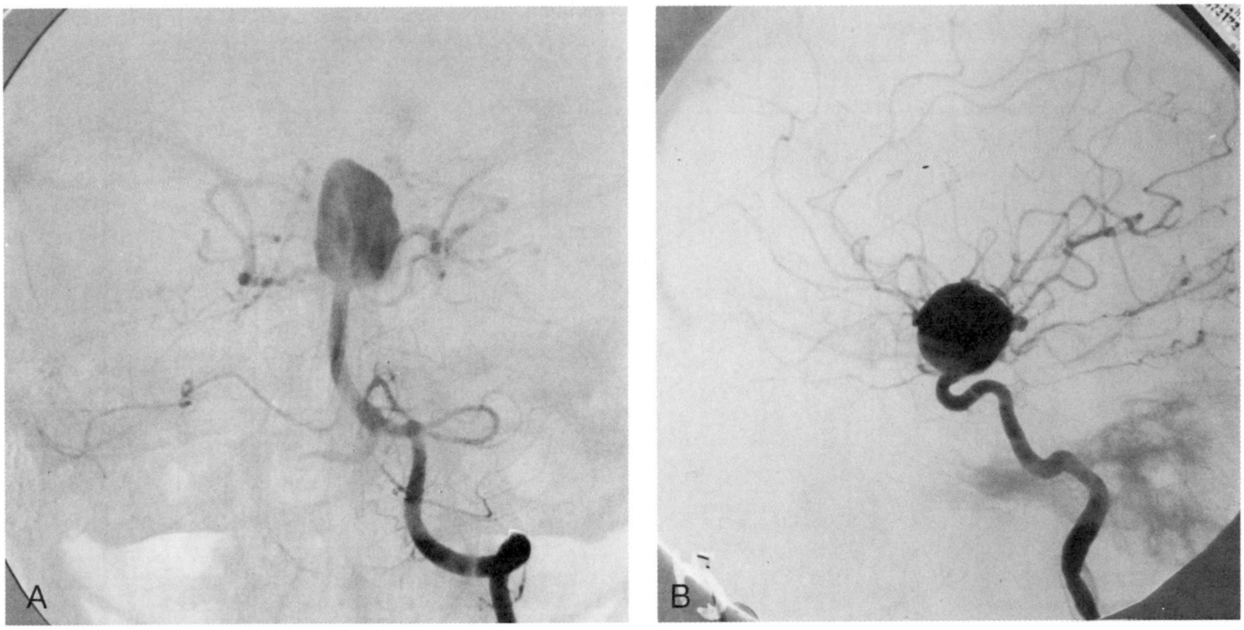


**Fig. 22-7.** (**A**) Anteroposterior view of left vertebral angiogram demonstrates a giant aneurysm of the basilar artery. (**B**) Lateral view of internal carotid artery angiogram showing a giant aneurysm in the same patient.

average survival after the first subarachnoid hemorrhage is 18 hours; (2) an intermediate group of 47 percent of the population, whose average survival is about 2 weeks; and (3) a "low-risk" group of 43 percent of the population, who tolerate the initial hemorrhage quite well and appear to have a low rate of subsequent late hemorrhage. Of particular neurosurgical significance is the finding that 90 percent of the patients dying within 72 hours of hemorrhage harbor an associated intracerebral, intracerebellar, or subdural hematoma and are the more severely affected. Striking differences have also been documented for the series from the early 1980s, with 3 to 5 percent death rates for delayed surgery in the group with the best preoperative clinical state versus 21 to 25 percent for those in the worst state.[110]

Rebleeding produces significant morbidity and mortality in the untreated patient. The risk of rebleeding within 1 month is approximately 33 percent, and the mortality rate for this second hemorrhage is 42 percent.[127] The risk of rebleeding is greatest between the 5th and 9th days, within 22 percent of all rebleeding episodes occurring within the first 2 weeks after hemorrhage. Thereafter, the risk of rebleeding diminishes, but it does not go to zero. Of long-term survivors, approximately 3 percent can be expected to rebleed annually.[257]

Pakarinen[171] calculated that of 589 patients with aneurysms who survived their first subarachnoid hemorrhage, 51 percent die within 5 years. For the 20 percent of patients with multiple aneurysms, the prognosis is considerably poorer.

Even considering the limitations of the information accumulated to date, it is not unreasonable to estimate that there is a mortality rate as high as 45 percent during the first year following rupture of a single aneurysm and a significant, continuing threat of rebleeding thereafter.

Alvord and colleagues[13] calculated the probabilities of future survival. In their analysis of the natural history of this disease, these authors noted that the probability of survival of a patient was not affected by the other deaths that had already occurred. In effect, the probability of survival at the time of observation is 100 percent, and the subsequent chances of survival can be expected to parallel those calculated for the entire population (Fig. 22-8). The parallel curves in Figure 22-8 mathematically define the expected survival for groups of patients (all grades) admitted to study at particular times after subarachnoid hemorrhage. To define the probability of survival for patients of a specific clinical grade, the authors applied the percentages of survival reported for conservative treatment in each of the clinical grades used by the Cooperative Study group proportionately to the results from each of Pakarinen's time intervals.[171] Table 22-1 provides the probability (rounded to the nearest 5 percent) that a patient classified at any grade at any point in time after his first or last hemorrhage will be alive 2 years later. Of convenience is the fact that the addition of 5 percentage points to each of the probabilities listed in Table 22-1 yields the prognosis for survival at 2 months. Thus, a grade 1 patient who has survived only 1 day after rupture has only a

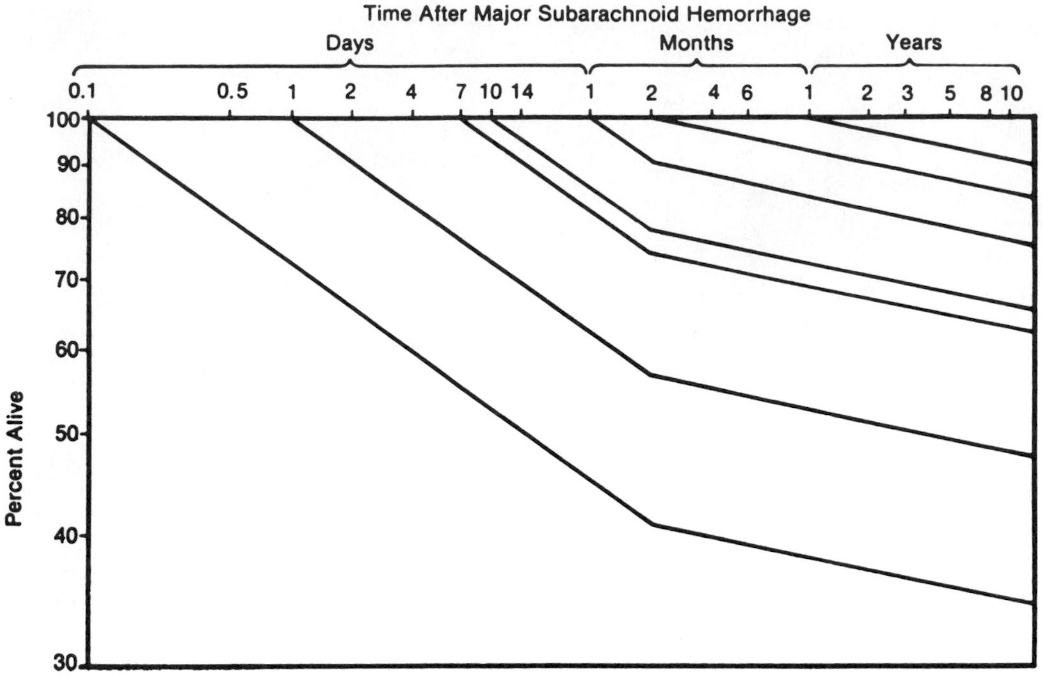


**Fig. 22-8.** Survival rates of patients admitted at varying intervals after their initial subarachnoid hemorrhage (conservative medical therapy). Note that the curves all parallel each other. In effect, one can restart the natural history by raising the probability of survival to 100 percent at the time of observation, and allowing the patients' probability of future survival to fall parallel with the original line. (From Alvord et al.,[13] with permission.)

65 percent probability of surviving for the same period. The particular advantage of an analysis such as this is that it readily permits the comparison of various reports in the literature and allows a physician to evaluate the results of his own medical or surgical treatments. Obviously, any new therapy would have to improve on these survival probabilities to be justified.

## PRODROMAL SYMPTOMS OF ANEURYSMAL RUPTURE

### Enlarging Aneurysm

Surgery is increasingly being recommended if there is clinical evidence that a saccular aneurysm is enlarging.[167,170] The onset of a 3rd cranial nerve palsy, particularly when associated with pupillary dilation and loss of light reflex, is highly suggestive of an expanding aneurysm at the junction of the posterior communicating artery and the distal internal carotid artery. The motor palsy of the lid and extraocular muscles may precede pupillary dilation and loss of light and accommodation reflexes. In some instances, aneurysmal dilation thus mimics diabetic 3rd cranial nerve palsy. Facial pain or pain around the eye are another possible indication of an expanding aneurysm. In 74 cases of expanding unruptured posterior communicating artery aneurysms prospectively studied,[215] painful 3rd cranial nerve palsy occurred in 59. The pain typically occurred above the brow and radiated back to the ear. It occurred in episodes of increasing intensity. With each attack of pain, the incidence of rupture increased. Without a 3rd cranial nerve palsy, up to seven attacks of pain occurred before rup-

**TABLE 22-1. Probabilities of Survival**

| | Number of Days After Subarachnoid Hemorrhage | | | | | | |
|---|---|---|---|---|---|---|---|
| Clinical Grade | 0 to 1 | 1 to 3 | 3 to 7 | 7 to 21 | 21 to 60 | 60+ | All Intervals |
| 1 | 65 | 80 | 90 | 95 | 95 | 95 | 90 |
| 2 | 55 | 70 | 75 | 90 | 95 | 95 | 75 |
| 3 | 45 | 55 | 65 | 75 | 85 | 95 | 65 |
| 4 | 30 | 40 | 45 | 50 | 60 | 70 | 45 |
| 5 | 5 | 5 | 5 | 5 | 5 | 5 | 5 |
| All grades | 45 | 55 | 65 | 75 | 85 | 95 | 65 |

ture in their series. When a 3rd cranial nerve palsy was present, however, no more than three attacks of pain occurred before rupture. In order for a 3rd cranial nerve palsy to occur, the aneurysm at the origin of the posterior communicating artery has to be 7 mm in size. If the 3rd cranial nerve palsy was present for more than 10 days, its chances of recovering are remote.[215]

Other cranial nerve palsies suggesting aneurysmal expansion include 6th nerve palsy in giant cavernous aneurysms, and visual field defects of an expanding supraclinoid carotid artery aneurysm. In some cases, focal headache involving the occipital and posterior cervical region when a posterior inferior cerebellar artery (PICA) or anterior/inferior cerebellar artery (AICA) aneurysm expand. Pain in or behind the eye and in the low temple can occur with middle cerebral artery aneurysm expansion. These same complaints may indicate arterial dissection and are not unique for aneurysm.

### Warning Leaks

Warning leaks of an aneurysm may cause focal frontal or occipital headache and stiff neck. Sudden headache with pain between the shoulder blades or at the back of the neck, accompanied by nausea and vomiting, is among the important symptoms. While these are often confused with migrainous headaches, patients usually state that they differ from their usual migraine headache. Computed tomography (CT) scan may be of diagnostic value without contrast to show blood in the subarachnoid space, after which contrast may show filling of the aneurysm. More often than not, however, the amount of blood from a warning leak will not be sufficient to be identified by CT scan. When suspicion of a warning leak arises and the patient has no focal neurologic signs that might be indicative of a mass effect, lumbar puncture is a safe and effective means of making the diagnosis. This should be done any time suspicion of a warning leak arises because of the devastating effects of major aneurysmal rupture. Auer[17] found that half of his patients with major hemorrhage (52 of 238, or 22 percent) had had warning leaks.

A variety of syndromes have been described.[4,115,133,168,248]

## SUBARACHNOID HEMORRHAGE

### Initial Clinical Presentation

At the moment of aneurysmal rupture, intracranial pressure approaches the mean arterial pressure and cerebral perfusion pressure falls.[161] This sudden surge in pressure and intracranial volume may account for the sudden but transient loss of consciousness that occurs in 45 percent of cases. While a brief moment of excruciating headache may occur just before loss of consciousness, the headache is usually reported upon regaining consciousness. In 10 percent of cases, aneurysmal bleeding may be severe enough to cause loss of consciousness for up to several days.[66] In 45 percent of cases, severe headache, without loss of consciousness, occurs as a presenting complaint.[66] Vomiting is another prominent symptom when the patient is awake, but it does not correlate well with headache severity. Rarely, a few cases may develop lightheadedness, followed by syncope within seconds, without headache; we have seen two such patients.

### Focal Deficits

Among cranial neuropathies, unilateral 3rd cranial nerve palsy after aneurysmal rupture suggests a posterior communicating artery aneurysm, while 6th cranial nerve palsy has no special localizing value.

Hemiparesis, aphasia of the dominant hemisphere, anosognosia (hemineglect) of the nondominant hemisphere, memory loss, and abulia are the more common hemispheric neurologic deficits. An aneurysm located at the bifurcation of the middle cerebral artery may rupture out into the temporal lobe and up into the frontal and parietal lobe (Fig. 22-9), less often into

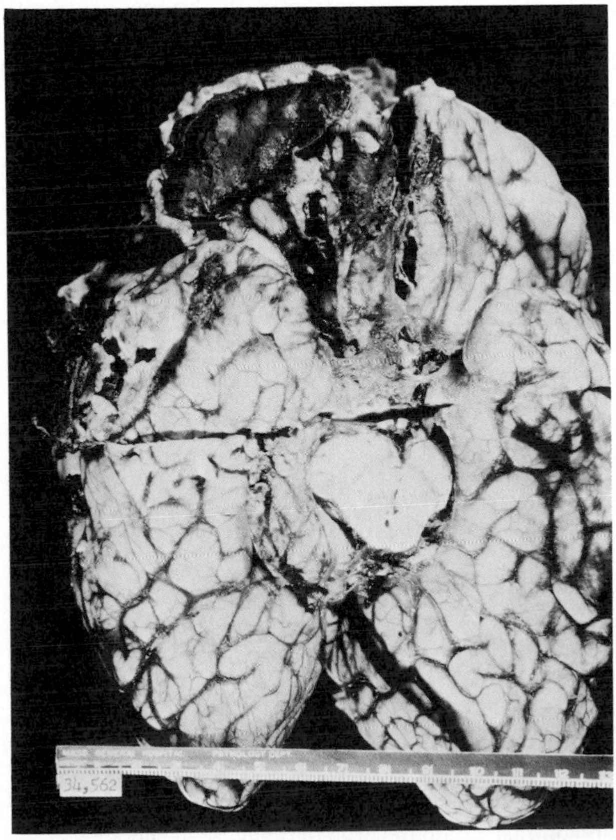

**Fig. 22-9.** Autopsy photograph of base of frontal lobe and circle of Willis showing diffuse subarachnoid hemorrhage and gross hemorrhage into frontal lobe.

the frontal or parietal region, and may occasionally be mistaken for primary parenchymatous hemorrhage.[46]

In many cases there is no adequate explanation for the initial neurologic deficits. In most cases, however, the deficits can be seen gradually to improve over a matter of days. The reason for brain edema is uncertain, but may be due to transient interruption of cerebral circulation in a given arterial territory during and immediately after aneurysmal rupture followed by recirculation.

## Grading Systems

The clinical grading system as modified by Botterell and colleagues,[28] Hunt and Hess,[106] and others have been widely used to categorize the clinical status of patients. They are reviewed in the Chapters 45 and 46 on medical and surgical management.

## Initial Laboratory Evaluation

Because saccular aneurysms that give rise to subarachnoid hemorrhage are located at the branch points of the large intracranial extracerebral arteries at the base of the brain, blood from the ruptured aneurysm is deposited as clots in the basal cisterns (Fig. 22-10). The specific location of the aneurysm and the severity and magnitude of the rupture determine the location and amount of blood in the various cisterns and fissures of the subarachnoid space.

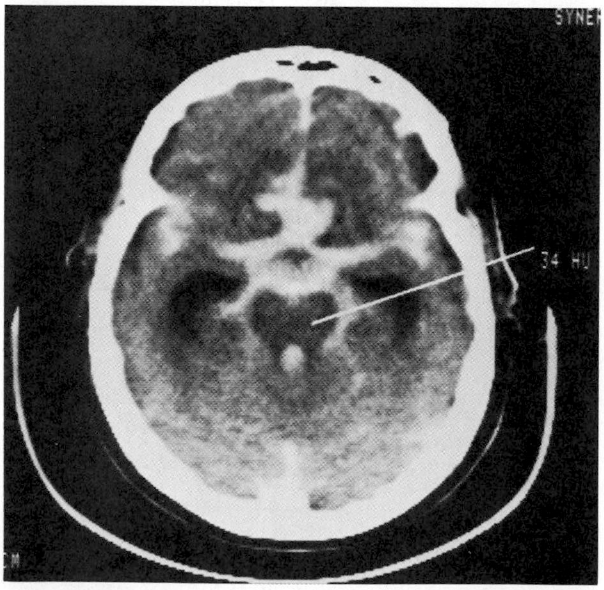


**Fig. 22-10.** Extensive subarachnoid hemorrhage shown on non-contrast computed tomography scan, flooding basilar cisterns with acute ischemic infarction of the midbrain. The patient died shortly thereafter.

## Computed Tomography Scan

About 75 percent of cases will have evidence of subarachnoid clot on non-contrast CT scan if the scan is obtained within the first 48 hours of aneurysmal rupture.[167] Furthermore, the extent and location of subarachnoid blood as seen on non-contrast CT scan may give useful information as to the location of the aneurysm and the cause of the initial neurologic deficit. It has been a useful means to predict those patients destined to develop delayed neurologic deficits because of symptomatic cerebral vasospasm[117]; in the study by Ohman et al.,[164] this is the most important in a logistic regression model. Using high-resolution CT scan after contrast, aneurysms down to 3 mm in size have been reported in 87 percent of 76 cases.[200] They are not as easily seen in the supraclinoid portion of the carotid artery and when bony or movement artifacts are present. In cases where the diagnosis of subarachnoid hemorrhage is uncertain, non-contrast scan should be done first, since contrast scans may show arterial enhancement in the basal cisterns that could be mistaken for clotted blood.

Arteriovenous malformations and mycotic aneurysms usually present with parenchymatous blood or subarachnoid blood located over the hemisphere rather than in the basal cistern.

## Magnetic Resonance Imaging

MR has been found as useful as CT for the diagnosis of subarachnoid hemorrhage.[131] In the future, MR may be developed to the point where it can reliably detect aneurysms of 0.5 mm or greater. MR angiography, because it is a flow study, may not be suitable for screening purposes.

Postoperatively, the use of ferromagnetic clips initially made MR imaging a risk for postoperative evaluations, but these risks have subsided considerably with the introduction of nonferromagnetic materials.

## Angiography

Cerebral angiography is still the crucial step in diagnosis. With the widespread use of early surgery, angiography has become common on the first day of symptoms. It is mandatory for diagnosis of intracerebral hematoma when emergency surgical evacuation is planned, as an occult aneurysm would be a disagreeable surprise to the surgical team evacuating an acute hematoma.

Where possible, selected angiography should be performed just prior to planned surgery, not only to localize the aneurysm, but to document its exact anatomy for approach. Rarely, despite the most thorough studies, a neck cannot be found suitable for clip placement or a tightly looped vessel misleads the team into a diagnosis of aneurysm.

Until recently, angiography was the only means to diagnose and follow the course of vasospasm.[69] Transcranial Doppler studies (see below) have greatly altered this approach. When angiography is used, angiographic evidence of severe vasospasm (i.e., middle cerebral artery stem or A1 segment of the anterior cerebral artery less than 1 mm or distal branch of the middle cerebral and anterior cerebral arteries at less than 0.5 mm) is present when symptoms of delayed ischemia occur in the territory of the internal carotid artery.[67]

If no aneurysm is found on the initial selected cerebral angiogram, the chance for repeat subarachnoid hemorrhage is quite low (1 to 2 percent.[24,93,175,212] Because selected cerebral angiography can miss a subtle aneurysm, particularly of the anterior communicating artery or in the posterior circulation, repeat four-vessel angiography is still a common practice after a week or so. However, recent challenges to this time-honored program have been made, citing the very low frequency of subsequent positive findings if an initial angiogram, in the absence of spasm, has shown no aneurysm.[40,79,83,114,128] Where no aneurysm is found it has been suspected that the aneurysm has obliterated itself in the clot after rupture. Other explanations of subarachnoid hemorrhage include rupture of a small superficial cortical artery,[100] spinal cord arteriovenous malformation (AVM),[87,96] an extramedullary aneurysm of the spinal cord, for example, a cervical reticular artery or an anterior spinal artery aneurysm,[101] or an artery of Adamkiewicz aneurysm.[63] Although they are rare, both a spinal cord AVM and an aneurysm of a cervical artery may appear together. In most cases back pain with minimal headache and subarachnoid blood suggests the diagnosis.

## Transcranial Doppler

A handy bedside and laboratory technique, transcranial Doppler has become a mainstay in the management of aneurysms, if for no other reason than it offers an excellent means of demonstrating the presence and severity of vasospasm. The details of the technique are found in Chapter 12 in this volume.

An excellent correlation has been found for angiographic evidence of spasm and Doppler velocities above 100 cm/s[43] to 120 mg/s.[214] The first appearance of increased velocity is typically on the 4th day after hemorrhage. Studies seeking signs of earlier or transient spasm have thus far been negative.[191] Flow velocities typically peak on the 11th and 18th days and normalize by the 3rd to 4th week.[208,214] The increase in velocities usually occurs before the appearance of delayed ischemic defects and mirrors the increase in angiographically evident vasospasm. Normal Doppler velocities have been shown to be associated with no spasm in the vessels insonated.[73]

Vasospasm within the territory of the middle cerebral artery can be detected reliably, while those in the anterior cerebral artery to the anterior communicating artery are usually undetected because of the sharp angulation of the artery out of the plane easily insonated by the Doppler.[123] For the same reason, the Doppler has also had difficulty in identifying spasm in vessels distal to the circle of Willis and middle cerebral artery stem.[157]

The Doppler velocity is inversely proportional to the concentration of formed elements in the blood, the hematocrit being the best biologic marker of the number of circulating formed elements. Volume expansion therapy to reduce spasm may result in hemodilution, which may reduce the density of circulating particles, improving flow, but producing a rise in Doppler velocity due to reduced hematocrit, which could be misinterpreted as increasing spasm.

## Cerebral Blood Flow, Single Photon Emission Computed Tomography, and Positron Emission Tomography

These techniques have had limited application because the patient must usually be transported from an intensive care unit and hold still for long periods of time. Although the application of the technology is difficult, when used they have correlated well with angiographic evidence of vasospasm and revealed evidence of tissue hypoperfusion in advance of symptoms.[50,107,217]

## Routine Laboratory Tests

The baseline electrocardiogram (ECG) is of value because peaked P waves, prolonged QT interval, and tall T waves are reported in patients with subarachnoid hemorrhage.[32,81] These changes have been linked to elevated catecholamine blood and urine levels and to hypothalamic dysfunction.[26,48,140,153,154] It has been hypothesized that $\alpha$-adrenergic receptors in the myocardium and coronary arteries are stimulated by norepinephrine-containing nerve terminals or circulating epinephrine, and result in prolonged muscle fiber contraction, which leads to myofibular necrosis. The $\alpha$-adrenergic receptors, which exist on the large coronary arteries could cause coronary spasm and lead to ischemic myocardial damage similar to Prinzmetal's angina.[81]

The clinical course correlates with body temperature and the white blood count (WC).[249] One explanation could be neurogenic hyperthermia.[213] Another is a system effect. An admission WBC above 15,000 or body temperature above 37.5°C had a 55 to 60 percent mortality compared with 25 to 35 percent for lower values, in both instances related to high frequencies of vasospasm. Baseline electrolytes have been of little predictive value for outcome,[55] but are of value because hyponatremia may develop later in the course—secondary to inappropriate antidiuretic hormone (ADH) secretion or an unknown factor, causing loss of salt and water in the urine, with subsequent volume depletion and dilutional hyponatremia. Platelet counts, bleeding time, and other clotting parameters should be documented. Serum viscosity increases with a hematocrit above 40 percent and a serum-fibrinogen level above 250 mg percent. High osmolality has also been related to poor outcome.[55]

## MEDICAL COMPLICATIONS OF SUBARACHNOID HEMORRHAGE

Although many medical complications can arise in a patient who is put to bed following subarachnoid hemorrhage, for example, thrombophlebitis with pulmonary embolism and perforated duodenal ulcer, two specific medical complications stand out as being related to subarachnoid hemorrhage. The first complication is ECG changes suggestive of myonecrosis and/or coronary arterial ischemia.[28,40,81,90] Here, the sympathetic nervous system is thought to be overactive,[154,162] and myofibrillar degeneration in focal areas of the myocardium has been documented.[78,183]

The second medical complication specifically related to subarachnoid hemorrhage is hyponatremia[155]: either from inappropriate antidiuretic hormone secretion or from secretion of atrial natriuretic factor.[55] Restriction of free water, while maintaining adequate intravascular volume, is an important management point.

## DELAYED NEUROLOGIC DEFICITS

There are three major causes of delayed neurologic deficits (i.e., those following stabilization or improvement of the initial neurologic symptoms or deficits after aneurysmal rupture): rebleeding, hydrocephalus, and cerebral vasospasm. Recognition of the onset, cause, and severity of each of these delayed neurologic deficits will be greatly aided by a precise knowledge of the cause and extent of the initial neurologic deficit and symptoms following subarachnoid hemorrhage. An accurate assessment of ventricular size and the extent and location of subarachnoid blood on early CT scan (24 to 48 hours after the hemorrhage) will be of great value in firmly establishing the diagnosis of each of these three complications.

### Rebleeding

While rerupture of an aneurysm is generally heralded by a sudden severe increase in headache and may be associated with nausea and vomiting, loss of consciousness, and new neurologic deficits, a sudden moderate to severe increase in headache is not in itself diagnostic. Repeat CT scan demonstrating an increase in the amount of blood in the subarachnoid space or a lumbar puncture showing new blood is essential to confirm the diagnosis.[82] Repeating a lumbar puncture in patients who have an increase in headache, however, may present some hazard and should only be done if the diagnosis of rebleed is mandatory. At present, it seems likely that increased morbidity of an aneurysmal rerupture is likely only if the CT scan shows new blood in the cisterns.[88]

The incidence of rebleeding may be as high as 30 percent of all cases.[158,257] Furthermore, rerupture carries a significant morbidity and mortality. In a study at the Mayo Clinic, 62 percent of patients who were drowsy or had headache, but no other neurologic deficit, sustained a major neurologic dysfunction upon rebleeding, and 31 percent of those patients died as a result of the rebleed.[228] The incidence of rerupture is highest in the first 3 weeks following aneurysmal rupture. By 6 months following aneurysmal rupture the rebleed rate has been estimated to be at 2 to 3 percent per year.[111]

### Antifibrinolytic Therapy

Because of the high early rebleeding rate and significant morbidity and mortality associated with it, considerable investigative interest has been directed toward the use of antifibrinolytic agents in the preoperative period.[3] Ramirez-Lassepas,[180] in a current extensive review of the subject, points out that of 25 published studies, only 13 were controlled and 9 were randomized. The results of all these studies are inconclusive. ε-Aminocaproic acid has been studied with conflicting results.[2,78,158,202,209] A recent effort[125] indicates that it may reduce the incidence of rebleeding, but may do so at the expense of a higher incidence of ischemic complications than that of controls. Similar experience has been had with a second antifibrinolytic agent, tranexamic acid (the transisomer of α-methylcyclohexane carboxylic acid).[68,112,132,244] An accurate diagnosis of rerupture for the purpose of any study is difficult. To establish firmly that a major rerupture has occurred, a worsening of the clinical status associated with an increased amount of blood seen on CT scan or evidence of an increased amount of blood in the cerebrospinal fluid on lumbar puncture must be evident. Such strict criteria would undoubtedly exclude minor moderate rebleeding episodes. To include all patients with an increase in headache without laboratory confirmation of increased blood would result in an overdiagnosis of recurrent hemorrhage. In the studies cited above, many patients did not have repeated lumbar puncture to establish the diagnosis, and CT scan criteria were not used to document the amount of rebleeding. Therefore, until more definitive evidence exists, antifibrinolytic therapy cannot be recommended in the preoperative period. Furthermore, the trend for early surgery makes it unnecessary. However, because of the often devastating effect of rerupture and the encouraging results in the most extensive study with ε-aminocaproic acid,[132] it should be considered if surgery is to be postponed. This plan seems useful especially when the extent and location of subarachnoid blood makes it unlikely spasm will occur. It is given as a continuous intravenous infusion of 30 to 36 g per day from the day of admission up to the day of surgery, but not longer than 3 weeks.

### Negative Angiographic Findings and Rebleeding

Hayward[94] estimated that in 9 percent of cases of subarachnoid hemorrhage, no aneurysm is found even with repeated four-vessel angiography. The incidence of rebleeding in these cases is low. Of the 41 patients with subarachnoid hemorrhage and no evidence of aneurysm on four-vessel angiography, none had evidence of rebleeding in a follow-up period from 3 months to 2½ years. It is possible that some of these patients had subarachnoid hemorrhages from causes other than rupture of a saccular aneurysm, for example, rupture of a small superficial artery.[101] The implication from the study by Hayward[94] is that most of the patients may have thrombosed their aneurysm, or the aneurysm was so small that it was destroyed at the time of rupture.

For perimesencephalic hemorrhage found on CT scan, the outlook seems especially good: none of the 37 patients studied by Rinkel et al.[187] rebled over the 18-month to 7-year follow-up.

When the initial angiogram fails to reveal an aneurysm, it seems prudent to keep the patient at rest for 1 to 3 weeks after the initial hemorrhage, then repeat the angiogram—an opinion no longer shared by all workers. If an aneurysm is found, then the patient may be mobilized. However, the utility of the bed rest program has not been adequately tested.

## Hydrocephalus

Communicating hydrocephalus with dilatation of the lateral ventricles and the 3rd and 4th ventricles may occur any time after aneurysmal rupture. In general, however, it occurs between 4 and 20 days following subarachnoid hemorrhage. Ventricular hemorrhage is a major risk factor for the development of hydrocephalus. Vasospasm seems unrelated to hydrocephalus or the need for shunt.[226]

Hydrocephalus may cause no detectable neurologic change, or it may be associated with profound stupor coming on in a matter of hours. Mild drowsiness, urinary incontinence, and inability to move the eyes above the equator are associated with early mild to moderate hydrocephalus. Often hydrocephalus is transient and may not require specific surgical intervention. In the past, frequent lumbar puncture was used in hopes of tiding the patient over a critical period until hydrocephalus subsided; at present, repeated lumbar puncture is considered hazardous because of the risk of rerupture, particularly with aneurysms lying in the posterior fossa. Obviously, when supratentoral mass effect exists, lumbar puncture is contraindicated. If significant neurologic deterioration occurs, and lumbar puncture is felt to be unsafe, then ventricular drainage or ventricular atrial shunting is advisable.

## Cerebral Vasospasm

It is now clearly established that narrowing of the caliber of the arteries at the base of the brain following subarachnoid hemorrhage from ruptured saccular aneurysm can lead to cerebral ischemia and infarction.[69] Compared to the other complications to which such patients are prone, vassospasm remains the most frightening and devastating even with advances in prevention and treatment. Reviews[210] appear often in the literature, the most persistent and thorough periodic reviewer being Wilkins.[255]

### Incidence and Prevalence

Vasospasm is now recognized as the major cause of delayed serious morbidity and death.[69,241] The severity and location of vasospasm are all-important in determining whether and where cerebral ischemia and/or cerebral infarction will develop.

The incidence of vasospasm in subarachnoid hemorrhage varies widely in the available literature. At one end of the spectrum is an incidence as low as 15 percent.[197,202] More often it has been reported in the range of 30 to 40 percent,[89,94,97,179,209] while a few papers showed higher values.[9,232] Higher incidences have been reported in population studies,[146,239] the highest is 76 percent.[146] Its onset is delayed 3 to 21 days after the initial hemorrhage, occurring most often 4 and 14 days.[69,71,116]

It has proved difficult to account for the wide variation in the incidence of spasm among centers. Some of the variation might reflect patterns of referral and differences in medical treatment programs. Given the wide spectrum for both of these variables, it seems likely that each institution does better to keep track of its own experience.

A separate matter is the incidence of delayed focal ischemic deficits attributed to vasospasm. In most patients there is a period of neurologic improvement or a period of clinical stability between the initial aneurysmal rupture and the onset of symptomatic vasospasm. The incidence of syndromes attributed to vasospasm also varies, and may be high in community hospitals,[146,239] but in major referral centers is reported with a frequency of some 30 percent.[229]

## Timing of Vasospasm

The onset and duration of vasospasm appears to follow a regular timetable. The few reports based on angiogram[109,197] and the increasing numbers based on Doppler suggest that the temporal course of vasospasm seems to be the same whether or not the vasospasm is later associated with delayed neurologic deficits.

Vasospasm has been documented *seconds or minutes* of vessel rupture in the experimental animal model, but only rarely has it been reported in man.[254] One case among the 5,484 cases of subarachnoid hemorrhage was reported in the Cooperative Study.[195] Wilkins and colleagues[256] found a mere 32 such cases in the literature, and in 13 most of the evidence suggested the cause was prior subarachnoid hemorrhage. Liliequist et al.[124] described a case whose acute spasm was documented on serial frames of an angiogram that documented acute rupture of the aneurysm during the procedure. Taneda et al.[238] found a similar case, angiogrammed within 12 hours of the initial rupture, who ruptured during the study with sudden spasm, which disappeared on repeat study after 14 minutes. Mohr and Kase[146] had a single case suffering from a syndrome consistent with a transient ischemic attack during the initial phase of aneurysm rupture. Their community-based study also showed vasospasm in 6 of the 20 angiograms done within the first 2 days after onset of subarachnoid hemorrhage severe enough to plunge the patient into coma. Others with a large experience with community cases[28] have had similar experiences. However, the vast majority of cases referred to a major medical center for surgery do not show these findings *before the third day* after a subarachnoid hemorrhage.[69,250,256] This late occurrence of the first signs of vasospasm has also been reported based on Doppler studies.[191]

The course of vasospasm may extend beyond 3 weeks. However, if vasospasm has not appeared by the end of the second week, there is little likelihood it will be of clinical significance.[250] Once vasospasm begins to subside, its recurrence in a given portion of an artery is not expected.[202]

Very late appearance of spasm, 7, 14, and 52 weeks after initial subarachnoid hemorrhage, has been described in rare instances.[118] In addition, transient spasm unexplained by ruptured aneurysm has also been described.[33]

## Distribution of Vasospasm

The topography varies somewhat, but usually affects the circle of Willis and stems of the major cerebral arteries.[130,179,211,256] In almost all instances the vasospasm begins in the proximal vessels, and spreads distally along the major CSF cylinders passing over the convexity in the general direction of the superior sagittal sinus.

This proclivity of vasospasm to affect the larger vessels may be a result of the differential responsiveness of larger vessels to sympathetic stimulation,[11] a result that is assumed to occur with subarachnoid hemorrhage. The spread of vasospasm through the arterial tree is controlled by factors not currently understood, but the process at least seems to develop in a centrifugal fashion.

## Types of Vasospasm

*Diffuse, segmental,* and *local forms* of vasospasm have been described over the years. In diffuse spasm, most of the arteries are affected by nearly uniform narrowing for long distances from their origin.[45] Segmental spasm presents with sausagelike bands of varying length. Local spasm is the short segments of narrowing seen in arteries in the vicinity of the aneurysm itself. Some surgeons argue[202] that the presence of the segmental or local varieties in the later stages of vasospasm is not a contraindication to surgery. However, diffuse vasospasm has been thought to have a more serious prognosis.[199,227]

## Predictors of Vasospasm

The incidence, severity, and location of cerebral vasospasm in patients following subarachnoid hemorrhage can be predicted by clotted blood in specific amounts at specific sites in the basal cisterns and fissures of the subarachnoid space as seen on CT scan.[67,104,116,144,146] A high incidence of cerebral vasospasm severe enough to produce symptoms has been found when the early CT scan shows globular subarachnoid clots larger than 5 × 3 mm in the basal cisterns or layers of blood 1 mm thick or greater in the cerebral fissures (see Fig. 22-10).

The location of the clot seen on CT scan carries a good correlation with the location of the spasm in the artery lying in the subarachnoid space adjacent to enveloped in the clot.[116] This correlation applies only for CT scans obtained later than 24 hours after the hemorrhage. Subarachnoid blood seen in the basal cisterns less than 24 hours after the rupture may dissipate during the 24- to 48-hour period following rupture. Because CT scan blood becomes attenuated over time, scans obtained more than 96 hours (4 days) after the rupture may not be reliable. If these observations prove reliable, then clotted blood, in sufficient amounts, at specific sites in the subarachnoid space, is the most important etiologic factor in the development of symptomatic cerebral vasospasm, and its removal or dispersal could be of crucial clinical importance.

Takemae et al.[236] were the first to indicate a correlation between high-density CT scan findings and subsequent vasospasm, a study that was updated and enlarged to 177 cases by Mizukami et al.[144] In this latter report, 85 percent of cases showing high density on the CT scan within 4 days of onset developed vasospasm, compared with none of eight whose CT scan was negative for high density during this period ($P < 0.01$), regardless of the location of the aneurysm. This correlation did not apply for cases whose scans were performed 5 days after onset. Fisher and Ojemann[69] independently quantitated the severity of the hemorrhage with the severity of the later vasospasm. Of their 47 cases, the CT scan showed either no evidence of blood or its diffuse distribution in 18 cases; only one experienced severe vasospasm. However, "in the presence of subarachnoid blood clots larger than 5 × 3 mm or layers of blood 1 mm or more thick in fissures and vertical cisterns, severe vasospasm followed almost invariably (23 of 24 cases)." When these CT scan criteria were applied prospectively to 50 cases, a strong correlation existed between extent and location of supratentorial subarachnoid blood and the location and severity of vasospasm and related symptoms. Mohr and Kase[146] had similar experience: all 15 of the angiogrammed cases among the 38 with massive bleeding shown on CT scan had vasospasm, among whom were 6 admitted in coma and angiogrammed the first day.

The occurrence of vasospasm was also significantly correlated with increased intracranial pressure ($P < 0.0001$) in the findings of the Cooperative Study.[195] Although the number of cases was too small for detailed analysis, local vasospasm occurred with equal frequency in cases with normal or increased intracranial pressure (3 of 14 vs 14 of 48), while diffuse vasospasm occurred only in those with increased intracranial pressure (0 of 13 vs 12 of 48). It seems likely that increased intracranial pressure is simply a reflection of the magnitude of the rupture.

A similar explanation probably applies to the relationship between vasospasm and the severity of the clinical picture. Although the incidence of vasospasm was rather low throughout the data of the Cooperative Study,[195] the small group of 63 cases with severe neurologic deficits had a remarkably high incidence of vasospasm.

## Proposed Mechanisms of Vasospasm

Work continues on the cause of cerebral vasospasm. There are so many candidates for vasospasm that it may be overly optimistic to assume any one of them can be the culprit.

Many available endogenous substances have been found to stimulate contraction of arterial smooth muscle.[216,246] They include serotonin,[10,39,182] prostaglandins,[52,173,252] catecholamines,[20,22,74,75] angiotensin,[15] and histamine.[11,252] All of these compounds are broken down quickly in vivo and they must be present in large, nonphysiologic amounts to produce or sustain spasm experimentally. Prolonged spasm has been produced by local hemostasis,[245] incubated whole blood,[61] a hemolysate of fresh whole blood,[174] and erythrocyte breakdown products, especially hemoglobin,[251] oxyhemoglobin,[113,240,242] and even bilirubin,[141] but not platelet-rich plasma alone.[174] Thromboxane inhibitors have not been found to reverse early or establish spasm, but patients with spasm have been found to have higher than normal circulating levels of thromboxane B2.[108]

The adventitial layer of pial vessels is innervated by adrenergic fibers containing dense core vesicles in their terminal varicosities,[34,60] which are believed to synthesize norepinephrine, and have been observed to disappear after subarachnoid hemorrhage[74,172] because they have been rendered more susceptible to circulating catecholamines.[98] Administration of 6-hydroxydopamine, which destroys catecholamine fiber, prevented acute and delayed spasm in an animal model.[234] Predepletion of substance P before injection of cisternal blood in the animal model has also been found to prevent vasospasm. Neuropeptide Y has been found in CSF at very high levels in a setting of spasm; the level is much lower in normals.[1] At the vascular level, vasoconstrictor products of the lipoxygenase, especially hydroperoxyeicosatetranenoic acids (HPETEs), have been shown to be produced by cerebral vessels, and their release could play a role in spasm,[203] and a role has even been proposed for substance P.[51]

Much of the animal work have been based on the recognition that persistence of the large subarachnoid clot is associated with spasm. The clot may create effects in addition to the blood products,[154] including the trapping of spasmogenic compounds in the cisterns,[252] which prevent their being carried off by the spinal fluid, and allow them to be absorbed by the pial vessels and the choroid plexus.[260] The coating of blood has been postulated to lead to local tissue acidosis and an anaerobic state, with inhibition of arterial wall synthesis of prostacyclin and overproduction of thromboxane A, resulting in vasospasm and platelet hyperaggregation.[233] Although the notion put forward by Mitzukami and coworkers[143] that the coating of blood over the adventitia of the major arteries may plug "vasa vasorum" has been refuted—there are no known vasa vasorum of the intracranial vessels[41]—but plugging has been demonstrated in adventitial "pores," possibly leading to the same result.[62]

At the cellular muscle level, under normal conditions, both contraction and relaxation of smooth muscle is an active process depending on the phosphorylation on a myosin light-chain kinase that is activated by binding a complex formed by calcium and calmodulin, a calcium-bonding regulatory protein.[98,218] When the calcium concentration in the sarcoplasm is greater than $10^{-5}$ $\mu$m or less than $10^{-7}$ $\mu$m the muscle is, respectively, fully contracted or relaxed, when these protein enzymes are available. Phosphorylation of myosin light chain responsible for muscle contraction is also dependent upon a cyclic adenosine monophosphate (AMP)-dependent protein kinase.[44] Beta-adrenergic stimulation[17] of the beta-adrenergic receptor in the cell membrane increases the availability of cyclic AMP in the sarcoplasm. This, in turn, decreases the affinity of the myosin light-chain kinase for calcium/calmodulin binding. This, in turn, reduces its ability to phosphorylate myosin light chains and to stimulate contraction. In order for relaxation to occur, the calcium ion concentration must decrease in the sarcoplasm, and it must be transported across the cell membrane into the extracellular space or into the intracellular organelles. This active process requires high-energy phosphate metabolism to be operational. Only when the calcium concentration in the sarcoplasm is reduced can there be disruption of the actin-myosin cross-bridges responsible for contracting utility. A reciprocal interaction has been shown between calcium and magnesium,[138] by which increased calcium or decreased magnesium causes constriction, while increased magnesium causes relaxation.[12,205] The increase in the calcium : magnesium ratio, from the usual 1 : 1 in spinal fluid to 3 : 1 after subarachnoid hemorrhage, provides a basis for speculating a role for calcium in vasospasm, against which the calcium antagonist, nimodipine, is directed.

## Histology of Spasm

Although popular, the term vasospasm may not correctly characterize the vascular changes that reduce lumen diameter. Alksne,[5,7] Fein et al.,[65] and Mizukami et al.[143] independently demonstrated fragmentation of myofilaments, destruction of the sarcolemma, and lipid inclusions within abnormal smooth muscle cells in the media close to the internal elastic lamina. Alksne and Branson[6] also documented endothelial cell loss and proliferation in the chronic arteriopathy in a monkey and dog model.[237] More recent work has expanded the idea of structural changes in other directions, with disagreements on the basic findings in microscopy: the process has been shown to be limited to corrugation of the endothelium, with desquamation of endothelial cells but no changes in the media,[206] to involve both endothelium and media,[65] and to involve all layers of the vascular wall.[134]

Other workers favor the notion of arterial constriction: canine basilar arteries in spasm between 2 and 28 days after subarachnoid injection of autogenous fresh blood showed no significant change in the radius or wall thickness when tested by strain gauge at various pressures, a finding that indicated that vascular smooth muscle constriction, not irreversible organic changes in the wall, were responsible for the luminal narrowing in vivo.[153]

A role for intraluminal thrombi, however, brought about, was suggested by autopsy studies in humans, showing white and fibrin microthrombi clustered along the intima and at the ostia of arterial branches, which fed regions of focal infarction.[233] This study brings back afresh the notion that thrombosis plays a role in delayed ischemic deficits, and with it the possibility of therapy with anticoagulants.[38]

## Clinical Syndromes of Vasospasm

A relationship between vasospasm and delayed clinical deficits was already widely accepted when Millikan,[142] after an extensive review of the literature, reported no acceptable clinical data bearing on the subject, and found no difference in the incidence of neurologic deficits between cases with vasospasm and those without in his series of 198 consecutive cases of subarachnoid hemorrhage from the Mayo Clinic. In the 81 patients with spasm, 48 (59 percent) showed neurologic abnormalities, among them 27 (33 percent) with focal signs. However, among the other 117 who showed no vasospasm, 83 (71 percent) had neurologic deficits, 44 (38 percent) of which were focal.

Although the overall thrust of Millikan's argument came under heavy criticism, his detailed literature review (up to 1975) well documented a remarkable paucity of clinical deficits attributable to vasospasm. His review covered 45 publications involving over 2,000 clinical cases from 1938 to 1974, and 198 cases in his own series. His clinical material contained 14 cases with hemiparesis-hemiplegia and 8 with dysphasia-aphasia present in the preoperative state at the time the angiogram showed spasm. In five of the cases with motor deficit and all of those with dysphasia-aphasia, the onset of the symptoms occurred 24 to 48 hours after the subarachnoid hemorrhage. Of the remaining cases, three were described in clinical sketches featuring sudden onset of focal symptoms with angiographic evidence of spasm. But the angiograms also showed occlusions attributed to emboli that involved branches serving the focally symptomatic territories of the middle cerebral artery. Disturbances of consciousness, another type of disorder considered linked to vasospasm, was more frequent in the cases with*out* vasospasm.

The findings of this paper sharpened interest in the subject[67,228] and in its therapy.[2,30,31,209] Fisher et al.[68] focused their 50 cases on the correlation between vasospasm severity and clinical deficits: of the 25 (50 percent) with delayed neurologic deficits, all showed severe vasospasm (3 to 4+ on his scale of severity). Another 19 had no focal signs, and in all of these cases the angiograms showed only 0 to 2+ spasm. Fisher and coworkers concluded that "blood localized in the subarachnoid space in sufficient amounts at specific sites is the only important etiological factor in vasospasm." The clinical deficits attributed to vasospasm were described in some detail. Among the 50 cases, right hemiplegia with aphasia occurred in the 10, 4 had right hemiparesis without aphasia, 5 had left hemiplegia, 2 each had right and left hemiplegia, aphasia, or initial paralysis of both legs. Signs referable to the middle cerebral artery on one or both sides were the most frequent, while in 8 cases the presence of abulia and leg weakness suggested that the anterior cerebral artery was affected.

In the years following Fisher's study clinical deficits have often been tabulated, but syndromes have only occasionally been described. Suzuki et al.[231] reported 20 cases of subarachnoid hemorrhage, of whom 9 had angiographic evidence of vasospasm. Two of the nine "displayed mild ischemic symptoms." Similarly, Sano and Saito[199] reported 68 to 443 cases with angiographic evidence of vasospasm at some point during the preoperative period. The clinical deficits included "disturbance of consciousness" in 58 cases, "motor disturbance" in 40, and "mental changes" in 24. A strong correlation existed between the location of severe vasospasm and the cerebral arterial territory in which delayed ischemic deficit occurred.[84] The neurologic deficits in that study included hemiparesis with or without aphasia when the dominant middle cerebral artery territory was involved and the middle cerebral artery stem or its immediate distal branches, upper and lower division, was involved. Hemiparesis with or without anosognosia and apractagnosia was present when the nondominant middle cerebral artery territory was involved. Anterior cerebral territory ischemic deficits were recognized as representing a quiet abulic state in which the patient may be awake but lies quietly with his eyes closed, responding to commands with delay. Such a patient may offer no spontaneous conversation, but is able to answer questions with short phrases in a whispered voice, again, often after a delay. Food is chewed for a prolonged period of time and often held between the cheek and gum. This state was associated with severe spasm in the A1 or A2 segment of the anterior cerebral artery. Homonymous hemianopic field defects have been seen in patients with severe spasm of the posterior cerebral artery. Focal brain stem dysfunction has been observed with severe spasm of the vertebral basilar artery, but that is rare. These focal neurologic symptoms have been observed to occur gradually over a few days or presented abruptly, coming to their full extent within a matter of minutes or an hour. They have been attributed to reduced blood flow in the arterial territory evolved. This has been amply documented along with an increase in blood volume.[87,148]

In earlier times, the appearance of these syndromes was taken as a sign of irreversible ischemic deficits and surgery was often delayed or canceled. Rare surprising examples of desperation therapy with extreme increases in blood pressure, followed by dramatic reversal of what looked like permanent deficits, were too infrequent to be considered typical of the chances for functional recovery. Yet recent work with angioplasty may be revising some of these notions. In some instances, stupor has been reversed by successful angioplasty,[120] as have some other neurologic deficits,[53] raising hopes that some deficits may prove to be reversible. But fatalities have been documented.[126]

If the brain becomes infarcted in a large enough area, cerebral edema may ensue and result in a fatal rise in intracranial pressure. Suggestion of such a severe outcome, that is, the entire middle cerebral artery territory becoming ischemic and infarcted, can be inferred from the early CT scan when a large clot is noted in the stem of the sylvian fissure and/or sylvian cistern, and a second significant clot is noted in the basal frontal inner hemispheric fissure.[119]

Simultaneous clots in these areas correlated well with severe spasm, both in the middle cerebral artery stem and/or the middle cerebral bifurcation and the corresponding anterior cerebral artery. Thus, when severe middle cerebral artery stem spasm reduced flow in that arterial territory, the chance for adequate collateral over the cortical surface into the distal middle cerebral branches from the anterior cerebral artery is eliminated. Likewise, a single large clot in the stem of the sylvian fissure or at the sylvian cistern where the middle cerebral artery stem bifurcates, may assure severe spasm in the middle cerebral artery stem or at its bifurcation. However, without a significant clot in the basal frontal inner hemispheric fissure, the proximal anterior cerebral artery would not be expected to develop severe vasospasm. Therefore, there would be a chance for adequate collateral flow to develop from the distal anterior cerebral branches into the middle cerebral artery territory. Patients with this particular location of subarachnoid blood may escape the development of ischemic middle cerebral artery territory symptoms or they may not be severe and may only be transient.[84]

In the series reported by Mohr and Kase,[146] delayed deficits attributed to vasospasm occurred in 29 of 37 cases (78 percent). The possibility of delayed ischemic syndromes could not be evaluated in another 23 patients who developed coma at onset and died without regaining consciousness. In only one of their cases was spasm documented angiographically in the absence of a delayed neurologic deficit: a woman with a 6 × 9 mm middle cerebral artery aneurysm with local spasm of the middle cerebral artery stem seen on angiogram performed 6 days later; she underwent surgery the 7th day and at no time pre- or postoperatively did a focal deficit occur. The *mode of onset* (whether sudden or gradual) in 19 of the 37 was imprecisely understood, since it developed to its fullest extent during a period between clinical observations. Yet, at the most, only a few hours elapsed between examinations. In another seven instances, a *sudden onset* of the deficit was clearly documented, since two observers encountered the patient within minutes of one another, and in every instance no further progression of the deficit occurred. In four others, the syndrome *worsened gradually,* stretching over a period of several days. In all cases, some focal deficit was present on admission. It remained unchanged until the 2nd to 6th day when other focal deficits made their appearance and the level of consciousness began to sink, first to obtundation, then to coma over the following 2 to 3 days.

The clinical deficits that we encountered and those reported in the literature range among surface branch syndromes that could be due to emboli, "distal field" or "watershed" infarcts attributable to perfusion failure, and huge infarcts encompassing both the deep and superficial portions of an entire arterial territory. It may be important that isolated deep infarcts of the lacunar type have not been encountered clinically, not have we seen these infarcts on CT scan, although they have been mentioned in the autopsy literature (16 isolated caudate infarcts in 119 cases described by Crompton[47]). The apparent infrequency of such infarcts is especially interesting, considering the high incidence of vasospasm confined to the stem of the anterior and middle cerebral arteries.

Autopsy reports have emphasized a variety of findings, but it has proved difficult to correlate specific ischemic lesions with the clinical picture, due to the changing nature of the clinical course. The study by Suzuki et al.[233] correlated microvascular thromboses with focal infarcts but not with syndromes.

The incidence of ischemic infarcts varies from 25 percent[185] to as high as 78 percent.[241] Most infarcts affected the arterial territory of the aneurysm, but also involved others. Some of the reports described widespread ischemic changes of the cerebrum, including the hypothalamus.[47] Others reported similar widespread neuronal loss with white matter edema, but no distinct large foci of infarction or lesions more proximal than the "watershed" regions. Ischemic zones ranged in size from small cortical foci to large infarcts in arterial territories distal to the site of the aneurysm,[188,241] usually with patent arteries.[103] Thrombi and emboli have been described in some reports,[23,47] and their potential role for symptoms attributable to vasospasm has been the source of considerable speculation.[142,188] Whether or not an embolic mechanism is frequent, its documentation has proved to be difficult and its occurrence seems intimately related to the process known as vasospasm. The possibility that emboli might arise from the intima of an artery in "vasospasm" is consistent with the hypothesis that endothelial thrombus formation set in motion by acidosis and platelet aggregation plays a more important role in symptoms than does spasm of the arteries.[231,233] However, Nagasawa et al.[153] found no thrombus within any of the freshly removed canine basilar arteries in spasm from 2 through 28 days.

## Outcome Long After Hemorrhage or Surgery

Cognitive deficits have been a nagging problem and are often mentioned by family more than they seem to be recognized by the professional staff. Detailed testing is uncommon. In Richardson's study[186] of 76 cases, a moderate impairment was found 6 weeks after hospitalization, unrelated to the site of aneurysm rupture, but especially common in patients who had experienced generalized vasospasm. By 6 months, the findings had mostly reverted to normal.

## REFERENCES

1. Abel PW, Han C, Noe BD, McDonald JK: Neuropeptide Y: vasoconstrictor effects and possible role in cerebral vasospasm after experimental subarachnoid hemorrhage. Brain Res 463:250, 1988
2. Acosta-Rua GJ: Familial incidence of ruptured intracranial aneurysms. Arch Neurol 35:675, 1978
3. Adams HP: Current status of antifibrinolytic therapy for treatment of patients with aneurysmal subarachnoid hemorrhage. Stroke 13: 256, 1982
4. Adams H, Jergenson DD, Kassell NF, Sahs AL: Pitfalls in the recognition of subarachnoid hemorrhage. JAMA 244:794, 1980
5. Alksne JF: Myonecrosis in chronic experimental vasospasm. Surgery 76:1, 1974
6. Alksne JF, Branson PJ: A comparison of intimal proliferation in experimental subarachnoid hemorrhage and atherosclerosis. Angiology 12:712, 1976
7. Alksne JF, Greenhoot JH: Experimental catecholamine-induced chronic cerebral vasospasm myonecrosis in vessel walls. J Neurosurg 41:440, 1974
8. Allcock J, Canham PB: Angiographic study of the growth of intracranial aneurysms. J Neurosurg 45:617, 1976
9. Allcock JM, Drake CG: Ruptured intracranial aneurysms: the role of arterial spasm. J Neurosurg 22:21, 1965
10. Allen GS, Gross CJ, Henderson LM, Chou SN: Cerebral arterial spasm. 4. In vitro effects of temperature, serotonin analogues, large nonphysiological concentrations of serotonin and extracellular calcium and magnesium on serotonin-induced contractions of the canine basilar artery. J Neurosurg 44:585, 1976
11. Allen GS, Henderson LM, Chow NS, French LA: Cerebral arterial spasm. I. In vitro contractile activity of vasoactive agents on canine basilar and middle cerebral arteries. J Neurosurg 40:433, 1974
12. Altura BT, Altura BM: Magnesium deficiency induces cerebral vasospasm, abstracted. Stroke 12:118, 1981
13. Alvord EC, Jr, Loeser JD, Bailey WL et al: Subarachnoid hemorrhage due to ruptured aneurysms: a simple method for estimating prognosis. Arch Neurol 27:273, 1972
14. Anderson RMD, Blackwood W: The association of arteriovenous angioma and saccular aneurysms of the arteries of the brain. J Pathol Bacteriol 77:101, 1959

15. Andrews P, Papadokis N, Garras H: Reversal of experimental acute cerebral vasospasm by angiotensin-converting enzyme inhibition. Stroke 13:480, 1982
16. Andrews RJ, Spiegel PK: Intracranial aneurysms: age, sex, blood pressure and multiplicity in an unselected series of patients. J Neurosurg 51:27, 1979
17. Auer LM: Unfavorable outcome following early surgical repair of ruptured cerebral aneurysms—a critical review of 238 patients. Surg Neurol 35:152, 1991
18. Bannerman RM, Ingall GB, Graf CJ: The familial occurrence of intracranial aneurysms. Neurology (NY) 20:283, 1970
19. Basset RC, Lemmen LJ: Subdural hematoma associated with bleeding intracranial aneurysms. J Neurosurg 9:443, 1952
20. Baumbach G, Heistad D: Effect of sympathetic nerves on segmental resistance of cerebral vessels, abstracted. (Presented at the Seventh Joint Meeting on Stroke and Cerebral Circulation, New Orleans, February 1982.) Stroke 13:5, 1982
21. Belber CJ, Hoffman RB: The syndrome of intracranial aneurysm associated with fibromuscular hyperplasia of the renal arteries. J Neurosurg 28:556, 1968
22. Bendict CR, Loach AB: Sympathetic nervous system activity in patients with subarachnoid hemorrhage. Stroke 9:237, 1978
23. Benoit BG, Wortman G: Traumatic cerebral aneurysms. J Neurol Neurosurg Psychiatry 36:127, 1973
24. Bequelin C, Seiler R: Subarachnoid hemorrhage with normal cerebral panangiography. Neurosurgery 13:409, 1983
25. Beumont PJV: The familial occurrence of berry aneurysms. J Neurol Neurosurg Psychiatry 31:399, 1968
26. Birse SH, Tom HI: Incidence of cerebral infarction associated with ruptured intracranial aneurysms. Neurology (NY) 10:101, 1960
27. Black BK, Hicks S: The relation of hypertension to arterial aneurysms of the brain. US Armed Forces Med J 3:1813, 1952
28. Botterell EH, Lougheed WM, Scott JW et al: Hypothermia, and interruption of carotid, or carotid and vertebral circulation, in the surgical management of intracranial aneurysm. J Neurosurg 13:1, 1956
29. Brass LM, Pavlakis S, Mohr JP: Transcranial Doppler measuremnts of the middle cerebral artery: the effect of hematocrit. Stroke 19:1446, 1988
30. Brisman R, Abbassioun K: Familial intracranial aneurysms. J Neurosurg 34:678, 1971
31. Brothers MF, Holgate RC: Intracranial angioplasty for treatment of vasospasm after subarachnoid hemorrhage: technique and modifications to improve branch access. AJNR 11:239, 1990
32. Brown FD, Hanlon K, Mullan S: Treatment of aneurysmal hemiplegia with dopamine and mannitol. J Neurosurg 49:525, 1978
33. Byer E, Ashman R, Toth LA: Electrocardiograms with large upright T waves and long QT intervals. Am Heart J 33:796, 1947
34. Call GK, Fleming MC, Sealfon S et al: Reversible cerebral segmental vasoconstriction. Stroke 19:1159, 1988
35. Candia CJ, Heros RC, Lavyne MH et al: Effects of intravenous sodium nitroprusside on cerebral blood flow and intracranial. Neurosurgery 3:50, 1978
36. Carmichael R: The pathogenesis of non-inflammatory cerebral aneurysms. J Pathol Bacteriol 62:1, 1950
37. Cates JE, Christ RV: Subacute bacterial endocarditis. Q J Med 20:93, 1951
38. Chason JL, Hindman WM: Berry aneurysms of the circle of Willis. Neurology (NY) 8:41, 1958
39. Chimowitz MI, Pessin MS: Is there a role for heparin in the management of complications of subarachnoid hemorrhage? Stroke 18:1169, 1987
40. Chow RWB, Newton TH, Smith MC, Adams JE: Cerebral vasospasm induced by subarachnoid blood and serotonin: an angiographic study. Invest Radiol 3:402, 1968
41. Cioffi F, Pasqualin A, Cavazzani P, DaPian R: Subarachnoid haemorrhage of unknown origin: clinical and tomographical aspects. Acta Neurochir (Wien) 97:31, 1989
42. Clower BR, Sullivan DM, Smith RR: Intracranial vessels lack vasa vasorum. J Neurosurg 61:44, 1984
43. Cohen MM: Cerebrovascular accidents: a study of two hundred cases. Arch Pathol 60:296, 1955
44. Compton JS, Redmond S, Symon L: Cerebral blood velocity in subarachnoid haemorrhage: a transcranial Doppler study. J Neurol Neurosurg Psychiatry 50:1499, 1987
45. Conti MA, Adelstein RS: Phosphorylations by cyclic adenosine 3′,5′-monophosphate-dependent protein kinase regulates myosin light chain kinase. Fed Proc 39:1569, 1980
46. Conway LW, McDonald LW: Structural changes of the intradural arteries following subarachnoid hemorrhage. J Neurosurg 37:715, 1972
47. Crompton MR: Intracerebral hematoma complicating ruptured cerebral berry aneurysm. J Neurol Neurosurg Psychiatry 25:378, 1962
48. Crompton MR: Cerebral infarction following the rupture of cerebral berry aneurysms. Brain 87:263, 1964
49. Cruickshank JW, Neil-Dwyer G, Stott AW: Possible role of catecholamines, corticosteroids, and potassium in production of electrocardiographic abnormalities associated with subarachnoid hemorrhage. Br Heart J 36:697, 1974
50. Dalgaard OZ: Bilateral polycystic disease of the kidneys: a follow-up of 284 patients and their families. Acta Med Scand, suppl. 328:186, 1957
51. Davis S, Andrews J, Lichtenstein M et al: A single photon emission computed tomography study of hypoperfusion after subarachnoid hemorrhage. Stroke 21:252, 1990
52. Delgado-Zygmunt TJ, Arbab MA, Edvinsson L et al: Prevention of cerebral vasospasm in the rat by depletion or inhibition of substance P in conducting vessels. J Neurosurg 72:917, 1990

53. Denton IC, Jr, White RP, Robertson JT: The effects of prostaglandins E1, A1, F2 on the cerebral circulation of dogs and monkeys. J Neurosurg 36:34, 1972
54. Dion JE, Duckwiler GR, Vinuela F et al: Preoperative microangioplasty of refractory vasospasm secondary to subarachnoid hemorrhage. Neuroradiology 32;232, 1990
55. Diringer MN, Lim JS, Kirsch JR, Hanley DF: Suprasellar and intraventricular blood predict elevated plasma atrial natriuretic factor in subarachnoid hemorrhage. Stroke 22:577, 1991
56. Disney L, Weir B, Grace M, Roberts P: Trends in blood pressure, osmolality and electrolytes after subarachnoid hemorrhage from aneurysms. Can J Neurol Sci 16:299, 1989
57. Drake CG: Management of cerebral aneurysms. Stroke 12:273, 1981
58. DuBoulay GH: Some observations on the natural history of intracranial aneurysms. Br J Radiol 38:721, 1965
59. Ebels EJ: Management of intracranial aneurysms. Lancet 1:692, 1975
60. Edelsohn L, Caplan L, Rosenbaum AE: Familial aneurysms and infundibular widening. Neurology (NY) 22:1056, 1972
61. Edvinsson L, Owman CH, Sjoberg N: Autonomic nerves, mast cells and amine receptors in human brain vessels: a histochemical and pharmacological study. Brain Res 115:377, 1976
62. Endo S, Suzuki J: Experimental cerebral vasospasm after subarachnoid hemorrhage—development and degree of vasospasm. Stroke 8:700, 1977
63. Espinosa F, Weir B, Shnitka T: Electron microscopy of simian cerebral arteries after subarachnoid hemorrhage and after the injection of horseradish peroxidase. Neurosurgery 19:935, 1986
64. Fairbaum B: "Twin" intracranial aneurysms causing subarachnoid hemorrhage in identical twins. Br Med J 1:210, 1973
65. Fein JM, Flor WJ, Cohan SL, Parkhurst J: Sequential changes of vascular ultrastructure in experimental vasospasm. J Neurosurg 41:49, 1974
66. Findlay JM, Weir BK, Kanamaru K, Espinosa F: Arterial wall changes in cerebral vasospasm. Neurosurgery 25:736, 1989
67. Fisher CM: Clinical syndromes in cerebral thrombosis, hypertensive hemorrhage and ruptured saccular aneurysm. Clin Neurosurg 22:117, 1975
68. Fisher CM, Kistler JP, Davis JM: Relation of cerebral vasospasm to subarachnoid hemorrhage visualized by computerized tomographic scanning. Neurosurgery 6;1, 1980
69. Fisher CM, Ojemann RG: Basal rupture of cerebral aneurysm—a pathological case report. J Neurosurg 48:642, 1978
70. Fisher CM, Roberson GH, Ojemann RG: Cerebral vasospasm with ruptured saccular aneurysm—the clinical manifestations. Neurosurgery 1:245, 1977
71. Fodstad H, Liliequist B, Schannong M, Thulin CA: Tranexamic acid in the preoperative management of ruptured intracranial aneurysms. Surg Neurol 10:9, 1978
72. Fogelholm R: Subarachnoid hemorrhage in middle Finland: incidence, early prognosis and indications for neurosurgical treatment. Stroke 12:296, 1981
73. Forbus WD: On the origin of miliary aneurysms of the superficial cerebral arteries. Bull Johns Hopkins Hosp 47:239, 1930
74. Fornezza U, Carraro R, Demo P et al: The transcranial Doppler ultrasonography in the evaluation of vasospasm and of intracranial hypertension after subarachnoid hemorrhage. Aggressologie 31:259, 1990
75. Fraser RAR, Stein BM, Barrett RE, Pool JL: Noradrenergic mediation of experimental cerebrovascular spasm. Stroke 1:356, 1970
76. Freytag E: Fatal rupture of intracranial aneurysms: survey of 250 medicolegal cases. Arch Pathol 81:418, 1966
77. Garcia CA, Dulcey S, Dulcey J: Ruptured aneurysm of the spinal artery of Adamkiewicz during pregnancy. Neurology (NY) 29:394, 1979
78. Gautier JC, Hauw JJ, Awada A et al: Artères cérébrales dolichoectasiques: association aux aneurysmes de l'aorte abdominale. Rev Neurol (Paris) 144:437, 1988
79. Gibbs JR, O'Gorman P: Fibrinolysis in subarachnoid hemorrhage. Postgrad Med J 43:779, 1967
80. Gilbert JW, Lee C, Young B: Repeat cerebral panangiogrpahy in subarachnoid hemorrhage of unknown etiology. Surg Neurol 33:19, 1990
81. Glynn LE: Medial defects in the circle of Willis and their relation to aneurysm formation. J Pathol Bacteriol 51:213, 1940
82. Goldman MR, Rogers EL, Rogers MC: Subarachnoid hemorrhage associated with unusual electrocardiographic changes. JAMA 234:957, 1975
83. Goldstein SL: Case reports and technical notes: ventricular opacification secondary to rupture of intracranial aneurysms during angiography. J Neurosurg 27:265, 1967
84. Gomez PA, Lobato RD, Rivas JJ et al: Subarachnoid haemorrhage of unknown aetiology. Acta Neurochir (Wien) 101:35, 1989
85. Graf CJ: Spontaneous carotid cavernous fistula: Ehlers-Danlos syndrome and related conditions. Arch Neurol 13:662, 1965
86. Graf CJ: Familial intracranial aneurysms: report of four cases. J Neurosurg 25:304, 1966
87. Grosman H, Fornasier VL, Bonder D et al: Dissecting aneurysm of the cerebral arteries: case report. J Neurosurg 53:693, 1980
88. Grubb RL, Raichle ME, Eichling JO, Gado MH: Effects of subarachnoid hemorrhage on cerebral blood volume, blood flow and oxygen utilization in humans. J Neurosurg 46:446, 1977
89. Gurus IN, Ghe MT, Richardson AE: The value of computerized tomography in aneurysmal subarachnoid hemorrhage, J Neurosurg 60:763, 1984

90. Hamer J, Penzholz H, Götte B: Time course and clinical significance of cerebral vasospasm after aneurysmal subarachnoid hemorrhage. Acta Neurochir 52:157, 1980
91. Hammermeister KE, Reichenbach DD: QRS changes, pulmonary edema and myocardial necrosis associated with subarachnoid hemorrhage. Am Heart J 78:94, 1969
92. Harrison MJG, Hampton JR: Neurologic presentation of bacterial endocarditis. Br Med J 2:148, 1967
93. Hassler O: Morphological studies on the large cerebral arteries with references to aetiology of subarachnoid hemorrhage. Acta Psychiatr Scand, suppl. 154:1, 1961
94. Hayward RD: Subarachnoid hemorrhage of unknown aetiology: a clinical and radiological study of 51 cases. J Neurol Neurosurg Psychiatry 40:926, 1977
95. Heilbrun MP: The relationship of neurological status and angiographical evidence of spasm to prognosis in patients with ruptured intracranial aneurysms. Stroke 4:973, 1973
96. Heiskanen O: Risk of bleeding from unruptured aneurysms in cases with multiple intracranial aneurysms. J Neurosurg 55:524, 1981
97. Herdt D, Jr, Chiro G, Doppman JL: Combined arterial and arteriovenous aneurysms of the spinal cord. Radiology 99:589, 1971
98. Heros RC, Zervas NT, Lavyne MH, Pickren KS: Reversal of experimental cerebral vasospasm by intravenous nitroprusside therapy. Surg Neurol 6:227, 1976
99. Heros RC, Zervas NT, Varsos V: Cerebral vasospasm after subarachnoid hemorrhage: an update. Ann Neurol 12:599, 1983
100. Hijdra A, Braakmanm R, vanGijn J et al: Aneurysmal subarachnoid hemorrhage: complications and outcome in a hospital population. Stroke 18:1061, 1987
101. Hochberg FH, Fisher CM, Roberson GH: Subarachnoid hemorrhage caused by rupture of a small superficial artery. Neurology (NY) 24:319, 1974
102. Hopkins CA, Wilkie FL, Vovis DC: Extramedullary aneurysm of the spinal cord. J Neurosurg 24:1021, 1966
103. Housepian EM, Pool JL: A systematic analysis of intracranial aneurysms from the autopsy file of the Presbyterian Hospital, 1914 to 1956. J Neuropathol Exp Neurol 17:409, 1958
104. Hughes JT, Schianchi PM: Cerebral artery spasm. J Neurosurg 48:515, 1978
105. Hunt HB, Schifrin BS, Suzuki K: Ruptured berry aneurysms and pregnancy. Obstet Gynecol 43:827, 1974
106. Hunt WE, Hess RM: Surgical risk as related to time of intervention in the repair of intracranial aneurysms. J Neurosurg 28:14, 1968
107. Hunt WE, Kosnik EJ: Timing and perioperative care in intracranial aneurysm surgery. Clin Neurosurg 21:79, 1974
108. Jakobsen M, Overgaard J, Marcussen E, Enevoldsen EM: Relation between angiographic cerebral vasospasm and regional CBF in patients with SAH. Acta Neurol Scand 82:109, 1990
109. Juvela S, Ohman J, Servo A et al: Angiographic vasospasm and release of platelet thromboxane after subarachnoid hemorrhage. Stroke 22:451, 1991
110. Kassell NF: Aneurysmal rebleeding: a preliminary report from the cooperative aneurysm study. Neurosurgery 13:479, 1983
111. Kassell NF, Peerless SJ, Durward QJ et al: Treatment of ischemic deficits from vasospasm with intravascular volume expansion and induced arterial hypertension. Neurosurgery 11:337, 1982
112. Kassell NF, Torner JC, Jane JA et al: The International Cooperative Study on the Timing of Aneurysm Surgery. 2. Surgical results.
113. Kaste M, Ramsey M: Transexamic acid in subarachnoid hemorrhage, a double-blind study. Stroke 10:519, 1979
114. Kawakami M, Kodama N, Toda N: Suppression of the cerebral vasospastic actions of oxyhemoglobin by ascorbic acid. Neurosurgery 28:33, 1991
115. Kawamura S, Yasui N: Clinical and long-term follow-up study in patients with spontaneous subarachnoid haemorrhage of unknown aetiology. Acta Neurochir (Wien) 106:110, 1990
116. Kindt GW, McGillicuddy J, Pritz M, Giammotta S: Hypertension and hypervolemia as therapy for patients with vasospasm. p. 659. In Cerebral Arterial Spasm. Proceedings of the Second International Workshop. Williams & Wilkins, Baltimore, 1980
117. King RB, Saba MI: Forewarnings of major subarachnoid hemorrhage due to congenital berry aneurysm. NY State J Med 74:638, 1974
118. Kistler JP: Management of subarachnoid hemorrhage from ruptured saccular aneurysm. p. 175. In Ropper AH et al (eds): Neurological and Neurosurgical Intensive Care. University Park Press, Baltimore, 1983
119. Kistler JP, Crowell RM, Davis KR et al: The relation of cerebral vasospasm to the extent and location of subarachnoid blood visualized by CT scan. Neurology (NY) 433:424, 1983
120. Kondziolka D, Bernstein M, Spiegel SM, terBrugge K: Symptomatic arterial luminal narrowing presenting months after subarachnoid hemorrhage and aneurysm clipping. J Neurosurg 69:494, 1988
121. Konishi Y, Maemura E, Sato E et al: A therapy against vasospasm after subarachnoidal haemorrhage: clinical experience of balloon angioplasty. Neurol Res 12:103, 1990
122. Krinsky CM, Merritt HH: Neurological manifestations of subacute bacterial endocarditis. N Engl J Med 218:563, 1938
123. Lennihan L, Petty GW, Mohr JP et al: Transcranial Doppler detection of anterior cerebral artery vasospasm. Stroke 20:151, 1989
124. Liliequist B, Lindqvist M, Probst F: Rupture of intracranial aneurysm during carotid angiography. Neuroradiology 11:185, 1976
125. Lindsay KW, Vermulen M, Murray G et al: Antifibrinolytic therapy in subarachnoid hemorrhage:

reduction of rebleeding without benefit to outcome. p. 9. Handbook of the American Association of Neurological Surgeons Annual Meeting, 1984
126. Linskey ME, Horton JA, Rao GR, Yonas H: Fatal rupture of the intracranial carotid artery during transluminal angioplasty for vasospasm induced by subarachnoid hemorrhage: case report. J Neurosurg 74:985, 1991
127. Locksley HB: Natural history of subarachnoid hemorrhage, intracranial aneurysm and arteriovenous malformation: based on 6368 cases in the cooperative study. (Parts I and II.) p. 37. In Sahs AL, Perret GE, Locksley HB, Nishioka H (eds): Intracranial Aneurysms and Subarachnoid Hemorrhage: A Cooperative Study. JB Lippincott, Philadelphia, 1969
128. Loiseau H, Castel JP, Stoiber HP: Aspects clinique, neuroradiologiques et evolutifs du syndrome d' "hemmoragie meninges benigne idiopathique" Neurochirurgie 35:2228, 1989
129. Martelli N, Colli BO, Assirati, JA, Machado HR: Cerebromeningeal hemorrhage: analysis of autopsies performed over a 10-year period. Arq Neurospiquiatr 46:166, 1988
130. Maspes PE, Marini G: Intracranial arterial spasm related to supraclinoid ruptured aneurysms. Acta Neurochirurg 10:630, 1962
131. Matsumura K, Matsuda M, Handa J, Todo G: Magnetic resonance imaging with aneurysmal subarachnoid hemorrhage: comparison with computed tomography scan. Surg Neurol 34:71, 1990
132. Maurice-Williams RS: Prolonged antifibrinolysis: an effective nonsurgical treatment for ruptured intracranial aneurysm? Br Med J 1:945, 1978
133. Mayberg MR: Warning leaks and subarachnoid hemorrhage. West J Med 153:549, 1990
134. Mayberg MR, Okada T, Bark DH: The significance of morphological changes in cerebral arteries after subarachnoid hemorrhage. J Neurosurg 72:626, 1990
135. McCormick F: Vascular diseases. p. 38. In Rosenberg RN et al (eds): The Clinical Neurosciences. Vol. 3. Churchill Livingston, New York, 1983
136. McCormick WF, Acosta-Rua GJ: The size of intracranial saccular aneurysms: an autopsy study. J Neurosurg 33:422, 1970
137. McCormick WF, Rosenfield DB: Massive brain hemorrhage: a review of 144 cases and an examination of their courses. Stroke 4:946, 1973
138. McCormick WF, Schmalotieg EJ: The relationship of arterial hypertension to intracranial aneurysms. Arch Neurol 34:285, 1977
139. McCussick VA: Heritable disorders of connective tissue. CV Mosby, St. Louis 1972
140. Melville KI, Blum B, Shister HL, Silver MD: Cardiac ischemic changes and arrhythmias induced by hypothalamic stimulation. Am J Cardiol 12:781, 1963
141. Miao FJ, Lee TJ: Effects of bilirubin on cerebral arterial tone in vitro. J Cereb Blood Flow Metab 9:666, 1989
142. Millikan CH: Cerebral vasospasm and ruptured intracranial aneurysm. Arch Neurol 32:433, 1975
143. Mizukami M, Kin H, Araki G et al: Is angiographic spasm real spasm? Acta Neurochirurg 34:247, 1976
144. Mizukami M, Takemae T, Tazawa T et al: Value of computed tomography in the prediction of the cerebral vasospasm after aneurysm rupture. Neurosurgery 7:583, 1980
145. Mohr JP, Caplan LR, Melski JS et al: The Harvard Cooperative Stroke Registry: a prospective registry. Neurology (NY) 28:754, 1978
146. Mohr JP, Kase CS: Cerebral vasospasm. Rev Neurol 139:99, 1983
147. Molinari GF, Smith L, Goldstein MN et al: Pathogenesis of cerebral mycotic aneurysms. Neurology (NY) 23:325, 1973
148. Montgomery EB, Jr, Grubb RL, Raichle ME: Cerebral hemodynamic and metabolism in postoperative cerebral vasospasm and treatment with hypertensive therapy. Ann Neurol 9:502, 1981
149. Morgan WL, Bland EF: Bacterial endocarditis in the antibiotic era. Circulation 19:753, 1959
150. Morley TP, Barr HWK: Giant intracranial aneurysms: diagnosis, course and management. Clin Neurosurg 16:73, 1968
151. Moskowitz MA, Rosenbaum AE, Tyler HR: Angiography monitored resolution of cerebral mycotic aneurysms. Neurology (NY) 24:1103, 1974
152. Nagamine Y, Takahashi S, Sonobe M: Multiple intracranial aneurysms associated with moyamoya disease: case report. J Neurosurg 54:673, 1981
153. Nagasawa S, Handa H, Naruo Y et al: Experimental cerebral vasospasm arterial wall mechanics and connective tissue composition. Stroke 13:595, 1982
154. Neil-Dwyer N, Cruickshank J, Doshi A et al: Systemic effects of subarachnoid hemorrhage. p. 256. In Wilkins RH (ed): Cerebral Arterial Spasm. Williams & Wilkins, Baltimore, 1980
155. Nelson PB, Seif SM, Maroon JC, Robinson AG: Hyponatremia in intracranial disease: perhaps not the syndrome of inappropriate secretion of antidiuretic hormone (SAIDH). J Neurosurg 55:938, 1981
156. New PFJ, Price DL, Carter B: Cerebral angiography in cardiac myxoma. Radiology 96:335, 1970
157. Newell DW, Grady MS, Eskridge JM, Winn HR: Distribution of angiographic vasospasm after subarachnoid hemorrhage: implications for diagnosis by transcranial Doppler ultrasonography. Neurosurgery 27:574, 1990
158. Nibbelink DW, Tormer JC, Henderson WG: Intracranial aneurysms and subarachnoid hemorrhage: a cooperative study—antifibrinolytic therapy in recent onset of subarachnoid hemorrhage. Stroke 6:622, 1975
159. Nicholls ES, Johansen HL: Implications of changing trends in cerebrovascular and ischemic heart disease mortality. Stroke 14:152, 1983
160. Nichols FT 3d, Mawad M, Mohr JP et al: Focal headache during balloon inflation in the internal carotid and middle cerebral arteries. Stroke 21:555, 1990

161. Nornes H, Magnaes B: Intracranial pressure in patients with ruptured saccular aneurysm. J Neurosurg 36:536, 1972
162. Norris JW: Effects of cerebrovascular lesions on the heart. Neurol Clin 1:87, 1983
163. O'Brien JG: Subarachnoid hemorrhage in identical twins. Br Med J 1:607, 1942
164. Ohman J, Servo A, Heiskanen O: Risk factors for cerebral infarction in good grade patients after aneurysmal subarachnoid hemorrhage and surgery: a prospective study. J Neurosurg 74:14, 1991
165. Ohno K, Suzuki R, Masaoka H et al: A review of 102 consecutive patients with intracranial aneurysms in a community hospital in Japan. Acta Neurochir (Wien) 94:23, 1988
166. Ojemann RG: Management of the unruptured intracranial aneurysm. N Engl J Med 304:725, 1981
167. Ojemann RG, Crowell RM: Intracranial aneurysms and subarachnoid hemorrhage: incidence, pathology, clinical features and medical management. p. 128. In: Surgical Management of Cerebrovascular Disease. Williams & Wilkins, Baltimore, 1983
168. Okawara SH: Warning signs prior to rupture of an intracranial aneurysm. J Neurosurg 38:575, 1973
169. Onuma T, Suzuki J: Surgical treatment of giant intracranial aneurysms. J Neurosurg 51:33, 1979
170. Osaka K: Prolonged vasospasm produced by the breakdown products of erythrocytes. J Neurosurg 47:403, 1977
171. Pakarinen S: Incidence, aetiology of primary subarachnoid haemorrhage. Acta Neurol Scand [Suppl] 29:43, 1967
172. Peerless SJ, Yasargil MG: Adrenergic innervation of the cerebral blood vessels in the rabbit. J Neurosurg 35:148, 1971
173. Penmink M, White RP, Cockavell JR: Role of prostaglandin F2 in the genesis of experimental cerebral vasospasm: angiographic study in dogs. J Neurosurg 37:398, 1972
174. Peterson JW, Roussos L, Kwun BD et al: Evidence of the role of hemolysis in experimental cerebral vasospasm. J Neurosurg 72:775, 1990
175. Phillips LH, Whisnant JP, O'Fallon MW, Sundt TM: The unchanging pattern of subarachnoid hemorrhage in a community. Neurology (NY) 30:1034, 1980
176. Pope FM, Nichols AC, Narcisi P et al: Some patients with cerebral aneurysms are deficient in type III collagen. Lancet, 1981
177. Popovic EA, Siu K: Ruptured intracranial aneurysms: a 12-month prospective study. Med J Aust 150:492, 496, 500, 1989
178. Post KD, Flamm ES, Goodgold A, Ransahoff J: Ruptured intracranial aneurysms: Case morbidity and mortality. J Neurosurg 46:290, 1977
179. Pritz MB, Giannotta SL, Kindt GW et al: Treatment of patients with neurological deficits associated with cerebral vasospasm by intravascular volume expansion. Neurosurgery 3:364, 1978
180. Ramirez-Lassepas M: Antifibrinolytic therapy in subarachnoid hemorrhage caused by ruptured intracranial aneurysm. Neurology (NY) 31:316, 1981
181. Ray BS, Wolff HG: Experimental studies on headache, pain sensitive structures of the head and their significance in headache. Arch Surg 41:813, 1940
182. Raynor RB, McMurtry JS, Pool JL: Cerebrovascular effects of topically applied serotonin in the cat. Neurology (NY) 11:190, 1961
183. Reichembach DD, Benedict EP: Catecholamines and cardiomyopathy: the pathogenesis and potential importance of myofibrillar degeneration. Hum Pathol 1:125, 1970
184. Reigh EE, Lemmen LJ: Cerebral aneurysms with other intracranial pathology. J Neurosurg 17:469, 1960
185. Reynolds AF, Shaw C-M: Bleeding patterns from ruptured intracranial aneurysms: an autopsy series of 205 patients. Surg Neurol 15:232, 1981
186. Richardson JT: Cognitive performance following rupture and repair of intracranial aneurysm. Acta Neurol Scand 83:110, 1991
187. Rinkel GJ, Wijdicks EF, Vermeulen M et al: Outcome in perimesencephalic (nonaneurysmal) subarachnoid hemorrhage: a follow-up study in 37 patients. Neurology (NY) 40:1130, 1990
188. Robertson EG: Cerebral lesions due to intracranial aneurysms. Brain 72:150, 1949
189. Robinson JL, Hall CS, Sedzimir CB: Arteriovenous malformations, aneurysms and pregnancy. J Neurosurg 41:63, 1974
190. Robinson RG: Coarctation of the aorta and cerebral aneurysm: report of two cases. J Neurosurg 26:527, 1967
191. Romner B, Ljunggren B, Brandt L, Saveland H: Transcranial Doppler sonography within 12 hours after subarachnoid hemorrhage. J Neurosurg 70:732, 1989
192. Ropper AH, Zervas NT: Outcome one year after subarachnoid hemorrhage from cerebral aneurysm. J Neurosurg 60:909, 1984
193. Rubenstein MK, Cohen NH: Ehlers-Danlos syndrome associated with multiple intracranial aneurysms. Neurology (NY) 14:125, 1964
194. Sahs AL: Preface. p. xvii. In Sahs AL, Nibbelink DW et al (eds): Aneurysmal Subarachnoid Hemorrhage. Report of the Cooperative Study. Urban and Schwarzenberg, Baltimore, 1981
195. Sahs AL, Nibbelink DW, Torner JC: Aneurysmal Subarachnoid Hemorrhage: Report of the Cooperative Study. Urban & Schwarzenberg, Baltimore, 1981
196. Sahs AL, Perret GE, Lockesley HB et al: Intracranial aneurysms and subarachnoid hemorrhage. JB Lippincott, Philadelphia, 1969
197. Saito I, Sano K: Vasospasm following rupture of cerebral aneurysms. Neurol Med Chir (Tokyo) 19:103, 1979
198. Sakoda K, Uozumi T, Oki S et al: A study of the treatment of multiple aneurysms. Hiroshima J Med Sci 38:151, 1989
199. Sano K, Saito I: Timing and indication of surgery for ruptured intracranial aneurysms with

regard to cerebral vasospasm. Acta Neurochir 41:49, 1978
200. Schmid UD, Steiger HJ, Huber P: Accuracy of high-resolution computed tomography in direct diagnosis of cerebral aneurysms. Neuroradiology 29:152, 1987
201. Schmidt M: Intracranial aneurysms. Brain 53:489, 1930
202. Schucart WA, Hussain SK, Cooper PR: epsilon-Aminocaproic acid and recurrent subarachnoid hemorrhage: a clinical trial. J Neurosurg 53:28, 1980
203. Schulz R, Jancar S, Cook DA: Cerebral arteries can generate 5- and 15-hydroxyeicosatetraenoic acid from arachidonic acid. Can J Physiol Pharmacol 68:807, 1990
204. Scott GE, Neubuerger KT, Denst J: Dissecting aneurysm of intracranial arteries. Neurology (NY) 10:22, 1960
205. Seelig JM, Wei EP, Kontos HA, Becker DP: Influence of magnesium ion on cat cerebral pial arterioles in vivo, abstracted. (Presented at the Seventh Joint Meeting on Stroke and Cerebral Circulation, New Orleans, February 1982.) Stroke 13:7, 1982
206. Seifert V, Stolke D, Reale E: Ultrastructural changes of the basilar artery following experimental subarachnoid haemorrhage: a morphological study on the pathogenesis of delayed cerebral vasospasm. Acta Neurochir (Wien) 100:164, 1989
207. Sekhar LN, Heros RC: Origin growth, and rupture of saccular aneurysms: a review. Neurosurgery 8:248, 1981
208. Sekhar LN, Wechsler LR, Yonas H et al: Value of transcranial Doppler examination in the diagnosis of cerebral vasospasm after subarachnoid hemorrhage. Neurosurgery 22:813, 1988
209. Senguptu RP, So SC, Villarego Ortega FJ: Use of epsilon-aminocaproic acid (EACA) in the preoperative management of ruptured intracranial aneurysms. J Neurosurg 44:479, 1976
210. Senter HJ, Sarwar M: Nontraumatic dissecting aneurysm of the vertebral artery: case report. J Neurosurg 56:128, 1982
211. Shepherd RH: Prognosis of spontaneous nontraumatic subarachnoid hemorrhage of unknown cause: a personal series 1958–1980. Lancet i:777, 1984
212. Shnider BI, Cotsonas NJ, Jr: Embolic mycotic aneurysms, a complication of bacterial endocarditis. Am J Med 16:246, 1953
213. Simpson RK, Jr, Fischer DK, Ehni BL: Neurogenic hyperthermia in subarachnoid hemorrhage. South Med J 82:157, 1989
214. Sloan MA, Haley EC, Jr, Kassell NF et al: Sensitivity and specificity of transcranial Doppler ultrasonography in the diagnosis of vasospasm following subarachnoid hemorrhage. Neurology (NY) 39:1514, 1989
215. Soni RC: Aneurysm of the posterior communicating artery and oculomolar paresis. J Neurol Neurosurg Psychiatry 37:475, 1974
216. Sonobe M, Suzuki J: Vasospasmogenic substance produced following subarachnoid haemorrhage, and its fate. Acta Neurochir (Wien) 44:97, 1978
217. Soucy JP, McNamara D, Mohr G et al: Evaluation of vasospasm secondary to subarachnoid hemorrhage with technetium 99m-hexamethylpropyleneamine oxime (HMPAO) tomoscintigraphy. J Nucl Med 31:972, 1990
218. Sparrow MP, Mrwa U, Hofmann H, Ruegg JC: Calmoduline is essential for smooth muscle contraction. FEBS Lett 125:141, 1981
219. Spetzler RF, Owen MP: Extracranial intracranial arterial bypass to a single branch of the middle cerebral artery in the management of a traumatic aneurysm. Neurosurgery 4:334, 1979
220. Spetzler RF, Zabramski JM: Revascularization of anterior and posterior circulation ischemia. Clin Neurosurg 29:575, 1982
221. Stehbens WE: Intracranial arterial aneurysms. Aust Ann Med 3:214, 1954
222. Stehbens WE: Histopathology of cerebral aneurysms. Arch Neurol 8:272, 1963
223. Stehbens WE: Haemodynamic production of lipid deposition, intimal tears, mural dissection, and thrombosis in the blood vessel wall. Proc R Soc Lond (Biol) 185:357, 1974
224. Stehbens WE: The ultrastructure of the anastomosed vein of experimental arteriovenous fistulae in sheep. Am J Pathol 76:363, 1974
225. Stehbens WE: Ultrastructure of aneurysms. Arch Neurol 32:798, 1975
226. Steinke D, Weir B, Disney L: Hydrocephalus following aneurysmal subarachnoid haemorrhage. Neurol Res 9:3, 1987
227. Stornelli SA, French JD: Subarachnoid hemorrhage: factors in prognosis and management. J Neurosurg 21:769, 1964
228. Sundt RM, Whisnant P: Subarachnoid Hemorrhage from intracranial aneurysms. N Engl J Med 299:116, 1978
229. Sundt TM, Jr: Management of ischemic complications after subarachnoid hemorrhage. J Neurosurg 43:418, 1974
230. Suzuki J, Onuma T: Intracranial aneurysms associated with arteriovenous malformations. J Neurosurg 50:742, 1979
231. Suzuki J, Sobata E, Iwabuchi T: Prevention of cerebral ischemic symptoms in cerebral vasospasm with trapidil, an antagonist and selective synthesis inhibitor of thrombaxane $A_2$. Neurosurgery 9, 679, 1981
232. Suzuki J, Yoshimoto T, Onuma T: Early operations for ruptured intracranial aneurysms: study of 31 cases operated on within the first four days of ruptured aneurysm. Neurol Med Chir (Tokyo) 18:82, 1978
233. Suzuki S, Kimura M, Souma M et al: Cerebral microthrombosis in symptomatic cerebral vasospasma quantitative histological study in autopsy cases. Neurol Med Chir (Tokyo) 30:309, 1990
234. Svendgaard NA, Delgado TJ, Brun A: Effect of selective lesions in the hypothalamicpituitary region on the development of cerebral vaso-

spasm following an experimental subarachnoid hemorrhage in the rat. J Cereb Blood Flow Metab 6:650, 1986
235. Sypert GW: Intracranial aneurysm: natural history and surgical management. Compr Ther 4:64, 1978
236. Takemae T, Mizukami M, Kin H et al: Computed tomography of ruptured intracranial aneurysms in acute stage: relationship between vasospasm and high density on CT scan. No To Shinkei 30:861, 1978
237. Tanabe Y, Sakata K, Yamada H et al: Cerebral vasospasm and ultrastructural changes in cerebral arterial wall. J Neurosurg 49:229, 1978
238. Taneda M, Otsuki H, Kumura E, Sakaguchi T: Angiographic demonstration of acute phase of intracranial arterial spasm following aneurysm rupture: case report. J Neurosurg 73:958, 1990
239. Tannenbaum H, Nadjmi M, Gruss P: Therapeutic considerations in the treatment of vasospasm in aneurysms. Acta Neurochir 52:158, 1980
240. Toda N, Kawakami M, Yoshida K: Constrictor action of oxyhemoglobin in monkey and dog basilar arteries in vivo and in vitro. Am J Physiol 260:420, 1991
241. Tomlinson BE: Brain changes in ruptured intracranial aneurysm. J Clin Pathol 12:391, 1959
242. Tsuji T, Weir BK, Cook DA: Time-dependent effects of extraluminally applied oxyhemoglobin and endothelial removal on vasodilator responses in isolated, perfused canine basilar arteries. Pharmacology 38:101, 1989
243. Turbull HM: Intracranial aneurysms. Brain 41:50, 1918
244. Van Rossum J, Wintzen AR, Endtz LJ et al: Effect of tranexamic acid on re-bleeding after subarachnoid hemorrhage: a double-blind controlled clinical trial. Ann Neurol 2:242, 1977
245. von Baumgarten FJ, Burkhard G, Englert D et al: Local hemostasis in subarachnoid hemorrhage. Eur Neurol 27:149, 1987
246. von Essen C: Effects of dopamine on the cerebral blood flow in the dog. Acta Neurol Scand 50:39, 1974
247. Waga S, Fijimato K, Morooka Y: Dissecting aneurysms of the vertebral artery. Surg Neurol 10:237, 1978
248. Waga S, Ohtsubo K, Handa H: Warning signs in intracranial aneurysms. Surg Neurol 3:15, 1975
249. Weir B, Disney L, Grace M, Roberts P: Daily trends in white blood cell count and temperature after subarachnoid hemorrhage from aneurysm. Neurosurg 25:161, 1989
250. Weir B, Grace M, Hansen J, Rothberg C: Time course of vasospasm in man. J Neurosurg 48:173, 1978
251. Wellum GR, Irvine TW, Zervas NT: Cerebral vasoactivity of heme proteins in vitro. J Neurosurg 56:777, 1982
252. White RP, Hagen AA, Morgan H et al: Experimental study of the genesis of vasospasm. Stroke 6:52, 1975
253. Wiebers DO, Whisnant JP, O'Fallen WM: The natural history of unruptured intracranial aneurysms. N Engl J Med 304:696, 1981
254. Wilkins RH: Aneurysm rupture during angiography: does acute vasospasm occur? Surg Neurol 5:299, 1976
255. Wilkins RH: Cerebral vasospasm. Crit Rev Neurobiol 6:51, 1990
256. Wilkins RH, Alexander JA, Odom GL: Intracranial arterial spasm; a clinical analysis. J Neurosurg 29:121, 1968
257. Winn HR, Richardson AE, Jane JA: The long-term prognosis in untreated cerebral aneurysms: 1. The incidence of late hemorrhage in cerebral aneurysm: a 10-year evolution of 364 patients. Ann Neurol 1:358, 1977
258. Wyllie E, Binkley FM, Paluhinska AS: Extrarenal fibromuscular hyperplasia. Am J Surg 112:149, 1966
259. Yonas H, Agamanolis D, Takaoka Y et al: Dissecting intracranial aneurysms. Surg Neurol 8:407, 1977
260. Ziment I: Nervous system complications of bacterial endocarditis. Am J Med 47:593, 1969

# 23
# ARTERIOVENOUS MALFORMATIONS AND OTHER VASCULAR ANOMALIES

J.P. Mohr
S.K. Hilal
Bennett M. Stein

Arteriovenous malformations (AVMs) are the most commonly recognized of the vascular malformations of the brain lesion because of their clinical and therapeutic implications. The other malformations are not easily visualized on an angiogram, and only recently have gained more attention because of the ability of magnetic resonance angiography to show the lesions.

## ARTERIOVENOUS MALFORMATIONS

AVMs are congenital, infrequently traumatic, in origin. They are composed of a coiled mass of arteries and veins partially separated by thin islands of sclerotic tissue, lying in a bed formed by displacement rather than invasion of normal brain tissue.[80] Although congenital, they usually take many years before they become clinically apparent. Some are more active than others, drawing huge collaterals to them, while others seem almost dormant.

### Classification

Many complex, sometimes confusing, schemes of classification for AVMs are in common use. McCormick[77] and McCormick and Schochet[81] have developed a useful and practical system based on pathology (Table 23-1), while Spetzler and Martin[132] proposed a system based on risks of mortality and morbidity associated with operative intervention.

Lesions not often recognized by the clinicians, including cavernous angiomas, telangiectasis, and venous malformations, are more frequent in routine autopsy evaluations, even though it is the AVM that attracts more clinical attention. A category of "cryptic" malformation is included, which is a clinically invisible form of AVM.[78] This type of malformation is thought to give rise to subcortical hemorrhage in young persons, which may destroy the original tangle of blood vessels and prevent its being shown by angiography.[12,21,23,57,74,79] Telangiectasis occur more often in the brain stem, cerebellum, or diencephalon than in the hemisphere or subcortical region.[30,79] Venous

**TABLE 23-1. Age of Onset of Symptoms**

| Year | Author | Ref. | Decade in Life | | | | | | |
|---|---|---|---|---|---|---|---|---|---|
| | | | <10 | <20 | <30 | <40 | <50 | <60 | <70 |
| 1980 | Parkinson | 109 | 4 | 10 | 7 | 15 | 10 | 4 | 2 |
| 1979 | Pertuiset | 116 | 10 | 27 | 43 | 44 | 21 | 15 | 2 |
| 1979 | Nornes | 97 | 4 | 18 | 10 | 9 | 11 | 6 | 5 |
| 1974 | Pia | 118 | 11 | 17 | 18 | 23 | 15 | 10 | 3 |
| 1970 | Moody & Poppen | 88 | 12 | 15 | 27 | 21 | 16 | 12 | 2 |
| 1969 | Perret & Nishioka | 113 | 15 | 56 | 66 | 70 | 48 | 39 | 10 |
| 1965 | Svien & McRae | 139 | 13 | 22 | 26 | 19 | 11 | 4 | |
| 1958 | Dinsdale | | 5 | 8 | 11 | 12 | 8 | 5 | 1 |
| 1956 | Paterson & McKissock | 110 | 11 | 38 | 26 | 23 | 7 | 4 | |
| 1953 | Mackenzie | 72 | 5 | 24 | 6 | 9 | 5 | 1 | |
| 1948 | Olivacrona & Riives | | 4 | 14 | 13 | 6 | 6 | | |

malformations are frequently noted in the cerebral white matter against the ventricular wall,[100] but also occur in the posterior fossa, usually the cerebellum. They have a characteristic angiographic appearance of vessels spreading away from the center like a "caput medusa." Their clinical significance is poorly understood because of the low frequency of clinical reports.[125,154]

Arteriovenous malformations are singled out for special attention by the clinician because of their frequent presentation in a young to middle-age group and the gross effects produced by hemorrhage or recurrent seizure disorder. They usually occur in isolation, unrelated to other disease states, but a few have been associated with the Rendu-Osler-Weber syndrome, and with the Wyburn-Mason syndrome.[155]

AVMs are made up of a tangle of vascular channels, some recognizable as arteries or veins, many merely twisted and convoluted vascular spaces. A characteristic histologic feature is the absence of capillaries (Fig. 23-1).[77,136,137] The arteries leading to and large draining veins draining from the malformation seem normal histologically, blending into the malformation near the fistula. The exact margin of the lesion is not often appreciated by angiography and sometimes cannot be discerned even at operation. AVMs vary in size from tiny, so-called cryptic, malformations[78] to massive anomalies which encompass a number of cerebral lobes (Fig. 23-2). On the convexity, AVMs are most frequently wedge-shaped, with the apex of the wedge directed toward the ventricular system. However, these lesions may assume cylindrical or globoid forms in the white matter (Fig. 23-3). The arterial supply also varies enormously, from the extremes of all major cerebral, brain stem, or cerebellar arterial systems to a single artery to the fistula drained by a single vein. The feeding arteries in the larger malformations are frequently abnormally enlarged and ectatic, reflecting the large loads they carry. Deep arterial feeders often feed the malformation as well. These deep vessels usually arise from branches or main trunks of the major cerebral arteries in the usual lenticulostriate, choroidal, or thalamoperforant arteries (Fig. 23-4), and reach the AVM after passing through healthy tissues. In the scant studies performed on feeding arteries, the muscularis and elastica are attenuated and perhaps nonfunctional, leading to the loss of autoregulation.[93] There is some evidence that the reactivity of the nutrient arteries is abnormal for a considerable distance proximal to the malformation proper.

The venous drainage of AVMs eventually reaches

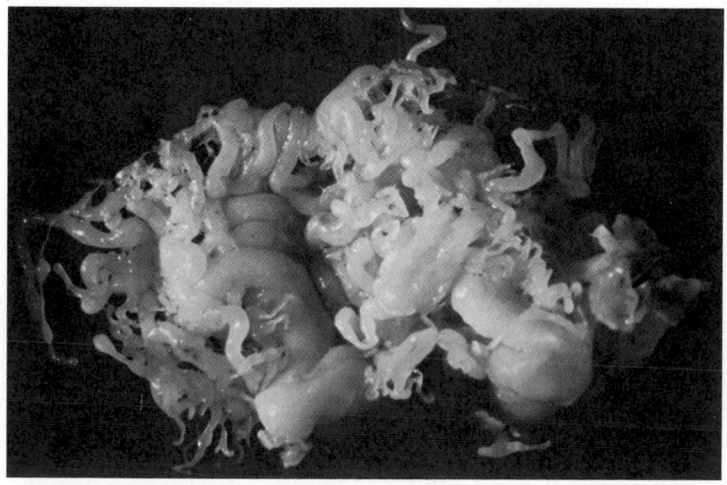

**Fig. 23-1.** Corrosion specimen of an arteriovenous malformation obtained after the injection of acrylate into the malformation and dissolution of the soft tissue by potassium hydroxide. The specimen reveals the three-dimensional anatomy of the malformation and the configuration of the large venous sinusoids.

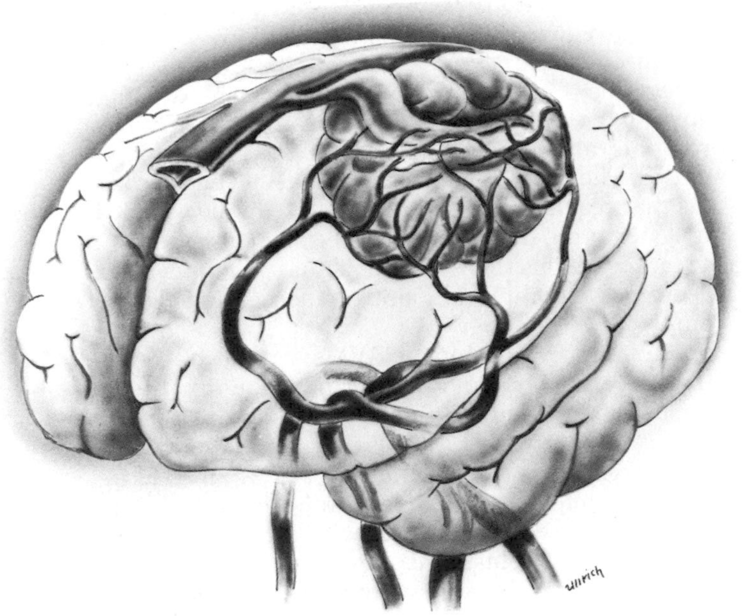

**Fig. 23-2.** Drawing of an arteriovenous malformation located in an eloquent area of the brain and supplied by the three major intracranial vascular systems.

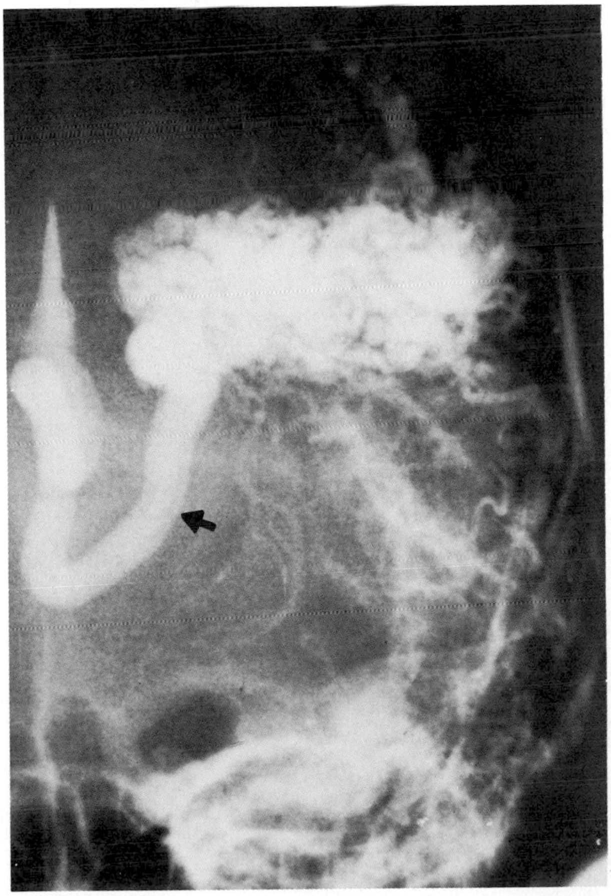

**Fig. 23-3.** Example of a large arteriovenous malformation with a component of deep arterial feeders (*arrows*).

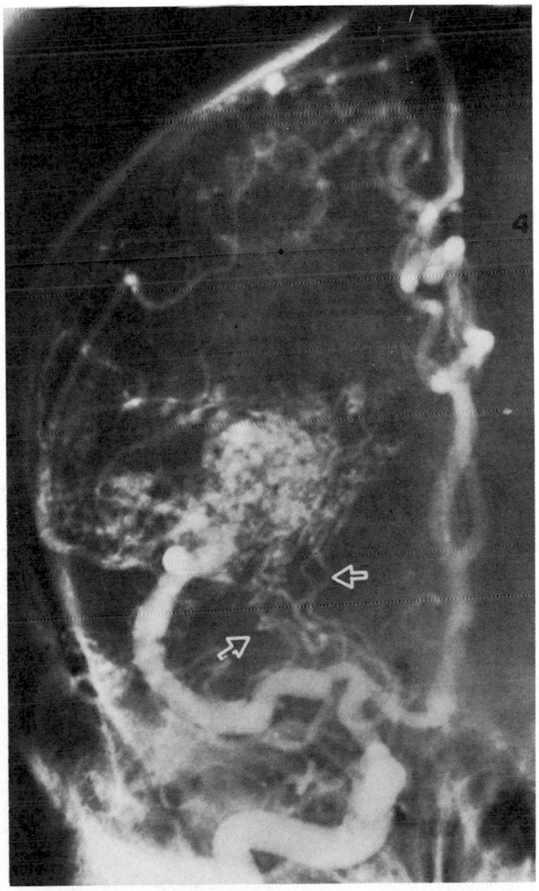

**Fig. 23-4.** Cylindrical-shaped arteriovenous malformation located in the frontal region and extended deep to the ventricle with a large vein draining to the ependyma (*arrow*).

recognizable venous channels, usually appearing as abnormally distended by the large volumes of blood flow through the shunt. The veins follow two basic routes, the most common by superficial drainage coursing over the cortex directly to the major sinuses or collateral venous channels that lead to the major sinuses. The other route is through deep venous channels that reach the ependymal surface of the ventricular system and, in turn, via the deep venous system. In the larger lesions there is often a dual venous network of drainage comprising both superficial and deep veins.

Histologic evaluation of AVMs demonstrates the large cavernous components of the malformation to be mostly devoid of elastica or significant muscularis in the walls (Fig. 23-5).[77,79] Within the malformation, the arteries show endothelial thickening, medial hypertrophy, and occasionally thrombosis; the veins are thin-walled and vary in size, with poorly developed muscular and elastic components. Spontaneous thrombosis may be seen within the confines of the malformation. Some vascular channels show hyalinization of the blood vessel wall with a deposit of collagenous tissue, probably related to spontaneous thrombosis and perhaps recanalization within the confines of the malformation. The exact site of the hemorrhage has never been demonstrated histologically. Where hemorrhage has occurred, hemosiderin-laden macrophages are found. Areas of gliosis surrounding old hemorrhagic cleavage planes and other evidence of previous hemorrhage are frequent findings.

Histologic studies of corrosion preparation of AVMs injected with inert substances after removal of the brain at autopsy have shown that there is virtually no normal cerebral tissue within the confines of an AVM (Figs 23-1 and 23-5). The intense gliosis suggests the neurons captivated within the margins of a malformation are probably nonfunctional. These findings support traditional views that these lesions are congenital and grow with the brain. Presumably, cerebral function, which should be located in the brain occupied by the malformation, is displaced to the margin of the malformation.[19]

## Location

No generally agreed method has been reached for defining the epicenter of an AVM. The huge size of the arterial and venous channels may dwarf whatever fistula can be found and make it absurd to speak of a precise center of the malformation. Yet some fistulas are discrete enough to determine if they are lobar, deep, etc.[4] When a center is said to be found, it is most often frontoparietal but recent work is documenting the occurrence of brain stem and cerebellar AVMs more frequently.[10,129] Careful volumetric studies suggest there is no special predilection for AVMs in any part of the brain. The locations encountered for the AVMs seem simply to reflect the relative volume of the brain represented by a given region. The frontal lobe, occupying 30 percent of the brain volume, is shown to have 30 percent of the AVMs. The posterior fossa, at 12 percent of brain volume, has some 12 to 14 percent of the malformations.[6] Location has not had a bearing on the tendency for hemorrhage, growth, regress, vascular complexity, or size.

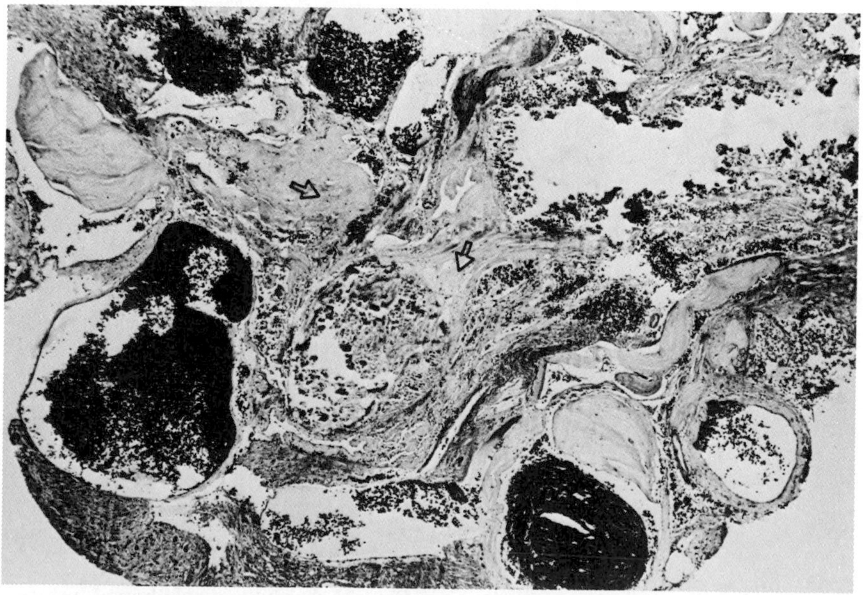

**Fig. 23-5.** Photomicrograph of an arteriovenous malformation at low power demonstrating areas of gliosis (*arrows*) between large thin-walled cavernous sinuses.

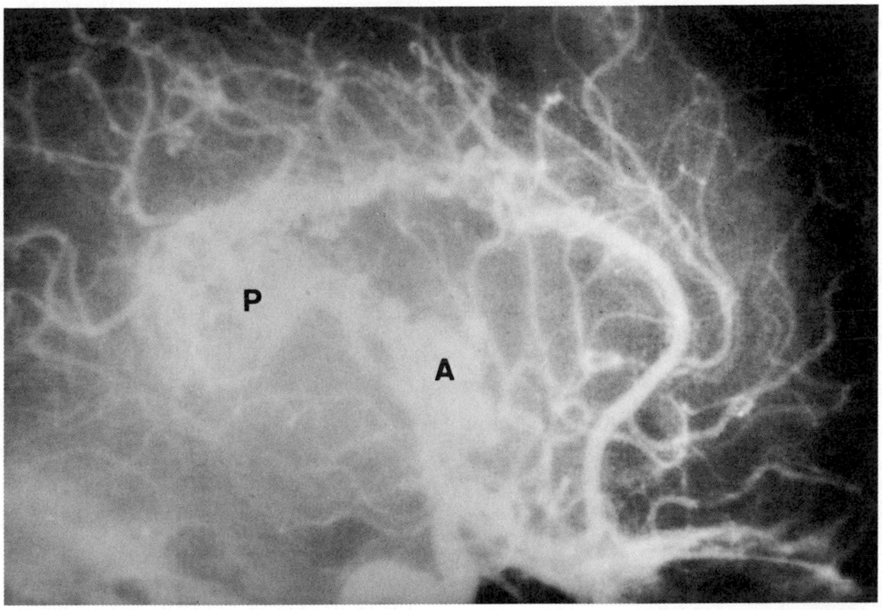


**Fig. 23-6.** Tandem arteriovenous malformations involving the anterior third ventricle (A) and the roof structures of the posterior third ventricle (P). Even though the draining vein is common to these two malformations, they are distinctly separate.

## Number

The vast majority of AVMs are single, but there has been an increasing frequency of cases with multiple AVMs (Fig. 23-6).[126,155] The most recent series, of 203 patients, reported a frequency of 19 (9 percent).[155] When multiple, the lesions are usually small.

## Angiographic Features

AVMs may also be classified by their angiographic appearance. Pertuiset et al.[115,116] devised a scheme of identifying AVMs according to the territories of their nutrient arteries. Luessenhop and Gennarelli[69] used their location and blood supply. The latter categorization relates an AVM to the three major arterial systems (anterior, middle, and posterior cerebral arteries), taking account of a dual or triple arterial supply, and whether the malformation is primarily superficial or deep in the hemisphere. Spetzler and Martin[132] suggested a classification based on a surgical approach. All three systems are useful in determining the operability of these lesions.

For this presentation, we prefer the scheme suggested by Parkinson and Bachers,[109] who described five angiographic patterns: (1) the most frequent (80 percent of cases) is the multiple-unit AVM, where more than one artery feeds a lesion drained by more than one vein; other forms of arteriovenous fistulas are distinctly less common, including (2) an AVM fed by a single artery and draining to a single vein AVM, (3) a straight-line connection between the artery and vein with almost no fistula, (4) AVM with both cerebral and extracerebral arterial supply, and (5) malformations made up predominantly of a venous sinus wall.

### Deep and Superficial Supply (Multiple-Unit Type)

In the type of AVM supplied by both deep and superficial vessels, the fistula is fed by vessels that originate separately from the brain surface or from deeper structures (e.g., in the cerebrum, the basal ganglia or diencephalon; in the posterior fossa, the brain stem). In some cases, the deep feeders are difficult to define angiographically, and may be obscured by the initial flush of contrast material from the surface feeders. The feeding arteries are branches of a major parent cerebral artery, arising in the usual fashion, then progressively changing in size, direction, and tortuosity as they approach the fistula. Usually, the fistula is drained by more than one vein. The venous drainage develops in two major directions, one involving ependymal veins of the ventricle and the other via the deep white matter to the cortex. The larger the AVM, the more numerous the feeders from both the deep and superficial arteries. The more branches of one cerebral artery that feed the fistula, the more likely similar branches from adjoining major cerebral arteries will also feed the fistula. This latter effect depends on the location of the main fistula: the closer to the arterial borderzones, the greater the probability of such feeders.

AVMs of this type usually have a pyramidal shape, that is, on the surface or subsurface, and penetrate deep into the hemispheral white matter. In the largest malformations, most of the hemisphere can be made up of these tortuous vessels, while in midline lesions supply may be drawn from branches of both carotid arteries and the basilar artery.

### Single-Vessel Source (Single-Unit Type)

In the infrequent (3 to 5 percent of cases) type of AVM supplied by one source, a single arterial feeder, arising from a surface vessel or a deep vessel, empties into a fistula drained by a single vein, a so-called straight-line AVM. The fistula may be so small that only the abnormal size of the artery and vein arouse suspicion. In others, the vein is aneurysmal; the best known being the vein of Galen malformation. This group is thought to be more easily approached surgically and may have a lower risk of hemorrhage.

### Cerebral and Extracerebral Arterial Supply

The cerebral and extracerebral AVM, varying in reported incidence from 3 percent to over 20 percent, has become increasingly recognized in recent years. Separate injection of the external carotid artery is required to demonstrate the extracranial feeders, a step not always taken in earlier days. Some feeders arise from muscular branches of the vertebral arteries. While such feeders are more often found in cerebellar or posterior fossa AVMs, the extracerebral and transdural supply to the fistula may be over the cerebrum, especially in those cases arising from trauma.[3]

### Venous Sinus Wall Type

The venous wall type of AVM represents an arterial supply directly to the venous sinus, in which case the arteries are usually extracerebral in origin, and drain directly into the wall of one of the venous sinuses.[5,18,62,148]

## Embryology

Although some lesions are acquired, it has long been accepted that AVMs represent a disorder of embryogenesis. Anomalies of the major extracranial and intracranial vessels are uncommon in patients with AVMs, forcing much of the histologic work to be done on the AVM vessels themselves. AVMs are presumed to result from "incomplete and abnormal resolution of the embryologic vascular network".[107] If this claim is true, some AVMs must represent static anomalies, while others have the potential to grow. What relation these two alternatives have to the risk of bleeding or progressive neurologic deficit is unknown. Some clues as to the significance of the various unusual angiographic findings known clinically as AVMs might be found in the details of vascular embryology as it applies to the cerebral circulation. Yet despite the progress in understanding of the embryogenesis of other vascular systems, remarkably little is known of the details as they apply to the surface and deep vessels of the cerebrum.

The standard studies of embryology, focused on the development of the major extracranial arteries, have largely been limited for intracranial arteries to the formation of the circle of Willis and its immediate branches. Until recent years only passing mention has been made of the growth of the branches of the major cerebral arteries and the vascular systems of the cortex and cerebral white matter. Moffat[86] made reference only to a capillary plexus in the 3.7-mm rat embryo. Mall's[73] eight embryo brains showed little development of the arteries in specimens less than 4 weeks old, but those older showed components of the circle of Willis and all the major vessels over the brain. He noted that all of the brain vessels arose at intervals so regular that they appeared segmental. Klosovskii[56] limited remarks on vascular malformations to a few cryptic statements under the heading "Fundamental Facts," and observed that primitive arteriovenous units began their penetration into the developing cerebrum in the second intrauterine month. The units penetrating the brain were tightly looped with the artery and vein more or less parallel. Tiny buds developed from the sides of the loop like tentacles, fusing with others from adjacent vessels to form the capillary bed. "The arteriovenous loops penetrate into the brain from the surface toward the germinal layer in radial fashion," while these same arteriovenous units were crosslinked, at right angles to the penetrating arteriovenous units, by the developing capillary system. These links created a net of vessels parallel to the plane of the cerebral surface. As development proceeds, the capillary network in the developing gray matter became more elaborate than that in the white matter. The author did not elaborate on what role, if any, these embryogenic principles might play in the development of AVMs.

The well-known work of Padget[107,108] was mainly devoted to the embryology of the major arteries and veins. However, in one publication[108] some reference was made to a possible embryologic basis of AVMs. The author speculated that both the deep and superficial AVMs had the same embryonic derivation, which

> primarily involves abnormal arterial influx into a relatively large vein on the neural tube. . . . Presuming an arteriovenous (AV) fistula between a definitive artery and vein, the sequence of resulting dilatations, namely, veins-to-capillaries-to-arteries, seems clear. The identity, size, and connections of the venous channels present, the subsequent development of veins and the amount of arterial influx may chiefly determine whether the resulting dilated coils are relatively localized or gradually spread to more remote parts.

The process could conceivably be set in motion at any point where the primitive arteries and veins cross one another. It should be possible to use embryologic observations to predict the spectrum of AVMs that could occur.

If this assumption is accepted, two broad categories of AVMs are possible. In one form the abnormality would continue to evolve, drawing to it collateral vessels, ever-enlarging and eventually rupturing. In another, the disorder might be static, conceivably even capable of regressing with time. Although such possibilities are easily envisioned, no useful criteria have as yet emerged to separate AVMs into these two classifications.

Within the last decade, other workers have added new ideas.[8,13,27,121] Bär[8] found the extrastriatal vessels of mouse cortex passed completely through the parenchyma of the telencephalon to the ventricle, and were at first simple channels with no media. With the steady outward growth of the telencephalon, the transcerebral vascular trunks elongate, but remain connected to the ventricle, while later vessels, increasingly appearing more like arteries, arose from the cortical mantle to penetrate roughly the same depth as did the original primitive vessels. However, this depth no longer brought the vessel to the ventricular wall, but left it in the centrum semiovale instead. With each new set of vessels the penetrating became progressively more less into the white matter, and the last of all appeared to arborize entirely within the surface gray matter. Kuban and Gilles[59] observed that some transcerebral vessels, originating in the operculum, curved over the striatal vascular territories to reach the ventricular wall, arguing that the transcerebral and lenticulostriate systems had no real linkage to one another.

To date no classification of AVMs has been developed according to their presumed disordered embryogenesis. This disappointing state of affairs may be preventing our understanding of the overall problem of the AVMs, or our separation of those representing mere static anomalies from those destined to rupture.

## Acquired Arteriovenous Fistulas

Some arteriovenous fistulas,[94] which appear angiographically to be AVMs, arise from trauma and thrombosis of large veins or sinuses. Two major causes have been identified: trauma and venous thrombosis.

### Trauma

Trauma to the brain surface[38] from closed head injury presumably may join or enlarge the existing arteriovenous shunts roughly 90 *u* in size near the superior sagittal sinus, and possibly in other sites. Once linked or enlarged, such fistulas would presumably lose their autoregulation and be subject to the same enlargement typical of any arteriovenous link. Such cases should have a history of or show evidence of prior head injury and be confined to the brain surface. To date, no ready classification for these lesions has been developed.

### Venous Thrombosis

Thrombosis of a large vein or sinus[38,62,140] may create a high enough resistance to normal arterial flow as to force creation of new pathways. The angiogram usually shows delayed filling of the carotid artery or vertebrobasilar artery, and those branches having access to a patent vein or sinus, such as the meningeal and other dural arteries, dilate and convolute in a manner seen in congenital AVMs. These shunts can develop in a fairly short time, possibly months. If sinus thrombosis occurs, a major hemorrhagic lesion may follow.[84] It is still unknown whether the hypertrophied channels become independent of autoregulation or can be expected to subside if the venous obstruction is relieved. Nor is it understood whether they have certain theoretical limits in size and extent or continue to develop until they hemorrhage. Lastly, it is unclear whether their proper treatment is ligation or neglect.

## Physiologic Studies

Physiologic evaluation of vascular malformations has been centered around the study of AVMs.[31,98,100,102,111,130,150,153] Cerebral blood flow (CBF) recordings indicate a varying degree of arteriovenous blood shunting within an AVM. This shunting depends upon the ratio of the feeding arteries to draining veins, the size of the lesion and the number of shunts within the lesion. When shunting is great enough, left ventricular cardiac failure can occur, as has been seen in children with larger AVMs. Intraoperative studies by Nornes and Grip[97] underscore the dynamic changes that occur in blood flow through these malformations during occlusion of the various nutrient arteries and with systemic changes of blood pressure and flow.[43]

Evidence is accumulating that the large feeding arteries lack autoregulation. Tarr et al.[142] found four types of responses in cerebral blood flow to challenge with acetazolamide (Diamox): (1) normal baseline and normal augmentation of CBF, (2) normal baseline and decreased augmentation, (3) low baseline, and (4) low baseline CBF and normal augmentation with acetazolamide. The largest number of patients fell in the fourth group, their data interpreted as showing decreased cerebral blood flow demand but with a normal vascular reserve. None of the patients studied showed abnormalities limited to the brain vascular system remote from the AVM.

Angiographic signs of disordered autoregulation postoperatively include enlargement of an artery proximal to an AVM in the days after the malformation is occluded by either embolization or by surgical

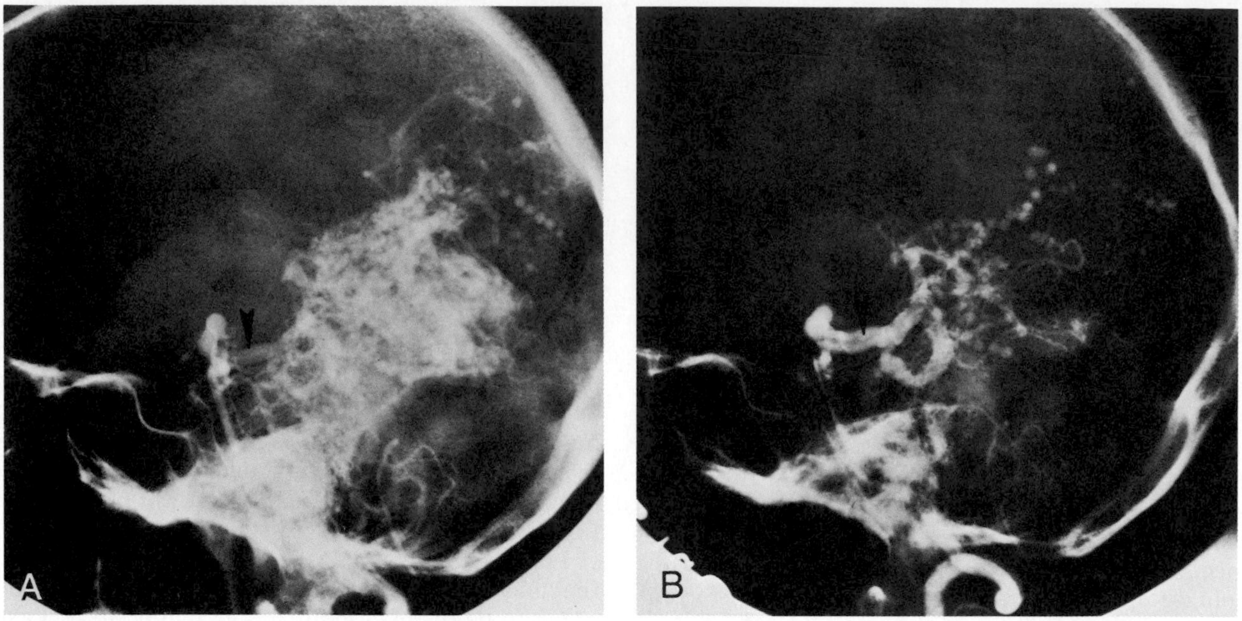


**Fig. 23-7.** (**A**) Large arteriovenous malformation fed by a posterior cerebral artery (*arrowhead*). (**B**) Enlargement of the posterior cerebral artery (*arrowhead*) after successful embolic occlusion of portions of the AVM and feeding artery with marked reduction of flow through the arteriovenous malformation, but with enlargement of the feeding artery.

ligation (Fig. 23-7). This postocclusion ectasia remains for days to weeks (Fig. 23-8). Persistent ectasia leads to decreased flow and stasis in the arterial system proximal to the AVM. Young et al.[158] studied 26 patients by cerebral blood flow before and after total AVM resection. There were no differences in baseline CBF and $CO_2$ reactivity between the AVM and six spinal surgical patients in a control group. CBF increased significantly, but did not show a hemispheric difference, indicating that obliteration of the shunt results in global increase in blood flow.

In the postoperative state, arterial stasis and even

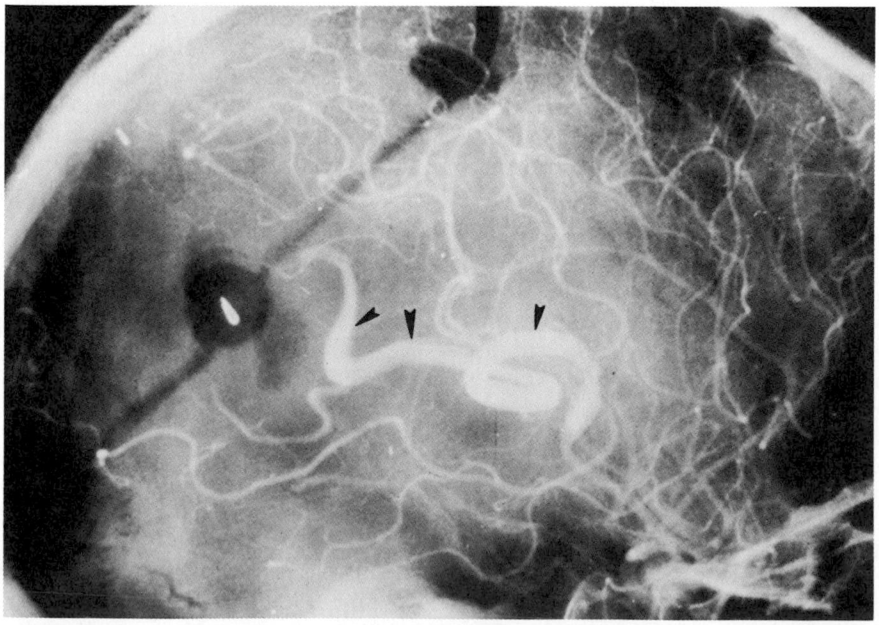

**Fig. 23-8.** Residual ectasia of an artery (*arrowheads*) feeding a malformation after successful obliteration of the malformation. This ectatic state of the feeding artery may remain for many weeks following surgery.

vein thrombosis and venous infarction in the normal brain have been described.[134,136] The pressure in the feeding arteries postoperatively is high initially, and may lead to hemorrhagic complications described by Spetzler et al.[134] as "perfusion pressure breakthrough." The pressure and flow that drives the nutrient blood to an AVM is thought to be redirected to the normal circulation following the obliteration of an AVM. This rerouted blood pressures the local arteries beyond their capacities, resulting in edema, then hemorrhage, in the area. Postoperative stasis, high arterial pressures, and/or hemorrhagic complications have been described by others as well.[10,61,90,92] Muraszko et al.[93] found support for this concept in their in-vitro study of feeding vessels removed at surgery. In 24 patients four nutrient vessels taken from the feeding vessels near the AVM showed no spontaneous activity in the perfusion chamber. The authors found that those with unreactive vessels had more postoperative edema and hemorrhage, suggesting that these vessels were subject to normal perfusion pressure breakthrough. The highest CBF increases in the study by Young et al.[158] were associated with postoperative brain swelling in one patient and fatal intracerebral hemorrhage in another. Both patients had normal $CO_2$ reactivity before excision. Similar experiences were reported by Batjer et al.[10]

## Incidence and Prevalence

In the Cooperative Study of Subarachnoid Hemorrhage,[113,114] still the largest such series to date, symptomatic AVMs were found in 549 to 6,368 cases, representing an incidence of 8.6 percent of subarachnoid hemorrhages. Since subarachnoid hemorrhage accounts for roughly 10 percent of strokes, AVMs make up approximately 1 percent of all strokes. These incidence figures for AVM are reflected in the most recent population-based prospective study of stroke, one carried out in south Alabama. In an eligible population of 100,000 studied over a period of 3 years, 9 AVMs occurred among 494 stroke cases, yielding an incidence of 1.8 percent.[41]

Data on the prevalence of AVMs are more difficult to obtain, but are equally important, especially in efforts to assess the risk for stroke in asymptomatic cases.[53,87] A high ratio of asymptomatic to symptomatic cases might encourage a less aggressive management for such cases, which are being encountered with increasing frequency. Through the use of computed tomography (CT) scanning there has been an increasing awareness of AVMs over the past few decades.[64] The early studies suggested a very low prevalence of AVMs. These figures were upgraded by McCormick,[80] who uncovered 196 AVMs among 4,530 consecutive autopsies, an incidence of 4.3 percent. While not a population-based study, McCormick's data are of special interest, since they represent a careful autopsy-based effort to document the prevalence of AVMs, symptomatic or asymptomatic. Only 24 of McCormick's 196 (12.2 percent) cases had been symptomatic from their AVM. This figure yields a symptomatic stroke incidence of 0.52 percent in this autopsied population, which is in the range of the 1 percent incidence found in purely clinical studies. Among the 24 symptomatic cases, 21 had suffered hemorrhage, 16 massive, while the remainder had epilepsy or "steal" phenomena. The distribution of AVMs in cerebral hemispheres was 118 (60 percent): 28 (14 percent) affected the brain stem, and the spinal cord was the site in 5 (3 percent). These distributions closely approximate those in clinically symptomatic series. Given the patterns of case referral, it is no surprise that the larger series of cases of AVMs come mainly from surgical clinics. The low frequency of the disorder prevents all but a few interested physicians and surgeons from having any but a passing encounter with such cases.

The largest single series is the 549 cases reported by the Cooperative Study,[113,114] itself a pooled effort involving many centers, and among the published series of AVMs uncovered in a literature survey carried back over almost half a century. Scarcely more than a dozen publications describe more than 100 cases per series.[20,33,46,49,104,110,115,139,144,152] The period of time required for each of the major contributors to accumulate such experience has usually been measured in decades. As referring physicians have become more aware that definitive therapy is possible, the database on the patient population for some of the clinical features has changed.

The presumably congenital nature of AVMs might be expected to yield many cases with a family history, but the familial incidence appears quite low.[9,16,26,36,131] Only 7 families had been reported through 1990, involving 15 people in all. The mode of inheritance is uncertain. In contrast to the male preponderance in general for AVMs reported in clinical surgical services, sexes are equally represented in the scanty family history data (Table 23-2). This constant is not easily explained by patterns of referral, and probably is a reliable finding. With increasing awareness of the successes in surgery, efforts at diagnosis have increased in the older population. In large centers, modern efforts at diagnosis have shifted the age of onset upward. Given that assumption, AVM is no longer to be considered a diagnosis mainly involving the young, even though most hemorrhages occur in the younger age group. Dural and extracerebral AVMs are the only types thought to be acquired usually from trauma.

## Natural History and Clinical Presentation

A large number of retrospective studies of AVMs have been accumulated to afford us some insight into the clinical presentation of these lesions; however, no definitive data are available on the natural history of

**TABLE 23-2. Sex**

| Year | Author | Ref. | Male > | Female | Ratio |
|---|---|---|---|---|---|
| 1981 | Guidetti & Delitala | 42 | 89 | 56 | 1.59 |
| 1979 | Pertuiset | 116 | 102 | 60 | 1.70 |
| 1979 | Nornes | 97 | 40 | 23 | 1.74 |
| 1973 | Morello & Borghi | 89 | 88 | 66 | 1.33 |
| 1972 | Forster | 33 | 99 | 51 | 1.94 |
| 1970 | Moody & Poppen | 88 | 65 | 40 | 1.63 |
| 1966 | Cooperative Study | 114 | 236 | 217 | 1.09 |
| 1958 | Tönnis | | 88 | 46 | 1.91 |
| 1956 | Paterson & McKissock | 110 | 63 | 47 | 1.34 |

a large group of AVMs as obtained through prospective studies.[20,33,46,49,104,110,112,115,139,144,152] This situation exists because these lesions are generally rare, and when symptomatic, are treated by the various therapeutic modalities that we now have available. Therefore, comments on the natural history of these disorders are anecdotal and are generally based on patients who are not suitable candidates for any form of treatment. Yet the clinical experience painstakingly accumulated at a few large centers is the only information available.

As the experience has accumulated, the remarkable variation of clinical material from center to center has become apparent, and with it a hesitancy to offer such experience for publication. In any uncommon condition, it is most important to have available data on the natural history of the condition in order to discuss risky and sometimes radical forms of treatment with the patient and relatives. Unfortunately, the rarity of these lesions has precluded any definitive prospective study of the natural history. Furthermore, the clinical picture of many of these lesions spans years if not decades. Therefore, it, has been difficult for any one center to accumulate an unmolested group of patients who have AVMs in various forms and locations and have been followed with arteriography for at least 1 to 2 decades.[52]

Anecdotal retrospective evaluations of a moderate number of patients, however, would indicate that these lesions are congenital, and, like many congenital lesions, do not manifest themselves until the middle decades when they are associated with a high incidence of incapacitating or fatal hemorrhages, perhaps as high as 40 to 50 percent as measured over the normal life expectancy of a young individual. There is another small group of individuals who present with a seizure or hemorrhage in the fifth and sixth decades. These individuals have been asymptomatic up to the event and in this context must be viewed in a different light from the situation of a younger individual. In the older individual who has lived asymptomatically with the malformation for many decades, caution is recommended against risky or radical forms of treatment. The overall risk is naturally diminished by the limitation in life expectancy after 50 years.

Estimates of the risk of first hemorrhage depend on the source of the clinical series. Ondra et al.[104] obtained a mean follow-up time of 23.7 years for 160 of 166 (96 percent) unoperated symptomatic patients and demonstrated a combined rate of mortality and major morbidity of 2.7 percent per year. The rate of rebleeding was 4 percent per year, and of mortality, 1 percent. The rates seemed fairly constant from year to year. Horton et al.[49] estimated a risk of 0.031 per patient years based on the course of 540 patients seen in referral at a major hospital. Crawford et al.[23] reported a 42 percent risk of rehemorrhage in 10.4 years, slightly more frequent among the smaller lesions. In all experienced groups, recurrent hemorrhage within hours to weeks seems quite rare, in contrast to that associated with aneurysms.

On the basis of available information and our own personal experience, young persons are told that they have a 40 to 50 percent risk of some major incapacitating or fatal hemorrhage from an AVM in their projected life span. This projection is made regardless of whether the patient presents with hemorrhage, seizure, migraine, or unrelated symptoms. With the frequent utilization of CT scans these lesions may be discovered quite by accident.

The fate of a treated AVM seems highly dependent on the form of treatment. Once an AVM has been removed as proven by postoperative angiography, recurrent hemorrhage should not occur. Therefore, in discussions with the patient and relatives, the surgical risk should be documented and the fact stressed that, if the lesion can be removed, the patient will be cured. Treatments that fall short of total obliteration of the AVM include embolization,[34] radiotherapy,[55] and partial surgical procedures[50] that have no valid statistical analysis that would document the degree of protection they offer. For embolization, Luessenhop and Presper[71] have stated the generally accepted view that, short of total obliteration of the malformation, embolization provides little protection from recurrent hemorrhage or progressive neurologic deficit. They note that seizures are easier to control following embolization, but this may be a factor of closer scrutiny of the patient rather than a direct effect of the embolization. We have a large series of patients who have only been embolized, but unfortunately a large number of these have not been followed for a sufficiently long period to draw any conclusions. It is our clinical impression that embolization affords some protection and amelioration of symptoms when there is a significant reduction in the AVM. Therefore, in frank discussions with the patient, the detriment of any form of incomplete therapy should be stressed and balanced with the risk of that therapy against the presumed natural risk of the malformation. In good faith, a physician could then recommend a form of incomplete therapy that has minimal risk, even though it might have little or no therapeutic effect for the patient; whereas any form of incomplete obliteration associated with a significant risk should be recommended with great reluctance. The risk of surgery as related to the configuration, location, and size of the malformation is discussed in Chapter 47. Suffice it to say that in our large series of operated AVMs, risk factors are under 2 percent mortality and 5 percent significant morbidity, with 12 percent minor morbidity following total obliteration of the lesion. Radiotherapy is becoming increasingly popular and has been shown to obliterate some of the smaller lesions,[55] but higher doses are required for the larger lesions, raising worries of radiation necrosis[135] and uncertainty of success.

In few studies has the course of the lesions been shown by repeat angiogram. Growth of the AVM has been documented, as has stability and even regression.[82,83,133,136,137] Minakawa et al.[83] repeated the angiogram 5 to 28 years after first discovery or treatment in 20 patients, 16 of whom were untreated, while the remaining were residual. The AVM was unchanged in 8, larger in 4, smaller in 4, and had disappeared in 4. The AVMs that disappeared were relatively small and fed by a single or few feeders. It remains to be seen whether such findings will be reproduced by others, but the possibility of estimation of AVM size by MR should provide opportunity for such studies in the future.

## CLINICAL SYNDROMES OF ARTERIOVENOUS MALFORMATIONS

### Hemorrhage

The vast majority of AVMs that become symptomatic present with hemorrhage.[72,75,89,109,137,145,151] Hemorrhage can be parenchymatous and subarachnoid. Unlike cerebral aneurysms, with which these lesions are often compared, the hemorrhage into the subarachnoid space is generally confined to local subarachnoid spaces and does not spread widely into the large cisterns.

The major clinical presentation is related to a parenchymal hemorrhage with focal neurologic deficits. Approximately half of the clinical presentations of AVMs are intracranial hemorrhage.[48,55,57,87,114] Primarily parenchymatous hemorrhage occurs most often (63 percent of cases), while subarachnoid hemorrhage occurs in 32 percent, and ventricular hemorrhage least often, at 6 percent.[48] Among 106 cases in 1 year at our institution, 40 percent had hemorrhage documented by CT scan at some time in the course of their illness. Although the malformation itself occupies space, it does not frequently present as a mass lesion in the absence of hemorrhage. In cases of stroke due to causes other than AVM, the brain tissue is essentially healthy and normal before its disruption. Stroke from AVMs is different; the lesion is embedded in the brain, surrounded by healthy tissue, and its disordered vessels may draw circulation from healthy brain or provide blood to healthy brain distal to the malformation. The degree of neurologic deficit depends on the location and size of the hemorrhage.

Those lesions located in polar regions of the brain may become apparent in the face of massive hemorrhage with little more than headache and nonfocal symptoms related to the mass effect and rise of intracranial pressure. However, those lesions located in deep structures, such as the diencephalon, basal ganglion, or motor, sensory, and speech areas, may present with devastating neurologic deficits secondary to involvement of these areas. Since the hemorrhages are often subcortical and into the white matter, there is frequently a separation of the fibers without lasting impairment of function. Many of these patients may make remarkable and often complete recovery from the initial hemorrhage, although this may be massive. Unfortunately, there is a group of patients, who have fixed and sometimes catastrophic neurologic deficits following the initial hemorrhage, and these remain for the life of the patient. As noted, the degree of subarachnoid blood varies and depends for the most part on two factors: (1) the extent of the hemorrhage and (2) the relationship of the AVM to large cisterns or to the ventricles. Many of the larger malformations project in a wedge-shaped fashion to the ventricle where the dilated tortuous loops of veins may lie free without ependymal covering. This is a source of hemorrhage in such malformations and may lead to massive amounts of intraventricular blood with acute hydrocephalus and spread of the blood throughout the cerebrospinal fluid (CSF).

Settings for the rupture may include the familiar exertional states commonly encountered with other causes of hemorrhage. However, a few authors have found no correlation with activity,[110] a point against advising asymptomatic patients to live a completely sedentary life. Pregnancy was once cautioned, but the bleeding rates of 0.031 per patient year during pregnancy compare favorably with the 0.031 risk for patient year for nonpregnant females,[49] indicating that pregnancy is not a greater risk for those without prior hemorrhage. It was thought that pregnancy, especially during the first trimester, held a greater risk of AVM hemorrhage, and some observers suggested cesarean section as a prudent measure to avoid complications during delivery.[49,54] There appears to be no greater risk to the mother during the various phases of pregnancy, and there seems to be no justification for abortion.

There has been a long-standing impression that the smaller AVMs appear to be more prone to hemorrhage than do the very large lesions.[23,24,33,34,46] In Morello and Borghi's series,[89] rupture had occurred in 86 percent of the small AVMs, in 75 percent of those of medium size, but in only 46 percent of the giant AVMs. These findings are consistent with those in other series, and suggest that the larger the lesion, the longer it has been present, and the less likely it is to rupture. At least 10 percent of AVMs at surgery show evidence of prior bleeding, more often encountered in the smaller AVMs.[42,89] This high prevalence of prior hemorrhage clearly indicates that many are small enough to escape clinical detection. In some cases, the hemorrhagic onset of symptoms related to these lesions is not recognized by the patient or the treating physician. It may be passed off as a migraine type of headache, severe tension headache, or when accompanied by a seizure, obscured. In a large series of AVMs that have been operated on, we have found approximately 15 percent with asymptomatic hemorrhages, identified by cystic encephalomalacia with pigmentation surrounding the site of hemorrhage and a review of the clinical history, which bears no indication of previous hemorrhage. Neither have these hemorrhages been documented by CT scan or lumbar puncture. This significant incidence of clinically silent hemorrhage raises a question about the authenticity of statements that indicate that AVMs are only dangerous if they have had previous hemorrhage.

Multiple hemorrhages associated with AVMs that have not been treated are common.[42] However, the time interval between these hemorrhages may span years or even decades. The course of recidivous hemorrhages is unpredictable. Experience dictates that the hemorrhages do not recur in the short time frame usually associated with the rupture of a cerebral aneurysm. Therefore, the evaluation of these patients may be carried out at a measured pace, and there is rarely the necessity for emergency operation on an AVM to protect against recurrent hemorrhage. Nevertheless, patients frequently inquire of the urgency of the treatment. No ready answer is available, but we say to the patients that these are congenital lesions, that they have existed for a number of years before the time of the hemorrhage, and practical experience would indicate that they are unlikely to rerupture in a relatively brief time frame. Therefore, the workup need not be completely predicated on the fear of recurrent hemorrhage. Because the hemorrhage from an AVM differs markedly from that of aneurysm and hypertension, it has long been believed they should be easily differentiated from one another clinically. While AVMs are buried in the brain, they are usually in continuity with the ventricle or cerebral surface. Thus, they can produce parenchymatous as well as subarachnoid and/or intraventricular hemorrhage. Since they are arteriovenous, the hemorrhage is less violent than from aneurysm, and evolves over a period of time longer than the usual few seconds characteristic of aneurysmal rupture. Since the hemorrhage arises in a malformation, it has a less disruptive impact on cerebral function than does the "hypertensive" hemorrhage. Vasospasm, that discouraging accompaniment of ruptured aneurysms, is less prevalent, since the subarachnoid hemorrhage of an AVM is located away from the base of the brain and is accompanied by a smaller volume of blood injected into the subarachnoid space.[7]

In our own experience, three distinct forms of hemorrhage are encountered: (1) The AVM bleeds mainly into the ventricular system, producing hydrocephalus rather than of parenchymatous damage (Fig. 23-9). About 10 percent of patients have this picture. An unrelenting course over minutes from the onset of headache to stupor is the typical presenting picture. (2) The hemorrhage affects the subarachnoid space in a fashion similar to ruptured aneurysm, potentially including severe vasospasm (Fig. 23-10). About 10 percent of patients have this presentation, some on several occasions. (3) A deficit due to a parenchymatous hemorrhage occurs followed by a satisfactory remis-

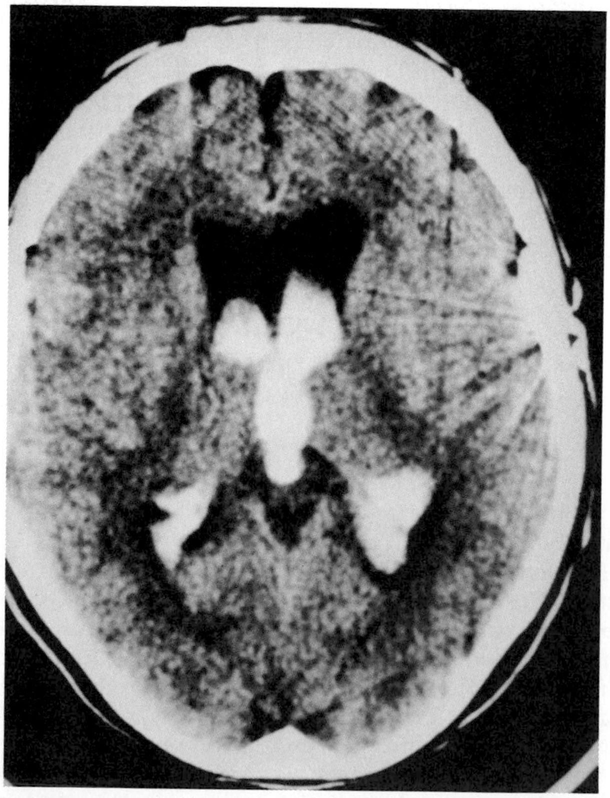

**Fig. 23-9.** Massive intraventricular hemorrhage observed on computed tomography scan following the rupture of a dural posterior fossa arteriovenous malformation.

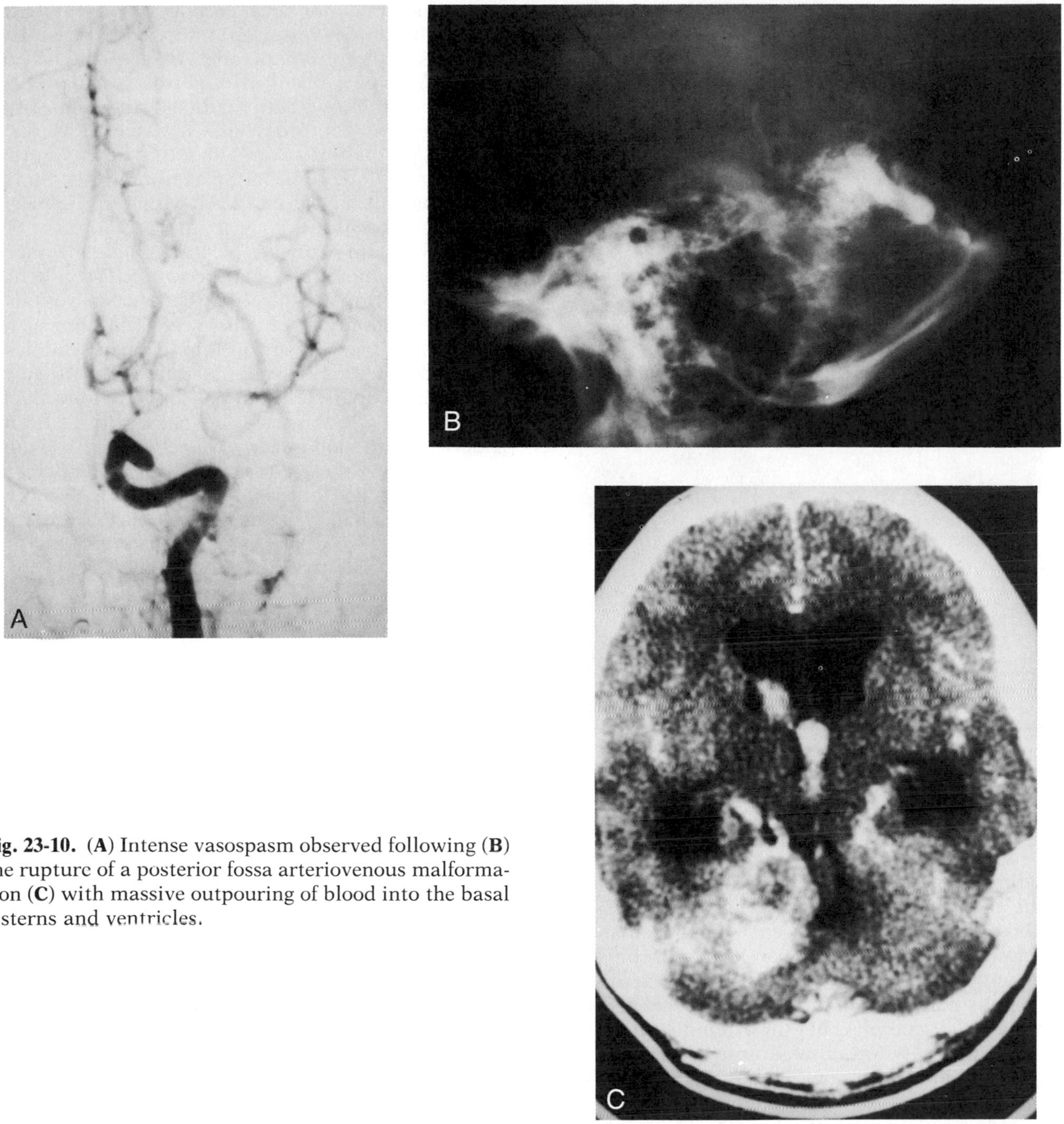


**Fig. 23-10.** (**A**) Intense vasospasm observed following (**B**) the rupture of a posterior fossa arteriovenous malformation (**C**) with massive outpouring of blood into the basal cisterns and ventricles.

sion (Fig. 23-11). This condition is decidedly uncommon save in the cases of lobar hemorrhage whose diagnosis as hemorrhage is increasingly documented by CT scan, after which they are not left alone to pursue their natural course. Little information can be found in the literature to corroborate these syndromes. However, a few cases are described well enough to create a characteristic clinical picture of AVM rupture. Mackenzie[72] stated that "in most cases there has been nothing remarkable about the history, the incident being simply one of sudden onset of severe headache, accompanied by neck stiffness, vomiting, and perhaps pyrexia." Deep hematomas in the basal ganglia[35] have been described with the same smooth onset, hemiparesis, sensory disturbance, ocular motility disorders, and language and mental defects that are encountered in hypertensive hemorrhage.[47] Three such cases in the series of Wilson and colleagues[156] were diagnosed only by surgical exploration, a finding that resurrects McCormick and Nofzinger's[78] long-

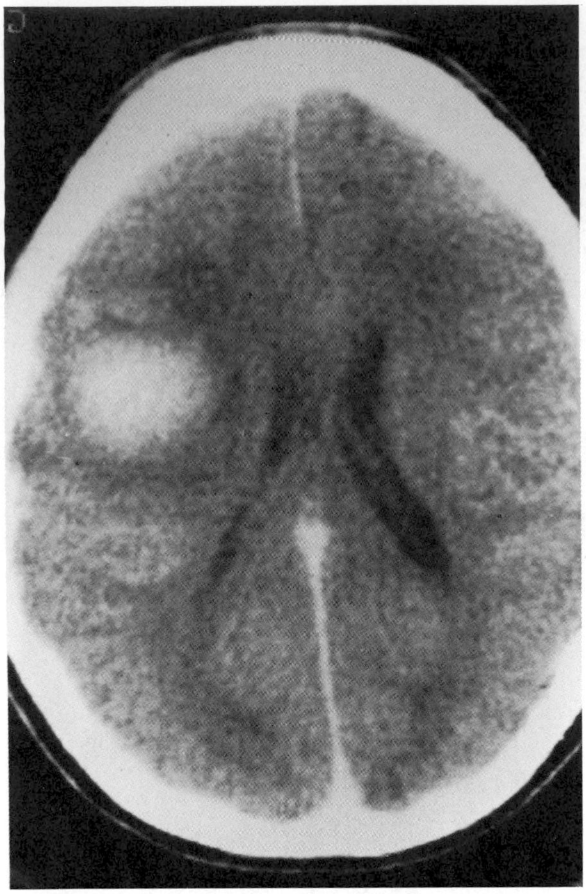

**Fig. 23-11.** Computed tomography scan demonstrating parenchymatous hemorrhage following the rupture of a previously unsuspected arteriovenous malformation.

standing contention that cryptic AVMs are more frequent than has been supposed. Data showing that AVMs cause as few as 10 percent[47] of parenchymatous hematomas may give some comfort to the physician faced with an etiologic diagnosis. Frequencies as high as 35 to 44 percent[114] in other series should promptly eliminate any complacency in attempts to make an etiologic diagnosis on clinical grounds alone. In the series of Pia et al.,[118] among 16 cases with hematomas of 100 to 250 $cm^3$ in size, only 1 died, and 14 fully regained complete capacity. Four had slight to moderate hemiparesis, while two were asymptomatic.

A few other reports have detailed cases who made remarkable functional improvements despite hemorrhage and extensive surgery. Garrido and Stein[35] described a 29-year-old man who had an extensive AVM fed by the lenticulostriate arteries. He developed a hemorrhage with left hemiparesis, hemianopia, and memory impairment. Following removal of this deep-seated lesion, he eventually improved enough to return to work. Other similar cases[50] have been described in which deep hemorrhages and the causative AVM have been removed with good results. However, the outlook may not be so encouraging for all hematoma syndromes: Pertuiset et al.[116] found that 19 of his cases with aphasia preoperatively made no postoperative improvement. It might be speculated that AVMs should have a better outlook, since some of the bleeding occurs into devitalized tissue. However, it may be premature to consider that such improvements are unique to hematomas from AVMs. Similar improvements have been shown with deep "hypertensive" hematomas if the size is small, as noted by Hier et al.[47] Ruff and Arbit[124] reported a single instance of acute minor motor aphasia precipitated by a hemorrhage from an AVM affecting the inferior frontal region of the dominant hemisphere. The clinical features and time course for improvement mimicked those documented in cases of infarction. As yet no study has compared the outlook for hematomas of the same size from AVMs and other causes. In the limited experience with lobar hemorrhage[53] and with caudate hemorrhage,[138] those due to AVM had features identical to those attributed to other causes. However, should AVMs have a better clinical outlook, more effort might be appropriate to deal aggressively with such hematomas than is routinely the case in many institutions.

Once hemorrhage has occurred, the risk of rehemorrhage is known to increase, but the extent and the timing are uncertain: in 81 cases of rehemorrhage in the Cooperative Study,[114] 13 were third hemorrhages and 4 were fourth. In a separate study, Krayenbühl and Yasargil[58] found 12 of 53 recurrent hemorrhages had occurred more than once. Graf et al.[39] reviewed the records of 191 patients with AVMs; however, the mean period of follow-up was a relatively short 2- to 5-year period. Nevertheless, there was a high rate of initial hemorrhage in the 11- to 35-year-old age group, and the rate of rebleeding was about 2 percent per year. Smaller lesions were more prone to hemorrhage, and approximately 13 percent of the patients died as a result of the hemorrhage. It is a generally accepted anecdote that approximately 15 percent of operated AVMs show evidence of prior but asymptomatic hemorrhage.[57]

## Vasospasm

The rarity of vasospasm, symptomatic or merely as an angiographic finding, has been a source of special commentary.[7,45,63] Although it is generally said that AVMs are associated with a smaller incidence of cerebral vasospasm than cerebral aneurysms, this statement may be based on artifact. The reasons are that these lesions hemorrhage with less frequency into the large basal cisterns than aneurysms, they are less frequent than cerebral aneurysms, and they may be evaluated in the acute stage by arteriography, whereas spasm is generally seen on follow-up arteriography done a few days after the subarachnoid hemorrhage to evaluate the progress of a cerebral aneurysm or its readiness for surgery. Such is not commonly the course of action taken with an AVM once it is identified. Anecdotal cases certainly have been observed where delayed cerebral vasospasm has been intense following the rupture of an AVM, and this spasm may go on to produce death or severe neurologic abnormalities (see Fig. 23-10).[7] It is our impression that cerebral vasospasm, when the quantity of blood is sufficient within the entire subarachnoid space, is probably of the same incidence following rupture of a cerebral AVM as in a comparable situation with cerebral aneurysm, but most AVMs do not rupture in ways that bring large amounts of blood into the basal cisterns. If present, vasospasm should be treated vigorously by whatever techniques are currently popular.

## Aneurysms and Arteriovenous Malformations

In approximately 10 percent of the cases, AVMs are associated with cerebral aneurysms.[45,85,105] It is important to recognize this possibility and to perform a complete angiography on all of these patients (Fig. 23-12). The question then arises as to which lesion has created the hemorrhage. It used to be thought that it was usually the AVM, but current experience would indicate the cerebral aneurysm. From an anatomic standpoint, the aneurysms are usually located on the feeding arteries proximal to an AVM and are often thin-walled and tenuous, not only at the dome, but also the neck. They apparently arise from abnormalities in the artery wall associated with the high flow and pressure related to the nourishment of an AVM. Rarely, the aneurysms are located on an arterial network distant and unrelated to the AVM. CT or magnetic resonance (MR) scanning, when the site of the hemorrhage is visible, will indicate which lesion has bled. Otherwise, it is pure speculation.

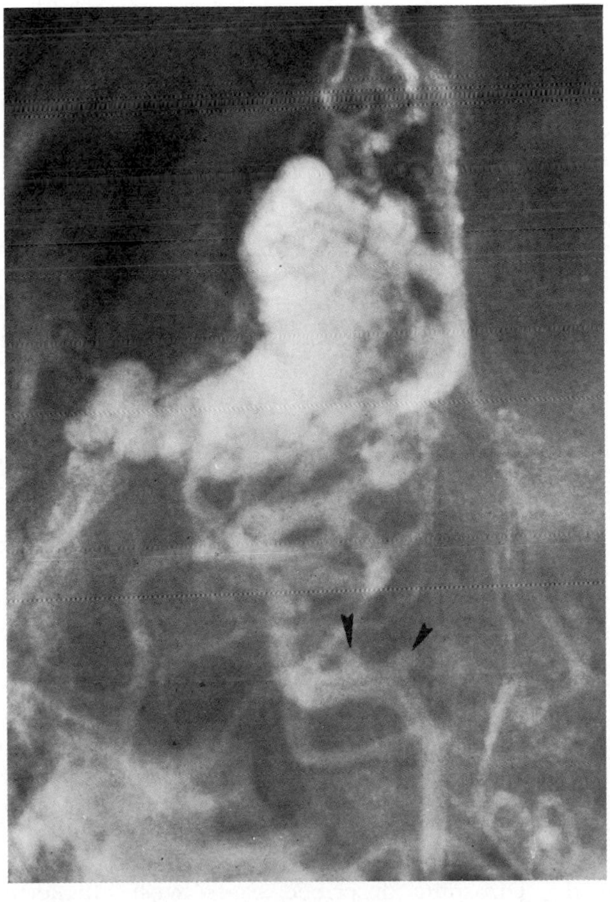

**Fig. 23-12.** Arteriovenous malformation associated with proximal aneurysms (*arrowheads*).

Sometimes the aneurysms are multiple. Which lesion to be operated on first is discussed in Chapter 47. Clinically, hemorrhage from cavernous and venous malformations is not as frequent as are hemorrhages from AVMs.[37,100,123,125,149] However, as these heretofore obscure conditions are recognized with increasing frequency by CT scans, it is realized that they can be the source of parenchymal and ventricular hemorrhage. Hemorrhages from telangiectasia are rarely recognized by the clinician, although some of these cases may fall under the category of hemorrhage from "cryptic malformations."[79] Contrariwise, pathologists have recognized a high incidence of microscopic hemorrhages associated with cavernous, venous, and telangiectatic malformations.

## Seizures

Seizures have attracted special attention because they may alert the physician to an AVM before rupture.[29,106,116,151,153] Some form of seizure disorder affected 32 percent of the cases of AVMs in our own series. In a study of 35 patients with AVM imaged by MR, the epileptogenic AVM seems more superficial in the cortex, had bled before, and was somewhat larger than does not non-epileptogenic.[146] The available literature documents a remarkable variation in incidence (Table 23-3). As a presenting feature of AVM, the incidence varies from 28 percent (Cooperative Study) to 67 percent.[114] Reports vary over too wide a range to be able to consider that the severity,[66] ease of control with medication, or prognosis for hemorrhage is fully understood. The frequency of seizures correlates so poorly with AVM location that at present no specific relationships can be claimed. None was found among our material.

The type of seizure is often unreported. In our experience, several types of attacks have been labeled as seizures by referring physicians. Among these are typical focal epilepsy not associated with loss of consciousness. Others have been of the Jacksonian type, with or without the loss of consciousness. Finally, several patients have experienced only a sudden loss of function, without tonic-clonic activity and without headache or loss of consciousness. Whether this latter

**TABLE 23-3. Seizures**

| Year | Author | Ref. | No. of Cases | Seizures as First sign of AVM in % Cases | | | | |
|---|---|---|---|---|---|---|---|---|
| | | | | Total(%) | Alone(%) | + Hemorrhage(%) | Generalized(%) | Focal(%) |
| 1981 | Stein | 136, 137 | 121 | 43.8 | 36.3 | 7.4 | | |
| 1980 | Parkinson | 109 | 100 | 67 | | | | |
| 1979 | Pertuiset | 16 | 162 | 37.6 | 25.3 | 12.3 | 41 | 59 |
| 1973 | Morello | 89 | 154 | 35.0 | 20.1 | 14.9 | | |
| 1969 | Troupp | 144 | 138 | 26 | | | | |
| 1966 | Cooperative | 114 | 406 | 28 | | | | |
| 1956 | Paterson | 109 | 110 | 46.4 | | | | |
| 1970 | Moody | 88 | 105 | 50.5 | 40 | 10.5 | 55 | 45 |
| 1967 | Tonnis | | 215 | 48.3 | | | | |
| 1958 | Krayenbuhl | 58 | 608 | 41.2 | | | | |

group represents epilepsy per se is difficult to determine. Where attacks have been described, focal spells predominate, varying from 45 to 59 percent.[114] In the Cooperative Study,[114] 102 cases had seizures, 45 percent of which were focal, 42 percent generalized, 8 percent psychomotor, and 7 percent unspecified. Ozer et al.[106] were unable to distinguish focal seizures from AVM from those of other etiology in their 14 cases of seizure among 65 AVMs. Earlier, Olivecrona and Ladenheim[103] were of the opinion that there was more variation in type and frequency of attacks in AVM seizures than in cryptogenic or traumatic epilepsy. Mackenzie[72] made three special observations: in all but one of 16 cases the attacks displayed focal features at some time or other; focal seizures had a wide periodicity up to 20 years; and when initially generalized, no remission for longer than 3 years was observed.

A small but separate literature applies to the occipital AVMs. Troost and Newton[143] reported 5 of 26 cases of occipital AVM with focal seizures. The aura varied widely, including "sudden dimming of everything in the right side of vision," "swirling spots of brightly colored lights," "dimming of vision," "red spots," and "frosted glass." Several were followed by generalized seizure. The subject is of interest because some of these attacks mimic the aura often encountered in migraine syndromes. Our experience includes six cases whose seizures have had unusual manifestations. In these cases, in addition to the more common grand mal and focal motor epilepsy, dystonic posturing of a limb (usually the arm) has occurred in brief episodes, affecting the limb(s) at other times by more conventional tonic-clonic epileptiform activity. In another three, the episodes took the form of sudden weakness, lasting between 30 seconds and many minutes. Whether these attacks represent ischemia (see below) or are examples of epilepsy is difficult to determine.

## Seizures and Hemorrhage

The incidence of seizures alone compared to seizures in association with hemorrhage varies from 36.3 to 7.4 percent, 25.3 to 12.3 percent, 20.1 to 14.9 percent, and 40.1 to 10.5 percent as is shown in Table 23-3. In the few reports that bear on the subject, the correlation is frequent in the AVMs involving the surface of the brain, especially centroparietal,[35,38,114] but is unusual for deep AVMs. Hemorrhage occurred within 1 year in only 15 percent of 90 cases of seizure in the Cooperative Study. Whether the character of the seizure differs when associated with hematoma is not certain.

## Headaches

AVMs are unusual forms of stroke in that they have been associated with premonitory symptoms and signs, the most common of which is headache. Because headache is such a common complaint in the population at large, it has proved difficult to determine if the headache associated with AVMs is unique to the condition.[2,24,28] The two most common claims for association are with migraine and with unilateral headache. Headache was a presenting complaint in roughly 10 percent of our patients.

Headaches having migrainous features are common among AVM patients. Mackenzie[72] emphasized the tendency of the headaches to occur before the aura and for the aura to persist beyond the few minutes that typifies migraine, a finding not confirmed by others. One of the earliest reported cases have atypical migraine. The patient reported by Hyland and Douglas[51] in 1930 experienced attacks over a period of 4 years. The attacks followed exertion, each commencing with numbness starting in the hands and spreading up the arms to the chest and neck. Then consciousness would be lost about 10 minutes after the onset. When she regained consciousness, she felt weak and drowsy.

Headaches identical to migraine also occur, sometimes in the same patients who experience atypical migraine in other attacks.[51,67,106] Similar experiences were documented in the early literature. Enoksson and Bynke[28] described a case with "luminous crosses replaced by curved flashing lights with convexity upward." Dimsdale described cases with "flickering lights."[25] Similarly, Lees[67] described cases with "flashing lights" and "flashes with black spots."

These and our own experiences force us to disagree with the opinion of Troost and Newton[143] that AVM headaches are unassociated with angular, scintillating figures typical of migraine. The association may well be purely coincidental. Paterson and McKissock[110] reviewed a series of AVMs with headache and suggested that the occurrence of migraine in AVMs was simply the incidence of the disorder in the normal population, and classic migraine in 2 percent, figures which approximate those with AVM. Some of the more recent authors have not been able to show any correlation with headache and AVMs.[42,67]

That recurrent unilateral headache should arouse suspicion of an ipsilateral AVM is an old concept. The notion of an ipsilateral feature to the AVM headache may have started with Northfield[98] whose 1940 report stated that the headache "may affect only one side of the head, usually the side on which the angioma is situated." There is very little evidence to support this claim. Based on their experience with 100 cases, Parkinson and Bachers[109] found no evidence that the incidence of headache has a specific relation to location of the AVM. Mackenzie[72] described 12 cases that were persistently unilateral, but other focal neurologic signs were present as well. Likewise, Lees[67] had only three cases whose headache was ipsilateral to the AVM among the 11 headache cases in his series of 70 AVMs. None of them had alternating headaches typical of migraine. Unilateral headache as a sign of AVM has not been borne out by our experience.

The disappearance of the migraine headaches postoperatively is not unusual, and may occur following any type of operation. Disappearance of migraine after operation was a common feature of the early literature, which was made up mostly of single case reports. The question is now raised as to whether all patients with migraine should be evaluated for an AVM. At the very least, CT scan with large bolus contrast should be carried out in these individuals. If anything suspicious is noted, then magnetic resonance scan should be performed.

## Arteriovenous Malformation as a Mass Lesion

Although AVMs occupy space they do not act as tumors and their bulk effect creating pressure on the brain is only recognized in terms of massive, distended draining veins. This phenomenon is most commonly noted in those malformations that occupy a site adjacent to the aqueduct of Sylvius. In such instances, the distended veins may block the aqueduct leading to hydrocephalus. In other instances, there is indirect evidence of a mass effect through the development of a raised intracranial pressure perhaps similar to that seen with otitic hydrocephalus, where the venous system is obstructed or carrying a higher pressure than it normally accommodates. Although rare, cases have been reported in which papilledema and raised intracranial pressures are a prominent part of the syndrome. Interestingly, this problem does not rapidly regress following the removal of the shunt. Nevertheless, there is a gradual resolution of the increased intracranial pressure and remission of the papilledema so that removal of the AVM to correct this dangerous state should be strongly considered.

Rarely, a large AVM may be placed close enough to the brain that symptoms arise from displacement of healthy tissue or hemorrhage into it. We saw a 44-year-old printer with progressive dystonia and myoclonus whose midbrain was rotated and compressed by the large size of the feeding artery; there had been no hemorrhage (Fig. 23-13). Nishino et al.[95] described a 64-year-old man with hemorrhage whose angiogram and MR showed part of the drainage from the AVM was a "varix" embedded in the pons. They found another 26 cases in the literature.

## Syndromes of Ischemia: Steal Syndromes

Clinical information on the subject of steal syndromes is still in the anecdotal stage. In suspect cases, it is presumed that the blood shunting through the fistula results in relative underperfusion of the adjacent brain, leading to focal or generalized symptoms. It is beyond doubt that shunting occurs. It has been amply documented by cerebral blood flow,[14] by radionuclide brain scanning,[31] by the preferential path of Silastic ball emboli,[136] and by the improved posttreatment perfusion of contrast to branches poorly filled.[137]

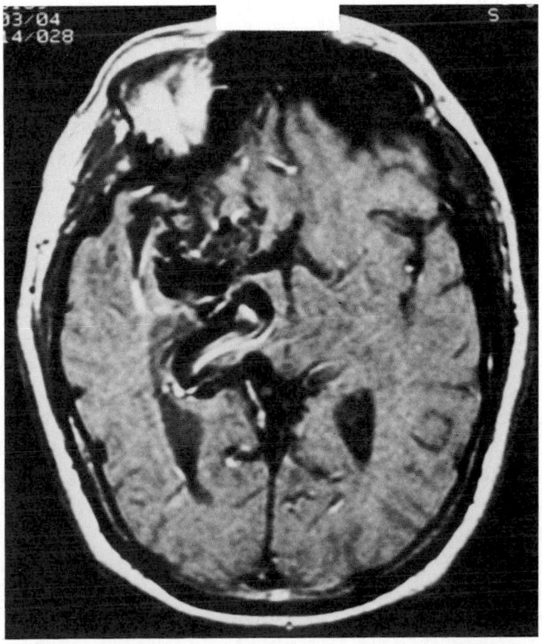


**Fig. 23-13.** Axial magnetic resonance imaging showing the large feeding artery and draining vein from an arteriovenous malformation acting as a mass and displacing the midbrain.

It is also apparent that the neuropathologic study of cases of AVM reveals many foci of infarction, suggesting that the shunting may lead to ischemic necrosis of tissue. Our own experience with "cerebral steal" approximates the findings reported in the literature. Roughly 6 percent have some focal deficits of gradual onset. In most, the neurologic deficit is limited to the region of the brain served by the AVM, and no instance occurred with neurologic deficits attributed to sites far distant to that of the AVM. In all cases, the AVM has been fed by both deep and superficial vessels and was quite large. The syndromes evolved over periods as short as 3 years or as long as 10 years. During this time the worsening occurred without notable sudden drops in function or obvious instances of hemorrhage. Some degree of hemiatrophy was present on examination in all cases; except for one patient, who also had a visual field disturbance with a large parietal AVM, the main complaints were motor. Sensory disturbance accompanied the motor in three instances, but language, memory, praxis, and other functions were normal.

In a report detailing large numbers, Paterson and McKissock[110] encountered eight patients among 110 AVMs with insidious deficits. The remaining literature represents isolated case reports. In a description of seven cases of large, deep AVMs, Leussenhop and Mujica[70] described one patient who had developed a slowly progressing hemiparesis 4 years before her first subarachnoid hemorrhage. A spastic left hemiplegia with no voluntary movements of the hand or ankle, hemihypesthesia, and hemianopia were prominent clinical findings. Two sessions of multiple embolization separated by an interval of approximately 2 weeks were necessary to obstruct the supply to the deep AVM from deep penetrating branches of the circle of Willis arising from anterior, middle, and posterior cerebral arteries. At first, no changes occurred. But by 3 weeks, she "could walk with a foreleg brace, and recovered voluntary flexion and extension of the fingers of her left hand." By 8 months "she was able to walk rapidly with a cane and had isolated movements of the wrist and fingers of the left hand which she could use for grasping and assisting." Sensory function was improved, but not fully restored.

Kusske and Kelly[60] reported two cases which were inferred to suffer symptoms of cerebral steal. One was a 43-year-old woman who suffered daily to weekly focal seizures and postictal left arm weakness. Atrophy of the left arm, palsy of the left face, and dysarthria was present prior to therapeutic embolization with Silastic balls for a right rolandic AVM. Postembolization, the seizure frequency declined to monthly intervals, and the left arm paresis improved. By 2 years, she had full use of the left hand, normal left facial strength, and improved speech. A second case, a 45-year-old man with progressive mental deterioration, incomplete hemiparesis, and aggression had an AVM of the sylvian region. After embolization for the AVM, the hemiparesis improved, the visual deficit regressed, the memory and personality changes reversed, and the patient returned to work. In Norlen's[96] case, a 19-year-old male had presented with left-sided spastic hemiparesis following hemorrhages 3 years and 1 year previously. Within 2 months following operative excision of the AVM, there was "pronounced improvement in the paresis and the patient was in good condition." He returned to regular work 2 years later. These dramatic cases leave little doubt that the steal phenomenon exists and may to some degree be reversible. Yet much work needs to be done to delineate the spectrum of syndromes that may prove reversible. Attempts to use the Luria battery[22] pre- and postoperatively are quantitative steps in the right direction. Amaurosis fugax has also been reported from a dural AVM,[15] but whether attributable to steal is unsettled.

## OTHER VASCULAR MALFORMATIONS

### Cavernous Malformations (Angiomas)

Because of their characteristic appearance on a magnetic resonance scan, less so on a CT scan, cavernous malformations are becoming more and more the subject of reports in the literature.[44,79,147,149] These lesions rarely occupy a clinically significant amount of space in the brain, but may be located in clinically important cortical or subcortical regions, and are occasionally multiple. Although they are masses, they do not produce displacements commensurable to that of a neoplasm. They are composed of cavernous channels with multiple areas of thrombosis. The flow through these lesions is minimal, therefore they are rarely seen on angiograms. Their characteristic configuration is recognized by contrast enhancement on CT scans. They are frequently associated with headache and seizures and occasionally with hemorrhage. Since the introduction of MRI, cavernous malformations have been diagnosed more frequently because the distinctive "cat's eye" that appears on MR scan is not readily identified on a CT scan. This appearance was once considered pathognomonic for cavernous angiomas, but no longer.[120]

Their clinical importance is unclear except in a differential diagnosis with tumor and other contrast-enhancing mass. Cavernous malformations most often present with a seizure disorder, and the same may be said for venous malformation.[7,32,37,89,118,119,151] These lesions may also be seen with headaches that may or may not be related to the lesion. It is often very difficult to determine a one-to-one relationship betwen lesion and symptoms. The lesions may occur anywhere, including the cortical surface or deep in the brain stem. Magnetic resonance imaging has allowed the study of family members, which in a small series of cases have suggested a hereditary basis for some instances of multiple cavernous malformations.[26,122]

### Telangiectasia

Telangiectasias are uncommon anomalies that appear as small clusters of capillarylike vessels located in the brain stem or cerebellum.[29,78,79] They are often deep and multiple. Their clinical significance is dubious. They rarely may be the source of a large hemorrhage, which, if located in a critical area, may cause death. Mostly they are curiosities noted at postmortem. Although frequently demonstrating small microhemorrhages on histologic examination, the size of the hemorrhage does not appear to be massive enough to create a clinical syndrome. When associated with the Rendu-Osler-Weber syndrome, the telangiectasias are recognized elsewhere in the body. The telangiectasias are generally curiosities for the pathologist to describe and rarely have clinical significance.[30] They are frequently found at postmortem, and may present clinically with hemorrhage at their common site of origin, which is the white matter of brain stem, cerebellum, and diencephalic regions. In such instances, the hemorrhages may be incapacitating or fatal, and postmortem examination may uncover the lesion as a thrombosed telangiectasia. The venous malformations are often deep within the white matter; however, they may extend to the cortical surface, presumably causing seizures. Both of these lesions rarely hemorrhage and are generally radiologic curiosities rather than threatening lesions that require radical treatment.

### Venous Malformations (Angiomas)

Venous malformations have come under increasing scrutiny because of the use of CT scans and sophisticated angiography.[32,91,99,100,123,125,129,154] They are represented by a deep prominent vein that shows late on the venous phase of an arteriogram, and is associated with a fingerlike projection from the main vein. This appearance is characteristic on an arteriogram. Pathologically, few studies have been done on these lesions; however, they appear to be abnormally distended veins located in an abnormal location, that is, deep in the white matter. There is some evidence that they represent anomalous venous drainage, which compensates for the absence of normal venous conduits. Rarely do these lesions hemorrhage. Very few of these have been resected, and intraoperative studies show that they are devoid of arterial blood. Curiously, they appear to be associated with headaches and occasionally with seizures.

## LABORATORY DIAGNOSIS

Because the clinical syndromes of AVM are not distinctive for the causes like those of subarachnoid hemorrhage from aneurysm, laboratory studies, especially brain imaging, plays an important role. In approximately 10 percent of the patients, the diagnosis is discovered in a serendipitous fashion.

### Computed Tomography Scan

In 85 percent of AVMs diagnosis can be made by CT scan,[64] a great improvement over the now-outmoded radionuclide scanning.[54] The CT scan done with contrast shows an enhancing lesion, which is usually at the cortical level extending deep, whose margins are irregular and, when viewed with the most sophisticated CT scanners, may be associated with serpentine vascular channels (Fig. 23-14). Large hemorrhages from one of these malformations can be recognized on the non-contrast scan, and these may be demonstrated in the ventricular system on in the subarachnoid cisterns at the base of the brain. A hemorrhage may partially obscure the malformation, which, how-

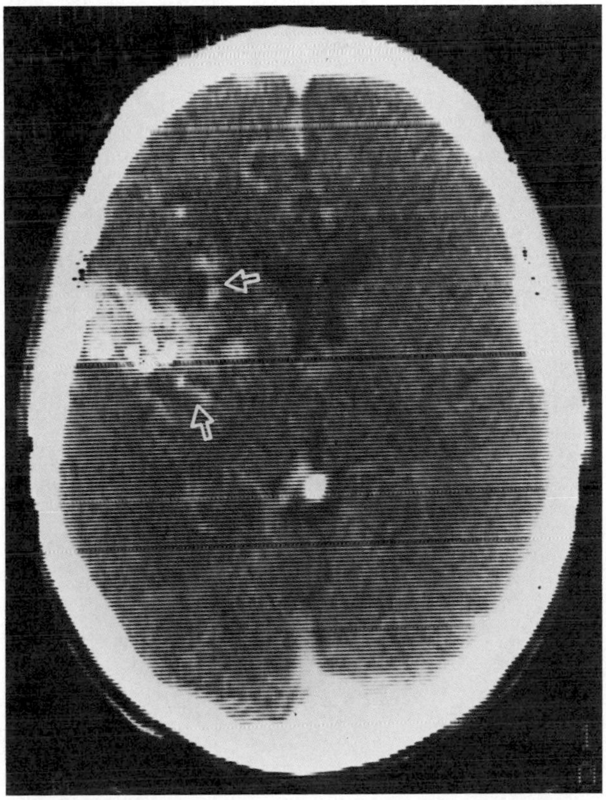

**Fig. 23-14.** Computed tomography scan with contrast enhancement demonstrating the typical serpentine channels characteristic of an arteriovenous malformation (*arrows*).

ever, should show up as an additional area of enhancement on the enhanced scan. When the malformation contains distended veins related to the aqueduct, hydrocephalus may be present. In those patients who have had previous hemorrhages that are now resolved, the CT scan will often show an area of encephalomalacia, a cleavage area between the nidus of the malformation and the normal brain. Calcium may occasionally be present with the AVM or associated with the encephalomalacia. Such areas of infarction or encephalomalacia may be extensive with minimal neurologic abnormalities. The more sophisticated fifth-generation CT and magnetic resonance imaging scanners are most important in identifying the exact location of the principal portion of the AVM and its relationship to brain components such as the cortex, the ventricular system, brain stem, and diencephalic regions (Fig. 23-15). Understanding these relationships significantly assists the surgeon in planning an approach. However, it must be recognized that even with the most sophisticated CT scan visualization of the exact vascular anatomy of a malformation is rarely possible. Such finite detail can only be determined by angiography.

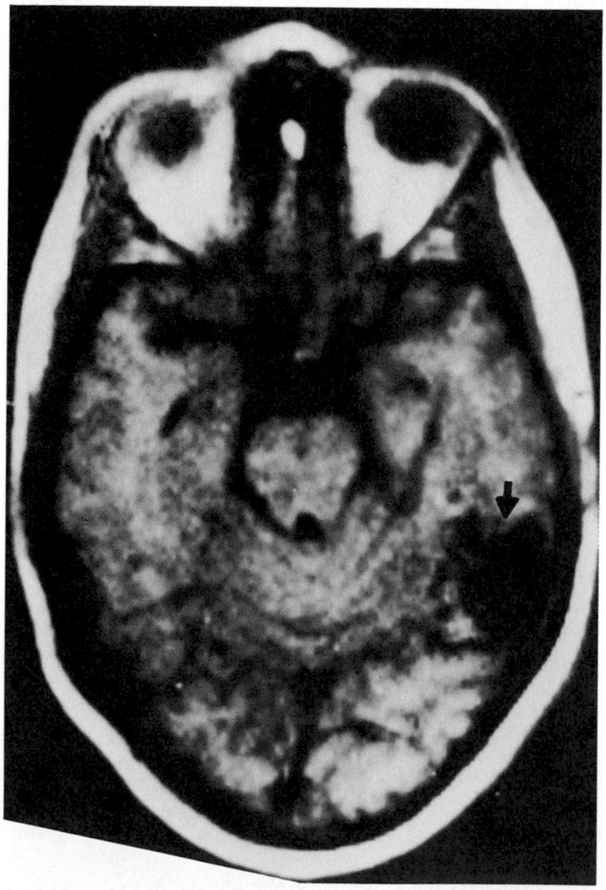

**Fig. 23-15.** Nuclear magnetic resonance evaluation of an arteriovenous malformation. The black areas represent an arteriovenous malformation (*arrow*) with rapid blood flow.

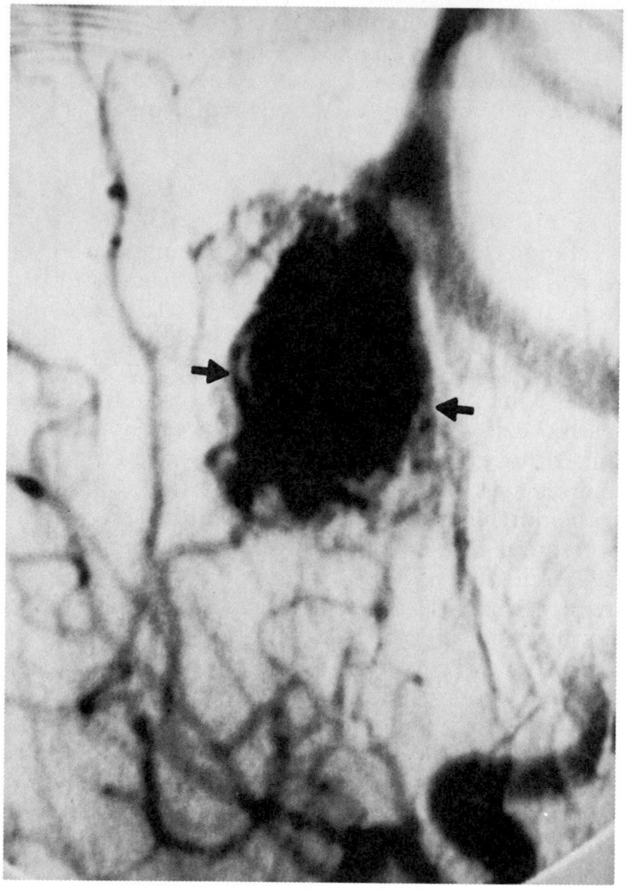

**Fig. 23-16.** Digital subtraction study demonstrating the anatomy of an arteriovenous malformation (*arrows*) of the temporal lobe.

The CT scan in cavernous malformations is typified by an extensive contrast-enhancing area, often involving the cortex and extending deep, which may be confused with a tumor except for the lack of displacement of adjacent structures. In the presence of venous malformations there is often a linear contrast-enhancing streak from the white matter, extending toward the cortical surface representing the major venous portion of the malformation. Telangiectasia may or may not be recognized. Presumably, small AVMs that have hemorrhaged, and for the most part destroyed themselves, may still be identified as pinpoint contrast-enhanced areas surrounded by cystic encephalomalacia on an enhanced CT scan (Fig. 23-16). They have a very characteristic appearance and often lie in a subcortical position. It should be emphasized that all these lesions may be mistaken for other types of pathology, most commonly tumors, and therefore angiography is definitive in establishing a diagnosis and identifying the anatomy of the contributing arteries.

## Magnetic Resonance Imaging

In the last 5 years, magnetic resonance imaging has almost eclipsed angiogram and far surpassed CT scanning for the diagnosis of AVM. MR has yet to replace angiography for the fine details needed by the surgeon, but for routine diagnosis and management planning, MR can now be relied upon as the first line of diagnosis. Early reports with low-field magnets[65,127] showed the high-flow vascular channels of an AVM as dark areas or regions of "reduced signal" (see Fig. 23-15). The intensity of the signal void is related to the flow rates, a finding that offers the opportunity to calculate blood flow noninvasively. As opposed to angiogram, which reveals nothing of the brain parenchyma, MR clearly shows the relationships to surrounding brain, and it has proved to be superior to angiography in defining the nidus.[101] Evidence of prior hemorrhage and its source,[76,141] the size of the nidus, the source of flow to the lesion, the course of draining veins, and the relation of the malformation to normal brain structures are now regularly shown. A central focus of a high-signal region, surrounded by hypointensity, once thought pathognomonic of cavernous angiomas, has been found to be due to AVM in 5 of 9 patients operated on,[120] and neoplasm in 18 of 24 patients.

## Regional Cerebral Blood Flow

Pre- and postoperative regional cerebral blood flow (rCBF) studies are increasingly being used to evaluate the flow patterns in AVMs.[157] Intraoperative rCBF evaluations have demonstrated that this technique may help in predicting those patients at risk for delayed complications presumably due to perfusion pressure breakthrough.[158] Positron emission tomography has also found application in localizing the nidus of an AVM recently. Leblanc and Mayer[66] described the first case.

## Doppler Insonation

Transcranial Doppler technology has increased the range of investigations for AVMs because the methodology has easy bedside use. Barely a decade old, the techniques for insonation of the inracranial vessels are now well described.[1,68] Using this method, investigators have demonstrated the principal sources of flow to the lesion.[17,40,128] This method has also been used to plan and evaluate embolization therapy.[117] It is being used in investigations of perfusion breakthrough. In our experience, the pattern of low resistance to arterial flow typical of AVMs has successfully predicted all angiographically obvious AVMs involving the cerebrum, missing only a handful of AVMs whose shunts required careful examination of the angiogram for their detection, or whose small feeders were exclusively from the anterior choroidal territory.

## Angiography

In spite of advances in other forms of diagnostic imaging, arteriography remains the foundation of the diagnosis of vascular abnormalities,[69] and has proved superior to MR in defining the details of the vascular supply.[101] However, a few examples of thrombosed, nonhemorrhagic AVMs have been found by brain imaging that were not shown by angiogram.[44,147]

Angiography plays a major role in preparing the patient for therapy. Full documentation of the lesion involves rapid-sequence filming, magnification of certain arterial territories, separate injection of the extracerebral vessels and stereoangiography done in the lateral series. Rapid-sequence filming at rates of five to six per second assists in the analysis of arterial supply in number, source, and size of the feeding arteries. This demonstration is especially important in those situations where the artery feeding the malformation also feeds healthy cerebrum in its more distal branches. It is recognized that the arterial contributions to an AVM are numerous, and not all may be identified by an angiogram; however, the major ones playing a role in the embolization or surgery of an AVM may be identified by conventional angiography. To provide the information of greatest help to the surgeon, stereoscopic angiograms should be obtained. This is carried out simply by performing an x-ray tube shift in an anteroposterior direction while performing the lateral angiogram. These paired angiograms can be visualized with or without the help of a stereoscopic viewer. The resultant stereoscopic image gives a more precise identification of the three-dimensional anatomy of an AVM and is extremely helpful in planning and carrying out an operative approach to these malformations. Other techniques that have proved to be useful are magnification angiography and large injections of contrast material with a prolonged venous phase. In terms of magnification angiography there are disadvantages to be considered. The malformation and its components are visualized in a somewhat distorted view, which makes exact measurements and the study of relationships difficult. However, magnification angiography will demonstrate small feeders to the malformation that may not be identified on standard angiography.

All forms of angiography should be as selective as possible. For practical purposes this means injection of the vertebral or internal carotid arteries, since techniques for injection directly into the distal feeding vessels of a vascular malformation are cumbersome and not yet readily available. External carotid artery injection is essential to document dural feeders, which are found the more they are sought, especially in posterior hemispheral and posterior fossa

AVMs. Angiotomography and cineangiography have not been of significant use in the evaluation of the more common vascular anomalies such as AVMs. Digital subtraction angiography, especially with arterial injection, provides a good survey, but does not give sufficient detail of these lesions to be of major help in planning an operation. Although multiple AVMs are infrequent,[96] the association with aneurysms is well recognized, so that comprehensive four-vessel angiography should be carried out in all patients. If severe arterial vasospasm is present, once the lesion has been identified the remainder of the arteriographic study should be deferred to a later date. The high volume injection of contrast agent and a prolonged venous phase are essential in identifying the somewhat ubiquitous and obscure venous malformations. Cavernous malformations rarely show at angiography because their arterial feeders are small and infrequent.

In planning embolization, it is frequently necessary to use a different catheter system for diagnosis than for interventional neuroradiology.[34,60,70] In such cases, angiography will be repeated at the time of embolization once this is selected as the course of treatment. Intraoperative arteriography is a difficult procedure and delays an already long operation; therefore it has thus far had limited use.

## REFERENCES


1. Aaslid R, Markwalde T-M, Nornes H: Noninvasive transcranial Doppler ultrasound recording of blood flow in basal cereral arteries. J Neurosurg 57:769, 1982
2. Adie WJ: Permanent hemianopsia in migraine and subarachnoid hemorrhage. Lancet 219:237, 1930
3. Agnoli AL: Extracranial and extra-intracranial arteriovenous angiomas. p. 66. In Pia HW, Gleave JRW, Grote E et al (eds): Cerebral Angiomas. Advances in Diagnosis and Therapy. Springer-Verlag, New York, 1975
4. Almeida GM, Shibata MK, Nakagawa EJ: Contralateral parafalcine approach for parasagittal and callosal arteriovenous malformations. Neurosurgery 14:744, 1984
5. Aminoff MJ: Vascular anomalies in the intracranial dura mater. Brain 96:601, 1973
6. Andoh T, Sakai N, Yamada H et al: Cerebellar AVM clinical analysis of 14 cases. No To Shinkei 42:913, 1990
7. Arutinov AI, Baron MA, Majorova NA: Experimental and clinical study of the development of spasm of the cerebral arteries related to subarachnoid hemorrhage. J Neurosurg 32:617, 1970
8. Bär Th: The vascular system of the cerebral cortex. Adv Anat Embryol Cell Biol 59:1, 1980
9. Barre RG, Suter GS, Rosenblum WI: Familial vascular malformations or chance occurrence? Neurology (NY) 28:98, 1978
10. Batjer HH, Devous MD, Sr, Meyer YJ et al: Cerebrovascular hemodynamics in arteriovenous malformation complicated by normal perfusion pressure breakthrough. Neurosurgery 22:503, 1988
11. Batjer H, Samson D: Arteriovenous malformations of the posterior fossa. J Neurosurg 64:849, 1986
12. Becker DH, Townsend JJ, Kramer RA, Newton TH: Occult cerebrovascular malformations: a series of 18 histologically verified cases with negative angiography. Brain 102:249, 1979
13. Bergh van den R, Eecken van der H: Anatomy and embryology of the cerebral circulation. Prog Brain Res 30:1, 1968
14. Bessman AN, Hayes GJ, Alman RW, Fazekas JR: Cerebral hemodynamics in cerebral arteriovenous vascular anomalies. Med Ann DC 21:422, 1952
15. Bogousslavasky J, Vinuela F, Barnett HJM, Drake CG: Amaurosis fugax as the presenting manifestation of dural arteriovenous malformation. Stroke 16:891, 1985
16. Boyd MC, Steinbok P, Paty DW: Familial arteriovenous malformations. J Neurosurg 62:597, 1985
17. Brass LR, Prohovnik I, Pavlakis S, Mohr JP: Transcranial Doppler examination of middle cerebral artery velocity versus xenon rCBF: two measures of cerebral blood flow. Neurology (NY) 37:85, 1987
18. Bruce DA: Surgery of the vein of Galen arteriovenous malformation. Contemp Neurosurg 3:1, 1981
19. Burchiel KJ, Clarke H, Ojemann GA et al: Use of stimulation mapping and corticography in the excision of arteriovenous malformations in sensorimotor and language related neocortex. Neurosurgery 24:322, 1989
20. Crawford PM, West CR, Chadwick DW, Shaw MDM: Arteriovenous malformations of the brain: natural history in unoperated patients. J Neurol Neurosurg Psychiatry 49:1, 1986
21. Cohen HCM, Tucker WS, Humphreys RP, Perrin RJ: Angiographically cryptic histologically verified cerebrovascular malformations. Neurosurgery 10:704, 1982
22. Conly FK, Moses JA, Helle TL: Deficits in higher cerebral function in two patients with posterior parietal arteriovenous malformations. Neurosurg 7:230, 1980
23. Crawford JV, Russell DS: Cryptic arteriovenous and venous hamartomas of the brain. J Neurol Neurosurg Psychiatry 19:1, 1956
24. Dandy WE: Arteriovenous aneurysm of the brain. Arch Surg (Chicago) 17:190, 1928
25. Dimsdale H: Discussion on the neuro-ophthalmological aspects of cerebral angiomas. Proc R Soc Med 50:85, 1957
26. Dobyns WB, Michels VV, Groover RV et al: Familial cavernous malformations of the central nervous system and retina. Ann Neurol 21:578, 1987
27. Duckett S: The establishment of internal vascu-

larization in the human telencephalon. Acat Anat 80:107, 1971
28. Ennoksson P, Bynke H: Visual field defects in arteriovenous aneurysms of the brain. Acta Ophthalmol 36:586, 1958
29. Epstein N, Epstein F: Arteriovenous malformation presenting as a first seizure in a 13-year-old child: surgical indications. Neurosurgery 7:391, 1980
30. Farrell DF, Forno LS: Symptomatic capillary telangiectasis of the brain stem without hemorrhage: report of an unusual case. Neurology (NY) 20:341, 1970
31. Feindel W, Yamamoto YL, Hodge CP: Red cerebral veins and the cerebral steal syndrome: evidence from fluorescein angiography and microregional blood flow by radioisotopes during excision of an angioma. J Neurosurg 35:167, 1971
32. Fierstein SB, Pribam HW, Hieshima G: Angiography and computed tomography in the evaluation of cerebral venous malformations. Neurology (NY) 17:137, 1979
33. Forster DMC, Steiner L, Hakanson S: Arteriovenous malformations of the brain: a long-term clinical study. J Neurosurg 37:562, 1972
34. Fox JL, Al Mefty O: Embolization of an arteriovenous malformation of the brain stem. Surg Neurol 8:7, 1977
35. Garrido E, Stein BM: Removal of an arteriovenous malformation from the basal ganglion. J Neurol Neurosurg Psychiatry 41:992, 1978
36. Gerosa M, Cappellotto P, Licata C et al: Cerebral arteriovenous malformations in children (56 cases). Childs Brain 8:356, 1981
37. Giombini S, Morello G: Cavernous angiomas of the brain: account of fourteen personal cases and review of the literature. Acta Neurochir (Wien) 40:61, 1978
38. Graeb DA, Dolman CL: Radiological and pathological aspects of dural arteriovenous fistulas. J Neurosurg 64:962, 1986
39. Graf CJ, Perret GE, Torner JC: Bleeding from cerebral arteriovenous malformations as part of their natural history. J Neurosurg 58:331, 1983
40. Grolimund P, Seiker RW, Aaslid R et al: Evaluation of cerebrovascular disease by combined extracranial and transcranial Doppler sonography: experience in 1039 patients. Stroke 18:1018, 1987
41. Gross CR, Kase CS, Mohr JP et al: Stroke in south Alabama: incidence and diagnostic features: population study. Stroke 15:249, 1984
42. Guidetti B, DeLitala A: Intracranial arteriovenous malformations: conservative and surgical treatment. J Neurosurg 53:149, 1980
43. Harders A, Bien S, Eggert HR et al: Haemodynamic changes in arteriovenous malformations induced by superselective embolization: transcranial Doppler evaluation. Neurol Res 10:239, 1988
44. Hashim ASM, Asakura T, Kiochi U et al: Angiographically occult arteriovenous malformations. Surg Neurol 16:431, 1985
45. Hayashi S, Arimoto T, Itakura T et al: The association of intracranial aneurysms and arteriovenous malformation of the brain. J Neurosurg 55:971, 1981
46. Henderson WR, Gomez RdeRL: Natural History of cerebral angiomas. Br Med J 4:571, 1967
47. Hier DB, Davis KR, Richardson EP, Mohr JP: Hypertensive putaminal hemorrhage. Ann Neurol 1:152, 1977
48. Höök O, Johanson C: Intracranial arteriovenous aneurysms: a follow-up study with particular attention to their growth. Arch Neurol Neurosurg Psychiatry 80:39, 1958
49. Horton JC, Chambers WA, Lyons SL et al: Pregnancy and the risk of hemorrhage from cerebral arteriovenous malformations. Neurosurgery 27:867, 1990
50. Hosobuchi Y: Electrothrombosis of carotid-cavernous fistula. J Neurosurg 42:76, 1975
51. Hyland HH, Douglas RP: Cerebral angioma arteriale: a case in which migrainous headache was the earliest manifestation. Arch Neurol Neurosurg Psychiatry 40:1220, 1938
52. Jane JA, Kassell NF, Torner JC, Winn HR: The natural history of aneurysms and arteriovenous malformations. J Neurosurg 62:321, 1985
53. Kase CS, Williams JP, Wyatt DA, Mohr JP: Lobar intracerebral hematomas: clinical and CT analysis of 22 cases. Neurology (NY) 32:1146, 1982
54. Kelly DL, Alexander E, Davis CH, Maynard DC: Intracranial AVMs: clinical review and evaluation of brain scans. J Neurosurg 31:422, 1969
55. Kjellberg RN, Hanamura T, Davis KR et al: Bragg-Peak proton beam therapy for arteriovenous malformations of the brain. N Engl J Med 5:269, 1983
56. Klosovskii N: The development of the brain and its disturbance by harmful factors. Macmillan, New York, 1963
57. Krayenbuhl E, Siebenmann R: Small vascular malformations as a cause of primary intracerebral hemorrhage. J Neurosurg 22:7, 1965
58. Krayenbuhl H, Yasargil G: L'aneurismo cerebral. Doc Geigy Ser Chir 4, 1959
59. Kuban KCK, Gilles FH: Human telencephalic angiogenesis. Ann Neurol 17:539, 1985
60. Kusske JA, Kelly WA: Embolization and reduction of the "steal" syndrome in cerebral AVMs. J Neurosurg 40:313, 1974
61. Kvam DA, Michelsen WJ, Quest DO: Intracerebral hemorrhage as a complication of artificial embolization. Neurosurgery 7:491, 1980
62. Lasjaunias P, Chiu M, Ter Brugge K et al: Neurological manifestations of intracranial dural arteriovenous malformations. J Neurosurg 64:724, 1986
63. Lazar ML, Watts CC, Kilgore B, Clark K: Cerebral angiography during operation for intracranial aneurysms and arteriovenous malformations: technical note. J Neurosurg 34:706, 1971
64. Leblanc R, Ethier R, Little JR: Computerized tomography findings in arteriovenous malformations of the brain. J Neurosurg 51:765, 1979
65. Leblanc R, Levesque M, Comair Y, Ethier R: Magnetic resonance imaging of cerebral arterio-

venous malformations. Neurosurgery 21:15, 1987
66. Leblanc R, Mayer E: Functional PET scanning in the assessment of cerebral arteriovenous malformations: case report. J Neurosurg 73:615, 1990
67. Lees F: The migrainous symptoms of cerebral angiomata. J Neurol Neurosurg Psychiatry 25:45, 1962
68. Lindegaard KF, Grolimund R, Asslid R, Nornes H: Evaluation of cerebral AVMs using transcranial Doppler ultrasound. J Neurosurg 65:335, 1986
69. Luessenhop AJ, Gennarelli TA: Anatomical grading of supratentorial arteriovenous malformations for determining operability. J Neurosurg 1:30, 1975
70. Luessenhop AJ, Mujica PH: Embolization of segments of the circle of Willis and adjacent branches for management of certain inoperable cerebral arteriovenous malformations. J Neurosurg 54:573, 1981
71. Luessenhop AJ, Presper JH: Surgical embolization of cerebral arteriovenous malformations through internal carotid and vertebral arteries: long-term results. J Neurosurg 42:443, 1975
72. Mackenzie I: The clinical presentation of cerebral angioma: a review of 50 cases. Brain 76:184, 1953
73. Mall FP: On the development of the blood-vessels of the brain in the human embryo. Am J Anat 4:1, 1905
74. Margolis G, Odom GL, Woodhall B: Further experiences with small vascular malformations as a cause of massive intracerebral bleeding. J Neuropathol Exp Neurol 20:161, 1961
75. Maspes PE, Marini G: Results of the surgical treatment of intracranial arteriovenous malformations. Vasc Surg 4:164, 1970
76. Mawad ME, Hilal SK, Silver AJ, Sane P: High resolution, high field MR imaging of cerebral arteriovenous malformations. Radiology 153:143, 1984
77. McCormick WF: The pathology of vascular ("arteriovenous") malformations. J Neurosurg 24:807, 1966
78. McCormick WF, Hardman JM, Boulter TR: Vascular malformations ("angiomas") of the brain with special reference to those occurring in the posterior fossa. J Neurosurg 28:241, 1968
79. McCormick WF, Nofzinger JD: "Cryptic" vascular malformations of the central nervous system. J Neurosurg 24:865, 1966
80. McCormick WF, Rosenfield DB: Massive brain hemorrhage: a review of 144 cases and an examination of their causes. Stroke 4:946, 1973
81. McCormick WF, Schochet SS, Jr: Atlas of Cerebrovascular Disease. WB Saunders, Philadelphia, 1976
82. Mendelow AD, Erfurth A, Grossart K, MacPherson P: Do cerebral arteriovenous malformations increase in size? J Neurol Neurosurg Psychiatry 50:980, 1987
83. Minakawa T, Tanaka R, Koike T et al: Angiographic follow up study of cerebral arteriovenous malformations with reference to their enlargement and regression. Neurosurgery 24:68, 1989
84. Mineta T, Fukiyama K, Koga H et al: Dural arteriovenous malformation associated with occlusion of the superior sagittal sinus case report. Neurol Med Chir (Tokyo) 31:41, 1991
85. Miyasaka K, Wolpert SM, Prager RJ: The association of cerebral aneurysms, infundibula, and intracranial arteriovenous malformations. Stroke 2:196, 1982
86. Moffat DB: The embryology of the arteries of the brain. Ann R Coll Surg Engl 30:368, 1962
87. Mohr JP, Caplan LR, Melski JW et al: The Harvard Cooperative Stroke Registry. Neurology (NY) 28:754, 1978
88. Moody RA, Poppen JL: Arteriovenous malformations. J Neurosurg 32:503, 1970
89. Morello G, Borghi GP: Cerebral angiomas: a report of the 154 personal cases and a comparison between the results of surgical excision and conservative management. Acta Neurochir (Wien) 28:135, 1973
90. Morgan MK, Johnston I, Besser M, Baines D: Cerebral arteriovenous malformations, steal and the hypertensive breakthrough threshold. J Neurosurg 66:563, 1987
91. Moritaka K, Handa H, Mori K et al: Venous angiomas of the brain. Surg Neurol 14:95, 1980
92. Mullan S, Brown FD, Patronas NJ: Hyperemic and ischemic problems of surgical treatment of arteriovenous malformations. J Neurosurg 51:757, 1979
93. Muraszko K, Wang HH, Pelton G, Stein BM: A study of the reactivity of feeding vessels to arteriovenous malformations: correlation with clinical outcome. Neurosurgery 26:190, 1990
94. Newton TH, Troost BT: Arteriovenous malformation and fistula: arteriovenous malformation and fistula. p. 2490. In Newton TH, Potts DG (eds): Radiology of the Skull and Brain: Angiography. Vol 2. CV Mosby, St. Louis, 1974
95. Nishino A, Sakurai Y, Takahashi A et al: Superior petrosal sinus dural arteriovenous malformation with varix indenting brain stem report of a case and review of the literature. No To Shinkei 43:62, 1991
96. Norlen G: Arteriovenous aneurysms of the brain: report of ten cases of total removal of the lesion. J Neurosurg 6:475, 1949
97. Nornes H, Grip A: Hemodynamic aspects of cerebral arteriovenous malformations. J Neurosurg 53:456, 1980
98. Northfield DWC: Angiomatous malformations of the brain. Guys Hosp Rep 90:149, 1940
99. Numaguchi Y, Kishikawa T, Fukui M et al: Prolonged injection angiography for diagnosing intracranial cavernous hemangiomas. Radiology 131:137, 1979
100. Numaguchi Y, Kitamura K, Fukui M et al: Intracranial venous angiomas. Surg Neurol 18:193, 1982
101. Nussel F, Wegmuller H, Huber P: Comparison of magnetic resonance angiography, magnetic resonance imaging and conventional angiogra-

phy in cerebral arteriovenous malformation. Neuroradiology 33:56, 1991
102. Okabe T, Meyer JS, Okayasu H et al: Xenon-enhanced CT CBF measurements in cerebral AVMs before and after excision: contribution to pathogenesis and treatment. J Neurosurg 59:21, 1983
103. Olivecrona H, Ladenheim J: Congenital arteriovenous aneurysms of the carotid and vertebral systems. Springer-Verlag, Berlin, 1957
104. Ondra SL, Troupp H, George ED, Schwab K: The natural history of symtpomatic arteriovenous malformations of the brain: a 24-year follow up assessment. J Neurosurg 73:387, 1990
105. Ostergaard JR: Association of Intracranial Aneurysm and Arteriovenous Malformation in Childhood: Congress of Neurological Surgeons. Neurosurgery 3:358, 1984
106. Ozer MN, Sencer W, Block J: A clinical study of cerebral vascular malformations: the significance of migraine. J Mt Sinai Hosp 31:403, 1964
107. Padget DH: The development of the cranial arteries in the human embryo. Contrib Embryol 32:205, 1948
108. Padget DH: The cranial venous system in man in reference to development, adult configuration, and relation to the arteries. Am J Anat 98:307, 1956
109. Parkinson D, Bachers G: Arteriovenous malformations: summary of 100 consecutive supratentorial cases. J Neurosurg 53:285, 1980
110. Paterson JH, McKissock W: A clinical survey of intracranial angiomas with special reference to their mode of progression and surgical treatment: a report of 110 cases. Brain 79:233, 1956
111. Patronas NJ, Marx WJ, Duda EE, Mullan JJ: Microvascular embolization of arteriovenous malformations: predicting success by cerebral angiography. Am J Neuroradial 1:459, 1980
112. Pellettieri L: Surgical versus conservative treatment of intracranial arteriovenous malformations: a study in surgical decision-making. Acta Neurochir, suppl. 29:1 1979
113. Perret G: The epidemiology and clinical course of arteriovenous malformations. p. 21. In Pia HW, Gleave JRW, Grote E, Zierski J (eds): Cerebral Angiomas. Advances in Diagnosis and Therapy. Springer-Verlag, New York, 1975
114. Perret G, Nishioka H: Report on the cooperative study of intracranial aneurysms and subarachnoid hemorrhage. VI. Arteriovenous malformations. J Neurosurg 25:467, 1966
115. Pertuiset B, Ancri D, Clergue F: Preoperative evaluation of hemodynamic factors in cerebral arteriovenous malformations for selection of a radical surgical tactic with special reference to vascular autoregulation disorders. Neurol Res 4:209, 1982
116. Pertuiset B, Sichez JP, Philippon J et al: Mortalité et morbidité après exerese chirurgicale totale et 162 malformation arterioveineuses intracraniennes. Rev Neurol (Paris) 35:319, 1979
117. Petty GW, TK Tatemichi, JP Mohr et al: Transcranial Doppler changes after treatment for arteriovenous malformations. Stroke 21:260, 1990
118. Pia HW, Gleave JRW, Grote E et al: Cerebral Angiomas: Advances in Diagnosis and Therapy. p. 285. Springer-Verlag, New York, 1975
119. Pool JL, Potts DG: Aneurysms and Arteriovenous Anomalies of the Brain. Diagnosis and Treatment. p. 463. Harper & Row, New York, 1965
120. Rapacki TF, Brantley MJ, Furlow TW, Jr et al: Heterogeneity of cerebral cavernous hemangiomas diagnosed by MR imaging. J Comput Assist Tomogr 14:18, 1990
121. Rhodes AJ, Hyde JB: Postnatal growth of arterioles in the human cerebral cortex. Growth 29:173, 1965
122. Rigamonti D, Hadley MN, Drayer BP et al: Cerebral cavernous malformations: incidence and familial occurrence. N Engl J Med 319:343, 1988
123. Rothfus WE, Albright A, Casey KF et al: Cerebellar venous angioma: "benign" entity? AJNR 5:61, 1984
124. Ruff RL, Arbit E: Aphemia resulting from a left frontal hematoma. Neurology (NY) 31:353, 1981
125. Saito Y, Kobayashi N: Cerebral venous angiomas. Radiology 139:87, 1981
126. Schlachter LB, Fleischer AS, Faria MA, Tindall GT: Multifocal intracranial arteriovenous malformations. Neurosurgery 7:440, 1980
127. Schoerner W, Bradac GB, Treisch J et al: Magnetic resonance imaging (MRI) in the diagnosis of cerebral arteriovenous angiomas. Neuroradiology 28:313, 1986
128. Schwartz A, Hennerici M: Noninvasive transcranial doppler ultrasound in intracranial angiomas. Neurology (NY) 36:626, 1986
129. Senegor M, Dohrmann GJ, Wollman RL: Venous angiomas of the posterior fossa should be considered anomalous venous drainage. Surg Neurol 19:26, 1983
130. Shenkin HA, Spitz EB, Grant FC, Kety SS: Physiologic studies of arteriovenous anomalies of the brain. J Neurosurg 6:165, 1948
131. Snead OC III, Acker JD, Morawetz R: Familial arteriovenous malformation. Ann Neurol 5:585, 1979
132. Spetzler RF, Martin NA: A proposed grading system for arteriovenous malformations. J Neurosurg 65:476, 1986
133. Spetzler RF, Wilson CB: Enlargement of an AVM documented by angiography: case report. J Neurosurg 43:767, 1975
134. Spetzler RF, Wilson CB, Weinstein P et al: Normal perfusion pressure breakthrough theory. Clin Neurosurg 25:651, 1978
135. Satham P, Macpherson P, Johnston R et al: Cerebral radiation necrosis complicating stereotactic radiosurgery for arteriovenous malformation. J Neurol Neurosurg Psychiatry 53:476, 1990
136. Stein BM, Wolpert SM: Arteriovenous malformations of the brain. I. Current concepts and treatment. Arch Neurol 37:1, 1980
137. Stein BM, Wolpert SM: Arteriovenous malformations of the brain. II. Current concepts and treatment. Arch Neurol 37:69, 1980
138. Stein RW, Kase CS, Hier DB et al: Caudate hemorrhage. Neurology (NY) 34:1549, 1984

139. Svien HJ, McRae JA: Arteriovenous anomalies of the brain: fate of patients not having definitive surgery. J Neurosurg 23:23, 1965
140. Sundt, Jr TF, Piepgras DG: The surgicalk approach to arteriovenous malformations of the lateral and sigmoid dural sinuses. J Neurosurg 59:32, 1983
141. Sze G, Harper PS, Galicich JH et al: Hemorrhagic neoplasms: MR mimics of occult vascular malformations. Am Soc Neuroradiol 10-15 May, p 125, 1987
142. Tarr RW, Johnson DW, Rutigliano M et al: Use of acetazolamide challenge xenon CT in the assessment of cerebral blood flow dynamics in patients with arteriovenous malformations. AJNR 11:441, 1990
143. Troost BT, Newton TH: Occipital lobe arteriovenous malformation. Arch Ophthalmol 93:250, 1975
144. Troupp H, Marttila I, Halonen V: Arteriovenous malformations of the brain: prognosis without operation. Acta Neurochir 22:125, 1970
145. Trumpy JH, Eldevik P: Intracranial arteriovenous malformations: conservative or surgical treatment? Surg Neurol 8:171, 1977
146. Trussart V, Berry I, Manelfe C et al: Epileptogenic cerebral vascular malformations and MRI. J Neuroradiol 16:273, 1989
147. Tsitsopoulos P, Andrew J, Harrison MJG: Occult cerebral arteriovenous malformations. J Neurol Neurosurg Psychiatry 50:218, 1987
148. Vinuela F, Fox AJ, Pelz DM, Drake CG: Unusual clinical manifestations of dural arteriovenous malformations. J Neurosurg 64:554, 1986
149. Voigt K, Yasargil MG: Cerebral cavernous haemangiomas or cavernomas. Incidence, pathology, localization, diagnosis, clinical features and treatment. Review of the literature and report of an unusual case. Neurochirurgia 19:59, 1976
150. Wallace JM, Nashold BS, Jr, Slewka AP: Hemodynamic effects of cerebral arteriovenous aneurysms. Circulation 31:696, 1965
151. Walter W: the influence of the type and localization of the angioma on the clinical syndrome. p. 271. In Pia HW, Gleave JRW, Grote E, Zierski J (eds): Cerebral Angiomas: Advances in Diagnosis and Therapy. Springer-Verlag, New York, 1975
152. Waltimo O: The change in size of intracranial arteriovenous malformations. J Neurol Sci 19:21, 1973
153. Waltimo O: The relationship of size, density, and localization of intracranial arteriovenous malformations to the type of initial symptom. J Neurol Sci 19:13, 1973
154. Wendling LR, Moore JS, Kieffer SA et al: Intracerebral venous angioma. Radiology 119:141, 1976
155. Willinsky RA, Lasjaunias P, Terbrugge K, Burrows P: Multiple cerebral arteriovenous malformations (AVMs): review of our experience from 203 patients with cerebral vascular lesions. Neuroradiology 32:207, 1990
156. Wilson CB, U HS, Dominque J: Microsurgical treatment of intracranial vascular malformations. J Neurosurg 51:446, 1979
157. Yamada S: Arteriovenous malformations in the functional area: surgical treatment and regional cerebral blood flow. Neurol Res 4:283, 1982
158. Young WL, Prohovnik I, Ornstein E et al: The effect of arteriovenous malformation resection on cerebrovascular reactivity to carbon dioxide. Neurosurgery 27:257, 1990

# 24

# *DISSECTIONS AND TRAUMA OF CERVICOCEREBRAL ARTERIES*

Jeffrey L. Saver
J. Donald Easton
Robert G. Hart

Cervicocerebral arterial dissections occur when blood extrudes into the wall of an artery supplying the brain. The resulting intramural hematoma may compromise the lumen and cause an aneurysmal dilation (dissecting pseudoaneurysm). Dissections are an uncommon cause of cerebral ischemia, except in young adults. They usually occur spontaneously, or are associated with trivial trauma to the artery. Major, nonpenetrating trauma of the cervical carotid and vertebral arteries may induce thrombosis, with or without associated dissection. Spontaneous dissections involving extracranial or intracranial arteries, and traumatic arterial injuries, have distinct clinical features that warrant their separate consideration. Cumulative case reports (totaling 192 patients) and series of patients (totaling 712 patients) were reviewed for this chapter and define the clinical spectrum of these arteropathies. The natural history of the milder cases may not be adequately reflected, as many may go unrecognized or unreported.

## EXTRACRANIAL CAROTID ARTERY DISSECTION

The cervical carotid artery is the most frequently reported site of cervicocerebral dissection. One to three cases per year are reported from large academic centers,[15,21,35,39,43,44,47,69,85,99,120] and in one series cervical carotid dissections accounted for 2.5 percent of first strokes.[18] Overall, these dissections account for perhaps 1 percent of cerebral ischemia. Cervical carotid dissection occurs predominantly in the middle adult years: 70 percent of patients are between ages 35 and 50, with a mean age of 44 years.[65] There is no sex predilection.

The major presenting features are stroke or transient ischemic attack (TIA) associated with pain in the ipsilateral neck, face, or head (Table 24-1). Transient monocular blindness constitutes approximately 35 percent of all transient ischemic attacks.[18,35,47,85,129] An ipsilateral oculosympathetic paresis (partial Horner syndrome) occurs in nearly 40 percent of the patients. Headache or neck pain often precedes the onset of ischemic symptoms by several hours to 2 to 3 days. The headache may be pounding, but more often it is nonthrobbing, and ipsilateral scalp tenderness may occur.[46] Pulsatile tinnitus or a subjective bruit are prominent complaints in one-third of patients. Ipsilateral lingual paresis, dysgeusia, and facial dysesthesia may occasionally be present.[49,62,86,113,143] Although individual features are nonspecific, constellations of these symptoms and signs, which are relatively unusual in atheroembolic ischemia, are present in about three-fourths of the patients with a cervical carotid dissection. Undue headache or neck pain in patients

**TABLE 24-1. Clinical Features of Extracranial Carotid Dissection[a]**

| Clinical Data | Percent |
|---|---|
| *Sex* | |
| Male | 54 |
| Female | 46 |
| *Laterality* | |
| Bilateral | 14 |
| Unilateral | 86 |
| Left | 60 |
| Right | 40 |
| *Major presenting complaint[b]* | |
| Transient ischemic attack | 33 |
| Cerebral infarction | 48 |
| Minor | 30 |
| Major or fatal | 18 |
| Neck or head pain | 14 |
| Pulsatile tinnitus only | 2 |
| Asymptomatic bruit only | 1 |
| *Associated features at diagnosis* | |
| Symptoms | |
| Neck pain | 21 |
| Headache | 67 |
| Neck or head pain | 69 |
| Tinnitus or subjective bruit | 33 |
| Signs | |
| Horner syndrome | 38 |
| Cervical bruit | 25 |
| Lingual paresis | 4 |
| Abducens paresis | 1 |
| *Outcome* | |
| Neurologically normal, or mild deficits only | 76 |
| Moderate or severe deficits/death | 18/5 |
| Normal or mildly stenotic vessel on follow-up imaging | 70 |
| Late stroke | 1 |
| Subsequent cervicocephalic dissection | 3 |

[a] Age of patients: mean, 44 years; range, 11 to 74 years.
[b] Major presenting complaint leading to evaluation, not necessarily the initial symptom.
(Aggregate data from 466 cases gathered from references 15, 18, 35, 39, 44, 56, 65, 69, 81, 99, 114, 116, 120, 129, 138, 142.)

with cerebral ischemia is often the initial clue suggesting a dissection.

Cervical carotid dissection may present with unilateral neck, face, or head pain and oculosympathetic paresis without ischemic symptoms, and thus may mimic an initial episode of Raeder's paratrigeminal syndrome or a migraine variant.[12,35,104,147]

There is an impressive temporal relationship of dissections to minimal neck torsion or trauma in many patients. If such activities as bowling or coughing can precipitate carotid dissections, perhaps few are truly spontaneous, and, for practical purposes, "spontaneous" dissection and dissection related to trivial trauma may be considered as one entity. Types of trivial trauma reported to antedate dissection include almost all varieties of sports activity, violent coughing, vigorous nose-blowing, sexual activity, chiropractic manipulation, and neck-turning while leading a parade.[47,65,85] Cervical rotation or extension can compress the cervical carotid artery against the transverse processes of the upper cervical vertebra, and this may precipitate a dissection in the predisposed person (Fig. 24-1).[137,152]

Spontaneous cervical carotid dissection usually occurs in otherwise healthy people. However, fibromuscular dysplasia of the artery is found in about 15 percent of patients, with a female preponderance.[6,10,18,31,35,39,43,44,51,65,73,82,99,122,124,126,129,145,146] Surprisingly, simultaneous bilateral carotid involvement accounts for 14 percent of all reported cases of dissection, at least half of which have associated fibromuscular dysplasia.[65,90,95,101,103] Cervical carotid dissections have occasionally been associated with atheromatous plaques, arterial coiling, Ehlers-Danlos disease or Marfan syndrome.[7,35,38,47,72,80,85,116,128] Dissections in more than one family member have been observed at least twice.[102] A history of migraine is present in only a minority of patients,[43,85,105,110,112,123] although one investigation[34] showed migraine, as well as oral contraceptives, to be a significant risk factor for dissection in a case-controlled study. Hypertension is reported in about one-third of patients. Early reports emphasized the association of these dissections with cystic medial necrosis, and O'Connell et al.[109] found an underlying arteropathy in 10 of 16 published cases examined pathologically. Nevertheless, dissection is reported to occur frequently in microscopically normal arteries or in arteries with minimal disorganization of elastic fibers.[22,43,47,85,110,139] We suspect that the majority of patients who have a dissection in the absence of substantial neck trauma have an as yet ill-defined underlying arteropathy.[66,103,148] Further pathologic studies may clarify this issue.

Pathologic specimens of cervical carotid dissection show hemorrhage into subintimal, medial, and, less often, subadventitial layers of the artery (Fig. 24-2).[51,109] Subintimal hemorrhage tends to result in luminal stenosis, while a hematoma in the outer media and subadventitia causes arterial dilatation (pseudoaneurysm).[85,109,116] Tortuous or coiled arterial segments may be more susceptible to aneurysm formation.[116] It is unclear whether a primary intimal tear allows dissection of blood to proceed from the lumen into the arterial wall or whether a primary intramedial hematoma secondarily ruptures into the true lumen. In some patients, no communication between the dissection cavity and the lumen can be demonstrated, while in others an intimal tear is present near the proximal extent of the dissection.

Thus, the pathogenesis of cervical carotid dissection is an enigma in most individuals, as they appear to have morphologically normal arteries. In those occurring below the C1 to C2 vertebral level, bony mechanical injury related to trivial trauma seems an unlikely mechanism. Recurrent or subsequent contralateral dissection is discussed below.

Cervical carotid dissection may result in cerebral ischemic symptoms owing to hemodynamic compromise from stenosis or occlusion, but more often from embolism of thrombotic fragments distally.[18,22] The

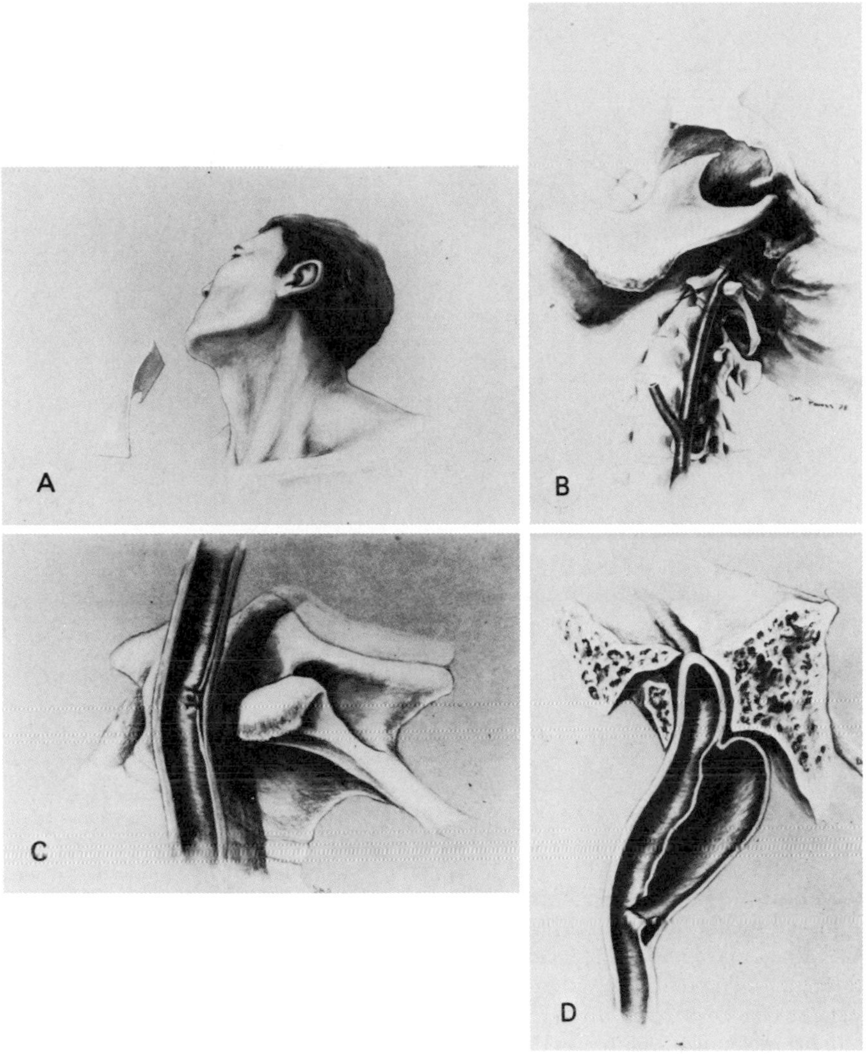


**Fig. 24-1.** Presumed mechanism of carotid injury induced by neck rotation. (**A**) Direction of hyperextension. (**B**) Impingement of artery on the process of the vertebra. (**C**) Intimal tear caused by impingement. (**D**) Progression of intimal tear to dissection. (From Stringer & Kelly,[137] with permission.)

importance of embolism is attested to by the occurrence of ischemic symptoms when stenosis is hemodynamically insignificant, by arteriographic evidence of distal emboli, and by the presence of friable intraluminal thrombus seen arteriographically and at surgery.

The diagnosis of cervical carotid dissection is based on a compatible clinical picture, coupled with the characteristic arteriographic features (Figs. 24-3 to 24-5).[21,47,73,110,129] Dissection usually begins 2 cm or more distal to the origin of the internal carotid artery and extends rostrally for a variable distance. It usually terminates before entry of the artery into the petrous bone, where mechanical support appears to limit further dissection in all but exceptional cases. Irregular narrowing of the artery is the most frequent finding, and it results in a "string sign" if it is severe (Fig. 24-5). A tapered occlusion beginning distal to the carotid sinus is less specific, but it occurs in about 20 percent of cases. Intimal flaps may be seen near the proximal margin of the dissection. An extraluminal pouch (dissecting pseudoaneurysm) may be visualized distally, usually near the base of the skull. Fibromuscular dysplasia of the contralateral carotid artery and embolic occlusion of intracranial arteries are sometimes seen. Rarely, dissections may begin in the common carotid artery or extend distally to involve the intracranial carotid and middle cerebral arteries (Fig. 24-6). Multiple dissections are more likely to be associated with fibromuscular dysplasia.[10,55,90,95,122]

Noninvasive imaging techniques, such as ultrasound, computed tomography (CT),[116] and magnetic resonance (MR), may be useful in several ways. They may suggest the presence of unsuspected dissection in

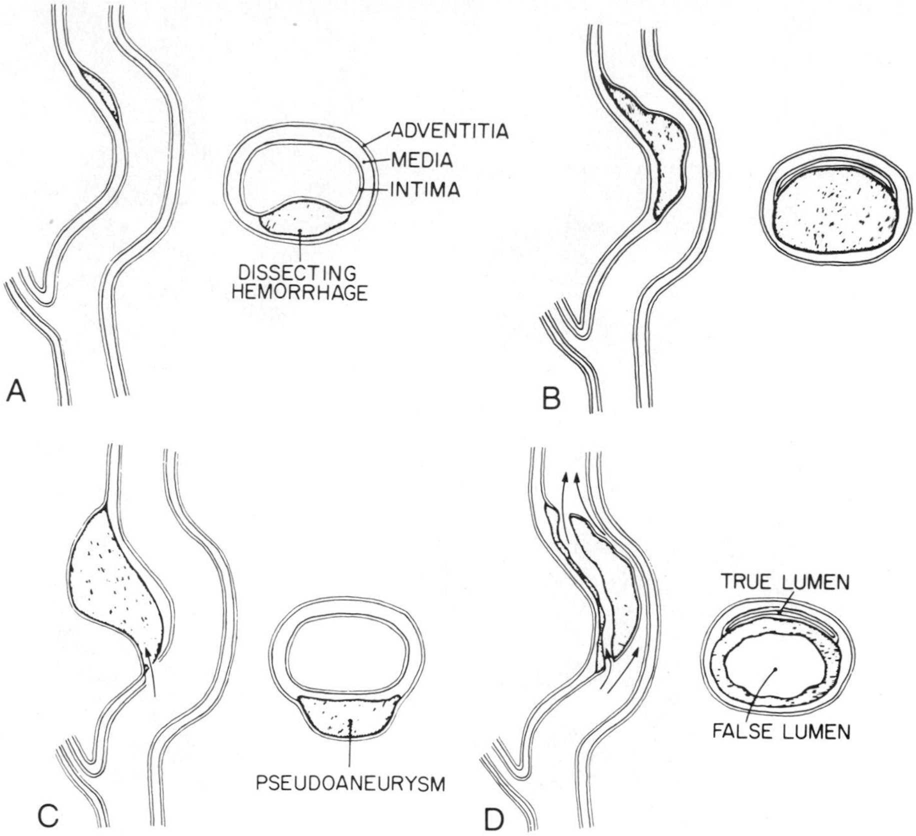


**Fig. 24-2.** Anatomy of dissections. (**A**) Lateral (*left*) and cross-sectional (*right*) schematic views of internal carotid artery demonstrate initial phase of intramedial and subintimal dissecting aneurysm; the three basic arterial layers (intima, media, and adventitia) are delineated. (**B**) Comparable views of progression of intramedial hemorrhage; arterial lumen is reduced in size. (**C**) Comparable views of an intramedial hemorrhage that dissects into the subadventitial, rather than the subintimal plane, as in Figs. A and B; large pseudoaneurysm results. (**D**) Dissecting hemorrhage ruptures through the intima, establishing communication with the true lumen; recanalization may occur, enlarging true and/or false lumen. (From Friedman et al.,[51] with permission.)

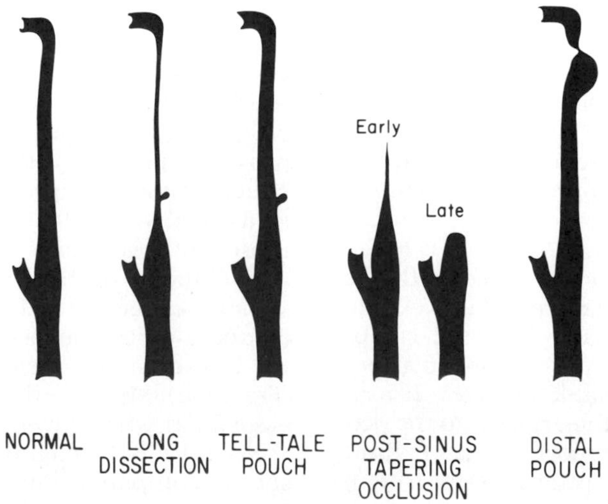


**Fig. 24-3.** Arteriographic features of carotid dissection. (From Fisher et al.,[47] with permission.)

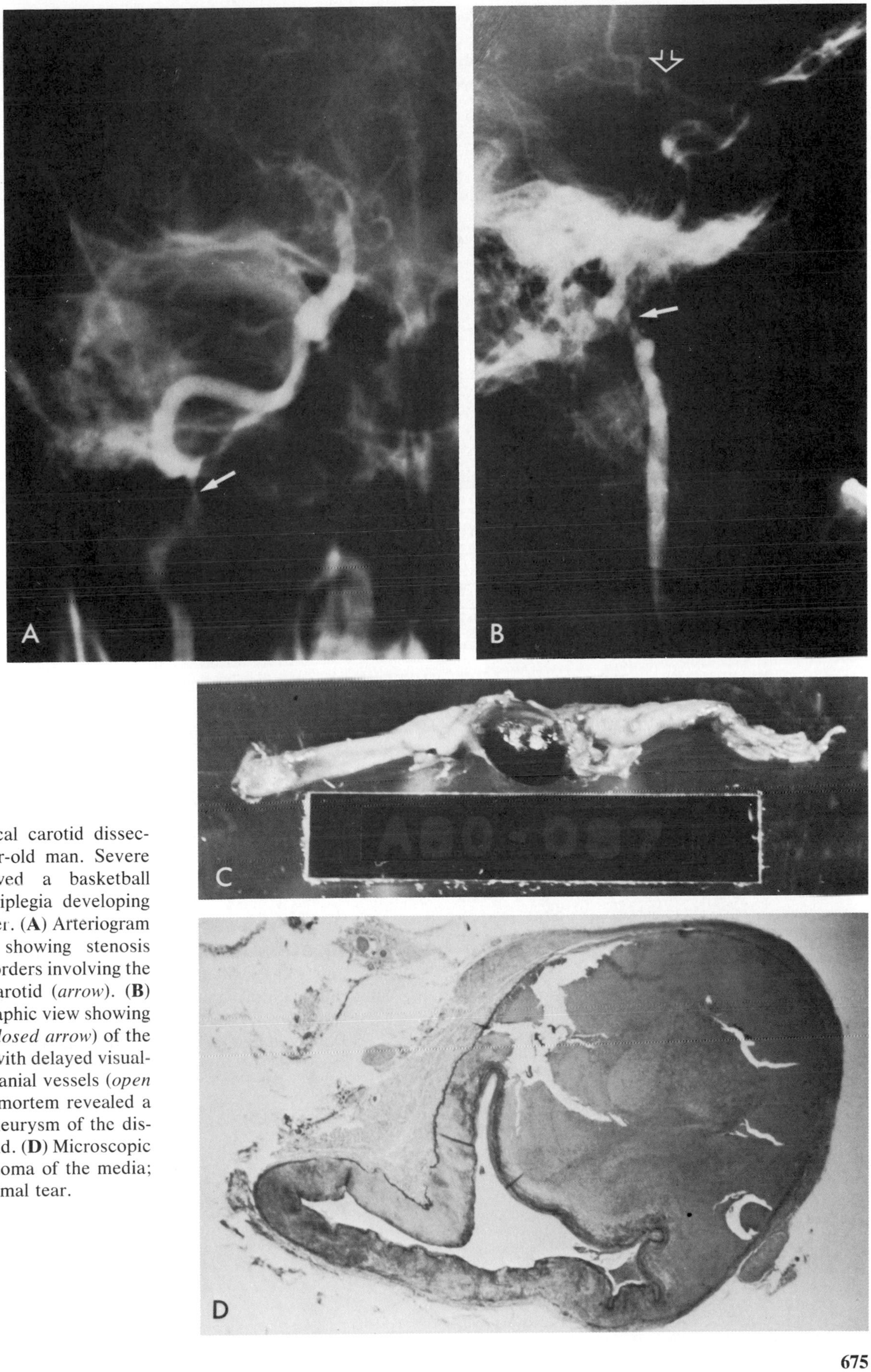


**Fig. 24-4.** Cervical carotid dissection in a 37-year-old man. Severe headache followed a basketball game, with hemiplegia developing several hours later. (**A**) Arteriogram (anterior view) showing stenosis with scalloped borders involving the distal cervical carotid (*arrow*). (**B**) Lateral arteriographic view showing distal stenosis (*closed arrow*) of the cervical carotid with delayed visualization of intracranial vessels (*open arrow*). (**C**) Postmortem revealed a 1.5-cm pseudoaneurysm of the distal cervical carotid. (**D**) Microscopic section of hematoma of the media; there was no intimal tear.

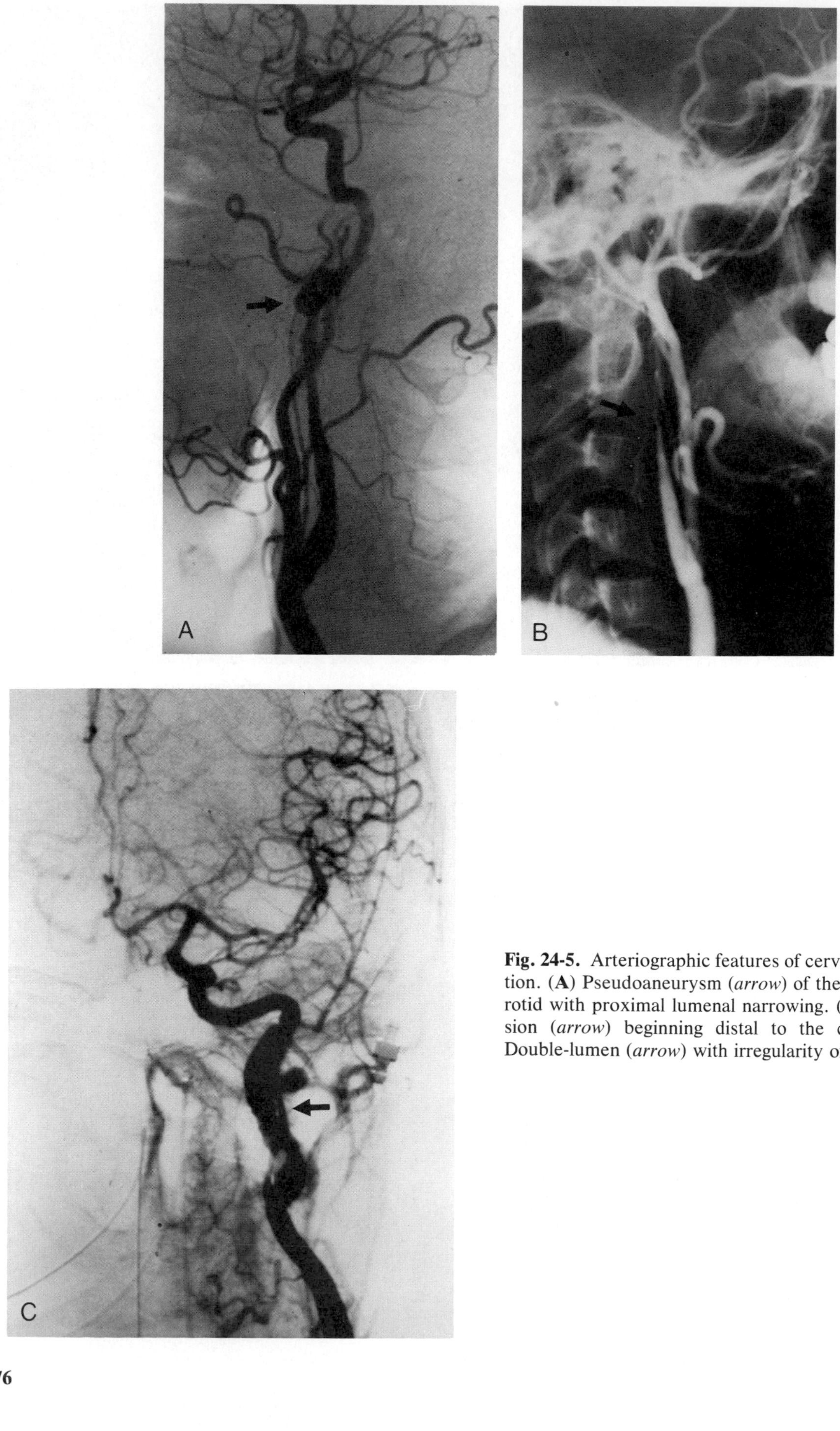


**Fig. 24-5.** Arteriographic features of cervical carotid dissection. (**A**) Pseudoaneurysm (*arrow*) of the distal cervical carotid with proximal lumenal narrowing. (**B**) Tapered occlusion (*arrow*) beginning distal to the carotid sinus. (**C**) Double-lumen (*arrow*) with irregularity of the entire lumen.

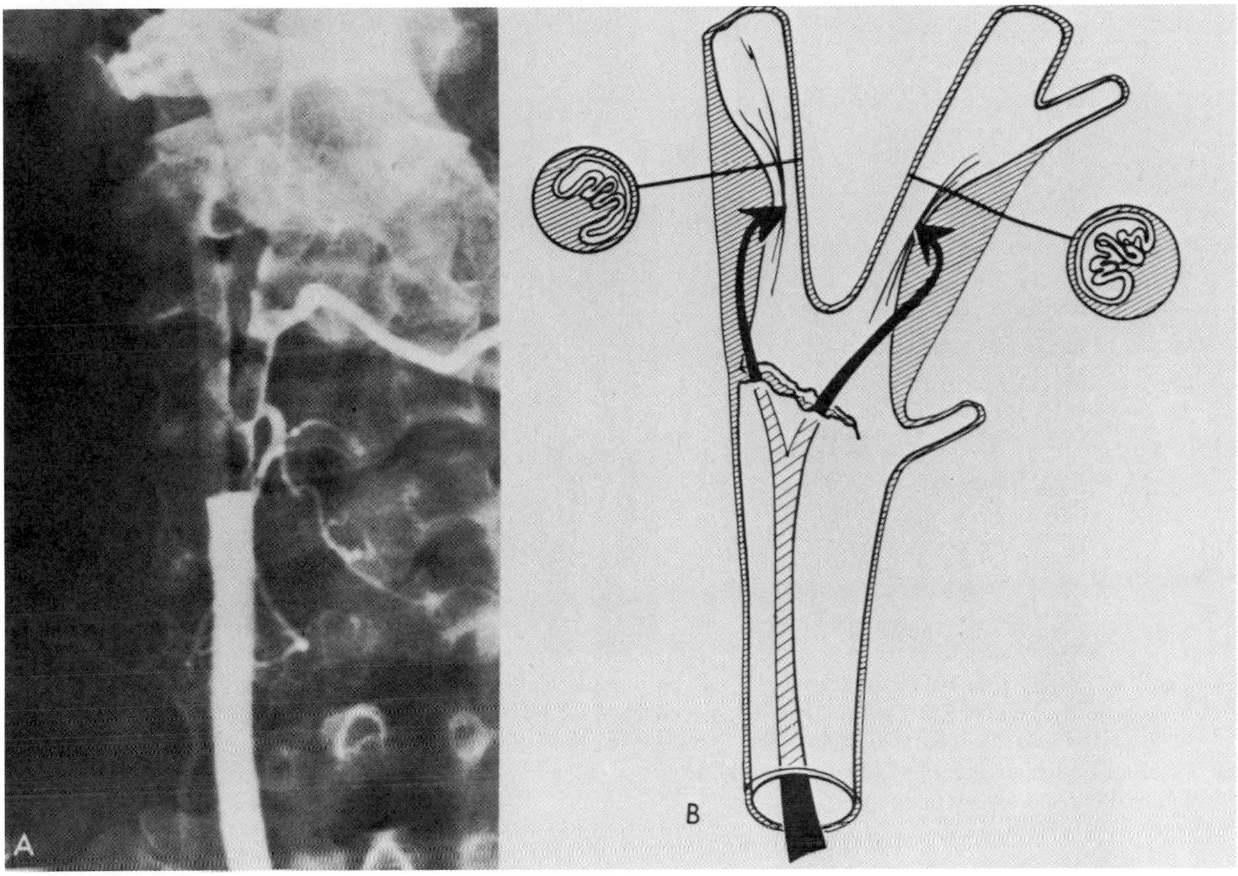


**Fig. 24-6.** A 32-year-old man experienced sudden hemiparesis. (**A**) Arteriography demonstrates a sharp cutoff of contrast at the common carotid bifurcation, with faint visualization of distal vessels. Exploration revealed a transverse intimal tear with subintimal dissection of blood. (**B**) Artist's concept of intimal tear with subintimal dissection of blood and occlusion of the lumen. The insets of the internal and external carotid arteries in cross-section graphically depict luminal compromise. (From Moore,[106] with permission.)

clinically atypical cases, supplement arteriographic diagnosis in confirmed dissection, and permit serial monitoring of lesion evolution. Extracranial Doppler studies typically show reduced or absent internal carotid artery flow at the level of the carotid bifurcation without evidence of atheroma, providing indirect evidence of distal stenosis or occlusion due to dissection.[18,39,44,69,125,138] Less often, sonographic duplex imaging may demonstrate directly a tapering luminal stenosis and/or a double lumen.[39,69,138] MR imaging shows particular promise in the diagnosis of dissection.[23,32,58,60,92,125,144] Because of its ability to visualize hematomas within the wall of dissected arteries in addition to luminal stenosis or occlusion, MR often may provide a more specific indication of dissection than conventional angiography (Fig. 24-7).[58,60]

Early reports emphasized major, often fatal, stroke as the sequel of cervical carotid dissection. Recent experience suggests a more benign outcome in most patients, with major stroke occurring in only 10 to 20 percent of patients (Table 24-2). Most ischemic symptoms evolve over a few hours to several days, and recurrent TIAs often precede major stroke. Dissections may present with hemicrania and oculosympathetic paresis without ischemic symptoms.[12,35,104,147]

Treatment of carotid dissections, as well as vertebral, is discussed below.

## TRAUMATIC INJURY OF THE CERVICAL CAROTID ARTERY

Major nonpenetrating trauma can damage the carotid artery either directly or by a rotational-stretch injury involving the upper cervical vertebra (Fig. 24-1).[9,27,36,37,59,78,99,152] Intimal or medial disruption may then result in thrombosis, with or without dissection.[48,127,137] Most nonpenetrating carotid injuries are associated with motor vehicle accidents, but bar fights, chiropractic manipulation, falls, strangulation and hanging have also caused traumatic carotid artery injury.[27,96,137] Although there may be associated

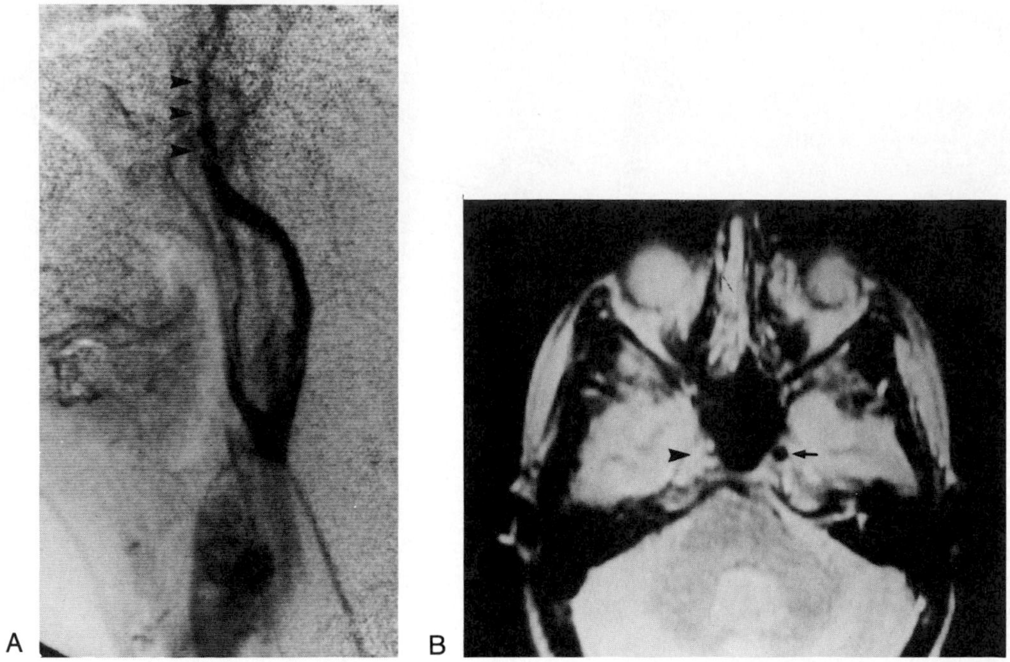


**Fig. 24-7.** Right internal carotid artery dissection in a 30-year-old woman. **(A)** Arteriogram demonstrates stenosis of the distal right internal carotid artery (arrowheads). **(B)** Axial T2-weighted MRI (TE 95 ms, TR 2000 ms) shows crescentic high intensity signal (arrowhead) from intramural hematoma surrounding the residual lumen of the right internal carotid artery. Compare with normal signal void from opposite, left internal carotid artery (arrow).

**TABLE 24-2. Survey of the Literature on Outcome of Management in 100 Patients**

| Presenting Feature[a] | Patients' Outcomes: Normal | Minor Deficit[b] | Major Deficit or Death |
|---|---|---|---|
| Major stroke (18 cases) | | | |
| No Rx or APT | 0/13 | 1/13 | 12/13 |
| Anticoagulant | 1/4 | 2/4 | 1/4 |
| Surgery | 0 | 1/1 | 0 |
| Single TIA or minor stroke (45 cases) | | | |
| No Rx or APT | 15/17 | 2/17 | 0 |
| Anticoagulant | 14/16 | 1/16 | 1/16 |
| Surgery | 6/12 | 5/12 | 1/12 |
| Multiple TIA (15 cases) | | | |
| No Rx or APT | 6/6 | 0 | 0 |
| Anticoagulant | 5/5 | 0 | 0 |
| Surgery | 3/4 | 1/4 | 0 |
| Other (pain, tinnitus) (22 cases) | | | |
| No Rx or APT | 18/20 | 1/20 | 1/20 |
| Anticoagulant | 2/2 | 0 | 0 |
| Surgery | 0 | 0 | 0 |
| Total in percent | 70% | 14% | 16% |

*Abbreviations:* Rx, medical therapy; APT, antiplatelet therapy; TIA, transient ischemic attack.

[a] Major complaint on presentation to physician, not necessarily the initial symptom.

[b] Nondisabling deficit, residual Horner syndrome considered normal.

(Data from 100 cases from English-language literature since 1975 on extracranial carotid dissection. Summarized in Hart and Easton[65] plus several recent studies given in references 11, 19, 55, 75, 90.)

subcutaneous hematomas, or fractures of the mandible or cervical spine, in about half of patients there is no evidence of neck injury.[27,137] In children, nonpenetrating carotid injury is frequently due to falls with blunt objects (e.g., toothbrushes, pencils) in the mouth contusing the artery.[48,118]

Frequently, nonpenetrating carotid artery injury occurs in association with a cerebral concussion or contusion, and the onset of symptoms is difficult to discern. Ipsilateral headache and neck pain are common. However, like spontaneous dissections, a lucid interval is the rule, with focal deficits occurring several hours to a few days after the trauma. Often, carotid occlusion or dissection is an unexpected finding in patients who deteriorate after head trauma and in whom a subdural hematoma or a delayed intracerebral hematoma is suspected. Based on the frequent finding of apparent embolic occlusion of distal vessels, embolism of thrombus from the site of injury is believed to be a common mechanism of cerebral ischemia in these dissections also. Delayed embolism may explain the lucid interval. Oculosympathetic paresis is common and, when present in obtunded trauma patients, should suggest traumatic carotid injury.

Angiography in patients with nonpenetrating carotid injury usually demonstrates occlusion of the distal cervical carotid artery, but the characteristic features of dissection may occasionally be present.[36] Intimal flaps and pseudoaneurysms may be more frequent with traumatic carotid dissection than with their spontaneous counterpart.[99,137] In a minority, intrapetrous carotid occlusion occurs, usually associated with basilar skull fractures.[1,4] Major stroke is the most commonly reported neurologic sequel of carotid artery trauma, possibly due to underrecognition of less afflicted patients.[1]

The optimal therapy of this disorder is controversial. Arteriotomy with thrombectomy and repair of intimal flaps has been advocated, especially in patients with submassive neurologic deficits.[27,111] An initial medical approach, using anticoagulation and follow-up arteriography, is a reasonable alternative.[137,152]

Penetrating injury to the carotid artery is more frequently reported than nonpenetrating trauma.[27,36,59] Most such injuries are caused by gunshot or knife wounds and result in tangential laceration of the carotid artery, with simultaneous involvement of the internal jugular vein in about one-fourth of patients. The carotid artery is occasionally injured, complicating local surgical procedures. Tonsillectomy, transphenoidal pituitary surgery, radical neck dissection, and percutaneous radiofrequency trigeminal rhizolysis have all been associated with symptomatic carotid injury. Penetrating carotid injuries may cause cerebral ischemia by either interruption of flow or distal embolism of thrombi. Resulting neck hematomas can cause tracheal compression. Brachial plexus injury, ipsilateral tongue weakness from hypoglossal nerve involvement, and oculosympathetic paresis may coexist. Formation of pseudoaneurysms and arteriovenous fistulas may result. There is controversy concerning whether angiography should precede immediate surgical exploration in suspected cases of penetrating carotid injury.[27,54] Primary arterial repair, with or without patch grafts, has supplanted carotid ligation as the preferred treatment.[83] However, proximal and distal ligation is often recommended for penetrating injury of the cervical vertebral artery[94] to prevent emboli.

## INTRACRANIAL CAROTID SYSTEM DISSECTION

Several clinical features warrant the distinction of dissections involving the intracranial carotid and middle cerebral arteries from those of the extracranial carotid artery. Intracranial dissections are infrequently reported.[108,150] Because specific angiographic features are lacking for these dissections, pathologic diagnosis has probably resulted in their underrecognition, especially of nonfatal cases. The age profile is younger than for cervical dissection, with the average age being the mid-20s, and perhaps half of the patients are under age 16.[65,150] Ipsilateral headache, usually severe, immediately precedes or coexists with the onset of neurologic deficit in almost all patients. Major stroke has been the rule, with evolution often occurring over several days. Aggregate reports show a 75 percent mortality. As noted, however, autopsied cases dominate the literature, and milder forms may be unrecognized. Subarachnoid hemorrhage can be associated with these dissections.[2,88] A relationship of intracranial arterial dissection to intense physical exertion or trivial trauma has been often noted. Bilateral intracranial carotid dissection has also been reported, separated by 6 weeks to 18 months.[3,28,88,107]

Arteriograms typically reveal irregular, scalloped stenosis of the arteries, resembling a string of beads, or total occlusion following irregular narrowing.[63,65,98] A double lumen is infrequently demonstrated but is specific for dissection. Intracranial dissection usually involves the middle cerebral or the supraclinoid carotid artery, and the latter occasionally extends into the anterior cerebral artery. Pseudoaneurysms are rarely seen in intracranial dissections, possibly due to the subintimal location of most hemorrhages. Arteriographic features usually do not allow the diagnosis of intracranial arterial dissection to be made with certainty. Arteritis, moyamoya disease, embolic occlusion, and fibromuscular dysplasia are often the initial radiologic considerations. MR may demonstrate intramural hemorrhage, enabling more definitive diagnosis.[23,58]

Intracranial carotid dissection has been associated with cystic medial necrosis, fibromuscular dysplasia, moyamoya disease, atherosclerosis, homocystinuria, and intimal fibroelastic abnormalities, but often no microscopic abnormalities are identified.[23,45,98,109,115,117] Intimal abnormalities, presumably developmental, have been recognized in some pathologic studies of intracranial dissection.[41,68,84,98,117,149] These intimal changes may represent a spectrum that underlies dissections, moyamoya disease, and intimal fibromuscular dysplasia. Despite the potential developmental predisposition, familial clustering has not been reported. The occurrence in patients with migraine has been occasionally reported.[134,135] Surprisingly, the association of intracranial dissections with oral contraceptive use, which may induce intimal proliferation of intracranial vessels, has been rarely noted.[24] Hypoperfusion as a direct result of luminal obstruction at the dissection site appears to be the usual mechanism of ischemia.

## VERTEBROBASILAR ARTERY DISSECTION

Dissection of the cervical and intracranial arteries of the posterior circulation is characterized by the sudden onset of pain, frequently severe and localized to the craniocervical region, followed by the abrupt, delayed, or progressive onset of ischemic symptoms.

Dissection of the cervical vertebral artery is most often related to sudden mechanical injury of the artery from rotational forces (Fig. 24-8).[52,53,91,131,132] Most cases have been associated with chiropractic or other

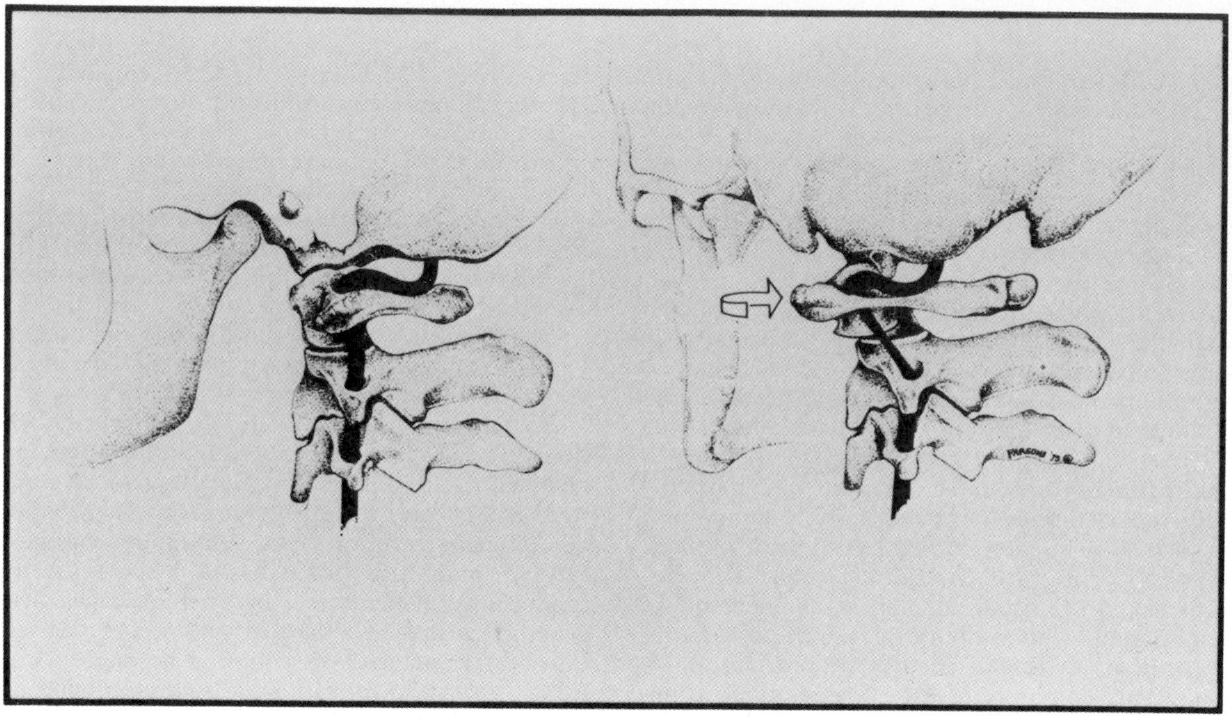

**Fig. 24-8.** Vertebral artery injury with abrupt cervical rotation. The vertebral artery is subject to stretch and mechanical trauma between C1 and C2 when the neck is vigorously rotated and extended. (From Barnett,[8] with permission.)

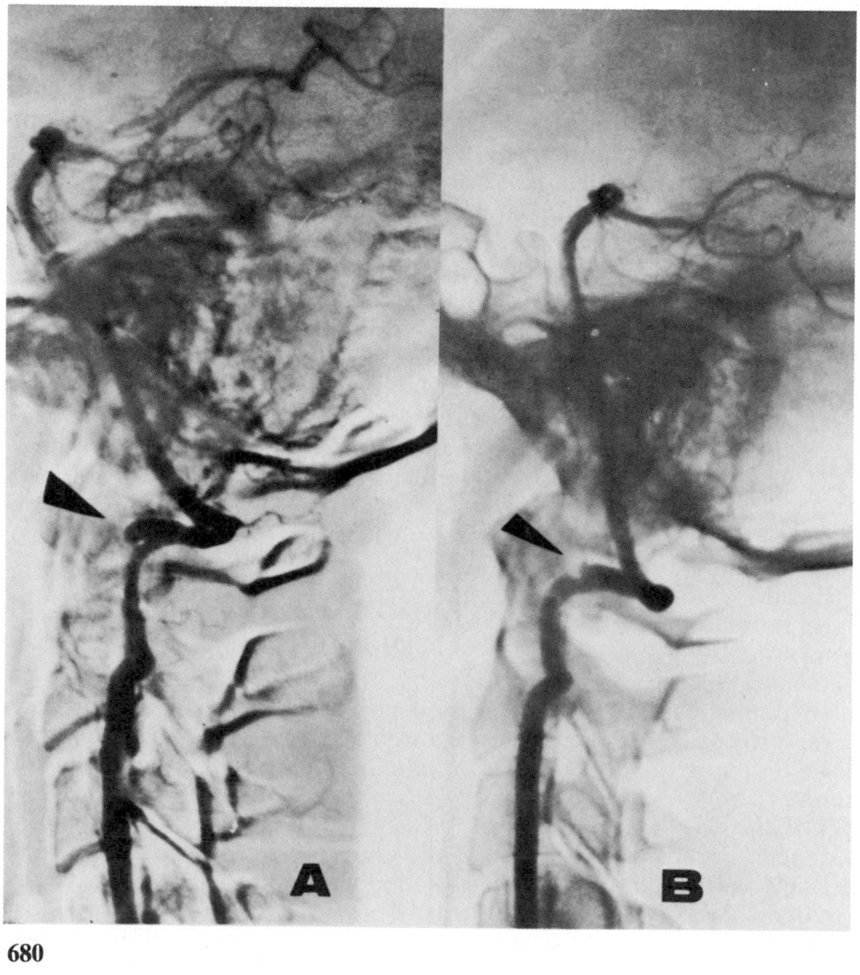


**Fig. 24-9.** Distal vertebral artery dissection associated with cervical chiropractic manipulation. (**A**) Irregular narrowing of the left vertebral artery at the level of C1 with pseudoaneurysm (*arrowhead*). (**B**) One month later, following anticoagulation, there is partial resolution (*arrowhead*). (From Sherman et al.,[131] with permission.)

neck manipulation, but minor falls, automobile accidents, ceiling painting, yoga, trampoline exercise, vigorously spanking a child, archery practice, and spontaneous, sudden head turning have all resulted in vertebral artery dissections.[77,131] Patient ages have ranged from the 1st through the 7th decades, with a mean age of 39 years.[52,70,131] Females may be affected slightly more often than males.[52,70] Narrowing or occlusion of the vessel, with associated pseudoaneurysm formation, is typically demonstrated at angiography (Fig. 24-9). The vertebral artery is most mobile, and thus most susceptible to mechanical injury, at the C1 to C2 level as it leaves the transverse foramen of the axis and abruptly turns to enter the intracranial cavity. The C1 to C2 site is involved in 80 to 90 percent of rotation-related dissections.[52,70]

Extracranial vertebral artery dissections that are not related to sudden cervical rotation are somewhat less common.[15,20,26,30,50,61,70,74,87,89,100,122,136] An association of these spontaneous dissections with cystic medial degeneration, arteritis, fibromuscular dysplasia, Marfan syndrome, and migraine has been reported.[16,30,34,70,89,122,130,134,136,151] Women are affected 2.5 times more frequently than men.[70] Dissection may affect the artery at any site, but the C1 to C2 level is most frequently involved, suggesting that mechanical factors may play a role even in cases with no apparent history of rotation or injury.[26,30,70,90,100]

The course and prognosis of extracranial vertebral artery dissection are variable (Table 24-3). Many patients suffer delayed or progressive infarction early in their course. The most frequent ischemic presentation is a lateral medullary syndrome, with cerebellar, occipital, or more extensive brain stem infarction possibly admixed. As unilateral vertebral artery occlusion, especially if proximal, may not cause ischemia due to adequate contralateral vertebral flow, it seems likely that unilateral vertebral artery dissections are underrecognized, explaining the surprisingly high prevalence in the literature of simultaneous bilateral vertebral dissections and concurrent vertebral and carotid dissections, accounting for one-half of all reported cases .[64] As experience with noninvasive ultrasound and MR diagnosis of vertebral artery dissection increases, a greater proportion of midly symptomatic cases may be recognized.[121]

**TABLE 24-3. Clinical Features of Extracranial Vertebral Dissection[a]**

| Clinical Data | Percent |
|---|---|
| *Sex* | |
| Male | 32 |
| Female | 68 |
| *Laterality* | |
| Bilateral | 35 |
| Unilateral | 65 |
| Left | 57 |
| Right | 43 |
| *Clinical features* | |
| Transient ischemic attack (not progressing to CVA) | 22 |
| Cerebral infarction | 69 |
| Neck pain | 50 |
| Headache | 59 |
| Neck or head pain | 74 |
| Preceding focal symptoms | 63 |
| Lateral medullary symptoms | 34 |
| *Outcome* | |
| Neurologically normal, or mild deficits only | 83 |
| Moderate or severe deficits/death | 7/9 |
| Normal or mildly stenotic vessel on follow-up imaging | 78 |
| Late stroke | 2.5 |
| Subsequent cervicocephalic dissection | 5 |

*Abbreviation:* CVA, cerebrovascular accident.
[a] Age of patients: mean, 39 years; range, 7 to 64 years.
(Aggregate data from 116 cases gathered from references 15, 26, 30, 53, 70, 89, 100, 151.)

In contrast to extracranial carotid and vertebral artery dissections, isolated intracranial vertebral artery dissections are more common in men than women.[17,25] The frequent occurrence of subarachnoid hemorrhage (more than half of reported cases) distinguishes the clinical picture from that of extracranial vertebral artery dissection.[13,50,133] Serious brain stem infarction occurs in less than one-third of patients, and occasionally patients present with aneurysms acting as mass lesions, compressing the brain stem and lower cranial nerves.[40,97] Angiography most commonly demonstrates aneurysmal dilation of the intracranial vertebral artery, at or near the origin of the posterior inferior cerebellar artery. Pathologic examination reveals subadventitial or transmural dissection with aneurysm formation in most cases of subarachnoid hemorrhage, while subintimal dissection with luminal compromise is more characteristic among the less frequent cases presenting with ischemia.

Primary dissections of the basilar artery are rare, and less is known about them than about other cervicocerebral dissections.[2,5,14,24,45,67,79,150] Intimal fibroelastic abnormalities have been reported.[2,14,24] Subadventitial or transmural hemorrhage may result in subarachnoid bleeding and the formation of large pseudoaneurysms.[2,5,45,61,88,150] The mean age of these patients is 35 years, and males and females are equally affected.[17] The initial symptoms are similar to those of distal vertebral dissections, save for the location of the resultant neurologic deficits.[76] The prognosis is much more guarded, with fatal issue in the large majority of cases.[17] Basilar artery dissection associated with chronic migraine has been reported.[5] Spontaneous dissection of the superior cerebellar artery associated with fibromuscular dysplasia has been reported.[76]

## RECURRENCE

The risk of recurrent dissection, or subsequent dissection in another artery, is small but real.[20,33] Review of case series published since 1983 uncovered nine patients who presented with extracranial cervicocephalic dissections and subsequent cervicocephalic or renal artery dissections. The recurrence rate of cervicocephalic dissection in our review, among patients followed for more than 1 year (mean 4 years), was 3 percent for carotid and 5 percent for vertebral system dissections.

Sellier et al.[129] reported two patients with dissection of the contralateral internal carotid artery 3 and 7 years after the initial dissection. D'Anglejan Chatillon et al.[35] described a patient with dissection of the contralateral internal carotid artery 3 years after the initial dissection in a patient with fibromuscular dysplasia treated with antiplatelet agents. They described another patient with bilateral dissection of the internal carotid arteries 14 years after the initial one in a woman without a known arteropathy, on no treatment at the time of the recurrence. Youl et al. reported an asymptomatic vertebral artery dissection[151] discovered incidentally in a patient with Marfan syndrome at the time of follow-up angiography 3 months after an internal carotid artery dissection. Bogousslavsky et al.[18] reported the recurrence of an internal carotid artery dissection 32 months after an initial one. Mokri and colleagues[100,105] reported an internal carotid artery dissection 5 years after a dissection of a vertebral artery, the dissection of a vertebral artery 2 years after a dissection of the contralateral vertebral artery, and the dissection of a renal artery 8 years after bilateral dissection of the internal carotid arteries.

Of these eight late cervicocephalic dissections, two were recurrent in the same vessel. Only one had a multiarterial dissection originally. The subsequent dissection occurred a mean of 4.6 years after the initial event.

## TREATMENT

The proper management of extracranial cervicocerebral dissections is controversial. Several medical and surgical treatments have been used in patients with cervical carotid dissection, precluding more than a general comparison of outcomes (Table 24-2). Most patients do well, either because of or despite treatment. While the use of heparin might seem to be contraindicated in a disorder involving hemorrhage into the arterial wall, most cerebral injury appears to result from secondary thrombotic and embolic complications of the dissection. Thus anticoagulation, with heparin followed by warfarin, is often recommended.[29,47,93] Repeat angiography is usually undertaken before discontinuing therapy.[145]

The time course of healing of the vessel wall guides the duration of therapy. Approximately 85 percent of extracranial carotid dissection-related stenoses, 51 percent of occlusions, and 43 percent of aneurysms are found to have improved or returned to normal at the time of follow-up angiography. Serial ultrasound studies show that the median time to resolution of carotid dissections is 6 weeks, most arteries recover by 3 months, and vessels that fail to reconstitute a normal lumen by 6 months are highly unlikely to improve thereafter.[18,21,42,43,47,56,57,69,85,110,119] A therapeutic algorithm for extracranial carotid dissection based on this emerging picture of lesion evolution is depicted in Figure 24-10. In general, once the dissection has largely resolved, the anticoagulant is discontinued over a 2-week period. If the artery is still abnormal, the anticoagulant is continued for several more weeks or months until the dissection has healed. Platelet antiaggregation agents, after an initial period of heparin administration, are recommended for patients in whom warfarin anticoagulation is not feasible. Consideration of surgery is reserved for patients with localized, accessible lesions who experience further ischemia despite medical therapy.

Activities predisposing to abrupt cervical rotation should probably be avoided in survivors of dissection. Estrogen-containing compounds, which are associated with fibromuscular and intimal arterial proliferation, are empirically discontinued.

We apply these same principles to patients with extracranial vertebral artery dissection. The less extensive data available suggests that the natural history of these dissections roughly parallels extracranial carotid dissections. We anticoagulate these patients if the dissection does not extend intracranially, or if the cerebrospinal fluid (CSF) does not contain blood.

Late strokes—infarctions occurring after discharge from the initial hospitalization—are infrequent among both extracranial carotid and vertebral dissections. Among 257 patients with long-term follow-up (mean 4 years), fewer than 2 percent experienced late cerebral infarction, and most of these occurred in the first year. While higher than might otherwise be expected in this relatively young population, this late stroke rate is low enough to suggest it will be difficult to obtain definitive information about the proper postacute treatment of arterial dissections. Even if the stroke rate were as high as 5 percent in the first year after dissection, a sample size of approximately 1,600 patients would be required to compare two treatments with an 80 percent chance of detecting a 50 percent reduction in events ($\alpha = 0.05$; 2-tailed). It seems unlikely that such a randomized trial will be carried out.

Several anecdotal reports of subarachnoid bleeding associated with *intracranial* dissections, as well as progression of deficits during treatment with heparin, suggest caution in the early anticoagulation of patients with these dissections.[2,63,71,88] However, radiographic distinction from embolic obstruction, which may warrant anticoagulation, is often difficult. Immediate anastomosis of the superficial temporal artery to the middle cerebral artery has been proposed for intracranial carotid dissections, but is of unproven value. Bed rest and observation may be a judicious

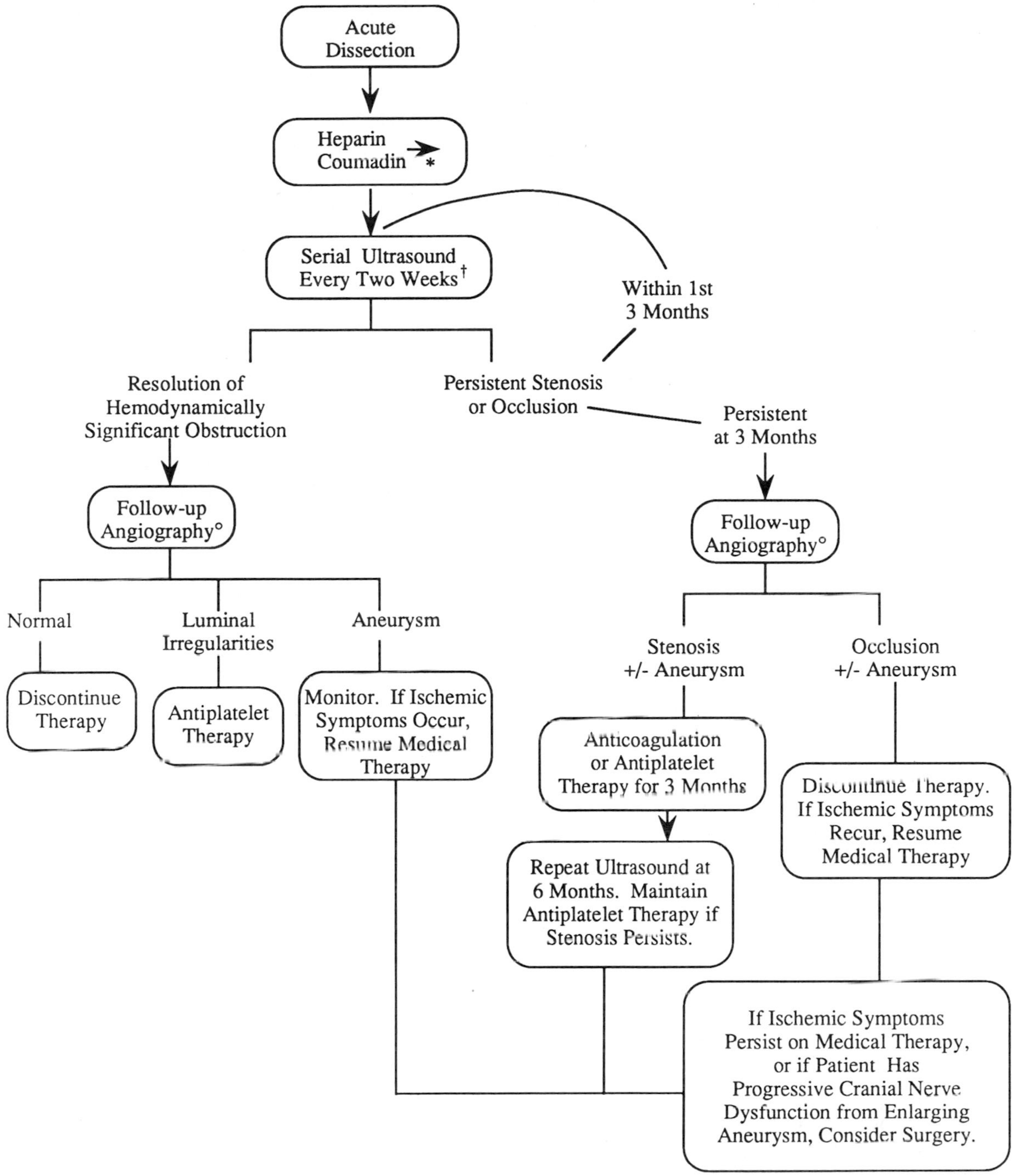


*Defer anticoagulation if patient has large or massive infarction, hemorrhagic infarction, intracranial extension with subarachnoid hemorrhage, or other contraindication.

†If ultrasound is not available, treat with anticoagulation and proceed to angiography at three months.

°As more experience is gained with MR, MR scanning and MR angiography may supplant conventional angiography at this decision point.

**Fig. 24-10.** Algorithm for the therapy of extracranial carotid artery dissection. MR, magnetic resonance.

initial approach. Though conservative treatment of dissections causing subarachnoid hemorrhage has been successful, fatal rebleeding is disturbingly common and urgent surgical management has been recommended.[25,45,50,64,133] Recurrent, contralateral intracranial dissections have been reported, but their frequency is uncertain. The impressive relationship of these dissections to intense exertion and minor trauma in many patients suggests that avoidance of vigorous activity and contact sports in survivors of dissection may be reasonable advice.

## REFERENCES


1. Aarabi B, McQueen JD: Traumatic internal carotid occlusion at the base of the skull. Surg Neurol 10:233, 1978
2. Adams HP, Jr, Aschenbrener CA, Kassell NF et al: Intracranial hemorrhage produced by spontaneous dissecting intracranial aneurysm. Arch Neurol 39:773, 1982
3. Adelman LS, Doe FD, Samat HB: Bilateral dissecting aneurysms of the internal carotid arteries. Acta Neuropathol 29:93, 1974
4. Ajir F, Tibbetts JC: Post-traumatic occlusion of the supraclinoid internal carotid artery. Neurosurgery 9:173, 1981
5. Alexander CB, Burger PC, Goree JA: Dissecting aneurysms of the basilar artery in 2 patients. Stroke 10:294, 1979
6. Anderson CA, Collins GJ, Jr, Rich NM et al: Spontaneous dissection of the internal carotid artery associated with fibromuscular dysplasia. Am Surg 4:263, 1980
7. Austin MG, Schaefer RF: Marfan's syndrome, with unusual blood vessel manifestations. Arch Pathol 64:205, 1957
8. Barnett HJM: Progress towards stroke prevention. Robert Wartenberg Lecture. Neurology (NY) 30:1212, 1980
9. Batzdorf U, Bentson JR, Machleder HI: Blunt trauma to the high cervical carotid artery. Neurosurgery 5:195, 1979
10. Bellot J, Gheradi R, Poirer J et al: Fibromuscular dysplasia of cervico-cephalic arteries with multiple dissections and a carotid-cavernous fistula. Stroke 16:255, 1985
11. Benoit BG, Russell NA, Grimes JD et al: Spontaneous dissection of carotid and vertebral arteries; management considerations. Can J Neurol Sci 11:328, 1984
12. Benrabah R, Bousser MG, Cabanis EA et al: Syndrome de Claude Bernard-Horner douloureux revelateur d'une dissection spontanée de l'artère carotide interne intérêt du bilan ultrasonique cervical: à propos de 2 observations. Bull Soc Ophthalmol France 6:763, 1988
13. Berger MS, Wilson CB: Intracranial dissecting aneurysms of the posterior circulation. J Neurosurg 61:882, 1984
14. Berkovic SF, Spokes RL, Anderson RM, Bladin PF: Basilar artery dissection. J Neurol Neurosurg Psychiatry 46:126, 1983
15. Biller J, Hingtgen WL, Adams HP, Jr et al: Cervicocephalic arterial dissections: a ten-year experience. Arch Neurol 43:1234, 1986
16. Bladin PF: Dissecting aneurysm of carotid and vertebral arteries. Vasc Surg 8:203, 1974
17. Bogousslavsky J: Dissections of the cerebral arteries: clinical effects. Curr Opin Neurol Neurosurg 1:63, 1988
18. Bogousslavsky J, Despland PA, Regli F: Spontaneous carotid dissection with acute stroke. Arch Neurol 44:137, 1987
19. Bogousslavsky J, Regli F, Despland PA: Aneurysmes disséquants spontanes de l'artère carotide interne. Rev Neurol (Paris) 11:625, 1984
20. Bostrom K, Liliequist B: Primary dissecting aneurysm of the extracranial part of the internal carotid and vertebral arteries. Neurology (NY) 17:179, 1967
21. Bradac GB, Kaernbach A, Bolk-Weischedel D et al: Spontaneous dissecting aneurysm of cervical cerebral arteries. Neuroradiology 21:149, 1981
22. Brice JG, Crompton MR: Spontaneous dissecting aneurysms of the cervical internal carotid artery. Br Med J 2:790, 1964
23. Brugieres P, Castrec-Carpo A, Heran F et al: Magnetic resonance imaging in the exploration of dissection of the internal carotid artery. J Neuroradiol 16:1, 1989
24. Bugiani O, Piola P, Tabaton M: Nontraumatic dissecting aneurysm of the basilar artery. Eur Neurol 22:256, 1983
25. Caplan LR, Baquis GD, Pessin MS et al: Dissection of the intracranial vertebral artery. Neurol 38:868, 1988
26. Caplan LR, Zarins CK, Hemmati M: Spontaneous dissection of the extracranial vertebral arteries. Stroke 16:1030, 1985
27. Chandler WF, Coon JV, Ericus MS: Carotid Arteries Injuries. Futura, Mt. Kisco, NY, 1982
28. Chang V, Rewcastle NB, Harwood-Nash DCF et al: Bilateral dissecting aneurysms of the intracranial internal carotid arteries in an 8-year-old boy. Neurology (NY) 25:573, 1975
29. Chapleau CE, Robertson JT: Spontaneous cervical carotid artery dissection: outpatient treatment with continuous heparin infusion using a totally implantable infusion device. Neurosurgery 8:83, 1981
30. Chiras J, Marciano S, Vega Molina J et al: Spontaneous dissecting aneurysm of the extracranial vertebral artery (20 cases). Neuroradiology 27:327, 1985
31. Collins GJ, Jr, Rich NM, Clagett GP et al: Fibromuscular dysplasia of the internal carotid arteries. Ann Surg 194:89, 1981
32. Cox LK, Bertorini T, Laster RE, Jr: Headaches due to spontaneous carotid artery dissection: magnetic resonance imaging evaluation and follow-up. Headache 31:12, 1991
33. Cusick JF, Daniels D: Spontaneous reversal of internal carotid artery occlusion. J Neurosurg 54:811, 1981

34. D'Anglejan-Chatillon J, Ribeiro V, Mas JL et al: Migraine—a risk factor for dissection of cervical arteries. Headache 29:560, 1989
35. D'Anglejan Chatillon J, Ribeiro V, Mas JL et al: Dissection de l'artère carotide interne extracranienne: soixante-deux observations. Presse Med 19:661, 1990
36. Davis JM, Zimmerman RA: Injury of the carotid and vertebral arteries. Neuroradiology 25:55, 1983
37. Davis JW, Holbrook TL, Hoyt DB et al: Blunt carotid artery dissection: incidence, associated injuries, screening and treatment. J Trauma 30:1514, 1990
38. De Baets P, Delanote G, Jackers G et al: Atherosclerotic dissection of the cervical internal carotid artery—a case report. Angiology 41:161, 1990
39. de Bray JM, Dubas F, Joseph PA et al: Étude ultrasonique de 22 dissections carotidiennes. Rev Neurol 145:702, 1989
40. De Busscher J: Aneurysme de l'artère vertébrale gauche chez un homme 45 ans. Acta Neurol Psychiatr Belg 52:1, 1952
41. Deck JHN: Pathology of spontaneous dissection of intracranial arteries. Can J Neurol Sci 14:88, 1987
42. Deramond H, Remond A, Rosat P et al: Spontaneous evolution of nontraumatic dissecting aneurysms of the cervical portion of the internal carotid artery. J Neuroradiology 17:167, 1980
43. Ehrenfeld WK, Wylie EJ: Spontaneous dissection of the internal carotid artery. Arch Surg 111:1294, 1976
44. Eljamel MSM, Humphrey PRD, Shaw MDM: Dissection of the cervical internal carotid artery. the role of Doppler/duplex studies and conservative management. J Neurol Neurosurg Psychiatry 53:379, 1990
45. Farrell MA, Gilbert JJ, Kaufmann JC: Fatal intracranial arterial dissection: clinical pathological correlation. J Neurol Neurosurg Psychiatry 48:111, 1985
46. Fisher CM: The headache and pain of spontaneous carotid dissection. Headache 22:60, 1982
47. Fisher CM, Ojemann RG, Roberson GH: Spontaneous dissection of cervico-cerebral arteries. Can J Neurol Sci 5:9, 1978
48. Fleming JFR, Petrie D: Traumatic thrombosis of the internal carotid artery with delayed hemiplegia. Can J Surg 11:166, 1968
49. Francis KR, Williams DP, Troost BT: Facial numbness and dyesthesia: new features of carotid artery dissection. Arch Neurol 44:345, 1987
50. Friedman AH, Drake CG: Subarachnoid hemorrhage from intracranial dissecting aneurysm. J Neurosurg 60:325, 1984
51. Friedman WA, Day AL, Quisling RG, Jr et al: Cervical carotid dissecting aneurysms. Neurosurgery 7:207, 1980
52. Frisoni GB, Anzola GP: Vertebrobasilar ischemia after neck motion. Stroke 22:1452, 1991
53. Frumkin LR, Baloh RW: Wallenberg's syndrome following neck manipulation. Neurology (NY) 40:611, 1990
54. Fry RE, Fry WJ: Extracranial carotid artery injuries. Surgery 88:581, 1980
55. Garcia-Merino JA, Gutierrez JA, Lopez-Lozano JJ: Double-lumen dissecting aneurysms of the internal carotid artery in fibromuscular dysplasia: a case report. Stroke 14:815, 1983
56. Gauthier G, Rohr J, Wildi E, Megret M: L'hématome disséquant spontane de l'artère carotide interne. 136:53, 1985
57. Gee W, Kaupp HA, McDonald KM et al: Spontaneous dissection of internal carotid arteries: spontaneous resolution documented by serial ocular pneumoplethysmography and angiography. Arch Surg 115:944, 1980
58. Gelbert F, Assouline E, Hodes JE et al: MRI in spontaneous dissection of vertebral and carotid arteries. Neuroradiology 33:111, 1991
59. George SM Jr, Croce MA, Fabian TC et al: Cervicothoracic arterial injuries: recommendations for diagnosis and management. World J Surg 15:134, 1991
60. Goldberg HI, Grossman RI, Gomori JM et al: Cervical internal carotid artery dissecting hemorrhage: diagnosis using MR. Radiology 158:157, 1986
61. Goldstein SJ: Dissecting hematoma of the cervical vertebral artery: case report. J Neurosurg 56:451, 1982
62. Goodman JM, Zink WL, Cooper DF: Hemilingual paralysis caused by carotid artery dissection. Arch Neurol 40:653, 1983
63. Grosman H, Fornasier VL, Bonder D et al: Dissecting aneurysm of the cerebral arteries. J Neurosurg 53:693, 1980
64. Hart RG: Vertebral artery dissection. Neurology (NY) 38:987, 1988
65. Hart RG, Easton JD: Dissections of cervical and cerebral arteries. Neurol Clin 1:155, 1983
66. Hartman JD, Eftychiadis AS: Medial smooth-muscle cell lesions and dissection of the aorta and muscular arteries. Arch Pathol Lab Med 114:50, 1990
67. Hayman JA, Anderson RM: Dissecting aneurysm of the basilar artery. Med J Aust 2:360, 1966
68. Hegedüs K: Reticular fiber deficiency in the intracranial arteries of patients with dissecting aneurysm and review of the possible pathogenesis of previously reported cases. Eur Arch Psychiatr Neurol Sci 235:102, 1985
69. Hennerici M, Steinke W, Rautenberg W: High-resistance Doppler flow pattern in extracranial carotid dissection. Arch Neurol 46:670, 1989
70. Hinse P, Thie A, Lachenmayer L: Dissection of the extracranial vertebral artery: report of four cases and review of the literature. J Neurol Neurosurg Psychiatry 54:863, 1991
71. Hochberg FH, Bean C, Fisher CM et al: Stroke in a 15-year old girl secondary to terminal carotid dissection. Neurology (NY) 25:725, 1975
72. Hodge CJ, Jr, Lee SH: Spontaneous dissecting cervical carotid artery aneurysm. Neurosurgery 10:93, 1982

73. Houser OW, Mokri B, Sundt TM, Jr et al: Spontaneous cervical cephalic arterial dissection and its residuum: angiographic spectrum. AJNR 5:27, 1984
74. Hugenholtz H, Pokrupa R, Montpetit VJA et al: Spontaneous dissecting aneurysm of the extracranial vertebral artery. Neurosurgery 10:96, 1982
75. Jackson MA, Hughes RC, Ward SP, McInnes EG: Headbanging and carotid dissection. Br Med J 287:1262, 1983
76. Kalyan-Raman UP, Kowalski RV, Lee RH, Fierer JA: Dissecting aneurysm of superior cerebellar artery: its association with fibromuscular dysplasia. Arch Neurol 40:120, 1983
77. Katirji MB, Reinmuth OM, Latchaw RE: Stroke due to vertebral artery injury. Arch Neurol 42:242, 1985
78. Krajewski LP, Hertzer NR: Blunt carotid artery trauma: report of two cases and review of the literature. Ann Surg 191:341, 1980
79. Kulla L, Deymeer F, Smith TW et al: Intracranial dissecting and saccular aneurysms in polycystic kidney disease. Arch Neurol 39:776, 1983
80. Lach B, Nair SG, Russell NA, Benoit BG: Spontaneous carotid-cavernous fistula and multiple arterial dissections in type IV Ehlers-Danlos syndrome: case report. J Neurosurg 66:462, 1987
81. Landre E, Roux FX, Cioloca C: Dissection spontanée de la carotide interne exocrânienne: aspects thérapeutiques. Presse Med 16:1273, 1987
82. Lederman RJ, Salanga V: Fibromuscular dysplasia of the internal carotid artery—a cause of Raeder's paratrigeminal syndrome. Neurology (NY) 26:353, 1976
83. Liekweg WG, Jr, Greenfield LJ: Management of penetrating carotid arterial injury. Ann Surg 188:587, 1978
84. Linden MD, Chou SM, Furlan AJ, Conomy JP: Cerebral arterial dissection: a case report with histopathologic and ultrastructural findings. Cleve Clin J Med 54:105, 1987
85. Luken MG, Ascherd GF, Jr, Correll JW et al: Spontaneous dissecting aneurysms of the extracranial internal carotid artery. Clin Neurosurg 26:353, 1979
86. Maitland CG, Black JL, Smith WA: Abducens nerve palsy due to spontaneous dissection of the internal carotid artery. Arch Neurol 40:448, 1983
87. Manz HJ, Lussenhop AJ: Dissecting aneurysm of intracranial vertebral artery: case report and review of the literature. J Neurol 230:25, 1983
88. Manz HJ, Vester J, Lavenstein B: Dissecting aneurysm of cerebral arteries in childhood and adolescence. Virchows Arch 384:325, 1979
89. Mas J-L, Bousser M-G, Hasboun D, Laplane D: Extracranial vertebral artery dissections: a review of 13 cases. Stroke 18:1037, 1987
90. Mas J-L, Goeau C, Bousser M-G et al: Spontaneous dissecting aneurysms of the internal carotid and vertebral arteries—two case reports. Stroke 16:125, 1985
91. Mas J-L, Henin O, Bousser et al: Dissecting aneurysm of the vertebral artery and cervical manipulation: a case report with autopsy. Neurology (NY) 39:512, 1989
92. Masaryk TJ, Ross JS, Modic MT et al: Carotid bifurcation: MR imaging. Radiology 166:461, 1988
93. McNeill DH, Jr, Dreisback J, Marsden RJ: Spontaneous dissection of the internal carotid artery: its conservation management with heparin sodium. Arch Neurol 37:54, 1980
94. Meier DE, Brink BE, Fry WJ: Vertebral artery trauma: acute recognition and treatment. Arch Surg 116:236, 1981
95. Milandre L, Perot S, Salamon G, Khalil R: Spontaneous dissection of both extracranial internal carotid arteries. Neuroradiology 31:435, 1989
96. Milligan N, Anderson M: Conjugal disharmony as a hitherto unrecognized cause of strokes. Br Med J 281:421, 1980
97. Miyazaki S, Yamaura A, Kamata K, Fukushima H: A dissecting aneurysm of the vertebral artery. Surg Neurol 21:171, 1984
98. Muzutani T, Goldberg HI, Parr J et al: Cerebral dissecting aneurysm and intimal fibroelastic thickening of cerebral arteries. J Neurosurg 56:571, 1982
99. Mokri B: Traumatic and spontaneous extracranial internal carotid artery dissections. J Neurol 237:356, 1990
100. Mokri B, Houser OW, Sandok BA, Piepgras DG: Spontaneous dissections of the vertebral arteries. Neurology (NY) 38:880, 1988
101. Mokri B, Houser OW, Stanson AW: Multivessel cervicocephalic and visceral arterial dissections: pathogenic role of primary arterial disease in cervicocephalic arterial dissections. J Stroke Cerebrovasc Dis 1:117, 1991
102. Mokri B, Piepgras DG, Wiebers DO, Houser OW: Familial occurrence of spontaneous dissection of the internal carotid artery. Stroke 18:246, 1987
103. Mokri B, Stanson AW, Houser OW: Spontaneous dissections of the renal arteries in a patient with previous spontaneous dissections of the internal carotid arteries. Stroke 16:959, 1985
104. Mokri B, Sundt TM, Jr, Houser OW: Spontaneous internal carotid dissection, hemicrania, and Horner's syndrome. Arch Neurol 36:677, 1979
105. Mokri B, Sundt TM, Houser OW, Piepgras DG: Spontaneous dissection of the cervical internal carotid artery. Ann Neurol 19:126, 1986
106. Moore WS: Pathology of extracranial cerebrovascular disease. p. 1206. In Rutherford RB (ed): Vascular Surgery. WB Saunders, Philadelphia, 1984
107. Nass R, Hays A, Chutorian A: Intracranial dissecting aneurysms in childhood. Stroke 13:204, 1982
108. Nedwich A, Haft H, Tellem M, Kauffman L: Dissecting aneurysm of cerebral arteries. Arch Neurol 9:477, 1963
109. O'Connell BK, Towfighi J, Brennan RW et al: Dissecting aneurysms of head and neck. Neurology (NY) 35:993, 1985

110. O'Dwyer JA, Moscow N, Trevor R et al: Spontaneous dissection of the carotid artery. Radiology 137:379, 1980
111. Oragon R, Saranchak H, Lakin P et al: Blunt injuries to the carotid and vertebral arteries. Am J Surg 141:497, 1981
112. Orgogozo JM, Henry PY, Pellerin R, Loiseau P: Ischemic strokes temporally related to migraine attacks. p. 292. In Meyer JS, Lechner H, Reivich M, Oh EO (eds): Cerebral Vascular Disease. Vol. 4. Proceedings of the World Federation of Neurology Eleventh International Conference. Excerpta Medica, Amsterdam, 1983
113. Panisset M, Eidelman BH: Multiple cranial neuropathy as a feature of internal carotid artery dissection. Stroke 21:141, 1990
114. Parenti G, Marconi F, Canapicchi R et al: Spontaneous recanalization of carotid artery occlusion following nontraumatic dissection. Ital J Neurol Sci 10:361, 1989
115. Pessin MS, Adelman LS, Barbas NR: Spontaneous intracranial carotid artery dissection. Stroke 20:1100, 1989
116. Petro GR, Witwer GA, Cacayorin ED et al: Spontaneous dissection of the cervical internal carotid artery: correlation of arteriography, CT, and pathology. Am J Radiol 148:393, 1987
117. Pilz P, Hartjes HJ: Fibromuscular dysplasia and multiple dissecting aneurysms of intracranial arteries: a further cause of moyamoya syndrome. Stroke 7:393, 1976
118. Pitner SE: Carotid thrombosis due to intraoral trauma: an unusual complication of a common childhood accident. N Engl J Med 274:764, 1966
119. Pozzati E, Gaist G, Poppi M: Resolution of occlusion in spontaneously dissected carotid arteries. J Neurosurg 56:857, 1982
120. Pozzati E, Giuliani G, Acciarri N, Nuzzo G: Long-term follow-up of occlusive cervical carotid dissection. Stroke 21:528, 1990
121. Quint DJ, Spickler EM: Magnetic resonance imaging demonstration of vertebral artery dissection: report of 2 cases. J Neurosurg 72:964, 1990
122. Ringel SP, Harrison SH, Norenberg MD et al: Fibromuscular dysplasia: multiple "spontaneous" dissecting aneurysms of the major cervical arteries. Ann Neurol 1:301, 1977
123. Roome NS Jr, Aberfeld DC: Spontaneous dissecting aneurysm of the internal carotid artery. Arch Neurol 34:251, 1977
124. Rossillon R, Six C, Dardenne G: Dysplasie et dissection spontanée bilatérale des carotides internes: à propos d'un cas intérêt du traitement chirurgical. Acta Chir Belg 90:97, 1990
125. Rothrock JF, Lim V, Press G, Gosink B: Serial magnetic resonance and carotid duplex examinations in the management of carotid dissection. Neurology (NY) 39:686, 1989
126. Sato S, Hata J: Fibromuscular dysplasia: its occurrence with a dissecting aneurysm of the internal carotid artery. Arch Pathol Lab Med 106:332, 1983
127. Scherman BM, Tucker WS: Bilateral traumatic thrombosis of the internal carotid arteries in the neck: a case report with review of the literature. Neurosurgery 10:751, 1982
128. Schievink WI, Limburg M, Dorthuys JW et al: Cerebrovascular disease in Ehlers-Danlos syndrome type IV. Stroke 21:626, 1990
129. Sellier N, Chiras J, Benhamou M, Bories J: Spontaneous dissection of the internal carotid artery: clinical, radiological and evolutive features: a study of 46 cases. J Neuroradiol 10:243, 1983
130. Senter HJ, Sarwar M: Nontraumatic dissecting aneurysm of the vertebral artery. J Neurosurg 56:128, 1982
131. Sherman DG, Hart RG, Easton JD: Abrupt change in head position and cerebral infarction. Stroke 12:2, 1981
132. Sherman MR, Smialek JE, Zane WE: Pathogenesis of vertebral artery occlusion following cervical spine manipulation. Arch Pathol Lab Med 111:851, 1987
133. Shimoji T, Bando K, Nakajima K, Ito K: Dissecting aneurysm of the vertebral artery: report of seven cases and angiographic findings. J Neurosurg 61:1038, 1984
134. Sinclair W, Jr: Dissecting aneurysm of the middle cerebral artery associated with migraine syndrome. Am J Pathol 29:1083, 1953
135. Spudis EV, Scharyj M, Alexander E et al: Dissecting aneurysms in the neck and head. Neurology (NY) 12:867, 1962
136. Stanley JC, Fry WJ, Seeger JF et al: Extracranial internal carotid and vertebral artery fibrodysplasia. Arch Surg 109:215, 1974
137. Stringer WL, Kelly DL, Jr: Traumatic dissection of the extracranial internal carotid artery. Neurosurgery 6:123, 1980
138. Sturzenegger M: Ultrasound findings in spontaneous carotid artery dissection: the value of duplex sonography. Arch Neurol 48:1057, 1991
139. Thapedi IM, Ashenhurst EM, Rozdilsky B: Spontaneous dissecting aneurysm of the internal carotid artery in the neck. Arch Neurol 23:549, 1970
140. Touboul P-J, Mas J-L, Bousser M-G, Laplane D: Duplex scanning in extracranial vertebral artery dissection. Stroke 18:116, 1987
141. Trattnig S, Schwaighofer B, Hubsch P et al: Color-coded Doppler sonography of vertebral arteries. J Ultra Med 10:221, 1991
142. Vanneste JAL, Davies G: Spontaneous dissection of the cervical internal carotid artery. Clin Neurol Neurosurg 86:307, 1984
143. Waespe W, Niesper J, Imhof H-G, Valavanis A: Lower cranial nerve palsies due to internal carotid dissection. Stroke 19:1561, 1988
144. Wagle WA, Dumoulin CL, Souza SP, Cline HE: 3DFT MR angiography of carotid and basilar arteries. AJNR 10:911, 1989
145. Welling RE, Taha A, Goel T et al: Extracranial carotid artery aneurysm. Surgery 93:319, 1983
146. Welsh P, Pradier R, Repetto R: Fibromuscular dysplasia of the distal cervical internal carotid artery. J Cardiovasc Surg 22:321, 1981

147. West TET, Davies RJ, Kelly RE: Horner's syndrome and headache due to carotid artery disease. Br Med J 1:818, 1976
148. Wirth FP, Miller WA, Russell AP: Atypical fibromuscular hyperplasia: report of two cases. J Neurosurg 54:685, 1981
149. Yamashita M, Tanaka K, Matsuo T et al: Cerebral dissecting aneurysms in patients with moyamoya disease. J Neurosurg 58:120, 1983
150. Yonas H, Agamanolis D, Takaoka Y et al: Dissecting intracranial aneurysms. Surg Neurol 8:407, 1977
151. Youl BD, Coutellier A, Dubois B et al: Three cases of spontaneous extracranial vertebral artery dissection. Stroke 21:618, 1990
152. Zelenock GB, Kasmers A, Whitehouse WM, Jr et al: Extracranial internal carotid artery dissections. Arch Surg 117:425, 1982

# IV

# *SPECIFIC MEDICAL DISEASES AND STROKE*

## J.P. Mohr, Section Editor

This section focuses on the major disease processes that cause stroke as part of the clinical picture. The chapters have been updated to reflect the advanced research and practical applications achieved most recently in the areas of cardiac disease, dissections, moyamoya, fibromuscular dysplasia, migraine, hypertensive encephalopathy, and substance abuse. The latter subject is also discussed extensively in the chapter on brain hemorrhage. The chapter on arteritis has been expanded to include the many arteritides in addition to giant cell arteritis. Authors appearing here for the first time discuss their challenging and promising investigations in this field.

Major advances in the understanding of platelet physiology have so expanded the subject of coagulopathy that disturbances of platelet function and therapy with platelet antiaggregants have been awarded a separate chapter. Meanwhile, the accumulation of information on disorders of thrombosis and thrombolysis, such as protein S, protein C, antithrombin III, lupus anticoagulant, antiphospholipid antibody, and the like, requires its own chapter. The chapter on cardiac arrest that appeared in the first edition has been reconsidered as less relevant to the overall focus of this edition, and therefore was deleted.

The management of the specific diseases discussed in this section is dealt with in Section V on Stroke Therapy.

# 25

# STROKE IN THE SETTING OF COLLAGEN VASCULAR DISEASE

George W. Petty
J.P. Mohr

## GIANT CELL ARTERITIS

Giant cell arteritis, also known as temporal arteritis, cranial arteritis, or Horton's disease, is an inflammatory disease that affects the medium- and large-sized arteries throughout the body, including the aorta and most of its major branches. Inflammation of the arteries of the head and neck are responsible for the major neurologic symptoms of headache and visual loss. Stroke, although uncommon, is a well-documented and potentially fatal complication.

The subject has a long history. It may have been the disease referred to in an ancient account in the Tadhkirat of Ali Ibn Isa,[7] a 10th century "oculist." In modern times, Hutchinson[188] published the first clinical description in 1890. Horton, Magath, and Brown[175,176] at the Mayo Clinic first described it as a distinct clinical and pathologic disease entity in 1932.

### Incidence

Giant cell arteritis is not a rare disease. The age- and sex-adjusted incidence of giant cell arteritis per 100,000 population, age 50 years or older, in Olmsted County, Minnesota, from 1950 to 1985, was 17.0.[250] There is a dramatic increase in incidence with age. The incidence in Olmsted County was only 2.6 per 100,000 for those in the 50- to 59-year age group, but rose to 44.6 per 100,000 in those over 80 years of age.[250] There is a threefold greater incidence in women than in men.[250] The incidence of giant cell arteritis may be up to seven times higher among whites than among blacks,[357] possibly related to the lower frequency of HLA-DR4 (D-related human leukocyte antigen) among blacks compared to whites.[244] The incidence of giant cell arteritis increased with time in the Olmsted County study, a phenomenon attributed in part to increased awareness of the disease and its varied manifestations on the part of clinicians.[250]

### Pathology

Giant cell arteritis primarily affects the medium and large elastic arteries, sparing the capillaries and veins. Although involvement of the temporal arteries is emphasized in clinical descriptions, the aorta and its branches are commonly involved as well[250,290]; in one study, 34 of 248 patients had evidence of large artery involvement.[220] The arterial wall is infiltrated with mononuclear cells (lymphocytes and plasma cells) and, to a lesser extent, with eosinophils and neutrophils predominantly in the media near the internal elastic lamina. Granulomas composed of multinucleated or foreign-body giant cells are found along with the inflammatory cells, but are not invariably present. The vessel may be necrotic in areas, especially in the media. Fibrinoid necrosis, characteristic of hypertension, usually is not present.[75,183,321] Intimal proliferation and fibrosis may result in lumen narrowing and thrombosis. The exact mechanism of thrombosis in temporal arteritis is uncertain. Anticardiolipin antibodies have been reported in one patient with arterial thrombosis in the setting of giant cell arteritis,[59] but no definite procoagulant state has been established.

The etiology of giant cell arteritis is unknown, but there is evidence that immunologic mechanisms are involved. Park et al.[295] and Papaioannou et al.[294] demonstrated circulating immune complexes in the sera of patients with biopsy-proven giant cell arteritis. Immunoglobulin has been found deposited in the temporal arteries.[37,58,239,295] Several studies have demonstrated an increased frequency of certain histocompatibility antigens, including HLA-B8 and HLA-DR4, among patients with giant cell arteritis,[13,46,157] although others have not.[185] Machado et al.[250] have noted that the highest incidence rates have been reported from regions with similar ethnic backgrounds: northern Europe and Minnesota.[26,33] Familial and conjugal cases have been reported.[120,371]

## General Clinical Features

If not known for any other feature, giant cell arteritis would be recognized for the wide variety of syndromes it produces. *Headache* is the most common presentation in most series.[131,147,157,160,186,201] It is usually constant, said to be especially common at night, and interferes with sleep. The headache is located predominantly in the temporal area, but may radiate to the scalp, face, jaw, or occiput.[101,147,265] Scalp tenderness is a frequent complaint, and many patients—but by no means all—have swollen, nodular, or pulseless temporal arteries.[157,187,332] Some consider jaw claudication pathognomonic for giant cell arteritis.[174] Other prominant symptoms include fever, weight loss, fatigue, and malaise. Many patients have arthralgias, but frank arthritis is uncommon.[147] Dementia, confusion, and psychiatric symptoms, such as depression, are reported.[49,51,131,382] Peripheral neuropathy and isolated or multiple mononeuropathies may occur in up to 14 percent.[50]

*Polymyalgia rheumatica* is a syndrome of limb girdle muscle pain and stiffness accompanied by systemic symptoms, including malaise, fever, weight loss, anorexia, and depression. Most patients with giant cell arteritis have symptoms of polymyalgia rheumatica for weeks to months before developing headache, jaw claudication, or visual loss.[2,25,101,187,291] Jones and Hazleman[202] found that 44 percent of patients who present with polymyalgia rheumatica alone develop overt giant cell arteritis, and 23 percent develop serious ophthalmologic or neurologic complications, such as visual loss, ophthalmoplegia, or stroke. Alestig and Barr,[2] Bengtsson and Malmvall,[26] and Fauchald et al.[101] demonstrated that patients with the clinical diagnosis of polymyalgia rheumatica frequently have giant cell arteritis on temporal artery biopsy, raising the possibility that polymyalgia rheumatica may not represent a distinct nosologic entity.

## Ophthalmologic Complications

Visual loss is the most feared complication of giant cell arteritis. Anterior ischemic optic neuropathy is the most common cause of visual loss in giant cell arteritis. It is a result of thrombosis of the involved posterior ciliary arteries.[26,158,171] Posterior ischemic optic neuropathy and central retinal artery occlusion also may cause visual loss in giant cell arteritis, but less frequently than does anterior ischemic optic neuropathy.[26,34,48,64,71,171] Homonymous hemianopia and cortical blindness may occur as a result of posterior circulation infarction (see below). Central retinal vein occlusion has also been reported.[51] Once established, the visual loss caused by giant cell arteritis rarely improves, despite treatment with corticosteroids.[158,171,201]

Large series report visual loss in 40 to 50 percent of patients with giant cell arteritis.[134,147,171,187,332] Hollenhorst et al.[171] noted loss of vision within 2 to 3 months of onset of giant cell arteritis symptoms in one-third of patients, and all of the remainder destined to have this symptom suffered loss of vision within 10 months after the onset of other symptoms.

Visual loss typically occurs suddenly, although 10 to 20 percent of patients with giant cell arteritis experience transient loss of vision (transient monocular blindness, amaurosis fugax) prior to development of fixed visual deficits.[51,171,187,201,332] It is usually monocular, but bilateral involvement occurred in 33 percent of patients with visual loss reported by Jonasson et al.[201] Visual loss in the second eye occurred simultaneously or within 24 hours after visual loss in the first eye in 36 percent of these patients; between the 2nd and 7th day in 36 percent; and between 1 week and 1 month in the remainder. Monocular or binocular positive visual phenomena ("scintillating scotoma") have been reported.[51]

Visual acuity is usually reduced to hand motion or light perception, and most patients have reduced color perception. The disc is swollen and usually pale, flame hemorrhages may be seen, and disc atrophy subsequently develops. Afferent pupillary defects are common. Field defects are usually altitudinal and inferior, although inferior nasal defects, arcuate defects, and scotomas may be seen.[158,269,390]

Diplopia or ophthalmoplegia, usually transient, occur in 10 to 15 percent of patients with giant cell arteritis.[134,171,187,265,332] Hollenhorst et al.[171] reported that weakness of an extraocular muscle was demonstrable in only 10 of 22 patients who had complained of double vision; the 10 diplopic patients eventually lost vision in one or both eyes, and 2 others had amaurosis fugax. Dimant et al.[86] found that 7 of 14 patients with biopsy-proven giant cell arteritis had ophthalmoplegia on examination, but only 1 complained of diplopia. Only one of their patients had a pattern of ophthalmoplegia that was compatible with a single nerve lesion (3rd cranial nerve). The other patients had patterns of ophthalmoplegia that did not conform to a lesion of a single nerve. Impairment of upward gaze was common.[86] Large clinical series have indicated that 3rd cranial nerve palsies and 6th cranial nerve palsies occur with roughly equal frequency in patients with giant cell arteritis.[134,265,332] Meadows[265] noted that, in his patients with ophthalmoplegias conforming to 3rd cranial nerve pareses, the pupils were spared.

In reviewing the subject of ophthalmoplegia in giant cell arteritis in 1959, Fisher[111] noted that ptosis was common and that ophthalmoplegia may be the only neurologic complication in some patients with the disease. He suggested that ophthalmoplegia in giant cell arteritis is caused by damage to the nerves supplying the extraocular muscles, a view shared by others[265] and supported by recent reports of oculomotor synkinesis[354] and tonic pupil[77] in the condition. However, in an autopsy study of a patient with giant cell arteritis and bilateral ophthalmoplegia, Barricks et al.,[22] who documented ischemic necrosis of the extraocular muscles, could find no lesion in the nerves to these muscles. They concluded that extraocular muscle ischemia, as opposed to nerve ischemia, is the mechanism of ophthalmoplegia in giant cell arteritis.

## Stroke In Giant Cell Arteritis

Stroke is an uncommon but potentially lethal complication of giant cell arteritis.[48,57,71,73,97,128,136,149,150,162,177,196,206,224,257,266,289,290,291,332,349,362,389,396,398] Although epidemiologic studies have not demonstrated an increased incidence of stroke among patients with giant cell arteritis,[25,187,201] studies from referral centers suggest that patients with giant cell arteritis may be at higher risk for stroke during the active phase of their disease. Paulley and Hughes[300] reported that 8 of their 76 patients with giant cell arteritis presented with stroke. Graham found that, of the eight patients who died within 6 weeks of diagnosis of giant cell arteritis, four had stroke.[134]

Elderly patients with giant cell arteritis are at greater risk for stroke, compared to the general population, by virtue of their age alone, and it is not always clear that giant cell arteritis actually causes the stroke in patients with cerebral infarction in this setting. In an effort to separate stroke due to giant cell arteritis from that which is merely incidental, the following discussion of the mechanisms of stroke in giant cell arteritis has been biased toward those reports in which full autopsy was performed or those in which the diagnosis was satisfactorily established.

Stroke caused by giant cell arteritis may occur as the first indication of the disease. In several well-documented autopsy-proven cases, stroke occurred on presentation, without known prior symptoms of giant cell arteritis (case 3 of Wilkinson and Russell,[398] case 2 of Ostberg,[289] case 8 of Säve-Söderbergh et al.,[338] and the cases of Bogousslavsky et al.[35] and Collado et al.[66]). However, the more easily recognized other symptoms, such as fever, weight loss, headache, and visual disturbance, frequently precede giant cell arteritis-related stroke for periods of weeks to months.[125,162,338,396,398] The erythrocyte sedimentation rate (ESR) is usually elevated in patients with stroke caused by giant cell arteritis, but temporal artery examination and biopsy may be normal.[177] In case 2 of Wilkinson and Russell,[398] stroke occurred after the ESR had returned to normal during treatment with corticosteroids. It is worrisome to note that several patients had strokes despite therapy with corticosteroids (case 14 of Heptinstall,[162] cases 1, 2, and 4 of Wilkinson and Russell,[398] case 9 of Säve-Söderbergh et al.,[338] and the case of Gibb et al.[125]) all within 2 weeks of initiation of treatment.

Stroke in patients with giant cell arteritis may occur in the carotid or vertebrobasilar circulation. Postmortem examination in such patients most often documents giant cell arteritis involving the extradural segments of the vessels only (Fig. 25-1),[35,66,128,162,177,291,338,396,398] although some have had evidence of intradural involvement as well.[125,138,195,218,270,275,338,382]

## Stroke Caused by Giant Cell Arteritis Involving Extracranial Arteries Only

### *Vertebrobasilar Territory Infarction*

In a brief report of a necropsy series, Missen[270] noted that obstruction of the arterial lumen due to giant cell arteritis was "three times as frequent in the vertebral arteries as in the internal carotids" and that "infarction was found more often in the hind-brain than in the forebrain." In the series of Graham,[134] the four patients who died with stroke soon after the diagnosis of giant cell arteritis all had brain stem infarction. In autopsy-proven cases of posterior circulation infarction caused by giant cell arteritis, the mechanism of stroke is arteritic involvement of the vertebral arteries with thrombosis and secondary infarction (frequently multifocal) in the vertebrobasilar territory.

Case 13 of Heptinstall et al.[162] was a 66-year-old man who was admitted for "fatigue, anorexia, and temporal headache, mainly left-sided, for three months, with recent drowsiness and weakness." The left temporal artery was thickened and pulseless. No detailed neurologic examination was reported. He

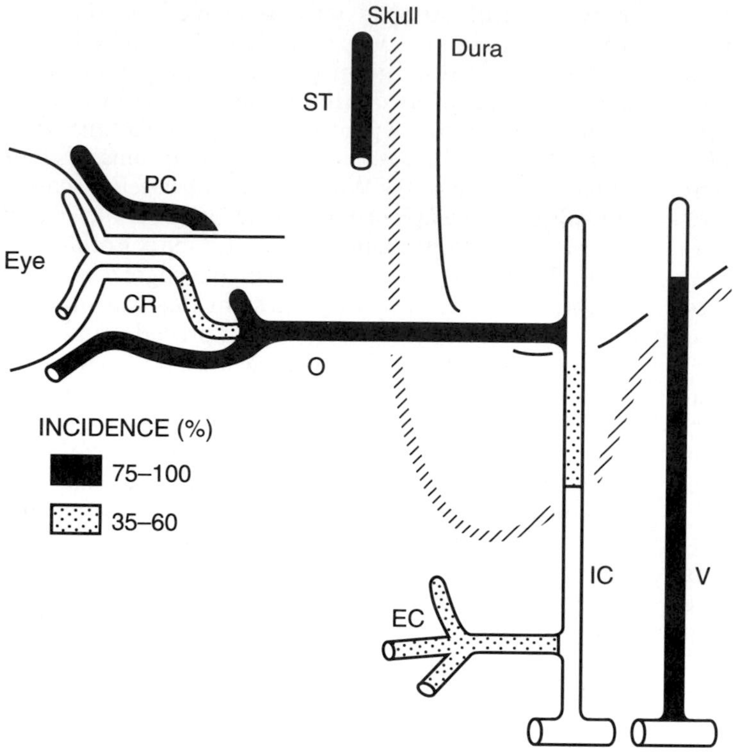


**Fig. 25-1.** Pattern of involvement of giant cell arteritis in head and neck arteries. Note high incidence of involvement of vertebral artery (v), superior temporal artery (st), ophthalmic artery (o), and posterior ciliary artery (pc). Intracranial arteries are rarely involved. CR, central retinal artery; EC, external carotid artery; IC, internal carotid artery. (From Wilkinson and Russell,[398] with permission.)

died in coma 3 weeks after admission. Postmortem examination demonstrated giant cell arteritis involving the following arteries: right and left facial, right and left temporal, right occipital, left external carotid, and right vertebral. The right vertebral artery was occluded by thrombus, and associated with this was an infarct of the right lobe of the cerebellum.

Case 14 of Heptinstall et al.[162] was a 60-year-old man with a 6-month history of sacral and shoulder pain, weight loss, malaise, and headache, transient diplopia, and blurring of vision. Both temporal arteries were thrombosed and the ESR was 62 mm/h. He became blind in both eyes shortly after temporal artery biopsies were obtained. There was no evidence of ischemic optic neuropathy, however. Treatment with adrenocorticotropic hormone (ACTH) and cortisone was initiated, but 10 days later he developed disorientation, left hemiparesis, and an extensor plantar response on the left. This was followed by development of a right hemiparesis, coma, and death. Autopsy demonstrated giant cell arteritis in the following cranial arteries: right and left temporal, right and left common carotid, right internal carotid, right and left ophthalmic, right and left vertebral. The vertebral arteries were occluded at their entry into the skull. Intracranially, thrombus was present in the posterior cerebral arteries as well. The brain demonstrated "extensive softening of both occipital poles." The brain stem and cerebellum were not mentioned. The optic nerves showed "little change." It would appear that this patient's sudden bilateral blindness was cortical in origin and related to bilateral posterior cerebral artery territory infarction.

The first case of Wilkinson and Russell[398] was a 74-year-old man who developed left-sided headaches 9 months prior to his stroke. One week before the stroke, he developed pain and blindness in the left eye. The right superficial temporal artery was thickened, and ophthalmologic examination demonstrated changes consistent with ischemic optic neuropathy involving the left eye. Mild ptosis was present bilaterally. Adduction was limited in the left eye. There was impaired adduction, elevation, and depression in the right eye. He had mild ataxia in both legs and the plantar response on the left was extensor. The ESR was 60 mm/h. Temporal artery biopsy demonstrated giant cell arteritis. Four days after admission he developed hoarseness and difficulty swallowing, followed by right-sided palatal weakness, right-sided pharyngeal numbness, and right arm ataxia, consistent with right lateral medullary infarction. Two days later he developed right facial weakness, tongue protrusion to the right, weakness and ataxia of all limbs, bilateral extensor plantar responses, and bilateral hyperreflexia, subsequently followed by coma and death. The autopsy demonstrated widespread giant cell arteritis involving the following cranial arteries: right and left external carotid, right and left temporal, both external carotid, right and left ophthalmic, right and left central retinal, right and left posterior ciliary and right and left internal carotid in the petrous and cavernous portions only. The right vertebral artery was involved in its cervical course up to a point 5 mm beyond perforation of the dura at the origin of the posterior inferior cerebellar artery. The left vertebral artery was involved in its cervical course up to a point just beyond its penetration of the dura. The right vertebral and posterior inferior cerebellar arteries were occluded with thrombus. Recent infarctions were found in the ventral aspect of the lower pons and in the right medulla. There was no giant cell arteritis in any intracranial artery.

Case 3 of Wilkinson and Russell[398] was a 79-year-old man who developed headaches, impaired vision, and episodic vertigo and falling 1 to 2 weeks prior to hospitalization. Admission examination demonstrated findings consistent with a "top of the basilar" syndrome. He was disoriented and amnesic. Visual acuity was markedly impaired, but he confabulated and denied blindness. Pupillary light reflexes were normal. The right fundus was normal, but the left fundus was obscured by a cataract. The ESR was 58 mm/h. Temporal artery biopsy demonstrated giant cell arteritis. Prednisone, 40 mg/day, was administered, but he became drowsy and disoriented, his eyes deviated down and to the right, and he subsequently expired. At autopsy, giant cell arteritis was found in the right temporal artery, left external carotid artery, and both vertebral arteries. The latter were involved to 5 mm beyond the point of dural penetration, extending just beyond the origin of the posterior inferior cerebellar artery on the left, but stopping short of the origin of the posterior inferior cerebellar artery on the right, and both cervical portions were occluded by thrombus. On the right, the thrombus extended into the intracranial portion of the vessel. Examination of the brain demonstrated recent infarcts in both cerebellar hemispheres. Old and recent infarcts were present in the right occipital lobe, and a recent infarct was present in the left occipital lobe. The posterior cerebral arteries were not occluded by thrombus. No giant cell arteritis was demonstrated in the intracerebral arteries. No abnormalities were found in the left eye. This case is similar to case 14 of Heptinstall et al.[162] in that decreased visual acuity was a manifestation of occipital lobe infarction and not anterior ischemic optic neuropathy.

The fourth case of Wilkinson and Russell[398] was a 75-year-old man with a history of impaired vision in the right eye. He developed headaches and scalp tenderness 3 weeks before stroke. He was started on prednisolone 5 mg twice a day 2 weeks prior to admission. One week prior to admission he developed persistent nausea and vomiting and more severe headache, followed by sensations of dizziness and unsteadiness. Admission examination demonstrated disorientation, decreased visual acuity in both eyes, normal fundi, a right Horner syndrome, normal pupillary light responses, nonsustained nystagmus on right and left gaze, decreased hearing in the right ear, a bovine cough, tongue deviation to the right, right hemiparesis, increased deep tendon reflexes on the right, bilateral extensor plantar responses, and ataxia in the right arm and right and left leg. Both temporal arteries were tender. The ESR was 45 mm/h. Shortly after admission he vomited, developed spontaneous nystagmus, lost consciousness, and died. Autopsy demonstrated giant cell arteritis in both temporal arteries, both internal carotid arteries in their cavernous segments, and the left external carotid artery. The left vertebral artery was involved but could not be traced beyond the first cervical vertebra. The right vertebral artery was involved by giant cell arteritis to a point 5 mm beyond its penetration of the dura and was occluded by thrombus. There were diffuse areas of ischemic changes in the pons and medulla. The optic nerves were normal.

The case presented before the Royal College of Physicians[396] was a 66-year-old man who developed headache and episodic loss of vision in the right eye 4 months prior to stroke. At that time the ESR was 31 mm/h. The episodes of loss of vision ceased spontaneously, and he was instructed to take aspirin as needed. Four months later he developed "unsteadiness on his feet" and diplopia, followed a week later by a headache and "loud noises in his head." Admission examination demonstrated dysarthria, dysphagia, horizontal nystagmus to the right on lateral gaze, small reactive pupils, a left ptosis, an absent gag reflex, deviation of the uvula to the left, deviation of the tongue to the right, sensory loss to pin over the right face, and left arm incoordination. The ESR was 33 mm/h. He died the morning after admission. Autopsy demonstrated giant cell arteritis and thrombosis of both vertebral arteries. There was acute infarction in the medulla.

The case of Collado et al.[66] was an 85-year-old man who was admitted for right hand discoordination, nausea, vomiting, hiccup, and ataxia. He had had a transient episode of visual blurring and unsteady gait 1 year previously. Examination on admission demonstrated findings consistent with right hemiparesis, decreased sensation in the right face and left side of the body, and right arm dysmetria. Temporal arteries were normal. Sedimentation rate was 30 mm/h. He subsequently developed impairment of consciousness, and died after developing pneumonia. Examination of the right vertebral artery demonstrated changes consistent with giant cell arteritis with thrombotic occlusion of the distal 2-cm segment extending into the ostium of the posterior inferior cerebellar artery. Infarction was noted in the right lateral medulla extending from the upper medulla to the pyramidal decussation. Infarction was also noted in the right posteroinferior region of the cerebellum with tonsillar herniation. A cystic infarct was also noted in the left calcarine area.

Although the clinical and autopsy findings were not

described in detail, cases 6, 8, and 9 in the series of Säve-Söderbergh et al.[338] probably represent instances of posterior circulation infarction secondary to arteritic involvement and thrombosis of the vertebral arteries.

### *Carotid Territory Infarction*

Thrombotic occlusion of the internal carotid arteries has also been described in a number of autopsy-proven cases. In each, the thrombus was found distal to the bifurcation.

The second case of Gilmour[128] was a 59-year-old woman who developed headache 4 months prior to stroke. Eight weeks prior to stroke the headaches became worse, and she developed persistent vomiting. Three weeks after admission she developed a flaccid left hemiplegia, became comatose, and died 8 days later. Autopsy demonstrated giant cell arteritis in the aorta and both internal carotid arteries. Both internal carotid arteries were occluded by thrombus in their intracranial segments, as were the "left middle cerebral arteries and small arteries" on the convexity.

The second case of Wilkinson and Russell[398] was an 80-year-old man who developed headache 3½ months prior to stroke. He lost vision in the right eye 2 weeks prior to stroke. Examination showed markedly decreased visual acuity in the right eye, a normal left fundus, a lens opacity in the right eye, obscuring the fundus, and thickened temporal arteries. The ESR was 80 mm/h. Prednisone was begun. A temporal artery biopsy demonstrated giant cell arteritis. Two weeks later he developed a right hemiplegia and dysphasia. Examination disclosed global aphasia, right hemiparesis, right hemisensory loss and findings consistent with ischemic optic neuropathy in the right eye. The ESR was normal. There was a left frontotemporal abnormality on EEG. He died 2 weeks after the onset of stroke. At autopsy, giant cell arteritis was demonstrated in the following arteries: right and left temporal, right and left ophthalmic, right and left posterior ciliary, right central retinal, right and left vertebral to a point 5 mm beyond their penetration of the dura, and right and left internal carotid in their cavernous segments. The left internal carotid artery was completely occluded with a thrombus that began at the level of the cavernous sinus and extended to the bifurcation. In the brain there was a large area of border-zone infarction in the left hemisphere involving the "cortex and subjacent white matter . . . between anterior and middle cerebral artery territories in the parietal region, and . . . between middle and posterior cerebral artery areas in the temporal and parieto-occipital regions." The brain stem and cerebellum were normal. There was anterior ischemia of the right optic nerve. In this case, visual disturbance initially was caused by anterior ischemic optic neuropathy in the right eye. The patient then developed a right hemianopia as a result of a stroke that occurred after treatment with corticosteroids and normalization of the ESR.

The patient of Howard et al.[177] was a 65-year-old woman with a history of chronic paranoid schizophrenia who was admitted to the hospital for "sudden onset of left facial drooping, left-sided weakness, and slurring of speech" after a 10-day history of difficulty walking, neglect of hygiene, dementia, and rigidity. Examination demonstrated impaired calculation and recent recall, perseveration, a right gaze preference, facial weakness on the left, paratonia in all limbs, movement of right side better than the left, increased deep tendon reflexes on both sides, good grasp, suck, and snout reflexes, bilateral extensor plantar responses, and normal temporal arteries. The gaze preference and focal weakness improved, but after 1 week in the hospital, she developed lethargy, slurred speech, inability to eat, and myoclonus. The ESR was 67 mm/h. After 1 month in the hospital she became less responsive and developed right facial weakness. CT scan demonstrated multiple infarcts. Although cerebral angiography demonstrated normal common carotid, vertebral, basilar, and temporal arteries, both internal carotid arteries were found to be occluded from 1.5 to 2 cm distal to their origins. This procedure was followed by development of signs of right temporal lobe herniation and death. Postmortem examination demonstrated giant cell arteritis and thrombosis in the cavernous segments of both internal carotid arteries. No giant cell arteritis was found in the intracranial vessels. Multiple areas of infarction, new and old, were found in the territories of the right anterior cerebral artery, the left middle cerebral artery, and the right middle and posterior cerebral arteries. There was cerebral edema and evidence of right uncal herniation.

### *Other Mechanisms of Cerebrovascular Disease Caused by Giant Cell Arteritis Involving Extracranial Arteries*

Four other cases in which giant cell arteritis of the extracerebral arteries resulted in cerebrovascular disease warrant mention. Bogousslavsky et al.[35] reported a case of giant cell arteritis with bilateral internal carotid artery siphon stenosis "related to internal hypertrophy and fibrosis, with infiltration of the media and elastic layer with lymphocytes and many giant cells" associated with infarction in the brain stem without arteritic involvement or thrombosis of the vertebral arteries. They postulated "steal phenomenon" as a mechanism.

Embolism was the mechanism of stroke in two cases. Case 2 of Ostberg[289] was a 73-year-old woman who developed a right hemiparesis and died shortly after a surgical procedure. No symptoms of giant cell arteritis were reported prior to stroke. Autopsy demonstrated giant cell arteritis in the ascending aorta with a mural thrombus just above the ostium. This thrombus was believed to have resulted in embolism "of the coronary, splenic, renal, and middle cerebral arteries with infarction. . . ." Spencer and Hoyt[362] reported an autopsy case in which giant cell arteritis involving the coronary arteries resulted in myocardial infarction, ventricular mural thrombus formation, and emboli to the brain and multiple infarcts. Pollack et al.[308] reported a case of subclavian steal associated with narrowing of a subclavian artery caused by giant cell arteritis.

## Stroke Caused by Giant Cell Arteritis Involving the Extracranial and Intracranial Arteries

Involvement of intracranial (intradural) vessels by giant cell arteritis is rare. In a detailed autopsy study of the pattern of arterial involvement in four patients with giant cell arteritis, Wilkinson and Russell[398] found that the vertebral arteries and the petrous and cavernous portions of the internal carotid arteries were consistently involved, but the abnormalities consistently ended at or just beyond the point of penetration of the dura, and intradural vessels were not involved (Fig. 25-1). In a brief report of 23 necropsy cases, Missen[270] found that the intracerebral vessels were involved by giant cell arteritis "infrequently," while involvement of the vertebral and carotid arteries was "virtually constant."

There are, however, a few autopsy cases that describe giant cell arteritis in the intracranial as well as extracranial vessels.[125,138,195,218,275,338,382] In the description of Verker's case,[382] only brief reference is made to "typical microscopic appearances of temporal arteritis" in the "temporal, cerebral, and superior thyroid arteries." Morrison and Abitol[275] mentioned that "all the arteries of the base of the brain (basilar, posterior, middle, and anterior cerebral) showed atherosclerosis and changes of granulomatous arteritis" in their case. Gibb et al.[125] reported a 76-year-old man who developed basilar artery thrombosis after presenting with spinal cord infarction. Autopsy demonstrated infarction of midbrain and pontine tegmentum. The basilar artery "demonstrated damage and reduplication of the internal elastic lamina and a segment of adventitia with chronic inflammatory cell infiltration" and thrombosis near its origin. A paramedian branch of the basilar artery was also said to have been involved. Cases 5 and 7 of Säve-Söderbergh et al.[338] also were said to have had arteritis in the intracranial portions of the basilar artery and the "basal cerebral arteries" respectively. Other cases are atypical in certain respects. In Greenfield's case,[138] granulomatous and lymphocytic infiltrations were present in the middle and anterior cerebral arteries, but only in the adventitia and not in the media. In the cases of Kjeldsen and Reske-Nielsen[218] and Ritama,[320] involvement of venules was described, which is atypical for giant cell arteritis, but is more often seen with granulomatous angiitis of the central nervous system (see below). In cases 1 and 2 of Jellinger,[195] visceral involvement appeared to be extensive.

Reports of giant cell arteritis confined to the intracranial vessels seem especially rare. The cases of Enzmann and Scott,[97] Hinck et al.,[168] Hirsch et al.,[169] McCormick and Neuberger,[262] and cases 3, 4, and 5 of Jellinger[195] may represent cases of isolated angiitis of the central nervous system. Reports of giant cell arteritis causing multiple intracranial aneurysms may actually be cases of Takayasu's disease or other as yet uncharacterized disease.[226,268]

## Diagnosis

The most common laboratory abnormality in patients with giant cell arteritis is a markedly elevated erythrocyte sedimentation rate. However, a normal ESR does not exclude the diagnosis.[208,403] Most patients have a mild to moderate normochromic or slightly hypochromic anemia. White blood cell counts are normal or moderately elevated.[147,157,171,332] Mild abnormalities of liver enzymes have been reported.[84,143]

Temporal artery biopsy is the most helpful diagnostic procedure.[146] Biopsy is recommended for all patients in whom giant cell arteritis is strongly suspected in order to avoid management dilemmas should patients relapse or develop complications while on steroids.[145] Yet the segmental nature of the disease means that a normal temporal artery biopsy does not exclude the diagnosis of giant cell arteritis.[219] In one series of biopsy proven cases, 86 percent were diagnosed by unilateral biopsy and the remaining 14 percent diagnosed only after biopsy of the second side.[145] Other types of vasculitis rarely may cause inflammation of the temporal arteries and mimic the disease.[148,274]

Angiographic signs are infrequently present. The superficial temporal arteriogram may demonstrate areas of dilation and constriction along the length of the artery.[93,127,182] Changes may also be seen in the internal carotid artery siphon segments.[386] Arteriography offers no advantage over the simple procedure of temporal artery biopsy,[187] and any findings are not specific. Angiographic abnormalities of intracranial arteries are rare, and possibly represent cases of isolated granulomatous angiitis of the central nervous system.[97,168,169]

## Treatment and Prognosis

Once the diagnosis of giant cell arteritis is suspected, the patient should be started on steroids, and a temporal artery biopsy should be obtained as soon as possible. An initial dose of 40 to 60 mg/day of prednisone is recommended for the first month, or until symptoms of the disease are controlled.[186] Symptoms usually respond promptly to steroids, although visual loss and stroke may occur after the initiation of treatment. Steroids may be tapered while monitoring symptoms and the ESR.[186] There is controversy over the duration of therapy. Rapid tapering is thought to lead to relapse more often than very slow tapering. Recurrence of symptoms or elevation of the ESR after initial control of the disease indicates relapse and should prompt resumption of higher doses of steroids. Relapse after withdrawal from steroids may not necessarily be accompanied by a rise in ESR, however.[388] In one series, the mean duration of steroid therapy was 5.8 years, 12.8 years being the maximum.[11] The relapse rate after withdrawal of treatment was 47 percent, 46 percent of these occurring within 1 month and 96 percent within 1 year after cessation of treatment. The relapse rate after withdrawal of steroid therapy bore little relationship to the duration of treatment.[11] Alternate-day treatment regimens are felt to be less effective than daily administration of steroids,[184] and carry not only the risk of relapses but also of blindness in the other eye. Some have advocated hospitalization and treatment with high-dose, pulsed intravenous methylprednisolone for patients with acute visual loss.[327]

Giant cell arteritis may cause death by stroke, myocardial infarction, or aortic rupture.[27,338] Epidemiologic studies and large clinical series, however, have not demonstrated that patients with giant cell arteritis have an increased mortality rate.[26,157,201]

## ISOLATED GRANULOMATOUS ANGIITIS OF THE CENTRAL NERVOUS SYSTEM

Isolated granulomatous angiitis of the central nervous system is an inflammatory arterial disease restricted to the cerebral circulation.* Unlike giant cell arteritis, isolated granulomatous angiitis of the central nervous system afflicts patients of any age, is characterized by neurologic disease out of proportion to systemic illness, preferentially involves smaller arteries and veins, responds poorly or not at all to steroids alone, and is frequently fatal. It would appear, therefore, that isolated granulomatous angiitis of the central nervous system is a condition distinct from giant cell arteritis.

### Pathology

Like giant cell arteritis, the pathologic process is segmental in character. Any of the vessels of the brain and spinal cord may be involved, but most reports have noted a predilection for the small leptomeningeal vessels. The precapillary arterioles are most often affected. Some reports, however, have noted predominance of venular involvement.[43,222] Occasionally the process may be quite focal, involving only one vessel or group of vessels.[259,353] The inflammatory infiltrate is composed of lymphocytes, plasma cells, granulomas with multinucleated giant cells, and occasionally neutrophils and eosinophils.[74,76] These infiltrates may involve any portion of the vessel wall. Some have noted more inflammation in the intima and adventitia than in the media.[43,70] Occasionally, thrombosis of larger intracranial arteries (internal carotid artery siphon, anterior cerebral, middle cerebral, posterior cerebral, basilar) is found.[14,259,278] Small aneurysms have also been reported.[168,335,353]

The etiology of granulomatous angiitis of the central nervous system is unknown. The available evidence suggests that an infectious agent or an immunologic mechanism may be involved. A necrotizing angiitis of the central nervous system has been observed in brains of turkeys infected with *Mycoplasma gallisepticum*.[61,373] "Viruslike" and "mycoplasmalike" particles in the brain and vascular lesions have been identified by electron microscopy, but no organisms have been cultured.[14,318] Other cases have been reported in association with Hodgkin's lymphoma, acquired immunodeficiency syndrome (AIDS), primary intracerebral lymphoma, varicella encephalitis, leukemia, sarcoid, or following varicella zoster infection.** The frequent association with another underlying disease and the pathologic heterogeneity of the lesions have lead some to conclude that isolated angiitis of the central nervous system is a "nonspecific reaction, not a unique disease."[408]

### Clinical and Pathologic Features and Autopsy Findings

Despite the hope authors usually entertain to present readers with a dependable "formula" for safely arriving at the diagnosis of the disease in question, the following analysis of 37 full autopsy cases of "idiopathic" isolated granulomatous angiitis of the central nervous system (not associated with infection or other underlying disease) reveals a discouragingly heterogeneous profile of clinical and diagnostic features with few *reliable* clues to the diagnosis short of brain biopsy or autopsy.†

The patients ranged in age from 3 years to 96 years. Twelve were women. The duration of illness from onset of symptoms to death was less than 6 months in

* References: 28, 30, 38, 43–45, 53, 54, 60, 70, 74, 76, 97, 100, 104, 106, 115, 129, 139, 151, 155, 168, 169, 180, 195, 197, 207, 222, 223, 227, 247, 259, 262, 272, 278, 281, 283, 288, 301, 305, 309, 313, 318, 333, 334, 335, 340, 343, 346, 348, 353, 378, 379, 380, 385, 405, 408.

** References: 32, 38, 47, 126, 137, 197, 243, 253, 288, 311, 317, 325, 326, 328, 356, 384, 405, 408.

† References: 14, 30, 43, 44, 53, 54, 70, 100, 104, 115, 155, 168, 180, 195, 222, 223, 259, 262, 278, 283, 309, 313, 315, 318, 333, 335, 353, 378, 408.

most. The briefest duration was 3 days.[278] Five patients, however, had courses greater than 1 year in duration, the longest being possibly 9 years.[309]

Headache, nausea, vomiting, dementia, amnesic states, disorientation, confusion, or somnolence occurred early in the course of the disease in many patients. Not uncommonly, brain tumor or stroke were initial diagnostic considerations. Systemic symptoms, such as fever and weight loss, were uncommon, occurring early in only four patients and seven patients, respectively.

Multifocal neurologic symptoms and signs developed in a stepwise progression, with episodes of quantitative and qualitative worsening, usually occurring after variable periods of stabilization from days to weeks or months. Seizures were common. Most developed hemiplegia or extensor plantar responses. Six patients had evidence of spinal cord involvement during their courses, including incontinence and paraplegia. Papilledema was noted in over 20 percent. Nearly all patients developed profound alteration of mental status or coma for variable periods of time prior to death.

The ESR, when reported, was elevated in 13 patients but normal in 7 patients. ESR elevations were not generally as high as seen in giant cell arteritis. Blood cell counts, electrolytes, and serologic tests for collagen vascular disease were usually normal. Spinal fluid examination was abnormal in 34 of 35 cases in which results were reported. The most consistent abnormality was an elevated protein (usually over 100 mg%), although occasionally it was normal. Elevated immunoglobulins were occasionally reported. Many patients had a moderate lymphocytic pleocytosis (usually less than 150 cells/mm$^3$). Isolated angiitis of the central nervous system may therefore present as "chronic meningitis."[315] Varying numbers of red cells were frequently present. Opening pressure was elevated in some but normal in others.

The EEG was abnormal in the 18 cases reported, usually demonstrating diffuse or occasionally focal slow wave activity. When computed tomography (CT) scans were performed, interpretations were remarkably heterogeneous, including single or multiple infarcts, single or multiple hemorrhages, tumor with mass effect, tumor with hemorrhage, ring-enhancing lesions suggestive of abscess, and multiple areas of increased attenuation with surrounding decreased attenuation suggestive of multiple metastatic lesions. Cerebral angiography was abnormal in 10 patients. Alternating segments of narrowing and dilatation (beading) were noted in five of these cases, while angiograms in other cases suggested mass lesions. However, fully seven patients had *normal* cerebral angiography.

At autopsy, examination of visceral structures revealed small discrete foci of angiitis in six cases. These small foci of angiitis were found in the lungs,[44,54,315] kidneys,[44,53] myocardium,[115] and prostate.[14] The most common neuropathologic finding (21 cases) was multiple small foci of infarction, followed by multiple foci of hemorrhage ("brain purpura," "petechiae") in 12 cases. Large infarcts were noted in only seven cases.[30,43,44,222,223,278,335] Large intraparenchymal hemorrhages were seen in three cases.[30,54,100] Large- or medium-vessel arterial occlusion by thrombus was uncommon[14,259,278]; subarachnoid blood was noted in four cases.[54,335,338,353] Small unruptured aneurysms were noted in two cases.[168,335] Herniation (uncal or cerebellar) was found in at least nine cases secondary to massive edema or hemorrhage.

Stroke was a presentation in a minority of cases. The case of Shuangshoti[353] was that of a young person who clinically presented with subarachnoid hemorrhage and died within 1 week. At autopsy there was a ruptured aneurysm in the involved portion of the left posterior cerebral artery.

Burger et al.[44] reported a 43-year-old man with "repetitive attacks of numbness on the left side of the body" for 2 months, followed by development of a left hemiparesis and left-sided numbness. A right carotid angiogram demonstrated "fusiform dilation" in the right parietal region. After the angiogram, the clinical impression was that the patient had a tumor as opposed to a stroke. The patient declined clinically over several months, developed uncal herniation, and died after exploratory craniotomy. Autopsy demonstrated a large infarct in the right frontoparietal area, and subfalcine and transtentorial herniation. In addition, there were older smaller infarcts within the larger area of recent infarction. Diffuse petechiae were noted as well.

The case of Nagaratnam and James[278] was a 15-year-old girl who developed headache, malaise, right hemiparesis, tonic-clonic seizure, and diminished consciousness over a 12-hour period. CT scan demonstrated a left parietal hypodense lesion with shift. The temporal, clinical, and radiographic profile was not inconsistent with massive cerebral infarction. She died within a few days and autopsy demonstrated angiitis involving the left middle cerebral artery, right posterior cerebral artery, a clot in the left internal carotid artery siphon, and a large infarction in the left temporoparietal territory of the left middle cerebral artery.

Case 4 of Koo and Massey[223] was a 78-year-old man who was found unresponsive and subsequently was witnessed to have a major motor seizure. Examination demonstrated a left hemianopia, left hemiparesis with hyperreflexia, and bilateral extensor plantar responses and frontal release signs. CT scan demonstrated bifrontal low attenuation changes, more on the right than the left, and a clinical diagnosis of "multi-infarct state" was made. Subsequent autopsy documented angiitis in arterioles and small arteries as well as some involvement of veins and venules. Vasculitic involvement was more marked in pial and penetrating vessels, and larger arteries appeared to be spared. "Patchy areas of ischemic changes" and "perivascular ring hemorrhages" were noted.

Case 1 of Biller et al.[30] was a 70-year-old man who had several weeks of altered mental status and at operation was found to have a subacute hemorrhage. The presentation was said to be that of a spontaneous intracranial hemorrhage. He subsequently developed inappropriate behavior and obtundation and eventually died 4 months later. Uncal herniation was demonstrated at autopsy. Microscopic findings were consistent with granulomatous angiitis. The brain "was variably hemorrhagic with nearly confluent acute and subacute cortical infarcts." There was also a large acute infarction in the cerebellum.

### Diagnosis

None of the standard laboratory tests are diagnostic for granulomatous angiitis, and normal findings do not exclude the diagnosis. Angiograms, in particular, may be normal[346]; a pattern of alternating dilation and constriction ("beading") is a nonspecific sign that may be seen in a variety of vasculitides and other conditions.[109,232,359,360,370] Laboratory tests may include blood cultures, spinal fluid cultures, viral titers (including human immunodeficiency virus), serologic tests for syphilis, coagulation studies (prothrombin time, partial thromboplastin time, lupus anticoagulant), anticardiolipin antibodies, antinuclear antibodies, rheumatoid factor, complement, cryoglobulins, immunofixation electrophoresis, and antineutrophil cytoplasmic autoantibodies (polyarteritis nodosa, Wegener's granulomatosis). Diagnostic studies or biopsies to exclude sarcoid, lymphoma, or systemic vasculitis should be performed as indicated. Brain biopsy may be necessary to differentiate between tumor, infection, and vasculitis. Since isolated granulomatous angiitis of the central nervous system has a predilection for leptomeningeal vessels, the procedure should include a leptomeningeal biopsy as well as a parenchymal biopsy. However, even these efforts are occasionally unrewarded: the biopsy has been negative in several subsequently autopsy-proven cases.[43,53,155,168,180,408]

### Treatment

There is no standard treatment. Progression of the disease and death has frequently occurred despite treatment with high-dose steroids.[14,155,195] Remissions have been reported using a combination of prednisone and cyclophosphamide,[76,272] In one patient with Hodgkin's disease, stabilization of granulomatous angiitis of the central nervous system occurred after treatment of the lymphoma.[137]

## TAKAYASU'S ARTERITIS

Takayasu's arteritis (pulseless disease, idiopathic aortitis) is a large-vessel granulomatous arteritis that affects the aorta, its main branches, and occasionally the pulmonary artery. Although pathologic changes in the arteries are similar to those found in giant cell arteritis,[280] Takayasu's arteritis tends to affect younger people, particularly women. Most cases have been reported from Asia, but the disease is found worldwide.[144] Like giant cell arteritis, constitutional symptoms (malaise, weight loss, fever) and elevated erythrocyte sedimentation rate are common.[144] Symptoms of arm claudication and syncope occur more frequently than retinal or cerebral ischemia.[144] Brachial pressures and pulses are frequently asymmetric, and there may be asymmetry between pressures in the arms and legs.[144]

Cerebrovascular complications occur in patients with more advanced disease, particularly in patients with retinopathy, hypertension secondary to renal artery stenosis, aortic regurgitation, and aortic aneurysms.[193] Cerebral infarction and retinal ischemia may occur consequent to stenosis or occlusion of the carotid or vertebral arteries, but the intracranial arteries are rarely, if ever, involved.[280] "Subclavian steal" may also occur, but this physiologic phenomenon is not always accompanied by symptoms of vertebrobasilar ischemia.[406] Intracerebral hemorrhage is usually related to hypertension.[192,387] Aneurysmal subarachnoid hemorrhage has been reported, although this could be a chance association in some cases. In one case, subarachnoid hemorrhage was attributed to an aneurysm of the distal intracranial segment of one of the vertebral arteries.[261]

Treatment may include corticosteroids, cytotoxic agents (cyclophosphamide), surgery, or a combination of these modalities.[348] Regression of carotid stenosis has been reported after administration of corticosteroids.[193] A variety of surgical reconstructive and bypass procedures have been employed,[322] including extracranial-intracranial bypass with saphenous vein grafts[117] and femoral artery to internal carotid artery bypass using synthetic grafts.[404] Some have advised delaying surgery until after the inflammatory process can be controlled with corticosteroids,[144] while others have not found this to be problematic.[348]

## HERPES ZOSTER OPHTHALMICUS AND DELAYED CONTRALATERAL HEMIPARESIS

Some patients with herpes zoster involving the first division of the trigeminal nerve (herpes zoster ophthalmicus) subsequently develop contralateral hemiparesis weeks to months later. The exact percentage of all patients with herpes zoster who are destined to develop this complication is unknown, but probably small. The onset of hemiparesis may be acute and undistinguishable from stroke syndromes caused by more conventional mechanisms, although some patients have more global mental status changes that suggest an underlying meningoencephalitic process.[121,167] Occasionally, the hemiparesis may progress, or may recur after a period of improvement.[167] Spinal fluid examination may disclose a mild to moderate pleocytosis and increased protein.[167]

Computerized tomograms have demonstrated large infarctions ipsilateral to the involved trigeminal nerve, most often in the lenticulostriate territory of the middle cerebral artery involving the capsule, striatum, and corona radiata.[167,228,381] Cerebral angiography may either be normal or document segmental narrowing or occlusion in the ipsilateral supraclinoid internal carotid artery siphon segment, middle cerebral artery M1 segment, anterior cerebral artery A1 segment, and the anterior cerebral artery A2 segment beneath the genu of the corpus callosum (pericallosal).[39,118,164,167,251] On rare occasions, the ipsilateral posterior cerebral artery P1 segment and contralateral anterior cerebral artery A1 segment have been involved.[39,164] Mycotic aneurysms and subarachnoid hemorrhage have been reported.[284] One patient developed aneurysmal dilatation of the intrapetrosal segment of the left internal carotid artery associated with ipsilateral Horner syndrome, hearing loss, and ear pain.[140] The predilection for involvement of the ipsilateral intracerebral arteries at the base of the brain have led some to suggest that the process may be due to viral spread to the involved arteries by route of the intracranial branches of the ophthalmic division of the trigeminal nerve.[252]

Postmortem examinations have most often documented cerebral infarction in the ipsilateral carotid or middle cerebral artery territory secondary to a necrotizing (not granulomatous) arteritis with or without thrombosis,[88,121,167] although one report has documented an occlusive thrombolic vasculopathy without frank vasculitis.[92] One patient has had cerebellar infarction ipsilateral to the involved trigeminal nerve, with a mild mononuclear infiltrate documented in the adventitia of the thrombosed superior cerebellar artery.[110] Large hematomas were found in the two cases of Mackenzie et al.[252] Swelling and lymphocytic infiltration of the ipsilateral trigeminal ganglion and nerve trunk have also been noted.[88,121,252] "Herpeslike" virions have been identified in middle cerebral artery smooth muscle.[88]

Therapy has included corticosteroids, acyclovir, and anticoagulants,[88,167,251] although recovery without treatment has been reported.

## POLYARTERITIS NODOSA

Polyarteritis nodosa is a necrotizing angiitis of the medium to small muscular arteries throughout the body. The peripheral nervous system is more commonly involved than the central nervous system, but in the series of Ford and Siekert,[113] fully 46 percent had symptoms and signs referable to the central nervous system. Central nervous system complications tend to occur late in the course of the disease in the setting of renal failure, fever, and other systemic manifestations.[113] Diffuse or multifocal cerebral symptoms and signs, such as headache, confusion or psychiatric syndromes, and generalized or focal seizures are more common than stroke. However, 13 percent of the patients in the series of Ford and Siekert[113] had cerebral infarction or hemorrhage. Cerebral angiography in patients with central nervous system manifestations may demonstrate multiple saccular-shaped aneurysms, similar to those visualized on visceral angiography.[374]

Necropsy has demonstrated the necrotizing vasculitic changes in large cerebral arteries (internal carotid, middle cerebral, posterior cerebral),[52,212,296,297] small meningeal arteries,[55,212,255,296,297] or both.[296,297] The size of the associated cerebral infarctions in these cases paralleled the size of the artery involved. In a particularly detailed study presented by Castaigne et al.,[52] arteritic involvement of one of the vertebral arteries resulted in thrombosis and infarction in the brain stem and cerebellum. Subarachnoid hemorrhage has been reported, and in one instance necropsy demonstrated massive subarachnoid hemorrhage in the region of the anterior cerebral and anterior communicating artery with dissection into the frontal lobe and rupture into the ventricular system.[124] A fusiform arteriosclerotic aneurysm of the anterior communicating artery was noted, but this was not the site of hemorrhage. Instead, the bleeding had emanated from a "longitudinal tear" in an arteritically involved segment of the right anterior cerebral artery.[124] Necropsy-proven cases of cerebral infarction associated with necrotizing arteritis of the cerebral arteries have been reported in the setting of polyarteritis nodosa associated with hepatitis B antigenemia.[347] The spinal cord may also be involved.[142,287]

Diagnostic studies in patients suspected of having polyarteritis nodosa should include serologic tests for hepatitis B, antineutrophil cytoplasmic autoantibody (ANCA), and may include visceral or cerebral angiography,[374] or biopsy of an organ system suspected of involvement.[65] Treatment consists of corticosteroids and cyclophosphamide.[103,233]

## WEGENER'S GRANULOMATOSIS

Wegener's granulomatosis is a necrotizing granulomatous vasculitis involving the upper and lower respiratory tracts and other organ systems in association with glomerulonephritis.[102] Nervous system complications include peripheral neuropathy and mononeuritis multiplex,[10,89] central nervous system infection,[10] local invasion by destructive granulomatous lesions causing cranial nerve palsies,[10,89,345] and central nervous system vasculitis.[10,89,267,337] Pathologically proven cerebrovascular complications have included infarction, hemorrhage (including subarachnoid hemorrhage), and cerebral venous thrombosis.[89,116,246,248,267,337,377] These complications typically occur in the setting of well-established extracranial disease. In one autopsied case reported by Drachman,[89] interhemispheric subarachnoid hemorrhage and cerebral infarction in the distribution of the anterior cerebral artery occurred consequent to panarteritic involvement of this artery. Lucas et al.[246] reported a patient who died of caudate hemorrhage with intraventricular rupture. At postmortem examination the hemorrhage appeared to originate from vessels affected by necrotizing vasculitis. The case of Satoh et al.[337] was a 67-year-old man who developed a clinical syndrome consistent with bifrontal infarction. At autopsy, the medium to large branches of the anterior cerebral artery were thrombosed and fibrinoid necrosis was noted. Necrotizing vasculitis and granulomatous lesions were present in the small arteries and veins in the frontal areas of the base of the brain where a suppurative meningitis was also noted. Necrotizing cerebral thrombophlebitis accounted for cortical vein thrombosis in the patient of Mickle et al.[267] Cavernous sinus invasion may occur, and internal carotid artery occlusion has been documented in one such case.[130]

The presence of antineutrophil cytoplasmic autoantibodies (ACPA, ANCA) may facilitate diagnosis of Wegener's granulomatosis.[361] Central nervous system complications may have become less frequent with the advent of protocols combining cyclophosphamide and corticosteroids, which appear to be more effective than corticosteroids alone.[102]

Occasional reports of amaurosis fugax, ischemic optic neuropathy,[394] subarachnoid hemorrhage,[238] and "strokelike" syndromes[400] have been reported in patients with various forms of necrotizing "allergic" angiitis.

## LYMPHOMATOID GRANULOMATOSIS

Lymphomatoid granulomatosis is an "angiocentric and angiodestructive lymphoreticular proliferative and granulomatous disease" that primarily involves the lungs and may involve the central nervous system in approximately 20 percent of cases.[242] The disease may mimic Wegener's granulomatosis,[241] and sometimes progression to lymphoma has occurred.[242] Clinical manifestations of central nervous system involvement usually consist of subacute, progressive syndromes of focal brain parenchymal or cranial nerve involvement that mimic neoplasm, encephalitis, or multiple sclerosis, but rarely cerebrovascular disease.[9,170,172,191,205,213,299,395] Primary central nervous system involvement has been reported.[221,339]

## CRYOGLOBULINEMIA

There are rare reports of central nervous system complications in patients with mixed cryoglobulinemia.[1,316,319] Central nervous system manifestations have included diffuse encephalopathic syndromes with focal signs, seizures, myelopathy, and occasionally stroke. Angiographic findings in these patients have included narrowing of the vertebral artery and occlusion of the posterior inferior cerebellar artery, and occlusion of the left middle cerebral artery without evidence of atherosclerosis elsewhere.[1] Postmortem findings in one patient demonstrated multiple small-vessel thrombotic occlusions.[1] The exact underlying pathophysiologic mechanisms of vascular occlusion are unknown.

## SYSTEMIC LUPUS ERYTHEMATOSUS

Reports on the neurologic and neuropathologic manifestations of systemic lupus erythematosus (SLE) have long emphasized the high frequency of central nervous system complications. However, specific clinical syndromes and pathophysiologic mechanisms of cerebrovascular disease in the setting of SLE have until recently largely remained obscure.[119] This has been due, in part, to the tendency in older clinical series to either lump stroke under broad categories along with other central nervous system manifestations ("neuropsychiatric disturbances," "neurologic lesions"), or to split neurologic manifestations into various signs and symptoms ("hemiplegia," "cranial nerve deficits," "aphasia").[119] Pathologic series have documented a variety of cerebrovascular lesions, but the point has recently been made that findings in the brain and cerebral vessels at autopsy infrequently correlate with clinical syndromes prior to death.[82] Over the last decade, however, a number of clinical and pathologic reports have called attention to potential embolic and prothrombotic mechanisms of stroke in systemic lupus erythematosus that were heretofore unrecognized or underemphasized.[82,114,119,133,153,217] These findings may have important therapeutic implications for some patients with SLE and stroke.[119]

The percentage of patients with SLE who develop stroke during their course is difficult to estimate from clinical series that often originate from referral centers. In a prospective series of 150 patients followed at Columbia-Presbyterian Medical Center, Estes and Christian[98] mention four patients who had fatal stroke. Feinglass et al.[107] reported that 5 (2.9 percent) of their 140 SLE patients had "typical cerebrovascular accidents." Two more recent clinical series focusing on the subject of stroke and SLE have documented clinical syndromes of cerebrovascular disease in 5.6 to 15 percent.[119,217] Certainly stroke is not the most common central nervous system manifestation of SLE. In the series of Feinglass et al.,[107] stroke occurred one-third as often as seizures, and one-fifth as often as "psychiatric illness." According to two recent series, stroke may be more likely to occur during the first 5 years after diagnosis of SLE.[119,217] Kitagawa et al.[217]

found renal involvement and high titers of anti-DNA antibodies significantly more frequently in SLE patients with stroke than in those without stroke. Among stroke "risk factors" (hypertension, hypercholesterolemia, heart disease, steroid therapy, diabetes), only hypertension was significantly more frequent in SLE patients with stroke than in those without stroke.[217] They associated hypertension with renal involvement. In their series, Futrell and Millikan[119] found a high risk of stroke (87 percent) among SLE patients with cardiac valvular disease. Few data exist on recurrence rates in patients with stroke in the setting of SLE, but in the series of Futrell and Millikan,[119] it was alarmingly high—64 percent.

## Mechanisms of Cerebrovascular Disease in Patients With Systemic Lupus Erythematosus

### Vasculitis

The sudden occurrence of central nervous system symptoms in a patient with SLE usually arouses diagnostic suspicions of "vasculitis" or "lupus cerebritis." However, if the numerous studies on the central nervous system complications of SLE published over the years have one feature in common, it is the strikingly low frequency of documented vasculitic changes in the vessels on postmortem examination.[82,94,119,199] Johnson and Richardson[199] documented a high frequency of destructive and proliferative lesions in arterioles and capillaries associated with microinfarction and hemorrhage, but vasculitis was found in only 3 of their 24 cases, and was felt to be either focal or reactive. Ellis and Verity[94] found vasculitis in only 7 percent in their series of 57 cases studied from 1955 to 1977. A recent report of clinical and neuropathologic findings in 50 patients with SLE presented by Devinsky et al.,[82] documented not a single instance of vasculitis involving the cerebral vessels!

### Cerebral Infarction

In the necropsy series of Johnson and Richardson,[199] widespread microinfarction in the cortex and brain stem occurred in the vast majority of patients (20 of 24 cases, 83 percent). This was felt to correlate with the predominant clinical features: seizures, "disturbances of mental function," and cranial nerve abnormalities. In contrast, macroscopically apparent areas of cerebral infarction, which would be expected to correlate with clinical stroke syndromes, occurred in only four cases (17 percent). The mechanisms of infarction in their few cases of macroscopic infarction were not apparent.[199] In the necropsy series of Ellis and Verity,[94] only 12 percent had large infarcts (greater than 1 cm) and these were "usually found in the distribution of the middle cerebral artery." Interestingly, in only one patient were they able to identify thrombosis in the responsible artery.[94] In this regard, it should be noted that angiographic studies have documented occlusions of large intracranial vessels (internal carotid artery, middle cerebral artery, anterior cerebral artery).[107,355,375] In Trevor's first case, a "rounded filling defect" was demonstrated in the supraclinoid segment of the right internal carotid artery, which 3 years later had recanalized.[375] Other patients have had tapering occlusions of the middle cerebral artery or internal carotid artery, a finding that was felt to be indicative of arteritis but no histologic confirmation was available.[375]

In their communication describing an "atypical verrucous endocarditis" in patients with SLE (Fig. 25-2), Libman and Sacks[240] suspected that cerebral embolism may have occurred in one of their patients (the brain was not examined at necropsy). However, only recently has attention been called to the possibility that cardiogenic brain embolism (with or without associated Libman-Sacks endocarditis) may be an important mechanism of stroke in patients with SLE.[82,114,119,133,217] In a necropsy series of 50 patients with SLE, Devinsky et al.[82] documented embolic brain infarcts in fully 10 patients (20 percent), cardiac sources being Libman-Sacks endocarditis in 5 patients, chronic valvulitis in 2 patients, and mural thrombus in 2 patients. Documentation of cardiac sources of emboli in patients with systemic lupus erythematosus and stroke might prompt treatment with anticoagulants.[119]

Thrombotic thrombocytopenic purpura, (thrombocytopenia, microangiopathic hemolytic anemia, fever, renal failure, central nervous system signs) may be an important but underdiagnosed mechanism of stroke in the terminal stages of SLE. Thrombotic thrombocytopenic purpura was documented in 7 (14 percent) of the 50 patients in the necropsy series of Devinsky et al.[82] Retrospectively, they found that 14 (28 percent) of their patients had a "clinical profile consistent" with thrombotic thrombocytopenic purpura during the terminal stages of the disease, but this diagnosis was made antemortem in only 1 patient.

The association of antiphospholipid antibodies (lupus anticoagulant, anticardiolipin antibody) with cerebrovascular disease in patients with and without SLE is discussed in a later section in this chapter.[153] The importance of a possible prothrombotic state associated with the lupus anticoagulant or anticardiolipin antibody as a mechanism of cerebral infarction in patients with SLE is underscored by a recent clinical series in which the lupus anticoagulant was detected in 38 percent and anticardiolipin antibody in 43 percent of SLE patients with stroke who were investigated for these abnormalities.[217] Documentation of an antiphospholipid antibody in a patient with SLE and stroke may have important treatment implications, anticoagulants having been recommended by some (see below).

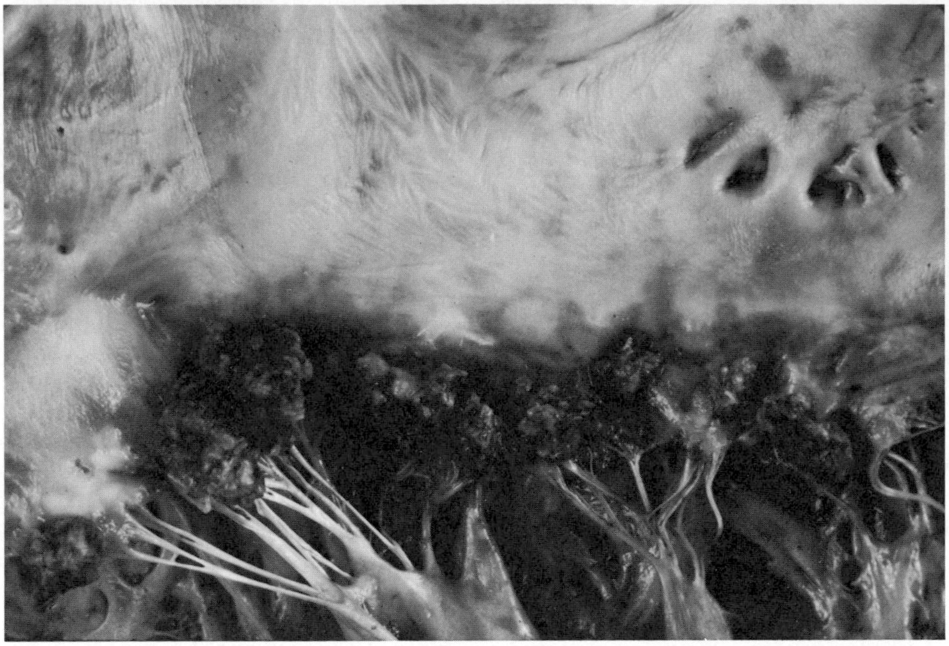

**Fig. 25-2.** Libman-Sacks endocarditis involving the mitral valve in a patient with systemic lupus erythematosus. (Courtesy of Dr. William D. Edwards, Department of Laboratory Medicine and Pathology, Mayo Clinic.)

## Hemorrhage

Hemorrhage as a cause of stroke in patients with SLE is well documented clinically, but appears to occur less often than infarction.[119,217,231] Intracerebral hemorrhage is sometimes, but not always, associated with hypertension and thrombocytopenia.[119,217,376] For example, in the series of Johnson and Richardson,[199] three patients died from intracerebral hemorrhage, but only one had hypertension, and none had thrombocytopenia. They could not establish the exact mechanism of hemorrhage in these three cases, but they did note that the hemorrhages were lobar, not in the typical location of hypertensive hemorrhage. Small hemorrhages were much more common in their series.[199] The more recent necropsy series of Devinsky et al.[82] did not document large intracerebral hematoma. Subarachnoid hemorrhage is frequently found at autopsy, but this may often be in association with intraparenchymal hemorrhage.[94] Some patients with SLE do develop clinical syndromes of subarachnoid hemorrhage. In some instances, the subarachnoid hemorrhage has been secondary to rupture of a berry aneurysm,[98,156,376] a possible chance association. On rare occasions, subarachnoid hemorrhage has occurred secondary to rupture of a fusiform aneurysm with associated transmural angiitis documented at necropsy.[211] In other instances of "primary subarachnoid hemorrhage," neither angiitis or berry aneurysm has been documented.[217] Subdural hematoma has also been reported, but mechanisms involved are uncertain.[82,108]

## Cerebral Venous Thrombosis

Cerebral venous thrombosis is an uncommon but well-documented cerebrovascular complication in SLE.[236,352,383] The mechanism of venous thrombosis in these patients may be multifactorial, lupus anticoagulant and anticardiolipin antibody having been detected in some, but not in all.[236,383] Clinical syndromes have included focal cerebral signs, including alternating hemiparesis, hemiplegia, and aphasia, but clinicians should be particularly alert to the fact that some patients have presented with headache, papilledema, and no focal neurologic signs ("pseudotumor cerebri").[383] Cerebral angiography, magnetic resonance imaging (MRI), or MRI angiography may be necessary to confirm this diagnosis.

### Antiphospholipid Antibodies and Stroke

Antiphospholipid antibodies, including anticardiolipin antibodies and the so-called "lupus anticoagulant," are a class of autoantibodies that bind to negatively charged phospholipid molecules.[123] Bowie and colleagues[40] noted the association of thrombotic events with the presence of the "circulating anticoagulant" in patients with lupus nearly 30 years ago, but it has only been in the last decade that attention has been called to the possible association of antiphospholipid antibodies with cerebrovascular disease, systemic thrombotic events, spontaneous abortion, and thrombocytopenia.[69,122,154,179,276] These phenomena may be associated with antiphospholipid antibodies either in the setting of SLE or as a "primary" antiphospholipid syndrome.[17] Antiphospholipid antibodies have been reported in patients with Behçet's disease,[181] Sneddon's syndrome,[135] acquired immunodeficiency syndrome,[63] and thymoma.[235] The exact cause of thrombosis in patients with antiphospholipid antibodies is unknown, but possible mechanisms include the binding of antiphospholipid antibody to platelet membranes or vascular endothelium, or the inhibition of various coagulation factors.[214]

There are currently no population-based studies that have defined the frequency with which antiphospholipid antibodies occur in the general population or in unreferred patients with stroke. Two recent studies from university-based referral institutions shed some light on this issue, however. Hess et al.[166] prospectively examined 110 consecutive patients with cerebrovascular disease over a 9-month period at a university medical center and found the presence of the IgG anticardiolipin antibody isotype in 8.2 percent, compared to only 1.6 percent of 122 age-matched controls. In a consecutive series of 46 patients with cerebrovascular disease under age 50 years, Brey et al.[41] found a significantly increased prevalence (45.7 percent) of antiphospholipid antibodies compared to controls (7.7 percent). Antiphospholipid antibodies may account for some familial cases of premature stroke.[112] Patients with IgM anticardiolipin antibody isotype may not be as prone to develop thrombotic events as those with IgG isotype.[154,166,234]

In three large clinical series of patients with cerebrovascular disease associated with antiphospholipid antibodies, 16 to 60 percent had systemic lupus erythematosus or a "lupuslike" syndrome.[12,42,234] Systemic thrombotic or thromboembolic events were reported in 14 to 46 percent.[12,42,234] A history of spontaneous abortion was reported in 16 to 29 percent of women in these series.[12,42,234]

A wide variety of cerebrovascular syndromes have been reported in association with antiphospholipid antibodies. Migraine has been a prominent feature in several reports,[12,42] although the prevalence of antiphospholipid antibodies among migraine patients appears to be low.[163] "Recurrent stereotypical events" were emphasized in the series of Levine et al.[234] Ocular manifestations have included amaurosis fugax, retinal artery occlusion, retinal artery branch occlusion, retinal vein occlusion, and acute ischemic optic neuropathy.[42,85,234]

Briley et al.[42] have called attention to a syndrome of "acute ischemic encephalopathy" in four patients who were "acutely ill," confused, and obtunded, with an asymmetrical quadriparesis, hyperreflexia, and bilateral extensor plantar responses" occurring in a setting of systemic illness and high anticardiolipin antibody levels. An autopsy in one of these patients demonstrated atherosclerotic changes in the carotid and middle cerebral arteries and multiple small-vessel occlusions with fibrin thrombi, but no vasculitis.[42]

Among those patients with cerebral infarction and antiphospholipid antibodies, the propensity for recurrent and multiple events has been emphasized. Of the patients reported by the Antiphospholipid Study Group,[12] 30 percent had evidence of prior cerebral infarction, and there was a 9.4 percent recurrence rate during an average 16.2-month mean follow-up. Levine et al.[234] reported multiple cerebral infarction in 70 percent of his patients with ischemic stroke, and a 1-year recurrence rate for cerebral infarction of 13 percent. Brain computed tomography and magnetic resonance imaging have demonstrated predominantly small cortical infarcts, rarely small deep infarcts.[42,234] Among patients undergoing cerebral angiography, intracranial lesions, including branch occlusions and stenoses or occlusions of the middle cerebral artery M1 segment, anterior cerebral artery A1 segment, and internal carotid artery, have been reported twice as frequently as extracranial carotid or vertebral stenoses or occlusions;[12] a finding opposite of what would be expected in patients with atherosclerotic cerebrovascular disease. The angiographic appearance of "vasculitis" was documented in only two of the 49 patients reported by the Antiphospholipid Study Group,[12] and in none of the patients in the series of Levine et al.[234] and Briley et al.[42] Other reports have called attention to possible association between antiphospholipid antibodies and syndromes of "multi-infarct dementia."[19,68] Potentially embologenic cardiac abnormalities, including valvular abnormalities and thrombus, have been reported in a number of patients with cerebrovascular disease and antiphospholipid antibodies.[12,16,78,277] Given the apparent potential for development of cerebral embolism in these patients, echocardiography may be particularly indicated in patients with cerebrovascular disease associated with antiphospholipid antibodies.[407] Autopsies have demonstrated small vessel occlusions with fibrin in the brain in one patient reported by Briley et al.,[42] and thrombi in large to medium-sized extracranial arteries (brain not examined) in the two cases of Levine et al.[234]

There is currently no standard treatment for ischemic cerebrovascular disease in association with antiphospholipid antibodies. Antiplatelet agents, anticoagulants, steroids, and immunosuppressants have been used.[15,42,234] The occurrence of "recurrent thrombosis" (deep vein thrombosis, myocardial infarction) in a series of six patients with anticardiolipin antibodies following warfarin withdrawal has prompted one group to recommend long-term anticoagulation.[15]

## SCLERODERMA

Scleroderma (progressive systemic sclerosis) rarely directly causes central nervous system manifestations.[132] Convulsions, stroke, and pathologic findings of arterial changes in the brains of patients with scleroderma are the result of hypertension consequent to renal disease.[132] However, the patient of Lee and Haynes[230] sustained a cerebral infarction associated with arteritic involvement of the ipsilateral internal carotid artery. She had a 10-year history of weight loss, intermittent fever, skin tightening, dysphagia, and Raynaud's phenomena, and developed a right hemiparesis and subsequent seizure. Blood pressure was normal on admission. Left carotid arteriogram demonstrated long segmental narrowing of the interosseous segment of the internal carotid artery siphon and occlusion of the anterior and middle cerebral arteries. At autopsy, the left carotid artery intima was thickened due to "fibrous proliferation." Muscle fibers in the media were "disorganized and indistinct." The vasa vasorum and medium-size arteries in the adventitia were surrounded by "inflammatory cells" and a few examples of "fibrinoid change" were seen. Examination of the brain demonstrated a large left cerebral hemisphere infarction with occlusion of the left anterior cerebral artery with recent thrombus and recanalized thrombus in the left middle cerebral artery. Degenerative changes attributable to scleroderma were not documented in these intracranial arteries, but the "surrounding connective tissue . . . showed inflammatory degenerative changes similar to those in the carotid sheath." The angiographic appearance of "cerebral arteritis" associated with mild CSF pleocytosis, increased CSF protein, and increased CSF opening pressure has been reported in a patient with scleroderma and seizures.[99]

## RHEUMATOID ARTHRITIS

Central nervous system manifestations of rheumatoid arthritis are rare, and tend to occur in the setting of long-established disease with either clinical (fever, weight loss, active arthritis) or laboratory (elevated rheumatoid factor, elevated erythrocyte sedimentation rate) evidence of disease activity. Rheumatoid meningitis ("pachymeningitis") has been reported as an asymptomatic finding at autopsy[363] or may cause a variety of central nervous system symptoms and signs, including headache, visual loss, seizures, altered mental status, hemiparesis, and spinal cord compression.[23,141,194,215,216,258,363] Findings at autopsy include thickening and distention of the meninges with a proteinaceous fluid.[194,363] The dura and leptomeninges demonstrate foci of inflammatory mononuclear cells and multinucleated giant cells.[194,215,216,258,363] Rheumatoid nodules similar to those found elsewhere in the body have been described in the meninges and the choroid plexus.[194,215,216]

Central nervous system vasculitis, either isolated[256,292,364,392] or in association with systemic rheumatoid vasculitis,[198,312,324] has been documented on rare occasions. Some of these cases had associated pachymeningitis. Usually the small vessels of the leptomeninges are affected by fibronoid necrosis, perivascular nodule formation (similar to polyarteritis nodosa), and "onion skin" proliferation. Small infarcts are the usual associated parenchymal findings, although hematoma formation has been associated with necrotizing vasculitis involving the small and medium-size arteries in at least one case,[392] and "patchy" subdural and subarachnoid hemorrhage was found in another instance, presumably related to vasculitis involving small vessels in the subarchnoid space.[364] Usually these patients have had encephalopathic syndromes, including seizures and altered mental status,[24,256,292,312,324] although the patient of Watson and coworkers[292] presented with acute signs and symptoms of stroke involving both the left frontal lobe and left pons, subsequently documented to be secondary to hematomas at autopsy.

One of the most feared neurologic complications of rheumatoid arthritis is compressive myelopathy secondary to C1–C2 vertebral subluxation. A well-documented and equally disasterous complication of C1–C2 subluxation is massive vertebrobasilar territory infarction as a result of vertebral artery thrombosis.[203,393] In two autopsy studies, patients presented with occipital headache and episodic vertigo with neck flexion or rotation, or "occasional blackouts."[203,393] The case of Jones and Kaufmann[203] subsequently developed an episode of unconsciousness, disorientation, nystagmus, bilateral extensor plantar responses, and bilateral leg weakness. He became comatose with decerebrate posturing and Cheyne-Stokes respirations, and gradually a "coma vigil" ensued prior to death. The patient of Webb et al.[393] had occipital headaches and occasional blackouts prior to being found unconscious with a flaccid left hemiparesis and bilateral extensor plantar responses. She died within 30 hours of onset of coma. Vertebral artery thrombosis was thought to have resulted from pinching of the vertebral artery between the odontoid and rim of the foramen magnum[203] or stretching of the vertebral arteries between the transverse foramina of the C1 and C2 vertebrae.[393] Precipitation of vertebrobasilar ischemic symptoms has been associated with neck flexion, extension, or rotation in patients with C1–C2 subluxation.[178,203,323,393] Some have had angiographic documentation of narrowing or occlusion of the vertebral arteries with these maneuvers.[178,323] Vertebral artery pseudoaneurysm formation has also been reported.[105]

Instances of cerebral and ocular ischemia in the setting of rheumatoid arthritis have been associated with thrombocytosis[91,307] and hyperviscosity syndromes secondary to polyclonal gammopathy.[336]

## SJÖGREN'S SYNDROME

Sjögren's syndrome (xerostomia and keratoconjunctivitis sicca) is frequently found in conjunction with other collagen vascular diseases which may result in central nervous system complications. There is some uncertainty over the frequency and severity with which central nervous system complications occur in patients with *primary* Sjögren's syndrome (i.e., Sjögren's syndrome not associated with another collagen vascular disease).[6,31,273,282] Multiple sclerosis-like[5] and strokelike[6] syndromes have been reported, along with a variety of CT and MRI findings.[3] However, the exact pathophysiologic mechanisms involved are unknown. Postmortem brain examination of three patients with primary Sjögren's syndrome demonstrated "diffuse polymorphous meningitis" in three patients, associated with microhemorrhages in two patients, but antemortem clinical correlations were uncertain.[81] Necrotizing arteritis and spinal subarachnoid hemorrhage has been reported in one patient with Sjögren's syndrome and cryoglobulinemia.[4]

## SNEDDON'S SYNDROME

Livedo reticularis is a cutaneous condition characterized by a "fixed, deep bluish-red, reticulated pattern" caused by impaired superficial venous drainage of the skin (Fig. 25-3).[310] This cutaneous sign is found in a number of diseases, including polyarteritis nodosa, systemic lupus erythematosus, rheumatoid arthritis, dermatomyositis, and cryoglobulinemia.[310] Cerebrovascular disease in association with livedo reticularis is known as Sneddon's syndrome.[56,358] Sneddon's original description also included hypertension as part of a triad.[358] Many, but not all, of these patients have antiphospholipid antibodies.[18,135,200,204,237]

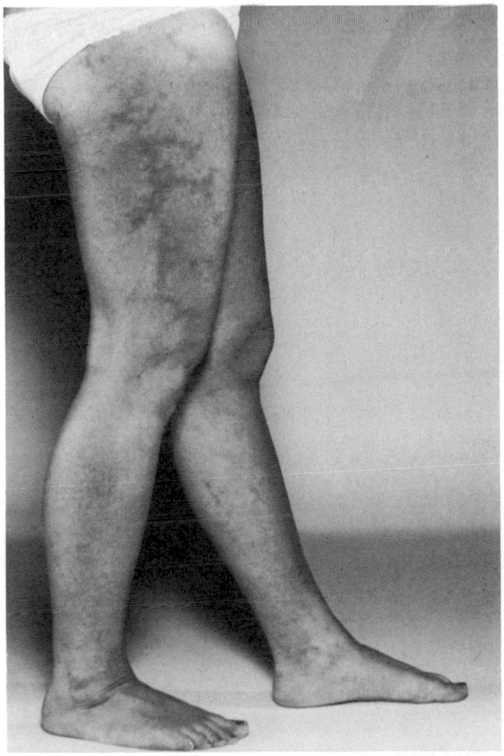

**Fig. 25-3.** Livedo reticularis in a patient with Sneddon's syndrome. (Courtesy of Department of Dermatology, Mayo Clinic.)

Livedo reticularis usually precedes neurologic involvement in these patients, but some present with stroke.[204] The most common cerebrovascular manifestation in this syndrome is recurrent cerebral infarction.[204,314,331,341,365,372] Transient ischemic attack, seizures, and dementia (possibly related to multiple infarctions) have been reported.[314,331,365] A variety of clinical stroke syndromes have been documented, frequently with prominent cortical signs.[314,331,365] The mechanism of infarction in these patients is for the most part unknown. Computerized tomograms have usually documented infarction involving the cortex (Fig. 25-4).[314,331,365,372] Angiograms have either been normal or demonstrated occlusions of medium-sized arteries and their branches, sometimes with moyamoya-type collateral networks.[302,314,331,358,365] Asherson et al.[18] found "heart valve lesions" in over a third of patients with levido reticularis associated with positive anticardiolipin antibodies. Skin biopsies have demonstrated "an occlusive and noninflammatory" vasculopathy involving the medium-sized arteries with focal and segmental intimal hyperplasia due to fibroelastic proliferation but no evidence of vasculititis.[314] In one autopsy case, Pĩnol Aquadé (quoted by Quimby and Perry)[310] found "vasculopathy with musculoelastic hyperplasia" with no vasculitis. Verrucous endocarditis was also documented. Various treatments have included antiplatelet agents, warfarin,[237] and plasmapheresis.[341]

## MALIGNANT ATROPHIC PAPULOSIS

Malignant atrophic papulosis (Degos' disease, Kohlmeier-Degos disease) is a progressive vasculopathy that affects the skin, cerebral circulation, and other organ systems.[80] Characteristic skin lesions consist of umbilicated raised papules with a white center (Fig. 25-5). The appearance of cutaneous lesions usually precedes neurologic manifestations, sometimes for years.[173,401] In some patients, however, neurologic manifestations may precede or accompany the development of cutaneous lesions.[263,343] Bowel perforations may occur.[21,367]

Neurologic complications are varied. In some patients, the initial neurologic manifestations have been symptoms and signs of transient ischemic attack[401] or stroke.[79] Others have had progressive focal or multifocal deficits with stepwise quantitative and qualitative worsening.[72,263,303,344,401] Others have had evidence of spinal cord involvement.[173,229,263,401] Angiographic

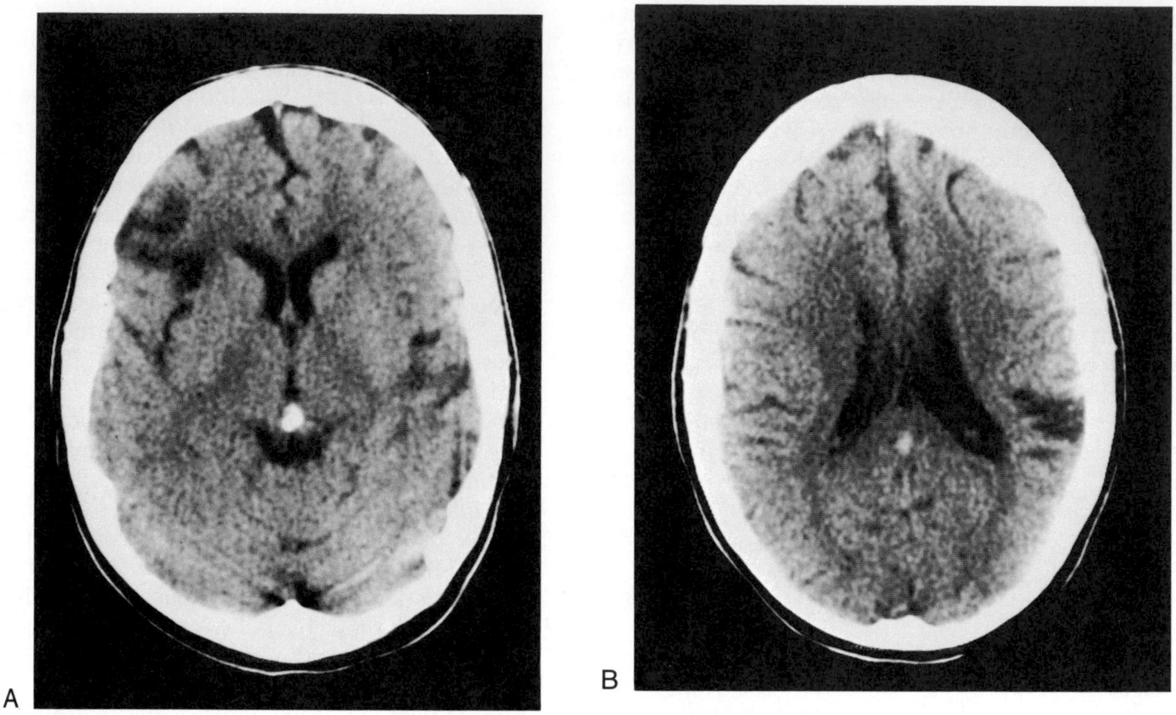

**Fig. 25-4.** Computerized tomogram demonstrating infarction in a patient with Sneddon's syndrome. (**A**) Right frontal cortex. (**B**) Left parietal cortex. (Courtesy of Dr. H. S. Luthra, Dr. A. J. D. Dale, Dr. J. Huston, and Department of Diagnostic Radiology, Mayo Clinic.)

findings have included multiple branch occlusions, and alternating segmental constriction and dilatation.[303,344] Computerized tomograms have demonstrated multifocal areas of infarction, hemorrhage, and even subdural hemorrhage.[303]

Pathologic examination of brain vessels has documented a peculiar "fibrous intimal proliferation" or "deposition of fibrous material" between endothelium and internal elastic lamina,[79,173,229,263,344,401] similar to vascular lesions in the skin. This may be accompanied by thrombosis. The small meningeal arteries are frequently involved,[263] but medium and even large arteries may also be affected.[173,401] Multiple small infarcts, either hemorrhagic or bland, are often

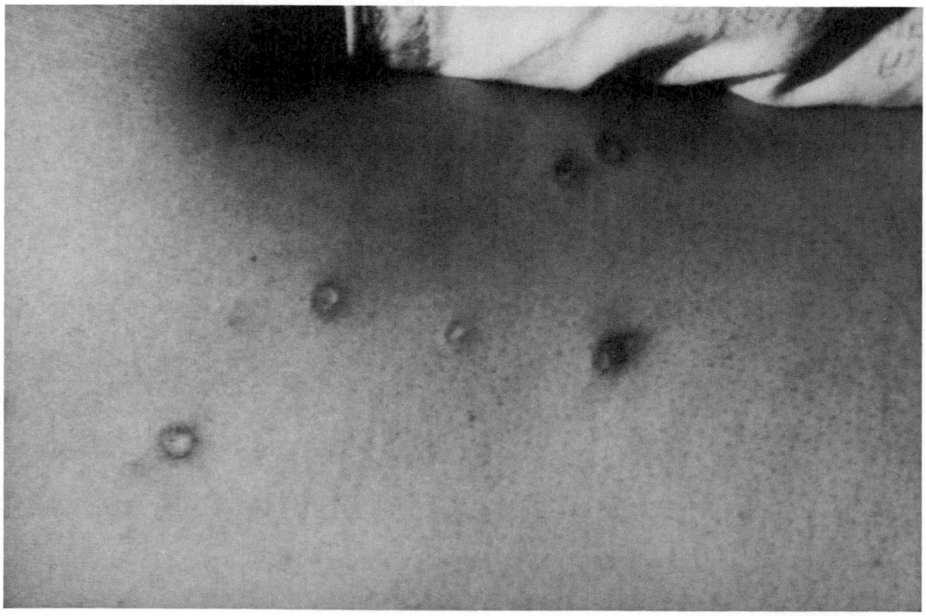

**Fig. 25-5.** Skin lesions of malignant atrophic papulosis (Degos' disease). (Courtesy of Department of Dermatology, Mayo Clinic.)

found.[72,229,263,344,401] These small infarcts may be confluent,[391] and involve the cortex,[263] or cortex and deeper structures.[173] Less often, large infarction with shift and herniation is documented.[21,344] Small parenchymal hemorrhages[79,173] and subarachnoid hemorrhage[263] are occasionally documented.

The exact etiology of this proliferative and occlusive vasculopathy has not been established. Some have reported increased platelet adhesiveness and aggregation,[90] although others have found no coagulation abnormalities.[254] The presence of anticardiolipin antibodies and lupus anticoagulant has been reported in at least one patient with Degos' disease.[96] A variety of therapies have been employed, usually ineffectively, including antiplatelet agents, anticoagulants, corticosteroids, and plasmapheresis.[229,263,350,401]

## BEHÇET'S DISEASE

Behçet's disease is an inflammatory condition of unknown etiology that is clinically typified by the triad of oral aphthous ulcers, genital ulcers, and uveitis. Other manifestations include arthritis, cutaneous vasculitis, thrombophlebitis, colitis, and central nervous system disease.[285,286] Central nervous system complications usually occur in patients who have established cutaneous or ocular disease, but there are well-documented instances of neurologic presentation.[87,190,225,368] Neurologic manifestations are varied, and few clinical features point to the underlying diagnosis in the absence of the cutaneous or ocular manifestations. Many patients present with a syndrome of aseptic meningitis or meningoencephalitis with fever and headache, with or without associated focal neurologic signs.[285,329] Many reports have emphasized a fluctuating course with exacerbations and remissions that are atypical for cerebrovascular disease.[209,245,285,330,402] Corticospinal tract signs, frequently bilateral, are common. Symptoms and signs of brain stem involvement and pseudobulbar palsy are frequently reported.[245,264,285,330,342,368] Less often, neurologic presentations may be sudden in onset and suggest stroke.[87,95,190,209,225] Some patients have presented with symptoms and signs of increased intracranial pressure, occasionally with minimal or no focal findings, due to angiographically documented cerebral venous sinus thrombosis.[20,62,152,189,293,329,366,397] Retinal ischemia and retinal "vasculitis" are also reported.[29,190,210,329]

Spinal fluid examination frequently demonstrates a moderate pleocytosis, predominantly lymphocytic, as well as increased protein, usually less than 100 mg/dl.[285,329] Anticardiolipin antibodies have been reported in patients with Behçet's disease, especially in patients with retinal ischemia or retinal "vasculitis."[181] Brain imaging with CT, and more recently MRI, has demonstrated a variety of lesions that, in some respects, are atypical for vascular disease.[165,210,298,399] Computerized tomograms demonstrate focal and circumscribed regions of decreased density that may enhance after contrast administration.[165,298,399] Findings on MRI usually consist of increased signal intensity on T2-weighted images.[210,298] These lesions usually are found in the deep structures, including brain stem, deep nuclei, and hypothalamus, but also in the hemispheric white matter.[165,210,298,399] Herskovitz et al.[165] have pointed out that, unlike vascular lesions, these findings tend to resolve over time after treatment and frequently do not conform to a single arterial territory. These features might be more suggestive of an inflammatory process as opposed to vascular occlusion.[165] Cerebral hemorrhage has been reported, but the mechanisms involved are unclear.[8,279] Cerebral angiography has usually been normal,[285] but occasional patients with a "vasculitic appearance" have been reported.[409] There is also a report of a large aneurysmal abnormality of the cervical segment of the internal carotid artery.[83]

Neuropathologic findings do not disclose clear-cut cerebrovascular mechanisms. The leptomeninges are frequently thickened and opacified.[245,264,330,368] Small regions of softening are most often found in the brain stem and basal ganglia, less often in the deep white matter, and least often in the cortex.[245,264,330,351,368] Gliosis has been prominent in some reports.[264,330,368] Many patients have had varying degrees of lymphocytic perivascular infiltration, usually mild to moderate,[264,330,351,368] sometimes perivenular. Small areas of perivascular necrosis and "scarring" are found, particularly in the brain stem, diencephalon, internal capsule, and basal ganglia.[330] Most reports have emphasized the paucity of arterial lesions and thromboses.[245,330,342,368] Small hemorrhages are also uncommonly documented.[209,279,342] Some reports have emphasized demyelination, perivenular and diffuse.[245,351,368] On rare occasions, large areas of infarction, either in the cortex or basal ganglia, with "endarteritis and postthrombotic recanalization" have been reported.[264] Granulomatous or necrotizing angiitis does not appear to be a commonly documented mechanism of central nervous system involvement in Behçet's disease.

A variety of therapies have been employed, including corticosteroids, cyclophosphamide, azathioprine, and chlorambucil.[286]

## RETINOCOCHLEOCEREBRAL VASCULOPATHY

Retinocochleocerebral vasculopathy is an unusual syndrome of small-vessel occlusions in the retina, cochlea, and brain affecting predominantly young women.[36,67,161,249,260,271,304,306,369] Fewer than 25 cases have been reported. Extracerebral clinical manifestations have included multiple episodes of visual loss related to retinal arteriolar occlusions, sensorineural hearing loss, and tinnitus. Funduscopic examination demonstrates occlusion of multiple retinal arterioles with peculiar "long columns of white material" oscillating with the pulse.[271,306] Neurologic manifestations include encephalopathy with prominent disturbances in cognition, memory and behavior, dysarthria, pseudobulbar affect, ataxia, vertigo, hemiparesis, and hemisensory loss.[36,67,161,260,271,304,369] Spinal fluid examinations may demonstrate a mild pleocytosis (predominantly lymphocytic) and elevated protein.[36,67,260,271,304,369] Cerebral angiography is usually normal.[36,304,369] Computerized tomograms are usually normal, but MRI may either be normal or demonstrate increased signal abnormalities on T2-weighted images in the white matter[36,260,271,304] or white matter and deep gray matter.[304] Brain biopsy has demonstrated gliosis, microinfarcts, small vessel "sclerosis," or "healed arteritis." Tests for anticardiolipin antibody, lupus anticoagulant, protein C deficiency, protein S deficiency, and antithrombin III deficiency have been negative.[304] No definite underlying connective tissue disease has been identified in these patients. Other patients with partial syndromes of characteristic retinal arteriolar occlusions and cerebral manifestations without cochlear or vestibular symptoms have been reported.[304] The etiology remains obscure. Some patients have appeared to respond to steroids and immunosuppressants,[271,369] while others have progressed despite these treatments.[36,304]

## REFERENCES


1. Abramsky O, Slavin S: Neurologic manifestations in patients with mixed cryoglobulinemia. Neurology (NY) 24:245, 1974
2. Alestig K, Barr J: Giant-cell arteritis: a biopsy study of polymyalgia rheumatica, including one case of Takayasu's disease. Lancet 1:1228, 1963
3. Alexander EL, Beall SS, Gordon B et al: Magnetic resonance imaging of cerebral lesions in patients with the Sjögren syndrome. Ann Intern Med 108:815, 1988
4. Alexander EL, Craft C, Dorsh C et al: Necrotizing arteritis and spinal subarachnoid hemorrhage in Sjögren syndrome. Ann Neurol 11:632, 1982
5. Alexander EL, Malinow K, Lejewski JE et al: Primary Sjögren's syndrome with central nervous system disease mimicking multiple sclerosis. Ann Intern Med 104:323, 1986
6. Alexander GE, Provost TT, Stevens MB, Alexander EL: Sjögren syndrome: central nervous system manifestations. Neurology (NY) 31:1391, 1981
7. Ali Ibn Isa: Memorandum book of a tenth-century oculist. (Translated by CA Wood.) Northwestern University Press, Chicago, 1936
8. Altinörs N, Senveli E, Arda N et al: Intracerebral hemorrhage and hematoma in Behçet's disease: case report. Neurosurgery 21:582, 1987
9. Amin SN, Gibbons CM, Lovell CR et al: A case of lymphomatoid granulomatosis with a protracted course and prominent CNS involvement. Br J Rheumatol 28:77, 1989
10. Anderson JM, Jamieson DG, Jefferson JM: Nonhealing granuloma and the nervous system. Q J Med 41:309, 1975
11. Andersson R, Malmvall BE, Bengtsson BA: Long-term corticosteroid treatment in giant cell arteritis. Acta Med Scand 220:465, 1986
12. Antiphospholipid Antibodies in Stroke Study Group: Clinical and laboratory findings in patients with antiphospholipid antibodies and cerebral ischemia. Stroke 21:1268, 1990
13. Armstrong RD, Behn A, Myles A et al: Histocompatibility antigens in polymyalgia rheumatica and giant-cell arteritis. J Rheumatol 10:659, 1983
14. Arthur G, Margolis G: Mycoplasma-like structures in granulomatous angiitis of the central nervous system: case reports with light and electron microscope studies. Arch Pathol Lab Med 101:382, 1977
15. Asherson RA, Chan JKH, Harris EN et al: Anticardiolipid antibody, recurrent thrombosis, and warfarin withdrawal. Ann Rheum Dis 44:823, 1985
16. Asherson RA, Gibson DG, Evans DW et al: Diagnostic and therapeutic problems in two patients with antiphospholipid antibodies, heart valve lesions, and transient ischaemic attacks. Ann Rheum Dis 47:947, 1988
17. Asherson RA, Khamashta MA, Ordi-Ros J et al: The "primary" antiphospholipid syndrome: major clinical and serological features. Medicine (Baltimore) 68:366, 1989
18. Asherson RA, Mayou SC, Merry P et al: The spectrum of livedo reticularlis and anticardiolipid antibodies. Br J Dermatol 120:215, 1989
19. Asherson RA, Mercey D, Phillips G et al: Recurrent stroke and multi-infarct dementia in systemic lupus erythematosus: association with antiphospholipid antibodies. Ann Rheum Dis 46:605, 1987
20. Bank I, Weart C: Dural sinus thrombosis in Behçet's disease. Arthritis Rheum 27:816, 1984
21. Barlow RJ, Heyl T, Simson IW, Schulz EJ: Malignant atrophic papulosis (Degos' disease): diffuse involvement of brain and bowel in an African patient. Br J Dermatol 118:117, 1988
22. Barricks ME, Traviesa DM, Glaser JS, Levy IS: Ophthalmoplegia in cranial arteritis. Brain 100:209, 1977
23. Bathon JM, Moreland LW, DiBartolomeo AG: Inflammatory central nervous system involvement in rheumatoid arthritis. Semin Arthritis Rheum 18:258, 1989
24. Beck DO, Corbett JJ: Seizures due to central nervous system rheumatoid meningovasculitis. Neurology (NY) 33:1058, 1983
25. Bengtsson BA, Malmvall BE: Prognosis of giant cell arteritis including temporal arteritis and polymyalgia rheumatica. Acta Med Scand 209:337, 1981
26. Bengtsson BA, Malmvall BE: The epidemiology of giant cell arteritis including temporal arteri-

tis and polymalgia rheumatica. Arthritis Rheum 24:899, 1981
27. Bengtsson BA, Malmvall BE: Giant cell arteritis. Acta Med Scand, suppl. 658:1, 1982
28. Beresford HR, Hyman RA, Shorer L: Self-limited granulomatous angiitis of the cerebellum. Ann Neurol 5:490, 1979
29. Besana C, Comi G, Del Maschio A et al: Electrophysiological and MRI evaluation of neurological involvement in Behçet's disease. J Neurol Neurosurgery Psychiatry 52:749, 1989
30. Biller J, Loftus CM, Moore SA et al: Isolated central nervous system angiitis first presenting as spontaneous intracranial hemorrhage. Neurosurgery 20:310, 1987
31. Binder A, Snaith ML, Isenberg D: Sjögren's syndrome: a study of its neurological complications. Br J Rheumatol 27:275, 1988
32. Blue MC, Rosenblum WI: Granulomatous angiitis of the brain with herpes zoster and varicella encephalitis. Arch Pathol Lab Med 107:126, 1983
33. Boesen P, Sorensen SF: Giant cell arteritis, temporal arteritis, and polymyalgia rheumatica in a Danish county: a prospective investigation, 1982–1985. Arthritis Rhem 30:294, 1987
34. Boghen DR, Glaser JS: Ischaemic optic neuropathy. Brain 98:689, 1975
35. Bogousslavsky J, Deruaz JP, Regli F: Bilateral obstruction of internal carotid artery from giant-cell arteritis and massive infarction limited to the vertebrobasilar area. Eur Neurol 24:57, 1985
36. Bogousslavsky J, Gaio JM, Caplan LR et al: Encephalopathy, deafness and blindness in young women: A distinct retinocochleocerebral arteriolopathy? J Neurol Neurosurg Psychiatry 52:43, 1989
37. Bonnetblanc JM, Adenis JP, Queroi M, Rammaert B: Immunofluoresence in temporal arteritis. N Engl J Med 298:458, 1978
38. Borenstein D, Costa M, Jannotta F, Rizzoli H: Localized isolated angiitis of the central nervous system associated with primary intracerebral lymphoma. Cancer 62:375, 1988
39. Bourdette DN, Rosenberg NL, Yatsu FM: Herpes zoster ophthalmicus and delayed ipsilateral cerebral infarction. Neurology (NY) 33:1428, 1983
40. Bowie EJW, Thompson JH, Jr, Pascuzzi CA, Owen CA, Jr: Thrombosis in systemic lupus erythematosus despite circulating anticoagulants. J Lab Clin Med 62:416, 1963
41. Brey RL, Hart RG, Sherman DG, Tegeler CH: Antiphospholipid antibodies and cerebral ischemia in young people. Neurology (NY) 40:1190, 1990
42. Briley DP, Coull BM, Goodnight SH, Jr: Neurological disease associated with antiphospholipid antibodies. Ann Neurol 25:221, 1989
43. Budzilovich GN, Feigin I, Siegel H: Granulomatous angiitis of the nervous system. Arch Pathol Lab Med 76:250, 1963
44. Burger PC, Burch JG, Vogel FS: Granulomatous angiitis: an unusual etiology of stroke. Stroke 8:29, 1977
45. Calabrese LH, Mallek JA: Primary angiitis of the central nervous system: report of 8 new cases, review of the literature, and proposal for diagnostic criteria. Medicine (Baltimore) 67:20, 1988
46. Calamia KT, Moore SB, Elveback LR, Hunder GG: HLA-DR locus antigens in polymyalgia rheumatica and giant cell arteritis. J Rheumol 8:993, 1981
47. Caplan L, Corbett J, Goodwin J et al: Neuro-ophthalmologic signs in the angiitic form of neurosarcoidosis. Neurology (NY) 33:1130, 1983
48. Cardell BS, Hanley T: A fatal case of giant-cell or temporal arteritis. J Pathol 63:587, 1951
49. Caselli RJ: Giant cell (temporal) arteritis: a treatable cause of multi-infarct dementia. Neurology (NY) 40:753, 1990
50. Caselli RJ, Daube JR, Hunder GG, Whisnant JP: Peripheral neuropathic syndromes in giant cell (temporal) arteritis. Neurology (NY) 38:685, 1988
51. Caselli RJ, Hunder GG, Whisnant JP: Neurologic disease in biopsy-proven giant cell (temporal) arteritis. Neurology (NY) 38:352, 1988
52. Castaigne P, Cambier J, Escourolle R, Brunet P: Les manifestations nerveuses centrales de la périartérite noueuse: à propos d'une observation anatomo-clinique. Ann Med Interne 121:375, 1970
53. Castleman B, McNeely BU: Case records of the Massachusetts General Hospital: case 41152. N Engl J Med 252:634, 1955
54. Castleman B, McNeely BU: Case records of the Massachusetts General Hospital: case 14-1967. N Engl J Med 276:741, 1967
55. Castleman B, McNeely BU: Case Records of the Massachusetts General Hospital: case 26-1967. N Engl J Med 276:1432, 1967
56. Champion RH, Rook A: Livedo reticularis. Proc R Soc Med 53:961, 1960
57. Chasnoff J, Vorzimer JJ: Temporal arteritis: a local manifestation of a systemic disease. Ann Intern Med 20:327, 1944
58. Chess J, Albert DM, Bhan AK et al: Serologic and immunopathologic findings in temporal arteritis. Am J Ophthalmol 96:283, 1983
59. Cid MC, Cervera R, Font J et al: Recurrent arterial thrombosis in a patient with giant-cell arteritis and raised anticardiolipin antibody levels. Br J Rheumatol 27:164, 1988
60. Clifford-Jones R, Love S, Gurusinghe N: Granulomatous angiitis of the central nervous system: a case with recurrent intracerebral haemorrhage. J Neurol Neurosurg Psychiatry 48:1054, 1985
61. Clyde WA, Thomas L: Pathogenesis studies in experimental mycoplasma disease: *M. gallisepticum* infections of turkeys. Ann NY Acad Sci 225:413, 1973
62. Cobby M, Hall CL, Higgs CMB: Behçet's syndrome presenting as intracranial hypertension in a Caucasian. J R Soc Med 81:478, 1988
63. Cohen AJ, Philips TM, Kessler CM: Circulating coagulation inhibitors in the acquired immunodeficiency syndrome. Ann Intern Med 104:175, 1986
64. Cohen DN, Damaske MM: Temporal arteritis: a

spectrum of ophthalmic complications. Ann Ophthalmol 7:1045, 1975
65. Cohen RD, Conn DL, Ilstrup DM: Clinical features, prognosis, and response to treatment in polyarteritis. Mayo Clin Proc 55:146, 1980
66. Collado A, Santamaria J, Ribalta T et al: Giant-cell arteritis presenting with ipsilateral hemiplegia and lateral medullary syndrome. Eur Neurol 29:266, 1989
67. Coppeto JR, Currie JN, Monteiro MLR, Lessell S: A syndrome of arterial-occlusive retinopathy and encephalopathy. Am J Ophthalmol 98:189, 1984
68. Coull BM, Bourdette DN, Goodnight SH, Jr et al: Multiple cerebral infarctions and dementia associated with anticardiolipin antibodies. Stroke 18:1107, 1987
69. Coull BM, Goodnight SH: Antiphospholipid antibodies, prethrombotic states, and stroke. Stroke 21:1370, 1990
70. Cravioto H, Feigin I: Non-infectious granulomatous angiitis with a predilection for the nervous system. Neurology (NY) 9:599, 1959
71. Crompton MR: The visual changes in temporal (giant cell) arteritis. Brain 82:377, 1959
72. Culicchia CF, Gol A, Erickson EE: Diffuse central nervous system involvement in papulosis atrophicans maligna. Neurology (NY) 12:503, 1962
73. Cull RE: Internal carotid artery occlusion caused by giant cell arteritis. J Neurol Neurosurg Psychiatry 42:1066, 1979
74. Cupps TR, Fauci AS: Central nervous system vasculitis: the vasculitides. Major Probl Intern Med 21:123, 1981
75. Cupps TR, Fauci AS: Giant cell arteritides: the vasculitides. Major Probl Intern Med 21:99, 1981
76. Cupps TR, Moore PM, Fauci AS: Isolated angiitis of the central nervous system. Am J Med 74:97, 1983
77. Currie J, Lessell S: Tonic pupil with giant cell arteritis. Br J Ophthalmol 68:135, 1984
78. D'Alton JG, Preston DN, Bormanis J et al: Multiple transient ischemic attacks, lupus anticoagulant and verrucous endocarditis. Stroke 16:512, 1985
79. Dastur DK, Singhal BS, Shroff HJ: CNS involvement in malignant atrophic papulosis (Kohlmeier-Degos disease): vasculopathy and coagulopathy. J Neurol Neurosurg Psychiatry 44:156, 1981
80. Degos R, Delort J, Tricot R: Dermatite papulosquameuse atrophiante. Bull Soc Franc Dermat Syph 49:148, 1942
81. de la Monte SM, Hutchins GM, Gupta PK: Polymorphous meningitis with atypical mononuclear cells in Sjögren's syndrome. Ann Neurol 14:455, 1983
82. Devinsky O, Petito CK, Alonso DR: Clinical and neuropathological findings in systemic lupus erythematosus: the role of vasculitis, heart emboli, and thrombotic thrombocytopenic purpura. Ann Neurol 23:380, 1988
83. Dhobb M, Ammar F, Bensaid Y et al: Arterial manifestations in Behçet's disease: four new cases. Ann Vasc Surg 1:249, 1986
84. Dickson ER, Maldonado JE, Sheps SG, Cain JA: Systemic giant-cell arteritis with polymyalgia rheumatica: reversible abnormalities of liver function. JAMA 224:1496, 1973
85. Digre KB, Durcan FJ, Branch DW et al: Amaurosis fugax associated with antiphospholipid antibodies. Ann Neurol 25:228, 1989
86. Dimant J, Grob D, Brunner NG: Ophthalmoplegia, ptosis, and myosis in temporal arteritis. Neurology (NY) 39:1054, 1980
87. Dobkin BH: Computerized tomographic findings in neuro-Behçet's disease. Arch Neurol 37:58, 1980
88. Doyle PW, Gibson G, Dolman CL: Herpes zoster ophthalmicus with contralateral hemiplegia: identification of cause. Ann Neurol 14:84, 1983
89. Drachman DA: Neurological complications of Wegener's granulomatosis. Arch Neurol 8:145, 1963
90. Drucker CR: Malignant atrophic papulosis: response to antiplatelet therapy. Dermatologica 180:90, 1990
91. Ehrenfeld M, Penchas S, Eliakim M: Thrombocytosis in rheumatoid arthritis: recurrent arterial thromboembolism and death. Ann Rheum Dis 36:579, 1977
92. Eidelberg D, Sotrel A, Horoupian DS et al: Thrombotic cerebral vasculopathy associated with herpes zoster. Ann Neurol 19:7, 1986
93. Elliott PD, Baker HL, Brown AL: The superficial temporal artery angiogram. Radiology 102:635, 1972
94. Ellis SG, Verity MA: Central nervous system involvement in systemic lupus erythematosus: a review of neuropathologic findings in 57 cases, 1955–1977. Semin Arthritis Rheum 4:253, 1979
95. Emura A, Takeuchi A, Hashimoto T et al: A case of Behçet's disease with Weber's syndrome. J Rheumatol 13:459, 1986
96. Englert HJ, Hawkes CH, Boey ML et al: Degos' disease: association with anticardiolipin antibodies and the lupus anticoagulant. Br Med J 289:576, 1984
97. Enzmann D, Scott WR: Intracranial involvement of giant-cell arteritis. Neurology (NY) 27:794, 1977
98. Estes D, Christian CL: The natural history of systemic lupus erythematosus by prospective analysis. Medicine (Baltimore) 50:85, 1971
99. Estey E, Lieberman A, Pinto R et al: Cerebral arteritis in scleroderma. Stroke 10:595, 1979
100. Faer MJ, Mead JH, Lynch RD: Cerebral granulomatous angiitis: case report and literature review. AJR 129:463, 1977
101. Fauchald P, Rygvold O, Oystese B: Temporal arteritis and polymyalgia rheumatica: clinical and biopsy finding. Ann Intern Med 77:845, 1972
102. Fauci AS, Haynes BF, Katz P, Wolff SM: Wegener's granulomatosis: prospective clinical and therapeutic experience with 85 patients for 21 years. Ann Intern Med 98:76, 1983
103. Fauci AS, Katz P, Haynes BF, Wolff SM: Cyclophosphamide therapy of severe systemic necrotizing vasculitis. N Engl J Med 301:235, 1979
104. Feasby TE, Ferguson GG, Kaufman JCE: Iso-

lated spinal cord vasculitis. Can J Neurol Sci 2:143, 1975
105. Fedele FA, Ho G Jr, Dorman BA: Pseudoaneurysm of the vertebral artery: a complication of rheumatoid cervical spine disease. Arthritis Rheum 29:136, 1986
106. Feinberg SB: Giant cell arteritis of the central nervous system: the place of roentgen diagnosis. Minn Med 47:656, 1964
107. Feinglass EJ, Arnett FC, Dorsch CA et al: Neuropsychiatric manifestations of systemic lupus erythematosus: diagnosis, clinical spectrum, and relationship to other features of the disease. Medicine (Baltimore) 55:323, 1976
108. Feit H, Frenkel EP, Dunn BR et al: Acute subdural hematomas with lupus anticoagulant (procoagulant inhibitor). Neurology (NY) 34:519, 1984
109. Ferris H: Cerebral Arteritis: classification. Radiology 109:327, 1973
110. Filloux F, Townsend J: Herpes zoster ophthalmicus with ipsilateral cerebellar infarction. Neurology (NY) 35:1531, 1985
111. Fisher CM: Ocular palsy in temporal arteritis. Minn Med 42:1258, 1959
112. Ford PM, Brunet D, Lillicrap DP, Ford SE: Premature stroke in a family with lupus anticoagulant and antiphospholipid antibodies. Stroke 21:66, 1990
113. Ford RG, Siekert RG: Central nervous system manifestations of periarteritis nodosa. Neurology (NY) 15:114, 1965
114. Fox IS, Spence AM, Wheelis RF, Healey LA: Cerebral embolism in Libman-Sacks endocarditis. Neurology (NY) 30:487, 1980
115. Frayne JH, Gilligan BS, Essex WB: Granulomatous angiitis of the central nervous system. Med J Aust 145:410, 1986
116. Fred HL, Lynch EC, Greenberg SD, Gonzalez-Angulo A: A patient with Wegener's granulomatosis exhibiting unusual clinical and morphologic features. Am J Med 37:311, 1964
117. Friedrich H, Laas J, Walterbusch G, Rickels E: Extra-intracranial bypass procedure with saphenous vein grafts. Thorac Cardiovasc Surgeon 34:57, 1986
118. Fryer DG, Crane R, Margolis MT: Angiographic changes in intracranial arteritis of ophthalmic herpes zoster. Ann Neurol 15:311, 1984
119. Futrell N, Millikan C: Frequency, etiology, and prevention of stroke in patients with systemic lupus erythematosus. Stroke 20:583, 1989
120. Galetta SL, Raps EC, Wulc AE et al: Conjugal temporal arteritis. Neurology (NY) 40:1839, 1990
121. Gasperetti C, Son SK: Contralateral hemiparesis following herpes zoster ophthalmicus. J Neurol Neurosurg Psychiatry 48:338, 1985
122. Gastineau DA, Kazmier FJ, Nichols WL, Bowie EJW: Lupus anticoagulant: an analysis of the clinical and laboratory features of 219 cases. Am J Hematol 19:265, 1985
123. Gharavi AE, Harris EN, Asherson RA, Hughes GRV: Anticardiolipin antibodies: isotype distribution and phospholipid specificity. Ann Rheum Dis 46:1, 1987
124. Gherardi GJ, Lee HU: Localized dissecting hemorrhage and arteritis: renal and cerebral manifestations. JAMA 199:187, 1967
125. Gibb WRG, Urry PA, Lees AJ: Giant cell arteritis with spinal cord infarction and basilar artery thrombosis. J Neurol Neurosurg Psychiatry 48:945, 1985
126. Gilbert GJ: Herpes zoster ophthalmicus and delayed contralateral hemiparesis: relationship of the syndrome to central nervous system granulomatous angiitis. JAMA 229:302, 1974
127. Gillanders LA, Strachan RW, Blair DW: Temporal arteriography. Ann Rheum Dis 28:267, 1969
128. Gilmour JR: Giant-cell chronic arteritis. J Pathol 53:263, 1941
129. Ginsberg L, Geddes J, Valentine A: Amyloid angiopathy and granulomatous angiitis of the central nervous system: a case responding to corticosteroid treatment. J Neurol 235:438, 1988
130. Goldberg AL, Tievsky AL, Jamshidi S: Wegener granulomatosis invading the cavernous sinus: a CT demonstration. J Comput Assist Tomogr 7:701, 1983
131. Goodman BW: Temporal arteritis. Am J Med 67:839, 1979
132. Gordon RM, Silverstein A: Neurologic manifestations in progressive systemic sclerosis. Arch Neurol 22:126, 1970
133. Gorelick PB, Rusinowitz MS, Tiku M et al: Embolic stroke complicating systemic lupus erythematosus. Arch Neurol 42:813, 1985
134. Graham E: Survival in temporal arteritis. Trans Ophthalmol Soc UK 100:108, 1980
135. Grattan CEH, Burton JL, Boon AP: Sneddon's syndrome (livedo reticularis and cerebral thrombosis) with livedo vasculitis and anticardiolipin antibodies. Br J Dermatol 120:441, 1989
136. Greaves DP: Ophthalmic manifestations of giant cell arteritis. Trans Ophthalmol Soc UK 81:427, 1961
137. Greco FA, Kolins J, Rajjoub RK, Brereton HD: Hodgkin's disease and granulomatous angiitis of the central nervous system. Cancer 38:2027, 1976
138. Greenfield JG: Giant cell arteritis. Proc R Soc Med 44:855, 1951
139. Griffin J, Price DL, Davis L, McKhann GM: Granulomatous angiitis of the central nervous system with aneurysms on multiple cerebral arteries. Trans Am Neurol Assoc 98:145, 1973
140. Gürsoy G, Aktin E, Bahar S et al: Post-herpetic aneurysm in the intrapetrosal portion of the internal carotid artery. Neuroradiology 19:279, 1980
141. Gutman L, Hable K: Rheumatoid pachymeningitis. Neurology (NY) 13:901, 1963
142. Haft H, Finneson BE, Cramer H, Fiol R: Periarteritis nodosa as a source of subarachnoid hemorrhage and spinal cord compression. J Neurosurg 14:608, 1957
143. Hall GH, Hargreaves T: Giant cell arteritis and raised serum alkaline phosphate levels. (Letter.) Lancet 2:48, 1972
144. Hall S, Barr W, Lie JT et al: Takayasu arteritis: a study of 32 North American patients. Medicine (Baltimore) 64:89, 1985

145. Hall S, Hunder GG: Is temporal artery biopsy prudent? Mayo Clin Proc 59:793, 1984
146. Hall S, Lie JT, Kurland LT et al: The therapeutic impact of temporal artery biopsy. Lancet 2:1217, 1983
147. Hamilton CR, Shelley WM, Tumulty PA: Giant cell arteritis: including temporal arteritis and polymyalgia rheumatica. Medicine (Baltimore) 50:1, 1971
148. Hammoudeh M, Khan M: Cranial arteritis as the initial manifestation of malignant histiocytosis. J Rheumatol 9:443, 1982
149. Hamrin B: Polymyalgia arteritica. Acta Med Scand [Suppl] 533:1, 1972
150. Hamrin B, Jonsson N, Hellsten S: "Polymyalgia arteritica": further clinical and histopathological studies with a report of six autopsy cases. Ann Rheum Dis 27:397, 1968
151. Harbitz F: Unknown forms of arteritis with special reference to their relation to syphillitic arteritis and periarteritis nodosa. Am J Med Sci 163:250, 1922
152. Harper CM Jr, O'Neill BP, O'Duffy JD, Forbes GS: Intracranial hypertension in Behçet's disease: demonstration of sinus occlusion with use of digital subtraction angiography. Mayo Clin Proc 60:419, 1985
153. Harris EN, Gharavi AE, Asherson RA, et al: Cerebral infarction in systemic lupus: association with anticardiolipin antibodies. Clin Exp Rheumatol 2:47, 1984
154. Harris EN, Hughes GRV, Gharavi AE: Antiphospholipid antibodies: an elderly statesman dons new garments. J Rheumatol, suppl, 13 14:208, 1987
155. Harrison PE: Granulomatous angiitis of the central nervous system. J Neurol Sci 29:335, 1976
156. Hashimoto N, Handa H, Taki W: Ruptured cerebral aneurysms in patients with systemic lupus erythematosus. Surg Neurol 26:512, 1986
157. Hauser WA, Ferguson RH, Holley KE, Kurland LT: Temporal arteritis in Rochester, Minnesota, 1951 to 1967. Mayo Clin Proc 46:597, 1971
158. Hayreh SS: Anterior ischemic optic neuropathy. Arch Neurol 38:675, 1981
159. Hazleman B, Goldstone A, Voak D: Association of polymyalgia rheumatica and giant cell arteritis with HLA-B8. Br Med J 2:989, 1977
160. Healey LA, Wilske KR: Manifestations of giant cell arteritis. Med Clin North Am 61:261, 1977
161. Heiskala H, Somer H, Kovanen J et al: Microangiopathy with encephalopathy, hearing loss and retinal arteriolar occlusions: two new cases. J Neurol Sci 86:239, 1988
162. Heptinstall RH, Porter KA, Barkley H: Giant cell (temporal) arteritis. J Pathol 67:507, 1954
163. Hering R, Couturier EG, Steiner TJ: Vascular headaches and anticardiolipin antibodies. Stroke 22:414, 1991
164. Herkes GK, Storey CE, Joffe R, Mackenzie RA: Herpes zoster arteritis: clinical and angiographic features. Clin Exp Neurol 64:169, 1987
165. Herskovitz S, Lipton RB, Lantos G: Neuro-Behçet's disease: CT and clinical correlates. Neurology (NY) 38:1714, 1988
166. Hess DC, Krauss J, Adams RJ, Nichols FT et al: Anticardiolipin antibodies: a study of frequency in TIA and stroke. Neurology (NY) 41:525, 1991
167. Hilt DC, Buchholz D, Krumholz A et al: Herpes zoster ophthalmicus and delayed contralateral hemiparesis caused by cerebral angiitis: diagnosis and management approaches. Ann Neurol 14:543, 1983
168. Hinck VC, Carter CC, Rippey GG: Giant cell (cranial) arteritis: a case with angiographic abnormalities. AJR 92:769, 1964
169. Hirsch M, Mayersdorf A, Lehman E: Cranial giant cell arteritis. Br J Radiol 47:503, 1974
170. Hogan PJ, Greenberg MK, McCarty GE: Neurologic complications of lymphomatoid granulomatosis. Neurology (NY) 31:619, 1981
171. Hollenhorst RW, Brown JR, Wagener HP, Shick RM: Neurologic aspects of temporal arteritis. Neurology (NY) 10:490, 1960
172. Hood J, Wilson ER Jr, Alexander CB et al: Lymphomatoid granulomatosis manifested as a mass in the cerebellopontine angle. Arch Neurol 39:319, 1982
173. Horner FA, Myers GJ, Stumpf DA et al: Malignant atrophic papulosis (Kohlmeier-Degos disease) in childhood. Neurology (NY) 26:317, 1976
174. Horton BT: Complications of temporal arteritis. Br Med J 1:105, 1966
175. Horton BT, Magath TB, Brown GE: An undescribed form of arteritis of the temporal vessels. Proc Mayo Clin 7:700, 1932
176. Horton BT, Magath TB, Brown GE: Arteritis of the temporal vessels, a previously undescribed form. Arch Intern Med 53:400, 1934
177. Howard GF, Ho SU, Kim KS, Wallach J: Bilateral carotid occlusion resulting from giant cell arteritis. Ann Neurol 15:204, 1984
178. Howell SJL, Molyneux AJ: Vertebrobasilar insufficiency in rheumatoid atlanto-axial subluxation: a case report with angiographic demonstration of left vertebral artery occlusion. J Neurol 235:189, 1988
179. Hughes GRV, Asherson RA, Khamashta MA: The antiphospholipid syndrome—from theory to discovery. Postgrad Med J 65:691, 1989
180. Hughes JT, Brownell B: Granulomatous giant celled angiitis of the central nervous system. Neurology (NY) 16:293, 1966
181. Hull RG, Harris N, Gharavi AE et al: Anticardiolipin antibodies: occurrence in Behçet's syndrome. Ann Rheum Dis 43:746, 1984
182. Hunder GG, Baker HL, Rhoton AL et al: Superficial temporal arteriography in patients suspected of having temporal arteritis. Arthritis Rheum 15:561, 1972
183. Hunder GG, Hazleman BL: Giant cell arteritis and polymyalgia rheumatica. In Kelly WN, Harris ED, Jr, Ruddy S, Sledge CB (eds): Textbook of Rheumatology. WB Saunders, Philadelphia, 1981
184. Hunder GG, Sheps SG, Allen GL, Joyce JW: Daily and alternate-day corticosteroid regimens in treatment of giant cell arteritis comparison in a prospective study. Ann Intern Med 82:613, 1975
185. Hunder GG, Taswell HF, Pineda AA, Elveback LR: HLA antigens in patients with giant cell ar-

teritis and polymyalgia rheumatica. J Rheumatol 4:321, 1977
186. Huston KA, Hunder GG: Giant cell (cranial) arteritis: a clinical review. Am Heart J 100:99, 1980
187. Huston KA, Hunder GG, Lie JT et al: Temporal arteritis: a 25-year-epidemiologic, clinical and pathologic study. Ann Intern Med 88:162, 1978
188. Hutchinson J: Diseases of the arteries. Arch Surg 1:323, 1890
189. Imaizumi M, Nukada T, Yoneda S, Abe H: Behçet's disease with sinus thrombosis and arteriovenous malformation in brain. J Neurol 222:215, 1980
190. Iraguli VJ, Maravi E: Behçet syndrome presenting as cerebrovascular disease. J Neurol Neurosurg Psychiatry 49:838, 1986
191. Ironside JW, Martin JF, Richmond J, Timperley WR: Lymphomatoid granulomatosis with cerebral involvement. Neuropathol Appl Neurobiol 10:397, 1984
192. Ishikawa K: Natural history and classification of occlusive thromboaortopathy (Takayasu's disease). Circulation 57:27, 1978
193. Ishikawa K, Yonekawa Y: Regression of carotid stenoses after corticosteroid therapy in occlusive thromboaortopathy (Takayasu's disease). Stroke 18:677, 1987
194. Jackson CG, Chess RL, Ward JR: A case of rheumatoid nodule formation within the central nervous system and review of the literature. J Rheumatol 11:237, 1984
195. Jellinger K: Giant cell granulomatous angiitis of the central nervous system. J Neurol 215:175, 1977
196. Jennings GH: Arteritis of the temporal vessels. Lancet 1:424, 1938
197. Johnson M, Maciunas R, Dutt P et al: Granulomatous angiitis masquerading as a mass lesion: magnetic resonance imaging and stereotactic biopsy findings in a patient with occult Hodgkin's disease. Surg Neurol 31:49, 1989
198. Johnson RL, Smyth CJ, Holt GW et al: Steroid therapy and vascular lesions in rheumatoid arthritis. Arthritis Rheum 2:224, 1959
199. Johnson RT, Richardson EP: The neurological manifestations of systemic lupus erythematosus: a clinical-pathological study of 24 cases and review of the literature. Medicine (Baltimore) 47:337, 1968
200. Jonas J, Kölble K, Völcker HE, Kalden JR: Central retinal artery occlusion in Sneddon's disease associated with antiphospholipid antibodies. Am J Ophthalmol 102:37, 1986
201. Jonasson F, Cullen JF, Elton RA: Temporal arteritis: a 14-year epidemiological, clinical and prognostic study. Scott Med J 24:111, 1979
202. Jones JG, Hazleman BL: Prognosis and management of polymyalgia rheumatica. Ann Rheum Dis 40:1, 1981
203. Jones MW, Kaufmann JCE: Vertebrobasilar artery insufficiency in rheumatoid atlantoaxial subluxation. J Neurol Neurosurg Psychiatry 39:122, 1976
204. Kalashnikova LA, Nasonov EL, Kushekbaeva AE, Gracheva LA: Anticardiolipin antibodies in Sneddon's syndrome. Neurology (NY) 40:464, 1990
205. Kapila A, Gupta KL, Garcia JH: CT and MR of lymphomatoid granulomatosis of the CNS: report of four cases and review of the literature. AJNR 9:1139, 1988
206. Katelaris CH, Walls RS: Fatal neurological complications in temporal arteritis: an unusual case. Aust NZ J Med 12:299, 1982
207. Kattah JC, Cupps TR, Di Chiro G, Manz HJ: An unusual case of central nervous system vasculitis. J Neurol 234:344, 1987
208. Kausu T, Corbett JJ, Savino P, Schatz NJ: Giant cell arteritis with normal sedimentation rate. Arch Neurol 34:624, 1977
209. Kawakita H, Nishimura M, Satoh Y, Shibata N: Neurological aspects of Behçet's disease: a case report and clinico-pathological review of the literature in Japan. J Neurol Sci 5:417, 1967
210. Kawi MZA, Bohlega S, Banna M: MRI findings in neuro-Behçet's disease. Neurology (NY) 41:405, 1991
211. Kelley RE, Stokes N, Reyes P, Harik SI: Cerebral transmural angiitis and ruptured aneurysm: a complication of systemic lupus erythematosus. Arch Neurol 37:526, 1980
212. Kernohan JW, Woltman HW: Periarteritis nodosa: a clinicopathologic study with special reference to the nervous system. Arch Neurol Neurosurg Psychiatry 39:655, 1938
213. Kerr RSC, Hughes JT, Blamires T, Teddy PJ: Lymphomatoid granulomatosis apparently confined to one temporal lobe: case report. J Neurosurg 67:612, 1987
214. Khamashta MA, Asherson RA, Hughes GRV: Possible mechanisms of action of the antiphospholipid binding antibodies. Clin Exp Rheumatol, suppl 3 7:85, 1989
215. Kim RC: Rheumatoid disease with encephalopathy. Ann Neurol 7:861, 1980
216. Kim RC, Collins GH, Parisi JE: Rheumatoid nodule formation within the choroid plexus: report of a second case. Arch Pathol Lab Med 106:83, 1982
217. Kitagawa Y, Gotoh F, Koto A, Okayasu H: Stroke in systemic lupus erythematosus. Stroke 21:1533, 1990
218. Kjeldsen MH, Reske-Nielsen E: Pathological changes of the central nervous system in giant cell arteritis. Acta Ophthalmol 46:49, 1968
219. Klein RG, Campbell RJ, Hunder GG, Carney JA: Skip lesions in temporal arteritis. Mayo Clin Proc 51:504, 1976
220. Klein RG, Hunder GG, Stanson AW, Sheps SG: Large artery involvement in giant cell (temporal) arteritis. Ann Intern Med 83:806, 1975
221. Kokmen E, Billman JK, Jr, Abell MR: Lymphomatoid granulomatosis clinically confined to the CNS. Arch Neurol 34:782, 1977
222. Kolodny EK, Rebeiz JJ, Caviness VS, Richardson EP: Granulomatous angiitis of the central nervous system. Arch Neurol 19:510, 1968
223. Koo EH, Massey EW: Granulomatous angiitis of the central nervous system protean manifestations and response to treatment. J Neurol Neurosurg Psychiatry 51:1126, 1988

224. Kott HS: Stroke due to vasculitis. Primary Care 6:771, 1979
225. Kozin F, Haughton V, Bernhard GC: Neuro-Behçet disease: two cases and neuroradiologic findings. Neurology (NY) 27:1148, 1977
226. Kozula S, Iguchi I, Furuse M et al: Cerebral granulomatous angiitis with atypical features. J Neurol 231:38, 1984
227. Kristoferitsch W, Jellinger K, Bock F: Cerebral granulomatous angiitis with atypical features. J Neurol 231:38, 1984
228. Kuroiwa Y, Furukawa T: Hemispheric infarction after herpes zoster ophthalmicus: computed tomography and angiography. Neurology (NY) 31:1030, 1981
229. Label LS, Tandan R, Albers JW: Myelomalacia and hypoglycorrhachia in malignant atrophic papulosis. Neurology (NY) 33:936, 1983
230. Lee JE, Haynes JM: Carotid arteritis and cerebral infarction due to scleroderma. Neurology (NY) 17:18, 1967
231. Lee P, Urowitz MB, Bookman AAM et al: Systemic lupus erythematosus: a review of 110 cases with reference to nephritis, the nervous system, infections, aseptic necrosis and prognosis. Q J Med 181:1, 1977
232. Leeds NE, Goldberg HI: Angiographic manifestations in cerebral inflammatory disease. Radiology 98:595, 1971
233. Leib ES, Restivo C, Paulus HE: Immunosuppressive and corticosteroid therapy of polyarteritis nodosa. Am J Med 67:941, 1979
234. Levine SR, Deegan MJ, Futrell N, Welch KMA: Cerebrovascular and neurologic disease associated with antiphospholipid antibodies: 48 cases. Neurology (NY) 40:1181, 1990
235. Levine SR, Diaczok IM, Deegan MJ et al: Recurrent stroke associated with thymoma and anticardiolipin antibodies. Arch Neurol 44:678, 1987
236. Levine SR, Kieran S, Puzio K et al: Cerebral venous thrombosis with lupus anticoagulants: report of two cases. Stroke 18:801, 1987
237. Levine SR, Langer SL, Albers JW, Welch KMA: Sneddon's syndrome: an antiphospholipid antibody syndrome? Neurology 38:798, 1988
238. Lewis IC, Philpott MG: Neurological complications in the Schönlein-Henoch Syndrome. Arch Dis Child 31:369, 1956
239. Liang GC, Simkin PA, Mammik M: Immunoglobulins in temporal arteritis. Ann Intern Med 81:19, 1974
240. Libman E, Sacks B: A hitherto undescribed form of valvular and mural endocarditis. Arch Intern Med 33:701, 1924
241. Liebow AA: Pulmonary angiitis and granulomatosis. Am Rev Respir Dis 108:1, 1973
242. Licbow AA, Carrington CRB, Friedman PJ: Lymphomatoid granulomatosis. Hum Pathol 3:457, 1972
243. Linneman CCJ, Alvira MM: Pathogenesis of varicella-zoster angiitis in the central nervous system. Arch Neurol 37:239, 1980
244. Love DC, Rapkin J, Lesser GR et al: Temporal arteritis in blacks. Ann Intern Med 105:387, 1986
245. Lu AT, Barasch S: Neurological involvement in Behçet's syndrome: a case report with neuropathological data and a summary of the reported autopsied cases. Bull Los Angeles Neurol Soc 28:85, 1963
246. Lucas FV, Benjamin SP, Steinberg MC: Cerebral vasculitis in Wegener's granulomatosis. Cleve Clin Q 43:275, 1976
247. Ludmerer KM, Kissane JM: Chronic meningitis in a 68-year-old man. Am J Med 85:407, 1988
248. MacFadyen DJ: Wegener's granulomatosis with discrete lung lesions and peripheral neuritis. Can Med Ass J 83:760, 1960
249. MacFadyen DJ, Schneider RJ, Chisholm IA: A syndrome of brain, inner ear and retinal microangiopathy. Can J Neurol Sci 14:315, 1987
250. Machado EBV, Michet CJ, Ballard DJ et al: Trends in incidence and clinical presentation of temporal arteritis in Olmsted County, Minnesota, 1950–1985. Arthritis Rheum 31:745, 1988
251. Mackenzie RA, Forbes GS, Karnes WE: Angiographic findings in herpes zoster arteritis. Ann Neurol 10:458, 1981
252. Mackenzie RA, Ryan P, Karnes WE, Okazaki H: Herpes zoster arteritis: pathological findings. Clin Exp Neurol 23:219, 1987
253. Magidson MA, Rajendran MM, Leutcher WM: Granulomatous angiitis of the central nervous system with an unusual angiographic feature. Surg Neurol 10:355, 1978
254. Magrinat G, Kerwin KS, Gabriel DA: The clinical manifestations of Degos' syndrome. Arch Pathol Lab Med 113:354, 1989
255. Malamud N, Foster DB: Periarteritis nodosa: a clinicopathologic report, with special reference to the central nervous system. Arch Neurol Psychiatr 47:828, 1942
256. Mandybur TI: Cerebral amyloid angiopathy: possible relationship to rheumatoid vasculitis. Neurology (NY) 29:1336, 1979
257. Manschot WA: A fatal case of temporal arteritis, with ocular symptoms. Ophthalmologica 149:121, 1965
258. Markenson JA, McDougal JS, Tsairis P et al: Rheumatoid meningitis: a localized immune process. Ann Intern Med 90:786, 1979
259. Marsden HB: Basilar artery thrombosis and giant cell arteritis, (Abstracted). Arch Dis Child 49:75, 1974
260. Mass M, Bourdette D, Bernstein W, Hammerstad J: Retinopathy, encephalopathy, deafness associated microangiopathy (the RED M Syndrome): three new cases, abstracted. Neurology (NY), suppl, 1 38:215, 1988
261. Masuzawa T, Shimabukuro H, Furuse M et al: Pulseless disease associated with a ruptured intracranial vertebral aneurysm. Neurol Med Chir 24:490, 1984
262. McCormick HM, Neuberger KT: Giant cell arteritis in involving small meningeal and intracerebral vessels. J Neuropathol Exp Neurol 17:471, 1958
263. McFarland HR, Wood WG, Drowns BV, Meneses ACO: Papulosis atrophicans maligna (Köhlmeier-Degos disease): a disseminated occlusive vasculopathy. Ann Neurol 3:388, 1978

264. McMenemey WH, Lawrence BJ: Encephalomyelopathy in Behçet's disease: report of necropsy findings in two cases. Lancet 2:353, 1957
265. Meadows SP: Temporal or giant cell arteritis. Proc R Soc Med 59:329, 1966
266. Meneely JK, Bigelow NH: Temporal arteritis. Am J Med 14:46, 1953
267. Mickle JP, McLennan JE, Chi JG, Lidden CW: Cortical vein thrombosis in Wegener's granulomatosis: case report. J Neurosurg 46:248, 1977
268. Milgram JW, Stecher K: Idiopathic arteritis with multiple intracranial aneurysms. Angiology 25:89, 1974
269. Miller NR: Anterior ischemic optic neuropathy: diagnosis and management. Bull NY Acad Med 56:643, 1980
270. Missen GA: Involvement of the vetebrocarotid arterial system in giant cell arteritis. J Pathol 106:ii, 1972
271. Monteiro MLR, Swanson RA, Coppeto JR et al: A microangiopathic syndrome of encephalopathy, hearing loss, and retinal arteriolar occlusions. Neurology (NY) 35:1113, 1985
272. Moore PM: Diagnosis and management of isolated angiitis of the central nervous system. Neurology (NY) 39:167, 1989
273. Moore PM, Lisak RP: Multiple sclerosis and Sjögren's syndrome: a problem in diagnosis or in definition of two disorders of unknown etiology? Ann Neurol 27:585, 1990
274. Morgan GJ Jr, Harris ED, Jr: Non-giant cell temporal arteritis. Arthritis Rheum 21:362, 1978
275. Morrison AN, Abitol M: Granulomatous arteritis with myocardial infarction. Ann Intern Med 42:691, 1955
276. Mueh JR, Herbst KD, Rapaport SI: Thrombosis in patients with the lupus anticoagulant. Ann Intern Med 92:156, 1980
277. Murphy JJ, Leach IH: Findings at necropsy in the heart of a patient with anticardiolipin syndrome. Br Heart J 62:61, 1989
278. Nagaratnam N, James WE: Isolated angiitis of the brain in a young female on the contraceptive pill. Postgrad Med J 63:1085, 1987
279. Nagata K: Recurrent intracranial haemorrhage in Behçet disease. J Neurol Neurosurg Psychiatry 48:190, 1985
280. Nasu T: Takayasu's truncoarteritis in Japan: a statistical observation of 76 autopsy cases. Pathol Microbiol 43:140, 1975
281. Newman W, Wolf A: Non-infectious granulomatous angiitis involving the central nervous system. Trans Am Neurol Assoc 77:114, 1952
282. Noseworthy JH, Bass BH, Vandervoort MK et al: The prevalence of primary Sjögren's syndrome in a multiple sclerosis population. Ann Neurol 25:95, 1989
283. Nurick S, Blackwood W, Mair WGP: Giant cell granulomatous angiitis of the central nervous system. Brain 95:133, 1972
284. O'Donohue JM, Enzmann DR: Mycotic aneurysm in angiitis associated with herpes zoster ophthalmicus. AJNR 8:615, 1987
285. O'Duffy JD, Goldstein NP: Neurologic involvement in seven patients with Behçet's disease. Am J Med 61:170, 1976
286. O'Duffy JD, Robertson DM, Goldstein NP: Chlorambucil in the treatment of uveitis and meningoencephalitis of Behçet's disease. Am J Med 76:75, 1984
287. Ojeda VJ: Polyarteritis nodosa affecting the spinal cord arteries. Aust NZ J Med 13:287, 1983
288. Ojeda VJ, Peters DM, Spagnolo DV: Giant cell granulomatous angiitis of the central nervous system in a patient with leukemia and cutaneous herpes zoster. Am J Clin Pathol 81:529, 1984
289. Ostberg G: Temporal arteritis in a large necropsy series. Ann Rheum Dis 30:224, 1971
290. Ostberg G: Morphological changes in the large arteries in polymyalgia arteritica. Acta Med Scand, suppl. 533:135, 1972
291. Ostberg G: On arteritis with special reference to polymyalgia arteritica. Acta Pathol Microbiol Scand, suppl A. 237:1, 1973
292. Ouyang R, Mitchell DM, Rozdilsky B: Central nervous system involvement in rheumatoid disease: report of a case. Neurology (NY) 17:1099, 1967
293. Pamir MN, Kansu T, Erbengi A, Zileli T: Papilledema in Behçet's syndrome. Arch Neurol 38:643, 1981
294. Papaioannou CC, Gupta RC, Hunder GG, McDuffie FC: Circulating immune complexes in giant cell arteritis and polymyalgia rheumatica. Arthritis Rheum 23:1021, 1980
295. Park JR, Jones JG, Harkniss GD, Hazleman BL: Circulating immune complexes in polymyalgia rheumatica and giant cell arteritis. Ann Rheum Dis 40:360 1981
296. Parker HL, Kernohan JW: The central nervous system in periarteritis nodosa. Trans Am Neurol Assoc 72:54, 1947
297. Parker HL, Kernohan JW: The central nervous system in periarteritis nodosa. Mayo Clin Proc 24:43, 1949
298. Patel DV, Neuman JM, Hier DB: Reversibility of CT and MR findings neuro-Behçet disease. J Comput Assist Tomogr 13:669, 1989
299. Patton WF, Lynch JP III: Lymphomatoid granulomatosis: clinicopathologic study of four cases and literature review. Medicine (Baltimore) 61:1, 1982
300. Paulley JW, Hughes JP: Giant cell arteritis or arteritis of the aged. Br Med J 2:1562, 1960
301. Peison B, Padlechas R: Granulomatous angiitis of the nervous system. IMJ 126:330, 1964
302. Pellat J, Perret J, Pasquier B et al: Étude anatomoclinique et angiographique d'une observation de thromboangiose disséminée a manifestations cérébrales prédominantes. Rev Neurol 132:517, 1976
303. Petit WA Jr, Soso MJ, Higman H: Degos disease: neurologic complications and cerebral angiography. Neurology (NY) 32:1305, 1982
304. Petty GW, Yanagihara T, Bartleson JD et al: Retinocochleocerebral vasculopathy, abstracted. Ann Neurol 30:245, 1991
305. Pezeshkpour G, Stuart TD, Estridge MN: Crystalline encephalopathy: cerebral immunopro-

tein deposits and isolated angiitis. Ann Neurol 17:96, 1985
306. Pfaffenbach DD, Hollenhorst RS: Microangiopathy of the retinal arterioles. JAMA 225:480, 1973
307. Pines A, Kaplinsky N, Olchovsky D et al: Recurrent transient ischemic attacks associated with thrombocytosis in rheumatoid arthritis. Clin Rheumatol 1:291, 1982
308. Pollack M, Blennerhasset JB, Clarke AM: Giant cell arteritis and the subclavian steal syndrome. Neurology (NY) 23:653, 1973
309. Probst A, Ulrich J: Amyloid angiopathy combined with granulomatous angiitis of the central nervous system: report on two patients. Clin Neuropathol 4:250, 1985
310. Quimby SR, Perry HO: Livedo reticularis and cerebrovascular accidents. J Am Acad Dermatol 3:377, 1980
311. Rajjoub RK, Wook JH, Ommaya AK: Granulomatous angiitis of the brain. A successfully treated case. Neurology (NY) 27:588, 1977
312. Ramos M, Mandybur TI: Cerebral vasculitis in rheumatoid arthritis. Arch Neurol 32:271, 1975
313. Rawlinson DG, Braun CW: Granulomatous angiitis of the nervous system first seen as relapsing myelopathy. Arch Neurol 38:129, 1981
314. Rebollo M, Val JF, Garijo F et al: Livedo reticularis and cerebrovascular lesions (Sneddon's syndrome): clinical, radiological and pathological features in eight cases. Brain 106:965, 1983
315. Reik L, Grunnett ML, Spencer RP, Donalson JO: Granulomatous angiitis presenting as chronic meningitis and ventriculitis. Neurology (NY) 33:1609, 1983
316. Reik L Jr, Korn JH: Cryoglobulinemia with encephalopathy: successful treatment by plasma exchange. Ann Neurol 10:488, 1981
317. Rawcastle NB, Tom MI: Non-infectious granulomatous angiitis of the nervous system associated with Hodgkin's disease. J Neurol Neurosurg Psychiatry 25:51, 1962
318. Reyes MG, Fresco R, Chokroverty S, Salud EQ: Virus-like particles in granulomatous angiitis of the central nervous system. Neurology (NY) 26:797, 1976
319. Ristow SC, Griner PF, Abraham GN, Shoulson I: Reversal of systemic manifestations of cryoglobulinemia: treatment with Melphalan and Prednisone. Arch Intern Med 136:467, 1976
320. Ritama V: Temporal arteritis. Ann Med Fenn 40:63, 1951
321. Robbins SL, Cotran RS: Blood vessels. p. 614. In: Pathological Basis of Disease. 2nd Ed. WB Saunders, Philadelphia, 1979
322. Robbs JV, Human RR, Rajaruthnam P: Operative treatment of nonspecific aortoarteritis (Takayasu's arteritis). J Vasc Surg 3:605, 1986
323. Robinson BP, Seeger JF, Zak SM: Rheumatoid arthritis and postitional vertebrovasilar insufficiency: a case report. J Neurosurg 65:111, 1986
324. Rodman GP: Clinical pathological conference. J Rheumatol 11:855, 1984
325. Rosenblum WI, Hadfield MG: Granulomatous angiitis of the nervous system in cases of herpes zoster and lymphosarcoma. Neurology (NY) 22:348, 1972
326. Rosenblum WI, Hadfield MG, Young HF: Granulomatous angiitis with preceding varicella-zoster. Ann Neurol 3:374, 1978
327. Rosenfeld SI, Kosmorsky GS, Klingele TG et al: Treatment of temporal arteritis with ocular involvement. Am J Med 80:143, 1986
328. Rottino A, Hoffman G: A sarcoid form of encephalitis in a patient with Hodgkin's disease: case report with review of the literature. J Neuropathol Exp Neurol 9:103, 1950
329. Rougemont D, Bousser MG, Wechsler B et al: Manifestations neurologiques de la maladie de Behçet: vingt-quatre observations. Rev Neurol 138:493, 1982
330. Rubinstein LJ, Urich H: Meningo-encephalitis of Behçet's disease: case report with pathological findings. Brain 86:151, 1963
331. Rumpl E, Neuhofer J, Pallua A: Cerebrovascular lesions and livedo reticularis (Sneddon's syndrome): a progressive cerebrovascular disorder? J Neurol 231:324, 1985
332. Russell RWR: Giant-cell arteritis: a review of 35 cases. Q J Med 28:471, 1959
333. Russi E, Kraus-Ruppert R, Mummenthaler M: Intracranial giant cell arteritis. J Neurol 221:219, 1979
334. Sabharwal UK, Keogh LH, Weiaman MH, Zvaifler NJ: Granulomatous angiitis of the nervous system: case report and review of the literature. Arthritis Rheum 25:342, 1982
335. Sandhu R, Alexander S, Hornabrook RW, Stehbens WE: Granulomatous angiitis of the CNS. Arch Neurol 36:433, 1979
336. Sarnat RL, Jampol LM: Hyperviscosity retinopathy secondary to polyclonal gammopathy in a patient with rheumatoid arthritis. Ophthalmology 93:124, 1986
337. Satoh J, Miyasaka N, Yamada T et al: Extensive cerebral infarction due to involvement of both anterior cerebral arteries by Wegener's granulomatosis. Ann Rheum Dis 47:606, 1988
338. Säve-Söderbergh J, Malmvall BO, Andersson R, Bengtsson BA: Giant cell arteritis as a cause of death: report of nine cases. JAMA 255:493, 1986
339. Schmidt BJ, Meagher-Villemure K, Del Carpio J: Lymphomatoid granulomatosis with isolated involvement of the brain. Ann Neurol 15:478, 1984
340. Schraeder PL, Lubar HS, Thorning DR, Dudley AW: Granulomatous arteritis presenting as an acute transverse myelopathy. Wis Med J 73:32, 1974
341. Schulze-Lohff E, Krapf F, Bleil L et al: IGM-containing immune complexes and antiphospholipid antibodies in patients with Sneddon's syndrome. Rheumatol Int 9:43, 1989
342. Scott D: Mucocutaneous-ocular syndrome (Behçet's syndrome) with meningoencephalitis: report of a case with autopsy. Acta Med Scand 161:397, 1958
343. Scully RE, Galdabini JJ, McNeely BU: Case records of the Massachusetts General Hospital: case 43-1976. N Engl J Med 295:944, 1976

344. Scully RE, Galdabini JJ, McNeely BU: Case records of the Massachusetts General Hospital: case 44-1980. N Engl J Med 303:1103, 1980
345. Scully RE, Mark EJ, McNeely WF, McNeely BU: Case records of the Massachusetts General Hospital: case 12-1988. N Engl J Med 318:760, 1988
346. Scully RE, Mark EJ, McNeely WF, McNeely BU: Case records of the Massachusetts General Hospital: case 8-1989. N Engl J Med 320:514, 1989
347. Sergent JS, Lockshin MD, Christian CL, Gocke DJ: Vasculitis with hepatitis B antigenemia: long-term observations in nine patients. Medicine (Baltimore) 55:1, 1976
348. Shelhamer JH, Volkman DJ, Parrillo JE et al: Takayasu's arteritis and its therapy. Ann Intern Med 103:121, 1985
349. Shillingford JP, Heard BE: A case of temporal arteritis: demonstrated at the Postgraduate Medical School of London. Br Med J 2:287, 1960
350. Shimazu S, Imai H, Kokubu S et al: Long-term survival in malignant atrophic papulosis: a case report and review of the Japanese literature. Nippon-Geka-Gakkai-Zasshi 89:1748, 1988
351. Shimizu T, Ehrlich GE, Inaba G, Hayashi K: Behçet's disease (Behçet syndrome). Semin Arthritis Rheum 8:223, 1979
352. Shiozawa Z, Yoshida M, Kobayashi K et al: Superior sagittal sinus thrombosis and systemic lupus erythematosus. Ann Neurol 20:272, 1986
353. Shuangshoti S: Localized granulomatous (giant cell) angiitis of brain with eosinophil infiltration and saccular aneurysm. J Med Assoc Thai 62:281, 1979
354. Sibony PA, Lessell S: Transient oculomotor synkinesis in temporal arteritis. Arch Neurol 41:87, 1984
355. Silverstein A: Cerebrovascular accidents as the initial major manifestation of lupus erythematosus. NY State J Med 5:2942, 1963
356. Sipe JC, Rosenberg JH: Granulomatous giant cell angiitis of the central nervous system. West J Med 127, 215:1977
357. Smith CA, Fidler WJ, Pinals RS: The epidemiology of giant cell arteritis: report of a ten year study in Shelby County, Tennessee. Arthritis Rheum 26:1214, 1983
358. Sneddon IB: Cerebro-vascular lesions and livedo reticularis: Br J Dermatol 77:180, 1965
359. Sole-Llenas J, Mercader JM, Mirosa F: Cerebral arteritis: angiographic and pathologic study. Angiology 29:713, 1978
360. Sole-Llenas J, Pons-Tortella E: Cerebral angiitis. Neuroradiology 15:1, 1978
361. Specks U, Wheatley CL, McDonald TJ et al: Anticytoplasmic autoantibodies in the diagnosis and follow-up of Wegener's granulomatosis. Mayo Clin Proc 64:28, 1989
362. Spencer WH, Hoyt WF: A fatal case of giant cell arteritis (temporal or cranial arteritis) with ocular involvement. Arch Ophthalmol 64:862, 1962
363. Spurlock RG, Richman AV: Rheumatoid meningitis: a case report and review of the literature. Arch Pathol Lab Med 107:129, 1983
364. Steiner JW, Gelbloom AJ: Intracranial manifestations in two cases of systemic rheumatoid disease. Arthritis Rheum 2:537, 1959
365. Stephens WP, Ferguson IT: Livedo reticularis and cerebro-vascular disease. Post Grad Med J 58:770, 1982
366. Stern JM, Kesler SM: Raised intracranial pressure in a 16-year-old boy: report of a case of Behçet's disease. S Afr Med J 75:243, 1989
367. Strole WE Jr, Clark WH Jr, Isselbacher KJ: Progressive arterial occlusive disease (Köhlmeier-Degos): a frequently fatal cutaneosystemic disorder. N Engl J Med 276:195, 1967
368. Strouth JC, Dyken M: Encephalopathy of Behçet's disease: report of a case. Neurology (NY) 14:794, 1964
369. Susac JO, Hardman JM, Selhorst JB: Microangiopathy of the brain and retina. Neurology (NY) 29:313, 1979
370. Tabbaa MA, Snyder BD: Vasospasm versus vasculitis in cases with "isolated benign cerebral vasculitis." Ann Neurol 21:109, 1987
371. Tanenbaum M, Tenzel J: Familial temporal arteritis. J Clin Neuro-ophthalmol 5:244, 1985
372. Thomas DJ, Kirby JDT, Britton KE, Galton DJ: Livedo reticularis and neurological lesions. Br J Dermatol 106:711, 1982
373. Thomas L, David S, McClusky RT: Studies of PPLO infection. I. The production of cerebral polyarteritis by *Mycoplasma gallispeticum* in turkeys, the neurotoxic property of the *Mycoplasma*. J Exp Med 123:897, 1966
374. Travers RL, Allison DJ, Brettle RP, Hughes GRV: Polyarteritis nodosa: a clinical and angiographic analysis of 17 cases. Semin Arthritis Rheum 8:184, 1979
375. Trevor RP, Sondheimer FK, Fessel WJ, Wolpert SM: Angiographic demonstration of major cerebral vessel occlusion in systemic lupus erythematosus. Neuroradiology 4:202, 1972
376. Tsokos GC, Tsokos M, le Riche NGH, Klippel JH: A clinical and pathologic study of cerebrovascular disease in patients with systemic lupus erythematosus. Semin Arthritis Rheum 16:70, 1986
377. Tuhy JE, Maurice GL, Niles NR: Wegener's granulomatosis. Am J Med 25:638, 1958
378. Urich H: Neurosarcoidosis or granulomatous angiitis: a problem of definition. Mt Sinai J Med 44:718, 1977
379. Valvanis A, Feiede R, Schubiger O, Hayek J: Cerebral granulomatous angiitis simulating brain tumor. J Comput Assist Tomogr 3:536, 1979
380. Vanderzant C, Bromberg M, MacGuire A, McCune J: Isolated small-vessel angiitis of the central nervous system. Arch Neurol 45:683, 1988
381. Vecht CJ, Sande JJ: Hemispheric infarction after herpes zoster ophthalmicus. Neurology (NY) 32:914, 1982
382. Verker R: Psychiatric aspects of temporal arteritis. J Mental Sci 98:280, 1952
383. Vidailhet M, Piett JC, Wechsler B et al: Cerebral venous thrombosis in systemic lupus erythematosus. Stroke 21:1226, 1990
384. Vilchez-Padilla JJ: CNS varicella-zoster vasculitis. (Letter.) Arch Neurol 39:785, 1982

385. Vincent FM: Granulomatous angiitis. N Engl J Med 296:452, 1977
386. Vincent FM, Vincent T: Bilateral carotid siphon involvement in giant cell arteritis. Neurosurgery 18:773, 1986
387. Vinijchaikul K: Primary arteritis of the aorta and its main branches (Takayasu's arteriopathy): a clinicopathologic autopsy study of eight cases. Am J Med 43:15, 1967
388. Von Knorring J: Treatment and prognosis in polymyalgia rheumatica and temporal arteritis: a ten-year survey of 53 patients. Acta Med Scand 205:429, 1975
389. Wadman B, Werner I: Thromboembolic complications during corticosteroid treatment of temporal arteritis. Lancet 1:907, 1972
390. Walsh FB, Hoyt WF: p. 213. In Miller NR (ed): Walsh and Hoyt's Clinical Neuro-ophthalmology. 4th Ed. Vol. 1. Williams & Wilkins, Baltimore, 1982
391. Warot P, Caron JC, Lehembre P, Houcke M: Maladie de Degos à forme cérébrale. Rev Neurol 133:353, 1977
392. Watson P, Fekete J, Deck J: Central nervous system vasculitis in rheumatoid arthritis. Can J Neurol Sci 4:269, 1977
393. Webb FWS, Hickman JA, Brew DSJ: Death from vertebral artery thrombosis in rheumatoid arthritis. Br Med J 2:537, 1968
394. Weinstein JM, Chui H, Lane S et al: Churg-Strauss syndrome (allergic granulomatous angiitis): neuro-ophthalmologic manifestations. Arch Ophthalmol 101:1217, 1983
395. Whelan HT, Moore P: Central nervous system lymphomatoid granulomatosis. Pediatr Neurosci 13:113, 1987
396. Whimster WF: Two neurological cases: demonstration at the Royal College of Physicians of London. Br Med J 1:727, 1979
397. Wilkins MR, Gove RI, Roberts SD, Kendall MJ: Behçet's disease presenting as benign intracranial hypertension. Post Grad Med J 62:39, 1986
398. Wilkinson IMS, Russell RWR: Arteries of the head and neck in giant cell arteritis: a pathological study to show the pattern of arterial involvement. Arch Neurol 27:378, 1972
399. Willeit J, Schmutzhard E, Aichner F et al: CT and MR imaging in neuro-Behçet disease. J Comput Assist Tomogr 10:313, 1986
400. Winkelmann RK, Ditto WB: Cutaneous and visceral syndromes of necrotizing or "allergic" angiitis: a study of 38 cases. Medicine 43:59, 1964
401. Winkelmann RK, Howard FM, Jr, Perry HO, Miller RH: Malignant papulosis of skin and cerebrum: a syndrome of vascular thrombosis. Arch Derm 87:94, 1963
402. Wolf SM, Schotland DL, Phillips LL: Involvement of nervous system in Behçet's syndrome. Arch Neurol 12:315, 1965
403. Wong RL, Korn JH: Temporal arteritis without an elevated erythrocyte sedimentation rate: case report and review of the literature. Am J Med 80:959, 1986
404. Yamamoto S, Nozawa T, Aoki H, Isobe Y: Femoro-internal carotid artery bypass for cerebral ischemia in Takayasu's arteritis. Arch Surg 119:1426, 1984
405. Yankner BA, Skolnik PR, Shoukimas GM et al: Cerebral granulomatous angiitis associated with isolation of human T-lymphotropic virus type III from the central nervous system. Ann Neurol 20:362, 1986
406. Yoneda S, Nukada T, Kunihiko T et al: Subclavian steal in Takayasu's arteritis: a hemodynamic study by means of ultrasonic Doppler flowmetry. Stroke 8:264, 1977
407. Young SM, Fisher M, Sigsbee A, Errichetti A: Cardiogenic brain embolism and lupus anticoagulant. Ann Neurol 26:390, 1989
408. Younger DS, Hays AP, Brust JCM, Rowland LP: Granulomatous angiitis of the brain: an inflammatory reaction of diverse etiology. Arch Neurol 45:514, 1988
409. Zelenski JD, Capraro JA, Holden D, Calabrese LH: Central nervous system vasculitis in Behçet's syndrome: angiographic improvement after therapy with cytotoxic agents. Arthritis Rheum 32:217, 1989

# 26
# MOYAMOYA DISEASE: DIAGNOSIS, TREATMENT, AND RECENT ACHIEVEMENT

Yasuhiro Yonekawa
Yasunobu Goto
Nobuyoshi Ogata

Moyamoya disease was previously believed to be peculiar to Japan, but recently a number of cases have been reported in other areas all over the world. In Japan there has been confusion concerning the disease, especially during the early period following its discovery. The purpose of this paper is to clarify the disease and its treatment, and to report recent achievements in clinical investigation.

## HISTORY

In 1955, at the fourteenth meeting of the Japan Neurosurgical Society, Takeuchi and Shimizu reported a case that is now considered to be moyamoya disease; the report was published in 1957 as a case of bilateral hypoplasia of the internal carotid artery.[141] The 29-year-old patient had suffered from visual disturbance and hemiconvulsive seizures since he was 10 years old, and he became blind at the age of 20. Carotid angiography revealed bilateral complete occlusion of the internal carotid arteries. Biopsy of the ascending pharyngeal artery revealed a slight proliferative change of the intima and media. They considered the occlusion to be congenital hypoplasia and to be different from the usual atheromatous occlusion of the internal carotid artery. Similar case reports were subsequently published by various authors. In 1960, Kudo[72] advocated the concept of occlusion of the circle of Willis for this disease.

For this disease, a variety of names have been proposed by various authors, including "cerebral juxtabasilar telangiectasia" by Sano, "cerebral arterial rete" by Handa, "rete mirabile" by Weidner, "cerebral basal rete mirabile" by Nishimoto, moyamoya disease (moyamoya means "puff of smoke" in Japanese) by Suzuki. "Nishimoto-Kudo disease" or "Nishimoto disease" has been used frequently in European countries, as this disease has been reported in English journals since its discovery.[74,105]

Nowadays, moyamoya disease or spontaneous occlusion of the circle of Willis are the names most fre-

This work is partly sponsored by the research committee on spontaneous occlusion of the circle of Willis, Ministry of Health and Welfare, Japan.

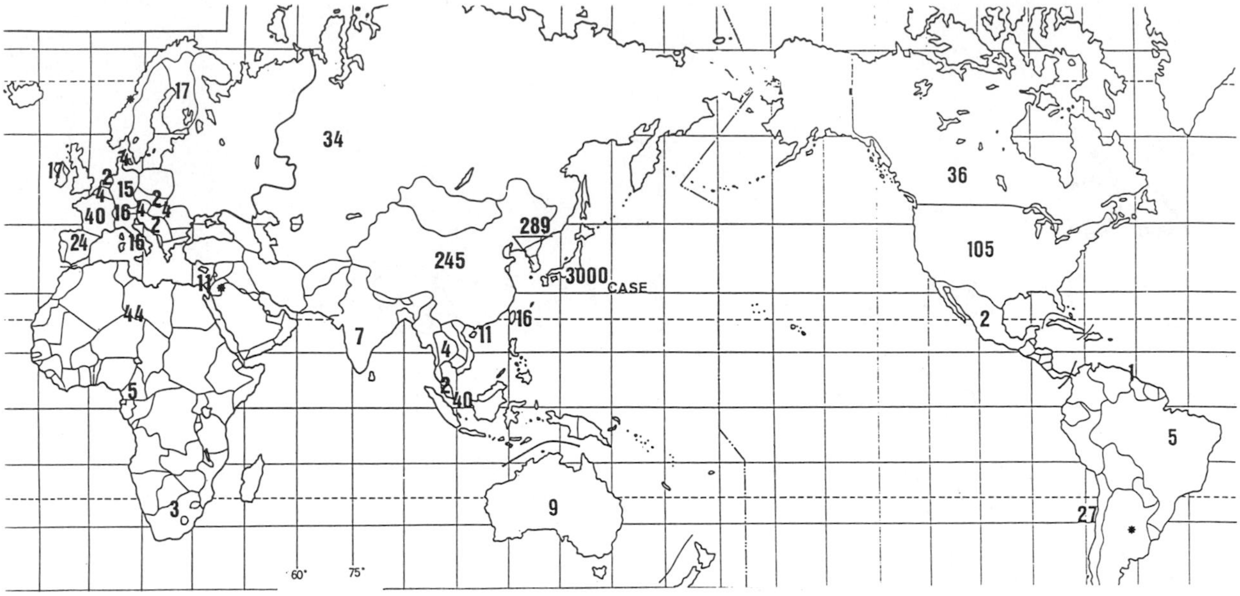


**Fig. 26-1.** Worldwide distribution of the moyamoya disease. Numerals indicate the number of the patients. (*) indicates there is a report from this country, but the number is not identified.

quently used. At the twenty-fifth annual meeting of the Japan Neurosurgical Society in 1966, Professor Kudo, as president of the society, focused upon the disease as a special theme, and the proceedings were published in 1967.[73] In 1977, a research committee on this disease, directed by Professor Gotoh, was organized and sponsored by the Ministry of Health and Welfare, Japan (MHWJ). Since then, this project has been carried out, directed by Professor Handa and then by one of the authors of this chapter (Yonekawa). Extensive investigations have been systematically organized in various fields: epidemiology, pathophysiology, clinical aspects, and pathology. Almost 2,000 cases were registered up to the end of 1990. Precise analyses have been published in the annual report of the research committee every year since 1977. The Research Committee of Etiology of Intractable Disease,[155] also sponsored by MHWJ, has estimated the number of patients in Japan to be 2,600 to 3,300 by a nationwide inquiry carried out in 1990.

In the United States and Europe, the disease has been only rarely reported. The cases of Weidner et al.[151] and Leed and Abbott[78] were Japanese patients,[53] but, following the report of Taveras[147] in 1969, moyamoya disease is now known to occur also in white and black races, and more and more cases have been reported in non-Japanese people.[4,6,8,10–12,27,29,34,43,44,45,76,106,114,115,118–120,149,152] In 1974, Picard and colleagues[116] summarized the worldwide status of the disease. We have calculated the number of cases in Figure 26-1 and Table 26-1 from the world literature between 1972 and 1990, except for the cases in Japan that have been estimated by the nationwide inquiry in 1990 mentioned above.[155] Many patients were found in Korea and the People's Republic of China. Although there are many other countries in which cases of moyamoya disease have been reported, Caucasian patients are rare.

## ETIOLOGY

The etiology of moyamoya disease is unknown. There is continuing debate concerning whether the disease is acquired or congenital. The similarity of the angiographic findings to those of embryonic brain vessels, the symmetrical abnormal vasculature, the frequent existence of abnormal vasculature without remarkable stenosis of the internal carotid artery, and the reported intrafamilial occurrence in combination with von Recklinghausen's disease, sickle cell anemia, and other disorders support the congenital theory. Suzuki et al.[133] and other investigators[92] considered the disease to be due to an autoimmune mechanism, since tonsillitis and other infections of the upper respiratory tract were frequently encountered in the anamnesis of the patient or for other reasons. They regarded the histologic findings in the vessels to be similar to the chronic inflammation changes observed in polyarteritis or Kawasaki's disease. In their experimental models, foreign protein of other animals was injected into one group of mongrel dogs and the toxin of $\beta$-hemolytic streptococcus into another group repeatedly for a certain period, so that a hyperimmune state could be obtained. Serial arterial specimens of both groups revealed exfoliation of intima, thickening

**TABLE 26-1. Reported Cases of Moyamoya Disease in the Literature Between 1972 and 1990, Japan Excluded**

| Location | No. of Cases |
|---|---|
| Asia | |
| Korea | 289 |
| People's Republic of China | 245 |
| Singapore | 40 |
| Taiwan | 16 |
| Hong Kong | 11 |
| Israel | 11 |
| India | 7 |
| Thailand | 4 |
| Malaysia | 2 |
| Lebanon | Unknown |
| Total | 625 |
| Europe | |
| France | 40 |
| USSR | 34 |
| Spain | 24 |
| England | 17 |
| Finland | 17 |
| Italy | 16 |
| Switzerland | 16 |
| Germany | 15 |
| Australia | 4 |
| Belgium | 4 |
| Denmark | 4 |
| Hungary | 4 |
| Czechoslovakia | 2 |
| Holland | 2 |
| Yugoslavia | 2 |
| Norway | Unknown |
| Total | 201 |
| America | |
| USA | 105 |
| Canada | 36 |
| Chile | 27 |
| Brazil | 5 |
| Mexico | 2 |
| Venezuela | 1 |
| Argentina | Unknown |
| Total | 176 |
| Africa | |
| North | 44 |
| Middle | 5 |
| South | 3 |
| Total | 52 |
| Oceania | |
| Australia | 9 |
| Total | 9 |
| Total | 1,063 |

of the intimal wall, fragmentation and winding of the internal elastic lamina, and muscle layer necrosis. The role of the sympathetic nerves was also emphasized, along with the inflammatory process, as the stenotic process has been considered to be confined to the anterior circulation.[63] However, a lack of other positive inflammatory findings, both histologically and biochemically, opposes this view. An autoimmune process has been implicated, but the inability to identify immune complexes using the complement method of C1q-binding and Raji cell radioimmunoassay in our study seems to refute this concept, at least its direct participation in the pathologic changes of moyamoya disease.[38] Various other etiologies have been suspected, including cranial trauma,[18] leptospirosis,[11] anaerobic bacteria such as *Propionibacterium acnes*,[153] and oral contraceptives. But these have not been convincing.

## EPIDEMIOLOGY

Cases of moyamoya disease are much more frequently encountered in Japan than in other areas, but they have been reported sporadically all over the world. No special regional predilection within Japan has been reported. This was also confirmed in the cooperative study of MHWJ.[31] The incidence seems to be approximately one in a million people per year. A female dominance (1:1.4) has been shown in the cooperative study of MHWJ.[31]

There seem to be two definite peaks of age incidence: children under 10 years old and young adults in the third decade (Fig. 26-2). The majority of cases are hospitalized within 2 years of the onset of the disease.

There is some evidence of a familial tendency. In the above-mentioned cooperative study of MHWJ, 13 out of 147 families showed a familial tendency.[31] Familial incidence is now about 7 to 12 percent in Japan,[22,31,64,102] and the ratio seems to be the same in other countries.[128] In descending order, familial occurrence of moyamoya disease is father-child, 5.77 percent; mother-child, 2.61 percent; and siblings, 2.22 percent.[22] Thirteen pairs of monovular twins have been reported as having the disease.[22,129,154] The mode of inheritance is by now considered to be a multifactorial one.[22]

In the same study, human leukocyte antigen (HLA) was investigated in 43 cases, and a remarkable difference in antigen type between juvenile and adult cases was observed. An increase in HLA-B40 in children under 10 years of age and in HLA-B54(20) in those over 11 years has been reported.[126] In another study, a significant association of the disease with the presence of HLA-A24, -B46, -B54, natural T-lymphocyte toxic antibody, and anti-double-stranded DNA antibody in patients' sera has been demonstrated.[65] However, how these antigens and antibodies contribute to the onset of moyamoya disease has not been clearly identified. Changes in lymphocyte function and complement reaction have been variously reported among investigators.[158] Further investigations are required to draw more concrete conclusions.

Various other diseases and disorders have been reported in conjunction with moyamoya disease, as shown in Table 26-2.[13,14,16,17,25,46,52,55,69,70,75,90,93,117,124,125,150] The association of aneurysm is discussed later in a separate section.

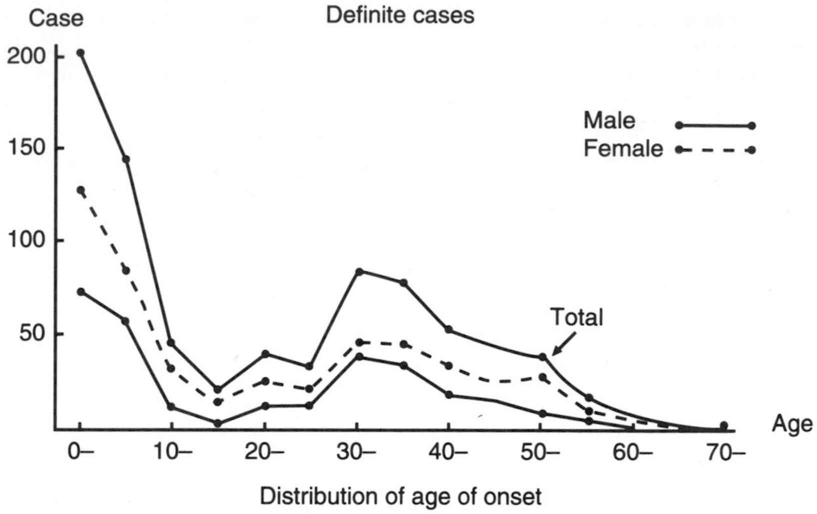


**Fig. 26-2.** Age distribution of moyamoya disease.

## CLINICAL SYMPTOMS AND SIGNS

There are no specific symptoms or signs related to moyamoya disease. The various clinical manifestations are generally caused by cerebrovascular accident, ischemia, or hemorrhage, and occasionally by epilepsy (Table 26-3).[37] The research committee of MHWJ has proposed four types of clinical manifestation: TIA, infarction, hemorrhage, and epilepsy.

In juvenile cases, the ischemic type of moyamoya disease, which includes transient ischemic attacks (TIAs) and infarction is dominant: 69 to 87 percent; TIAs are more prevalent than infarction: TIAs, 40 percent; infarction, 29 percent (Table 26-4).[37] Different kinds of deficits are encountered in ischemic cases. They are sometimes progressive, such that cortical blindness, motor aphasia, or even a vegetative state are observed within several years of the onset. They are usually preceded by TIAs or reversible ischemic neurologic deficits (RINDs). These transient weaknesses or pareses are provoked by some condition of hyperventilation, such as blowing wind instruments, blowing to cool something hot, or crying. They are considered to be induced by decreased $Pa_{CO_2}$, therefore by decreased cerebral blood flow (CBF). Ischemic deterioration is often precipitated by infection of the upper respiratory tract. Mental retardation is reported to be found in about half the patients.[113,132] Children with moyamoya disease have problems in school: they are incapable of concentrating on the lectures and fall seriously behind the class. A low intelligence quotient (IQ) is frequently seen among the cases (71 percent).[21,24] Usually, the earlier the onset of the disease and, therefore, the longer the period of suffering, the lower the mental function and intelligence quality. Cases with the onset under 4 years of age seem to have a poor functional prognosis.[38,97] By contrast, juvenile cases with TIAs of relatively late onset seem to have a better prognosis. In adult cases, the hemorrhage is more prevalent,[77,89] and occurring in 66 percent of the cases of the cooperative study. A predominance of the hemorrhagic disorders is noticed especially in females (Table 26-4). Previously, subarachnoid hemorrhage was considered to be the major type of bleeding, but now ventricular hemorrhage and/or intracerebral hemorrhage seems to be more common, judging from CT[139] and autopsy findings.[145] Of 29 adult cases of bleeding, 9 had recurrent bleeding at an interval from several days to more than 10 years.[163]

Epilepsy was observed in about 5 percent of all cases.[37] More than 80 percent of cases with epilepsy have been reported to be children less than 10 years old.[31]

A fatal outcome has been frequently encountered in cases with massive bleeding. In the series of Tanaka and colleagues,[145] 20 out of 22 autopsied cases had been bleeding.

Although prognosis of moyamoya disease is generally considered to be benign (75 to 80 percent of cases), the natural history of the disease is still unclear. It is unknown whether both the juvenile and adult types belong to the same entity, and whether unilateral involvement can evolve into bilateral. The clinical manifestations, as shown in Table 26-4, are not constant but are interchangeable.[160] The pathologic process seems to be active until about 10 years of age, when it appears to stabilize.

## PATHOLOGY

The first autopsy case of moyamoya disease was reported by Maki et al.[82] in 1965. It was a 9-year-old child who died of hemorrhage. He enumerated the following important findings:

**TABLE 26-2. Combined Disorders of Moyamoya Disease, as Reported in the Literature**

| |
|---|
| Infectious Disease |
| Leptospirosis |
| Meningitis (tuberculosis etc.) |
| Arteritis |
| Nephritis |
| Tonsillitis |
| Hematological Disorders |
| Sickle cell anemia |
| Fanconi's anemia |
| Thalassemia |
| Metabolic Disorders |
| Hyperlipoproteinemia (type 2A) |
| Glycogen storage disease (type 1) |
| Lipohyalinosis |
| Pseudoxanthoma elasticum |
| Hyperthyroidism |
| Impaired NADH-CoQ reductase activity |
| Genetic, Chromosomal Disorders |
| Neurofibromatosis |
| von Recklinghausen's disease |
| Tuberous sclerosis |
| Down syndrome (21-trisomy) |
| Turner syndrome |
| Retinitis pigmentosa |
| Congenital Anomalies |
| Cloverleaf skull |
| Transposition of the great arteries |
| Neoplasms |
| Parasellar tumor (craniopharyngioma, etc.) |
| Wilm's tumor |
| Drug Abuse |
| Phenobarbital |
| Oral contraceptives |
| Other Disorders |
| Cardiomyopathy |
| Progressive myopathy |
| Autoimmune disease |
| Renal artery stenosis |
| Fibromuscular dysplasia |
| Cranial trauma |
| Cranial irradiation |
| Arteriovenous malformation |
| Cerebral aneurysm (saccular, dissecting) |
| Identical twins |
| Harlequinism |
| Growth failure |
| Allagille syndrome |
| Polycystic kidney and eosinophilic granuloma |
| Hydrocephalus |
| Perforation of the small intestine |

1. Narrowing of main trunks of the intracranial skull base arteries.
2. Many abnormal small vessels originating from the circle of Willis.
3. Undifferentiated small arteries and veins in the subarachnoid space and in the cerebral parenchyma.
4. Secondary parenchymatous changes such as infarction and necrosis, encountered in the temporal and occipital lobes.

Later, autopsy cases were reported by various authors,[9,35,48,79,107,108] including Handa et al.,[36] Suzuki et al.,[134] Tanaka et al.,[145] and Hosoda et al.[49] Most of the autopsy cases had died of intracranial hemorrhage. The youngest autopsy case seems to be that of a 2-year-old boy reported by Carlson et al.[9] in 1973. The pathologic findings that typify this disease have been summarized in the diagnostic manual of spontaneous occlusion of the circle of Willis proposed by the research committee of MHWJ, as shown in Table 26-5. It should be noted that the lipid deposit in the thickened intima seems to be frequently noted, and this finding does not necessarily differentiate moyamoya disease from atherosclerotic occlusion.

**TABLE 26-3. Symptomatology of Moyamoya Disease**

| Symptom | Children (0–9 Years Old) $N$ = 431 | Adults (30–39 Years Old) $N$ = 235 |
|---|---|---|
| Motor paresis | 338 | 83 |
| Disturbance of consciousness | 56 | 123 |
| Headache | 37 | 137 |
| Convulsion | 113 | 25 |
| Psycho-organic syndrome | 7 | 17 |
| Speech disturbance | 83 | 32 |
| Sensory disturbance | 44 | 24 |
| Involuntary movement | 7 | 1 |
| Mental retardation | 38 | 8 |
| Visual disturbance | 15 | 11 |
| Visual field defect | 9 | 13 |

(Data from Handa et al.[37])

Previously it was believed that the intracranial bleeding was due to subarachnoid hemorrhage[77,89] originating from ruptured cortical moyamoya vessels.[94] However, accumulated autopsy cases and the development of CT scan revealed intraventricular hemorrhage originating from the ventricular wall,[58] basal ganglia, or thalamus to be the major source of bleeding.

The following are considered to be the main causes of bleeding:[110,145]

1. Rupture of dilated and stressed perforating arteries.
2. Fibrinoid necrosis of the arterial wall in the basal ganglia.

**TABLE 26-4. Clinical Manifestations of Moyamoya Disease in Children and Adults[a]**

| | Children (0–9 Years Old) $N$ = 431 | Adults (30–39 Years Old) $N$ = 235 |
|---|---|---|
| Hemorrhage | 21 | 161 |
| Epilepsy | 107 | 11 |
| Infarction | 137 | 40 |
| TIA | 194 | 23 |
| Others | 23 | 8 |

[a] Numerals in clinical manifestations were multiple counted in case registration.
(Data from Handa et al.[37])

**TABLE 26-5. Guidelines for the Diagnosis of Moyamoya Disease[a]**

I. A. 1. Age of onset varies, but is more prevalent in youth and in females. Familial occurrence is sometimes reported.
2. Symptoms and types of progression vary, namely, an asymptomatic type or a type with transient or persistent neurologic deficits of slight or severe degree.
3. Cerebral ischemia is observed, usually in juvenile patients, and hemorrhage in adult patients.
B. In juveniles, hemiparesis, monoparesis, sensory disturbance, involuntary movement, headache, and convulsions appear with recurrence, sometimes on alternating sides. Mental retardation or persistent neurologic deficits are also observed. The hemorrhagic type is rare, however.
C. In adults, symptoms similar to those observed in juveniles may appear, but most of them have a sudden onset of intraventricular, subarachnoid, or intracerebral hemorrhage. Patients usually recover from the bleeding with or without persistent deficits, but deaths have also been noted in severe cases.

II. Angiography is indispensable for the diagnosis. The following findings are observed.
A. Stenosis or occlusion is observed at the terminal portion of the intracranial ICA and/or at the proximal portion of the ACA and/or the MCA.
B. Abnormal vascular moyamoya networks are observed in the vicinity of the above-mentioned areas in the arterial phase.
C. These findings are recognized bilaterally.

III. Etiology is unknown, and an underlying disease (such as atherosclerosis, meningitis, Down syndrome, neoplasms, von Recklinghausen's disease, postirradiation) is ruled out.

IV. Pathologic findings helpful for the diagnosis:
A. Intimal thickening and resulting stenosis or occlusion are observed around the intracranial terminal portion of the ICA, usually bilaterally. They are sometimes associated with lipoid degeneration.
B. In the main arteries (ACA, MCA, Pcom) that construct the circle of Willis, various degrees of stenosis and occlusion are observed in association with intimal fibrous thickening and widening of the internal elastic lamina and tunica media.
C. Many small vascular channels (perforators and anastomotic branches) are observed around the circle of Willis.
D. Small vessels of networks are observed in the pia mater.

*Abbreviations*: ACA, anterior cerebral artery; ICA, internal carotid artery; MCA, middle cerebral artery; Pcom, posterior communicating artery.

[a] Diagnostic criteria are divided in two groups: as follows, in reference to I.

1. Definite case: fulfills all the findings described in II and III simultaneously. Juvenile cases fulfill IIA and IIB on one side and remarkable stenosis at the terminal portion of the intracranial internal carotid artery on the other side.
2. Probable case: does not fulfill the criteria in IIC, but fulfills the other criteria mentioned for the definite cases.

Autopsy cases in which angiography was not performed will be investigated separately, in reference to IV.

(From Research Committee on Spontaneous Occlusion of the Circle of Willis, Ministry of Health and Welfare, Japan, 1988.)

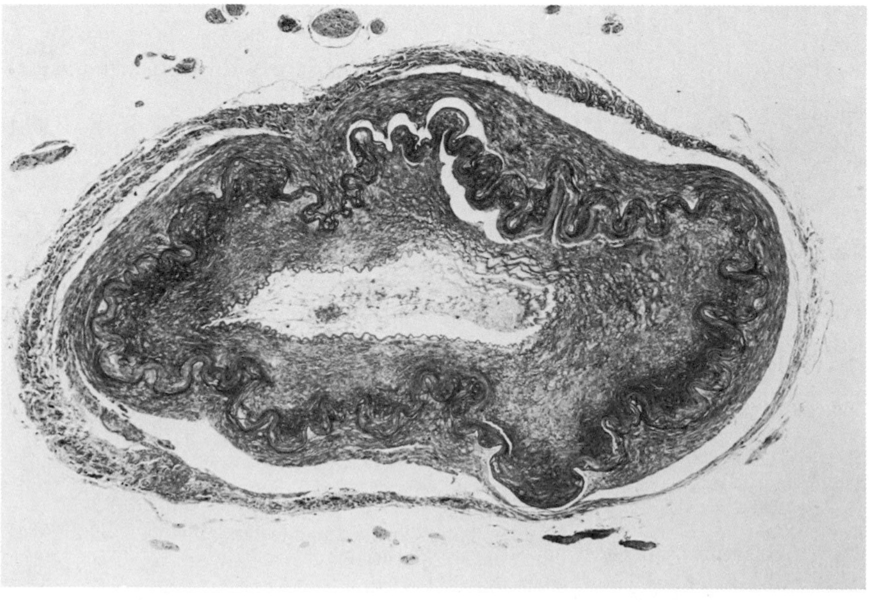

**Fig. 26-3.** Typical intimal thickening of the right internal carotid artery of a patient with moyamoya disease. (Terminal portion, Mallory trichrome stain, × 64.) (Courtesy of Dr. Y. Hosoda.)

3. Rupture of microaneurysms in the periventricular region, especially around the superior-lateral wall of the lateral ventricles.

Severe stenosis at the carotid fork has been reported to be due to concentric lamellar intimal thickening by cellular fibrous tissue.[9] The internal elastic lamina is frequently partly stratified, while the tunica media and adventitia are usually normal. Pathologic changes in the perforating arteries of moyamoya can be classified into three types: stenosis dilatation, and mixed[9] (Fig. 26-3). Lipohyalinosis and multiple microaneurysms have also been reported in these small vessels (50 to 1,500 $\mu$m) and are presumed to be the origin of hemorrhage.[88]

Thrombus formation is found at the distal portion of the occluded artery and is composed of white thrombus, consisting mainly of platelets, of fibrin thrombus, or of mixed thrombus. This thrombus may play an essential role in moyamoya disease, or it may participate in the progress of the disease and in the development of cerebral ischemia.[50] So far, there has been little description of the histologic findings in the vertebrobasilar system, although there have been sporadic reports of intimal thickening or calcium deposits on the internal elastic lamina.[56]

Similar lesions, such as intimal thickening and other characteristic findings observed in the major cerebral vessels, have been observed also in vessels of the heart, kidney, and other organs, and moyamoya disease is believed to be a systemic vascular disease.[35,51]

## CLINICAL EXAMINATION

No remarkable findings appear in the laboratory data,[132] except for the platelet aggregation test, in which an increase of nondissociative patterns and an increase of maximum aggregation has been reported to be observed in a patient group compared with controls.[84]

### Angiography

Cerebral angiography is indispensable in the diagnosis of this disease, but it should be performed with great care. The complication rate is considered to be higher than in the more usual atherosclerotic occlusive disease. A postangiographic death due to infarction occurred in our hospital several years ago. The following measures have been undertaken to prevent angiographic complications in our department:

1. Selective angiography with Seldinger's method is applied by a trained hand.
2. Unnecessary intravascular wedging of the catheter, especially at the internal carotid artery, is avoided.
3. General anesthesia is administered to children and infants to maintain hemodynamics and stable blood gases.
4. An intravenous drip is always established, to avoid intraoperative hypotension even in adult cases.
5. Low molecular weight dextran is administered intraoperatively, and the catheter with heparin-containing saline is irrigated frequently to prevent clot formation around the catheter.
6. Preoperative dehydration should be avoided.
7. Preoperative administration of steroids is advisable, especially in children.

The characteristic angiographic findings of moyamoya disease (Fig. 26-4) are as follows:

1. Stenosis or occlusion beginning at the termination of the intracranial internal carotid artery, and also at the origin of the anterior and middle cerebral arteries.
2. Abnormal vascular network in the region of the basal ganglia.
3. Findings (1) and (2) symmetrical on both sides.
4. Transdural anastomosis (rete mirabile).

The first three items are included in the diagnostic criteria of moyamoya disease proposed by the research committee of MHWJ.[31] Suzuki et al.[133] classified the progression of disease into six phases, according to angiographic findings:

1. Stenosis of the intracranial bifurcation of the internal carotid artery.
2. First appearance of moyamoya (dilatation of the intracerebral arteries).
3. Increasing of moyamoya (disappearing process of the middle and anterior cerebral arteries).
4. Finer formation of moyamoya (disappearing process of the posterior cerebral artery).
5. Shrinking of moyamoya (disappearance of the intracerebral arteries).
6. Disappearance of moyamoya and collateral circulation only from the external carotid system.

These changes, however, have not always been observed in our series, nor in others, although some remarkable changes, such as the progression of stenosis in the main trunks and decreased visualization of cortical arteries, were noticed in accordance with progression of symptoms, especially in juvenile cases.[39,109] Abnormal networks, named moyamoya, in the region of basal ganglia appear to function as collateral pathways (intraparenchymatous anastomosis) in relation to the cortical arteries.[78] They can be precisely visualized by a serial magnification angiography.[136]

Besides this type of collateral circulation in the basal ganglia, *ethmoidal moyamoya* or a moyamoyalike network in the frontobasal region may also be visualized. In our series, some juvenile cases revealed this type of moyamoya, which is believed to function as a

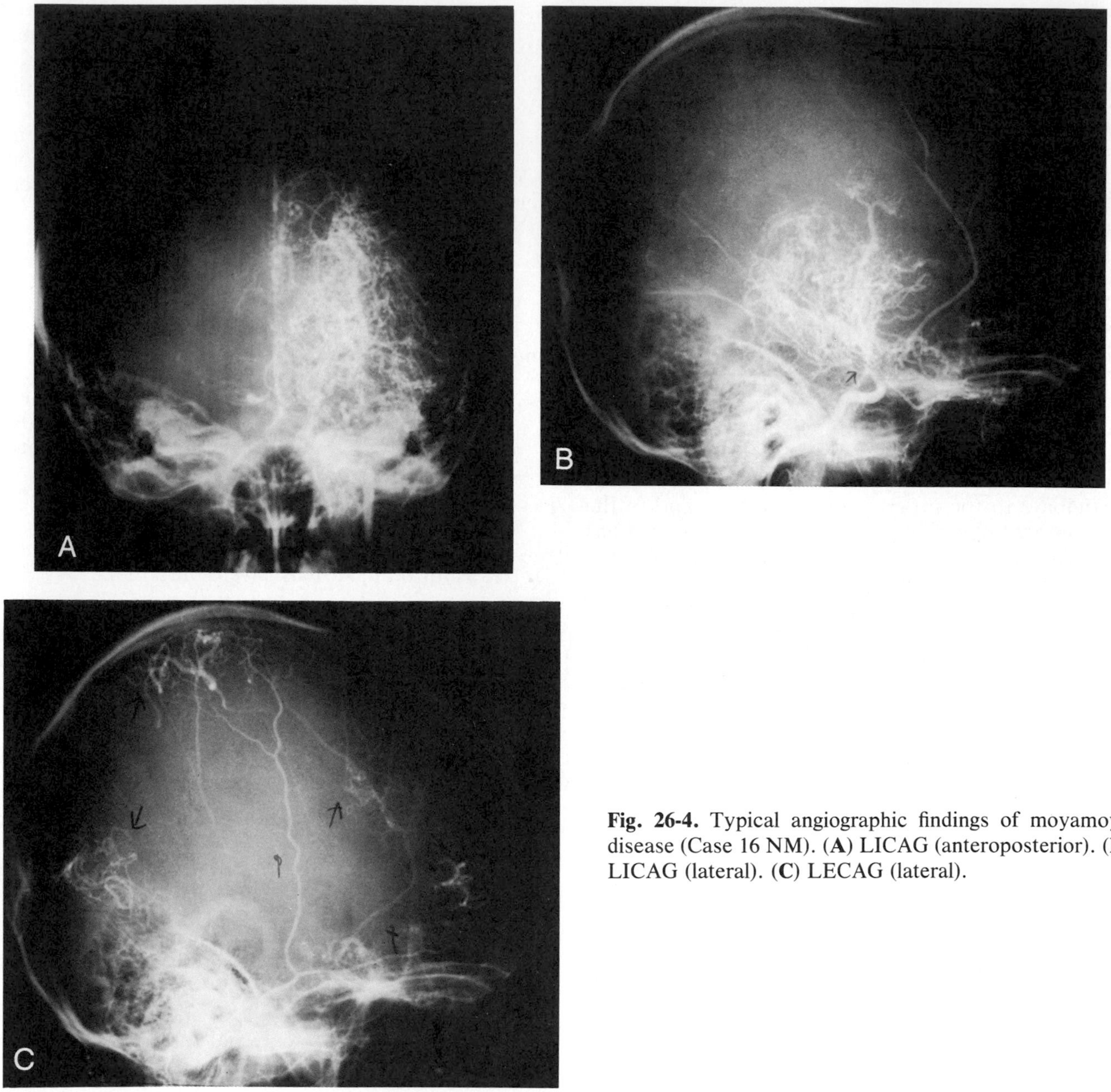


**Fig. 26-4.** Typical angiographic findings of moyamoya disease (Case 16 NM). (**A**) LICAG (anteroposterior). (**B**) LICAG (lateral). (**C**) LECAG (lateral).

collateral pathway to the forebrain via the ethmoid sinus through branches of the internal maxillary artery.

Transdural anastomosis, termed *rete mirabile,* is abundant[42,106] and may also be named *vault moyamoya.*[67] The contributing arteries to this anastomosis are as follows: anterior falcial artery, middle meningeal artery, ethmoidal arteries, occipital artery, tentorial artery, and superficial temporal arteries. Of these, the first three are considered to be main contributing arteries. According to Kodama et al.,[67] the appearance of vault moyamoya seems to be confined to specific localities, of which there are nine in juvenile cases and six in adults. These transdural anastomoses appear to play a significant role as collateral pathways.

From the surgical point of view, cortical arteries deserve more attention. The territory of the middle cerebral artery (MCA) might be divided into two (or three) segments: the candelabra (anterior part) and the rest, including the angular artery and the posterior temporal artery (posterior part). About half of our moyamoya cases revealed nonvisualization of the posterior part of the MCA. Scarceness of collateral circulation due to the nonvisualization of the cortical artery seems to be closely related with computed tomography (CT) findings (low-density areas [LDAs]). In our children's cases the entire territory of the MCA and the posterior cerebral artery (PCA) seems to be more involved than in the adult cases. It is not yet known whether such changes in the cortical artery are due to secondary ischemic changes or to a primary process inherent to the disease.

The vertebrobasilar system has rarely been reported to be involved in this disease.[131,132] There have been two cases of children followed in our department, in which the trunk of the basilar artery occluded completely.

Aneurysms in combination with moyamoya disease have been frequently reported.[3,26,68,99,111,112,157,167] There seem to be three types of aneurysm combinations: (1) aneurysm at the usual sites, for example, the circle of Willis; (2) aneurysm of peripheral arteries, such as the posterior choroidal artery, the anterior choroidal artery, the posterior cerebral artery, and Heubner's artery; (3) aneurysm localized in the area of moyamoya vessels. The latter two have been reported to be false aneurysms, in view of their location and form.[26] But the true aneurysm might also be included. They may rupture and are probably one of the origins of cerebral hemorrhage. A case with multiple aneurysms originating from all three groups has been reported.[99] Magnification angiography has been reported to be very effective in visualizing these aneurysms.[137]

## Computed Tomography Scan

Up to 40 percent of the ischemic cases of moyamoya disease are reported to have normal CT findings.[31] Positive CT scan findings of moyamoya disease of the ischemic type reported by Handa et al.[40,41] and others[29,91,138] are as follows (Fig. 26-5):

1. Low-density areas confined to the cerebral cortex and subcortex.
2. Dilated cerebral sulci and fissures.
3. Slight ventricular dilation.

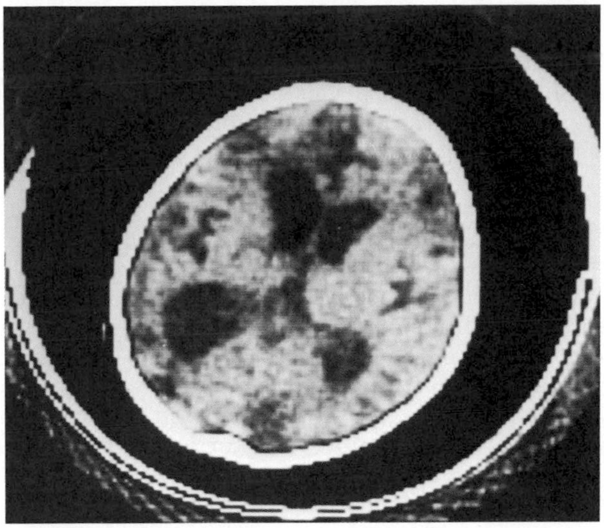

**Fig. 26-5.** Typical computed tomography findings of an advanced moyamoya disease. Note multiple low-density areas in the cortex and subcortex, as well as dilated sulci.

LDAs are not usually observed in the basal ganglia, in contrast to acute infantile hemiplegia and/or atherosclerotic occlusive disease. In our series, LDAs have been rather more frequently observed in children, in the territory of the posterior cerebral artery rather than in any other territory, and this seems to be related to the scarceness of the collateral supply through the affected PCA.[160]

In the hemorrhagic type, high-density areas (HDAs) may be observed in the basal ganglia and thalamus,[101] ventricular system[139] (including subependymal hemorrhage[58]), subcortex, and cortex, in that order of frequency[31] (Fig. 26-6).

Contrast study often visualizes tortuous or curvilinear vessels and moyamoya vessels in the basal ganglia. The most proximal segment of the anterior and

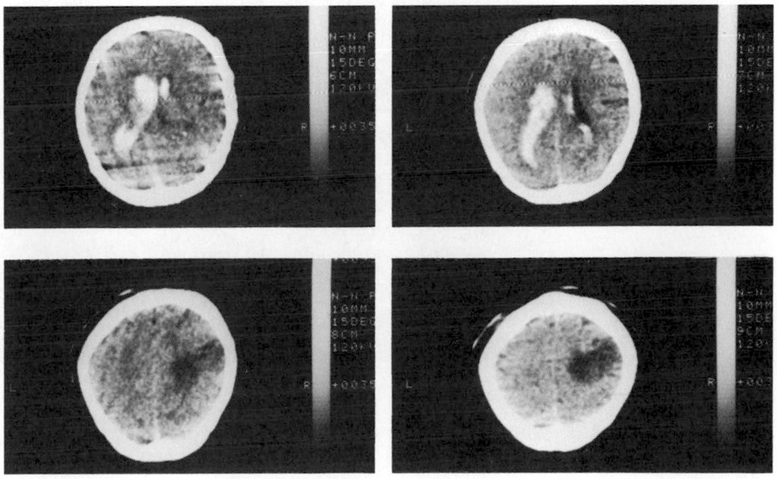

**Fig. 26-6.** Typical intraventricular hemorrhage observed in an adult female case.

middle cerebral arteries are often poorly opacified.[138] Although these all are nonspecific findings, attempts are being made to use the CT scan as a screening test, in combination with newer methods such as biplane computed cerebral angiotomometry[5] or dynamic CT scan (Fig. 26-7), which seems to be very promising.[160]

## Magnetic Resonance Imaging Scan

Magnetic resonance imaging (MRI) can demonstrate a small subcortical lesion that cannot be detected by CT. Cerebral infarctions due to moyamoya are bilateral, multiple, often small, and asymptomatic, affecting predominantly the carotid circulation in cortical watershed regions. Subcortical infarctions in the centrum semiovale and large hemispheric infarctions in hemodynamically compromised areas are the predominant findings. Brain atrophy and slight ventricular dilatation can also be demonstrated in some cases.

Stenosis or occlusion of the carotid fork is also visualized in most of the cases. Multiple, small, round, or tortuous low-intensity areas extending from the suprasellar cistern to the basal ganglia can be demonstrated in the majority of cases. These areas are thought to represent abnormal networks of parenchymal collaterals, the so-called moyamoya vessels seen on angiogram (Fig. 26-8).[19]

Magnetic resonance angiography (MRA) might obviate routine catheter angiography in the near future as the definite diagnostic tool. Although the resolution of the MRA is not enough at present to visualize abnormal moyamoya vessels, abnormality in the vicinity of the internal carotid artery (ICA) terminal portion can be well detected.[2]

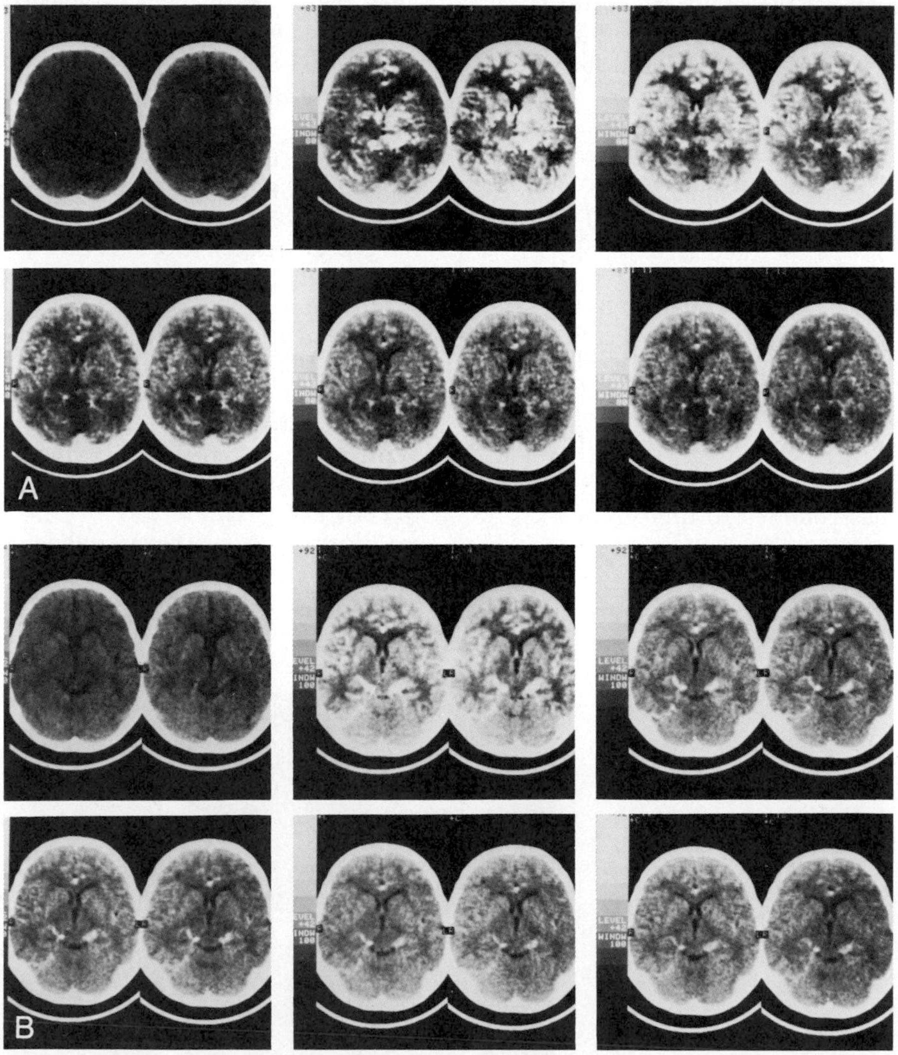


**Fig. 26-7.** Preoperative and postoperative dynamic computed tomography (CT) scan (Case NM). (**A**) Preoperative CT scan (**B**) postoperative CT scan. Note decreased opacification of abnormal vasculature in the basal ganglia and increased blood flow in the cerebral cortex.

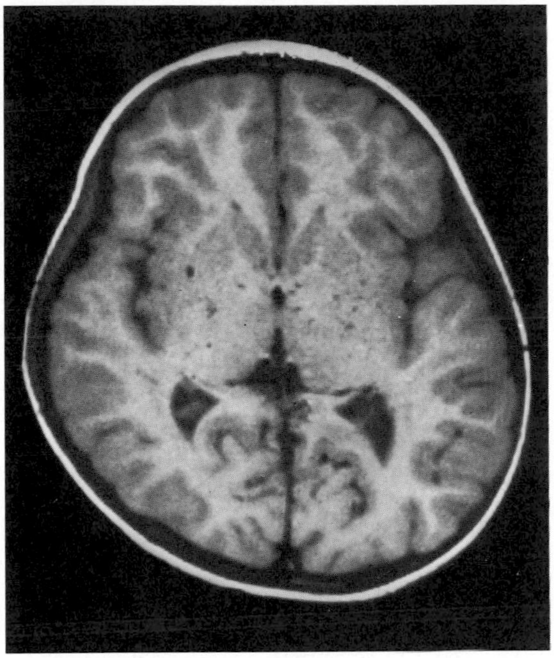

A

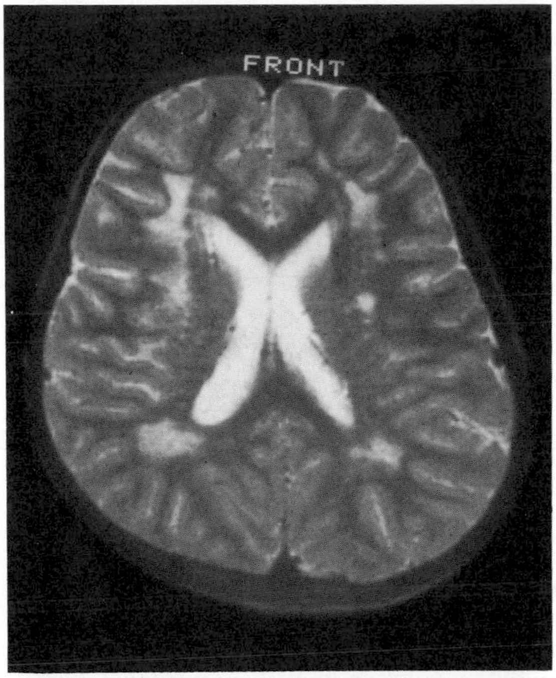


B

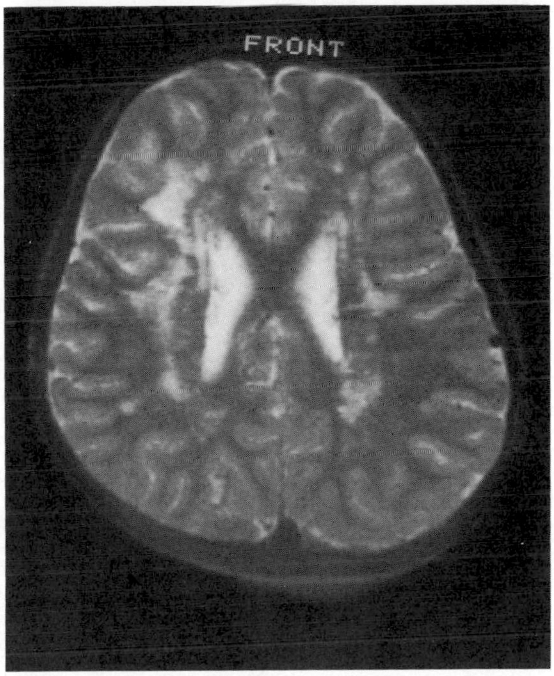


C

**Fig. 26-8.** (**A**) Many small punctous low-intensity areas were shown in the basal ganglia: representing dilated perforating arteries. (**B & C**) Many high-intensity areas are demonstrated in the periventricular areas: representing areas of small infarctions.

## Cerebral Blood Flow Measurement

Early studies of regional cerebral blood flow (rCBF) measurement using the $^{133}Xe$ inhalation system Cerebrograph-R (Novo Co. Ltd) in patients with moyamoya disease revealed decreased response to $CO_2$ changes, postoperative increase of rCBF, and postoperative changes in the rCBF distribution.[160] These results, however, were based on two-dimensional images with the disadvantage of extracranial contamination; rCBF in the deep structure such as basal ganglia could not be evaluated.

Recently three-dimensional images of rCBF can be obtained by the new method such as stable xenon-enhanced CT (XeCT), positron emission CT (PET), and single photon emission CT (SPECT). These techniques can evaluate hemodynamics of moyamoya disease more topographically and quantitatively. Vascular response to $CO_2$ or acetazolamide also can be studied in detail by these methods. Although they are very useful tools for evaluating hemodynamics in moyamoya disease, it must be stated that there are still some disagreements about the results among investigators.[32,146,148] This is partly due to the limited number of patients available with various types and stages of the disease and partly because these methods are still in a developing stage.

Outlines of these techniques and their results are as follows.

## Stable Xenon-Enhanced Computed Tomography and Dynamic Computed Tomography

Stable XeCT provides a rCBF image of high resolution and has the advantage that the study can be repeated after a short period. These characteristics make it suitable for studying vascular response in moyamoya patients. Regional cerebral blood flow (rCBF) and cerebrovascular reactivity to acetazolamide can be measured by stable Xe-enhanced CT. The mean transit time (MTT) is measured by dynamic CT, which enables the clinician to assess regional cerebral blood volume (rCBV).[159] Although there are some reports emphasizing the relative preservation of rCBF and vascular response to hypercapnia, our data generally support the above-mentioned findings obtained by the two-dimensional method. In the moyamoya brain, the regions of delayed MTT were distributed heterogeneously. In these areas, cerebrovascular reactivity (CVR) to acetazolamide was reduced and rCBV was increased. This tendency was marked in the patients of ischemic type. rCBF was decreased, especially in the frontal region, having delayed MTT and increased rCBV. In the basal ganglia rCBF was relatively preserved and rCBV was high, indicating a well-developed collateral circulation in accordance with the abnormal moyamoya vessels (Fig. 26-9).

## Positron Emission Computed Tomography

Positron emission computed tomography (PET) has the advantage of measuring not only rCBF, but also regional cerebral metabolism of oxygen ($rCMRO_2$), which makes it an ideal method for determining indications for surgery and for assessing its effectiveness.[143] In the pediatric cases, decrease of rCBF was marked in the parietal region and preserved in the basal ganglia and in the cerebellum. In the adult

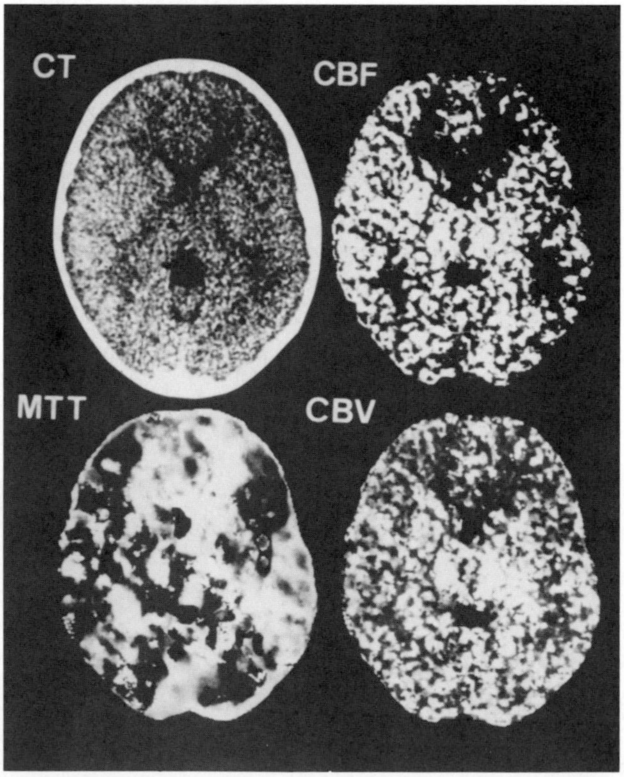


A

**Fig. 26-9.** (**A**) Images of regional cerebral blood flow (rCBF), regional mean transit time (rMTT) and regional cerebral blood volume (rCBV) of 7-year-old moyamoya patient obtained by Xe-enhanced computed tomography and dynamic computed tomography. Decrease of rCBF was shown in the bilateral frontal areas and in the left hemisphere; rMTT increased in the same region. Increase of rCBV was demonstrated in the bilateral basal ganglia. (*Figure continues.*)

cases, rCBF was decreased in the whole brain. But the degree of decrease of rCBF reported is different among investigators. Regional oxygen extraction fraction (rOEF) is reported to be increased in the early stage of some juvenile cases, but is generally not elevated significantly. In these cases, $rCMRO_2$ and rOEF have been reported to show a gradual decrease with a lapse of time, while they remain unchanged in the adult cases. Probably the most consistent finding of the PET study of moyamoya disease is increased rCBV.[144] rCBV was increased in the whole brain region, and rCBF/rCBV (an indicator of cerebral perfusion pressure) was decreased. These findings are remarkable in the children, but are also found in the adult. These results suggest that the brain of a moyamoya patient is in a chronic low-perfusion state. Vascular response to hypercapnia was impaired in both adult and juvenile cases, but the tendency is more remarkable in the adult cases.

## Single Photon Emission Computed Tomography

Single photon emission computed tomography (SPECT), using *N*-isopropyl-*p*-($^{123}$iodoamphetamine) ($^{123}$I-IMP), $^{99m}$Tc-hexamethylpropyleneamineoxime ($^{99m}$Tc-HM-PAO),[98] or $^{133}$Xe inhalation can provide a three-dimensional image of regional cerebral blood

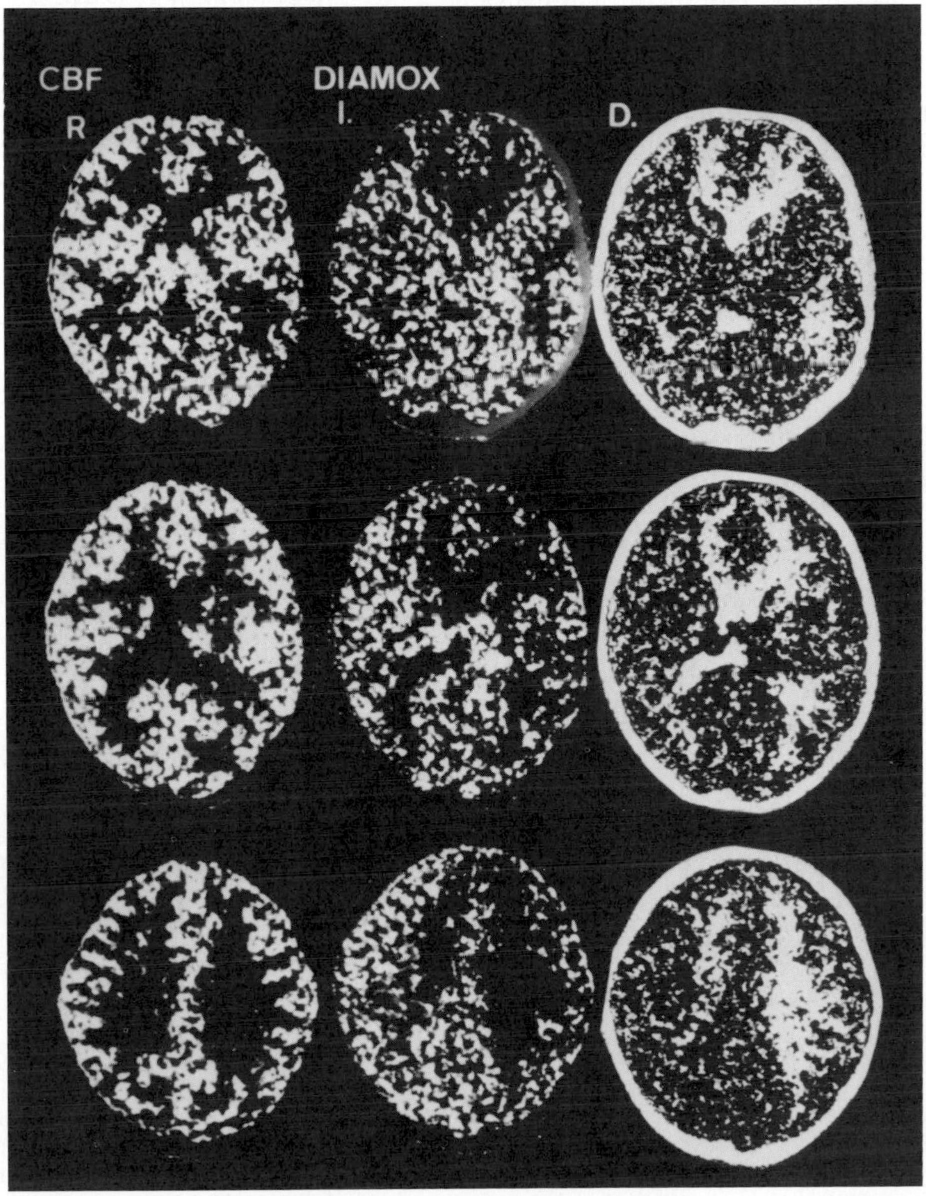


B

**Fig. 26-9** (*Continued*). (**B**) Changes of rCBF of the same patient by acetazolamide (Diamox) administration. Responsiveness to acetazolamide was demonstrated as a subtracted image in the right side.

flow. Abnormalities seen on SPECT have been reported to appear more extensively than those revealed by CT scanning, reflecting the areas of hemodynamic disturbances (Fig. 26-10). This method is considered to provide a simple and noninvasive method of measuring rCBF, enabling the clinician to evaluate the pathophysiology of moyamoya disease and its response to therapy.

## Doppler Sonography

Doppler sonography is well known as one of the most useful noninvasive methods of detecting extracranial stenotic and occlusive lesions. We have registered the change of flow pattern of moyamoya disease preoperatively, intraoperatively, and postoperatively.[96] The special flow patterns in moyamoya disease include decreased or absent flow in the cervical portion of the internal carotid artery on both sides, and flow pattern changes of the external carotid artery, especially of the superficial temporal artery into the pattern of the internal carotid artery. This finding is well-correlated with the angiographic findings of rete mirabile through transdural anastomosis. A method of visualizing stenotic sites with color displays by scanning Doppler flow signals has become available recently.

## Electroencephalogram

Abnormal electroencephalogram (EEG) findings in moyamoya disease are nonspecific. The EEG shows low voltage or slow waves, such as hemispheric posterior slowing (HP-slowing) or centrotemporal slowing (CT-slowing), with or without an asymmetry.[66,105,113] They are related to permanent ischemic change or to transient hemodynamic changes due to a $PaCO_2$ variation. Depression of sleep spindles has also been reported to be one of the pathologic EEGs observed in moyamoya disease. Yoshii and Kudo[166] summarized EEG changes in moyamoya disease as follows:

1. Abnormal EEG changes are more frequently observed in juvenile cases than in adult cases.
2. Diffuse and/or bilateral slow waves are observed usually as abnormal waves and occasionally as spike waves.
3. "Buildup" occurs with the appearance of delta waves during hyperventilation.
4. Polymorphous slow waves appear a few minutes after hyperventilation ("rebuildup") and are characteristic of juvenile cases, related to TIAs in more than half of the cases, but are observed less frequently in adult cases.
5. Photic stimulation usually has no effect on the EEG.

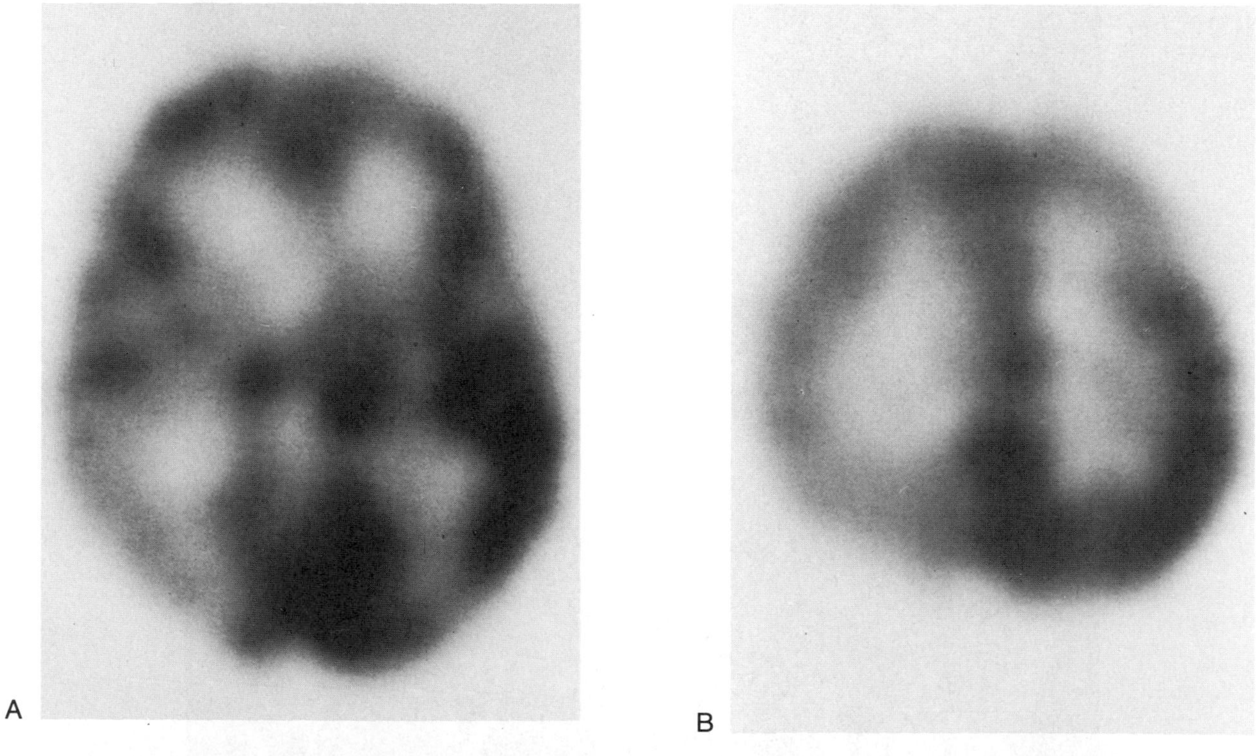


**Fig. 26-10.** *N*-isopropyl-*p*-($^{123}$iodoamphetamine) single photon emission computed tomography of the same patient as Figure 26-8A. Diffuse decrease of regional cerebral blood flow (rCBF) was shown in the right hemisphere. Decrease of rCBF in the periventricular region of left hemisphere was also revealed in this film; rCBF in the basal ganglia was relatively preserved. Compared to Figure 26-8B, the regions of decreased rCBF was found to be more profound than shown in the magnetic resonance imaging as areas of infarction.

### Somatosensory Evoked Response

Among other kinds of examinations somatosensory evoked response (SER) deserves to be mentioned. The SER reflects neuronal function in somatosensory centrifugal pathways. An abnormality of the SER is reported to be better correlated with clinical fixed neurologic deficits than CT findings. By contrast, auditory brain stem response (ABR) is reported to reveal no abnormality in moyamoya disease, except in patients with vertebrobasilar occlusion.

## DIAGNOSIS

The revised diagnostic criteria for moyamoya disease have been proposed by the research committee of MHWJ, as described in Table 26-5. In this revision of 1988, there are two important points to distinguish these from the previous criteria: (1) to consider those cases as definite that have typical findings unilaterally but atypical findings contralaterally and (2) to exclude cases even with typical findings when the symptoms are combined with Down syndrome or with any other diseases. The differential diagnoses that should be taken into consideration include atherosclerotic occlusive disease, acute infantile hemiplegia, angiographic differentials, and vasospasm.

### Atherosclerotic Occlusive Disease

The occlusive processes of atherosclerotic occlusive disease are observed mainly at the cervical bifurcation and, next in order of frequency, at the carotid siphon. They do not usually reach the carotid fork, so that blood supply from the vertebrobasilar system, via the posterior communicating artery, is usually present without moyamoya vessel formation. The CT findings are also different: LDAs are observed in the basal ganglia, as well as the cortex and subcortex, while LDAs in moyamoya disease are confined to the cortex and subcortex and are frequently multiple. Probable cases, according to criteria of the research committee of MHWJ, particularly those with unilateral lesions, should be followed up carefully as an unfinished or incomplete type.

### Acute Infantile Hemiplegia

Sudden onset of hemiplegia is characteristically observed in both diseases, but preceding reversible ischemic episodes are frequently observed in moyamoya disease and not in acute infantile hemiplegia (AIH).[28] The two diseases can also be differentiated on CT findings: LDAs appear in the basal ganglia as well as in the cortex and subcortex in AIH, in contrast to multiple cortical LDAs in moyamoya disease. Finally, the characteristic angiographic findings of moyamoya disease are the key points of the differential diagnosis.[18]

### Angiographic Differentials

Confusing angiographic findings similar to moyamoya disease have been reported in certain brain tumors such as craniopharyngioma, which may occlude the terminal portion of the internal carotid artery.[15,76,95,123] However, clinical and CT findings will easily differentiate one from the other.

### Vasospasm

Vasospasm after a subarachnoid hemorrhage or meningitis sometimes shows marked stenosis of the main trunks of the cerebral arteries. However, these findings are usually transient and improve after a time. The clinical manifestations are also usually different. There are some confusing terminologies that should be clarified: moyamoya phenomenon[140] and moyamoya syndrome.[71] Moyamoya phenomenon should be interpreted as formation of the abnormal vasculature "puff of smoke," especially in the region of the basal ganglia, and moyamoya syndrome should be interpreted as a syndrome consisting of moyamoya phenomenon in combination with acquired occlusions of the internal carotid artery of known etiology: atherosclerosis, skull base tumor, basal meningitis, vasospasm,[140] and postirradiation.[15,121,127]

## TREATMENT

### Medical Treatment

Although no effective specific medical treatment for moyamoya disease has been reported hitherto, steroids are considered to be effective in certain cases, especially (1) in cases with involuntary movements and (2) in the active phase of recurrent ischemic attacks. The mechanism of their effectiveness is unknown, although influences on vasculitis, edema, and CBF have all been presumed.

Acetylsalicylic acid (ASA) and ticlopidine chloride, a platelet antiaggregant, may also be prescribed, as platelets appear to play an important role in the progressive thrombotic occlusions of the main vascular trunk in moyamoya disease.[50]

Other drugs, such as vasodilators, antifibrinolytics, and fibrinolytics, are occasionally used. But no study has supported the definite efficacy of these drugs. Other symptomatic medication, for bleeding, epilepsy, and headache, will not be mentioned here.

### Surgical Treatment

Superficial temporal artery-middle cerebral artery (STA-MCA) bypass, encephalomyosynangiosis (EMS), omentum transplantation, and cervical sympathectomy including stellate ganglionectomy are options. For treatment of hemorrhage, ventricular drainage, and hematoma evacuation are considered to be the main methods of surgical treatment.

## Superficial Temporal Artery-Middle Cerebral Artery Bypass

STA-MCA bypass, pioneered by Yasargil and Donaghy[156] in 1967, was independently applied to moyamoya disease with success by Reichman et al.,[122] Karasawa and Kikuchi and colleagues,[58] and later by Yonekawa and Yasargil.[164] The purpose of the bypass procedure is to give additional collateral flow to the ischemic brain and to prevent or minimize irreversible brain damage on progression of the disease. Also, it might be expected to reduce hemodynamic stress to the moyamoya vascular network, and therefore might eventually prevent the hemorrhage.

It was Professor Krayenbuehl, during the International Symposium of Extracranial/Intracranial (EC/IC) Bypass in 1976, who told us (Yonekawa) to pay attention to Dr. Tew's skepticism regarding the application of the bypass procedure to the treatment of moyamoya disease. Dr. Peerless was also skeptical, as cases of complication with postoperative hemiplegia, in spite of patent bypass, had been recorded. Professor Suzuki is of the same opinion, and that seems to be the reason why he resorts to cervical sympathectomy as surgical treatment of this disease.[135]

From bitter experiences with ischemic complications in our earlier series, we have investigated perioperative hemodynamic changes with various monitoring parameters, such as measurement of the intra-arterial pressure (IAP) of the middle cerebral artery, Doppler sonography, and power EEG.

The important points to know in performing a revascularization procedure in order to avoid complications include the following:

1. Suitable cortical arteries of about 1 mm in diameter may be few, in spite of extensive craniotomy, or may be hidden relatively deep in the sulci. There may be a rich supply of small branches to the cortex, making preparation of a cortical branch for bypass difficult. If a suitable cortical branch cannot be found, EMS or omentum transplantation should be considered as alternative methods for revascularization procedure.
2. The middle meningeal artery and frontal branches of the superficial temporal artery should be preserved as much as possible when performing craniotomy in cases in which marked transdural anastomoses are observed, or when Doppler sonography reveals the pattern of the internal carotid artery in these arteries. These transdural anastomoses make an important contribution to collateral circulation.
3. In combination with STA-MCA bypass, encephalomyosynangiosis or double bypasses (one is for the candelabra and the other for the angular artery or the posterior temporal artery) may be applied to prevent harmful changes in blood flow and its distribution, which have been frequently recorded by CBF measurement and angiography in some cases following bypass.
4. Intraoperative hypotension should be carefully avoided, as the collateral circulation through basal moyamoya and rete mirabile seems to be critical in cases with active ischemia, and hypotension might lead to ischemic complications. The intra-arterial pressure of the cortical arteries is extremely low in comparison with cerebrovascular occlusive disease of atherosclerotic origin. Intraoperative Doppler sonography may reveal a weak flow signal, even when a suitable recipient artery is present on the cortex.
5. Hyperventilation or a low $Paco_2$ level should be also avoided. Collateral pathways are affected by low $Paco_2$, increasing the danger of ischemic complications. Furthermore, with the brain shrinkage due to hyperventilation and cerebrospinal fluid (CSF) drainage after opening of the arachnoidea, a considerable volume of the air will remain in the subdural space after craniotomy closure. This might induce delicate hemodynamic changes. Subgaleal or epidural drainage with negative pressure may also reduce CBF. As a rule, we use inhalation anesthesia and maintenance of $Paco_2$ around 40 mmHg, so that sufficient CBF and expansion of the brain can be accomplished.
6. The duration of clamping of the middle cerebral artery during the anastomotic procedure should be as short as possible. Because of the complicated mode of collateral circulation, prolonged clamping might induce a cardinal decrease of rCBF. Power EEG revealed marked decrease of fast waves toward the end of the clamping in several cases.
7. The day before the operation, when oral intake is prohibited, continuous parenteral fluid administration is initiated to prevent hemoconcentration and hypotension, which might induce further deterioration of hemodynamics. Steroids are sometimes used for the reasons mentioned in the section on medical treatment.

## Encephalomyosynangiosis

Encephalomyosynangiosis (EMS) was first reported by Henschen[47] in 1950. His intention was to divert blood flow from the external carotid artery into the internal carotid system by applying temporal muscle to the brain surface of a patient with bilateral internal carotid stenosis. This method has been revived and applied to moyamoya disease by Karasawa and Kikuchi and their colleagues.[57] It is felt that new vascularization via temporal muscle takes place much more effectively in juvenile cases than in adult cases, and when the arachnoidea has been opened extensively. EMS was thus routinely performed in our earlier juvenile series, EMS alone when suitable recipient arteries could not be found, or in combination with the usual STA-MCA bypass, to prevent the ischemic complications due to change of blood flow distribution after the STA-MCA bypass alone. Indirect revascularization procedures, such as EMS and encephalodurosynangiosis (EDAS), do not always induce production of sufficient collateral pathways, which would fail to improve existing symptoms. No preoperative examination can predict the degree and efficacy of indirect vascularization. Occasionally, direct bypass procedures were necessary to obtain effective vascularization, as the indirect method failed to be effective.[100]

## Omentum Transplantation

Pedicled omentum application[30] has been investigated and evaluated as an effective treatment for lymphedema of the upper extremity after radical mastectomy, ischemia of the lower extremity, postirradiation carotid rupture after radical neck surgery, and cerebral ischemia. Autogenic free graft transplantation of the greater omentum has been performed, for example, in a patient with extensive scalp defect in plastic surgery. The capability of fluid absorption and vascularization by the transplanted greater omentum was reevaluated by Yonekawa and Yasargil.[165] The method has been described in detail elsewhere. Omentum has a greater potential for vascularizing ischemic tissues than does muscle. We have applied this method to four juvenile cases with success. However, this method has two disadvantages as compared to EMS: it is technically difficult, and it requires laparotomy. Our four cases were boys, and no suitable recipient artery could be found. A 2-year follow-up result has also been reported about the clinical application of the method.[59] This method is considered to be most suitable to treat cases with TIAs presenting with visual field disturbance, as augmentation of the cerebral blood flow in the occipital or occipitomedial area can be obtained, which is difficult by a direct revascularization procedure.

The method of pedicled omentum transposition on the brain surface, reported by Goldsmith, has been performed frequently in China and is reported to be effective for cerebral ischemia.

## Other Methods

Durapexia (Tsubokawa) and encephalodurosynangiosis (EDAS) (Matsushima et al.[85–87]) belong to the same category of operation as EMS, namely, introduction of external carotid flow into the internal carotid system via newly developed vascularization. Cervical sympathectomy, including stellate ganglionectomy, was advocated by Suzuki et al.[135] to improve CBF, but this method has not been widely acknowledged as a method of improving CBF permanently. It is well known that construction of a burr hole induces revascularization of an ischemic brain later through the hole. The mechanism is the same with the durapexia or with the EDAS. Ventricular drainage for intraventricular hemorrhage and evacuation of intracerebral hematoma for the hemorrhagic type of moyamoya disease will not be mentioned here.

## Results of Operative Treatment

Results of operative treatment for moyamoya disease in our 38 patients (27 children and 11 adults) were reported.[160] A summary of the results is as follows:

1. About two-thirds of the patients received surgical treatment on both sides.
2. Most of the surgery was the STA-MCA bypass (usually double bypass), one for the candelabra, the other for the angular or posterior temporal artery, with or without EMS.
3. EMS without bypass and omentum transplantation was performed only in two cases, respectively, because no proper recipient artery could be found.
4. There were no mortalities, but two morbidities with persisting neurologic deteriorations. One of them was connected with a malignant hyperthermia.
5. New LDAs appeared postoperatively in five cases, with or without permanent neurologic deficits.
6. Improvement of ischemic symptoms were observed on the operated side usually, but TIAs were sometimes observed on the contralateral side of the bypassed brain.
7. Recurrent ventricular hemorrhage was noticed in one case.

Our series showed that the revascularization procedure could prevent or minimize the progression of cerebral ischemia. This result coincides well with the recent report of the research committee with larger series reported as follows.[162]

Effectiveness of surgical and medical therapies was evaluated in 595 patients who had been registered from 1983 through 1990 and intensively followed up. Of these 595 cases, 541 were definite moyamoya disease cases. The mean duration of follow-up for these cases was 4.3 years. A detailed analysis of patients who underwent surgical treatment (revascularization) revealed that the activity of daily living (ADL) was better in patients who received both direct and indirect revascularization irrespective of ischemic or hemorrhagic type (Fig. 26-11). Above all, the proportion of patients with ADL-1 increased during the follow-up period. By contrast, patients who received only indirect revascularization or medication failed to show this tendency.

For the prevention of recurrence of bleeding (recurrence rate: about 10 percent) or ischemia, surgical treatment tended to be more effective. A decrease in frequency of TIAs (cases with TIAs reduced from 30

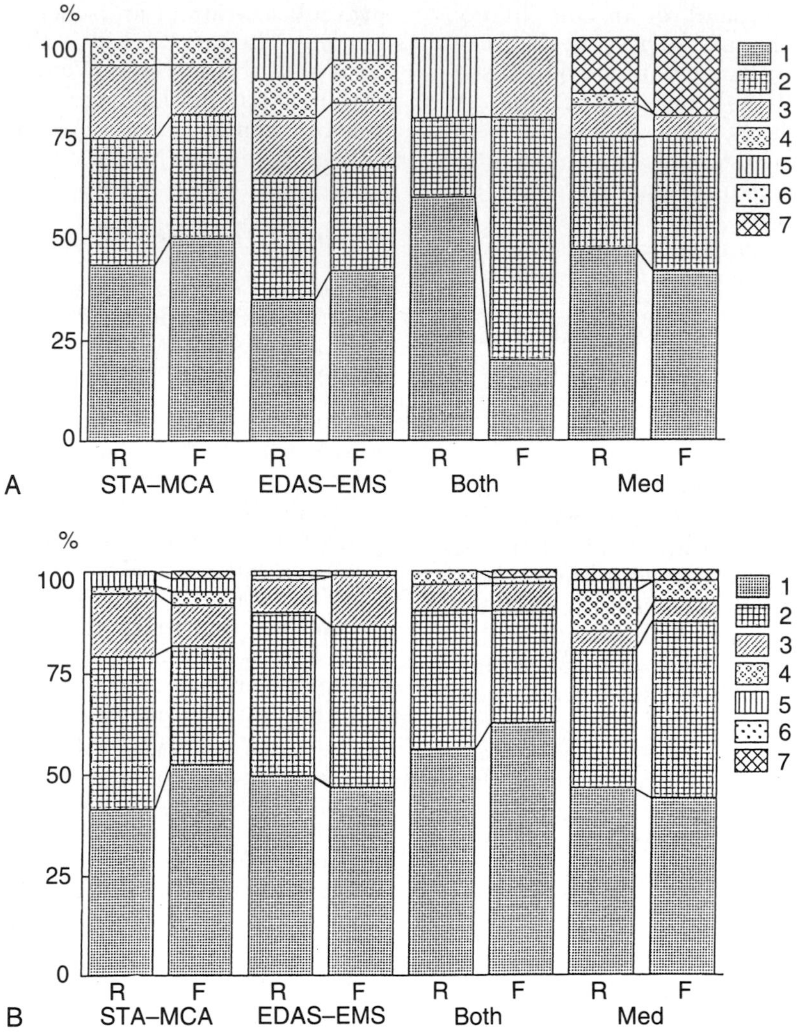


**Fig. 26-11.** Changes of activities of daily living (ADL) of (**A**) hemorrhagic and (**B**) ischemic types of moyamoya disease during follow-up periods. Upper figure means changes of ADL in hemorrhagic type and lower one, in ishemic type. (*1*) ADL in good health; (*2*) ADL in almost full independence; (*3*) ADL in independent though minor deficit; (*4*) ADL in partly dependent; (*5*) ADL in completely dependent; (*6*) ADL in vegetative state; (*7*) dead. ADL-R, ADL at the time of registration; ADL-F, ADL at the time of follow-up (4.3 years on average). (Data for Fig. B from Yonekawa et al.[161])

percent to 16 percent of the series surgically treated over a 5-year period) was also confirmed.[162]

Patients with moyamoya disease generally show good prognosis; more than 80 percent of them are in good health (ADL-1) or in a state of independence (ADL-2), irrespective of treatments received. But recent reports are emphasizing that many patients are not well accommodated in social or school life due to lowered IQ, psychological impairment, and/or personality changes.[1,24] Although there are some reports that surgical treatment improves CBF and IQ,[1,54,87] more meticulous and finer assessment is necessary in this matter.

## Perioperative Procedures

### Angiography

Follow-up angiography is usually performed after 2 months. The patency rate in our personal series is over 95 percent (Fig. 26-12). Visualization of cortical middle cerebral arteries was also possible in cases in which EMS alone was performed. Other findings, such as dilatation of deep muscular arteries, dural arteries, and arteriolar or capillary blushes, indirectly indicate the contribution of these vessels as collateral pathways. These "blushes" may originate from vasa vasorum or periadventitial vessels preserved at the

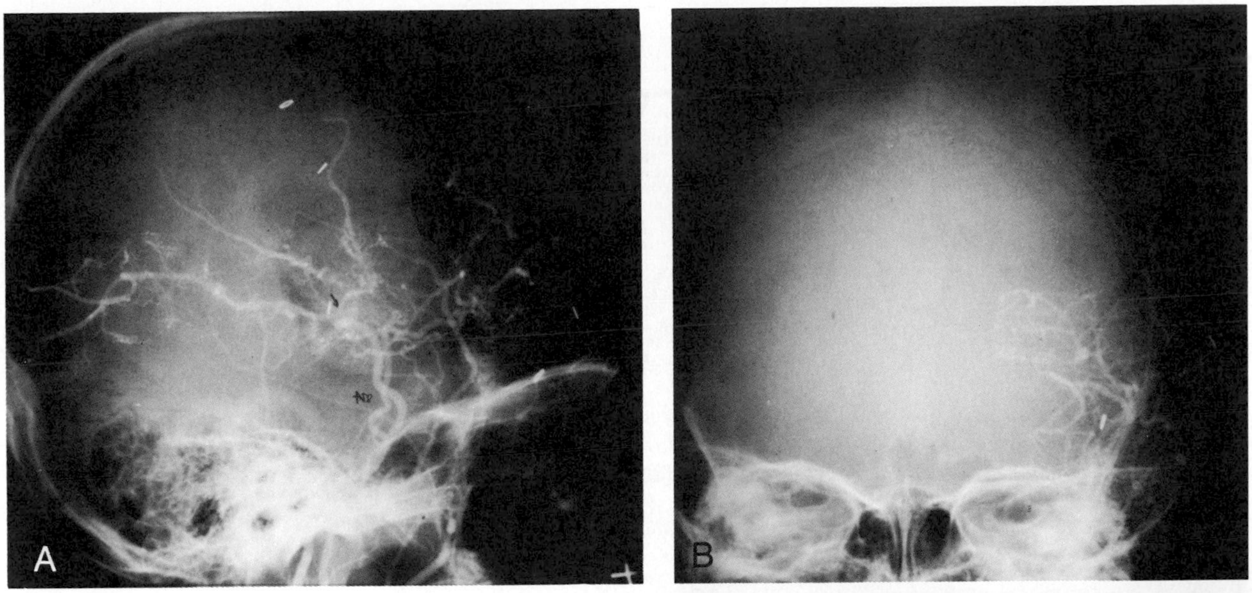


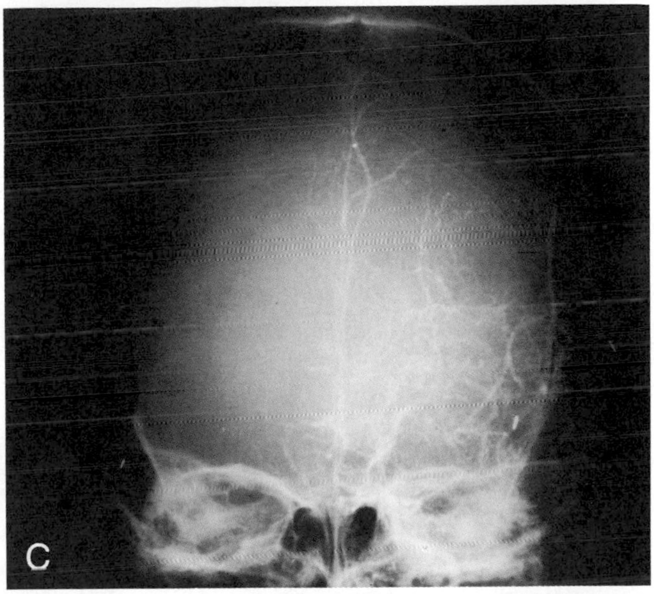


**Fig. 26-12.** Example of postoperative angiography with patent double bypass (Case NM). (**A**) LECAG (lateral). (**B**) LECAG (AP). (**C**) LICAG (AP).

time of STA dissection. In contrast to the postoperative angiographic findings of occlusive atherosclerotic disease, visualization of the entire territory of the middle cerebral artery through STA-MCA bypass is a rather infrequent finding in advanced moyamoya disease. In a few cases, the flow pattern within the territory of the middle cerebral artery changed remarkably postoperatively. Figure 26-13 indicates a case in our earlier series in which the posterior part of the middle cerebral artery was clearly visualized through the bypass, while the anterior part, which had been opacified by the preoperative internal carotid angiography, was visualized neither via the bypass nor via the internal carotid artery. Postoperative CT scan revealed a new LDA accordingly associated with temporary deterioration of neurologic deficits (Fig. 26-14). This is why we are performing the double bypass, so that various territories of the MCA can be irrigated by the newly constructed collaterals. Frequent reduction of moyamoya after the revascularization procedure has been reported by Karasawa et al.[62] Cases with such marked reduction of moyamoya in a few months seems to be limited.

## Regional Cerebral Blood Flow Measurement

Hemodynamic assessment of moyamoya disease has been reported with various methods, including SPECT, dynamic scintigraphy, and argon-CBF measurement.[60,61,80,81,83,103,142]

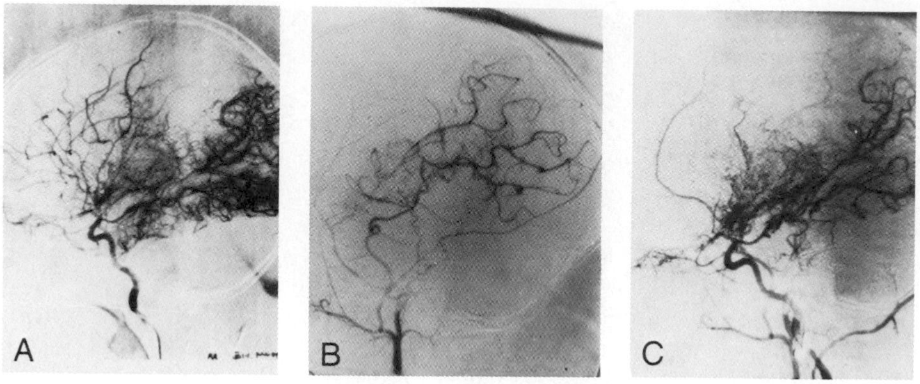


**Fig. 26-13.** Example of postoperative change of blood flow distribution (Case NT). (**A**) Preoperative ICAG. (**B**) Postoperative ECAG. (**C**) Postoperative ICAG.

Note nonvisualization of the anterior part of middle cerebral artery postoperatively neither from the ECAG nor from the ICAG.

Two-dimensional data of rCBF ($^{133}$Xe inhalation method) in moyamoya disease were also reported:[7,160]

1. Preoperative decreased rCBF on the symptomatic side
2. Increased rCBF on the operated side
3. Improved rCBF distribution on the operated side
4. Decreased $CO_2$ response or even paradoxical response.

These were tendencies and were without statistical significance.

Using stable Xe-enhanced CT and acetazolamide, the rCBF of 12 juvenile cases was examined pre- and postoperatively (Fig. 26-15). Surgical revascularization enhanced rCBF mainly in the vicinity of the operative field. Before the operation, reactivity to acetazolamide was decreased in almost all regions of interest (ROI). Bypass flow contributed to the improvement of the reactivity to acetazolamide, perhaps by reducing the state of preoperative vasodilatation.[33] rCBF patterns or distributions peculiar to this disease were normalized and equalized by the operation. These postoperative changes were more remarkable in juvenile cases and less so in adult cases.[103,104]

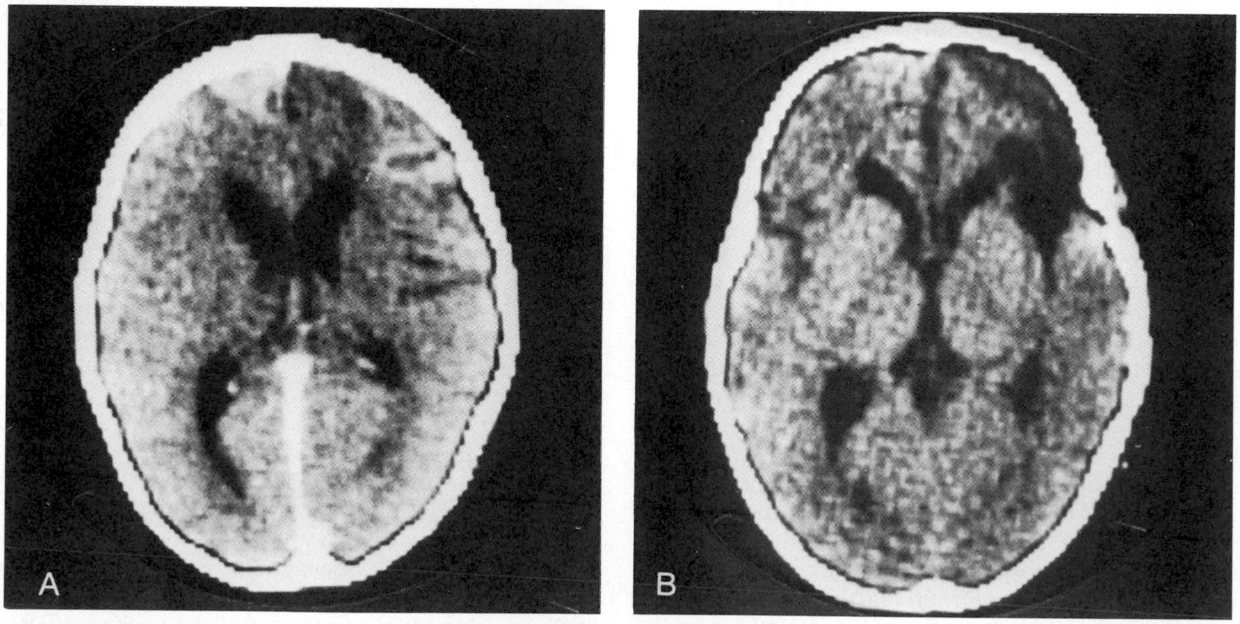


**Fig. 26-14.** Newly developed postoperative low-density area in the same case (Case NT). (**A**) Preoperative computed tomography scan. (**B**) Postoperative computed tomography scan.

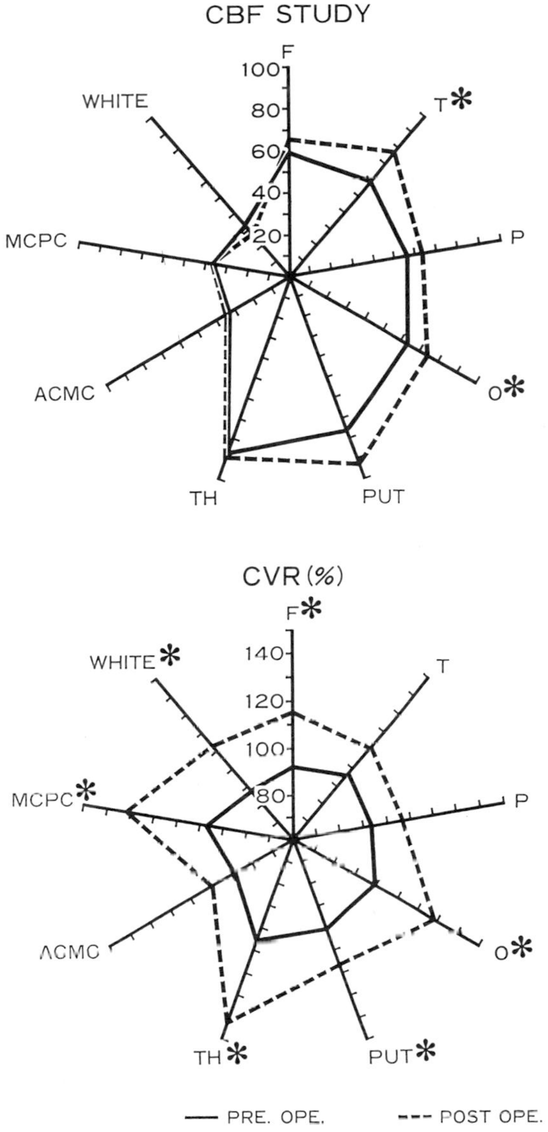


**Fig. 26-15.** Regional cerebral blood flow (rCBF, ml/100 g · min) and reactivity to acetazolamide (cerebrovascular reactivity, CVR,%) before and after operation in juvenile type moyamoya disease. (*), statistical significance ($P < 0.05$). (From Gotoh et al., with permission.[33])

## Doppler Sonography

The flow pattern of the internal carotid artery in branches of the external carotid artery has already frequently been observed in moyamoya disease preoperatively, and it correlated well with the angiographic findings of transdural anastomoses. Postoperative patency of the STA-MCA bypass by Doppler sonography has been assessed from the following findings:[96]

1. Marked increase of the blood flow of the STA as the donor artery in comparison with preoperative findings.
2. Marked difference in the flow volume, compared with the unoperated side.
3. A flow pattern change of the STA to that of the internal carotid artery.

These changes could be observed more or less in accordance with angiographic patency. Remarkable improvement of blood flow through the STA could be observed only in half our series with angiographically confirmed patency. This is in good contrast with constant marked postoperative increase of the STA flow in atherosclerotic occlusions.

Intraoperative Doppler sonography revealed absent or weak flow signals in cortical arteries in almost half our cases, indicating decreased cortical flow.

Transcranial Doppler sonography revealed increased flow velocity in the ophthalmic artery and in the basilar artery, while decreased velocity in the middle cerebral artery indicated its usefulness as a screening and follow-up measure of the disease.[21]

## Intra-arterial Pressure Measurement

The method of intra-arterial pressure (IAP) measurement was reported elsewhere.[164] This value is considered to reflect cortical flow and the capacity of the collateral circulation. IAP in moyamoya disease was far lower than in the usual cerebrovascular occlusive lesion of atherosclerotic origin, and may be below the theoretical opening pressure of 10 mmHg. Again, these findings indicate decreased cortical flow in moyamoya disease.

## Computed Tomography Scanning

The postoperative appearance of a new LDA has been noticed in five cases in our early series, as mentioned above. In the four juvenile cases, one is due to malignant hyperthermia, three revealed one watershed zone infarction and two wedge-shaped infarctions in the frontal region, in spite of patent bypasses. The latter two LDAs seem to have resulted either from change of blood flow distribution following bypass construction or from temporary occlusion of the cortical artery during the anastomotic procedure.

# CONCLUSION

Moyamoya disease has been discovered relatively recently in Japan. At first, it was believed to be confined to Japan, but was later acknowledged to occur all over the world. The etiology is still unknown. The angiographic findings are characteristic, classically revealing symmetrical stenosis or occlusion of both carotid forks, which are associated with an abnormal vascular network, called moyamoya, in the basal ganglia. In the juvenile type, cerebral ischemia is the typical clinical presentation, while cerebral hemorrhage predominates in the adult type. One-third of the cases have been reported to show progressive deterioration. Although no definite effective treatment has been found hitherto, surgical therapy to augment collateral circulation seems to be promising as treatment for relapse of ischemia and hemorrhage. However, complications have been occasionally encountered in the surgical series of the juvenile type. From the viewpoint of the cerebral hemodynamics peculiar to this disease, we have proposed several measures to prevent ischemic complications.

# ACKNOWLEDGMENTS

The authors express their gratitude to Professor H. Handa for his thoughtful suggestion for the clinical investigation of the disease.

The authors are deeply indebted to Dr. J.P. Mohr for correcting and editing the manuscript.

# REFERENCES

1. Abe H, Kamiyama H, Takigawa S et al: Intellectual development of children with moyamoya disease. p. 126. In Yonekawa Y (ed): Annual Report (1989) by Research Committee on Spontaneous Occlusion of the Circle of Willis. Ministry of Health and Welfare, Japan, 1990
2. Abe H, Matsuzawa H, Kamiyama H et al: Magnetic Resonance Angiography in Moyamoya Disease. p. 102. In Yonekawa Y (ed): Annual Report (1989) by Research Committee on Spontaneous Occlusion of the Circle of Willis. Ministry of Health and Welfare, Japan, 1990
3. Adams HP, Jr, Kassell NF, Wisoff HS et al: Intracranial saccular aneurysm and moyamoya disease. Stroke 10:174, 1979
4. Adelman LS, Doe FD, Sarnat HB: Bilateral dissecting aneurysms of the internal carotid arteries. Acta Neuropathol (Berl) 29:93, 1974
5. Asari S, Satoh T, Sakurai M et al: Biplane computed cerebral angiotomography of moyamoya disease. Brain Nerve (Tokyo) 33:1201, 1981
6. Austin JH, Sters JC: Familial hypoplasia of both internal carotid arteries. Arch Neurol 24:1, 1971
7. Baba H, Moriyama T, Ono H et al: A study of regional cerebral blood flow by intravenous injection method of xenon-133. Neurol Surg (Tokyo) 7:1061, 1979
8. Bruno A et al: Cerebral infarction due to moyamoya disease in young adults. Stroke 19:826, 1988
9. Carlson CB, Harvey FH, Loop J: Progressive alternating hemiplegia in early childhood with basal arterial stenosis and telangiectasia (moyamoya syndrome). Neurology (Minneapolis) 23:734, 1973
10. Chen ST et al: Moyamoya disease in Taiwan. Stroke 19:53, 1988
11. Cheng MK: A review of cerebrovascular surgery in the People's Republic of China. Stroke 13:249, 1982
12. Choi KS: Moyamoya disease in Korea—a cooperative study. p. 107. In Suzuki J (ed): Advances in Surgery for Cerebral Stroke. Springer-Verlag, Tokyo, 1988
13. Coakham HB, Duchen LW, Scaravilli F: Moyamoya disease: clinical and pathological report of a case with associated myopathy. J Neurol Neurosurg Psychiatry 42:289, 1979
14. Cohen N, Berant M, Simon J: Moyamoya and Fanconi's anemia. Pediatrics 65:804, 1980
15. Debrun G, Sauvergrain J, Aicardi J et al: Moyamoya, a nonspecific radiological syndrome. Neuroradiology 8:242, 1975
16. Ellison PH, Largent JA, Popp AJ: Moyamoya disease associated with renal artery stenosis. Arch Neurol (Chicago) 38:467, 1981
17. Erickson RP, Wooliscroft J, Allen RJ: Familial occurrence of intracranial arterial occlusive dis-

ease (Moyamoya) in neurofibromatosis. Clin Genet 18:191, 1980
18. Fernandes-Alvares E, Pineda M, Royo C et al: Moyamoya disease caused by cranial trauma. Brain Dev 1:133, 1979
19. Fujisawa I, Asato R, Nishimura K et al: Moyamoya disease: MR imaging. Radiology 164:103, 1987
20. Fujiwara S, Kodama N, Sakurai Y, Hori S: CT scan in moyamoya disease of children. Brain Dev (Tokyo) 10:446, 1978
21. Fukuyama Y, Mitsuishi Y, Umezu R: Intellectual prognosis of children with TIA type of spontaneous occlusion of the circle of Willis: with special reference to Wechsler's intelligence test and Benton's visual aretention test. p. 43. In Handa H (ed): Annual Report (1986) of Research Committee on Spontaneous Occlusion of the Circle of Willis. Ministry of Health and Welfare, Japan, 1987
22. Fukuyama Y, Sugahara N, Osawa M: A genetic study of idopathic spontaneous multiple occlusion of the circle of Willis. p. 139. In Yonekawa Y (ed): Annual Report (1990) by Research Committee on Spontaneous Occlusion of the Circle of Willis. Ministry of Health and Welfare, Japan, 1991
23. Fukuyama Y, Umezu R, Mitsuishi Y et al: Evaluation of idiopathic occlusion of the circle of Willis with transcranial Doppler sonography. p. 55. In Handa H (ed): Annual Report (1987) of the Research Committee on Spontaneous Occlusion of the Circle of Willis. Ministry of Health and Welfare, Japan, 1988
24. Fukuyama Y, Utsumi H, Umezu R: Intellectual prognosis of children with TIA type of spontaneous occlusion of the circle of Willis: special emphasis on IQ and soft neurological signs. p. 29. In Handa H (ed): Annual Report (1985) by Research Committee on Spontaneous Occlusion of the Circle of Willis: Ministry of Health and Welfare, Japan, 1986
25. Funk K, Kurakawa T, Nishimura M et al: A case of cerebral arterial occlusion with retinitis pigmentosa. Neuropediatrics 13:158, 1982
26. Furuse S, Matsumoto S, Tanaka Y et al: Moyamoya disease associated with a false aneurysm. Neurol Surg (Tokyo) 10:1005, 1982
27. Galligioni F, Andrioli GC et al: Hypoplasia of the internal carotid artery associated with cerebral pseudoangiomatosis: report of 4 cases. Am J Roentgenol 112:251, 1971
28. Gold AP, Carter S: Acute hemiplegia of infancy and childhood. Pediatr Clin North Am 23:413, 1976
29. Goldberg HJ: Moyamoya associated with peripheral vascular occlusive disease. Arch Dis Child 49:964, 1974
30. Goldsmith HS, De Los Santos R, Beattie EJ, Jr: Relief of chronic lymphedema by omental transposition. Ann Surg 196:572, 1967
31. Gotoh F: Annual Report (1982) of the Research Committee on Spontaneous Occlusion of the Circle of Willis (Moyamoya Disease). Ministry of Health and Welfare, Japan, 1983
32. Gotoh F, Fukuchi Y, Shinohara T et al: Comparison of local cerebral blood flow and $CO_2$ responsiveness between patients with moyamoya disease and those with atherosclerotic occlusion of the major cerebral arterial trunk. p. 70. In Yonekawa Y (ed): Annual Report (1989) of the Research Committee on Spontaneous Occlusion of the Circle of Willis (Moyamoya Disease). Ministry of Health and Welfare, Japan, 1990
33. Gotoh Y, Yonekawa Y, Tanaka K: Determination of CBF and Diamox reactivity by stable Xe-CT before and after operation: special reference to ischemic type of childhood moyamoya disease. p. 76. In Yonekawa Y (ed): Annual Report (1990) by Research Committee on Spontaneous Occlusion of the Circle of Willis. Ministry of Health and Welfare, Japan, 1991
34. Halonen H, Halonen V et al: Occlusive disease of intracranial main arteries with collateral networks in children. Neuropädiatrie 4:187, 1973
35. Hanakita J, Kondo A, Ishikawa J et al: An Autopsy case of moyamoya disease. Neurol Surg 1982: 10:531, 1982
36. Handa H, Tani K, Kajikawa H et al: Clinicopathological study on an adult case with cerebral arterial rete. Brain Nerve (Tokyo) 21:181, 1969
37. Handa H, Yonekawa Y, Goto Y et al: Analysis of the filing data bank of 1500 cases of spontaneous occlusion of the circle of Willis and follow-up study of 200 cases for more than 5 years. p. 14. In Handa H (ed): Annual Report (1984) by Research Committee on Spontaneous Occlusion of the Circle of Willis, Ministry of Health and Welfare, Japan, 1985
38. Handa H, Yonekawa Y, Suda K et al: Postoperative appearance of newly developed LDA on CT scan. Research on the immune complex. p. 124. In Gotoh F (ed): Annual report of the research committee on spontaneous occlusion of the circle of Willis. Ministry of Health and Welfare, Japan, 1981
39. Handa J, Handa H: Progressive cerebral arterial occlusive disease: analysis of 27 cases. Neuroradiology 3:119, 1974
40. Handa J, Handa H, Nakano Y, Okuno T: Computed tomography in moyamoya: analysis of 16 cases. Comput Tomogr 1:165, 1977
41. Handa J, Nakano Y, Okukno T et al: Computerized tomography in moyamoya syndrome. Surg Neurol 7:315, 1977
42. Handa J, Waga S, Handa H: Dural-cortical arterial anastomosis as a collateral channel in carotid occlusive disease. Clin Radiol 22:302, 1971
43. Harwood-Nash DC, Fita CR: Neuroradiology in Infants and Children. p. 948. CV Mosby, St Louis, 1976
44. Harwood-Nash DC, McDonald P, Argent W: Cerebral arterial disease in children. Am J Roentgenol 3:672, 1971
45. Hately W, Shapiro R: Carotid rete mirabile: an unusual example associated with diffuse bilateral cerebral telangiectasia. Clin Radiol 20:32, 1969
46. Hell K, Bachmann B, Erne P et al: Perforation of

the small intestine in systemic disease. Helv Chir Acta 43:569, 1976

47. Henschen C: Operative Revascularization des zirkulatorisch geschädigten Gehirns durch Auflage gestielten Muskellappen (Encephalo-myo-synangiose). Langerbecks Arch Klin Chir 264:392, 1950
48. Hirayama A, Kowada M, Fukasawa H et al: Cerebrovascular moyamoya disease: a case report and review of 12 autopsy cases in Japan. Brain Nerve (Tokyo) 26:1215, 1974
49. Hosoda Y: A pathomorphological analysis of so-called "spontaneous occlusion of the circle of Willis" (cerebrovascular moyamoya disease). Brain Nerve (Tokyo) 26:471, 1974
50. Hosoda Y: A pathological study of so-called "spontaneous occlusion of the circle of Willis" (cerebrovascular moyamoya disease). Folia Angiol 24:85, 1976
51. Hosoda Y, Ikeda E: Extracranial Vascular changes in spontaneous occlusion of the circle of Willis. p. 179. In Yonekawa Y (ed): Annual Report (1990) by Research Committee on Spontaneous Occlusion of the Circle of Willis. Ministry of Health and Welfare, Japan, 1991
52. Imaizumi M, Nukada T, Yoneda S et al: Tuberous sclerosis with moyamoya disease: case report. Med J Osaka Univ 28:345, 1978
53. Iraci G, Martin G et al: Further observations on the so-called "Japanese cerebrovascular disease." Ann J Roentogenol 115:35, 1972
54. Ishii R, Takeuchi S, Ibayashi K, Tanaka R: Intelligence in children with moyamoya disease: evaluation after surgical treatments with special reference to changes in blood flow. Stroke 15:873, 1984
55. Izawa M, Beppu T, Kitamura K: Three cases of moyamoya disease in childhood complicated with other disorders. J Tokyo Wom Med Coll 46:505, 1976
56. Kaneko H, Okamura A, Nishida K et al: An autopsy case of intracranial rete mirabile. Brain Nerve (Tokyo) 23:1381, 1971
57. Karasawa J, Kikuchi H, Furuse S: A surgical treatment of moyamoya disease Encephalomyosynangiosis. Neurol Med Chir (Tokyo) 17:29, 1977
58. Karasawa J, Kikuchi H, Furuse S: Subependymal hematoma in moyamoya disease. Surg Neurol 13:118, 1980
59. Karasawa J, Kikuchi H, Kawamura J et al: Intracranial transplantation of the omentum for cerebrovascular Moyamoya disease. a two-year follow-up study. Surg Neurol 14:444, 1980
60. Karasawa J, Kikuchi H, Kuriyama Y et al: Cerebral hemodynamics in moyamoya disease. I. Dynamic brain scintigraphy before and after bypass surgery. Neurol Med Chir (Tokyo) 21:923, 1981
61. Karasawa J, Kikuchi H, Kuriyama Y et al: Cerebral hemodynamics in moyamoya disease. II. Measurement of cerebral circulation and metabolism by use of the argon desaturation method in pre- and postneurosurgical procedures. Neurol Med Chir 21:1161, 1981
62. Karasawa J, Kikuchi H, Furuse S et al: Treatment of moyamoya disease with STA-MCA anastomosis. J Neurosurg 49:679, 1978
63. Kasai N, Fujiwara S, Kodama N et al: The experimental study on causal genesis of moyamoya disease: correlation with immunological reaction and sympathetic nerve influence for vascular changes. Neurol Surg (Tokyo) 10:251, 1982
64. Kitahara T, Ariga N, Yamaura A et al: Familial occurrence of moyamoya disease: report of three Japanese families. J Neurol Neurosurg Psychiatry 42:208, 1979
65. Kitahara T, Okumura K, Semba T et al: Genetic and immunologic analysis of moyamoya disease. J Neurol Neurosurg Psychiatry 45:1048, 1982
66. Kodama N, Aoki Y, Hiraga H et al: Electroencephalographic findings in children with moyamoya disease. Arch Neurol (Chicago) 36:16, 1979
67. Kodama N, Fujiwara S, Horie Y et al: Transdural anastomosis in moyamoya disease: vault moyamoya. Neurol Surg (Tokyo) 8:729, 1980
68. Kodama N, Suzuki J: Moyamoya disease associated with aneurysm. J Neurosurg 48:55, 1978
69. Koo AH, Newton TH: Pseudoxanthoma elasticum associated with carotid rete mirabila: case report. Am J Roentgenol 116:16, 1972
70. Kramer HH, Karsch D, Seibert H: Moyamoya-like vascular disease in tuberous sclerosis. Monatsschr Kinderheilkd 129:595, 1981
71. Krayenbuhl HA: The moyamoya syndrome and the neurosurgeon. Surg Neurol 4:353, 1975
72. Kudo T: Occlusion of the internal carotid artery and the type of recovery of cerebral blood circulation. Clin Neurol (Tokyo) 1:199, 1960
73. Kudo T: General aspects. p. 1. In Kudo T (ed): A Disease with Abnormal Intracranial Vascular Networks. Spontaneous occlusion of the circle of Willis (in Japanese). Igaku Shoin, Tokyo, 1967
74. Kudo T: Spontaneous occlusion of the circle of Willis: a disease apparently confined to Japanese. Neurology (NY) 18:485, 1968
75. Lamas E, Diez Lobato R, Cabello A et al: Multiple intracranial arterial occlusions (Moyamoya disease) in patients with neurofibromatosis: one case report with autopsy. Acta Neurochir 45:133, 1978
76. Lee KF, Hodes PHJ: Intracranial ischemic lesions. Radiol Clin North Am 5:363, 1967
77. Lee KLK, Cheung EMT: Moyamoya disease as a cause of subarachnoid hemorrhage in Chinese. Brain 96:623, 1973
78. Leed NK, Abbott KH: Collateral circulation in cerebrovascular occlusive disease in childhood via rete mirabile and perforating branches of anterior chorioidal and posterior cerebral arteries. Radiology 85:628, 1965
79. Mabuchi A, Tanabe H, Fujikawa Y et al: An autopsy case of the abnormal network of the intracranial artery: congenital dysplasia of the cerebral artery. Brain Nerve (Tokyo) 25:1759, 1973
80. Maeda T, Matsuda H, Tonami N et al: Regional cerebral blood flow image by the method of single photon emission computed tomography:

continuous carotid injection of krypton-81m. Jpn J Nucl Med (Tokyo) 17:829, 1980
81. Maeda T, Mori H, Hisada K et al: Radionuclide cerebral angiography in moyamoya disease. Clin Nucl Med 4:513, 1979
82. Maki Y, Nakata Y: Autopsy of a case with an anomalous hemangioma of the internal carotid artery at the skull base. Brain Nerve (Tokyo) 17:764, 1965
83. Maki Y, Nakata Y et al: Clinical and radioisotopic follow-up study moyamoya. Childs Brain 2:257, 1976
84. Maki Y, Nose T, Tanoue K et al: Platelet aggregation in patients with moyamoya disease. Angiology 32:522, 1981
85. Matsushima Y, Fukai N, Tanaka K et al: A new surgical treatment of moyamoya disease in children: a preliminary report. Surg Neurol 15:313, 1981
86. Matsushima Y, Inaba Y: Moyamoya disease in children and its surgical treatment. Childs Brain 11:155, 1984
87. Matsushima Y, Tomita H, Takei H et al: Changes in Symptoms after Encephalo-duro-arterio-synangiosis (EDAS) in Pediatric Moyamoya Disease. p. 578. Cerebral Revascularization for Stroke. Thieme-Stratton, New York, 1985
88. Mauro AJ, Johnson ES, Chikos PM et al: Lipohyalinosis and miliary microaneurysms causing hemorrhage in a patient with moyamoya disease: a clinicopathological study. Stroke 11:405, 1980
89. Meriwether RP, Barnett HJM, Echolos DH: Moyamoya disease as a cause of subarachnoid hemorrhage in a Negro patient. J Neurosurg 44:620, 1976
90. Merkel KHH, Ginsberg PL, Parker JC, Jr et al: Cerebrovascular disease in sickle cell anemia: a clinical, pathological and radiological correlation. Stroke 9:45, 1978
91. Miyasaka K, Takei H, Nakagawa Y et al: A disease showing moyamoya vascular networks in base of brain: evaluation of angiography and cranial computed tomography. Brain Nerve (Tokyo) 30:1083, 1978
92. Miyazaki M, Takeshiro A, Sugawa M et al: Aortitis syndrome associated with so-called intracranial moyamoya phenomenon: case report. Neurol Med (Tokyo) 12:53, 1980
93. Mizukawa N, Iwatsuki K: A case of cerebral basal rete mirabile combined with brain tumor. Clin Neurol (Tokyo) 13:650, 1973
94. Mori K, Miyazaki H, Yasunaga A et al: A case of moyamoya syndrome with subdural and intracerebral hematoma due to different bleeding sources. Acta Med Nagasaki 24:48, 1979
95. Mori K, Takeuchi J, Ishikawa M et al: Occlusive arteriopathy and brain tumor. J Neurosurg 49:22, 1978
96. Moritake K, Handa H, Yonekawa Y et al: Ultrasonic Doppler assessment of hemodynamics in superficial temporal artery-middle cerebral artery anastomosis. Surg Neurol 13:249, 1980
97. Moritake K, Handa H, Yonekawa Y, Taki W, Okuno T: Follow-up study on the relationship between age at onset of illness and outcome in patients with "moyamoya disease." Neurol Surg 14:957, 1986
98. Mountz JM, Foster NL, Ackermann RJ et al: SPECT imaging of moyamoya disease using $^{99m}$Tc-HM PAO. J Comput Tomog 12:247, 1988
99. Nagamine Y, Takahashi S, Sonobe M: Multiple intracranial aneurysms associated with moyamoya disease: case report. J Neurosurg 54:673, 1981
100. Nagata I, Kikuchi H, Miyamoto S: Additional reconstructive surgery in the patients of moyamoya disease pretreated with unsuccessful encephaloduroarterio-synangiosis (EDAS). p. 95. In Handa H (ed): Annual Report (1987) by Research Committee on Spontaneous Occlusion of the Circle of Willis. Ministry of Health and Welfare, Japan, 1988
101. Nakagawara K, Fujishima M, Numaguchi Y et al: Thalamic hemorrhage in moyamoya disease: a case report. Angiology 30:856, 1979
102. Narumi S, Nishimura K, Fuchizawa K et al: Three cases of the moyamoya disease found in an inbred family. Brain Nerve (Tokyo) 28:1201, 1976
103. Nishikawa M, Handa H: Effect of surgical revascularization on cerebral blood flow in patients with moyamoya disease: second report. p. 94. In Yonekawa Y (ed): Annual Report (1989) by Research Committee on Spontaneous Occlusion of the Circle of Willis. Ministry of Health and Welfare, Japan, 1990
104. Nishimoto A, Niimi H, Kinugasa K et al: Comparison between medical treatment and surgical treatment for "moyamoya" disease: antiplatelet therapy and vascular reconstructive surgery. p. 111. In Handa H (ed): Annual Report (1987) by Research Committee on Spontaneous Occlusion of the Circle of Willis. Ministry of Health and Welfare, Japan, 1988
105. Nishimoto A, Takeuchi S: Abnormal cerebrovascular network related to the internal carotid arteries. J Neurosurg 29:255, 1968
106. Numaguchi Y, Balsys R, Marc JA et al: Some observations in progressive arterial occlusions in children and young adolescents (Moyamoya disease). Surg Neurol 6:283, 1976
107. Ogawa Y, Hosoda Y, Matsuyama H: An autopsy case of occlusion of the circle of Willis in a child. Brain Nerve (Tokyo) 26:483, 1974
108. Ohashi T, Ueda K, Mizukawa N et al: Autopsy cases of moyamoya disease. Brain Nerve (Tokyo) 27:1017, 1975
109. Ohno K, Fujimoto T, Komatsu K et al: Spontaneous successive occlusion of the circle of Willis with the growth of abnormal vascular networks at the base of brain: in relation to the pathogenesis of so-called moyamoya disease. Brain Nerve (Tokyo) 29:37, 1971
110. Oka K, Yamashita M, Sadoshima S et al: Cerebral hemorrhage in moyamoya disease at autopsy. Virchows Arch 392:247, 1981
111. Okamoto J, Mukai K, Kashihara M et al: A case of atypical moyamoya vessel. Neurol Surg (Tokyo) 10:897, 1982

112. Okuma A, Oshita H, Funakoshi T et al: A case of aneurysm in the cerebral moyamoya vessel: aneurysmal rupture during cerebral angiography and spontaneous regression of the aneurysm. Neurol Surg (Tokyo) 8:181, 1980
113. Okuno T, Hojyo H, Nakano Y et al: Clinical analysis and computed tomography of cerebrovascular Moyamoya disease in childhood. Ann Paediatr Jpn (Tokyo) 7:175, 1977
114. Olds MV et al: The surgical treatment of childhood moyamoya disease. J Neurosurg 66:675, 1987
115. Peh WC et al: Moyamoya disease in Singapore. Ann Acad Med Singapore 14:71, 1985
116. Picard L, Levesque M, Crouzet G et al: The moyamoya syndrome. J Neuroradiol 1:47, 1974
117. Pilz P, Hartjes HJ: Fibromuscular dysplasia and multiple dissecting aneurysms of intracranial arteries: a further cause of moyamoya syndrome. Stroke 7:393, 1976
118. Poblete R: Moyamoya disease in South Africa. p. 129. Advances in Surgery for Cerebral Stroke. In Suzuki J (ed): Springer-Verlag, Tokyo, 1988
119. Poor GY, Gacs GY: The so-called moyamoya disease. J Neurol Neurosurg Psychiatry 37:370, 1974
120. Prensky AL, Davis DO: Obstruction of major cerebral vessels in early childhood without neurological signs. Neurology (NY) 20:945, 1970
121. Rajakulasingam K, Cerullo LJ, Raimondi AJ: Childhood moyamoya syndrome: postradiation pathogenesis. Childs Brain 5:469, 1979
122. Reichmann Ott, Anderson RE, Roberts TC et al: The treatment of intracranial occlusive cerebrovascular disease by STA-cortical MCA anastomosis. p. 31. In Handa H (ed): Microneurosurgery. Igaku Shoin, Tokyo, 1975
123. Rosengreen K: Moyamoya vessels collateral arteries of the basal ganglia: malignant occlusion of the anterior cerebral arteries. Acta Radiol Diagn 15:145, 1974
124. Schrager GO, Cohen SJ, Vigman MP: Acute hemiplegia and cortical blindness due to moyamoya disease: report of a case in a child with Down's syndrome. Pediatrics 60:33, 1977
125. Seeler RA, Royal JE, Powe L et al: Moyamoya in children with sickle cell anemia and cerebrovascular occlusion. J Pediatr 93:808, 1978
126. Sekiguchi S, Kobayashi K, Hattori M et al: HLA antigen in spontaneous occlusion of the circle of Willis. p. 76. In Gotoh F (ed): Annual Report (1979) of the Research Committee on Spontaneous Occlusion of the Circle of Willis. Ministry of Health and Welfare, Japan, 1979
127. Servo A, Puranen M: Moyamoya syndrome as a complication of radiation therapy: case report. J Neurosurg 48:1026, 1978
128. Sogaard I, Jorgensen J: Familial occurrence of bilateral intracranial occlusion of the internal carotid arteries (moyamoya). Acta Neurochir 31:245, 1975
129. Sonobe M, Takahashi S, Urakawa Y et al: Moyamoya disease found in identical twins. Neurol Surg (Tokyo) 8:1183, 1980
130. Sunder TR: Moyamoya disease in a patient with type I glycogenosis. Arch Neurol (Chicago) 38:251, 1981
131. Suzuki J, Kodama N, Mineura K: Mechanism of symptomatic occurrence in cerebrovascular moyamoya disease. Brain Nerve (Tokyo) 28:459, 1976
132. Suzuki J, Takaku A: Cerebrovascular moyamoya disease: disease showing abnormal net-like vessels in base of brain. Arch Neurol 20:288, 1969
133. Suzuki J, Takaku A, Asahi M: The disease showing the abnormal vascular network at the base of brain, particularly found in Japan. Brain Nerve (Tokyo) 18:897, 1966
134. Suzuki J, Takaku A, Fukasawa H: Cerebrovascular Moyamoya disease among Japanese, on study of an autopsy case. p. 97. In Kudo T (ed): A disease with abnormal intracranial vascular networks. Igaku Shoin, Tokyo, 1967
135. Suzuki J, Takaku A, Kodama N et al: An attempt to treat cerebrovascular moyamoya disease in children. Childs Brain 1:193, 1975
136. Takahashi M: Magnification angiography in moyamoya disease: new observations on collateral vessels. Radiology 136:379, 1980
137. Takahashi M: Magnification angiography of cerebral aneurysms associated with moyamoya disease. Am J Neuroradiol 1:547, 1980
138. Takahashi M, Miyauchi T, Kowada M: Computed tomography of moyamoya disease: demonstration of occluded arteries and collateral vessels as important diagnostic signs. Radiology 134:671, 1980
139. Takahashi M, Saito Y, Konno K: Intraventricular hemorrhage in childhood moyamoya disease. J Comput Assist Tomogr 4:117, 1980
140. Takeuchi K, Hara M, Yokota H et al: Factors influencing the development of moyamoya phenomenon. Acta Neurochir 59:79, 1981
141. Takeuchi K, Shimizu K: Hypoplasia of the bilateral internal carotid arteries. Brain and Nerve (Tokyo) 9:37, 1957
142. Takeuchi S, Tanaka R, Ishii R et al: Cerebral hemodynamics in patients with moyamoya disease. Surg Neurol 23:468, 1985
143. Taki W, Handa H, Yonekawa Y et al: Cerebral blood volume, blood flow and oxygen utilization in moyamoya disease. J Cereb Blood Flow Metab, Suppl. 5:439, 1985
144. Taki W, Yonekawa Y, Kobayashi A et al: Cerebral circulation and oxygen metabolism in moyamoya disease of ischemic type in children. Childs Nerv Syst 4:259, 1988
145. Tanaka K, Oka K, Yamashita M: Intracranial and systemic vascular lesion and intracranial hemorrhage in spontaneous occlusion of the circle of Willis. p. 86. In Gotoh F (ed): Annual Report (1981) of the Research Committee on Spontaneous Occlusion of the Circle of Willis. Ministry of Health and Welfare, Japan, 1981
146. Tatemichi TK, Prohovnik I, Mohr JP et al: Reduced hypercapnic vasoreactivity in moyamoya disease. Neurology (NY) 38:1575, 1988
147. Taveras JM: Multiple progressive intracranial arterial occlusion: a syndrome of children and young adults. Am J Roentgenol 106:235, 1969

148. Uemura K, Yamaguchi K, Kojima S et al: Regional cerebral blood flow on cerebrovascular moyamoya disease. Brain Nerve (Tokyo) 27:385, 1975
149. Urbanek H, Farkova H et al: Nishimoto-Takeuchi-Kudo disease. J Neurol Psychiatry 33:671, 1970
150. Van Damme W, Beeckman P, Verbruggen R: Moyamoya syndrome probably associated with hydrocephalus. Neuroradiology (Berl) 9:39, 1975
151. Weidner W, Hanafee W, Markham C: Intracranial collateral circulation via leptomeningeal and rete mirabile anastomosis. Neurology (Minneapolis) 15:39, 1965
152. Wen HL, Mehal ZD, Kwok JCK, Chan YW, Kay CS: Moyamoya Disease in Hong Kong. In Suzuki J (ed): Advances in Surgery for Cerebral Stroke. Springer-Verlag, Tokyo, 1988
153. Yamada H, Deguchi K, Sakai N et al: Relationship between moyamoya disease and anaerobic bacterium *Propionibacterium acnes* infection. p. 33. In Handa H (ed): Annual Report (1987) by Research Committee on Spontaneous Occlusion of the Circle of Willis. Ministry of Health and Welfare, Japan, 1988
154. Yamada H, Nakamura S, Kageyama N: Moyamoya disease in monovular twins: case report. J Neurosurg 53:109, 1980
155. Yanagawa H: Annual Report by Research Committee on Epidemiology of Intractable Disease, 1991
156. Yasargil MG: Microsurgery Applied to Neurosurgery. Thieme, Stuttgart, 1969
157. Yasargil MG, Smith RD: Association of middle cerebral anomalies with saccular aneurysms and moyamoya disease. Surg Neurol 6:37, 1976
158. Yonekawa Y (ed): Annual Report (1990) by Research Committee on Spontaneous Occlusion of the Circle of Willis. Ministry of Health and Welfare, Japan, 1991
159. Yonekawa Y, Gotoh Y, Yamashita K et al: Determination of cerebral blood flow and volume by stable Xe-CT and dynamic CT in moyamoya disease. p. 87. In Yonekawa Y (ed): Annual Report (1989) of the Research Committee on Spontaneous Occlusion of the Circle of Willis (Moyamoya Disease). Ministry of Health and Welfare, Japan, 1990
160. Yonekawa Y, Handa H, Okuno T: Moyamoya Disease: diagnosis, treatment, and recent achievement. p. 805. In Barnett HJM, Stein BM, Mohr JP, Yatsu FM (eds): Stroke: Pathophysiology, Diagnosis, and Management. 1st Ed. Churchill Livingstone, New York, 1986
161. Yonekawa Y, Kawano T: Follow-up study of 546 cases in spontaneous occlusion of the circle of Willis registered from 1983 to 1989. p. 14. In Yonekawa Y (ed): Annual Report (1989) by Research Committee on Spontaneous Occlusion of the Circle of Willis. Ministry of Health and Welfare, Japan, 1990
162. Yonekawa Y, Kawano T: Follow-up study of 595 cases in spontaneous occlusion of the circle of Willis registered from 1983 to 1990. p. 23. In Yonekawa Y (ed): Annual Report (1990) by Research Committee on Spontaneous Occlusion of the Circle of Willis. Ministry of Health and Welfare, Japan, 1991
163. Yonekawa Y, Yamashita K, Taki W, Kikuchi H: Clinical features of hemorrhagic type of moyamoya disease: Special emphasis on cases with rebleeding. p. 81. In Handa H (ed): Annual Report (1987) by Research Committee on Spontaneous Occlusion of the Circle of Willis. Ministry of Health and Welfare, Japan, 1988
164. Yonekawa Y, Yasargil MG: Arterial extracranial intracranial anastomosis: Technical and clinical aspects. results. p. 47. In Krayenbuhl H (ed): Advances and Technical Standards of Neurosurgery. Vol. 3. Springer, Wien, 1976
165. Yonekawa Y, Yasargil MG: Brain vascularization by transplanted omentum: a possible treatment of cerebral ischemia. Neurosurgery 1:256, 1977
166. Yoshii N, Kudo T: Electroencephalographical study on occlusion of the Willis arterial ring. Clin Neurol (Tokyo) 8:301, 1968
167. Yuasa H, Tokito S, Izumi K et al: Cerebrovascular moyamoya disease associated with an intracranial pseudoaneurysm: case report. J Neurosurg 56:131, 1982

# 27
# CEREBROVASCULAR FIBROMUSCULAR DYSPLASIA

Edward B. Healton

## DEFINITION AND HISTORICAL REVIEW

Fibromuscular dysplasia (FMD) is an uncommon, idiopathic, systemic vascular disease characterized by nonatherosclerotic abnormalities of smooth muscle and fibrous and elastic tissue in small and medium-sized arteries. FMD is multifocal, affecting renal, cephalic, visceral, iliac, femoral, axillary, subclavian, and internal mammary arteries and the aorta.[97,175] There has been only one report of venous involvement.[141] Cephalic vessels are affected in 25 percent of reported cases of FMD, the most common location after the renal arteries.[101] Although FMD may be widespread, one or two arterial territories are usually involved in each patient.

In 1938, Leadbetter and Burkland[95] first described the condition in a 5-year-old hypertensive boy with renal artery stenosis caused by a "smooth muscle plug." Subsequent investigators reported patients with similar renal artery lesions and introduced the terms *fibromuscular hyperplasia*[107] and, later, *fibromuscular dysplasia*[62,89] to describe the proliferative, disruptive arterial changes. In these early reports,[88,124,177] FMD was established as a unique radiologic and pathologic entity and an important, surgically curable cause of hypertension, but it was believed to be confined to the renal artery.

In 1964, Palubinskas and Ripley[123] first reported angiographic and histologic evidence of FMD outside the renal arteries. One of these patients, an apparently asymptomatic woman, had angiographic "changes in the extracranial internal carotid artery indistinguishable from the classical appearance of fibromuscular hyperplasia." FMD was histologically proven in the internal carotid artery 1 year later,[27,72] and subsequently described in the vertebral, external carotid, and intracranial arteries. Angiographic criteria for distinguishing this disease from other extracranial and intracranial arterial abnormalities were also established.[15,75,118,121,122,174]

There was disagreement, however, about the relationship between FMD and neurologic symptoms. Some authors believed that FMD was usually diagnosed coincidentally and caused neurologic abnormalities infrequently. Others attributed focal or generalized neurologic symptoms to FMD and advocated surgical treatment. In 1965, Connett and Lansche[27] first reported surgical resection of internal carotid artery FMD in a patient with cerebral infarction. Graduated intraluminal dilation was introduced 3 years later and has become the most frequently used surgical procedure.[115]

Although there are now over 600 reported cases of cerebrovascular FMD, the etiology, frequency and pathogenesis of clinical symptoms, and the proper management of this disease remain controversial.[2,7,8,10,13,19,23,34,40,50,76,77,87,102,104,111,125,133,165,179]

## EPIDEMIOLOGY

The true incidence of cephalic FMD in the general population is unknown. In 819 consecutive autopsies, FMD of the renal artery occurred in 1.1 percent;[70] a similar study of cerebrovascular FMD has not been reported. In several large retrospective reviews of consecutive angiograms (totaling approximately 22,000 studies),[28,64,118,156,160] FMD was diagnosed in less than 1 percent of cases (range: 0.25 to 0.61 percent). In one other review of 936 cephalic angiograms, the incidence of internal carotid artery FMD was 3.7 percent.[172]

FMD is considerably more common among women, constituting up to 85 percent of those with cerebrovascular FMD. FMD also may be more common among white ethnic groups.[157] Although it has occurred in patients aged 2 to 83 years, cerebrovascular FMD is usually diagnosed in the 4th or 5th decade and rarely occurs in children.[6,39,96,130,153,169]

## ETIOLOGY

Ultrastructural studies of FMD have shown that, independent of histologic type, arterial lesions are identical at the subcellular level and "differ only in their intensity and localization."[21,55] Smooth muscle transformation into fibroblastlike cells (myofibroblasts) and increased collagen synthesis are fundamental processes in the morphogenesis of these lesions. The etiology of this process and the stimulus for smooth muscle differentiation are unknown, but several hypotheses have been proposed. Genetic factors in FMD have been suggested in reports of familial FMD among siblings or identical twins.[59,61,103,114,119] The mode of inheritance was consistent with an autosomal dominant trait with reduced penetrance in males.[54,109,145] In some of these studies, however, relatives with only a history of unexplained hypertension, stroke, or acute myocardial infarction were considered to have FMD. Only a few families with angiographic or histologic confirmation of FMD have been reported.[119] Because of an association between FMD and skeletal deformities or features of Ehlers-Danlos syndrome in a few patients, an hereditary mesenchymal defect has been proposed.[146,147] Because renal angiograms have been normal up to 12 years before diagnosis of renal FMD,[11] a hereditary abnormality must be associated with other factors to account for the delayed expression in some patients.

Because of the predominance of FMD in women and the stimulatory effect of estrogen on smooth muscle cells, hormonal influences are probably important.[81,142,143,159] Ischemia of the arterial wall also may cause dysplastic abnormalities in humans.[127] Lesions very similar to human FMD have been produced in dogs by experimental occlusions of the vasa vasorum,[116,158] and the renal and internal carotid arteries receive fewer of these nutrient branches than other muscular arteries of similar caliber. Vascular lesions resembling FMD have also been reported in ergotism.[41,42,128]

Because there are vessel wall abnormalities associated with the rubella syndrome, and a disease similar to FMD occurs in domestic turkeys,[82] a viral etiology has been proposed. Stretch-traction stresses on the arterial wall have also been considered, but not uniformly supported by[30,98] experimental evidence.[144]

FMD may have several different etiologies, each acting on vulnerable areas of the arterial wall in hereditarily predisposed individuals when there is an hormonally conducive environment.

## PATHOLOGY AND ANATOMIC DISTRIBUTION OF LESIONS

The pathology of FMD is characterized by smooth muscle hyperplasia or thinning, elastic fiber destruction, fibrous tissue proliferation, and arterial wall disorganization.[62,63,161] Inflammation, necrosis, lipid accumulation, and calcification are absent. Although there is not complete agreement about terminology, FMD can be classified into three histologic types based on the arterial layer in which lesions predominate.[63,161] Medial FMD occurs in 90 to 95 percent of cases, much more commonly in women. Concentric rings of fibrous proliferation or smooth muscle hyperplasia cause medial thickening and destruction of the internal or external elastic lamina. These fibromuscular ridges can occur singly, extend for a variable length along the artery, or alternate sequentially with areas of medial thinning and arterial dilatation. Based on location within the media and the predominant histologic abnormality, medial FMD has been subdivided into medial or perimedial fibroplasia and medial hyperplasia.[68]

Intimal fibroplasia is present in approximately 5 percent of cases and occurs equally between men and women.[166] Fibrous tissue proliferation causes intimal thickening and destruction of the internal elastic lamina. In periarterial (adventitial) fibroplasia, the least common histologic type, there is fibrosis of the adventitia and surrounding periarterial tissue.

The internal carotid artery is affected in approximately 95 percent of patients with cephalic FMD, and is bilateral in 60 to 85 percent of affected individuals.[25,47,101,118,156] The abnormalities characteristically occur in the midportion of the artery, opposite the second cervical vertebra, and they extend 0.5 to 7 cm proximally or distally, usually sparing the proximal 2.5 cm. Only 17 patients have been reported with proximal internal carotid artery disease,[113] and FMD of the common carotid artery has been reported in three patients.[173] FMD has occasionally involved the intraosseous carotid artery, either alone or as an extension of cervical abnormalities.[156,173,180] External carotid artery FMD has also been reported.[24,43]

The incidence of vertebral artery FMD is uncertain because complete angiography has not always been performed in patients with cephalic FMD. For this reason, the reported incidence of vertebral artery FMD has varied from 12 to 43 percent of affected patients, usually in association with internal carotid artery disease.[76,110] Vertebral artery FMD is also commonly located opposite the second cervical vertebra and may extend for 1 to 2 cm. There are no reports of FMD at the origin of the vertebral artery.

Intracranial FMD is uncommon. Angiographic abnormalities consistent with FMD have been identified in the intracranial segments of the internal carotid and vertebral arteries, and the anterior cerebral, middle cerebral, posterior cerebral, basilar and anterior inferior, and superior cerebellar arteries, but the abnormalities rarely have been verified histologically.[1,5,38,46,56,151,154,167] All but four patients with intracranial disease also had extracranial FMD.

The histologic abnormalities may cause three patterns of pathology of the arterial wall.[28,75,118] Multifocal stenoses, alternating with mural dilatations (beaded appearance), is the most common pattern and occurs in 80 to 90 percent of patients. In 6 to 12 percent of patients there is a longitudinal stenosis (tubular appearance). When FMD involves the arterial wall in a noncircumferential manner, there may be an outpouching or diverticulum of the wall (4 to 6 percent of patients) or, rarely, an asymmetrical septal appearance, leading to a weblike stenosis. Lesions with a septal appearance have occurred only in the proximal internal carotid artery, and there are only three histologically proven cases.[113]

Vessels affected by FMD may become very elongated or kinked. Severe stenosis is uncommon in cephalic FMD, and complete occlusion has been reported in only 14 patients.[3]

Progressive disruption of the arterial wall by FMD may lead to several complications. FMD-related arterial disease has been reported in up to 20 percent of cervical carotid artery dissections.[4,22,36,44,65,112,150] FMD may also underlie arterial dissection in the vertebral, middle cerebral, anterior cerebral, or superior cerebellar arteries and may be the cause of unexplained "spontaneous" dissection in some patients.[58,78,84,106] Multiple arterial dissections associated with FMD have also been reported.[65,140]

Expansion of a dilated arterial segment may cause local saccular or giant aneurysms reported in the midcervical, skull base, or cavernous sinus portions of the internal carotid artery.[16,69,86,180] Similarly, carotid-cavernous sinus and vertebral-perivertebral vein arterial venous fistulas also have been caused by FMD.[52,71]

Intracranial "berry" aneurysms in association with cerebrovascular FMD have been reported in 21 to 51 percent of affected patients, depending on completeness of cerebral angiography.[60,73,83,109,118] These aneurysms have the same arterial distribution and histology as in patients without FMD. There has been one report of FMD associated with a cerebral arterial venous malformation.[85]

Cerebrovascular and renal FMD may coexist in as many as 50 percent of patients when complete angiography is performed.[35,105,118]

## CLINICAL FEATURES AND PATHOGENESIS OF SYMPTOMS

Neurologic abnormalities associated with cerebrovascular FMD (Table 27-1) have been attributed to focal cerebral ischemia, global cerebral hypoperfusion, and the direct compressive or disruptive effects of the arterial wall lesion. Focal neurologic abnormalities such as hemiparesis, hemisensory impairment, aphasia, or neglect have usually been attributed to transient cerebral ischemia or cerebral infarction.[149] A causal relationship between FMD and focal cerebral ischemia has been established in a minority of patients, however. In some patients there was severe stenosis or occlusion of the internal carotid artery or vertebral artery.[1,3,9,66,76,139] In others there was nonocclusive thrombus formation at the site of internal carotid artery FMD or distal intracranial or retinal artery branch occlusions, and cerebral embolization seemed likely.[12,26,80,109] Cerebral embolization may be more likely in patients with septal lesions involving the proximal internal carotid artery.[113] In other patients with cephalic FMD and transient ischemic attacks or cerebral infarction there was dissection of the internal carotid, vertebral, or intracranial arteries.[65] Head-turning precipitated transient ischemic attacks in one patient with internal carotid artery FMD,[136] and neck trauma preceded cerebral infarction in three others.[100,110,178] Focal and generalized neurologic abnormalities also have been reported in patients with cerebrovascular FMD following a subarachnoid hemorrhage because of the association between intracranial aneurysms and FMD.

In most patients with cerebrovascular FMD and symptoms of focal cerebral ischemia, however, the relationship between the two conditions is uncertain. In various reports, therefore, the initial incidence of stroke or transient ischemic attacks was zero to 20 percent and 7 to 67 percent, respectively (Table 27-1). In these reports the authors understandably reached widely divergent conclusions regarding the relationship between FMD and focal cerebral ischemia, indicating that it occurred commonly, infrequently, or that the relationship between the two conditions was usually coincidental. This discrepancy is explained in part by the methods of patient selection. In some studies all patients with FMD diagnosed in consecutive angiograms were reviewed, including cases in

**TABLE 27-1. Neurologic Diagnoses in Patients with Cerebrovascular Fibromuscular Dysplasia[a]**

| Ref. | Total Patients | Method of Patient Selection | Asymptomatic Bruit | Cerebral Infarction | Transient Ischemic Attack | Unilateral Facial Pain or Horner Syndrome | Nonlocalizing Neurologic Symptoms[b] | Intracranial Aneurysm | Coincidental Fibromuscular Dysplasia[c] |
|---|---|---|---|---|---|---|---|---|---|
| 28 | 79 | e | 8 (10.1)[d] | 7 ( 8.9) | 6 ( 7.6) | 0 (0 ) | 3 ( 3.8) | 10 (12.7) | 45 (56.9) |
| 110 | 37 | f | 1 ( 2.7) | 3 ( 8.1) | 4 (10.8) | 3 (8.1) | 0 ( 0 ) | 19 (51.4) | 7 (18.9) |
| 172 | 30 | g | 5 (16.7) | 3 (10 ) | 16 (53.3) | 0 (0 ) | 4 (13.3) | 0 ( 0 ) | 2 ( 6.7) |
| 170 | 17 | h | 2 (11.7) | 0 ( 0 ) | 9 (52.9) | 0 (0 ) | 6 (35.4) | 0 ( 0 ) | 0 ( 0 ) |
| 157 | 32 | i | 2 ( 6.3) | 9 (28.1) | 9 (28.1) | 3 (9.4) | 4 (12.5) | 5 (15.6) | 0 ( 0 ) |
| 164 | 49 | i | 11 (22.4) | 3 ( 6.1) | 17 (34.7) | 0 (0 ) | 15 (30.6) | 7 (14.3) | 3 ( 6.1) |
| 33 | 86 | j | 7 ( 8.1) | 19 (22.1) | 58 (67.5) | 0 (0 ) | 2 ( 2.3) | 0 ( 0 ) | 0 ( 0 ) |
| 162 | 40 | k | 6 (15.0) | 4 (10.0) | 11 (27.5) | 0 (0 ) | 19 (47.5) | 0 ( 0 ) | 0 ( 0 ) |
| 26 | 18 | l | 0 ( 0 ) | 3 (16.7) | 6 (33.3) | 0 (0 ) | 9 (50.0) | 0 ( 0 ) | 0 ( 0 ) |
| 160 | 15 | m | 1 ( 6.7) | 1 ( 6.7) | 3 (20.0) | 0 (0 ) | 2 (13.4) | 4 (26.6) | 4 (26.6) |
| 118 | 25 | m | 0 ( 0 ) | 6 (24.0) | 8 (32.0) | 0 (0 ) | 2 ( 8.0) | 9 (36.0) | 0 ( 0 ) |

[a] Reported series of 10 or more patients (English language).
[b] Dizziness, vertigo, syncope, generalized seizure, scintillating scotomata, or unspecified.
[c] Head trauma, intracranial mass lesion, or unspecified.
[d] Numbers in parenthesis indicate percent.
[e] Review of 13,955 consecutive cerebral angiograms.
[f] Review of 4,000 consecutive cerebral angiograms.
[g] Review of 936 consecutive angiograms.
[h] Review of "radiographic and clinical records."
[i] Review of "medical records and cerebral angiographic registry."
[j] Surgical series: all patients had surgery.
[k] Surgical series: 25 of 40 patients had surgery.
[l] Surgical series: 13 of 18 patients had surgery.
[m] Uncertain.

which FMD was a coincidental abnormality. The incidence of stroke and transient ischemic attack was low in these reports. Other studies have been more selective, excluding patients with coincidental FMD or including predominantly patients with surgical treatment. In some reports selection criteria were not clearly stated.

In most reports, moreover, it is uncertain how carefully other causes of focal neurologic symptoms have been sought. Some patients with stroke or transient ischemic attack and FMD were taking birth control pills, including two patients with cerebral infarction and complete thrombotic occlusion of the internal carotid artery or vertebral artery.[66,139] Carotid artery or vertebral artery atherosclerosis coexisted with FMD in 12 to 35 percent of patients with symptoms of cerebral ischemia.[26,28,33,172] In a few of these patients, recurrent transient ischemic attacks stopped after surgical resection of an atherosclerotic plaque.[74]

FMD should be considered, therefore, in the differential diagnosis of stroke or transient ischemic attack, especially in young or middle-aged patients, but other more common causes also must be excluded.

Syncope, generalized convulsions, episodic dizziness, vertigo, and scintillating scotomata in patients with cerebrovascular FMD have been attributed to global cerebral hypoperfusion. A few of these patients had bilateral internal carotid artery FMD and syncope, dizziness, or vertigo following head-turning.[93,117,136,168] These positional symptoms presumably were caused by temporary occlusion of the carotid artery or vertebral artery, further compromising cerebral perfusion already reduced by FMD-related stenosis. In most reports, however, the mechanism of cerebral hypoperfusion is unclear, and the causal relationship between these nonfocal neurologic symptoms and FMD is unproven.

Neurologic abnormalities also may be caused by the direct effect of the arterial wall lesions or their associated complications. Cervical bruits caused by turbulent flow through affected arteries are sometimes the only neurologic abnormality. Bruits are frequently audible to the patient and may be reported as troublesome pulsatile tinnitus.[29] Arterial dilatation and disruption of sympathetic nerve fibers may cause anterior cervical pain or tenderness, unilateral facial pain, Horner syndrome, or a fully developed Raeder syndrome.[129,156] Giant internal carotid artery aneurysms caused by FMD have been reported in the cavernous sinus in association with cavernous sinus syndrome, at the base of the skull in patients with lower cranial nerve impairment, and in the midcervical area in one patient with an enlarging neck mass.[69,92,94,137] A cavernous sinus syndrome has also been caused by carotid-cavernous sinus fistulae in patients with intracavernous carotid FMD.[71,86,180] Vertebral artery-paravertebral venous fistulas have been reported in patients with progressive cervical myelopathy and in two patients with only a cervical bruit.[18,52,138]

Finally, cerebrovascular FMD has also been diagnosed coincidentally in patients with neurologic symptoms associated with head trauma, neoplasm, or other mass lesion.

A few patients with FMD have had associated pes cavus, pectus excavatum, scoliosis, hallux valgus, endocardial fibroelastosis, otosclerosis, and retinal degeneration.[5,48,109] There was no evidence, however, that these abnormalities were other than coincidental.

## ANGIOGRAPHY AND OTHER DIAGNOSTIC TESTS

The angiographic appearance of affected vessels is based on the arterial wall morphology previously described.[20] In the most common pattern, irregularly spaced areas of sharply localized concentric narrowing usually reduce the lumen caliber less than 40 percent and alternate with areas of dilatation, which are always wider than the normal lumen (Fig. 27-1). This appearance, termed the "string of beads," occurs in 80 to 90 percent of patients. Other less common patterns are tubular stenosis (Fig. 27-2), diverticulum (Fig. 27-3), and, rarely, weblike stenosis (septum). Severe stenosis is uncommon. When FMD is bilateral, the angiographic pattern occasionally may be different on the two sides.

Angiography may also identify arterial complications of FMD: embolic occlusion of distal vessels, local saccular or giant aneurysms, and arterial dissections. The typical angiographic appearance of dissection is severe linear narrowing (string sign), but complete occlusion and "double barrel" lumen (when the dissecting channel reenters the lumen) have also been described in FMD. A basal "moyamoya" angiographic pattern has been reported in two patients

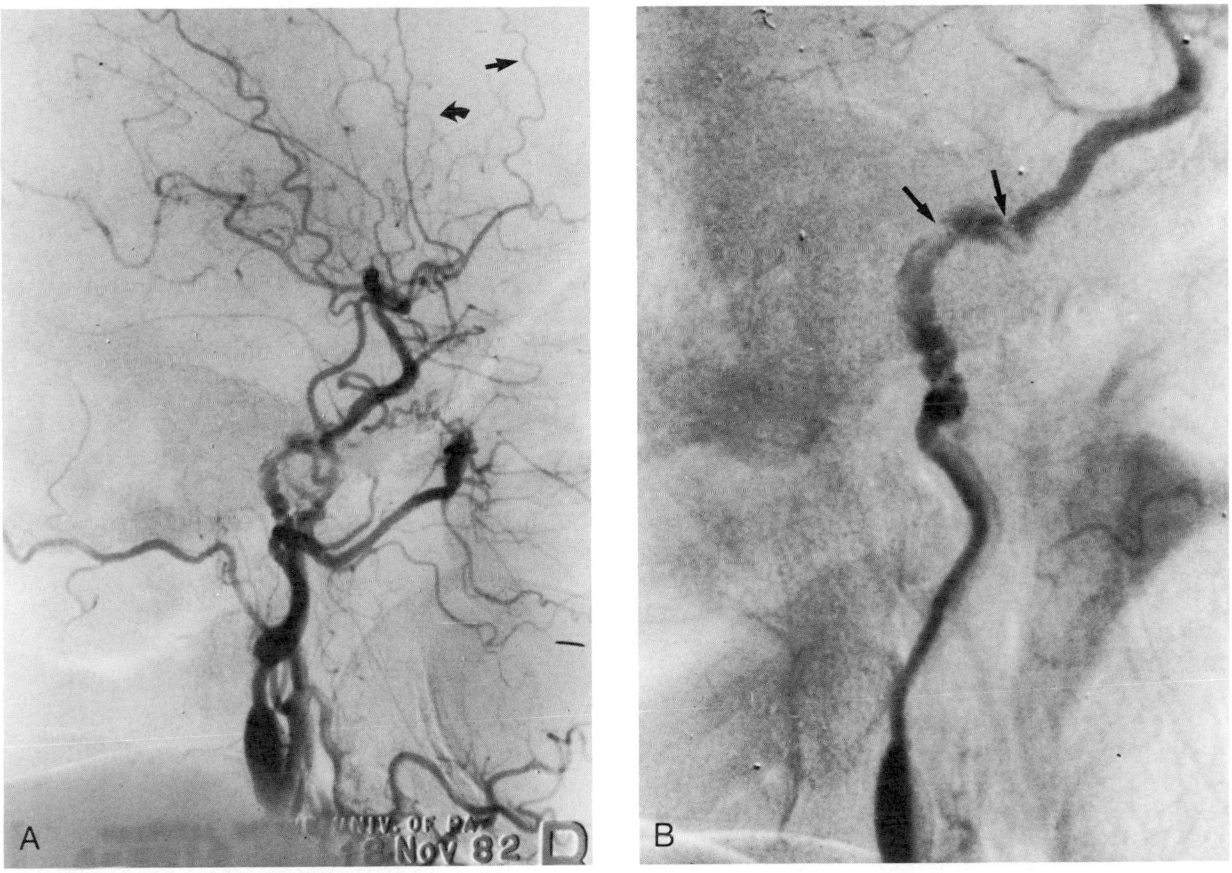


**Fig. 27-1.** Hemodynamically significant fibromuscular dysplasia in the distal cervical segment of internal carotid artery and petrous portion. (**A**) Lateral head and neck projection of carotid angiogram demonstrates typical "string of beads" configuration of fibromuscular dysplasia in the distal cervical and proximal petrous portion of internal carotid artery. Circulation in distal branches of superficial temporal artery (*straight arrow*) leads circulation in middle cerebral artery branches (*curved arrow*) indicating hemodynamic significance of carotid stenosis. (**B**) Delayed lateral carotid angiogram shows close-up view of internal carotid artery. Several severe bandlike regions of narrowing (*arrows*) are present between the dilated regions of fibromuscular dysplasia.

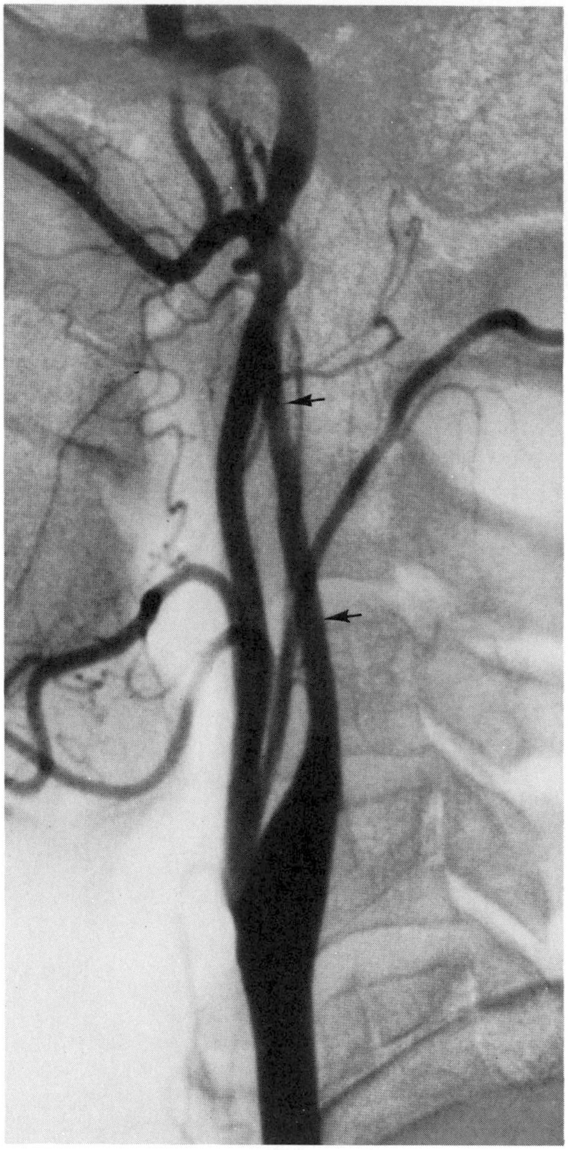

Fig. 27-2. Internal carotid artery fibromuscular dysplasia: tubular stenosis (*arrows*). (From Osborne and Anderson,[118] with permission.)

with internal carotid artery and proximal middle cerebral artery stenosis caused by FMD.[120,132]

The angiographic appearance of cerebrovascular FMD must be differentiated from similar arterial patterns: carotid artery stationary arterial waves produced by distal arterial occlusion, increased intracranial pressure, or subarachnoid hemorrhage; arterial spasm or circular spastic contractions at the site of catheterization; Takayasu's arteritis; arterial hypoplasia resembling tubular stenosis; posttraumatic or atherosclerotic aneurysm of the internal carotid; and, in intracranial FMD, cerebral vasculitis.[53,57,76,90,118]

When FMD involves the proximal segments of the internal carotid artery, the arterial abnormalities must be differentiated from atherosclerotic cerebrovascular disease. When FMD is diagnosed, full cerebral angiography should be performed.

Doppler ultrasonography and B-mode echotomography can detect carotid artery FMD and differentiate these abnormalities from atherosclerosis in some patients.[17,31,91,152] Although reported infrequently, noninvasive hemodynamic studies have been normal or consistent with mild stenosis in most patients.[26,45,170] Superficial temporal artery biopsy may show diagnostic dysplastic abnormalities.[5,96,134]

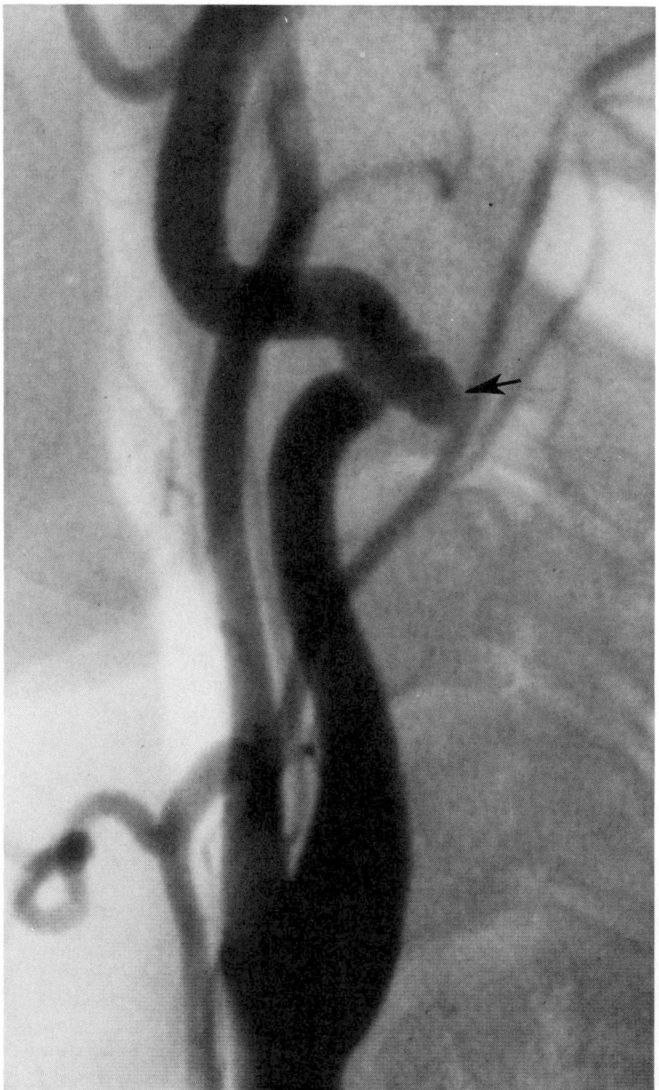

Fig. 27-3. Internal carotid artery fibromuscular dysplasia: diverticulum (*arrow*). (From Osborne and Anderson,[118] with permission.)

## TREATMENT CONSIDERATIONS

Because there has been no prospective study of the natural history of untreated cerebrovascular FMD, there is limited information available about anatomic or clinical progression in untreated patients. In renal artery FMD anatomic progression of arterial lesions has been reported in 8.3 to 37.5 percent of patients when serial angiographic studies were performed 6 months to 8 years after the initial diagnosis, but progression was usually mild.[14,37,108] A limited number of studies have reported serial angiography in patients with cerebrovascular FMD in whom the angiogram was repeated because of recurrent symptoms or for uncertain reasons. In 31 such selected patients with repeat angiography 3 months to 7 years after the initial diagnosis, there was no anatomic progression in 18 patients, and progressive stenosis of mild to moderate degree occurred in 7.[4,76,164,170,171] Other abnormalities reported were the development of FMD in the contralateral carotid artery in 1, aneurysm formation at the site of a diverticulum related to FMD in 1, and resolution of spontaneous carotid artery dissection in 3. Progression of cerebrovascular FMD lesions, defined as increasing stenosis or anatomic complication of the arterial lesion, does occur, therefore, in a minority of selected patients.

Information regarding the clinical natural history of FMD is also limited. In two retrospective clinical outcome studies, prognosis was usually benign.[28,170] In the largest such series, 79 patients with FMD diagnosed in association with focal cerebral ischemia (13), intracranial mass lesion (29), intracranial aneurysm (10), or miscellaneous disorders (27) were followed for an average of 5 years. There was no treatment in 64 cases. Antiplatelet therapy or anticoagulation was started in 11 patients, and 3 patients had surgical treatment. In the untreated group one patient, aged 71, had a stroke in the same vascular territory as the fibromuscular dysplastic lesion 216 months after diagnosis. A stroke occurred in two other patients in that group (aged 65 and 75) 50 and 136 months after diagnosis, but the clinical symptoms did not correspond with the FMD lesion. Stroke or transient ischemic attack did not occur in the treated group. In a smaller study of 17 patients with cerebrovascular FMD followed for an average of 3.8 years, 9 patients were not treated, 7 patients received anticoagulation or antiplatelet therapy, and 1 patient had surgery. In two untreated patients (aged 60 and 79) with severe cerebral atherosclerosis, cerebral infarction occurred 18 months and 5 years after diagnosis.

In untreated patients, therefore, the incidence of stroke or transient ischemic attack clearly related to cephalic FMD appears to be quite low.

Medical treatment using antiplatelet medication or anticoagulation and surgical therapy have been advocated in the initial management of cerebrovascular FMD. Graduated intraluminal dilation has been the most frequently performed surgical procedure, but some patients have had percutaneous transluminal angioplasty, resection of the FMD lesion, arterial bypass, extraction of stenotic rings, or incision of adventitial fibrosis.[49,67,99,155] Because of the frequent association of FMD with atherosclerosis, endarterectomy has also been performed together with these surgical procedures. A controlled trial of medical or surgical therapy has not been performed and retrospective uncontrolled studies have provided conflicting results. For example, in a retrospective study of 30 patients with cerebrovascular FMD in association with focal cerebral ischemia (19), global or unlocalized neurologic symptoms (4), or no neurologic symptoms (7), followed for an average of 21.5 months (range 1 to 96 months), there was significant benefit to arterial dilation or antiplatelet therapy when compared with no therapy in patients with focal neurologic symptoms.[172] There was also a trend in favor of surgical intervention, but the overall results did not achieve statistical significance. In another report of 45 patients with angiographically proven cerebrovascular FMD, cerebral or retinal infarction did not occur in the 35 patients treated with antiplatelet therapy or followed without therapy.[163] In two of these patients, graduated intraluminal dilation was performed because of persistent nonfocal neurologic symptoms (syncope and vertigo). Stroke also did not occur in the 10 other patients in whom graduated intraluminal dilation was carried out because of persistent neurologic symptoms.

Overall, however, aggregate data from other reports indicate that the incidence of subsequent stroke or transient ischemic attack in medically treated patients is 0 to 4 percent.[28,126,164,170] Operative mortality for patients treated with graduated intraluminal dilation has been zero or not reported, but operative and perioperative morbidity has ranged from 3 to 6 percent.[101,164] In two studies with long-term follow-up after surgery, there was a 5 to 8 percent incidence of stroke when perioperative morbidity was included.[26,33,164]

Because of the low incidence of stroke, transient ischemic attack, or other serious outcome in untreated or medically managed patients, a conservative approach to treatment has been recommended, and seems warranted, based on available information.[148] Prior to therapy, all patients with neurologic symptoms should be carefully evaluated for etiologies other than FMD. Patients with associated atherosclerosis should receive appropriate medical or surgical management as indicated for that disorder. Patients with no neurologic symptoms, a cervical bruit alone, or nonlocalizing neurologic abnormalities should receive antiplatelet therapy only. Most patients with stroke or transient ischemic attack attributed to FMD also should receive antiplatelet therapy, which carries less risk than surgery. Patients with focal ischemic symptoms and a high-grade hemodynamically significant stenosis or recurrent symptoms while medically treated may require surgery. Surgical treatment has also been recommended for patients with proximal septal lesions because of the possibly increased risk of thromboembolism.[113]

Management of dissecting aneurysms is difficult because both spontaneous aneurysm resolution and recurrent ischemic symptoms have occurred in untreated patients. An initial trial of antiplatelet therapy or anticoagulation followed by surgery if symptoms continue has been recommended.

Finally, all patients with cephalic FMD should have complete cerebral angiography to identify all FMD lesions and associated intracranial aneurysms. Antiplatelet therapy or anticoagulation should be avoided in patients with aneurysms until appropriate management is completed. All patients should also have long-term blood pressure monitoring and angiographic investigation for renal artery FMD if hypertension occurs.[79,176]

## ACKNOWLEDGMENTS

I thank Mrs. Florine C. Lee for her assistance in preparation of this manuscript.

## REFERENCES

1. Abdul-Rahman AM, Abu-Salih Brun A et al: Fibromuscular dysplasia of the cervicocephalic arteries. Surg Neurol 9:217, 1978
2. Alvarez-Amandi MR, Berciano-Blanco JA, Combarros-Pascual O et al: Fibromuscular dysplasia of the cervicocephalic arteries: report of two cases and review of the literature. Med Clin (Barc) 74:98, 1980
3. Andersen CA, Collins GJ, Rich NM et al: Internal carotid artery occlusions associated with fibromuscular dysplasia. Vasc Surg 13:349, 1979
4. Andersen CA, Collins GJ, Rich NM et al: Spontaneous dissection of the internal carotid artery associated with fibromuscular dysplasia. Am Surg 46:263, 1980
5. Andersen PE: Fibromuscular hyperplasia of the carotid arteries. Acta Radiol [Diagn] (Stockh) 10:90, 1970
6. Andersen PE: Fibromuscular hyperplasia in children. Acta Radiol [Diagn] (Stockh) 10:203, 1970
7. Angelini C, Brunoro N, Gallucci V: Report of two patients with fibromuscular dysplasia of the internal carotid artery. Riv Patol Nerv Ment 101:139, 1981
8. Antunes ACM, Borges ACG, DaCosta JC et al: Dysplasia fibromuscular de vasos cerebrais. Arq Neuropsiquiat (Sao Paulo) 32:118, 1974
9. Appleberg M: Graduated internal dilatation in the treatment of fibromuscular dysplasia of the internal carotid artery. S Afr Med J 51:244, 1977
10. Arnott G, Clarisse J, Houcke M et al: Dysplasia fibromusculaire d'artéres cervicales et encéphaliques (a'propos d'un cas d'hémorragie cérébroméningée par rupture d'anévrysme intra-carnien dysplasique). Lille Med 21:308, 1976
11. Aurell M: Fibromuscular dysplasia of the renal arteries. Br Med J 1:1180, 1979
12. Balaji MR, DeWeese JA: Fibromuscular dysplasia of the internal carotid artery. Arch Surg 115:984, 1980
13. Barbizet J, Debrun G, Brunet P et al: Hyperplasie fibromusculaire de la carotide interne. Ann Med Interne (Paris) 122:537, 1971
14. Belan A, Vesela M, Vanek I et al: Percutaneous transluminal angioplasty of fibromuscular dysplasia of the internal carotid artery. Cardiovasc Inervent Radiol 5:79, 1982
15. Bergan JJ, MacDonald JR: Recognition of cerebrovascular fibromuscular hyperplasia. Arch Surg 98:332, 1969
16. Bergentz SE, Ericsson BF, Olivecrona H: Bilateral fibromuscular hyperplasia in the internal carotid arteries with aneurysm formation. Acta Chir Scand 142:501, 1976
17. Boespflug OJ: Ultrasonography of supraaortic trunks. Neuroradiology 27:544, 1985
18. Bonduelle M, Ruscalleda J, Zalzal P: Dysplasie fibromusculaire avec fistule arterioveineuse de l'artére vertébrale extracranienne. Rev Neurol 128:204, 1973
19. Boudin G, Guillard A, Romion A: Dysplasies fibromusculaires des artéres carotides et vertébrales. Ann Med Interne 125:863, 1974
20. Bradac GB, Haymat F: Considerations concerning a case of fibromuscular hyperplasia of the carotid arteries. Neuroradiology 1:217, 1970
21. Bragin MA, Cherkasov AP: On the morphogenesis of fibrous-muscular dysplasia of renal arteries (an ultrastructural study). Arkh Patol 41:46, 1979
22. Brown OL, Arnitage JL: Spontaneous dissecting aneurysms of the cervical internal carotid artery. Am J Radiol 118:648, 1973
23. Caes F, Van der Niepen P, Cham B: Fibromuscular dysplasia of the internal carotid artery. Acta Chirurg Belg 86:153, 1986
24. Cina C, Williamson C, Ameli FM: Fibromuscular dysplasia of the posterior auricular artery: an unusual aneurysmal lesion. J Cardiovasc Surg (Torino) 29:56, 1989
25. Claiborne TS: Fibromuscular hyperplasia: report of a case with involvement of multiple arteries. Am J Med 49:103, 1970
26. Collins GJ, Rich NM, Clagett GP et al: Fibromuscular dysplasia of the internal carotid arteries: clinical experience and follow-up. Ann Surg 194:89, 1981
27. Connett MC, Lansche JM: Fibromuscular hyperplasia of the internal carotid artery: report of a case. Ann Surg 162:59, 1965
28. Corrin LS, Sandok BA, Houser OW: Cerebral ischemic events in patients with carotid artery fibromuscular dysplasia. Arch Neurol 38:616, 1981
29. Dufour JJ, Layigne F, Plante R: Pulsatile tinni-

tus and fibromuscular dysplasia of the internal carotid. J Otolaryngol 14:293, 1985
30. Duncan CE, Buck K, Lynch A: The effect of pressure and stretching on the passage of labeled albumin into canine aortic wall. J Atheroscler Res 5:69, 1965
31. Edell SL, Huang P: Sonographic demonstration of fibromuscular hyperplasia of the cervical internal carotid artery. Stroke 12:518, 1981
32. Effeney DJ, Ehrenfeld WK, Stoney et al: Fibromuscular dysplasia of the internal carotid artery. World J Surg 3:179, 1979
33. Effeney DJ, Ehrenfeld WK, Stoney RJ et al: Why operate on carotid fibromuscular dysplasia? Arch Surg 115:1261, 1980
34. Ehrenfeld WK, Stoney RJ, Wylie EJ: Fibromuscular hyperplasia of the internal carotid artery. Arch Surg 95:284, 1967
35. Ehrenfeld WK, Wylie EJ: Fibromuscular dysplasia of the internal carotid artery: surgical management. Arch Surg 109:676, 1974
36. Ehrenfeld WK, Wylie EJ: Spontaneous dissection of the internal carotid artery. Arch Surg 111:1294, 1976
37. Ekelund L, Gerlock J, Molin J et al: Roentgenologic appearance of fibromuscular dysplasia. Acta Radiol [Diagn] (Stockh) 19:433, 1978
38. Elias WS: Intracranial fibromuscular hyperplasia. JAMA 218:254, 1971
39. Emparanza JI, Aldamiz-Echevarria L, Perez-Yarza E: Ischemic stroke due to fibromuscular dysplasia. Neuropediatrics 20:181, 1989
40. Ennis JT, Bateson EM: Fibromuscular dysplasia of the internal carotid arteries: a report of three cases. Br J Radiol 43:452, 1970
41. Fievez M: Relations ergotisme—hyperplasie fibromusculaire. Nouv Presse Med 4:1753, 1975
42. Fievez M, Koerperich G, Dulieu J: Arterial fibromuscular dysplasia and ergotism. Ann Anat Pathol 20:357, 1975
43. Fiore DL, Pardatscher K, Fiore D et al: Persistant dorsal ophthalmic artery: report of a case with associated fibromuscular hyperplasia of the extracranial internal carotid artery and multiple cerebral aneurysms. Neurochirurgia (Stuttg) 24:106, 1981
44. Fisher CM, Ojemann RG, Roberson GH: Spontaneous dissection of cervico-cerebral arteries. Can J Neurol Sci 5:9, 1978
45. Fitzer PM, Rinaldi I: Abnormal radionuclide angiogram in proven intracranial fibromuscular dysplasia: case report. J Nucl Med 17:190, 1975
46. Frens DB, Petajan JH, Anderson R et al: Fibromuscular dysplasia of the posterior cerebral artery: report of a case and review of the literature. Stroke 5:161, 1974
47. Galligioni F, Iraci G, Marin G: Fibromuscular hyperplasia of the extracranial internal carotid artery. J Neurosurg 34:647, 1971
48. Garcia-Merino JA, Gutierrez JA, Lopez-Lozano JJ et al: Double lumen dissecting aneurysm of the internal carotid artery in fibromuscular dysplasia: case report. Stroke 14:815, 1983
49. Garrido E, Montoya J: Transluminal dilatation of internal carotid artery in fibromuscular dysplasia: a preliminary report. Surg Neurol 16:469, 1981
50. Gee W, Burton R, Stoney RJ: Atypical fibromuscular hyperplasia involving the internal carotid artery. Ann Surg 7:136, 1974
51. George B, Zerah M, Mourier KL et al: Ruptured intracranial aneurysms: the influence of sex and fibromuscular dysplasia upon prognosis. Acta Neurochir (Wien) 97:20, 1989
52. Geraud J, Manelfe C, Caussanel JP et al: Fistule arterioveineuse spontaneé del artére-vertébrale: role eventuel de la dysplasie fibromusculaire dans sa pathogeneie. Rev Neurol 128:206, 1973
53. Gibbons RB, Ashton AL: Buerger's disease and multicentric fibromuscular hyperplasia mimicking Takayasu's arteritis. Arthritis Rheum 23:1067, 1980
54. Gladstein K, Rushton AR, Kidd KK: Penetrance estimates and recurrence risks for fibromuscular dysplasia. Clin Genet 17:115, 1980
55. Golosovskaia MA, Spiridonov AA, Cherkasov AP: Fibromuscular dysplasia of the renal arteries. Arkh Patol 39:19, 1977
56. Green PM, Letellier MA: Fibromuscular dysplasia of the infratentorial circulation: discussion of two cases and treatment. Wis Med J 77:99, 1978
57. Grollman JH, Lecky JW, Rosch J: Miscellaneous diseases of arteries, or all arterial lesions aren't fatty. Semin Roentgenol 5:306, 1970
58. Grotta JC, Ward RE, Flynn TC et al: Spontaneous internal carotid artery dissection associated with fibromuscular dysplasia. J Cardiovasc Surg (Torino) 23:512, 1982
59. Halpern HH, Sanford HS, Viamonte M: Renal artery abnormalities in three hypertensive sisters. JAMA 194:124, 1965
60. Handa J, Kamijyo Y, Handa H: Intracranial aneurysm associated with fibromuscular hyperplasia of renal and internal carotid arteries. Br J Radiol 43:483, 1970
61. Hansen J, Holter C, Thorberg JV: Hypertension in two sisters caused by so-called fibromuscular hyperplasia of the renal arteries. Acta Med Scand 178:461, 1965
62. Harrison EG, Hunt JC, Bernatz PE: Morphology of fibromuscular dysplasia of the renal artery in renovascular hypertension. Am J Med 43:97, 1967
63. Harrison EG, McCormack LJ: Pathologic classification of renal arterial disease in renovascular hypertension. Mayo Clin Proc 46:161, 1971
64. Harrington OB, Crosby VG, Nicholas L: Fibromuscular hyperplasia of the internal carotid artery. Ann Thorac Surg 9:516, 1970
65. Hart RG, Easton JD: Dissections. Stroke 16:925, 1985
66. Hartman JD, Young I, Bank A et al: Fibromuscular hyperplasia of internal carotid arteries. Arch Neurol 25:295, 1971
67. Hasso AN, Bird CR, Zinke DE et al: Fibromuscular dysplasia of the internal carotid artery: Percutaneous transluminal angioplasty. Am J Neuroradiol 2:175, 1981
68. Hata J, Hosoda Y: Perimedial fibroplasia of the

renal artery: a light and electron microscopic study. Arch Pathol Lab Med 103:220, 1979
69. Havelius U, Hindfelt B, Brismar J et al: Carotid fibromuscular dysplasia and paresis of lower cranial nerves (Collect-Sicard syndrome): case report. J Neurosurg 56:850, 1982
70. Heffelfinger MJ, Holley KE, Harrison EG et al: Arterial fibromuscular dysplasia studied at autopsy. Am J Clin Pathol 54:274, 1970
71. Hieshima GB, Cahan LD, Mehringer CM et al: Spontaneous arteriovenous fistulae of cerebral vessels in association with fibromuscular dysplasia. Neurosurgery 18:454, 1986
72. Hill LD, Antonius JI: Arterial dysplasia: an impotant surgical lesion. Arch Surg 90:585, 1965
73. Hirsch CS, Roessman U: Arterial dysplasia with ruptured basilar artery aneurysm: report of a case. Hum Pathol 6:749, 1975
74. Hooshmand H, Boykin ME, Vines FS et al: Fibromuscular dysplasia of the extracranial internal carotid arteries associated with an ulcerative plaque. Stroke 3:67, 1972
75. Houser OW, Baker HL, Jr: Fibromuscular dysplasia and other uncommon diseases of the cervical carotid artery: angiographic aspects. Am J Roentgenol 104:201, 1968
76. Houser OW, Baker HL, Jr, Sandok BA et al: Fibromuscular dysplasia of the cephalic arterial system. p. 366. In Vinken PJ, Bruyn GW (eds): Handbook of Clinical Neurology. Vol. 11. North-Holland Publishing, Amsterdam, 1972
77. Huber P, Fuchs WA: Gibt es eine fibromuskuläre hyperplasie zerebraler arterien? Fortschr Rontgenstr 107:119, 1967
78. Hugenholtz H, Pokrupa R, Montpetit VJA et al: Spontaneous dissecting-aneurysm of the extracranial vertebral artery. Neurosurgery 10:96, 1982
79. Hunt JC, Harrison EG, Kincaid OW et al: Idiopathic fibrous and fibromuscular stenoses of the renal arteries associated with hypertension. Mayo Clin Proc 37:181, 1962
80. Iosue A, Kier EL, Ostrow D: Fibromuscular dysplasia involving the intracranial vessels. J Neurosurg 37:749, 1972
81. Irey NS, Manion WC, Taylor HB: Vascular lesions in women taking contraceptives. Arch Pathol 89:1, 1970
82. Julian LM: The occurrence of fibromuscular dysplasia in the arteries of domestic turkeys. Am J Pathol 101:415, 1980
83. Kalyan-Raman UP, Elwood PW: Fibromuscular dysplasia of intracranial arteries causing multiple intracranial aneurysms. Hum Pathol 11:481, 1980
84. Kalyan-Raman UP, Kowalski RV, Lee RH et al: Dissecting aneurysm of superior cerebellar artery: its association with fibromuscular dysplasia. Arch Neurol 40:120, 1983
85. Kaufman HH: Fibromuscular hyperplasia of the carotid artery in a case associated with an arteriovenous malformation. Arch Neurol 22:299, 1970
86. Kaufman HH, Lind TA, Mullan S: Spontaneous carotid-cavernous fistula with fibromuscular dysplasia. Acta Neurochir (Wien) 40:123, 1978
87. Kelly TF, Morris GC, Jr: Arterial fibromuscular disease: observations on pathogenesis and surgical management. Am J Surg 143:232, 1982
88. Kincaid OW, Davis GD: Renal arteriography in hypertension. Mayo Clin Proc 36:689, 1961
89. Kincaid OW, Davis GD, Hallermann FJ et al: Fibromuscular dysplasia of the renal arteries: arteriographic features, classification, and observations on natural history of the disease. Am J Roentgenol 104:271, 1968
90. Kishore PRS, Lin JP, Kricheff II: Fibromuscular hyperplasia and stationary waves of the internal carotid artery. Acta Radiol [Diagn] (Stockh) 11:619, 1971
91. Kliewer MA, Carroll BA: Ultrasound case of the day. Internal carotid artery web (atypical fibromuscular dysplasia). Radiographics 11:504, 1991
92. Kramer W: Hyperplasie fibromusculaire et anévrisme extracranien de la carotide interne avec syndrome parapharyngien typique. Rev Neurol 120:239, 1969
93. Lamis PA, Carson WP, Wilson JP et al: Recognition and treatment of fibromuscular hyperplasia of the internal carotid artery. Surgery 69:498, 1971
94. Lane RJ, Weisman RA, Savino PJ et al: Aneurysm of the internal carotid artery at the base of the skull: an unusual cause of cranial neuropathies. Otolaryngol Head Neck Surg 88:230, 1980
95. Leadbetter WF, Burkland CE: Hypertension in unilateral renal disease. J Urol 39:611, 1938
96. Lemahieu SF, Marchau MM: Intracranial fibromuscular dysplasia and stroke in children. Neuroradiology 18:99, 1979
97. Letsch R, Kantartzis M, Sommer T et al: Arterial fibromuscular dysplasia: report of a case with involvement of the aorta and review of the literature. Thorac Cardiovasc Surg 28:206, 1980
98. Leung DYM, Glagov S, Mathews MB: Cyclic stretching stimulates synthesis of matrix components by arterial smooth muscle cells in vitro. Science 191:475, 1976
99. Levin SM, Sondheimer F: Surgical technique in fibromuscular disease of the carotid arteries. Angiology 22:463, 1971
100. Llorens-Terol J, Sole-Llenas J, Lura A: Stroke due to fibromuscular hyperplasia of the internal carotid artery. Acta Paediatr Scand 72:299, 1983
101. Luscher TF, Stanson AW, Hauser OW et al: Arterial fibromuscular dysplasia. Mayo Clin Proc 62:931, 1987
102. Maiuri F, Gallicchio B, Gangemi M: Fibromuscular dysplasia of the carotid arteries. Clin Neurol Neurosurg 90:57, 1988
103. Major P, Genest J, Cartier P et al: Hereditary fibromuscular dysplasia with renovascular hypertension. Ann Intern Med 86:583, 1977
104. Manelfe C, Clairesse J, Fredy D: Dysplasies fibromusculaires des arteres cervicocephalique. J Neuroradiol 1:149, 1974
105. Manns RA, Nanda KK, Mackie G: Fibromuscular dysplasia of the cephalic and renal arteries. Clin Radiol 38:427, 1987
106. Mas JL, Bousser MG, Hasboun D et al: Extracra-

nial vertebral artery dissections: a review of 13 cases. Stroke 18:1037, 1987
107. McCormack LJ, Hazard JB, Poutasse EF: Obstructive lesions of the renal artery associated with remediable hypertension. Am J Pathol 34:582, 1958
108. Meaney TF, Dustan HP, McCormack LJ: Natural history of renal arterial disease. Radiology 91:881, 1968
109. Mettinger KL: Fibromuscular dysplasia and the brain: current concepts of the disease. Stroke 13:53, 1982
110. Mettinger KL, Erickson K: Fibromuscular dysplasia and the brain: observations on angiographic, clinical, and genetic characteristics. Stroke 13:46, 1982
111. Momose KJ, New PFJ: Non-atheromatous stenosis and occlusion of the internal carotid artery and its main branches. AJR 118:550, 1973
112. Monfort JC, Degos JO, Eizenbaum JF et al: Dissecting aneurysm of the carotid artery in a patient with angiographic evidence of fibromuscular dysplasia. Ann Med Interne 132:333, 1981
113. Morgenlander JC, Goldstein LB: Recurrent transient ischemic attacks and stroke in association with an internal carotid artery web. Stroke 22:94, 1991
114. Morimoto S, Kuroda M, Uchida K et al: Occurrence of renovascular hypertension in two sisters. Nephron 17:314, 1976
115. Morris GC, Lechter A, Debakey ME: Surgical treatment of fibromuscular disease of the carotid arteries. Arch Surg 96:636, 1968
116. Nakata Y: An experimental study on the vascular lesions caused by obstruction of the vasa vasorum. Jpn Circ J 31:275, 1967
117. Nunn DB: Fibromuscular hyperplasia of the internal carotid artery. Am Surg 40:309, 1974
118. Osborne AG, Anderson RE: Angiographic spectrum of cervical and intracranial fibromuscular dysplasia. Stroke 8:617, 1977
119. Ouchi Y, Tagawa H, Yamakado M et al: Clinical significance of cerebral aneurysm in renovascular hypertension due to fibromuscular dysplasia: two cases in siblings. Angiology 40:581, 1989
120. Overgaard J, Laursen B, Ingstrup HM: Oligophrenia in a case of late onset in cerebral fibromuscular hyperplasia. Dan Med Bull 17:19, 1970
121. Palubinskas AJ, Perloff P, Newton TH: Fibromuscular hyperplasia: an arterial dysplasia of increasing clinical importance. AJR 98:907, 1966
122. Palubinskas AJ, Newton TH: Fibromuscular hyperplasia of the internal carotid arteries: Radiol Clin Biol 34:365, 1965
123. Palubinskas AJ, Ripley HR: Fibromuscular hyperplasia in extra-renal arteries. Radiology 82:451, 1964
124. Palubinskas AJ, Wylie EJ: Roentgen diagnosis of fibromuscular hyperplasia of the renal arteries. Radiology 76:634, 1961
125. Pappada G, Panzarasa G, Sani R: Intracranial fibromuscular dysplasia: report of two cases and review of the literature. J Neurosurg Sci 31:13, 1987
126. Patman RD, Thompson JE, Talkington CM: Natural history of fibromuscular dysplasia of the carotid artery. Stroke 11:135, 1980
127. Paule WJ, Zemplenyi TK, Rounds DE et al: Light and electronmicroscopic characteristics of arterial smooth muscle cell cultures subjected to hypoxia or carbon monoxide. Atherosclerosis 25:111, 1976
128. Paulson GW: Fibromuscular dysplasia antiovulent drugs and ergot preparations (Letter.) Stroke 9:172, 1978
129. Paulson GW, Boesel CP, Evans WE: Fibromuscular dysplasia. Arch Neurol 35:287, 1978
130. Perez-Hiqueras A, Alvarez-Ruiz F, Martinez-Bermejo A et al: Cerebeller infarction from fibromuscular dysplasia and dissecting aneurysm of the vertebral artery: report of a child. Sroke 19:521, 1988
131. Perry DO: Fibromuscular disease of the carotid artery. Surg Gynecol Obstet 134:57, 1972
132. Pilz P, Hartjes HJ: Fibromuscular dysplasia and multiple dissecting aneurysms of intracranial arteries: a further cause of moyamoya syndrome. Stroke 7:393, 1976
133. Polin SG: Carotid artery fibromuscular hyperplasia: three cases and review of the literature. Am Surg 35:501, 1969
134. Pollock M, Jackson BM: Fibromuscular dysplasia of the carotid arteries. Neurology (NY) 21:1226, 1971
135. Probst C: Fibromuscular hyperplasia of cerebral arteries in childhood. Monatsschr Kinderheilkd 119:604, 1971
136. Rainer WG, Cramer GG, Newby JP et al: Fibromuscular hyperplasia of the carotid artery causing positional cerebral ischemia. Ann Surg 167:444, 1968
137. Rebello M, Quintana F, Combarros O et al: Giant aneurysm of the intracavernous carotid artery and bilateral carotid fibromuscular dysplasia. (Letter.) J Neurol Neurosurg Psychiatry 46:284, 1983
138. Reddy SVR, Karnes WE, Earnest F et al: Spontaneous extracranial vertebral arteriovenous fistula with fibromuscular dysplasia. J Neurosurg 54:399, 1981
139. Rinaldi I, Harris WO, Kopp JE et al: Intracranial fibromuscular dysplasia: report of two cases, one with autopsy verification. Stroke 7:511, 1976
140. Ringel SP, Harrison SH, Norenberg MD et al: Fibromuscular dysplasia: multiple "spontaneous" dissecting aneurysms of the major cervical arteries. Ann Neurol 1:301, 1977
141. Rosenberger A, Alder O, Lichtig H: Angiographic appearance of the renal vein in a case of fibromuscular dysplasia of the artery. Radiology 118:579, 1976
142. Ross R, Klebanoff SJ: Fine structural changes in uterine smooth muscle and fibroblasts in response to estrogen. J Cell Biol 32:155, 1967
143. Ross R, Klebanoff SJ: The smooth muscle cell. I. In vivo synthesis of connective tissue proteins. J Cell Biol 50:159, 1971
144. Rothfield NJH: Experimental fibromuscular arterial dysplasia. Radiology 93:1291, 1969

145. Rushton AR: The genetics of fibromuscular arterial dysplasia. Arch Intern Med 140:233, 1980
146. Russo LS, Jr: Fibromuscular hyperplasia of the extracranial arteries: report of a case associated with intracranial aneurysm and skeletal deformities and a brief review of the literature. Mt. Sinai J Med (NY) 40:60, 1973
147. Sanchez-Torres G, Contreras R: Fibromuscular dysplasia: a genetic entity related to Ehlers-Danlos syndrome. Arch Inst Cardiol Mex 44:571, 1974
148. Sandok BA: Fibromuscular dysplasia of the internal carotid artery. p. 17. In Barnett HJM (ed): Neurology Clinics. Vol. 1. WB Saunders, Philadelphia, 1983
149. Sandok BA, Houser OW, Baker HL, Jr et al: Fibromuscular dysplasia: neurologic disorders associated with disease involving the great vessels in the neck. Arch Neurol 24:462, 1969
150. Sato S, Hata J: Fibromuscular dysplasia: its occurrence with a dissecting aneurysm of the internal carotid artery. Arch Pathol Lab Med 106:332, 1982
151. Saygi S, Bolay H, Tekkok IH et al: Fibromuscular dysplasia of the basilar artery: a case with brainstem stroke. Angiology 41:658, 1990
152. Schlagenhauff RE, Khatri A: Fibromuscular dysplasia of internal carotid arteries with Doppler ultrasonic studies. NY State J Med 83:234, 1983
153. Shields WD, Ziter FA, Osborn AG et al: Fibromuscular dysplasia as a cause of stroke in infancy and childhood. Pediatrics 59:899, 1977
154. Slagsvold JE, Bergsholm P, Larsen JL: Fibromuscular dysplasia of intracranial arteries in a patient with multiple enchondromas (Ollier disease). Neurology (NY) 27:1168, 1977
155. Smith LL, Smith DC, Killeen JD et al: Operative balloon angioplasty in the treatment of internal carotid artery fibromuscular dysplasia. J Vasc Surg 6:482, 1987
156. So EL, Toole JF, Dalal P et al: Cephalic fibromuscular dysplasia in 32 patients. Arch Neurol 38:619, 1981
157. So EL, Toole JF, Moody DM et al: Cerebral embolism from fibromuscular dysplasia of the common carotid artery. Ann Neurol 6:75, 1979
158. Sottiurai V, Fry WJ, Stanley JC: Ultrastructural characteristics of experimental arterial medial fibroplasia induced by vasa vasorum occlusion. J Surg Res 24:169, 1978
159. Sottiurai VS, Fry WJ, Stanley JC: Ultrastructure of medial smooth muscle and myofibroblasts in human arterial dysplasia. Arch Surg 113:1280, 1978
160. Stanley JC, Fry WJ, Seeger JF et al: Extracranial internal carotid and vertebral artery fibrodysplasia. Arch Surg 109:215, 1974
161. Stanley JC, Gewertz BL, Bove EL et al: Arterial fibrodysplasia: histopathologic character and current etiologic concepts. Arch Surg 110:561, 1975
162. Starr DS, Lawrie GM, Morris GC, Jr: Fibromuscular dysplasia of carotid arteries: long-term results of graduated internal dilation. Stroke 12:196, 1981
163. Stewart DR, Price RA, Nebesar R et al: Progressive peripheral fibromuscular hyperplasia in an infant: a possible manifestation of the rubella syndrome. Surgery 73:374, 1973
164. Stewart MT, Moritz MW, Smith RB et al: The natural history of carotid fibromuscular dysplasia. J Vasc Surg 3:305, 1986
165. Strian F, Backmund H: Fibromusculäre Dysplasie der Carotiden: neurologische and atiologische Aspekte. Nervenartz 43:557, 1972
166. Sukoff MH, Dorsey TJ, Johnson DA et al: Intimal fibroplasia of the internal carotid arteries. Stroke 2:483, 1971
167. Tomasello F, Cioff FA, Albanese V: Fibromuscular dysplasia of the basilar artery. Neurochirurgia 19:29, 1976
168. Upson J, Raza ST: Fibromuscular dysplasia of internal carotid arteries: graduated internal dilatation by arterial Fogarty catheter. NY State J Med 76:972, 1976
169. Vies JS, Hendriks JJ, Lodder J et al: Multiple vertebrobasilar infarctions from fibromuscular dysplasia related dissecting aneurysm of the vertebral artery in a child. Neuropediatrics 21:104, 1990
170. Wells RP, Smith RR: Fibromuscular dysplasia of the internal carotid artery: a long term follow-up. Neurosurgery 10:39, 1982
171. Welsh P, Pradier R, Repetto R: Fibromuscular dysplasia of the distal cervical internal carotid artery. J Cardiovasc Surg (Torino) 22:321, 1981
172. Wesen CA, Elliot BM: Fibromuscular dysplasia of the carotid arteries. Am J Surg 151:448, 1986
173. Wirth FP, Miller WA, Russell AP: Atypical fibromuscular hyperplasia: report of two cases. J Neurosurg 54:685, 1981
174. Wylie EG, Binkley FM, Palubinskas AJ: Extrarenal fibromuscular hyperplasia. Am J Surg 112:149, 1966
175. Wylie EJ, Perloff D, Wellington JS: Fibromuscular hyperplasia of the renal arteries. Ann Surg 156:592, 1962
176. Wylie EJ, Wellington JS: Hypertension caused by fibromuscular hyperplasia of the renal arteries. Am J Surg 100:183, 1960
177. Yamamoto I, Kageyama N, Usui K et al: Fibromuscular dysplasia of the internal carotid artery: unusual angiographic changes with progression of clinical symptoms. Acta Neurochir 50:293, 1979
178. Young PH, Smith KR, Crafts DC et al: Traumatic occlusion in fibromuscular dysplasia of the carotid artery. Surg Neurol 16:432, 1981
179. Zeumer H, Hauke R, Kotlarek F: Fibromuscular dysplasia of the internal carotid and intracerebral arteries. Dtsch Med Wochenschr 100:132, 1975
180. Zimmerman R, Leeds NE, Naidich TP: Carotid-cavernous fistula associated with intracranial fibromuscular dysplasia. Radiology 122:725, 1977

# 28
# MIGRAINE AND STROKE

Thomas K. Tatemichi
J.P. Mohr

Migraine is among the most common neurologic disorders encountered in clinical practice,[100] estimated to affect 9.1 percent of men and 16.1 percent of women in adult samples studied primarily in the United Kingdom.[107,277] In the general United States population, the annual incidence has been calculated to be approximately 250/100,000 with a point prevalence of 10 percent.[155] Frequency estimates have varied widely, in part because well-defined diagnostic criteria have been lacking. The definition provided in 1962 by the Ad Hoc Committee on Classification of Headache[3] has been supplanted by the nomenclature proposed in 1988 by the Headache Classification Committee of the International Headache Society (IHS).[127] Application of this operationalized classification should improve diagnostic consistency and specificity for both clinical and research purposes.[212] In this system migraine is defined as follows:

> Idiopathic headache disorder manifesting in attacks lasting 4–72 hours. Typical characteristics of headache are unilateral location, pulsating quality, moderate or severe intensity, aggravation by routine physical activity, and association with nausea, photo-, and phonophobia.

Various forms of migraine are recognized, generally classified according to the transient, though sometimes persistent neurologic deficits that may precede, accompany, or outlast the headache phase. In the first edition of this book, this review proposed a classification of migraine subtypes based on the duration of neurologic symptoms and their presumed topographic origin in the central nervous system. This approach is reflected to some extent in the newer definitions contained in the IHS classification (Table 28-1), which will be adopted in this chapter as a guide to the discussion on the relationship between migraine and stroke. The most fundamental taxonomic change is the distinction between *migraine without aura* (or "common migraine," as defined above) and *migraine with aura,* which includes the older terms migraine accompagnée, hemiplegic,[22] complicated,[13] ophthalmic, hemisensory, aphasic, basilar, and confusional migraine.[94,212]

For the vascular neurologist, three migraine syndromes have proved troublesome from the diagnostic standpoint, since they each mimic conventional cerebrovascular syndromes: *retinal migraine,*[43] *basilar migraine,* and *migraine, with prolonged aura.*[53,135,220,269,273] When cerebral symptoms persist beyond 1 week (as defined operationally in the IHS classification), or if brain imaging reveals an ischemic lesion, *migrainous cerebral infarction*[20,21,65,71,209,230] is a possible diagnosis, but other causes of stroke must be excluded by appropriate investigations. How often, under what circumstances, and by what mechanism(s) migraine leads to ischemic stroke has been a subject of contention.

## EPIDEMIOLOGY

Few epidemiologic studies have addressed the association between migraine and cerebrovascular disease. Leviton et al.[170] carried out a retrospective cohort study of middle-aged and elderly subjects who were parents of migraineurs, one with and the other without migraine. The risk of stroke was not elevated

**TABLE 28-1. Classification of Migraine Subtypes**

| IHS Terminology[a] (Previously Used Terms) | Main Features |
|---|---|
| Migraine without aura (common migraine) | Headache without focal neurologic symptoms |
| Migraine with aura | Headache with attacks of neurologic symptoms localizable to cerebral cortex or brain stem, developing gradually over 5–20 minutes and lasting <1 hour |
| Migraine with typical aura (ophthalmic, hemiparesthetic, hemiparetic, hemiplegic, or aphasic migraine, migraine accompaignée) | Aura consisting of homonymous visual disturbances, hemisensory symptoms, hemiparesis or dysphasia, or combinations thereof |
| Migraine with prolonged aura (complicated migraine, hemiplegic migraine) | Aura symptoms lasting >1 hour and ±7 days with normal brain imaging |
| Familial hemiplegic migraine[102] | At least one first-degree relative has identical attacks |
| Basilar migraine (basilar artery migraine, Bickerstaff's migraine, syncopal migraine) | Aura symptoms originate from brain stem or both occipital lobes |
| Migraine aura without headache (migraine equivalents, acephalgic migraine) | Aura unaccompanied by headache; when the onset is after 40 years, distinction from TIAs may be difficult |
| Migraine with acute-onset aura | Aura developing fully in <5 minutes |
| Ophthalmoplegic migraine[95] | Repeated attacks of headache associated with paresis of one or more ocular cranial nerves |
| Retinal migraine | Repeated attacks of monocular scotomata or blindness lasting <1 hour with headache |
| Childhood periodic syndromes that may be precursors to or associated with migraine | Poorly defined disorders of childhood, including benign paroxysmal vertigo and alternating hemiplegia |
| Complications of migraine | |
| Status migrainosus | Headache lasting >72 hours with or without treatment and headache-free interval <4 hours |
| Migrainous infarction (complicated migraine) | Aura symptoms not fully reversible without 7 days, and/or associated infarct on brain imaging |

[a] From the Headache Classification Committee of the International Headache Society.[127]

among the parents with migraine compared to those without, although hypertension was more frequent among migraineurs. In a case-control study of migraine as a risk factor for thromboembolic stroke in young persons (aged 15 to 65 years), Henrich and Horwitz[130] determined that a history of migraine with aura occurred in 13 percent of 89 cases and 5 percent of 178 controls, giving an odds ratio of 2.6 (confidence interval: 1.1 to 6.6). When hypertension, diabetes, or tobacco exposure was present, however, the risk of migraine was nonsignificant. In the group who had migraine and stroke, none of the strokes occurred in relation to the migraine attack; in addition, the side and vascular territory did not correlate with the neurologic symptoms occurring in previous attacks of migraine. These observations suggest that the occurrence of migraine with aura may increase the risk of stroke *unrelated* to an attack of migraine. Although this study did not find an interaction between migraine and vascular risk factors, others[48] have found that migraineurs are more likely to smoke, and that among migraineurs who smoke, the probability of ischemic heart disease is increased.

The etiologic importance of migraine in stroke can be inferred from series of young patients evaluated for ischemic stroke. Most of these studies reflect the experience of referral centers; criteria for the diagnosis of migraine or migraine-related stroke were often not well-defined; and exposure information was often obtained by retrospective review. The likely result is an overestimation of the risk. Among 1,680 young stroke patients found in 17 reports (Table 28-2), an average of 10 percent gave a history of migraine. This figure appears reasonable, as it approximates the frequency of migraine in the general population. Some of the studies made an effort to identify those cases whose infarct occurred during the course of migraine attack; among those which provided this information, an average of 7 percent (range, 0 and 20 percent) had stroke directly related to migraine, an estimate inflated slightly by the high rates reported in a few studies.[18,260] Our own experience at the Neurological Institute approximates that of Adams et al.[1] and Lisovoski and Rousseaux,[174] who found a frequency between 2 and 3 percent.

In a community-based sample, the frequency of stroke directly attributable to migraine appears to be low. Among 244 cases of first cerebral infarction encountered in Oxfordshire,[131] 18 percent gave a history of migraine, but only 3 percent were considered to have a migrainous stroke, corresponding to an annual incidence rate of 3.36/100,000 persons when extrapolated to the population at large. Based on the available epidemiologic information on disabling headache up until 1982, the conclusion of Goldstein and Chen[107] still applies today: the relationship between migraine and cerebral infarction has yet to be clearly demonstrated.

**TABLE 28-2. Frequency of Cerebral Infarction in Young Adults Associated with Migraine and Occuring During the Course of Migraine**

| Author (Ref.) | Total Cases | Age Range | History of Migraine *N* (%) | Stroke During Migraine Attack *N* (%) |
|---|---|---|---|---|
| Hindfelt & Nilsson, 1977 (138) | 64 | 16–40 | 7 (11) | 4 ( 6) |
| Grindal et al., 1978 (111) | 58 | 15–40 | 0 ( 0) | 0 ( 0) |
| Snyder & Ramirez-Lassepas, 1980 (257) | 61 | 16–49 | ( 2) | NS |
| Marshall, 1982 (179) | 114 | 10–49 | 0 ( 0) | 0 ( 0) |
| Hart & Miller, 1983 (123) | 100 | <40 | 5 ( 5) | NS |
| Hillbom & Kaste, 1983 (136) | 100 | 15–55 | 24 (24) | 9 ( 9) |
| Spaccavento & Solomon, 1984 (260) | 15 | 20–40 | 4 (27) | 3 (20) |
| Milton-Jones & Warlow, 1985 (137) | 75 | ±45 | 10 (13) | 9 (12) |
| Adams et al., 1986 (1) | 144 | 15–45 | 20 (14) | 4 ( 3) |
| Bogousslavksy & Regli, 1987 (18) | 41 | 16–29 | 6 (15) | 6 (15) |
| Alvarez et al., 1989 (6) | 386 | <50 | 19 ( 5) | 19 ( 5) |
| Gautier et al., 1989 (103) | 112 | 9–45 | 16 (14) | NS |
| Sacquena et al., 1989 (242) | 61 | ±40 | 6 (10) | 6 (10) |
| Bevan et al., 1990 (10) | 48 | 15–45 | 1 ( 2) | 1 ( 2) |
| Federico et al., 1990 (78) | 56 | 17–45 | 10 (18) | 2 ( 4) |
| Milandre et al., 1990 (190) | 100 | 16–45 | 2 ( 2) | NS |
| Lisovoski & Rousseaux, 1991 (174) | 145 | 5–40 | 25 (17) | 3 ( 2) |
| Totals (average %) | 1,680 | | 156 (10) | 66 ( 7) |

*Abbreviation:* NS, not specified in report.

While the association between migraine and stroke from the epidemiologic standpoint has been difficult to prove, it is likely that migraine with aura, perhaps with coexisting risk factors, increases the risk of ischemic stroke in some patients. Clinical evidence and the few examples from autopsy material argue for the existence of migraine-related infarction affecting the cerebral hemispheres, retina, and brain stem. Through a survey of the literature, an effort was made to identify reported cases of persisting neurologic sequelae attributed to migraine with emphasis given to those cases supported by pathologic studies or laboratory investigation.

## POTENTIAL MECHANISMS OF MIGRAINOUS INFARCTION BASED ON PATHOLOGY

Although rare, permanent hemispheral deficits ascribable to migraine have long been recognized. In 1881, Fere,[81] working with Charcot at the Salpêtrière hospital, provided one of the earliest comprehensive descriptions of the problem. He reviewed 12 patients suffering from classic migraine who also experienced language and sensorimotor symptoms. Fere[82] later reported Charcot's fatal case of a 53-year-old man with classic migraine since adolescence who developed permanent aphasia and right faciobrachial paralysis, offering the following explanation:

> Dans la migraine il existe une constriction passagère d'abord des vaisseaux sous l'influence d'un trouble du système nerveux sympathique; peu à peu la constriction devient permanente et arrive jusqu'à l'oblitération prèsque complète des vaisseaux et détermine une thrombose d'ou résulte la mort des tissus compris dans le térritoire vasculaire atteint.

Charcot[47] again emphasized this notion of cerebral ischemia as a result of vasospasm in his discussion of a case of ophthalmoplegic migraine. Among the fatal cases of migrainous cerebral infarction that have been studied at autopsy, characteristic pathologic changes have not been consistently identified. In one instance, the brain was normal,[163] including one patient subjected to craniotomy;[203] in another, nonspecific changes were reported.[200] In the 10 cases reviewed below, various abnormalities were found, suggesting multiple potential mechanisms in the pathogenesis of this cerebrovascular syndrome.

### Vasospasm With or Without Secondary Thrombosis

Buckle et al.[32] reported a fatal case whose angiogram just prior to death showed widespread narrowing. A 16-year-old girl had a 4-month history of episodic unresponsiveness during which she was restless, pale, and cold, followed by a dull headache upon regaining consciousness. She was admitted because of vomiting and progressive lethargy over 4 days, evolving into coma, accompanied by spontaneous writhing movements of all limbs and teeth grinding. Cerebrospinal fluid was normal except for a protein level of 125 mg/dl. She later developed decerebrate rigidity with eye deviation to the right. About 25 hours after the onset of coma, right carotid angiography was performed, showing severe narrowing of the supraclinoid internal carotid artery (ICA) and the anterior cerebral artery (ACA), middle cerebral artery (MCA) and posterior cerebral arteries (PCAs). The cavernous and extracranial ICAs were normal in caliber. The left ACA and MCAs were visualized with cross-compression and found to be narrowed. The patient became hypotensive and died 7 hours later. At necropsy the brain was swollen, with evidence of central and uncal herniation. No aneurysm or hematoma was found, nor was there evidence of primary vascular disease in the vessels of the white matter or cortex. Severe ischemic changes were found in the cortex, and the underlying white matter showed swollen, irregular axons. The cerebellum and brain stem were normal. The neuropathologic changes were not attributable to hypotension, since laminar necrosis was not seen. Although the exact clinical diagnosis was not firm, alternative explanations were lacking and the authors considered the previous attacks possibly migrainous.

Two other cases support the possibility of vasospasm, but the conclusions are inferential. Lindboe et al.[173] studied a 50-year-old woman who had a severe, week-long attack of migraine treated with ergotamine, followed by the abrupt onset of left hemiparesis and somnolence. Early CT scanning revealed slight edema in the region supplied by the right MCA, progressing over days to midline shift and herniation. Angiography was not performed. Pathologic examination showed severe edema and acute infarction involving the basal ganglia and overlying cortex. The right ACA territory was spared. Both extracranial and intracranial arteries were free of pathologic changes. The heart and systemic vessels were normal. The authors proposed the mechanism of thrombosis superimposed on vasospasm due to the combination of migraine and ergotamine, with spontaneous fibrinolysis explaining the absence of occlusive disease on postmortem examination.

Thrombosis of the middle cerebral artery was found in the case of Selby and Fryer,[246] which they felt was a secondary to vasospasm. A 58-year-old woman had suffered frequent attacks of migraine with visual aura since her youth. A typical attack occurred while playing bowls, accompanied by flexor spasms of the left hand. After sleeping for an hour, she awoke with a left faciobrachial paresis and anosognosia, which worsened after admission to the hospital. The following day she was stuporous, and developed conjugate eye deviation to the right with left hemiplegia. Computed tomography (CT) revealed an extensive low-density area in the right frontoparietal cortex with midline shift. Despite antiedema therapy, her condition progressed to coma with decerebrate posturing. At autopsy the hemispheres were swollen with evidence of central and uncal herniation. A large, pale infarct was evident in the right MCA and adjacent territories with features indicating ischemic damage of several days duration. All major vessels of the circle of Willis were unremarkable except for the right MCA, which contained a thrombus of recent origin (estimated 2 days) without evidence of organization, inferred to have developed from stasis related to vasospasm. No systemic or cardiovascular disease was identified.

## Arteriopathy, Including Vascular Hyperplasia

Oppenheim's case[216] as cited by Hunt[143] was that of a 35-year-old woman who suffered from migraine since childhood. Four months after pregnancy, she had an attack of migraine accompanied by transient aphasia, followed by four similar attacks. During the last episode, she was aphasic and delirious with a right hemiplegia. Autopsy showed infarction of the left cerebral hemisphere, produced by thrombosis of the left ICA near the origin of the MCA. Microscopic examination of the vessel wall showed a distinct endarteritis, with thickening of the adventitia. Hunt proposed a preexisting organic defect in the vessel wall, which could not withstand the acute vascular disturbances associated with migraine.

The only other instance demonstrating a possible vasculopathy was a patient with familial hemiplegic migraine, who died following a respiratory arrest. Neligan et al.[206] reported a 41-year-old woman who suffered from repeated, hour-long episodes of unilateral frontal headache followed by numbness and weakness of the contralateral face and limbs, accompanied by dysphasia. About 36 hours before admission she awoke with severe right temporal headache, followed within minutes by left arm weakness. On admission she was drowsy, irritable, and photophobic with a stiff neck and a moderate left hemiparesis. She developed frequent seizures. Spinal fluid examination and bilateral cerebral angiography were normal. She remained in a persistent vegetative state until death 4 months later. At autopsy cystic infarcts in the head of the left caudate nucleus and putamen and a granular infarct in the head of the right caudate nucleus were found. Histologic examination confirmed the varying ages of the infracts. Most of the small arteries were normal, but within or near the infarcts some vessels were thick-walled and showed subintimal hyperplasia and reduplication of elastic lamina in vessel walls. Examination of the heart and extracranial arteries was unremarkable. The deep microinfarcts were attributed to the previous attacks of migrainous hemiplegia, presumed to be a result of spasm.

These reports raise the possibility that repeated attacks of severe migraine, presumably accompanied by vasospasm may lead to focal arterial injury, whether an "endarteritis" or intimal proliferation and media myonecrosis, comparable to that observed as a result of spasm induced by subarachnoid hemorrhage.[54,79,141] These arterial changes may in turn predispose to thrombosis (as suggested above), or in some cases distal embolization (see below). The autopsied case of familial hemiplegic migraine is exceptional for its demonstration of small, deep infarcts, a distinctly uncommon site of migrainous cerebral infarction, indicating that lenticulostriate arteropathy may be one mechanism, a hypothesis favored by Bruyn.[29–31]

## Embolism

Cases clinically resembling cerebral embolism have been amply described, in many instances with acute hemiplegia so swift in onset that patients reported falling.[15,49,286] The clinicopathologic features of the patient reported by Guest and Woolf,[114] a frequently cited example of the malignant consequences of migraine, are consistent with this mechanism. A 28-year-old man had a 2-year history of severe headaches associated with nausea but unaccompanied by neurologic symptoms. He suddenly became unresponsive with right-sided weakness while having a meal; death occurred 20 hours after the onset of coma. At autopsy the cortex of the left superior and middle frontal convolutions were stippled with petechial hemorrhage and showed ischemic changes microscopically. Widespread ischemic changes were also seen in the left insula, paracentral lobule, and postcentral gyrus. Patchy areas of ischemic changes were found in the brain stem, including the substantia nigra, both pontine reticular nuclei, and the spinal tract of the 5th nerve. The left ICA was patent up to its bifurcation; the left ACA and MCA were also normal. Guest and Wolf concluded that infarction occurred in the territory of the left ACA, presumably due to migrainous vasospasm with no structural abnormalities of the blood vessels.

Another example of pathologically verified cerebral infarction associated with migraine, but clinically compatible with embolism, is Polyak's report.[227] In his late twenties, Dr. Frank B. Mallory began to suffer recurrent attacks of scintillating scotoma in the left visual field, sometimes accompanied by nausea. "At the approximate age of forty-seven, on a Sunday in the summer of 1910 while at dinner, immediately after the reflection from a white surface of bright sunlight into the patient's eyes, he began to complain of brilliant flashes recurring at very frequent intervals, leaving within a few hours—at any rate in less than a day—a visual field defect. The defect, according to the patient's estimate, was at first large, but subsequently it "cleared." The duration of this attack was approximately from 20 to 40 minutes." One year after this episode an ophthalmologist, consulted for another reason, found a large hemianopic scotoma in the left upper field. At age 71, another ophthalmologic examination disclosed an absolute left upper homonymous quadrantic defect extending from the fixation point along the vertical meridian for 10 degrees and along the horizontal meridian for 20 degrees. At autopsy an old infarct confined to the lower calcarine lip on the right was found. Serial sections of the main stem of the calcarine artery and its continuation revealed no occlusions.

One of Shuabib's five cases[249] was a 42-year-old woman who experienced the sudden onset of right hemiparesis and aphasia while being examined for a bout of severe migraine headaches. There was a history of migraine without aura. Initial echocardiographic studies suggested mitral valve thickening, but this was not confirmed on two subsequent examinations. Cerebral angiogram revealed occlusion of a left MCA branch. A second infarction involving the right cerebral hemisphere occurred 2 weeks later complicated by disseminated intravascular coagulation, leading to death. At autopsy no sign of cerebral atherosclerotic or other occlusive disease was evident. However, systemic examination showed advanced carcinoma of the cervix with marantic endocarditis and evidence of embolization to other organs.

Despite the lack of pathologically verified arterial thromboembolism in any of the cases, the abrupt onset during activity (in one case with premonitory headache), the presence of hemorrhagic infarction in one case, and evidence for a cardiac source of embolism in another case are consistent with cerebral embolism. How often cerebral infarction in the setting of migraine is related to cardiogenic embolism is uncertain, although Centonze et al.[46] have argued that prolapsed mitral valve accounts for the majority of ischemic focal deficits in migraineurs. Moreover, it is unclear if the pathophysiology of migraine itself can account for embolism, although hemispheral stroke syndromes resembling embolism have also been recognized in instances of vasospasm complicating subarachnoid hemorrhage,[195] suggesting a possible parallel mechanism in some cases of migrainous vasospasm.

## Arterial Dissection

Sinclair[253] reported a 27-year-old migraineur with a nontraumatic dissecting aneurysm of the MCA, which he ascribed to migraine in the absence of pathologic evidence for congenital vascular anomaly, arteriosclerosis, arteritis, or cystic medial necrosis. The patient had been affected for several years with episodes of right-sided facial and retro-ocular pain refractory to ergot medication. At 16 hours before admission, she experienced her usual headache, followed 8 hours later by paresthesias of all limbs, weakness of both hands, and tongue numbness. Initially lethargic and confused without lateralizing signs, she developed a flaccid left hemiplegia within 24 hours and died 3 days later. At autopsy the right frontal and parietal lobes showed recent infarction. The right MCA, 1 cm from its origin, showed dark red discoloration for a 2-cm distance and was enlarged, firm, and stiff. Microscopically, there was dissection of the media without medial necrosis; the elastic lamina was intact, and there was no intimal tear. Sinclair considered the local vascular alterations in the course of a migraine attack, in particular, the vasodilatory phase as suggested by early experimental studies[271] contributed to the development of dissection.

Shuabib[249] described a 29-year-old man who had a long history of migraine with and without aura. He developed a typical unilateral headache, prompting him to leave work. Several hours later, the headache intensified, accompanied by involuntary spasms of the left limbs. Initially awake and alert, he showed intermittent decerebrate posturing on the left. By the next day, he became comatose. Initial CT of the head was normal. Angiography was also normal, except for an uncertain irregularity in the lumen of the basilar artery. Subsequent CT revealed bilateral superior cerebellar infarcts, confirmed at autopsy, which was performed when he died from sepsis 6 weeks later. In addition, there were bilateral pontine infarcts. The basilar artery at the junction of its upper and lower two-thirds showed a 5-mm region of hemorrhagic discoloration, accounted for by a small dissection in the media, seen on cross section, reducing the lumen to 10 percent of its original size.

Whether dissection occurs as part of the migrainous process, serves as the trigger for the migraine attack or is an unrelated, coincidental phenomenon, cannot be determined from these cases. One unconfirmed report suggests that migraineurs may be predisposed to arterial dissection.

## CLINICAL STUDIES OF MIGRAINOUS INFARCTION WITH LABORATORY INVESTIGATIONS

Scattered clinical examples were reported prior to the 1950s describing serious neurologic consequences of migraine, usually permanent visual field defects[35,120,143,217,234,236,268,280,290] suspected but not documented to be ischemic in origin. Not only was thrombosis related to vasoconstriction considered a sequelae of migraine, but also intracerebral and subarachnoid hemorrhage, presumed related to repeated vasodilation,[68] were recorded,[68,106] in some instances documented by autopsy.[4,38,61,223] Despite the demonstration of aneurysm in some of these latter reports, the link between migraine and cerebral hemorrhage is currently thought to be coincidental, having little biologic plausibility and no support from large series defining the prevalence of migraine among patients with documented aneurysm[276] or angioma.[16] (For headaches associated with arteriovenous malformations, see Ch. 23.)

Clinical reports in the last 40 years, however, have provided more convincing demonstration of the association between migraine and cerebral infarction, especially those cases documented with the use of angiography and CT. Metabolic imaging has been used rarely, and studies with transcranial Doppler,[267] while promising, are still preliminary and difficult to interpret.[213] Unfortunately, little corroborating evidence has been accrued to support fully any of the possible mechanisms inferred from pathologic data, and many of the early reports fail to describe an exclusionary evaluation, limiting our confidence in assigning a causal relationship.

### Angiographic Case Reports and Series

Cerebral angiography has typically revealed *no abnormalities,*[19,44] depending partly on the timing of the study, or *intracranial arterial occlusions.*[77] Among the earliest reports, Symonds[265] described two cases with hemiplegia and one with persisting hemianopia. The latter patient, a 54-year-old man with classic migraine since childhood, awoke with a typical visual aura consisting of wavy lines in the right visual field. Instead of spreading across the whole field, the lines were confined to the right and persisted for 6 months. Unlike the usual attacks, no headache ensued in the acute phase of the deficit. Angiography performed at 6 months later showed no abnormality. Myhrman's case[204] was subjected to angiography on two separate occasions, once after a partial field defect and then a year later when the patient presented with generalized seizures. In both instances the study was normal. Pearce and Foster[220] reported 40 cases, investigated for various symptoms, including persisting visual field or sensorimotor disturbances, ophthalmoplegia, recurrent unilateral headaches confined to the same side, carotid or intracranial bruit, meningeal symptoms, or epilepsy occurring during an attack. Hemispheral symptoms occurred in 19 patients, 12 of whom had deficits persisting beyond 24 hours. Ten patients had visual symptoms, six with field defects consistent with occipital ischemia.[219] Among 29 angiograms performed, 2 vascular malformations were detected, but these cases had unusual features, including loss of consciousness and seizures.

Brain[23] described five cases with permanent hemianopia attributed to migraine among a total of 200 patients admitted to the hospital with a stroke syndrome. In one case, not described clinically, angiography revealed a *PCA occlusion.* Connor's[53] report of 18 cases identified three groups of patients with "complicated migraine," a term he originated. Five patients had retinal deficits, ten had hemispheral deficits, and three had deficits localized to the brain stem. Among the eight hemispheral cases studied by angiography, two showed occlusions. One of these cases was a 26-year-old man who suffered attacks of vertigo, teichopsia, frontal headache, and vomiting. On one occasion, he experienced left focal paresthesias with weakness. After a week-long period of constant headache, he developed giddiness, abrupt left hemiplegia, and homonymous hemianopia. Angiography of the carotid and vertebral arteries failed to fill the right PCA. Seven months later, he developed focal motor epilepsy; examination showed residual sensorimotor deficits and an incomplete left field cut. Repeat angiography showed normal filling of both PCAs. An investigation for cardiac disease was not described. Among the remaining cases most developed a defect (7 of 10) during the course of a migrainous attack and most (7 of 10) experienced preceding transient neurologic symptoms similar to the persisting deficit. Connor observed, as others prior to him remarked, that there was a predilection for occipital cortex involvement (6 of 10). In only one case was the use of ergotamine considered a causative factor.

In correlating angiographically defined arterial occlusions in the PCA territory with permanent visual field defects, Kaul et al.[153] reported a series of 19 patients, 4 of whom had syndromes attributed to migraine. One of their patients was a 42-year-old woman who had an occlusion of the main trunk of the PCA presenting with right hemianopia, hemianesthesia, spontaneous pain, transient amnesia, and dysphasia. The remaining three had branch *occlusions of the calcarine artery*, producing pure quadrantic defects. In each case, a prominent, though transient, visual disturbance was a feature of the previous migraine attacks, and the permanent deficit occurred during the course of a severe migraine. Among the 35 patients with occipital infarction reported by Pessin et al.,[222] five had strokes attributed to migraine; in two patients, *intraluminal thrombus* in the PCA was demonstrated angiographically, a finding also reported in the single case encountered by Moen et al.[193]

Despite the increasing refinement in angiographic techniques, the report by Boisen[20] demonstrates the difficulty of interpreting abnormal radiographic findings in the context of permanent migrainous deficits. A 47-year-old patient had carotid stenosis whose migraine attacks improved with anticoagulation, and another patient had vertebral artery occlusion in the setting of thrombocytosis. Similarly, among the nine cases presented by Davis-Jones et al.[62] a 40-year-old hypertensive woman with visual spells developed aphasia with angiography showing a left MCA occlusion; no cardiac evaluation was specified.

Rare instances of *vasospasm* documented by angiogram have been reported, among the first by Dukes and Vieth.[67] A 44-year-old man suffered from episodes of left hemianopia and hemianesthesia, followed by a throbbing right-sided headache. The patient underwent angiography at a time when he was asymptomatic. Initial right carotid artery views showed good intracranial filling. Following this injection, he developed scotoma in both visual fields without sensory loss, reaching a peak at 15 minutes. At that point, repeat filming revealed decreased filling of the internal carotid artery system. Over the ensuing 30 minutes, symptoms cleared completely followed by a typical right-sided headache. A third set of films then showed good intracranial filling. Fifteen minutes later, he developed a left hemiplegia, clearing within an hour. Thus, at a time when the focal deficit was maximal, there was evidence of vasospasm with reversal to normal vessel caliber during the headache phase. Another example of reversible vasospasm, involving the extracranial ICAs bilaterally as well as MCA branches, was documented by Lieberman et al.,[171] whose patient was a 39-year-old woman with attacks of headaches and left-sided weakness. Although the right ICA occlusion demonstrated initially had the appearance of carotid dissection, repeat angiography 4 days later revealed reopening of the previously occluded artery, with focal narrowing of the left ICA.

An anomolous finding was reported by Masuzawa et al.,[180] whose patient, a 27-year-old postpartum migraineur, was studied because of severe recurrent headache with vomiting. Angiography on the right revealed widespread *vasodilation* of the intracranial ICA, but no abnormalities of the external carotid. Repeat studies when the headache had subsided showed segmental narrowing of the ACA and MCA. Garnic and Schellinger[99] recounted their unusual experience demonstrating vasospasm-induced headache in a 33-year-old woman whom they considered to have cluster headaches. She had severe, sharp, brief retro-orbital pain unaccompanied by autonomic symptoms. Vertigo and nystagmus were present on right lateral gaze. After four vessel-selective injections were uneventfully performed, a repeat right internal carotid artery injection led to spasm of the ICA, MCA, and ACA accompanied by retro-orbital pain.

Other unusual cases, similar to those above, have been brought to attention by Call et al.,[39] who summarized 19 patients in the literature, including four of their own, with a clinical-angiographic syndrome labeled *reversible cerebral segmental vasoconstriction.* The salient clinical feature was sudden, high-intensity headache resembling the headache of aneurysmal rupture associated with nausea, vomiting, and photophobia occurring in young women. Seizures were sometimes observed around the time of headache onset, followed by resolving sensorimotor disturbances, although a few had persisting focal deficits. Most had a normal cerebrospinal fluid, and in no case was an infectious or aneurysmal cause uncovered. In the six who underwent autopsy or biopsy, including one of their own cases, histopathology was normal. Angiographic findings were characteristic, showing severe narrowing of the arteries leading to or emerging from the circle of Willis, alternating with regions of dilatation or normal vessel caliber. In some cases smaller cortical arteries were similarly involved. These findings appeared fully reversible on repeat angiography, and did not always correlate with the headaches. An unusually severe form of migraine was suspected, possibly precipitated by hormonal factors.

## Clinical Studies with Anatomic and Metabolic Brain Imaging

The widespread use of CT scanning beginning in the mid-1970s permitted documentation of lesions compatible with *cerebral infarction,* in many cases correlated with angiogram. Reports of single cases[150,199,237] or small series[34,59,184,245,262] have all shown low-density lesions of the cerebral cortex, most commonly in the occipital lobe. In radiologic series of selected migrainous patients with or without focal neurologic deficits (Table 28-3), the frequency of low-density lesions consistent with stroke has averaged about 4 percent (range, 0 to 19 percent). Cala and Mastaglia[37] examined 94 patients with a history of "recurrent migrainous headaches" of whom six showed evidence of cerebral infarction. Four of these patients had fixed visual field defects with mesial occipital low densities. *Cerebral edema,* particularly in the periventricular white matter, was evident in another six patients, a finding they had emphasized in an earlier report.[36] Of the 49 migrainous patients studied, 21 had evidence of low attentuation in the white matter, most extensive in the hemisphere on the side of the headache and contralateral to the sensory aura or signs. This finding corroborated the initial report by Baker,[8] who described diffuse low-density zones during a migraine attack, which disappeared on subsequent CT examination.

Hungerford et al.[142] studied 53 patients who had "exceptionally severe" migraine or serious clinical complications, including hemiplegia. The most frequently encountered abnormality was *cerebral atrophy,* seen in 14 patients, of whom 8 showed focal changes. Infarction was seen in six patients. Among 13 patients who had permanent neurologic deficits, 11 had abnormal scans. The high frequency of cerebral atrophy was confirmed in the series of du Boulay et al.[66] Mathew and coworkers[181,182] found abnormal scans in 12 of 31 patients with various migraine types. Of the three with common migraine, one had evidence of multiple infarction and two showed mild to moderate *hydrocephalus.* Two of the three patents with classical migraine showed focal cortical atrophy, and the third had mild ventricular enlargement. Two patients with basilar migraine both showed moderately severe hydrocephalus and one also showed multiple infarction. All four patients with migraine and hemiparesis showed low-density lesions in regions of the cerebral cortex consistent with their clinical syndrome.

Studies using magnetic resonance imaging (MRI) have generally corroborated these earlier findings. Among 17 migraineurs with and without aura examined by Sorges et al.,[259] 41 percent had parenchymal abnormalities consisting of focal regions of increased signal intensity in the cerebral white matter on T2-weighted studies. The lesions resembled those seen in multiple sclerosis or small-vessel atherosclerotic disease. In seven patients with complicated migraine, four showed unilateral cerebral or cerebellar lesions. Using a case-control method, Ferbert et al.[80] showed that "subcortical patchy lesions" were more frequent in patients suffering from more than 20 attacks of migraine with aura compared to age-matched subjects free of migraine.

Although cerebral edema has been invoked as one cause of transient focal deficits related to migraine,[121,181] those cases demonstrating infarcts and arterial occlusions should dispel any doubts about the pathologic process involved in permanent focal deficits. Bousser et al.[21] provided confirmatory and novel evidence for an ischemic process using positron emission tomography in their study of a 45-year-old man with a long history of classic migraine. In this instance the focal deficit, a pure right hemianopia, occurred on awakening followed by severe generalized headache. CT showed a contrast-enhancing low-density lesion in the left occipital lobe, and an unenhanced lesion in the left temporal cortex, suggesting a subclinical old infarct. Cerebral angiography, performed 21 days after onset, was normal. Oxygen extraction and cerebral blood flow (CBF) (to a lesser

**TABLE 28-3. Frequency of Computed Tomography Scan Abnormalities in Migraineurs**

| Author (Ref.) | Total Cases | Migraine Type | Focal or Diffuse Atrophy *N* (%) | Low-Density Regions *N* (%) | Cerebral Edema *N* (%) | Other *N* (%) |
|---|---|---|---|---|---|---|
| Baker, 1975 (8) | 11 | NS | 2 (18) | 0 ( 0) | 2 ( 2) | 0 ( 0) |
| Cala and Mastaglia, 1976 (36) | 49 | NS | 8 (16) | 6 (12) | 21 (43) | 2 ( 4) |
| Hungerford et al., 1976 (142) | 53 | ± Aura | 14 (26) | 6 (11) | 1 ( 2) | 5 ( 9) |
| Mathew, 1978 (181) | 31 | ± Aura | 11 (35) | 6 (19) | 0 ( 0) | 0 ( 0) |
| Cala and Mastaglia, 1980 (37) | 94 | NS | 11 (12) | 6 ( 6) | 6 ( 6) | 2 ( 2) |
| Ruiz et al., 1982 (241) | 22 | ± Aura | 8 (36) | 0 ( 0) | 0 ( 0) | 0 ( 0) |
| Sargent and Solbach, 1983 (244) | 88 | ± Aura | 10 (11) | 2 ( 2) | 0 ( 0) | 2 ( 2) |
| du Boulay et al., 1983 (66) | 53 | ± Aura | 36 (68) | 4 ( 8) | 0 ( 0) | 3 ( 6) |
| Cuetter and Aita, 1983 (60) | 435 | ± Aura | 0 ( 0) | 0 ( 0) | 0 ( 0) | 1 (0.2) |
| Totals (average %) | 836 | | 100 (12) | 30 ( 4) | 30 ( 4) | 15 ( 2) |

*Abbreviations:* NS, not specified in report; ± Aura, with and without aura.

extent) were reduced in the left occipital cortex, typical of recent infracts, while in the temporal lobe, CBF was increased with normal oxygen extraction. The former finding was considered compatible with luxury perfusion and the latter with reactive hyperemia. Unexplained supernormal oxygen extraction occurred in the asymptomatic right occipital lobe. Intriguing evidence for a primary vascular process was reported by Herold et al.,[132] who found focally *increased oxygen extraction* but reduced blood flow and normal metabolism in a 23-year-old patient experiencing a migraine attack with aura. Further clarification of the migrainous ischemic process will depend on more detailed studies, however difficult they are to perform, defining the relationship among cerebral metabolism, flow, and clinical symptoms.

## Case Series of Migrainous Infarction

Perhaps the most convincing reports of migrainous cerebral infarction documented by CT scanning, angiography, and, where appropriate, a cardiac and hematologic evaluation were initially reported by Dorfman et al.[65] and Rascol et al.[230] In the first series, four adults ranging in age from 16 to 32 years were evaluated among 66 cases of CT-confirmed cerebral infarction. One case, a 25-year-old man with a 5-year history of headaches associated with left visual obscuration, is especially well documented. Following the onset of an episode with characteristic photophobia and right temporal headaches, he went to sleep and awoke 2 hours later, noticing weakness and numbness of the limbs on the left and visual difficulty to the left. Examination showed no behavioral disturbance except mild irritability, a left hemianopia, and a mild left sensorimotor deficit. The cerebrospinal fluid (CSF) was normal. An electroencephalogram (EEG) showed posterior slowing on the right. CT scan 4 days after onset revealed a low density in the posterior medial portion of the right temporal lobe, becoming less prominent with enhancement. A cerebral angiogram showed a branch occlusion of the right PCA, and no other abnormalities. Other studies, including echocardiography, collagen vascular screening, routine coagulation profile, and blood cultures, were all negative. CT in the remaining three patients showed a large, deep infarct in one, an enhancing insular cortex lesion in another, and a hemorrhagic infarct in the third.

Rascol and colleagues[230,231] reported 10 cases (mean age, 33 years) with CT-confirmed cerebral infarction occurring in the course of a migraine attack. Three conditions were required for the diagnosis of migrainous cerebral infarction: (1) a previous history of migraine attacks conforming to the Ad Hoc Committee's definition, (2) close chronologic relationship between the migraine attack and the prolonged or persisting neurologic disorder, and (3) exclusion of other vascular diseases or predisposing disorders, such as vascular malformation, atherosclerotic risk factors (e.g., hypertension, diabetes, hyperlipidemia), atherosclerotic lesions on cerebral angiography, exposure to oral contraceptives, signs of ergotism, and infectious, inflammatory, hematologic or immunologic diseases associated with cerebral thrombosis. Six cases had MCA syndromes, while four had hemianopic defects due to PCA territory infarctions. Angiogram was performed in each patient between 2 days and 6 months from stroke onset and was abnormal in nine, showing ICA occlusion in one case, MCA or PCA stem occlusions in four cases, and branch occlusions in four cases.

In the past 5 years, interest in migrainous infarction has burgeoned. Among three recent reports,[19,26,239] 64 patients are newly described but investigated with a variable degree of completeness. Inclusion criteria have differed, and none has strictly conformed to the new IHS definitions. In the Mayo Clinic series,[26] 7 of their 20 patients (mean age, 28 years) developed migraine after the stroke; the remaining patients with either classic or common migraine were included if the attending neurologist attributed the stroke to the migraine attack. Echocardiography was performed in only four patients, and vascular risk factors were evident in several patients, including tobacco exposure (7), hypertension (2), hyperlipidemia (1), oral contraceptive use (3), and pregnancy or recent childbirth (2). Angiography revealed a range of findings similar to those previously cited: normal (7), single-branch occlusions (1), multiple-branch occlusion (1), and intraluminal thrombus (1). There was a predilection for the PCA territory. Using the Rochester, Minnesota population under 50 years of age as a base, these investigators estimated that migraine accounted for 25 percent (3 of 12) of all incident cases of cerebral infarction in young patients, and that the recurrence rate was 1 to 2 percent per year. Given the limitations in the data, Broderick and Swanson[26] acknowledged that "it is more accurate to say that a patient had a stroke of unknown cause in conjunction with a migraine attack rather than a stroke secondary to migraine."

Rothrock et al.[240] reported 22 patients (mean age, 35 years) using criteria similar to that of Rascol et al.[230] The series included patients with hypertension (4), tobacco exposure (6), oral contraceptive (3) or ergotamine use (3), and mitral valve prolapse (1). Angiography was performed in 12 patients, revealing abnormalities in 5: ICA stenosis at C2; bilateral ACA, MCA, and vertebral spasm (in a patient with right thalamic hematoma); distal CCA occlusion; "luxury perfusion"; and "beading of the PCA" with delayed filling of the calcarine branch. Based on these findings, we agree with the authors' conclusions that "the diagnosis of migrainous stroke should . . . require . . . a healthy dose of skepticism."

The controlled and systematic investigations reported by Bogousslavksy et al.[19] in 22 patients with classic migraine (mean age, 33 years) who suffered a stroke during the course of an attack warrant serious attention. Detailed cardiac and vascular studies were performed prospectively in most of their cases. Two control groups were also studied, including stroke patients with a history of migraine temporally unrelated to the stroke (22 patients) and stroke subjects without a migraine history (22 subjects). Vascular risk factors were evident in all groups, but did not differ between cases and controls. Those with migrainous infarction more often showed evolution of deficits over 1 to 2 hours compared to the controls, with the PCA territory more frequent in cases than controls (41 percent vs 9 percent). Surprisingly, mitral valve prolapse occurred more frequently in controls than cases (45 percent vs 9 percent). Cerebral angiogram was normal in 19 of the 22 cases studied, while dissection (27 percent) and distal intracranial arterial occlusion (32 percent) were the most frequent findings in controls. While referral bias could account for these latter differences, the conclusion is inescapable that "migraine itself was the most important phenomenon causing cerebral infarction" in the study group.

Finally, *migrainous infarction in childhood* has also been described. Ment et al.[188] reported three children aged 8 to 14 who developed stroke syndromes attributed to migraine with headache as a prominent feature. Angiography in one patient showed a PCA occlusion. The patient reported by Castaldo et al.[45] was a 7-year-old boy who presented with a gradually progressive syndrome consisting of dysphasia and right hemiplegia preceded by severe headaches. An occlusion of the MCA was visualized on angiography. Rossi et al.[239] identified seven children aged 4 to 14 with stroke attributed to migraine, using the criteria of Bogousslavsky et al.[19] Transient segmental narrowing was seen in two cases subjected to serial angiography. Three patients had PCA territory infarctions.

## Critique and Synthesis

Ample evidence has accumulated from both the autopsy literature and recent laboratory-supported case reports indicating that persistent neurologic deficits associated with migraine are the result of cerebral infarction. Whether vasospasm is the primary and only mechanism involved is unsettled. The view that migraine is a vasospastic disorder seems now so well entrenched in neurologic thinking that consideration of alternative mechanisms to account for ischemic complications might be regarded as a challenge to central dogma.[108,134] Nonetheless, direct evidence for vasospasm, of the larger arteries at least, is limited, depending on the weight given to the few angiographic reports reviewed above. Although it is clear that reductions in cerebral blood flow occur,[117,183,208,211,243,254,255] flows below levels critical for normal neuronal metabolism have only rarely been documented.[161,162] It has been suggested that flow reductions have been underestimated because of technical reasons,[256] but more importantly, that there may be an instability of vascular tone during a migraine attack, which may lead to ischemic flow declines intermittently.[93] The relevance of spreading neuronal depression, a phenomenon described by Leao,[165] and considered by Milner[192] to be a possible explanation for the migrainous aura based on Lashley's descriptions[160] of his own attacks, has also been reinvestigated.[30] The recent demonstration[161,214] of spreading oligemia[215] or hypoperfusion,[213] using the cerebral blood flow methods as a wave passing from the occipital cortex anteriorly at a rate of 2 mm/min beginning before the onset of focal neurologic symptoms, suggests that flow reductions may be a secondary effect of a primary neurogenic process whose origins possibly lie in dysfunction of the hypothalamus or lower brain stem centers, including the locus ceruleus.[158] Presumably, flow alterations occur at the level of arterioles or capillaries,[157] a concept supported by the absence of significant caliber changes in large arteries seen on angiography during attacks with aura,[93,148,161,215] and recent studies showing reduction in flow velocity in the ipsilateral MCA measured by transcranial Doppler unaccompanied by changes in cerebral blood flow.[92] Neurogenic control of the cerebral microcirculation in vasospastic disorders including migraine, subarachnoid hemorrhage, and possibly eclampsia and hypertensive encephalopathy, is likely mediated by a variety of neuropeptides, including 5-hydroxytryptamine, which also play a role in central nociception.[250,252]

Whether these pathophysiologic considerations can fully account for the focal infarctions related to migraine seems doubtful. Migrainous infarction is likely the consequence of diverse pathophysiologic events,[284] including "migraine-mimics."[249] Some examples of large-artery occlusions in the extracranial arteries or stems of the major cerebral vessels seem best explained by cardiogenic embolism or arterial dissection. In other instances, it is likely that an unrelated thromboembolic episode triggers spreading hypoperfusion and migrainous aura symptoms. To what extent vasospasm also plays a role in large-artery occlusions is uncertain, including whether superimposed thromboembolism may occur in this setting. In most cases of infarction evolving during a migraine attack, it seems more plausible to consider that occlusions occur primarily in smaller vessels, either from small particle thromboembolism, in situ thrombosis, or vasospasm, exacerbating (or even provoked by) the ischemic flow levels in the microcirculation induced by spreading oligemia. It has been suggested that occlusion of these smaller vessels, invisible to angiography, may lead to increased downstream resistance and stasis in proximal feeding arteries, perhaps accounting indirectly for some examples of large-artery occlusions in migrainous infarction with major territorial damage.[193] Other factors predisposing to thrombosis may be contributory. The syndrome of migraine with aura represents not only hypothalamic and brain stem dysfunction, but also a platelet disorder, at least in certain individuals.[119] Hyperaggregability, manifested by a lower threshold for the platelet release reaction and increased stickiness, has been documented in migraineurs compared to a control group[56] as well as in subjects with migraine complications.[151] During attacks of migraine, whether or not complicated by neurologic symptoms, both plasma coagulability and platelet aggregability are increased.[152] Prodromal changes in aggregability have also been observed.[63] Thus, it is reasonable to suppose that release of vasoactive substances from platelets or some other prothrombotic tendency could further aggravate the cascade of ischemic events, leading to cerebral infarction.[282]

## RETINAL OR OCULAR MIGRAINE

While transient homonymous scintillations or fortification scotoma are well-recognized cortical migrainous phenomena, monocular visual loss from retinal involvement is less often a manifestation of migraine.[55] It is nonetheless a differential diagnostic problem in the patient presenting with amaurosis fugax.[105] Since both retinal and ciliary circulations may be affected, the term "ocular migraine" has been preferred by some authors,[55] as distinguished from the term "ophthalmic migraine" referring to any migrainous disturbance of vision whether ocular or cortical.[73,182] In addition, optic nerve dysfunction may occur as well, prompting Troost[272] to suggest the broader term "anterior visual pathway migraine." The ambiguity resulting from these overlapping terms has been addressed in part by the IHS classification[127] which recognizes only "retinal migraine" as a distinct entity, defined by repeated attacks of fully reversible monocular scotoma or blindness lasting less than 1 hour, associated with headache following (or preceding) the attack within an hour, with appropriate investigations excluding ocular or structural vascular disorders but especially embolism. In some cases headache may not occur.

Carroll[43] considered the syndrome of retinal migraine an uncommon disorder, usually occurring in a young adult who experiences recurrent and unaccompanied episodes of visual loss or dimness in one or both eyes almost never exceeding 10 minutes in duration, but rarely persisting for an hour or more. He emphasized the usual absence of preceding fortification spectra, the invariable absence of headache and the nearly invariable return to normal visual function, although with repeated attacks a permanent visual defect may develop. While typical attacks of classic or common migraine occasionally occur at other times, the visual disturbance without headache may be the predominant or sole manifestation of a migrainous disorder.

Subsequent reports have generally corroborated these points; the co-occurrence of headache or the presence of scintillations in other cases have helped to stamp the disorder as migrainous. In children Hachinski and colleagues[118] encountered 7 out of 100 cases with monocular symptoms in the setting of headache. Except for their unilateral occurrence, the visual disturbances consisted of obscurations and scotomas similar to those in patients with binocular symptoms. Among 83 young adults with a mean age of 26 years who were studied retrospectively, Tippin et al.[270] found headache temporally associated with transient monocular visual loss in 41 percent; an additional 25 percent had headaches apart from the visual loss. In follow-up, none of the 42 patients who were reexamined after a mean period of 5.8 years had cerebrovascular complications, leading to the conclusion that transient blindness, presumably of migrainous origin in most of their patients, was a benign disorder. On the other hand, among a group of older adults, Hedges[128,129] identified 33 patients with a mean age of 53 years who had purely monocular attacks from 129 cases with ophthalmic symptoms. Interestingly, when followed for periods of between 5 and 10 years, the patients with monocular symptoms had a 45 percent incidence of vascular complications (not further specified), in contrast to 13 percent seen in the group with homonymous complaints. This observation serves as a cautionary note: while migrainous transient monocular blindness may occur for the first time in a patient over 50, carotid atherosclerosis is probably the more likely cause.[2]

The pathophysiology of transient monocular visual loss occurring in the setting of migraine is poorly understood. Walsh and Hoyt[275] have asserted that "the eye itself can be involved in the angiospastic circulatory disturbance of a migraine attack." Only a few examples of funduscopic abnormalities photographed *during* an episode of transient monocular visual loss have been reported. Wolter and Burchfield[293] observed disc hyperemia and diffuse retinal opacity with a cherry-red macular spot considered to represent retinal edema. Moreover, although the authors did not believe that a change in vessel caliber occurred, Troost[272] felt that there was *venous* vasoconstriction, based on his review of the fundus photographs. Kline and Kelly[154] documented transient funduscopic changes occurring in a 48-year-old man with a long-standing history of cluster headaches and recurrent transient monocular visual reduction lasting for 1 to 2 minutes. They observed venous narrowing during an attack and subsequent venous dilatation; no retinal arteriolar vasospasm or embolic material was evident. Despite prompt filling of two cilioretinal vessels seen on fluorescein angiography, there was a delay in the appearance of dye in branches of the central retinal artery. In addition, during an attack, pattern-reversal visual evoked potentials showed diminution of amplitude with only a small effect on latency. The authors interpreted the retinal venous narrowing as a phenomenon secondary to reduced arterial flow, although "venous spasm" is an alternative explanation.[5] More recently, Burger et al.[33] examined five patients during an attack of monocular blindness, two of whom were also photographed. A 59-year-old man had sudden, painless "white-out" of vision lasting for 2 minutes, which recurred several times. During a subsequent attack, ophthalmoscopy disclosed multifocal narrowing of retinal arteries and slight narrowing of veins, accompanied by slight pallor of the optic disc and enhancement of the foveal color. No further episodes occurred during 6 years of follow-up. One of their five patients had episodic headaches, although two others had temporal arteritis.

Another case, photographed after the episode of amaurosis, also appeared to show retinal *arteriolar* narrowing.[133] Repots of funduscopic examination during an attack have confirmed the observation of arteriolar spasm,[113,238,275,278,289] despite one negative report of five patients, most having binocular visual symptoms.[149] In Fisher's seminal report[84] on transient monocular blindness, 26 cases in the literature of ophthalmoscopically observed narrowing of retinal vessels were reviewed, some of which were quite likely of migrainous origin.

Whatever mechanism is involved, whether arteriolar or venous spasm or platelet emboli possibly inducing spasm, prolonged ischemia in the retinal or choroidal circulations has rarely led to permanent monocular visual defects. In the first edition of this book, we identified 32 cases of permanent monocular visual disturbance ascribed to migraine. These and additional cases have since been summarized in detail from the ophthalmologic standpoint in a review by Hupp et al.[144] The defects in vision included central or centrocecal scotomas, altitudinal defects, monocular constriction, and complete blindness. The mean age of the patients was in the late 30s, with four times as many women as there were men. The presence of a family history of migraine was variable. The mean duration of migraine was approximately 13 years with diverse migraine subtypes, the most frequent being migraine with aura, followed by retinal migraine unaccompanied by headache. Other headache types included retinal migraine with headache, migraine without aura, retinal migraine, and migraine with aura, and cluster headache. The visual loss almost always occurred abruptly usually in the setting of a headache that appeared as often before or following the onset of the visual disturbance. In a few cases local eye pain was a prominent symptom. A variety of funduscopic abnormalities were reported, as reviewed below. In the few instances where carotid angiography was performed, no abnormalities were evident. Only a small number of cases were fully investigated to exclude alternative causes of abrupt visual loss, although most cases appeared to fulfill the requirements of a prior history of migraine and abrupt visual loss occurring in the context of a migrainous headache.

Many of the cases cited here were reported before modern diagnostic techniques were available, particularly to pursue an embolic etiology, the cause likeliest to confound a diagnosis of permanent visual loss resulting from retinal migraine. Transient or permanent monocular visual obscurations of migrainous origin, even when accompanied by specific funduscopic abnormalities, is not a syndrome clinically distinguishable from amaurosis fugax or retinal infarction due to embolism. Goodwin et al.[109] concluded after a review of 170 attacks in 32 patients with angiographically proven carotid artery disease or cardiogenic emboli that the clinical syndrome of amaurosis fugax was sufficiently variable to preclude definitive distinction from migraine. Other authors have concurred with this view,[55,73] although Corbett[55] has suggested that one clinical subtype of amaurosis is characteristic of retinal migraine. A specific instance is described as follows: gradual monocular constriction beginning as spotty darkening in the periphery, later coalescing into a ring, followed by more spots in the darkened area until only small clear spots remain in the center. The eye remains blind for 1 to 2 minutes with clearing from the periphery to the center. This pattern of lobular constriction appears conveniently explained by ischemia in the choroidal circulation, which Hayreh[126] has shown to have a segmental, cobblestone architecture.

Galezowski[97] was first to describe *central retinal artery occlusion* as a consequence of migrainous attacks. At the time of his report he had seen 76 cases of "ophthalmic megrim" and detailed the features of four cases, two of whom had central retinal artery occlusion. A recent, single case reported briefly by Crowell et al.[59] is worthy of mention because of its atypical features and the failure of an extensive evaluation to reveal a nonmigrainous cause. In only two other cases[53,203] have ocular and cerebral deficits occurred in the same patient closely linked in time. Ordinarily such a combination, though uncommon, can be considered a sign highly predictive for carotid atherostenosis.[221] An unusual example of bilateral central retinal artery occlusions associated with disc drusen in a 25-year-old woman with migraine has been recently documented.[207]

Several examples of *branch retinal arterial occlusions* have been reported.[62,97,110,113,143,279] Gronvall's case[113] of an 18-year-old woman is particularly well documented. Typical attacks began with a sensation of dimness before her eyes consisting of grayish-white patches with a colored margin superimposed on an intact background visual field. After 1 to 2 minutes, a boring pressure in one temple supervened, sometimes accompanied by nausea and vomiting. During one such attack with the usual spots, she experienced sudden right monocular blindness. Ten minutes later she was able to see in the lower half of the visual field, vision returning in the course of a half-minute, but a grayish black defect persisted in the superior half. Ophthalmologic examination 24 hours later showed a complete upper nasal defect extending into an upper temporal crescent. A patch of retinal edema was evident inferior to the macula and the inferior temporal artery was threadlike. Routine cardiac examination and hematologic studies were normal.

Brown et al.[28] studied 27 patients under 30 years old with central or branch arterial occlusions. The most common associated finding was a history of migraine, occurring in eight patients. All had a previous history of scintillating scotomata associated with headaches, usually unilateral but not consistently lateralized to the side of the affected eye. Only one patient experienced a headache at the time of the occlusion.

*Central retinal vein occlusion* has been less frequently encountered. Lohlein[177] and Wegner[279] followed the disturbing developments in the case of a 46-year-old man with a 25-year history of migraine who suffered recurrent amaurosis in either eye. He sustained permanent visual loss on three occasions associated with hemorrhage into the optic nerve head on the left, retinal venous occlusion on the right, and later central retinal artery occlusion also on the right. Friedman's single case[96] of central retinal venous occlusions occurred during the course of a severe migraine headache; no abnormalities were found on carotid angiogram.

The recent recognition of *ischemic optic neuropathy* as a complication of migraine has served to broaden our conception of the presumed site of microcirculatory disturbance in "ocular migraine." Seven cases, with a mean age of 44, are known in the literature,[57,143,186,274,281] each presenting with abrupt visual loss in the form of a central scotoma or arcuate defect occurring during the course of a typical headache. Disc swelling, in some cases accompanied by peripapillary hemorrhages was seen acutely, while optic disc pallor occurred in the later stages; in either situation, the funduscopic appearance was indistinguishable from cases of idiopathic ischemic optic neuropathy. The two patients reported by Weinstein and Feman[281] appear the most exhaustively investigated, revealing no other apparent causative factor, including temporal arteritis, collagen vascular disease, syphilis, hyperviscosity or hypercoaguable states, multiple sclerosis, or a compressive nerve lesion. Neither patient had hypertension and in the one patient undergoing carotid angiography, no abnormalities were detected. Fluorescein angiography, performed acutely in the one patient reported by McDonald and Sanders[186] showed normal arterial filling but a delay in filling of the peripapillary plexus in the upper pole and, in the venous phase, dilatation of the superficial peripapillary plexus.

Ischemic susceptibility of the prelaminar portion of the optic nerve might be related to its "watershed" position between the retinal and choroidal systems. While the surface of the optic disc derives its blood supply primarily from branches of the central retinal artery, the prelaminar and laminar portions are supplied through an anastomotic arterial circle receiving contributions from the posterior ciliary arteries, pial vessels, and choroidal arterioles.[125,172] Microcirculatory disturbances affecting any of these three vascular sources can be implicated in the pathogenesis of migrainous ischemic optic neuropathy. The short posterior ciliary arteries, possessing a muscular coat, have been favored as the site of vasoconstriction, producing impaired perfusion of the optic nerves.[281] Examples of unilateral[164] and bilateral[145] cilioretinal artery occlusions in the setting of migraine have been documented. On the other hand, there is little doubt that the choroidal circulation may be affected, given the evidence from fluorescein angiography, and the demonstration of *retinal pigmentary changes*. Among Connor's five cases[53] with permanent retinal lesions, two patients with hemicranial headache, accompanied by teichopsia, developed monocular visual loss with retinal pigment having "the appearance and distribution of that found in retinitis pigmentosa."

## BASILAR MIGRAINE

Isolated diplopia as part of a migrainous disorder was recognized by Liveing,[176] and others have suggested that attacks of vertigo as well as a full labyrinthine syndrome indistinguishable from Menière's disease may be a migrainous disorder.[265,292] It was Bickerstaff,[11] however, who described a characteristic clinical syndrome accompanied by severe headache and coined the term "basilar artery migraine," referring to the premonitory symptoms of a migrainous attack, which he believed was a result of transient ischemia in the territory of the basilar artery. In the IHS classification, the syndrome is called *basilar migraine,* in order to avoid an implied vascular mechanism for a disorder whose pathogenesis is still uncertain.

Whatever the underlying mechanism, it is clear that a variant of migraine exists with brain stem symptoms as the predominant feature. Reviewing a personal series of 300 cases, Bickerstaff identified 34 patients whose attacks were usually heralded by visual disturbances, either complete visual loss or positive phenomena such as teichopsia so dazzling as to obscure the entire field of vision. Other basilar symptoms followed, including dizziness or vertigo, gait ataxis, dysarthria, tinnitus, bilateral acral, perioral and lingual numbness, or paresthesias. These symptoms persisted for 2 to 60 minutes, ending abruptly, although the visual loss generally recovered more gradually. After the premonitory phase subsided, a severe throbbing occipital headache supervened and was accompanied by vomiting. These patients recovered completely, and between such attacks many had episodes of classical migraine. Typically affected were young adolescent girls. Attacks were usually infrequent but strongly related to menstruation. In Bickerstaff's series, all but two were under 23 years of age and 26 of 34 were girls. Bickerstaff[14] later noted that it was not rare for subjects with migraine earlier in life to develop symptoms of basilar migraine as "they enter the atheromatous age groups." A clear-cut family history of migraine in close relatives was obtained in 82 percent of cases.

Lapkin and Golden[159] encountered this entity in a younger population, reporting a group of 30 children with a mean age at onset of 7 years (range 7 months to 14 years). The duration of episodes ranged from minutes to many hours; one patient was symptomatic for nearly 3 days. Unlike the adolescent cases, the most common complaint was vertigo (73 percent), while visual disturbances occurred in 43 percent of cases. In children more severely affected, pyramidal tract dysfunction was observed as well as cranial nerve abnormalities, including internuclear ophthalmoplegia and facial nerve paresis. A family history of migraine was obtained in 86 percent of patients. During the follow-up period of 6 months to 3 years, none of the patients showed signs of progressive neurologic dysfunction, although one child was mentioned as having developed a permanent oculomotor nerve paralysis. A favorable outcome was also noted in the series of Hockaday.[139]

The definition of basilar migraine was later expanded to include alteration in consciousness. Bickerstaff[12] cited 4 cases in detail and recorded a total of 8 among 32 patients with previously diagnosed basilar migraine. The onset of impaired consciousness occurred in the context of other basilar symptoms with a leisurely onset, not causing the patient to fall or incur self-injury, and was sometimes preceded by a dreamlike state. Ranging from drowsiness to stupor, the altered consciousness was akinetic and usually brief, lasting up to several minutes and not accompanied by rigidity, posturing, tongue-biting, urinary incontinence, or changes in the respiratory pattern. Like the usual basilar migraine, a throbbing headache occurred on recovery. Laboratory investigations were generally unrevealing with normal cerebrospinal fluid and EEG. However, more recent examples of patients with basilar migraine and abnormal EEGs have been reported, including severe epileptiform discharges[40] and a photoconvulsive response recorded during an actual attack.[264] Angiogram was normal in three of Bickerstaff's cases[12] and in subsequently reported cases as well, except in one instance (see below). Finally, in a single patient described by Petersen et al.[224] atrial fibrillation occurred during three documented episodes of basilar migraine with impaired consciousness and was considered to reflect brain stem sympathetic dysfunction in the course of the attack.

Lee and Lance[166] encountered seven patients with a similar syndrome of altered consciousness, using the term "migraine stupor." Unlike the brief episodes observed by Bickerstaff,[12] the duration of stupor ranged from 2 hours to 5 days. Four patients showed aggressive and hysterical behavior during the attacks, leading to initial psychiatric diagnoses. A confusional state lasting up to several hours has also been reported as a major feature of juvenile migraine.[101] In adults, the syndrome of transient global amnesia is possibly a variant of migraine in the vertebrobasilar territory.[42] A locked-in syndrome occurring in a 29-year-old woman has also been attributed to basilar artery migraine.[263]

Permanent brain stem deficits occurring as a result of basilar artery migraine have been reported rarely. None of Bickerstaff's cases[11,12] had persisting neurologic disturbances; indeed, he stressed the return to complete normality as a criterion for the diagnosis. Among the cases of migraine-associated stroke uncovered in the literature, few have occurred in the vertebrobasilar territory, excluding the posterior cerebral artery. In Connor's series[53] of 18 cases with complicated migraine, three were considered to have lesions in the brain stem. In no instance did the transient episodes clearly resemble basilar migraine as defined above. The one case described in the text was a 42-year-old man whose attacks consisted of "right-sided teichopsia, hemianopia, frontal headache and sickness which had occurred every 3 months for 4 years." During the course of an unusually severe attack lasting 2 days, he experienced paresthesias in all limbs. On admission to the hospital, he had a temperature of 104 degrees, complete ophthalmoplegia, palatal weakness, and left hemiataxia, but normal sensation. The CSF was acellular with a protein level of 86 mg/dl. An EEG, pneumoencephalogram, and carotid and vertebral angiogram were all normal. The second patient, a 36-year-old man who had teichopsia, visual loss, hemiparesis, and vomiting during his transient attacks, was left with nystagmus on lateral gaze and a sensorimotor deficit following a migraine attack. Angiography was normal. The third patient, a 35-year-old woman who had a 12-year history of headaches with vomiting, presumably common migraine, developed left facial palsy and right hemiparesis during the course of an attack. Angiography in this case was also normal.

Solomon and Spaccavento[258] reported an unusual patient, an otherwise healthy 21-year-old man who had a 2-year history of occipital headaches preceded by ataxia, vertigo, and visual disturbances. Treatment with propranolol led to an "excellent response." Following discontinuation of this medication, the patient experienced a recurrence of basilar migraine attacks. At some point after the second attack, he abruptly developed vertigo, nausea, and gait ataxia. The neurologic examination revealed a complete lateral medullary syndrome. Blood pressure and routine laboratory studies were unremarkable. Angiography revealed a total occlusion of the left vertebral artery. "The tapering of the vessel just proximal to the obstruction was considered highly suggestive of vasospasm" according to the authors, but the published angiogram pictures are more consistent with arterial dissection.

The patient reported by Cohen and Taylor[50] suffered a series of devastating strokes in both carotid and vertebrobasilar territories. At the age of 20, he developed episodic throbbing occipital headache preceded by diplopia, dysarthria, perioral and left arm numbness, left arm paresis, and scotoma lasting for 2 hours. The first episode of prolonged neurologic dysfunction occurred at the age of 29, when he presented with left hemiparesis, hemianesthesia, hemiataxia, tinnitus, dysarthria accompanied by headache, nausea, and vomiting. The blood pressure was 236/142 and the electrocardiogram showed evidence of an old inferior wall myocardial infarction. The hemiparesis disappeared in several weeks. A four-vessel angiogram was normal. About 17 months later, he had an episode of left hemiparesis, slurred speech, photophobia, and occipital headache. Blood pressure was 140/100 and he had minimal left-sided incoordination. He was treated with propranolol. Then 16 months later, 2 days after the propranolol dosage was reduced, he experienced a 1-hour episode of perioral paresthesia and photophobia; 1 month later, he abruptly developed left hemiplegia, sensory loss, and hemianopia. The blood pressure was 170/100. CT scan revealed nonenhancing low densities in the left frontal, left cerebellar, and right parieto-occipital areas on the first day, with enhancement of the latter lesion on day 8. A four-vessel angiogram performed on the seventh hospital day was again normal. Laboratory studies for hypercoagulability, vasculitis, homocystinuria, sickle cell disease, and hyperlipidemia were all unremarkable.

The nine patients reported by Caplan[41] with vertebrobasilar ischemia attributed to migraine are noteworthy because they illustrate the difficulties in assigning a causal relationship between migraine and brain infarction. The two patients with multiple attacks resembling TIAs were otherwise typical of basilar migraine in their clinical features except that migraine with aura occurred 4 years after the onset of attacks in one patient, and developed concurrently with the attacks in the other patient. CT and angiography were normal. Unusual profiles occurred in the six patients with permanent deficits. In only one of them, a 6-year-old boy with a family history of migraine, did the stroke evolve in the setting of migraine headache. Among the remainder, one patient developed migraine with aura 5 months *after* the basilar stroke (normal angiogram), while five patients had migraine with aura diagnosed historically, but which did not occur *during* any stroke episode (angiogram showing basilar occlusion in three, occlusion of distal superior cerebellar artery in one, and diffuse basilar artery narrowing in one). Whether or not migraine was involved in the pathogenesis of these latter cases is unclear. If these cases are representative of basilar migraine, then Caplan's conclusion that this disorder is not benign is certainly correct, though contrary to prevailing views.

## PROBLEMS IN THE DIAGNOSIS OF MIGRAINOUS INFARCTION

When the clinician is confronted with the migrainous patient presenting for the first time with focal neurologic symptoms and signs, the quandary arises of establishing a causal relationship between migraine and the neurologic deficit. If the neurologic syndrome resembles that experienced in previous migraine attacks, and if the stroke evolves in the setting of a migraine attack, the diagnosis can be made with more confidence. Otherwise, as suggested in the IHS classification,[127] the event should be classified as either *cerebral infarction of other cause coexisting with migraine, or cerebral infarction of other cause presenting with symptoms resembling migraine.* In evaluating the problem, exclusion of underlying comorbid conditions or other potential causes of ischemic stroke is essential. It is worth reviewing several points that might be considered before invoking the diagnosis of migrainous infarction.

### Ischemic Cerebrovascular Disease of Thromboembolic Mechanism Accompanied by Severe Headache

The landmark experiments of Ray and Wolff[233] demonstrated that sensitivity to pressure, traction, and faradization occurred in the intracranial ICA, the first 1 to 2 cm of the MCA stem, the first several centimeters of the ACA just beyond the A2 segment, and 1 to 2 cm of the vertebral, anterior and posterior inferior cerebellar, and pontine arteries. These sensitive structures, when electrically stimulated, provoke pain, which was localized to specific areas of the scalp and face.

Fisher's clinicopathologic observations[83,85,86] have extended these findings. A study of the headache syndromes due to ischemic cerebrovascular disease showed that most complained of the symptom at the onset of a persisting neurologic deficit, although in some cases headache was premonitory or accompanied TIAs, findings also noted by others.[72,112,187,205,285] The headache was usually nonthrobbing, often localized, and frequently lateralized ipsilateral to the presumed arterial occlusion; it was occasionally severe. Of especial interest was the relatively high frequency of headache in PCA territory infarctions compared to that seen in carotid or basilar disease. Headache was the exception in lacunar strokes with pure motor or pure sensory syndromes, and none occurred in any of the 58 patients with transient monocular blindness. Overall, the frequency of headache was 31 percent in carotid artery and 42 percent in vertebrobasilar disease. Other series, less detailed in their classification of vascular distribution, have reported headache with a frequency as low as 9 percent for anterior and posterior circulations[194] and as high as 50 percent for vertebrobasilar ischemia in two studies.[74,205] Reviewing the possible mechanisms of headache due to thromboembolism, Fisher[86] and Edmeads[72] both provided arguments against many of the traditional and prevailing views, including (1) dilatation of collaterals, an idea proposed originally by Willis[291] in 1664 and promulgated by Symonds,[266] (2) focal distension of the artery,[285] (3) local ischemia of the arterial muscle, (4) irritation of pain-sensitive wall by atheroma,[25] and (5) severe hypertension or ischemic edema accompanying an acute stroke. Evidence has been accumulating showing no correlation between ischemic vascular disease with headache and the presence of hypertension, focal edema on CT, collateral circulation on angiography, or cerebral hyperperfusion assessed by dynamic technetium brain scan and intracarotid $^{133}$Xe regional cerebral blood flow studies.[72,205] Rather, the role of platelet aggregation with release of prostaglandins, serotonin, and other vasoactive peptides has recently become the focus of attention,[72] consistent with emerging views on the role of the trigeminovascular system in the pain syndrome of migraine.[201] An alternative hypothesis postulates that neurotransmitter depletion occurring in acute stroke[202,283] produces an alteration in pain threshold[251,252] or cerebral blood flow.[226] In the context of these biochemical changes occurring in acute stroke, it is not implausible to consider the possibility that a stroke may provoke an attack of migraine headache in certain susceptible individuals.[213]

The issue of *spontaneous carotid artery dissection* is relevant to this discussion. Although the mechanism of pain production is not clearly understood, the occurrence of headache is an expected finding, present in 60 percent of patients[122] along with a variable incidence of ischemic complications, a combination that may mimic migrainous infarction. Fisher[90] analyzed 21 selected cases of angiographically documented cervical carotid dissection, observing that almost all patients (19 of 21) had ipsilateral pain in one or more regions of the head, including forehead, orbit, temple, retro-orbit, side of head, and the frontal region. In addition, 12 patients had neck pain as well, usually in the upper neck and localized to a region including the mastoid, upper carotid, behind or below the angle of the jaw, and along the sternocleidomastoid muscle. The pain was usually severe, often sudden in onset, described equally as steady or throbbing, and occasionally accompanied by alterations in ipsilateral scalp sensation. The duration ranged from several hours to 2 years, with most lasting no longer than 3 to 4 weeks. About three-fourths of Fisher's patients experienced ischemic complications and in half of them the headache preceded the ischemic event from a few hours to 4 days. Other common diagnostic findings were the Horner syndrome, subjective bruit, dysgeusia, and visual scintillations. Given this clinical picture, it is difficult to avoid considering the possibility that cases formerly diagnosed as carotidynia[104,232] paratrigeminal syndrome,[88] or migraine cluster with miosis or transient focal deficits[76,147] may have been instances of carotid dissection. Similarly, in the series of Gautier et al.,[103] examining 133 young persons with ischemic stroke, 7 of the 16 patients who had a history of migraine had dissecting aneurysms discovered on angiography.

## Migraine Attacks Without Headache

Adding to the potential for diagnostic confusion is the occurrence of migraine attacks consisting of visual disturbances or other focal deficits but not accompanied by typical headache. Although not universally accepted as a diagnostic entity,[191] "acephalgic migraine"[210] is likely familiar to many clinicians and recognized by authorities on headache.[58,73,292] In the IHS classification, it is regarded as a separate entity, *migraine aura without headache.* Charcot[47] identified an incomplete form of ophthalmic migraine, "migraines ophthalmiques frustes" consisting only of "les troubles oculaires." More controversial has been the entity of accompanied migraine without headache, originally described by Whitty.[287] Fisher[87,89,91] emphasized that the migrainous syndrome, despite the absence of headache could be diagnosed based on characteristic clinical features. Syndromes included transient visual manifestations (blindness, homonymous hemianopia, blurred vision) either alone or accompanied by paresthesias, speech disturbances (dysarthria or aphasia), speech disturbances and paresis, or brain stem symptoms. In some cases, only the latter symptoms occurred without the visual effects. The duration of attacks ranged from minutes to 3 days or more.[91] Follow-up studies[91,210] suggest that the disorder is benign.

## Ischemic Focal Deficits in Migraineurs Caused by Cardiogenic Embolism

There are several studies that argue for an association between migraine and mitral valve prolapse (MVP), evidence sufficiently suggestive that perhaps all migraineurs with aura should be evaluated for the presence of this valvular abnormality. Litman and Friedman[175] in a retrospective study of 230 unselected patients with MVP found a 28 percent frequency of migraine, which they considered excessive when compared to the expected frequency of 10 percent[17] among the general female population. Amat et al.[7] studied the problem conversely, examining 88 patients with vascular headaches for echocardiographic evidence of MVP, compared to a group of 102 patients with tension headaches. The prevalance of MVP was 20 percent in the former group, while no patient in the latter group was found to have MVP. The frequency of MVP in the vascular headache group exceeded by about threefold the 6 percent prevalence encountered in the general population.[229] Similarly, in case-control study, Spence et al.[261] found the odds of having MVP was 2.7 in migraineurs compared to controls. Gamberini et al.[98] prospectively corroborated the 20 percent prevalence of MVP in migraineurs. They studied 100 consecutive patients with migraine looking for MVP and 100 consecutive patients with MVP; among the latter group, 51 suffered from migraine.

Whatever the mechanism for focal cerebral symptoms in the patient with MVP, whether due to microemboli arising from myxomatous valves[7,9] or intravascular platelet thromboemboli, it appears to be a risk factor for cerebral ischemia in a subgroup of patients as yet undefined, although the evidence cited above suggests that migraineurs with MVP may be especially stroke prone, a notion supported by the data indicating that platelet disorders may be a feature of the migraine syndrome as well. Centonze et al.[46] illustrated this point in their series of 10 patients with migraine presenting with transient hemispheric deficits, retinal artery or vein occlusions, and ischemic optic neuropathy. Each patient on subsequent evaluation had echocardiographic evidence of MVP. The authors argued that cerebrovascular accidents in migraineurs might commonly be due to coexisting MVP and that such patients represent a subgroup "haute-risque."

## Effect of Ergot Therapy on Focal and Diffuse Cerebral Dysfunction

The peripheral vascular and central nervous system effects of ergot alkaloids in toxic doses have long been recognized, consisting of gangrene, seizures, encephalopathy, and coma.[189] The mechanism responsible for diffuse cerebral dysfunction is not settled and may be the result of either a direct central nervous system (CNS) toxic effect or severe cerebral vasoconstriction, although in therapeutic doses ergotamine usually has no effect on cerebral blood flow.[75,116] Scattered reports have appeared, linking ergotamine use to focal disturbances in the ophthalmic and cerebral circulations, manifested by transient monocular blindness,[189] bilateral papillitis,[115] and sensorimotor deficits.[27,235,248]

## Increased Risk of Stroke in Migraineurs Using Oral Contraceptives

The Colloborative Study Group in Young Women used a case-control method to evaluate the risk of cerebrovascular disease in users of oral contraceptives[51] and later reported the effect of other risk factors including hypertension, smoking, and migraine.[52] The risk of cerebral thrombosis among women using oral contraceptives was 9.5 times greater than among nonusers. The relative risk for hemorrhagic stroke was lower, though significant. The role of migraine was assessed in both users and nonusers of contraceptives. Among migraineurs not exposed to birth control pills, the risk of stroke was equivocal, depending on the control group used for comparison. The use of oral contraceptives in combination with migraine, however, increased the relative risk for thrombotic stroke from 2.0 to 5.9, but not for hemorrhagic stroke. Although other studies have disputed the association with ischemic strokes, a recent review of the best available literature by Longstreth and Swanson[178] concluded that oral contraceptives alone increases the ischemic stroke risk. Of particular interest in relation to the interactive role of migraine is the pathologic finding of intimal hyperplasia associated with thrombosis in three fatal cases of stroke in young women exposed to contraceptives.[146] Patients with migraine who use oral contraceptives probably represent a high-risk subgroup for ischemic cerebrovascular disease.[169,185]

Several studies indicate that oral contraceptives may exacerbate migraine attacks.[64,225,288]

## Role of Lupus Anticoagulant in Thrombotic Stroke and Migraine

The association between cerebral ischemic events in young persons and the presence of the lupus anticoagulant and other antiphospholipid antibodies has recently been emphasized,[24,124,167,228] although prospective validation of its risk is still awaited. Moreover, an association between lupus anticoagulant and migraine has also been proposed, providing a link between ischemic events and migraine through a prothrombotic mechanism.[140,168] Among 48 patients with antiphospholipid antibodies encountered by Levine et al.,[167] 16 (33 percent) had severe vascular headache or recurrent stereotypic headache resembling migraine. Among 46 patients examined by Brey et al.,[24] 12 (26 percent) had vascular headaches, two of whom had complicated migraine. Even though this association needs further study, these antibodies should be sought in migraine patients with prolonged aura or evidence of infarction.

## Relationship of Migraine Headaches to the Mitochondrial Cytopathies

An unusual constellation of symptoms, collectively referred to as the "malignant migraine syndrome" consisting of classical migraine, occipital seizures, and alternating strokes were described in 1984 by Dvorkin et al.[70] Eight patients were reported, of whom four died because of intractable seizures. The one autopsied case showed cortical infarcts and the pathologic studies of cerebral biopsies revealed normal large vessels and focal cortical lesions with vascular hyperplasia. A second report by these investigators followed,[69] relating this syndrome to mitochondrial encephalopathy, even though some of their patients lacked the expected muscle enzyme abnormalities found in the disorder comprising MELAS (mitochondrial myopathy, encephalopathy, lactic acidosis, and strokelike episodes).[218] In that disorder, the episodes of stroke are often preceded by prolonged migrainous headaches, accompanied by nausea and vomiting occurring in clusters over a few days.[196] Brain infarction is said to be "nonterritorial" and not usually associated with vascular occlusions, although Lach et al.[156] have described mitochondrial abnormalities in the smooth muscle of cerebral blood vessels, representing a "mitochondrial microangiopathy".[247]

Subsequent studies have suggested that impaired mitochondrial energy metabolism may be a general finding in migraine. Montagna et al.[198] studied nine women (16 to 48 years old), four of whom had migraine with prolonged aura and five with migrainous infarction. Cerebral angiography was normal among the eight performed, and none of the subjects had physical signs of a mitochondrial disorder (i.e., no evidence of ophthalmoplegia, peripheral neuropathy, or myopathy). Lactate was significantly elevated during the effort in all subjects compared to controls; some subjects showed reduced activity of mitochondrial enzymes in platelets and muscles; and one of the seven patients undergoing muscle biopsy showed "ragged-red" fibers. Conceivably, these enzyme deficits could also involve neural and neurovascular tissue. One proposal[197] is that the energy failure in the endothelial and smooth muscle cells of blood vessels leads to diminished calcium-binding, generalized cell failure, and vasospasm. Reduced perfusion coupled with brain oxidative metabolism failure, triggered by environmental factors, could in theory lead to the ischemic deficits seen in MELAS, providing a model for migraine with ischemic complications. Migraine is a prominent feature of MELAS;[196] when strokelike episodes occur, there is a predilection for the posterior cerebrum, particularly the occipital lobes. The putative link between these disorders is provocative though preliminary.

## SUMMARY

While transient focal disturbances of migrainous origin are commonly encountered, persistent deficits from infarction of the cerebral hemisphere, retina, and brain stem as a direct consequence of migraine are rare. The mechanisms involved are probably multiple, including vasospasm, local arteropathy, embolism, arterial dissection, secondary consequences of spreading depression and platelet dysfunction. Because migraine is such a common disorder, it often coexists with another disorder directly responsible for the ischemic process rather than being causal itself. Migraine may also be a syndromic manifestation of another disorder (e.g., mitral valve prolapse, lupus anticoagulant, MELAS) that leads to stroke. In the presence of permanent sequelae, exclusion of other causes of cerebral or retinal infarction appears prudent, since there are no criteria to permit the diagnosis to be made reliably on clinical grounds alone. Most likely, true migrainous infarction is overdiagnosed.

## REFERENCES

1. Adams HP, Butler MJ, Biller J, Toffol GJ: Nonhemorrhagic cerebral infarction in young adults. Arch Neurol 43:793, 1986
2. Adams HP, Putnam SF, Corbett JJ et al: Amaurosis fugax: the results of arteriography in 59 patients. Stroke 5:742, 1983
3. Ad Hoc Committee on Classification of Headache: A classification of headache. Neurology (NY) 12:378, 1962
4. Adie WJ: Permanent hemianopia in migraine and subarachnoid hemorrhage. Lancet 2:237, 1930
5. Aellig WH: Agonists and antagonists of 5-hydroxytryptamine on veno-motor receptors. Adv Neurol 33:321, 1982
6. Alvarez J, Matias Guiu J, Sumalla J et al: Ischemic stroke in young adults. I. Analysis of etiologic subgroups. Acta Neurol Scand 80:28, 1989
7. Amat G, Jean Louis P, Lorsy C et al: Migraine and the mitral valve prolapse syndrome. Adv Neurol 33:27, 1983
8. Baker HL: Computerized transaxial tomography (EMI scan) in the diagnosis of cerebral vascular disease: experience at the Mayo Clinic. p. 195. In Whisnant JP (ed): Cerebral Vascular Diseases. Proceedings of the Ninth Conference. Grune & Stratton, New York, 1975
9. Barnett HJM, Jones MV, Boughner DR, Kostuk WJ: Cerebral ischemic events associated with prolapsing mitral valve. Arch Neurol 33:777, 1976
10. Bevan H, Sharma K, Bradley W: Stroke in young adults. Stroke 21:382, 1990
11. Bickerstaff ER: Basilar artery migraine. Lancet 1:15, 1961

12. Bickerstaff ER: Impairment of consciousness in migraine. Lancet 2:1057, 1961
13. Bickerstaff ER: Complicated migraine. p. 83. In Rose FC (ed): Progress in Migraine Research. Vol. 2. Pitman, London, 1984
14. Bickerstaff ER: Basilar artery migraine. p. 135. In Rose FC (ed): Handbook of Clinical Neurology. Elsevier, New York, 1986
15. Blau JN, Whitty CWM: Familial hemiplegic migraine. Lancet 2:1115, 1955
16. Blend R, Bull JWD: The radiological investigation of migraine. p. 1. In Smith RA (ed): Background to Migraine. Proceedings of the First Migraine Symposium. Heinemann, London, 1967
17. Blumenthal LS: Introduction. p. 6. In Vinken PJ, Bruyn GW (eds): Handbook of Clinical Neurology. Vol. 5. North-Holland Publishing, Amsterdam, 1968
18. Bogousslavsky J, Regli F: Ischemic stroke in adults younger than 30 years of age. Arch Neurol 44:479, 1987
19. Bogousslavsky J, Regli F, Van Melle G et al: Migraine stroke. Neurology (NY) 38:223, 1988
20. Boisen E: Strokes in migraine: report on seven strokes associated with severe migraine attacks. Dan Med Bull 22:100, 1975
21. Bousser MG, Baron JC, Iba-Zizen MT et al: Migrainous cerebral infarction: a tomographic study of cerebral blood flow and oxygen extraction fraction with the oxygen-15 inhalation technique. Stroke 11:145, 1980
22. Bradshaw P, Parsons M: Hemiplegic migraine: a clinical study. Q J Med 34:65, 1965
23. Brain R: Cerebral vascular disorders. Lancet 2:831, 1954
24. Brey RL, Hart RG, Sherman DG, Tegeler CH: Antiphospholipid antibodies and cerebral ischemia in young people. Neurology (NY) 40:1190, 1990
25. Bright R: Cases illustrative of the effects produced when the arteries of the brain are diseased: selected chiefly with a view to the diagnosis in such affections. Guys Hosp Rep (Series 1) 1:9, 1836
26. Broderick JP, Swanson JW: Migraine-related strokes. Arch Neurol 44:868, 1987
27. Brohult J, Forsberg O, Hellstrom R: Multiple arterial thrombosis after oral contraceptives and ergotamine. Acta Med Scand 181:453, 1967
28. Brown GC, Magargal LE, Shields JA et al: Retinal arterial obstruction in children and young adults. Ophthalmology 88:18, 1981
29. Bruyn GW: Complicated migraine. p. 59. In Vinken PJ, Bruyn GW (ed): Handbook of Clinical Neurology. Vol. 5. North-Holland Publishing, Amsterdam, 1968
30. Bruyn GW: Cerebral cortex and migraine. Adv Neurol 33:151, 1982.
31. Bruyn GW, Weenink HR: Migraine accompagnée: a critical evaluation. Headache 6:1, 1966
32. Buckle RM, du Boulay G, Smith B: Death due to vasospasm. J Neurol Neurosurg Psychiatry 27:440, 1964
33. Burger SK, Saul RF, Selhorst JB, Thurston SE: Transient monocular blindness caused by vasospasm. N Engl J Med 325:870, 1991
34. Burns RJ, Blumbergs PC, Sage MR: Brain infarction in young men. Clin Exp Neurol 16:69, 1979
35. Butler TH: Scotoma in migrainous subjects. Br J Ophthalmol 17:83, 1933
36. Cala LA, Mastaglia FL: Computerized axial tomography findings in patients with migrainous headaches. Br Med J 2:149, 1976
37. Cala LA, Mastaglia FL: Computerized tomography in the detection of brain damage. 2. Epilepsy, migraine, and general medical disorders. Med J Aust 2:616, 1980
38. Caldwell A, Kennedy R: Migraine headaches with preheadache retinal and visual disturbances in a case of congenital vascular anomaly and subarachnoid hemorrhage. Arch Neurol Psychiatry 61:397, 1953
39. Call GK, Fleming MC, Sealfon S et al: Reversible cerebral segmental vasoconstriction. Stroke 19:1159, 1988
40. Camfield PR, Metrakos K, Andermann F: Basilar migraine, seizures, and severe epileptiform EEG abnormalities. Neurology (NY) 28:584, 1978
41. Caplan LR: Migraine and vertebrobasilar ischemia. Neurology (NY) 41:55, 1991
42. Caplan LR, Chedru F, Lhermitte F, Mayman C: Transient global amnesia and migraine. Neurology (NY) 31:1167, 1981
43. Carroll D: Retinal migraine. Headache 10:9, 1970
44. Castaigne P, Brunet P, Peirrot-Deseilligny C, Roullet E: Accidents déficitaires neurologiques centraux et migraine. Ann Med Interne (Paris) 134:306, 1983
45. Castaldo JE, Anderson DMS, Reeves AG: Middle cerebral artery occlusion with migraine. Stroke 13:308, 1982
46. Centonze V, Amat G, Loisy C et al: Considerations sur les accidents vasculaires cérébraux chez les migraineux. Sem Hop Paris 56:1908, 1980
47. Charcot JM: Sur un cas de migraine ophtalmologique (paralysie oculomotrice périodique). Progr Med 18:83, 1890
48. Chen TC, Leviton A, Edelstein S, Ellenberg JS: Migraine and other diseases of women of reproductive age. Arch Neurol 44:1024, 1987
49. Clarke JM: On recurrent motor paralysis in migraine, with a report in which recurrent hemiplegia accompanied the attacks. Br Med J 2:1534, 1910
50. Cohen RJ, Taylor JR: Persistent neurologic sequelae of migraine: a case report. Neurology (NY) 29:1175, 1979
51. Collaborative Group for the Study of Stroke in Young Women: Oral contraception and increased risk of cerebral ischemia or thrombosis. N Engl J Med 288:871, 1973
52. Collaborative Group for the Study of Stroke in Young Women: Oral contraceptives and stroke

in young women: associated risk factors. JAMA 231:718, 1975
53. Connor RCR: Complicated migraine: a study of permanent neurological and visual defects caused by migraine. Lancet 2:1072, 1962
54. Conway LW, McDonald LW: Structural changes of the intradural arteries following subarachnoid hemorrhage. J Neurosurg 37:715, 1972
55. Corbett JJ: Neuro-ophthalmic complications of migraine and cluster headaches. p. 973. In Packard, RC (ed): Neurologic Clinics. Vol. 1. WB Saunders, Philadelphia, 1983
56. Couch JR, Hassanein RS: Platelet aggregability in migraine. Neurology (NY) 27:843, 1977
57. Cowan CL, Knox DL: Migraine optic neuropathy. Ann Ophthalmol 14:164, 1982
58. Critchely M, Fergusen FR: Migraine. Lancet 1:123, 1933
59. Crowell GF, Carlin L, Biller J: Neurologic complications of migraine. Am Fam Physician 26:139, 1982
60. Cuetter AC, Aita JF: CT scanning in classic migraine. (Letter.). Headache 4:195, 1983
61. Dassen R: Jacqueca oftalmoplejica con paralisis recidivante del III par craneano: muerte en el segundo ataque: necropsia. Sem Med 1:1049, 1931
62. Davis-Jones A, Gregory MC, Whitty CWM: Permanent sequelae in the migraine attack. p. 25. In Cummings JN (ed): Background to Migraine. Proceedings of the Fifth Symposium. Springer-Verlag, New York 1972
63. Deshmukh SV, Meyer JS: Cyclic changes in platelet dynamics and the pathogenesis and prophylaxis of migraine. Headache 17:101, 1977
64. Desrossiers JJ: Headaches related to contraceptive therapy and their control. Headache 13:117, 1973
65. Dorfman LJ, Marshall WH, Enzmann DR: Cerebral infarction and migraine: clinical and radiologic correlations. Neurology (NY) 29:317, 1979
66. du Boulay GH, Ruiz JS, Rose FC et al: CT changes associated with migraine. AJNR 4:472, 1983
67. Dukes HT, Vieth RG: Cerebral arteriography during migraine prodrome and headache. Neurology (NY) 14:636, 1964
68. Dunning HS: Intracranial and extracranial vascular accidents in migraine. Arch Neurol Psychiatry 48: 392, 1942
69. Dvorkin GS, Andermann F, Carpenter S et al: Classical migraine, intractable epilepsy, and multiple strokes: a syndrome related to mitchondrial encephalopathy. p. 203. In Andermann F, Lugaresi F (eds): Migraine and Epilepsy. Butterworth's, Boston, 1987
70. Dvorkin G, Andermann F, Melancank D et al: Malignant migraine syndrome: classical migraine, occipital seizures, and alternating strokes, abstracted. Neurology (NY) 34:245, 1984
71. Editorial: Migrainous cerebral infarction. Br Med J 1:532, 1977
72. Edmeads J: The headaches of ischemic cerebrovascular disease. Headache 19:127, 1979
73. Edmeads J: Complicated migraine and headache in cerebrovascular disease. Neurol Clin 1:385, 1983
74. Edmeads J, Barnett HJM: La cephalea en las affeciones cerebrovasculares occlusivas. p. 89. In Friedman AP, Poch GF (eds): Cephaleas y Jacquecas. Eudeba, Buenos Aires, 1973
75. Edmeads JG, Hachinski VC, Norris JW: Ergotamine and the cerebral circulation. Hemicrania 7:6, 1976
76. Ekbom K: A clinical comparison of cluster headache and migraine. Acta Neurol Scand, suppl 41. 46:7, 1968
77. Featherstone HJ: Clinical features of stroke in migraine: a review. Headache 26:128, 1986
78. Federico F, Calvario T, Di Turi N, Paradiso F: Ischaemic cerebral infarction in young adults. Acta Neurol (Napoli) 12:101, 1990
79. Fein JM, Flor WJ, Cohan SL, Parkhurst J: Sequential changes of vascular ultrastructure in experimental cerebral vasospasm. J Neurosurg 41:49, 1974
80. Ferbert A, Busse D, Thron A: Microinfarction in classic migraine?—a study with magnetic resonance imaging findings. Stroke 22:1010, 1991
81. Fere C: Contribution à l'étude de la migraine ophtalmique. Rev Med Paris 1:40, 1881
82. Fere C: Note sur un cas de migraine ophthalmique a access répètes suivis de mort. Rev Med Paris 3:194, 1883
83. Fisher CM: Occlusion of the internal carotid artery. Arch Neurol Psychiatry 65:346, 1951
84. Fisher CM: Observations of the fundus oculi in transient monocular blindness. Neurology (NY) 9:333, 1959
85. Fisher CM: Clinical syndromes in cerebral arterial occlusion. p. 126. In Fields WS (ed): Pathogenesis and Treatment of Cerebrovascular Disease. Thomas, Springfield, IL, 1961
86. Fisher CM: Headache in cerebrovascular disease. p. 124. In Vinken PJ, Bruyn GW (eds): Handbook of Clinical Neurology. Vol. 5. North-Holland Publishing, Amsterdam, 1968
87. Fisher CM: Migraine accompaniments versus arteriosclerotic ischemia. Trans Am Neurol Assoc 93:211, 1968
88. Fisher CM: Raeder's benign paratrigeminal syndrome with dysgeusia. Trans Am Neurol Assoc 96:234, 1972
89. Fisher CM: Late-life migraine accompaniments as a cause of unexplained transient ischemic attacks. Can J Med Sci 7:9, 1980
90. Fisher CM: The headache and pain of spontaneous carotid dissection. Headache 22:60, 1982
91. Fisher CM: Late-life migraine accompaniments—further experiences. Stroke 17:1033, 1986
92. Friberg L, Olesen J, Iversen HK, Sperling B: Migraine pain associated with middle cerebral artery dilatation: reversal by sumatriptan. Lancet 338:13, 1991
93. Friberg L, Skyhoj Olsen T, Roland PE, Lassen N:

Focal ischemia caused by instability of cerebrovascular tone during attacks of hemiplegic migraine: a regional cerebral blood flow study. Brain 110:917, 1987
94. Friedman AP: Overview of migraine. Adv Neurol 33:1, 1982
95. Friedman AP, Harter DH, Merritt HH: Ophthalmoplegic migraine. Arch Neurol 7:320, 1962
96. Friedman MW: Occlusion of the central retinal vein in migraine. Arch Ophthalmol 45:678, 1951
97. Galezowski X: Ophthalmic megrim. Lancet 1:176, 1882
98. Gamberini G, D'Alessandro R, Labriola E et al: Further evidence on the association of mitral valve prolapse and migraine. Headache 24:39, 1984
99. Garnic JD, Schellinger D: Arterial spasm as a finding intimately associated with onset of vascular headache. Neuroradiology 24:273, 1983
100. Garrison LP, Bowman MA, Perrin MB: Estimating physician requirements for neurology: a needs based approach. Neurology (NY) 34:1218, 1984
101. Gascon G, Barlow C: Juvenile migraine, presenting as an acute confusional state. Pediatrics 45:628, 1970
102. Gastaut JL, Yermenos E, Bonnefoy M, Cros D: Familial hemiplegic migraine: EEG and CT scan of two cases. Ann Neurol 10:392, 1981
103. Gautier JC, Pradat-Diehl P, Loron P et al: Accidents vasculaires cérébraux des sujets jeunes: une étude de 133 patients agés de 9 à 45 ans. Rev Neurol 145:437, 1989
104. Gelmers HJ: The pericarotid syndrome: a combination of hemicrania, Horner's syndrome, and internal carotid artery wall lesion. Acta Neurochir 57:37, 1981
105. Glaser JS: Neuro-ophthalmology. Vol. 2. Harper & Row, New York 1978
106. Goldflamm S: Beitrag zur Ätiologie und Symptomatologie der spontanen subarachnoidealen Blutungen. Dtsch Z Nervenheilkd 76:158, 1923
107. Goldstein M, Chen TC: The epidemiology of disabling headache. Adv Neurol 33:377, 1982
108. Goltman AM: The mechanism of migraine. J Allergy 7:351, 1936
109. Goodwin JA, Gorelick P, Hegalson C: Symptoms of amaurosis fugax in atherosclerotic carotid artery disease. Neurology 37:892, 1987
110. Graveson GS: Retinal arterial occlusion in migraine. Br Med J 2:838, 1949
111. Grindal A, Cohen RJ, Saul RF, Taylor JR: Cerebral infarction in young adults. Stroke 9:39, 1978
112. Grindal A, Toole J: Headache and transient ischemic attacks. Stroke 5:603, 1975
113. Gronvall H: On changes in the fundus oculi and persisting injuries to the eye in migraine. Acta Ophthalmol, suppl, 14-16 16:602, 1938
114. Guest IA, Woolf AL: Fatal infarction of the brain. Br Med J 1:225, 1964
115. Gupta DR, Strobos RJ: Bilateral papillitis associated with cafergot therapy. Neurology (NY) 22:793, 1972
116. Hachinski VC, Norris JW, Cooper PW, Edmeads JG: Ergotamine tartrate and cerebral blood flow. Can J Neurol Sci 2:333, 1975
117. Hachinski VC, Norris JW, Cooper PW, Edmeads JG: Migraine and the cerebral circulation. p. 11. In Greene R (ed): Current Concepts in Migraine Research. Raven Press, New York, 1978
118. Hachinski VC, Porchawka J, Steele JC: Visual symptoms in the migraine syndrome. Neurology (NY) 23:570, 1973
119. Hanington E: Migraine, a blood disorder. Lancet 2:501, 1978
120. Harrington DO: Ophthalmoplegic migraine: a discussion of its pathogenesis: report of the pathological findings in a case of recurrent oculomotor palsy. Arch Ophthalmol 49:643, 1953
121. Harrison MJG: Hemiplegic migraine. (Letter.). J Neurol Neurosurg Psychiatry 44:652, 1981
122. Hart RG, Easton JD: Dissection of cervical and cerebral arteries. Neurol Clin 1:155, 1983
123. Hart RG, Miller VT: Cerebral infarction in young adults: a practical approach. Stroke 14:110, 1983
124. Hart RG, Miller VT, Coull B et al: Cerebral infarction associated with lupus anticoagulants—preliminary report. Stroke 15:114, 1984
125. Hayreh SS: Pathogenesis of visual field defects: role of ciliary circulation. Br J Ophthalmol 54:289, 1970
126. Hayreh SS: Segmental nature of the choroidal vasculature. Br J Ophthalmol 59:631, 1975
127. Headache Classification Committee of the International Headache Society: Classification and diagnostic criteria for headache disorders, cranial neuralgias and facial pain. Cephalalgia, suppl 8. 7:1, 1988
128. Hedges TR: An ophthalmologist's view of headache. Headache 19:151, 1979
129. Hedges TR, Lackman R: Isolated ophthalmic migraine in the differential diagnosis of cerebro-ocular ischemia. Stroke 7:379, 1976
130. Henrich JB, Horwitz RI: A controlled study of ischemic stroke risk in migraine patients. J Clin Epidemiol 42:773:1989
131. Henrich JB, Sandercock PA, Warlow CP et al: Stroke and migraine in the Oxfordshire Community Stroke Project. J Neurol 233;257, 1986
132. Herold S, Gibbs JM, Jones AKP et al: Oxygen metabolism in migraine. J Cereb Blood Flow Metab, suppl 1. 5:S445, 1985
133. Heyck H: Die neurologischen Begleiterscheinungen der Migraine und des Problems des "angiospastischen Hirninsults." Nervenarzt 33:193, 1962
134. Heyck H: Pathogenesis of migraine. Res Clin Stud Headache 2:1, 1969
135. Heyck H: Varieties of hemiplegic migraine. Headache 12:135, 1973
136. Hillbom M, Kaste M: Ethanol intoxication: a risk factor for cerebral infarction in young adults. Stroke 11:694, 1983
137. Hilton-Jones D, Warlow CP: The cause of stroke in the young. J Neurol 232:137, 1985
138. Hindfelt B, Nilsson O: Brain infarction in young adults. Acta Neurol Scand 55:145, 1977

139. Hockaday JM: Basilar migraine in childhood. Dev Med Child Neurol 21:455, 1979
140. Hogan MJ, Brunet DG, Ford PM, Lillicrap D: Lupus anticoagulant, antiphospholipid antibodies and migraine. Can J Neurol Sci 15:420, 1988
141. Hughes JT, Schianchi M: Cerebral artery spasm: a histological study at necropsy of the blood vessels in cases of subarachnoid hemorrhage. J Neurosurg 48:515, 1978
142. Hungerford GD, du Boulay GH, Zilkha KJ: Computerized axial tomography in patients with severe migraine: a preliminary report. J Neurol Neurosurg Psychiatry 39:990, 1976
143. Hunt JR: A contribution to the paralytic and other persistent sequelae of migraine. Am J Med Sci 150:313, 1915
144. Hupp SL, Kline LB, Corbett JJ: Visual disturbances in migraine. Surv Ophthalmol 33:221, 1989
145. Hykin PG, Gartry D, Brazier DJ, Graham E: Bilateral cilioretinal artery occlusion in classic migraine. Postgrad Med J 67:282, 1991
146. Irey NS, McAllister HA, Henry JM: Oral contraceptives and stroke in young women. Neurology (NY) 28:1216, 1978
147. Jacobsen HH: The naso-ocular reflex in migrainous subjects. Acta Psychiatr Scand 27:63, 1952
148. Janzen R, Taner A, Zschocke ST et al: Postangiographische Spätreaktionen der Hirngefasse bei Migranekranken. Z Neurol 201:24, 1972
149. Joffe SN: Retinal blood vessel diameter during migraine. Eye, Ear, Nose Throat Monthly 52:338, 1973
150. Julien J, Laguey A, Darriet D: Infarctus cerebral au cours d'un accès migraineux. Sem Hop Paris 55:810, 1979
151. Kalendovsky Z, Austin JH: "Complicated migraine": its association with increased platelet aggregability and abnormal plasma coagulation factors. Headache 15:18, 1975
152. Kalendovsky Z, Austin JH: Changes in blood clotting systems during migraine attacks. Headache 16:293, 1977
153. Kaul SN, du Boulay GH, Kendall BE, Russel WR: Relationship between visual field defect and arterial occlusion in the posterior cerebral circulation. J Neurol Neurosurg Psychiatry 37:1022, 1974
154. Kline LB, Kelly CL: Ocular migraine in a patient with cluster headaches. Headache 20:253, 1980
155. Kurtzke JF: The current neurologic burden of illness and injury in the United States. Neurology (NY) 32:1207, 1982
156. Lach B, Preston D, Servidei S et al: Maternally inherited mitochondrial encephalomyopathy: a vasculopathy, abstracted. Muscle Nerve, suppl. 9:180, 1986
157. Lance JW: What is migraine? Adv Neurol 33:21, 1982
158. Lance JW, Lambert GA, Goadsby PJ, Duckworth JW: Brainsteam influences on the cephalic circulation: experimental data from cat and monkey of relevance to the mechanism of migraine. Headache 23:258, 1983
159. Lapkin ML, Golden GS: Basilar artery migraine: a review of 30 cases. Am J Dis Child 132:278, 1978
160. Lashley KS: Patterns of cerebral integration indicated by the scotomas of migraine. Arch Neurol Psychiatry 46:331, 1941
161. Lauritzen M, Olsen TS, Lassen NA, Paulson OB: Changes in regional cerebral blood flow during the course of classic migraine attacks. Ann Neurol 13:633, 1983
162. Lauritzen M, Olsen TS, Paulson OB: Regional cerebral blood flow in classic migraine: a possible relationship to the spreading depression of Leao? p. 117. In Rose FC (ed): Advances in Migraine Research and Therapy. Raven Press, New York, 1982
163. Lavitry M, Riser A, Dreyfus R, Grezes-Rueff C: Migraine ophtalmique accompagnée et epilepsie. Toulouse Med 55:37, 1954
164. Lawton-Smith J. Permanent infarctions complicating ocular migraine. J Clin Neuro Ophthalmol 6:74, 1986
165. Leao AAP: Spreading depression of activity in the cerebral cortex. J Neurophysiol 8:33, 1944
166. Lee CH, Lance JW: Migraine stupor. Headache 17:32, 1977
167. Levine SR, Deegan MJ, Futrell N, Welch KMA: Cerebrovascular and neurologic disease associated with antiphospholipid antibodies: 48 cases. Neurology (NY) 40:1181, 1990
168. Levine SR, Joseph R, D'Andrea G, Welch KMA: Migraine and the lupus anticoagulant: case reports and review of the literature. Cephalalgia 7:93, 1987
169. Leviton A: Epidemiology of headache. Adv Neurol 19:341, 1978
170. Leviton A, Malvea B, Graham JR: Vascular diseases, mortality, and migraine in the parents of migraine patients. Neurology (NY) 24:669, 1974
171. Lieberman AN, Jonas S, Hass WK et al: Bilateral cerebral carotid and intracranial vasospasm causing cerebral ischemia in a migrainous patient: a case of diplegic migraine. Headache 24:245, 1984
172. Lieberman MF, Maumenee AE, Green RW: Histologic studies of the vasculature of the anterior optic nerve. Am J Ophthalmol 82:405, 1968
173. Lindboe CF, Dahl T, Rostad B: Fatal stroke in migraine: a case report with autopsy findings. Cephalalgia 9:277, 1989
174. Lisovoski F, Rousseaux P: Cerebral infarction in young people: a study of 148 patients with early cerebral angiography. J Neurol Neurosurg Psychiatry 54:596, 1991
175. Litman GI, Freidman HM: Migraine and the mitral valve prolapse syndrome. Am Heart J 96:610, 1978
176. Liveing E: On Megrim, Sick Headache and Some Allied Disorders. Churchill, London, 1873
177. Lohlein W: Erblindung durch Migräne. Dtsch Med Wochenschr 48:1408, 1922

178. Longstreth WT, Swanson PD: Oral contraceptives and stroke. Stroke 15:747, 1984
179. Marshall J: The cause and prognosis of strokes in people under 50 years. J Neurol Sci 53:473, 1982
180. Masuzawa T, Shinoda S, Furuse M et al: Cerebral angiographic changes on serial examination of a patient with migraine. Neuroradiology 24:277, 1983
181. Mathew NT: Computerized axial tomography in migraine. p. 63. In Greene R (ed): Current Concepts in Migraine Research. Raven Press, New York, 1978
182. Mathew NT: Complicated migraine and differential diagnosis of migraine. p. 9. In Mathew RJ (ed): Treatment of Migraine. Pharmacological and Biofeedback Considerations. Spectrum, New York, 1981
183. Mathew NT, Krastnik F, Meyer JS: Regional cerebral blood flow in the diagnosis of vascular headache. Headache 15:252, 1976
184. Mathew NT, Meyer JS, Welch KMA, Neblett CR: Abnormal CT-scans in migraine. Headache 16:272, 1977
185. Matias Guiu J, Alvarez J, Insa R et al: Ischemic stroke in young adults. II. Analysis of risk factors in the etiological subgroups. Acta Neurol Scand 81:314, 1990
186. McDonald WI, Sanders MD: Migraine complicated by ischemic papillopathy. Lancet 1:521, 1971
187. Medina J, Diamond S, Rubino S: Headaches in patients with transient ischemic attacks. Headache 15:194, 1975
188. Ment LR, Duncan CC, Parcells PR, Collins FC: Evaluation of complicated migraine in childhood. Childs Brain 7:261, 1980
189. Merhoff GC, Porter JM: Ergot intoxication: historical review and description. Ann Surg 180:773, 1974
190. Milandre L, Ceccaldi M, Ali Cherif A, Khalil R: Cerebral arterial ischemic complications in young adults: etiology and prognosis. Rev Med Interne (Paris) 11:29, 1990
191. Millikan C: The differential diagnosis of transient focal cerebral attacks and migraine accompaniments. Trans Am Neurol Assoc 105:118, 1980
192. Milner PM: Note on a possible correspondence between the scotomas of migraine and spreading depression of Leao. EEG Clin Neurophysiol 10:705, 1958
193. Moen M, Levine SR, Newman DS et al: Bilateral posterior cerebral artery strokes in a young migraine sufferer. Stroke 19:525, 1988
194. Mohr JP, Caplan LR, Melski JW et al: The Harvard Cooperative Stroke Registry: a prospective registry. Neurology (NY) 28:754, 1978
195. Mohr JP, Kase CS: Cerebral vasospasm. I. In cerebral vascular malformations. Rev Neurol (Paris) 139:99, 1983
196. Montagna P, Gallassi R, Medori R et al: MELAS syndrome: characteristic migrainous and epileptic features and maternal transmission. Neurology (NY) 38:751, 1988
197. Montagna P, Sacquegna T, Cortelli P, Lugaresi E: Migraine as a defect of brain oxidative metabolism. J Neurol 236:124, 1989
198. Montagna P, Sacquegna T, Martinelli P et al: Mitochondrial abnormalities in migraine: preliminary findings. Headache 28:477, 1988
199. Moorehead MT, Movius HJ, Moorehead JR et al: Classic migraine with cerebral cortical infarction causing permanent hemianopsia. South Med J 72:821, 1979
200. Morenas L, Dechaume J: Migraine aphasique et monoplégique: étude anatomo-clinique: les rapports de la migraine avec l'epilepsie. J Med Lyon 10:259, 1929
201. Moskowitz MA: The neurobiology of vascular head pain. Ann Neurol 16:157, 1984
202. Mrsulja BB, Mrsulja BJ, Spatz M, Klatzo I: Brain serotonin after experimental vascular occlusion. Neurology (NY) 26:785, 1976
203. Murphy JP: Cerebral infarction in migraine. Neurology (NY) 5:359, 1955
204. Myhrman G: Migrainous attacks with persistent brain lesions. Acta Med Scand 181:583, 1967
205. Nappi G, Bono G: Headaches and transient cerebral ischemia: comments on Welch's report. Adv Neurol 33:41, 1982
206. Neligan P, Harriman DGF, Pearce J: Respiratory arrest in familial hemiplegic nigraine: a clinical and neuropathological study. Br Med J 2:732, 1977
207. Newman NJ, Lessell S, Brandt EM: Bilateral central retinal artery occlusions, disk drusen, and migraine. Am J Ophthalmol 107:236, 1989
208. O'Brien MD: Cerebral blood flow changes in migraine. Headache 10:139, 1971
209. O'Connor PJ: Strokes in migraine. p. 40. In Cummings JN (ed): Background to Migraine. Proceedings of the Fifth Symposium. Springer-Verlag, New York, 1972
210. O'Connor PS, Tredici TJ: Acephalgic migraine: fifteen years experience. Ophthalmology 88:999, 1981
211. Olesen J: The ischemic hypothesis of migraine. Arch Neurol 44:321, 1987
212. Olesen J: The classification and diagnosis of headache disorders. Neurol Clin 8:793, 1990
213. Olesen J: Cerebral and extracranial circulatory disturbances in migraine: pathophysiological implications. Cerebrovasc Brain Metab Rev 3:1, 1991
214. Olesen J, Frisberg L, Olsen TS et al: Timing and topography of cerebral blood flow, aura, and headache during migraine attacks. Ann Neurol 28:791, 1990
215. Olesen J, Larsen B, Lauritzen M: Focal hyperemia followed by spreading oligemia and impaired activation of rCBF in classic migraine. Ann Neurol 9:344, 1981
216. Oppenheim H: Casuistischer Beitrag zur Prognose der Hemikranie. Charite Ann 15:298, 1890
217. Ormond AW: Two cases of permanent hemianopsia following severe attacks of migraine. Ophthalmol Rev 32:192, 1913
218. Pavlakis SG, Phillips PC, DiMauro S et al: Mito-

chondrial myopathy, encephalopathy, lactic acidosis, and strokelike episodes: a distinctive clinical syndrome. Ann Neurol 16:481, 1984
219. Pearce J: The ophthalmological complications of migraine. J Neurol Sci 6:73, 1968
220. Pearce JMS, Foster JB: An investigation of complicated migraine. Neurology (NY) 15:323, 1965
221. Pessin MS, Duncan GW, Mohr JP, Poskanzer DC: Clinical and angiographic features of carotid transient ischemic attacks. N Engl J Med 296:358, 1977
222. Pessin MS, Lathi ES, Cohen BM et al: Clinical features and mechanism of occipital infarction. Ann Neurol 21:209, 1987
223. Peters R: Tödliche Gehirnblutung bei menstrueller Migräne. Beitr Pathol 93:209, 1934
224. Peterson J, Scruton D, Downie AW: Basilar artery migraine with transient atrial fibrillation. Br Med J 2:1125, 1977
225. Phillips BM: Oral contraceptives and migraine. Br Med J 2:99, 1968
226. Pickard JD, Mackenzie ET, Harper AM: Serotonin and prostaglandins: intracranial and extracranial effects with reference to migraine. p. 101. In Greene R (ed): Current Concepts in Migraine Research. Raven Press, New York, 1978
227. Polyak S: The Vertebrate Visual System. University of Chicago Press, Chicago, 1957
228. Pope JM, Canny CL, Bell DA: Cerebral ischemic events associated with endocarditis, retinal vascular disease, and lupus anticoagulant. Am J Med 90:299, 1991
229. Procacci PM, Savran SV, Schreiter SL, Bryson AL: Prevalence of clinical mitral-valve prolapse in 1,169 young women. N Engl J Med 294:1086, 1976
230. Rascol A, Cambier J, Guiraud B et al: Accidents ischémiques cérébraux au cours de crises migraineuses: à propos des migraines compliquées. Rev Neurol (Paris) 135:867, 1979
231. Rascol A, Clanet M, Rascol O: Cerebrovascular accidents complicating migraine attacks. p. 110. In Rose FC, Amory WK (eds): Cerebral Hypoxia in the Pathogenesis of Migraine. Pitman, London, 1982
232. Raskin NE, Prusiner S: Carotidynia. Neurology (NY) 27:43, 1977
233. Ray BS, Wolff HG: Experimental studies on headache: pain-sensitive structures of the head and their significance in headache. Arch Surg 41:813, 1940
234. Rich WM: Permanent quadrantanopsia after migraine. Br Med J 116:592, 1948
235. Richter AM, Banker VP: Carotid ergotism. Radiology 106:339, 1973
236. Robinson BE: Permanent homonymous migrainous scotomata. Arch Ophthalmol 53:566, 1955
237. Romain LF: Stroke as a complication of migraine disease. J Indiana State Med Assoc 74:506, 1981
238. Rosenstein AM: Beitrag zu den beiderseitigen Verdunkelungen des Sehvermögens mit vorübergehenden ophthalmoskopischen Befund bei Herzklappenfehler. Klin Monatsbl Augenheilkd 75:357, 1925
239. Rossi LN, Penzien JM, Deonna T et al: Does migraine-related stroke occur in childhood? Dev Med Child Neurol 32:1005, 1990
240. Rothrock JF, Walicke P, Swenson MR: Migrainous stroke. Arch Neurol 45:63, 1987
241. Ruiz JS, du Boulay GH, Zilkha KJ, Rose FC: The abnormal CT scan in migraine patients. In Rose FC, Amery WK (eds): Cerebral Hypoxia in the Pathogenesis of Migraine. Pitman, London, 1982
242. Sacquena T, Andreoli A, Baldrati A et al: Ischemic stroke in young adults: the relevance of migrainous infarction. Cephalalgia 9:255, 1989
243. Sakai F, Meyer JS: Regional cerebral hemodynamics during migraine and cluster headaches measured by the $^{133}$xenon inhalation method. Headache 18:122, 1978
244. Sargent JD, Solbach P: Medical evaluation of migraineurs: review of the value of laboratory and radiological tests. Headache 23:62, 1983
245. Saudeau D, Larmande P, Odier F, Autret A: Migraine compliquée, epilepsie et hypodensite tomodensitometrique. Rev Neurol (Paris) 138:787, 1982
246. Selby G, Fryer JA: Fatal migraine. Clin Exp Neurol 20:85, 1984
247. Sengers R, Sadhonders A, Bastiensen L: Ragged red fibre pathology due to micro-angiopathy?, abstracted. Muscle Nerve 55:184, 1986
248. Senter HJ, Lieberman AN, Pinto R: Cerebral manifestations of ergotism: report of a case and review of the literature. Stroke 7:88, 1976
249. Shuabib A: Stroke from other etiologies masquerading as migraine-stroke. Stroke 22:1068, 1991
250. Sicuteri F: Vasoneuroactive substances and their implications in vascular pain. Res Clin Stud Headache 1:6, 1967
251. Sicuteri F: Migraine, a central biochemical dysnociception. Headache 16:145, 1976
252. Sicuteri F: The nature of pain in headache and central panalgesia. p. 295. In Beers RF, Jr, Bassett EG (eds): Mechanism of pain and analgesic compounds. Raven Press, New York, 1979
253. Sinclair W: Dissecting aneurysm of the middle cerebral artery associated with migraine syndrome. Am J Pathol 29:1083, 1953
254. Skinhoj E: Regional cerebral blood flow in internal carotid distribution during migraine attack. Br Med J 3:569, 1969
255. Skinhoj E: Hemodynamic studies within the brain during migraine. Arch Neurol 29:95, 1973
256. Skyhoj-Olsen TS, Griberg L, Lassen NA: Ischemia may be the primary cause of the neurologic deficits in classic migraine. Arch Neurol 44:156, 1987
257. Snyder B, Ramirez-Lassepas M: Cerebral infarction in young adults: long term prognosis. Stroke 11:149, 1980
258. Solomon GD, Spaccavento LJ: Lateral medullary syndrome after basilar migraine. Headache 22:171, 1982

259. Sorges LJ, Cacyorin ED, Petro GR, Ramachandran T: Migraine: evaluation by MR. AJNR 9:425, 1988
260. Spaccavento LJ, Solomon GD: Migraine as an etiology of stroke in young adults. Headache 24:19, 1984
261. Spence JD, Wong DG, Melendez LJ et al: Increased prevalence of MVP in patients with migraine. Can Med Assoc J 131:1457, 1984
262. Stone GM, Burns RJ: Cerebral infarction caused by vasospasm. Med J Aust 1:556, 1982
263. Sulkava R, Kovanen J: Locked-in syndrome with rapid recovery: a manifestation of basilar artery migraine? Headache 23:238, 1983
264. Swanson JW, Vick NA: Basilar artery migraine: 12 patients, with an attack recorded electroencephalographically. Neurology (NY) 28:782, 1978
265. Symonds C: Migrainous variants. Trans Med Soc Lond 67:237, 1952
266. Symonds C: The circle of Willis. Br Med J 1:119, 1956
267. Thie A, Fuhlendorf A, Spitzer K, Kunze K: Transcranial Doppler evaluation of common and classic migraine. II. Ultrasonic features during attacks. Headache 30:109, 1990
268. Thomas JJ: Migraine and hemianopsia. J Nerv Ment Dis 34:153, 1907
269. Tinuper P, Cortelli P, Sacquegna T, Lugaresi E: Classic migraine attack complicated by confusional state: EEG and CT study. Cephalalgia 5:63, 1985
270. Tippin J, Corbett JJ, Kerbr RE et al: Amaurosis fugax and ocular infarction in adolescents and young adults. Ann Neurol 26:69, 1989
271. Torda C, Wolff HG: Experimental studies on headache. transient thickening of walls of cranial arteries in relation to certain phenomena of migraine headache and action of ergotamine tartrate on thickened walls. Arch Neurol Psychiatry 53:329, 1945
272. Troost BT: Migraine. In Glaser JS (ed): Neuro ophthalmology. Vol. 2. Harper & Row, New York, 1978
273. Troost BT: Migraine and facial pain. p. 288. In Lessell S, Van Dalen JTW (eds): Neuro-ophthalmology. Vol. 2. Excerpta Medica, Princeton, 1982
274. Victor DI, Welch RB: Bilateral retinal hemorrhages and disk edema in migraine. Am J Ophthalmol 84:555, 1977
275. Walsh WB, Hoyt WF: Clinical Neuro-ophthalmology. Vol. 2. Williams & Wilkins, Baltimore, 1969
276. Walton JN: Subarachnoid Hemorrhage. Livingstone, London, 1956
277. Waters WE, O'Connor PJ: Prevalence of migraine. J Neurol Neurosurg Psychiatry 38:613, 1975
278. Weber LW, Runge W: Störungen und Veränderungen des Sehappartas bei Pychosen und Neurosen. p. 800. In Schieck R, Bruckner A (eds): Kurzes Handbuch der Ophthalmologie. Vol. 6. J Springer, Berlin, 1931
279. Wegner W: Augenspiegelbefunde bei Migrane. Klin Monatsbl Augenheilkd 76:194, 1926
280. Weiner A: A case of permanent homonymous hemianopia following an attack of migraine. Med Rec 99:849, 1921
281. Weinstein JM, Feman SS: Ischemic optic neuropathy in migraine. Arch Ophthalmol 100:1097, 1982
282. Welch KMA. Migraine: a biobehavioral disorder. Arch Neurol 44:323, 1987
283. Welch KMA, Chabi JH, Nell K et al: Biochemical comparison of migraine and stroke. Headache 16:160, 1976
284. Welch KMA, Levine SR: Migraine-related stroke in the context of the International Headache Society Classification of Head Pain. Arch Neurol 47:458, 1990
285. Wells C: Premonitory symptoms in cerebral embolism. Arch Neurol 5:490, 1961
286. Whitty CWM: Familial hemiplegic migraine. J Neurol Neurosurg Psychiatry 16:172, 1953
287. Whitty CWM: Migraine without headache. Lancet 2:283, 1967
288. Whitty CWM, Hockaday JM, Whitty MM: The effect of oral contraceptives in migraine. Lancet 1:856, 1966
289. Wilbrand H, Saenger A: Neurologic des Auges. Vol. 3. JF Bergmann, Weisbaden, 1906
290. Williams TA: Variable migrainous recurrent paralyses followed by permanent incomplete lateral homonymous hemianopsia. Proc Philadelphia Neurol Soc 99:187, 1911
291. Willis T: Cerebri anatome, cui accessit nervorum descripto et usus. London, 1664. (As translated by Samuel Pordage, 1681, and reproduced in facsimile in Willis T: The Anatomy of the Brain and Nerves. McGill University Press, Montreal, 1965)
292. Wolff HG: Headache and other head pain. 2nd Ed. Oxford University Press, New York, 1963
293. Wolter JR, Burchfield WJ: Ocular migraine in a young man resulting in unilateral transient blindness and retinal edema. J Pediatr Ophthalmol 8:173, 1971

# 29
# *HYPERTENSIVE ENCEPHALOPATHY*

Henry B. Dinsdale

The term *hypertensive encephalopathy* refers to an acute cerebral syndrome precipitated by sudden, severe hypertension.[30] It is a medical emergency requiring prompt, effective treatment. Its incidence has declined in recent years, presumably due to improved treatment of hypertension, but this makes it even more important for clinicians to be alert to the condition, as it may be fatal if undiagnosed. Hypertensive encephalopathy is not to be confused with uremic encephalopathy or the various cerebrovascular complications of chronic, sustained hypertension;[18] indeed, it develops more easily in patients who are normotensive before the acute hypertensive episode.

## PATHOGENESIS

Cerebral blood flow remains constant under normal circumstances, despite wide variations of systemic blood pressure. This autoregulation depends primarily on a myogenic response of brain resistance vessels to elevations in arterial pressure and is essentially independent of control by the autonomic nervous system in normal circumstances. The mean systemic arterial blood pressure in a healthy adult is 90 mmHg, and the lower limit of normal autoregulation is approximately 60 mmHg. Long-standing hypertension causes a shift of the cerebral blood flow/blood pressure curve to the right due presumably to thickening of vessel walls and diminished responsiveness of resistance vessels.[40] Therefore, sudden elevations to relatively higher blood pressure levels are required to produce hypertensive encephalopathy in a patient with chronic hypertension, as compared to a normotensive person. Children may have the curve shifted to the left,[19] leaving them more at risk for the development of hypertensive encephalopathy. Adults rarely develop hypertensive encephalopathy at levels below 250/150 mmHg unless they were previously normotensive. The rate and the extent of rise of blood pressure are the most important factors determining the development of hypertensive encephalopathy, but it is difficult clinically and experimentally to evaluate them independent of each other.

Some patients show a "breakthrough of autoregulation" when systemic blood pressure is raised suddenly by angiotensin infusion, and it is suggested this is due to forced dilation of cerebral resistance vessels.[23] However, animal studies, which allow more detailed examination of regional cerebral blood flow, demonstrate that patterns of blood flow with acute hypertension are complex with both low and high flow areas coexisting in adjacent cortical regions.[6] Numerous studies have documented surface pial artery behavior in response to systemic hypertension with emphasis on regions either of vascular narrowing (spasm)[37] or dilation.[15] During initial blood pressure elevation there is a generalized decrease in diameter of surface cerebral arteries and maintenance of autoregulation, but when mean systemic arterial pressure exceeds 170 mmHg, dilation accompanied by a focal increase in cerebral blood flow is seen in some arteries that had resting diameters 100 $\mu$m or less. The largest component of cerebrovascular resistance is provided by penetrating, parenchymal arterioles, which are unavailable for in vivo visual inspection. Less is known about their physiologic behavior, but in some circumstances they show changes in flow and caliber opposite to that found in surface vessels.[16]

Retinal vessels possess interendothelial tight junctions and a blood-retinal barrier providing a model for comparison with cerebral vessels. Experiments in monkeys demonstrate that when systolic pressure becomes greater than 150 mmHg, retinal precapillary arterioles are markedly constricted with focal leakage of fluorescein.[11] Maximal vascular reactivity in response to hypertension is observed in the small precapillary arterioles, some of which become narrowed due to fibrin deposition in their walls. Dilated necrotic arterioles are uncommon.

Brain swelling, occasionally sufficient to cause herniation of cerebellar tonsils through the foramen magnum, is well documented at autopsy in patients dying during the hypertensive crisis[1,4] and in animal models of hypertensive encephalopathy.[2] Brain weight is increased, gyri are flattened and ventricles compressed, with microscopic examination revealing both generalized and patchy areas of edema,[1] providing autopsy confirmation of the computerized tomographic appearance of areas of diminished density in the white matter in patients with hypertensive encephalopathy.[34]

Hypertensive permeability changes in penetrating cerebral vessels have been carefully studied by Nag et al.[28] Within 90 seconds of angiotensin-induced hypertension, penetrating cerebral arterioles show abnormal permeability to protein-bound dyes and swelling of astrocytes limited to permeable regions. These changes are most pronounced at the level of the second and third cortical cell layers (Fig. 29-1) and are mediated by enhanced pinocytosis, which provides a means of rapid transport of macromolecules from blood through vessel walls to the neuropil. Pinocytosis probably is an important mechanism leading to the extravasation of protein-rich fluid into brain and the subsequent development of brain edema. Structural damage to cerebral vessels is not necessary for the production of brain edema, but vascular permeability presumably is increased further in the presence of the frequently associated findings of acute fibrinoid change of vessel walls, thrombosis, and microinfarction. In addition to osmotic changes, hydrostatic factors may alter the water content of the brain; central noradrenergic mechanisms, neuropeptides,[33] and sympathetic stimulation[14] have been shown to influence brain water permeability.

Extensive fibrin deposits (fibrinoid necrosis) is found in medium- and small-sized arteries throughout the brain. Similar vascular lesions are common in kidney and retina. If hypertensive encephalopathy develops in a patient with long-standing hypertension, a variety of additional hypertensive cerebrovascular changes may be found, including medial atrophy, hyperplasia, hyalinization, microinfarcts, and microaneurysms.

## CLINICAL FEATURES

Hypertensive encephalopathy may present at any age from the newborn[25] to the elderly but is most common in the second to fourth decades of life. Sometimes the syndrome will develop in the setting of acute or chronic renal disease, disseminated vasculitis (e.g., polyarteritis nodosa), or pheochromocytoma. Other less common but well-documented causes include autonomic stimulation secondary to bladder or gastrointestinal distention in patients with spinal cord injuries and rebound hypertension with substantial elevation of plasma catecholamines following discontinuation of clonidine[35] or other antihypertensive drugs. Rebound hypertension causing hypertensive encephalopathy has also been reported in

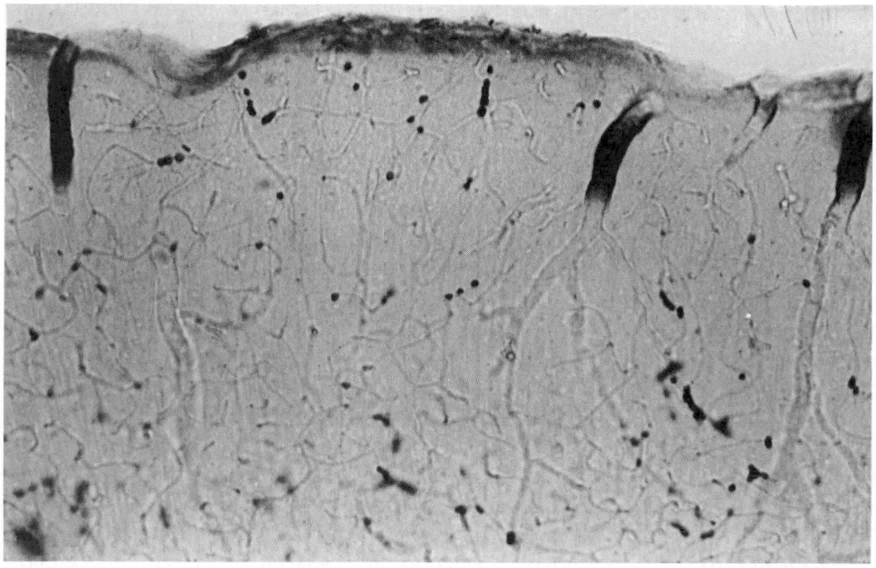

**Fig. 29-1.** Rat cerebral cortex 90 seconds after onset of hypertension. Horseradish peroxidase is present in the walls of three penetrating arterioles at level of lower portion of molecular layer and 2nd and 3rd cortical layers. (× 80.) (Courtesy of Dr. S. Nag.)

children after withdrawal of minoxidil, especially if withdrawal was rapid and total cumulative dose of the drug relatively high.[26] Patients taking monoamine oxidase inhibiting drugs may induce a hypertensive crisis if they ingest food high in tyramine content. Hypertensive encephalopathy can develop in infants with renal artery stenosis, thrombosis, or coarctation of the aorta.[25] Systemic arterial hypertension sufficient to cause hypertensive encephalopathy is a well-documented complication of thermal injury in children, particularly in males, and increasing with the magnitude of the thermal injury. Scorpion envenomation is another rare but well-documented cause.[39]

Severe acute hypertension can produce symptoms of headache, nausea, and vomiting within a few hours, presumably as the result of increasing intracranial pressure. There may be a variety of visual symptoms, including blurring or dimness, scintillating scotomata, or visual loss. Cortical blindness, color blindness, and dyslexia have been documented.[20] In the early stages of encephalopathy, patients may be anxious, agitated, and complaining of headache, while others are drowsy, confused, or disoriented. Generalized or focal convulsions or both may occur early, especially in children. Blood pressure is elevated to high levels. Bradycardia may reflect increasing intracranial pressure. A variety of changes of respiratory rhythm can develop, especially if the patient is showing neurologic deterioration. Optic disc swelling can reflect either increasing intracranial pressure or local ischemia of the nerve head, which can occur with normal intracranial pressure, progress to optic nerve infarction, and leave a permanent visual field defect. Visual acuity may be impaired due to subhyaloid hemorrhages or bullous retinal detachment.[41] Initial swelling of the optic disc can be masked by retinal edema. Fibrinoid necrosis of retinal arterioles may produce focal hemorrhage and serosanguineous exudates. Retinal ischemia leads to focal edema and collections of swollen neurons that appear as cotton-wool spots.

Although casual reference is often made to diffuse or focal "narrowing" or "spasm" of retinal arteries, there are few convincing reports of such "spasm" in hypertensive encephalopathy, especially with return to normal diameter following treatment. Vessel narrowing noted on funduscopic examination is usually due to the structural changes of arteriosclerosis.

Generalized hyperreflexia is a common early finding. Focal or lateralizing motor or sensory signs are sometimes present, which may be postictal or reflect focal cerebral ischemia. If hypertensive encephalopathy goes undiagnosed and untreated, the patient's condition may deteriorate within a few hours, with stupor progressing to coma and death.

*Lumbar puncture should be avoided.*

Computed tomography may show regions of decreased density in the cerebral or cerebellar white matter that disappear with reduction of blood pressure, suggesting reversal of cerebral edema.[21] MRI provides even better documentation of these changes.[17] Computed tomography may reveal evidence of brain swelling or ischemia. *The most important diagnostic factor is awareness by the responsible clinician of the association between severely elevated blood pressure and the patient's neurologic status.*

Hypertension accompanies many types of cerebrovascular disease, and the diagnosis of cerebral infarction, cerebral hemorrhage, or subarachnoid hemorrhage is considered in some patients with hypertensive encephalopathy, but the degree of elevation of blood pressure in hypertensive encephalopathy is usually much greater than that encountered with other cerebrovascular events. The diagnosis of hypertensive encephalopathy is supported by the absence of computed tomographic evidence of cerebral hemorrhage or infarction and the resolution of the neurologic syndrome when blood pressure is returned to normal.

Eclampsia can be considered a special example of hypertensive encephalopathy. Hypertension is a complication of 5 to 7 percent of pregnancies.[32] Approximately one-fourth of patients with essential hypertension who become pregnant develop superimposed preeclampsia as defined by the development, after the 24th week of pregnancy, of blood pressure greater than 145/90 mmHg, proteinuria, and persisting peripheral edema. If hypertension is not managed carefully, the patient will enter the eclamptic phase, with weight gain and increasing ankle and pretibial edema. The patient becomes restless, complains of headache and visual blurring, and often has an epileptic convulsion at home, after which she is brought to the hospital. Convulsions develop before labor in 50 percent of eclamptic patients, during labor in 25 percent, and within 24 hours of delivery in the remainder.

## TREATMENT

The Joint National Committee on Detection, Evaluation and Treatment of High Blood Pressure in its 1984 report[22] divided the treatment of severe hypertension into two categories: (1) hypertensive emergencies in which severe elevation of blood pressure results in acute end organ damage and represents an acute threat to vital organs or to the patient's survival, and (2) hypertensive urgencies in which severe elevation of blood pressure represents a potential threat but acute end organ damage is not present. The patient with hypertensive encephalopathy belongs in the first category and must be treated in the hospital where blood pressure, seizures, level of consciousness, and airway patency can be monitored closely.

Under normal conditions, symptoms of cerebral hypoperfusion develop when mean arterial pressure is reduced to 40 percent of baseline levels. Therefore, a patient with a blood pressure of 225/150 mmHg will have a reduction of cerebral blood flow if pressure is lowered to 140/100 mmHg, and develop symptoms of cerebral anoxia if pressure drops to 110/70 mmHg or less. Patients with chronic hypertension have their lower limit of autoregulation set at a higher level than normotensive patients,[24,40] which may explain reports of boundary zone infarction after rapid treatment of chronic hypertension.[12]

An ideal drug to lower blood pressure rapidly in an emergency would have rapid reversible action that is predictable and controlled, low toxic-to-therapeutic ratio, and no depressant effects on the central nervous system. Such an ideal drug is not yet available, but those currently favored are the vasodilators nitroprusside, diazoxide, and hydralazin. Vasodilators elevate intracranial pressure in some circumstances depending upon the extent of brain swelling, level of preexisting blood pressure, $PaCO_2$, and method of administration.[5,27,42,43] Concern has therefore been expressed that vasodilators might be harmful by increasing intracranial pressure; however, clinical experience strongly suggests that the benefits of prompt reduction of blood pressure outweigh other considerations. Some authors advocate the continuous monitoring of intracranial pressure throughout treatment.[13]

Sodium nitroprusside is given intravenously (0.5 to 0.8 $\mu$g/kg/min) and requires skillful and constant supervision. The rate of infusion is adjusted according to response, and its hypotensive effect is potentiated by a head-up tilt of the patient. Its effect is seen within a few minutes through venous relaxation and increased venous capacitance while maintaining an unchanged cardiac output.

Diazoxide must be given rapidly intravenously, but the effect is less predictable and controlled than with sodium nitroprusside. The recommended dose is 150 mg given in 15 to 30 seconds. This usually produces a dramatic lowering of blood pressure within 1 to 2 minutes. It causes sodium retention and also interferes with carbohydrate metabolism, which could be a disadvantage as suggested by evidence of increased CNS damage in the presence of hyperglycemia.[38]

Hydralazine may increase cardiac work and therefore must be given cautiously to patients with coronary artery disease. It increases heart rate, stroke volume, and cardiac output and appears to be less effective than sodium nitroprusside or diazoxide in treating encephalopathy.

Captopril, an angiotensin-converting enzyme inhibitor, is effective in acutely reducing blood pressure and reversing encephalopathy in some patients treated under carefully controlled conditions.[3]

Oral drugs lower blood pressure less rapidly than parenteral drugs and may be used in urgent situations to treat patients who have not yet developed encephalopathy or severe cardiac complications. Nifedipine, an oral calcium channel blocking agent[8] has been compared with intravenous sodium nitroprusside in patients with severe (diastolic blood pressure greater than 130 mmHg) uncomplicated (free of focal neurologic signs or coma) hypertension.[10] Treatment with nifedipine resulted in less time in the intensive care unit for the patient without an increase in morbidity or mortality. Nifedipine was administered as a 10-mg oral dose and repeated within 2 hours if diastolic blood pressure had not fallen below 120 mmHg. The average total dose required was 20 mg with the onset of effect within 1 hour and peak effect at 1.5 or 2 hours following the initial dose. Blood pressure was lowered immediately with sodium nitroprusside, but it took longer to stabilize the diastolic blood pressure at an acceptable lower level. Nifedipine is effective in the treatment of hypertensive urgencies and some emergencies, but caution is required using this medication in the elderly, those with coronary disease, and in patients whose volume is depleted because of vomiting.[29] Absorption of nifedipine from the oral cavity is slow and incomplete. The capsule should be bitten and the contents swallowed if a rapid effect is required.

During the acute phase of hypertensive encephalopathy it may be necessary to attempt to lessen cerebral edema directly, in addition to lowering blood pressure. Dexamethasone 4 to 6 mg intramuscularly every 4 to 6 hours reduces cerebral edema.[36] Steroids probably have multiple modes of action on central nervous system function, including effects on neurotransmitters and other systems,[9] as well as restoring normal permeability to cerebral vessels. Hyperosmolar agents such as mannitol or glycerol may also be given to treat cerebral edema in the absence of renal disease.

Anticonvulsants will usually be required from the outset. Intravenous administration ensures rapid loading doses of drugs such as phenytoin. Diazepam is much favored as an anticonvulsant drug in emergency situations, but its central depressant action, including the risk of respiratory arrest, dictates that it be used with caution. The hypotensive effect of diazepam can also complicate assessment of the efficacy of other hypotensive agents.

Parenteral agents can be discontinued and oral antihypertensive drugs commenced when blood pressure is reduced to target levels, which will be slightly higher for patients with long-standing hypertension than with normotensives. Treatment with a diuretic is often combined with a beta-blocker such as propanolol. If there is impairment of renal function, a loop diuretic such as furosemide will be required.

Eclamptic patients require stabilization of vital signs achieved by controlling convulsions, lowering blood pressure, and maintaining renal output. Pregnancy can then be terminated, at which time one may have to treat hypovolemia, disseminated microvascular coagulation, and the cumulative effects of various medications.

There is a general clinical impression that patients who survive hypertensive encephalopathy make a complete neurologic recovery. A minority of patients, however, are left with focal neurologic deficits such as occipital lobe infarction. It is also possible that general disturbances might remain due to multiple small infarcts of the cerebral cortex and white matter. A multicenter follow-up study with careful neurologic and psychometric evaluation would help to determine the long-term consequences of this illness, but with improved treatment of hypertension it is unlikely that any single hospital will develop a sizeable number of such patients in the future.

The quality of follow-up care and treatment of blood pressure in patients with hypertensive encephalopathy has been demonstrated to be as poor as the management of hypertension in the general population.[7]

## REFERENCES


1. Adams RD, VanderEecken HM: Vascular diseases of the brain. Annu Rev Med 4:213, 1953
2. Byrom FB: The pathogenesis of hypertensive encephalopathy and its relation to the malignant phase of hypertension: Experimental evidence from the hypertensive rat. Lancet 2:201, 1954
3. Case DB, Atlas SA, Sullivan PA, Laragh JH: Acute and chronic treatment of severe and malignant hypertension with the oral angiotensin converting enzyme inhibitor captopril. Circulation 64:765, 1981
4. Chapmen K, Karimi R: A case of postpartum eclampsia of late onset confirmed by autopsy. Am J Obstet Gynecol 117:858, 1978
5. Cottrell JE, Patel K, Turndorf H, Ransohoff J: Intracranial pressure changes induced by sodium nitroprusside in patients with intracranial mass lesions. J Neurosurg 48:329, 1978
6. Dinsdale HB, Robertson DM, Haas RA: Cerebral blood flow in acute hypertension. Arch Neurol 31:80, 1974
7. Dollery CT: The care of patients with malignant hypertension in London 1974–1975. p. 37. In McLachlan G (ed): A Question of Quality. Oxford University Press, London, 1976
8. Ellrodt AG, Ault MJ, Riedinger MS, Murata GH: Efficacy and safety of sublingual nifedipine in hypertensive emergencies. Am J Med 79:19, 1985
9. Fishman RA: Steroids in the treatment of brain edema. N Engl J Med 306:359, 1982
10. Franklin C, Nightingale S, Mamdani B: A randomized comparison of nifedipine and sodium nitroprusside in severe hypertension. Chest 90:500, 1986
11. Garner A, Ashton N, Tripathi R et al: Pathogenesis of hypertensive retinopathy: an experimental study in the monkey. Br J Ophthalmol 59:3, 1975
12. Graham DI: Ischaemic brain damage of cerebral perfusion type after treatment of severe hypertension. Br Med J 4:739, 1975
13. Griswold WP, Viney J, Mendoza SA, James HE: Intracranial pressure monitoring in severe hypertensive encephalopathy. Crit Care Med 9:573, 1981
14. Grubb RL, Raichle ME, Eichling JO: Peripheral sympathetic regulation of brain water permeability. p. 264. In Ingvar DH, Lassen NA (eds): Cerebral Function, Metabolism and Circulation. Munksgaard, Copenhagen, 1977
15. Haggendal E, Johansson B: On the pathophysiology of the increased cerebrovascular permeability in acute arterial hypertension in cats. Acta Neurol Scand 48:265, 1972
16. Harper AM, Deshmukh VD, Rowen JO, Jennett WB: The influence of sympathetic nervous activity on cerebral blood flow. Arch Neurol 27:1, 1972
17. Hauser RA, Lacey M, Knight MR: Hypertensive encephalopathy: magnetic resonance imaging demonstration of reversible cortical and white matter lesions. Arch Neurol 45:1078, 1988
18. Healton EB, Brust JC, Feinfeld DA, Thomson GE: Hypertensive encephalopathy and the neurologic manifestations of malignant hypertension. Neurology (NY) 32:127, 1982
19. Hulse JA, Taylor DSI, Dillon MJ: Blindness and paraplegia in severe childhood hypertension. Lancet 2:553, 1979
20. Jellinek EH, Painter M, Prineas J, Ross Russell RW: Hypertensive encephalopathy with cortical disorders of vision. QJ Med 33:239, 1964
21. Jespersen CM, Rasmussen D, Hennild V: Focal intracerebral oedema in hypertensive encephalopathy visualized by computerized topographic scan. J Intern Med 225:349, 1989
22. Joint National Committee on Detection, Evaluation and Treatment of High Blood Pressure: The 1984 Report of the Joint National Committee. Arch Intern Med 144:1045, 1984
23. Lassen NA, Agnoli A: Scand J Clin Lab Invest 30:113, 1972
24. Ledingham JGG, Rajagopalan B: Cerebral complications in the treatment of accelerated hypertension. QJ Med 48:25, 1979
25. Mace S, Hirschfeld S: Hypertensive encephalopathy. Am J Dis Child 137:32, 1983
26. Makker SP, Moorthy B: Rebound hypertension following minoxidil withdrawal. J Pediatr 96:762, 1980
27. Marsh ML, Shapiro HM, Smith RW, Marshall LF: Changes in neurologic status and intracranial pressure associated with sodium nitroprusside administration. Anesthesiology 51:336, 1979
28. Nag S, Robertson DM, Dinsdale HB: Cerebral cortical changes in acute experimental hypertension: an ultrastructural study. Lab Invest 36:150, 1977
29. O'Mailia J, Sander G, Giles T: Nifedipine-associated myocardial ischemia or infarction in the treatment of hypertensive urgencies. Ann Intern Med 107:85, 1987
30. Oppenheimer BS, Fishberg AM: Hypertensive encephalopathy. Arch Intern Med 41:264, 1928
31. Popp MB, Friedberg DL, MacMillan BG: Clinical characteristics of hypertension in several children. Ann Surg 191:473, 1980
32. Pritchard JA, MacDonald PC: Hypertensive disor-

ders in pregnancy. p. 666. In Williams Obstetrics. 16th Ed. Appleton & Lange, E. Norwalk, CT, 1980
33. Raichle ME, Grubb RL, Eichling JO: Central neuroendocrine regulation of brain water permeability. Ciba Found Symp 56:219, 1977
34. Rail DL, Perkin GD: Computerized tomographic appearance of hypertensive encephalopathy. Arch Neurol 37:310, 1980
35. Reid JL, Wing LMH, Dargie HJ et al: Clonidine withdrawal in hypertension: changes in blood pressure and plasma and urinary noradrenaline. Lancet 1:1171, 1977
36. Reulen HJ, Hadjidimos A, Shermann K: The effect of dexamethasone on water electrolyte content and on rCBF in perifocal brain edema in man. p. 239. In Reulen HJ, Shermann K (eds): Steroids and Brain Edema. Springer-Verlag, New York, 1972
37. Rodda R, Denny-Brown D: The cerebral arteries in experimental hypertension. I. The nature of arteriolar constriction and its effects on the collateral circulation. Am J Pathol 49:53, 1966
38. Siemkowicz E, Hansen AJ: Brain extracellular ion composition and EEG activity following 10 minutes' ischemia in normotensive and hyperglycemic rats. Stroke 12:236, 1981
39. Sofes S, Gueron M: Vasodilators and hypertensive encephalopathy following scorpion envenomation in children. Chest 97:118, 1990
40. Strandgaard S, Olesen J, Skinhoj E, Lassen NA: Autoregulation of brain circulation in severe arterial hypertension. Br Med J 1:507, 1973
41. Stropes LL, Luft SC: Hypertensive crisis with bilateral bullous retinal detachment. JAMA 238:1948, 1977
42. Stullken EH Jr, Sokoll MD: Intracranial pressure during hypotension and subsequent vasopressor therapy in anesthetized cats. Anesthesiology 42:425, 1975
43. Turner JM, Powell D, Gibson RM, McDowall DJ: Intracranial pressure changes in neurosurgical patients during hypotension induced with sodium nitroprusside or trimethaphan. Br J Anaesth 49:419, 1977

# 30
# *MULTI-INFARCT DEMENTIA: AN EXPANDING CONCEPT*

Shirish M. Hastak
Vladimir C. Hachinski

In 1694, Malpighi was affected by a stroke involving the right side of his body.[67] About 40 days later "he got clear of apoplexy and palsie"; however, he continued to suffer "in his memory and reason and melted into tears on the slightest occasion." This may have been the first case of vascular dementia in the literature, but, as late as 1883, when Kraeplin[61] published his classification of mental disorders, few higher function disorders had a clearly established etiology, with the notorious exception of neurosyphilis. This was despite the suggestion by Wilks[109] in 1864 that there could be a pathologic substrate to mental disorders. Dementia remains, in spite of all advances, a clinical diagnosis, even though underlying structural changes are generally implied.

It was Otto Binswanger[14] in 1894 who wrote on the differential diagnosis of general paralysis of the insane and differentiated an entity he called "encephalitis subcorticalis chronica progressiva." This was based on the clinicopathologic observations of eight cases, but he failed to publish microscopic descriptions. Binswanger had noted a subcortical white matter atrophy which was associated with dementia, and he postulated this white matter change to be secondary to arteriosclerosis and the resultant deficient blood supply. Interestingly, it was Alois Alzheimer[4] who first introduced the name "Binswanger's disease" and gave the first microscopic description of the change in the white matter. In 1899 Alzheimer,[3] after having done a pathologic evaluation of the cortex in arteriosclerosis, postulated that macrovascular disease produced strokes, while microvascular disease produced dementia.

The term *arteriosclerotic dementia* was coined by Alvarez,[2] a gastroenterologist. The concept of arteriosclerotic dementia long survived, despite vigorous attacks by Wertham and Wertham[108] in 1934 and by Fields[31] in 1972. Later it became increasingly clear that the idea of arteriosclerotic dementia with slow strangulation of the blood vessels and chronic ischemic damage was untenable, as there was no evidence of any ischemic damage over a prolonged period of time in a dementing process. In 1974 Hachinski et al.[47] coined the term *multi-infarct dementia* (MID) arguing that brain infarction is the necessary pathogenetic substrate for a vascular dementia.

The pathologic work of Tomlinson et al.[99] supported the concept of multi-infarct dementia and suggested that a minimal quantitative brain damage (more than 100 ml brain tissue) was a prerequisite for the production of dementia. This overemphasis on quantitative threshold for production of dementia has since been questioned.[26] Strategically situated brain infarctions with much less tissue damage can also produce a dementing disorder.[20,28,44,59,71] Even to date, controversy prevails as to the contribution of white matter in a dementing process and whether this white matter change is vascular in origin. It remains unproved whether, apart from the classical quantal brain damage due to infarction, subtle cellular or subcellular

**TABLE 30.1. Ischemic Threshold (Experimental)**

| Threshold | Cerebal Blood Flow (ml/100 g/min) | Ref. |
|---|---|---|
| Protein synthesis | 40 | 110 |
| Reversible neurologic deficits | 23 | 58 |
| Cessation of spontaneous neuronal spikes | 18 | 51 |
| Evoked potentials absent | 15 | 15 |
| White matter damage | >14 | 69 |
| Gray matter damage | 10–12 | 69 |
| Intracellular $K^+$ release | 8 | 7 |

damage to the brain due to ischemia occurs, which individually may be clinically silent but cumulatively could lead to dementia.

Ischemic damage to the brain may not only be *histologic brain infarction* with destruction of all elements as defined by pathologic observation. The spectrum of ischemic damage to the brain is broad (see Table 30-1) and, experimentally, when brain blood flow is gradually reduced, a functional threshold is initially reached below which the neurons do not function but remain morphologically intact. Further reduction of blood supply leads to morphologic damage (presumed infarction).[9,50] It is also necessary to take into account, apart from flow values of blood, the duration of reduction of blood flow and the difference in ischemic vulnerability of the brain tissue.[52] It may well be that histologic brain infarction is the end result of this chain of ischemic injury and we are looking at the "devastation done," having completely missed the route that this process has taken. This does not mean that the concept of multi-infarct dementia is being challenged, as this is based on a firm foundation of histologic brain infarction, but that this concept probably needs expansion to include ischemic damage that occurs prior to definite brain infarction. It must be admitted that in the human brain at autopsy there is no morphologic correlate of ischemia other than histologic brain infarction; hence the concept at present remains speculative. Certain guidelines will be considered to put things into perspective.

## DEFINITIONS

### Dementia

According to DSM-III,[5] dementia refers to a deterioration in multiple cognitive abilities that exceeds the decline expected with normal aging and occurs in a state of clear consciousness. The lengthy criteria laid down in DSM-IIIR (see Table 30-2)[6] are useful for research purposes, but in clinical practice the operational definition of Cummings and Benson[24] is useful: "Dementia is an acquired persistent impairment of intellectual function with compromise in at least three of the following spheres of mental activity: memory, cognition, emotion or personality, visuospatial skills, and language." Impairment in any one sphere indicates focal brain dysfunction and is not sufficient to diagnose dementia, which is a global brain deficit.

DSM-IIIR[6] also lays down certain guidelines for indicating the severity of dementia into mild, moderate, and severe.

*Mild Dementia:* Although work or social activities are significantly impaired, the capacity of independent living remains with adequate personal hygiene and relatively intact judgment.

*Moderate Dementia:* Independent living is hazardous, and some degree of supervision is necessary.

**TABLE 30-2. Diagnostic Criteria for Dementia**

A. Demonstrable evidence of impairment in short- and long-term memory. Impairment in short-term memory (inability to learn new information) may be indicated by inability to remember three objects after 5 minutes. Long-term memory impairment (inability to remember information that was known in the past) may be indicated by inability to remember past personal information (e.g., what happened yesterday, birthplace, occupation) or facts of common knowledge (e.g., past presidents, well-known dates).
B. At least one of the following:
   1. Impairment in abstract thinking, as indicated by inability to find similarities and differences between related words, difficulty in defining words and concepts, and other similar tasks.
   2. Impaired judgment, as indicated by inability to make reasonable plans to deal with interpersonal, family, and job-related problems and issues.
   3. Other disturbances of higher cortical function, such as aphasia (disorder of language), apraxia (inability to carry out motor activities despite intact comprehension and motor function), agnosia (failure to recognize or identify objects despite intact sensory function), and "constructional difficulty" (e.g., inability to copy three-dimensional figures, assemble blocks, or arrange sticks in specific designs).
   4. Personality change (i.e., alteration or accentuation of premorbid traits).
C. The disturbance in A and B significantly interferes with work or usual social activities or relationships with others.
D. Not occurring exclusively during the course of delirium.
E. Either 1 or 2:
   1. There is evidence from the history, physical examination, or laboratory tests of a specific organic factor (or factors) judged to be etiologically related to the disturbance.
   2. In the absence of such evidence, an etiologic organic factor can be presumed if the disturbance cannot be accounted for by any nonorganic mental disorder (e.g., major depression accounting for cognitive impairment).

(From American Psychiatric Association,[6] with permission.)

*Severe Dementia:* Activities of daily living are so impaired that continual supervision is required.

### Multi-infarct Dementia (Vascular Dementia)

It may be thought of as an acquired persistent mental impairment as a result of brain injury secondary to vascular disease.

DSM-IIIR[6] has proposed certain criteria for the diagnosis of multi-infarct dementia (vascular dementia):

1. Dementia
2. Stepwise deteriorating course with patchy distribution of deficit early in the course
3. Focal neurologic signs and symptoms
4. Evidence from history, physical examination, or laboratory tests of significant cerebrovascular disease that is judged to be etiologically related to the disturbance

## EPIDEMIOLOGY

Vascular dementia is at present the second commonest cause for a dementing disorder after Alzheimer's disease, and we suspect that with increasing recognition of mixed form of dementia this is likely to go down in the list. Its prevalence in patients seen for dementia ranges from 8[38,70] to 12 percent.[13,68,94] Clinicopathologic studies have shown that in an elderly population with dementing disorder 50 to 65 percent are likely to have Alzheimer's disease, 12 to 20 percent vascular dementia, and 15 to 20 percent show mixed features.[60,99] These series are likely to be biased; but we must accept their conclusions until more precise studies are carried out. The figure of 20 percent as due to vascular factors may not be an exaggeration of the problem, as a substantial number of mixed cases may have predominant vascular component as a basis of their dementia. It is increasingly being recognized that clinically diagnosed degenerative dementia may show mixed pathology and may have a potentially preventable vascular component.

Since the age at onset of a dementing disorder cannot be ascertained objectively, it is likely to have an examiner, patient, or family bias. Some original reports stated that vascular dementia affects the younger age group than dementia of the Alzheimer type, but it is felt that recent findings are less conclusive.[12,23,90,99] Interestingly, mixed dementia is more likely to start at a later age than vascular dementia or Alzheimer's disease alone.[12,23] In relation to the sex difference the analysis of various studies makes one conclude that a demented male is more likely to have vascular dementia, while a woman has more chance of suffering from Alzheimer's disease, although the power of this effect is not great.[75]

In a recent study[98] 927 patients with acute ischemic stroke, aged above 60 years, were analyzed in relation to epidemiologic variables in dementia. Though the basic framework of the study has definite limitations and it is not a population-based study, these investigators have presented some interesting findings. Based on logistic regression analyses, the probability of new-onset dementia at 1 year was 5.4 percent for a 60-year-old patient and 10.4 percent for a patient who was 90 years old. They observed that incidence of dementia in this selected population was related to age and not to sex. They felt that the most important predictors of incidence of a dementing disorder were a previous stroke and the presence of cortical atrophy at stroke onset.

## PATHOGENESIS AND THE CONTROVERSY OF THE WHITE MATTER

The classical work of Tomlinson et al.[99,100] was instrumental in generating a concept that quantity of brain destroyed is the critical factor in a vascular dementing process. They observed that more than 100 ml of brain tissue destruction was invariably associated with dementia, and this came to be considered later as a quantitative threshold for the production of cognitive decline. They concluded from their work that "important pathological differences exist between nondemented and demented old people and these are largely quantitative and not qualitative." Their sample was biased, and no indication as to the severity of dementia and vascular risk factors were given in the study. In spite of a clear description of the changes in the white matter in patients with vascular dementia, no speculation as to the contribution of this process to the cognitive decline was made. In another study[91] it was observed that within the group of patients with vascular dementing process there was a relationship between volume of the infarcted brain tissue and degree of dementia.

Later case reports showed that strategically located vascular lesions (e.g., mesencephalic or diencephalic), though involving minimal brain tissue, could produce a dementing syndrome.[20,28,44,59,71] In a recent clinicopathologic study[26] 40 patients with vascular dementia were studied. The number of strokes, neurologic and neuropsychological disturbances, volume of infarction specifically in the frontal, occipital and basal regions, lacunar state, and white matter lesions were found to be significantly greater in demented patients. The authors write: "thereby it cannot be generally stated that vascular dementia is due to the loss of a volume of brain tissue larger than a critical threshold of 50 or 100 ml. The importance previously attributed to multiple gross cortical lesions can be challenged and the role of other minute lesions mainly subcortical must be considered." They conclude that the volume of macroscopic infarction, the white matter lesion, and the lacunar state showed equal contribution to the cognitive impairment. Thus it seems likely that the quantity of brain destroyed may not be as critical a factor contributing to cognitive impairment as believed previously.

If the volume of destroyed brain tissue is not critical, and, except for case reports, the majority of vascular lesions of the brain seen in dementing disorders are not strategically placed, what then is the real pathogenetic substrate of a vascular cognitive change in humans? Can there be a link between the radiologic change in the density of white matter (termed leuko-araiosis from *leuko,* white, *araiosis,* diminution of density)[48] and cognitive impairment? If this is so then what exactly is the pathogenesis of this change? Is this change in the white matter vascular in origin? These are some of the recent controversies in vascular dementia to which a substantial amount of recent research work has been directed.

We studied[96] 105 "normal" elderly volunteers, investigated with CT scans, psychometric testing [extended scale for dementia (ESD)] and neurologic examination. After doing item analysis of the ESD, it was found that subjects with leuko-araiosis performed poorly on time orientation, sentence construction, and memory tasks. It was concluded that leuko-araiosis may represent a marker for early vascular dementia and that white matter abnormalities play a significant role in development of cognitive impairment. The white matter change seen on CT scan may not reflect the white matter change seen on MRI either temperospatially or pathogenetically. Thus, when one considers the change in the white matter it is important to take into account the radiologic technique used to observe this change. Interestingly, most studies using CT scan[25,41,101] point toward an association between changes in the white matter and cognition, whereas a number of MRI studies have been unable to show such an association.[10,53,85] It is now accepted that MRI has the capacity to study brain water distribution well beyond the capabilities of a CT scan. Thus we suspect that MRI picks up white matter changes so early that no correlation with cognitive change can be established with the present neuropsychological testing methods.

DeReuck and his colleagues,[27] in their study of the brain, have shown a vulnerability of the subcortical areas of the brain to ischemic insult. It is felt that the periventricular region is a watershed area between the central penetrating and the deep perforating vessels. It has been suggested[21] that given the high incidence of cerebrovascular risk factors in patients with white matter changes and its frequent association with *état criblé* and perivascular demyelination with areas of infarction and hyalinized cortical vessels all point toward a vascular pathogenetic mechanism for this change in the brain. Some workers have found an association between leuko-araiosis and arteriosclerosis,[78] while others have related it to cerebral amyloid angiopathy.[43] Cerebral blood flow studies do provide some support that this change in the white matter could be related to vascular factors.[17,30] Recently Hijdra and colleagues[55] studied the relation of the white matter change in the brain to the type of vascular lesion (lacune, infarct, hemorrhage). It was found that leuko-araiosis was associated with lacunar infarcts and brain hemorrhages (not related to aneurysms or arteriovenous malformations). They thus concluded that these findings suggest that leuko-araiosis is associated with small vessel disease.

Initial pathologic studies of the white matter were done using gross observation as a guideline, and later CT scan and MRI were used as markers. Janota[56] in patients with dementia has reported an ischemic destruction predominantly of the white matter of the brain resembling that seen in infarction. He was careful to observe that neuropathologically there was no evidence of Alzheimer's disease or any other organic dementing process. Microscopically the white matter showed diffuse patchy lack of myelin, axons, and fibrillary gliosis. The white matter also showed areas of reactive gemistocytic astrocytes, fibrillary astrocytes, microglia, compound granular corpuscles with neutral lipid and edema. The wall of the blood vessels in the white matter was thickened and fibrous. He postulated from his study that the white matter may suffer from reduced blood supply due to a relatively poor anastomotic system combined with pathologic changes in the small arteries.

In a pathologic study[78] of four patients with CT scan showing periventricular white matter changes it was reported that these brains microscopically showed demyelination without inflammatory cells, infarctions in the periventricular white matter, lacunar infarctions, and marked arteriosclerosis. In a remarkable work, Brun and Englund[19] studied the white matter changes in patients with Alzheimer's disease. They stated "we have observed in addition to grey matter degeneration a lesion that has a character of an incomplete infarction confined to the white matter." This white matter lesion was characterized by partial loss of myelin, axons and oligodendroglial cells, mild reactive astrocytic gliosis and sparsely distributed macrophages with stenosis resulting from hyaline fibrosis of arterioles and smaller vessels. They felt that this white matter change was due to hypoperfusion of the white matter and was vascular in origin. Similar pathologic findings were noted in a study[41] in which five patients with Alzheimer's disease and white matter changes (leuko-araiosis) seen on CT scan were studied. The authors felt that the white matter change histopathologically represented typical features of subcortical vascular disease. It was observed that all five patients were severely demented prior to death, but only one brain showed pathologic changes typical of severe Alzheimer's disease and it was postulated that white matter lesions (presumably vascular in origin) may contribute to the cognitive change. A detailed histologic analysis of the pericapillary nerve plexus was done in five patients with senile dementia of the Alzheimer type (SDAT) and compared to five age-matched controls.[92] Surprisingly, there was no trace of the perivascular nerve plexus in patients with SDAT, and this was present in controls. The workers thus felt that "denervation microangiopathy" may lead to a profound alteration in blood-brain barrier function and may act as a pathogenetic factor in SDAT. In a recent study[15] blood-brain barrier function (as measured by albumin ratio) was found to be disturbed in patients with Alzheimer's disease and this was said to be related to clinical vascular factors. This leads to an interesting hypothesis that in Alzheimer's disease a part of the cognitive change may be related to vascular involvement and thus is likely to be reversible.

Wallin et al.[107] studied the composition of the white matter from the centrum semiovale in patients with vascular dementia and in some cases of Alzheimer's disease. They found that in both these disorders the content of phospholipids and cholesterol was reduced in the white matter, the diminution of cerebrosides and sulfatides was more pronounced, while the concentration of gangliosides was normal. In the white matter, the axonal membrane has the highest ganglioside content, while the cerebrosides are mainly restricted to the myelin. This study indicated that the primary structure involved in the white matter was myelin. Based on their observations they felt that in vascular dementia the subcortical white matter is involved not only in the areas of infarction but more generally. It has been postulated that, considering the ratio of cell body surface membrane to the myelin membrane,[84] the oligodendrocyte is likely to have a large metabolic requirement[107] and thus be vulnerable to ischemic insult. These findings are in line with the evidence put forward by Brun and Englund[19] that a white matter involvement occurs in Alzheimer's disease and this is likely to be vascular in origin. It was shown in vascular dementia[106] that the albumin ratio (CSF/serum) is elevated as compared to controls, indicating an alteration of the blood-brain barrier. Since in the group with vascular dementia there was no clinical evidence of TIA/stroke in the 3 months prior, the authors felt that this altered blood-brain barrier was unlikely to be due to brain infarction and was related to chronically disturbed function of the small vessels. A previous study had also reported an altered blood-brain barrier in patients with vascular dementia.[64]

Another interesting thought was that immunologic factors may be involved in the pathogenesis of a vascular dementing process. The intrathecal synthesis of immunoglobulin G was evaluated by analyzing CSF and serum IgG and oligoclonal band in CSF.[105] In vascular dementia intrathecal synthesis of IgG was shown, and the authors also noted a correlation between IgG index and hypertension. They felt that the elevated IgG index was not a consequence of brain infarction, but was an indication of a small vessel disorder as hypertension is related to small vessel disease. Alafuzoff et al.[1] studied the changes in the cerebral cortex by an immunocytologic technique in cases of vascular dementia. They found the presence of heavy deposits of serum proteins around capillaries of the gray matter in cases of vascular dementia. They suggest that this may indicate a defect of the cortical capillary system, which might play a role in the development of vascular dementia. They add that the enrichment of C1q in the perivascular deposit supports a likely immunologic process underlying the deposit of proteins.

The evidence that multiple lacunes in the brain lead to a dementing disorder is weak. Fisher,[32–35] who did the pioneering work in this field, considered dementia to be rare even in the presence of multiple lacunes. It should be appreciated that commonly lacunes occur at sites in the brain functionally unrelated to cognition. Roman[88] states that dementia usually does not occur even in cases with severe involvement and multiple lacunes. It is clear from previous studies that the presence of vascular lesion in the brain does not imply that the dementing disorder is secondary to a vascular insult unless Alzheimer's disease has been carefully ruled out, and not even then can a direct relationship be established. Most of the studies that claim an entity of lacunar dementia on pathologic grounds have failed to take this fact into account.[93]

Neurotransmitter changes in vascular dementia were studied[104] in nine patients with macroscopic signs of brain infarcts and no clinical evidence of senile dementia of the Alzheimer's type. The mean volume of brain infarction was 6.8 ml. Marked disturbances of the serotoninergic and cholinergic systems were noted in the subcortical and cortical regions. It was felt that this widespread neurotransmitter change could not be explained by localized infarcts. It was thus hypothesized that in severely demented patients there is a capillary defect that is precipitated by hemodynamic factors such as changes in heart rhythm or blood pressure. This general disturbance of the vessels is responsible for the widespread neurotransmitter disturbance. Interestingly, a similar neurotransmitter disturbance has been observed in cases of Alzheimer's disease.[42] Neuron-specific enolase (NSE) in the CSF is a marker of active injury to the central nervous system.[76] This fact was utilized by Sulkava et al.[97] who studied CSF-NSE in 35 patients with multi-infarct dementia and compared this to controls. They found that patients with vascular dementia without history suggestive of recent stroke had lower CSF-NSE levels as compared to controls. This is in keeping with the prevailing opinion that vascular dementia is caused by multiple infarcts and is not due to a chronic neuronal ischemia.

## DIAGNOSIS

The diagnosis of vascular dementia consists of the following two steps.

**Clinical Diagnosis of Dementia.** Here the guidelines as given by DSM-IIIR[6] may be used, but as pointed out previously, this is useful mainly for research purposes. Clinically we have found the approach outlined by Cummings and Benson[24] to be extremely useful. In all our patients we try to evaluate if there is an acquired persistent impairment of intellectual function, with impairment in at least three of the following five: memory, cognition, emotion or personality, visuospatial skills, or language.[24] The mini-mental state examination (Folstein et al.[36]) is a useful screening test in clinical practice provided its limitations are considered.[7,40] Once the diagnosis of dementia is established, it becomes necessary to define to what extent the underlying changes in the brain are vascular in origin. Dementia secondary to depression (pseudodementia), drugs, and metabolic factors must be ruled out in each case as these are common reversible causes of a cognitive impairment.[22]

**Ischemic Score.** The ischemic score was proposed by Hachinski et al.[46] by giving numerical values to the clinical features of vascular dementia (Table 30-3). Wade and Hachinski[102] have attempted to clarify the clinical features in the ischemic score so as to enhance its application unambiguously. *Abrupt onset* means the onset of cognitive change and should be carefully differentiated from sudden recognition of a change that had taken place previously. *Stepwise deterioration* refers to the intellectual function characterized by stable plateaus and short periods of steep decline. A *fluctuating course* refers to the overall temporal course of the disorder which is like a "sawtooth" with improvement following one vascular insult followed by deterioration caused by the next. *Nocturnal confusion* also implies a relative daytime lucidity and should be differentiated from nocturnal exacerbation, which is common to all types of dementias. *Relative preservation of personality* reflects the tendency for insight and emotional responsiveness to be preserved in multi-infarct dementia as compared to Alzheimer's disease. The more frequent occurrence of *depression* is also perhaps related to this preserved personality. *Somatic complaints* refer to vague symptoms such as dizziness, unsteadiness, or headache that do not have a definite physical correlate. *Emotional incontinence* means a rapid, inappropriate, and inconsequential change in mood and usually occurs with bilateral corticobulbar lesions, commonly vascular. *Hypertension* is a known risk factor for stroke as is the presence of *associated atherosclerosis* (ischemic heart disease, claudication, carotid bruit, absent foot pulses). *History of stroke* is obviously relevant to a vascular dementing process but does not necessarily imply this diagnosis as a patient with Alzheimer's disease may also suffer from a stroke. *Focal neurologic symptoms or signs* should be used in the score with the understanding that aphasia, apraxia, agnosia, acalculia, cortical sensory loss, primitive reflexes, and lower motor neuron features have little discriminant value in relation to vascular dementia and hence are excluded from the score. The presence of focal visual, motor or sensory symptoms, or signs or reflex asymmetrics favor a diagnosis of multi-infarct dementia.

**TABLE 30-3. Ischemic Score**

| Clinical Feature | Score |
|---|---|
| 1. Abrupt onset | 2 |
| 2. Stepwise deterioration | 1 |
| 3. Fluctuating course | 2 |
| 4. Nocturnal confusion | 1 |
| 5. Relative preservation of personality | 1 |
| 6. Depression | 1 |
| 7. Somatic complaints | 1 |
| 8. Emotional incontinence | 1 |
| 9. History of hypertension | 1 |
| 10. History of strokes | 2 |
| 11. Evidence of associated atherosclerosis | 1 |
| 12. Focal neurologic symptoms | 2 |
| 13. Focal neurologic signs | 2 |

(From Hachinski et al.,[46] with permission.)

The principal value of the score is to differentiate dementing disorders due to multiple infarcts with a score more than 7 from a group that is presumed predominantly to be degenerative with a score below 4.[46] It should be noted that the score does not offer a linear scale of severity and, for example, a total of maximum 18 does not mean that the dementia is more severe or the diagnosis of multi-infarct state more certain than a score of 8. The limitations of the score should be understood, in order to apply it properly. The score separates patients with dementia into two groups: the "infarct group" and the "everything else" group, which would include noninfarction causes of vascular dementia and mixed causes of dementia apart from patients with Alzheimer's disease. The ischemic score also does not differentiate pure vascular dementias from dementias with a mixed contribution of vascular and degenerative changes to the disease process.[89,103]

Rosen et al.[89] in a neuropathologic study of 14 elderly demented subjects have confirmed the discriminant utility of the ischemic score. In another neuropathologic study[77] the value of the ischemic score in differentiating vascular dementia from Alzheimer's disease was also well demonstrated. In a logistic regression model these workers note that fluctuating course, nocturnal confusion, and focal neurologic symptoms had the best discriminating value and helped to diagnose vascular dementia in 71 percent and Alzheimer's disease in 89 percent of cases correctly. Loeb and Gandolfo[65] in a study found that four features (abrupt onset, history of stroke, focal symptoms, focal signs) were most relevant to the diagnosis of multi-infarct dementia. They suggested a modified ischemic score using these four items of the original scale and, in addition, using CT scan findings. In another study done by Portera-Sanchez et al.,[82] seven variables (hypertension, abrupt onset, previous history of stroke, focal motor disturbances, pyramidal signs, focal CT atrophy, and focal EEG slowing) were found relevant, and when weighted by discriminant function analysis, the most important single factor was previous history of stroke. Unfortunately no pathologic data were included in these studies.

## INVESTIGATIONS

### Routine

The investigations in a clinically suspected vascular dementia are directed with two objectives in mind: (1) to further support the diagnosis of vascular dementia and (2) to find out the cause of the vascular process that has led to the dementing disorder. With this in perspective the following investigations are advised: complete blood count (including hematocrit and platelets), blood smear, erythrocyte sedimentation rate, serum urea and electrolytes, serum calcium, plasma protein electrophoresis, thyroid function tests, serum folate, serum B12, and VDRL. If vascular dementia is suspected, especially in a young patient, a screen for collagen-vascular disease and lupus anticoagulant (PTT) may be done. We have found chest x-rays to be useful as it looks at two major organs—heart and lungs. Cardiac enlargement occurs with hypertensive, ischemic, or valvular heart disease. Lungs may show a primary or secondary growth. An ECG is useful in that it shows arrhythmias and also indicates ischemic heart disease or chamber enlargement. If an arrhythmia is suspected, Holter monitoring may be useful. Though precordial 2D echocardiography has been used in the past, recently it has been shown that transesophageal echocardiography may be more useful in case an intracardiac embolic source is suspected in patients with TIA;[81] however, this modality is not widely available at present and its advantage over precordial model in evaluating vascular dementia is unexplored.

EEG is useful in a dementing disorder provided its limitations are kept in view. In a study of EEG in dementia[29] it was reported that this electrophysiologic modality is useful in differentiating normal elderly from cases of dementia. It was also pointed out that a normal EEG is not incompatible with the diagnosis of dementia especially in mild cases. The EEG is a useful guide indicating the rate and severity of the pathologic process and is a useful tool to follow-up a case of dementia. In another study[95] the MID group differed from controls in all EEG parameters including asymmetric findings. Patients with senile dementia of Alzheimer type differed from MID group only in asymmetric findings which were more common in the MID cases. It was felt that EEG was valuable in differentiating dementia patients from the normal elderly, but EEG alone cannot differentiate MID from senile dementia of the Alzheimer type with any great degree of certainty.

With the widespread availability of CT scanners, a CT of the head has become a part of routine workup in a case of suspected vascular dementia. It must be emphasized that the presence of multiple infarcts on CT scan does not necessarily mean that the dementing process is vascular but that this should be taken only as supportive evidence of a vascular pathology, the diagnosis of vascular dementia being mainly on clinical grounds. In one study[62] 60 percent of patients with vascular dementia had multiple infarcts seen on CT scan, while in another study[57] brain infarcts were seen in 93 percent of patients with multi-infarct dementia, but they were observed in only 10 percent of controls. It was also shown that cerebral atrophy correlated with the presence of dementia.[57] It is our opinion that in the presence of white matter hypodensity on CT scan (leuko-araiosis) a vascular contribution to the dementing process is more likely; this, however, remains controversial at present. Magnetic resonance imaging (MRI) has a sensitivity much higher than CT scan and this at times leads to a lower specificity. This has resulted in a much higher detection rate of white matter changes but the value of this finding in any given patient is even less specific. Enlargement of the central CSF space was the only MRI radiologic feature seen more commonly in vascular dementia when compared to nondemented persons with ischemic cerebrovascular disease.[54] Further work is necessary to define the role of imaging techniques in vascular dementia.

### Special Investigations

There was a lot of initial enthusiasm in cerebral blood flow (CBF) studies in vascular dementia. Most studies indicate that global cerebral blood flow is reduced in dementia of all types,[11,39,46,63,79,80,86] and the reduction mainly depends on the severity of the dementing disorder rather than on the underlying etiology.[45,49] An interesting study[87] of 181 neurologically normal elderly with a 7-year prospective follow-up with CBF and neuropsychological testing was done. It was reported that in patients who later developed vascular dementia, CBF values began to decline 2 years before onset of symptoms, while in patients with Alzheimer's disease, CBF values remained within normal ranges until symptoms of dementia appeared, declining rapidly thereafter. In another study[73] it was observed that in multi-infarct dementia, cognition and CBF fluctuate together, while in Alzheimer's disease no such fluctuation is seen and a progressive deterioration in cognition and CBF occurs. PET studies were done in 22 demented persons of whom 9 were considered vascular and 13 degenerative.[37] The critical point is that if chronic brain hypoperfusion is a mechanism for production of dementia then one would expect a rise in oxygen extraction fraction. There was no increase in oxygen extraction in this study thus strengthening the previous conclusion that chronic cerebral ischemia does not play a major role in a vascular dementing process.[47]

Recently transcranial Doppler sonography was evaluated as a diagnostic tool in vascular dementia.[83] The rest flow velocity and vasomotor response to hypercapnia was lower in patients with vascular dementia as compared to patients with Alzheimer's disease or control group. These findings were neither exclusive nor homogeneous in the group with vascular dementia, and further work is required to define the role of this diagnostic modality.

## MANAGEMENT

Epidemiologic studies in North America indicated a downward trend in the incidence of stroke until its stabilization in the 1970s, and in 1980 to 1984 the incidence rate was 17 percent higher than that for 1975 to 1979.[18] The decline in incidence was correlated with introduction of effective antihypertensive therapy and the increase in incidence of the early 1980s to the introduction of CT scan and increased detection of minor strokes.[18] Though vascular dementia is thought to result principally from multiple infarcts, there are no studies to the best of our knowledge indicating such a trend in this disorder. The management of vascular dementia, at present, basically hinges around the treatment of the etiologic factor(s) and elimination or correction of risk factor(s) of stroke.

This is a good theory but is this really true in clinical practice? Meyer et al.[72] did a study in which 52 patients with multi-infarct dementia were followed up prospectively for a period of 22.2 months. They found that among hypertensive patients with MID, control of blood pressure within upper limits of normal range (135 to 150 mmHg) correlated with improved cognition, but if the systolic BP fell below this level patients deteriorated. They also found that in patients with MID who were normotensive, cessation of smoking improved cognition. In another study[74] 70 MID patients were assigned to treatment and no-treatment groups to investigate the effect of one aspirin tablet daily on cognitive function and cerebral blood flow (CBF) carried out in a blinded fashion. Patients were evaluated at yearly intervals. Significant improvement was observed in the cognitive function and CBF in patients treated with aspirin as compared to the control group. The same group[74] studied 41 elderly hypertriglyceridimic individuals with cognitive impairment and treated them with gemfibrosil. They found that gemfibrosil-treated individuals had a lower triglyceride levels and maintained a significantly higher CBF and, more importantly, cognitive performance improved 4 to 6 months later.

These initial studies tend to indicate that treatment of the etiologic factor(s) or correction of risk factors improves cognitive function in vascular dementia though larger and better controlled clinical trials are needed to prove this point.[66] Thus a patient with vascular dementia should be evaluated from the stroke point of view of etiology and prevention and put on antiplatelets, anticoagulants or antihypertensives as required in an individual case and control of risk factors be considered.

## CONCLUSION

The complexity of MID stems from the fact that neither ischemic brain damage nor the clinical syndrome of dementia are all-or-none phenomena. Despite rapidly advancing technology, MID remains a clinical diagnosis. The only common denominator to this poorly defined, increasingly accepted, nonhomogeneous group is that a vascular mechanism is invoked as a predominant factor for the change in cognition. At this point in our understanding of vascular dementia it seems clear that chronic cerebral ischemia is unlikely to be a mechanism of any significance and cerebral infarction either overt (macroscopic) or subtle (microscopic) seems to be the most likely pathogenetic substrate. It is possible that episodic ischemia affects the selectively vulnerable cells, such as oligodendrocyte,[107] which may result in damage to the white matter. The concept of a "multi-infarct dementia" should be extended as a hypothesis to include not only "macro" but "micro" infarcts and not only wholesale damage to all elements of a part of the brain but selective damage to some of its components. The challenge is to transform these postulates into proof.

## REFERENCES

1. Alafuzoff I, Adolfsson R, Grundke-Iqbal I et al: Perivascular deposits of serum proteins in cerebral cortex in vascular dementia. Acta Neuropathol (Berl) 66:292, 1985
2. Alvarez WC: Cerebral arteriosclerosis with small commonly unrecognized apoplexies. Geriatrics 1:159, 1946
3. Alzheimer A: Beitrag zur pathologischen Anatomie der Seelenstörungen des Griesenalters. Neurol Zentralbl 18:95, 1899
4. Alzheimer A: Die Seelenstörungen auf arteriosclerotischer Grundlage. Allg Z Psychiatr Psych Gericht Med 59:695, 1902
5. American Psychiatric Association, Committee on Nomenclature and Statistics: Diagnostic and Statistical Manual of Mental Disorders. 3rd Ed.

American Psychiatric Association, Washington, DC, 1980
6. American Psychiatric Association: DSM-IIIR Diagnostic and Statistical Manual of Mental Disorders. 3rd Ed. (Revised.) American Psychiatric Association, Washington, DC, 1987
7. Anthony JC, Le Resche L, Niaz U et al: Limits of the mini-mental state as a screening test for dementia and delirium among hospital patients. Psychol Med 12:397, 1982
8. Astrup J: Energy-requiring cell functions in the ischemic brain: their critical supply and possible inhibition in protective therapy. J Neurosurg 56:482, 1982
9. Astrup J, Siesjo BK, Symon L: Thresholds in cerebral ischemia—the ischemic penumbra. Stroke 12:723, 1981
10. Awad IA, Spetzler RP, Hodak JA et al: Incidental subcortical lesions identified on MRI in the elderly. 1. Correlation with age and cerebrovascular risk factors. Stroke 17:1084, 1986
11. Barclay L, Zemcov A, Blass JP et al: Rates of decrease of cerebral blood flow in progressive dementias. Neurology (NY) 34:1555, 1984
12. Barclay LL, Zemcov A, Blass JP et al: Survival in Alzheimer's disease and vascular dementias. Neurology (NY) 35:834, 1985
13. Beck JC, Benson DF, Scheibel AB et al: Dementia in the elderly: the silent epidemic. Ann Intern Med 97:231, 1982
14. Binswanger O: Die Abgrenzung des allgemeinen progressiven Paralysie. Berl Klin Wochenschr 31:1103, 1894
15. Blennow K, Wallin A, Fredman P et al: Blood-brain barrier disturbance in patients with Alzheimer's disease is related to vascular factors. Acta Neurol Scand 81:323, 1990
16. Branston NM, Symon L, Crockard HA et al: Relationship between the cortical evoked potential and local cortical blood flow following acute middle cerebral artery occlusion in the baboon. Exp Neurol 45:195, 1974
17. Brown MM, Pelz DM, Hachinski V: White matter vasodilatory reserve is impaired in patients with cerebrovascular disease and diffuse periventricular lucency. J Neurol 237:157, 1990
18. Broderick JP, Phillips SJ, Whisnant JP et al: Incidence rates of stroke in the eighties: the end of the decline in stroke? Stroke 20:577, 1989
19. Brun A, Englund E: A white matter disorder in dementia of the Alzheimer type: a pathoanatomical study. Ann Neurol 19:253, 1986
20. Castaigne P, Lhermitte F, Buge A et al: Paramedian thalamic and midbrain infarction: clinical and neuropathological study. Ann Neurol 10:127, 1981
21. Chimowitz MI, Awad IA, Furlan AJ: Periventricular lesions on MRI—facts and theories. Stroke 20:963, 1989
22. Clarfield AM: The reversible dementias: do they reverse? Ann Intern Med 109:476, 1988
23. Corsellis JAN: Mental Illness and the Ageing Brain. Oxford University Press, London, 1962
24. Cummings JL, Benson DF: Dementia. A Clinical Approach. p. 5. Butterworth, Boston, 1983
25. Delpla P, Meyer E, Zatorre R et al: Metabolic and neuropsychological correlates of periventricular lucencies. J Cereb Blood Flow Metab, suppl 1. 9:5569, 1989
26. del Ser T, Bermejo F, Portera A et al: Vascular dementia: a clinicopathological study. J Neurol Sci 96:1, 1990
27. DeReuck JL: The human periventricular arterial blood supply and the anatomy of cerebral infarctions. Eur Neurol 5:321, 1971
28. Dunne JW, Leedman PJ, Edis RH: Inobvious stroke: a cause of delirium and dementia. Aust NZ J Med 16:771, 1986
29. Erkinjuntii T, Larsen T, Sulkava L et al: EEG in the differential diagnosis between Alzheimer's disease and vascular dementia. Acta Neurol Scand 77:36, 1988
30. Fazekas F, Niederkorn K, Schmidt R et al: White matter signal abnormalities in normal individuals: correlation with carotid ultrasonography, cerebral blood flow measurements, and cerebrovascular risk factors. Stroke 19:1285, 1988
31. Fields WS: Cerebral arteriosclerosis: A "non-cause" of dementia. In Meyer JS, Lechner H, Reivich M et al (eds): Cerebrovascular Disease. Proceedings of the Sixth International Conference. Thieme, Stuttgart, 1973
32. Fisher CM: Lacunes: small deep cerebral infarcts. Neurology (NY) 15:774, 1954
33. Fisher CM: Dementia in cerebral vascular disease. p. 232. In Siekert R, Whisnant J (eds): Cerebral Vascular Disease. Sixth Conference. Grune & Stratton, Orlando, FL, 1968
34. Fisher CM: Arterial lesions underlying lacunes. Acta Neuropathol 12:1, 1969
35. Fisher CM: Lacunar strokes and infarcts: a review. Neurology (NY) 32:871, 1982
36. Folstein MF, Folstein S, McHugh PR: Mini-mental state: a practical method for grading the cognitive state of patients for the clinician. J Psychiatr Res 12:189, 1975
37. Frackowiak RSJ, Pozzilli IC, Legg NJ et al: Regional cerebral oxygen supply and utilisation in dementia: a clinical and physiological study with oxygen-15 and positron tomography. Brain 104:753, 1981
38. Freemon FR: Evaluation of patients with progressive intellectual deterioration. Arch Neurol 33:658, 1976
39. Freyhan FA, Woodford RB, Kety SS: Cerebral blood flow and metabolism in psychoses of senility. J Nerv Ment Dis 113:449, 1951
40. Gagnon M, Letenneur L, Dartigues J-F et al: Validity of the mini-mental state examination as a screening instrument for cognitive impairment and dementia in French elderly community residents. Neuroepidemiology 9:143, 1990
41. George AE, DeLeon MJ, Gentes CI et al: Leukoencephalopathy in normal and pathologic aging. Am J Neuroradiol 7:561, 1986
42. Gottfries CG, Adolfsson R, Aquilonius SM et al: Biochemical changes in dementia disorders of Alzheimer type (AD/SDAT). Neurobiol Aging 4:261, 1983
43. Gray F, Dubas F, Roullet E et al: Leukoencepha-

lopathy in diffuse hemorrhagic cerebral amyloid angiopathy. Ann Neurol 18:54, 1985
44. Guberman A, Stuss D: The syndrome of bilateral paramedian thalamic infarction. Neurology (Cleveland) 33:540, 1983
45. Gustafson L, Risberg J: Regional cerebral blood flow related to psychiatric symptoms in dementia with onset in the presenile period. Acta Psychiatry Scand 50:516, 1974
46. Hachinski VC, Iliff LD, Zilkha E et al: Cerebral blood flow in dementia. Arch Neurol 32:632, 1975
47. Hachinski VC, Lassen NA, Marshall J: Multi-infarct dementia: a cause of mental deterioration in the elderly. Lancet 2:207, 1974
48. Hachinski VC, Potter P, Merskey H: Leukoaraiosis. Arch Neurol 44:42, 1987
49. Hagberg B, Ingvar DH: Cognitive reduction in presenile dementia related to regional abnormalities in the cerebral blood flow. Br J Psychiatry 128:209, 1976
50. Heiss WD: Flow thresholds of functional and morphological damage of brain tissue. Stroke 14:329, 1983
51. Heiss WD, Hayakawa T, Waltz AG: Cortical neuronal function during ischemia. Arch Neurol 33:813, 1976
52. Heiss WD, Rosner G: Duration versus severity of ischemia as critical factors of cortical cell damage. p. 225. In Reivich M, Hurtig HI (eds): Cerebrovascular Diseases: Thirteenth Research (Princeton) Conference. Raven Press, NY, 1982
53. Hendrie HC, Farlow MR, Austrom MG et al: Foci of increased $T_2$ signal intensity on brain MR scans of healthy elderly subjects. AJNR 10:703, 1989
54. Hershey LA, Modic MT, Greenbough PG et al: Magnetic resonance imaging in vascular dementia. Neurology (NY) 37:29, 1987
55. Hijdra A, Verbeeten Jr. B, Verhulst JAP: Relation of leukoaraiosis to lesion type in stroke patients. Stroke 21:890, 1990
56. Janota I: Dementia, deep white matter damage and hypertension: "Binswanger's disease." Psychol Med 11:39, 1981
57. Jayakumar PN, Taly AB, Shanmugam V et al: Multi-infarct dementia: a computed tomographic study. Acta Neurol Scand 73:292, 1989
58. Jones TH, Morawetz RB, Crowell RM et al: Thresholds of focal cerebral ischemia in awake monkeys. J Neurosurg 54:773, 1981
59. Katz DI, Alexander MP, Mandell AM: Dementia following strokes in the mesencephalon and diencephalon. Arch Neurol 44:1127, 1987
60. Katzman R, Terry RD: The Neurology of Aging. p. 1. FA Davis, Philadelphia, 1983
61. Kraepelin E: Compendium der Psychiatrie. Barth, Leipzig, 1883
62. Ladurner G, Iliff LD, Lechner H: Clinical factors associated with dementia in ischemic stroke. J Neurol Neurosurg Psychiatry 45:97, 1982
63. Lassen NA, Munk O, Tottey ER: Mental function and cerebral oxygen consumption in organic dementia. Arch Neurol Psychiatry 77:126, 1957
64. Leonardi A, Gandolfo C, Caponnetto C et al: The integrity of the blood-brain barrier in Alzheimer's type and multi-infarct dementia evaluated by the study of albumin and IgG in serum and cerebrospinal fluid. J Neurol Sci 67:253, 1985
65. Loeb C, Gandolfo C: Diagnostic evaluation of degenerative and vascular dementia. Stroke 14:399, 1983
66. Loeb C, Gandolfo C: Methodological problems of clinical trials in multi-infarct dementia. Neuroepidemiology 9:223, 1990
67. Major RH: Classic Descriptions of Disease. p. 476. Charles C Thomas, Springfield, IL, 1945
68. Maletta GJ, Pirizzolo FJ, Thompson G et al: Organic mental disorders in a geriatric out-patient population. Am J Psychiatry 139:521, 1982
69. Marcoux FW, Morawetz RB, Crowell RM et al: Differential regional vulnerability in transient focal cerebral ischemia. Stroke 13:339, 1982
70. Marsden CD, Harrison MJG: Outcome of investigation of patients with presenile dementia. Br Med J 2:249, 1972
71. Meissner I, Shapir S, Kokmen E et al: The paramedian diencephalic syndrome: a dynamic phenomenon. Stroke 18:380, 1987
72. Meyer JS, Judd BW, Tawaklna T et al: Improved cognition after control of risk factors for multi-infarct dementia. JAMA 256:2203, 1986
73. Meyer JS, Rogers RL, Judd BW et al: Cognition and cerebral blood flow fluctuate together in multi-infarct dementia. Stroke 19:163, 1988
74. Meyer JS, Rogers RL, Mortel KF: Multi-infarct dementia: demography, risk factors, and therapy. In Ginsberg MD, Dietrich WD (eds): Cerebrovascular Diseases. Raven Press, New York, 1989
75. Mirsen T, Hachinski V: Epidemiology and classification of vascular and multi-infarct dementia. In Meyer JS, Lechner H, Marshall J et al (eds): Vascular and Multi-infarct Dementia. Future Publishing, Mount Kisco, NY, 1988
76. Mokuno K, Kato K, Kawai K et al: Neuron-specific enolase and S-100 protein levels in cerebrospinal fluid of patients with various neurological diseases. J Neurol Sci 60:443, 1983
77. Molsa PK, Paljarvi L, Rinne JO et al: Validity of clinical diagnosis in dementia: a prospective clinicopathological study. J Neurol Neurosurg Psychiatry 48:1085, 1985
78. Naheedy MH, Gupta SR, Young JC et al: Periventricular white matter changes and subcortical dementia: clinical, neuropsychological, radiological, and pathological correlation. AJNR 6:468, 1985
79. Obrist W, Chivian E, Cronqvist S et al: Regional cerebral blood flow in senile and presenile dementia. Neurology (NY) 20:315, 1970
80. Perez F, Mathew NT, Stump DA et al: Regional cerebral blood flow, statistical patterns and psychological performance in multi-infarct dementia and Alzheimer's disease. CJNS 4:53, 1977
81. Pop G, Sutherland GR, Koudstaal PJ et al: Transesophageal echocardiography in the detection of intracardiac embolic sources in patients

with transient ischemic attacks. Stroke 21:560, 1990
82. Portera-Sanchez A, del Ser T, Bermejo F et al: Clinical diagnosis of senile dementia of Alzheimer type and vascular dementia. In Terry RD, Bolis CL, Toffano G (eds): Neurological Pathology. Aging. Vol. 18. Raven Press, New York, 1982
83. Provinciali L, Minciotti P, Ceravolo G et al: Transcranial doppler sonography as a diagnostic tool in vascular dementia. Eur Neurol 30:98, 1990
84. Raine CS: Neurocellular anatomy. p. 5. In Albers RW, Siegel GJ, Katzman R et al (eds): Basic Neurochemistry. 2nd Ed. Little, Brown, Boston, 1976
85. Rao SM, Mittenberg W, Bernardin L et al: Neuropsychological test findings in subjects with leuko-araiosis. Arch Neurol 46:40, 1989
86. Risberg J, Gustafson L: 133-Xe cerebral blood flow in dementia and in neuropsychiatric research. p. 151. In Magistretti PL (ed): Functional Radionuclide Imaging of the Brain. Raven Press, New York, 1983
87. Rogers RL, Meyer JS, Mortel KF et al: Decreased cerebral blood flow precedes multi-infarct dementia, but follows senile dementia of Alzheimer type. Neurology (NY) 36:1, 1986
88. Roman GC: Lacunar dementia. p. 131. In Hutton JT, Kenny AD (eds): Senile Dementia of the Alzheimer's Type. Alan R. Liss, New York, 1985
89. Rosen WG, Terry RD, Fuld PA et al: Pathologic verification of ischemic score in differentiation of dementias. Ann Neurol 7:486, 1979
90. Roth M: The natural history of mental disorder in old age. J Ment Sci 110:281, 1955
91. Roth M: Classification and aetiology in mental disorders of old age: some recent developments. p. 1. In: Recent Developments in Psychogeriatrics. Br J Psychiatry, spec publ 6, 1971
92. Scheibel AB, Duong T, Tomiyasu U: Denervation microangiopathy in senile dementia, Alzheimer type. Alzheimer Dis Associated Disord 1:19, 1987
93. Scheinberg P: Dementia due to vascular disease—a multifactorial disorder. Stroke 19:1291, 1988
94. Smith JS, Kiloh LG: The investigation of dementia: results in 200 consecutive admissions. Lancet 1:824, 1981
95. Soininen H, Partanen VJ, Helkala EL et al: EEG findings in senile dementia and normal aging. Acta Neurol Scand 65:59, 1982
96. Steingart A, Hachinski VC, Lau C et al: Cognitive and neurologic findings in subjects with diffuse white matter lucencies on CT scan. Arch Neurol 44:32, 1987
97. Sulkava R, Viinikka L, Erkinjuntti T et al: Cerebrospinal fluid neuron-specific enolase is decreased in multi-infarct dementia, but unchanged in Alzheimer's disease. J Neurol Neurosurg Psychiatry 51:549, 1988
98. Tatemichi TK, Foulkes MA, Mohr JP et al: Dementia in stroke survivors in the stroke data bank cohort: prevalence, incidence, risk factors, and computed tomographic findings. Stroke 21:858, 1990
99. Tomlinson BE, Blessed G, Roth M: Observations on the brains of demented old people. J Neurol Sci 11:205, 1970
100. Tomlinson BE, Henderson G: Some quantitative cerebral findings in normal and demented old people. In Terry RD, Gershon S (eds): Neurobiology of Aging. Vol. 3. Raven Press, New York, 1976
101. Valentine AR, Moseley IF, Kendall BE: White matter abnormality in cerebral atrophy: clinicoradiological correlations. J Neurol Neurosurg Psychiatry 43:139, 1980
102. Wade JPH, Hachinski VC: Multi-infarct dementia. p. 209. In Pitt B (ed): Dementia. Churchill Livingstone, London, 1987
103. Wade JPH, Mirsen TR, Hachinski VC et al: The clinical diagnosis of Alzheimer's disease. Arch Neurol 44:24, 1987
104. Wallin A, Alafuzoff I, Carlsson A et al: Neurotransmitter deficits in a non-multi-infarct category of vascular dementia. Acta Neurol Scand 79:397, 1989
105. Wallin A, Blennow K, Fredman P et al: Intrathecal synthesis of immunoglobulin G in vascular dementia. Acta Neurol Scand 81:168, 1990
106. Wallin A, Blennow K, Fredman P et al: Blood-brain barrier function in vascular dementia. Acta Neurol Scand 81:318, 1990
107. Wallin A, Gottfries CG, Karlsson I et al: Decreased myelin lipids in Alzheimer's disease and vascular dementia. Acta Neurol Scand 80:319, 1989
108. Wertham F, Wertham F: The Brain as an Organ. Macmillan, New York, 1934
109. Wilks S: Clinical notes on atrophy of the brain. J Ment Sci 10:381, 1864
110. Xie Y, Mies G, Hossmann KA: Ischemic threshold of brain protein synthesis after unilateral carotid artery occlusion in gerbils. Stroke 20:620, 1989

# 31 *BINSWANGER'S DISEASE*

Julien Bogousslavsky

## HISTORICAL BACKGROUND

Otto Binswanger (October 14, 1852 to July 15, 1929) (Fig. 31-1) was born and died in Switzerland, where his father was director of an insane asylum, but he made his neurologic career in Germany. He studied under Von Recklinghausen and Westphal, and was subsequently appointed in Jena, where he had many pupils, including Theodor Ziehen, Oskar Vogt, Hans Berger, and K. Brodmann.[15] In 1894 he published in the *Berliner Klinische Wochenschrift*[19] a three-part paper entitled "Die Abgrenzung der allgemeinen progressiven Paralyse" (the frontier of general paresis), in which he introduced the term *encephalitis subcorticalis chronica progressiva* to describe a clinicopathologic entity characterized by slow progression of mental deterioration beginning between 50 and 65 years, with aphasia, hemianopia, hemiparesis, and hemianesthesia, as well as apoplectiform attacks, epileptic fits, and periods of psychomotor excitation, corresponding at autopsy to a pronounced atrophy of the white matter predominating posteriorly, with enlarged ventricles and thickened ependyma, but little changes in the cortex (Fig. 31-2). Binswanger stated that " it is very likely that the subcortical loss of fibers is caused by the deficiency of the blood resulting from arteriosclerosis," though the only case that he reported in detail only had "insignificant isolated whitish plaques" on the arteries at the base of the brain. Actually, though Binswanger mentioned that he had observed eight cases, only one was reported in the paper, and, as Olszewski[141] stated in his 1962 review, "the history of syphilitic infection in this case, the presence of thickened ependyma, and the clinical course all point to the possibility of neurosyphilis"; he added, "whether all 8 cases that Binswanger observed belong to the same entity remains unknown." No new information appeared in a short abstract published by Binswanger[20] in 1895, in his 1904 *Lehrbuch der Psychiatrie*,[21] and in a long paper published in 1924 on pathology and pathogenesis of neurosyphilis.[22] Despite these uncertainties, Binswanger's contribution has been regularly acknowledged over the following 100 years and the term *Binswanger's disease* has become established in the literature. This may be due in part to the impact of two papers, published in 1898 and 1902 by Alois Alzheimer,[5,6] who emphasized "Binswanger's encephalitis subcorticalis chronica progressiva," which corresponded to a "particular form of subcortical atrophy due to atherosclerosis of cerebral arteries, which differs from other arteriosclerotic cerebral atrophies" (Fig. 31-3), a view subsequently accepted by prominent neuropathologists early this century.[83,138,160] We do not know how many cases Alzheimer studied, but his main contribution was the addition of microscopic details confirming that the cortex was little involved, and, above all, his description of a severe arteriosclerosis involving the long arteries of the hemispheres' white matter. Subsequent studies included those by Buchholz[39] (1905), who reported five patients with "Encephalitis subcorticalis chronica Binswangers," by Ladame[111] (1912), who reported the first patient with "encéphalite sous-corticale chronique" in the French literature, by Nissl[138] (1920), who reported one patient with "Encephalitis subcorticalis," and by Kashida[103] (1924 to 1925), who showed seven cases before the first paper in English literature appeared in 1932 by Frederic

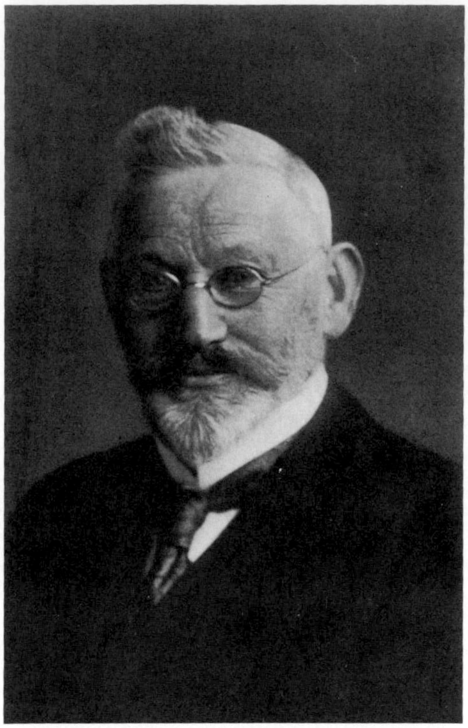

**Fig. 31-1.** Otto Binswanger (born October 14, 1852; died July 15, 1929).

Farnell and Joseph Globus,[66] who introduced the term *chronic progressive vascular subcortical encephalopathy.* Before Olszewski's 1962 famous review on "subcortical arteriosclerotic encephalopathy,"[142] only six further papers with pathologic cases were published.[7,48,57,75,145,173] Atypical cases without arteriosclerosis were also reported,[1,12,56,58,71,134,143] but they were more likely related to a leukodystrophy or to a primary degenerative disorder.

In 1962 Olszewski[142] reported on two new patients and reviewed extensively the literature on the 34 reported "typical cases"; he concluded that there was "little justification for speaking about 'Binswanger's disease' since we are dealing only with a peculiar form of cerebral arteriosclerosis," and he suggested the term "Binswanger's type of subcortical arteriosclerotic encephalopathy." Since that time, several clinicopathologic reports have appeared, mainly since CT and more recently MRI have renewed interest in this condition,[4,10,18,40,44,49,50,54,59,60,75,81,90,96–98,100,101,119,123,127,131,139,146,153,165,166,169,170,175,181,182] so that in 1989, at least 146 cases with an adequate neuropathologic study had been reported under various labels: encephalitis subcorticalis chronica progressiva,[19] subcortical encephalitis Binswanger,[5] chronic progressive vascular subcortical encephalopathy,[66] Binswanger's disease,[48] subcortical arteriosclerotic encephalopathy,[142] encephalopathia subcorticalis chronica,[100] subcortical arteriosclerotic encephalopa-

**I. Die Abgrenzung der allgemeinen progressiven Paralyse.**

Von

Prof. Dr. **Otto Binswanger**, Jena.

(Referat, erstattet auf der Jahresversammlung des Vereins Deutscher Irrenärzte zu Dresden am 20. September 1894.)

Die Aufgabe, mit welcher der Vorstand unseres Vereins mich betraut hat, die Discussion über die Abgrenzung der allallgemeinen progressiven Paralyse durch Kennzeichnung der maassgebenden Gesichtspunkte einzuleiten, lässt sich in drei Theile zerlegen:

1. Erwägung der anatomischen Kriterien,
2. die Aetiologie,
3. der klinische Verlauf.

Ich will versuchen, die differentiell-diagnostischen Merkmale, welche die progressive Paralyse gegenüber anderen ihr nahestehenden Krankheitsformen darbietet, nach diesen drei Richtungen hin kurz zu beleuchten. Ich bemerke hierzu aber, dass es mir in dem knappen Rahmen eines kurzen Referates nur möglich sein wird, die Skizze des Bildes zu zeichnen, und dass ich die genauere Ausführung des Ganzen oder einzelner Theile desselben von der Discussion erhoffe.

I. Die erste Frage über die anatomischen Kriterien der allgemeinen progressiven Paralyse ist gerade in den letzten Jahren Gegenstand lebhafter Controversen gewesen. Ich rufe Ihnen nur die Debatten auf dem internationalen Congress in Berlin in's Gedächtniss zurück, welche die grundsätzlichen Meinungsverschiedenheiten, die hierüber noch vorhanden sind, am klarsten wiedergeben. Ich habe selbst vor Kurzem in einer ausführlicheren Bearbeitung der histologischen Befunde, soweit dieselben die Grosshirnrinde betreffen, versucht, die primären

**Fig. 31-2.** First lines of Binswanger's original paper in the *Berliner Klinische Wochenschrift* in 1894.

Alzheimer, Neuere Arbeiten über die Dementia senilis etc.

**Neuere Arbeiten über die Dementia senilis und die auf atheromatöser Gefässerkrankung basierenden Gehirnkrankheiten**

referiert von

A. ALZHEIMER

in Frankfurt a. M.

Nicht in dem gleichen Masse wie die Dementia paralytica ist die Dementia senilis in den letzten Jahren Gegenstand klinischer und histologischer Untersuchungen gewesen. Immerhin lässt sich über eine Reihe von Arbeiten berichten, welche uns teils neue interessante Gesichtspunkte eröffnet, teils unsere symptomatologischen und anatomischen Kenntnisse wesentlich vertieft haben. Zum Teil handelt es sich dabei um Untersuchungen, welche die Dementia senilis im engeren Sinne zwar nicht behandeln, die aber psychische Störungen des Seniums zum Gegenstande haben, die gleichfalls mit der Arteriosclerose des Gefässsystems im Zusammenhange stehen und deswegen am besten im Zusammenhang mit dem Greisenblödsinn besprochen werden.

**Fig. 31-3.** Paper published in 1898 by Alzheimer in the *Monatsschrift für Psychiatrie und Neurologie,* confirming Binswanger's findings and emphasizing arteriosclerosis of the perforating arterioles of white matter.

thy of Binswanger type,[93] Binswanger's subacute arteriosclerotic encephalopathy,[137] senile dementia of Binswanger's type,[151] or Binswanger's encephalopathy.[70]

## CLINICAL PICTURE OF BINSWANGER'S DISEASE

The incidence of Binswanger's disease is unknown, but in Japan, Tomonaga et al.[169] reported a prevalence of 45 cases among 1,000 autopsies. The disease may be more prevalent in men than in women.[44] Age at onset is usually in the sixth or seventh decade[10,44] with a mean age of 57 years in the review of Babikian and Ropper.[10] A familial trend has been suggested only exceptionally.[72,173]

Most of the patients who had clinicopathologic correlation presented clinically with the combination of dementia and stroke events, usually evolving in a subacute pattern, with stepwise progression followed by a plateau phase.[10,19,40,44,59,60,81,98,101,127,153,169] The average duration of illness before death was 5 years, but occasionally up to 22 years.[10] Death was usually related to intercurrent diseases (myocardial infarct, pneumonia), less often to a new stroke, which followed angiography in two instances.[59]

### Dementia

Dementia is the cardinal clinical feature of Binswanger's disease.[10,42,43,137,151] It may be its only manifestation,[40,98] sometimes with rapid progression, which can falsely suggest Creutzfeldt-Jakob disease, especially when associated with myoclonus and periodic complexes on EEG.[40] *Subcortical features* with apathy, abulia, mutism, depression, decreased attention, and memory may predominate over speech and gnosia disturbances.[42,43,169] It is possible that the severity of dementia has often been overestimated, mainly in patients with pseudobulbar features due to iterative small deep strokes. In rare instances, personality changes may be the presenting features.[50]

### Stroke

Most authors have emphasized the occurrence of focal neurologic disturbances, which, when iterative, can give a picture of a subacutely evolving encephalopathy. Binswanger himself reported "apoplectiform" events in the course of the disease.[19] In a review of 47 cases, Babikian and Ropper[10] found that stroke may be the presenting manifestation of Binswanger's disease in up to one third of the patients. Most of these strokes correspond to small deep infarcts, though some patients may also have cortical infarcts.[59,144] For that reason, repetition of strokes usually generates a classical picture of pseudobulbar syndrome with bilateral corticobulbar and corticospinal tract signs.[44,51,59,81,101,127,153,169] Frank hemiplegia may occur,[127,175] but it is uncommon. Dementia may be related in part to stroke repetition (multi-infarct dementia), but it is likely that the white matter changes themselves also contribute to dementia because many patients with multiple deep infarcts and pseudobulbar features are not demented at all.[23]

### Other Manifestations

Seizures and syncopes have been reported during evolution.[44,50,153] Parkinsonian features were mentioned by Tomonaga et al.,[169] but a coincidental finding cannot be ruled out. A gait disorder combining ataxic and Parkinsonian features with a "difficulty in using their legs to walk out of proportion to that of other movements of the lower limbs when lying or seating" was emphasized recently,[167] but the patients did not have autopsy verification. In rare instances, diagnosis has been made at autopsy in the absence of a significant neurologic history in patients who died rapidly from severe systemic diseases (renal failure, myocardial infarct).[74]

### Nemoto's Syndrome

Since Nemoto et al.[133] in 1966, four Japanese and one English reports of younger (26 to 49 years) men with alopecia, spondylitis deformans and lumbago, and the clinical pathologic features of Binswanger's disease have been published.[73,109,117,120,178] No patient had hypertension or metabolic disturbances, but a familial trend could be present.

## NEUROPATHOLOGY OF BINSWANGER'S DISEASE

The pathology of Binswanger's disease is much more characteristic than its clinical manifestations.[144] Macroscopically, no or only moderate atrophy may be present, while the deep white matter of the cerebral hemispheres appears shrunk and softened, with diffuse discoloration of the centrum semiovale (Fig. 31-4); some infarcts, usually deep, but sometimes involving the cortex may be seen. Examination of the white matter shows confluent, patchy, greyish, softened areas which may predominate in the periventricular and occipital region of the centrum semi-ovale (Fig. 31-5), but not always. U-fibers, internal capsules, and above all the corpus callosum are markedly spared. In more than 90 percent of the cases, the ventricles are enlarged and small deep cystic cavities are present.[10,59,144] Microscopically, on myelin stains, there is a pallor and swelling of myelin sheaths, with loss and swelling of oligodendrocytes, and to a lesser extent some axonal loss, and prominent astrocytic gliosis, sometimes with cavitation. The foci of myelin loss are typically irregular and they decrease toward

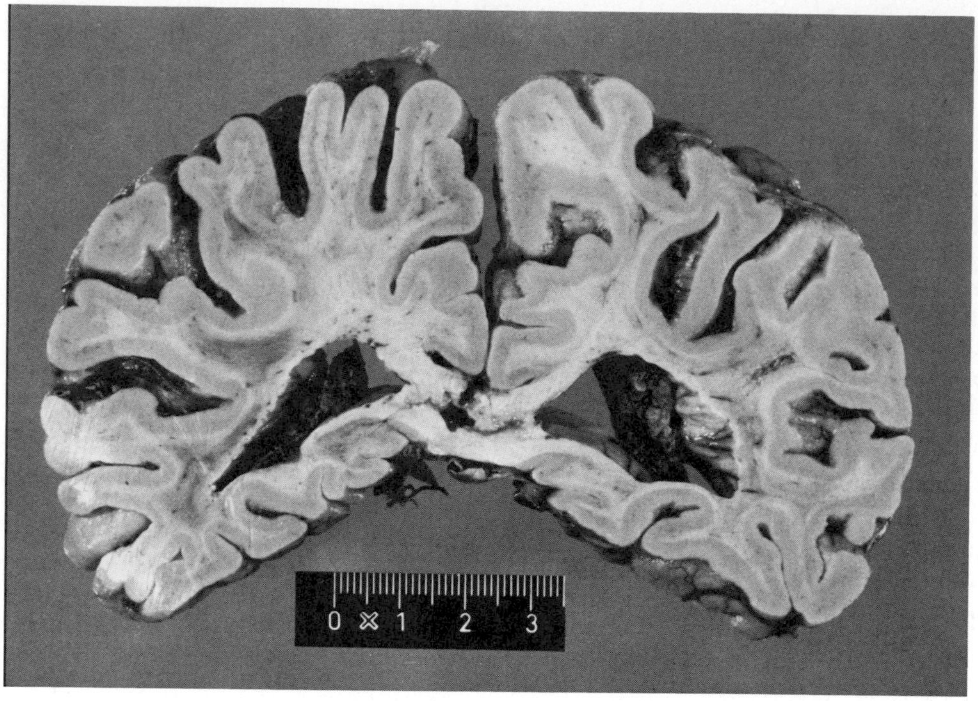


**Fig. 31-4.** Severe atrophy and discoloration of white matter with small deep infarcts and enlarged ventricles. (Courtesy of J.P. Deruaz, Lausanne.)

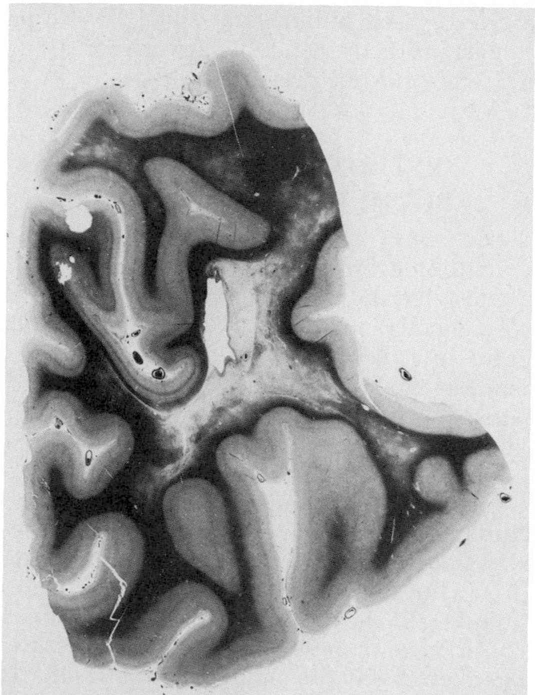

**Fig. 31-5.** Occipital lobe, Loyez stain. Severe demyelination in the periventricular region and core of white matter. (Courtesy of J.P. Deruaz, Lausanne.)

the cortex. Small holes within the deep white matter and basal ganglia are compatible with lacunar infarcts, dilatation of perivascular spaces, or *état criblé* (periarteriolar dilatations without surrounding parenchymatous changes).[10,14,51,97,100] Occasionally, larger infarcts involving the cortex may be present.[59] The association with segmental changes in the medullary arterioles of the hemisphere white matter was first emphasized by Alzheimer[5] and is typical: the adventitia is severely thickened, and the media may show lipohyalinosis.[10,81,92,117,122,123] It has also been suggested that a decrease in arteriolar branching may be present.[124] Large-artery atheroclerosis was reported in 40 of 43 cases reviewed by Babikian and Ropper,[10] but severe stenosis or occlusion of the carotid arteries is almost unreported in patients whose autopsy data give sufficient details.[10,40,44,59,74,75,98,127,142,144,175,181,182]

## CONTROVERSIES

Because the clinical picture described by Binswanger and in subsequent reports is nonspecific among the dementias in general, and because cerebral atrophy with hypodensity of the white matter and multiple lacunar infarcts is not an uncommon finding on CT in elderly people,[35,135,179,184] the autonomization of Binswanger's disease as a distinct clinicopathologic entity has been questioned.[51,137,172] On the other hand, other authors have continued to maintain that Binswanger's disease is likely to be a distinct disease, different from multi-infarct dementia as a whole and from lacunar state in particular.[10,24,25,27,43,59,60]

This controversy derives mainly from the expansion of neuroimaging since the mid-seventies, as it was found that a decreased density of white matter on CT or increased signal on T2-weighted MRI could be observed in many patients, much more often than Binswanger's disease used to be diagnosed at autopsy before the CT era. Though "cerebral arteriosclerosis" was considered common, the pathologic changes of Binswanger's disease were exceedingly rare in neuropathologic practice.[83,134,143] For instance, Binswanger's disease was not reported in 50 demented patients who underwent an autopsy, though 12 percent of them showed findings suggesting a vascular origin for dementia, including one patient with "extensive white matter softening."[168] On the other hand, there are recent papers without pathologic confirmation, which report large series of patients with "Binswanger's disease" seen over a short period of 1 year.[79,114,125,180]

## LEUKO-ARAIOSIS

An attenuation of the cerebral white matter density on CT is nonspecific and can be seen in several neurologic diseases, such as Reye syndrome, Canavan's disease, aminoacidurias, mitochondrial cytopathies, leukodystrophies, multiple sclerosis, irradiation, methotrexate toxicity, and progressive multifocal leukoencephalopathy.[137] In order to clarify confusion related to this increase of radiologic diagnoses of Binswanger's disease in elderly patients with or without mental impairment and hypodense white matter on CT (hyperintense on T2-weighted MRI), Hachinski et al.[85] introduced the term *leuko-araiosis* (literally from the Greek, white rarefaction) to describe the neuroimaging findings of this rarefaction of the white matter, sometimes also involving the brain stem,[155] whatever its underlying etiology. Thus, leuko-araiosis is—and should remain—a purely descriptive term with no pathophysiologic implications. However, it is unfortunate that the same people who used to make a diagnosis of Binswanger's disease just on CT or MRI pictures now diagnose leuko-araiosis as if it were a particular disease of the central nervous system.

The concept of rarefaction of the hemisphere white matter is not new. Hauw[88] recently pointed out that Durand-Fardel[62] had already reported a "rarefied white matter" which he differentiated from état criblé on neuropathologic findings in people with cerebrovascular disease in the middle of the nineteenth century. On CT, leuko-araiosis has been defined as a patchy, diffuse hypodensity (increased signal on T2-weighted MRI) limited to the white matter of the cerebral hemispheres, with ill-defined margins.[85,94]

In fact, leuko-araiosis has been increasingly reported in "normal" nondemented people,[32,76,78,89,147,149,184] in whom it may be related to age[34,76,78] and to associated risk factors such as hypertension[67,113] (Fig. 31-6). According to the selectivity of the radiologic criteria used for diagnosis, the prevalence of leuko-araiosis on CT has been comprised between less than 1 percent and more than 25 percent.[35,46,94,107,126,147,182,183] Criteria differentiating "normal" and "abnormal" leuko-araiosis have not been developed, though severe periventricular rims, focal areas of increased T2-signal in the centrum semiovale ("unidentified bright objects" or UBOs), and caps at the frontal and occipital horns on MRI have been reported to be "pathologic"[105,171] (Fig. 31-7).

### Leuko-araiosis in Non-Binswanger's Dementia

Though some authors did not find an association between dementia and leuko-araiosis,[9,148] others reported that the prevalence of dementia increased markedly (up to more than 50 percent) in patients in whom leuko-araiosis was discovered on CT.[35,91,107,162] In the London Ontario Dementia Study,[88] leuko-

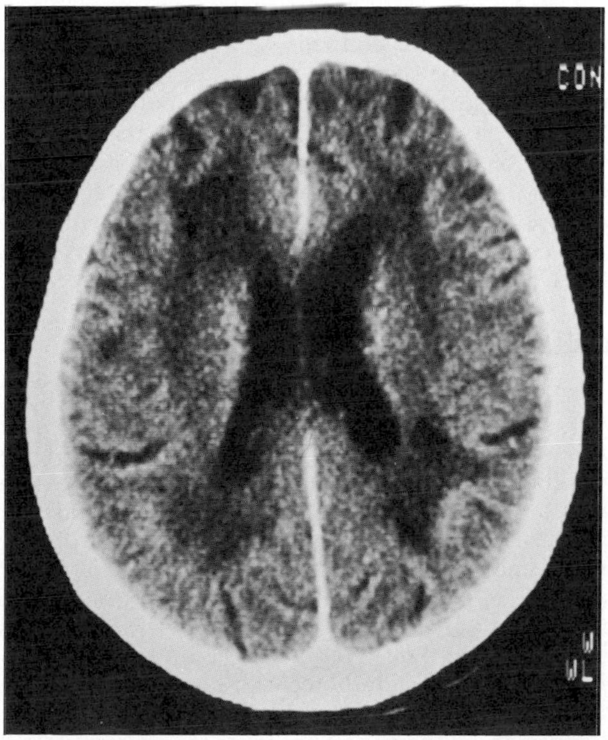


**Fig. 31-6.** Leuko-araiosis on CT in a 62-year-old hypotensive woman with normal neurologic and neuropsychological findings. (Preoperative CT before coronary bypass surgery, courtesy of A. Uské, Lausanne.)

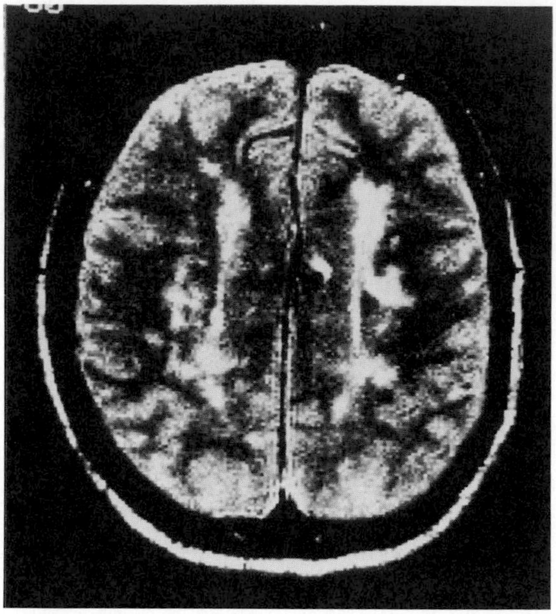

**Fig. 31-7.** White matter rims and "unidentified bright objects" (UBO) on MRI in a 70-year-old man admitted after transient weakness in the right hand.

araiosis on CT was seen in 49 of 110 (35.5 percent) dementia patients, as compared with 12 of 110 (10.9 percent) sex- and age-matched nondemented controls. Moreover, as the controls with leuko-araiosis had lower dementia scores and an increased prevalence of abnormal gait, Babinski sign, and palmomental reflex, it was suggested that leuko-araiosis may be a marker of early dementia with neurologic dysfunction.[161] In the patients with dementia and leuko-araiosis, "subcortical" features of the dementia have been emphasized (impaired attention, depression, apathy).[54,84]

## Leuko-araiosis in Alzheimer's Disease

In 1986 George et al.[76,78] reported one patient with leuko-araiosis who had autopsy-proven Alzheimer's disease. Other reports with CT/MRI-neuropathologic correlation have followed.[123,149] In series of patients with a clinical diagnosis of Alzheimer's disease, 7 to 55 percent had leuko-araiosis,[3,162,176] a proportion which may be dependent on age.[176] In a pathologic series of 84 patients with Alzheimer's disease, 60 percent had a white matter encephalopathy, with gliosis and partial loss of myelin, axons, and oligodendroglia.[36] Recent neuropathologic data suggest that white matter changes may even precede cortical atrophy in Alzheimer's disease.[129] The pathophysiology of leuko-araiosis in Alzheimer's disease remains unclear. Based on an autopsied case, Besson et al.[17] suggested that it may correspond to reduction in neural elements in regions of white matter rarefaction with an increase in water content. On the other hand, Brun and Englund[36,64] emphasized ischemic changes due to hyalinized and thickened white matter arterioles, on the basis of an extensive neuropathologic study. These authors made biochemical analyses of the abnormal white matter and could not relate the changes to an increased water content or to wallerian degeneration. They suggested the term *selective incomplete white matter infarction* (SIWI)[64] to explain the white matter changes, and emphasized hypoperfusion-hypoxic disturbances related to white matter local arteriolopathy associated with systemic heart disease and hypotension and lacunar infarcts. These findings in Alzheimer's disease are very provocative, and remain controversial, as other recent studies failed to demonstrate arteriolar thickening in the white matter.[149] Also, the relationship between amyloid angiopathy and white matter changes in Alzheimer's disease have not been cleared. Leuko-araiosis and white matter abnormalities similar to those of Binswanger's disease have been reported in cerebral amyloid angiopathy.[59,82,116] As more than three-quarters of patients with Alzheimer's disease may have amyloid angiopathy,[16,102,177] it is possible that in Alzheimer's disease an association may exist between leuko-araiosis and amyloid changes in the cerebral arterioles, but this point has not been studied as yet.

## Leuko-araiosis in Multi-infarct Dementia

We mentioned earlier that some authors think that Binswanger's disease may not differ from multi-infarct dementia.[51,137,172] In clinical series of multi-infarct dementia, the prevalence of leuko-araiosis on CT or MRI has been reported to be 32 to 100 percent.[3,65,99,162] Because the clinical diagnosis of multi-infarct dementia is controversial,[31,37] the interpretation of these data on leuko-araiosis remains unclear.

## Leuko-araiosis in Other Dementias

Hypodensity of the periventricular white matter on CT has been considered as a feature of *normal pressure hydrocephalus* with transependymal transsudation of CSF. However, the exact nature of leuko-araiosis associated with normal pressure hydrocephalus had not been elucidated by appropriate pathologic studies, and an association with local arteriolar changes has been suspected in several reports.[45,63,86,93,110,136,159] Leuko-araiosis on CT may be found in three-quarters of patients with biopsy-proven *amyloid angiopathy*.[116] Neuropathologic correlates include a diffuse patchy loss of myelin with edema and astrocytic gliosis in the hemisphere white matter.[59,82,154] Clinically, the patients show dementia and focal signs with subacute worsening, and lobar hemorrhages. These hemorrhages are likely to be related to amyloid changes in the cortical vessels, but the causal relationship between the white matter changes and amyloid angiopathy is more uncertain, as the white matter arterioles may be thickened by fibrohyalinous material, but do not show amyloid deposits.[30,102] In *progressive subcortical gliosis* ("Pick type II dementia"),[106,135] global cerebral atrophy is more common on CT than leuko-araiosis,[106] though the white matter is affected primarily. *AIDS-dementia complex* may sometimes be associated with leuko-araiosis on CT or MRI.[115]

### Leuko-araiosis in Stroke

Though leuko-araiosis has been discussed mainly in dementia, it may be discovered in patients admitted primarily for stroke.[2,24,107] The significance of this finding in acute stroke patient was assessed in the Lausanne Stroke Registry, a prospective registry of first-ever stroke patients admitted consecutively to a population-based primary care center.[29] In this study, 31 or 1,000 patients with ischemic stroke had leuko-araiosis on CT.[28] In 15 of the 31, stroke corresponded to a small deep infarct. Among the 1,000 patients with stroke, leuko-araiosis was more prevalent in those with a small deep infarct (8 percent) than in those with cortical involvement (0.8 percent). A history of hypertension and elevated blood pressure on admission were significantly more common in patients with leuko-araiosis than in controls with stroke but without leuko-araiosis, matched for age, sex, and infarct topography and size. On the other hand, large-vessel disease was significantly less common in patients with leuko-araiosis than in controls. The prevalence of diabetes, high cholesterol, hematocrit above 0.45, smoking, and prior myocardial infarct did not differ between patients with leuko-araiosis and controls. A history of progressive intellectual impairment (23 percent) and neuropsychological findings on dementia (84 percent) were more common in patients with leuko-araiosis than in controls. In this study, it was concluded that in patients with acute stroke, leuko-araiosis on CT is not a fortuitous finding as it is associated with small deep infarcts but not with large-vessel disease, with hypertension but no other risk factors, and with overt or mild dementia. In patients with cerebral hemorrhage, leuko-araiosis may be present in up to 12 percent of the cases;[158] it may be associated with a lobar topography of hemorrhage,[95] which may suggest underlying amyloid angiopathy.

It has also been claimed that leuko-araiosis may be a marker of stroke. In the London Ontario Dementia Study,[94] demented patients with leuko-araiosis had four times more strokes than demented patients without leuko-araiosis.

### Neuropathology of Unselected Leuko-araiosis

Only a few studies with MRI-pathologic correlations of leuko-araiosis in the elderly are available. In 1986 Awad et al.[8] reported one patient with multiple incidental white matter foci on MRI, who showed at autopsy multiple dilatations of the perivascular spaces, probably due to "shrinkage and atrophy of the parenchyma around ectatic blood vessels" with a "network of tunnels filled with extracellular water." These alterations are those of état criblé of Durand-Fardel,[61,62] in which multifocal perivascular cavitation of the white matter occurs without overt alterations of the nervous tissue. They may explain several cases of leuko-araiosis in "normal" people.[11] In another study,[108] 8 of 12 patients with patchy white matter changes in MRI showed atrophic perivascular demyelinating lesions at autopsy; other lesions included "small vascular malformations" in the centrum semiovale in 4 patients, diverticula of lateral ventricles into white matter in 3, and isolated central white matter infarct in 1. In fixed brains of 23 deceased patients older than 60 years, MRI showed 15 hyperintense white matter foci;[33] at pathologic examination these foci corresponded to infarction in 6, small areas of gliosis with noncavitated infarct in 2, congenital diverticule of the lateral ventricle in 1, and in 3 instances no lesion was found. In four other patients with leuko-araiosis, demyelination without inflammatory changes and small infarcts in the basal ganglia and periventricular region were found at autopsy.[84] In many instances, the area of prolonged T2 on MRI may be larger than actual demyelination because reactive astrocytes along axons may be found at distance (isomorphic gliosis).[121]

These findings in unselected cases with leuko-araiosis, with varied or no neurologic dysfunction, confirm the nonspecificity of leuko-araiosis as a radiologic finding, though most of the underlying lesions appear to be related to vascular pathology.

## PATHOPHYSIOLOGY OF BINSWANGER'S DISEASE

Because the white matter changes of Binswanger's disease are not just demyelination secondary to remote infarcts,[144] and as they are associated with thickened and stenosed medullary arterioles in the white matter, most authors have suggested that the pathophysiology of Binswanger's disease is ischemic and is related in some way to arterial hypertension.[10,42,43,87,141,142] However, the main lesion of Binswanger's disease, that is, the patchy white matter changes, is not an infarct per se, and it is highly questionable to implicate chronic hypoperfusion due to arteriolar stenosis, as ischemia itself is not a chronic phenomenon. The term *incomplete infarction* has been used to explain the white matter pallor with demyelination, edema, and gliosis.[59] However, the concept of incomplete infarction is also controversial, and within the brain it has mainly been applied to selective neuronal necrosis, not to demyelinating lesions.[112,140] Because it is difficult to explain the white matter changes by a purely ischemic mechanism, associated phenomena have been advanced, with "chronic edema"[69,146] and of a disturbed hematoencephalic barrier,[80] which could be related to local hypoxia and acidosis.[44,90,139,174] Actually, an edematous leukoencephalopathy has been observed as a consequence of acute ischemia-hypoxia.[69] The role of acute hypotensive and hypertensive phenomena has been emphasized in patients with Binswanger's disease, as they typically have chronic hypertension. It is certainly important to emphasize the not uncommon occurrence of hypotensive events in patients with cardiac failure and disturbed cerebral autoregulation due to chronic hypertension.[51,98,101,118] The role of hypotension related to cardiac arrhythmia, orthostatism, and diuretic-induced hypovolemia has also been emphasized in multi-infarct dementia in general.[164] Okeda[139] mentioned that hypertension alone could not be rendered responsible for the lesions of Binswanger's disease, as the small vessels of the white matter are in fact more severely involved in subjects with hypertensive encephalopathy and hypertensive hemorrhage than in patients with Binswanger's disease. Nutritional factors,[101] increased blood viscosity,[150,157] and impaired venous drainage[163] have also been mentioned, but there are few data to support such mechanisms.

The concept of watershed ischemia of the white matter has been advanced to explain at least some of the white matter lesions of Binswanger's disease.[51,54] Selective infarcts of the white matter have been reported,[26,38,41,152] but they are "watershed" only when they occur at the border zone between the territory of the deep perforators and the territory of the pial system.[26] On the other hand, the medullary arterioles involved in Binswanger's disease are endarterioles, and it is likely that ischemia in their territory would not occur in a watershed pattern. The periventricular watershed leukomalacia, which has been reported in patients with severe carotid disease and heart failure,[4,52,53,152] is likely to be a completely different entity from Binswanger's disease, although it has often been misclassified with it.

With reference to the vascular changes seen in Binswanger's disease, thickening and stenosis of the medullary arterioles of the hemisphere white matter has usually been related to chronic hypertension.[10,44,59,137] However, similar arteriolar changes have rarely been reported in younger patients with the pathology of Binswanger's disease; in the absence of hypertension,[73,109,117,120,133,178] these patients also had alopecia-spondylitis deformans and it is likely that they can be grouped into a "syndrome," but the underlying cause of their arteriolar changes remains unknown. Also, hypertension is common and Binswanger's disease is rare, and it is not possible to consider that hypertension is anything but a risk factor.

The topography of white matter involvement may be an argument favoring an ischemic phenomenon associated with specific arteriolar changes. Actually, the corpus callosum, which is typically spared in Binswanger's disease, appears to have a completely different pattern of vascular supply from the centrum semiovale,[128] which is typically involved in Binswanger's disease: the central zone and genu of the corpus callosum are supplied by short penetrating arterioles in a way very similar to the cerebral cortex. Unique features of this supply include arteriole-venule pairs, perivascular fibrous alae, and recurrent companion arterioles. On the other hand, the extremely lateral part of the corpus callosum and the adjacent centrum semiovale are supplied by the long medullary endarterioles, precisely those involved in Binswanger's disease. Patterns of vascular supply may also explain sparing of U-fibers in Binswanger's disease, because these fibers receive their supply together with the central cortex from the pial system.[160]

In summary, it is likely that an ischemic phenomenon related to arteriosclerosis of the medullary arterioles of the hemispheric deep white matter plays a significant role in the pathophysiology of Binswanger's disease, but associated hypoxic-hypotensive phenomena from cardiac failure, hypovolemia and hypertension-induced impairment of autoregulation, and possibly other mechanisms should also be emphasized; a genetic susceptibility is not impossible, but it has not been studied.

## RISK FACTORS ASSOCIATED WITH BINSWANGER'S DISEASE

Chronic arterial hypertension is the most common risk factor associated with autopsy-verified Binswanger's disease.[40,44,50,51,59,60,68,98,101,153,169] In most series in which the data are available, the prevalence of hypertension approaches 100 percent,[44,51] though isolated cases without hypertension have been reported.[74] Nonhypertensive patients with the pathology of Binswanger's disease are usually younger and show associated features (spondylitis, alopecia), maybe in the context of a specific syndrome.[73,109,117,120,133,178] Hypertension is also the most common risk factor present in patients with leuko-araiosis on CT or MRI from different series.[9,28,35,47,67,84,91,94,126,172] Other risk factors for leuko-araiosis, associated or not with neurologic dysfunction, include age,[9,47,177] less often diabetes mellitus,[35,105] hyperviscosity,[150] and heart disease.[35,67] On the other hand, risk factors other than hypertension and age have not been associated with Binswanger's disease. The sole other factors reported in the series of 45 patients of Tomonaga et al.[169] were cardiac disease and malnutrition.

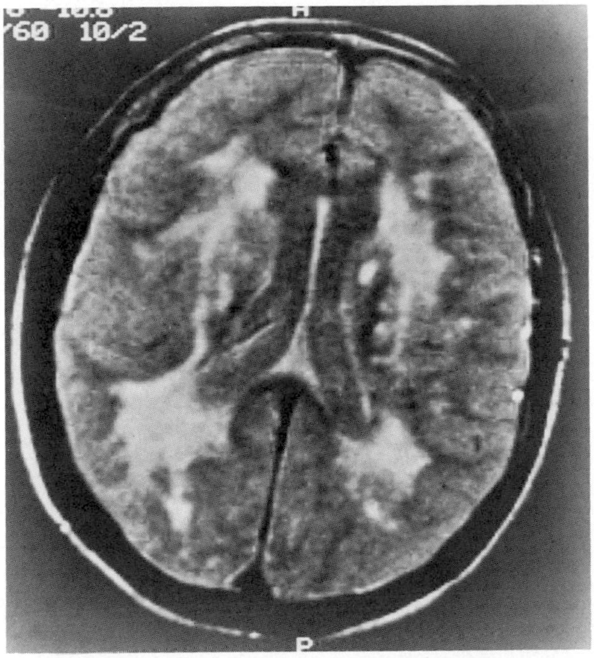
A

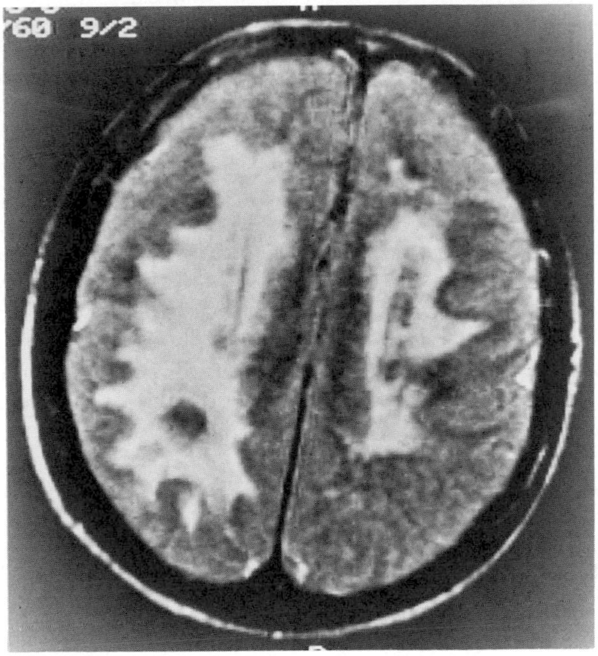
B

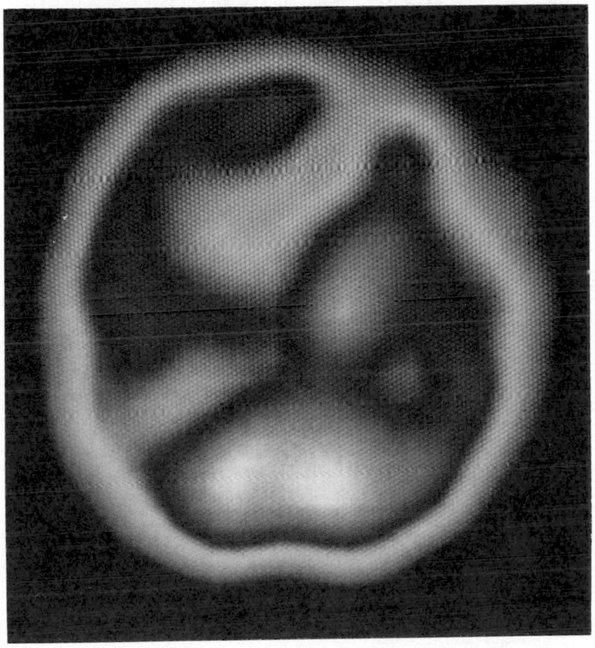
C

**Fig. 31-8. (A & B)** Prolonged T2-signal in cerebral white matter of a 73-year-old woman with hypertension and stepwise progression of dementia with repeated strokes. ($^{95m}$Tc-HMPAO SPECT.) (Courtesy of B. Delaloye, Lausanne.) **(C)** Heterogeneously reduced blood flow in subcortical and cortical regions. Binswanger's disease is possible, but not definite, in the absence of pathologic confirmation.

## CLINICAL DIAGNOSIS OF BINSWANGER'S DISEASE

Binswanger's disease is mainly a neuropathologic diagnosis, and, at best, it can only be suspected during life, in the absence of histopathologic studies. This problem of clinical diagnosis is a general problem in dementia, and there are convincing data that show that in patients with a clinical diagnosis of dementia, the etiology cannot be accurately predicted during life.[31] There may be good reasons to suspect Binswanger's disease in an elderly patient with longstanding hypertension and stepwise evolution of dementia with multiple lacunar strokes, leuko-araiosis, and small deep infarcts on CT or MRI. However, confirmation of the white matter changes and arteriosclerosis will require postmortem studies. In the absence of a definite therapy that can significantly alter evolution, brain biopsy has no indication in principle.

CT and MRI findings of leuko-araiosis can be misleading, as discussed in this chapter, although I have attempted to delineate characteristics that suggest Binswanger's disease among CT/MRI scans showing leuko-araiosis. In Binswanger's disease confirmed at autopsy, leuko-araiosis on MRI (best evaluated on spin-echo sequences with long repetition time) usually involves almost the entire white matter of the corona radiata;[55] contrary to other forms of leuko-araiosis, the core of the white matter is more involved than the periventricular region. Other features include centering at the angle of frontal horns, ill-defined margins, and marked sparing of corpus callosum and of white matter medial to ventricular trigone.[119] There seems to be a correlation between the intensity of the T2 signal on MRI and the severity of the histologic process of demyelination-gliosis.[122,123] On CT, the decrease in density of white matter averages only 5.5 HU,[81] so that the findings are less prominent than on MRI. The presence of markedly enlarged ventricles[44] and of cortical infarcts[59,144] does not rule out the diagnosis.

Other imaging techniques have not been assessed in pathologically proven Binswanger's disease. Metabolic studies with PET and CBF evaluations in patients with leuko-araiosis have shown white matter hypoperfusion, usually heterogeneous, which may also involve the cortex.[67,72,118]

EEG may be normal[44,48,75] or show slowing that may be diffuse[10,75] or focal,[18,153] rarely with a periodic[40] or triphasic activity. CSF is usually normal or shows mildly elevated proteins.[10]

Doppler ultrasounds and angiographic studies usually show only mild nonstenosing lesions in large arteries. As mentioned above, leuko-araiosis in general seems to be rarely associated with carotid stenosis or occlusion,[28,183] except in some instances of periventricular leukomalacia.[52,53]

## TREATMENT OF BINSWANGER'S DISEASE

No specific treatment has been advocated in patients suspected to have Binswanger's disease, but in those with hypertension, it is advised to control blood pressure with appropriate drugs. However, it must be remembered that hypotensive events have also been implicated in the pathogenesis of Binswanger's disease, so that they should be avoided. It is likely that the earlier the treatment of hypertension and other risk factors, the better the prevention of the disease. The role for platelet antiaggregant therapy is unknown in Binswanger's disease.

## CONCLUSION

Although controversies may persist and the intrusion of leuko-araiosis into medical terminology does not seem to have much stabilized the confusion between other terms such as leukoencephalopathy and Binswanger's dementia, there is enough evidence in our view to maintain Binswanger's disease as a separate, though rare, clinicopathologic entity, in which typical white matter changes showing uniform progression, small deep infarcts, thickened hyalinized white matter arterioles, high blood pressure, and a rather stereotyped, though not specific, clinical picture are associated.[70] However, one should remember (1) that Binswanger's disease can at best only be suspected during life (Fig. 31-8), and (2) that most demented patients with leuko-araiosis on CT or MRI do not have Binswanger's disease. As for Alzheimer's disease, "a definite diagnosis of Binswanger's disease requires pathologic confirmation and exclusion of other dementing illness."[13]

## REFERENCES

1. Acevedo M: Demencia for reblandecimientos multiplex subcorticales. Rev Soc Med Argentina 17:873, 1909
2. Agnoli A, Ruggieri S, Denaro A et al: White matter disease (Binswanger's encephalopathy) in chronic cerebrovascular disorders. Monogr Neural Sci 11:144, 1984
3. Aharon-Peretz J, Cummings JL, Hill MA: Vascular dementia and dementia of the Alzheimer type: cognition, ventricular size, and leuko-araiosis. Arch Neurol 45:719, 1988
4. Ali Chérif A, Labrecque R, Pellissier JF et al: Encéphalopathie sous-corticale de Binswanger: étude d'un cas comportant une atteinte hémisphérique gauche nettement prédominante. Rev Neurol 135:665, 1979
5. Alzheimer A: Neure Arbeiten über die Dementia senilis und die auf atheromatöser Gefässerkrankung basierenden Gehirnkrankheiten. Monatsschr Psychiatr Neurol 3:101, 1898
6. Alzheimer A: Die Seelenstörungen auf arteriosclerotischer Grundlage. Allg Z Psychiatr Psychisch (Ger Med) 59:695, 1902
7. Antunes IL: Lésions de la substance blanche dans l'artériosclérose cérébrale. p. 199. In: Proceedings of the First International Congress of Neuropathology. Vol 3. Rosenberg & Sellier, Torino, 1952
8. Awad IA, Johnson PC, Spetzler RF, Hodak JA: Incidental subcortical lesions identified on MRI in the elderly. II. Postmortem pathological correlations. Stroke 17:1090, 1986
9. Awad IA, Spetzler RF, Hodak JA et al: Incidental subcortical lesions identified on MRI in the elderly. I. Correlation with age and cerebrovascular risk factors. Stroke 17:1084, 1986
10. Babikian V, Ropper AH: Binswanger's disease: a review. Stroke 18:2, 1987
11. Ball MJ: "Leukoaraiosis" explained. Lancet 1:612, 1989
12. Behr H: Ein Beitrag zur Frage der Encephalitis subcorticalis chronica. Monatsschr Psychiatr Neurol 19:498, 1906

13. Benett DA, Wilson RS, Gilley DW, Fox JH: Clinical diagnosis of Binswanger's disease (BD). Neurology (NY), suppl 1. 39:253, 1989
14. Benhaïem-Sigaux N, Gray F, Gherardi R et al: Expanding cerebellar lacunes due to dilatation of the perivascular space associated with Binswanger's subcortical arterioclerotic encephalopathy. Stroke 18:1087, 1987
15. Berger H: Otto Binswanger. Arch Psychiatr Nervenkr 89:1, 1930
16. Bergeron C, Ranalli PJ, Miceli PN: Amyloid angiopathy in Alzheimer's disease. Can J Neurol Sci 14:564, 1987
17. Besson JAO, Ebmeier KP, Best PV, Smith FW: Do white matter changes on MRI and CT differentiate vascular dementia from Alzheimer's disease? J Neurol Neurosurg Psychiatry 51:318, 1988
18. Biemond A: On Binswanger's subcortical arteriosclerotic encephalopathy and the possibility of its clinical recognition. Psychiatr Neurol Neurochir 73:413, 1970
19. Binswanger O: Die Abgrenzung der allgemeinen progressiven Paralyse. Berl Klin Wochenschr 49:1103, 50:1137, 52:1180, 1894
20. Binswanger O: Die Begrenzung der allgemeinen Paralyse. Allg Z Psychiatr 51:804, 1895
21. Binswanger O, Siemering E: Lehrbuch der Psychiatrie. Fischer, Jena, 1904
22. Binswanger O: Die Pathologie und Pathogenese der Paralyse. Arch Psychiatr Nervenkr 72:341, 1924
23. Bogousslavsky J: Les démences "traitables." Med Hyg 44:2710, 1986
24. Bogousslavsky J: Leucoencéphalopathie, leucoaraiose et infarctus cérébraux. Rev Neurol 144:11, 1988
25. Bogousslavsky J: Lacunar stroke, Binswanger's disease and atherosclerosis. p. 523. In Crepaldi G, Gotto AM, Manzato E, Baggio G (eds): Atherosclerosis. Excerpta Medica, Amsterdam, 1989
26. Bogousslavsky J, Regli F: Unilateral watershed cerebral infarcts. Neurology (NY) 36:373, 1986
27. Bogousslavsky J, Regli F: Micro-angiopathies cérébrales, lacunes et leucoaraiose. Schweiz Rundschau Med (Praxis) 76:1318, 1987
28. Bogousslavsky J, Regli F, Uske A: Leucoencephalopathy in patients with ischemic stroke. Stroke 18:896, 1987
29. Bogousslavsky J, Regli F, Van Melle G, for the Lausanne Stroke Registry Group: The Lausanne Stroke Registry: analysis of 1000 consecutive patients with first stroke. Stroke 19:1083, 1988
30. Bogucki A, Papierz W, Szymanska R, Staniaszczyk R: Cerebral amyloid angiopathy with attenuation of the white matter on CT scans: subcortical arteriosclerotic encephalopathy (Binswanger) in a normotensive patient. J Neurol 235:435, 1988
31. Boller F, Lopez OL, Moossy J: Diagnosis of dementia: clinicopathologic correlations. Neurology (NY) 39:76, 1989
32. Bradley WG, Jr, Waluch V, Braut-Zawadzki M: Patchy, periventricular white matter lesions in the elderly: a common observation during NMR imaging. Noninv Med Imag 1:35, 1984
33. Braffman BH, Zimmerman RA, Trojanowski JQ et al: Pathologic correlation with gross and histopathology. 2. Hyperintense white-matter foci in the elderly. AJR, 151:559, 1988
34. Brant-Zawadzki M, Fein G, Van Dyke C et al: MRI of the aging brain: patchy white matter lesions and dementia. AJNR 6:675, 1985
35. Brott T, Mouradin M, Uthman B: Dementia, ventricular enlargement, and hypertension associated with periventricular hypodensity by CT. Ann Neurol 20:129, 1986
36. Brun A, Englund E: A white matter disorder in dementia of the Alzheimer type: a pathoanatomical study. Ann Neurol 19:253, 1986
37. Brust JCM: Dementia and cerebrovascular disease. p. 131. In Mayeux R, Rosen WG (eds): The Dementias. Raven Press, New York, 1983
38. Buchan GC, Alvord EC, Jr: Diffuse necrosis of subcortical white matter associated with bacterial meningitis. Neurology (NY) 19:1, 1969
39. Buchholz K: Über die Geistesstörungen bei Arteriosklerose und ihre Beziehungen zu den psychiscehn Erkrankungen des Seniums. Arch Psychiatr Nervenkr 39:499, 1106, 1905
40. Burger PC, Burch JG, Kunze U: Subcortical arteriosclerotic encephalopathy (Binswanger's disease): a vascular etiology of dementia. Stroke 7:626, 1976
41. Burger PC, Vogel FS: Hemorrhagic white matter infarction in three critically ill patients. Hum Pathol 8:121, 1977
42. Caplan LR: Binswanger's disease. p. 317. In Vinken PJ, Bruyn GW, Klawans ML (eds): Handbook of Clinical Neurology. Vol 46. Neurobehavioral Disorders. Elsevier, New York, 1985
43. Caplan LR: Binswanger's disease. Curr Opinion Neurol Neurosurg 1:57, 1988
44. Caplan LR, Schoene WC: Clinical features of subcortical arteriosclerotic encephalopathy (Binswanger disease). Neurology (NY) 28:1206, 1978
45. Casimiro M, D'Alessandro R, Cacciatore FM et al: Risk factors for the syndrome of ventricular enlargement with gait apraxia (idiopathic normal pressure hydrocephalus): a case-control study. J Neurol Neurosurg Psychiatry 52:847, 1989
46. Chimowitz MI, Awad IA, Furlan AJ: Periventricular lesions on MRI: facts and theories. Stroke 20:963, 1989
47. Clark C, Welsh K, Earl N: The association of T2 signals on MRI with cognitive impairment in patients with clinical Alzheimer's disease. Ann Neurol 24:161, 1988
48. Davison C: Progressive subcortical encephalopathy (Binswanger's disease). J Neuropathol Exp Neurol 1:42, 1942
49. Delay J, Brion S: Les démences tardives. Masson, Paris, 1962
50. Delong GR, Kemper TL, Pogacar S, Lee HY: Clinical neuropathological conference. Dis Nerv Syst 35:286, 1974
51. De Reuck J, Crevits L, De Coster W et al: Pathogenesis of Binswanger chronic progressive subcortical encephalopathy. Neurology (NY) 30:920, 1980
52. De Reuck J, Schaumburg HH: Periventricular

atherosclerotic leukoencephalopathy. Neurology (NY) 22:1094, 1972
53. De Reuck J, van der Eecken HM: Periventricular leukomalacia in adults. Arch Neurol 35:517, 1978
54. Deris MMA, Hijdra A, Verbeeten BWJ, Jr: Mental changes in subcortical arteriosclerotic encephalopathy. Clin Neurol Neurosurg 89:71, 1987
55. De Witt LD, Kistler JP, Miller DC et al: NMR-neuropathologic correlation in stroke. Stroke 18:342, 1987
56. Dickmann H: Über Encephalitis subcorticalis chronica progressiva. Z Ges Neurol Psychiatr 49:1, 1919
57. Dimitri V, Aranovich J: Sobre los aspectos leucoencefalósicos de la arteriosclerosis cerebral. Rev Neurol Buenos Aires 10:290, 1945
58. Donegani G, Grattarola FR: Considerazioni anatomo-cliniche sulla encefalopatia sottocorticale cronica di Binswanger. Schweiz Arch Neurol Psychiatr 81:132, 1958
59. Dubas F, Gray F, Roullet E, Escourolle R: Leucoencephalopathies artériopathiques (17 cas anatomo-cliniques). Rev Neurol 141:93, 1985
60. Dupuis M, Brucher JM, Gonsette RE: Observation anatomo-clinique d'une encéphalite souscorticale artérioscléreuse ("maladie de Binswanger") avec hypodensité de la substance blanche au scanner cérébral. Acta Neurol Belg 94:131, 1984
61. Durand-Fardel M: Mémoire sur une altération particulière de la substance cérébrale. Gaz Méd Paris 10:23, 33, 1842
62. Durand-Fardel M: Traité Clinique et Pratique des Maladies des Vieillards. p. 12. Baillière, Paris, 1854
63. Earnest MP, Fahn S, Karp JH, Rowland LP: Normal pressure hydrocephalus and hypertensive cerebrovascular disease. Arch Neurol 31:262, 1974
64. Englund E, Brun A, Alling C: White matter changes in dementia of Alzheimer's type: biochemical and neuropathological correlates. Brain 111:1425, 1988
65. Erkinjuntti T, Ketonen L, Sulkava R et al: Do white matter changes on MRI and CT differentiate vascular dementia from Alzheimer's disease. J Neurol Neurosurg Psychiatry 50:37, 1987
66. Farnell FJ, Globus JH: Chronic progressive vascular subcortical encephalopathy: chronic progressive subcortical encephalitis of Binswanger. Arch Neurol Psychiatry 27:593, 1932
67. Fazekas F, Niederhorn K, Schmidt R et al: White matter signal abnormalities in normal individuals: correlation with carotid ultrasonography, CBF measurements, and cerebrovascular risk factors. Stroke 19:1285, 1988
68. Feigin I, Budzilovich G, Weinberg S, Ogata J: Degeneration of white matter in hypoxia, acidosis and edema. J Neuropathol Exp Neurol 32:125, 1973
69. Feigin I, Popoff N: Neuropathological changes late in cerebral edema; the relationship to trauma, hypertensive disease and Binswanger encephalopathy. J Neuropathol Exp Neurol 22:500, 1963
70. Fisher CM: Binswanger's encephalopathy: a review. J Neurol 236:65, 1989
71. Foix C, Chavany JA: Pallilalie syllabique: sclérose intracérébrale en foyers disséminés. Rev Neurol 1:61, 1926
72. Friedland RP, Koss E, Jagust WJ, Borcich J: Familial subcortical arteriosclerotic encephalopathy (SAE) in two families: studies with x-ray, CT, NMR and PET. Neurology (NY), suppl 1. 36:102, 1986
73. Fukutake T, Hattor T, Kita K, Hirayama K: Familial juvenile encephalopathy (Binswanger type) with alopecia and lumbago. Clin Neurol (Tokyo) 25:949, 1985
74. Garcia-Albea E, Cabello A, Franch O: Subcortical arteriosclerotic encephalopathy (Binswanger's disease): a report of five patients. Acta Neurol Scand 75:295, 1987
75. Garcin R, Lapresle J, Lyon G: Encéphalopathie sous-coricale chronique de Binswanger: etude anatomo-clinique de 3 observations. Rev Neurol 102:423, 1960
76. George AE, de Leon MJ, Gentes CI et al: Leukoencephalopathy in normal and pathologic aging. 1. CT of brain lucencies. AJNR 7:561, 1986
77. George AE, de Leon MJ, Kalnin A et al: Leukoencephalopathy and pathologic aging. 2. MRI of brain lucencies. AJNR 7:567, 1986
78. Gerard G, Weisberg LA: MRI periventricular lesions in adults. Neurology (NY) 36:998, 1986
79. Gilley DW, Wilson RS, Bennett DA, Fox JH: Depression in putative Binswanger's disease. Ann Neurol 26:134, 1989
80. Ginsberg MD, Hedley-White ET, Richardson EP, Jr: Hypoxic-ischemic leukoencephalopathy in man. Arch Neurol 33:5, 1976
81. Goto K, Ishii N, Fukasawa H: Diffuse white matter disease in the geriatric population: a clinical, neuropathological and CT study. Radiology 141:687, 1989
82. Gray F, Dubas F, Roullet E, Escourolle R: Leukoencephalopathy in diffuse hemorrhagic cerebral amyloid angiopathy. Ann Neurol 18:54, 1985
83. Grünthal E: Zur Klinik und Anatomie des arteriosklerotischen Grosshirnmarkschwundes. Arch Psychiatr Nervenkr 88:849, 1929
84. Gupta SR, Naheedy MH, Young JC et al: Periventricular white matter changes and dementia: clinical, neuropsychological, radiological, and pathological correlation. Arch Neurol 45:637, 1988
85. Hachinski VC, Potter P, Merskey H: Leukoaraiosis. Arch Neurol 44:21, 1987
86. Haidri NH, Modi SM: Normal pressure hydrocephalus and hypertensive cerebrovascular disease. Dis Nerv Syst 38:918, 1977
87. Harrison MGJ, Marshall J: Hypoperfusion in the etiology of subcortical arteriosclerotic encephalopathy (Binswanger type). J Neurol Neurosurg Psychiatry 47:754, 1984

88. Hauw JJ: Leuko-araiosis: the brain interstitial atrophy (atrophie interstitielle du cerveau) of Durand-Fardel. Arch Neurol 45:140, 1988
89. Hershey LA, Modic MT, Greenough PG, Jaffé DF: MRI in vascular dementia. Neurology (NY) 37:29, 1987
90. Huang K, Wu L, Luo Y: Binswanger's disease: progressive subcortical encephalopathy or multi-infarct dementia. Can J Neurol Sci 12:88, 1985
91. Hurwitz BJ, Heyman A, Drayer B, Utley C: Cerebral white matter hypodensity in CT scans: an indication of Binswanger's disease? Ann Neurol 16:155, 1984
92. Iglesias-Rozas JR, Ebhardt G: Alterations of microvasculature in progressive subcortical encephalopathy (Binswanger). p. 454. In Cervas-Navarro J (ed): Pathology of Cerebral Microcirculation. De Guyter, Berlin, 1974
93. Inzitari D, Bracco L, Capparelli R et al: CSF dynamics, white matter degeneration and mental deterioration in subcortical arteriosclerotic encephalopathy of Binswanger type. Monogr Neural Sci 11:150, 1984
94. Inzitari D, Diaz JF, Fox AJ et al: Vascular risk factors and leuko-araiosis. Arch Neurol 44:42, 1987
95. Inzitari D, Giordano GP, Ancona AL et al: Leukoaraiosis and intracerebral hemorrhage: a CT study. Stroke 20:135, 1989
96. Ishino H, Higashi H, Hayara T et al: A case of subcortical arteriosclerotic encephalopathy (Binswanger's disease). Folia Psychiatr Neurol Jpn 26:39, 1972
97. Ishisaki K: Coexistence of état lacunaire and subcortical arteriosclerotic encephalopathy in old age. Clin Neurol (Tokyo) 15:618, 1975
98. Janota I: Dementia, deep white matter damage and hypertension: "Binswanger's disease." Psychol Med 11:39, 1987
99. Jayakumar PN, Taly AB, Shanmugam V et al: Multi-infarct dementia: a CT study. Acta Neurol Scand 73:292, 1989
100. Jelgersma HC: A case of encephalopathia subcorticalis chronica (Binswanger's disease). Psychiatr Neurol (Basel) 147:81, 1964
101. Jellinger K, Neumayer E: Progressive subcorticale vasculare Encephalopathie Binswanger: eine klinische neuropathologische Studie. Arch Psychiatr Nervenkr 205:523, 1964
102. Joachim CL, Morris JH, Selkoe DJ: Amyloid angiopathy in 100 cases of Alzheimer's disease. Neurology (NY), suppl 1. 37:225, 1987
103. Johnson KA, Davis KR, Buonanno FS et al: Comparison of MR and Roentgen ray CT in dementia. Arch Neurol 44:1075, 1987
104. Kashida: Über Gehirnarteriosklerose des frühen Alters und über die Kombination von kortikalen, pyramidalen und extrapyramidalen Symptomen bei der Gehirnarteriosklerose. Z Ges Neurol Psychitr 94:659, 1924–1925
105. Kertesz A, Black SE, Tokar G et al: Periventricular and subcortical hyperintensities on MRI: rims, caps, and unidentified bright objects. Arch Neurol 45:404, 1988
106. Khoubesserian P, Davous P, Bianco C et al: Démence familiale type Neumann (gliose sous-corticale). Rev Neurol 141:706, 1985
107. Kinkel WR, Jacobs L, Polachini I et al: Subcortical arteriosclerotic encephalopathy (Binswanger's disease): CT, NMR and clinical correlations. Arch Neurol 42:951, 1985
108. Kirkpatrick JB, Hayman LA: White-matter lesions in MR imaging of clinically healthy brains of elderly subjects: possible pathologic basis. Radiology 162:509, 1987
109. Kondo S, Ogasawara N, Ito T, Tsunoda T: Über einen autoptischen Fall von der im ZNS lokalisierten nekrotisierenden Angiitis (Periarteritis nodosa?). Adv Neurol Sci (Tokyo) 14:274, 1970
110. Koto A, Rosenberg A, Zindesser H et al: Syndrome of normal pressure hydrocephalus: possible relation to hypertensive and arteriosclerotic vasculopathy. J Neuropathol Exp Neurol 40:73, 1977
111. Ladame C: Encéphalopathie sous-corticale clinique: un cas de psychose d'origine arterioscléreuse. L'Encéphale 7:13, 1912
112. Lassen NA: Incomplete cerebral infarction—focal incomplete ischemic tissue necrosis not leading to emollision. Stroke 13:522, 1982
113. Lechner H, Schmidt R, Bertha G et al: Nuclear MRI white matter lesions and risk factors for stroke in normal individuals. Stroke 19:263, 1988
114. Lee A, Yu YL, Tsoi M et al: Subcortical arteriosclerotic encephalopathy: a controlled psychometric study. Clin Neurol Neurosurg 91:235, 1989
115. Levy RM, Rosenbloom S, Perrett LV. Neuroradiologic findings in AIDS: a review of 200 cases. AJR 147:977, 1986
116. Loes D, Biller J, Yuh W et al: MRI of cerebral amyloid angiopathy. Ann Neurol 24:160, 1988
117. Loizou LA, Jefferson JM, Smith TW: Subcortical arteriosclerotic encephalopathy (Binswanger's type) and cortical infarcts in a young normotensive patient. J Neurol Neurosurg Psychiatry 45:409, 1982
118. Loizou LA, Kendall BE, Marshall J: Subcortical arteriosclerotic encephalopathy: a chemical and radiological investigation. J Neurol Neurosurg Psychiatry 50:294, 1987
119. Lotz PR, Ballinger WE, Jr, Quisling RG: Subcortical arteriosclerotic encephalopathy: CT spectrum and pathologic correlation. AJR, 147:1209, 1986
120. Maeda S, Nakayama H, Isaka K et al: Familial unusual encephalopathy of Binswanger's type without hypertension. Folia Psychiatr Neurol Jpn 30:165, 1976
121. Marshall VG, Bradley WG, Jr, Marshall CE et al: Deep white matter infarction: correlation of MR imaging and histopathologic findings. Radiology 167:517, 1988
122. Mascalchi M, Inzitari D, Baratti E et al: In vitro MRI-pathologic correlations in a case of Binswanger's encephalopathy. Neurology (NY), suppl 1. 37:300, 1987
123. Mascalchi M, Inzitari D, Marini P et al: Leuko-

araiosis and Binswanger's disease: a CT-pathological study. Neurology (NY), suppl 1. 38:372, 1988
124. Masden JC, Horiuchi K, Dickson D, Wolfson L: Small-vessel changes in white matter disease of the elderly. Neurology (NY), suppl 1. 39:123, 1989
125. Mathers SE, Chambers BR, Merory JR, Alexander I: Subcortical arteriosclerotic encephalopathy: Binswanger's disease. Clin Exp Neurol 23:67, 1987
126. McQuinn BA, O'Leary DH: White matter lucencies on CT, subacute arteriosclerotic encephalopathy (Binswanger's disease), and blood pressure. Stroke 18:900, 1987
127. Mikol J: Maladie de Binswanger et formes apparentées: contribution à l'étude des leucoencéphalopathies artérioscléreuses. Rev Neurol 118:111, 1968
128. Moody DM, Bell MA, Challa VR: The corpus callosum, a unique white-matter tract: anatomical features that may explain sparing in Binswanger disease and resistance to flow of fluid masses. AJNR 9:1051, 1988
129. Monte de la SM: Quantitation of cerebral atrophy in preclinical and end-stage Alzheimer's disease. Ann Neurol 15:450, 1989
130. Morris JC, Gado MH, Grant EA, Rezek DL: Periventricular white matter lucencies: no effect on the natural history of senile dementia of the Alzheimer type. Ann Neurol 24:159, 1988
131. Naheedy MH, Gupta SR, Young JC et al: Periventricular white matter changes and subcortical dementia: clinical, neuroradiological, radiological, and pathological correlation. AJNR 6:468, 1985
132. National Multiple Sclerosis Society Working Group on Neuroimaging for the Medical Advisory Board: Use of MRI in the diagnosis of multiple sclerosis: policy statement. Neurology (NY) 36:1575, 1986
133. Nemoto S: Einige Beiträge zur Encephalitis subcorticalis chronica progressiva (Binswanger) p. 51. In: Festschrift zum Zurücktritt von Professor Toshimi Ishibachi. Sendai, 1966
134. Neumann MA: Chronic progressive subcortical encephalopathy: report of a case. J Gerontol 2:57, 1947
135. Neumann MA, Colin R: Progressive subcortical gliosis: a rare form of presenile dementia. Brain 90:405, 1967
136. Newton H, Pickard JP, Weller RO: Normal pressure hydrocephalus and cerebrovascular disease: findings of post-mortem. J Neurol Neurosurg Psychiatry 52:804, 1989
137. Nichols FT III, Mohr JP: Binswanger's subacute arteriosclerotic encephalopathy. In Barnett HJM, Stein BM, Mohr JP, Yatsu FM (eds): Stroke: Pathophysiology. Diagnosis and Management. Vol. 2. p. 875. Churchill Livingstone, New York, 1986
138. Nissl F: Zur Kasuistik der arteriosklerotischen Demenz (ein Fall von sog. "Encephalitis subcorticalis"). Z Ges Neurol Psychiatr 19:438, 1920
139. Okeda R: Morphometrische Vergleichsuntersuchungen an Hirtarterien bei Binswangerscher Encephalopathie und Hochdruckencephalopathie. Acta Neuropathol 26:23, 1973
140. Olsen TS: Regional CBF after occlusion of the middle cerebral artery. Acta Neurol Scand 73:321, 1986
141. Olszewski J: The myth of Binswanger disease. J Neuropathol Exp Neurol 20:312, 1961
142. Olszewski J: Subcortical arteriosclerotic encephalopathy: review of the literature on the so-called Binswanger's disease and presentation of two cases. World Neurol 3:359, 1962
143. Orlando R, Orlando JC: Contribucion al conocimiento de las leucoencefalosis tipo Binswanger. p. 60. In: Proceedings of the Fifth International Congress of Neurology. Vol 4. 1954
144. Pellissier JF: Binswanger's encephalopathy. In Vinken PJ, Bruyn GW, Klawans HC (eds): Handbook of Clinical Neurology. Vascular Diseases. Vol. 54 p. 221. Elsevier, Amsterdam, 1989
145. Pilleri G, Risso M: Das klinische Bild und die pathologischen Veränderungen eines Falles von schwerem subkortikalem Markabbau auf arterio-sklerotischer Grundlage (Encephalopathia subcorticalis chronica, Binswanger). Psychiatr Neurol 131:209, 1959
146. Poppe W, Tennstedt A: Ein Beitrag zur Encephalopathia subcorticalis Binswanger. Psychiatr Clin (Basel) 145:27, 1963
147. Pullicino P, Eskin T, Ketonen L: Prevalence of Binswanger's disease. Lancet 1:939, 1983
148. Rao SM, Mittenberg W, Bernardin L, Haughton V, Leo GJ: Neuropsychological test findings in subjects with leukoaraiosis. Arch Neurol 46:40, 1989
149. Rezek DL, Morris JC, Fulling KH, Gado MH: Periventricular white matter lucencies in SDAT and normal aging. Neurology (NY) 37:1365, 1987
150. Ringelstein EB, Manckner A, Schneider R et al: Effects of enzymatic blood defibrination in subcortical arteriosclerotic encephalopathy. J Neurol Neurosurg Psychiatry 51:1051, 1988
151. Roman GC: Senile dementia of the Binswanger type: a vascular form of dementia in the elderly. JAMA 258:1782, 1987
152. Romanul FCA: Selective infarction of gray or white matter caused by occlusion of large arteries. Clin Dev Med 39/40:41, 1971
153. Rosenberg GA, Kornfeld M, Stovring J, Bicknell JM: Subcortical arteriosclerotic encephalopathy (Binswanger): CT. Neurology (NY) 29:1102, 1979
154. Roullet E, Baudrimont M, Hauw JJ et al: Leukoencephalopathy in cerebral amyloid angiopathy: clinical, radiologic, and pathologic study of six cases. Neurology (NY), supp 1. 38:325, 1988
155. Salomon A, Yeates AE, Burger PC, Heinz ER: Subcortical arteriosclerotic encephalopathy: brain stem findings with MR imaging. Radiology 165:625, 1987
156. Sarpel G, Chaudry F, Hindo W: MRI of peri-

ventricular hyperintensity in a veterans administration hospital population. Arch Neurol 44:725, 1987
157. Schneider R, Ringelstein EB, Zeumer H et al: The role of plasma hyperviscosity in subcortical arteriosclerotic encephalopathy (Binswanger's disease). J Neurol 234:67, 1987
158. Selekler K, Erzen C: Leukoaraiosis and intracerebral hematoma. Stroke 20:1016, 1989
159. Shukla D, Singh DM, Strobos RJ: Hypertensive cerebrovascular disease and normal pressure hydrocephalus. Neurology (NY) 30:998, 1980
160. Spielmeyer H: Histopathologie des Nervensystems. Berlin, 1922
161. Steingart A, Hachinski VC, Lau C et al: Cognitive and neurologic findings in subjects with diffuse white matter lucencies on CT scan (leuko-araiosis). Arch Neurol 44:32, 1987
162. Steingart A, Hachinski VC, Lau C et al: Cognitive and neurologic findings in demented patients with diffuse white matter lucencies on CT scan (leuko-araiosis). Arch Neurol 44:36, 1987
163. Stochdorph O, Meesen H: Die arteriosklerotische und die hypertonische Hirnerkrankung. p. 1167. In Scholz W (ed): Handbuch der spezielle pathologischen Anatomie und Histologie. Vol 13/1B. Springer-Verlag, Berlin, 1957
164. Sulkava R, Erkinjuntti T: Vascular dementia due to cardiac arrhythmias and systemic hypotension. Acta Neurochir 76:23, 1987
165. Takayama K, Kato Y, Sasaki S: White matter change in cerebral arteriosclerosis: especial reference on the relation to Binswanger's disease. Adv Neurol Sci (Tokyo) 2:358, 1966
166. Tanaka M, Ikuta F, Oyake H: Report of a case of chronic progressive subcortical encephalopathy (Binswanger's disease) unassociated with hypertension. Clin Neurol (Tokyo) 9:398, 1969
167. Thomson PD, Marsden D: Gait disorder of subcortical arteriosclerotic encephalopathy: Binswanger's disease. Movement Disord 2:1, 1987
168. Tomlinson BE, Blessed G, Roth M: Observations on the brains of demented old people. J Neurol Sci 11:205, 1970
169. Tomonaga M, Yamanouchi H, Tohgi H, Kameyama M: Clinicopathologic study of progressive subcortical vascular encephalopathy (Binswanger type) in the elderly. J Am Geriatr Soc 30:524, 1982
170. Ueno T, Takahata N, Ishijima H: Clinical and pathological study with Binswanger's disease: correlation of the white matter involvement with cerebral arteriosclerotic dementia. Clin Psychiatry (Tokyo) 16:69, 1974
171. Uhlenbrock D, Sehlen S: The value of T1-weighted images in the differentiation between MS, white matter lesions, and subcortical arteriosclerotic encephalopathy (SAE). Neuroradiology 31:203, 1989
172. Valentine AR, Moseley IF, Kendall BE: White matter abnormality in cerebral atrophy: clinicoradiological correlations. J Neurol Neurosurg Psychiatry 43:139, 1980
173. Van Bogaert L: Encéphalopathie sous-corticale progressive (Binswanger) à évolution rapide chez deux soeurs. Greek Med 24:3, 1955
174. Van Bogaert L, Martin JJ: Analyse critique de la pathologie de l'angiomatose cérébroméningée diffuse non calcifiante et de l'encéphalopathie de Binswanger. J Neurol Sci 14:301, 1971
175. White JC: Periodic EEG activity in subcortial ats encephalopathy (Binswanger's type). Arch Neurol 36:485, 1979
176. Wilson RS, Bennett D, Fox JH et al: Alzheimer's disease: prevalence and clinical significance of white matter lesions on MRI. Ann Neurol 24:160, 1988
177. Yamada M, Tsukagoshi H, Otomo E, Hayakawa M: Cerebral amyloid angiopathy in the aged. J Neurol 234:371, 1987
178. Yamamura T, Nishimura M, Shirabe T, Fujita M: Subcortical vascular encephalopathy in a normotensive, young adult with premature baldness and spondylitis deformans: a clinicopathological study and review of the literature. J Neurol Sci 78:175, 1987
179. Young IR, Randell CP, Kaplan PW et al: NMR imaging in white matter disease of the brain using spin-echo sequences. J Comput Assist Tomogr 7:290, 1983
180. Yu YL, Yeung DWC, Woo E et al: Subcortical arteriosclerotic encephalopathy: a clinical and radionuclide brain scintiscan study. Acta Neurol Scand 77:486, 1988
181. Yvonneau M, Vital C, Lafforgue J, Kinsala MS: L'encéphalopathie sous-corticale chronique de Binswanger. Etude anatomo-clinique d'une observation. Bordeaux Med 2:1135, 1969
182. Zeumer H, Hacke W, Kolmann HL, Ringelstein EB: Subcortical arteriosclerotic encephalopathy (Binswanger's disease). Exp Brain Res, suppl. 5:272, 1982
183. Zeumer H, Schonsky B, Sturm KW: Predominant white matter involvement in subcortical arteriosclerotic encephalopathy (Binswanger disease). J Comput Assist Tomogr 4:14, 1980
184. Zimmerman RD, Fleming CA, Lee BC et al: Periventricular hyperintensity as seen by magnetic resonance: prevalence and significance. AJNR 7:13, 1986

# 32

# *CEREBRAL AMYLOID ANGIOPATHY*

Harry V. Vinters

Cerebral amyloid angiopathy (CAA), synonyms for which include *cerebral congophilic angiopathy* and *cerebrovascular amyloidosis*, describes and defines a group of clinical and neuropathologic conditions, in the course of which cerebral and cerebellar microvessels—arterioles, venules, and capillaries—become infiltrated by a hyaline eosinophilic substance with characteristic tinctorial properties.[67,228] Though its existence has been recognized for several decades, its importance as a nosologic entity has emerged within the last 10 to 20 years for a variety of reasons. As risk factors for forms of cerebrovascular disease that were especially prominent during early parts of this century come under increasingly effective control, and as people live to an ever more advanced age, atherosclerotic and hypertensive cerebrovascular disease have decreased in relative importance, even as cerebral hemorrhages (and possibly infarcts) related to CAA have taken on a relatively greater significance. Primary intraparenchymal hemorrhage, ischemia (including lacunar infarcts), and cardiogenic embolism are all important causes of stroke in the geriatric population.[136] CAA has been implicated as the cause of primary nontraumatic intracerebral hemorrhage in as many as 15 percent of patients over the age of 60 and almost 20 percent of patients over the age of 70.[136] Its importance as a cause of ischemic lesions is less clearly defined. Unfortunately, as will be described in the section Possible Treatment Modalities, CAA is likely to prove refractory to therapeutic intervention in the immediate future, barring new and revolutionary findings related to its pathogenesis. Several excellent clinical and clinicopathologic reviews have placed CAA in its proper context as a cause of hemorrhagic and ischemic stroke and cerebrovascular disease.[4,136,232]

A more basic reason for the broadened interest in the pathophysiology of CAA is the recognition that this microangiopathic lesion is an important component of the neuropathologic changes that occur in the brains of patients with senile dementia of Alzheimer type (SDAT) or Alzheimer disease (AD).[233] In the text to follow, the neuropathologic substrates of AD and SDAT will be assumed to be similar if not identical (possibly an oversimplification), and both entities will often be referred to by the abbreviation AD. The recognition that the amyloidotic protein present in age-associated CAA-related microangiopathy is almost identical to the amyloidotic protein present in senile plaques (which are an important component of the neuropathologic substrate of AD) has led to exciting hypotheses regarding the deposition of these two proteins within the aging brain. Recent reviews summarize the morphologic and immunohistochemical findings that have emerged from numerous studies on CAA and related brain amyloids.[175,229] It is a reasonable simplification to state that any disorder in which amyloid is seen to be deposited in the central nervous system (CNS) will be one that has CAA as a component. The relative frequency of CAA-related stroke in these different disorders, however, is extremely vari-

---

This chapter is dedicated to Miss Laurel Reed on the occasion of her retirement from the Division of Neuropathology, June 1991.

Work in the author's laboratory has been supported since 1985 by UCLA BRSG grants, a John Douglas French/Wilson Foundation Fellowship, and NS 26312.

able. Important findings relevant to morphology, immunohistochemistry, and molecular biology of CNS amyloidotic proteins have emerged from the remarkable technology (developed over the past 30 years) that allows for separation and resolution of brain proteins and characterization of the genes that encode them. (See the Sections Biochemical and Immunohistochemical Studies and Theories of Pathogenesis of Cerebral Amyloid Angiopathy later in this chapter.)

Although a detailed discussion of the biochemistry and molecular biology of amyloidoses in general is beyond the scope of this chapter, several excellent reviews summarize recent important findings and historical milestones in this field.[25,56,61,195,207] Emphasis throughout this chapter will be placed on the most common form of CAA encountered, namely, that associated with aging and AD. However, all known forms of CAA and their relative importance in stroke and cerebrovascular disease will be considered. They are summarized briefly in Table 32-1.

## CLINICAL PRESENTATION

There is solid epidemiologic evidence (reviewed elsewhere in this book) to show that the frequency and severity of cerebrovascular disease in general have decreased in the past two decades. This probably relates to control of important stroke-related risk factors.[72] Detailed epidemiologic studies from the Mayo Clinic showed a declining incidence of primary intracerebral intraparenchymal hemorrhage in residents of Rochester, Minnesota, for the 32-year period extending from 1945 to 1976.[48] A subsequent slight increasing incidence (observed 1975 to 1979) was attributed at least in part to more frequent identification of small intraparenchymal hemorrhages by computerized tomographic (CT) scanning.[37] At the time these studies were carried out, CAA as a cause of primary intraparenchymal hemorrhage was as yet relatively poorly understood. A declining incidence of intracere-

**TABLE 32-1. Neuropathologic Conditions Associated with Cerebral Amyloid Angiopathy**

| Condition[a] | Brain Parenchymal Amyloid | Biochemical Subtype |
|---|---|---|
| Brain aging and AD/SDAT | ++ (Variable) | A4 (± gamma-trace)[b] |
| Down syndrome | ++ (Variable) | A4 |
| Age-related cerebral hemorrhage (± AD/SDAT) | ++ (Variable) | A4 + gamma-trace |
| Familial cerebral hemorrhage | | |
| Icelandic (HCHWA-I) | — | Gamma-trace |
| Dutch (HCHWA-D) | ± | A4 |
| Spongiform encephalopathy (incl Creutzfeldt-Jakob disease, Gerstmann-Sträussler, scrapie) | Variable | PrP[c] |
| Non-AD neurodegenerative conditions (incl. pediatric) | Variable | ? |
| Leukoencephalopathy | Variable | A4 ± gamma-trace |
| Vasculitis (e.g., granulomatous angiitis) | Variable | A4 (demonstrated rarely) |
| Within cerebral vascular malformations | Variable | A4 |
| Postradiation therapy | Variable | ? |
| Oculoleptomeningeal amyloidosis | ± | Transthyretin (prealbumin) |
| Systemic amyloidosis | ± | Prealbumin, A4 |

*Abbreviations*: AD, Alzheimer's disease; SDAT, senile dementia of Alzheimer type; HCHWA-I, HCHWA-D, hereditary cerebral hemorrhage with amyloidosis–Icelandic type; –Dutch type.

[a] Conditions are listed in *approximately* decreasing order of frequency of clinically significant CAA (usually as a cause of stroke).

[b] A4 = Alzheimer A4 or beta protein (see the sections in text on Neuropathologic Features, Biochemical, Immunohistochemical Studies, and Theories of Pathogenesis of Cerebral Amyloid Angiopathy).

[c] PrP = protease resistant prion protein (see the section Neuropathologic Features in text).

bral hemorrhage in Japanese populations has also been attributed to a reduced prevalence of hypertension.[222] Other clinical, radiologic, and neuropathologic studies of peripheral or lobar primary intracerebral hemorrhages, even those from the early and mid-1980s, have paid relatively little attention to CAA as a possible etiologic mechanism in the causation of such hematomas.[177,212,246] Nevertheless, these studies recognized that patients with peripherally placed or lobar hematomas were frequently normotensive. Over the past decade, CAA as a cause of peripherally placed cerebral hemorrhages has been recognized and carefully described.[143,219] Although CAA is the likely cause of a lobar hemorrhage in an elderly patient, other etiologic factors must be considered in the differential diagnosis, including anticoagulant therapy or thrombocytopenia, vascular malformations (especially arteriovenous malformations), primary or metastatic brain tumor, a blood dyscrasia, and hypertension.[143]

## Cerebral Amyloid Angiopathy-Related Intraparenchymal Hemorrhage

Several clinicopathologic studies and case reports have documented clinical and neuropathologic findings in CAA-related primary intracranial hemorrhage. The findings from these studies will be summarized, in order to illustrate the common themes that run through the investigations. The studies have emerged over the last 20 years from laboratories with various approaches to the study of patients and brain tissue affected by stroke, but sufficient information exists in all of the publications to allow for reasonable generalizations.[2,20,32,44,45,52,53,87,89,90,96,97,99,111,125,132,171,173,176,220,221] In an earlier review, demographic characteristics of patients shown to have well-documented CAA-related brain hemorrhage were summarized, as were the relevant neuropathologic findings. Table 32-2 summarizes the data abstracted from the relevant literature.[228] I emphasize that this analysis pertains only to AD or age-related cerebral hemorrhage resulting from CAA. Familial stroke syndromes related to this entity will be discussed separately.

CAA-related intracerebral hemorrhage is seen most commonly in the elderly, though significant numbers of cases are reported to occur in persons in the sixth or seventh decade of life. No sex preponderance exists among the patients, and hemorrhage tends to occur at the same age in men and women, the mean age of hemorrhage being in the early seventies. Some patients have a "mixed microangiopathy" (see the section Neuropathologic Features), with features of both hypertensive and amyloid angiopathy-related microvascular alterations—not surprising when one considers that a significant proportion (approximately one-third) of patients with CAA-related intraparenchymal hemorrhage have clinically documented hypertension. One concludes that high blood pressure may exacerbate the tendency to CAA-related hemorrhage or vice versa. In some patients, morphologic sequelae of high blood pressure (e.g., left ventricular hypertrophy, cardiomegaly, nephrosclerosis) are found at autopsy when clinical hypertension has not been documented during the patient's life.[228] Almost 50 percent of patients with CAA-related parenchymal brain hemorrhage show some degree of dementia during life, and at least a similar proportion show histopathologic changes of AD at necropsy. The issue of the pathologic criteria used to make or confirm the clinical diagnosis of AD/SDAT will be addressed below. Changes of AD may be difficult to diagnose on a small cortical biopsy that otherwise shows florid CAA as the cause of an intracerebral hemorrhage. As well, it is common to find AD changes in a patient at necropsy when relatively normal or, at most, borderline mental function was observed during the patient's life.

**TABLE 32-2. Neuropathologic Features of Cerebral Amyloid Angiopathy-Related Encephalic Hematomas[a]**

| Location | Percentage |
|---|---|
| Frontal lobe | 35.1 |
| Temporal lobe | 14.0 |
| Parietal lobe | 26.3 |
| Occipital lobe | 18.7 |
| Deep central gray matter | 4.1 |
| Cerebellum | 1.8 |
| Corpus callosum | <1 |
| *Associated Features* | |
| Hypertension | |
| By clinical history | 31.8 |
| Evidence at autopsy | 11.2 |
| Dementia | |
| Clinical | 40.2 |
| AD/SDAT changes at autopsy | 43.9 |
| "Miliary" or petechial hemorrhages | Frequently observed |
| Microinfarcts | Frequently observed |

*Abbreviations*: AD, Alzheimer's disease; SDAT, senile dementia of Alzheimer type.
[a] Sex: 51.4% female, 48.6% male. Mean age: females, 73; males, 71.
(Adapted from Vinters,[228] with permission.)

CAA-related brain parenchymal hemorrhage tends to occur in a clinically consistent fashion. It presents in elderly, frequently demented people as a cerebral (peripheral) lobar hemorrhage, and over time several lobes on both sides of the brain may be affected. Rarely, multiple simultaneous intraparenchymal hemorrhages result from CAA. In a previous review,[228] a total of 171 hematomas were identified in over 100 patients. With rare exceptions, hematomas affect the cortex and subcortical white matter. Only one se-

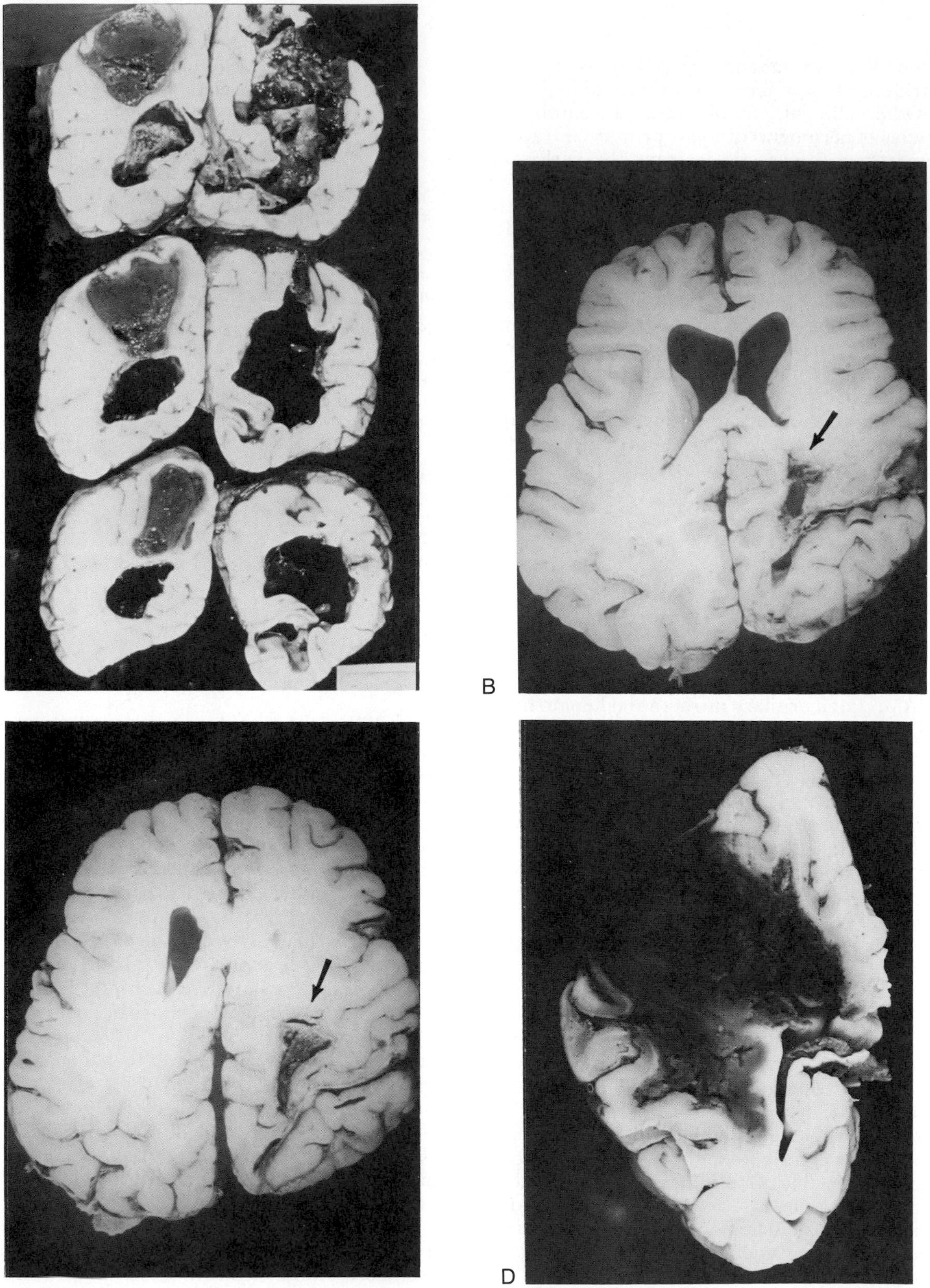


**Fig. 32-1.** Autopsy specimens of fixed brain from patients with primary intracerebral hemorrhage(s) related to severe cerebral amyloid angiopathy. (**A**) Multiple bihemispheric hematomas in an elderly demented patient have extended into both the subarachnoid space and the lateral ventricles. (**B & C**) Two horizontal levels from brain of a 53-year-old man with mental retardation (possible Down syndrome) show right parieto-occipital hematoma (*arrows*) with extensive adjacent encephalomalacia and collapse of brain substance. For microscopic details, see Figure 32-11. (**D**) Massive left parietal hematoma in a 72-year-old woman with senile dementia of Alzheimer type showing prominent extension into the subarachnoid space. (Fig. A from Vinters and Mah,[232] with permission; Fig. D from Ferreiro et al.,[42] with permission.)

ries[111] has described predominantly ganglionic or deeply situated hematomas as being most commonly related to CAA, but this is exceptional in my experience. Deep central grey structures, deep white matter structures (e.g., corpus callosum), and the cerebellum are primarily involved on rare occasions, though these cases can be instructive (see case summary below). CAA is virtually never found as a cause of primary brain stem hematomas. Because CAA-related hemorrhages are usually peripheral in the brain, blood may course directly into the subarachnoid space (an extremely rare occurrence with hypertensive intraparenchymal bleeds) as well as into the ventricles. Figure 32-1 illustrates the appearances of brain examined at necropsy from patients with CAA-related parenchymal hemorrhage. Unusual sites of hemorrhage resulting from CAA are discussed separately later in this chapter. Although most CAA-related hemorrhages are large, miliary and petechial hemorrhages may be noted within affected brain, and scattered microinfarcts may be present. Despite the now well-established association between CAA and brain hemorrhage, the actual site of bleeding from an amyloid-infiltrated arteriole or venule is rarely identified, although this is less than surprising in view of the extensive tissue destruction that occurs in and around regions of brain hemorrhage in general.

Despite its relative rarity, a recent example of cerebellar hemorrhage related to CAA highlights the importance of recognizing this type of hemorrhage even within posterior fossa structures (though virtually never the brain stem itself). The case is briefly summarized below.

A 72-year-old woman, who was under treatment for hypertension, experienced the sudden onset of headache, dizziness, imbalance, and vomiting. On admission to hospital the morning after the ictus, she was alert and had normal vital signs, but was mildly disoriented and had poor recent memory. She had mild meningismus, nystagmus, and ataxia of the left upper and lower limbs. There was no paresis and plantar responses were flexor. A lumbar puncture revealed bloody spinal fluid under normal pressure. A CT scan showed moderate dilatation of the lateral and third ventricles, while the fourth ventricle was not visualized. A hypodense lesion was seen in the left cerebellar hemisphere. An angiogram was consistent with a space-occupying lesion in the left cerebellar hemisphere and an aneurysm was not seen. The patient was managed conservatively and experienced full neurologic recovery.

She remained asymptomatic until 2 years later when she again suffered a sudden attack of dizziness, nausea, and headache. In hospital, she rapidly became comatose and was intubated. Blood pressure was 170/65 mmHg. She responded slightly to noxious stimuli and had no clear localizing signs. Plantar responses were extensor. A CT scan showed a persisting obstructive hydrocephalus and the fourth ventricle could not be visualized. There were two small crescentic hemorrhagic lesions in the posterior aspect of both cerebellar hemispheres. A shunt was placed in the right lateral ventricle and the cerebrospinal fluid was blood-tinged. She died 25 days later without regaining consciousness.

General autopsy findings included a 300-g heart with a left ventricular wall thickness of 1.3 cm and normal kidneys. The 1420-g brain showed bilateral cerebellar tonsillar herniation. Horizontal sections of the cerebral hemispheres disclosed a hematoma around the site of insertion of the ventricular catheter in the right frontal lobe, and the lateral ventricles were slightly dilated. Three cerebellar hematomas were identified (Fig. 32-2). The oldest was a pigmented scar, 1.5 × 1 cm, in the left lobe 3 cm from the midline, which most likely corresponded to the lesion that had precipitated the first hospital admission. Medial to this was a recent hematoma measuring 2 cm in diameter. A horseshoe-shaped hematoma extended from the right cerebellar lobe across the vermis. It was surrounded by a well-defined resorption membrane consistent with 3 weeks duration. All hematomas were superficial and extended into the subarachnoid space. Microscopic sections of the cerebellum showed severe amyloid angiopathy involving mostly the small vessels of the leptomeninges, as demonstrated using conventional Congo red staining and immunohistochemical techniques incorporating primary antibodies to the Alzheimer A4 or $\beta$-peptide, as described in the sections Neuropathologic Features and Biochemical and Immunohistochemical Studies. Less frequently, heavily amyloid-laden vessels were seen in the molecular layer of the cerebellar folia. Electron-microscopic examination confirmed the presence of 9 nm nonparallel nonbranching fibrils in the vascular media. This intriguing patient emphasizes that CAA should be considered as a source of cerebellar hemorrhage in elderly people. As with hematomas in the supratentorial compartment, multiple hemorrhagic episodes distributed in space and time within the cerebellum may occur. (This case was studied by the kind courtesy of Dr. Françoise Robert, Department of Pathology, Hôpital Notre-Dame, Montréal, Quebec.)

Familial syndromes of cerebral hemorrhage related to CAA have also been described. Hereditary cerebral hemorrhage with CAA had been recognized in areas of Iceland since the 1930s, though hereditary cerebral hemorrhage with amyloidosis of Icelandic type (HCHWA-I) became defined as a nosologic entity in the early 1970s.[74,91,202] Hemorrhage in affected people in this population presents at a much younger age than age-related or AD-related CAA.[228] Patients in their twenties or thirties frequently succumb to multiple intraparenchymal (cerebral) hemorrhages, which are peripherally situated in the brain substance as are age-related CAA hematomas.[74] Neuropathologic features of HCHWA—I will be presented

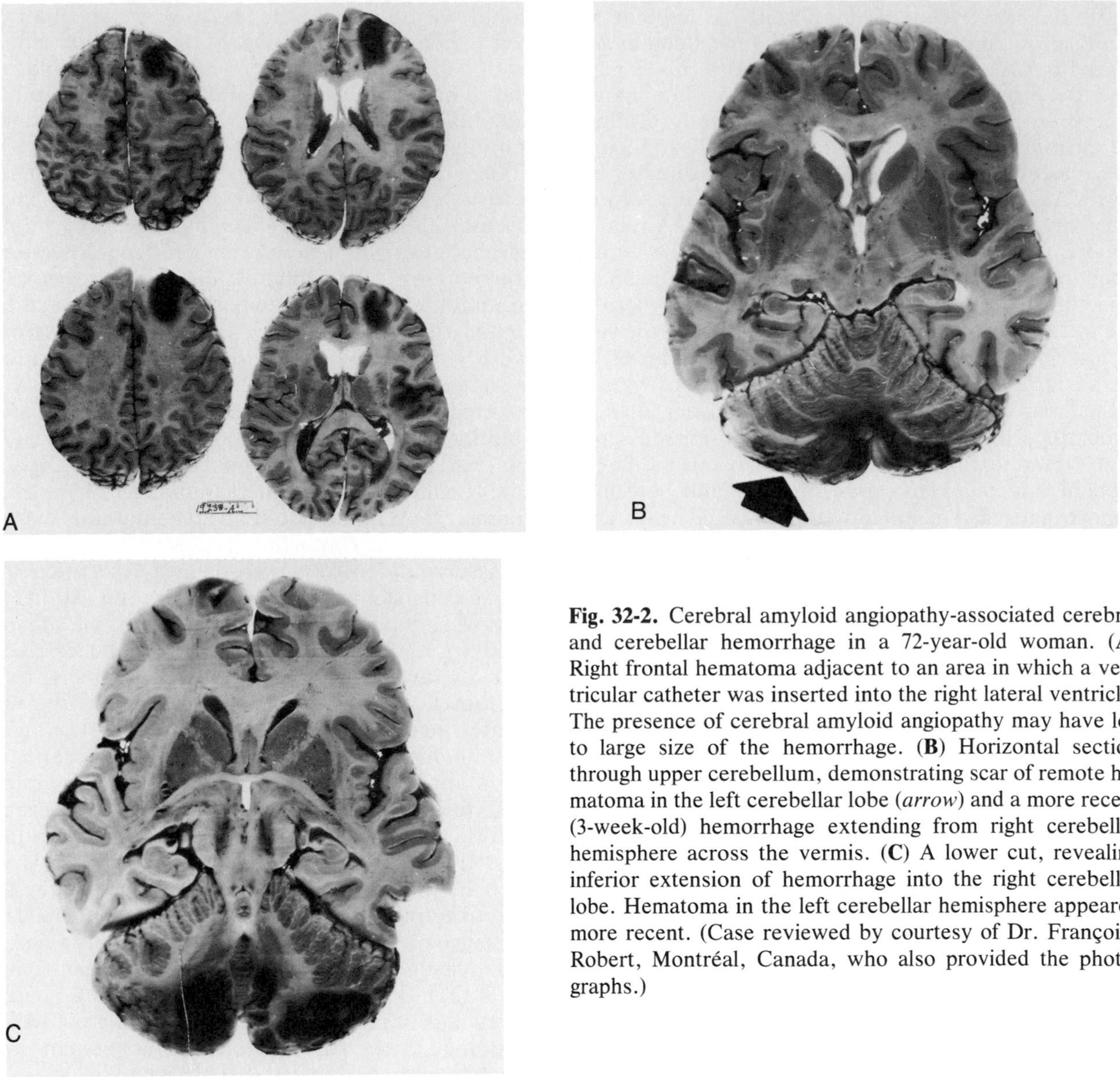


**Fig. 32-2.** Cerebral amyloid angiopathy-associated cerebral and cerebellar hemorrhage in a 72-year-old woman. (**A**) Right frontal hematoma adjacent to an area in which a ventricular catheter was inserted into the right lateral ventricle. The presence of cerebral amyloid angiopathy may have led to large size of the hemorrhage. (**B**) Horizontal section through upper cerebellum, demonstrating scar of remote hematoma in the left cerebellar lobe (*arrow*) and a more recent (3-week-old) hemorrhage extending from right cerebellar hemisphere across the vermis. (**C**) A lower cut, revealing inferior extension of hemorrhage into the right cerebellar lobe. Hematoma in the left cerebellar hemisphere appeared more recent. (Case reviewed by courtesy of Dr. Françoise Robert, Montréal, Canada, who also provided the photographs.)

below, but the importance of this entity in understanding the molecular genetics and biochemical basis of CAA-related hemorrhage cannot be overstated. HCHWA-I is inherited as an autosomal dominant trait.

A familial tendency to cerebral hemorrhage related to CAA has also been observed in the Netherlands.[75,118,245] In affected persons, multiple cerebral hematomas and infarcts have been described. Cerebellar hemorrhages have also been noted. The entity occurs in the Katwijk region of the Netherlands, and to date over 130 patients with the entity (abbreviated as hereditary cerebral hemorrhage with amyloidosis–Dutch type, HCHWA-D) have been described. Inheritance of this disorder is also as an autosomal dominant trait. Another pocket of HCHWA-D was discovered in the Dutch coastal village of Scheveningen. A connection between the pedigrees from Iceland, Scheveningen, and Katwijk has not been established. Affected patients are usually in their midforties or older, that is, they present at a more advanced age than patients who suffer from HCHWA-I. Biochemically (see the sections Biochemical and Immunohistochemical Studies and Theories of Pathogenesis of Cerebral Amyloid Angiopathy), HCHWA-D is more closely associated with age- or AD-related CAA.[118]

A few practical clinical and diagnostic points merit consideration. It is clear that patients with CAA are at increased risk for primary intraparenchymal brain hemorrhage when thrombolytic agents or anticoagulants are administered. Recent case reports and clinical series suggest that a synergistic relationship may exist between CAA and intracranial intraparenchymal hemorrhage induced by fibrinolytic agents, and that thrombolytic agents may induce intraparenchymal brain hemorrhage in conditions associated with a high incidence of CAA, specifically, advanced age and AD. The importance of autopsy examination of patients with intracerebral hemorrhage (particularly elderly persons) has been emphasized.[47,156,170] One series concludes that in patients older than 50 years of age, the risk of intracerebral hemorrhage during anticoagulant treatment increases approximately eight-fold but seems unrelated to the degree of anticoagulation.[47]

Controversy has existed as to the relative merits of confirming the diagnosis of CAA-related hemorrhage and/or treating the patient by brain biopsy or evacuation of the clotted blood.[70,217] Early reports based on small numbers of patients suggested that a neurosurgical procedure might eventuate in subsequent massive CAA-related brain hemorrhage.[217] Subsequent investigations suggest that, with modern neurosurgical techniques, patients with CAA-related hemorrhage may safely undergo operative procedures, and that patients who present with CAA-related intraparenchymal hemorrhage may improve neurologically following evacuation of the hematoma.[70] In any event, it is incumbent on the surgical neuropathologist to carefully examine blood clot and associated brain paren-

**TABLE 32-3. Clinical Features of Spontaneous Cerebral Hemorrhage in Six Patients with Cerebral Amyloid Angiopathy**

| Case | Age[a]/ Sex | HTN/ Smoker | Dementia at Onset | Clinical Presentation | Subsequent Symptoms | Location of Hemorrhages (Onset/ Subsequent) | Surgical Procedures |
|---|---|---|---|---|---|---|---|
| 1 | 54/M | ?/+ | No | Loss of consciousness<br>(h/o TIAs?, R hemiparesis, 1 yr?) | Seizures<br>Dementia<br>Depression<br>Blindness<br>Obtundation | L,R periventricular[b]<br>R occipitoparietal (×2)<br>R temporal<br>L occipital<br>R hemisphere | R temporal biopsy |
| 2 | 58/F | −/+ | Yes | Confusion<br>Difficulty walking<br>Urinary incontinence<br>Aphasia<br>HA, N/V<br>(h/o depression, 38 yr) | Memory loss<br>Irritability<br>Depression<br>Paranoia | L,R frontal/<br>None | L frontal biopsy |
| 3 | 60/F | −/+ | No | L hemiparesis<br>HA, N/V<br>Progressive lethargy<br>(h/o TIAs with R hemiparesis, 7 yr, L hemiparesis, 6 mo) | Seizures<br>Aphasia<br>L hemiparesis<br>L paresthesias | R frontal/<br>None | R frontal evacuation of hematoma |
| 4 | 71/M | +/+ | Yes | HA<br>Confusion<br>Ataxia<br>L homonymous hemianopsia<br>L hemiplegia (h/o carotid & peripheral vascular disease) | Confusion<br>L hemiparesis<br>L paresthesia<br>Memory loss<br>Irritability | R frontal<br>L cerebellar/<br>L occipital<br>R cerebellar | R frontal biopsy |
| 5 | 82/F | −/− | No | HA<br>Slurred speech<br>R hemiparesis<br>Obtundation | No change | L occipital/<br>None | L occipital evacuation of hematoma |
| 6 | 86/M | ?/? | No | Malaise<br>N/V<br>Ataxia<br>Obtundation<br>L hemiparesis | L hemiparesis<br>L homonymous hemianopsia | R parieto-occipito-temporal/<br>None | R parieto-occipito-temporal evaucation of hematoma |

*Abbreviations*: L left; R, right; M, male; F, female; HTN, hypertension; HA, headache; N/V, nausea/vomiting; h/o, history of.
[a] Age given in table is at onset of first hemorrhage.
[b] The periventricular lucencies probably represented infarcted and demyelinated areas.
(From Yong et al.,[257] copyright 1992, American Medical Association, with permission.)

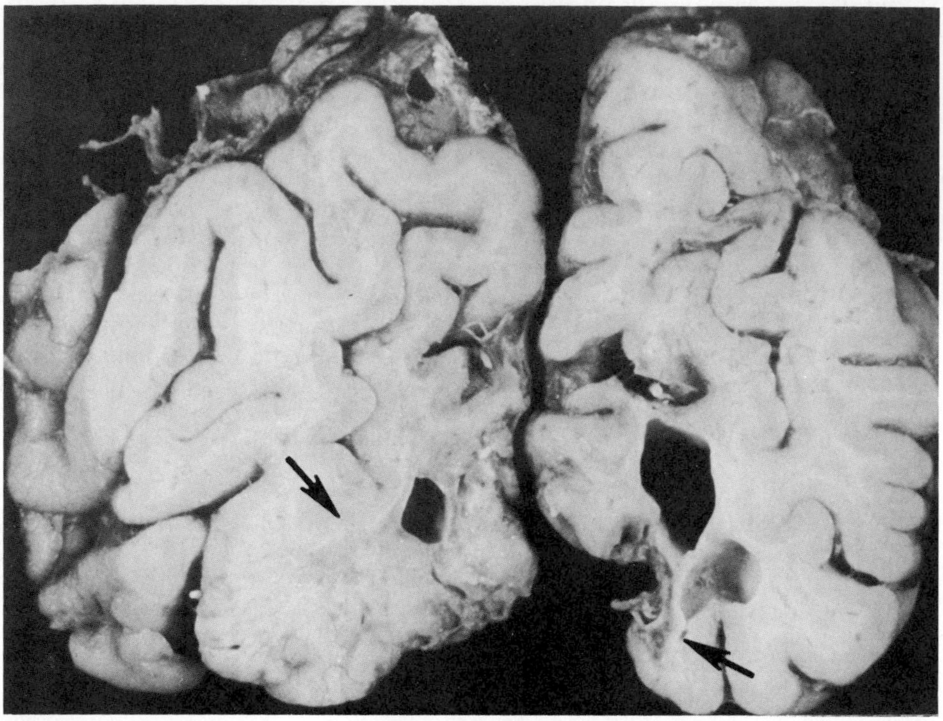

A

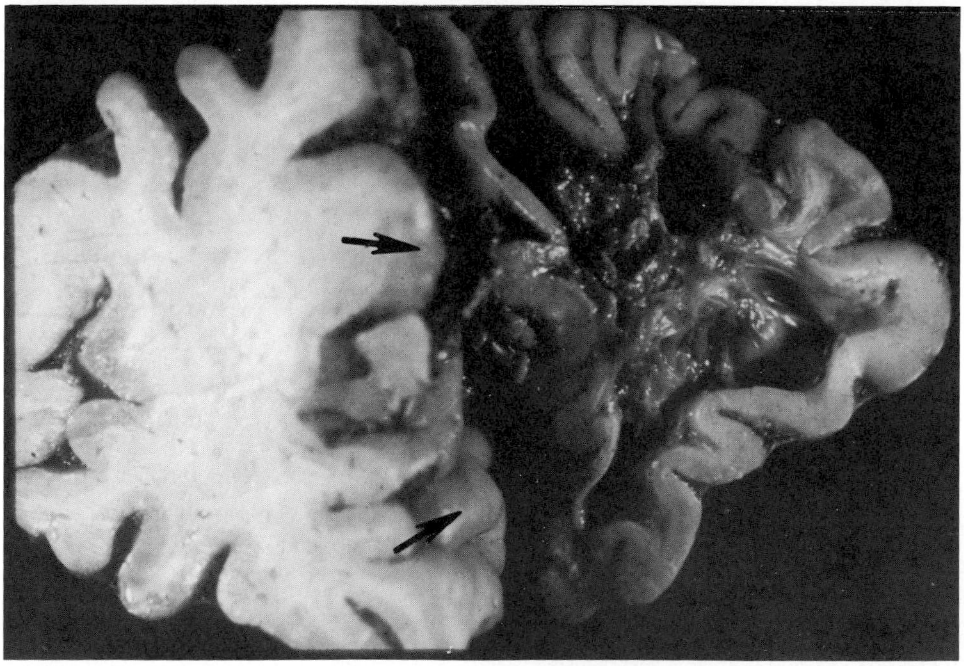

B

**Fig. 32-3.** Encephalomalacia associated with (though not necessarily caused by) cerebral amyloid angiopathy. (**A**) Coronal section of parieto-occipital region of fixed brain shows bilateral mesial and inferior (old) cystic infarcts (*arrows*). Microvessels in these areas were densely infiltrated by amyloid, though the infarcts appear to be in the posterior cerebral artery territories bilaterally. (**B**) Right frontal lobe (*arrows*) shows severe cystic encephalomalacia of the subcortical white matter—overlying cortex had severe cerebral amyloid angiopathy, but cortical integrity appears relatively well preserved. (Material studied courtesy of Dr. Linda Ansbacher, Columbia, Missouri.) (*Figure continues.*)

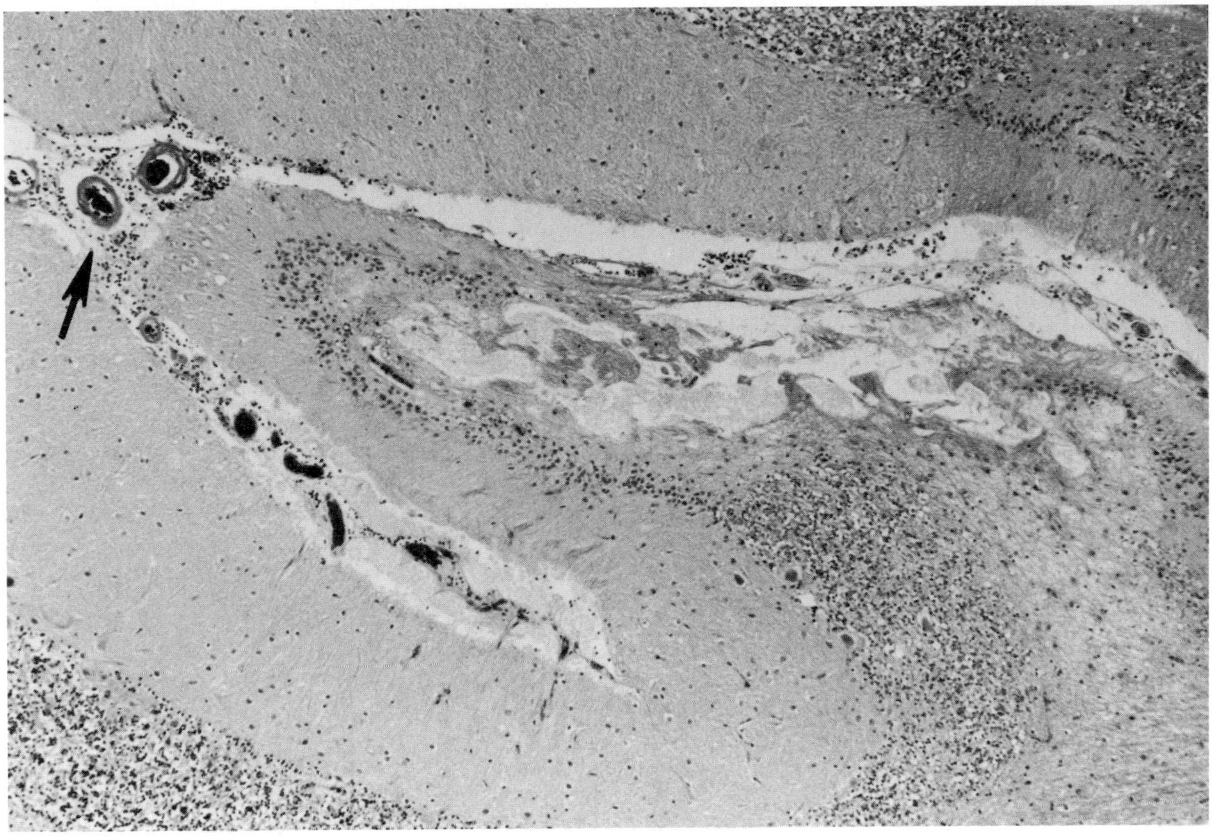

C

**Fig. 32-3** (*Continued*). **(C)** Section of cerebellum shows an old cystic infarct adjacent to leptomeningeal vessels (*arrow*) heavily infiltrated by amyloid. The vessels are not occluded, however. (Hematoxylin & eosin; × 75, approximate.)

chyma resected in the course of a neurosurgical procedure, particularly in a patient who has experienced a peripherally placed intraparenchymal intracerebral hematoma.[83,243,257] Unexpected diagnoses that have been made[83] include primary or metastatic neoplasm, but CAA is a surprisingly common diagnosis, especially when the clot and associated brain parenchyma are derived from a patient in an age group at risk for this entity (usually over 65 years of age). Table 32-3 summarizes my own experience with brain biopsy findings from six patients with well-documented CAA-related primary brain parenchymal hemorrhage.[257]

### Infarcts and Transient Ischemic Attacks

The association between CAA and regions of encephalomalacia within the brain has never been as clearly established as that between CAA and primary encephalic hemorrhage. Nevertheless, cerebral infarcts are frequently seen in the brains of patients with CAA.[42] This may in part relate to the fact that CAA occurs with increasing frequency in the aging population, a group also prone to show the complications of hypertensive microvascular disease and atherosclerosis, even though the incidence of the latter appears to be declining. A retrospective postmortem analysis of 25 patients with CAA in the setting of AD or SDAT showed that seven patients experienced clinically significant cerebral infarcts or hemorrhages or both. There did not appear to be a statistically significant difference in the incidence of infarcts or hemorrhages in hypertensive as opposed to normotensive persons. It was concluded that hypertension does not appear to be an additional risk factor in the causation of cerebral infarct or hemorrhage associated with CAA of AD. Many of the patients studied showed atherosclerosis of the circle of Willis, sometimes in the context of severe disseminated atheromatous disease.[42]

Transient ischemic attacks have also been described in patients with CAA,[196] although again the association is largely anecdotal. Detailed analysis of clinical histories in several patients with surgically proven CAA-related brain hemorrhage revealed a history of transient ischemic attack-like episodes in at least one of the patients.[257]

The brains of elderly, demented patients with or without AD may contain large areas of encephalomalacia (infarcts), and microvessels within these regions of infarction may be heavily laden with amyloid (Fig. 32-3). The association between these two sets of findings, however, does not prove that the CAA caused the infarct. The association is especially tenuous when the infarct is within the territory of supply of one of the large cerebral arteries.

## Dementia and the Relation of Multi-infarct Dementia to Cerebral Amyloid Angiopathy

CAA occurs commonly in the brains of patients with AD/SDAT, though it frequently occurs in the brains of individuals of advanced age who show normal mentation.[120,228] Most experts in the field recognize CAA as being one of the four primary microscopic hallmarks by which the clinical diagnosis of AD is confirmed using neuropathologic studies.[100,157,166,233] The other key histologic markers that represent the morphologic correlate of AD (discussed at greater length below) include senile plaques, neurofibrillary tangles and granulovacuolar degeneration, the latter finding usually confined to the hippocampal formation.[233] Some have proposed that, since the finding of amyloidotic lesions (including primarily microvascular amyloid and senile plaques) within the brains of patients with AD is so common and such a pathognomonic feature, AD/SDAT should be considered a form of amyloidosis in which amyloid deposits are confined to the CNS.[58] Some degree of CAA is seen in 85 to 100 percent of brains from patients who die with the clinical syndrome of AD/SDAT,[60,233] though it is a relatively frequent finding in the brains of elderly individuals who show normal mentation.[228,233] Indeed, as recently as 1985, consensus criteria for the neuropathologic diagnosis of AD made little mention of the significance of CAA in arriving at a firm neuropathologic diagnosis of AD.[104] Although CAA of some degree is common in the vast majority of brains from AD patients, there are individuals in whom microvascular amyloid deposition is the overwhelming neuropathologic finding, whereas there are others in whom relatively minimal or negligible degrees of CAA are encountered, though a diligent search through multiple specimen blocks with appropriate stains is usually rewarded by the discovery of some microvessels with CAA. It is possible, indeed likely, that the neuropathologic substrate of AD/SDAT is heterogeneous, which explains why some patients have a pronounced degree of microvascular amyloid, whereas many others have extensive cortical and hippocampal neurofibrillary tangles or senile plaques in the absence of CAA. Indeed, studies aimed at understanding the reasons for this heterogeneity might lead to a greater understanding of the morphologic substrate of dementia rather than increasing confusion, as some fear. Clinical and morphologic heterogeneity of AD subgroups is thus the subject of increasing numbers of clinicopathologic and genetic studies of AD/SDAT.[16,24]

CAA may also play a role in the pathogenesis of multi-infarct dementia (MID). Traditionally, MID has been assumed to represent a syndrome in which patients become demented on the basis of sequential discrete infarcts within the brain parenchyma (usually involving the cerebral hemispheres.)[43,76] Clearly dementias exist in which causal factors include microscopic lesions associated with AD as well as multiple areas of encephalomalacia within brain. Pitfalls in making the clinical diagnosis of MID as opposed to primary degenerative dementia (usually AD) have been emphasized.[113,114] It is possible that MID is a diagnosis of exclusion—one that can be made fairly easily using currently available neuroimaging techniques. Depending on one's viewpoint, vascular dementia (usually MID) is either underdiagnosed[139] or overdiagnosed.[21] Even in patients with neuropathologically well-defined AD/SDAT, the existence of CAA of a severe degree may lead to superimposed micro- or macrohemorrhages within the brain, or (less likely) regions of encephalomalacia.[182] Thus, patients with AD may show a component of vascular dementia as a simple function of the severity of amyloidotic microvascular change within their brain parenchyma.

## Vasculitis

Whereas CAA is commonly recognized as an important cause of primary brain hemorrhage in the elderly, and the microvascular amyloidotic change is a frequent finding in the brains of patients with AD/SDAT, vasculitis in association with (and possibly caused by) the presence of CAA is a rare phenomenon. A handful of case reports have described CAA associated with vasculitis.[55,69,121,124,135,168,172,193] The dozen or so cases described do not allow for detailed demographic analysis. Most of the patients have been in the seventh decade of life. Clinical features were relatively nonspecific, including a deterioration in higher cerebral cortical functions and unsteadiness of gait. The diagnosis was usually made at autopsy or biopsy, and generally came as a surprise to the examining neuropathologist. The histologic patterns of vasculitis differed from case to case, though in general the findings resembled rheumatoid vasculitis[121] or a giant cell (granulomatous) angiitis.[55,69,124,135,168,172,193] In a patient that we have reviewed,[69] Alzheimer A4 peptide could be demonstrated immunohistochemically within the walls of many of the affected microvessels and even within the cytoplasm of many of the giant cells, supporting the hypothesis that the granulomatous angiitis (Fig. 32-4) may represent, in part, a foreign body giant cell reaction to the deposition of amyloid A4 protein (see the section Biochemical and Immunohistochemical Studies). It is of clinical interest that on rare occasions, affected patients showed significant

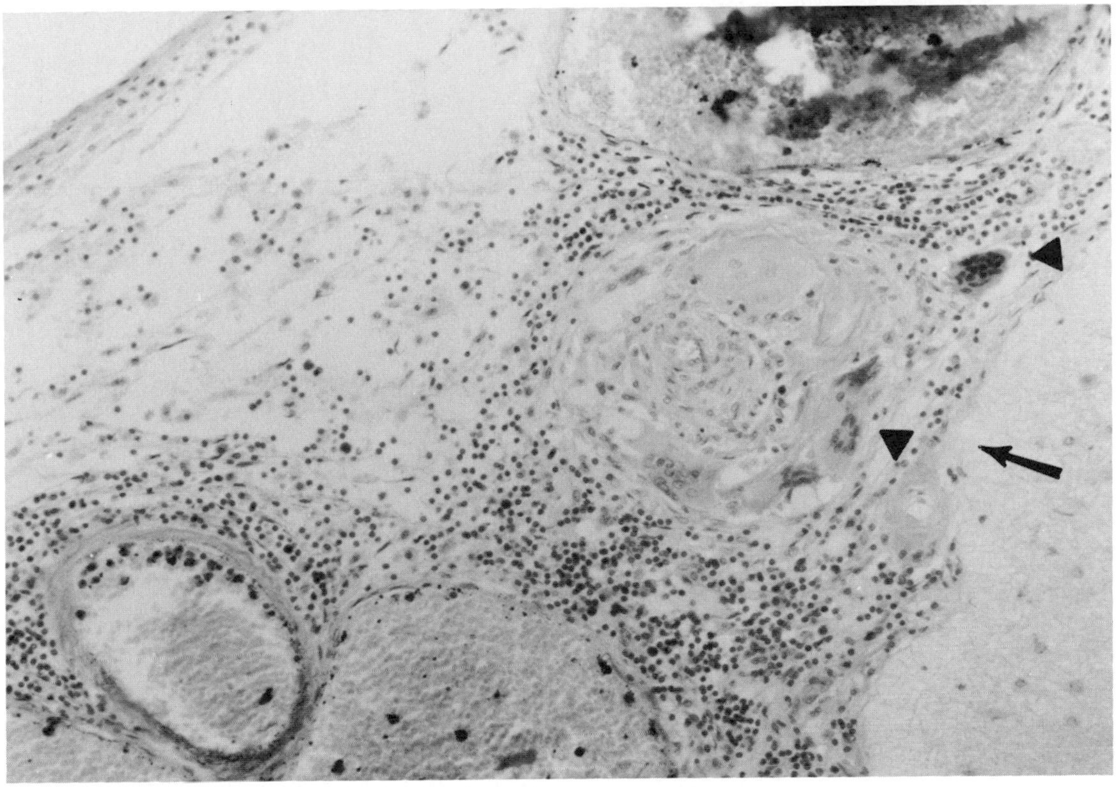

A

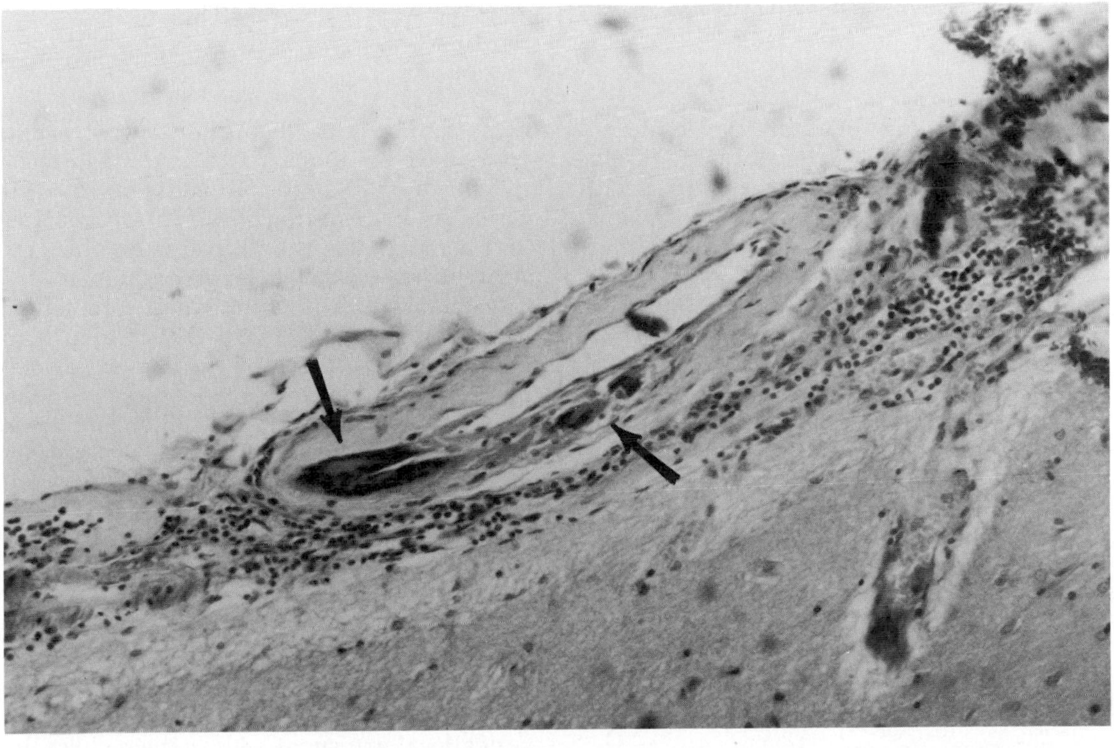

B

**Fig. 32-4.** Granulomatous angiitis associated with cerebral amyloid angiopathy. (**A**) A leptomeningeal vessel (*arrow*) shows thickening, with adventitial multinucleated giant cells (*arrowheads*). A mononuclear infiltate is noted in the adjacent subarachnoid space. (**B**) Another thickened meningeal vessel demonstrates multinucleated cells within media (*arrows*). (Figs. A & B: hematoxylin & eosin, × 205). (*Figure continues.*)

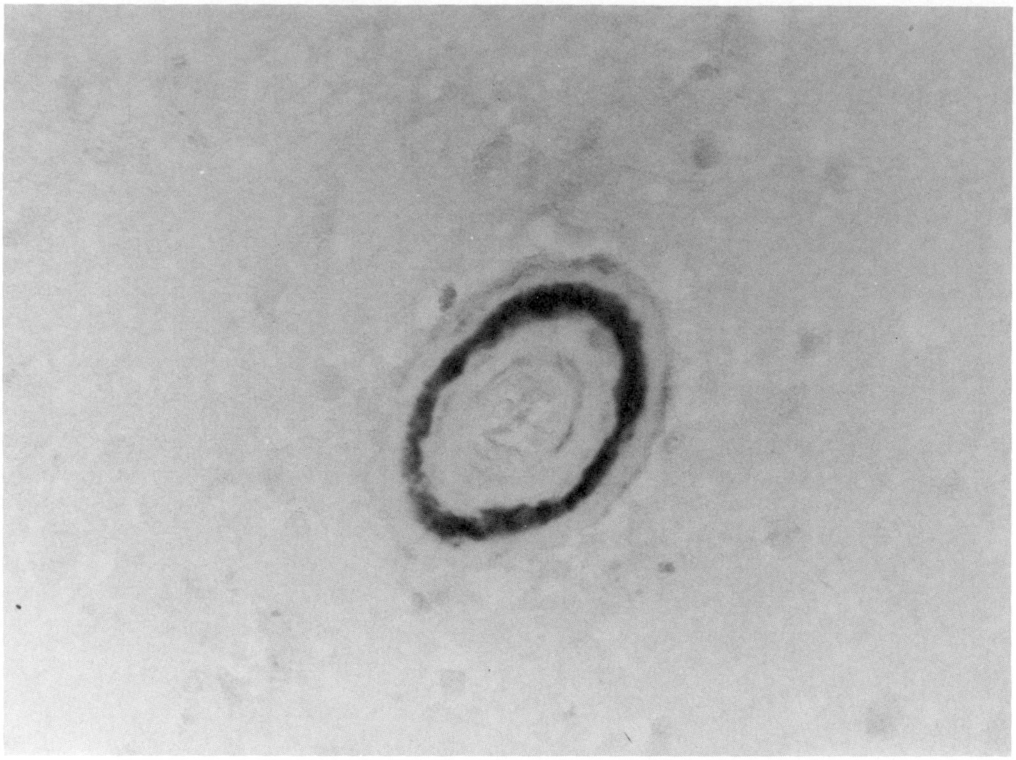
C

**Fig. 32-4** (*Continued*). (**C**) Anti-A4 immunohistochemistry (see Vinters et al.[237,238]) shows Alzheimer A4/$\beta$-peptide within wall of a parenchymal microvessel ($\times$ 525). (For details of the case, see Gray et al.[69])

amelioration of symptoms following corticosteroid therapy.[55,124] Such reports, while encouraging insofar as they suggest a therapeutic avenue for patients with at least one complication or variant of CAA, must be regarded at the present time as anecdotal.

### Miscellaneous Presentations of Cerebral Amyloid Angiopathy

Whereas intraparenchymal hemorrhage related to CAA is relatively common, in rare instances direct bleeding into the subarachnoid space may occur in patients who have extensive CAA largely confined to the leptomeningeal vessels.[142] CAA may present as a mass lesion, for example, in a 55-year-old patient who presented with signs and symptoms suggestive of a brain tumor. Brain biopsy conclusively established the diagnosis of CAA.[18]

## RADIOGRAPHIC FEATURES

The diagnosis of CAA in the brain of an aging or demented patient is almost impossible to make using CT or magnetic resonance imaging (MRI) scans, though the finding of an atrophic brain in a patient who has experienced a slowly progressive dementing illness strongly suggests that some degree of CAA will be present within this brain tissue.[228,233] Excellent reviews have summarized CT and MRI appearances of the normal and abnormal aging brain.[35,36] If CAA declares itself, resulting in an intraparenchymal cerebral hemorrhage, the diagnosis becomes much more straightforward. The neuropathologic features of CAA-related brain hemorrhage predict the radiographic findings.[19,155,201,242] CAA-related hemorrhages are usually visualized on the CT scan as peripherally placed lobar hemorrhages, with or without mass effect. Hemorrhage may be seen in an otherwise atrophic brain. As predicted by the neuropathologic findings, the hemorrhage may extend directly into the lateral ventricle or into the subarachnoid space. Rarely, CAA-related hemorrhages occur in atypical locations (e.g., the corpus callosum).[242] Otherwise, superficial location of the hematoma, irregular borders, and surrounding edema are characteristic features on CT scanning. Ring enhancement is sometimes seen. Findings on cerebral angiography have included opercular branch occlusion and irregularity of the pericallosal artery, as well as mass effect in the areas of hemorrhage.[242] Since the size of vessel involved by CAA is usually too small to be visualized by angiography, no specific patterns of vascular change attributable to CAA have been described. MRI scanning has added a new dimension to the neuroradiologist's ability to diagnose pathophysiologic mechanisms important in the genesis of acute intracerebral and subarachnoid hemorrhage.[81] As well, high-resolution MRI techniques allow for the detection of multiple incidental subcortical lesions within the aging brain, which possibly result from chronic cerebrovascular disease (including CAA?) and resultant changes in the brain parenchyma that occur over a period of many years.[6,7]

In general, white matter disease detectable by CT is increasingly recognized as one of the hallmarks of patients with AD/SDAT.[85,203,204] One group has referred to this finding as leuko-araiosis, and has shown a strong association between leuko-araiosis and dementia, which could in part be explained by a history of stroke and cerebrovascular disease. However, stroke alone did not account for the radiographic finding.[85] It is reasonable to hypothesize that, if the white matter abnormality detected by MRI or CT scanning represents an incomplete form of infarction, the incomplete ischemic lesion may result from overlying cortical involvement by variable degrees of CAA.[236] Study of the neuropathologic correlates of leuko-araiosis has shown that, while there is a coexistence of white matter lesions (primarily pallor on sections stained to demonstrate myelin) with CAA in the brains of patients with AD, there is no evidence that the CAA causes or produces the white matter abnormality.[88] MRI studies of leukoencephalopathy associated with CAA have shown that, in a majority of patients, white matter signal hyperintensities on T2-weighted spin-echo pulse sequences were present. The authors concluded, however, that the white matter lesions associated with CAA were nonspecific but rather reflected hypoperfusion of distal white matter resulting from vascular disease.[115] Figure 32-5 shows CT and MRI images of brain in patients who subsequently had biopsy-confirmed CAA (see also Table 32-3). Among the unusual presentations was a picture of ring enhancement in symmetrical bifrontal cerebral hematomas related to CAA.

Recent advances in the clinician's ability to image systemic amyloidosis include scintigraphy after injection of $^{123}$I-serum amyloid P component.[26,80] Given an increasingly sophisticated understanding of the biochemistry and immunohistochemistry of various forms of CAA (see the sections Biochemical and Immunohistochemical Studies and Theories of Pathogenesis of Cerebral Amyloid Angiopathy), it is conceivable that injection of radiolabeled precursors that are destined to be incorporated into amyloidotic microvessel walls may lead to potentially valuable techniques for imaging brain amyloid as well, although to the present time this has not been achieved.

## NEUROPATHOLOGIC FEATURES

Because subtle yet important differences exist in the neuropathologic findings associated with different subtypes of CAA, these are described and discussed in separate sections below. Obviously, a consideration of the biochemistry and immunohistochemistry of these forms is also highly germane to an understanding of CAA in a global neuropathologic context.

### Alzheimer Disease/Age-Related Cerebral Amyloid Angiopathy

The recognition of CAA as a distinct neuropathologic phenomenon, especially in the context of AD/SDAT, began in the late 1940s and early 1950s. Clinicopathologic studies extending into the 1960s and 1970s described the microscopic features of microvascular amyloid, although the significance of CAA-related brain hemorrhage was not well appreciated until the 1970s.[14,138,151,183,208,224] More recent investigations have focused on the incidence and topography of CAA as a function of age and dementia, especially AD/SDAT. CAA can be detected in histologic sections of the brain using conventional stains, usually Congo red (with application of polarization microscopy) and thioflavin S or T used in conjunction with fluorescence microscopy (Fig. 32-6). The latter techniques, though they have been superseded by the immunohistochemical methods described below, remain a valuable method for screening histologic sections suspected of showing CAA.[228,233]

Most studies in which brain tissue has been examined using these conventional techniques concur that occurrence of the most common form of CAA is strongly correlated with increasing age of the patient.[109,131,216,230,252] The likelihood of discovering CAA in a given brain from an aged individual depends largely on how extensively the brain is sampled, because the angiopathy may be very focal and asymmetrical within the neocortex. In the age- or AD-related form of CAA, the microvascular change is essentially confined to the neocortical and overlying leptomeningeal vessels. The exact incidence of CAA found in various investigations is thus variable. In one study, it was found in 36 percent of all brains examined from patients over the age of 60.[230] In a Japanese study, CAA was found in 18 percent of men and almost 30 percent of women over the age of 40. The most severe degrees of CAA are found in brain tissue from patients who are demented as a result of AD, and the presence and severity of CAA have shown significant correlations (in some studies) with the numbers of senile plaques and neurofibrillary tangles present, the latter two being other important microscopic hallmarks of AD/SDAT.[252] Nevertheless, significant degrees of CAA can be found in patients who have relatively normal mentation at the time of death despite their advanced age.[230] There is no significant association between the presence of CAA or senile plaque amyloid in the brain and extracerebral amyloid, although in any population of aged individuals non-CNS amyloids may frequently be found, for example, in the pituitary gland, pancreas, or heart.[253]

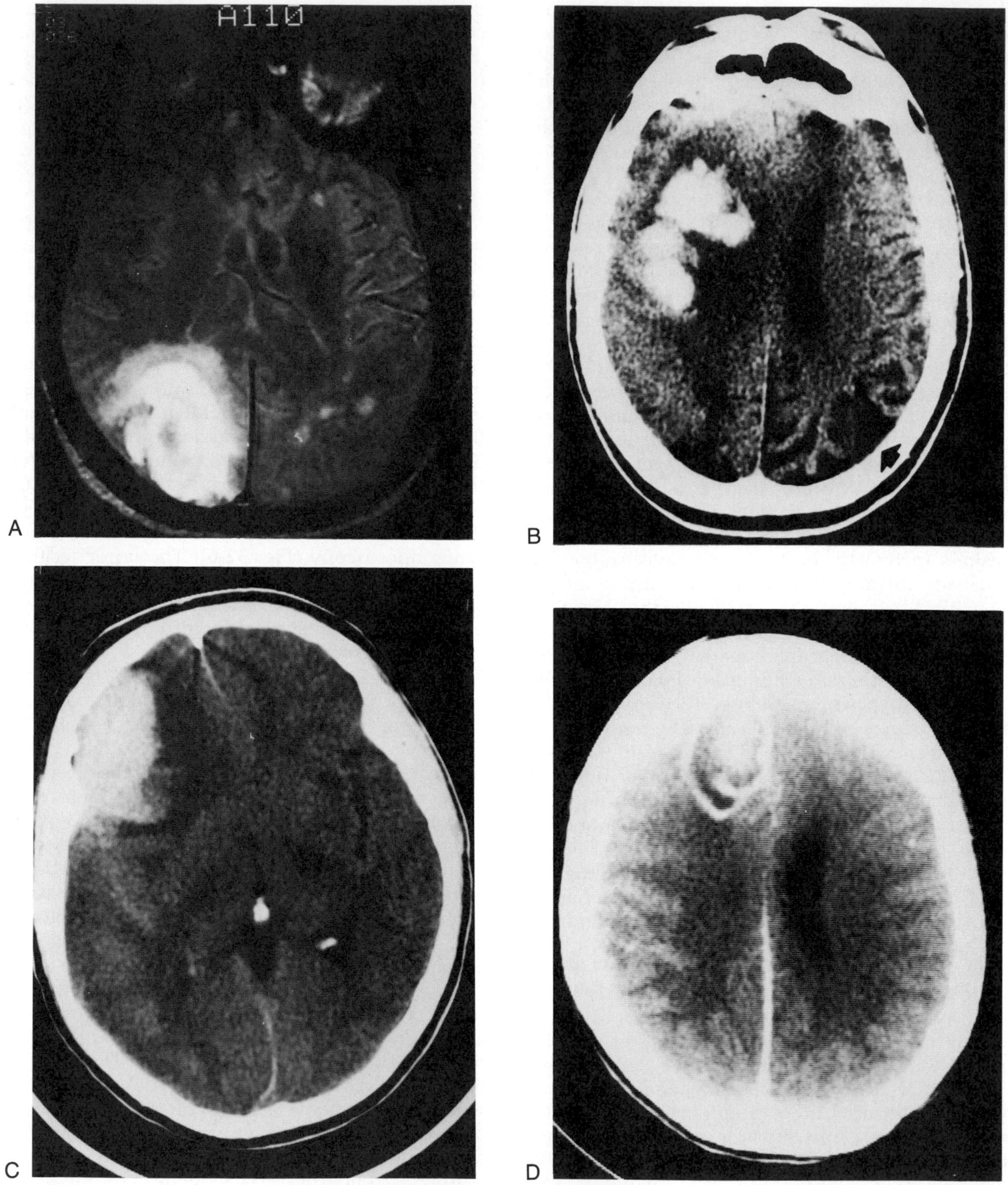


**Fig. 32-5.** Radiographic appearances of cerebral amyloid angiopathy-associated intracerebral hemorrhage. (**A**) MRI study (TR 2,800, TE 30) shows large parieto-occipital hemorrhage with central lucency. (**B**) CT scan (without contrast) demonstrates large right cerebral hematoma with surrounding edema. Note cerebral atrophy with possible focal encephalomalacia in the opposite parieto-occipital region (*arrow*). (**C**) CT scan (without contrast) shows a large right frontal hematoma with surrounding edema and mass effect. (**D**) CT scan with contrast shows a right frontal hematoma with ring enhancement. In all cases, cerebral amyloid angiopathy was established as cause of the hemorrhage by brain biopsy/clot evacuation. (For details, see Yong et al. (Panel D),[257] copyright 1992, American Medical Association.)

Microscopically, amyloid deposits can be strongly suspected on routine hematoxylin and eosin-stained sections of the brain, in which the microvascular lesion presents as effacement of the normal microvessel wall by a hyaline eosinophilic material (Fig. 32-6). CAA can involve arteries and arterioles, venules, and capillaries. There may be some value in making the distinction among involvement of different sizes of vessels because in our experience only patients with extensive arteriolar amyloid deposition are prone to develop brain hemorrhage. Capillary amyloid is frequently (though not invariably) associated with adjacent senile plaques containing amyloid cores; quantitative studies of this association are discussed below.

Detailed clinicopathologic investigations have examined the reasons why patients with CAA may develop microvascular weakening that can in turn lead to intraparenchymal and even subarachnoid hemorrhage. Though amyloid usually infiltrates the media, intima and adventitia of severely involved microvessels, luminal stenosis is not always present, though it may be observed.[145] Furthermore, small arteries may be diffusely infiltrated with resultant fibrinoid degeneration of the vessel wall and the formation of miliary aneurysms that resemble more traditionally defined Charcot-Bouchard aneurysms seen in association with hypertensive microvascular disease of the brain.[228] These latter microvascular abnormalities may precipitate intracerebral (intraparenchymal) hemorrhage, especially if rapid changes in systemic blood pressure occur.[145,240] Mandybur[122,123] has analyzed microvascular changes that appear to be secondary to the deposition of mural amyloid within vessels, referring to these as CAA-associated vasculopathies (Fig. 32-7). These changes include clustering of multiple arteriolar lumina ("glomerular formations"), aneurysmal dilatation of vessels, and obliterative intimal changes as well as "double-barreling." Chronic inflammatory perivascular or transmural infiltrates may be seen, and when these are severe the diagnosis of CAA-associated vasculitis may be rendered in a given specimen (see the section Vasculitis, earlier in this chapter).[122] The deposition of amyloid within a vessel wall may lead to injury or separation of smooth muscle cells, rendering the affected vessel weak and prone to hemorrhage.[123] The elastica in larger (leptomeningeal) amyloidotic vessels is remarkably well preserved, and when amyloid deposition is present in the walls of larger vessels of the leptomeninges is usually seen on the adventitial component of such vessels. Ultrastructural analysis of microvascular amyloid has often been carried out on suboptimal necropsy material, but usually the existence of 7- to 9-nm filaments that compose the amyloid material can be discerned.[146,227] Thickening of the associated vascular basement membrane with accumulation of cellular debris may be found.[146] In capillary amyloid deposition ("plaque-like degeneration") the basement membrane of capillaries was seen to be enlarged, and the cytoplasm of endothelial cells appeared to contain amyloid fibrils, though we have not been able to confirm this observation in more optimally preserved biopsy material.[133,184] In five biopsy specimens from patients with AD, optimally preserved for ultrastructural study, amyloid fibrils present within vessel walls (which were strongly labeled by Congo red using light microscopy and A4 immunohistochemistry) were seen interspersed with degenerate smooth muscle cells in the media, while the endothelial cells were largely unremarkable (Fig. 32-8).[184] Amyloid fibrils were seen in close apposition to collagen bundles and (in arteriolar vessels) were clearly separate from tightly packed neurites and astrocytic processes within the adjacent brain parenchyma. The detailed cellular relationships of *capillary* amyloid with respect to the surrounding brain parenchyma may be different, as has been suggested.[133]

The relationship between microvascular amyloid and senile plaque amyloid (which are virtually identical biochemically and immunohistochemically) has been examined in careful morphometric studies. As expected, CAA was more common and extensive in patients with dementia.[13] Surprisingly, senile plaques containing amyloid cores were not closely associated with amyloidotic vessels. As well, distributions of senile plaques in AD subjects with and without CAA differed, plaque density being greatest in those without CAA.[13] Other recent studies, using a variety of markers for capillaries and associated basement membranes, suggest that, although a small number of capillaries in brains from patients with AD show amyloid deposition beneath the basement membrane, the capillaries appear to play only a limited direct role (if any) in the formation of amyloid plaques. Thus the apparent association of senile amyloid plaques and capillaries may represent a fortuitous occurrence, and capillary degeneration may have little to do with senile plaque formation in the neocortex.[102] All studies have focused attention on cortical microvessels because the finding of CAA is extremely unusual in the subcortical white matter, deep central grey structures, or brain stem, although varying degrees of CAA may be seen in the cerebellar cortex and overlying leptomeninges.[42,228,229] Deposition of Alzheimer-type amyloid has also been noted within the walls of cerebral and spinal cord vascular malformations from elderly individuals.[78,158]

The exact role of CAA in the pathogenesis of AD/SDAT remains a significant mystery. CAA is essentially a constant finding in the brain tissue of patients with AD.[94] It is thus widely accepted as one of the microscopic diagnostic features by which the clinical diagnosis of AD/SDAT can be confirmed, although relatively few laboratories quantify CAA or any of the other microscopic lesions of AD in arriving at a firm neuropathologic diagnosis.[250] While debate as to the topography of the earliest lesions in AD continues,[126] the relative role of microvascular amyloid in the pathogenesis of AD is unclear. For example, significant numbers of neuritic plaques can occur in the cortex in the absence of CAA. While vascular and plaque amyloid are usually of comparable severity in many cases, significant discrepancies are observed, with preferential deposition of stainable amyloid in either microvessel walls or senile plaques.[15] The possibility of phenotypic heterogeneity manifesting as different types of neuropathologic change, all of which underlie the clinical syndrome of AD/SDAT, has already been discussed. Recent studies, using sophisticated immunohistochemical and ultrastructural imaging techniques, conclude that abnormal neurites and neurofibrillary tangles seen in the brains of AD patients may represent a widespread alteration of cytoskeletal components rather than an effect of chronic amyloid deposition.[209] The initial events important in the formation of neurities and deposition of parenchymal amyloid may be entirely independent of the appearance of vascular amyloid.[31] Finally, immunohistochemical studies using antibodies to synapse-specific proteins in the cortex suggest that the neuropathologic change associated with AD may begin with synapse loss and degeneration rather than with the deposition of amyloidotic proteins in the brain parenchyma or vessel walls.[129] Nevertheless, rare patients are described in whom syndromes of dementia are associated with purely microvascular deposition of amyloid (i.e., CAA).[137] The debate is complicated by the claims of some that the hippocampal formation (a

A B

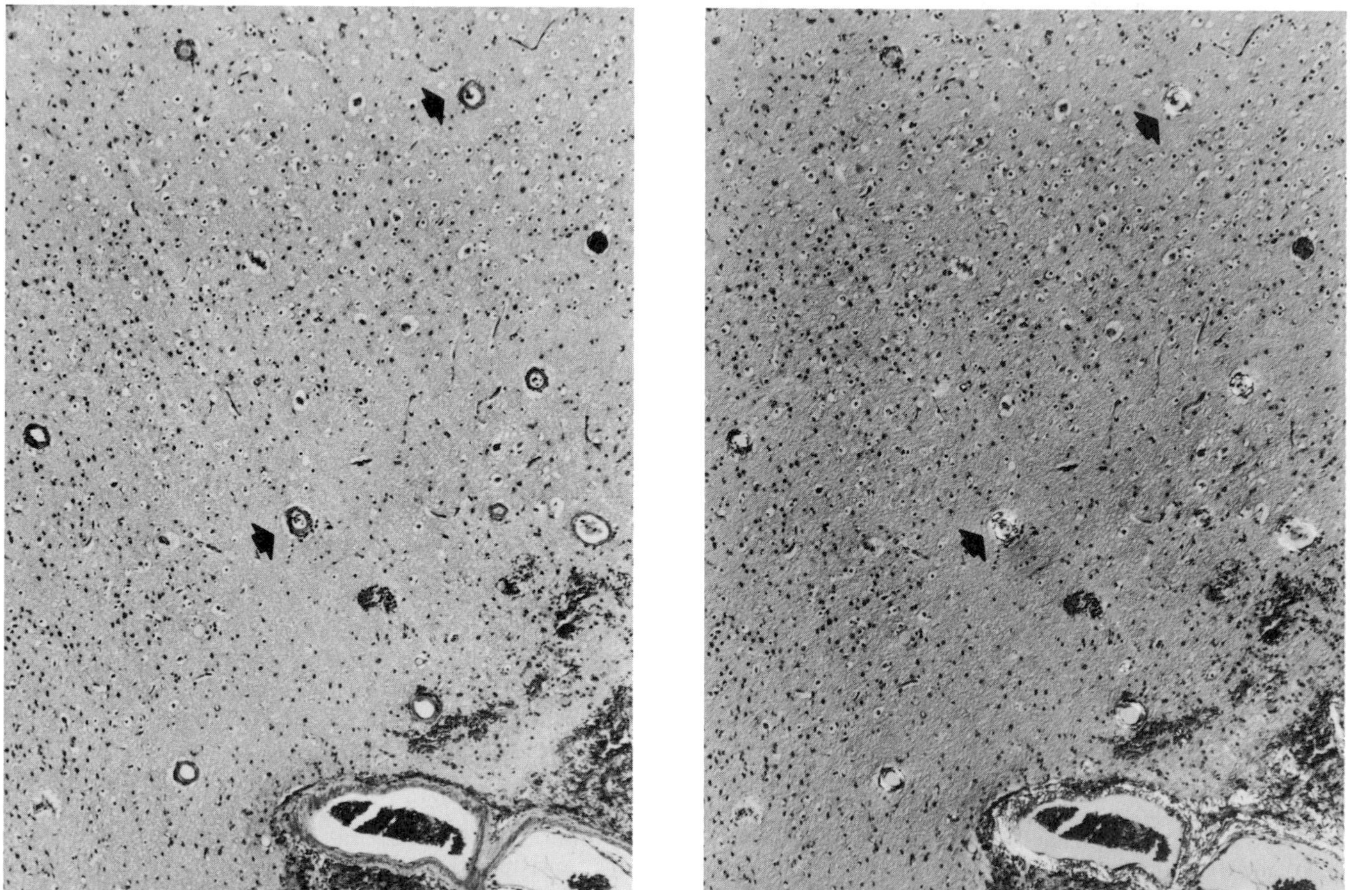

**Fig. 32-6.** Routine histologic study of cerebral amyloid angiopathy. (**A**) Brain biopsy from an elderly patient with lobar cerebral hemorrhage. Congo red-stained section shows thickened arterioles (*arrows*), viewed with nonpolarized light. (**B**) Same section viewed with polarized light shows birefringent vessels (**arrows**) but virtually no parenchymal amyloid deposits. (Figs. A & B × 95.) (**C**) Brain parenchyma and blood vessels evacuated with intracerebral blood clot from a right frontal hematoma in a 60-year-old female. Note markedly thickened and ectatic vessels with hyaline material in their walls (*arrow*). (**D**) Detail of vessel wall. Note relatively normal endothelium (*arrows*). (Figs. C & D: hematoxylin & eosin; Fig. C, × 190; Fig. D, × 495.) (**E & F**) Congo red-stained sections of thickened vessels show characteristic birefringence (apple green) of mural amyloid. (Fig. E viewed without polarized light, Fig. F with polarized light; × 190.) (Figs. E & F from Vinters,[229] with permission.) (*Figure continues.*)

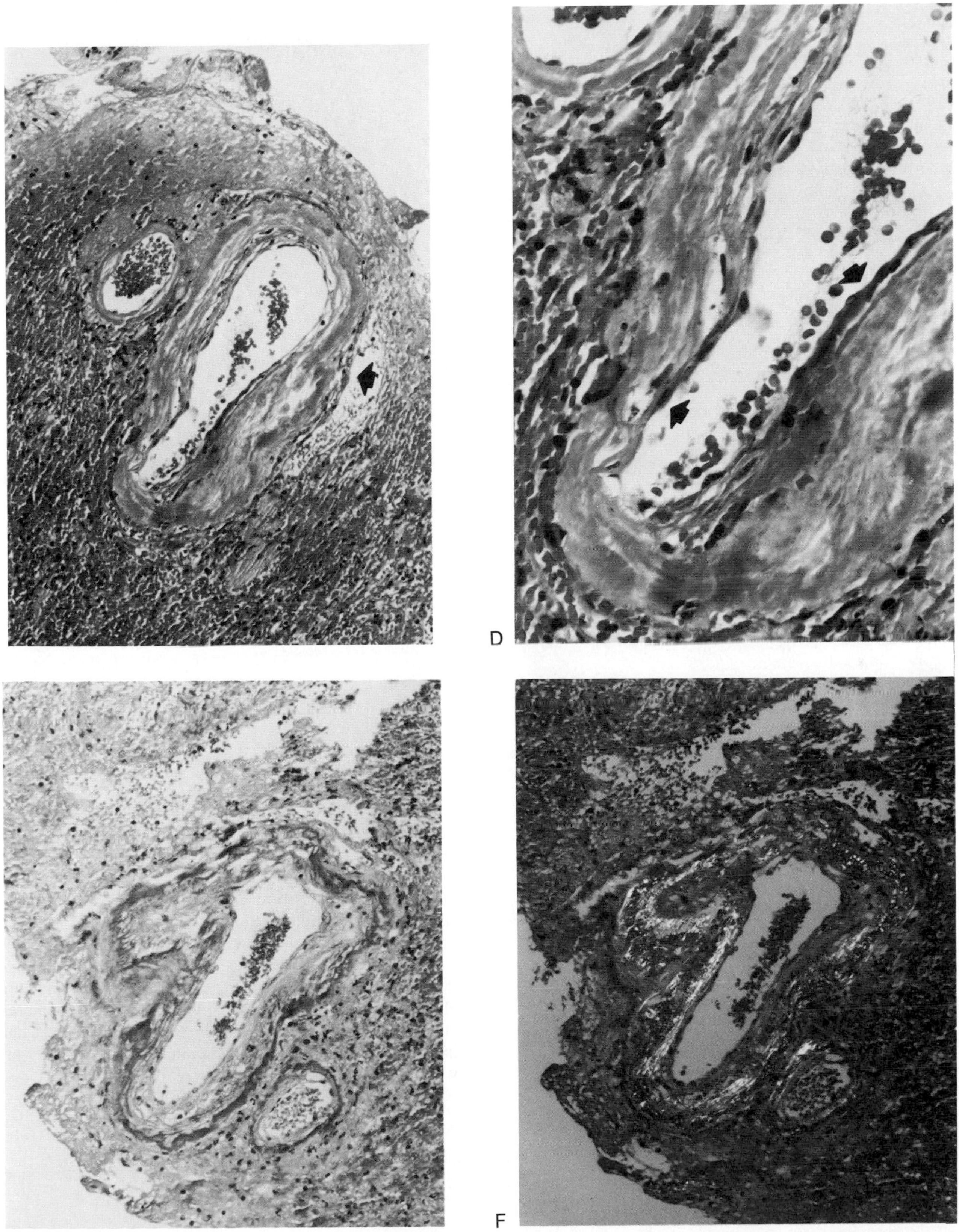
C D E F

**Fig. 32-6** (*Continued*).

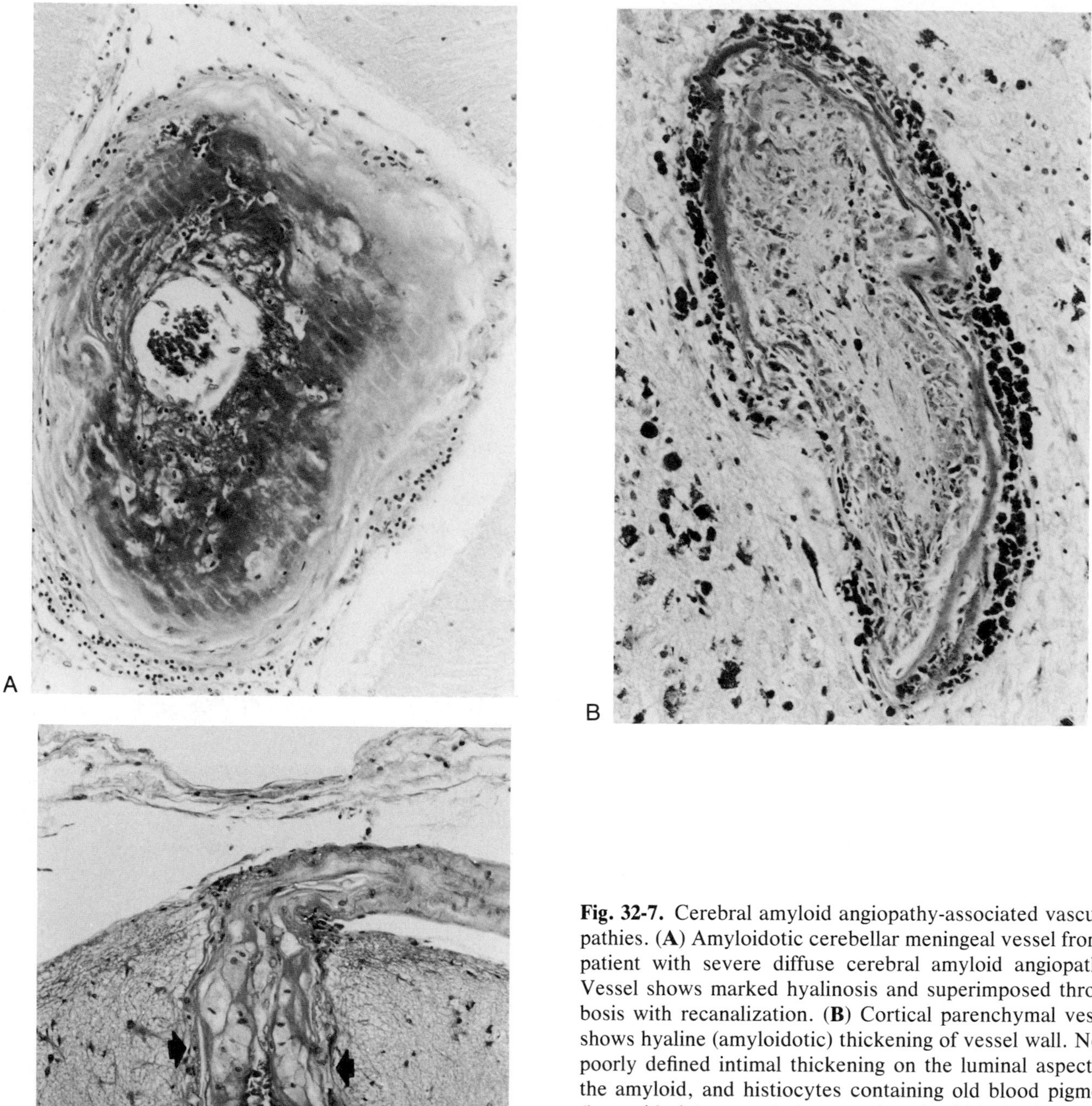

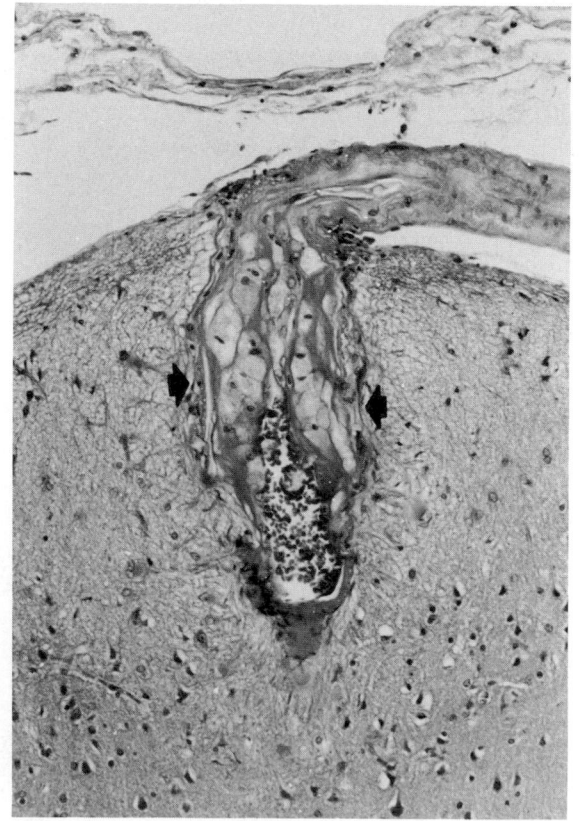


**Fig. 32-7.** Cerebral amyloid angiopathy-associated vasculopathies. (**A**) Amyloidotic cerebellar meningeal vessel from a patient with severe diffuse cerebral amyloid angiopathy. Vessel shows marked hyalinosis and superimposed thrombosis with recanalization. (**B**) Cortical parenchymal vessel shows hyaline (amyloidotic) thickening of vessel wall. Note poorly defined intimal thickening on the luminal aspect of the amyloid, and histiocytes containing old blood pigment (hemosiderin) around the vessel and within brain parenchyma. (Figs. A & B: hematoxylin & eosin; × 190; material studied by kind permission of Dr. Linda Ansbacher, Columbia, Missouri.) (**C**) Focal thickening of amyloidotic vessel wall by foamy histiocytes (*arrows*). (Hematoxylin & eosin; × 190.) (*Figure continues.*)

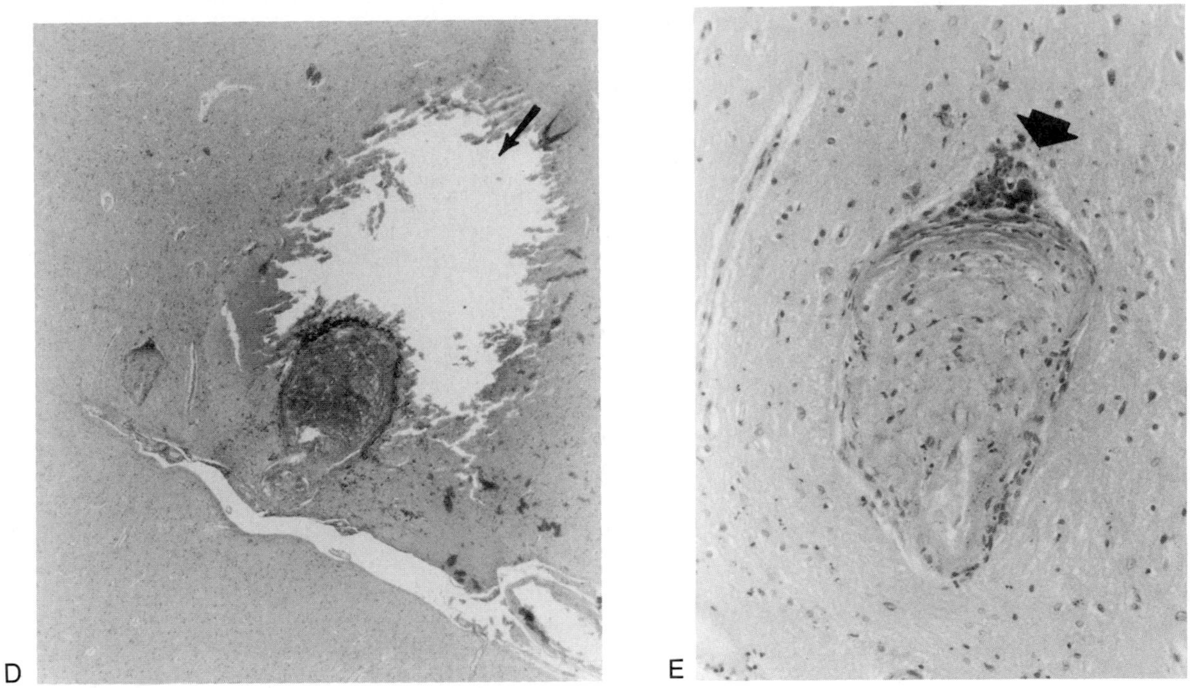


**Fig. 32-7** (*Continued*). (**D & E**) Cerebral amyloid angiopathy-associated microaneurysms resembling typical Charcot-Bouchard-type aneurysms. The larger of the two aneurysms is surrounded by old and recent (*arrow*) hemorrhage (Fig. D). Detail of the smaller aneurysm is shown in Fig. E. Note old hemorrhage on adventitial aspect of the aneurysm (*arrow*, E). (Figs. D & E: hematoxylin & eosin; Fig D: × 25; Fig. E: × 165.) (Figs. A & B from Vinters,[229] with permission; Fig. E from Vinters and Mah,[232] with permission.)

site in which CAA is usually negligible or of minimal severity)[230] may be the site at which the most significant or primary neuropathologic lesions of AD/SDAT occur.[9]

White matter changes are increasingly appreciated as a neuropathologic component of AD.[41] Occasionally, extensive leukoencephalopathy in demented patients is associated with severe CAA in the overlying neocortex and leptomeninges.[38,68,181] Such cases may be related to subcortical arteriosclerotic encephalopathy of the Binswanger type, though most patients with this rare disorder show minimal or negligible degrees of neocortical and meningeal CAA.[8,46,147] A rare demyelinating disorder resembling multiple sclerosis has been described in association with CAA, but has not been studied using immunohistochemical techniques.[82]

## Familial Syndromes of Cerebral Amyloid Angiopathy (Hereditary Cerebral Hemorrhage with Amyloidosis: Icelandic and Dutch Types)

These entities have briefly been described earlier in this chapter.[74,75,91,118,202,245] The only points that bear reemphasis are that the Dutch form of CAA, which leads to familial cerebral hemorrhage, is both morphologically and immunohistochemically closely related to the age- or AD-related variant of CAA described above.[226] The major difference is that in HCHWA-D, relatively few parenchymal senile plaques are identified, but we have already stated that relatively few plaques may be seen in the neocortex of some patients with AD/SDAT. Nevertheless, in HCHWA D, the overwhelming majority of the amyloid is deposited within the walls of arterioles and small arteries.

In HCHWA-I, amyloid is deposited exclusively in leptomeningeal and parenchymal arterioles and capillaries (most commonly the former), although the amyloidotic microvascular change is much more widely distributed throughout the cortex, white matter and even deep central grey structures than is the case in age- or AD-related CAA. However, virtually no parenchymal (plaque type) amyloid is seen in this disorder.

## Spongiform Encephalopathy (Creutzfeldt-Jakob Disease)

A wealth of research has been published over the last decade on spongiform encephalopathies in both man and animals (e.g., scrapie in sheep), neurodegenerative diseases now thought to be caused by "infectious" agents referred to as *prions*.[169] Amyloid deposition within the brain parenchyma may be a

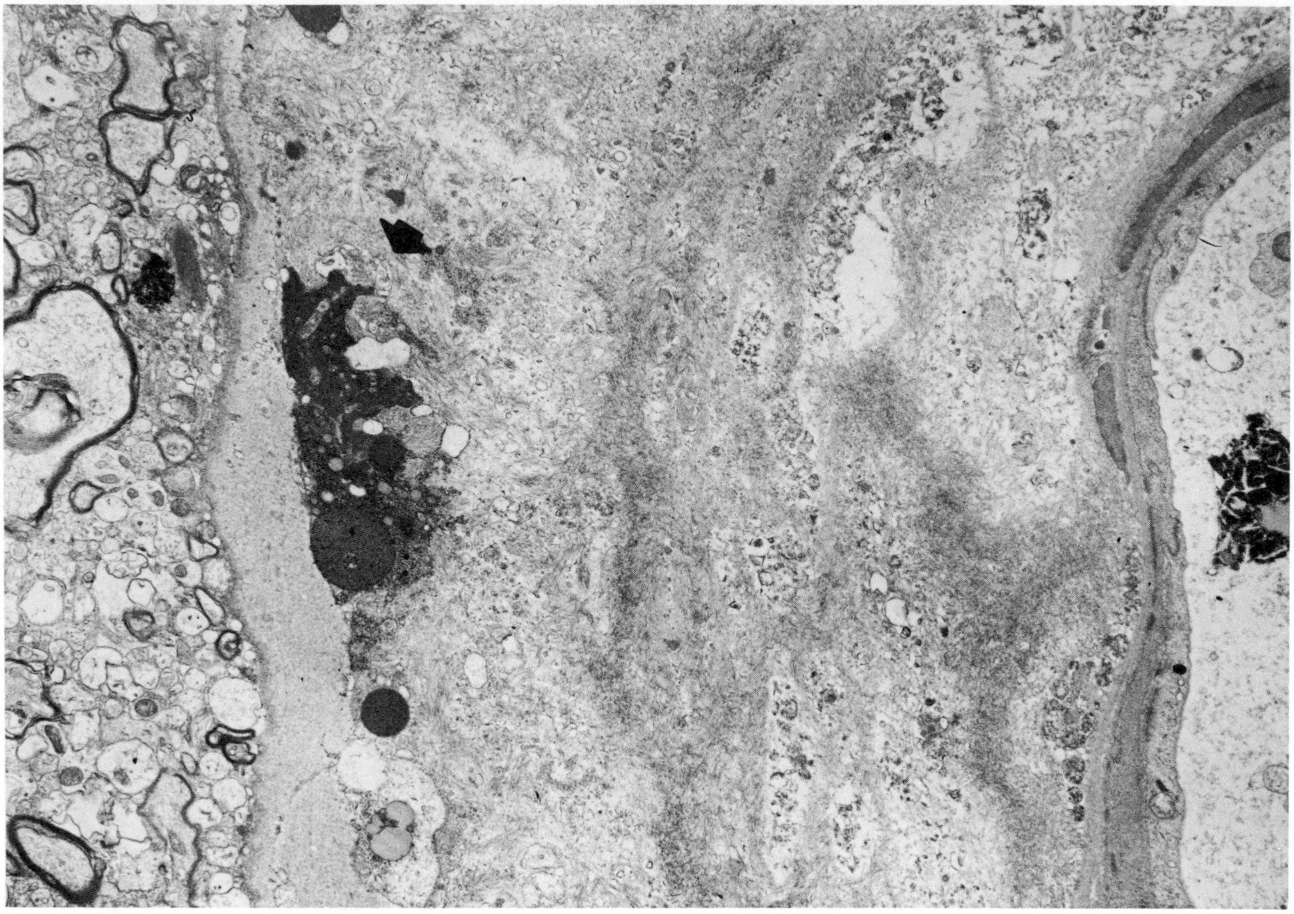

**Fig. 32-8.** Ultrastructure of cerebral amyloid angiopathy. Brain biopsy, plastic-embedded tissue from a patient with severe cerebral amyloid angiopathy and Alzheimer's disease. Wall of arteriole shows intact endothelium at right, fibrillar amyloid material replacing media, and clear distinction between mural amyloid and brain parenchyma (at left). Cellular debris (*arrow*), possibly representing degenerate smooth muscle cell, is present among the amyloid fibrils. Collagenlike basement membrane substance is seen between amyloid deposits and brain parenchyma. Vascular lumen is at right. (× 8700.) (From Vinters,[229] with permission.)

prominent component of some of these disorders, especially the Gerstmann-Sträussler-Scheinker variant.[231] Nevertheless, *microvascular* amyloid deposition is relatively unusual in these conditions, and the author is unaware of a single report of fatal cerebral hemorrhage or stroke in a patient with any variant of spongiform encephalopathy. Familial cerebral amyloidosis has been described in association with spongiform encephalopathy.[3] Rapidly progressive dementia secondary to CJD was associated with extensive amyloid infiltration of cerebral vessels in the absence of neuritic plaques in one reported patient.[103] Cerebrovascular amyloid, which by light-microscopic examination resembles age-related or AD-related CAA, has been observed in scrapie-affected sheep,[54] and the vascular amyloid in this disorder reacts with antibodies to the prion protein.[5]

## Oculoleptomeningeal Amyloidosis

A familial disorder described in Japanese and North American kindreds is characterized by widespread deposition of amyloid within the vitreous and retinal vessels, with unusually heavy meningovascular amyloid deposition adjacent to the brain though generally not within it.[65,140,144,223] Perivascular tissue throughout the body is also infiltrated by amyloid, and there may be associated peripheral nerve degeneration. Patients frequently experience extensive seizures, cerebral infarcts and even cerebral hemorrhages. The strokes are thought to result from adventitial infiltration of meningeal vessels with associated intimal thickening or weakening of the vessel wall. The infiltrating amyloid shows characteristic ultrastructural appearances of 7- to 9-nm filaments, but biochemically the material has been found to represent transthyretin (prealbumin). Plasmapheresis has been suggested as one treatment for this disorder.[223]

### Miscellaneous Syndromes of Cerebral Amyloid Angiopathy

Several familial syndromes in which CAA plays a prominent role have been described, most from the United Kingdom. Griffiths et al.[71] reported siblings who died in their late fifties or early sixties in whom neuropathologic findings included severe CAA present in the spinal cord, brain, and leptomeninges. Multiple cerebral hemorrhages or areas of encephalomalacia were discovered, and there were numerous amyloid-containing "plaques" found mainly in the hippocampus and cerebellar cortex. The disorder was thought to show autosomal dominant transmission. Love and Duchen[117] reported a 49-year-old woman with familial cerebellar ataxia but no dementia, in whom widespread CAA of the CNS was found at necropsy. Particularly heavy infiltration of capillaries by amyloid was found in the hippocampus and cerebellum.[117] More recently, Plant et al.[160] described novel studies on members of two families in whom individuals showed features of a familial CAA with nonneuritic plaque formation inherited as an autosomal dominant trait. Clinical features included dementia, ataxia, and spastic paralysis. A total of 26 affected individuals in five generations have been described.[160] The relationship of these unusual conditions, in which CAA is a prominent component of the neuropathologic change, to AD/SDAT remains to be determined, though the authors of many of the reports feel strongly that these represent distinct and unusual diseases that should be considered separately from AD/SDAT. Shaw[192] has described a young boy (with no significant family history) in whom widespread microvascular and parenchymal amyloid was seen throughout the CNS (Fig. 32-9). Encephalomalacia and cerebral hemorrhage were not a prominent component of the neuropathologic findings, however.

Although CAA usually occurs without an associated pattern of systemic amyloid deposition, cerebrovascular amyloid (CAA) has been found in the leptomeninges and cerebral cortex of six patients with systemic amyloidosis, including two patients with amyloid A protein amyloidosis, one with AL amyloidosis related to immunoglobulin light chains, and two patients with familial amyloidotic polyneuropathy.[86] When vascular amyloid was noted in the pituitary glands and choroid plexus of affected patients, the type of amyloid was found to be biochemically identical to that seen in the viscera of the afflicted persons. However, CAA (when present in the leptomeninges and cortex of two patients with AA amyloidosis and one with AL amyloidosis) was shown to react with the Alzheimer A4 or $\beta$-protein. The authors concluded that the AA and AL amyloid proteins do not readily accumulate in meningeal or cortical vessels even though the proteins are found in the circulation.[86]

### Animal Models of Cerebral Amyloid Angiopathy

CAA of varying severity has been found in a number of species of vertebrates.[34] Using modern immunohistochemical techniques (see the section Biochemical and Immunohistochemical Studies), the cerebrovascular amyloid in aged monkeys, orangutans, polar bears, and dogs has been shown to cross-react with the Alzheimer amyloid protein.[191] Alzheimer-type amyloid has been found within intracerebral and meningeal capillaries and arterioles in aged squirrel monkeys, with a pattern of distribution similar to that observed in the aging human brain.[244] CAA has been well described in aged canines.[51,249] Stroke in the form of cerebral hemorrhage or encephalomalacia does not appear to occur in relation to CAA in any of these species. Thus, while the finding of brain (including microvascular) amyloid in aging animal populations is of biologic interest, the likelihood of developing an animal model for CAA-related stroke seems remote at this time.

## BIOCHEMICAL AND IMMUNOHISTOCHEMICAL STUDIES

One of the most important steps leading to our current understanding of the biochemistry and molecular biology of CAA and related brain amyloids occurred with the isolation and characterization of cerebrovascular amyloid from patients with AD (and subsequently Down syndrome) by Glenner's group[62,63] in 1984. Subsequently, amyloidotic microvessels were isolated from the neocortex of a patient with AD (Fig. 32-10) and studied, using comparable biochemical techniques.[154] The amyloidotic cores of senile plaques have been isolated and analyzed.[130] Both the microvascular and the plaque core amyloid were found to be composed of a polypeptide with a molecular weight of approximately 4,200 Da, showing a unique amino acid composition and sequence which differed substantially from that of other known amyloid proteins. The peptide was named the Alzheimer $\beta$ or A4 protein. Molecular biologic techniques allowed for the characterization of the A4 precursor molecule (subsequently referred to as A4P), which was found to consist of 695 amino acid residues and to show features characteristic of a glycosylated cell-surface receptor.[98] The gene encoding this A4P molecule was mapped to chromosome 21.[64,98,174,213] Eventually, sub-

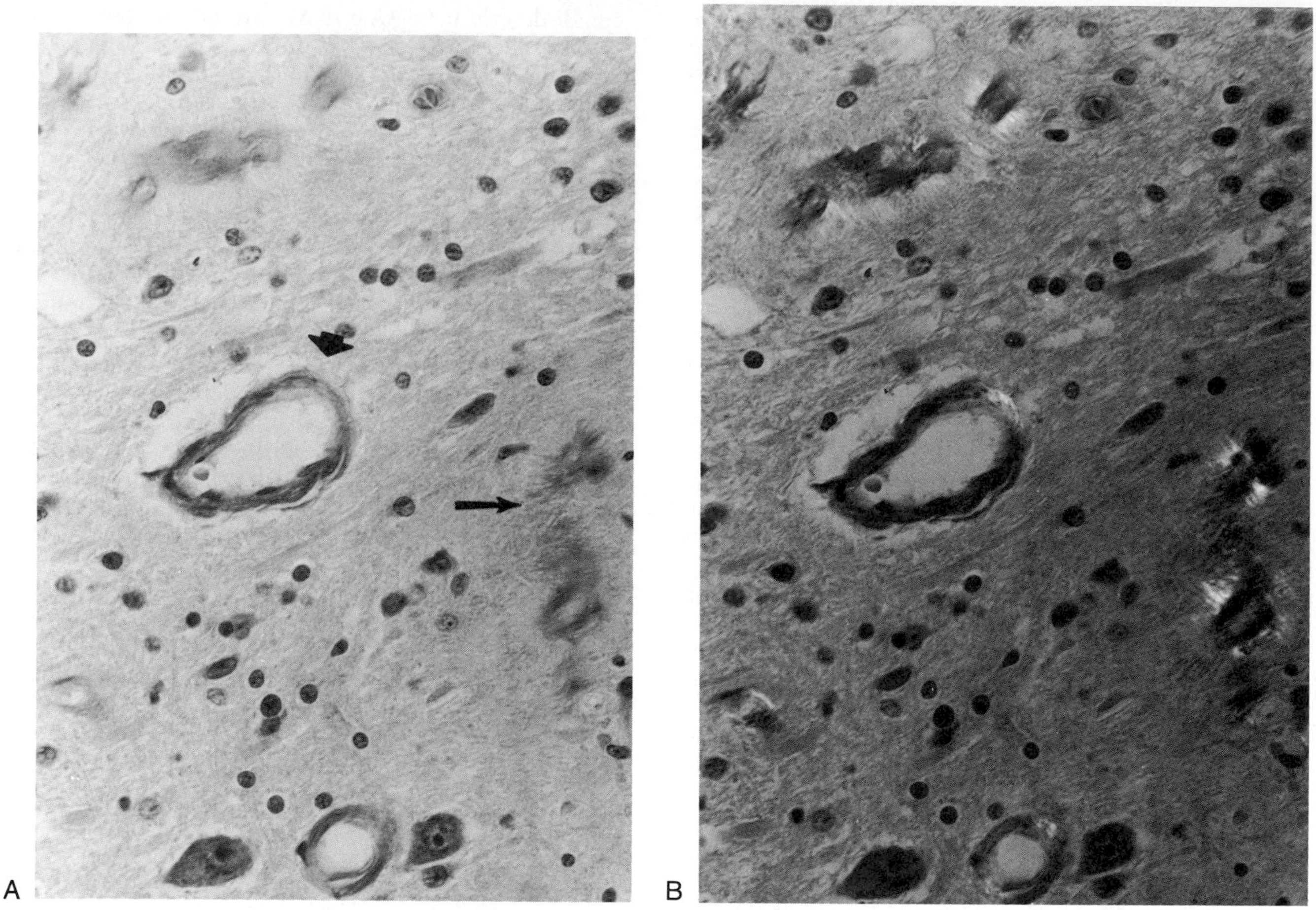


**Fig. 32-9.** (**A & B**) Micrographs of the same section, showing unusual neurodegenerative disorder in a 14-year-old boy. Widespread capillary (*thin arrow*) and arteriolar (*thick arrow*) amyloid was identified throughout the nervous system. Fig. A viewed without polarized light, Fig. B with polarized light to show birefringence. (× 495.) (Tissue generously provided by Dr. Cheng-Mei Shaw, Seattle, Washington.) (For details of the case, see Shaw.[192]) (Fig. B from Vinters et al.,[237] with permission.)

tle differences between the vascular and plaque core amyloids were discovered,[164] the cerebrovascular amyloid being composed of 39 amino acids, the plaque amyloid of 42. Other important components of cerebral amyloids (including $\alpha$-1-antichymotrypsin) were discovered.[159] Nevertheless, the close kinship and amino acid sequence homology between senile plaque and cerebrovascular amyloid of AD was intriguing.[251] Amyloid fibrils could be formed in vitro from synthetic peptides homologous to the Alzheimer A4 or $\beta$-protein.[23] The pivotal discoveries that led to our current relatively sophisticated (though as yet incomplete) understanding of the biochemistry of AD and related brain amyloid proteins have been reviewed by Selkoe.[188]

Comparable advances in biochemical and molecular technology allowed for a detailed analysis of microvascular amyloidotic proteins important in the pathogenesis of HCHWA-D and HCHWA-I. The Dutch form of CAA related to the pathogenesis of familial cerebral hemorrhage was shown to be biochemically closely related to the AD form of microvascular amyloidosis.[165,226] In contrast, the microvascular amyloid seen in patients with HCHWA-I was found to be composed of a variant protein of gamma-trace (cystatin C), consisting of 110 amino acid residues, and showing a molecular weight of approximately 11,000 to 12,000 Da. The gamma-trace protein was entirely different from the Alzheimer A4 or $\beta$-peptide.[27,49,50,73] Cystatin C is recognized as an inhibitor of lysosomal cysteine proteases, suggesting that in this form of CAA peptide processing might be extremely important in the molecular events that eventually lead to microvascular degeneration leading to stroke. Patients with HCHWA-I could be distinguished from healthy subjects and from patients with other diseases by measurement of the gamma-trace concentration in the cerebrospinal fluid, suggesting a relatively noninvasive diagnostic test that could be used to predict which patients are at risk for cerebral hemorrhage among the Icelandic population.[73]

Advances in understanding the biochemical fea-

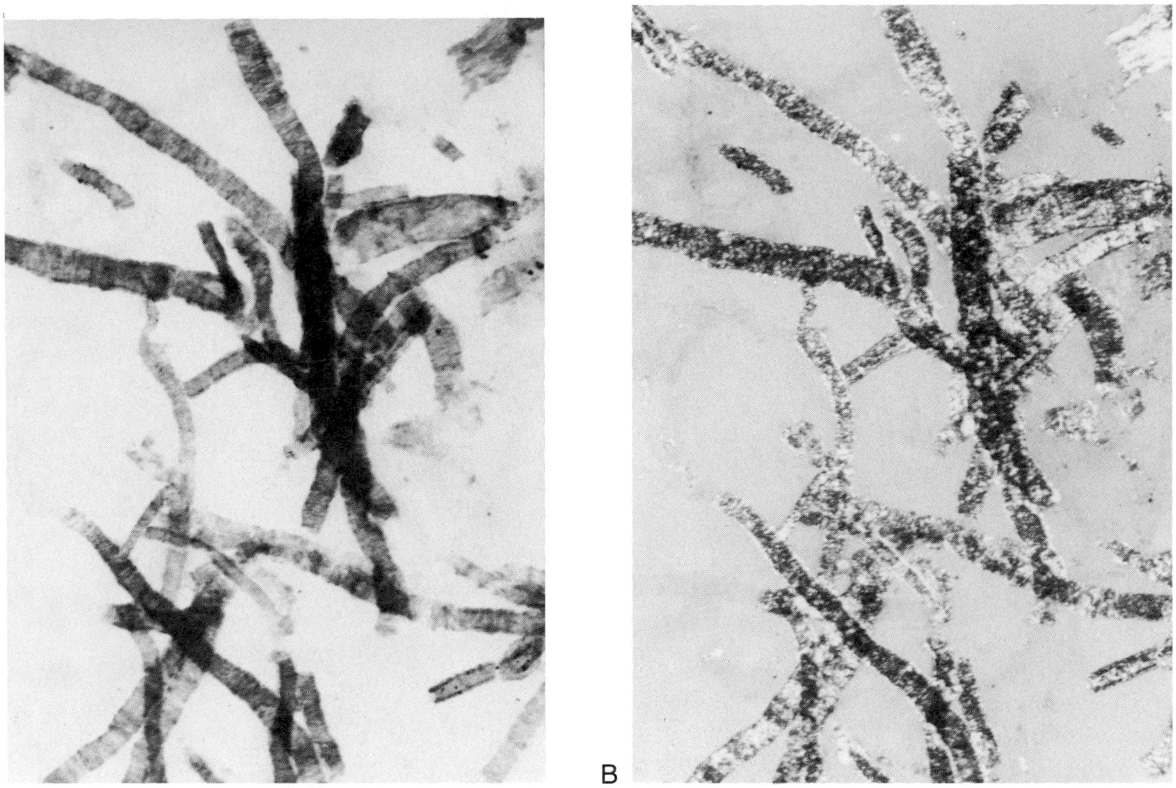


**Fig. 32-10.** (**A & B**) Amyloidotic brain cortical parenchymal arterioles, isolated as described in Pardridge et al.[154] and stained with Congo red. (Fig. A photographed with routine illumination, Fig. B under polarized light.) (× 75.)

tures of various types of CAA have led to novel strategies for demonstrating these peptides within amyloidotic blood vessel walls in the brains of patients with relevant stroke syndromes and/or dementia. Earlier cytochemical and immunohistochemical studies had used conventional procedures to demonstrate suspected materials or peptides within amyloidotic blood vessel walls.[40,66,163,167,194,218,241] These investigations concluded that a variety of serum and non-serum proteins were present in amyloidotic plaques and microvessels. Histochemically identified components of these structures included lysozyme, fibrinogen, albumin, IgA and IgG, haptoglobin, macroglobulin, microglobulin, and prealbumin. A monoclonal antibody was also generated that reacted intensely with congophilic elements in AD brain.[119]

Knowledge of the amino acid sequence of the AD, Dutch, and Icelandic variants of CAA based on direct microvessel isolation techniques allowed for the preparation of monoclonal or polyclonal antibodies to artificially synthesized subsequences of the larger peptides and use of these antibodies in standard avidin-biotin peroxidase and peroxidase-antiperoxidase methods to demonstrate amyloid proteins in blood vessel walls (as well as parenchyma) in brain sections. Moreover, most of the techniques could be applied to formalin-fixed paraffin-embedded tissues, allowing for extensive study of archival material using these methodologies. Anti-A4 or anti-$\beta$-protein immunohistochemistry has thus been utilized to highlight amyloid plaques and microvessels in aging and AD brain (Fig. 32-11), as demonstrated in numerous studies from multiple laboratories.[17,28,30,92,141,205,238,255] It has been the experience of most investigators that anti-A4 or anti-$\beta$-peptide antibodies fail to label neurofibrillary tangles.[11,237] This suggests that the neurofibrillary tangle (paired helical filament) constituent protein differs from the senile plaque core and microvascular amyloid proteins. Modifications of the immunohistochemical procedures, for example, pretreatment of tissue sections with "solubilizing agents" such as formic acid or proteases, enhances the neuropathologist's ability to detect amyloidotic proteins.[108,237] These immunohistochemical techniques have allowed for detailed assessment of the histotopography of A4 protein within aging and AD brain.

In addition to labeling of senile plaques and amyloidotic microvessels, anti-A4 immunohistochemistry allows for identification of perivascular coronas of immunoreactive A4 material in many patients (Fig. 32-11). It also shows parenchymal deposits of A4 situated at the pial membrane in some patients with large amounts of intraparenchymal amyloid (Fig. 32-11). Anti-A4 antibodies may also decorate diverse cell

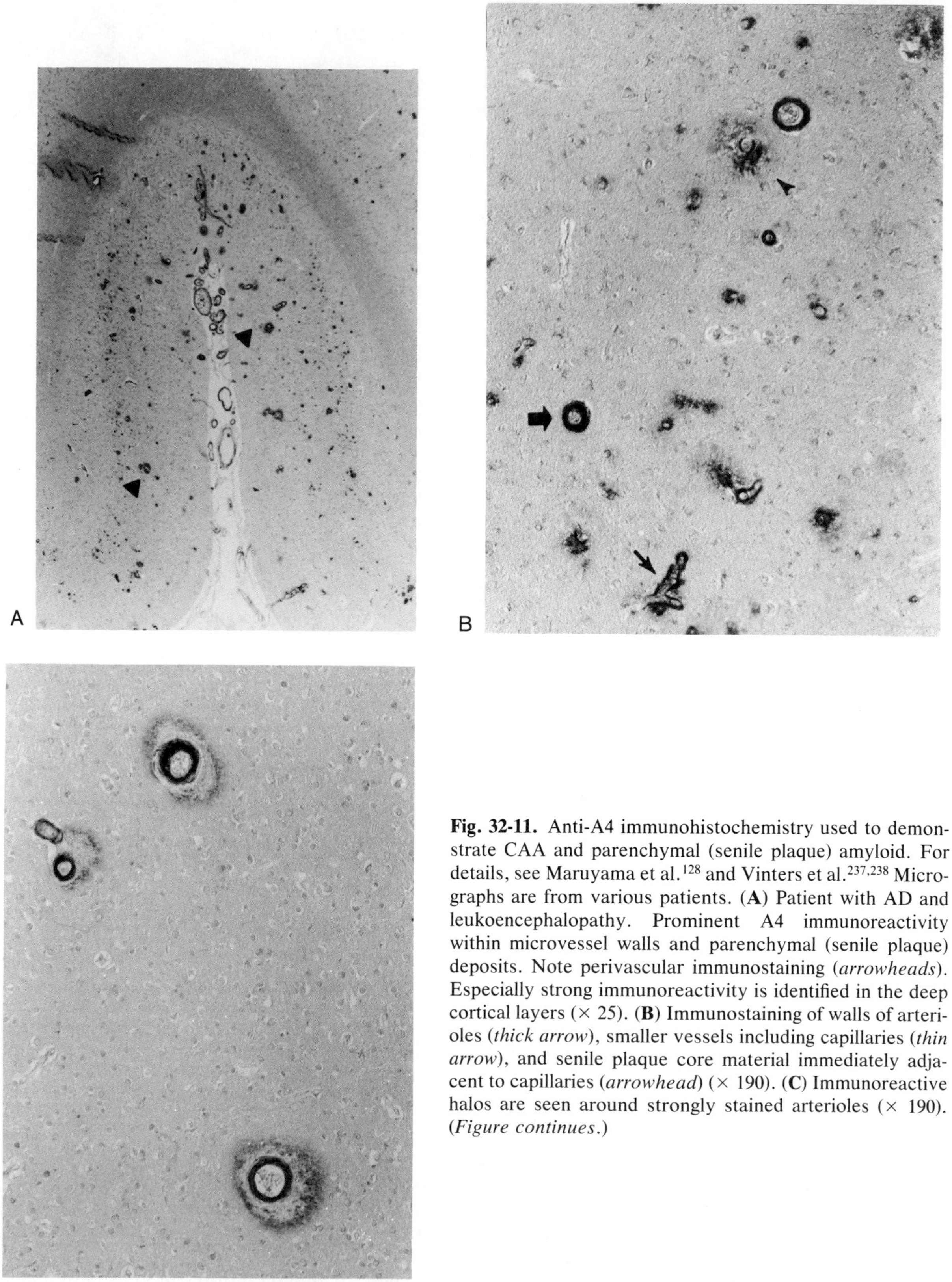


**Fig. 32-11.** Anti-A4 immunohistochemistry used to demonstrate CAA and parenchymal (senile plaque) amyloid. For details, see Maruyama et al.[128] and Vinters et al.[237,238] Micrographs are from various patients. (**A**) Patient with AD and leukoencephalopathy. Prominent A4 immunoreactivity within microvessel walls and parenchymal (senile plaque) deposits. Note perivascular immunostaining (*arrowheads*). Especially strong immunoreactivity is identified in the deep cortical layers (× 25). (**B**) Immunostaining of walls of arterioles (*thick arrow*), smaller vessels including capillaries (*thin arrow*), and senile plaque core material immediately adjacent to capillaries (*arrowhead*) (× 190). (**C**) Immunoreactive halos are seen around strongly stained arterioles (× 190). (*Figure continues.*)

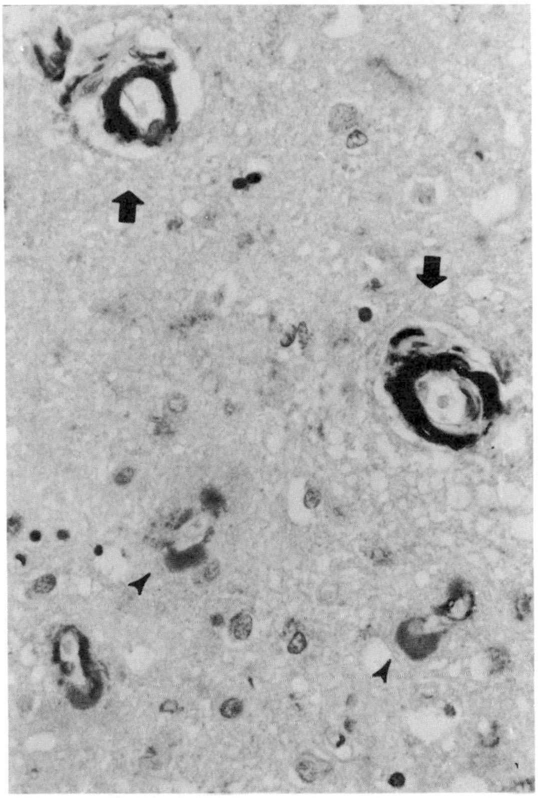

D

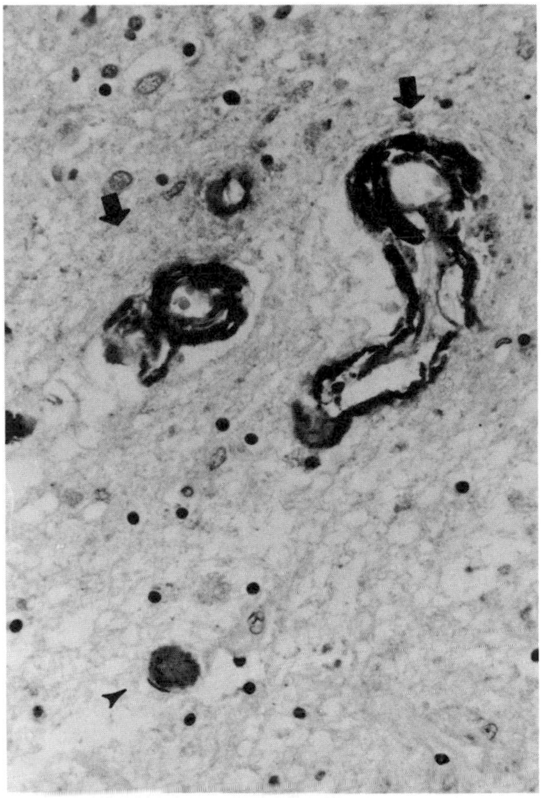

E

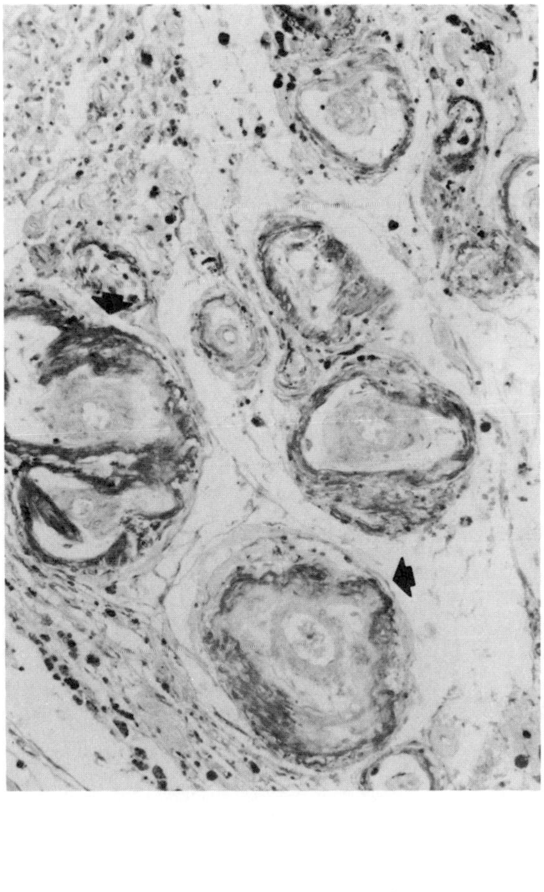

F

**Fig. 32-11** (*Continued*). (**D & E**) Antibody labels parenchymal microvessels (*arrows*) and senile plaque cores (*arrowheads*) in brain from a patient with long-standing dementia. In Fig. D, plaques are seen adjacent to capillaries, whereas in Fig. E, a large plaque (*arrowhead*) is present in brain parenchyma. (× 490.) (**F & G**) Tissue from brain illustrated in Figure 1B and C. Macrophages containing hemosidern are seen in the leptomeninges. Meningeal vessels show "double-barrel" lumen. (*Figure continues.*)

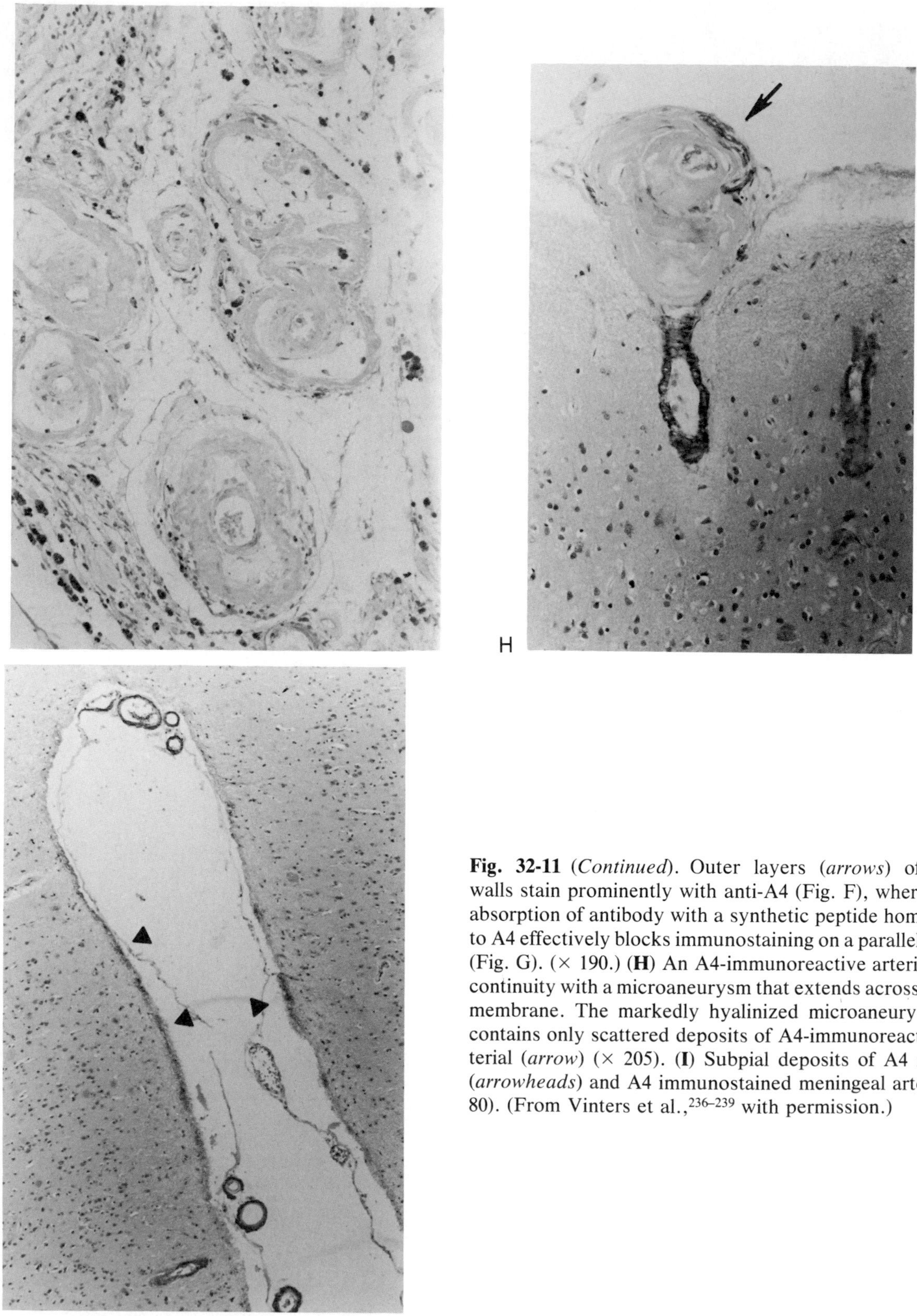

G

H

I

**Fig. 32-11** (*Continued*). Outer layers (*arrows*) of vessel walls stain prominently with anti-A4 (Fig. F), whereas preabsorption of antibody with a synthetic peptide homologous to A4 effectively blocks immunostaining on a parallel section (Fig. G). (× 190.) (**H**) An A4-immunoreactive arteriole is in continuity with a microaneurysm that extends across the pial membrane. The markedly hyalinized microaneurysm wall contains only scattered deposits of A4-immunoreactive material (*arrow*) (× 205). (**I**) Subpial deposits of A4 material (*arrowheads*) and A4 immunostained meningeal arteries (× 80). (From Vinters et al.,[236–239] with permission.)

types in the CNS (e.g., neuronal, astrocytic, and ependymal elements) in specially treated tissues.[205] Larger leptomeningeal vessels, when they are immunolabeled using anti-A4, frequently show an abundance of reaction product on their adventitial aspect (Fig. 32-11), suggesting the possibility of circulation of the amyloid protein within the subarachnoid space and adherence of the peptide to the external aspects of larger vessels. Conversely, parenchymal vessels (especially arterioles) usually show deposition of amyloid in their media and adventitia, sometimes extending into the adjacent brain parenchyma. The immunohistochemical techniques to demonstrate AD amyloid peptide are now so commonplace that commercial antibodies to perform the studies have become available. Many investigators have suggested that anti-A4 immunohistochemistry is more sensitive than traditional silver (e.g., Bielschowsky) staining techniques to demonstrate amyloidotic lesions within brain parenchyma.[33,84] The immunohistochemical studies have also confirmed the biochemical similarity between AD microvascular amyloid and the amyloid seen in the brains of patients with HCHWA-D (Fig. 32-12). However, more refined genetic analyses of the HCHWA-D kindred have found that a single amino acid substitution at position 22 of the amyloid protein may be a consequence of a point mutation that causes deposition of the amyloid protein in the walls of cerebral blood vessels of affected patients leading to stroke in these individuals.[112] Other investigations suggest that the A4P gene (described above) is very tightly linked to HCHWA-D and may represent the site of a causal mutation in this familial stroke syndrome.[225]

Further refinements of A4 or $\beta$-peptide immunohistochemistry indicate that the AD amyloid may be present within not only cortex but also subcortical white matter of patients with parenchymal amyloid deposition.[12] An abundance of $\alpha$-1 antichymotrypsin has been found within senile plaque cores and cerebrovascular amyloid.[1,211]

Whereas most immunohistochemical studies have utilized antibodies to portions of the A4 molecule, which is near the C-terminal end of the A4P (A4 precursor), antibodies have also been generated to the near N-terminal end of the AD amyloid precursor. Using this strategy, A4P has been detected immunohistochemically in senile plaques and amyloidotic microvessels.[149,210] Such studies imply that the blood vessel wall may represent a source of A4P and that the processing of A4P into insoluble amyloidotic fibrils in AD may take place within the vessel wall itself.[210] A very recent study shows that the smooth muscle cells within blood vessel walls may represent the site of synthesis of the A4P.[101]

Comparable immunohistochemical studies have been carried out on amyloidotic vessels derived from brain tissue of patients with HCHWA-I (the Icelandic variant of CAA). Cystatin C or gamma-trace variant protein can be demonstrated immunohistochemically in affected blood vessel walls (Fig. 32-13), and is rarely seen in extra-CNS locations (e.g., a submandibular lymph node).[116] A further intriguing finding has emerged. Whereas cystatin C/gamma-trace CAA was previously thought to be entirely distinct from A4 or $\beta$-peptide (Alzheimer-related) CAA,[254] several laboratories have now confirmed that A4 or $\beta$-peptide may colocalize with cystatin C or gamma-trace protein in the microvessel walls of brain tissue from elderly patients and those with AD/SDAT.[128,234,239] In our experience, gamma-trace peptide is likely to be especially prominent within amyloidotic arterioles in brain tissue from patients prone to stroke in the form of cerebral hemorrhage. This preliminary finding may lead to new avenues in research on mechanisms of stroke related to CAA.

Amyloid P component has also been found in microvascular lesions of CAA as well as in senile plaque and neurofibrillary tangle structures of AD patients.[29,39,178] Other workers, however, find amyloid P component only within amyloidotic microvessels[247] and not in other AD microscopic lesions.

Proteoglycans including sulfated glycosaminoglycans have been demonstrated immunohistochemically in various amyloidotic lesions of AD, including CAA.[106,197–200] Whereas different amyloids throughout the body have different protein components—the uniqueness of age- or AD-related A4 or $\beta$-protein has been stressed throughout this review—the almost universal finding of proteoglycans and amyloid P component in multiple biochemically diverse forms of amyloid suggests an interaction between proteoglycans and amyloidogenic proteins that may be important in the final deposition of amyloid in a given organ or tissue substructure. Glycolytic pretreatment of tissue sections enhances immunolabeling of amyloid plaques and CAA by anti-A4 immunohistochemistry.[10] This suggests that, although the precise interaction between complex carbohydrates and brain A4 amyloid protein is unknown, such treatment exposes "buried epitopes" within the amyloid and allows for enhancement of immunohistochemical demonstration of the brain amyloid protein.

## THEORIES OF PATHOGENESIS OF CEREBRAL AMYLOID ANGIOPATHY

The reader can infer from the foregoing extensive discussion that the pathogenesis of CAA and other forms of brain amyloid (whether related to AD, other stroke syndromes, or non-stroke-related deposition of CNS amyloid) is far from settled—this despite the monumental advances that have been a function of refinements in biochemical and molecular biologic technology. A discussion of the very extensive and

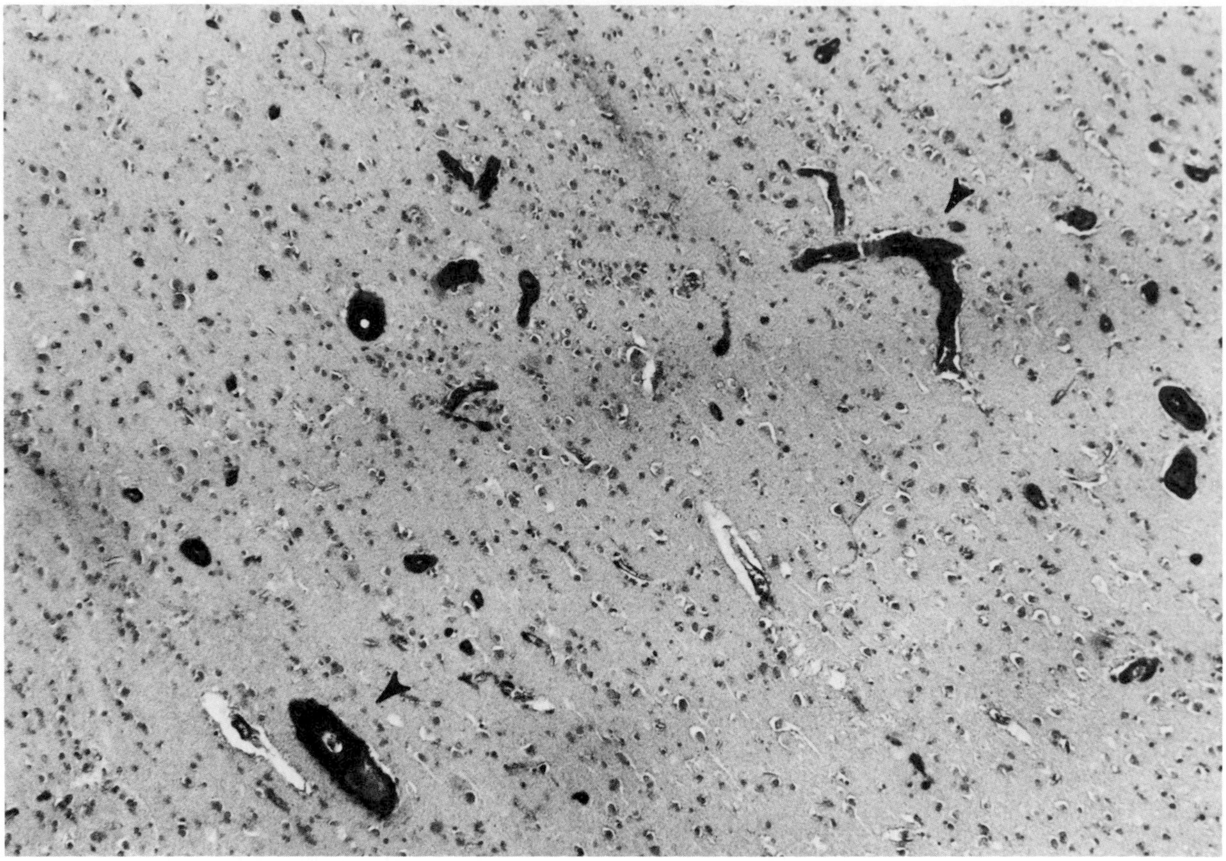

**Fig. 32-12.** Immunocytochemistry of hereditary cerebral hemorrhage with amyloidosis–Dutch type. Brain tissue from a patient with familial cerebral hemorrhage. Almost exclusively microvascular staining (*arrowhead*) shown with anti-A4 immunohistochemisty. (× 90.) (Tissue studied by courtesy of Dr. G.T.A.M. Bots, Leiden, The Netherlands.) (From Vinters et al.,[237] with permission.)

complex literature in this area is well beyond the scope of this chapter, which has highlighted clinical and diagnostic considerations. The controversies in the field relate to precise mechanisms of amyloid deposition, specifically molecular and cellular events that lead to the precipitation of these insoluble proteins in CNS parenchyma. The reader is referred to several excellent reviews that present different viewpoints and emphasize varying themes on the subject.[22,59,77,79,95,134,185–187,189,190,215] Genetically transformed cells in tissue culture can be engineered to overexpress A4P (amyloid precursor protein).[127] Synthetic peptides showing homology to the Alzheimer A4 or $\beta$-protein can be manipulated to form amyloid-like fibrils in vitro.[105] Unfortunately, in vitro studies on the A4 and A4P proteins have also led to apparently conflicting and somewhat confusing results. For example, the amyloid A4 or $\beta$-protein has been found to enhance the survival of hippocampal neurons in tissue culture,[248] whereas fragments of the A4P may show significant neurotoxicity.[256] A continuing and increasingly amplified theme in brain amyloid research is that of deranged peptide processing, either at the blood vessel wall or within the brain parenchyma itself. For example, cDNA segments closely related to the DNA that encodes the A4P protein codes for a peptide that is very similar to molecules found in the Kunitz family of serine protease inhibitors,[162,214] and another cDNA closely related to that encoding the A4P codes for a protein which is highly homologous to the basic trypsin inhibitor family.[107] The recurring theme that presents itself is one of abnormal proteolysis of the A4P molecule or protease inhibition, which leads to accumulation of A4 or $\beta$-peptide within tissues, possibly including the blood vessel wall. The secreted form of the AD amyloid precursor protein containing the Kunitz domain has been further characterized to be protease nexin-II.[148] It is hoped that an understanding of the pathogenesis of AD/SDAT will, almost by definition, lead to an understanding of the pathogenesis of A4- or $\beta$-peptide-related forms of CAA and possible treatments for the condition.[57] This may be an overly optimistic view, given the theme presented throughout this chapter of the phenotypic heterogeneity of AD and the multiplicity of predominating microscopic lesions that might be present in any

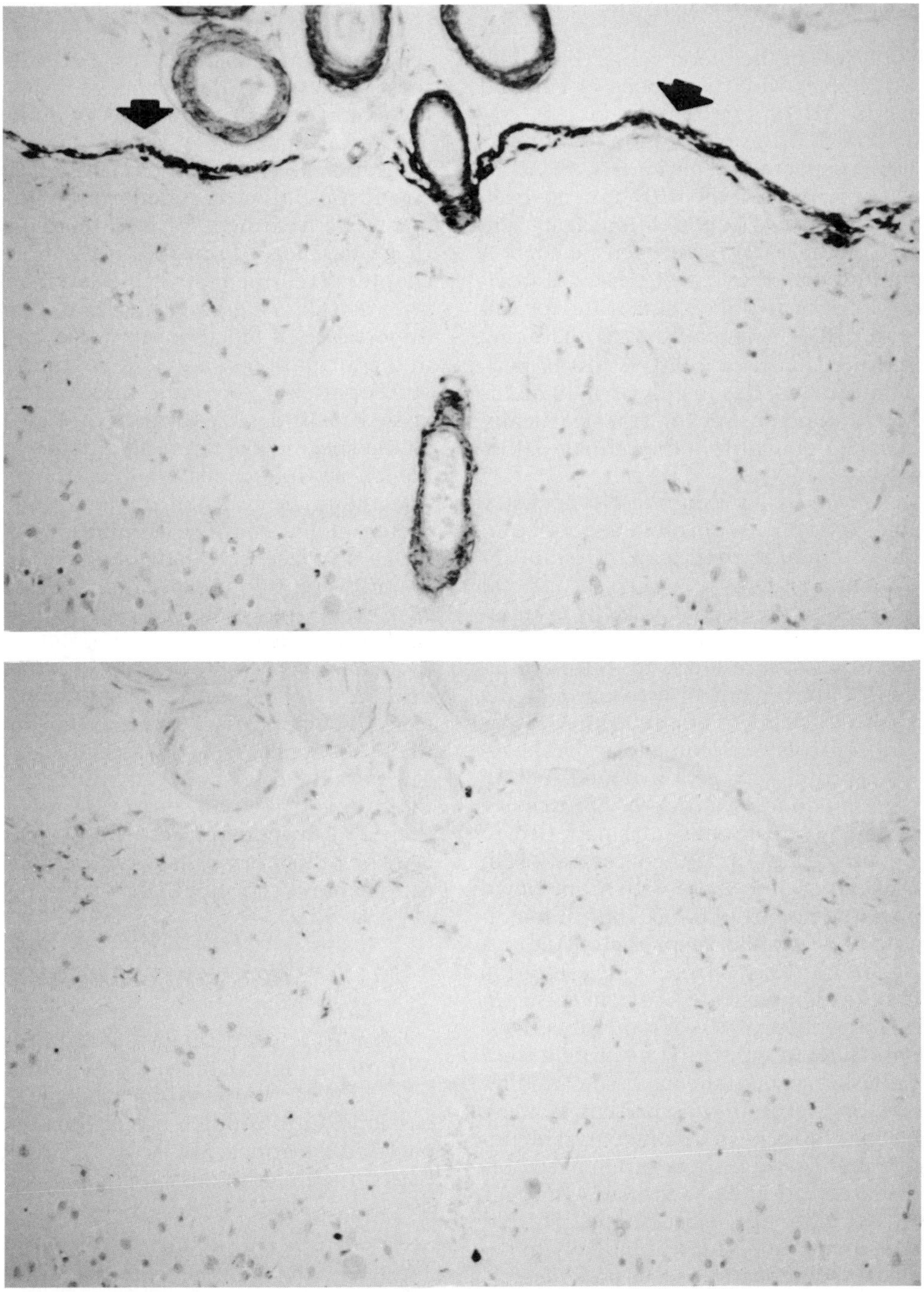

A

B

**Fig. 32-13.** Hereditary cerebral hemorrhage with amyloidosis–Icelandic type. Anti-gamma-trace antibody was utilized to immunostain sections of brain tissue from a patient with HCHWA-I. (**A**) Arteriolar wall and pial (*arrows*) staining with anti-gamma-trace. (**B**) Lack of immunoreactivity in a parallel section stained with anti-A4. (× 160.) (Brain tissue kindly supplied by Dr. Olafur Jensson, Reykjavik, Iceland.) (From Vinters et al.,[234] with permission.)

given brain from a patient with the clinical disorder. An understanding of primary as opposed to secondary cellular events in amyloid deposition (both within the blood vessel wall and brain parenchyma) is imperative.[179]

Given the pivotal role of the blood vessel (including capillary and arteriolar) wall as a locus of amyloid protein, whether in AD or one of the non-AD syndromes of CAA, abnormalities of the blood-brain barrier (BBB) may be suspected in patients with AD.[235] While specific abnormalities of the BBB have not been identified in patients with AD, age-related changes in the fine structure of the BBB have been noted.[206] A characteristic finding was the loss of pericytes in elderly patients. No morphologic substrate for increased nonspecific BBB permeability in the aging human was discovered, but the relative loss of pericytes suggested that the barrier in elderly individuals may be less able to compensate for transient leaks, which may in turn be important in the cellular pathogenesis of CAA.[206]

Major advances in understanding the biochemistry and molecular biology of AD A4 protein and A4P protein led to studies that had as their goal the establishment of simple diagnostic tests by which the clinical diagnosis of AD/SDAT could be confirmed by examining body fluids (blood or CSF) or extra-CNS tissues. Unfortunately, whereas serum levels of A4P were increased significantly above control levels in patients with Down syndrome, levels in patients with AD were similar to those in controls.[180] Soluble forms of the A4 amyloid precursor protein have been found in CSF and plasma.[150,161] A double antibody immunoradiometric assay for A4P in human plasma failed to show significant differences of A4P concentration in control patients as opposed to those with AD or Down syndrome.[153] Thus, the potential to use this radiometric assay to confirm a clinical suspicion of AD in a given patient seems remote. A recent investigation has been the first to demonstrate amyloid A4 or $\beta$-protein deposits in nonneural tissues and blood vessels of AD patients. Loci in which the A4 protein were found included the skin, subcutaneous tissues, and intestines.[93] The A4 or $\beta$-protein was present in these various locations in relatively small amounts, and unfortunately the protein could be detected in aged normal and aged diseased individuals without AD/SDAT as well as AD/SDAT patients, again suggesting that skin or gastrointestinal tract biopsy is unlikely to become a confirmatory diagnostic test in patients suspected to have AD or CAA.[93]

## POSSIBLE TREATMENT MODALITIES FOR CEREBRAL AMYLOID ANGIOPATHY

The brevity of this section will attest to the frustrations inherent in any attempt to diminish the severity of CAA in a given patient or arrest its progression. The first difficulty arises insofar as the amount of CAA in given patient cannot be realistically assessed during the patient's life using any currently available diagnostic modality. Possible future approaches to quantifying CAA in AD patients (during life) have been described in previous sections, but at the present time these are only theoretical possibilities. Unfortunately, the extent and severity of CAA can be assessed most accurately at necropsy, though the severity of the vascular change in a given topographic brain region can be substantially estimated from a generous brain biopsy. The treatment for CAA-related cerebral hemorrhage has been discussed in the first section of this chapter. Treatment strategies are likely to emerge as scientists gain a greater understanding of the relative importance of blood-borne versus brain-derived A4P in the formation of amyloid peptides within the CNS of AD patients, including microvascular localization of such peptides.[152] Advances are also likely to come as the specific events in peptide processing responsible for amyloid deposition (i.e., conversion of the A4P into the microvascular amyloidotic peptide) become better understood. The cellular localization of the putative proteases that have this hypothesized function is not currently known. Manipulation of such proteases, when they are discovered and their location becomes clear, is likely to yield to therapeutic strategies that can at least slow the deposition of microvascular brain amyloid if not lead to removal of the peptide from the blood vessel wall and thus diminish the likelihood of stroke from CAA-related microangiopathy. The possible role of novel methods of drug delivery to the brain is likely to impact on this process, though their role in potential amelioration of the effects of CAA or other forms of brain amyloid at the present time is purely speculative.[110]

## ACKNOWLEDGMENTS

I am grateful to Diana Lenard Secor and Gregory Nishimura for assistance with immunochemical studies, and to Dr. William M. Pardridge for extensive discussions. Carol Appleton and Stephen Kaufman prepared illustrations. Mr. Scott D. Brooks prepared and edited the final manuscript.

## REFERENCES

1. Abraham CR, Selkoe D, Potter H: Immunochemical identification of the serine protease inhibitor alpha 1-antichymotrypsin in the brain amyloid deposits of Alzheimer's disease. Cell 52:487, 1988
2. Ackerman RH, Richardson EP Jr, Heros RC: Case 49-1982. N Engl J Med 307:1507, 1982
3. Adam J, Crow TJ, Duchen LW: Familial cerebral amyloidosis and spongiform encephalopathy. J Neurol Neurosurg Psychiatry 45:37, 1982

4. Adams JH, Graham DI: Cerebrovascular disease. Recent Adv Histopathol 14:205, 1989
5. Allsop D, Ikeda S, Bruce M, Glenner GG: Cerebrovascular amyloid in scrapie-affected sheep reacts with antibodies to prion protein. Neurosci Lett 92:234, 1988
6. Awad IA, Johnson PC, Spetzler RF, Hodak JA: Incidental subcortical lesions identified on magnetic resonance imaging in the elderly. II. Postmortem pathological correlations. Stroke 17:1090, 1986
7. Awad IA, Spetzler RF, Hodak JA et al: Incidental subcortical lesions identified on magnetic resonance imaging in the elderly. I. Correlation with age and cerebrovascular risk factors. Stroke 17:1084, 1986
8. Babikian V, Ropper AH: Binswanger's disease: a review. Stroke 18:2, 1987
9. Ball MJ, Hachinski V, Fox A et al: A new definition of Alzheimer's disease: a hippocampal dementia. Lancet 1:14, 1985
10. Behrouz N, Defossez A, Delacourte A et al: Alzheimer's disease: glycolytic pretreatment dramatically enhances immunolabeling of senile plaques and cerebrovascular amyloid substance. Lab Invest 61:576, 1989
11. Behrouz N, Defossez A, Delacourte A et al: An antiserum to the N-terminal subsequence of the Alzheimer amyloid beta protein does not react with neurofibrillary tangles. J Gerontol 44:B156, 1989
12. Behrouz N, Defossez A, Delacourte A, Mazzuca M: Cortical beta-amyloid. Nature 344:497, 1990
13. Bell MA, Ball MJ: Neuritic plaques and vessels of visual cortex in aging and Alzheimer's dementia. Neurobiol Aging 11:359, 1990
14. Benedek S, McGovern VJ: A case of Alzheimer's disease with amyloidosis of the vessels of the cerebral cortex. Med J Aust 2:429, 1949
15. Bergeron C, Ranalli PJ, Miceli PN: Amyloid angiopathy in Alzheimer's disease. Can J Neurol Sci 14:564, 1987
16. Bird TD, Sumi SM, Nemens EJ et al: Phenotypic heterogeneity in familial Alzheimer's disease: a study of 24 kindreds. Ann Neurol 25:12, 1989
17. Bobin SA, Currie JR, Merz PA et al: The comparative immunoreactivities of brain amyloids in Alzheimer's disease and scrapie. Acta Neuropathol (Berl) 74:313, 1987
18. Briceno CE, Resch L, Bernstein M: Cerebral amyloid angiopathy presenting as a mass lesion. Stroke 18:234, 1987
19. Brown RT, Coates RK, Gilbert JJ: Radiographic-pathologic correlation in cerebral amyloid angiopathy: a review of 12 patients. J Can Assoc Radiol 36:308, 1985
20. Bruni J, Bilbao JM, Pritzker KPH: Vascular amyloid in the aging central nervous system: clinico-pathological study and literature review. Can J Neurol Sci 4:239, 1977
21. Brust JCM: Vascular dementia is overdiagnosed. Arch Neurol 45:799, 1988
22. Castaño EM, Frangione B: Human amyloidosis, Alzheimer disease and related disorders. Lab Invest 58:122, 1988
23. Castaño EM, Ghiso J, Prelli F et al: In vitro formation of amyloid fibrils from two synthetic peptides of different lengths homologous to Alzheimer's disease beta-protein. Biochem Biophys Res Commun 141:782, 1986
24. Chui HC: The significance of clinically defined subgroups of Alzheimer's disease. J Neural Transm [Suppl] 24:57, 1987
25. Cohen AS, Connors LH: The pathogenesis and biochemistry of amyloidosis. J Pathol 151:1, 1987
26. Cohen AS, Skinner M: New frontiers in the study of amyloidosis. N Engl J Med 323:542, 1990
27. Cohen DH, Feiner H, Jensson O et al: Amyloid fibril in hereditary cerebral hemorrhage with amyloidosis (HCHWA) is related to the gastroentero-pancreatic neuroendocrine protein, gamma trace. J Exp Med 158:623, 1983
28. Coria F, Castaño EM, Frangione B: Brain amyloid in normal aging and cerebral amyloid angiopathy is antigenically related to Alzheimer's disease beta-protein. Am J Pathol 129:422, 1987
29. Coria F, Castaño, E, Prelli F et al: Isolation and characterization of amyloid P component from Alzheimer's disease and other types of cerebral amyloidosis. Lab Invest 58:454, 1988
30. Coria F, Prelli F, Castaño EM et al: Beta-protein deposition: a pathogenetic link between Alzheimer's disease and cerebral amyloid angiopathies. Brain Res 463:187, 1988
31. Cork LC, Masters C, Beyreuther K, Price DL: Development of senile plaques: relationships of neuronal abnormalities and amyloid deposits. Am J Pathol 137:1383, 1990
32. Cosgrove GR, Leblanc R, Meagher-Villemure K, Ethier R: Cerebral amyloid angiopathy. Neurology (NY) 35:625, 1985
33. Davies L, Wolska B, Hilbich C et al: A4 amyloid protein deposition and the diagnosis of Alzheimer's disease: prevalence in aged brains determined by immunocytochemistry compared with conventional neuropathologic techniques. Neurology (NY) 38:1688, 1988
34. Dayan AD: Comparative neuropathology of ageing: studies on the brains of 47 species of vertebrates. Brain 94:31, 1971
35. Drayer BP: Imaging of the aging brain. I. Normal findings. Radiology 166:785, 1988
36. Drayer BP: Imaging of the aging brain. II. Pathologic conditions. Radiology 166:797, 1988
37. Drury I, Whisnant JP, Garraway WM: Primary intracerebral hemorrhage: impact of CT on incidence. Neurology (NY) 34:653, 1984
38. Dubas F, Gray F, Roullet E, Escourolle R: Leucoencéphalopathies artériopathiques. (17 cas anatomo-cliniques). Rev Neurol (Paris) 141:93, 1985
39. Duong T, Pommier EC, Scheibel AB: Immunodetection of the amyloid P component in Alzheimer's disease. Acta Neuropathol 78:429, 1989
40. Eikelenboom P, Stam FC: An immunohistochemical study on cerebral vascular and senile plaque amyloid in Alzheimer's dementia. Virchows Arch [Cell Pathol] 47:17, 1984
41. Englund E, Brun A, Alling C: White matter changes in dementia of Alzheimer's type: bio-

chemical and neuropathological correlates. Brain 111:1425, 1988
42. Ferreiro JA, Ansbacher LE, Vinters HV: Stroke related to cerebral amyloid angiopathy: the significance of systemic vascular disease. J Neurol 236:267, 1989
43. Fields WS: Multi-infarct dementia. Neurol Clin 4:405, 1986
44. Filloux FM, Townsend JJ: Congophilic angiopathy with intracerebral hemorrhage. West J Med 143:498, 1985
45. Finelli PF, Kessimian N, Bernstein PW: Cerebral amyloid angiopathy manifesting as recurrent intracerebral hemorrhage. Arch Neurol 41:330, 1984
46. Fisher CM: Binswanger's encephalopathy: a review. J Neurol 236:65, 1989
47. Franke CL, de Jonge J, van Swieten JC et al: Intracerebral hematomas during anticoagulant treatment. Stroke 21:726, 1990
48. Furlan AJ, Whisnant JP, Elveback LR: The decreasing incidence of primary intracerebral hemorrhage: a population study. Ann Neurol 5:367, 1979
49. Ghiso J, Jensson O, Frangione B: Amyloid fibrils in hereditary cerebral hemorrhage with amyloidosis of Icelandic type is a variant of gamma-trace basic protein (cystatin C). Proc Natl Acad Sci USA 83:2974, 1986
50. Ghiso J, Pons-Estel B, Frangione B: Hereditary cerebral amyloid angiopathy: the amyloid fibrils contain a protein which is a variant of cystatin C, an inhibitor of lysosomal cysteine proteases. Biochem Biophys Res Commun 136:548, 1986
51. Giaccone G, Verga L, Finazzi M et al: Cerebral preamyloid deposits and congophilic angiopathy in aged dogs. Neurosci Lett 114:178, 1990
52. Gilbert JJ, Vinters HV: Cerebral amyloid angiopathy: incidence and complications in the aging brain. I. Cerebral hemorrhage. Stroke 14:915, 1983
53. Gilles C, Brucher JM, Khoubesserian P, Vanderhaeghen JJ: Cerebral amyloid angiopathy as a cause of multiple intracerebral hemorrhages. Neurology (NY) 34:730, 1984
54. Gilmour JS, Bruce ME, Mackellar A: Cerebrovascular amyloidosis in scrapie-affected sheep. Neuropathol Appl Neurobiol 11:173, 1985
55. Ginsberg L, Geddes J, Valentine A: Amyloid angiopathy and granulomatous angiitis of the central nervous system: a case responding to corticosteroid treatment. J Neurol 235:438, 1988
56. Glenner GG: Amyloid deposits and amyloidosis: the beta-fibrilloses. N Engl J Med 302:1283, 1333, 1980
57. Glenner GG: On causative theories in Alzheimer's disease. Hum Pathol 16:433, 1985
58. Glenner GG: Alzheimer's disease. The commonest form of amyloidosis. Arch Pathol Lab Med 107:281, 1988
59. Glenner GG: Alzheimer's disease: its proteins and genes. Cell 52:307, 1988
60. Glenner GG, Henry JH, Fujihara S: Congophilic angiopathy in the pathogenesis of Alzheimer's degeneration. Ann Pathol 1:120, 1981
61. Glenner GG, Murphy MA: Amyloidosis of the nervous system. J Neurol Sci 94:1, 1989
62. Glenner GG, Wong CW: Alzheimer's disease and Down's syndrome: sharing of a unique cerebrovascular amyloid fibril protein. Biochem Biophys Res Commun 122:1131, 1984
63. Glenner GG, Wong CW: Alzheimer's disease: initial report of the purification and characterization of a novel cerebrovascular amyloid protein. Biochem Biophys Res Commun 120:885, 1984
64. Goldgaber D, Lerman MI, McBride OW et al: Characterization and chromosomal localization of a cDNA encoding brain amyloid of Alzheimer's disease. Science 235:877, 1987
65. Goren H, Steinberg MC, Farboody GH: Familial oculoleptomeningeal amyloidosis. Brain 103:473, 1980
66. Goust J-M, Mangum M, Powers JM: An immunologic assessment of brain-associated IgG in senile cerebral amyloidosis. J Neuropathol Exp Neurol 43:481, 1984
67. Gray F: L'angiopathie amyloïde cérébrale. Nouv Presse Med 18:1818, 1989
68. Gray F, Dubas F, Roullet E, Escourolle R: Leukoencephalopathy in diffuse hemorrhagic cerebral amyloid angiopathy. Ann Neurol 18:54, 1985
69. Gray F, Vinters HV, Le Noan H et al: Cerebral amyloid angiopathy and granulomatous angiitis: immunohistochemical study using antibodies to the Alzheimer A4 peptide. Hum Pathol 21:1290, 1990
70. Greene GM, Godersky JC, Biller J et al: Surgical experience with cerebral amyloid angiopathy. Stroke 21:1545, 1990
71. Griffiths RA, Mortimer TF, Oppenheimer DR, Spalding JMK: Congophilic angiopathy of the brain: a clinical and pathological report on two siblings. J Neurol Neurosurg Psychiatry 45:396, 1982
72. Grotta JC: Current medical and surgical therapy for cerebrovascular disease. N Engl J Med 317:1505, 1987
73. Grubb A, Jensson O, Gudmundsson G et al: Abnormal metabolism of gamma-trace alkaline microprotein: the basic defect in hereditary cerebral hemorrhage with amyloidosis. N Engl J Med 311:1547, 1984
74. Gudmundsson G, Hallgrímsson J, Jónasson TA, Bjarnason Ó: Hereditary cerebral haemorrhage with amyloidosis. Brain 95:387, 1972
75. Haan J, Algra PR, Roos RAC: Hereditary cerebral hemorrhage with amyloidosis–Dutch type: clinical and computed tomographic analysis of 24 cases. Arch Neurol 47:649, 1990
76. Hachinski VC, Lassen NA, Marshall J: Multi-infarct dementia: a cause of mental deterioration in the elderly. Lancet 2:207, 1974
77. Hardy JA, Mann DMA, Wester P, Winblad B: An integrative hypothesis concerning the pathogenesis and progression of Alzheimer's disease. Neurobiol Aging 7:489, 1986
78. Hart MN, Merz P, Bennett-Gray J et al: Beta-

amyloid protein of Alzheimer's disease is found in cerebral and spinal cord vascular malformations. Am J Pathol 132:167, 1988
79. Hauw J-J, Duyckaerts C, Delaere P, Chaunu MP: Hypothese: maladie d'Alzheimer, amyloïde, microglie et astrocytes. Rev Neurol (Paris) 144:155, 1988
80. Hawkins PN, Lavender JP, Pepys MB: Evaluation of systemic amyloidosis by scintigraphy with $^{123}$I-labeled serum amyloid P component. N Engl J Med 323:508, 1990
81. Hayman LA, Pagani JJ, Kirkpatrick JB, Hinck VC: Pathophysiology of acute intracerebral and subarachnoid hemorrhage: applications to MR imaging. AJNR 10:457, 1989
82. Heffner RR Jr, Porro RS, Olson ME, Earle KM: A demyelinating disorder associated with cerebrovascular amyloid angiopathy. Arch Neurol 33:501, 1976
83. Hinton DR, Dolan E, Sima AAF: The value of histopathological examination of surgically removed blood clot in determining the etiology of spontaneous intracerebral hemorrhage. Stroke 15:517, 1984
84. Ikeda S-I, Allsop D, Glenner GG: Morphology and distribution of plaque and related deposits in the brains of Alzheimer's disease and control cases: an immunohistochemical study using amyloid beta-protein antibody. Lab Invest 60:113, 1989
85. Inzitari D, Diaz F, Fox A et al: Vascular risk factors and leuko-araiosis. Arch Neurol 44:42, 1987
86. Ishihara T, Nagasawa T, Yokota T et al: Amyloid protein of vessels in leptomeninges, cortices, choroid plexuses, and pituitary glands from patients with systemic amyloidosis. Hum Pathol 20:891, 1989
87. Ishii N, Nishihara Y, Horie A: Amyloid angiopathy and lobar cerebral haemorrhage. J Neurol Neurosurg Psychiatry 47:1203, 1984
88. Janota I, Mirsen TR, Hachinski VC et al: Neuropathologic correlates of leuko-araiosis. Arch Neurol 46:1124, 1989
89. Jellinger K: Cerebral hemorrhage in amyloid angiopathy. Ann Neurol 1:604, 1977
90. Jellinger K: Cerebrovascular amyloidosis with cerebral hemorrhage. J Neurol 214:195, 1977
91. Jensson O, Gudmundsson G, Arnason A et al: Hereditary cystatin C (gamma-trace) amyloid angiopathy of the CNS causing cerebral hemorrhage. Acta Neurol Scand 76:102, 1987
92. Joachim CL, Duffy LK, Morris JH, Selkoe DJ: Protein chemical and immunocytochemical studies of meningovascular beta-amyloid protein in Alzheimer's disease and normal aging. Brain Res 474:100, 1988
93. Joachim CL, Mori H, Selkoe DJ: Amyloid beta-protein deposition in tissues other than brain in Alzheimer's disease. Nature 341:226, 1989
94. Joachim CL, Morris JH, Selkoe DJ: Clinically diagnosed Alzheimer's disease: autopsy results in 150 cases. Ann Neurol 24:50, 1988
95. Joachim CL, Selkoe DJ: Amyloid protein in Alzheimer's disease. J Gerontol 44:B77, 1989
96. Julien J, Vital C, Lagueny A et al: Hémorragie cérébrale récidivante et angiopathie amyloide. Rev Neurol (Paris) 139:763, 1983
97. Kalyan-Raman UP, Kalyan-Raman K: Cerebral amyloid angiopathy causing intracranial hemorrhage. Ann Neurol 16:321, 1984
98. Kang J, Lemaire H-G, Unterbeck A et al: The precursor of Alzheimer's disease amyloid A4 protein resembles a cell-surface receptor. Nature 325:733, 1987
99. Kase CS, Davis KR, Richardson EP Jr et al: Case 10-1988. N Engl J Med 318:623, 1988
100. Katzman R: Alzheimer's disease. N Engl J Med 314:964, 1986
101. Kawai M, Cras P, Siedlak S et al: Role of vascular smooth muscle cells in amyloid deposition in cerebral amyloid angiopathy. J Neuropathol Exp Neurol 49:331, 1990
102. Kawai M, Kalaria RN, Harik SI, Perry G: The relationship of amyloid plaques to cerebral capillaries in Alzheimer's disease. Am J Pathol 137:1435, 1990
103. Keohane C, Peatfield R, Duchen LW: Subacute spongiform encephalopathy (Creutzfeldt-Jakob disease) with amyloid angiopathy. J Neurol Neurosurg Psychiatry 48:1175, 1985
104. Khachaturian ZS: Diagnosis of Alzheimer's disease. Arch Neurol 42:1097, 1985
105. Kirschner DA, Inouye H, Duffy LK et al: Synthetic peptide homologous to beta protein from Alzheimer disease forms amyloid-like fibrils in vitro. Proc Natl Acad Sci USA 84:6953, 1987
106. Kisilevsky R: Theme and variations on a string of amyloid. Neurobiol Aging 10:499, 1989
107. Kitaguchi N, Takahashi Y, Tokushima Y et al: Novel precursor of Alzheimer's disease amyloid protein shows protease inhibitory activity. Nature 331:530, 1988
108. Kitamoto T, Ogomori K, Tateishi J, Prusiner SB: Methods in laboratory investigation: formic acid pretreatment enhances immunostaining of cerebral and systemic amyloids. Lab Invest 57:230, 1987
109. Kurucz J, Charbonneau R, Kurucz A, Ramsey P: Quantitative clinicopathologic study of cerebral amyloid angiopathy. J Am Geriatr Soc 29:61, 1981
110. Langer R: New methods of drug delivery. Science 249:1527, 1990
111. Lee S-S, Stemmermann GN: Congophilic angiopathy and cerebral hemorrhage. Arch Pathol Lab Med 102:317, 1978
112. Levy E, Carman MD, Fernandez-Madrid IJ et al: Mutation of the Alzheimer's disease amyloid gene in hereditary cerebral hemorrhage, Dutch type. Science 248:1124, 1990
113. Liston EH, La Rue A: Clinical differentiation of primary degenerative and multi-infarct dementia: a critical review of the evidence. I. Clinical studies. Biol Psychiatry 18:1451, 1983
114. Liston EH, La Rue A: Clinical differentiation of primary degenerative and multi-infarct dementia: a critical review of the evidence. II. Pathological studies. Biol Psychiatry 18:1467, 1983

115. Loes DJ, Biller J, Yuh WTC et al: Leukoencephalopathy in cerebral amyloid angiopathy: MR imaging in four cases. AJNR 11:485, 1990
116. Löfberg H, Grubb AO, Nilsson EK et al: Immunohistochemical characterization of the amyloid deposits and quantitation of pertinent cerebrospinal fluid proteins in hereditary cerebral hemorrhage with amyloidosis. Stroke 18:431, 1987
117. Love S, Duchen LW: Familial cerebellar ataxia with cerebrovascular amyloid. J Neurol Neurosurg Psychiatry 45:271, 1982
118. Luyendijk W, Bots GTAM, Vegter-van der Vlis M et al: Hereditary cerebral haemorrhage caused by cortical amyloid angiopathy. J Neurol Sci 85:267, 1988
119. Macdonald SM, Esiri MM: Monoclonal antibody binding to congophilic elements in human Alzheimer brain. J Clin Pathol 39:1199, 1986
120. Mandybur TI: The incidence of cerebral amyloid angiopathy in Alzheimer's disease. Neurology (NY) 25:120, 1975
121. Mandybur TI: Cerebral amyloid angiopathy: possible relationship to rheumatoid vasculitis. Neurology (NY) 29:1336, 1979
122. Mandybur TI: Cerebral amyloid angiopathy: the vascular pathology and complications. J Neuropathol Exp Neurol 45:79, 1986
123. Mandybur TI: Structural changes in cerebral vessels following amyloid deposition. Can J Neurol Sci 17:350, 1990
124. Mandybur TI, Balko G: Cerebral amyloid angiopathy with granulomatous angiitis ameliorated by steroid treatment. Can J Neurol Sci 17:344, 1990
125. Mandybur TI, Bates SRD: Fatal massive intracerebral hemorrhage complicating cerebral amyloid angiopathy. Arch Neurol 35:246, 1978
126. Mann DMA, Esiri MM: The site of the earliest lesions of Alzheimer's disease. N Engl J Med 318:789, 1988
127. Marotta CA, Chou W-G, Majocha RE et al: Overexpression of amyloid precursor protein A4 (beta-amyloid) immunoreactivity in genetically transformed cells: implications for a cellular model of Alzheimer amyloidosis. Proc Natl Acad Sci USA 86:337, 1989
128. Maruyama K, Ikeda S-I, Ishihara T et al: Immunohistochemical characterization of cerebrovascular amyloid in 46 autopsied cases using antibodies to beta protein and cystatin C. Stroke 21:397, 1990
129. Masliah E, Terry RD, Mallory M et al: Diffuse plaques do not accentuate synapse loss in Alzheimer's disease. Am J Pathol 137:1293, 1990
130. Masters CL, Simms G, Weinman NA et al: Amyloid plaque core protein in Alzheimer disease and Down syndrome. Proc Natl Acad Sci USA 82:4245, 1985
131. Masuda J, Tanaka K, Ueda K, Omae T: Autopsy study of incidence and distribution of cerebral amyloid angiopathy in Hisayama, Japan. Stroke 19:205, 1988
132. Michel B, Gastaut JL, Gambarelli D, Chave B: Hématomes intracérébraux lobaires récidivants au cours de l'angiopathie amyloïde cérébrale: un cas clinico-pathologique. Rev Neurol (Paris) 144:503, 1988
133. Miyakawa T, Sumiyoshi S, Murayama E, Deshimaru M: Ultrastructure of capillary plaque-like degeneration in senile dementia. Acta Neuropathol (Berl) 29:229, 1974
134. Müller-Hill B: Molecular biology of Alzheimer's disease. Annu Rev Biochem 58:287, 1989
135. Murphy MN, Sima AAF: Cerebral amyloid angiopathy associated with giant cell arteritis: a case report. Stroke 16:514, 1985
136. Nadeau SE: Stroke. Med Clin North Am 73:1351, 1989
137. Nadeau SE, Bebin J, Smith E: Nonspecific dementia, cortical blindness, and congophilic angiopathy: a clinicopathological report. J Neurol 234:14, 1987
138. Neumann MA: Combined amyloid vascular changes and argyrophilic plaques in the central nervous system. J Neuropathol Exp Neurol 19:370, 1960
139. O'Brien MD: Vascular dementia is underdiagnosed. Arch Neurol 45:797, 1988
140. Ogata J, Okayama M, Goto I et al: Primary familial amyloidosis with vitreous opacities: report of an autopsy case. Acta Neuropathol (Berl) 42:67, 1978
141. Ogomori K, Kitamoto T, Tateishi J et al: Beta-protein amyloid is widely distributed in the central nervous system of patients with Alzheimer's disease. Am J Pathol 134:243, 1989
142. Ohshima T, Endo T, Nukui H et al: Cerebral amyloid angiopathy as a cause of subarachnoid hemorrhage. Stroke 21:480, 1990
143. Ojemann RG, Heros RC: Spontaneous brain hemorrhage. Stroke 14:468, 1983
144. Okayama M, Goto I, Ogata J et al: Primary amyloidosis with familial vitreous opacities: an unusual case and family. Arch Intern Med 138:105, 1978
145. Okazaki H, Reagan TJ, Campbell RJ: Clinicopathologic studies of primary cerebral amyloid angiopathy. Mayo Clin Proc 54:22, 1979
146. Okoye MI, Watanabe I: Ultrastructural features of cerebral amyloid angiopathy. Hum Pathol 13:1127, 1982
147. Olszewski J: Subcortical arteriosclerotic encephalopathy: review of the literature on the so-called Binswanger's disease and presentation of two cases. World Neurol 3:359, 1962
148. Oltersdorf T, Fritz LC, Schenk DB et al: The secreted form of the Alzheimer's amyloid precursor protein with the Kunitz domain is protease nexin-II. Nature 341:144, 1989
149. Palmert MR, Podlisny MB, Witker DS et al: Antisera to an amino-terminal peptide detect the amyloid protein precursor of Alzheimer's disease and recognize senile plaques. Biochem Biophys Res Commun 156:432, 1988
150. Palmert MR, Podlisny MB, Witker DS et al: The beta-amyloid protein precursor of Alzheimer disease has soluble derivatives found in human brain and cerebrospinal fluid. Proc Natl Acad Sci USA 86:6338, 1989

151. Pantelakis S: Un type particulier d'angiopathie sénile du système nerveux central: l'angiopathie congophile: topographie et fréquence. Monatsschr Psychiatr Neurol 128:219, 1954
152. Pardridge WM: Amyloid angiopathy: future treatment strategies. p. 339. In Cummings JL, Miller BL (ed): Alzheimer's Disease: Treatment and Long-Term Management. Marcel Dekker, New York, 1990
153. Pardridge WM, Buciak JL, Yang J et al: Measurement of amyloid peptide precursor of Alzheimer disease in human blood by double antibody immunoradiometric assay. Alzheimer Dis Associated Disord 5:12, 1991
154. Pardridge WM, Vinters HV, Yang J et al: Amyloid angiopathy of Alzheimer's disease: amino acid composition and partial sequence of a 4,200-dalton peptide isolated from cortical microvessels. J Neurochem 49:1394, 1987
155. Patel DV, Hier DB, Thomas CM, Hemmati M: Intracerebral hemorrhage secondary to cerebral amyloid angiopathy. Radiology 151:397, 1984
156. Pendlebury WW, Iole ED, Tracy RP, Dill BA: Intracerebral hemorrhage related to cerebral amyloid angiopathy and t-PA treatment. Ann Neurol 29:210, 1991
157. Perl DP, Pendlebury WW: Neuropathology of dementia. Neurol Clin 4:355, 1986
158. Peterson EW, Schulz DM: Amyloid in vessels of a vascular malformation in brain. Arch Pathol 72:118, 1961
159. Picken MM, Larrondo-Lillo M, Coria F et al: Distribution of the protease inhibitor alpha 1-antichymotrypsin in cerebral and systemic amyloid. J Neuropathol Exp Neurol 49:41, 1990
160. Plant GT, Révész T, Barnard RO et al: Familial cerebral amyloid angiopathy with nonneuritic amyloid plaque formation. Brain 113:721, 1990
161. Podlisny MB, Mammen AL, Schlossmacher MG et al: Detection of soluble forms of the beta-amyloid precursor protein in human plasma. Bio chem Biophys Res Commun 167:1094, 1990
162. Ponte P, Gonzalez-DeWhitt P, Schilling J et al: A new A4 amyloid mRNA contains a domain homologous to serine proteinase inhibitors. Nature 331:525, 1988
163. Powers JM, Schlaepfer WW, Willingham MC, Hall BJ: An immunoperoxidase study of senile cerebral amyloidosis with pathogenetic considerations. J Neuropathol Exp Neurol 40:592, 1981
164. Prelli F, Castaño E, Glenner GG, Frangione B: Differences between vascular and plaque core amyloid in Alzheimer's disease. J Neurochem 51:648, 1988
165. Prelli F, Castaño EM, van Duinen SG et al: Different processing of Alzheimer's beta-protein precursor in the vessel wall of patients with hereditary cerebral hemorrhage with amyloidosis–Dutch type. Biochem Biophys Res Commun 151:1150, 1988
166. Price DL: New perspectives on Alzheimer's disease. Annu Rev Neurosci 9:489, 1986
167. Probst A, Heitz Ph U, Ulrich J: Histochemical analysis of senile plaque amyloid and amyloid angiopathy. Virchows Arch [A] 388:327, 1980
168. Probst A, Ulrich J: Amyloid angiopathy combined with granulomatous angiitis of the central nervous system: report on two patients. Clin Neuropathol 4:250, 1985
169. Prusiner SB: Prions and neurodegenerative diseases. N Engl J Med 317:1571, 1987
170. Ramsay DA, Penswick JL, Robertson DM: Fatal streptokinase-induced intracerebral haemorrhage in cerebral amyloid angiopathy. Can J Neurol Sci 17:336, 1990
171. Regli F, Vonsattel J-P, Perentes E, Assal G: L'angiopathie amyloïde cérébrale: une maladie cérébro-vasculaire peu connue: étude d'une observation anatomo-clinique. Rev Neurol (Paris) 137:181, 1981
172. Reid AH, Maloney AFJ: Giant cell arteritis and arteriolitis associated with amyloid angiopathy in an elderly Mongol. Acta Neuropathol (Berl) 27:131, 1974
173. Rengachary SS, Racela LS, Watanabe I, Abdou N: Neurosurgical and immunological implications of primary cerebral amyloid (congophilic) angiopathy. Neurosurgery 7:1, 1980
174. Robakis NK, Ramakrishna N, Wolfe G, Wisniewski HM: Molecular cloning and characterization of a cDNA encoding the cerebrovascular and the neuritic plaque amyloid peptides. Proc Natl Acad Sci USA 84:4190, 1987
175. Roberts GW, Lofthouse R, Allsop D et al: CNS amyloid proteins in neurodegenerative diseases. Neurology (NY) 38:1534, 1988
176. Roosen N, Martin J-J, de la Porte C, Van Vyve M: Intracerebral hemorrhage due to cerebral amyloid angiopathy: case report. J Neurosurg 63:965, 1985
177. Ropper AH, Davis KR: Lobar cerebral hemorrhages: acute clinical syndromes in 26 cases. Ann Neurol 8:141, 1980
178. Rowe IF, Jensson O, Lewis PD et al: Immunohistochemical demonstration of amyloid P component in cerebro-vascular amyloidosis. Neuropathol Appl Neurobiol 10:53, 1984
179. Rozemuller JM, Eikelenboom P, Stam FC et al: A4 protein in Alzheimer's disease: primary and secondary cellular events in extracellular amyloid deposition. J Neuropathol Exp Neurol 48:674, 1989
180. Rumble B, Retallack R, Hilbich C et al: Amyloid A4 protein and its precursor in Down's syndrome and Alzheimer's disease. N Engl J Med 320:1446, 1989
181. Salama J, Gherardi R, Amiel H et al: Post-anoxic delayed encephalopathy with leukoencephalopathy and non-hemorrhagic cerebral amyloid angiopathy. Clin Neuropathol 5:153, 1986
182. Scheinberg P: Dementia due to vascular disease—a multifactorial disorder. Stroke 19:1291, 1988
183. Schlote W: Die Amyloidnatur der kongophilen, drusigen Entartung der hirnarterien (Scholz) im Senium. Acta Neuropathol 4:449, 1965
184. Secor DL, Read SL, Frazee JG et al: Brain biopsies from patients with Alzheimer disease: im-

munohistochemical and ultrastructural study. J Neuropathol Exp Neurol 48:326, 1989
185. Selkoe DJ: Altered structural proteins in plaques and tangles: what do they tell us about the biology of Alzheimer's disease? Neurobiol Aging 7:425, 1986
186. Selkoe DJ: Aging, amyloid, and Alzheimer's disease. N Engl J Med 320:1484, 1989
187. Selkoe DJ: Amyloid beta protein precursor and the pathogenesis of Alzheimer's disease. Cell 58:611, 1989
188. Selkoe DJ: Biochemistry of altered brain proteins in Alzheimer's disease. Annu Rev Neurosci 12:493, 1989
189. Selkoe DJ: Deciphering Alzheimer's disease: the amyloid precursor protein yields new clues. Science 248:1058, 1990
190. Selkoe DJ, Abraham CR: Isolation of paired helical filaments and amyloid fibers from human brain. Methods Enzymol 134:388, 1986
191. Selkoe DJ, Bell DS, Podlisny MB et al: Conservation of brain amyloid proteins in aged mammals and humans with Alzheimer's disease. Science 235:873, 1987
192. Shaw C-M: Primary idiopathic cerebrovascular amyloidosis in a child. Brain 102:177, 1979
193. Shintaku M, Osawa K, Toki J et al: A case of granulomatous angiitis of the central nervous system associated with amyloid angiopathy. Acta Neuropathol (Berl) 70:340, 1986
194. Shirahama T, Skinner M, Westermark P et al: Senile cerebral amyloid: prealbumin as a common constituent in the neuritic plaque, in the neurofibrillary tangle, and in the microangiopathic lesion. Am J Pathol 107:41, 1982
195. Skinner M, Cohen AS: Amyloidosis: clinical, pathologic, and biochemical characteristics. p. 97. In Wagner BM, Fleischmajer R, Kaufman N (eds): Connective Tissue Diseases. IAP Monograph. Williams & Wilkins, Baltimore, 1983
196. Smith DB, Hitchcock M, Philpott PJ: Cerebral amyloid angiopathy presenting as transient ischemic attacks: case report. J Neurosurg 63:963, 1985
197. Snow AD, Lara S, Nochlin D, Wight TN: Cationic dyes reveal proteoglycans structurally integrated within the characteristic lesions of Alzheimer's disease. Acta Neuropathol 78:113, 1989
198. Snow AD, Mar H, Nochlin D et al: The presence of heparan sulfate proteoglycans in the neuritic plaques and congophilic angiopathy in Alzheimer's disease. Am J Pathol 133:456, 1988
199. Snow AD, Wight TN: Proteoglycans in the pathogenesis of Alzheimer's disease and other amyloidoses. Neurobiol Aging 10:481, 1989
200. Snow AD, Willmer JP, Kisilevsky R: Sulfated glycosaminoglycans in Alzheimer's disease. Hum Pathol 18:506, 1987
201. Sobel DF, Baker E, Anderson B, Kretzschmar H: Cerebral amyloid angiopathy associated with massive intracerebral hemorrhage. Neuroradiology 27:318, 1985
202. Stefansson K, Antel JP, Oger J et al: Autosomal dominant cerebrovascular amyloidosis: properties of peripheral blood lymphocytes. Ann Neurol 7:436, 1980
203. Steingart A, Hachinski VC, Lau C et al: Cognitive and neurologic findings in demented patients with diffuse white matter lucencies on computed tomographic scan (leuko-araiosis). Arch Neurol 44:36, 1987
204. Steingart A, Hachinski VC, Lau C et al: Cognitive and neurologic findings in subjects with diffuse white matter lucencies on computed tomographic scan (leuko-araiosis). Arch Neurol 44:32, 1987
205. Stern RA, Otvos L Jr, Trojanowski JQ, Lee VMY: Monoclonal antibodies to a synthetic peptide homologous with the first 28 amino acids of Alzheimer's disease beta-protein recognize amyloid and diverse glial and neuronal cell types in the central nervous system. Am J Pathol 134:973, 1989
206. Stewart PA, Magliocco M, Hayakawa K et al: A quantitative analysis of blood-brain barrier ultrastructure in the aging human. Microvasc Res 33:270, 1987
207. Stone MJ: Amyloidosis: a final common pathway for protein deposition in tissues. Blood 75:531, 1990
208. Surbek B: L'angiopathie dyshorique (Morel) de l'écorce cérébrale: étude anatomoclinique et statistique, aspect génétique. Acta Neuropathol 1:168, 1961
209. Tabaton M, Mandybur TI, Perry G et al: The widespread alteration of neurites in Alzheimer's disease may be unrelated to amyloid deposition. Ann Neurol 26:771, 1989
210. Tagliavini F, Ghiso J, Timmers WF et al: Coexistence of Alzheimer's amyloid precursor protein and amyloid protein in cerebral vessel walls. Lab Invest 62:761, 1990
211. Takahashi H, Hirokawa K, Tsukagoshi H: Immunohistological study on the distribution of alpha 1-antichymotrypsin in Alzheimer's brain, compared to beta-amyloid precursor protein and beta-amyloid protein. J Neurol Sci 99:301, 1990
212. Tanaka Y, Furuse M, Iwasa H et al: Lobar intracerebral hemorrhage: etiology and a long-term follow-up study of 32 patients. Stroke 17:51, 1986
213. Tanzi RE, Gusella JF, Watkins PC et al: Amyloid beta protein gene: cDNA, mRNA distribution, and genetic linkage near the Alzheimer locus. Science 235:880, 1987
214. Tanzi RE, McClatchey AI, Lamperti ED et al: Protease inhibitor domain encoded by an amyloid protein precursor mRNA associated with Alzheimer's disease. Nature 331:528, 1988
215. Tanzi RE, St George-Hyslop PH, Gusella JF: Molecular genetic approaches to Alzheimer's disease. TINS 12:152, 1989
216. Tomonaga M: Cerebral amyloid angiopathy in the elderly. J Am Geriatr Soc 29:151, 1981
217. Torack RM: Congophilic angiopathy complicated by surgery and massive hemorrhage: a light and electron microscopic study. Am J Pathol 81:349, 1975

218. Torack RM, Lynch RG: Cytochemistry of brain amyloid in adult dementia. Acta Neuropathol (Berl) 53:189, 1981
219. Trouillat R, Bogousslavsky J, Regli F, Uske A: Hémorragies intracérébrales supratentorielles. Schweiz Med Wochenschr 120:1056, 1990
220. Tucker WS, Bilbao JM, Klodawsky H: Cerebral amyloid angiopathy and multiple intracerebral hematomas. Neurosurgery 7:611, 1980
221. Tyler KL, Poletti CE, Heros RC: Cerebral amyloid angiopathy with multiple intracerebral hemorrhages. J Neurosurg 57:286, 1982
222. Ueda K, Hasuo Y, Kiyohara Y et al: Intracerebral hemorrhage in a Japanese community, Hisayama: incidence, changing pattern during long-term follow-up, and related factors. Stroke 19:48, 1988
223. Uitti RJ, Donat JR, Rozdilsky B et al: Familial oculoleptomeningeal amyloidosis: report of a new family with unusual features. Arch Neurol 45:1118, 1988
224. Ulrich G, Taghavy A, Schmidt H: Zur Nosologie und Ätiologie der kongophilen Angiopathie (Gefässform der cerebralen Amyloidose). Z Neurol 206:39, 1973
225. van Broeckhoven C, Haan J, Bakker E et al: Amyloid beta-protein precursor gene and hereditary cerebral hemorrhage with amyloidosis (Dutch). Science 248:1120, 1990
226. van Duinen SG, Castaño EM, Prelli F et al: Hereditary cerebral hemorrhage with amyloidosis in patients of Dutch origin is related to Alzheimer disease. Proc Natl Acad Sci USA 84:5991, 1987
227. Vanley CT, Aguilar MJ, Kleinhenz RJ, Lagios MD: Cerebral amyloid angiopathy. Hum Pathol 12:609, 1981
228. Vinters HV: Cerebral amyloid angiopathy: a critical review. Stroke 18:311, 1987
229. Vinters HV: Amyloid and the central nervous system: the neurobiology, genetics and immunocytochemistry of a process important in neurodegenerative diseases and stroke. p. 55. In Cancilla PA, Vogel FS, Kaufman N (eds): Neuropathology. Williams & Wilkins, Baltimore, 1990
230. Vinters HV, Gilbert JJ: Cerebral amyloid angiopathy: incidence and complications in the aging brain. II. The distribution of amyloid vascular changes. Stroke 14:924, 1983
231. Vinters HV, Hudson AJ, Kaufmann JCE: Gerstmann-Sträussler-Scheinker disease: autopsy study of a familial case. Ann Neurol 20:540, 1986
232. Vinters HV, Mah VH: Vascular diseases. p. 20. In Duckett S (ed): The Pathology of the Aging Human Nervous System. Lea and Febiger, Philadelphia, 1991
233. Vinters HV, Miller BL, Pardridge WM: Brain amyloid and Alzheimer disease. Ann Intern Med 109:41, 1988
234. Vinters HV, Nishimura GS, Secor DL, Pardridge WM: Immunoreactive A4 and gamma-trace peptide colocalization in amyloidotic arteriolar lesions in brains of patients with Alzheimer's disease. Am J Pathol 137:233, 1990
235. Vinters HV, Pardridge WM: The blood-brain barrier in Alzheimer's disease. Can J Neurol Sci 13:446, 1986
236. Vinters HV, Pardridge WM, Secor DL et al: Vascular dementia: immunocytochemical study of brain microvascular and parenchymal lesions associated with Alzheimer's disease. p. 213. In Ginsberg MD, Dietrich WD (eds): Cerebrovascular Diseases. Proceedings of the Sixteenth Research Conference. Raven Press, New York, 1989
237. Vinters HV, Pardridge WM, Secor DL, Ishii N: Immunohistochemical study of cerebral amyloid angiopathy. II. Enhancement of immunostaining using formic acid pretreatment of tissue sections. Am J Pathol 133:150, 1988
238. Vinters HV, Pardridge WM, Yang J: Immunohistochemical study of cerebral amyloid angiopathy: use of an antiserum to a synthetic 28-amino-acid peptide fragment of the Alzheimer's disease amyloid precursor. Hum Pathol 19:214, 1988
239. Vinters HV, Secor DL, Pardridge WM, Gray F: Immunohistochemical study of cerebral amyloid angiopathy. III. Widespread Alzheimer A4 peptide in cerebral microvessel walls colocalizes with gamma trace in patients with leukoencephalopathy. Ann Neurol 28:34, 1990
240. Vonsattel JP, Hedley-Whyte ET, Ropper AH, Richardson EP Jr: Coincidence of fibrinoid necrosis with amyloid angiopathy as the cause of cerebral hemorrhage. J Neuropathol Exp Neurol 43:316, 1984
241. Vuia O: Paraproteins and amyloidosis of the cerebral vessels and senile plaques. J Neurol Sci 39:37, 1978
242. Wagle WA, Smith TW, Weiner M: Intracerebral hemorrhage caused by cerebral amyloid angiopathy: radiographic-pathologic correlation. AJNR 5:171, 1984
243. Wakai S, Nagai M: Histological verification of microaneurysms as a cause of cerebral haemorrhage in surgical specimens. J Neurol Neurosurg Psychiatry 52:595, 1989
244. Walker LC, Masters C, Beyreuther K, Price DL: Amyloid in the brains of aged squirrel monkeys. Acta Neuropathol 80:381, 1990
245. Wattendorff AR, Bots GThAM, Went LN, Endtz LJ: Familial cerebral amyloid angiopathy presenting as recurrent cerebral haemorrhage. J Neurol Sci 55:121, 1982
246. Weisberg L: Multiple spontaneous intracerebral hematomas: clinical and computed tomographic correlations. Neurology (NY) 31:897, 1981
247. Westermark P, Shirahama T, Skinner M et al: Immunohistochemical evidence for the lack of amyloid P component in some intracerebral amyloids. Lab Invest 46:457, 1982
248. Whitson JS, Selkoe DJ, Cotman CW: Amyloid beta protein enhances the survival of hippocampal neurons in vitro. Science 243:1488, 1989
249. Wisniewski H, Johnson AB, Raine CS et al: Senile plaques and cerebral amyloidosis in aged dogs: a histochemical and ultrastructural study. Lab Invest 23:287, 1970

250. Wisniewski HM, Rabe A, Zigman W, Silverman W: Neuropathological diagnosis of Alzheimer disease. J Neuropathol Exp Neurol 48:606, 1989
251. Wong CW, Quaranta V, Glenner GG: Neuritic plaques and cerebrovascular amyloid in Alzheimer disease are antigenically related. Proc Natl Acad Sci USA 82:8729, 1985
252. Yamada M, Tsukagoshi H, Otomo E, Hayakawa M: Cerebral amyloid angiopathy in the aged. J Neurol 234:371, 1987
253. Yamada M, Tsukagoshi H, Otomo E, Hayakawa M: Systemic amyloid deposition in old age and dementia of Alzheimer type: the relationship of brain amyloid to other amyloid. Acta Neuropathol 77:136, 1988
254. Yamada M, Tsukagoshi H, Wada Y et al: Absence of the cystatin C amyloid in the cerebral amyloid angiopathy, senile plaque, and extra-CNS amyloid deposits of aged Japanese. Acta Neurol Scand 79:504, 1989
255. Yamaguchi H, Hirai S, Morimatsu M et al: A variety of cerebral amyloid deposits in the brains of the Alzheimer-type dementia demonstrated by beta protein immunostaining. Acta Neuropathol 76:541, 1988
256. Yankner BA, Dawes LR, Fisher S et al: Neurotoxicity of a fragment of the amyloid precursor associated with Alzheimer's disease. Science 245:417, 1989
257. Yong WH, Robert ME, Secor DL et al: Cerebral hemorrhage with biopsy-proven amyloid angiopathy Arch Neurol 49:51, 1992

# 33 ANTIPHOSPHOLIPID ANTIBODIES AND COAGULATION DISORDERS IN ISCHEMIC STROKE

Bruce M. Coull
Scott H. Goodnight

Activation of blood coagulation with thrombosis is an obligatory event in almost all ischemic strokes. The formation of thrombus, which precedes the acute stroke, most often ensues from the sudden and pathologic activation of hemostasis as may be found with endothelial injury within an atherosclerotic precerebral artery. Whereas many well-defined defects in hemostasis are associated with hemorrhagic stroke, most coagulation disorders that favor ischemic stroke remain less well characterized. The coagulation disturbances, however, which are associated with conditions predisposing to stroke, such as malignancy, perioperative states, infection, and pregnancy are now becoming better defined. Most often these coagulation abnormalities are a relatively nonspecific activation of coagulation, but in some instances certain distinct abnormalities of coagulation are known to predispose to vascular thrombotic events, including brain infarction. A predisposition to thrombotic events is often termed a "hypercoagulable" state by clinicians, but a better terminology when thrombosis is favored is a prethrombotic state, which may involve activated blood coagulation, increased platelets reactivity, or impaired fibrinalysis.[13]

## PATHOGENESIS OF THROMBOSIS

### Vascular Injury

As shown in Figure 33-1, prevention of intravascular thrombosis involves a dynamic interplay between the normal blood vessel and certain plasma proteins, platelets, fibrin formation, and fibrinolysis. Interactions between three plasma proteins, protein C, protein S, and antithrombin III (ATIII), and normal vascular endothelial cells form a particularly important barrier to thrombosis. A key glycoprotein, thrombomodulin, expressed on the endothelial surface, promotes the activation of protein C, a vitamin K-dependent plasma glycoprotein. When complexed with another potent natural anticoagulant, protein S, the activated protein C-S complex can rapidly destroy activated factors V and VIII. By blocking a plasminogen

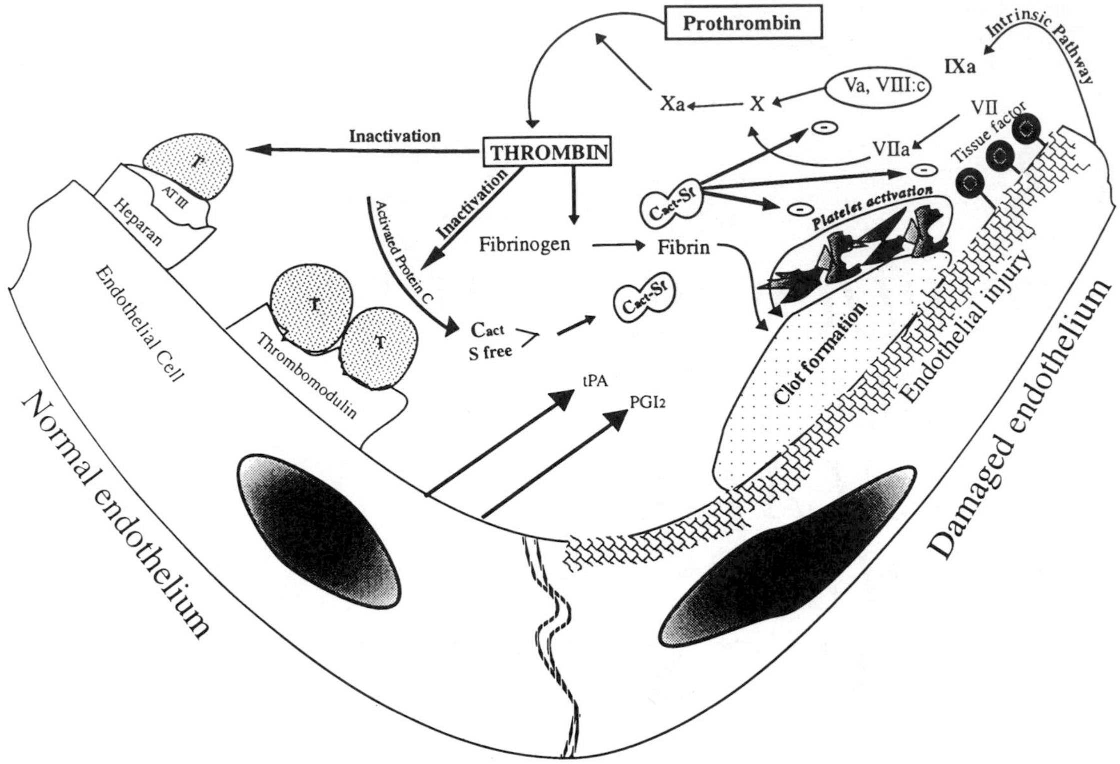


**Fig. 33-1.** When vascular endothelium is injured, clot formation is instigated by expression of tissue factor, and activation of platelets and the coagulation pathways. The pivotal reaction is transformation of prothrombin to thrombin (T) with cleavage of fibrinogen to fibrin. The normal endothelium limits thrombosis by inactivating thrombin, and by releasing prostacycline ($PGL_2$), and tissue plasminogen activator (tPA). Activated protein C (Cact) when complexed with free protein S (S free) antagonizes platelet and factor X activation. See text for details.

activator inhibitor (PAI-1), activated protein C may also have an indirect fibrinolytic effect. Protein S is found in the plasma as both an active (free) and an inactive (C4b binding protein bound) form. A glycosaminoglycan, heparan, is also widely distributed on the normal endothelial surface, which can bind and enhance the anticoagulant function of ATIII. Once bound to endothelial heparan, ATIII rapidly neutralizes the clotting enzyme thrombin, as well as activated factor X and other prothrombotic serine proteases.

Vascular endothelial cells may also inhibit platelet adhesion and platelet aggregation. When the endothelium is activated by local injury, inflammation, or other thrombogenic stimuli, prostacyclin ($PGI_2$), which causes vasodilation and inhibits platelet plug formation, may be released. Under appropriate circumstances, blood vessels may also markedly enhance local fibrinolysis via the synthesis and release of tissue plasminogen activator (tPA).

Although usually a barrier against thrombosis, the normal vascular endothelium may become a potent stimulus to thrombosis when injured. Mediators of inflammation such as interleukin 1(IL-1), tumor necrosis factor (TNF), and immune complexes may induce endothelial cells to express tissue factor, expose binding sites for clotting factors, and downregulate thrombomodulin expression.[42,62,134] With more severe injury, endothelial cells may be lost from the vascular surface altogether. For example, the rupture of an atherosclerotic plaque within a carotid or vertebral artery may expose a thrombogenic surface which promotes mural thrombus formation. The ultimate size of the intravascular clot may be limited by the antithrombotic potential of the surrounding intact endothelium. A similar sequence of events may occur within damaged cerebral arterioles or an abnormal structure in the heart. Platelets and fibrin rapidly accumulate at the area of vascular injury leading to arterial occlusion and/or cerebral thromboembolism with stroke.

## Antithrombin III, Protein C, and Protein S Deficiencies

### Hereditary Deficiencies

Hereditary deficiencies of ATIII, protein C, and protein S are identified by various laboratory assays showing either low concentrations of the protein or low functional activity (e.g., 50 percent or less).[14,42] Both activity and concentration may be required, since some antigenic assays do not detect mutations producing dysfunctional molecules. Since there are multiple categories of protein S deficiency, both the free and bound forms should be measured.[41] Hereditary ATIII deficiency occurs in roughly 1:2,000 to 1:5,000 people and is three to seven times less common than hereditary protein C or protein S deficiency. About 20 percent of patients with prior venous thrombosis or with a strong family history of thromboemboli will be found to have a deficiency of one of these natural anticoagulant proteins.[40] The prevalence of stroke among persons with hereditary deficiencies of these proteins is unknown, but children and young adults seem to be most often affected. In young subjects whose anticoagulant proteins are reduced or dysfunctional, TIAs, amaurosis fugax, and occlusive arterial strokes have all been reported, but a predisposition to cerebral venous thrombosis appears to be more common.[4,22,48,58,96,107,120,161,182] It is likely, moreover, that the genetic abnormalities that produce the partial reductions in levels of anticoagulant proteins may thereby produce a prethrombotic state.[13] The risks of thrombotic events in persons with lesser deficiencies of ATIII, protein C, or protein S, probably as a consequence of aging, the use of oral contraceptives or pregnancy, tobacco abuse, or following surgery may also be increased.[93]

### Acquired Deficiencies

Acquired deficiencies of ATIII and proteins C and S, have also been reported to produce a prethrombotic state related to brain infarction.[51] Although extensive epidemiologic studies have not yet been performed, acquired anticoagulant protein deficiencies usually are associated with stroke in special clinical settings. Many of these clinical situations are outlined Table 33-1. Reduced levels of the anticoagulant proteins have been found in perioperative settings in women who are pregnant or taking oral contraceptives, and in patients with malignancies, hepatic failure, or the nephrotic syndrome.[104] Acute fluctuations of anticoagulant protein levels can also follow plasmapheresis and hemodialysis. When TIA, stroke, or amaurosis fugax is encountered in patients with any of these conditions, careful evaluation may uncover one of these prethrombotic states.

The contributions of the anticoagulant proteins to the pathogenesis of stroke remain to be clarified. Two studies, one of them retrospective, have failed to document deficiencies in the natural anticoagulant proteins in most patients who experience stroke.[37,131] A recent prospective study found free protein S deficiency in 23 percent of young patients with stroke of uncertain cause.[154] All but one patient in this series were under age 55. In another prospective study D'Angelo and colleagues[50] reported that a reduced protein C level measured at the time of acute stroke was correlated with a poor outcome, but no differences in ATIII levels were found between survivors and nonsurvivors of stroke. To date, there has not been a prospective examination of the possible relationship between acquired long-term deficiencies of these antithrombotic proteins and the occurrence of stroke.

**TABLE 33-1. Acquired Deficiencies of Antithrombin III and Proteins C and S**

| |
|---|
| Consumption coagulopathy |
| Disseminated intravascular coagulation (shock, sepsis) |
| Surgery |
| Preeclampsia |
| Liver dysfunction |
| Acute hepatic failure |
| Cirrhosis |
| Renal disease |
| Nephrotic syndrome |
| Hemolytic-uremic syndrome |
| Malignancies |
| Leukemia (acute promyelocytic leukemia) |
| Malnutrition or gastrointestinal loss |
| Vascular reconstruction (diabetes, age) |
| Protein-calorie deprivation |
| Inflammatory bowel disease |
| Drugs |
| Estrogens-progestins |
| Heparin |
| L-asparginase |
| Other |
| Vasculitis (? systemic lupus erythematosis) |
| Infection-neutropenia |
| Hemodialysis |
| Plasmapheresis |

## Reduced Blood Flow

Sluggish or reduced cerebral blood flow as seen with tight carotid stenosis, severe congestive heart failure, or with increased blood viscosity may greatly enhance the likelihood of stroke. Many clinical studies have demonstrated abnormalities of blood viscosity parameters in persons with TIA and stroke, but the relationship of high blood viscosity to activation of platelets or coagulation remains unknown.[61,78,157] Most studies suggest that the effects of severe atherosclerosis, cardiac failure, or hemorheologic abnormalities on blood coagulation are likely to be a nonspecific augmentation.[44,68,140,179] Furthermore, in circumstances of reduced blood flow, the supply of inhibitors such as ATIII or protein C from inflowing blood to an area of local vascular or brain injury will be reduced, and activated clotting factors may tend to accumulate rather than being washed away into the circulation where they can be cleared by the liver.

## Activated Clotting Factors

Clotting proteins such as prothrombin or factor X normally circulate in their nonactivated or zymogen form. However, certain stimuli may convert them to an activated state, greatly increasing the possibility of thrombosis. Examples include surgical procedures, tissue necrosis due to infarction, malignancy, infections, or inflammatory reactions with the release of thrombogenic cytokines such as interleukin 1 or tumor necrosis factor. The acute and chronic reactions to these stimuli may alter the plasma concentrations of clotting proteins.[44] Epidemiologic studies suggest that high concentrations of fibrinogen, and excess concentrations of factor V, factor VIII coagulant activity (VIII:C), and factor VII may all be risk factors for stroke, but their role is ischemic brain infarction remains uncertain,[102,171,180] as illustrated in the upper portion of Figure 33-1.

### Fibrinolytic Defects

The fibrinolysis balance may be depressed in patients with cerebrovascular disease leading to an increased likelihood or thrombosis. Feinberg and colleagues[66] found evidence of increased thrombin activity for 4 weeks after acute stroke, whereas endogenous fibrinolytic activity was either inhibited or slowed. Most often decreased fibrinolytic activity is a result of increased levels of plasminogen activator inhibitor (PAI-1). For example, a group of young men have been shown to have increased PAI-1 levels, following myocardial infarction but systematic studies in stroke have not been performed.[82] Recently, a newly appreciated atherogenic lipoprotein, Lp(a), has been shown to inhibit fibrinolysis in vitro. Lp(a) has substantial structural homology with plasminogen, the precursor to the fibrinolytic enzyme plasmin. Lp(a) has been shown to stimulate the release of PAI-1 from endothelial cells, and to effectively compete with plasminogen for binding either to fibrin or to the surface of vascular endothelial cells, inhibiting fibrinolysis.[63,80] Lp(a) levels have recently been found to be elevated in selected populations with cerebrovascular disease.[98,184,186]

### Heightened Platelet Reactivity

The concept that increased platelet reactivity may contribute to arterial thrombosis has not been thoroughly tested, in part due to the lack of sensitive and specific laboratory assays for platelet activation. However, patients with extensive peripheral atherosclerosis have been shown to have increased platelet-vascular interactions as evidenced by the excretion of increased quantities of platelet and vascular prostaglandin metabolites in the urine.[70] Enhanced platelet reactivity has also been found in patients with acute stroke and TIA.[55,158] Patients with marked hypercholesterolemia were reported several years ago to have increased platelet reactivity, as measured by an increased sensitivity to platelet aggregating agents such as epinephrine.[36] Finally, several studies have suggested that essential thrombocythemia, a myeloproliferative disease in which platelets are sometimes large and hyperreactive is frequently associated with stroke.[97,136]

### Antiphospholipid Antibodies

Antiphospholipid antibodies (aPL), including the lupus anticoagulant (LA) and anticardiolipin antibodies (aCL), are associated with both arterial and venous thromboses that have been reported to involve virtually every organ in the body.[86,116,117,118,155] This association is particularly well established for stroke and TIA.[10,30,87,89,113] The LA is defined by the prolongation of phospholipid-dependent coagulation tests such as the activated partial thromboplastin time (APTT), which is not due to a coagulation factor deficiency. An aPL that affects coagulation tests in this manner is termed a LA. Bowie et al.[21,23] first recognized that patients with LA developed thrombotic complications despite the presence of "circulating anticoagulants," an observation now amply confirmed by others. The LA rarely produces a bleeding tendency, even in surgical patients.[122,123,156,159] Another assay for aPL employs cardiolipin as an antigen in an enzyme-linked immunosorbent assay (ELISA).[85,115] Although aCL and LA are both aPL, they are clearly distinct antibodies that can be separated using a polyacrylamide gel-phospholipid affinity column.[64,127]

## EPIDEMIOLOGY

Despite many case reports, the prevalence of aPL in unselected patients with cerebrovascular disease remains unknown, but some data are available for selected populations. Most studies suggest a prevalence of 2 to 5 percent, but if very sensitive tests are used, antiphospholipid antibodies may be found in up to 16 percent of normal people with quite variable frequencies in elderly subjects.[57,67,122,160] aPL antibodies are often detected in patients with rheumatic diseases such as systemic lupus erythematosus (SLE), Sjögren syndrome, Behçet syndrome, mixed connective tissue disease, rheumatoid arthritis, and autoimmune thrombocytopenia purpura.[81,88,116,121,165] The frequency of aPL in SLE is about 40 percent with concordance of both the LA and aCL in 45 to 70 percent of these patients.[116] In a series of retrospective analyses, the presence of LA or aCL in SLE patients imparted a significant increased frequency of thrombosis.[128] In one series of more than 1,000 patients with SLE, neurologic disorders were strongly associated with the presence of either the LA or aCL.[116] The association of aPL with thrombosis in patients without a clear diagnosis of an autoimmune disorder has been termed the *primary antiphospholipid antibody syndrome*.[8,118]

Although patients with aPL most often experience venous thrombosis, arterial thrombosis is likely to involve the brain.[11,30,87,89,113] Briley and colleagues[30] found that in 80 subjects with aPL, 25 (31 percent), had neurologic symptoms caused by cerebral ischemia. In this study the patients with neurologic dysfunction were young, with an average age of 42 years. Depending upon the sensitivity of the tests employed, the prevalence of aPL in young patients with stroke varied from 4 to 46 percent.[27,89] Trimble et al.[173] found aPL in 3 of 51 (6 percent) unselected stroke patients whose ages ranged from 17 to 78 years. Hess and colleagues,[92] in a prospective study of 110 patients (average age 58 years), who were admitted to a single medical center with a diagnosis of stroke or TIA, found an 8.2 percent prevalence of IgG aCL, compared to 1.6 percent in age-matched healthy blood donors. Only a few studies have been published of stroke recurrence or mortality rates in subjects with aPL. In one small study with limited numbers of young patients, the yearly stroke rate was 6.75 percent, with an estimated stroke recurrence rate of 13 to 14 percent.[111] Mortality was estimated to be as much as 10 percent per year.[111] Taken together, these reports suggest that aPL may be present in roughly 10 percent of all strokes, and that the association is greater for stroke in the young, and especially in subjects with unexplained recurrent stroke. aPL may be found in high prevalence in other select populations with stroke such as those with rheumatic diseases, and underlying human immunodeficiency virus (HIV) or *Mycoplasma pneumoniae* infections.[19,60,164,168]

## CLINICAL ASPECTS

Stroke and TIA with rather variable presentations have been reported in persons with aPL.[11,30,87,111,113] Thromboses have involved large and small arteries and veins in both the anterior and posterior circulations. Especially common are visual disturbances and ischemic eye or optic nerve events.[23,49,56,76,111] Amaurosis fugax, retinal vein or artery occlusion, ischemic retinopathy and ophthalmoplegia from a cranial neuropathy and migrainelike positive or negative visual phenomena, with or without headache, have all been reported. Although deep lacunar infarctions and isolated white matter signal-enhancing lesions on magnetic resonance imaging (MRI) scanning and large brain infarctions occur, most strokes are relatively small and involve cortex and subadjacent white matter. No single mechanism for stroke associated with aPL has been established, but a few pathologic reports have demonstrated nonspecific microvascular platelet-fibrin plugs, suggesting possible thrombosis in situ.[52] However, cardiac lesions, including mitral-valve degeneration and nonbacterial thrombotic endocarditis, often accompany the aPL syndrome and could be responsible for these lesions as well.[6,9]

Several more or less well-defined stroke syndromes, such as Sneddon syndrome and vascular dementia, are particularly characteristic of aPL-related stroke, but atypical migraine, encephalopathy, chorea, epilepsy, and myelopathy have also been reported.[112,113] Sneddon syndrome, with stroke and livedo reticularis of the skin in the absence of systemic disease is a commonly encountered aPL relationship.[31,45,99,112,163] Besides livedo reticularis, patients often have Raynaud's phenomenon and demonstrate acrocyanosis. Recent reports indicate that Sneddon syndrome is more common in women then in men and tobacco use is frequent in both. In one case, skin biopsy demonstrated focal epidermal ulceration with chronic inflammatory infiltrates in the dermis, without evidence of vasculitus.[112] Despite various treatments, vascular dementia often ensues in patients with this syndrome. While not all subjects with Sneddon syndrome harbor aPL, it appears likely that these antibodies are often present among persons with Sneddon syndrome who go on to develop dementia.[31] This view is coincident with data of Kalashnikova et al., which showed increased disability in patients with aPL.[99]

As in Sneddon syndrome, recurrent stroke and vascular dementia are a feared consequence of aPL. Literally dozens of patients with aPL and vascular dementia have now been reported.[11,29,45] These subjects distinguish themselves by a typically younger age than the general stroke population with multi-infarction dementia, and by higher aPL levels than less symptomatic cohorts. In a recent report of 29 subjects with vascular dementia and aPL, the average age of 52 years was a decade younger than aPL negative subjects with vascular dementia.[29] These aPL positive subjects also had fewer stroke risk factors than the cohort of older subjects. Several cases have been documented in which cognitive deterioration progressed in the absence of a history of strokelike episodes and despite antithrombotic therapy. This clinical course is reminiscent of the insights of both Sneddon[163] and Rebollo et al.[147a] who emphasized that stroke with Sneddon syndrome often left little neurologic deficit, but the patients gradually became demented nonetheless. Unfortunately, except for the possible relationship to high aPL levels, no specific findings identify those subjects who experience recurrent ischemic events and progressive decline in intellectual function.

The vast majority of migraineurs do not have aPL or aPL-related features. However, many subjects with aPL describe prominent migrainelike headaches and visual symptoms.[24,30,113] The patient with typical migraine does not require laboratory screening for aPL, but further evaluation is warranted when the clinical course is complicated by symptoms such as monocular amaurosis or other monocular visual disturbances, when a hemisensory syndrome is present, or when small infarctions or white matter signal-enhancing lesions are seen on computed tomography (CT) or MRI. Patients with SLE or other connective tissue disorders who have thrombocytopenia and migrainelike headache should also be considered for evaluation. Unlike typical migraine, headaches with aPL are often a relatively recent onset. In addition, the subjects may complain of vertigo and fail to respond to typical migraine prophylaxes.

Seizures, both focal and generalized, are occasionally encountered[94,113] in patients with aPL who do not have a prior history of stroke. It is possible that in some of these cases aPL was induced by the anticonvulsant drugs themselves. Nevertheless, most seizures are probably of ischemic origin. Certain syndromes seem to have a predilection for seizures or epilepsy. Thus, in one retrospective series of patients with aPL and dementia the prevalence of epilepsy was higher than in aPL negative dementia, or individuals with aPL and less severe symptoms.[29] Generalized seizures and status epileptics are a cardinal feature of the syndrome of ischemic encephalopathy, which includes altered mental status, diffuse systemic involvement of pulmonary and cardiac function and dermatologic manifestations.[30,95]

Myelopathy, especially in patients with SLE, has been associated with the aPL syndrome, and may have a clinical presentation indistinguishable from the myelopathic form of multiple sclerosis.[73,111] Hence the term "lupoid sclerosis" has been suggested for this entity.[95] One peculiar form of dermatologic disease associated with myelopathy, brain infarction, and dementia is the Kohlmeier-Degos syndrome. The vascular pathology appears to be identical to that described in Sneddon and other aPL syndromes, where the skin signs are[53,59,110] characterized by papules with a porcelain-white center distributed over the trunk and extremities. This illness has a predilection for men, unlike Sneddon syndrome, and may frequently involve the gastrointestinal trait as well as the central nervous system.

## EFFECTS OF ANTIPHOSPHOLIPID ANTIBODIES ON THE COAGULATION SYSTEM

The pathologic features of microvascular occlusion by platelet fibrin plugs observed in patients with aPL suggest that endothelial cell reactions may be implicated in the production of thromboses. This notion would be supported by observations that some aPL bind to endothelial cells in vitro,[90,176,177] although in vivo binding seems unlikely, since negatively changed phospholipids are located on the inner surface of the cell membrane. aPL might alter normal endothelial cell function so that the surface promotes rather than retards thrombosis. Specific endothelial cell activation functions such as prostacyclin ($PGI_2$) production, antithrombin III, or placental anticoagulant protein (PAP) binding, the proteins C and S, complement activation, or fibrinolysis are all possible targets for aPL.[33–35,43,132,138] Cariou and colleagues have demonstrated that sera from patients with LA interferes with the activation of protein C,[33,34] and others have shown that aPL may inhibit the ability of protein C to destroy the clotting factors Va. Protein S deficiency has been observed in a few patients with LA, but this has been an inconsistent finding.[132] Other studies have suggested that LA binds to thrombomodulin and thereby interferes with the protein C-S complex.[43,177] So far, there is little evidence that ATIII is involved in aPL-mediated thromboses.[46,138]

Although the role of placental anticoagulant proteins (PAP) in the regulation of coagulation within the cerebral microcirculation is uncertain, competitive inhibition of PAP by aPL is postulated.[69,148,170] Thus, the pathologic role of aPL in thrombosis may occur after protein C activation,[5,71,72] and more than one action in the functional pathway of proteins C and S may be impaired by interactions with aPL. This issue may ultimately be resolved as more is learned about $\beta_2$-glycoprotein I.[74,124,129,138] This glycoprotein appears to be a target antigen for anticardiolipin antibodies, and may also play an important role in the inhibition of coagulation and platelet activation.

### Platelets

Platelet membrane is another possible target for aPL binding, since platelet membranes are rich in phospholipids, and thrombocytopenia is frequently found during thrombotic episodes associated with aPL.[105,174] An indirect relationship between aPL levels and platelet count has been reported. One study found binding of aPL to several platelet phospholipids when platelet membranes were disrupted, but no binding was found to intact platelets.[75] A recent study found that the urinary secretion of prostoglandin metabolites (i.e., thromboxan and prostacyclin) were increased in a group of patients with aPL, suggested chronic platelet activation in those individuals.

### Complement Activation

Some aPL have been known to bind complement.[52] Low levels of C3 and C4, have been observed in patients with aPL and thrombosis implying depletion of these factors during complement activation.[91] Davis and Brey[52] described a significant increase in complement activation in young stroke patients with aPL compared to those without these antibodies. Thus, complement activation occurs in young stroke patients with aPL, but its relationship to thrombosis remains unknown.

## DIAGNOSIS OF THE ANTIPHOSPHOLIPID ANTIBODY SYNDROME

A diagnosis of the primary antiphospholipid antibody syndrome may be established by both clinical and laboratory findings. Prominent systemic manifes-

**TABLE 33-2. Laboratory Findings**

| |
|---|
| Coombs test: positive (hemolytic anemia) |
| Thrombocytopenia |
| Positive ANA test (low titer) |
| False-positive VDRL test |
| Antimitochondrial antibodies (type M5) |
| Reduced serum complement C4 level |
| Prolonged phospholipid-dependent coagulation tests (aPTT,PT) |

*Abbreviations:* ANA, antinuclear antibodies; VDRL, Venereal Disease Research Laboratory; aPTT, activated partial thromboplastin time; PT, prothrombin time.

tations include livedo reticularis, cardiac value lesions, pulmonary hypertension, adrenal insufficiency and a history of spontaneous abortion in women. The laboratory features that are most consistently associated with aPL are listed in Table 33-2. Young patients with stroke or patients of any age who lack a clear cause for their ischemic cerebrovascular symptoms should be tested for aPL. Likewise, aPL testing should be obtained if the laboratory features shown in Table 33-2 are present in stroke patients. To identify aPL, both aCL and LA assays should be used, since these immunoglobulins have different specificities and antigenic recognition sites.[64,127] The concordance of aPL and LA among patients with aPL are not 100 percent. For example, when aCL is present, LA coexist in approximately 50 percent and, conversely, when the LA is present, aCL activity can be detected in approximately 70 to 80 percent.[3] It still remains unclear, however, whether the association with thrombosis is stronger with the LA or aCL. Several assays of various sensitivity and specificity are currently available to test individual patients for the presence of aPL.[65,114]

## TREATMENT OF ANTIPHOSPHOLIPID ANTIBODY SYNDROME

Not only is it now known whether treatment of any kind benefits patients with aPL, the "natural history" of patients with aPL, whether or not they have experienced cerebral ischemic event, is ill-defined. Some individuals with aPL remain asymptomatic, whereas other experience recurring stroke and subsequently become severely demented or disabled. Unfortunately, there are few hard and fast rules for approaching treatment of patients with aPL at the present time. Thrombotic events are probably more likely when aCL levels are high, when aCL and the LA coexist, or when SLE or other connective tissue disease is present.

Patients with aPL should most certainly receive treatment for coexisting risk factors, such as hypertension and cigarette smoking, since these may very likely contribute to a worse prognosis. Subjects with minimal symptoms or a single mild event can be given aspirin treatment, although the optimal dose is unknown. Patients who experience serious or recurrent events, or who have livedo reticularis, high levels particularly of the IgG aCL or multiple antibody types, including both the LA and aCL, should be considered for oral anticoagulant therapy. Warfarin treatment may be particularly useful in subjects with cardiac vascular lesions or other evidence for cardiac emboli.

The LA can sometimes be suppressed with prednisone, but aCL is often not steroid responsive. In patients who experience recurrent cerebral ischemic events despite warfarin therapy, prednisone or other forms of immunosuppressive therapy might be considered, although there is no evidence as yet that this form of therapy may prevent thromboses. Other treatments may be directed at coexisting SLE or other connective tissue diseases diagnosed by the American Rheumatologic Association criteria.[172] For subjects who experience acute encephalopathy seizures or disseminated coagulation, plasmaphoresis and immunosuppression therapy has been of apparent benefit in a few instances.[95]

## HEPARIN-ASSOCIATED THROMBOCYTOPENIA

Heparin-associated thrombocytopenia (HAT) may provide some additional insight into immune mechanisms that promote thrombosis. There are several forms of HAT of which so-called type II has been associated with arterial thrombosis.[7] Individuals developing this syndrome experience a high risk for arterial thrombotic events, including stroke, and a high mortality rate.[16,106] HAT is often encountered in postsurgical settings. Atkinson and Sundt and colleagues[12] have emphasized the relationship between HAT and ischemic stroke after carotid endarterectomy. Somewhere between 5 and 10 percent of patients who receive heparin develop thrombocytopenia, but the incidence of arterial thrombosis as a result of heparin treatment is no more than 1 to 2 percent. In a typical case, moderate to severe thrombocytopenia develops 5 to 10 days after heparin therapy is instituted for the first time. Although platelet counts may fall as low as 20,000/cu mm, with HAT, hemorrhagic complications are relatively uncommon. Cines and colleagues,[38] who studied sera from 27 patients with this syndrome, suggested that the HAT antibody may bind to the heparan on the surface of endothelial cells and stimulate the production of tissue factor on the endothelial cell surface. Becker and Miller[15] have reviewed 29 patients with HAT-related stroke reported in the literature. Few of these patients had previous cerebrovascular disease and most patients either died (25 percent) or remained severely disabled from their strokes. Cerebral venous thrombosis has also been reported with HAT.[109]

## HOMOCYSTINURIA AND HOMOCYSTEINEMIA

Homocystinuria and probably mild homocysteinemia are independent risk factors for ischemic stroke. In homocystinuria, the 20-fold or more increases in plasma homocysteine, homocystine, and cysteine-homocysteine mixed disulfide produce the well-recognized complications of premature atherosclerosis and brain infarction from carotid or other large intracranial arterial occlusions.[134,135] Recent studies now indicate that modest (2 to 5 times) increases in plasma homocysteine also impart a significant risk for stroke.[18,20,25,47,118] Usually one of several inborn errors of metabolism that impair cystathionine β-synthase (CBS) or other of the related enzyme systems for methionine metabolism that cause homocystinuria (Fig. 33-2). As autosomal recessive traits, persons homozygous for CBS deficiency usually experience premature atherosclerosis and thromboembolic complications including stroke by age 30. Children with homocystinuria often have abnormalities of the eye, vascular, skeletal, and nervous systems. Thus a marfanoid habitus with arm spans greater than body height, setting-sun lenticular dislocations and cognitive impairment, malar flush, and livedo reticularis may be present, but these are not consistent features.[32,134] About 0.3 to 1.5 percent of the general population may be heterozygous for CBS deficiency, and the estimated incidence of homocystinuria is approximately 1 in 332,000 live births.[20,134] In obligate heterozygotes, CBS activity is reduced by 50 percent.

Although controversial, in the absence of elevated plasma homocysteine and related compounds, heterozygosity for CBS deficiency per se does not impart an increased risk for premature atherosclerosis.[133] In contrast, several others report that heterozygosity for CBS deficiency does increase risk for premature atherosclerosis and stroke.[20,39] This interpretation remains open to question, since an accurate genetic marker to detect the carrier state is currently not available, and studies have not always included known obligate heterozygotes for CBS deficiency.[39,126] The use of fibroblast cultures and oral methionine loading for detection of genetic causes of homocysteinemia are equally likely to detect acquired defects in methionine metabolism.[126] Environmental factors may unmask subtle enzymatic deficiencies in persons heterozygous for hyperhomocysteinemia. Thus, moderate hyperhomocysteinemia and cerebrovascular disease in young adults may be genetically linked, whereas in elderly patients homocysteinemia is more likely to be acquired.

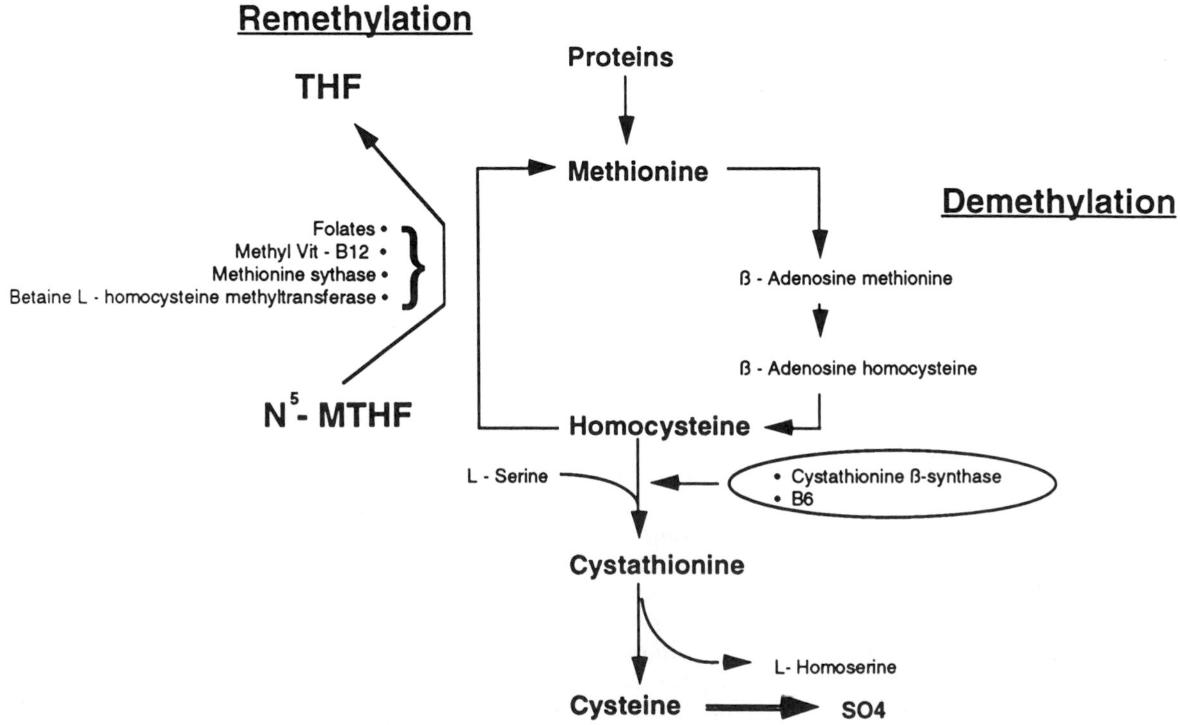


**Fig. 33-2.** Plasma homocysteine levels may increase because of genetic or acquired metabolic deficiencies in pathways of methionine metabolism. The principal causes include dysfunction of the cystathionine β-synthase enzyme system for cysteine metabolism and because of dysfunction of remethylation tetrahydrofolate pathway (THF) as may occur with folate or vitamin $B_{12}$ deficiencies. See text for details. $N^5$-MTHF, methyltetrahydrofolate.

Regardless of a genetic predisposition, many individuals are at risk for hyperhomocysteinemia because of acquired defects in methionine metabolism. As shown in Figure 33-2, decreased CBS activity and reduced remethylation of homocysteine may produce hyperhomocysteinemia via abnormalities in folate-, cobalamine-, or betaine-dependent metabolic pathways.[101,134] Clarke et al.[39] found plasma homocysteine levels to be inversely related to red-cell folate and serum vitamin $B_{12}$ levels. Others have found a direct relationship between plasma homocysteine levels and serum uric acid concentration.[47,100] A high prevalence of abnormalities in methionine metabolism in cerebrovascular disease is suggested by a roughly 30 percent prevalences of homocysteinemia in young subjects with stroke reported by Boers et al.[25] and Brattstrom et al.[27] and a similar prevalence in randomly selected subjects with stroke whose average age was 65 years reported by Coull et al.[47]

A not altogether satisfying view, but one that is generally held, is that homocysteinemia promotes the development of premature atherosclerosis and therefore stroke. Pathologic studies of large arteries from subjects with homocysteinemia demonstrate features typical of atherosclerosis such as fibrous intimal plaques, medial fibrosis, and disruption of the internal elastic membranes.[14,125] Accumulation of lipids are less conspicuous, and despite the documentation of premature atherosclerosis, the vascular occlusive events appear disproportionate to the severity of arterial pathology. More compelling are several lines of evidence that implicate a toxic effect of homocysteine on vascular endothelial cells, perhaps via peroxide production.[54,83,84,167] Endothelial damage may be pivotal for inducing thrombosis, since coagulation or platelet reactivity may also be activated via this mechanism.[147,150,175]

Since the development of sensitive assays for plasma homocysteine and related compounds, it is now possible to easily test for elevated levels of homocysteine in appropriate patients.[100,119,162] Probably all young persons with unexplained stroke should be tested. If elevated levels are present, their siblings and other related family members should also be examined. Additional epidemiologic studies are needed to better define whether elderly people with cerebrovascular disease may also benefit from testing for hyperhomocysteinemia. Older patients with stroke and TIA and underlying atherosclerosis in the absence of diabetes mellitus, hypercholesterolemia, or tobacco smoking have been found to have moderate hyperhomocysteinemia. As indicated in Figure 33-2, when an elevated level of homocysteine is detected, serum folate and vitamin $B_{12}$ levels should also be measured.[166] Establishing the presence of hyperhomocysteinemia may well be worthwhile, since many abnormalities of methionine metabolism (Fig. 33-2) respond to treatment with dietary supplements of folic acid, biotin, or vitamin $B_{12}$.[26,101,166]

## SICKLE CELL DISEASE

The single-point mutation in the hemoglobin $\beta$-chain produces the disease sickle cell anemia (SSA). The substitution of valine for glutamic acid in the $\beta^{s\ globin}$ chain markedly lowers the solubility of deoxyhemoglobin S, thereby promoting hemoglobin polymerization when erythrocytes are exposed to environments such as acidosis or hypoxemia.[77,79,103] The HbSS polymerization produces a rigid RBC with the characteristic sickle shape. This biophysical change and the resulting tremendous increase in blood viscosity induces RBC sludging in the microcirculation during sickle crises.[155] Initially, much of the pathology of sickle cell disease (SSD) was thought to be a result of this phenomenon, but clinical and pathologic studies now indicate that this does not provide an adequate explanation for the complex processes that underlie SSD.[28,79,143] Rather, the hallmark of SSD is a progressive systemic vasculopathy, which involves many organs including the brain[130,152,185] Although never benign, for unknown reasons, only about 30 percent of patients with SSA develop SSD as children and young adults.[143] These individuals with SSD experience vascular occlusive events, often recurrent, which lead to failure of the kidney, lung, bone, skin, eye, and the brain. The remainder of persons with SSA have a less fulminant course, and many live into early or middle adulthood before manifesting symptoms.

In black Americans the prevalence of sickle trait (HbSA) is about 8.5 percent, hemoglobin HbSS is approximately 0.03 to 0.16 percent, and the variant HbSC is 0.21 percent. Stroke incidence with HbSS is roughly 10 percent, but population statistics vary between 8 and 17 percent.[79,139] These estimates of stroke prevalence may be low, since a recent study of asymptomatic subjects with SSA undergoing MRI scanning of brain found a 10 percent incidence of asymptomatic brain infarction.[187] The incidence of stroke in HBSC is roughly 2 to 5 percent, whereas brain infarction is very uncommon in sickle trait and usually occurs in extraordinary circumstances such as severe hypoxia, heat stress, or dehydration. However, over a dozen well-documented cases of stroke with HbSA have now been reported.[146,149]

Although the rheologic properties of the sickled RBC suggest a predilection for microvascular occlusion, the major cerebral arterial pathology in patients with SSD is segmental narrowing of the distal internal carotid artery and portions of the circle of Willis and proximal branches of the major vessels of the brain.[169] This large-vessel arteriopathy is characterized by intimal proliferation and an increase in fibroblasts and smooth muscle cells within the arterial wall. The progressive nature of this occlusive arteriopathy is evidenced by the occasional development of the moyamoya phenomenon. Besides large arterial pathology sickled cell plugging of the microcirculation and venous thromboses are also well documented.[108,142] Presumably the major arterial pathology underlies most large brain infarctions in SSD.[2,168]

Both brain infarction and intracerebral hemorrhage (ICH) are consequences of SSD, but the incidence of aneurysmal subarachnoid hemorrhage is probably not increased. Brain infarction has been reported to occur around age 10 in young children and outnumbers ICH by a ratio of 3 to 1, which is more often encountered in older subjects. Infarctions include both deep and subcortical types, with no region of the brain being spared. Brain stem, spinal cord infarction, and central retinal artery occlusion, retinal hemorrhages, and dural sinus thrombosis have all been reported. Pavlakis and colleagues[141] have emphasized that watershed infarctions particularly in territories of the middle cerebral artery are often found in SSD. They speculate that a combination of occlusive arteriopathy and perfusion failure produce these strokes. Brain infarctions, however, may also occur in subjects who have little demonstrable arteriopathy. Finally, a satisfactory explanation for ICH has not been advanced, but either medial necrosis of arterioles with subsequent vascular rupture, or venous thrombosis are possible mechanisms. Increased cerebral blood flow, only partially explained by underlying anemia, and increased cerebral blood volume may provide additional clues to the predisposition to ICH.[145]

It is not currently possible to predict who with SSA will develop the ravages of SSD. MRI scanning, including MRI angiography, may identify presymptomatic individuals with asymptomatic stroke or vasculopathy who may benefit from aggressive therapeutic intervention.[183] Transcranial Doppler studies have proved useful for identifying persons with the distal cerebral arteriopathy.[1] These methods maybe particularly suitable for following patients who have experienced stroke or other neurologic symptoms and who are receiving ongoing treatment.

The mainstay of treatment for SSD is repeated exchange transfusion to maintain the concentration of HbS at less than 30 percent. Some have suggested that in asymptomatic persons or in persons who are neurologically, stable HbS of up to 50 percent may be tolerated. Others have suggested that repeated transfusions may decrease vascular lesions in SSD.[153] If not treated, the risk of recurrent stroke in children is exceedingly high. Powars et al.[144] reported a 67 percent recurrence in untreated persons, compared with a 10 percent incidence of recurrent stroke in those receiving repeated transfusions. Studies of individuals receiving repeated transfusions over 1 to 10 years indicate that, in persons at risk, it may not be safe to discontinue transfusions, since even after 10 years the risk of stroke recurrence was 50 percent per year.[178,181] Because of the coincidence of complications of repeated transfusions, recent enthusiasm has developed for bone marrow transplantation.

## REFERENCES

1. Adams RJ, Aaslid R, El Gammal T et al: Detection of cerebral vasculopathy in sickle cell disease using transcranial Doppler ultrasonography and magnetic resonance imaging. Stroke 19:518, 1988
2. Adams RJ, Nichols FT, McKie K et al: Cerebral infarction in sickle cell anemia: mechanism based on CT and MRI. Neurology (NY) 38:1012, 1988
3. Alving BM, Barr CF, Tang DB: Correlation between lupus anticoagulants and anticardiolipin antibodies in patients with prolonged activated partial thromboplastin times. Am J Med 88:112, 1990
4. Ambruso DR, Jacobson LJ, Hathaway WE: Inherited antithrombin III deficiency and cerebral thrombosis in a child. Pediatrics 65:125, 1980
5. Amer L, Kisiel W, Searles RP, Williams RC, Jr: Impairment of the protein C anticoagulant pathway in a patient with systemic lupus erythematosus, anticardiolipin antibodies and thrombosis. Thromb Res 57:247, 1990
6. Anderson D, Bell D, Lodge R et al: Recurrent cerebral ischemia and mitral valve vegetation in a patient with antiphospholipid antibodies. J Rheumatol 14:839, 1989
7. Ansell J, Deykin D: Heparin-induced thrombocytopenia and recurrent thromboembolism. Am J Hematol 8:325, 1980
8. Asherson RA: A "primary" antiphospholipid syndrome. J Rheumatol 15:1742, 1988
9. Asherson RA, Hughes GRV: The expanding spectrum of Libman Sacks endocarditis: the role of antiphospholipid antibodies. Clin Exp Rheum 7:255, 1989
10. Asherson RA, Khamashta MA, Gil A et al: Cerebrovascular disease and antiphospholipid antibodies in systemic lupus erythematosus lupus-like disease, and the primary antiphospholipid antibody syndrome. Am J Med 86:391, 1989
11. Asherson RA, Mercay D, Phillips G et al: Recurrent stroke, multi-infarct dementia in systemic lupus erythematosus associated with antiphospholipid antibodies. Ann Rheum Dis 46:605, 1987
12. Atkinson JLD, Sundt TM, Kazmier FJ et al: Heparin-induced thrombocytopenia and thrombosis in ischemic stroke. Mayo Clin Proc 63:353, 1988
13. Bauer KA, Rosenberg RD: The pathophysiology of prethrombotic state in humans: insights gained from studies using markers of hemostatic system activation. Blood 70:343, 1987
14. Baumgartner R, Wick H, Onacker H et al: Vascular lesions in two patients with congenital homocystimuria due to different defects of remethylation. J Inher Metab Dis 3:101, 1980

15. Becker PS, Miller VT: Heparin-induced thrombocytopenia. Stroke 20:1449, 1989
16. Bell WR: Heparin-associated thrombocytopenia and thrombosis. J Lab Clin Med 111:600, 1988
17. Bertina RM: Hereditary protein S deficiency. Haemostasis 15:241, 1985
18. Bienvenu T, Ankri A, Chadefaux B, Kamoun P: Dosage de l'homocysteine plasmatique dans l'exploration des thromboses du sujet jeune. Presse Med 20:985, 1991
19. Bloom EJ, Abrams DI, Rodgers G: Lupus anticoagulant in the acquired immunodeficiency syndrome. JAMA 256:491, 1986
20. Boers GHJ, Smals AGH, Trijbels FJM et al: Heterozygosity for homocystinuria in premature peripheral and cerebral occlusive arterial disease. N Engl J Med 313:709, 1985
21. Boey ML, Colaco CB, Gharavi AE et al: Thrombosis in SLE: striking association with the presence of circulating "lupus" anticoagulant. Br Med J 287:1021, 1983
22. Bousser MG, Chiras J, Bories J, Castaigne P: Cerebral venous thrombosis—a review of 38 cases. Stroke 16:199, 1985
23. Bowie WEJ, Thompson JH, Pasacuzzi CA et al: Thrombosis in systemic lupus erythematosus despite circulating anticoagulants. J Clin Invest 62:416, 1963
24. Brandt KD, Lessel S, Cohen AS: Cerebral disorders of vision in systemic lupus erythematosis. Ann Intern Med 83:163, 1975
25. Brattstrom LE, Hardebo JE, Hultberg BL: Moderate homocysteinemia—a possible risk factor for arteriosclerotic cerebrovascular disease. Stroke 15:1012, 1984
26. Brattstrom LE, Israelsson B, Jeppson J-O, Hultberg BL: Folic acid—an innocuous means to reduce plasma homocysteine. Scand J Clin Lab Invest 48:215, 1988
27. Brey RL, Hart RG, Sherman DG et al: Antiphospholipid antibodies and cerebral ischemia in young people. Neurology (NY) 40:1190, 1990
28. Bridges W: Cerebral vascular disease accompanying sickle cell anemia. Am J Pathol 15:353, 1939
29. Briley DP, Coull BM: Antiphospholipid antibodies and vascular dementia. Stroke, suppl. 7. 41:296, 1991
30. Briley DP, Coull BM, Goodnight SH: Neurological disease associated with antiphospholipid antibodies. Ann Neurol 25:221, 1989
31. Bruyn RPM, VanderVeen JPW, Donker AJM et al: Sneddon's syndrome: case report and literature review. J Neurol Sci 79:243, 1987
32. Cacciari E, Salardi S: Clinical and laboratory features of homocystineimia Halmostasis, suppl 1. 19:10, 1989
33. Cariou R, Tobelen G, Bellucci S et al: Effect of lupus anticoagulant on antithrombogenic properties of endothelial cells: inhibition of thrombomodulin-dependent protein C activation. Thromb Haemost 60:54, 1988
34. Cariou R, Tobelem G, Soria C et al: Inhibition of protein C activation by endothelial cells in the presence of lupus anticoagulant. (Letter.) N Engl J Med 314:1193, 1986
35. Carreras LO, Veraylan JG: "Lupus" anticoagulant and thrombosis—possible role of inhibition of prostacyclin formation. Thromb Haemost 48:38, 1982
36. Carvalho ACA, Colman RW, Lees RS: Platelet function in hyperlipoproteinemia. N Engl J Med 290:434, 1974
37. Chancellor AM, Glasgow GL, Ockelford PA et al: Etiology, prognosis, and hemostatic function after cerebral infarction in young adults. Stroke 20:477, 1989
38. Cines DB, Tomaski A, Tannenbaum S: Immune endothelial-cell injury in heparin-associated thrombocytopenia. N Engl J Med 316:581, 1987
39. Clarke R, Daly L, Robinson K et al: Hyperhomocysteinemia: an independent risk factor for vascular disease. N Engl J Med 324:1149, 1991
40. Comp PC: Hereditary disorders predisposing to thrombosis. Prog Hemost Thromb 8:71, 1986
41. Comp PC: Laboratory evaluation of protein S status. Sem Thromb Hemost 16:177, 1990
42. Comp PC: Overview of the Hypercoagulable states. Sem Thromb Hemost 16:158, 1990
43. Comp PC, DeBault LE, Ramon NL et al: Human thrombomodulin is inhibited by IgG from two patients with nonspecific anticoagulants, abstracted. Blood 62:299a, 1983
44. Coull BM, Beamer N, de Garmo P et al: Chronic blood hyperviscosity in subjects with acute stroke, transient ischemic attack, and risk factors for stroke. Stroke 22:162, 1991
45. Coull BM, Bourdette DN, Goodnight SH et al: Multiple cerebral infarctions and dementia associated with anticardiolipin antibodies. Stroke 18:1107, 1987
46. Coull BM, Goodnight SH, Jr: Antiphospholipid antibodies, prethrombotic states, and stroke. Stroke 31:1370, 1990
47. Coull BM, Malinow MR, Beamer N et al: Elevated plasma homocyst(e)ine concentration as a possible independent risk factor for stroke. Stroke 21:572, 1990
48. Cros D, Comp PC, Beltran G, Gum G: Superior sagittal sinus thrombosis in a patient with protein S deficiency. Stroke 21:633, 1990
49. D'Alton JG, Preston DN, Bormaris J et al: Multiple transient ischemic attacks, lupus anticoagulant and verrucous endocarditis. Stroke 16:512, 1985
50. D'Angelo A, Landi G, D'Angelo SV et al: Protein C in acute stroke. Stroke 19:579, 1988
51. D'Angelo A, Vigano-D'Angelo S, Esmon CT, Comp PC: Acquired deficiencies of protein S. J Clin Invest 81:1445, 1988
52. Davis WD, Brey RL: Complement activation in stroke associated with antiphospholipid antibodies. (Abstract.) Neurology (NY) 41:296, 1991
53. Degos R, Kalis B: La papulose atrophiante maligne. Rev Pract 19:4335, 1969
54. De Groot P, Willems C, Boers GHJ et al: Endothelial dysfunction in homocystinuria. Eur J Clin Invest 13:405, 1983

55. Dougherty JH, Jr, Levy DE, Weksler BB: Platelet activation in acute cerebral ischemia. Lancet 1:821, 1977
56. Elias M, Eldor A: Thromboembolism in patients with "lupus"-type circulating anticoagulant. Arch Intern Med 144:510, 1984
57. El-Roeiy A, Gleicher N: Definition of normal autoantibody levels in an apparently healthy population. Obstet Gynecol 72:596, 1988
58. Engesser L, Broekmans AW, Briet E et al: Hereditary protein S deficiency: clinical manifestations. Ann Intern Med 106:677, 1987
59. Englert H, Hawkes CH, Boey ML et al: Degos' disease: association with anticardiolipin antibodies and the lupus anticoagulant. Br Med J 289:576, 1984
60. Engstrom JW, Lowenstein DH, Bredesen DE: Cerebral Infarctions and transient neurologic deficits associated with acquired immunodeficiency syndrome. Am J Med 86:528, 1989
61. Ernst E, Matrai A, Marshall M: Blood rheology in patients with transient ischemic attacks. Stroke 19:634, 1988
62. Esmon CT: The regulation of natural anticoagulant pathways. Science 235:1348, 1987
63. Etingin OR, Hajjar DP, Hajjar KA et al: Lipoprotein (a) regulates plasminogen activator inhibitor-1 expression in endothelial cells: a potential mechanism in thrombogenesis. J Biol Chem 266:2459, 1991
64. Exner T, Sahman N, Trudinger B: Separation of anticardiolipin antibodies from lupus anticoagulant on a phospholipid-coated polystyrene column. Biochem Biophys Res Commun 1:1001, 1988
65. Exner T, Triplett DA, Taberner D, Machin SJ: Guidelines for testing and revised criteria for lupus anticoagulants. Thromb Haemost 65:320, 1991
66. Feinberg WM, Bruck DC, Ring ME, Corrigan JJ, Jr: Hemsotatic markers in acute stroke. Stroke 20:592, 1989
67. Fields RA, Toubbeh H, Searles RP et al: The prevalence of anticardiolipin antibodies in a healthy elderly population and its association with antinuclear antibodies. J Rheumatol 16:623, 1989
68. Fisher M, Meiselman HJ: Hemorheological factors in cerebral ischemia. Stroke 22:1164, 1991
69. Fisherty MJ, West S, Heimark R et al: Placental anticoagulant protein 1: measurement in the extracellular fluids and cells of the hemostatic system. J Clin Lab Med 115:174, 1990
70. FitzGerald GA, Smith B, Pedersen AK, Brash AR: Increased prostacyclin biosynthesis in patients with severe atherosclerosis and platelet activation. N Engl J Med 310:1065, 1984
71. Freyssinet JM, Cazenave JP: Lupus-like anticoagulants, modulation of the protein C pathway and thrombosis. Thromb Haemost 88:679, 1987
72. Freyssinet JM, Gauchy J, Cazenave JP: The effect of phospholipids on the activation of protein C by the human thrombin-thrombomodulin complex. Biochem J 238:151, 1986
73. Fulford KWM, Catterall RD, Delhinty JJ et al: A collagen disorder of the nervous system presenting as multiple sclerosis. Brain 95:373, 1972
74. Galli M, Comfurius P, Maassen C et al: Anticardiolipin antibodies directed not to cardiolipin but to a plasma protein cofactor. Lancet 335:1544, 1990
75. Galli M, Cortelazzo S, Viero P et al: Interaction between platelets and lupus anticoagulant, Eur J Haematol 41:88, 1988
76. Gastineau DA, Kazmer FJ, Nichols WL et al: Lupus anticoagulant: an analysis of the clinical and laboratory features of 219 cases. Am J Hematol 19:265, 1985
77. Green MA, Noguchi CT, Marwah SS et al: Polymerization of sickle cell hemoglobin at arterial oxygen saturation impairs erythrocyte deformability. J Clin Invest 81:1669, 1988
78. Grotta J, Ackerman R, Correia J et al: Whole blood viscosity parameters and cerebral blood flow. Stroke 13:296, 1982
79. Grotta JC, Manner C, Pettigrew C, Yatsu FM: Red blood cell disorders and stroke. Stroke 17:811, 1986
80. Hajjar KA, Gavish D, Breslow JL, Nachman RL: Lipoprotein (a) modulation of endothelial cell surface fibrinolysis and its potential role in atherosclerosis. Nature 339:303, 1989
81. Hall RG, Harris EN, Gharavi AE et al: Anticardiolipin antibodies: occurrence in Behcet's syndrome. Ann Rheum Dis 43:746, 1984
82. Hamsten A, Winman B, de Faire U, Blomback M: Increased plasma levels of a rapid inhibitor of tissue plasminogen activator in young survivors of myocardial infarction. N Engl J Med 313:1557, 1985
83. Harker LA, Ross R, Slichter SJ, Scott CR: Homocysteine-induced arteriosclerosis: the role of endothelial cell injury and platelet response in its genesis. J Clin Invest 58:731, 1976
84. Harker LA, Slichter SJ, Scott CR, Ross R: Homocysteinemia vascular injury and arterial thrombosis. N Engl J Med 291:537, 1974
85. Harris EN: The second international anti-cardiolipin standardization workshop/the Kingston anti-phospholipid antibody study (KAPS) group. Am J Clin Pathol 94:476, 1990
86. Harris EN, Asherson RA, Hughes GRV: Antiphospholipid antibodies—autoantibodies with a difference. Ann Rev Med 39:261, 1988
87. Harris EN, Gharavi AE, Asherson RA, Boey ML, Hughes GRV: Cerebral infarction in systemic lupus: association with anticardiolipin antibodies. Clin Exp Rheumatol 2:47, 1984
88. Harris EN, Gharavi AE, Hughes GRV: Antiphospholipid antibodies. Clin Rheum Dis 11:591, 1985
89. Hart RG, Miller VT, Coull BM, Bril V: Cerebral infarction associated with lupus anticoagulants—preliminary report. Stroke 15:114, 1984
90. Hasselaar P, Derksen RHWM, Blokzijl L, de Groot PG: Cross-reactivity of antibodies directed against cardiolipin, DNA, endothelial cells and blood platelets. Thromb Haemost 63:169, 1990
91. Hazeltine M, Rauch J, Danoff D et al: Antiphos-

pholipid antibodies in systemic lupus erythematosus: evidence of an association with positive Coombs' and hypocomplementemia. J Rheumatol 15:80, 1988
92. Hess DC, Krauss J, Adams RJ et al: Anticardiolipin antibodies: a study of frequency in TIA and stroke. Neurology (NY) 41:525, 1991
93. High KA: Antithrombin III, protein C, and protein S. Arch Pathol Lab Med 112:28, 1988
94. Hughes GRV, Harris EN, Gharavi AE: The anticardiolipin syndrome. J Rheumatol 13:486, 1986
95. Ingram S, Goodnight SH, Bennett RM: An unusual syndrome of a devastating noninflammatory vasculopathy associated with anticardiolipin antibodies: report of two cases. Arthritis Rheum 30:1167, 1987
96. Israels SJ, Seshia SS: Childhood stroke associated with protein C or S deficiency. J Pediatrics 111:562, 1987
97. Jabaily J, Iland HJ, Laszlo J et al: Neurologic manifestations of essential thrombocythemia. Ann Intern Med 99:513, 1983
98. Jurgens G, Koltringer P: Lipoprotein (a) in ischemic cerebrovascular disease: a new approach to the assessment of risk for stroke. Neurology (NY) 37:513, 1987
99. Kalashnikova LA, Nasonov EL, Kushakbaeva AE, Gracheva LA: Anticardiolipin antibodies in Sneddon's syndrome. Neurology (NY) 40:464, 1990
100. Kang SS, Wong PWK, Cook HY et al: Protein-bound homocyst(e)ine: a possible risk factor for coronary artery disease. J Clin Invest 77:1482, 1986
101. Kang S, Zhou J, Wong PWK et al: Intermediate homocysteinemia: a thermolabile variant of methylenetetrahydrofolate reductase. Am J Hum Genet 43:414, 1988
102. Kannel WB, Wolf PA, Castelli WP, D'Agostino RB: Fibrinogen and risk of cardiovascular disease. JAMA 258:1183, 1987
103. Keidan AJ, Sowter MC, Johnson CS et al: Effect of polymerization tendency of haematological, rheological and clinical parameters in sickle cell anemia. Br J Haematol 71:551, 1989
104. Kessler CM, Strickland DK: Protein C and protein S clinical perspectives. Clin Chim Acta 170:25, 1987
105. Khamashta MA, Harris EN, Gharavi AE et al: Immune mediated mechanism for thrombosis: antiphospholipid antibody binding to platelet membranes. Ann Rheum Dis 47:849, 1988
106. King DJ, Keltron JG: Heparin-associated thrombocytopenia. Ann Intern Med 100:535, 1984
107. Kohler J, Kasper J, Witt I, von Reutern G-M: Ischemic stroke due to protein C deficiency. Stroke 21:1077, 1990
108. Kurantsin-Mills J, Klug PP, Lessin LS: Vaso-occlusion in sickle cell disease: pathophysiology of the microvascular circulation. Am J Pediatr Hematol Oncol 10:357, 1988
109. Kyritsis AP, Williams EC, Schutta HS: Cerebral venous thrombosis due to heparin-induced thrombocytopenia. Stroke 21:1503, 1990
110. Label LS, Tandan R, Albers JW: Myelomalacia and hypoglycorrhachia in malignant atrophic papulosis. Neurology (NY) 33:936, 1983
111. Levine SR, Deegan MJ, Furtell N, Welch KMA: Cerebrovascular and neurologic disease associated with antiphospholipid antibodies: 48 cases. Neurology (NY) 40:1181, 1990
112. Levine SR, Langer SL, Albers JW, Welch KMA: Sneddon's syndrome: an antiphospholipid antibody syndrome? Neurology (NY) 38:798, 1988
113. Levine SR, Welch KMA: The spectrum of neurologic disease associated with antiphospholipid antibodies: lupus anticoagulants and anticardiolipin antibodies. Arch Neurol 44:876, 1987
114. Lo SCL, Oldmeadow MJ, Howard MA, Firkin BG: Comparison of laboratory tests used for identification of lupus anticoagulant. Am J Hematol 30:213, 1989
115. Loizou S, McCrea JD, Rudge AC et al: Measurement of anti-cardiolipin antibodies by an enzyme-linked immunosorbent assay (ELISA): standardization and quantitation of results. Clin Exp Immunol 62:738, 1985
116. Love PE, Santoro SA: Antiphospholipid antibodies: anticardiolipin and the lupus anticoagulant in systemic lupus erythematosus (SLE) and in non-SLE disorders. Ann of Intern Med 112:682, 1990
117. Mackworth-Young CG, Loizou S, Walport MJ: Antiphospholipid antibodies and disease. QJ Med 269:767, 1989
118. Mackworth-Young CG, Loizou S, Walport MJ: Primary antiphospholipid syndrome: features of patients with raised anticardiolipin antibodies and no other disorder. Ann Rheum Dis 48:362, 1989
119. Malinow MR, Kang SS, Taylor LM et al: Prevalence of hyperhomocyst(e)inemia in patients with peripheral arterial occlusive disease. Circulation 79:1180, 1989
120. Mannucci PM, Tripodi A, Bertina RM: Protein S deficiency associated with "juvenile" arterial and venous thromboses. Thromb Haemost 55:440, 1986
121. Manoussakis MN, Gharavi AE, Drosos AA et al: Anticardiolipin antibodies in unselected autoimmune rheumatic disease patients. Clin Immun Immunopathol 44:297, 1987
122. Manoussakis MN, Tzioufas AG, Silis MP et al: High prevalence of anti-cardiolipin and other autoantibodies in a healthy elderly population. Clin Exp Immunol 69:557, 1987
123. Margolius A, Jackson DP, Ratnoff OD: Circulating anticoagulants: a study of 40 cases and a review of the literature. Medicine (Baltimore) 40:145, 1961
124. Matsuura E, Igarashi Y, Fujimoto M et al: Anticardiolipin cofactor(s) and differential diagnosis of autoimmune disease. (Letter.) Lancet 336:177, 1990
125. McCully KS: Vascular pathology of homocysteinemia: implications for the pathogenesis of arteriosclerosis. Am J Pathol 56:111, 1969
126. McGill JJ, Metler G, Rosenblatt DS, Scriver CR: Detection of heterozygotes for recessive alleles:

homocyst(e)inemia: paradigm of pitfalls in phenotypes. Am J Med Genet 36:45, 1990
127. McNeil HP, Chesterman CN, Krilis SA: Binding specificity of lupus anticoagulants and anticardiolipin antibodies. Thromb Res 52:609, 1988
128. McNeil HP, Chesterman CN, Krilis SA: Immunology and clinical importance of antiphospholipid antibodies. Adv Immun 49:193, 1991
129. McNeil HP, Simpson RJ, Chesterman CN et al: Antiphospholipid antibodies are directed against a complex antigen that includes a lipid-binding inhibitor of coagulation: beta-2-glycoprotein I (aproprotein H). Proc Natl Acad Sci USA 87:4120, 1990
130. Merkel KH, Ginsberg PL, Parker JC et al: Cerebrovascular disease in sickle cell anemia: a clinical, pathological and radiological correlation. Stroke 9:45, 1978
131. Mettinger KL, Nyman D, Kjellin KG et al: Factor III-related antigen, antithrombin III, spontaneous platelet aggregation and plasminogen activator in ischemic cerebrovascular disease: a study of stroke before 55. J Neurol Sci 41:31, 1979
132. Moreb J, Kitchens CS: Acquired functional protein S deficiency, cerebral venous thrombosis, and coumarin akin necrosis in association with antiphospholipid syndrome: report of two cases. Am J Med 87:207, 1989
133. Mudd SH, Haulik R, Levy HL et al: A study of cardiovascular risk in heterozygotes for homocystinuria. Am J Hum Genet 33:883, 1981
134. Mudd SH, Levy HL, Skouby F: Disorders of transsulfuration. p. 693. In Scriver C, Beaudet AL, Sly WS, Valle D (eds): The Metabolic Basis of Inherited Disease. 6th Ed. Vol 1. McGraw-Hill, New York, 1989
135. Mudd SH, Skouby F, Levy HL et al: The natural history of homocystinuria due to cystathionine $\beta$-synthase deficiency. Am J Hum Genet 37:1, 1985
136. Murphy S, Iland H, Rosenthal D, Laszlo J: Essential thrombocythemia: an interim report from the Polycythemia Vera Study Group. Semin Hematol 23:177, 1986
137. Nawroth PP, Handley DA et al: Interleukin 1 induces endothelial cell procoagulant while suppressing cell-surface anticoagulant activity. Proc Natl Acad Sci USA 83:3460, 1986
138. Nelson D, Goodnight S: Pathology of antiphospholipid antibodies and thrombosis. Thrombosis and haemostasis check samples 10, No. TH88-6(TH-60). Am Soc Clin Pathol 10:1, 1988
139. Ohene-Frempong K: Stroke in sickle cell disease: demographic, clinical, and therapeutic considerations. Semin Hematol 28:213, 1991
140. Ono N, Koyama T, Suchiro A et al: Clinical significance of new coagulation and fibrinolytic markers in ischemic stroke patients. Stroke 22:1369, 1991
141. Pavlakis SG, Bello J, Prohovnik I et al: Brain infarction in sickle cell anemia: magnetic resonance imaging correlates. Ann Neurol 23:125, 1988
142. Portnoy BA, Herion JC: Neurological manifestations in sickle-cell disease. Ann Intern Med 76:643, 1972
143. Powars D, Chan LS, Schroeder WA: The variable expression of sickle cell disease is genetically determined. Semin Hematol 27:360, 1990
144. Powars D, Wilson B, Imbus C et al: The natural history of stroke in sickle cell disease. Am J Med 65:461, 1978
145. Prohovnik I, Pavlakis SG, Piomelli S et al: Cerebral hyperemia, stroke and transfusion in sickle cell disease. Neurology (NY) 39:334, 1989
146. Radhakrishnan K, Thacker AK, Maloo JC, El-Mangoush MA: Sickle cell trait and stroke in the young adult. Postgrad Med J 66:1078, 1990
147. Ratnoff OD: Activation of hageman factor by L-homocystine. Science 162:1007, 1968
147a. Rebello M, Val JF, Garijo F et al: Livedo reticularis and cerebrovascular lesions (Sneddon's syndrome). Brain 106:965, 1983
148. Reutalingsperger CPM, Hornstra G, Henker HC: Purification and characterisation of a novel protein from bovine aorta that inhibits coagulation. Eur J Biochem 151:625, 1985
149. Reyes MG: Subcortical cerebral infarctions in sickle cell trait. J Neurol Neurosurg Psychiatry 52:516, 1989
150. Rodgers GM, Kane WH: Activation of endogenous factor V by a homocysteine-induced vascular endothelial cell activator. U Clin Invest 77:1909, 1986
151. Rodgers GP, Schechter AN, Noguchi CT et al: Periodic microcirculatory flow in patients with sickle cell disease. N Engl J Med 311:1534, 1984
152. Rothman SM, Fulling KH, Nelson JS: Sickle cell anemia and central nervous system infarction: a neuropathological study. Ann Neurol 20:684, 1986
153. Russell MO, Goldberg HI, Hodson A et al: Effect of transfusion therapy on arteriographic abnormalities and on the recurrence of stroke in sickle cell disease. Blood 63:162, 1984
154. Sacco RL, Owen J, Mohr JP et al: Free protein S deficiency: a possible association with cerebrovascular occlusion. Stroke 20:1657, 1989
155. Sammaritano LR, Gharavi AE, Lockshin MD: Antiphospholipid antibody syndrome: immunologic and clinical aspects. Semin Arthritis Rheum 20:81, 1990
156. Schleider MA, Nachman RL, Jaffe EA et al: A clinical study of the lupus anticoagulant. Blood 48:499, 1976
157. Schmid-Schonbein H: Macrorheology and microrheology of blood in cerebrovascular insufficiency. Eur Neurol, suppl 1. 22:2, 1983
158. Shah AB, Beamer N, Coull BM: Enhanced in vivo platelet activation in subtypes of ischemic stroke. Stroke 16:643, 1985
159. Shapiro SS, Thiagarajan P: Lupus anticoagulants. Prog Hemost Thromb 6:263, 1982
160. Shi W, Gordon S, Krilis SA et al: Prevalence of lupus anticoagulant and anticardiolipin antibodies in a healthy population. Aust NZ J Med 20:231, 990
161. Smith DB, Ens GE: Protein C deficency: a cause

of amaurosis fugax? J Neurol Neurosurg Psychiatry 50:361, 1986
162. Smolin LA, Schneider JA: Measurement of total plasma cysteamine using high-performance liquid chromatography with electrochemical detection. Anal Biochem 168:374, 1988
163. Sneddon IB: Cerebrovascular lesions and livedo reticularis. Br J Dermatol 77:180, 1965
164. Snowden N, Wilson PB, Longson M et al: Antiphospholipid antibodies and *Mycoplasma pneumoniae* infection. Postgrad Med J 66:356, 1990
165. Sontheimer RD: The anticardiolipin syndrome. Arch Dermatol 123:590, 1985
166. Stabler SP, Marcell PD, Podell ER et al: Elevation of total homocysteine in the serum of patients with cobalamin or folate deficiency detected by capillary gas chromatography-mass spectrometry. J Clin Invest 81:466, 1988
167. Starkebaum G, Harlan JM: Endothelial cell injury due to copper-catalyzed hydrogen peroxide generation from homocysteine. J Clin Invest 77:1370, 1976
168. Stimmler MM, Quismorio FP, McGehee WG et al: Anticardiolipin antibodies in acquired immunodeficiency syndrome. Arch Intern Med 149:1833, 1989
169. Stockman JA, Nigro MA, Miskin NM et al: Occlusion of large cerebral vessels in sickle cell anemia. N Engl J Med 287:846, 1972
170. Tait JF, Gibson D, Fujikawa J: Phospholipid binding properties of human placental anticoagulant 1, a member of lipocortin family. J Biol Chem 264:7944, 1989
171. Takano K, Yamaguchi T, Okada Y et al: Hypercoagulability in acute ischemic stroke: analysis of the extrinsic coagulation reactions in plasma by a highly sensitive automated method. Thromb Res 58:481, 1990
172. Tan EM, Cohen AS, Fries JT et al: The 1982 revised criteria for the classification of systemic lupus erythematosus. Arthritis Rheum 25:1271, 1982
173. Trimble M, Bell DA,Brien W et al: The antiphospholipid syndrome: prevalence among patients with stroke and transient ischemic attacks. Am J Med 88:593, 1990
174. Tsakiris DA, Settas L, Makris PE, Marbet GA: Lupus anticoagulant-antiphospholipid antibodies and thrombophilia: relation to protein C-protein S-thrombomodulin. J Rheum 17:785, 1990
175. Uhlemann ER, TenPas JH, Lucky AW et al: Platelet survival and morphology in homocystinuria due to cystathionine synthase deficiency. N Engl J Med 295:1283, 1976
176. Vismara A, Meroni L, Tincani A et al: Relationship between anti-cardiolipin and anti-endothelial cell antibodies in systemic lupus erythematosus. Clin Exp Immunol 74:247, 1988
177. Walker TS, Triplett DA, Javed N, Musgrave K: Evaluation of lupus anticoagulants: antiphospholipid antibodies, endothelium associated immunoglobulin, endothelial prostacyclin secretion, and antigenic protein S levels. Thromb Res 51:267, 1988
178. Wang WC, Kovnar EH, Tonkin IL et al: High risk of recurrent stroke after discontinuance of five to twelve years of transfusion therapy in patients with sickle cell disease. J Pediatr 118:377, 1991
179. Weiller C, Ringelstein EB, Reiche W, Buell U: Clinical and hemodynamic aspects of low-flow infarcts. Stroke 22:1117, 1991
180. Wilhelmsen L, Svardsudd K, Korsan-Bengtsen K et al: Fibrinogen as a risk factor for stroke and myocardial infarction. N Engl J Med 311:501, 1976
181. Wilimas J, Goff JR, Anderson HR, Jr et al: Efficacy of transfusion therapy for one to two years in patients with sickle cell disease and cerebrovascular accidents. Pediatrics 96:205, 1980
182. Wintzen AR, Broekmans AW, Bertina RM et al: Cerebral hemorrhagic infaction in young patients with hereditary protein C deficiency: evidence for "spontaneous" cerebral venous thrombosis. Br Med J 290:350, 1985
183. Wiznitzer M, Ruggieri PM, Masaryk TJ et al: Diagnosis of cerebrovascular disease in sickle cell anemia by magnetic resonance angiography. J Pediatr 17:551, 1990
184. Woo J, Lau E, Lam CW et al: Hypertension, lipoprotein (a), and apolipoprotein A-1 as risk factors for stroke in the Chinese. Stroke 22:203, 1991
185. Wood DH: Cerebrovascular complications of sickle cell anemia. Stroke 9:73, 1978
186. Zenker G, Koltringer P, Bone G et al: Lipoprotein (a) as a strong indicator for cerebrovascular disease. Stroke 17:942, 1986
187. Zimmerman RA, Gill F, Goldberg HI et al: MRI of sickle cell cerebral infarction. Neuroradiology 29:232, 1987

# 34
# STROKE AND SUBSTANCE ABUSE

John C.M. Brust

According to the World Health Organization, drug dependence is "a state of psychic or physical dependence, or both, on a drug, arising in a person following administration of that drug on a periodic or continuous basis."[103] Drug abuse, on the other hand, implies a social judgment, whether or not the substance is taken continuously, periodically, or infrequently, and whether or not it is legally available. When alcohol and tobacco are included, millions of Americans are substance abusers, and many of them are at increased risk of stroke, occlusive or hemorrhagic.[306] Mechanisms vary, including an increased incidence of atherosclerotic infarction in alcohol drinkers, cerebral complications of endocarditis common in parenteral drug abusers, and vasculitides affecting users of particular substances.[44,45]

## OPIATES

There are currently about a half million heroin abusers in the United States,[42] whose commonest causes of death are violence, overdose, acute adverse reactions, and AIDS.[41,43,154] Other medical complications include stroke. Heroin must be taken parenterally (and in addicts more than once a day), and so infectious endocarditis is common,[16,62,256,308,309,330] especially with *Staphylococcus aureus* and *Candida*.[392] It affects in equal frequency the mitral, aortic, and tricuspid valves,[176] and cerebral emboli are common.

Stroke may be occlusive or hemorrhagic. Infarction follows embolic vessel occlusion or, less often, bacterial or fungal meningitis. Cerebral or subarachnoid hemorrhage usually follows rupture of a septic ("mycotic") aneurysm.[7,123,184] Unlike saccular ("berry") aneurysms, septic aneurysms are more likely to present with subtle or insidiously progressive neurologic or systemic symptoms (e.g., headache, fever, syncope, hemiparesis, aphasia) than with a sudden onset suggesting subarachnoid hemorrhage; and cerebrospinal fluid (CSF) white cell pleocytosis may occur in asymptomatic endocarditis patients days before a mycotic aneurysm ruptures.[46] The infrequency with which these aneurysms spontaneously disappear during antimicrobial therapy, the high mortality associated with their rupture, and the relative ease (compared to berry aneurysms) of surgical removal support the view that cerebral angiography should be performed in endocarditis patients with either unexplained neurologic symptoms or abnormal CSF, and that, once found, most mycotic aneurysms should be promptly excised.[46,112] Mycotic aneurysms in heroin users have also occurred on the carotid[235] and subclavian arteries.[173]

Heroin abusers may also have hemorrhagic stroke secondary to hepatitis, liver failure, and deranged clotting, or to heroin nephropathy with uremia or malignant hypertension. Nine heroin addicts were reported from Harlem Hospital Center with stroke unassociated with endocarditis.[48] In three, age 41 to 45, the relation of stroke to heroin was uncertain: one, while using heroin, had an intracerebral hemorrhage in the presence of probable heroin nephropathy and malignant hypertension; another, normotensive, had a basal ganglia hemorrhage 3 days after beginning methadone detoxification; the third, mildly hypertensive, had a probable capsular infarct 6 weeks after starting methadone maintenance. In six other patients, age 25 to 38, heroin appeared more directly causal. Four, all normotensive, had probable cerebral infarcts in association with loss of consciousness after intravenous heroin. Cerebral angiography in one of these was normal but in another showed stenosis of the internal carotid artery at the siphon and of the early anterior cerebral artery, plus occlusion of the middle cerebral artery; the changes suggested primary vessel disease more than emboli. Cerebral infarctions occurred in two other patients who were using heroin at the time, although the strokes were not related to overdose, nor did they follow a recent injection. In one of these patients, who was normotensive, cerebral angiography suggested widespread small vessel arteritis. None of these patients was using oral contraceptives or had other illnesses that would predispose to stroke. Consistent with hypersensitivity, one patient had 10 percent eosinophilia, serum hypergammaglobulinemia, and a positive direct Coombs test, and another had an ESR of 94 mm and two positive latex fixation tests. Except for cocaine in one patient (whose stroke followed an acute reaction to heroin), no other drugs were being used.

Other reports of stroke in heroin abusers include that of a 19-year-old man who had taken heroin intravenously weekly for a year, plus intermittent LSD, and developed sudden global aphasia;[251] cerebral angiography suggested diffuse angiitis. A 21-year-old woman developed hemiparesis 2 weeks after starting daily heroin use and 6 hours after an intravenous injection.[415] Symptoms began with vomiting, headache, sweating, and shortness of breath, suggesting anaphylaxis, and cerebral angiography showed narrowing and irregularity of the distal internal carotid artery, suggesting arteritis. Eosinophilia and the fact that her husband had shared her heroin were consistent with hypersensitivity to heroin or an adulterant. A normotensive 20-year-old man who had used heroin occasionally for 2 years took his first intravenous injection in 8 months and developed sudden left homonymous hemianopia and incoordination; cerebral angiography showed "beading" of the right posterior cerebral artery.[210] A 34-year-old man developed hemiparesis while sniffing heroin; cerebral angiography was normal.[163] Within minutes of intravenous heroin a young German had an intracerebral hemorrhage.[217]

Heroin could cause stroke by a number of possible mechanisms.[48,57] Following heroin overdose, hypoventilation and hypotension have produced permanent brain damage with bilateral cerebral leukoencephalopathy,[124] and hemiplegia has appeared upon awakening from nalorphine-responsive coma.[48] Delayed postanoxic encephalopathy has also occurred.[74,319,323] Bilateral globus pallidus infarction, commonly associated with shock, has been reported in over 2 percent of heroin addict autopsies,[309,375] and hemichorea was present in one patient with heroin stroke.[48] In no stroke patient has hypotension been documented, however, nor has any had bibracheal palsy or other signs suggestive of border-zone ("watershed") infarction.[3,40]

Direct toxic injury from either heroin or an adulterant is another possibility. Heroin is usually mixed with quinine and lactose or mannitol, as well as, on occasion, talc, starch, curry powder, Ajax, Vim, caffeine, or even strychnine.[57] Quinine caused amblyopia in a heroin addict,[47] and may contribute to acute adverse reactions with pulmonary edema or sudden death following parenteral injection.[14,241] There is no evidence linking quinine to stroke, however.

Embolization of foreign material to the brain has not been observed in parenteral heroin users (even though the jugular vein is frequently used, with occasional accidental arterial injection), but has been documented at autopsy in abusers of other agents,[12,281,352] including opiates. Probably because of restricted heroin supply, pentazocine (Talwin) and tripelennamine (Pyribenzamine) ("Ts and Blues") were widely abused in Chicago and other midwestern cities during the 1970s.[227,400] Oral tablets were crushed, suspended in water, passed through cotton or a cigarette filter, and injected intravenously, and cerebral infarcts and hemorrhages occurred in users.[59] Common at autopsy was pulmonary arteriolar occlusion by microcrystalline cellulose[174] or particulate magnesium silicate (talc),[377] used to bind pentazocine and tripelennamine. Such microemboli also reached the brain, especially when multiple lung emboli produced pulmonary hypertension and opened "functional pulmonary arteriovenous shunts."[57] "Beaded arteries" were seen at cerebral angiography in Ts and Blues stroke patients, consistent with vasculitis, in turn secondary to "a granulomatous or immune process provoked by the injection of foreign material."[57]

Talc microemboli were also found at autopsy in the liver, spleen, and central nervous system of a parenteral paregoric abuser.[52] A young man who several times a day injected pulverized unfiltered meperidine tablets intravenously had occasional seizures following injection and then developed difficulty concentrating, impaired memory, and visual blurring; fundal hemorrhages and areas of arterial occlusion were seen, and his symptoms improved with abstinence.[236]

Some heroin strokes have followed the first injection in weeks or months, and laboratory studies have further suggested an immunologic cause. Heroin nephropathy may be immunologically mediated;[80,116,140,208] the C3 component of complement is reduced in patients with heroin pulmonary edema; and heroin addicts frequently have hypergammaglobulinemia[19,309] (including elevated IgM independent of IgG and IgA levels[81,177,294,300]), circulating immune complexes,[300] antibodies to smooth muscle and lymphocyte membranes,[177] false positive serology,[19,30] and lymph node hypertrophy.[57] Opium, morphine, codeine, and meperidine, moreover, have caused urticaria, angioneurotic edema, and anaphylaxis.[356]

Whether the offending antigen is the opiate or a contaminant is unclear, but morphine binding by gamma globulin has been reported in addicts[329,349] and experimental animals.[24,333,398]

Relevant to heroin stroke and its possible mechanisms is heroin myelopathy. Acute paraparesis, sensory loss, and urinary retention have been reported in at least 16 heroin users, occurring shortly after injection and frequently following a period of abstinence.[239,310,330,331,334,355,384] In some, symptoms were present upon awakening from coma. Proprioception and vibratory sense were often preserved relative to loss of spinothalamic sensory modalities, suggesting infarction in the territory of the anterior spinal artery.[91,119,159,394] Autopsy in one patient showed necrosis "confined almost entirely" to the upper thoracic spinal cord gray matter and in another demonstrated additional involvement of the anterior aspect of the posterior columns and a pyramidal tract in the lower thoracic cord. If these lesions were cord infarcts, their possible causes, as with cerebral stroke in heroin users, include "watershed" infarction during a period of coma, hypoventilation, and hypotension,[159] as well as hypersensitivity reaction. Consistent with the latter, a young man, remaining conscious, had several episodes of numbness and weakness of both legs for a few minutes after injection.[331] An adolescent developed, 11 days after injection, a rash on the chest and feet and then, 6 days later, became paraplegic following a second injection.[355] Cord biopsy in another patient, moreover, showed vasculitis affecting mainly small arteries and arterioles, with "double refractile fragments" in inflamed tissue, including vessel walls.[186] (Such foreign particles have also been seen in the skin of heroin addicts.[172]) A patient at Harlem Hospital had heroin injected into a vessel over his midthoracic spine and within 30 minutes developed paraparesis and then urinary retention and sensory loss below that level. Myelography was normal. Whether the vessel injected was arterial or venous, the common intercostal origins of the posterior cutaneous and spinal arteries or veins would have allowed access of injected material directly to the spinal cord,[9,318] but that would not explain whether the damage was direct toxicity, hypersensitivity, or embolism of foreign material.

A man using intravenous heroin for the first time in 2 years became comatose and apneic; receiving nalorphine, he developed over several hours quadriplegia, anarthria, dysphagia, and sensory loss consistent with a ventral pontine lesion.[143] Recovery was partial, and whether or not the lesion was vascular was not determined.

A heroin addict with unexplained clotting abnormalities was found to have high circulating levels of heparin, presumably added to her drug mixture;[268] if heparin becomes a common adulterant, addicts will obviously be at increased risk for hemorrhagic stroke.

## AMPHETAMINE AND RELATED AGENTS

Although their manufacture was greatly reduced after the 1972 Controlled Substances Act, amphetamine and similar stimulants are still produced in huge quantities.[389] There are two patterns of abuse. Housewives, truck drivers, or students may take it orally, often with sedatives or alcohol. Addicts more often take it intravenously, sometimes in doses of up to 300 mg every few hours over days. Strokes common to any parenteral drug abuse are therefore encountered. There are also strokes that may be unique to these agents.

Acutely, amphetamine can cause excitement, hypertension, and a rectal temperature of over 109°F, followed by coma, vascular collapse, and death;[24,138,185,247,322,423] at autopsy there are diffuse cerebral edema and petechiae, without large infarcts or hematomas.[24,33,150,185,423] In dogs[422] or rabbits[201] given lethal doses of amphetamine there was severe hyperpyrexia and, at autopsy, subendocardial and epicardial hemorrhage, myocardial fiber necrosis, and, in the brain, neuronal degeneration in the cerebral cortex and cerebellum.[201,421,422] Curare prevented the fever and the fatal course, suggesting that the hyperpyrexia was secondary to muscle hyperactivity and that death was secondary to heat stroke. Fever may have also contributed to similar brain pathological findings in cats receiving chronic methedrine over 2 weeks, although in that study neuronal catecholamine depletion was suspected as the primary cause.[81,99]

Significant brain hemorrhage was not present in these experimental animals but has been found, along with focal neurologic signs, in animal and human cases of heat stroke,[69,108,114,225] often with severe clotting abnormalities, including decreased prothrombin activity, thrombocytopenia, hypofibrinogenemia, and fibrinolysis.[360] Hyperpyrexia and disturbed clotting have not been reported, however, with intracranial hemorrhage after amphetamine use. Over 30 patients have been reported, aged 16 to 60.[53,66,73,86,98,104,121,129,142,148,192,206,252,253,259,262,269,273,299,320,362,386,406,418,419,420] Eighteen had taken the drug orally, nine intravenously, two orally and intravenously, one nasally and intravenously, and two by uncertain route. Most were chronic users, but in five patients stroke followed a first exposure. The dose was usually unknown, but in one case was as low as 80 mg. Except for one instance each of diethylpropion and pseudoephedrine, all took amphetamine or methedrine; seven also took methylphenidate, LSD, dimethoxymethylamphetamine ("STP"), cocaine, heroin, or barbiturates. Severe headache usually occurred within minutes of drug use. Blood pressure was elevated in 15 of the 26 in whom it was recorded, with diastolic pressures as high as 120 mmHg in five. Eight patients died, usually soon after admission. Computerized tomography

(CT), done on 14 patients, showed, variably, intracerebral hemorrhage (frequently lobar), subarachnoid hemorrhage, or no abnormality. In 12 patients at angiography, irregular narrowing ("beading") of distal cerebral arteries suggested vasculitis; three of these patients had taken the drug only orally. Such vessel changes were present at autopsy in three (including one whose angiogram showed only an avascular mass). In another patient a cerebral vascular malformation was seen by both angiography and CT.

Thus, some of these amphetamine-induced intracranial hemorrhages seem to have been secondary to acute hypertension, some to cerebral vasculitis, and some to a combination of the two, but in others neither feature was apparent. While acute hypertension secondary to amphetamine could be causal, in some patients it might have been a transient result of the stroke.[85] Conversely, in others, fleeting blood pressure elevations could have been missed.

Amphetamine-induced cerebral vasculitis, which has caused occlusive as well as hemorrhagic strokes, appears to be of more than one type. Necrotizing angiitis, sometimes affecting the nervous system, occurred in 14 Los Angeles abusers of multiple drugs, including amphetamine, methedrine, barbiturates, chlordiazepoxide, diazepam, marijuana, hydroxyzine, LSD, heroin, meperidine, mescaline, oxycodone, oxymorphone, dimethoxymethylamphetamine, and strychnine.[67] All but two patients used intravenous methedrine, and one used it exclusively. Five patients were asymptomatic, and in the others there was fever, weight loss, malaise, weakness, skin rash, pneumonitis, pulmonary edema, hematuria, proteinuria, renal failure, abdominal pain, pancreatitis, gastrointestinal hemorrhage, arthralgia, myalgia, peripheral neuropathy, anemia, leukocytosis, and hemolysis. One patient had renal failure, severe hypertension, papilledema, retinal detachment, "progressive encephalopathy," and, at autopsy, vasculitis affecting pontine arterioles. Another, with "mental obtundation" and hypertension, had at autopsy "recent and resolving cerebral and pontine infarction," "marked cerebellar hemorrhage," and vasculitis in the cerebrum, cerebellum, and brain stem. Vessel lesions consisted acutely of fibrinoid necrosis of the media and intima, with infiltration by neutrophils, eosinophils, lymphocytes, and histiocytes; later there was destruction of muscular and elastic components, replacement by collagen, and often "a nodular (nodose) bulge with nearly aneurysmal dilatation." The authors considered these lesions, which affected only muscular arteries and arterioles, typical for polyarteritides nodosa and distinguished them from hypersensitivity angiitis, which involves small arteries, capillaries, and venules. They further noted that more than one drug or adulterant could have caused them, and that, in contrast to polyarteritis nodosa,[125,126] they were not associated with the presence of Australia antigen.[68]

While such brain lesions have been found pathologically in other polydrug (including amphetamine) abusers,[36,206] in some, cerebral arteritis has been presumed on the basis of cerebral angiography,[53,66,104,269,344,346,418,420] and sometimes the relation to amphetamine abuse has been tenuous.[285] In a report of three young men who developed ischemic strokes in association with intranasal methamphetamine, cerebral angiography revealed in one supraclinoid beading of the internal carotid artery, in another occlusion of the internal carotid artery near its origin, and in the third supraclinoid occlusion of the internal carotid artery.[340] A radiographic study of 19 young drug abusers, most taking intravenous methedrine and hospitalized for coma or stroke, revealed widespread segmental constrictions of large and medium-sized cerebral arteries and stenosis or occlusion of many penetrating arterioles, consistent with either multiple emboli or vasculitis and thrombosis.[344] The same authors then gave rhesus monkeys intravenous methedrine, 1.5 mg/kg (considered the lower limit of dosage for most abusers), and did serial cerebral angiograms for 2 weeks.[345] Several animals studied 10 minutes after receiving the drugs showed irregularly decreased caliber of small cerebral vessels, with a return to normal at 24 hours. In others these changes occurred in both small and large vessels and persisted for the 2-week period, in one actually worsening. Clinically there was hypertension and behavioral change. Postmortem examination at 2 weeks revealed subarachnoid hemorrhage in some animals, with numerous brain petechial hemorrhages, infarcts, edema, microaneurysms, and perivascular white blood cell cuffing. In a later study monkeys received intravenous methedrine three times weekly.[347] After either a month or a year serial angiograms showed occlusions and slow blood flow in small cerebral arteries, and at autopsy there were attenuated and fragmented brain arterioles and capillaries, microaneurysms, dilated venules, petechiae, neuronal loss, and gliosis. Talc crystals were present in capillaries (the drug was given as crushed methamphetamine hydrochloride (Desoxyn) tablets); but against such particles playing a critical role in the vasculitis was the fact that in the animals receiving crushed placebo tablets containing all the ingredients of Desoxyn except methedrine vasculitis was minimal or absent.

In rats receiving 2 weeks of intravenous methedrine, brain capillaries had, by electron microscopy, abnormal "budding" from the luminal walls of endothelial cells and vesicles within the endothelial cell cytoplasm.[347] These changes affected vessels smaller than 100 $\mu$m and would therefore be missed angiographically. (The vulnerability of small vessels might be related to their separate innervation: large cerebral vessels are innervated by the peripheral sympathetic nervous system, but nerve terminals on smaller arteries appear to be from central noradrenergic neurons.)[149]

Of three monkeys receiving intravenous methylphenidate (Ritalin) for a month, all had "a moderate degree of vascular change" angiographically, but only one had "some chromatolysis" histologically.[347] Rats receiving methylphenidate, however, had the same severe degree of histologic brain damage as those receiving methedrine.

These lesions are different from polyarteritis nodosa, in which elastic arteries, capillaries, and veins are spared. Whether they are the result of direct toxicity or of hypersensitivity is unclear, nor can the possibility be excluded that the early angiographic findings are secondary to subarachnoid hemorrhage (although beading of distal pial arteries in subarachnoid hemorrhage is rare[66]). In an adolescent amphetamine abuser with mononeuritis multiplex, sural nerve biopsy showed apparent hypersensitivity angiitis of medium and small muscular arteries, arterioles, venules, and veins, with fibrinoid necrosis and infiltration by polymorphonuclear leukocytes, lymphocytes, eosinophils, and plasma cells.[367] The central nervous system was clinically unaffected, however.

Federal restrictions on amphetamine do not apply to phenylpropanolamine (PPA), a similar but less potent drug found, sometimes with ephedrine or caffeine, in over-the-counter decongestants (e.g., Contac) and diet pills (e.g., Dex-a-diet, Dexatrim, Anorexin, Maxi-slim), as well as in drugs made deliberately to resemble amphetamine ("look-alike pills").[29,288] Although the FDA has restricted over-the-counter combinations of phenylpropanolamine, ephedrine, and caffeine, an estimated five billion doses of phenylpropanolamine are used in the United States annually.[234] Acute hypertension, severe headache, psychiatric symptoms, seizures, and hemorrhagic stroke have occurred in users.[25,111,191,209,258,288–290,301,347,353,408] PPA with caffeine, from a commercial diet preparation, produced subarachnoid hemorrhage in rats receiving it intraperitoneally in three to six times the recommended dose.[289]

Ephedrine and pseudoephedrine are present in over-the-counter decongestants and bronchodilators. Complications have included headache, tachyarrhythmia, hypertensive emergency, and hemorrhagic stroke.[118,253,270,312,373]

A young man who had previously used "speed" and LSD had a subarachnoid hemorrhage within an hour of ingesting pills that turned out to be ephedrine.[416] Cerebral angiography was initially normal but a week later showed beading and branch occlusions suggesting arteritis; a biopsy from grossly normal skin showed deposits of IgM and the C3 component of complement periluminally in dermal vessels, consistent with circulating immune complexes.

A young woman who injected crushed methylphenidate tablets into her jugular veins developed immediate right hemiplegia after a left injection and two months later left hemiplegia after a right injection; presumably the injections were inadvertently into the carotid artery, but the exact mechanism of stroke was not determined.[63] Intraretinal talc microemboli have been seen in the fundi of intravenous methylphenidate abusers.[12,391] In some there were retinal vascular and choroidal abnormalities, neovascularization, and vitreous hemorrhage,[391] and in one, who had not had a clinical stroke, talc and cornstarch emboli were also present in arterioles, capillaries, and veins of brain and lung.[12] Infarction of the medial medulla in a young woman occurred a few minutes after intravenous methylphenidate; at autopsy there was systemic granulomatosis due to talc and talc deposits in small vessels around the medullary infarct.[281]

Mycotic subclavian and carotid aneurysms developed following inadvertant intra-arterial injection of the diet compound phentermine.[144]

Death has followed parenteral[8] or oral[332] abuse of propylhexedrine from "Benzedrex" inhalers; stroke has not yet been reported in such patients, and the cause of death has been uncertain.

## COCAINE

In the 1980s cocaine use became widespread in the United States. In 1982 it was estimated that 28 percent of people aged 18 to 25 had used cocaine hydrochloride, usually intranasally but often parenterally (including cocaine-heroin mixtures—so-called "speedballs").[45] In 1985 the appearance of commercially prepared alkaloidal cocaine ("crack") led to acceleration of the epidemic, with increasing addictive use and widespread illegal trafficking and social disruption. Smokable "crack" produces a psychological "high" even more intense than that which follows intravenous cocaine hydrochloride and is taken in larger and more frequent doses. The result has been increasing morbidity and mortality, including stroke.[190,407]

Parenteral cocaine users are at risk for stroke related to infection, including endocarditis, AIDS, and hepatitis. They also develop strokes caused directly by the drug itself, whether taken intranasally, intravenously, or intramuscularly or smoked as "crack."[242] The first report of a cocaine-related stroke was in 1977: a middle-aged, mildly hypertensive man after drinking a bottle of wine injected cocaine intramuscularly and an hour later abruptly developed aphasia and right hemiparesis; CSF was normal, and cerebral angiography was refused.[49] The same year fatal rupture of a cerebral saccular aneurysm occurred in a young man sniffing cocaine.[263] Further cases were not reported until the mid-1980s, but by the early 1990s over 200 cases of stroke had been described, about half occlusive and half hemorrhagic.[4,58,61,76,77,84,88,89,90,105,127,137,156,182,189,204,216,223,240,245,246,248,260,266,278–281,284,293,296,314,317,335,341,342,354,357,366,382,389,403,411]

Ischemic strokes have included transient ischemic attacks and infarction of cerebrum, thalamus, brain stem, spinal cord, and retina.[89,223,282] Infarction has occurred in newborns whose mothers used cocaine shortly before delivery[61] and in pregnant women.[242] In some cases cerebral infarction has been attributed to vasculitis on the basis of angiographic findings;[204] such changes, however, may have represented vasospasm following undiagnosed subarachnoid hemorrhage.[243] Autopsies have usually shown histologically normal cerebral vessels,[242,246] although in two cases mild cerebral vasculitis was observed at biopsy or autopsy.[223] A young crack smoker had middle cerebral artery branch occlusion, cardiomyopathy, and a left atrial thrombus.[317] A 20-year-old with no other risk factors had superior cerebellar artery occlusion six months after last use, raising the possibility of delayed effects.[88] In a 27-year-old occasional cocaine sniffer with "heaviness and paresthesias" in the legs and occasional "forgetfulness" magnetic resonance imaging revealed multiple periventricular white matter lesions.[403]

Intracerebral or subarachnoid hemorrhage has occurred during or within hours of cocaine use or has had less clear temporal relationship. In some instances there has been other substance use, especially ethanol. Nearly half of those undergoing angiography have had saccular aneurysms or vascular malformations. Other hemorrhages have included bleeding into embolic infarction or glioma.[411] Cerebral hemorrhages have occurred in newborns and postpartem women.[156,242,278] In a patient with multiple cerebral hemorrhages after smoking crack autopsy revealed histologically normal cerebral vessels.[137]

The mechanisms of cocaine-related stroke are unclear.[336] Striking, considering that cocaine and amphetamine have similar actions and effects, are the high frequency of underlying aneurysm or vascular malformation in hemorrhagic strokes of cocaine users compared to amphetamine users and, conversely, the frequency of vasculitis in amphetamine users compared to cocaine users. Cocaine hydrochloride is more often associated with hemorrhagic than occlusive stroke, whereas hemorrhagic and occlusive strokes occur with roughly equal frequency in "crack" users, but the rising prevalence of stroke since the appearance of "crack" is probably attributable to wider use and higher dosage rather than to a peculiarity of "crack" itself. By blocking reuptake of norepinephrine from sympathetic nerve endings (and probably also by affecting calcium flux) cocaine is a vasoconstrictor.[175,181] Acute hypertension can result, leading to intracranial hemorrhage, especially in subjects with underlying aneurysms or vascular malformations. Coronary artery vasoconstriction has been documented during cardiac catheterization,[64,231] and there are numerous reports of angina pectoris and myocardial infarction during or following cocaine use.[64,364] Cocaine also causes cardiac arrhythmia and cardiomyopathy, which, like myocardial infarction, carries the potential risk for embolic stroke.[65,200,402] Cerebral vasoconstriction may cause occlusive stroke, and it is possibly significant that cocaine metabolites, which in some chronic users are detectable in urine for weeks, have also been reported to cause cerebral vasospasm.[321,405] The situation is complex, however, for cerebral and peripheral vessels frequently respond differently to similar stimuli. Whereas intraluminal cocaine constricted cat and rat pial vessels in vitro, topical cocaine dilated pial vessels in living cats.[92,175,321] Cocaine enhances the response of platelets to arachidonic acid, possibly promoting aggregation.[388] In rabbits repeated cocaine injections caused arteriosclerotic aortopathy.[232] In a cocaine user with symptoms of coronary artery disease protein C and antithrombin III were depleted and returned to normal, with clearing of symptoms, when use was discontinued.[65]

## PHENCYCLIDINE

Phencyclidine (PCP, "angel dust") became a widely abused American street drug in the 1970s; it can be smoked, eaten, or injected, and is often misrepresented as marijuana or mescaline. One to 5 mg produce euphoria, emotional lability, and a feeling of diffuse numbness; 5 to 15 mg cause confusion, excitation, decreased sensory perception, and body distortion; higher doses cause psychosis, myoclonus, nystagmus, seizures, coma, and sometimes fatal respiratory and circulatory collapse.[43,50,205,274,295] Hypertension can occur both early and late during intoxication[78,102,274] and may be related to enhancement of the action of catecholamines and serotonin.[179] However, contractile responses to phencyclidine of isolated basilar and middle cerebral arteries were not prevented or reversed by methysergide, phentolamine, atropine, diphenhydramine, or indomethacin, raising the possibility of phencyclidine receptors on cerebral blood vessels.[5]

A 13-year-old boy became comatose after taking phencyclidine; admission blood pressure was normal, and he became more alert, but 3 days later his condition deteriorated with a blood pressure of 220/130 mmHg. At autopsy there was an intracerebral hemorrhage.[102] A 6-year-old boy became unresponsive with seizures and right hemiparesis; urine contained phencyclidine. CT demonstrated left parieto-occipital lucency and vessel enhancement suggesting a vascular malformation. He recovered, and cerebral angiography was not done.[78] A young man collapsed after smoking phencyclidine; blood pressure was 180/100 mmHg, and at autopsy there was subarachnoid hemorrhage without parenchymal hematoma. A 17-year-old boy with phencyclidine in his blood died following perforation of the ventral surface of his basilar artery.[38] Hypertensive encephalopathy followed phencyclidine ingestion in a young woman with systemic lupus erythematosus and a history of migraine.[51]

## LSD

Lysergic acid diethylamide (LSD) in high doses causes severe hypertension, obtundation, and convulsions.[37,72,371] In vitro spasm of cerebral vessel strips immersed in LSD-containing solution was prevented or reversed by methysergide.[5] Following ingestion of four LSD capsules, a 14-year-old boy developed seizures and, 4 days later, left hemiplegia; carotid angiography showed progressive narrowing of the internal carotid artery from its origin to the siphon, with occlusion at its bifurcation.[365] A young woman developed sudden left hemiplegia a day after oral LSD; angiography showed marked constriction of the internal carotid artery at the siphon; 9 days later the vessel was occluded at that level.[250] A 19-year-old with acute aphasia and cerebral angiographic findings consistent with arteritis had used both LSD and heroin, and the time relationship of either drug to the stroke was not stated.[251] Another patient with angiographic evidence of vasculitis had used both LSD and "diet pills."[344]

## BARBITURATES

Usually abused orally, barbiturates and other sedatives and tranquilizers can cause cerebral infarction in association with overdose and diffusely decreased brain perfusion, but occlusive or hemorrhagic stroke has not otherwise been reported. A 20-year-old man taking orally a combination of secobarbital and strychnine ("M and Ms") became comatose with right hemiplegia, and cerebral angiography showed widespread segmental vascular irregularity consistent with arteritis; he had been taking other drugs as well for at least 10 years.[346] Cerebral vasculitis was also found in four other barbiturate abusers; two also abused chlorpromazine, one took other unidentified drugs, and the fourth apparently used only barbiturates, but whether orally or parenterally was not revealed.[344]

Monkeys receiving dissolved secobarbital (Seconal) capsules, 1.5 mg/kg intravenously three times a week for a year, had at cerebral angiography narrowing of small arteries. Histologically there were scattered talc crystals in brain capillaries, without cellular reaction; one animal had a frontal lobe microinfarct.[346]

## INHALANTS

Inhalation of vapors to achieve euphoric intoxication is common in the United States, especially among children. Substances include aerosals, enamels, paint thinners, lighter fluid, cleaning fluid, glues, cements, gasoline, and anesthetics. Death results from violence, accidents, suffocation, aspiration, or cardiac arrhythmia. Clinical stroke has not been reported, but radioisotope brain scan in a boy with status epilepticus after toluene sniffing showed several wedge-shaped areas of increased uptake in both cerebral hemispheres, consistent with infarcts.[228]

## ALCOHOL

Coronary artery disease and myocardial infarction may be less prevalent in those who drink alcohol than in those who do not. The increased risk of coronary artery disease in heavy drinkers becomes an indirect risk for cardioembolic stroke secondary to cardiac wall hypokinesia or arrhythmia. Alcohol intoxication and withdrawal are also directly associated with cardiac arrhythmia ("holiday heart"),[106,261,385] and thromboembolism is a prominent feature of alcoholic cardiomyopathy.[58]

A large literature has addressed whether acute or chronic alcohol use is a risk factor for stroke independent of its cardiac effects or other risk factors.[15,203,211,223,237,297,338] Retrospective studies, most notably from Finland, have found an association between recent heavy alcohol use and both occlusive and hemorrhagic stroke.[165,167–169,376] The Finnish studies, however, used population prevalence data as controls, and other similarly designed analyses have either not found such an association,[171] or, as in the NINCDS Data Bank, only for intracerebral hemorrhage.[286] A study from Chicago found that the association between alcohol intoxication and stroke disappeared when corrected for cigarette smoking.[134,135]

Numerous case-control and cohort studies have addressed the relationship of stroke to chronic alcohol use.[39,79,122,130,161,207,215,249,298,304,307,359,370,383,398] Contradictory findings are not surprising, for studies have differed in endpoints chosen (e.g., total stroke, occlusive stroke, hemorrhagic stroke, or stroke mortality), amount and duration of alcohol consumption, correction for other risk factors (especially hypertension and smoking), and ethnicity and socioeconomics of populations being studied. Among cohort studies, the Yugoslavia Cardiovascular Disease Study found increased stroke mortality among drinkers, and, although the association was especially strong for hypertensives, it persisted with adjustment for blood pressure.[221,222] A reduced risk was found for modest drinkers. In the Honolulu Heart Study heavy drinkers had an increased risk of hemorrhagic stroke independent of other risk factors including hypertension and smoking.[27,96,187,378] There was no comparable risk for occlusive stroke. Early reports from the Framingham Study found both positive[414] and negative[131,194,198,199] associations; a later report described lower than expected stroke incidence among "moderate" drinkers and higher rates in both heavy drinkers and nondrinkers.[413] In the Nurses' Health Study independent of smoking and hypertension there was an inverse association between modest alcohol intake (less than two drinks daily) and occlusive stroke, with a positive association at higher intake; subarachnoid hemorrhage was associated with both low and high alcohol intake.[368] In the Lausanne Stroke Registry severity of internal carotid artery stenosis inversely correlated with "light-to-moderate" alcohol intake; there were too few patients to assess heavy intake.[31] The Japanese Hisayama Study initially reported positive correlations,[202] but later found no independent association between alcohol and occlusive or hemorrhagic stroke after adjusting for other variables.[395] A study of Japanese physicians found a positive association between stroke mortality and alcohol intake.[219,220] Three other Japanese studies found either independent associations between alcohol and hemorrhagic but not occlusive stroke,[380] no association between alcohol and hemorrhagic or occlusive stroke,[166] and no association between alcohol and occlusive stroke.[379]

In a review of 62 epidemiologic studies that examined the relation between stroke and "moderate" alcohol consumption (less than two drinks, or 1 oz. of absolute ethanol) it was concluded that ethnicity played a role in the disparate results.[54] Among whites moderate doses of alcohol seemed to protect against ischemic stroke, whereas higher doses increased risk. (This pattern is similar to that for alcohol and coronary artery disease.) Among the Japanese little association seemed to exist between alcohol and ischemic stroke. In both populations all doses of alcohol seemed to increase the risk of both intracerebral and subarachnoid hemorrhage. Some studies have suggested that the risk of hemorrhagic stroke declines with abstinence, but the evidence is insufficient to draw an association between stroke and recent intoxication per se.

As with coronary artery disease several mechanisms might explain the association between alcohol and stroke. Alcohol acutely and chronically raises blood pressure,[20,27,100,197,213,221,264,265,271,272,325,348] perhaps related to increased adrenergic activity and to increased blood levels of cortisol, renin, aldosterone, and vasopressin.[132] With abstinence blood pressure may become normal.[254]

Perhaps related to its protective effects, alcohol lowers blood levels of low-density lipoproteins and elevates levels of high-density lipoproteins.[17,55,60,152] One study found that alcohol seemed preferentially to protect large vessels from atherosclerosis, perhaps accounting for ethnic differences in patterns of protection or risk.[326] The relationship is uncertain, however, for alcohol may not raise blood levels of the more protective HDL-2 subfraction.[13,133]

Acutely alcohol decreases fibrinolytic activity, increases factor VIII, increases platelet reactivity to ADP, and shortens bleeding time.[164,170,230,238,276] On the other hand, moderate doses of alcohol increase levels of prostacyclin,[183,229] and some studies have found decreased platelet function following alcohol.[75,107,153,193,311,324,328,374] In chronic alcoholics decreased levels of clotting factors, excessive fibrinolysis, and platelet abnormalities appear to be secondary to liver disease.[132] During or following ethanol withdrawal "rebound thrombocytosis" and platelet hyperaggregability have been observed.[151,178]

Acute alcohol intoxication had been accompanied by cerebral vasodilatation[275,404] and blood-brain barrier leakage of albumin,[313] perhaps contributing to the severity of traumatic intracerebral hemorrhage during drinking.[109,363] Increased cerebral blood flow has also been observed during alcohol withdrawal.[155] Chronic drinking is associated with reduced cerebral blood flow, mainly from reduced cerebral metabolism.[23] In vitro, however, alcohol causes constriction of both large and small cerebral vessels.[6] Alcohol-related hemoconcentration may also contribute to reduced cerebral blood flow.[132]

## TOBACCO

Epidemiologic studies have shown smoking to be a major risk factor for coronary artery and peripheral vascular disease.[10,94,195,305] Although a few reports have been negative or demonstrated only insignificant trends toward increased risk of stroke among smokers,[82,160,196] most case control and cohort studies have shown that smoking does increase the risk for both occlusive and hemorrhagic stroke.[1,2,28,34,35,56,87,93,95,110,135,145–147,162,188,218,226,257,283,302,303,339,351,361,393,414] In women smokers the risk of occlusive and hemorrhagic stroke is greater in those taking oral contraceptives.[71,113,128,315,343] In a prospective cohort study of middle-aged women smoking increased stroke risk in a dose-dependent fashion; for those smoking 25 or more cigarettes daily, the relative risk for all stroke was 3.7 and for subarachnoid hemorrhage 9.8 independent of other risk factors, including oral contraceptives, hypertension, and alcohol.[70] In another report smoking in hypertensive men and women carried a 15-fold risk for subarachnoid hemorrhage and was a greater risk than hypertension itself.[34] In another study the treatment of hypertension reduced stroke incidence in nonsmokers but not in smokers.[277] In the Honolulu Heart Program stroke risk was independent of coronary artery disease.[1] The Framingham Study found smoking to be a risk factor for subarachnoid hemorrhage and, independent of age and hypertension, for both occlusive and hemorrhagic stroke; this risk was dose-dependent and disappeared when smoking ceased.[350,412] Others have confirmed reduction of risk with cessation of smoking.[218,339]

Several possible mechanisms could underlie tobacco's risk for stroke. Smoking aggravates atherosclerosis; in a study of identical twins discordant for smoking, carotid plaques were significantly more prominent in the smokers, and in other reports smoking correlated in dose-related fashion with severity of extracranial carotid atherosclerosis.[31,141,409] The reversibility of stroke risk with cessation of smoking is against such a mechanism being paramount, however.[291,337,412] Carbon monoxide in cigarette smoke reduces blood's oxygen carrying capacity, and nicotine constricts coronary arteries.[22,267] In animals nicotine damages endothelium, and increased numbers of circulating endothelial cells are found in smokers.[83,424] Smoking acutely raises blood pressure, systole more than diastole; cerebral blood flow is reduced even after such acute effects have worn off.[224,255] Smoking is not a risk factor for chronic hypertension, but it accelerates the progression of chronic hypertension to malignant hypertension.[136,180] Smokers become tachycardic, and atrial fibrillation has followed nicotine gum chewing.[22] Smoking increases platelet reactivity and inhibits prostacyclin formation.[21,291,292,327,358] It also raises blood fibrinogen, a linkage noted in several stroke studies.[21,195,196,410] The increased risk of subarachnoid hemorrhage in smokers has been blamed on increased elastolytic activity in the serum.[110]

Progressive multifocal symptoms occurred in four young women who smoked and used oral contraceptives. Cerebral angiography demonstrated moyamoya, and abnormal studies included elevated ESR, positive antinuclear antibodies, and elevated CSF IgG. Disease progression ceased with discontinuation of oral contraceptives and reduction in smoking.[244]

## REFERENCES


1. Abbott RD, Reed DM, Yano K: Risk of stroke in male cigarette smokers. N Engl J Med 315:717, 1986
2. Abu-Zeid HAH, Choi NW, Maini KK et al: Relative role of factors associated with cerebral infarction and cerebral hemorrhage: a matched pair case-control study. Stroke 8:106, 1977
3. Adams JH, Brierley JB, Connor RCR, Treip CS: The effects of systemic hypotension upon the human brain: clinical and neuropathological observations in 11 cases. Brain 89:235, 1966
4. Altes-Capella J, Cabezudo-Artero JM, Forteza-Rei J: Complications of cocaine abuse. Ann Intern Med 107:940, 1987
5. Altura B, Altura BM: Phencyclidine, lysergic acid diethylamide, and mescaline: cerebral artery spasms and hallucinogenic activity. Science 212:1051, 1981
6. Altura BM, Altura BT, Gebrewold A: Alcohol-induced spasms of cerebral blood vessels: relations to cerebrovascular accidents and sudden death. Science 220:331, 1983
7. Amine AB: Neurosurgical complications of heroin addiction: brain abscess and mycotic aneurysm. Surg Neurol 7:385, 1977
8. Anderson RJ, Garza H, Garriott JC, Dimaio V: Intravenous propylhexedrine (Benzedrex) abuse and sudden death. Am J Med 67:15, 1979
9. Anson BJ: p. 728. Morris's Human Anatomy. McGraw-Hill, New York, 1966
10. Aronow WS, Kaplan NM: Smoking. p. 50. In Kaplan NM, Stamler (eds): Prevention of Coronary Heart Disease. Philadelphia, WB Saunders, 1983
11. Ashley MJ: Alcohol consumption, ischemic heart disease, and cerebrovascular disease. J Stud Alcohol 43:869, 1982
12. Atlee W: Talc and cornstarch emboli in eyes of drug abusers. JAMA 219:49, 1972
13. Avogaro P, Cazzolato G, Belussi F, Bittolo Bon G: Altered apoprotein composition of HDL-2 and HDL-3 in chronic alcoholics. Artery 10:317, 1982
14. Baden MM: Pathology of the addictive states. p. 189. In Richter RW (ed): Medical Aspects of Drug Abuse. Harper & Row, Hagerstown, MD, 1975
15. Balow J, Alter M, Resch J: Cerebral thromboembolism: a clinical appraisal of 100 cases. Neurology (NY) 16:559, 1966
16. Banks T, Fletcher R, Ali N: Infective endocarditis in heroin addicts. Am J Med 55:444, 1973
17. Barboriak JJ, Anderson AJ, Hoffman RG: Interrelationships between coronary artery occlusion, high-density lipoprotein cholesterol, and alcohol intake. J Lab Clin Med 94:348, 1979
18. Barenek JT: Morphine binding by serum globulins from morphine-treated rabbits. Fed Proc 33:474, 1974
19. Becker C: Medical complications of drug abuse. Adv Intern Med 24:183, 1979
20. Beevers DG: Alcohol and hypertension. Lancet 2:114, 1977
21. Belch JJ, McArdle BM, Burns P et al: The effects of acute smoking on platelet behavior, fibrinolysis, and haemorheology in habitual smokers. Thromb Haemost 51:6, 1984
22. Benowitz NL: Pharmacologic aspects of cigarette smoking and nicotine addiction. N Engl J Med 319:1318, 1988
23. Berglund M: Cerebral blood flow in chronic alcoholics. Alcoholism Clin Exp Res 5:295, 1981
24. Bernheim J, Cox JN: Heat stroke and amphetamine intoxication in a sportsman. Schweiz Med Wochenschr 90:322, 1960
25. Bernstein E, Diskant B: Phenylpropanolamine, a potentially hazardous drug. Ann Emerg Med 11:315, 1982
26. Besson HA: Intracranial hemorrhage associated with phencyclidine abuse. JAMA 248:585, 1982
27. Blackwelder WC, Yano K, Rhoads GC et al: Alcohol and mortality: the Honolulu Heart Study. Am J Med 68:164, 1980
28. Bloch C, Richard JL: Risk factors for atherosclerotic diseases in the Prospective Parisan Study. I. Comparison with foreign studies. Rev Epidemiol Sante Publique 33:108, 1985
29. Blum A: Phenylpropanolamine: an over-the-counter amphetamine? JAMA 245:1346, 1981
30. Boak RA, Carpenter CM, Miller JN: Biologic false-positive reactions for syphilis among narcotic addicts: a report on the incidence of BFP reactions as measured by the TPI test. JAMA 175:326, 1961
31. Bogousslavsky J, Van Melle G, Despland PA,

Regli F: Alcohol consumption and carotid atherosclerosis in the Lausanne Stroke Registry. Stroke 21:715, 1990
32. Bohmfalk GL, Story JL, Wissinger JP, Brown WE: Bacterial intracranial aneurysm. J Neurosurg 48:369, 1978
33. Bonhoff C, Lewrenz H: Über Werkamine. p. 144. Springer-Verlag, Berlin, 1954
34. Bonita R: Cigarette smoking, hypertension, and the risk of subarachnoid hemorrhage: a population-based case-control study. Stroke 17:831, 1986
35. Bonita R, Scragg R, Stewart A et al: Cigarette smoking and risk of premature stroke in men and women. Br Med J 293:6, 1986
36. Botwick DG: Amphetamine induced cerebral vasculitis. Hum Pathol 12:1031, 1981
37. Bourne PG: Acute Drug Abuse Emergencies. Academic Press, San Diego, CA, 1976
38. Boyko OB, Burger PC, Heinz ER: Pathological and radiological correlation of subarachnoid hemorrhage in phencyclidine abuse: case report. J Neurosurg 67:446, 1987
39. Boysen G, Nyboe J, Appleyard M et al: Stroke incidence and risk factors for stroke in Copenhagen, Denmark. Stroke 19:1345, 1988
40. Brierley JB: The neuropathology of brain hypoxia. p. 243. In Critchley M, O'Leary JL, Jennett B (eds): Scientific Foundations of Neurology. Heinemann, London, 1972
41. Brust JCM: Drug abuse and nervous system toxins. p. 540. In Rosenberg R (ed): Neurology. Vol. 5: The Science and Practice of Clinical Medicine, Dietschy JM (ed-in-chief). Grune & Stratton, Orlando FL, 1980
42. Brust JCM: The non-impact of opiate research on opiate abuse. Neurology (NY) 33:1327, 1983
43. Brust JCM: Neurology and drug abuse. Neurology and Neurosurgery Update Series 4/29:1, 1983
44. Brust JCM: Stroke and drugs. p. 517. In Toole JF (ed): Vascular Diseases, Part III, Vol 55 of Handbook of Clinical Neurology, Rev Series II. Elsevier, Amsterdam, 1989
45. Brust JCM: Drug dependence. In Joynt RJ (ed): Clinical Neurology. Harper & Row, New York, 1991
46. Brust JCM, Dickinson PCT, Hughes JEO, Holtzman RNN: The diagnosis and treatment of cerebral mycotic aneurysms. Ann Neurol 27:238, 1990
47. Brust JCM, Richter RW: Quinine amblyopia related to heroin addiction. Ann Intern Med 74:84, 1971
48. Brust JCM, Richter RW: Stroke associated with addiction to heroin. J Neurol Neurosurg Psychiatry 39:194, 1976
49. Brust JCM, Richter RW: Stroke associated with cocaine abuse? NY State J Med 77:1473, 1977
50. Burns RS, Lerner SE: Causes of phencyclidine-related deaths. Clin Toxicol 12:463, 1978
51. Burns RS, Lerner SE: The effects of phencyclidine in man: a review. p. 449. In Domino EF (ed): PCP (Phencyclidine): Historical and Current Perspectives. NPP Books, Ann Arbor, MI, 1981
52. Butz WC: Disseminated magnesium and silicate associated with paregoric addiction. J Forensic Sci 15:581, 1970
53. Cahill DW, Knipp H, Mosser J: Intracranial hemorrhage with amphetamine abuse. Neurology (NY) 31:1058, 1981
54. Camargo CA: Moderate alcohol consumption and stroke: the epidemiologic evidence. Stroke 20:1611, 1989
55. Camargo CA, Williams PT, Vranizan KM et al: The effect of moderate alcohol intake on serum apolipoproteins A-I and A-II: a controlled study. JAMA 253:2854, 1985
56. Candelise L, Bianchi F, Galligoni F et al: Italian multicenter study on cerebral ischemic attacks. III. Influence of age and risk factors on cerebral atherosclerosis. Stroke 15:379, 1984
57. Caplan LR, Hier DB, Banks G: Stroke and drug abuse. Stroke 13:869, 1982
58. Caplan LR, Hier DB, DeCruz I: Cerebral embolism in the Michael Reese Stroke Registry. Stroke 14:530, 1983
59. Caplan LR, Thomas C, Banks G: Central nervous system complications of addiction to "T's and Blues." Neurology (NY) 32:623, 1982
60. Castelli WP, Gordon T, Hjortland MC et al: Alcohol and blood lipids: the Cooperative Lipoprotein Phenotyping Study. Lancet 2:153, 1977
61. Chasnoff IJ, Bussey ME, Savich R, Stack CM: Perinatal cerebral infarction and maternal cocaine use. J Pediatr 108:456, 1986
62. Cherubin CE: The medical sequelae of narcotic addiction. Ann Intern Med 67:23, 1967
63. Chillar RK, Jackson AL: Reversible hemiplegia after presumed intracarotid injection of Ritalin. N Engl J Med 304:1305, 1981
64. Chokshi SK, Miller G, Rongione A, Isner JM: Cocaine and cardiovascular disease: the leading edge. Cardiology 3:1, 1989
65. Chokshi SK, Moore R, Pandian NG, Isner JM: Reversible cardiomyopathy associated with cocaine intoxication. Ann Intern Med 111:1039, 1989
66. Chynn KY: Acute subarachnoid hemorrhage. JAMA 233:55, 1973
67. Citron BP, Halpern M, McCarron M et al: Necrotizing angiitis associated with drug abuse. N Engl J Med 283:1003, 1970
68. Citron BP, Peters RL: Angiitis in drug abusers. N Engl J Med 284:112, 1971
69. Clowes GHA, O'Donnell TF: Heat stroke: N Engl J Med 291:564, 1974
70. Colditz GA, Bonita R, Stampfer MJ et al: Cigarette smoking and risk of stroke in middle-aged women. N Engl J Med 318:937, 1988
71. Collaborative Group for the Study of Stroke in Young Women: oral contraception and increased risk of cerebral ischemia or thrombosis. N Engl J Med 288:871, 1973
72. Corales RL, Maull KI, Becker DP: Phencyclidine abuse mimicking head injury. JAMA 243:2323, 1980
73. Coroner's Report: Amphetamine overdose kills boy. Pharm J 198:172, 1967
74. Courville CN: The process of demyelination in

the central nervous system. IV. Demyelination as a delayed residual of carbon monoxide asphyxia. J Nerv Ment Dis 125:534, 1957
75. Cowan DH: Effect of alcoholism on hemostasis. Semin Hematol 17:137, 1980
76. Cregler LL, Mark H: Medical complications of cocaine abuse. N Engl J Med 315:1495, 1986
77. Cregler LL, Mark H: Relation of stroke to cocaine abuse. NY State J Med 87:128, 1987
78. Crosley CJ, Binet EF: Cerebrovascular complications in phencyclidine intoxication. J Pediatr 94:316, 1979
79. Cullen K, Stenhouse NS, Wearne KL: Alcohol and mortality in the Busselton study. Int J Epidemiol 11:67, 1982
80. Cunningham EE, Brentjens JR, Zielezny MA et al: Heroin nephropathy: a clinicopathologic and epidemiologic study. Am J Med 68:47, 1980
81. Cushman P, Grieco MH: Hyperimmunoglobulinemia associated with narcotic addiction: effects of methadone maintenance treatment. Am J Med 54:320, 1973
82. Davanipour Z, Sobel E, Alter M et al: Stroke/transient ischemic attack in the Lehigh Valley: evaluation of smoking as a risk factor. Ann Neurol 24:130, 1988
83. Davis JW, Shelton L, Eigenberg DA et al: Effects of tobacco and non-tobacco cigarette smoking on endothelium and platelets. Clin Pharmacol Ther 37:529, 1985
84. DeBroucker T, Verstichel P, Cambier J, De-Truchis P: Accidents neurologiqes après prise de cocaine. Presse Med 18:541, 1989
85. Delaney P: Intracranial hemorrhage associated with amphetamine use. Neurology (NY) 31:923, 1981
86. Delaney P, Estes M: Intracranial hemorrhage with amphetamine abuse. Neurology (NY) 30:1125, 1980
87. Department of Health and Human Services: The Health Consequences of Smoking: Nicotine Addiction. A Report of the Surgeon General. (DHHS Publ No (CDC) 88-8406.) US Government Printing Office, Washington, DC, 1988
88. Deringer PM, Hamilton LL, Whelan MA: A stroke associated with cocaine use. Arch Neurol 47:502, 1990
89. Devenyi P, Schneiderman JF, Devenyi RG, Lawby L: Cocaine-induced central retinal artery occlusion. Can Med Assoc J 138:129, 1988
90. Devore RA, Tucker HM: Dysphagia and dysarthria as a result of cocaine abuse. Otolaryngol Head Neck Surg 98:174, 1988
91. DiChiro G, Fried LC: Blood flow currents in spinal arteries. Neurology (NY) 21:1088, 1971
92. Dohi S, Jones D, Hudak ML, Traystman RJ: Effects of cocaine on pial arterioles in cats. Stroke 21:1710, 1990
93. Doll R, Gray R, Hafner B et al: Mortality in relation to smoking: twenty-two years observations on female British doctors. Br Med J 1:967, 1980
94. Doll R, Hill AB: Mortality of British doctors in relation to smoking: observations on coronary thrombosis. Natl Cancer Inst Monogr 19:205, 1966
95. Doll R, Peto R: Mortality in relation to smoking: 20 year's observations on male British doctors. Br Med J 2:1525, 1976
96. Donahue RP, Abbott RD, Reed DM, Yano K: Alcohol and hemorrhagic stroke: the Honolulu Heart Study. JAMA 255:2311, 1986
97. Doyle JT, Heslin AS, Hilleboe HE et al: A prospective study of degenerative cardiovascular disease in Albany: report of three years' experience. 1. Ischemic heart disease. Am J Public Health 47:25, 1957
98. D'Souza T, Shraberg D: Intracranial hemorrhage associated with amphetamine use. Neurology (NY) 31:922, 1981
99. Duarte Escalante O, Ellinwood EH: Central nervous system cytopathological changes in cats with chronic methedrine intoxication. Brain Res 21:151, 1970
100. Dyer A, Stamler J, Paul O et al: Alcohol consumption, cardiovascular risk factors, and mortality in two Chicago epidemiologic studies. Circulation 56:1067, 1977
101. Dyer AR, Stamler J, Paul O et al: Alcohol consumption and 17-year mortality in the Chicago Western Electric Company. Prev Med 9:78, 1980
102. Eastman JW, Cohen SN: Hypertensive crisis and death associated with phencyclidine poisoning. JAMA 231:1270, 1975
103. Eddy NB, Halbach H, Isbell H, Seevers MH: Drug dependence: its significance and characteristics. Bull WHO 32:721, 1965
104. Edwards K: Hemorrhagic complications of cerebral arteritis. Arch Neurol 34:549, 1977
105. Engstrand BC, Daras M, Tuchman AJ et al: Cocaine-related ischemic stroke. Neurology (NY), suppl 1. 39:186, 1989
106. Ettinger PO, Wu CF, DeLa Cruz C et al: Arrhythmias and the "holiday heart": alcohol-associated cardiac rhythm disorders. Am Heart J 95:555, 1978
107. Fenn CG, Littleton JM: Inhibition of platelet aggregation by ethanol: the role of plasma and platelet membrane lipids. Br J Pharmacol 73:305P, 1981
108. Ferris EB, Blankenhorn MA, Robinson HW et al: Heat stroke: clinical and chemical observations on 44 cases. J Clin Invest 17:249, 1938
109. Flamm ES, Demopoulos HB, Seligman ML et al: Ethanol potentiation of central nervous system trauma. J Neurosurg 46:328, 1977
110. Fogelholm R: Cigarette smoking and subarachnoid hemorrhage: a population-based case-control study. J Neurol Neurosurg Psychiatry 50:78, 1987
111. Forman HP, Levin S, Stewart B et al: Cerebral vasculitis and hemorrhage in an adolescent taking diet pills containing phenylpropanolamine: case report and review of the literature. Pediatrics 83:737, 1989
112. Frazee JG, Cahan LD, Winter J: Bacterial intracranial aneurysms. J Neurosurg 53:633, 1980
113. Frederiksen H, Ravenholt RT: Thromboembolism, oral contraceptives, and cigarettes. Public Health Rep 85:197, 1970
114. Freeman W, Dumoff S: Cerebellar syndrome fol-

lowing heat stroke. Arch Neurol Psychiatry 51:67, 1944
115. Friberg L, Cederlof R, Lorich U et al: Mortality in twins in relation to smoking habits and alcohol problems. Arch Environ Health 27:294, 1973
116. Friedman EA, Sreepada Rao TK, Nicastri AD: Heroin-associated nephropathy. Nephron 13:421, 1974
117. Friedman GD, Dales LG, Ury HK: Mortality in middle-aged smokers and non-smokers. N Engl J Med 300:213, 1979
118. Garcia-Albea E: Subarachnoid hemorrhage and nasal vasoconstrictor abuse. J Neurol Neurosurg Psychiatry 46:875, 1983
119. Garland H, Greenburg J, Harriman DGF: Infarction of the spinal cord. Brain 89:645, 1966
120. Gay GR, Inaba DS, Sheppard CW et al: Cocaine: history, epidemiology, human pharmacology, and treatment: a perspective on a new debut for an old girl. Clin Toxicol 8:149, 1975
121. Gericke OL: Suicide by ingestion of amphetamine sulfate. JAMA 128:1098, 1945
122. Gill JS, Zezulka AV, Shipley MJ et al: Stroke and alcohol consumption. N Engl J Med 315:1041, 1986
123. Gilroy J, Andaya L, Thomas VJ: Intracranial mycotic aneurysms and subacute bacterial endocarditis in heroin addiction. Neurology (NY) 23:1193, 1973
124. Ginsberg MD, Hedley-Whyte ET, Richardson EP: Hypoxic-ischemic leukoencephalopathy in man. Arch Neurol 33:5, 1976
125. Gocke DJ, Christian CL: Angiitis in drug abusers. N Engl J Med 284:112, 1971
126. Gocke DJ, Morgan C, Lockshin M et al: Association between polyarteritis and Australia antigen. Lancet 2:1149, 1970
127. Golbe LI, Merkin MD: Cerebral infarction in a user of free-base cocaine ("crack"). Neurology (NY) 36:1602, 1986
128. Goldbaum GM, Kendrick JS, Hogelin GC, Gentry EM: The relative impact of smoking and oral contraceptive use on women in the United States. JAMA 258:1339, 1987
129. Goodman SJ, Becker DP: Intracranial hemorrhage associated with amphetamine abuse. JAMA 212:480, 1970
130. Gordon T, Doyle JT: Drinking and mortality: the Albany Study. Am J Epidemiol 125:263, 1987
131. Gordon T, Kannel WB: Drinking habits and cardiovascular disease: the Framingham Study. Am Heart J 105:667, 1983
132. Gorelick PB: Alcohol and stroke. Stroke 18:268, 1987
133. Gorelick PB: The status of alcohol as a risk factor for stroke. Stroke 20:1607, 1989
134. Gorelick PB, Rodin MB, Langenberg P et al: Is acute alcohol ingestion a risk factor for ischemic stroke?—results of a controlled study in middle-aged and elderly stroke patients at three urban medical centers. Stroke 18:359, 1987
135. Gorelick PB, Rodin MB, Langenberg P et al: Weekly alcohol consumption, cigarette smoking, and the risk of ischemic stroke: results of a case-control study at three urban medical centers in Chicago, Illinois. Neurology (NY) 39:339, 1989
136. Green MS, Jucha E, Luz Y: Blood pressure in smokers and non-smokers: epidemiologic findings. Am Heart J 111:932, 1986
137. Green R, Kelly KM, Gabrielson T et al: Multiple intracerebral hemorrhages after smoking "crack" cocaine. Stroke 21:957, 1990
138. Greenwood R, Peachey RS: Acute amphetamine poisoning: an account of three cases. Br Med J 1:742, 1957
139. Grieg M, Pemberton J, Hay I, MacKensie G: A prospective study of the development of coronary heart disease in a group of 1202 middle-aged men. J Epidemiol Community Health 34:23, 1980
140. Grishman E, Churg J, Porush JG: Glomerular morphology in nephrotic heroin addicts. Lab Invest 35:415, 1976
141. Haapanen A, Koskenvuo M, Kaprio J et al: Carotid arteriosclerosis in identical twins discordant for cigarette smoking. Circulation 80:10, 1989
142. Hall CD, Blanton DE, Scatliff JH, Morris CE: Speed kills: fatality from the self administration of methamphetamine intravenously. South Med J 66:650, 1973
143. Hall JH, Karp HR: Acute progressive ventral pontine disease in heroin abuse. Neurology (NY) 23:6, 1973
144. Hamer R, Phelp D: Inadvertent intra-arterial injection of phentermine: a complication of drug abuse. Ann Emerg Med 10:148, 1981
145. Hammond EC: Smoking in relation to mortality and morbidity: finding in the first 34 months of follow-up in a prospective study started in 1959. JNCI 32:1161, 1964
146. Hammond EC: Smoking in relation to death rates of 1 million men and women. Natl Cancer Inst Monogr 19:127, 1966
147. Harmsen P, Rosengren A, Tsipogianni A, Wilhelmsen L: Risk factors for stroke in middle-aged men in Göteborg, Sweden. Stroke 21:223, 1990
148. Harrington H, Heller HA, Dawson D et al: Intracerebral hemorrhage and oral amphetamine. Arch Neurol 40:503, 1983
149. Hartman BK, Zide D, Udenfriend A: The use of dopamine beta-hydroxylase as a marker for the central noradrenergic nervous system in rat brain. Proc Natl Acad Sci USA 69:2722, 1972
150. Harvey JK, Todd CW, Howard JW: Fatality associated with Benzedrine ingestion: a case report. Del Med 21:111, 1949
151. Haselager EM, Vreeken J: Rebound thrombocytosis after alcohol abuse: a possible factor in the pathogenesis of thromboembolic disease. Lancet 1:774, 1977
152. Haskell WJ, Camargo C, Williams PT et al: The effect of cessation and resumption of moderate alcohol intake on serum high-density lipoprotein subfractions: a controlled study. N Engl J Med 310:805, 1984
153. Haut MJ, Cowan DH: The effect of ethanol on hemostatic properties of human blood platelets. Am J Med 56:22, 1974
154. Helpern M, Rho Y-M: Deaths from narcotism in New York City. NY State J Med 66:2391, 1966

155. Hemmingsen R, Barry DL, Hertz MM, Klinken L: Cerebral blood flow and oxygen consumption during ethanol withdrawal in the rat. Brain Res 173:259, 1979
156. Henderson CE, Torbey M: Rupture of intracranial aneurysm associated with cocaine use during pregnancy. Am J Perinatol 5:142, 1988
157. Hennekens CH, Rosner B, Cole DS: Daily alcohol consumption and fatal coronary heart disease. Am J Epidemiol 107:196, 1978
158. Hennekens CH, Willett W, Rosner B et al: Effects of beer, wine, and liquor in coronary deaths. JAMA 242:1973, 1979
159. Henson RA, Parsons M: Ischemic lesions of the spinal cord: an illustrated review. Q J Med 36:205, 1967
160. Herman B, Leyten ACM, van Luuk JH et al: An evaluation of risk factors for stroke in a Dutch community. Stroke 13:334, 1982
161. Herman B, Schmintz PIM, Leyten ACM et al: Multivariate logistic analysis of risk factors for stroke in Tilburg, the Netherlands. Am J Epidemiol 118:514, 1983
162. Herrschaft H: Prophylaxe zerbraler Durchblutungsstörungen. Fortschr Neurol Psychiatr 53:337, 1985
163. Herskowitz A, Gross E: Cerebral infarction associated with heroin sniffing. South Med J 66:778, 1973
164. Hillbom M, Kangasaho M, Kaste M et al: Acute ethanol ingestion increases platelet reactivity: is there a relationship to stroke? Stroke 16:19, 1985
165. Hillbom M, Kaste M: Does ethanol intoxication promote brain infarction in young adults? Lancet 2:1181, 1978
166. Hillbom M, Kaste M: Does alcohol intoxication precipitate aneurysmal subarachnoid hemorrhage? J Neurol Neurosurg Psychiatry 44:523, 1981
167. Hillbom M, Kaste M: Ethanol intoxication: a risk factor for ischemic brain infarction in adolescents and young adults. Stroke 12:422, 1981
168. Hillbom M, Kaste M: Alcohol intoxication: a risk factor for primary subarachnoid hemorrhage. Neurology (NY) 32:706, 1982
169. Hillbom M, Kaste M: Ethanol intoxication: a risk factor for ischemic brain infarction. Stroke 14:694, 1983
170. Hillbom M, Kaste M, Rasi V: Can ethanol intoxication affect hemocoagulation to increase the risk of brain infarction in young adults? Neurology (NY) 33:381, 1983
171. Hilton-Jones O, Warlow CP: The cause of stroke in the young. J Neurol 232:137, 1985
172. Hirsch CS: Dermatopathology of narcotic addiction. Hum Pathol 3:37, 1972
173. Ho K, Rassekh Z: Mycotic aneurysm of the right subclavian artery: a complication of heroin addiction. Chest 74:116, 1978
174. Houck RJ, Bailey G, Daroca P et al: Pentazocine abuse. Chest 77:227, 1980
175. Huang QF, Gebrewold A, Altura BT, Altura BM: Cocaine-induced cerebral vascular damage can be ameliorated by $Mg^{2+}$ in rat brain. Neurosci Lett 109:113, 1990
176. Hubbell G, Cheitlin MD, Rapaport E: Presentation, management, and follow-up evaluation of ineffective endocarditis in drug addicts. Am Heart J 102:85, 1981
177. Husby G, Pierce PE, Williams RL: Smooth muscle antibody in heroin addicts. Ann Intern Med 83:801, 1975
178. Hutton RA, Fink FR, Wilson DT, Marjot DH: Platelet hyperaggregability during alcohol withdrawal. Clin Lab Haematol 3:223, 1981
179. Illett KF, Jarrott B, O'Donnell SR et al: Mechanism of cardiovascular actions of 1-(1-phenylcyclohexyl)piperidine hydrochloride (phencyclidine). Br J Pharmacol Chemother 28:73, 1966
180. Isles C, Brown JJ, Cumming AM et al: Excess smoking in malignant phase hypertension. Br Med J 1:579, 1979
181. Isner JM, Chokshi SK: Cocaine and vasospasm. N Engl J Med 321:1604, 1989
182. Jacobs IG, Roszler MH, Kelly JK et al: Cocaine abuse: neurovascular complications. Radiology 170:223, 1989
183. Jakubowski JA, Vaillancourt R, Deykin D: Interaction of ethanol, prostacyclin, and aspirin in determining human platelet reactivity in vitro. Arteriosclerosis 8:436, 1988
184. Jara FM, Lewis JF, Magilligan DJ: Operative experience with infective endocarditis and intracerebral mycotic aneurysm. J Thorac Cardiovasc Surg 80:28, 1980
185. Jordan SC, Hampson F: Amphetamine poisoning associated with hyperpyrexia. Br Med J 2:844, 1960
186. Judice DJ, LeBlanc HJ, McGarry PA: Spinal cord vasculitis presenting as spinal cord tumor in a heroin addict. J Neurosurg 48:131, 1978
187. Kagan A, Popper JS, Rhoads GG, Yano K: Dietary and other risk factors for stroke in Hawaiian Japanese men. Stroke 16:390, 1985
188. Kahn HA: The Dorn study of smoking and mortality among US veterans: report on $8\frac{1}{2}$ years of observations. Natl Cancer Inst Monogr 19:i, 1966
189. Kaku DA, Lowenstein DH: Recreational drug use: a growing risk factor for stroke in young people. Neurology (NY), suppl 1. 39:161, 1989
190. Kaku DA, Lowenstein DH: Emergence of recreational drug abuse as a major risk factor for stroke in young adults. Ann Intern Med 113:821, 1990
191. Kane FJ, Greene BQ: Psychotic episodes associated with the use of common proprietary decongestants. Am J Psychiatry 123:484, 1966
192. Kane FJ, Keeler MH, Reifler CB: Neurological crisis following methamphetamine. JAMA 210:556, 1969
193. Kangasaho M, Hillbom M, Kaste M, Vapaatalo H: Effects of ethanol intoxication and hangover on plasma levels of thromboxane $B_2$ and 6-keto-prostaglandin $F_1\alpha$ and on thromboxane $B_2$ formation by platelets in man. Thomb Haemost 48:232, 1982
194. Kannel WB: Current status of the epidemiology of brain infarction associated with occlusive arterial disease. Stroke 2:295, 1971
195. Kannel WB, D'Agostino RB, Belanger AL: Fi-

brinogen, cigarette smoking, and risk of cardiovascular disease: insights from the Framingham Study. Am Heart J 113:1006, 1987
196. Kannel WB, Dawber TR, Cohen ME et al: Vascular disease of the brain-epidemiologic aspects: the Framingham Study. Am J Public Health 55:1355, 1965
197. Kannel WB, Sorlie P: Hypertension in Framingham. p. 553. In Paul O (ed): Epidemiology and Control of Hypertension. Symposia Specialists, Miami, 1975
198. Kannel WB, Wolf PA, Dawber TR: An evaluation of the epidemiology of atherothrombotic brain infarction. Milbank Mem Fun Q 53:405, 1975
199. Kannel WB, Woosley P: Alcohol and cardiovascular risk. Circulation, suppl II. 52:200, 1975
200. Karch SB, Billingham ME: The pathology and etiology of cocaine-induced heart disease. Arch Pathol Lab Med 112:225, 1988
201. Kasirsky G, Zaidi IH, Tansy MF: LD50 and pathologic effects of acute and chronic administration of methamphetamine HCl in rabbits. Res Commun Chem Pathol Pharmacol 3:215, 1972
202. Katsuki S: Hisayama study. Jpn J Med 10:167, 1971
203. Katsuki S, Omae T: Stroke prone profiles in the Japanese. p. 215. In Engel A, Larsson T (eds): Frist Thule International Symposium on Stroke, 1966. Nordiska Bokhandein, Stockholm, 1967
204. Kaye BR, Fainstat M: Cerebral vasculitis associated with cocaine abuse. JAMA 258:2104, 1987
205. Kessler GF, Demers LM, Brennan RW: Phencyclidine and fatal status epilepticus. N Engl J Med 291:979, 1974
206. Kessler JT, Jortner BS, Adapon BD: Cerebral vasculitis in a drug abuser. J Clin Psychiatry 39:559, 1978
207. Khaw AL, Barrett-Connor E: Dietary potassium and stroke-associated mortality: a 12-year prospective study. N Engl J Med 316:235, 1987
208. Kilkoyne MM, Daly JJ, Gocke DJ et al: Nephrotic syndrome in heroin addicts. Lancet 1:17, 1972
209. King J: Hypertension and cerebral hemorrhage after Trimolers ingestion. Med J Aust 2:258, 1979
210. King J, Richards M, Tress B: Cerebral arteritis associated with heroin abuse. Med J Aust 2:444, 1978
211. Klassen AC, Loewenson RB, Resch JA: Cerebral atherosclerosis in selected chronic disease states. Atherosclerosis 18:321, 1973
212. Klatsky AJ, Friedman GD, Siegelaub AB: alcohol consumption before myocardial infarction: results from the Kaiser-Permanente epidemiologic study of myocardial infarction. Ann Intern Med 81:294, 1974
213. Klatsky AL, Friedman GD, Siegelaub AB et al: Alcohol consumption and blood pressure: Kaiser-Permanente Multiphasic Health Examination data. N Engl J Med 296:1194, 1977
214. Klatsky AJ, Friedman GD, Siegelaub AB: Alcohol use, myocardial infarction, sudden cardiac death, and hypertension. Alcoholism Clin Exp Res 3:33, 1979
215. Klatsky AL, Friedman GD, Siegelaub AB: Alcohol and mortality: a ten-year Kaiser-Permanente experience. Ann Intern Med 95:139, 1981
216. Klonoff DC, Andrews BT, Obana WG: Stroke associated with cocaine use. Arch Neurol 46:989, 1989
217. Knoblauch AL, Buchholz M, Koller MG, Kistler H: Hemiplegie nach Injektion von Heroin. Schweiz Med Wochenschr 113:402, 1983
218. Koch A, Reuther R, Boos R et al: Risikofactoren bei cerebralen Durchblutungesstörungen. Verh Dtsch Ges Inn Med 83:1773, 1977
219. Kono S, Ikeda M, Ogata M et al: The relationship between alcohol and mortality among Japanese physicians. Int J Epidemiol 12:437, 1983
220. Kono S, Ikeda M, Tokudome S et al: Alcohol and mortality: a cohort study of male Japanese physicians. Int J Epidemiol 15:527, 1986
221. Kozaravic D, McGee D, Vojvodic N et al: Frequency of alcohol consumption and morbidity and mortality: the Yugoslavia cardiovascular disease study. Lancet 1:613, 1980
222. Kozarevic DJ, Vodvodic N, Gordon T et al: Drinking habits and death: the Yugoslavia Cardiovascular Disease Study. Int J Epidemiol 12:145, 1983
223. Krendel DA, Ditter SM, Frankel MR, Ross WK: Biopsy-proven cerebral vasculitis associated with cocaine abuse. Neurology (NY) 40:1092, 1990
224. Kubota K, Yamaguchi T, Abe Y: Effects of smoking on regional cerebral blood flow in neurologically normal subjects. Stroke 14:720, 1983
225. Kumar P, Rathore CK, Nagar AM et al: Hyperpyrexia with special reference to heat stroke: an analysis of 108 cases. J Indian Med Assoc 43:213, 1964
226. Kurtzke JF: Epidemiology of Cerebrovascular Disease. Springer-Verlag, New York, 1969
227. Lahmeyer HW, Steingold RG: Pentazocine and tripelennamine: a drug abuse epidemic? Int J Addict 15:1219, 1980
228. Lamont CM, Adams FG: Glue-sniffing as a cause of a positive radio-isotope brain scan. Eur J Nucl Med 7:387, 1982
229. Landolfi R, Steiner M: Ethanol raises prostacyclin in vivo and in vitro. Blood 64:679, 1984
230. Lang WE: Ethyl alcohol enhances plasminogen activator secretion by endothelial cells. JAMA 250:772, 1983
231. Lange RA, Cigarroa RG, Yancy CW et al: Cocaine-induced coronary artery vasoconstriction. N Engl J Med 321:1557, 1989
232. Langner RO, Bement CL, Perry LE: Arteriosclerotic toxicity of cocaine. Natl Inst Drug Abuse Res Monogr Ser 88-1585:325, 1987
233. LaPorte RE, Cresanta JL, Kuller LH: The relationship of alcohol consumption to atherosclerotic heart disease. Prev Med 9:22, 1980
234. Lasagna L: Phenylpropanolamine: A Review. Wiley, New York, 1988
235. Ledgerwood AM, Lucas CE: Mycotic aneurysm of the carotid artery. Arch Surg 109:496, 1974
236. Lee J, Sapira JD: Retinal and cerebral microem-

bolization of talc in a drug abuser. Am J Med Sci 265:75, 1973
237. Lee K: Alcoholism and cerebral thrombosis in the young. Acta Neurol Scand 59:270, 1979
238. Lee K, Nielsen JD, Zeeberg I, Gormsen J: Platelet aggregation and fibrinolytic activity in young alcoholics. Acta Neurol Scand 62:287, 1980
239. Lee MC, Randa DC, Gold LH: Transverse myelopathy following the use of heroin. Minn Med 59:82, 1976
240. Lehman LB: Intracerebral hemorrhage after intranasal cocaine use. Hosp Physician 7:69, 1987
241. Levine LH, Hirsch CS, White LW: Quinine cardiotoxicity: a mechanism for sudden death in narcotic addicts. J Forensic Sci 18:167, 1973
242. Levine SR, Brust JCM, Futrell N et al: Cerebrovascular complications of the use of the "crack" form of alkaloidal cocaine. N Engl J Med 323:699, 1990
243. Levine SR, Brust JCM, Welch KMA: Cerebral vasculitis associated with cocaine abuse or subarachnoid hemorrhage. JAMA 259:1648, 1988
244. Levine SR, Fagan SC, Floberg J et al: Moyamoya, oral contraceptives, and cigarette use. Ann Neurol 24:155, 1988
245. Levine SR, Washington JM, Jefferson MF et al: "Crack" cocaine-associated stroke. Neurology (NY) 37:1849, 1987
246. Levine SR, Welch KM: Cocaine and stroke. Stroke 19:779, 1988
247. Lewis E: Hyperpyrexia with antidepressant drugs. Br Med J 2:1671, 1965
248. Lichtenfield PJ, Rubin DB, Feldman RS: Subarachnoid hemorrhage precipitated by cocaine snorting. Arch Neurol 41:223, 1984
249. Lieber CS: To drink (moderately) or not to drink. N Engl J Med 310:846, 1984
250. Lieberman AN, Bloom W, Kishore PS, Lin JP: Carotid artery occlusion following ingestion of LSD. Stroke 5:213, 1974
251. Lignelli GJ, Buchheit WA. Angiitis in drug abusers. N Engl J Med 284:112, 1971
252. Lloyd JTA, Walker DRH: Death after combined dexamphetamine and phenylzine. Br Med J 2:168, 1965
253. Loizou LA, Hamilton JG, Tsementzis SA: Intracranial hemorrhage in association with pseudoephedrine overdose. J Neurol Neurosurg Psychiatry 45:471, 1982
254. Longstreth WT, Koepsell TD, Yerby MS, van Belle G: Risk factors for subarachnoid hemorrhage. Stroke 16:377, 1985
255. Longstreth WT, Swanson PD: Oral contraceptives and stroke. Stroke 15:747, 1984
256. Louria DB, Hensle T, Rose J: The major medical complications of heroin addiction. Ann Intern Med 67:1, 1967
257. Love BB, Biller J, Jones MP et al: Cigarette smoking. A risk factor for cerebral infarction in young adults. Arch Neurol 47:693, 1990
258. Lovejoy FH: Stroke and phenylpropanolamine. Pediatr Alert 12:45, 1981
259. LoVerme S: Complications of amphetamine abuse. p. 5. In Culebras A (ed): Clini-Pearls. Vol. 2, No. 8. Creative Medical Publications, Syracuse, NY, 1979
260. Lowenstein DH, Massa SM, Rowbotham MC et al: Acute neurologic and psychiatric complications associated with cocaine abuse. Am J Med 83:841, 1987
261. Luck JC: Arrhythmias and social drinking. Ann Intern Med 93:253, 1983
262. Lukes SA: Intracerebral hemorrhage from an arteriovenous malformation after amphetamine injection. Arch Neurol 40:60, 1983
263. Lundberg GD, Garriott JC, Reynolds PC et al: Cocaine-related death. J Forensic Sci 22:402, 1977
264. MacMahon S: Alcohol consumption and hypertension. Hypertension 9:111, 1987
265. MacMahon SW, Norton RN: Alcohol and hypertension: implications for prevention and treatment. Ann Intern Med 105:124, 1986
266. Mangiardi JR, Daras M, Geller ME et al: Cocaine-related intracranial hemorrhage: report of nine cases and reviews. Acta Neurol Scand 77:177, 1988
267. Maouad J, Fernandez F, Barrillon A et al: Diffuse or segmental narrowing (spasm) of coronary arteries during smoking demonstrated on angiography. Am J Cardiol 53:354, 1984
268. Maqbool Z, Billett HH: Unwitting heparin abuse in a drug addict. Ann Intern Med 96:790, 1982
269. Margolis MT, Newton TH: Methamphetamine ("speed") arteritis. Neuroradiology 2:179, 1971
270. Mariani PJ: Pseudoephedrine-induced hypertensive emergency: treatment with labetalol. Am J Emerg Med 4:141, 1986
271. Mathews JD: Alcohol use, hypertension, and coronary heart disease. Clin Sci 51:661, 1976
272. Mathews UD: Alcohol and hypertension. Aust NZ J Med 9:158, 1979
273. Matick H, Anderson D, Brumlik J: Cerebral vasulitis associated with oral amphetamine overdose. Arch Neurol 40:523, 1983
274. McCarron MM, Schultze BW, Thomspon GA et al: Acute phencyclidine intoxication: incidence of clinical findings in 1000 cases. Ann Emerg Med 10:237, 1981
275. McQueen JD, Sklar FK, Posey JB: Autoregulation of cerebral blood flow during alcohol infusion. J Stud Alcohol 39:1477, 1978
276. Meade TW, Chakrabarti R, Haines AP et al: Characteristics affecting fibrinolytic activity and plasma fibrinogen concentrations. Br Med J 1:153, 1979
277. Medical Research Council Working Party: MRC Trial of treatment of mild hypertension: principle results. Br Med J 291:97, 1985
278. Mercado A, Johnson G, Calver D, Sokol RJ: Cocaine, pregnancy, and postpartum intracerebral hemorrhage. Obstet Gynecol 73:467, 1989
279. Meza I, Estrad CA, Montalvo JA et al: Cerebral infarction associated with cocaine use. Henry Ford Hosp Med J 37:50, 1989
280. Mittleman RE, Wetli CV: Cocaine and sudden "natural" death. J Forensic Sci 32:11, 1987
281. Mizutami T, Lewis R, Gonatas N: Medial medul-

lary syndrome in a drug abuser. Arch Neurol 37:425, 1980
282. Mody CK, Miller BL, McIntyre HB et al: Neurologic complications of cocaine abuse. Neurology (NY) 38:1189, 1988
283. Molgaard CA, Bartok A, Peddercord KM et al: The association between cerebrovascular disease and smoking: a case-control study. Neuroepidemiology 5:88, 1986
284. Moore PM, Peterson PL: Nonhemorrhagic cerebrovascular complications of cocaine abuse. Neurology (NY), suppl 1. 39:302, 1989
285. Moore RD, Pearson TA: Moderate alcohol consumption and coronary artery disease: a review. Medicine (Baltimore) 65:242, 1986
286. Moorthy G, Price TR, Tuhrim S et al: Relationship between recent alcohol intake and stroke type?—the NINCDS Stroke Data Bank. Stroke 17:141, 1986
287. Morris JN, Kagan A, Pattison DC et al: Incidence and prediction of ischemic heart disease in London busmen. Lancet 2:553, 1966
288. Mueller SM: Neurologic complications of phenylpropanolamine use. Neurology (NY) 33:650, 1983
289. Mueller SM, Ertel PJ: Subarachnoid hemorrhage associated with over-the-counter diet medications. Stroke 14:16, 1983
290. Mueller SM, Solow EB: Seizures associated with a new combination "pick-me-up" pill. Ann Neurol 11:322, 1982
291. Murchison LE, Fyfe T: Effects of cigarette smoking on serum lipids, blood glucose, and platelet adhesiveness. Lancet 2:182, 1966
292. Nadler JL, Velasso JS, Horton R: Cigarette smoking inhibits prostacyclin formation. Lancet 1:1248, 1983
293. Nalls G, Disher A, Darabagi J et al: Subcortical cerebral hemorrhages associated with cocaine abuse: CT and MR findings. J Comput Assist Tomogr 13:1, 1989
294. Nickerson DS, Williams RL, Boxmeyer M et al: Increased opsonic capacity of serum in chronic heroin addiction. Ann Intern Med 72:671, 1970
295. Noguchi TT, Nakamura GR: Phencyclidine-related deaths in Los Angeles County, 1976. J Forensic Sci 23:503, 1978
296. Nolte KB, Gelman BB: Intracerebral hemorrhage associated with cocaine abuse. Arch Pathol Lab Med 113:812, 1989
297. Okada H, Horibe H, Ohno Y et al: A prospective study of cerebrovascular disease in Japanese rural communities, Akabane and Asahi. I: Evaluation of risk factors in the occurrence of cerebral hemorrhage and thrombosis. Stroke 7:599, 1976
298. Oleckno WA: The risk of stroke in young adults: an analysis of the contribution of cigarette smoking and alcohol consumption. Public Health 102:45, 1988
299. Olsen ER: Intracranial hemorrhage and amphetamine usage. Angiology 28:464, 1977
300. Ortona L, Laghi V, Cauda R: Immune function in heroin addicts. N Engl J Med 300:45, 1979
301. Ostern S, Dodson WH: Hypertension following Ornade ingestion. JAMA 194:472, 1965
302. Paffenbarger RS, Williams JL: Chronic disease in former college students. XI. Early precursers of nonfatal stroke. Am J Epidemiol 94:524, 191
303. Paffenbarger RS, Wing A: Characteristics in youth predisposing to fatal stroke in later years. Lancet 1:753, 1967
304. Paganini-Hill A, Ross RK, Henderson BE: Postmenapausal oestrogen treatment and stroke: a prospective study. Br Med J 297:519, 1988
305. Palmer JR, Rosenberg, Shapiro S: "low yield" cigarettes and the risk of nonfatal myocardial infarction in women. N Engl J Med 320:1569, 1989
306. Patel AN: Self-inflicted strokes. Ann Intern Med 76:823, 1972
307. Peacock PB, Riley CP, Lampton TD et al: The Birmingham stroke, epidemiology, and rehabilitation study. p. 231. In Stewart G (ed): Trends in Epidemiology: Applications to Health Service Research and Training. Charles C Thomas, Springfield, IL, 1972
308. Pearson J, Richter RW: Neuropathological effects of opiate addiction. p. 308. In Richter RW (ed): Medical Aspects of Drug Abuse. Harper & Row, Hagerstown, MD, 1975
309. Pearson J, Richter RW: Addiction to opiates: neurologic aspects. p. 365. In Vinken PJ, Bruyn GW (eds): Handbook of Clinical Neurology. Vol. 37: Intoxications of the Nervous System. North-Holland Publishing, Amsterdam, 1979
310. Pearson J, Richter RW, Baden MM et al: Transverse myelopathy as an illustration of the neurologic and neuropathologic features of heroin addiction. Hum Pathol 3:109, 1972
311. Pennington SN, Smith CP: The effect of ethanol on thromboxane synthesis by blood platelet. Prostaglandins 2:43, 1979
312. Pentel P: Toxicity of over-the-counter stimulants. JAMA 252:1898, 1984
313. Persson LI, Rosengren LE, Johansson BB, Hansson HA: Blood brain barrier dysfunction to peroxidase after air embolism, aggravated by acute ethanol intoxication. J Neurol Sci 42:65, 1979
314. Peterson PL, Moore PM: Hemorrhagic cerebrovascular complications of crack cocaine abuse. Neurology (NY), suppl 1. 39:302, 1989
315. Pettiti DB, Wingerd J: Use of oral contraceptives; cigarette smoking, and risk of subarachnoid hemorrhage. Lancet 2:234, 1978
316. Petitti DB, Wingerd J, Pellegrin F, Ramcharan S: Risk of vascular disease in women: smoking, oral contraceptives, non-contraceptive estrogens, and other factors. JAMA 242:1150, 1979
317. Petty GW, Brust JCM, Tatemichi TK, Barr ML: Embolic stroke ofter smoking "crack" cocaine. Stroke 21:1632, 1990
318. Pick TP, Howden R: Gray's Anatomy. p. 548. Running Press, Philadelphia, 1974
319. Plum F, Posner JB, Hain RF: Delayed neurologic deterioration after anoxia. Arch Intern Med 110:18, 1962
320. Poteliakhoff A, Roughton BC: Two cases of amphetamine poisoning. Br Med J 1:26, 1956
321. Powers RH, Madden JA: Vasoconstrictive effects

of cocaine, metabolites and structural analogs on cat cerebral arteries. FASEB 4:A1095, 1990
322. Pretorius HPJ: Dexedrine intoxication of children: two cases, one fatal. S Afr Med J 27:945, 1953
323. Protass LM: Delayed postanoxic encephalopathy after heroin use. Ann Intern Med 74:738, 1971
324. Quintana RP, Lasslo A, Dugdale ML et al: Effects of ethanol and of other factors on ADP-induced aggregation of human blood platelets in vitro. Thromb Res 20:405, 1980
325. Ramsey LE: Liver dysfunction in hypertension. Lancet 2:111, 1977
326. Reed DM, Resch JA, Hayashi T et al: A prospective study of cerebral artery atherosclerosis. Stroke 19:820, 1988
327. Renaud S, Blache O, Dumont E et al: Platelet function after cigarette smoking in relation to nicotine and carbon monoxide. Clin Pharmacol Ther 36:389, 1984
328. Rhoads GG, Blackwelder WC, Stemmerwan GN et al: Coronary risk factors and autopsy findings in Japanese-American men. Lab Invest 38:304, 1978
329. Richter RW, Pearson J: Heroin addiction related neurological disorders. p. 320. In Richter RW (ed): Medical Aspects of Drug Abuse. Harper & Row, Hagerstown, MD, 1975
330. Richter RW, Pearson J, Bruun B et al: Neurological complications of addiction to heroin. Bull NY Acad Med 49:3, 1973
331. Richter RW, Rosenberg RN: Transverse myelitis associated with heroin addiction. JAMA 206:1255, 1968
332. Riddick L, Reisch R: Oral overdose of propylhexedrine. J Forensic Sci 26:834, 1981
333. Ringle DA, Herndon BL: In vitro morphine binding by sera from morphine-treated rabbits. J Immunol 109:174, 1972
334. Rodriguez E, Smokvina M, Sokolow J, Grynbaum BB: Encephalopathy and paraplegia occurring with use of heroin. NY State J Med 71:2879, 1971
335. Rogers JN, Henry TE, Jones AM et al: Cocaine related deaths in Pima Country, Arizona, 1982–1984. J Forensic Sci 31:1404, 1986
336. Rogers KJ, Nahorski SR: Depression of cerebral metabolism by stimulant doses of cocaine. Brain Res 57:255, 1973
337. Rogers RL, Meyer JS, Shaw TG et al: Cigarette smoking decreases cerebral blood flow suggesting increased risk for stroke. JAMA 250:2796, 1983
338. Ramanova MV, Romanov NS: Cerebral circulation disturbance in patients with chronic alcoholism. Sov Med 7:148, 1978
339. Rogot E: Smoking and General Mortality Among US Veterans, 1954–1969. National Heart and Lung Institute, Bethesda MD, 1974
340. Rothrock JF, Rubenstein R, Lyden PD: Ischemic stroke associated with methamphetamine inhalation. Neurology (NY) 38:589, 1988
341. Rowbotham MC: Neurologic aspects of cocaine abuse. West J Med 149:442, 1988
342. Rowley HA, Lowenstein DH, Rowbotham MC, Simon RP: Thalamomesencephalic strokes after cocaine abuse. Neurology (NY) 39:428, 1989
343. Royal College of General Practitioners: Oral Contraceptives and Health. Pitman, London, 1974
344. Rumbaugh CL, Bergeron RT, Fang HCH, McCormick R: Cerebral angiographic changes in the drug abuse patient. Radiology 101:335, 1971
345. Rumbaugh CL, Bergeron T, Scanlon RL et al: Cerebral vascular changes secondary to amphetamine abuse in the experimental animal. Radiology 101:345, 1971
346. Rumbaugh CL, Fang HCH: The effects of drug abuse on the brain. p. 37s. Med Times, March, 1980
347. Rumbaugh CL, Fang HCH, Higgins RE et al: Cerebral microvascular injury in experimental drug abuse. Invest Radiol 11:282, 1976
348. Russell M, Cooper ML, Frone M et al: Drinking patterns and blood pressure. Am J Epidemiol 128:917, 1988
349. Ryan JJ, Parker CW, Williams RL: Gamma-globulin binding of morphine in heroin addicts. J Lab Clin Med 80:155, 1972
350. Sacco RL, Wolf PA, Bharucha NE et al: Subarachnoid and intracerebral hemorrhage: natural history, prognosis, and precursive factors in the Framingham Study. Neurology (NY) 34:847, 1984
351. Salonen JT, Puska P, Tuomilehto J et al: Relation of blood pressure, serum lipids, and smoking to the risk of cerebral stroke: a longitudinal study in eastern Finland. Stroke 13:327, 1982
352. Sapira JD: The narcotic addict as a medical patient. Am J Med 45:555, 1968
353. Schaffer CB, Pauli MW: Psychotic reaction caused by proprietary oral diet agents. Am J Psychiatry 137:1256, 1980
354. Schwartz ICA, Cohen JA: Subarachnoid hemorrhage precipitated by cocaine snorting. Arch Neurol 41:705, 1984
355. Schein PS, Yessayun L, Mayman CI: Acute transverse myelitis associated with intravenous opium. Neurology (NY) 21:101, 1971
356. Schoenfeld MR: Acute allergic reactions to morphine, codeine, meperidine hydrochloride, and opium alkaloids. NY State J Med 60:2591, 1960
357. Seaman ME: Acute cocaine abuse associated with cerebral infarction. Ann Emerg Med 19:34, 1990
358. Seiss W, Lorenz R, Roth P, Weber PC: Plasma catecholamines, platelet aggregation and associated thromboxane formation after physical exercise, smoking, or norepinephrine infusion. Circulation 66:44, 1982
359. Semenciw RM, Morrison MI, Mao Y et al: Major risk factors for cardiovascular disease mortality in adults: results from the Nutrition Canada Survey Study. Int J Epidemiol 17:317, 1988
360. Shibolet S, Coll R, Gilat T, Sohar E: Heatstroke: its clinical picture and mechanism in 36 cases. Q J Med 36:525, 1967
361. Shinton R, Beevers G: Meta-analysis of relation

between cigarette smoking and stroke. Br Med J 298:789, 1989

362. Shukla D: Intracranial hemorrhage associated with amphetamine use. Neurology (NY) 32:917, 1982
363. Simonsen J: Traumatic subarachnoid hemorrhage in alcohol intoxication. J Forensic Sci 8:97, 1963
364. Smith HWB, Liberman HH, Brody SL et al: Acute myocardial infarction temporally related to cocaine use: clinical, angiographic, and pathophysiologic observations. Ann Intern Med 107:13, 1987
365. Sobel J, Espinas OE, Friedman SA: Carotid artery obstruction following LSD capsule ingestion. Arch Intern Med 127:290, 1971
366. Spires MC, Gordon EF, Choudhuri M, Maldonado E, Chan R: Intracranial hemorrhage in a neonate following prenatal cocaine exposure. Pediatr Neurol 5:324, 1989
367. Stafford CR, Bogdanoff BM, Green L, Spector HB: Mononeuropathy multiplex as a complication of amphetamine angiitis. Neurology (NY) 25:570, 1975
368. Stamfer MJ, Coditz GA, Willett WC et al: A prospective study of moderate alcohol consumption and the risk of coronary disease and stroke in women. N Engl J Med 319:267, 1988
369. Stason WB, Neff RK, Miettinen OS, Jick H: Alcohol consumption and nonfatal myocardial infarction. Am J Epidemiol 104:603, 1976
370. Stemmermann GN, Hayashi T, Resch JA et al: Risk factors related to ischemic and hemorrhagic cerebrovascular disease at autopsy: the Honolulu Heart Study. Stroke 15:23, 1984
371. Stimmel B: Cardiovascular Effects of Mood-altering Drugs. Raven Press, New York, 1979
372. St. Leger AS, Cochrane AL, Moore F: Factors associated with cardiac mortality in developed countries with particular reference to the consumption of wine. Lancet 1:1017, 1979
373. Stoessl AJ, Young G, Feasby TE: Intracerebral hemorrhage and angiographic beading following ingestion of catecholaminergics. Stroke 16:734, 1985
374. Stuart M: Ethanol inhibited platelet prostaglandin synthesis in vitro. J Stud Alcohol 40:1, 1979
375. Sturner WQ, Stressman G, Helpern M: Bilateral symmetrical encephalomalacia in the globus pallidus in drug addicts. Paper read at the meeting of the American Academy of Forensic Sciences, Chicago, February, 1968
376. Syrjanen J, Valtonen VV, Ivananainen M et al: Association between cerebral infarction and increased serum bacterial antibody levels in young adults. Acta Neurol Scand 73:273, 1986
377. Szwed JJ: Pulmonary angiothrombosis caused by "blue velvet" addiction. Ann Intern Med 73:771, 1970
378. Takeya Y, Popper JS, Shimizu Y et al: Epidemiologic studies of coronary heart disease and stroke in Japanese men living in Japan, Hawaii, and California: incidence of stroke in Japan and Hawaii. Stroke 15:15, 1984
379. Tanaka H, Hayaski M, Date C et al: Epidemiologic studies of stroke in Shibata, a Japanese provincial city: preliminary report on risk factors for cerebral infarction. Stroke 16:773, 1985
380. Tanaka H, Ueda Y, Hayashi M et al: Risk factors for cerebral hemorrhage and cerebral infarction in a Japanese rural community. Stroke 13:62, 1982
381. Tarasyuk IK: The effect of alcohol misuse on the development and course of acute brain circulation disorders. Zh Nevropatol Psikhiatr 76:1777, 1976
382. Tardiff K, Gross E, Wu J et al: Analysis of cocaine-positive fatalities. J Forensic Sci 34:53, 1989
383. Taylor JR, Combs-Orme T: Alcohol and strokes in young adults. Am J Psychiatry 142:116, 1985
384. Thompson WR, Waldman MB: Cervical myelopathy following heroin administration. J Med Soc NJ 67:223, 1970
385. Thornton JR: Atrial fibrillation in healthy nonalcoholic people after an alcoholic binge. Lancet 2;1013, 1984
386. Tibbetts JC, Hinck VC: Conservative management of a hematoma in the fourth ventricle. Surg Neurol 1:253, 1973
387. Tibblin G, Wilhelmsen L, Werko L: Risk factors for myocardial infarction and death due to ischemic heart disease and other causes. Am J Cardiol 35:514, 1975
388. Togna G, Tempesta E, Togna AR et al: Platelet responsiveness and biosynthesis of thromboxane and prostacyclin in response to in vitro cocaine treatment. Haemostasis 15:100, 1985
389. Toler KA, Anderson B: Stroke in an intravenous drug user secondary to the lupus anticoagulant. Stroke 19:274, 1988
390. Treffert DA, Joranson D: Restricting amphetamines. JAMA 245:1336, 1981
391. Tse DT, Ober RR: Talc retinopathy. Am J Ophthalmol 90:624, 1980
392. Tuazon CU, Sheagren JN: Staphylococcal endocarditis in parenteral drug abusers: source of the organism. Ann Intern Med 82:788, 1975
393. Tuomilehto J, Bonita R, Stewart A et al: Hypertension, cigarette smoking, and the decline in stroke incidence in eastern Finland. Stroke 22:7, 1991
394. Turnbull IM: Microvasculature of the human spinal cord. J Neurosurg 35:141, 1971
395. Ueda K, Hasuo Y, Kiyohara Y et al: Hisayama: incidence, changing pattern during long-term follow up, and related factors. Stroke 19:48, 1988
396. US National Institute on Alcohol Abuse and Alcoholism: Alcohol and health. Second special report to the Congress. DHEW Pub No ADM 75-212, US Government Printing Office, Washington, DC, 1975
397. Van Dyuke C, Byck R: Cocaine. Sci Am 246:128, 1982
398. Van Vanukis H, Wasserman E, Levine L: Specificities of antibodies to morphine. J Pharmacol Exp Ther 180:514, 1972
399. Von Arbin M, Britton M, De Faire U, Tisell A: Circulatory manifestations and risk factors in

patients with acute cerebrovascular disease and in matched controls. Acta Med Scand 218:373, 1985
400. Wadley C, Stillie GD: Pentazocine (Talwin) and tripelennamine (Pyribenzamine): a new drug abuse combination or just a revival? Int J Addict 15:1285,1980
401. Walbran BB, Nelson JS, Taylor JR: Association of cerebral infarction and chronic alcoholism: an autopsy study. Alcoholism 5:531, 1981
402. Weiner RS, Lockhart JT, Schwartz RG: Dilated cardiomyopathy and cocaine abuse: report of two cases. Am J Med 81:699, 1986
403. Weingarten KO: Cerebral vasculitis associated with cocaine abuse or subarachnoid hemorrhage? JAMA 259:1658, 1988
404. Weiss MH, Craig JR: The influence of acute ethanol intoxication on intracranial physical dynamics. Bull Los Angeles Neurol Soc 43:1, 1978
405. Weiss RD, Gawin FH: Protracted elimination of cocaine metabolites in long-term, high-dose cocaine abusers. Am J Med 85:879, 1988
406. Weiss SR, Raskind R, Morganstern NL et al: Intracerebral and subarachnoid hemorrhage following use of methamphetamine ("speed"). Int Surg 53:123, 1970
407. Wetli C, Wright RK: Death caused by recreational cocaine use. JAMA 241:2519, 1979
408. Wharton BK: Nasal decongestants and paranoid psychosis. Br J Psychiatry 117:429, 1970
409. Whisnant JP, Homer D, Ingall TJ et al: Duration of cigarette smoking is the strongest predictor of severe extracranial carotid atherosclerosis. Stroke 21:707, 1990
410. Wilhelmsen L, Svardsudd K, Korsan-Bengsten K et al: Fibrinogen as a risk factor for stroke and myocardial infarction. N Engl J Med 311:501, 1984
411. Wojak JC, Flamm ES: Intracranial hemorrhage and cocaine use. Stroke 18:712, 1987
412. Wolf PA, D'Agostino RB, Kannel WB et al: Cigarette smoking as a risk factor for stroke: the Framingham Study. JAMA 259:1025, 1988
413. Wolf PA, D'Agostino RB, Odell P et al: Alcohol consumption as a risk factor for stroke: the Framingham Study. Ann Neurol 24:177, 1988
414. Wolf PA, Kannel WB, Verter J: Current status of risk factors for stroke, p. 317. In Barnett HJM (ed): Neurologic Clinics. Vol. 1: Symposium on Cerebrovascular Disease. WB Saunders, Philadelphia, 1983
415. Woods BT, Strewler GJ: Hemiparesis occurring six hours after intravenous heroin injection. Neurology (NY) 22:863, 1972
416. Wooten MR, Khangure MS, Murphy MJ: Intracerebral hemorrhage and vasculitis related to ephedrine abuse. Ann Neurol 13:337, 1983
417. Yano K, Rhoads GG, Kagan V: Coffee, alcohol and risk of coronary heart disease among Japanese men living in Hawaii. N Engl J Med 297:405, 1977
418. Yarnell PR: "Speed" headache and hematoma. Headache 17:69, 1977
419. Yatsu FM, Wesson DR, Smith DE: Amphetamine abuse. p. 50. In Richter RW (ed): Medical Aspects of Drug Abuse. Harper & Row, Hagerstown, MD, 1975
420. Yu YJ, Cooper DR, Wellenstein DE, Block B: Cerebral angiitis and intracerebral hemorrhage associated with methamphetamine abuse: case report. J Neurosurg 58:109, 1983
421. Zalis EG, Kaplan G, Lundberg GD, Knutson RA: Acute lethality of the amphetamines in dogs and its antagonism with curare. Proc Soc Exp Biol Med 18:557, 1965
422. Zalis EG, Lundberg GD, Knutson RA: The pathophysiology of acute amphetamine poisoning with pathologic correlation. J Pharmacol Exp Ther 158:115, 1967
423. Zalis EG, Parmley LF: Fatal amphetamine poisoning. Arch Intern Med 112:822, 1963
424. Zimmerman M, McGreachie J: The effect of nicotine on aortic endothelium: a quantitative ultrastructural study. Atherosclerosis 63:33, 1987

# 35
# STROKE IN YOUNG ADULTS

Julien Bogousslavsky

The potential devastating consequences of stroke can be particularly dramatic when a young, previously healthy, person experiences acute cerebral infarction or hemorrhage. Apart from the dramatic consequences on the patient himself, the burden can be extremely heavy on the spouse, family, and society in general when permanent sequelae remain for the whole life, that is, another 30 to 50 years. In contrast to a common but erroneous view, a significant proportion of strokes occur in active young adults. Experience from the Lausanne Stroke Registry, which surveys stroke patients admitted to a population-based primary care center in Switzerland, shows that 225 (13.5 percent) of 1661 patients with first-ever stroke were not older than 45 years. More than 25 specific studies on stroke in people below 55 years have been published.[1–5,12,16,21,23,26–29,31–33,36,37,39,43,44,48–50,55,64,66]

## EPIDEMIOLOGY

In 1970 estimates from the Mayo Clinic gave an annual incidence of stroke of 10.4 per 100,000 in women between 15 and 29 years of age. In people between 15 and 49 years, the infarct rate was calculated to be 87 per 100,000 per year between 1945 and 1954, and 62 per 100,000 per year between 1955 and 1966.[62] A 10-year survey among infants under 15 years old from the same institution found 38 cases with ischemic stroke and 31 cases with cerebral or subarachnoid hemorrhage; the annual stroke incidence in Rochester, Minnesota residents was 2.5 per 100,000.[61] In the Stockholm County, Sweden, a 5-year survey suggested an annual stroke incidence of 34 per 100,000 in adults younger than 55 years.[51] In Demark, stroke incidence in people from 15 to 44 years was reported to be 14.4 per 100,000 per year in men and 15.5 per 100,000 per year in women.[47] In Libya, the annual stroke incidence in people from 15 to 40 years was reported to be 40.3 per 100,000 in women and 39.3 per 100,000 in men.[56]

Most of the strokes in the young appear to be ischemic, though there is one report with a proportion of hemorrhages that was superior to that of infarcts.[51] For that reason, ischemic stroke in young people has been far better studied than cerebral hemorrhage. In the Lausanne Stroke Registry, 5 percent of strokes under 30 years of age and 12 percent of strokes between 30 and 45 years (the same percentage as in older patients) were cerebral hemorrhages. Within the group of ischemic events, infarcts form about two-thirds and transient ischemic attacks (TIAs) one-third[47] of the total. TIAs were reported by 16 women and 10 men among 501 people between 20 and 54 years from Tromsø, Norway. It is interesting that all these individuals remained stroke-free over 55 months, so the authors suggested that TIA in the young may constitute a separate group, with a very low risk of developing permanent strokes.[40]

The sex ratio usually shows a female predominance in very young adults (under 30 years),[15,21,28,31,50] while there may be a male predominance above 30 years. This is likely to reflect differences in etiologies among the different age groups.[15,28]

## CEREBRAL INFARCT IN THE YOUNG

It is difficult to give an accurate hierarchy of causes of infarct based on their frequency because most studies come from secondary or tertiary care centers, so that the results are invariably biased toward uncommon causes. Table 35-1 shows the etiologic spectrum given by Hart and Miller[33] from their experience with young patients. In this series, stroke associated with migraine or mitral valve prolapse was classified as "uncertain etiology." Table 35-2 shows the more recent study of arterial infarct by Gautier et al.[29] in 1989. Table 35-3 shows our 1989-updated survey from the Lausanne Stroke Registry.

The differences between these series are not only related to referral patterns but also to the local geographic emphasis that has been put on some of the presumed etiologies, such as oral contraceptives[29] or migraine,[12] which remain controversial.

Overall, the causes of stroke in the young adult do not really differ from those in the older individual; it is only their relative frequency that is not the same. Thus, each of the chapters in this book devoted to stroke etiology may sometimes apply to strokes in the young; we do not review here all the potential causes extensively, but clinical aspects relevant to this chapter are discussed.

## ATHEROSCLEROSIS

The prevalence of arterial atherosclerosis increases with age, and it is not surprising that atherosclerosis has been associated with stroke more often in young adults above 30 years than below.[2,12,29,33,55] Overall, atherosclerosis (including large-artery and small-artery disease) has been considered to be the cause of stroke in 7 to 27 percent of patients younger than 50 years.[2,3,27,29,33,37,43,44,50,64] The patients with large-artery disease usually have classical risk factors, such as hypertension, diabetes, cigarette smoking, and, above all, hyperlipidemia.[1,17,26,27,37,50,56] Fogelholm and Aho[26] emphasized hypertriglyceridemia rather than hypercholesterolemia. Bansal et al.[6] found that 60 percent of 25 adults not older than 40 years with stroke had hyperlipidemia, most commonly type IIb, familial in two-thirds of the cases. The association between stroke and familial lipoprotein disorders was also emphasized by Daniels et al.[22] in children.

In patients with hypertension and small infarct in the territory of a deep perforator, small-artery disease may be suspected, in the absence of an alternative etiology; presumed small-artery disease associated

**TABLE 35-1. Etiology of Cerebral Infarct: Based on 100 Patients Under 40 Years of Age**

| Cause | No. of Cases |
|---|---|
| Embolism: cardiac | 27 |
| Paradoxical/pulmonary source | 4 |
| Aortitis, cholesterol, fat, unruptured aneurysm | |
| Atherosclerosis | 18 |
| Other arteriopathy | 10 |
| Inflammatory (Takayasu's disease, infection, allergy, etc.) | |
| Noninflammatory (dissection, radiotherapy, dysplasias, etc.) | |
| Hematologic disturbances: hyperviscosity, coagulopathies | 9 |
| Peripartum | 5 |
| Uncertain etiology | 27 |

(Data from Hart and Miller.[33])

**TABLE 35-2. Etiology of Cerebral Infarct: Based on 112 Patients from 9 to 45 Years of Age**

| Cause | Percentage |
|---|---|
| Dissection | 20.5 |
| Atherosclerosis | 15 |
| Cardioembolism | 12 |
| Rare causes: Takayasu's disease, Behçet's disease, Sneddon-Wilkinson disease, infectious arteritis, radiotherapy, sickle cell disease, etc. | 8 |
| Possible causes: oral contraceptives, peripartum, migraine, trauma, dysplasia, alcohol intoxications, etc. | 36 |
| Unknown cause | 9 |

(Data from Gautier et al.[29])

**TABLE 35-3. Etiology of Cerebral Infarct: Based on 202 Patients from 16 to 45 Years of Age**

| Cause | Percentage |
|---|---|
| Cardioembolism | 23 |
| Dissection | 21 |
| Other arterial diseases | |
| Extracranial | |
| Atherosclerosis | 5 |
| Dysplasia | 2 |
| Intracranial | |
| Arteritis | 4 |
| Hypertensive small-artery disease | 2 |
| Dolichoectasia | 1 |
| Reversible angiopathy (toxemia, peripartum, ergotism) | 2 |
| Migraine stroke | 15 |
| Cerebral venous thrombosis | 1 |
| Other (aortography, MELAS[a] syndrome) | 1 |
| Undetermined | 23 |

[a] Mitochondrial encephalomyopathy with lactic acidosis and strokelike episodes.

with hypertension was the most likely cause of infarct in 2 percent of patients 45 years old or younger (all were older than 30 years) in the Lausanne Stroke Registry.

## CARDIOEMBOLISM

Cardioembolism has been found to be the cause of stroke in 12 percent to one-third of adults younger than 50 years,[2,3,12,20,27,29,31,43,55,66] according to variable diagnostic criteria for cardioembolism and the extent of investigations. Overall, cardioembolism is one of the three most common causes of stroke in the young.[2,12,29,33]

The type of the potential cardiac sources of embolism may show geographic variations. For instance, rheumatic heart disease is a much more prevalent cause of stroke in India and developing countries than in occidental countries.[67] In Europe and North America, mitral valve prolapse and patent foramen ovale with or without interatrial septum aneurysm have often been considered to be the most common "occult" cardiopathies associated with stroke.[7,12,44,45,71] However, this issue is controversial, as a low prevalence of such abnormalities has been reported in series of young patients with ischemic stroke.[2,25,29,37] It has become obvious that very strict criteria should be used for the diagnosis of "pathologic" mitral valve prolapse, and it is likely that the morphology of the valves, that is, redundance of the leaflets, is also important.[54] A patent foramen ovale is not uncommon in healthy young adults, and is not "emboligenic" by itself; on the other hand, a paradoxical embolic phenomenon may be considered when the patient also has a documented peripheral venous thrombosis or when stroke was triggered by a Valsalva maneuver.[9,41,45,71] Thus, the discovery of a mild prolapse of the mitral valve or of an isolated patent foramen ovale in a young adult with recent cerebral infarct may be more an incidental finding than the origin of stroke, and the clinician should be encouraged to look for alternative causes.

It is our opinion that echocardiography is a useful screening procedure in young adults with stroke, but any possible "pathologic" finding should be carefully assessed before attributing stroke to cardioembolism. The main screening interest of echocardiography is to detect mitral valve prolapse with redundant valves, a patent foramen ovale when paradoxical embolism is suspected, and atrial myxoma in patients without cardiac symptoms and with unclear auscultation. Otherwise, echocardiology is mainly a tool for better delineating an already suspected cardiac abnormality, as in older patients. The potential role of continuous electrocardiographic (ECG) monitoring as a screening test in young adults with stroke has not been well established, and at the present time, we believe that it should be performed only in selected instances.

## ARTERIAL DISSECTION

In the large series by Gautier et al.[30] and in our experience from the Lausanne Stroke Registry, dissection of the cervicocerebral arteries were, respectively, the first and second causes of stroke in a total of 323 patients not older than 45 years. These findings suggest that one in every four to five young adults with stroke may have arterial dissection, though previous reports gave lower figures.[33,64] A survey of 1,200 patients of all ages admitted to a primary care center for acute stroke showed that 30 (2.5 percent) had carotid artery dissection; the mean age was 41 years.[10] In other large series, the mean age of patients was also around 40 years.[8,24,53] Vertebrobasilar dissection is less commonly recognized, probably because posterior circulation angiography is less widely performed than carotid angiography in many centers. One unresolved question is the quasi-specific occurrence in young individuals; if a defect in a component of the arterial wall plays a role in the genesis of dissections, it is possible that progressive increasing wall rigidity with aging may preclude the development of arterial dissection.

## MIGRAINE STROKE

Diagnosis of migraine stroke is primarily based on exclusion of other conditions, and it is essential to use strict criteria, otherwise a diagnosis of migraine stroke will be made in every migraineur who suffers a stroke. The diagnosis of migraine stroke can be made reliably only in known migraineurs who develop a cerebral infarct during a typical attack of migraine.[14,18,34,59]

Between 5 and 25 percent of cerebral infarcts in the young have been attributed to migraine stroke.[14,18,33,34,55] In a recent survey of 202 patients 45 years old or younger with ischemic stroke from the Lausanne Stroke Registry, 20 percent of the patients younger than 30 years and 12 percent of the patients between 30 and 45 years, had the diagnosis of migraine stroke. It is likely that migraine stroke also occurs in older patients, but as atherosclerotic concomitants are likely to be also present, diagnosis may remain more uncertain. In our own experience, cerebral infarct during a migraine attack is not associated with cardioembolism or arterial disease,[14] and it is likely to be related to a prolongation of the migrainous process itself—whatever it is—beyond usual limits.

In a recent study on amaurosis fugax and optic nerve infarction in 83 patients younger than 45 years, 41 percent had headaches or orbital pain and another

25 percent had remote headaches, in the absence of abnormal investigations for arterial, cardiac, or hematologic disease.[68] The authors suggested that a migrainous phenomenon was likely.

## REVERSIBLE CEREBRAL ANGIOPATHIES

Recently the concept of reversible angiopathy with transient segmental narrowing of the middle-sized intracerebral arteries has progressively emerged. Initially these cases were reported as a form of "benign cerebral vasculitis,"[65] but recent studies are more consistent with a transient vasoconstriction phenomenon without inflammatory changes.[19,52,60,63] Case reports have been nearly limited to patients, usually women, younger than 50 years. The clinical picture is rather stereotyped, although nonspecific, with severe headaches, nausea, and vomiting, sometimes with seizures and reversible neurologic deficits. This may suggest subarachnoid hemorrhage, but the cerebrospinal fluid (CSF) is normal or shows only a few red and white cells. Characteristically, the segmental narrowings seen on angiography disappear within a few days to a few months, and clinical recovery is complete. The exact nature of these reversible multiple narrowings of the cerebral vessels is not fully explained, but, in many cases, they may correspond to a vasoconstriction response to intermittent or prolonged bursts of severe hypertension, in the absence of chronic hypertension. There are cases without reported acute rise of blood pressure, but the hypertensive phenomena may be labile and easily missed when no continuous monitoring of blood pressure is available.

In some cases, no obvious cause for this angiopathy can be found, but in a few instances, a cause of paroxysmal hypertension (pheochromocytoma)[4] was present, or a previous "viral" illness has been observed.[52,60] In other patients, predisposing conditions are present:

*Toxic angiopathies* (cocaine-crack, amphetamine-like substances, phenylpropanolamine, ergot derivatives).[30,35,46,58,73]

*Cerebral angiopathy of toxemia*,[57,70,72] in which the response to hypertensive crisis is obvious.

*Peripartum angiopathy*[11,16,57,60] was first reported in 1979 by Rascol et al.,[57] but the first report in the English literature appeared only in 1988.[16] It develops during the last days of delivery in the absence of toxemia. Although this has not always been demonstrated, it is likely to be associated with hypertensive peaks. Sometimes it seems to be triggered by the administration of ergot derivatives, like methylergonovine,[11,60] but not always. In one personal case, transcranial Doppler monitored very well improvement and normalization of intracranial flow changes over a few weeks.[11] The clinical picture of this angiopathy may mimic that of peripartum cerebral venous thrombosis, which should always be excluded by appropriate angiograms.

## OTHER ETIOLOGIES

Potential causes of ischemic stroke in the young are summarized in Table 35-4. Every specific etiology is discussed in the corresponding chapter of this book.

It may be emphasized that the prevalence of some etiologies was particularly high in individual series. For instance, acute alcoholic intoxication within the preceding 24 hours was reported in 40 percent of people 55 years old and younger from a Finnish population.[36] A traumatic factor was present in 13 (22 percent) of 60 patients under 45 years old from Oxford Community.[37] Gautier et al.[29] considered that the contraceptive pill was the "cause" of 43 percent of ischemic stroke in young women from a Parisian series. In India, meningovascular syphilis may form 15 percent and cerebral venous thrombosis 20 percent of strokes in the young.[21,67]

The antiphospholipid syndrome has been emphasized recently as a possible cause of stroke in the young; however, we are still lacking the controlled studies to demonstrate an etiologic role for antiphospholipid antibodies in stroke, and the issue remains, in our view, controversial.

Unknown etiology was reported in as many as one-third of young adults with ischemic stroke.[3,31,43] In the Lausanne Stroke Registry, 46 (23 percent) of 202 adults 45 years old and younger had an undetermined etiology of stroke after extensive arterial, hematologic, and immunologic testing.

## INVESTIGATIONS

In our institution, brain computed tomography (CT), ECG, echocardiography, standard hematologic and other blood tests, and extracranial and transcranial Doppler ultrasounds are performed in every young adult with suspected ischemic stroke. Cerebral angiography is usually also performed in every patient, except when another nonarterial etiology is obvious or in typical migraine stroke, which in our experience is invariably negative.[14] More specific investigations, including sophisticated hematologic tests (antithrombin III, protein C, protein S), immunologic tests (autoantibodies, antiphospholipid antibodies, microbiologic tests, etc.), Holter monitoring, and CSF studies are performed only in selected cases. Of course, this policy may be adapted according to the prevalence of a specific disease (e.g., syphilis) in a particular geographic area. A brain biopsy may sometimes be indicated in suspected cerebral arteritis, but is rarely performed in practice.

**TABLE 35-4. Potential and Possible Causes of Ischemic Stroke in the Young**

- Arterial Disease
  - Large-artery atherosclerosis (including postactinic disease and cholesterol embolism)
  - Small-artery disease (hypertension-associated)
  - Nonatherosclerotic disease
    - Noninflammatory
      - Dissection, fibromuscular dysplasia, moyamoya and variants, neoplastic angioendotheliosis, Bürger's disease, neurofibromatosis, Köhlmeyer-Degos disease, AIDS, homocystinuria, Marfan syndrome, Fabry's disease, Sneddon syndrome and Van Bogaert-Divry syndrome, pseudoxanthoma elasticum, dolichoectasia, Grönblad-Strandberg disease, contraceptive-induced hyperplasia, reversible cerebral angiopathies (toxemia, peripartum, some toxic angiopathies, subarachnoid hemorrhage vasospasm, paroxysmal hypertension, hyperparathyroidism, idiopathy)
    - Inflammatory
      - Takayasu's disease, granulomatous arteritides, aortoarteritis, infective arteritis (syphilis, tuberculosis, rickettsiosis, neuroborreliosis, brucellosis, mycoses, AIDS, herpes zoster, mycoplasma pneumoniae, malaria), Eales disease, some toxic angiopathies, systemic arteritides (Wegener syndrome, rheumatoid arthritis, sarcoidosis, collagen disease, polyarteritis nodosa, Behçet's disease, relapsing polychondritis, ulcerative colitis)
- Migraine Stroke
- Trauma (Dissection, In Situ Thrombosis)
- Venous Thrombosis
- Hematologic Conditions
  - Hyperviscosity (myeloproliferative syndromes, dysproteinemia)
  - Coagulopathy (Moschcowitz disease, disseminated intravascular coagulation, paraneoplastic, paroxysmal nocturnal hemoglobinuria, thrombocytosis, sickle cell disease, hemoglobin sickle cell disease, thalassemia, hemoglobin C disease, protein C deficiency, protein S deficiency, antithrombin III deficiency, prekallikrein deficiency, factor XII deficiency, heparin cofactor II deficiency, $C_2$ deficiency, antiphospholipid syndrome, alcohol intoxication, platelet hyperaggregability, vitamin K or antifibrinolytic therapy, snake bite)
  - Anemia
- Heart Disease
  - Valvular (mitral stenosis, prosthetic valve, infective endocarditis, marantic endocarditis, Libman-Sacks endocarditis, mitral annulus calcification, mitral valve prolapse, rheumatic heart disease)
  - Atrial fibrillation and sick sinus syndrome
  - Acute myocardial infarct, left ventricular akinesia/aneurysm, atrial septal aneurysm
  - Left (right) atrial myxoma, cardiac rhabdomyomas (tuberous sclerosis), cardiac papillary fibroelastoma, left ventricular cavernous angiectasia
  - Dilated cardiomyopathy (with/without myopathy)
  - Chagas disease
  - Cardiac surgery/catheterism
  - Atrial (including patent foramen ovale) and ventricular septal defects with shunt (paradoxical embolism)
- Pulmonary Disease
  - Arteriovenous malformation/fistula, Rendu-Osler-Weber syndrome
  - Pulmonary vein thrombosis
- Other Embolic Phenomena
  - Fat embolism
  - Fibrocartilaginous embolism
  - Air embolism (divers)
  - Foreign particle embolism (iatrogenic)
  - Embolism distal to saccular aneurysm
  - Tumor embolism
- Other Disorders
  - Neuroleptic malignant syndrome
  - Congenital odontoid aplasia, atlantoaxial subluxation
  - Mediastinal mass (tumor, thyroid mass)
  - Osteopetrosis
  - MELAS (mitochondrial encephalomyopathy with lactic acidosis and strokelike episodes) syndrome

## PROGNOSIS

Prognosis and recurrence rate is obviously a function of the underlying etiology. Overall, death during the acute phase may vary from 1.5 to 7.3 percent.[12,49] In most series with an adequate follow-up, at least three-quarters of the patients improved markedly or completely and could return to their previous activities.[5,12,31,38] The annual incidence of recurrent stroke seems to be less than 1 percent.[12,38]

## CEREBRAL HEMORRHAGE IN THE YOUNG

Intraparenchymal hemorrhage has been poorly studied in young adults. Only one single study was specifically devoted to this condition.[69] It dealt with 72 patients from 15 to 45 years, 61 of whom had angiography. The most common site of bleeding was lobar (41 cases). A presumed cause was diagnosed in 55 (76 percent) patients and included the following conditions: arteriovenous malformation (21 cases), hypertension (11 cases), aneurysm (7 cases), use of sympathicomimetic agents (5 cases). In a study on nonhypertensive causes of cerebral hemorrhages, arteriovenous malformations, tumors, anticoagulant therapy, and amphetaminelike agents were emphasized as the main causes in young patients.[42]

Cerebral hemorrhage is certainly much more uncommon than ischemic stroke in young adults.[13] Gautier et al.[29] reported that 12 (9 percent) of 133 patients 45 years old and under with stroke had a hemorrhage. In the Oxford study, 15 (20 percent) of 75 patients under 45 years old had a hemorrhage.[37] In the Toronto Stroke Unit, only 3 of 54 patients under 45 years had a hemorrhage.[32] In our own experience from the Lausanne Stroke Registry, 23 (10.2 percent) of 225 patients aged 16 to 45 years had CT-proven cerebral hemorrhage. The mean age was 38 years, and only 3 patients were younger than 30 years, contrary to 28 percent of 202 patients with cerebral infarct. Only 3 (13 percent) of the 23 patients were women (vs 56 percent of patients with infarct). Hypertension (43 percent) was much more prevalent than in the infarct cases (8 percent). Early death and persisting severe disability were more common than with cerebral infarct (48 percent vs 17 percent).

## REFERENCES


1. Abraham J, Shetty G, Jose CJ: Strokes in the young. Stroke 2:258, 1971
2. Adams HP, Jr, Butler MJ, Biller J, Toffol GJ: Nonhemorrhagic cerebral infarction in young adults. Arch Neurol 43:793, 1986
3. Alvarez J, Matias-Guin J, Sumalla J et al: Ischemic stroke in young adults. I. Analysis of the etiological subgroups. Acta Neurol Scand 80:28, 1989
4. Armstrong FS, Hayes GJ: Segmental cerebral arterial construction associated with pheochromocytoma. J Neurosurg 18:843, 1961
5. Auff E, Schnaberth G, Zeiler K: Langzeit-prognose von Patienten mit juvenilem Insult: katamnestische Ergebnisse. Eur Arch Psychiatr Neurol Sci 234:275, 1984
6. Bansal BC, Good AK, Bonsal CB: Familial hyperlipidemia in stroke in the young. Stroke 17:1142, 1986
7. Barnett HJM, Boughner DR, Taylor DW et al: Further evidence relating mitral valve prolapse to cerebral ischemic events. N Engl J Med 302:139, 1980
8. Biller J, Hingtgen WL, Adams HP, Jr et al: Cervicocephalic arterial dissections: a ten-year experience. Arch Neurol 43:1234, 1986
9. Biller J, Johnson MR, Adams HP, Jr et al: Echocardiographic evaluation of young adults with nonhemorrhagic cerebral infarction. Stroke 17:608, 1986
10. Bogousslavsky J, Despland PA, Regli F: Spontaneous carotid dissection with acute stroke. Arch Neurol 44:137, 1987
11. Bogousslavsky J, Despland PA, Regli F, Dubuis PY: Postpartum cerebral angiopathy: reversible vasoconstriction assessed by transcranial Doppler ultrasounds. Eur Neurol 29:102, 1989
12. Bogousslavsky J, Regli F: Ischemic stroke in adults younger than 30 years of age: cause and prognosis. Arch Neurol 44:479, 1987
13. Bogousslavsky J, Regli F: Klinik der intrazerebralen Blutungen. In Hopf HC, Poeck K, Schliack H (eds): Neurologie in Praxis und Klinik. Vol. 3. Thieme, Stuttgart, 1992
14. Bogousslavsky J, Regli F, Van Melle G et al: Migraine stroke. Neurology (NY) 38:223, 1988
15. Bogousslavsky J, Van Melle G, Regli F, for the Lausanne Stroke Registry Group: The Lausanne Stroke Registry: analysis of 1000 consecutive patients with first stroke. Stroke, 19:1083, 1988
16. Brick JF: Vanishing cerebrovascular disease of pregnancy. Neurology (NY) 38:804, 1988
17. Brick JF, Riggs JE: Ischemic cerebrovascular disease in the young adult: emergence of oral contraceptive use and pregnancy as the major risk factors in the 1980s. Ann Neurol 18:125, 1985
18. Broderick JP, Swanson JW: Migraine-related stroke clinical profile and prognosis in 20 patients. Arch Neurol 44:868, 1987
19. Call GK, Fleming MC, Sealfon S et al: Reversible cerebral segmental vasoconstriction. Stroke 19:1159, 1988
20. Cardiac Embolism Task Force: Cardiogenic brain embolism: the second report of the cerebral embolism task force. Arch Neurol 46:727, 1989
21. Chopra JS, Prabhakar S: Clinical features and risk factors in stroke in young. Acta Neurol Scand 60:289, 1979
22. Daniels SR, Bates S, Lukin RR et al: Cerebrovascular arteriopathy (arteriosclerosis) and ischemic childhood stroke. Stroke 13:360, 1982
23. Dizinger HG, Ringelstein EB: Die Diagnostik des Schlaganfalls bei jungen Erwachsenen. Dtsch Med Wochenschr 110:1759, 1985
24. Duché B: Dissections spontanées des artères cervico-cérébrales: analyse de 52 cas et revue de la littérature. Thèse, Bordeaux, 1986
25. Egeblad H, Soelberg Sørensen P: Prevalence of mitral valve prolapse in younger patients with cerebral ischaemic attacks: a blinded controlled study. Acta Med Scand 216:385, 1985
26. Fogelholm R, Aho K: Ischaemic cerebrovascular disease in young adults. Acta Neurol Scand 49:415 and 428, 1973
27. Franck G, Doyen P, Grisar T et al: Les accidents ischémiques cérébraux du sujet jeune, âgé de moins de 45 ans. Sem Hop Paris 59:2642, 1983
28. Gandolfo C, Loeb C, Moretti C et al: Patient characteristics in the cooperative controlled study of focal cerebral ischemia in young adults. In Meyer JS, Lechner H, Reivich M, Otto EO (eds): Cerebral Vascular Disease. Vol. 6. p. 77. Excerpta Medica, Amsterdam, 1987
29. Gautier JC, Pradat-Diehl P, Loron P et al: Accidents vasculaires cérébraux des sujets jeunes: une étude de 133 patients âgés de 9 à 45 ans. Rev Neurol 145:437, 1989
30. Golbe LI, Merkin MD: Cerebral infarction in a user of free-base cocaine ("crack"). Neurology (NY) 36:1602, 1986

31. Grindal AB, Cohen RJ, Saul RF, Taylor JR: Cerebral infarction in young adults. Stroke 9:39, 1978
32. Hachinski VC, Morris J: The acute stroke. p. 141. FA Davis, Philadelphia, 1985
33. Hart RG, Miller VT: Cerebral infarction in young adults: a practical approach. Stroke 14:110, 1983
34. Henrich JB, Sandercock PAG, Warlow CP et al: Stroke and migraine in the Oxfordshire Community Stroke Project. J Neurol 233:257, 1986
35. Henry PY, Larre P, Aupy M et al: Reversible cerebral arteriopathy associated with the administration of ergot derivatives. Cephalalgia 4:171, 1984
36. Hillbom M, Kaste M: Ethanol intoxication: a risk factor for ischemic brain infarction. Stroke 14:694, 1983
37. Hilton-Jones D, Warlow CP: The causes of stroke in the young. J Neurol 232:137, 1985
38. Hindfelt B, Nilsson O: The prognosis of ischaemic stroke in young adults. Acta Neurol Scand 55:123, 1977
39. Hindfelt B, Nilsson O: Brain infarction in young adults with particular reference to pathogenesis. Acta Neurol Scand 55:145, 1977
40. Johnson SE, Skre H: Transient cerebral ischemic attacks in the young and middle aged: a population study. Stroke 17:662, 1986
41. Jones HR, Caplan LR, Come PC et al: Cerebral emboli of paradoxical origin. Ann Neurol 13:314, 1983
42. Kase CS: Intracerebral hemorrhage: non-hypertensive causes. Stroke 17:590, 1986
43. Klein GM, Seland TP: Occlusive cerebrovascular disease in young adults. Can J Neurol Sci 11:302, 1984
44. Kouvaras G, Bacoulas G: Association of mitral valve leaflet prolapse with cerebral ischaemic events in the young and early middle-aged patient. Q J Med 55:387, 1985
45. Lechat P, Mas JL, Lascault G et al: Prevalence of patent foramen ovale in patients with stroke. N Engl J Med 318:1148, 1988
46. Le Coz P, Woimant F, Rougemont D et al: Angiopathies cérébrales bénignes et phénylpropanolamine. Rev Neurol 144:295, 1988
47. Lidegaard O, Sol M, Andersen MVN: Cerebral thromboembolism among young women and men in Denmark 1977–1982. Stroke 17:670, 1986
48. Logan WR, Tegeler CH, Keniston WD, Hart RG: Migraine and stroke in young adults. Neurology (NY), suppl 1. 34:206, 1984
49. Marshall J: The cause and prognosis of strokes in people under 50 years. J Neurol Sci 53:473, 1982
50. McDowell FH, Louis S, Heyman A, Arons M: Nonembolic cerebral infarction in young adults. In Took JF, Siekert RG, Whisnant JP (eds): Cerebrovascular Diseases. Proceedings of the Sixth Research Conference. p. 23. Grune & Stratton, Orlando, FL, 1968
51. Mettinger KL, Söderström CE, Allander E: Epidemiology of acute cerebrovascular disease before the age of 55 in the Strockholm county 1973–1977. I. Incidence and mortality rates. Stroke 15:795, 1984
52. Michel D, Vial C, Antoine JC et al: Angiopathie cérébrale aiguë bénigne: quatre cas. Rev Neurol 141:786, 1985
53. Mokr B, Sundt TM, Jr, Houser OW, Piepgras DG: Spontaneous dissection of the cervical internal carotid artery. Ann Neurol 19:126, 1986
54. Nishimura RA, McGoon MD, Shub C et al: Echocardiographically documented mitral-valve prolapse. N Engl J Med 313:1305, 1985
55. Pereira Monteiro JM, Leite Carneiro A, Bastos Lima AF, Castro Lopes JR: Migraine and cerebral infarction; three case studies. Headache 25:429, 1985
56. Radhakrishnan K, Ashok PP, Sridharan R, Monsa ME: Stroke in the young: incidence and pattern in Benghazi, Libya. Acta Neurol Scand 73:434, 1986
57. Rascol A, Guiraud B, Manelfe C, Clanet M: Accidents vasculaires cérébraux de la grossesse et du post partum. p. 84. In: Deuxième Conférence de la Salpêtrière sur les Maladies Vasculaires Cérébrales. Baillère, Paris, 1980
58. Rothrock JF, Rubenstein R, Lyden PD: Ischemic stroke associated with methamphetamine inhalation. Neurology (NY) 38:589, 1988
59. Rothrock JF, Walicke P, Swenson MR et al: Migrainous stroke. Arch Neurol 45:63, 1988
60. Rousseaux P, Scherpereel B, Bernard MH, Guyot JF: Angiopathie cérébrale aiguë bénigne: six observations. Nouv Pressee Med 12:2163, 1983
61. Schoenberg BS, Mellinger JF, Schoenberg DG: Cerebrovascular disease in infarcts and children: a study of incidence, clinical features, and survival. Neurology (NY) 28:763, 1978
62. Schoenberg BS, Whisnant JP, Taylor WF, Kenyers RD: Strokes in women of childbearing age—a population study. Neurology (NY) 20:187, 1970
63. Serdaru M, Chiras J, Cujas M, Lhermitte F: Isolated benign cerebral vasculitis or migrainous vasospasm. J Neurol Neurosurg Psychiatry 47:73, 1984
64. Smoker WRK, Biller J, Hingtgen WL et al: Angiography of nonhemorrhagic cerebral infarction in young adults. Stroke 18:708, 1987
65. Snyder BD, McClelland RR: Isolated benign cerebral vasculitis. Arch Neurol 35:612, 1978
66. Snyder BD, Ramirez-Lassepas M: Cerebral infarction in young adults—long-term prognosis. Stroke 11:149, 1980
67. Srinivasan K: Ischemic cerebrovascular disease in the young—two common causes in India. Stroke 15:733, 1984
68. Tippin J, Corbett JJ, Kerber RE et al: Amaurosis fugax and ocular infarction in adolescents and young adults. Ann Neurol 26:69, 1989
69. Toffol GJ, Biller J, Adams HP, Jr: Nontraumatic intracerebral hemorrhage in young adults. Arch Neurol 44:483, 1987
70. Trommer BL, Homer D, Mikhael MA: Cerebral vasospasm and eclampsia. Stroke 19:326, 1988
71. Webster MWI, Chancellor AM, Smith HJ et al: Patent foramen ovale in young stroke patients. Lancet 2:11, 1988
72. Will AD, Lewis KL, Hinshaw DB, Jr et al: Cerebral vasoconstriction in toxemia. Neurology 37:1555, 1987
73. Zumstein V, Uske A, Regli F: Angiopathie cérébrale diffuse sur ergotisme avec troubles neurologiques persistants. Schweiz Rundschau Med 76:1315, 1987

# V

# *STROKE THERAPY*

## Henry J.M. Barnett and Bennett M. Stein, Section Editors

Therapy for stroke prevention has advanced since the first edition. The evidence that stroke continues to decline in all developed countries probably reflects an increased awareness of the importance of risk factors on the part of the medical profession and the public. Public educational programs find a diminishing number of people in these countries ignoring hypertension or dietary advice and even warnings about cigarette smoking. The battle in the area of primary preventive measures is heading toward a tangible victory.

Secondary medical and surgical stroke prevention measures may never have the same impact on stroke incidence as has been witnessed by the assault that has occurred in the last 30 years on these primary factors. Nevertheless, encouraging evidence has been accumulating that establishes treatment strategies with a surety that had not existed when the first edition of this work appeared: We know for sure now of the benefit of two platelet-inhibiting agents (aspirin and ticlopidine) in patients with transient ischemic attacks or prior stroke. We can state with assurance that anticoagulants and platelet inhibitors reduce the risk of stroke in patients with atrial fibrillation, and that anticoagulants are indicated in patients threatened with cardiac thromboembolism. Finally, we know that carotid endarterectomy is not purely empirical—it is clearly indicated in patients with very severe carotid stenosis causing focal hemisphere and retinal symptoms.

Thus we are reporting real progress in both primary and secondary stroke prevention measures. Life-style changes, antithrombotics, and surgery have defined roles. For individual patients, their application often will be combined. The third requirement arises when the first two have failed and the circulation to the brain has been interfered with in a focal or diffuse fashion. We must try to reduce the amount of brain that does not recover its function. Efforts at this "ischemic resuscitation" have been intense in the laboratory and in early clinical trials. We cannot make solid claims here as yet. However, strategies for dealing with thrombi in the cerebral arteries, including the use of thrombolysins, and the use of a variety of methods to protect the ischemic brain cells will be watched with great anticipation. We hope that the third edition of this book will report in a positive way about work now in progress for this.

The struggle to reduce the toll of death and disability from aneurysm moves ahead at a pace that remains disappointing. Better imaging and new interventional techniques are beginning to take away some of the shadows. The next decade may be the critical one for this lingering problem. Evidence that vasospasm can be dealt with is emerging. The improvement for survival and reduction of disability for patients with arteriovenous and other nonaneurysmal malformations is yielding slowly to new technological advances both of a diagnostic and of a therapeutic nature.

This section presents an account of these successes, deals with some failures, and makes some promises for the future.

# 36
# FUNDAMENTALS OF ANTICOAGULANT ACTION AND ADMINISTRATION

Jack Hirsh

## FUNDAMENTALS OF ACTION OF VITAMIN K ANTAGONISTS

Warfarin is the most widely used vitamin K antagonist because its onset and duration of action is predictable and it has excellent bioavailability.[8,12,13,35,44,47] The mean half-life of a single dose of warfarin is 40 hours. The concentration of warfarin in plasma shows a poor correlation with its anticoagulant effect because its metabolism and excretion varies greatly between individuals.[7,35] The absorption, metabolism, and excretion of warfarin sodium is influenced by diet, drugs, and disease. Ninety-seven percent of warfarin sodium is bound to the albumin fraction of plasma at therapeutic doses. Only the free warfarin is therapeutically active; therefore, drugs that influence the binding of warfarin to albumin can have marked effects on the anticoagulant effect of warfarin.

Warfarin inhibits the effect of vitamin K on a postribosomal step in the hepatic synthesis of factors II, VII, IX, and X, and of the anticoagulant proteins known as protein C and protein S. This results in the synthesis of biologically inactive but immunologically detectable forms of these proteins.[17,18,33,37,43,55,56]

Warfarin inhibits vitamin K in a complex manner. The function of vitamin K is to promote carboxylation of factors II, VII, IX, X, and protein C, which increases their affinity for calcium and facilitates their binding to phospholipids, a process that is necessary for their effective participation in the coagulation process.[3,18] The vitamin K antagonists induce their anticoagulant effect by interfering with the cyclic interconversion of vitamin K and its 2,3-epoxide (vitamin K epoxide) and result in an increased ratio of vitamin K epoxide to vitamin K in the liver.[56,63]

Protein C is a proenzyme activated by thrombin to form activated protein C.[16,38] The ability of thrombin to activate protein C is enhanced by its binding to an endothelial-bound thrombin receptor called thrombomodulin. Thrombomodulin-bound thrombin loses its ability to cleave fibrinogen and to activate factors V and VIII. Activated protein C inhibits factors Va and VIIIa by a proteolytic step and is an important anticoagulant.[16,38] The anticoagulant effect of warfarin is delayed until the normal clotting factors are cleared from the circulation.[46] An anticoagulant effect occurs within 24 hours due to suppression of factor VII, but peak anticoagulant activity is delayed for 72 to 96 hours because of the longer half-lives of factors II, IX, and X.[7,9,12,13,24,35] Protein C has a short half-life similar to factor VII (6 to 7 hours), and so for the first 24 to 48 hours after initiating oral anticoagulant therapy, the antithrombotic effect is limited to suppression of factor VII, while there is a potentially important thrombogenic effect caused by the suppression of protein C activity.[61]

When warfarin is administered as a loading dose it begins to prolong the prothrombin time (PT) within 24 hours by reducing the level of factor VII; however, peak anticoagulant activity is delayed for up to 96 hours because of the longer half-life of factors II, IX, and X. The use of a daily maintenance dose tends to avoid overdosage and unopposed reduction of protein C, especially in patients who are sensitive to warfarin, and this is the preferred approach.[45] The use of a 4- to 5-day overlap of heparin and warfarin provides the patient with protection (by heparin) against thrombus extension until the levels of factors II, IX, and X are reduced into an acceptable range.[45]

## ORAL ANTICOAGULANT THERAPY

### The Therapeutic Range for the Control of Oral Anticoagulant Therapy

The optimal therapeutic range for monitoring oral anticoagulant therapy has been reviewed recently,[1,25] and recommendation to reduce the therapeutic range for a number of indications were made. Until recently, the recommendations for the therapeutic range for oral anticoagulant therapy had been made empirically and lacked validity by current methodologic standards.

### Monitoring Oral Anticoagulant Therapy

The prothrombin time test, introduced by Quick[50] in 1935, is the most common method used for monitoring oral anticoagulant therapy. This test is responsive to reductions in three of the vitamin K-dependent clotting factors: factors II, VII, and X. The interpretation of the PT result has been confused because thromboplastins prepared by different methods and derived from different species vary markedly in their response to reduction of the vitamin K-dependent clotting factors by coumarinlike drugs.[49,67] In general, thromboplastins prepared from human brain are more responsive to reduction of these clotting factors than those prepared from rabbit brain, although some human brain thromboplastins are relatively nonresponsive, and it is possible to prepare highly responsive thromboplastins from rabbit brain.[36]

As a consequence of the variability in responsiveness of different thromboplastins, PT results obtained from patients on oral anticoagulant therapy may not be interchangeable between laboratories and as a consequence could produce potential problems for anticoagulant control. The differences in responsiveness of various thromboplastins to the therapeutic reduction of vitamin K-dependent clotting factors has also been associated with and possibly responsible for clinically important differences in the dosage of anticoagulant used between countries.[67]

### Standardization of the Prothrombin Time

Over the years, a number of attempts have been made to standardize the reporting system for the PT. The history of standardization has been reviewed by Poller[49] and by Kirkwood.[36] In the United Kingdom, a standardized human brain thromboplastin reagent, the Manchester Comparative Reagent (MCR), was produced in 1964, and a supply of reference batches was made available to a large number of hospitals in the United Kingdom.

Attempts were made to standardize PT reagents in the United States by the College of American Pathologists in 1969 by the introduction of plasmas artificially depleted of vitamin K-dependent clotting factors,[49] but this approach was not widely adopted.

In 1977 the World Health Organization (WHO) designated a single batch of human brain thromboplastin as the First International Reference Preparation (IRP).[36,49] Secondary reference thromboplastins were also developed to ensure that supplies of IRP would not be depleted. The calibration model based on the first WHO reference thromboplastin had a number of limitations[36,49] and was replaced by a revised system of calibration and by new primary and secondary reference thromboplastins. The revised model assumes a linear relationship between the logarithm of the PT ratios of the reference and test thromboplastins. This calibration model adopted by the WHO in 1982 is used to standardize the reporting of the PT by converting the PT ratio observed with the local thromboplastin into an International Normalized Ratio (INR). The INR is calculated as follows: INR = observed ratio$^c$ where $c$ is the constant that represents the International Sensitivity Index (ISI). The INR, therefore, is the PT ratio that reflects the result that would have been obtained if the WHO reference thromboplastin had been used to perform the test.[36,49] It has been suggested[25,49] that manufacturers calibrate their thromboplastin reagent against the WHO reference standard and provide the user with an ISI value. If this was done, individual hospital laboratories could report the results in a standard way based on the INR.

A number of commercial manufacturers are now providing ISI values and INRs with their reagents. The ISI values for the commercial rabbit brain thromboplastin used in North America vary between 2.0 and 2.6.[49]

The conversion of the observed PT into the INR loses reliability if the local thromboplastin is much less responsive to reduction of vitamin K-dependent clotting factors than the reference thromboplastin and when the PT is performed on plasma from patients in the early stages of therapy.[49] Despite these imperfections there appears to be general agreement that the INR system of reporting should be adopted internationally, but this recommendation has been adopted by only a very small number of laboratories throughout North America.

## The Optimal Therapeutic Range for the Control of Oral Anticoagulant Therapy

The optimal therapeutic range for laboratory control of oral anticoagulant therapy has been debated for more than 30 years and, until recently, has remained unresolved. Resolution of this important issue requires randomized studies in which patients have their PT titrated to obtain different intensities of oral anticoagulant effect and by relating the results of the anticoagulant effect to clinically relevant outcomes.[1]

In the early 1950s, Wright and associates[65,66] recommended a therapeutic range of 2.0 to 2.5 control for oral anticoagulant therapy. The recommendation of a PT ratio of 2.0 to 2.5 was accepted and has been adhered to in North America for the last 30 years. In 1984 the British Society of Haematology recommended different levels of therapeutic ranges, which varied in intensity depending on the indication for oral anticoagulant therapy.[1,49] These recommendations, which were modified by the ACCP/NHLBI committee, are summarized in Table 36-1 which shows the ratios expressed as an INR and as the corresponding PT ratio for a thromboplastin with an ISI value of 2.4, which represents the commonly used commercial rabbit brain thromboplastins in North America.

There is good evidence based on critical review of the literature that effective protection against thromboembolism and its recurrence can be achieved for most indications by using the less intense ranges (by current North American standards). Hull and associates[29-31] performed a series of randomized studies using clinically relevant endpoints (bleeding and thrombosis) that addressed the issue of the optimal therapeutic range for prothrombin time control for the treatment of patients with deep venous thrombosis. They demonstrated that venous thrombosis could be treated effectively and more safely by using a less intense anticoagulant regimen (INR of 2).[31] These conclusions were based on the results of three randomized studies that were performed sequentially. In all three studies patients randomized into the standard sodium warfarin group were monitored to maintain their prothrombin time using a less responsive rabbit brain thromboplastin (ISI = 2.3) at 1.5 to 2 times control (INR, 2.5 to 5.0). At this range, there was a high frequency of bleeding in the sodium warfarin group in all studies. The first two studies demonstrated that patients with proximal vein thrombosis were at high risk of recurrence if the initial course of intravenous heparin was followed by a course of low-dose heparin[30] but that protection from recurrence could be achieved by using adjusted-dose heparin.[29] The third study demonstrated that the less intense anticoagulant regimen (with a targeted INR of 2) was effective against recurrent venous thromboembolism but produced significantly less bleeding than the (then) standard (more intense) regimen.[31]

Taberner and associates,[57] using a human brain thromboplastin (ISI = 1.1) and Francis and associates,[21] using a less responsive rabbit brain thromboplastin (assumed ISI = 2.3), used less intense anticoagulant regimens and reported that vitamin K an-

**TABLE 36-1. Recommended Therapeutic Range for Oral Anticoagulant Therapy***

| Indication | INR | Corresponding PT Ratios with Less Responsive Thromboplastins: ISI 2.0 | ISI 2.3 | ISI 2.6 |
|---|---|---|---|---|
| Prophylaxis: venous thromboembolism (high-risk surgery) | 2.0–2.5 | 1.4–1.6 | 1.4–1.5 | 1.3–1.4 |
| Prophylaxis: venous thromboembolism (hip surgery) | 2.0–3.0 | 1.4–1.7 | 1.4–1.6 | 1.3–1.5 |
| Treatment of deep-vein thrombosis or pulmonary embolism | | | | |
| Prevention of systemic embolism in patients with atrial fibrillation, valvular heart disease, tissue heart valves, or acute myocardial infarction | | | | |
| Mechanical prosthetic heart valves, recurrent systemic embolism | 3.0–4.5 | 1.7–2.1 | 1.6–1.9 | 1.5–1.8 |

*Abbreviations*: INR, international normalized ratio; ISI, international sensitivity index; PT, prothrombin time.

* Modified by the ACCP/NHLBI, American College of Chest Physicians/National Health, Lung and Blood Institute.

tagonists are effective in preventing venous thrombosis in high-risk surgical patients. The results of these two studies strongly support the effectiveness of less intense anticoagulant therapy for prevention of venous thrombosis in high-risk patients.

Three randomized trials have evaluated the effectiveness of oral anticoagulants in patients with acute myocardial infarction.[15,40,60] There was a significant reduction in stroke in two studies[40,60] and in the third the reduction in stroke was nonsignificant.[15] There was also a reduction in incidence of clinically diagnosed pulmonary embolism in all three studies. All three studies. All three studies used a less intense anticoagulant regimen.[1]

Bjerkelund and Orning[5] reported the results of a cohort study in patients with atrial fibrillation undergoing direct current cardioversion in which there was a substantial reduction in systemic embolism in patients who received anticoagulant therapy at a targeted therapeutic range of 10 to 25 percent with the thrombotest (equivalent to an INR of 1.45 to 2.8). This study provides the most convincing evidence to date that anticoagulant therapy reduces the risk of systemic embolism in patients with atrial fibrillation.

In summary, there is good evidence that a less intense oral anticoagulant regimen with a targeted therapeutic range of an INR of 2 to 3 is effective in the prevention of venous thrombosis, in the treatment of venous thrombosis after an initial course of heparin, and in the prevention of systemic embolism in patients with acute myocardial infarction. There is also suggestive evidence that this less intense regimen is effective in preventing systemic embolism in patients with atrial fibrillation who undergo direct current conversion.

The dose of warfarin that is currently used in North America to prolong the PT to a ratio of 2 to 2.5 times control is higher than the dose that was used to produce an identical prolongation in the prothrombin time in the 1940s, 1950s, and 1960s. This increase in dose of oral anticoagulants has occurred because the thromboplastins that are now used to monitor oral anticoagulant therapy in North America are less responsive to reduction of vitamin K-dependent clotting factors than the reagents that were used in North America prior to the 1970s.

When the PT was introduced to monitor oral anticoagulant therapy in the 1940s, clinical laboratories in North America used locally prepared thromboplastin reagents that were more responsive to the reduction of vitamin K-dependent clotting factors by warfarin than the commercially prepared thromboplastins in current use in North America.[15,50,60,65,67] In the late 1960s, more and more hospitals and clinical laboratories turned to commercial sources for their thromboplastin supply; this change from more responsive to less responsive thromboplastins was not accompanied by a change in the recommended therapeutic range. At present, approximately 90 percent of all of the thromboplastin reagents used in North America are provided by three manufacturers: Dade, General Diagnostics, (Origon Teknika), and Ortho;[1,25] all three manufacturers produce relatively less responsive thromboplastins (with an ISI value which varies between 2.0 and 2.6) than the domestically produced thromboplastin of the 1950s and 1960s and the WHO reference thromboplastin.[36,49] As a result many clinicians have unknowingly increased the dose of warfarin that they use to treat patients. It is of interest that the special committee of the American Heart Association on anticoagulant therapy recommended a therapeutic range based on the use of a thromboplastin that is more responsive than the commonly used commercial rabbit brain thromboplastins.[65] Thus, in North America we have come full circle. The initial recommendation made by the American Heart Association was for a relatively low dose (less intense) anticoagulant regimen. The dose of oral anticoagulants was increased with the introduction of less responsive thromboplastins, which was not accompanied by a corresponding lowering of the therapeutic range. The recommended dosage has now been adjusted downward by the Special Committee on Antithrombotic Therapy of the ACCP and NHLBI who now recommend a less intense regimen for most indications. These latest recommendations are based on evidence from randomized trials and are similar to the dosage regimens that have been used in the United Kingdom and other parts of Europe for the last 4 decades.

## FUNDAMENTALS OF ACTION OF HEPARIN

Heparin is an anionic mucopolysaccharide consisting of molecular chains of D-glucuronic acid, L-iduronic acid, and D-glucosamine. Commercial heparin is highly heterogeneous with a molecular weight range of 3,000 to 30,000 (mean 16,000). Heparin is marketed as either a sodium or a calcium salt and is effective as an anticoagulant when administered parenterally.

Heparin inhibits blood coagulation by three independent mechanisms and has an additional effect on hemostasis through its interaction with blood platelets.

The major anticoagulant effect of heparin is through catalysis of the inhibition of activated coagulation factors, thrombin, and factor Xa by antithrombin III. Heparin also catalyzes the inhibition of factors IXa, XIa, and XIIa by antithrombin III,[51] but these effects are relatively minor in comparison to its effect on thrombin and factor Xa. The arginyl residue in antithrombin III esterifies the active serine residue in these factors, which are serine proteases. Heparin binds to specific lysyl residues of antithrombin III, causing a conformational change, thereby catalyzing the inhibitory effect of antithrombin III on the activated coagulation factors.[51] Heparin then dissociates from the complex and can be reutilized. Inhibition of thrombosis by heparin requires a minimum chain length of 18 sugar units, while inhibition of factor Xa can be achieved by a 5-sugar unit (pentasaccharide) with a unique sequence. At much higher concentrations, heparin has an additional anticoagulant effect by catalyzing the inhibition of thrombin by heparin cofactor II.[59] Heparin also inhibits the generation of factor Xa and the activation of prothrombin by factor Xa in the absence of antithrombin III by disrupting the alignment of coagulation factors on the platelet surface.[42] Finally, heparin impairs hemostasis by inhibiting platelet function in vivo.[20]

Heparin prolongs the bleeding time in man[23] and experimental animals[10] probably by inhibiting platelet function in vivo.[20]

Heparin can cause thrombocytopenia, which may or may not be accompanied by major arterial thrombosis.

## Pharmacokinetics

Heparin kinetics have been studied using bioassays that measure the ability of heparin to inhibit the enzymatic activity of factor Xa or thrombin (factor IIa). The enzymatic activity of factors Xa and IIa can be measured by coagulation assays (using the natural substrate for these clotting enzymes) or by chromogenic or fluorometric assays (using artificial substrates). Other assays are based on chemical titration with positively charged compounds, such as protamine and hexadimethrine bromide.[6]

Heparin is not absorbed orally. It is absorbed through the respiratory tract, but this is not a practical route of administration.[34] It is absorbed well after subcutaneous injection and is effective both prophylactically and therapeutically by this route.[2,4,14,27,30,62] Peak heparin levels are usually obtained at 4 to 5 hours after subcutaneous administration, and the effect lasts for 12 hours or longer, depending on the dose.[27,30]

The half-life ($t_{1/2}$) of heparin has been reported to vary from 23 minutes to 2.48 hours. McAvoy[39] has shown that much of this discrepancy is due to the method of heparin analysis used.

Bjornsson and associates,[6] using three different assays (two based on coagulation tests and one based on heparin neutralization with hexadimethrine bromide), evaluated kinetic parameters in four normal subjects at three dose levels of heparin. They demonstrated dose-dependent kinetics for heparin, irrespective of the assay method used. Thus, the biologic half-life increased, the total clearance decreased, and the apparent volume of distribution remained the same, with increasing doses.

Heparin clearance is increased in patients with pulmonary embolism compared to patients with deep-vein thrombosis and normal controls.[28,54]

## Antithrombotic Effects

Heparin has a narrow therapeutic range. The drug is monitored, using either a global blood coagulation test such as the partial thromboplastin time or heparin level.

Two important issues relate to laboratory monitoring of heparin therapy that have not been resolved: (1) Should monitoring be performed using a global test such as the activated partial thromboplastin time (APTT) or a test that measures the effect of heparin on a specific step in blood coagulation? (2) If a global test is used, should the projected increment in the clotting time test value be based on the patient's own preheparin value or on the results obtained using a normal laboratory control?

The answers to these questions are best addressed through randomized trials. One such trial demonstrated that prevention of the recurrence of venous thromboembolism is dependent on maintaining the APTT above one and a half times the laboratory control, particularly in the first few days after the acute thromboembolic event.[32]

The APTT is a global test that is affected by factor VIII levels and the levels of other plasma factors. Factor VIII is an acute-phase reactant that increases following trauma or inflammation. Patients with these concomitant conditions have a short APTT that may be only minimally prolonged at heparin levels that consistently double a normal baseline APTT. There is experimental animal evidence that venous thrombosis can be prevented at heparin levels (by protamine titration) of 0.3 to 0.4 U $ml^{-1}$ even when the APTT, which has been short prior to heparin administration, is not prolonged to twice a normal control value.[11] There is also experimental animal evidence that heparin-induced bleeding is dose-related.[10] These observations suggest that it may be safer to adjust the APTT result to the patient's own pretreatment level or to use the heparin level to monitor heparin therapy.

The bleeding side effect may not be simply related to anticoagulant effect of heparin measured either as the APTT or the heparin level. There is evidence that a high molecular weight heparin inhibits placebo function more than a low molecular weight fraction.[53] This contention is supported by research on the low molecular weight heparins[26] and on the demonstration in animals that heparin with no affinity to antithrombin III and with no measurable anticoagulant activity potentiates bleeding.[41]

## Metabolism

Heparin has a very short half-life. The most likely explanation for such a short half-life is the transfer of heparin to an extravascular space, probably the reticuloendothelial system.[19]

Although patients with severe renal impairment sometimes demonstrated a prolonged half-life for heparin,[48] this does not necessarily support a renal route of elimination for heparin. Various groups have postulated other explanations, such as loss of antithrombin III[58] and a decreased[54] half-life for heparin. There is no good evidence that the liver is a site of metabolism of heparin, and the contradictory results cited above require that further studies be conducted.

## Contraindications

For contraindications, see Table 36-2.

## Mode of Use

For prophylaxis, heparin is usually administered in doses of 5,000 units subcutaneously every 8 or 12 hours. The injections should be administered into the fat of the subcutaneous tissue of the lower abdominal wall or laterally above the iliac crest. If it is not possible to use these sites, a site on the lateral aspect on the upper thigh or upper arm may be used. Bruising can be minimized by using concentrated heparin (25,000 U/ml), a narrow-gauge needle (size 25), and by applying pressure for at least 5 minutes after the injection.

For treatment purposes, heparin can be administered by a continuous infusion, by intermittent intravenous injection, or by subcutaneous injection.

**TABLE 36-2. Contraindications for Heparinization**

| |
|---|
| *Absolute Contraindications* |
| Cerebral or subarachnoid hemorrhage |
| Abdominal or thoracic bleeding into a closed space |
| Severe traumatic bleed |
| Hepatic, renal, splenic, or arterial injury |
| Recent liver or renal biopsy |
| Recent cerebrospinal surgery (including lumbar puncture and epidural anesthesia) |
| Recent eye surgery |
| Severe hemostatic defect |
| Major bleeding during anticoagulant therapy |
| Arterial thrombosis with heparin-associated thrombocytopenia |
| Heparin-associated severe thrombocytopenia |
| Recent bleed from proven peptic ulcer |
| *Relative Contraindications* |
| Patients with active bleeding or predisposition to severe hemorrhage |
| Hypertension |
| Proven peptic ulcer disease |
| Previous bleeding during anticoagulant therapy |
| Hypersensitivity or idiosyncratic reaction, including heparin-associated mild thrombocytopenia (consider switching to alternative heparin or other anticoagulant) |

### Continuous Intravenous Infusion

When administered as a continuous infusion, heparin is given as an initial bolus injection (5,000 units) followed by a maintenance infusion. The laboratory test used for monitoring heparin is performed approximately 6 hours after the bolus injection and then at least once more in the first 24 hours. Monitoring is continued twice daily until the desired effect is achieved and the dose-response relationship is stable. Monitoring is then continued on a once-daily basis.

The anticoagulant effect of heparin should then be maintained at a level that is equivalent to 0.3 to 0.4 units of heparin per ml by protamine titration. This corresponds to APTT of approximately twice the normal laboratory control value. The use of a normal laboratory control value to adjust the patient's dose can occasionally lead to unnecessary high heparin doses. If a heparin dose in excess of 40,000 U/24 h is required to double the normal control APTT, the heparin level should be checked, and if it is in excess of 0.4 U/ml, no further increase in dose is necessary.

If the monitoring test is above the therapeutic range, the dose of heparin should be reduced and the test repeated. If the result of the monitoring test is below the therapeutic range, a second bolus can be given and the dose of heparin increased.

### Intermittent Intravenous Injection

Intermittent intravenous injections of heparin can be used as an alternative to full-dose continuous intravenous heparin infusions. This approach has been reported to produce a greater frequency of bleeding.[22,52,64] Intermittent injection of heparin should be administered every 4 hours in a dose of between 5,000 and 7,000 units per injection. It is desirable to demonstrate that an effect of heparin is obtained and that this effect is not cumulative. This can be achieved by performing a laboratory test within 1 hour of the initial injection and then once or twice daily for the first few days before the next injection is due.

### Subcutaneous Injection

Heparin is also effective when given by subcutaneous injection in full therapeutic doses. It is usually administered twice daily and the dose adjusted to obtain an APTT of twice control (a heparin level of 0.3 to 0.4 U/mg) 6 hours after injection. This can usually be achieved with an initial 12-hourly dose of 20,000 units, which can usually be reduced to 15,000 units every 12 hours.[2,4,14,62]

## REFERENCES

1. ACCP/NHLBI National Conference on Antithrombotic Therapy: Chest, 89:suppl. February 1986

2. Andersson G, Fagrell B, Holmgren K et al: Subcutaneous administration of heparin: a randomised comparison with intravenous administration of heparin to patients with deep vein thrombosis. Thromb Res 27:631, 1982
3. Bell RG: Metabolism of vitamin K and prothrombin synthesis: anticoagulant and the vitamin K-epoxide cycle. Fed Proc 37:2599, 1978
4. Bentley PG, Kakkar VV, Scully MF et al: An objective study of alternative methods of heparin administration. Thromb Res 18:177, 1980
5. Bjerkelund CJ, Orning OM: The efficacy of anticoagulant therapy in preventing embolism related to D.C. electrical conversion of atrial fibrillation. Am J Cardiol 23:208, 1969
6. Bjornsson T, Wolfram KM, Kitchell BB: Heparin kinetics determined by three assay methods. Clin Pharmacol Ther 31:104, 1982
7. Breckenridge AM: Interindividual differences in the response of oral anticoagulants. Drugs 14:367, 1977
8. Breckenridge AM: Oral anticoagulant drugs: pharmacokinetic aspects. Semin Hematol 15:19, 1978
9. Brozovic M: Oral anticoagulants in clinical practice. Semin Hematol 15:27, 1978
10. Carter CJ, Kelton JG, Hirsh J et al: The relationship between haemorrhagic and antithrombotic properties of low molecular weight heparin in rabbits. Blood 59:1239, 1982
11. Chiu HM, Hirsh J, Yung WL: Relationship between the anticoagulant and antithrombotic effects of heparin in experimental venous thrombosis. Blood 49:171, 1977
12. Deykin D: Warfarin therapy. N Engl J Med 283:691, 801, 1970
13. Douglas AS: Management of thrombotic diseases. Semin Hematol 8:94, 1971
14. Doyle DJ, Turpie AGG, Hirsh J et al: Adjusted subcutaneous heparin or continuous intravenous heparin in patients with acute deep vein thrombosis: a randomized trial. Ann Intern Med 107:441, 1987
15. Drapkin A, Merskey C: Anticoagulant therapy after acute myocardial infarction. JAMA 222:541, 1972
16. Esmon CT, Owen WG: Identification of endothelial cell cofactor for thrombin-catalyzed activation of protein C. Proc Natl Acad Sci USA 78:2249, 1981
17. Esmon CT, Sadowski MA, Suttie JW: A new carboxylation reaction. J Biol Chem 250:4744, 1975
18. Esmon CT, Suttie JW, Jackson CM: The functional significance of vitamin K action: difference in phospholipid between normal and abnormal prothrombin. J Biol Chem 250:4095, 1975
19. Estes JW: Clinical pharmacokinetics of heparin. Clin Pharmacokinet 5:204, 1980
20. Fernandez F, Nguyen P, Van Ryn J et al: Hemorrhagic doses of heparin and other glycosaminoglycans induce a platelet defect. Thromb Res 43:491, 1986
21. Francis CW, Marder VJ, McCollister EC et al: Two-step warfarin therapy. JAMA 249:374, 1983
22. Glazier RL, Crowell EB: Randomized prospective trial of continuous vs intermittent heparin therapy. JAMA 236:1365, 1976
23. Heiden D, Mielke CH, Rodvien R: Impairment by heparin of primary haemostasis and platelet ($^{14}C$) 5-hydroxytryptamine release. Br J Haematol 36:427, 1977
24. Hellemans J, Vorlat M, Verstraete M: Survival time of prothrombin and factors VII, IX, and X after complete synthesis blocking doses of coumarin derivatives. Br J Haematol 9:506, 1963
25. Hirsh J: Is the dose of warfarin prescribed by American physicians unnecessarily high? Arch Intern Med 147:769, 1987
26. Hirsh J, Ofosu F, Buchanan MR: Rationale behind the development of low molecular weight heparin derivatives. Semin Thromb Hemostas 11:13, 1985
27. Hirsh J, O'Sullivan EF, Gallus AS, Martin M: Evaluation of subcutaneous calcium heparin therapy in the treatment of thromboembolic disease. Med J Aust 1:15, 1970
28. Hirsh J, Van Aken WG, Gallus AS et al: Heparin kinetics in venous thrombosis and pulmonary embolism. Circulation 53:691, 1976
29. Hull R, Delmore T, Carter C et al: Adjusted subcutaneous heparin versus warfarin sodium in the long-term treatment of venous thrombosis. N Engl J Med 306:189, 1982
30. Hull R, Delmore T, Genton E et al: Warfarin sodium versus low dose heparin in the long-term treatment of venous thromboembolism. N Engl J Med 301:855, 1979
31. Hull R, Hirsh J, Jay R et al: Different intensities of anticoagulation in the long-term treatment of proximal venous thrombosis. N Engl J Med 307:1676, 1982
32. Hull RD, Raskob G, Hirsh J et al: Continuous intravenous heparin compared with intermittent subcutaneous heparin in the initial treatment of proximal-vein thrombosis. N Engl J Med 315:1109, 1986
33. Jackson CM, Suttie JW: Recent developments in understanding the mechanism of vitamin K and vitamin K antagonist drug action and the consequences of vitamin K action in blood coagulation. Prog Hematol 10:333, 1977
34. Kavanagh LW, Jacques LB: A new route of heparin administration—the lung. Drug Res 26:398, 1976
35. Kelly JG, O'Malley K: Clinical pharmacokinetics of oral anticoagulant. Clin Pharmacokinet 4:1, 1979
36. Kirkwood TBL: Calibration of reference thromboplastins and standardisation of the prothrombin time ratio. Thromb Haemost 49:238, 1983
37. Kisiel W: Human plasma protein C: isolation, characterization, and mechanism of activations by a-thrombin. J Clin Invest 64:761, 1979
38. Kisiel W, Canfield WM, Cricsson LHG, Davie EW: Anticoagulant properties of bovine plasma protein C following activation by thrombin. Biochemistry 16:5824, 1977
39. McAvoy TJ: The biologic half-life of heparin. Clin Pharm Ther 25:372, 1979
40. Medical Research Council: Assessment of short-

term anticoagulant administration after cardiac infarction. Br Med J 1:335, 1969
41. Ockelford P, Carter CJ, Cerskus A et al: Comparison of the in vivo haemorrhagic and antithrombotic effects of a low antithrombin III affinity heparin fractions. Thromb Res 27:679, 1982
42. Ofosu FA, Blajchman MA, Hirsh J: The inhibition of heparin of the intrinsic pathway activation of factor X in the absence of antithrombin III. Thromb Res 20:391, 1980
43. Olson RE, Suttie JW: Vitamin K and carboxyglutamate biosynthesis. Vitamin Horm 35:59, 1977
44. O'Reilly RA: Vitamin K and other oral anticoagulant drugs. Annu Rev Med 27:245, 1976
45. O'Reilly RA, Aggeler PM: Studies on coumarin anticoagulant drugs: initiation of therapy without a loading dose. Circulation 38:169, 1968
46. O'Reilly RA, Aggeler PM: Determinants of the response to oral anticoagulant drug in man. Pharmacol Rev 22:35, 1970
47. O'Reilly RA, Welling PR, Wagner JG: Pharmacokinetics of warfarin following intravenous administration to man. Thromb Haemost 25:178, 1971
48. Perry PJ, Herron GR, King JC: Heparin half-life in normal and impaired renal function. Clin Pharmacol Ther 16:514, 1979
49. Poller L: Progress in standardisation in anticoagulant control. Hematol Rev 1:225, 1987
50. Quick AJ: The prothrombin time in haemophilia and in obstructive jaundice. J Biol Chem 109:73, 1935
51. Rosenberg RD, Damus RS: The purification and mechanism of action of human antithrombin-heparin cofactor. J Biol Chem 248:6490, 1973
52. Salzman EW, Deykin D, Shapiro RM, Rosenberg R: Management of heparin therapy. N Engl J Med 292:1046, 1975
53. Salzman EW, Rosenberg RD, Smith MH et al: Effect of heparin and heparin fractions on platelet aggregation. J Clin Invest 65:64, 1980
54. Simon TL, Hyers TM, Gaston JP, Harker LA: Heparin pharmacokinetics: increased requirements in pulmonary embolism. Br J Haematol 39:111, 1978
55. Stenflo J, Suttie JW: Vitamin K dependent formation of y-carboxyglutamic acid. Annu Rev Biochem 46:157, 1977
56. Suttie JW. How coumarin anticoagulants work. Drug Ther 9:63, 1979
57. Taberner DA, Poller L, Burslem RW, Jones JB: Oral anticoagulants controlled by the British comparative thromboplastin versus low-dose heparin in prophylaxis of deep venous thrombosis. Br Med J 1:272, 1978
58. Teien A: Heparin elimination in patients with liver cirrhosis. Thromb Haemostas (Stuttgart) 38:701, 1977
59. Tollefsen DM, Blank MK: Detection of a new heparin-dependent inhibitor of thrombin in human plasma. J Clin Invest 68:589, 1981
60. Veterans Administration: Anticoagulants in acute myocardial infarction. JAMA 225:724, 1973
61. Vigano S, Mannucci PM, Solinas S et al: Early fall of protein C during short-term anticoagulant treatment, abstracted. Thromb Haemost 50:310, 1983
62. Walker MG, Shaw JW, Thomson GJL et al: Subcutaneous calcium heparin versus intravenous sodium heparin in treatment of established acute deep vein thrombosis of the legs: a multicentre prospective randomized trial. Br J Med 294:1190, 1987
63. Whitlon DS, Sadowski JA, Suttie JW: Mechanism of coumarin action: significance of vitamin K epoxide reductase inhibition. Biochemistry 17:1371, 1978
64. Wilson JE, Bynum LJ, Parkey RW: Heparin therapy in venous thromboembolism. Am J Med 70:808, 1980
65. Wright IS: Recent developments in antithrombotic therapy. Ann Intern Med 71:823, 1969
66. Wright IS, Beck DF, Marple CD: Myocardial infarction and its treatment with anticoagulants: summary of findings in 1031 cases. Lancet 1:92, 1954
67. Zucker S, Cathey MH, Sox PJ, Hallec EC: Standardisation of laboratory tests for controlling anticoagulant therapy. Am J Clin Pathol 53:348, 1970

# 37
# *PLATELET FUNCTION AND ANTIPLATELET THERAPY IN ISCHEMIC CEREBROVASCULAR DISEASE*

Babette B. Weksler

## PATHOGENESIS OF THROMBOSIS IN THE CENTRAL NERVOUS SYSTEM

Cerebral ischemia producing either transient or permanent cerebral damage is most frequently the consequence of arterial obstruction that results from the occlusion of atherosclerotic, inflamed, or otherwise abnormal vessels by thrombus. The hemostatic process becomes activated on an abnormal or damaged vascular surface. Activation of blood platelets on the wall of a diseased artery has been recognized for many years as an initiating step in the formation of arterial thrombi in the absence of vascular stasis.[68] The occluding thrombus may form in situ on a cerebral arterial atherosclerotic plaque or, more frequently, may embolize into intracerebral end-arteries from a more proximal location such as the carotid arteries.[40] Because platelet activation is often a key initial step in the development of cerebral arterial ischemia, therapy directed against the primary, platelet-dependent steps of the hemostatic process, rather than anticoagulation, has proved to be useful in preventing episodes of cerebral ischemia in the setting of atherosclerosis.[2,37]

Occluding emboli in cerebral arteries, however, need not have platelets as a major component. Emboli often consist of other materials derived from atherosclerotic plaque such as cholesterol crystals liberated from an ulcerated plaque or fragments of the plaque itself that do not involve platelets; in such cases, antiplatelet therapy is not useful. Moreover, cerebral embolism from intracardiac or heart valve thrombus in patients with arrhythmias, valvular heart disease, or cardiac ventricular aneurysm, a less

This work was supported by a SCOR in Thrombosis NIH HL18828.

common cause of cerebral ischemia than atherosclerosis at the present time (approximately 15 percent of all cerebral ischemia), also represents a different pathogenesis of thrombosis that is more closely related to vascular stasis than to platelet activation and that contains major components of fibrin and erythrocytes rather than platelets. Anticoagulation, rather than antiplatelet therapy, is more effective to prevent this type of thrombus. Therefore, antiplatelet therapy will be effective prophylaxis against some but not all types of cerebral ischemia.[23,39,84]

It cannot be overstressed that cerebral arterial thrombosis tends to occur on vascular endothelial surfaces that have already been damaged or are diseased, since the normal endothelial lining of blood vessels is equipped with multiple mechanisms to promote thromboresistance and to enhance blood fluidity. Damage, inflammatory changes, or involvement with disease alters the function state of the endothelium (this may occur in the absence of morphologic change) to produce a thrombogenic, rather than a thromboresistant surface.

A logical approach to the pathogenesis and treatment of cerebral thrombosis and cerebral ischemia should therefore address platelet function, endothelial function, and contributions from other blood cells or plasma components. Abnormalities in any one of these areas—platelets, vessel wall, or blood—may predispose to cerebral ischemia or may alter the functioning of the other key components in a prothrombotic direction.

## ROLE OF THE VASCULAR ENDOTHELIUM IN HEMOSTASIS AND THROMBOSIS

The vascular endothelium has been called the ideal blood-compatible surface because of its normal lack of reactivity toward blood cells. Indeed, the endothelial surface facing the blood not only fails to activate the hemostatic process, but it promotes blood fluidity by a number of mechanisms (Fig. 37-1). First, endothelial cells are negatively charged and repel negatively charged platelets, red cells, and leukocytes. The endothelium secretes antiplatelet substances with vasodilating properties such as prostacyclin, endothelium-derived relaxing factors (EDRF, recently identified as nitric oxide) and adenosine diphosphate (ADP)-metabolizing enzymes.[24,59,78,102] The surface of endothelial cells is rich in heparan sulfate proteoglycans that activate antithrombin III[15] to inhibit thrombin and other serine protease procoagulants. Endothelial cells also synthesize and contain thrombomodulin, a protein that binds thrombin and alters its substrate specificity so that it ceases to activate coagulation but instead activates protein C, a natural anticoagulant.[24]

Moreover, the endothelium participates actively in the initiation and potentiation of fibrinolysis. Components of the fibrinolytic enzyme cascade are assembled on the endothelial surface by binding to specific receptors.[42] Endothelium protects the bound fibrinolytic components from proteolytic degradation or inactivation by plasma factors, and also amplifies the biologic effects of the bound fibrinolytic components. Endothelial cells also secrete plasminogen activators and plasminogen activator-inhibitors; their synthesis and release is regulated by thrombin and growth factors. These profibrinolytic activities of the vascular endothelium contribute to the control of thrombosis by favoring the clearance of incipient thrombi and activated coagulation factors. The importance of these endothelial activities is underlined by the association of elevated plasma levels of lipoprotein (a), an enzymatically inactive plasminogen homologue that may competitively block endothelial cell fibrinolytic systems, with early cardiac and cerebral ischemia.[41]

In contrast to the activities of normal endothelium, endothelium that is damaged, ischemic, or exposed to inflammatory cytokines loses many of its thromboresistant properties. The production of thrombomodulin, EDRF, and prostacyclin are suppressed,[91,92] increased amounts of plasminogen activator inhibitor are produced, and the endothelium supports the binding and activation of plasma procoagulant factors.[9,75,92] The altered endothelium also becomes adhe-

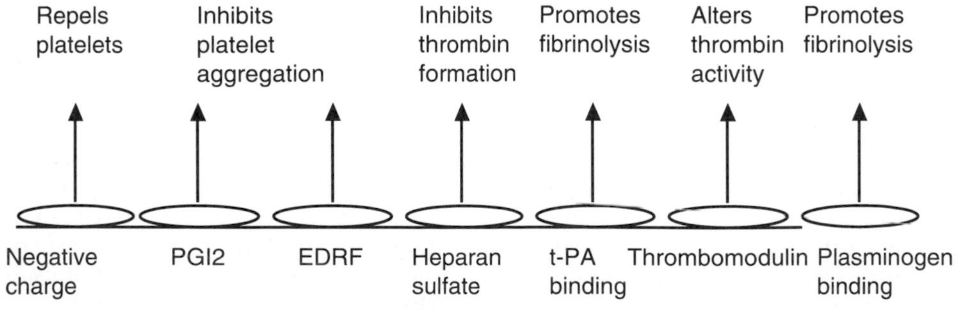


**Fig. 37-1.** Functions of normal vascular endothelium that contribute to nonthrombogenicity: these include effects on platelets, blood coagulation, and fibrinolysis.

sive for leukocytes, developing specific adhesion receptors for these cells.[35,75] Curiously, one product made by ischemic endothelium, the vasoconstrictor peptide endothelin, does not appear to affect the function of human platelets.[68] All of these events produce alterations in endothelial cell function, potentiate local thrombin production, decrease local fibrinolysis, and favor thrombosis. In turn, thrombin—the terminal enzyme in the coagulation cascade—is itself a potent activator of platelets, and activated platelets further catalyze coagulation.

Receptors for coagulation factors appear on intact endothelial cells when the latter are exposed to tumor necrosis factor (TNF), endotoxin, or interleukin-1 (IL-1) as well as to thrombin.[91,92] These cells also develop the capacity to produce and express IL-1.[4] The same inflammatory stimuli induce the production of tissue factor, the cofactor for the extrinsic pathway of coagulation, on the endothelial surface.[19] Endothelial cells that are so stimulated generate fibrin at the endothelial surface but still resist platelet aggregation.[105] However, the subendothelial matrix produced by cells subjected to such stimulation attracts platelet aggregation and furthers fibrinopeptide generation, the latter process dependent upon tissue factor and factor VIIa.[105] Fibrin deposition was particularly pronounced at low shear rates, suggesting that turbulent flow or stasis would further enhance a thrombotic tendency at the luminal surface of activated endothelial cells.

## PARTICIPATION OF PLATELETS IN HEMOSTASIS AND THROMBOSIS

Blood platelets are anucleate fragments of megakaryocytes and, after their maturation in the bone marrow, enter the bloodstream, and circulate for 7 to 10 days. Circulating platelets are packed with vasoactive substances, yet are normally unreactive with one another, with other blood cells, or with the vascular endothelium as they traverse the bloodstream. Only when specifically activated do platelets adhere to surfaces, change shape from flat discs to spiny spheres and spread out, aggregate into clumps that directly occlude small wounds, release their vasoactive contents, and catalyze on their activated plasma membranes the enzymatic cascade of coagulation.

The major signal for platelet activation is disruption of the continuity of the endothelial surface with exposure of subendothelial components. However, more subtle damage to the endothelium can also initiate platelet activation. The common causes for endothelial damage are direct injury (e.g., wounds), disturbed blood flow, or inflammation; but contact of platelets with a foreign surface, as in extracorporeal circulation or prosthetic vascular grafts, can also lead to platelet activation. While the endothelial lining of blood vessels is normally nonthrombogenic (as detailed above), its collagen- and fibronectin-rich substratum contains numerous substances that support rapid platelet activation. The process of platelet activation following contact with a stimulus contains a number of sequential steps that are sensitive to different pharmacologic interventions. These steps include adhesion, spreading, aggregation, the release reaction, and clot retraction.

Platelets respond to a variety of physiologic and pathologic stimuli, including mechanical stimuli, that may interact to augment platelet responsiveness. Some of these stimuli are released by the platelets themselves. Physiologic stimuli for platelet activation include ADP, epinephrine, serotonin, collagen, vasopressin, and thrombin. Pathologic stimuli include vascular turbulence, hypotonicity, foreign surfaces, tumor cells, viruses, and bacteria. Weak stimuli, for example, serotonin or epinephrine, or low concentrations of strong stimuli, for example, collagen or thrombin, cause reversible platelet aggregation that must trigger the release of endogenous platelet agonists, such as ADP or thromboxane $A_2$ ($TXA_2$), in order to lead to irreversible aggregation and the release of granule contents. Strong stimuli directly induce aggregation (and usually release) without the mediation of platelet-derived agonists. Thus, combinations of stimuli, which probably occur often under physiologic conditions, have greater activation effects than do single stimuli.

### Adhesion

Adhesion is the first major step in the sequence of platelet activation. Platelets adhere rapidly via specific membrane receptors to subendothelial collagen or fibronectin that is exposed to the blood after endothelial damage. The major membrane receptors involved in platelet activation are glycoproteins (GP) that belong to the integrin or selectin superfamilies of adhesion receptors present on the surface membranes of many different types of cells besides platelets, including leukocytes and endothelial cells.[14] These integrins mediate many of the interactions between different cell types and between cells and the extracellular matrix and thereby link the processes of hemostasis, inflammation, and immune recognition.[70]

Platelet integrins that are important in hemostasis and thrombosis include GPIa, a collagen receptor; GP1b, a receptor for von Willebrand factor; the GPIIb-IIIa complex, a major receptor for fibrinogen, fibronectin, and von Willebrand factor; and GPIV, a receptor for thrombospondin, a glycoprotein crucial for irreversible platelet aggregation. Many of the adhesive glycoproteins that bind these receptors share a small peptide sequence, RGD: arginine (R), glycine (G), and aspartic acid (D) that plays a critical role in cell-cell adhesion.[70,74] These receptors are functionally present on resting platelets except for GPIIb-IIIa, which is made available by stimuli for aggregation and therefore assembles upon platelet activation.[16,83] This fact is central to the use of certain new therapeutic approaches to antiplatelet therapy that utilize the strategy of blocking or preventing function of GPIIb-IIIa (see below).

The importance of these receptors in normal hemostasis is exemplified by the bleeding disorders that occur in their absence, abnormal structure, or blockade. For example, congenital absence of GPIb produces the Bernard-Soulier syndrome in which platelets cannot adhere to sites of vascular injury, and severe bleeding ensues. Similarly, the lack or abnormality of either of the GPIIb or GPIIIa, which normally function in a complex, leads to the severe hemorrhagic disorder thrombasthenia, in which platelets fail to adhere or aggregate. Efficient surface expression of both GPIIb and GPIIIa at the same time appears essential for normal platelet function.[69]

Normally adherent platelets rapidly form pseudopods, spread out in a flat monolayer over the damaged vascular surface, and, depending on the intensity of the inciting stimulus, begin to recruit other platelets into aggregates by releasing vasoactive and platelet-stimulatory substances. These substances are either stored preformed in platelet granules or are synthesized at the moment of activation. A key hemostatic component for normal platelet adhesion is the macromolecule von Willebrand factor, which not only circulates in the blood, but is secreted by endothelial cells into the subendothelial extracellular matrix, and is released by platelets from their alpha granules. Inherited lack of von Willebrand factor leads to a very common hemorrhagic disorder, von Willebrand's disease, characterized by a long bleeding time, bruising, and mucosal hemorrhage. This condition affects both sexes equally. In contrast, stress and inflammation can enhance blood levels of von Willebrand factor.

The entire process of platelet activation, including recruitment of platelets into aggregates and the release of their contents sufficient to stop bleeding in injured microvessels, is measured as the *bleeding time* and is normally less than 6 to 7 minutes. This process constitutes *primary hemostasis.* If the activation or release process is impaired or defected, as in the congenital disease noted above, or after administration of drugs such as aspirin or ticlopidine, the bleeding time is much prolonged, reflecting the impaired hemostasis. Conversely, a short bleeding time, although difficult to quantitate precisely, reflects enhanced platelet activation and can be associated with a thrombotic tendency.

## Platelet Aggregation

Platelet aggregation is the key phase of platelet activation. In this process, clumps of platelets form as "white thrombi" and halt bleeding from injured microvessels. Platelet aggregation takes place via three different physiologic pathways that are separately controlled and differently responsive to antiplatelet drugs. The first pathway involves an initial activation of platelets by stimuli that cause the release of ADP from platelet dense granules and induce the generation of $TXA_2$ (Fig. 37-2); both ADP and $TXA_2$ markedly enhance the aggregation process and the recruitment of nearby unactivated platelets. This pathway of activation depends upon the normal release of platelet-derived vasoactive substances and upon normal activity of the cyclooxygenase enzyme system and is blocked by aspirin and related drugs. In general, platelet agonist interaction with the surface membrane is transduced to activate phospholipase C, which cleaves phosphatidylinositol, liberating inosine triphosphate (IP3), which releases ionic calcium from storage in the dense tubular system, and diacylglycerol, which activates protein kinase C and initiates phosphorylation of platelet proteins. The released calcium activates phospholipase A, which releases arachidonic acid from its stored esterified form and permits its oxygenation into eicosanoid metabolites.[64] This pathway is also opposed by stimulators of adenylate cyclase, since raised cyclic adenosine monophosphate (cAMP) inhibits calcium release within platelets, and inhibits both aggregation and secretion.

The second pathway of platelet aggregation depends upon ADP, that can derive from extraplatelet sources (such as red cells), which aggregates platelets directly without requiring release or thromboxane generation. This pathway thus operates in the presence of aspirin.

The third pathway is initiated by thrombin via direct stimulation of phospholipases A and C and produces irreversible aggregation and release independent of arachidonic acid metabolism and thus is unaffected by aspirin. Moreover, the phosphorylcholine derivative, platelet-activating factor (PAF), that is produced by leukocytes or disturbed endothelial cells can directly activate platelets also by an aspirin-insensitive mechanism. The existence of these separate pathways for platelet aggregation can be regarded as a fail-safe mechanism against hemorrhage.

In practical terms, these multiple pathways of aggregation mean that drugs that inhibit only one pathway—for example, aspirin—can be expected to inhibit platelet activation only in situations where the thromboxane-related pathway is important. Natural mechanisms that limit platelet aggregation include plasma ADPases that break down ADP and prostacyclin (prostaglandin $I_2$ [$PGI_2$]), produced by endothelium and by blood monocytes, which stimulates adenylate cyclase and raises cAMP levels in platelets.[32,63] Increase in cyclic guanosine monophosphate (cGMP), which occurs in response to aggregating agents, has recently been shown also to be involved in inhibiting platelet aggregation. A soluble guanylate cyclase in platelets is stimulated by production of nitric oxide (NO) from L-arginine, in a manner similar

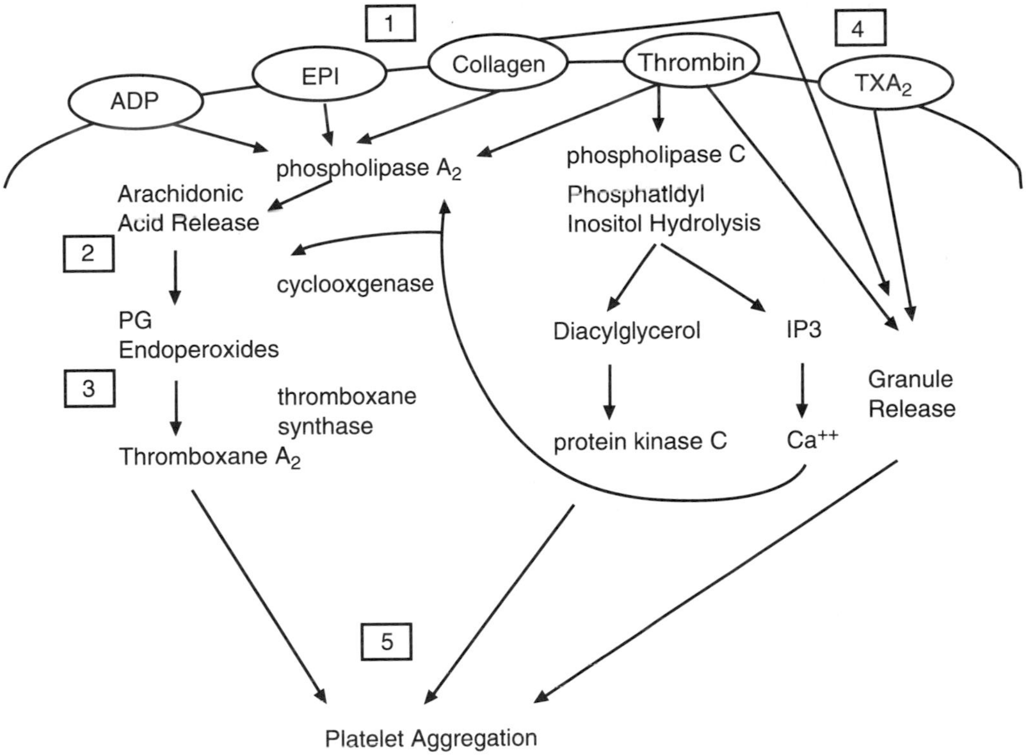


**Fig. 37-2.** Pathways leading to platelet aggregation. Stimulation of specific receptors on platelet surface activate the arachidonic acid pathway, phosphatidyl inositol hydrolysis, or granule release singly or in combination. The products synthesized or released further augment activation. Not shown here is the activation of the glycoprotein (GP) IIb-IIIa receptor on the platelet surface by epinephrine, collagen, thrombin, or thromboxane (TX) $A_2$. Inhibition of platelet activation results from blocking expression of GPIIb-IIIa receptors (*1*); arachidonic acid conversion by cyclo-oxygenase (*2*); $TXA_2$ production (*3*); $TXA_2$ receptor function (*4*); or by raising cAMP (*5*).

to the production of EDRF in endothelium or leukocytes, with a subsequent rise in intraplatelet cGMP and inhibition of aggregation.[76] In vitro, L-arginine itself has been shown to inhibit platelet aggregation, while inhibitors of NO synthase potentiated the effects of L-arginine, suggesting that the mechanisms of inhibition occurs via NO synthesis and consequent stimulation of guanylate cyclase. It is known that $PGI_2$ and NO synergistically block platelet aggregation. The possibility therefore should be considered that altering dietary L-arginine could affect platelet aggregability.[76]

At the present time, the only agents that inhibit all three pathways of platelet activation are those that block expression of the key membrane receptor GPIIb-IIIa on the platelet surface.[17] Experimental thrombosis systems have shown that antibodies to GPIIb-IIIa have powerful antithrombotic effects in the short term by inducing a temporary thrombasthenic state. Other means of blocking GPIIb-IIIa include synthetic peptides containing the arginine-glycine-aspartic acid sequence, or the gamma-chain carboxyl terminal sequence of fibrinogen.[18,34,38,74] All of these block GPIIb-IIIa receptor function, prevent the binding of fibrinogen to platelets, and thus inhibit platelet aggregation. While such therapeutic approaches may have important future clinical implications for situations of acute thrombotic risk, at present they are not feasible for chronic treatment because, in a sense, they are too efficacious.

Platelet aggregation appears to be enhanced in numerous situations where an acute cardiovascular event has occurred, for example, shortly after a stroke, after myocardial infarction, and in unstable angina (but not in chronic stable angina).[30] Many factors appear to enhance platelet aggregability, including stress, elevated plasma lipids and free fatty acids, and smoking. It is known that catecholamines, although weak direct platelet agonists, by augmenting platelet aggregability can oppose the effect of natural antiplatelet agents such as prostacyclin[68] and can overcome some effects of aspirin. These same clinical settings are associated with increases in plasma fibrinogen and factor VIII, both of which are important in platelet activation. Increased plasma fibrinogen has been noted to be an independent risk factor for stroke, perhaps in part through effects on platelet aggregation.

### Platelet Release Reaction

The platelet release reaction usually accompanies and enhances platelet aggregation and its consequences. Platelets contain several distinct types of granules rich in substances that participate in the processes of blood coagulation and wound repair. These include coagulation factors, cellular adhesion molecules, calcium, vasoactive amines, growth factors, and nucleotides. The granules are functionally distinguished both by contents and by ease of release and are classified as dense granules, alpha granules, lysosomes, and peroxisomes. The dense granules, which release their contents after platelet exposure to weaker stimuli, contain ADP, serotonin, and calcium. The alpha granules, which require stronger stimulation for release, contain fibrinogen, fibronectin, von Willebrand factor, thrombospondin, coagulation factor V, platelet-derived growth factor (PDGF), epidermal growth factor (EGF), insulin-like growth factor (IGF), and transforming growth factor beta (TGF-$\beta$) the antiplatelet peptide platelet factor 4, and many other substances. Lysosomes contain proteases, and peroxisomes, catalase. These substances are released within seconds to a few minutes after platelet activation, depending upon the stimulus.

Additional vasoactive substances produced by platelets are not stored in granules but are synthesized and immediately released during platelet activation. Most of these substances are oxygenated metabolites of arachidonic acid. They include $TXA_2$, a potent platelet agonist and vasoconstrictor that is a major platelet product of arachidonic acid oxygenation by the cyclooxygenase pathway. Specific receptors for $TXA_2$ are present on platelets and many other cell types, such as those in the vascular wall. These receptors also bind prostaglandin endoperoxides. Platelets also release 12-hydroxyeicosatetraenoic acid (12-HETE), an inflammatory mediator, produced from arachidonic acid by the lipoxygenase pathway. 12-HETE can be further converted to other bioactive products by neutrophils. Arachidonic acid itself or prostaglandin endoperoxides is also released by activated platelets and can be transformed by nearly endothelial cells or leukocytes into other vasoactive substances, such as $PGI_2$. Platelets can also release cholesterol that may be incorporated into the atherosclerotic plaque.

The release of granule contents by platelets responding to strong activation stimuli, in particular, collagen, $TXA_2$ or thrombin, leads to the formation of the primary hemostatic plug and at the same time promotes efficient catalysis of blood coagulation at the surface of activated platelets. By providing a specific site and specific lipid cofactors for the assembly of the prothrombin complex of procoagulants, the activated platelet membrane enhances the rate of thrombin generation 200,000-fold. Platelets have specific receptors for factors Xa and V, and release factor V from their granules during aggregation. Since thrombin itself is a strong stimulus for platelet activation, the release reaction and production of vasoactive eicosanoids such as $TXA_2$, initial formation of thrombin at the site of injury further enhances platelet activation in addition to enhancing coagulation.

Several substances released by platelets are directly chemotactic to polymorphonuclear leukocytes (e.g., 12-HETE, the antiheparin peptide, platelet factor 4, and PDGF), while platelet cathepsins can cleave the complement protein C5 to release chemotactic fragment C5a and can potentiate C3a formation. Thus several pathways link platelet activation with the initiation of inflammatory responses. Indeed, hemostasis/thrombosis and inflammation are physiologically intertwined processes, with activation of either potentiating the activity of the other. In this regard, the products of arachidonic acid metabolism have strong proinflammatory effects on vascular permeability and neutrophil activation.

Adhesive proteins released by platelets, such as von Willebrand factor, crucial for normal primary hemostasis in high-flow systems; thrombospondin, important in stabilizing platelet aggregates, and fibronectin all potentiate the formation and stabilization of the primary hemostatic plug and the interaction of blood cells with the injured vessel wall. Clot retraction, the process of consolidating the permanent fibrin clot that follows the platelet plug, is also dependent upon platelet function and requires the contraction of a specific platelet actomyosin.

Growth factors for fibroblasts, smooth muscle cells, and other cell types are abundant in platelet alpha granules and are released during platelet aggregation, and sometimes upon platelet adhesion alone. These factors, which include PDGF, EGF, and TGF-$\beta$, are chemotactic factors for leukocytes as well as important initiators and stimuli for cell division in the process of wound healing. PDGF has recently also been found to be a vasoconstrictor.[3] The growth factors released by platelets are very stable polypeptides that adhere well to the vascular substratum. It is clear that these factors, when inappropriately released, promote atherogenesis. Therefore, antiplatelet therapy, which diminishes the release of platelet granule contents, has potential antiatherosclerotic value.

## ROLE OF PLATELETS IN CARDIOVASCULAR DISEASE

Thrombosis is an important component of many types of cardiovascular disorder, particularly those associated with atherosclerosis. The normal participation of platelets in the hemostatic process after vascular injury is considered to be exaggerated or enhanced in patients with atherosclerosis and certain other thrombotic processes, such as collagen vascular disease. Since platelet activation is promoted by abnormal vascular surfaces such as are commonly found in atherosclerotic arteries, the interaction between normally functioning platelets and an abnormal surface may suffice to potentiate thrombosis. Thus platelet function and survival often appear normal in persons with cardiovascular disease. In some situations, evidence for enhanced platelet function reflecting inflammation, lipid abnormalities, or turbulent blood flow may enhance platelet activation on relatively normal vascular surfaces. It is clear that enhanced platelet aggregability or turnover is not required for platelets to contribute to thrombosis.

In situations where platelet destruction is enhanced, compensatory increase in megakaryocyte size and DNA content may result in the release of platelets that are more hemostatically active than usual, which may augment the process of atheroma formation.[54] It is known that the concentration of platelet-derived mitogens (e.g., PDGF) in blood is elevated in young patients with coronary atherosclerosis or hypercholesterolemia.[67] It is likely that these mitogens contribute to enhancement of atherosclerosis.

There is a circadian rhythm of acute myocardial infarction and of sudden cardiac death that is documented as being the highest in the morning, shortly after arising.[66] Investigations of the mechanism indicate that platelet aggregability is highest at this time, concomitant with a rise in plasma catecholamine levels and free fatty acids.[94] Both types of substances are known to potentiate platelet aggregation. Recently, a similar matinal pattern in the incidence of acute stroke has been described.[60] Platelet aggregation patterns have not yet been verified for stroke-prone patients, but earlier studies have suggested that circulating platelet aggregates are increased in the first days following an episode of acute cerebral ischemia.

## THE ROLE OF PLATELETS IN FIBRINOLYSIS

Elucidation of the involvement of platelets in the process of fibrinolysis, or clot resolution, has been greatly aided by the clinical interest in thrombolytic therapy by streptokinase and tissue plasminogen activators. Platelets participate both in profibrinolytic and antifibrinolytic activities. First, platelets can bind plasminogen as well as tissue and urokinase-type plasminogen activators[62] by mechanisms involving the glycoprotein complex GPIIb-IIIa. Activated platelets express surface thrombospondin (derived from release of alpha-granule thrombospondin), which binds plasminogen[85] and enhances its activation. Therefore platelets act to localize plasminogen in a fashion parallel to their localization of procoagulants. Platelet-bound plasminogen is more readily activated by tissue plasminogen activator and by streptokinase,[93] suggesting that platelets can enhance local fibrinolysis.

At the same time, platelets contain and secrete two fibrinolytic antagonists: plasminogen activator inhibitor-1 (PAI-1) and $\alpha_2$-antiplasmin.[55,73] They also release factor XIII, fibrin-stabilizing factor, that cross-links fibrin to enhance its stability. The net effect of these different activities seems to be that platelet-rich thrombi resist thrombolysis, and that platelets are activated during clinical thrombolysis,[29,31,52] even though plasmin itself can both activate and depress platelet function, depending upon concentration.[81] Clinical complications of fibrinolytic therapy include both hemorrhage and reocclusion, probably reflecting different types of effects both on platelet function and on the vessel wall. While aspirin has been used in combination with fibrinolytic agents to decrease platelet activation, it may only be of limited efficacy, since it blocks only one of the several pathways of platelet activation and is not inhibitory to thrombin-mediated platelet aggregation. Recently, the combination of other antiplatelet agents with thrombolytic therapy has suggested improved outcome, that is, decreased reocclusion rates without undue hemorrhage. Agents used in this combined therapy include monoclonal antibodies against GPIIb-IIIa,[38] thromboxane synthase inhibitors,[61] or prostacyclin analogues,[51] all agents with profound effects upon platelet function. Since thrombolysis is under study for treatment of acute stroke, these combined modality approaches are of great interest, especially if hemorrhagic side effects are minimized, as early results suggest.

## PHARMACOLOGIC BASES FOR THE USE OF PLATELET INHIBITORY DRUGS IN PREVENTION OF CEREBRAL ISCHEMIA

Several reviews comparing the efficacy of drugs that inhibit platelet function in different types of vascular disease, including myocardial infarction, unstable and chronic angina pectoris, peripheral vascular disease, cardiovascular surgery, and vascular grafting, as well as in cerebrovascular disease, have been recently updated and can be consulted for evaluation of particular drug regimens in particular settings.[2,23,39,44,48,72,78,90] This section will concentrate on the pharmacologic rationale for and applicability of such drugs in cerebrovascular disease (Table 37-1).

### Aspirin

By 1968 it was established that aspirin could prolong the bleeding time and that this effect involved a depression of platelet aggregation;[26,100,101] in 1971 these effects were linked to aspirin's capacity irrevers-

**TABLE 37-1. Mechanisms of Action of Antiplatelet Drugs**

| Action | Effects on Platelets | Type of Drug |
|---|---|---|
| Inhibition of surface membrane receptor | Prevent ADP and fibrinogen binding; blocks adhesion and aggregation | Ticlopidine<br>Penicillins[a]<br>Monoclonal antibodies to GPIIb-IIIa[b]<br>Dextrans |
| | Prevent thrombin binding | Antithrombin peptides |
| Alteration of arachidonic acid metabolism | Blocks PG endoperoxide and $TXA_2$ synthesis; inhibits platelet aggregation and secretion; prevents $TXA_2$-induced vasoconstriction | Aspirin<br>NSAIDs<br>Sulfinpyrazone |
| | Inhibit $TXA_2$ synthesis alone; effects as above; permits endoperoxide conversion to $PGI_2$ by endothelium | $TXA_2$ synthase blockers[b] |
| | Generate $TXA_3$; decrease $TXA_2$ synthesis, enhance $PGI_2$ | Fish oils (omega-3 fatty acids)[b] |
| Inhibition of $TXA_2$ receptors | Prevent $TXA_2$ and PG endoperoxide binding; block aggregation, release, and vasoconstriction | $TXA_2$ receptor antagonists[b] |
| Increase cAMP | Stimulate adenylate cyclase to increase cAMP; block platelet aggregation and secretion | Prostacyclin<br>$PGE_1$, $PGD_2$[b] |
| | Maintain raised cAMP; same effects | Phosphodiesterase inhibitors<br>Dipyridamole<br>Methylxanthines[a] |
| Increase cGMP | Stimulate platelet NO synthesis; block aggregation | L-Arginine[a] |
| | Provide source of NO; block aggregation | Nitrates[a]<br>Nitroprusside[a] |
| Inhibit $CA^{2+}$ channels | Decrease aggregation and release | $Ca^{2+}$ channel blockers[a]<br>Local anesthetics[a]<br>Beta blockers[a] |
| Inhibit thrombin generation or action | Inhibit aggregation and release; block thrombus formation | Low molecular weight heparin[b]<br>Antithrombin peptides[b] |

*Abbreviations:* ADP, adenosine diphosphate; cAMP, cyclic adenosine monophosphate; GP, glycoprotein; NO, nitric oxide; PG, prostaglandin; $TXA_2$, thromboxane $A_2$; NSAIDs, nonsteroidal anti-inflammatory drugs.
[a] Limited or adjunct therapeutic effects.
[b] Under development for clinical usage; effective in experimental thrombosis systems.

ibly to inhibit the platelet enzyme cyclo-oxygenase, thereby preventing the formation of proaggregatory $TXA_2$.[86,96] Cyclo-oxygenase, or prostaglandin endoperoxide synthase, is the rate-limiting enzyme in the conversion of the unsaturated fatty acid arachidonic acid into oxygenated eicosanoid metabolites, prostaglandin endoperoxides, which are then further converted into prostaglandins and thromboxanes. $TXA_2$, the major eicosanoid produced by blood platelets, is a strong stimulus for platelet aggregation and one of the most potent vasoconstrictor substances known. $TXA_2$ is, however, very unstable under physiologic conditions of temperature and pH, and is converted to inactive $TXB_2$ within seconds. Aspirin irreversibly acetylates the active site of cyclo-oxygenase, rendering the enzyme incapable of catalyzing the attachment of molecular oxygen to this fatty acid to form prostaglandin endoperoxides.[79] All subsequent conversions of endoperoxides to eicosanoid products are thus blocked. Since platelets do not carry out protein synthesis, they cannot make new cyclo-oxygenase during their lifespan in the circulation and therefore, once treated with aspirin, can no longer generate $TXA_2$. Without production of $TXA_2$, one major pathway of platelet activation is markedly impaired, and platelet aggregation and release induced by numerous stimuli are decreased.

Other cell types, such as vascular endothelium, kidney, lung, or monocytes, rapidly resynthesize cyclo-oxygenase, so that the inhibitory effect of aspirin on eicosanoid synthesis in these tissues is much briefer, in contrast to the prolonged inhibitory effect on platelet cyclo-oxygenase. Therefore intermittent dosage with aspirin can achieve a "selective" inhibition of platelet function without impairing the production of vasoprotective prostaglandins such as prostacyclin because resynthesis of cyclo-oxygenase in the vessel wall can maintain prostacyclin production.[50] Aspirin has little direct effect upon the lipoxygenase pathway of arachidonic acid metabolism; conflicting reports suggest that it may limit or enhance production of 12-HETE, the major lipoxygenase product of platelets, depending upon the conditions employed. Although the beneficial effects of aspirin as an antithrombotic agent have been demonstrated more frequently in men than in women, there is no evidence for a sex-related difference in antiplatelet effect.

Aspirin is rapidly absorbed after oral administration and reaches a peak plasma level within 30 minutes. It is rapidly deacetylated in the liver, releasing salicylate, which has very little antiplatelet effect. Following a single oral dose of aspirin, blood levels are negligible within about 3 hours. However, because platelet cyclo-oxygenase is inactivated by aspirin within minutes, even a brief exposure of platelets to acetylsalicylate suffices to produce maximal aspirin effects.[10] If administered at very low doses, such as 1 mg/h orally, aspirin is virtually completely deacetylated on first pass through the liver, so that a blood level of acetylsalicylate is only achieved in the portal circulation, while there is no detectable aspirin in the peripheral blood. Since platelets traverse the portal circulation, complete inactivation of platelet cyclo-oxygenase can be achieved within a few hours of such low-dose therapy without any effect of aspirin on peripheral tissues.[78] Thus, very low-dose, slow-release aspirin can have good antiplatelet potency. In clinical studies it has been recognized that, to maintain antiplatelet effects in vivo, only small daily doses of aspirin (20 to 325 mg/day) were required,[56,71] since the platelet inhibition was cumulative over time both in normal[71] and atherosclerotic[104] subjects. Higher or more frequent doses of aspirin may have negative effects on antithrombotic mechanisms in blood vessels.[103] High doses of aspirin have significant noxious side effects,[48] especially gastrointestinal tract irritation and bleeding. However, inhibition of $TXA_2$ formation, was observed to be significantly less impaired (70 percent) after 20 to 40 mg/day aspirin, compared to 325 mg/day.[77] Fitzgerald has shown that, unless 95 percent or greater inhibition of $TXA_2$ formation is achieved, clinically significant amounts of $TXA_2$ continue to be produced and maximal inhibition of platelet aggregation is not achieved.[77] Aspirin prolongs the bleeding time when used in doses of 325 mg/day or greater, but only to about twice the baseline level. Large doses of aspirin do not further prolong the bleeding time, indeed may shorten it slightly. Gastric irritation and bleeding caused by aspirin do not correlate well with bleeding time prolongation.

In contrast to its rapid and profound effects on platelet aggregation, aspirin does not alter platelet adhesion to vascular surfaces, does not prolong abnormally short platelet survival, fails to decrease secretion of vascular growth factors from platelets (especially when secretion is produced by thrombin), and fails to inhibit the release of PDGF-like factors from monocytes or damaged endothelium. Consequently, aspirin has antithrombotic effects but does not prevent the progression of atherosclerosis. Moreover, because the action of thrombin on platelets is unaffected by aspirin, the antiplatelet effect of aspirin is limited to inhibition of only one of the three possible means of activating platelets. This fact, which itself restricts the bleeding tendency produced by aspirin, probably also accounts for the limited beneficial antithrombotic effects of aspirin in clinical practice.

Regardless of the dose of aspirin administered, platelet aggregation and formation of $TXA_2$ in blood return to predosing levels within 7 to 10 days of stopping the drug, following a linear recovery pattern after a 1- to 2-day initial lag. This lag probably represents megakaryocyte acetylation by aspirin.

Aspirin was approved by the FDA in 1980 for prevention of transient ischemic attacks (TIAs) and stroke and in 1985 for the prevention of unstable angina and secondary prevention of myocardial infarction. In numerous controlled clinical trials, the overall decrease in incidence of these vascular endpoints with aspirin therapy has ranged from about 20 percent for stroke or secondary myocardial infarction to 40 to 50 percent for progression of unstable angina to acute myocardial infarction or death.[2,78] In addition, aspirin treatment has decreased the incidence of pulmonary embolism after hip surgery and the rate of coronary artery reocclusion following coronary artery bypass graft surgery. Curiously, although some of the first positive clinical trials with aspirin were those showing that aspirin therapy prevented TIA and stroke in patients who had previously had cerebral ischemia,[8,12,13,25,28] the recently concluded Physicians' Health Study of aspirin as primary prevention of myocardial infarction in healthy males suggested no reduction in stroke risk in this group, and indeed a slight increase in hemorrhagic strokes was observed.[88,89] It must be remembered that this primary prevention study involved healthy male subjects with no evidence of cerebrovascular disease, whereas the many studies using aspirin for the secondary prevention of cerebral ischemia have dealt with a patient population at high risk of stroke, a population in which enhanced platelet activation has been frequently documented.

In addition to its effects upon platelet activation, aspirin has been reported to affect fibrinolysis;[65] large amounts can produce hypoprothrombinemia. At high concentrations, such as those used to treat acute rheumatic fever, aspirin can inhibit the synthesis of vitamin K-dependent coagulation factors; this is most likely an effect of salicylate and the effect is reversed by vitamin K. There is no significant depression of vitamin K-dependent clotting factors by usual antiplatelet doses of aspirin.

The mechanisms by which aspirin affects fibrinolysis are not well elucidated, and conflicting effects have been reported. Chronic aspirin administration is associated with shortening of the plasma clot lysis time by 40 to 50 percent and by enhancement of thrombin-induced fibrin aggregation.[65] Aspirin acetylates fibrinogen in vitro to form ε-*N*-acetyllysine groups.[65] This process may impede factor XIII-induced fibrin cross-linking, permitting fibrinolysis to occur more easily. The clinical importance of this effect of aspirin has not yet been established. Independent studies have suggested that large, but not small, doses of aspirin may decrease fibrinolysis in vivo by inhibiting the release of tissue plasminogen activator from veins following venous occlusion.[5,58] Release of plasminogen activator inhibitor, which is also induced by venous occlusion, was unchanged after aspirin treatment.

## Other Nonsteroidal Anti-inflammatory Drugs

Aspirin represents one member of a class of nonsteroidal anti-inflammatory drugs (NSAID) that act to inhibit eicosanoid synthesis by blocking cyclo-oxygenase; it is the only member of this class that is a truly irreversible inhibitor rather than a competitive inhibitor. Other NSAIDs such as indomethacin or ibuprofen are on a molar basis more potent inhibitors of cyclo-oxygenase but only during the time a critical blood level of drug is maintained. Therefore antiplatelet effects of indomethacin or ibuprofen require high steady-state blood levels of drug and have a much shorter duration than aspirin because they lack the ability to permanently inactivate platelet cyclo-oxygenase. This difference in duration of action requires multiple daily doses and thus makes compliance a clinical problem for the use of nonaspirin NSAIDs as antiplatelet therapy. However, in certain settings, such as before surgical procedures, where a brief duration of action is desirable, these drugs (especially ibuprofen) may be useful because of their short-term activity.

## Sulfinpyrazone

Sulfinpyrazone is a uricosuric agent related to phenylbutazone but possessing little anti-inflammatory activity. It is a weak competitive inhibitor of cyclo-oxygenase, has slow onset of action, and must be administered in multiple daily doses for effect. The active moiety is a sulfide metabolite. Sulfinpyrazone has been shown to decrease platelet adhesion to subendothelium or to artificial surfaces and to have endothelial protective activity,[49] possibly related to scavenging of oxygen-free radicals. It may prolong platelet survival in patients with shortened platelet survival times.[87] Although an early study suggested that sulfinpyrazone was useful to prevent sudden death in patients with myocardial ischemia, it has not been shown to decrease rates of vascular reocclusion in patients with unstable angina or stroke,[12,13,25] either alone or in combination with aspirin, and it is generally no longer used for antithrombotic purposes.

## Dipyridamole

Interest in the pyrimidopyrimidine derivative dipyridamole as an antiplatelet and antithrombotic agent has been based on several theoretical considerations. Dipyridamole has been used to prevent thrombosis in a number of experimental models (for a detailed review, see Fitzgerald[32]). The principal mechanisms suggested to underlie its antithrombotic effects are inhibition of phosphodiesterase, inhibition of cellular uptake of adenosine, interaction with aspirin, vasodilatation, and platelet survival.

Elevation of intracellular cAMP levels prevents platelet activation;[7,63] for example, prostacyclin, by stimulating adenylate cyclase in platelets, raises cAMP and blocks intracellular calcium release, platelet aggregation, and the release reaction. Therefore prevention of breakdown of cAMP should enhance inhibition of platelet activation. Dipyridamole can be shown to inhibit cAMP phosphodiesterase in platelet homogenates, but does not itself raise cAMP levels in intact platelets. Platelets from subjects receiving oral dipyridamole do not show inhibition of platelet aggregation as do platelets from subjects treated with aspirin or prostacyclin. Moreover, the concentrations of dipyridamole required to maintain an elevated cAMP level, once the level has been raised by another mechanism, are much higher than those that can be achieved in vivo.[32] The possibility that dipyridamole would augment the effect of prostacyclin on inhibition of platelet activation has not been directly demonstrated. Neither is dipyridamole a stimulator of prostacyclin biosynthesis by the blood vessel wall, as tested by incubation of vascular tissue or cells with the drug, or by measuring urinary excretion of prostacyclin metabolites following dipyridamole administration. Therefore the attractive hypothesis that the phosphodiesterase blocking action of dipyridamole accounts for antiplatelet or antithrombotic activity has not been upheld by experimental evidence.

A second possible mechanism of action of dipyridamole is to block cellular uptake of adenosine, a metabolite of adenosine triphosphate (ATP) and ADP.[7] Circulating adenosine is a vasodilator and directly stimulates cellular adenylate cyclase, thereby acting as an inhibitor of platelet activation. Adenosine can be derived from released platelet ADP, endothelial cells, or red cells. Dipyridamole prevents the uptake of adenosine by vascular cells and its subsequent metabolism to inosine, so that in the presence of dipyridamole a higher concentration of adenosine can be maintained at the blood-vascular wall interface. In vitro studies suggest that under circumstances involving release of ADP, dipyridamole can block ADP-induced platelet aggregation and can potentiate the effects of adenosine. For example, dipyridamole might potentiate in vivo the antiplatelet effect of adenosine derived from erythrocyte leakage of ADP that is normally metabolized to adenosine by endothelial cells.

As a vasodilator, dipyridamole has mild antihypertensive effects. Indeed, its major noxious side effect is headache, which results from vasodilatation. It lacks any effect upon the bleeding time. This permits its usage without inducing additional hemorrhagic risk in combination with oral anticoagulants to prevent thromboembolism in patients with prosthetic cardiac valves who are not controlled by anticoagulants alone.

There is also evidence that dipyridamole can affect the pharmacokinetics of other antiplatelet agents such as aspirin.[32] It is known that the absorption of dipyridamole after oral ingestion is very variable among different subjects. No consistent patterns have been discerned. Some studies have suggested that dipyridamole can correct toward normal pathologically shortened platelet survival, possibly by preventing platelet activation and adhesion on abnormal vascular surfaces.[45,82] The results of several clinical studies comparing aspirin to the combination of aspirin and dipyridamole in preventing thrombosis have not shown that dipyridamole provides additional benefit. These studies include secondary prevention of stroke or myocardial infarction and arterial reocclusion following coronary bypass surgery.[1,72]

## Dextran

Intravenous dextran infusion inhibits platelet function and can prolong the bleeding time, probably by binding to the platelet membrane and preventing platelet-platelet interactions or platelet binding to von Willebrand factor.[99] Its primary use has been as prophylaxis against pulmonary embolism after surgery, such as hip replacement, where anticoagulation has been considered to be associated with an excess of wound hematoma formation. Dextran can cause anaphylactic reactions on repeated exposure.

## Ticlopidine

Ticlopidine (5-[*O*-chlorobenzyl]-4,5,6,7-tetrahydrothieno-[3,2-c]pyridine hydrochloride) is an antithrombotic drug unrelated to other known platelet inhibitors, although its mechanism of action has not yet been completely elucidated.[80] In vivo activity is delayed several days after starting oral dosage and is prolonged in duration after stopping the drug, suggesting that drug metabolites are important.[22] In addition, normal platelets incubated in plasma from subjects taking ticlopidine show altered function. These findings suggest that ticlopidine has good steady-state effects but cannot be used to induce rapid inhibition of platelet function. Ticlopidine inhibits ADP-dependent platelet activation and release, with variable effects on other types of platelet activation. Its effects are much more pronounced in vivo than in vitro, again reflecting presumed metabolite formation. It appears to decrease the binding of ADP and of fibrinogen to the platelet membrane but does not inhibit the cyclo-oxygenase pathway nor platelet thromboxane production. It has been suggested that ticlopidine induces a mild functional "thrombasthenic state."[22] Ticlopidine prolongs the bleeding time in vivo in a dose-dependent manner, having in this regard a much more profound effect than aspirin; its effect on bleeding time is additive to that of aspirin. Ticlopidine decreases platelet adhesion to artificial surfaces and tends to lengthen abnormally short platelet survival toward normal. It also decreases blood viscosity and enhances red cell deformability, suggesting a possible rheologic component of its clinical effects. In many different experimental thrombosis systems, ticlopidine has been shown to decrease thrombosis and improve outcome whether or not platelets are important in the pathogenesis of thrombosis.[80] Several large clinical studies of ticlopidine in the prevention of stroke have shown it to be an effective prophylactic agent not only in patients with previous transient cerebral ischemia but also in patients with a previous completed stroke.[36,46] Moreover, both sexes appeared to benefit. In one study, ticlopidine appeared to be slightly more effective than aspirin, to which it was compared.[36] Ticlopidine has also been reported to reduce neurologic deficit after subarachnoid hemorrhage without directly affecting vasospasm. A recent small study comparing the combination of low-dose ticlopidine and low-dose aspirin with either drug alone or placebo showed that the drug combination markedly inhibited platelet aggregation by ADP, arachidonate, and PAF and reduced plasma concentrations of platelet factor 4 and $\beta$-thromboglobulin released by platelets in vivo.[95] Similarly, only the drug combination lengthened platelet survival. Bleeding time was more prolonged by the combination than by either drug alone. These results suggested that a more potent antiplatelet effect, inhibiting multiple pathways of platelet activation, might be achieved by combining low doses of aspirin and ticlopidine. It remains to be tested whether this combination will have good therapeutic efficacy and diminished side effects.

At usual clinical doses for antiplatelet therapy (about 500 mg/day) ticlopidine has significant side effects that include diarrhea, rash, and marked neutropenia. In published studies of ticlopidine prophylaxis for cerebral ischemia, 50 percent of subjects discontinued treatment before the end of the study because of side effects, necessity for other treatment modalities, or cerebrovascular ischemic events.[36,46] Severe neutropenia is reported in about 1 percent of subjects, usually occurs during the first 3 months of therapy, and has been reversible upon stopping the drug. Careful monitoring of the blood count during early months of treatment is recommended. Because of the effect on bleeding time, hemorrhage may also occur, and patients must be cautioned to avoid taking nonsteroidal anti-inflammatory drugs during ticlopidine therapy because of possible further prolongation of bleeding time and enhanced hemorrhagic risk. Case reports have indicated that desmopressin may reverse bleeding time prolongation in emergent situations.

## Inhibitors of Thromboxane Synthesis and Blockade of Thromboxane Receptors

Imidazole analogues and other chemical species have been developed that specifically block the activity of the enzyme thromboxane synthase. These compounds are designed to achieve two interacting therapeutic goals: to prevent the synthesis of $TXA_2$ and to permit increased transformation of prostaglandin endoperoxides to $PGI_2$ by nearby vascular endothelium or leukocytes.[33] Experimental models have shown that these goals can be achieved, but clinical trials have been disappointing in that only transient blockade of thromboxane synthesis and prevention of progression of atherosclerosis have been achieved. Large-scale clinical trials of the efficacy of these compounds in this area have not yet been carried out.

It now appears that prostaglandin endoperoxides themselves may bind the same receptors as $TXA_2$ and therefore have thromboxanelike effects, that is, promotion of platelet aggregation. More recently, combinations of thromboxane synthase inhibitors and thromboxane receptor blockers have been developed, sometimes in the same molecule, which are undergoing early trials. For example, one of these combined molecules, R 68070, is reported to produce more than 90 percent inhibition of $TXA_2$ for 48 hours after a single dose to human subjects, to increase serum levels of $PGI_2$ metabolites, to reduce markedly platelet aggregation by several stimuli, and to prolong bleeding time without affecting coagulation or fibrinolysis.[21] In animal experiments this compound reduces experimental coronary thrombosis and reperfusion-induced arrhythmias. Whether such agents will be more efficacious than aspirin remains to be determined.

## Other Potential Antiplatelet Agents

Many drugs that are used to treat cardiovascular disease have weak antiplatelet effects, including diuretics, calcium channel blockers,[6] nitrates, and $\beta$-adrenergic blockers. Similarly, compounds with local anesthetic properties, such as chlorpromazine or lidocaine have mild antiaggregating effects. Drugs that inhibit epinephrine binding or are $\alpha$-adrenergic antagonists (e.g., phentolamine) also decrease platelet aggregation. Penicillin-type antibiotics in large doses also inhibit platelet function by competing for platelet surface receptors. None of these compounds directly suppresses platelet function at clinically useful doses, but they may enhance activity of the commonly used platelet antagonist drugs.

Antibodies to platelet integrins, such as antibodies to the GPIIb-IIIa complex, or peptides that compete with the key peptide sequence RGD on platelet integrins, can block platelet aggregation and produce a temporary thrombasthenic state.[18,38] As mentioned above, these compounds have been successfully applied to prevent thrombosis in experimental models, but no long-term studies have been undertaken. (See discussion above of platelets and fibrinolysis.) Finally, antithrombin peptides, which block the procoagulant and platelet agonist function of thrombin, have shown good antithrombotic potential in short-term experimental models of thrombosis and may eventually also find implementation for short-term inhibition of platelet aggregation and for reduction of ischemic events after coronary angioplasty or thrombolysis.[61] Iloprost and other synthetic analogues of prostacyclin are chemically more stable and therefore are potentially useful for short-term antithrombotic therapy.

## Fish Oils

Interest has been developed in the antiplatelet and antithrombotic activity of highly polyunsaturated fatty acids, usually derived from oils in cold-water fish that are rich in eiciosapentaenoic and docosahexaenoic acids.[57] These fatty acids compete with arachidonic acid for cyclo-oxygenase, and they form eicosanoids of the omega-3 series (the last double bond in the fatty acid chain is 3-carbons from the C-terminus) in place of omega-6 eicosanoids derived from arachidonic acid.[97,98] The product $PGI_3$ is similar to prostacyclin in antiaggregatory and vasodilatory properties, whereas $TXA_3$ is a very weak platelet agonist. Administration of these omega-3 fatty acids has been shown to decrease platelet aggregation, decrease $TXA_2$ production, prolong bleeding time, and decrease triglyceride levels in humans and to impede the development of atherosclerosis in a number of experimental models.[53,57] These substances also reduce inflammatory responses of leukocytes. The omega-3 fatty acids also can induce increased production of prostacyclin in human vascular tissue.[20] As inhibitors of platelet aggregation, omega-3 fatty acids are much weaker than aspirin, but they may be useful as adjuncts to antiplatelet therapy and may be important in the antithrombotic effects have been minimal in tests of a large variety of such agents.[27]

## Prostacyclin and Its Analogues

$PGI_2$ (prostacyclin) and $PGE_1$ are direct inhibitors of platelet aggregation by virtue of their stimulation of adenylate cyclase, leading to increased platelet cAMP. No oral preparations are available. Intravenous $PGI_2$ is a potent vasodilator at the concentrations needed to inhibit platelet aggregation and thus its use is limited by hypotension as well as by its instability under physiologic conditions. It has been successfully used to support hemodialysis in bleeding patients where heparin could not be given and as a substitute for heparin during cardiac surgery. A synthetic analogue, iloprost, has been used in prevention of thrombosis.[34,74] These peptides either can bind nascent thrombin on the platelet surface or can form complexes with thrombin that occupy and block thrombin receptors.[43] In contrast, heparin, which has potent activity against thrombin, has generally not been useful in preventing platelet-initiated thrombosis. Standard clinical heparin frequently has platelet-activating effects that may contribute to this lack of efficacy despite its capacity to prevent thrombin generation and inhibit thrombin action. Another possibility for the failure of heparin therapy in these settings is the inability of standard heparin to reach thrombin protected within platelet aggregates. Recently, low molecular weight heparin[11] or hirudin[47] have been shown to exert antithrombotic effects in platelet-dependent thrombosis systems, with less risk of hemorrhagic side effects.

## REFERENCES


1. American-Canadian Co-operative Study Group: Persantine aspirin trial in cerebral ischemia. II. Endpoint results. Stroke 14:5, 1985
2. Antiplatelet Trialists' Collaboration: Secondary prevention of vascular disease by prolonged antiplatelet treatment. Br Med J 296:320, 1988
3. Berk BC, Alexander RW, Brock TA et al: Vasoconstriction: a new activity for platelet-derived growth factor. Science 232:87, 1986
4. Bevilacqua MP, Pober JS, Majno GR et al: Interleukin-1 biosynthesis and cell surface expression of procoagulant activity in human vascular endothelial cells. J Exp Med 60:618, 1984
5. Bjornsson TD, Schneider DE, Berger H Jr: Aspirin acetylates fibrinogen and enhances fibrinolysis: fibrinolytic effect is independent of changes in plasminogen activator levels. J Pharm Exp Ther 250:154, 1989
6. Block LH, Emmons LR: A new perspective on the antiatherosclerotic activity of calcium-channel blockers. Eur J Clin Invest 20:236, 1990
7. Born GV, Mills DC: Potentiation of the inhibitory effect of adenosine on platelet aggregation by drugs that prevent its uptake. J Physiol 202:41, 1969
8. Bousser MG, Eschwege E, Haguenau M et al: "AICLA" controlled trial of aspirin and dipyridamole in the secondary prevention of atherothrombotic cerebral ischemia. Stroke 14:5, 1983
9. Brenner BM, Troy JL, Balterman BJ: Endothelium-dependent vascular responses: mediators and mechanisms. J Clin Invest 84:1373, 1989
10. Burch JW, Stanford N, Majerus PW: Inhibition of platelet prostaglandin synthetase by oral aspirin. J Clin Invest 61:314, 1978
11. Cadroy F, Harker LA, Hanson SR: Inhibition of platelet-dependent thrombosis by low molecular weight heparin (CY222): comparison with standard heparin. J Lab Clin Med 114:349, 1989
12. Canadian Cooperative Study Group: A randomized trial of aspirin and sulfinpyrazone in threatened stroke. N Engl J Med 299:53, 1978
13. Candelise L, Landi G, Perrone P et al: A randomized trial of aspirin and sulfinpyrazone in patients with TIA. Stroke 13:175, 1982
14. Cheresh DA, Berliner SA, Vicente V, Ruggeri ZM: Recognition of distinct adhesive sites on fibrinogen by related integrins on platelets and endothelial cells. Cell 58:945, 1989
15. Colburn P, Buonassisi V: Anti-clotting activity of endothelial cell cultures and heparan sulfate proteoglycans. Biochem Biophys Res Commun 15:220, 1982
16. Coller BS: Activation affects access to the platelet receptor for adhesive glycoproteins. J Cell Biol 103:451, 1986
17. Coller BS: Platelets and thrombolytic therapy. N Engl J Med 322:33, 1990
18. Coller BS, Scudder LE, Berger HJ, Iuliucci JD: Inhibition of human platelet function in vivo with a monoclonal antibody: with observations on the newly dead as experimental subjects. Ann Intern Med 109:635, 1988
19. Colucci M, Balconi G, Lorenzet R et al: Cultured human endothelial cells generate tissue factor in response to endotoxin. J Clin Invest 71:1893, 1983
20. DeCaterina R, Giannessi D, Mazzone A et al: Vascular prostacyclin is increased in patients taking fish oil n-3 polyunsaturated fatty acids prior to coronary bypass surgery. Circulation 82:428, 1990
21. De Clerck F, Beetens J, Van de Water A et al: R 68070: thromboxane A2 synthetase inhibition and thromboxane A2/prostaglandin endoperoxide receptor blockade combined in one molecule. II. Pharmacologic effects in vivo and ex vivo. Thromb Haemost 61:43, 1989
22. Di Minno G, Cerbone AM, Mattioli PL et al: Functionally thrombasthenic state in normal platelets following the administration of ticlopidine. J Clin Invest 75:328, 1985
23. Easton JD, Hart RG, Sherman DG, Kaste M: Diagnosis and management of ischemic stroke. I. Threatened stroke and its management. Curr Probl Cardiol 8:1, 1983
24. Esmon N, Owen W, Esmon C: Isolation of a membrane-bound cofactor for thrombin-catalyzed activation of protein C. J Biol Chem 257:859, 1982
25. ESPS Group: The European stroke prevention study (ESPS). Lancet 2:1351, 1987
26. Evans G, Packham MA, Nishizawa EE et al: The effect of acetylsalicylic acid on platelet function. J Exp Med 128:877, 1968
27. Fiddler GI, Lumley P: Preliminary clinical studies with thromboxane synthase inhibitors and thromboxane receptor blockers: a review. Circulation, suppl I. 81:I69, 1990
28. Fields WS, Lemak NA, Frankowski M et al: Controlled trial of aspirin in cerebral ischemia. I. Stroke 8:301, 1977
29. Fitzgerald DJ, Catella F, Roy L, Fitzgerald GA: Marked platelet activation in vivo after intravenous streptokinase in patients with acute myocardial infarction. Circulation 77:142, 1988

30. Fitzgerald DJ, Roy L, Catella F, Fitzgerald GA: Platelet activation in unstable coronary disease. N Engl J Med 315:983, 1986
31. Fitzgerald DJ, Wright F, Fitzgerald GA: Increased thromboxane biosynthesis during coronary thrombolysis: evidence that platelet activation and thromboxane A2 modulate the response to tissue-type plasminogen activator in vivo. Circ Res 65:83, 1989
32. Fitzgerald GA: Dipyridamole. N Engl J Med 316:1247, 1987
33. Fitzgerald GA, Reilly IA, and Pedersen AK: The biochemical pharmacology of thromboxane synthase inhibition in man. Circulation 72:1194, 1985
34. Gartner TK, Bennett JS: The tetrapeptide analogue of the cell attachment site of fibronectin inhibits platelet aggregation and fibrinogen binding to activated platelets. J Biol Chem 260:11891, 1985
35. Geng JG, Bevilacqua MP, Moore KL et al: Rapid neutrophil adhesion to activated endothelium mediated by GMP-140. Nature 343:757, 1990
36. Gent M, Easton JD, Hachinski VC et al: The Canadian-American Ticlopidine Study (CATS) in thromboembolic stroke. Lancet 1:1215, 1989
37. Genton E, Barnett JJ, Fields WS et al: Cerebral ischemia: the role of thrombosis and of antithrombotic therapy: study group on antithrombotic therapy. Stroke 8:150, 1977
38. Gold HK, Gimple L, Yasuda T et al: Phase I human trial of the potent antiplatelet agent 7E-F(ab')2, a monoclonal antibody to the GPIIb/IIIa receptor. Circulation, suppl II. 80:267, 1989
39. Grotta JC: Current medical and surgical therapy for cerebrovascular disease. N Engl J Med 317:1505, 1987
40. Gunning AJ, Pickering GW, Robb-Smith AH, Russell RR: Mural thrombosis of the internal carotid artery and subsequent embolization. Q J Med 33:155, 1964
41. Hajjar KA, Gavish D, Breslow JL, Nachman RL: Lipoprotein (a) modulation of endothelial cell surface fibrinolysis and its potential role in atherosclerosis. Nature 339:303, 1989
42. Hajjar KA, Nachman RL: Endothelial cell mediated conversion of glu-plasminogen to lys-plasminogen: further evidence for assembly of the fibrinolytic system on the endothelial cell surface. J Clin Invest 82:1769, 1988
43. Hanson SR, Harker LA: Interruption of acute platelet-dependent thrombosis by the synthetic antithrombin D-phenylalanyl-L-prolyl-L-arginyl chloromethyl ketone. Proc Natl Acad Sci USA 85:3184, 1988
44. Harker LA, Fuster V: Pharmacology of platelet inhibitors. J Am Coll Cardiol 8:21b, 1986
45. Harker LA, Slichter SJ: Platelet and fibrinogen consumption in man. N Engl J Med 287:999, 1972
46. Hass WK, Easton JD, Adams HP et al: A randomized trial comparing ticlopidine hydrochloride with aspirin for the prevention of stroke in high-risk patients. N Engl J Med 321:501, 1989
47. Heras M, Chesebro JH, Penny WJ et al: Effects of thrombin inhibition on the development of acute platelet-thrombus deposition during angioplasty in pigs: heparin versus recombinant hirudin, a specific thrombin inhibitor. Circulation 79:657, 1989
48. Hirsh J, Salzman EW, Harker L et al: Aspirin and other platelet active drugs: relationship among dose, effectiveness and side effects. Chest suppl 2. 95:12S, 1989
49. Hladovec J: Is the antithrombotic activity of "antiplatelet" drugs based on protection of endothelium. Thromb Haemost 41:774, 1979
50. Jaffe EA, Weksler BB: Recovery of endothelial cell prostacyclin production after inhibition by low doses of aspirin. J Clin Invest 63:532, 1979
51. Kerins DM, Fitzgerald GA, Fitzgerald DJ: Interaction of a prostacyclin analog and tissue plasminogen activator (tPA) during coronary thrombolysis. Clin Res 37:321A, 1989
52. Kerins PM, Roy L, Fitzgerald GA, Fitzgerald DJ: Platelet activation and depressed prostacyclin ($PGI_2$) biosynthesis following reperfusion with tissue-type plasminogen activator (tPA) in man. Circulation suppl II. 78:508, 1988
53. Knapp HR, Reilly IAG, Alessandrini P, Fitzgerald GA: In vivo indexes of platelet function and vascular function during fish-oil administration in patients with atherosclerosis. N Engl J Med 314:937, 1986
54. Kristensen SD, Roberts KM, Kishk YT, Martin JF: Accelerated atherogenesis occurs following platelet destruction and increases in megakaryocyte size and DNA content. Eur J Clin Invest 20:239, 1990
55. Kruithof EK, Tran-Thang C, Bachmann F: Studies on the release of plasminogen activator inhibitor from human platelets. Thromb Haemost 55:201, 1986
56. Kyrle PA, Eichler HG, Jager U, Lechner K: Inhibition of prostacyclin and thromboxane $A_2$ generation by low-dose aspirin at the site of plug formation in man in vivo. Circulation 75:1025, 1987
57. Leaf A, Weber PC: Cardiovascular effects of n-3 fatty acids. N Engl J Med 318:549, 1988
58. Levin RI, Harpel PC, Harpel JG, Recht PA: Inhibition of tissue plasminogen activator activity by aspirin in vivo and its relationship to levels of tissue plasminogen activator antigen, plasminogen activator inhibitor and their complexes. Blood 74:1635, 1989
59. Loskutoff D, Edgington T: Synthesis of a fibrinolytic activator and inhibitor by endothelial cells. Proc Natl Acad Sci USA 74:3903, 1977
60. Marler JR, Price TR, Clark GL et al: Morning increase in onset of ischemic stroke. Stroke 20:473, 1989
61. Mickelson JK, Simpson PJ, Gallas MT, Lucchesi BR: Thromboxane synthase inhibition with CGS 13080 improves coronary blood flow after streptokinase-induced thrombolysis. Am Heart J 113:1345, 1987
62. Miles LA, Ginsberg MH, White JG, Plow EF:

Plasminogen interacts with human platelets through two distinct mechanisms. J Clin Invest 77:2001, 1986
63. Mills DC, Smith JB: The influence on platelet aggregation of drugs that affect the accumulation of adenosine 3′ : 5′-cyclic monophosphate in platelets. Biochem J 121:185, 1971
64. Moncada S, Vane JR: Arachidonic acid metabolites and the interactions between platelets and blood-vessel walls. N Engl J Med 300:1142, 1979
65. Moroz L: Increased blood fibrinolytic activity after aspirin ingestion. N Engl J Med 296:525, 1977
66. Muller JE, Ludmer PL, Wilich SN et al: Circadian variation in the frequency of sudden cardiac death. Circulation 75:131, 1987
67. Nilsson J, Svensson J, Hamsten A, de Faire U: Increased platelet-derived mitogenic activity in plasma of young patients with coronary atherosclerosis. Atherosclerosis 61:237, 1986
68. Ohlstein EH, Storer B, Nambi P et al: Endothelin and platelet function. Thromb Res 57:967, 1990
69. O'Toole TE, Loftus JC, Plow EF et al: Efficient surface expression of platelet GPIIb-IIIa requires both subunits. Blood 74:14, 1989
70. Parmentier S, Kaplan C, Catimel B, McGregor J: New families of adhesion molecules play a vital role in platelet functions. Immunol Today 11:225, 1990
71. Patrignani P, Filabozzi P, Patrono C: Selective cumulative inhibition of platelet thromboxane production by low-dose aspirin in healthy subjects. J Clin Invest 69;1366, 1982
72. Pfisterer M, Jockers G, Regenass S et al: Trial of low-dose aspirin plus dipyridamole versus anticoagulants for prevention of aortocoronary vein graft occlusion. Lancet 2:1, 1989
73. Plow EF, Collen D: The presence and release of $alpha_2$-antiplasmin from human platelets. Blood 58:1069, 1981
74. Plow EF, Pierschbacher MD, Ruoslahti E et al: The effect of Arg-Gly-Asp-containing peptides on fibrinogen and von Willebrand factor binding to platelets. Proc Natl Acad Sci USA 82:8057–8061, 1985
75. Pober JS: Cytokine-mediated activation of vascular endothelium: physiology and pathology. Am J Pathol 133:426, 1988
76. Radomski MW, Palmer RM, Moncada S: An L-arginine/nitric oxide pathway present in human platelets regulates aggregation. Proc Natl Acad Sci USA 87:5193, 1990
77. Reilly IA, Fitzgerald GA: Inhibition of thromboxane formation in vivo and ex vivo; implications for therapy with platelet inhibitory drugs. Blood 69:180, 1987
78. Reilly IA, Fitzgerald GA: Aspirin in cardiovascular disease. Drugs 35:154, 1988
79. Roth GJ, Stanford N, Majerus PW: Acetylation of prostaglandin synthetase by aspirin. Proc Natl Acad Sci USA 72:3073, 1975
80. Saltiel E, Ward A: Ticlopidine: a review of the pharmacodynamic and pharmacokinetic properties and therapeutic efficacy in platelet-dependent disease states. Drugs 34:222, 1987
81. Schafer AI, Adelman B: Plasmin inhibition of platelet function and of arachidonic acid metabolism. J Clin Invest 75:456, 1985
82. Schbath J, Boissel JP, Mathy B et al: Drug effects on platelet survival times: comparison of two pyrimido-pyrimidine derivatives in patients with aortic or mitral replacement. Thromb Haemost 51:45, 1984
83. Shattil SJ, Brass LP: Induction of the fibrinogen receptor on human platelets by intracellular mediators. J Biol Chem 262:992, 1987
84. Sherman DG, Dyken ML, Fisher M et al: Antithrombotic therapy for cerebrovascular disorders. Chest, suppl. 95:140S, 1989
85. Silverstein RL, Leung LL, Harpel PC, Nachman RL: Complex formation of platelet thrombospondin with plaminogen: modulation of activation by tissue activator. J Clin Invest 74:1625, 1984
86. Smith JB, Willis AL: Aspirin selectively inhibits prostaglandin production in human platelets. Nature 231:235, 1971
87. Steele P, Carroll J, Overfield D, Genton E: Effect of sulphinpyrazone on platelet survival time in patients with transient cerebral ischemic attacks. Stroke 8:396, 1977
88. Steering Committee of the Physicians' Health Study Research Group: Final report on the aspirin component of the ongoing Physicians' Health Study. N Engl J Med 321:129, 1989
89. Steering Committee of the Physician's Health Study Research Group Preliminary Report: Findings from the aspirin component of the ongoing Physicians' Health Study. N Engl J Med 318:262, 1988
90. Stein B, Fuster V, Israel DH et al: Platelet inhibitor agents in cardiovascular disease: an update. J Am Coll Cardiol 14:813, 1989
91. Stern DM, Nawroth PP: Modulation of endothelial cell hemostatic properties by tumor necrosis factor. J Exp Med 163:740, 1986
92. Stern DM, Nawroth PP, Handley D, Kisiel W: An endothelial cell dependent pathway of coagulation. Proc Natl Acad Sci USA 82:2523, 1985
93. Stricker RB, Wong D, Shiu DT et al: Activation of plasminogen by tissue plasminogen activator on normal and thrombasthenic platelets: effects on surface proteins and platelet aggregation. Blood 68:275, 1986
94. Tofler GH, Brezinski D, Schafer AI et al: Concurrent morning increase in platelet aggregability and the risk of myocardial infarction and sudden cardiac death. N Engl J Med 316:1514, 1987
95. Uchiyama S, Sone R, Nagayama T et al: Combination therapy with low-dose aspirin and ticlopidine in cerebral ischemia. Stroke 20:1643, 1989
96. Vane JR: Inhibition of prostaglandin synthesis as a mechanism of action for aspirin-like drugs. Nature 231:232, 1971
97. von Schacky C, Fischer S, Weber PC: Long-term effects of dietary marine omega-3 fatty acids

upon plasma and cellular lipids, platelet function, and eicosanoid formation in humans. J Clin Invest 76:1626, 1985
98. von Schacky C, Weber PC: Metabolism and effects on platelet function of the purified eicosapentaenoic and docosahexaenoic acids in humans. J Clin Invest 76:2446, 1985
99. Weiss HJ: The effect of clinical dextran on platelet aggregation, adhesion and ADP release in man: in vivo and in vitro studies. J Lab Clin Med 69:37, 1967
100. Weiss HJ, Aledort LM: Impaired platelet-connective tissue reaction in man after aspirin ingestion. Lancet 2:495, 1967
101. Weiss HJ, Aledort LM, Kochwa S: The effects of salicylate on the hemostatic properties of platelets in man. J Clin Invest 47:2169, 1968
102. Weksler BB, Marcus AJ Jaffe EA: Synthesis of prostaglandin I2 (prostacyclin) by cultured human and bovine endothelial cells. Proc Natl Acad Sci USA 74:3922, 1977
103. Weksler BB, Pett SB, Alonso D et al: Differential inhibition by aspirin of vascular and platelet prostaglandin synthesis in atherosclerotic patients. N Engl J Med 308:800, 1983
104. Weksler BB, Tack-Goldman K, Subramanian VA, Gay WA Jr: Cumulative inhibitory effect of low dose aspirin on vascular prostacyclin and platelet thromboxane production in patients with atherosclerosis. Circulation 71:332, 1985
105. Zwaginga JJ, Sixma JJ, De Groot PG: Activation of endothelial cells induces platelet thrombus formation on their matrix. Arteriosclerosis 10:49, 1990

# 38
# ANTITHROMBOTIC THERAPY IN CEREBRAL ARTERIAL DISEASE

Henry J.M. Barnett

The majority of vascular strokes are accompanied by thrombosis, with or without an embolic component. Therefore, it was natural that the discovery and introduction of the preparations that alter coagulation, heparin and warfarin, would stimulate attempts to use them in order to prevent and treat ischemic strokes. Two decades later, a new series of drugs that affect the process of thrombosis by altering platelet aggregation were identified and thereby appeared as additional agents to evaluate in the prevention of stroke. Although the collective observations on these two classes of drugs have been made over a 35-year period, complete understanding about the appropriate indications for all of them is still evolving.

The final acceptance of anticoagulants and platelet-inhibiting therapy for any disease process involving thrombosis demands that trials of their effectiveness be conducted by strict and methodologically sound protocols. Carefully calculated samples of patients must be properly identified and scrupulously evaluated. Only in this way can it be assured that a major error will not occur and that neither efficacy will be denied when in fact it exists nor the equally disastrous conclusion be reached that no value in the treatment has been obtained when it is present. The randomized double-blind study is the gold standard for acceptable studies. The mere existence of a double-blind component and randomized assignment in these studies does not automatically confer validity upon the results; attention must be directed to all other aspects of the design, execution, and analysis of such a trial to avoid mistakes. The evidence that has accumulated about antithrombotic agents in ischemic central arterial disease is related in this chapter. The existing studies are examined critically, and the areas in which more work is needed are outlined.

## ANTICOAGULANTS

Anticoagulants have theoretical worth in several circumstances: transient ischemic attacks (TIAs), reversible ischemic neurologic disability (RIND) of atherotherombotic origin, progressing stroke, completed stroke, cardiogenic stroke, and certain other uncommon conditions.

### Reversible Ischemic Neurologic Disability and Transient Ischemic Attacks

No randomized trials addressing the problem of benefit from warfarin or heparin have been conducted in patients with reversible ischemic neurologic disease (RIND). The efficacy and usefulness of anticoagulants in the prevention of stroke in patients with transient ischemic attacks (TIAs) due to atherothrombotic disease in the major cerebral arteries is uncertain and probably best described as unknown. Decisions about their usefulness cannot be drawn from the many anecdotal observations reported in the literature and based on the physicians' experiences. The course of cerebral ischemic events is much too variable and unpredictable. Nor can they be drawn from comparisons with contemporary nonrandomized studies. These are flawed invariably by the incomparability of the populations with which the treated patients were compared. Many comparisons have been attempted using data from populations, which, unfortunately, are most probably not comparable in such important features as age, sex, ethnic origin, and the exact pathogenesis of the events. The decade in which the observations were conducted is vital. The baseline for stroke occurrence and stroke mortality has been changing dramatically over the past few years, with some reduction extending as far back as 35 years ago. No conclusion about efficacy of therapy can be derived from comparisons with prognostic studies conducted in the past. Natural history and prognostic studies cannot serve as denominators for treatment comparisons.

A few small, randomized studies were conducted in the 1950s and 1960s and an aggregate of 185 patients drawn from 4 studies, totaling 90 in the treated category and 95 in the control category, were treated for an average of 19 and 21 months, respectively.[5–7,53] During this time 18 strokes occurred, 10 in the placebo- and 8 in the warfarin-treated groups. Death was more frequent in the treated than in the placebo groups (15 vs 10); cerebral hemorrhage was the explanation for the increased risk of death in the warfarin-treated group. These early randomized evaluations were flawed in many ways.[38] The major faults resulted from the immaturity of the disciplined design and execution of clinical trials: the entry characteristics were not precise by today's standards; a variety of ischemic events of varying pathogenesis undoubtedly were included; definition and evaluation of end-points, the mixture of patients with atherothrombotic and cardiogenic stroke, attention to risk factors, particularly hypertension, concern for compliance and contaminating therapy, strictness of follow-up, and avoidance of crossover were reported in less detail than would be demanded today. No attempt was made to blind the investigations. The most obvious flaws were in the sample size: by modern biostatistical calculations the aggregate of patients entered into all the anticoagulant studies represents a sampling that falls short of the ideal by approximately 95 percent.[64]

The conclusion is inevitable: the place, if any, for warfarin in the treatment of patients with threatened stroke of atherothrombotic origin has not been established. This state of continuing ignorance is about to be addressed by a major multicenter trial that has been designed to compare, in patients with TIA and minor stroke, the relative value of warfarin, aspirin, or ticlopidine in stroke and vascular death. Until this study is completed, any recommendations about the use of anticoagulants in TIA or RIND patients must be considered speculative.

At the bedside or in the clinic, a pragmatic approach can be justified when facts are not available for patients who are threatened with serious and distressing illness such as a major stroke. Therefore, it is reasonable to make a recommendation that for patients with TIA or RIND due to atherothrombotic disease of the carotid or vertebral basilar arteries that 3 months of anticoagulant therapy may be administered when platelet antiaggregants fail to reduce the ischemic attacks, or when these agents are not tolerated, and when surgery is not indicated.

## Progressing Stroke

It has been common practice to consider that heparin followed by warfarin is indicated if there is clear evidence, under observation, that ischemic neurologic disability is recognizably worsening.[6,22] This conclusion has been based on mostly incomplete and largely anecdotal data. Many of the reports have not included a strict definition of progressing stroke.

The incidence of the entity remains to be clarified; the pathogenesis needs further study. Diagnostic tests to clarify the mechanism in any given patient need to be perfected. Only then will a background exist against which a convincing clinical trial can be conducted. If a subgroup can be identified with exactitude in which progressing thrombus formation or thromboembolic phenomena are recognizable by objective study, the rationale for anticoagulant therapy will be on firm ground. These patients will probably include most of those with a stepwise progressive worsening. Conversely, in patients who are progressing apparently because of the immediate or delayed accumulation of excitatory neurotoxins with recognizably increasing edema and the herniations secondary to it, identified by computed tomography (CT) examination, the use of anticoagulants will be disappointing, and to withhold them is rational. Until we have effective measures to correct the molecular abnormalities accompanying ischemia, many patients with an edematous infarction will continue to experience this type of worsening over several days after an ictus. Stroke in evolution is by no means synonymous with thrombosis in evolution.

Before considering any unproven treatment for the progressing stroke patient, a CT examination is essential. It will identify the presence of substantial edema and will ensure the recognition of instances of intracerebral hemorrhage—both hemorrhagic infarction and intracerebral hematoma. Some instances of intracerebral hemorrhage probably went unrecognized and contaminated the early studies, which constituted the first reports relating to anticoagulant therapy administered for progressing stroke patients.

Two recent studies, one randomized, one observational, have been neither conclusive nor encouraging in regard to the indications for anticoagulants in progressing stroke. The trial in which patients were randomized involved 225 patients with recent onset of ischemic stroke.[27] As many went on to progress in the heparin-treated group as in those receiving the placebo. In the observational trial, 50 percent of 36 patients with progressing symptoms deteriorated despite receiving heparin.[42]

With all these uncertainties now in focus, the use of heparin followed by warfarin in patients with progressing stroke must be regarded as an empirical strategy. It is a reasonable but neither a proven nor a "standard" therapy. Once initiated, the duration of such therapy must be regarded as unknown, but a few weeks is a common and rational period. This is the period when worsening is common. Thrombogenesis is an intermittent phenomenon. These facts added to the dangers of anticoagulants influence the recommendation that warfarin should be used only for a limited time if possible.

## Completed Stroke

Anticoagulants serve no purpose and carry a decided risk after a major infarction has produced a severe and disabling stroke.[38] It is known, however, that a patient with a more modest ischemic disability of recent origin could subsequently experience a more damaging and disabling additional infarction. No data exist to confirm or deny the usefulness of anticoagulants for such patients. Despite this ignorance of their benefit they are commonly administered in this situation. Their superiority to aspirin or ticlopidine therapy is unknown. At the moment, many would favor the use of platelet inhibitors. However, if the decision is made to use anticoagulants on empirical grounds, this therapy should be limited to a few weeks up to 3 months. The patients so treated should then be switched to, and maintained on, long-term platelet inhibitors.

## Thrombi Visible in Extracranial Cerebral Arteries and Carotid Stumps

Patients under investigation for TIA or partial stroke commonly are submitted to arteriography. On infrequent occasions, a thrombus is seen in the carotid or vertebral arteries appropriate to the ischemic events. Many of the recognized examples have been detected in association with tight stenoses of the involved arteries. Experimental studies have demonstrated the precipitation of thrombus in experimental lesions producing arterial stenosis.[39] Other patients have had no detectable underlying disease in the artery containing the thrombus and have systemic disorders or have been utilizing agents, including the contraceptive pill, known to increase the tendency toward coagulability.[9]

Some regard the finding of an intraluminal thrombus as an indication for emergency endarterectomy. This is an uncertain strategy for a variety of reasons. First, the surgical creation of a denuded endothelium over a long extent of the artery and the operative release of thromboplastin may add to the possibility of further and extending thrombosis. Second, there are examples where thrombus is visible in the artery in the neck coexisting with thrombus within the cavernous portion of the same internal carotid artery (Fig. 38-1). Any attempt to remove the thrombus from the neck will not improve the likelihood of lysis of the intracranial thrombus. Furthermore, in my experience, there is an increased hazard to the management of this condition by thromboendarterectomy. Of 29 patients recognized with thrombus in the extracranial portion of stenosed carotid arteries, an additional postoperative ischemic deficit was detected in 25 percent of those submitted to urgent surgery. No worsening was seen in those receiving anticoagulant or platelet antiaggregant therapy alone.[19] Twenty-five percent is an unacceptably high perioperative complication rate.

Finally, it is improbable that a thrombotic tendency with a so-called hypercoagulable state will benefit from the isolated surgical removal of one thrombus located in an otherwise normal artery. It is known that such thrombi are subject to spontaneous lysis; disappearance of thrombi in these locations has been observed to occur on a number of occasions without progression of the neurologic deficit.

The empirical but rational recommendations for patients in whom a thrombus is radiologically visible in an extracranial artery is for 3 months of anticoagulant therapy, beginning with heparin and proceeding with the simultaneous and subsequent administration of warfarin. When the prothrombin time is at acceptable levels, the heparin will be discontinued. In the patients with carotid stenosis and a thrombus beyond it, a repeat arteriogram after 4 to 6 weeks of anticoagulation therapy should be performed, provided the other clinical findings and the operative risk are within reasonable limits. In those with systemic or iatrogenic disorders, the decision to continue anticoagulation treatment will rest with the ability of the physician to alter this unnatural process.

A variant of the situation in which intraluminal thrombi are visualized in the stenosed internal carotid artery occurs when such clots are identified in the "stump" of the totally occluded internal carotid artery[14] (Fig. 38-2). Thrombi in the stump may be carried up in the collateral channels supplying the brain through the external carotid artery. They are an un-

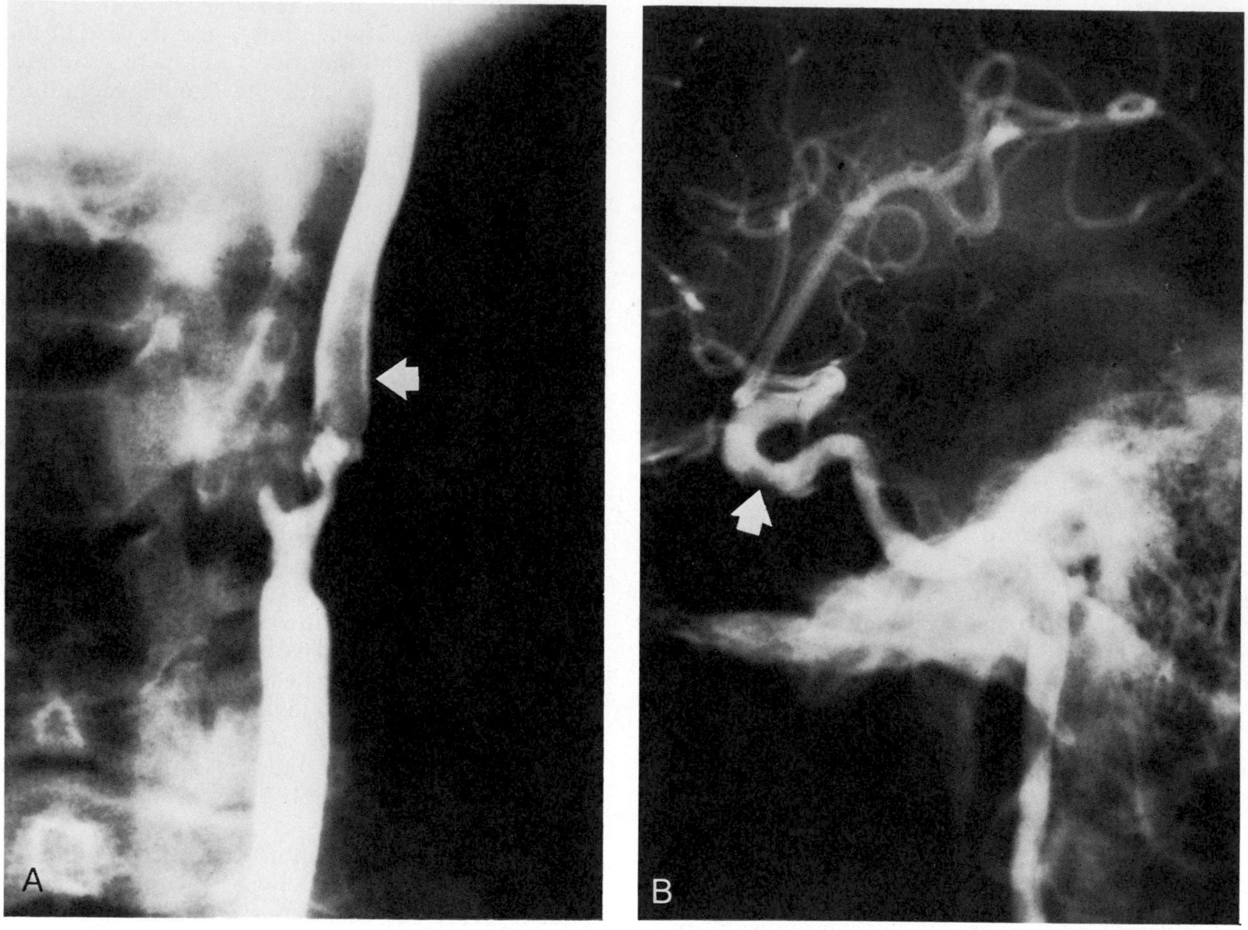


**Fig. 38-1.** (**A**) A thrombus (*arrow*) streaming up internal carotid artery beyond stenosis of terminal common carotid and proximal internal carotid artery segments. External carotid artery is occluded. (**B**) The same patient with simultaneous occurrence of thrombus (*arrow*) in cavernous sinus portion of the internal carotid artery. The patient received anticoagulation therapy, had no further ischemic events, and refused further investigation. (From Barnett,[10] with permission.)

common but proven cause of ischemic events beyond an artery known to be occluded.

The recognition of these thrombi presents two difficulties. First, because a stump is common, occurring in two-thirds of the patients who have occluded an internal carotid artery, it is important to be as certain as possible that the stump is the cause of the continuing ischemic events in a given patient. Second, the angiographic visualization of thrombus may be very difficult, and its existence is no more than by inference when an irregular stump, a stump with changing length or shape, or a stump with a central shadow intruding into the contrast suggest the presence of a thrombus. When this syndrome was recognized initially, we recommended that patients with these findings should be considered for surgery. Our own subsequent experience and that of others has identified this as a high-risk situation for surgery; 4 to 6 months of anticoagulant treatment, followed by an indefinite period of aspirin treatment, is preferred.[11,63]

## Summary of Anticoagulant Usefulness

A summary of the recommended uses for anticoagulants in noncardiac disorders is presented in Table 38-1. All have been discussed above except for the coagulation abnormalities (Ch. 36), venous and sinus disease (Ch. 19), and for cerebral emboli from pulmonary vein thrombosis. This is a rare complication of severe chest trauma or pulmonary sepsis. In the unusual circumstances when this condition can be clinically identified, anticoagulants are indicated until the primary process is controlled. Anticoagulants for patients with cerebral ischemic events related to *cardiac conditions* are discussed in Chapter 41.

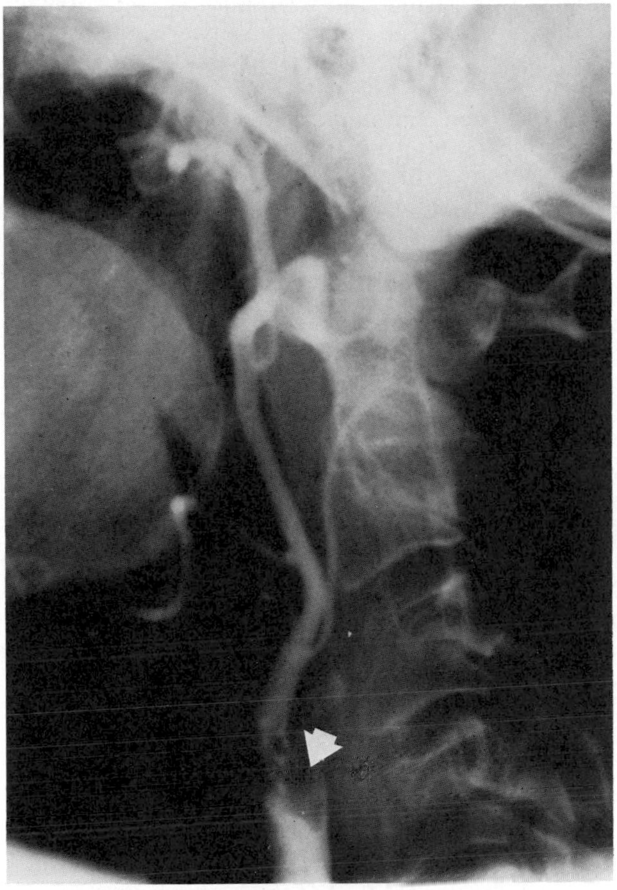

**Fig. 38-2.** Thrombus within "stump" of internal carotid artery (*arrow*). Some thrombus visible in irregular lumen of external carotid artery.

## PLATELET ANTIAGGREGANTS

A description of the physiology, pathophysiology, and pharmacologic responses of the platelets is given in Chapter 37.

Interest in platelet antiaggregants in stroke prevention began at about the time when the intensive search for the pathogenesis of transient cerebral and retinal ischemic events had narrowed to define the two causative mechanisms: those of a hemodynamic nature and those related to thromboembolic events. For the latter, the commoner mechanism, the platelet inhibitor appeared as an important prospect. Studies of platelet physiology were focusing attention on the importance of the platelet in initiation of thrombosis in fast-flowing arterial systems. Experimental studies determined that the platelets adhered to irregular surfaces, discharged their contents, and thereby triggered aggregation with the attraction of other platelets, the addition of fibrin, and the formation of a whitish-gray platelet-fibrin thrombus. Clinical observations were made of material passing through the retinal arterioles in a few patients with monocular amaurosis fugax, and it was hypothesized that the material was platelet-fibrin in nature.[34,41] Eventually, by fortuitous postmortem study, this speculation was proved to be correct.[4] Such material has since been observed at surgical procedures, passing through cortical branches of the middle cerebral artery at craniotomy (Fig. 38-3).

Nonsteroidal anti-inflammatory drugs that alter platelet function were identified: within 2 years sulfinpyrazone, acetylsalicylic acid, and dipyridamole were all discovered to have such properties.[31,51,57,67] Their mechanisms of action differed, but all were submitted to experimental evaluation in situations involving arterial thrombosis. They appeared to be worthy of clinical studies in patients with stroke-

**TABLE 38-1. Empirical Recommendations for Anticoagulants in Noncardiac Disorders Producing Embolic Cerebral Ischemia**

| |
|---|
| Failure to prevent ischemia by using platelet inhibitors in patients who have transient ischemic attacks or reversible ischemic neurologic disability |
| Patients with transient ischemic attacks or reversible ischemic neurologic disability unable to tolerate platelet-inhibiting drugs |
| Progressing stroke in the absence of massive edema or hemorrhage |
| Thrombi visualized by arteriography in cerebral arteries |
| Coagulation abnormalities |
| Cerebral vein and sinus occlusion |
| Thrombi suspected in pulmonary veins |

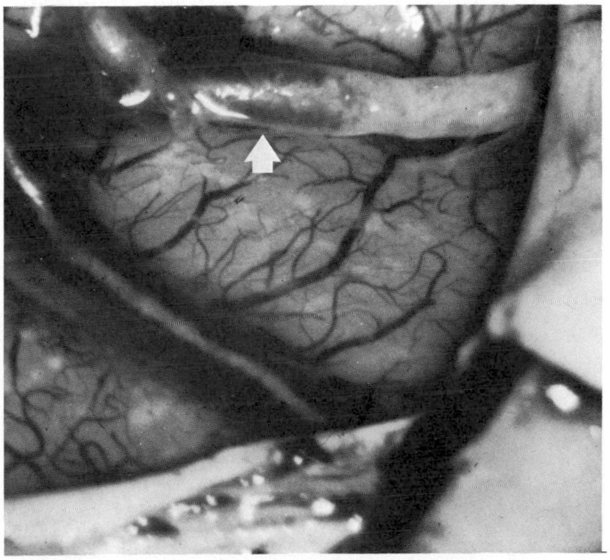

**Fig. 38-3.** Platelet fibrin material (*arrow*), which arrived in middle cerebral artery leptomeningeal branch during exposure for extracranial/intracranial anastomosis. (Courtesy of Dr. Howard Reichman.)

threatening symptoms. The initial anecdotal observations, made in patients with frequent recurrent events of amaurosis fugax, with and without thrombocytosis, were exciting and led to clinical trials.[8]

The first clinical trial involved a heterogeneous group of patients, probably with a variety of pathogenic mechanisms.[1] It included 169 patients with transient cerebral ischemia (TIA) and stroke, used dipyridamole in moderate and then in large daily dosage, but showed negative results after an average of 25 months of treatment.

Unlike the early clinical evaluation of anticoagulants, most of the subsequent trials of platelet antiaggregants have been conducted in the era of more advanced methodology and biostatistics, and have been conducted on patients with specific stroke-threatening symptoms. Attempts have been made in the later studies to select for treatment those patients whose TIAs, within the limits of clinical evaluation, were of artery-to-artery type rather than of cardiac origin or lacunar in nature. By this more refined process the selected patients were more likely to have been experiencing platelet thrombogenesis as distinct from a heterogeneous group of causes of TIA such as existed in the patients entered into the warfarin trials. In most of these antiplatelet trials, the entry characteristics and endpoints were defined; risk factors were identified and treated when possible; loss to follow-up was minimized; inviolate randomization procedures were used; adequate sample size, proper data management, and modern biostatistical methods were utilized in a way that was neither usual nor possible during the evaluation of anticoagulants two decades earlier.

The first trial launched to evaluate aspirin against placebo in stroke prevention in TIA and minor stroke patients was designed in 1970 and patient entry was begun in 1971. The conclusions were published in 1978, and a benefit for aspirin was found but only detected in males.[21] Ten trials with placebo control have now been completed and reported randomizing an aggregate of 7,684 patients with cerebral ischemic events (Table 38-2) comparing the benefit of aspirin with or without another platelet inhibitor.[16–18,21,27,32,33,40,56,58,66] One of these[32] utilized two platelet-inhibiting drugs simultaneously. The other trial, which tested two agents, utilized a factorial design.[21] A total of 1,311 patients were studied in the negative trials. One of them used a maximum of 75 mg, which, despite experimental data to the contrary, may not be an adequate dose.[58] One of the other negative trials did not detect benefit from aspirin in patients who had already experienced a major stroke and did not evaluate this treatment in patients with TIA or minor stroke.[18]

Considering collectively all the trials utilizing aspirin, the evidence strongly confirms the fact that aspirin prevents stroke. Because the outcome events and analyses were not always clearly identified and the trials not conducted in a uniform manner, and because some of the trials were too small, it is not easy to compare the relative risk reductions for all 10 of the trials. Table 38-3 identifies the risk reductions reported in the four largest trials that have tested aspirin against placebo.

## Sex Differential

The sex differential found in the Canadian study was totally unexpected and has since been the subject of considerable inquiry. Certain laboratory data identify differing responsiveness between males and fe-

**TABLE 38-2. Aspirin and Placebo-Controlled Secondary Prevention Trials[a]**

| Trial | Ref. | Publication Year | No. of Patients | Dose (mg) | Entry Criteria[b] | Outcome Events | Overall Benefit | Female Benefit |
|---|---|---|---|---|---|---|---|---|
| American | 33 | 1977 | 178 | ASA 1,300 | TIA, stroke | TIA, stroke & death | Yes | Not shown |
| Canadian | 21 | 1978 | 585 | ASA 1,300 | TIA, stroke | Stroke & death | Yes | Not shown |
| German | 56 | 1978 | 58 | ASA 1,500 | TIA, stroke | TIA, stroke & death | Yes | |
| Toulouse | 40 | 1982 | 302 | ASA 900<br>Persantine 150<br>Hydergine 3 | TIA, stroke | Stroke & death | No | |
| Paris | 27 | 1983 | 604 | ASA 1,000<br>Persantine 225 | TIA, stroke | Stroke, death | Yes | Yes |
| Danish | 58 | 1983 | 203 | ASA 1,000 | TIA, stroke | Stroke & death | No | |
| Swedish | 18 | 1987 | 505 | ASA 1,500 | Stroke[c] | Stroke | No | |
| European | 32 | 1987 | 2,500 | ASA 1,200<br>Persantine 225 | TIA, stroke | Stroke, death | Yes | Yes |
| Danish | 17 | 1988 | 301 | ASA 50–75 | TIA, stroke | Stroke & death | No | |
| British | 66 | 1988 | 2,448 | ASA 1,200 or<br>ASA 300 | TIA, stroke | Stroke & death | Yes | Not shown |

*Abbreviations:* ASA, acetylsalicylic acid; TIA, transient ischemic attack.

[a] The 10 trials testing aspirin against placebo in 7,684 patients who had experienced transient ischemic attacks, reversible ischemic neurologic disability, minor stroke, and, in one instance,[18] a major stroke.

[b] Minor stroke, recovered stroke.

[c] Major stroke.

**TABLE 38-3. The Four Large Acetylsalicylic Acid Trials in Patients with TIA or Minor Stroke[a]**

| Trial Placebo | *N* | Daily Dose (mg) | Endpoints | Relative Risk Reduction (%) | Female Benefit | Annual Stroke Rate (%) | Ref. |
|---|---|---|---|---|---|---|---|
| Canada | 585 | 1,300 | S, D | 30 | Not shown | 5.9 | 21 |
| France | 600 | 1,000 | S, SD | 50 | Yes | 6.0 | 40 |
| Europe | 2,500 | 975 + Pers | S, SD | 35 | Yes | 7.3 | 32 |
| Britain | 2,435 | 1,200 or 300 | S, Vasc D | 20 | Not shown | 3.2 | 66 |

*Abbreviations:* S, stroke; D, death; Vasc, vascular; Pers, Persantine (dipyridamole).

[a] Four trials have tested aspirin against placebo in sufficient numbers to be important. The British trial entered an unusually low-risk group of patients.

males in other species, which conceivably supports this finding in human subjects.[47,48] An alternative explanation may be found in the prognostic difference, which has been identified in a number of randomized treatment studies in which female patients threatened with stroke have a substantially better prognosis for stroke and vascular death than do males.[12,25,30,50] Additionally, this better prognosis for women after TIA or stroke has been observed in several community studies, including the Oxford Community and the Framingham studies.[43,68] The total number of female patients in the Canadian study was approximately 200, and because women are at a low risk compared to male patients, a benefit might have been missed by chance, which was likely to have been detected had a larger population been studied. Subsequent studies add to this speculative explanation (Table 38-3). The French trial with 200 women and 400 men found equal benefit for both. The European Stroke Prevention Study (ESPS) trial, involving 2,500 patients, confirmed benefit for both sexes. The British trial was large (2,435 patients) but reported no female benefit. The paradox presented by differences found in the two largest trials may be explained by the fact that the British trial entered patients of both sexes at lower risk than the other largest trial. In the Canadian, French, and European trials, the annual risk of stroke in the placebo groups was 5.9, 6.0, and 7.2 percent, respectively. In the British trial, the annual risk was merely 3.2 percent. This unexpectedly low risk to the total British study population may possibly have neutralized the strong statistical probability of showing benefit that might have been expected from such a large total number. It has been proved that women with unstable angina given aspirin benefit as well as do men with a reduced risk from fatal and nonfatal myocardial infarction.[20,49,65] On balance, for stroke-threatened patients, it is probable that aspirin benefits women as well as men, but that there is a lessened risk to start with for women experiencing cerebral ischemic events.

## Optimal Dosage of Aspirin

The optimal dosage of aspirin has been the subject of major debate. The concern is that aspirin inhibits prostacyclin in the endothelial cells by its inhibition of cyclo-oxygenase. This enzyme is common to the production not only of this antithrombotic and vasodilating substance in the endothelium cell but also to the thrombogenic and vasoconstricting substance thromboxane, released from the platelet. From the theoretical point of view, it is an attractive hypothesis that a smaller dosage will interfere less with the prostacyclin production than with the platelet inhibition. Extrapolation of this information from the laboratory to the bedside requires clinical trials.

Undoubtedly, a smaller dosage is effective as an antithrombotic: in preventing thrombus formation in the plastic tubing of dialysis shunts, 165 mg aspirin daily was beneficial when compared with placebo.[44] Unfortunately, in this study the comparative benefit of a larger daily dosage was not assessed. Unstable angina is a platelet-dependent symptom known to be associated with aggregation of platelets in the intramyocardial arterioles supplied from the coronary arteries.[26] A dosage of 325 mg of aspirin daily compared to placebo control was shown to reduce by 51 percent the risk of fatal and nonfatal myocardial infarction in 1,200 patients presenting with unstable angina.[49] A subsequent report on 555 patients with the same disorder had similar results. A reduced risk of 51 percent was achieved with a dosage of 1,300 mg aspirin/day.[20] A third study determined a reduced risk of 72 percent utilizing 650 mg daily.[65] The smaller dosage conferred equal benefit, but was accompanied by a reduction in gastrointestinal side effects. If this low dosage is proved to be best in stroke-threatened patients, it will be much more desirable than a 1 g/day dosage, with its resultant intolerable side effects in approximately 15 percent of patients. Whether these data from one arterial system and disease process can be transposed to the disorders of the blood supply of another organ is at best a speculation.

The evidence accumulated about the best dose fails to provide a completely satisfactory and clearly definitive answer. Taking all clinical trials where any platelet-inhibiting drugs have been evaluated against placebo, whether the disease targeted for study was heart disease or cerebral ischemia, the metanalyses have led to a conclusion that a dose of 300 o 325 mg daily is as effective as a dose of 1,200 to 1,300 mg daily.[3,13] More than 90 percent of the patients in these trials were randomized after presenting with evidence of heart disease, not with cerebral ischemic events. The analyses included data from trials of drugs which by themselves have not been shown to prevent stroke (sulfinpyrazone, dipyridamole, suloctidil). From the aggregate of this very heterogeneous group, the risk of ischemic stroke was reduced 25 percent. How much dilution if any of the true benefit of aspirin in stroke-threatened patients results from this mode of analysis is uncertain. When the four large trials that entered a minimum of approximately 600 patients presenting with TIA or stroke are considered, the benefits from aspirin in reducing the outcome events varied from 50 percent relative risk reduction for stroke and stroke death down to 20 percent reduction in stroke and vascular death. The lowest figure was that obtained in the British trial, in which there was an entire population at peculiarly low risk and in which half of the active-treatment patients received 300 mg/day, and the other half 1,200 mg. The conclusion of the investigators in the British trial was that there was equal benefit from either dose schedule. Dyken,[29] reviewing their data, remarked on the low incidence of events in both the two treatment groups and the placebo group and commented on a trend (8.9 percent) toward a better response from 1,200 mg than 300 mg.

A Dutch trial, treating a large (3,131) number of patients with a mean follow-up of 2.6 years utilized either 30 mg or 300 mg of aspirin as the daily dose.[28] They concluded that the prevention of vascular events (death from vascular causes, nonfatal stroke, nonfatal myocardial infarction) was no less in the group receiving either dose. They did not compare the treatment against placebo nor against the higher dose of 975 to 1,300 mg of aspirin daily.

A recent Swedish trial has involved 1,360 patients, given by random assignment, either 75 mg daily of acetylsalicylic acid (ASA) or placebo. The early report has stated that 7.3 percent of the patients on ASA had vascular events compared with 9.5 percent in the placebo group. Benefit was equal in the sexes. No comparison was made with a larger dose (Britton, personal communication).

Preliminary unpublished observations from the North American Symptomatic Carotid Endarterectomy Trial (NASCET), referred to in Dyken's reflective paper[29] on the dose of aspirin in stroke prevention, are highly suggestive of the probability that a 1,300 mg daily dose of aspirin is superior to 325 mgms in the postendarterectomy subjects.

Opinion about dosage remains divided. In Britain and Europe and among many cardiologists, the evidence from the unstable angina trials, from the Dutch and Swedish trials, and from the metanalyses, is used to sway recommendations for stroke-threatened patients toward a lower dose. Among North American neurologists, including the author of this chapter, the common opinion remains that for patients threatening with a stroke because of recent TIA or recent minor infarction, the optimum recommended dose of aspirin must remain at 975 to 1,300 mg daily until harder evidence emerges than has been forthcoming from present clinical trials. Reduced amounts are recommended in the event of gastrointestinal upsets. An enteric-coated variety is desirable for most individuals for long-term use. It is equally effective as a platelet inhibitor as the standard buffered or uncoated varieties of acetylsalicylic acid.

## Other Platelet Antiaggregants

Several other platelet antiaggregants have been shown not to reduce the occurrence of stroke in patients with TIA or who have experienced stroke. Sulfinpyrazone alone in the Canadian study was of no more benefit than placebo. A trial of suloctidil in 438 patients who had experienced a recent cerebral infarction produced no benefit in stroke reduction when a dosage of 600 mg daily was compared with placebo in a random assignment and follow-up study of 20 months.[37] The one trial of dipyridamole alone against placebo was not able to establish benefit.[1]

A new platelet-inhibiting drug useful in stroke prevention, ticlopidine, has been tested and given approval by drug regulating agencies in most countries. It acts by a different mechanism not completely understood. It interferes with the platelet membrane function by inhibiting adenosine diphosphate (ADP)-induced platelet-fibrinogen binding and platelet-platelet interactions.

The drug was evaluated in two populations: 3,069 patients with TIA or recent minor stroke were given 250 mg of ticlopidine bid or aspirin (1,200 mg daily) by random assignments; 1,047 recent major stroke victims were given the same dose of ticlopidine or placebo.[36,45] In the first instance, ticlopidine was given to TIA patients and the result was described as "somewhat better" in preventing stroke and death than was aspirin; in the stroke patients of the second study, ticlopidine was significantly better than placebo. Side effects include a 2.4 percent chance of any degree of neutropenia, a 0.8 percent risk of serious neutropenia, and a 12 percent risk of inducing a disturbing diarrhea. Ticlopidine lengthens the bleeding time and gastrointestinal bleeding has occurred but with less frequency than with aspirin. An occasional fatal occurrence of thrombotic thrombocytopenic purpura has been noted. A few patients have developed cholestatic jaundice so that it is contraindicated in patients with hepatic dysfunction. During its administration blood counts and liver function tests are mandatory. With any indication of liver function abnormality or bone marrow suppression, the drug must be discontinued.

Ticlopidine is recommended for patients who cannot tolerate aspirin, or who fail to experience a reduction or an elimination of continuing ischemic events despite aspirin.

## Combined Antiaggregants

The administration of combinations of platelet antiaggregants has been studied with no evidence yet of any synergistic benefit. The rationale for such attempts lies in the fact that the mechanisms of action of the known platelet antiaggregants are disparate. Compared with aspirin, sulfinpyrazone has been shown to have a competitive inhibiting action and to alter the survival time of circulating platelets. Whatever significance this pharmacologic difference may have, the combination of aspirin with sulfinpyrazone was not better than aspirin alone in the Canadian study. Dipyridamole (Persantine) is an inhibitor of phosphodiesterase rather than cyclo-oxygenase. Three trials have failed to establish that dipyridamole added to aspirin is superior to aspirin alone.[2,27,40] In the Paris trial, one-third of 600 patients were randomly assigned to receive placebo, one-third to receive aspirin alone, and one-third to receive aspirin with 400 mg Persantine/day. No added benefit accompanied the combination. Similarly, in an American-Canadian multicenter trial in which 890 patients were stratified so that one-half randomly received 1.3 g aspirin alone and one-half a combination of 1.3 g aspirin with 300 mg Persantine, and were evaluated for a median time of 25 months, an identical number of endpoints occurred in the two groups. In the third trial, 100 patients received hydergine, 100 received hydergine plus 900 mg daily of ASA, 100 received both of these plus 150 mg daily of dipyridamole. No difference in stroke event was detected in any of the groups. The event rates were lower than anticipated. Ticlopidine combined with aspirin has not been tested, and the altered bleeding time and gastrointestinal side effects of each drug individually do not encourage such a trial. Neither aspirin nor ticlopidine should be given with warfarin. In conclusion, no evidence exists as yet that any combination of platelet antiaggregants is superior to aspirin alone.

## Platelet Antiaggregants versus Anticoagulant

The relative benefit of platelet antiaggregants and anticoagulants in stroke prevention has been addressed on a few occasions. Some studies on cerebral and systemic embolism after the insertion of a prosthetic valve have compared the benefit of warfarin alone with the addition of dipyridamole to warfarin.[2,62] The evidence favored the combination, but the results cannot be regarded as conclusive for today's needs because they were carried out prior to the use of the bioprosthetic valve.

Two small Scandinavian studies have compared the use of anticoagulants and platelet antiaggregants in TIA patients. The first study examined the benefit of two therapies in 156 patients with TIA or RIND.[52] All patients were given anticoagulants for 2 months, and then 135 of the patients who were available for long-term follow-up in the trial were randomized to receive either continued anticoagulants or 1 g aspirin/day combined with 150 mg dipyridamole for a total period of 12 months. One of the patients in the preliminary anticoagulant phase experienced an ischemic stroke. In the second phase of the trial, two strokes occurred in the 68 patients on continued anticoagulent therapy, one a fatal hemorrhage, the other an infarction. Three cerebral infarctions occurred in the 67 patients given platelet antiaggregants. Lethal myocardial infarction occurred in four of those on anticoagulants and one in the group taking aspirin and dipyridamole. The authors concluded that they had demonstrated a prophylactic effect against cerebral infarction with both treatment strategies, but, in the absence of a placebo, this conclusion must be regarded as tentative. There was no convincing evidence that subsequent to the 2-month period of anticoagulant therapy either therapy utilized thereafter was better than the other, but the numbers were small enough that this conclusion could be in error.

The second study compared warfarin used in standard dosage with 1 g/day aspirin in a randomized study of 155 male and 86 female patients with TIA and minor stroke evaluated for 20 months.[35] Among the 114 patients randomized to receive anticoagulant, 3.5 percent had a cerebral infarct, 12.3 percent further TIA or RIND, and 2.6 percent died. The comparable figures for those randomized to receive aspirin were 3.1 percent, 8.7 percent, and 2.4 percent, respectively. The conclusion was drawn that there was no demonstrable superiority between the two treatment strategies. No placebo group existed and the study involved a small sample size and a brief follow-up.

A pilot study has looked at the question of possible superiority of heparin over aspirin in 55 hospitalized TIA patients where the TIAs were of recent origin.[15] The study confirmed the fact that recency of TIA is of prognostic importance for recurrent TIA and for ischemic stroke. No definite evidence of superiority of heparin over aspirin was forthcoming. There were recurrent TIA in eight of the patients receiving heparin and in seven of those assigned to aspirin; there were four infarctions (three brain, one retina) in the aspirin and one infarction (brain) in the heparin group. The numbers are too small for any conclusion, but a large study is clearly indicated.

In TIA patients, existing evidence therefore does not favor anticoagulants over platelet-inhibiting therapy, and controlled trials of sufficiently large size must be conducted. The greater hazard of warfarin and heparin therapy casts doubt on the wisdom of using warfarin as the first line of therapy rather than aspirin in TIA when they appear to arise from arterial as compared to cardiac sources. A major North American trial has been designed with a view to comparing anticoagulant against platelet-inhibiting drugs in a large number of TIA patients. This trial may resolve this long-standing issue.

## Aspirin in Primary Stroke Prevention

No trial has been designed to determine specifically whether or not there is benefit from platelet-inhibitors in preventing stroke in populations without any evidence of symptomatic cardiovascular and cerebrovascular disease. The design of the two primary prevention trials that have been done was ideal to evaluate benefit for myocardial infarction or peripheral vascular disease. The outcome of stroke was noted, but the age of the patients averaged a decade below that of the average age of occurrence of stroke.

Stroke was not reduced in the two large primary prevention population studies conducted in the United States and Great Britain. In both studies, 325 mg of aspirin was administered every other day to 22,071 and 5,139 normal individuals.[54,59] The American trial raised the possibility of an increase in the number of hemorrhagic strokes related to aspirin use. Editorial commentary warned of this risk of brain hemorrhage.[55] When the longer follow-up was reported 1 year later, this trend to hemorrhage was less impressive, and the numbers both of strokes and hemorrhagic strokes were small.[60] A similar concern about hemorrhagic stroke was raised in the British secondary prevention trial. Nine hemorrhagic strokes occurred in the patients in the aspirin groups, compared with one hemorrhagic stroke in those receiving the placebo. The unsatisfactory part of these reports is that in neither instance were the definitions and criteria of cerebral hemorrhage identified, nor was the mode of determining the presence of hemorrhage disclosed. No indication was given as to the confirmatory use or otherwise of CT scanning in validating the hemorrhage.

By contrast, in the American Atrial Fibrillation Study, fewer end points of hemorrhagic stroke occurred in the aspirin-treated group (325 mg daily) than with the placebo.[61] In the ISIS.2 study, hemorrhagic stroke occurred in only five of the 4,250 patients receiving both streptokinase and aspirin.[46] No hemorrhagic strokes were identified in approximately 4,250 patients who received aspirin alone in a daily dosage of 162.5 mg. In the ongoing NASCET study, a CT scan is required, and an external adjudication is carried out for all stroke outcome events. The patients are advised to take 1,300 mg of aspirin per day. Among the 143 stroke endpoints reported in the severely stenotic patients, and evaluated by the combination of a clinical and CT examination, only three hemorrhagic infarctions have occurred. All of them were in the postoperative period, and one had never taken aspirin (NASCET, unpublished data). It is not possible to claim that the last word has been written on the subject, but it is unlikely that aspirin poses a risk of consequence in causing hemorrhagic stroke.

The failure to determine reduction in stroke despite a reduction in myocardial infarction in the American and British primary prevention trials is of great interest. It may be explained in two ways. First, it might be speculated that the dose of 325 mg every other day may have been inadequate to reduce stroke. The assumption that the primary vascular processes are identical in ischemic stroke and ischemic heart disease may be incorrect. Second, the trials involved populations at risk for myocardial infarction, but the patients on average were a decade younger than is known to be the peak age incidence for stroke expectancy. They were a low-risk group, and benefit may simply have been missed. There the matter rests until such time as there is a trial of platelet-inhibitors designed and conducted specifically to determine the possible benefit of aspirin in primary stroke prevention.

## Further Areas of Uncertainty in the Use of Platelet Inhibitors

The gaps in accurate knowledge of platelet-inhibiting agents in stroke prevention are considerable but are narrowing slowly.

Data are lacking about the use of platelet antiaggregants in a number of conditions in which their use might be thought reasonable (Table 38-4). In many of these conditions, the possibility is slight that a meaningful trial could be mounted because the conditions are sufficiently uncommon and their identification sufficiently difficult that a study with sufficient numbers would scarcely be attainable, even if a multicenter strategy were adopted. This constraint applies especially to the nonarteriosclerotic arteriopathies affecting the major arterial supply of the brain and to the cardiac valvular lesions specified. Nevertheless, in the case of prolapsing mitral valve and of nonbacte-

**TABLE 38-4. Clinical Conditions in Which Platelet Antiaggregants Appear to Be Indicated but in Which No Trials Have Been Conducted**

| |
|---|
| Arterial lesions of nonarteriosclerotic variety |
| Fibromuscular dysplasia |
| Carotid dissection, with and without aneurysm formation |
| Post-traumatic arteriopathy |
| Postirradiation arteriography |
| Prophylaxis before angiography |
| Postendarterectomy |
| Post-extracranial/intracranial anastomosis |
| Asymptomatic bruit and stenosis |
| Cardiac valvular lesions |
| Prolapsing mitral valve |
| Mitral annulus calcification |
| Nonbacterial thrombotic endocarditis |

rial endocarditis, the usual pathologic process that has been recognized is a small lesion with small collections of platelets and fibrin with the potential for thromboembolic behavior (Fig. 38-4). The usefulness of platelet antiaggregants remains speculative, but they are recommended as first treatment when symptoms occur in these disorders. Good clinical trials of prophylactic platelet antiaggregants as a prelude to angiography, or in patients with bruit and known asymptomatic stenoses are obviously needed but have not been done. Many subjects, and therefore multicenter cooperation, would be demanded to achieve a convincing answer. After carotid endarterectomy, the NASCET observations provide a compelling reason to launch a trial utilizing two doses of aspirin for comparison. There are few remaining indications for extracranial-intracranial anastomoses but those that are done may remain patent more frequently with postoperative platelet inhibitors. A trial is improbable due to the rarity of the use of the procedure.

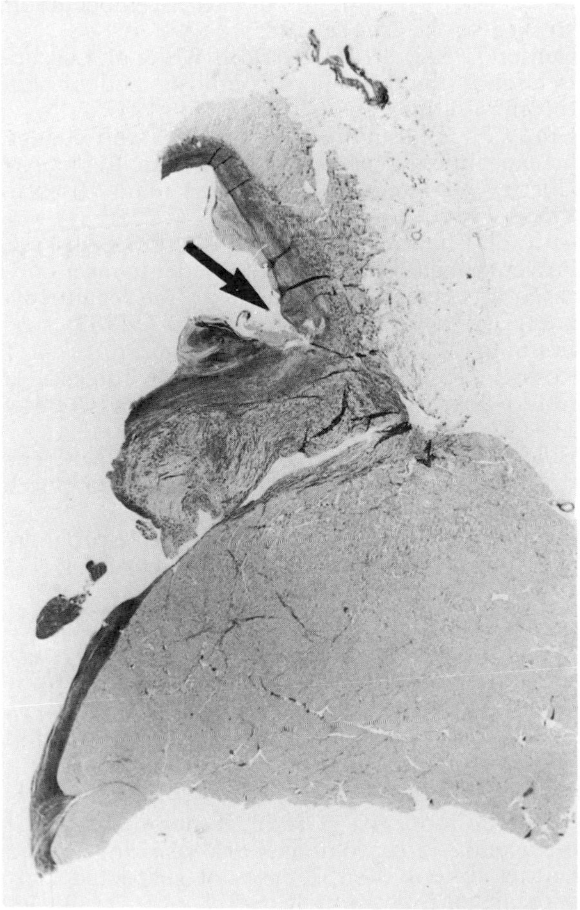

**Fig. 38-4.** Myxomatous degeneration of prolapsing mitral valve with ulcerative lesion at junction of valve to atrium. Granular deposition in base of ulcer is platelet fibrin material (*arrow*). (From Chesler et al.,[23] with permission.)

## Conclusions Concerning the Use of Platelet-Inhibiting Drugs

The evidence is now convincing that aspirin is of value in stroke prevention when given to those patients with TIA and minor stroke of cerebral arterio-sclerotic origin. The management of stroke-threatened patients will involve aspirin and the use of ticlopidine if aspirin fails to reduce recurring events or cannot be tolerated. All TIA and minor stroke patients will require evaluation for possible lesions that will benefit from surgery. All patients, whether treated by antithrombotic therapy or by surgery, must be given scrupulous risk factor management.[24] Better and safer platelet inhibitors are still needed.

## REFERENCES

1. Acheson J, Danta G, Hutchinson EC: Controlled trial of dipyridamole in cerebral vascular disease. Br Med J 1:614, 1969
2. The American-Canadian Cooperative Study Group, Fields W: Persantine aspirin trial in cerebral ischaemia. II. End-point results. Stroke 16:406, 1985
3. Antiplatelet Trialists' Collaboration: Secondary prevention of vascular disease by prolonged antiplatelet treatment. Br Med J 296:320, 1988
4. Ashby BM, Oakley N, Lorentz I, Scott D: Recurrent monocular blindness. Br Med J 2:894, 1963
5. Baker RN: An evaluation of anticoagulant therapy in the treatment of cerebrovascular disease: report of the Veterans Administration Cooperative Study of Atherosclerosis. Neurology (NY) 11:132, 1961
6. Baker RN, Broward JA, Fang HC et al: Anticoagulant therapy in cerebral infarction: report on cooperative study. Neurology (NY) 123:823, 1962
7. Baker RN, Schwartz WS, Rose AS: Transient ischemic strokes: a report of a study of anticoagulant therapy. Neurology (NY) 16:841, 1966
8. Barnett HJM: Transient cerebral ischemia: pathogenesis, prognosis and management. Ann R Coll Physicians Surgeons Can 7:153, 1974
9. Barnett HJM: Platelet and coagulation function in relation to thromboembolic stroke. 16:45, 1977
10. Barnett HJM: Problems in the therapy of stroke prevention—antithrombotic drugs and surgical considerations. p. 243. In Barnett HJM, Paoletti P, Flamm ES, Brambilla G (eds): Cerebrovascular Diseases: New Trends in Surgical and Medical Aspects. Elsevier/North-Holland, Amsterdam, 1981
11. Barnett HJM: The stump syndrome. p. 295. In Smith R (ed): Stroke and the Extracranial Vessels. Raven Press, New York, 1984
12. Barnett HJM: Stroke prevention and treatment: milestones, perspectives and challenges. p. 27. In Plum F, Pulsinelli W (eds): Cerebrovascular Disease. Proceedings of the Fourteenth Research Conference. Raven Press, New York, 1985
13. Barnett HJM: 35 years of stroke prevention: chal-

lenges, disappointments and successes. Cerebrovasc Dis 1:61, 1991
14. Barnett HJM, Peerless SJ, Kaufmann JCE: "Stump" of internal carotid artery—a source for further cerebral embolic ischemia. Stroke 9:48, 1978
15. Biller J, Bruno A, Adams HP et al: A randomized trial of aspirin or heparin in hospitalized patients with recent transient ischemic attacks. Stroke 20:441, 1989
16. Bousser MG, Eschwege E, Haguenau M et al: "AICLA" controlled trial of aspirin and dipyridamole in the secondary prevention of atherothrombotic cerebral ischemia. Stroke 14:5, 1983
17. Boysen G, Sorenson PS, Juhler M et al: Danish very-low-dose aspirin after carotid endarterectomy trial. Stroke 19:1211, 1988
18. Britton M, Helmers C, Samuelsson K: High-dose acetylsalicylic acid after cerebral infarction—a Swedish cooperative study. Stroke 18:325, 1987
19. Buchan AM, Barnett HJM: Vascular malformations and hemorrhage of the spinal cord. p. 721. In Stroke: Pathophysiology, Diagnosis and Management. Barnett HJM, Mohr JP, Stein BM (eds): Churchill Livingstone, New York, 1985
20. Cairns J, Gent M, Singer J et al: A study of aspirin and/or sulfinpyrazone in unstable angina. Circulation, suppl II. 70:415, 1984
21. Canadian Cooperative Study Group: A randomized trial of aspirin and sulfinpyrazone in threatened stroke. N Engl J Med 299:53, 1978
22. Carter AB: Use of anticoagulants in patients with progressive cerebral infarction. Neurology (NY) 11:601, 1961
23. Chesler E, King RA, Edwards JE: The myxomatous mitral valve and sudden death. Circulation 67:632, 1983
24. Collins R, Peto R, MacMahon S et al: Blood pressure, stroke and coronary heart disease. 2. Short-term reductions in blood pressure: overview of randomized drug trials in their epidemiological context. Lancet 335:827, 1990
25. Conneally PM, Dyken ML, Futty DE et al: Cooperative study of hospital frequency and character of transient ischemic attacks. VIII. Risk factors. JAMA 240:742, 1978
26. Davies MJ, Thomas AC, Knapman PA, Hangartner JE: Intramyocardial platelet aggregation in patients with unstable angina suffering sudden ischemic cardiac death. Circulation 73:418, 1986
27. Duke RJ, Bloch RF, Turpie AGG et al: Intravenous heparin for the prevention of stroke progression in acute partial stable stroke: A randomized controlled trial. Ann Intern Med 105:825, 1986
28. The Dutch TIA Trial Study Group: A comparison of two doses of aspirin (30 mg vs. 283 mg a day) in patients after a transient ischemic attack or minor ischemic stroke. N Engl J Med 325:1261, 1991
29. Dyken M: Meta analyses in the assessment of therapy of stroke prevention. Cerebrovasc Dis. In press.
30. Dyken ML: Antiplatelet aggregating agents in transient ischemic attacks and the relationship of risk factors. p. 141. In Breddin K, Loew D, Uberla K et al (eds): Prophylaxis of Venous, Peripheral Cardiac and Cerebral Vascular Diseases with Acetylsalicylic Acid. Schattauer Verlag, Stuttgart, 1981
31. Emmons PR, Harrison MJ, Honour AJ, Mitchell JR: Affect of a pyrimido pyrimidine derivative on thrombus formation in the rabbit. Nature 208:255, 1965
32. The ESPS Group: The European Stroke Prevention Study (ESPS): principal endpoints. Lancet 2:1351, 1987
33. Fields WS, Lemak NA, Frankowski RF, Hardy RJ: Controlled trials of aspirin in cerebral ischemia. Stroke 8:301, 1977
34. Fisher CM: Observations of the fundus oculi in transient monocular blindness. Neurology (NY) 9:333, 1959
35. Garde A, Samuelsson K, Fahlgren H et al: Treatment after transient ischemic attacks: a comparison between anticoagulant drug and inhibition of platelet aggregation. Stroke 14:677, 1983
36. Gent M, Blakely J, Easton JD et al: The Canadian-American Ticlopidine Study (CATS) in thromboembolic stroke. Lancet 1:1215, 1989
37. Gent M, Blakely JA, Hachinski V et al: A second prevention, randomized trial of suloctidil in patients with a recent history of thromboembolic stroke. Stroke 16:416, 1985
38. Genton E, Barnett HJM, Fields WS et al: Cerebral ischemia: the role of thrombosis and of antithrombotic therapy. Stroke 8:150, 1977
39. Grady PA, Blaumanis OR: Arterial wall changes in experimental stenosis. p. 347. In Reivich M, Hurtig HD (eds): Cerebrovascular Diseases. Raven Press, New York, 1983
40. Guiraud-Chaumeil B, Rascol AD, Boneu B et al: Prévention des récidives des accidents vasculaires cérébraux ischemiques parles anti-agrégants plaquettaires. Rev Neurol (Paris) 5:367, 1982
41. Gunning AJ, Pickering GW, Robb-Smith AHT, Russell RR: Mural thrombosis of the internal carotid artery and subsequent embolism. Q J Med 33:155, 1964
42. Haley EC, Kassell NF, Torner JC: Failure of heparin to prevent progression in progressing ischemic infarction. Stroke 19:10, 1988
43. Hankey FJ, Warlow CP, Slattery J: The prognosis of transient ischaemic attacks. J Neurol 237:142, 1990
44. Harter HR, Burch JW, Majerus PW et al: Prevention of thrombosis in patients on hemodialysis by low dose aspirin. N Engl J Med 301:577, 1978
45. Hass WK, Easton JD, Adams HP, Jr et al: A randomized trial comparing ticlopidine hydrochloride with aspirin for the prevention of stroke in high-risk patients. N Engl J Med 321:501, 1989
46. ISIS-2 Collaborative Group: Randomized trial of intravenous streptokinase, oral aspirin, both, or neither among 17,187 cases of suspected acute myocardial infarction. ISIS-2. Lancet 2:349, 1988
47. Kelton JG, Hirsh J, Carter CJ, Buchanan MR: Sex differences in the antithrombotic effects of aspirin. Blood 52:1973, 1978
48. Kelton JG, Powers P, Julian J et al: Sex-related differences in platelet aggregation: influence of hematocrit. Blood 56:38, 1980

49. Lewis HD, Jr, Davis JW, Archibald DG et al: Protective effects of aspirin against acute myocardial infarction and death in men with unstable angina. N Engl J Med 309:396, 1983
50. Marshall J, Wilkinson IMS: The prognosis of carotid transient ischemic attacks in patients with normal angiograms. Brain 94:395, 1971
51. Mustard JF, Rowsell HC, Smythe HA et al: The effect of sulfinpyrazone on platelet economy and thrombus formation in rabbits. Blood 29:859, 1967
52. Olsson J-E, Brechter C, Backlund H et al: Anticoagulant vs. anti-platelet therapy as prophylactic against cerebral infarction in transient ischemic attacks. Stroke 11:4, 1980
53. Pearce JMS, Gubbay SS, Walton JN: Long-term anticoagulant therapy in transient cerebral ischaemic attacks. Lancet 1:6, 1965
54. Peto R, Gray R, Collins R et al: Randomized trial of prophylactic daily aspirin in British male doctors. Br Med J 296:313, 1988
55. Relman AS: Aspirin for the primary prevention of myocardial infarction. (Editorial.) N Engl J Med 318:245, 1988
56. Reuther R, Domdorf W, Loew D: Behandlung transitorisch-ischämischer Attacken mit Acetylsalizylsaure Ergebnisse einer Doppelblindstudy. Munch Med Wochenschr 122:795, 1980
57. Smythe HA, Ogryzlo MD, Murphy EA, Mustard JF: Effect of sulpinpyrazone (Anturan) on platelet economy and blood coagulation in man. JAMA 92:818, 1965
58. Sorenson PS, Pedersen H, Marquardsen J et al: Acetylsalicylic acid in the prevention of stroke in patients with reversible cerebral ischemic attacks: a Danish cooperative study. Stroke 14:15, 1983
59. The Steering Committee of the Physician's Health Study Research Group: Special report: preliminary report: findings from the aspirin component of the ongoing physician's health study. N Engl J Med 318:262, 1988
60. The Steering Committee of the Physician's Health Study Research Group: Final report on the aspirin component of the ongoing physician's health study. N Engl J Med 321:129, 1989
61. Stroke Prevention in Atrial Fibrillation Study Group Investigators: Special report: preliminary report of the stroke prevention in atrial fibrillation study. N Engl J Med 322:386, 1990
62. Sullivan J, Harken DE, Gorlin R: Pharmacologic control of thromboembolic complications of cardiac-valve replacement. N Engl J Med 284:1391, 1971
63. Sundt TM, Jr, Dyken ML, Jr: Surgical treatment for ischemic vascular disease. p. 284. In Harrison MJG, Dyken ML (eds): Cerebral Vascular Disease. Butterworth's, London, England, 1983.
64. Taylor DW, Sackett DL, Haynes RB: Sample size for randomized trials in stroke prevention: how many patients do we need? Stroke 15:968, 1984
65. Theroux P, Ouimet H, McCans J et al: Aspirin, heparin, or both to treat acute unstable angina. N Engl J Med 349:1105, 1988
66. UK-TIA Study Group: United Kingdom transient ischaemic attack (UK-TIA) aspirin trial: interim results. Br Med J 296:316, 1988
67. Weiss HJ, Aledort LM: Impaired platelet connective-tissue in man after aspirin ingestion. Lancet 2:495, 1967
68. Wolf PA, Kannel WB, Cupples LA, D'Agostino RB: Risk factor interaction in cardiovascular and cerebrovascular disease. In Furlan AJ (ed): The Heart and Stroke—Exploring Mutual Cerebrovascular and Cardiovascular Issues. Springer-Verlag, London, 1987

# 39 PHARMACOLOGIC MODIFICATION OF ACUTE CEREBRAL ISCHEMIA

James C. Grotta

Treatment of cerebral ischemic disease is advancing rapidly. Recently completed and ongoing large randomized controlled studies have been based on an improving understanding of the pathophysiology of coagulation and fibrinolysis, cerebral blood flow, and ischemic neuronal injury. This chapter covers recent advances in therapy and some experimental approaches that are just beginning to have clinical evaluation.

Therapy of acute cerebral infarct has focused on three main strategies: prevention of thrombosis (anticoagulation), augmenting cerebral blood flow (reperfusion), and neuronal protection. Recent clinical trials have suggested a role for all three strategies, but one consistent finding in most trials is that, to be effective, any pharmacotherapy must be started very early, probably within the first 6 hours after the onset of symptoms.

## ANTICOAGULATION AND ANTITHROMBOTIC THERAPY

There is still no consensus on the use of anticoagulants in the setting of acute cerebral infarct, even though a recent survey found that heparin is administered to 38 to 73 percent of all stroke patients (Adams HP, personal communication). Studies to date have had conflicting or inconclusive results, or were performed before the development of modern neuroimaging techniques, which have improved our ability to exclude patients with cerebral hemorrhage. Current practice is to rely heavily on unproven empiric criteria for selecting patients. Presumably, those who have already completed a thrombotic event would not benefit from antithrombotic therapy. On the other hand, patients with a prothrombotic state, such as lupus anticoagulant, ongoing thrombosis formation, or underlying cardiac conditions likely to cause recurrent embolization, would be more logical candidates. In an attempt to evaluate anticoagulation therapy in these subgroups, investigators have recorded the rate of stroke progression and of recurrent embolization in patients treated with heparin compared to untreated patients. A recent study found a slight nonsignificant reduction of progression in patients with acute partial thrombotic stroke treated with heparin.[20] Slightly more convincing benefit has been reported in patients with major brain stem infarction.[86] Based on these data, there is inconclusive evidence supporting the use of anticoagulation in patients with suspected basilar artery occlusion or partial thrombotic stroke. The selection of such patients may be aided by newer diagnostic techniques, such as carotid and transcranial Doppler ultrasound and magnetic resonance angiography. If heparin therapy is chosen for such patients, it should be undertaken with the following caveats: a high-resolution computed tomography (CT) scan should be done to exclude hemorrhage; lumbar puncture is not necessary to detect hemorrhage if a high-resolution CT is negative; it is logical to begin heparin with an initial bolus of 1,000 units followed by a constant infusion of 800 to 1,200 U/h to result in an immediate 1.5 to 2.0 times prolongation of the partial thromboplastin time; and the platelet count should be followed daily to detect heparin-induced thrombocytopenia, which may lead to systemic vascular occlusion.[7,61] Heparin should be stopped if the platelet count falls below 100,000. The optimal duration of heparin treatment is not known, but it should be carefully withdrawn only after the patient has been stable for 72 hours and reintroduced if further worsening occurs.

Studies using heparin for preventing recurrent cardioembolic strokes have been slightly more suggestive, though still not conclusive. The arguments for and against anticoagulation for various cardiac conditions have recently been reviewed.[15] A collaborative study estimated that the risk of reembolization after a stroke associated with atrial fibrillation or myocardial infarction was as high as 1 percent/day or 14 to 16 percent over the first 2 weeks[14] and that heparin followed by coumadin will reduce this risk by approximately 66 percent.[13] However, this latter study was terminated prematurely before conclusive results were obtained. Because of the natural tendency toward hemorrhagic transformation of embolic infarcts, the benefits of anticoagulation may be outweighed by injudicious use. Again, the risks of anticoagulation are debated, since some investigators have found hemorrhagic complications in up to 24 percent of treated patients,[46,70] but others have found a much lower rate that did not differ from untreated patients.[68] As with treating progressing stroke, anticoagulation can be recommended for preventing recurrent cardioembolism, but, because of the risks and uncertainties in studies performed to date, there are several caveats that should be followed:[88] heparin should be delayed for at least 48 hours after stroke and hemorrhagic transformation excluded by a high-resolution CT scan; anticoagulation should not be carried out in patients with cerebral edema seen on CT; and, unlike treating progression, a bolus of heparin should not be administered. Again the optimal duration of treatment is unknown but should last as long as the underlying cardiac condition predisposing to embolism exists.

It is obvious that a carefully planned prospective trial of antithrombotic therapy is urgently needed to determine its role in cerebral infarct and, in particular, for preventing progression or recurrent embolization. Recent development of *low molecular weight heparinoids* and pilot studies demonstrating their safety and efficacy make it logical to employ these instead of heparin in such trials. Heparinoids have an antithrombotic affect by blocking factor Xa, but have less antithrombin III activity than heparin, do not significantly prolong the partial thromboplastin time, and therefore do not produce a net anticoagulant effect. They also do not seem to cause thrombocytopenia. Recent pilot studies of intravenous heparinoid determined the dose needed to produce therapeutic plasma anti-factor Xa levels[10] and found favorable outcome and a low risk of hemorrhagic complications compared to historical controls.

## REPERFUSION

Since infarction is caused by an interruption of blood supply to the brain, efforts to restore perfusion after stroke are logical, but to be effective such therapy probably must be employed within the first few minutes. Until recently, clinical trials did not incorporate this feature. Studies of middle cerebral artery occlusion in animals have shown that reopening the artery after more than 3 hours will not reduce infarct volume.[39] There are four strategies for improving reperfusion: vasodilation, increasing perfusion pressure, improving blood rheology, and removing the arterial obstruction.

### Vasodilation

Clinical studies of vasodilators have largely been negative probably because vasodilators have a major effect on vessels in normal brain, and less effect on vessels in ischemic regions that might already be dilated due to local tissue acidoses. An example is *prostacyclin,* which is a potent vasodilator as well as platelet antiaggregant, but which failed to improve outcome after stroke.[35] *Calcium channel blockers* are also vasodilators. While they are effective in treating vasospasm, which obviously may be associated were vasoconstriction in ischemic regions (see below), their efficacy in acute cerebral infarct remains to be proved, though the results of one clinical trial was positive.[26] If calcium blockers are proved effective, it is possible that some of their benefit may be the result of direct neuronal protection from calcium influx (see below).

### Increasing Perfusion Pressure and Improving Blood Rheology

Efforts to optimize perfusion pressure and blood rheology have also had mixed results. *Vasopressor therapy* increases perfusion pressure but also increases hydrostatic pressure and can aggravate cerebral edema. It is common clinical experience, however, that rapid lowering of perfusion pressure by injudicious use of antihypertensive drugs results in clinical worsening. *Isovolemic hemodilution* accomplished by phlebotomy associated with isovolemic volume replacement improves blood rheology by decreasing hematocrit and viscosity but has not improved outcome in large well-executed clinical trials.[37,69] Similarly, *pentoxifylline* improves rheology by improving red blood cell deformability but did not improve outcome.[55] *Hypervolemic hemodilution,* accomplished by raising intravascular volume monitored by pulmonary artery catheterization, results in both increased perfusion pressure and improved rheology. Increased left ventricular filling and consequent increased cardiac output increases cerebral perfusion, and dilutional lowering of hematocrit lowers viscosity. A pilot study of this therapy demonstrated improved outcome in patients treated early (within 12 hours) whose cardiac output responded to therapy, but also demonstrated cerebral edema in patients with large infarcts.[32] While the utility and safety of hypervolemic therapy must be proved by subsequent clinical evaluation in selected patients, it can be recommended that clinicians make every effort to maintain at least normovolemia and normotension in all patients. Future studies of hypervolemic hemodilution should include patients with high hematocrit, absence of brain edema on CT scan, and should be started within 6 hours of the onset of symptoms.

### Removing the Arterial Obstruction

*Thrombolysis* has now been proved effective in the coronary circulation and is under evaluation for very early strokes where obstruction of vessels by thrombus or embolism is still present. Preliminary studies have evaluated both intra-arterial streptokinase and urokinase[17,49] and intravenous tissue plasminogen activator (tPA), which is more clot-specific and results in less systemic fibrinolysis than streptokinase.[22] Because of its ease of administration, thereby allowing earlier intervention, tPA may be safer for stroke and is now the focus of several ongoing studies in the United States. A pilot study has demonstrated the feasibility and safety of up to 90 mg of tPA within 180 minutes of stroke onset,[11] and one positive preliminary controlled trial has been reported from Japan.[50] Despite early concerns that thrombolysis may not succeed or may result in cerebral hemorrhage or edema, preliminary reports from animal studies indicate that recanalization can occur without unacceptable side effects if treatment is begun within the first 1 to 3 hours.[90] Furthermore, tPA subfractions under development may be equally effective and safer.

The efficacy of thrombolytic therapy in stroke patients remains to be established. In addition, many questions exist about choice and route of agent, dose, need for associated antiplatelet or anticoagulant therapy to prevent reocclusion, and interval after stroke during which this therapy can be safely and effectively administered. While present practice patterns would limit thrombolytic therapy to that small subpopulation of stroke patients in whom arterial occlusion can be documented within the first few hours, the promise of effective treatment may increase patient awareness of stroke symptoms and treatment and galvanize clinicians toward earlier referral and evaluation of stroke patients, which would result in a higher yield of candidates for thrombolysis.

## NEURONAL PROTECTION

### Calcium Channel Blockers

Calcium channel blocker therapy has received wide attention because free calcium is normally excluded from the intracellular environment, but intracellular calcium levels rise within minutes after ischemia because of ion flux into neurons and liberation of intracellular stores. Calcium-activated proteases and phospholipases produce cytotoxic free radicals and leukotrienes, and persistent calcium-calmodulin binding in neurons for 2 to 4 hours after ischemia predicts irreversible damage.[29,58,60,87] The trigger for calcium entry into neurons after ischemia is unknown, but some calcium channels open after membrane depolarization (voltage-operated channels), and others may be forced open by the release of excitatory neurotransmitters such as glutamate (receptor-operated channels). One strategy for interrupting this cytotoxic chain of events is the administration of calcium channel blockers, especially the dihydropyridines (nifedipine, nimodipine, nicardipine, and nitrendipine) and diphenylalkylaminines (flunarizine, cinnarizine), which prevent calcium flux through one of three known voltage-operated channels.

Laboratory studies in animals indicate that these drugs may reduce delayed neuronal damage during reperfusion and increase cerebral blood flow by causing relaxation of vascular smooth muscle.[27,41,74] However, their ability to prevent calcium influx into neurons is probably limited by their action on only one calcium channel.[80] Moreover, there is great variability between these drugs in their effect on the cerebral circulation versus peripheral vascular bed. For instance, nifedipine has substantial peripheral but limited central activity, while nicardipine has both, and nimodipine has chiefly central activity. Furthermore, the potency of these drugs may differ in their effect on neuronal membrane channels. These considerations may explain the wide variability in results found in experimental stroke studies with this category of drugs.

Human studies to date have had mixed results. At least four studies have proved that nimodipine reduces morbidity from vasospasm after subarachnoid hemorrhage.[5,47,57] Consequently, nimodipine has been approved for this use and is the first pharmacotherapy ever approved primarily for a cerebrovascular indication (see below). A controlled prospective clinical trial of oral nimodipine 30 mg every 6 hours for 28 days was carried out in the Netherlands for acute ischemic stroke and demonstrated reduced morbidity and mortality when treatment was begun within 24 hours.[26] Nimodipine was not associated with significant hypotension or other serious side effects, although 14 patients were dropped from the study or did not complete the course of therapy in the nimodipine group versus 8 with placebo. Similar positive results were reported in a Spanish study,[82] but German and British nimodipine trials were negative.[33,81]

A recently completed study compared three doses of nimodipine (60, 120, and 240 mg daily) to placebo in 1,064 patients. Oral therapy was started within 48 hours of acute infarct and continued for 21 days. While there was no difference in mortality or outcome between any of the four groups overall, patients starting treatment with 60 or 120 mg daily within 12 hours of stroke did significantly better than placebo patients who demonstrated a net deterioration in score over the first 4 days of observation. This deterioration was not seen in treated patients.[48] In a study of 60 patients treated with intravenous nicardipine (2 to 7 mg/h) within 12 hours of stroke, 41 percent had little or no disability after 3 months, and patients starting treatment within 6 hours did better than those starting between 6 and 12 hours. There were no placebo controls in this study, and hypotension significantly limited the dose of nicardipine that could be given.[66] A randomized controlled study of IV nicardipine 2 mg/h started within 8 hours of stroke in Spain also suggested benefit in treated patients.[16] These results suggest that further studies of calcium channel blockers for acute cerebral infarct are justified but that treatment must be started within 6 to 12 hours to be effective, and that associated hypotension will probably limit therapy to relatively low doses, which most likely have more of an effect by raising cerebral blood flow than by limiting calcium influx into neurons.

## Glutamate Inhibitors and Antagonists

Glutamate inhibitors and antagonists are under evaluation because receptor-operated channels also provide a conduit for calcium entry into neurons after a variety of stimuli, including seizures, trauma, and ischemia. Among these is the *N*-methyl-*d*-aspartate (NMDA) ion channel, which is activated by glutamate and antagonized by noncompetitive (ketamine, phencyclidine [PCP], MK-801, dextrorphan) and competitive (CGS 19755, CPP) antagonists. The NMDA receptor has been the focus of recent research because it controls a major conduit for calcium and because it can be so easily manipulated pharmacologically.[67]

Delayed neuronal damage can be prevented by sectioning glutamatergic afferents to hippocampal neurons and by intraventricular administration of inhibitors of glutamate release such as cyclohexyl adenosine.[59,83] However, systemically administered baclofen provided no protection to hippocampal neurons, although measured levels of glutamate were elevated, indicating less glutamate release in treated animals.[56]

Since it may be difficult to prevent the massive release of glutamate after brain injury, the most intensive efforts have been directed at blocking the action of glutamate at the receptor level. These investigations have been encouraged by some striking results with MK-801 and related drugs that are very lipophilic and can be administered systemically. Numerous studies in animal models of focal ischemia have demonstrated protection in ischemic brain regions,[42,54,71,77] but one study suggests that these drugs may cause transient cytologic changes in normal neurons.[51] Also, noncompetitive NMDA antagonists may have prolonged action and other central effects besides those on the NMDA receptor, resulting in sedation and possibly memory disturbances. Therefore, there is great interest in less toxic agents such as dextrorphan[75] and in synthesizing and evaluating specific competitive NMDA antagonists. We have found that one such agent, CGS 19755, improves outcome and reduces cellular injury in a global ischemia model even when drug administration is begun after ischemia during the reperfusion phase.[28] Pilot human studies are underway to evaluate the toxicity and possible application of these drugs to such clinical situations as acute stroke, cardiac arrest, intraoperative brain protection, and cerebral trauma.[3]

## Free Radical Scavengers

Free radical scavengers are under evaluation because calcium entry into neurons and consequent activation of proteases and phospholipases results in formation of numerous potentially damaging byproducts of membrane lipid breakdown. These include arachidonic acid metabolites, which, in the presence of oxygen during reperfusion, provide a source of superoxide and hydroxyl free radical formation. Once these free radicals saturate endogenous antioxidants, they cause peroxidation of membrane lipids and a consequent disruption of blood-brain barrier and neuronal integrity. The free radical scavenger superoxide dismutase improves cerebral blood flow and reduces ischemic cerebral edema in animal models of reperfusion after stroke.[12,36] Since high doses of glucocorticosteroids also inhibit lipid peroxidation, there is much interest in 21-aminosteroids, which have no corticosteroid activity but strongly inhibit lipid peroxidation. In experimental models, these drugs reduce cerebral edema, neuronal injury, and mortality when begun before or after ischemia.[31]

## Gangliosides

Gangliosides are components of neuronal membranes that are important in cellular repair and are known to improve recovery of peripheral nerve lesions. Gangliosides may work in part by preventing membrane inositol hydrolysis. Inositol triphosphate is a "second messenger," and its production after a variety of stimuli results in release of intracellular calcium stores. Ganglioside $GM_1$, administered 30 minutes after middle cerebral artery (MCA) occlusion in cats, improved outcome and reduced neuronal damage.[43] However, a recent small clinical evaluation was negative,[38] and a large controlled trial in Italy had equivocal results. In this study 502 patients were randomized to receive either placebo or ganglioside $GM_1$ for 15 days. While the treated patients showed more improvement during the period of treatment, this difference was no longer evident at the end of follow-up (4 months).[6] Further studies of more prolonged therapy are planned.

### Opiate Antagonists and Agonists

Opiate antagonists and agonists have been evaluated following preliminary observations that the nonselective opiate antagonist naloxone improved outcome after spinal cord injury and experimental cerebral ischemia.[21,34,89] Consequently, there was considerable interest in the hypothesis that neuronal damage might be caused by activation of opiate receptors. Clinical studies in stroke patients, however, have been inconclusive. Naloxone can be given safely in large doses,[2] but its efficacy was never thoroughly demonstrated.

Recently, investigators have focused on stimulation or inactivation of the kappa opiate receptor subtype. Synthetic kappa opiate agonists have been studied in animal models of cerebral ischemia with encouraging results.[78] Kappa-related compounds are under intensive investigation in spinal cord trauma, and, if studies are positive, it is hoped they be evaluated more thoroughly in stroke patients.

## OTHER THERAPY

### Steroids

There is no evidence supporting the routine use of *glucocorticosteroids* for acute cerebral infarct.[18] Theoretically, steroids have some free radical scavenging effect and may reduce vasogenic edema, but this is usually not a major contributor to cerebral edema after acute infarction. In a study of 100 patients with middle cerebral artery distribution infarction randomized to 100 mg dexamethasone IV daily for 7 days versus placebo, there was no difference in the patients after 1 year of follow-up. However, over the short term there was more rapid improvement in the steroid-treated patients, especially in those with large strokes and presumably worse cerebral edema.[52] If edema does occur, dehydrating agents such as *glycerol* are probably preferable to steroids. In a recent study, intravenous glycerol reduced mortality after acute cerebral infarct, probably because it reduced cerebral edema.[9]

One condition for which steroids are probably of value is cerebral arteritis. Steroids have been used as the first line of treatment for both systemic rheumatic diseases affecting the brain and for isolated central nervous system (CNS) angiitis. Though prospective studies are lacking, it is conventional practice to administer the equivalent of 80 to 100 mg prednisone daily until the patient's clinical course is stabilized. *Cyclophosphamide* may be added if deterioration continues, but most authorities now recommend that a pulse of this drug should be given along with prednisone as initial therapy. Therapy should be continued until disease activity disappears either by serologic markers or by arteriography, and then slowly withdrawn. If the vasculitis is due to infection such as meningovascular lues, tuberculosis, or herpes zoster, appropriate *antimicrobial or antiviral therapy* should be administered.

### Heparin

Subcutaneous heparin, 5,000 units every 12 hours, will prevent deep-vein thrombosis (DVT) and presumably pulmonary emboli. In one randomized study of 104 patients, Gelmers found DVT in 23 percent of placebo and 2 percent of heparin-treated patients and reported no bleeding complications or increase in hemorrhagic transformation of the infarct. Two patients had fatal pulmonary emboli in the placebo group and none in the heparin group.[25]

### Antidepressants

Depression has been recognized in 30 to 50 percent of patients during the first year after stroke but may not occur until the patient leaves the hospital and rehabilitation setting.[63] Such depression is often associated with an abnormal dexamethasone suppression test[23] and shows a gratifying response to tricyclic antidepressant therapy. *Nortriptyline* 100 mg QHS is effective for poststroke emotional lability as well as depression.[45,53,62] Both the biochemical basis of poststroke depression as well as our emerging understanding of the role of neurotransmitters and opiates in the worsening of ischemic injury argue against the widespread and unselective use of CNS depressant drugs such as hypnotics, tranquilizers, and some antihypertensive agents during the poststroke period. Finally, recent reports, suggesting the benefit of *bromocriptine* for poststroke aphasia, and *dopamine agonists* for neglect,[4,24] underscore the potential of neurotransmitter manipulation during stroke rehabilitation.

## Physical, Occupational, and Speech Therapy

Physical, occupational, and speech therapy are of value, although studies have had conflicting results.[19,44,72,76,85] One recent anecdotal report emphasizes that frequent and prolonged therapy can result in improved language function.[84]

## Increased Intracranial Pressure

For the neurologist, management of raised intracranial pressure (ICP) (ICP above 15 mmHg or 20 $cmH_2O$) is a major challenge, and attention has been focused on the value of ICP monitoring in patients with strokes associated with brain swelling.[65] Timely ventriculostomy allows measurement of ICP as well as drainage of cerebrospinal fluid (CSF) and should be considered for patients who are deteriorating from increased ICP. If the ventricles are not large enough to accommodate a catheter, a subarachnoid monitor can be substituted.

When uncontrolled ICP is associated with decreasing level of consciousness or other signs of herniation, the patient should be carefully intubated and hyperventilated to a $PCO_2$ of 25 to 30 mmHg, remembering that excessive coughing or straining associated with intubation causes a dramatic increase in ICP. The assistance of experienced nursing, respiratory therapy, and anesthesia personnel is invaluable. Morphine sulfate 2 to 10 mg intravenously every 2 hours can allay agitation in patients requiring intubation who are still conscious and is a useful adjunct in controlling ICP. Muscular paralysis with metacurine 0.3 mg/kg may be necessary and is a better choice than pancuronium, which is a sympathomimetic and may cause hypertension and tachycardia. The head should be elevated 30 degrees in all patients with increased ICP.

Appropriate management of blood pressure frequently poses a dilemma, because many patients have severe underlying systemic hypertension aggravated by sympathetic overactivity and reflex hypertension in response to elevated ICP. It may be necessary to lower mean arterial blood pressure (MABP) to prevent renal and cardiac injury. However, cerebral perfusion pressure (MABP-ICP) must be maintained above 50 mmHg to insure adequate CBF. In controlling dangerously increased MABP, the best approach is first, make every effort to lower ICP, and then carefully titrate intravenous antihypertensive drugs if necessary once adequate cerebral perfusion is assured. Though nitroprusside has been used most frequently, parenteral beta blockers (labetalol 20 to 60 mg IV each 20 minutes until blood pressure is controlled) prevent associated sympathetic overactivity. The newer parenteral calcium channel blockers may also be useful. Diuretics are often given, but it is essential to avoid volume depletion or hemoconcentration, and careful volume expansion with isotonic fluids may be indicated to maintain optimal cardiac output and tissue perfusion. Hypotonic fluids should not be used.

Osmotic therapy with mannitol should be given acutely for uncontrolled increased ICP, and can be used repetitively (0.25 to 1 g/kg every 4 hours) to help control ICP on a longer-term basis. Serum osmolality should be monitored and maintained between 300 to 320 mOsm. The value of corticosteroid therapy is still debated. Studies have not proved that these drugs are useful acutely,[18,52,79] but they may prevent delayed vasogenic edema. High-dose barbiturate therapy (pentobarbital 3 to 30 mg/kg intravenously followed by 1 to 2 mg/kg/h) is heroic, but as yet unproved treatment.[64]

# VASOSPASM

The most common cause of morbidity after aneurysmal subarachnoid hemorrhage (SAH) is cerebral ischemia resulting from arterial spasm. Three recent large controlled studies confirmed Allen's original observation that *nimodipine* reduced mortality and bad outcome due to vasospasm compared to placebo,[5,47,57] and this drug is now approved for noncomatose patients. The approved dose is 60 mg orally or per nasogastric tube every 4 hours for 21 days begun within 96 hours of SAH. Side effects include hypotension, headache, edema, and muscle cramps, but the drug is generally well tolerated. An intravenous preparation of a related drug, nicardipine, is under evaluation,[1] and preliminary results have shown reduced angiographic and clinical vasospasm.[30] Adjunctive therapy for vasospasm, namely, *volume expansion* can be carried out once the aneurysm is successfully clipped,[8,40,73] and raising perfusion pressure by *vasopressors* if necessary, should be considered for symptomatic patients. Appropriate monitoring of intravascular volume, cardiac output, and intracranial pressure are important if these treatments are instituted.

# REFERENCES


1. Adams H, Flamm E, Beck D et al: A study of nicardipine in prevention of infarction after subarachnoid hemorrhage. Stroke 18:281, 1987
2. Adams HP, Olinger CP, Barsan WG et al: A dose-escalation of study of large doses of naloxone for treatment of patients with acute cerebral ischemia. Stroke 17:404, 1986
3. Albers GW, Goldberg MP, Choi DW: *N*-methyl-*d*-aspartate antagonists: ready for clinical trial in brain ischemia? Ann Neurol 25:398, 1989
4. Albert ML, Bachman DL, Morgan A, Helm-Estabrooks N: Pharmacotherapy for aphasia. Neurology (NY) 38:877, 1988
5. Allen GS, Ahn HS, Preziosi TJ et al: Cerebral arterial spasm—a controlled trial of nimodipine in

patients with subarachnoid hemorrhage. N Engl J Med 308:619, 1983

6. Argentino G, Sacchetti ML, Toni D et al: $GM_1$ ganglioside therapy in acute ischemic stroke. Stroke 20:1143, 1989
7. Atkinson JLD, Sundt TM Jr, Kazmier FJ et al: Heparin-induced thrombocytopenia and thrombosis in ischemic stroke. Mayo Clin Proc 63:353, 1988
8. Awad IA, Carter LP, Spetzler RF et al: Clinical vasospasm after subarachnoid hemorrhage: response to hypervolemic hemodilution and arterial hypertension. Stroke 18:365, 1987
9. Bayer AJ, Pathy MSJ, Newcome R: Double-blind randomised trial of intravenous glycerol in acute stroke. Lancet 405, 1987
10. Biller J, Massey ED, Marler JR et al: A dose escalation study of ORG 10172 (low molecular weight heparinoid) in stroke. Neurology (NY) 39:262, 1989
11. Brott T, Haley C, Levy D et al: Safety and potential efficacy of tissue plasminogen activator (tPA) for stroke. Stroke 21:181, 1990
12. Cerchiari EL, Hoel TM, Safar P, Sclabassi RJ: Protective effects of combined superoxide dismutase and desferoxamine on recovery of cerebral blood flow and function after cardiac arrest in dogs. Stroke 18:869, 1987
13. Cerebral Embolism Study Group: Immediate anticoagulation of embolic stroke: a randomized trial. Stroke 14:668, 1983
14. Cerebral Embolism Task Force: Cardiogenic brain embolism. Arch Neurol 43:71, 1986
15. Cerebral Embolism Task Force: Cardiogenic brain embolism. Arch Neurol 46:727, 1989
16. Davalos A, Cendra E, Gonzalez B et al: Double-blind randomized clinical trial of nicardipine vs placebo in acute ischemic stroke: clinical, radiological and biochemical evaluation of the ischemic area: preliminary results. (Presented at the Fourteenth World Congress of Neurology, New Delhi, October 27, 1989.)
17. Del Zoppo GJ, Zeumer H, Harker LA: Thrombolytic therapy in stroke: possibilities and hazards. Stroke 17:595, 1986
18. De Reuck J, Vandekerckhove T, Bosma G et al: Steroid treatment in acute ischaemic stroke. Eur Neurol 28:70, 1988
19. Dignan MB, Howard G, Toole JF et al: Evaluation of the North Carolina Stroke Care Program. Stroke 17:817, 1986
20. Duke RJ, Bloch RF, Turpie AGG et al: Intravenous heparin for the prevention of stroke progression in acute partial stable stroke: a randomized controlled trial. Ann Intern Med 105:825, 1986
21. Faden AI, Jacobs TP, Holaday JW: Opiate antagonist improves neurologic recovery after spinal injury. Science 211:493, 1981
22. Fears R: Biochemical pharmacology and therapeutic aspects of thrombolytic agents. Pharmacol Rev 42:201, 1990
23. Finklestein S, Benowitz LI, Baldessarini RJ et al: Mood, vegetative disturbance and dexamethasone suppression test after stroke. Ann Neurol 12:463, 1982
24. Fleet WS, Valenstein E, Watson RT, Heilman KM: Dopamine agonist therapy for neglect in humans. Neurology (NY) 37:1765, 1987
25. Gelmers HJ: Effects of low-dose subcutaneous heparin on the occurrence of deep vein thrombosis in patients with ischemic stroke. Acta Neurol Scand 61:313, 1980
26. Gelmers HJ, Gorter K, de Weerdt CJ, Wiezer JHA: A controlled trial of nimodipine in acute ischemic stroke. N Engl J Med 318:203, 1988
27. Grotta JC, Pettigrew LC, Rosenbaum D et al: Efficacy and mechanism of action of a calcium channel blocker after global cerebral ischemia in rats. Stroke 19:447, 1988
28. Grotta JC, Picone CM, Ostrow PT: The glutamate antagonist CGS-19755 improves behavior and cellular damage after ischemia. J Cereb Blood Flow Metab, suppl 1. 9:S303, 1989
29. Haas WK: Beyond cerebral blood flow, metabolism and ischemic thresholds: an examination of the role of calcium in the initiation of cerebral infarction. p. 3. In Meyer JS, Lechner H, Reivich M et al (eds): Cerebral Vascular Disease. Vol. 3. Proceedings of the Tenth International Conference. Excerpta Medica, Amsterdam, 1981
30. Haley EC, Kassell NF, Torner JC, Kongable G: Nicardipine ameliorates angiographic vasospasm following subarachnoid hemorrhage (SAH). Neurology (NY), suppl 1. 41:346, 1991
31. Hall E, Pazara K, Braugher JM: 21-Aminosteroid lipid peroxidation inhibitor U74006F protects against cerebral ischemia in gerbils. Stroke 19:997, 1988
32. The Hemodilution in Stroke Study Group: Hypervolemic hemodilution treatment of acute stroke: results of a randomized multicenter trial using pentastarch. Stroke 20:317, 1989
33. Hornig CR, Kaps M, Hacke W et al: Nimodipine in acute ischemic stroke. Stroke 22:29, 1991
34. Hosobuchi Y, Baskin WS, Woo SK: Reversal of induced ischemic neurologic deficit in gerbils by the opiate antagonist naloxone. Science 215:69, 1982
35. Hsu CY, Faught RE Jr, Furlan AJ et al: Intravenous prostacyclin in acute nonhemorrhagic stroke: a placebo-controlled double-blind trial. Stroke 18:352,1987
36. Imaizumi S, Woolworth V, Fishman RA, Chan PH: Superoxide dismutase activities and their role in focal cerebral ischemia. J Cereb Blood Flow Metab, suppl 1. 9:S217, 1989
37. Italian Acute Stroke Study Group: Haemodilution in acute stroke: results of the Italian haemodilution trial. Lancet 1:318, 1988
38. Jamieson DG, Reivich M, Alves W et al: Ganglioside ($GM_1$) treatment of acute ischemic infarction: a randomized, double-blind study using positron emission tomography. Neurology (NY), suppl 1. 39:217, 1989
39. Kaplan BA, Wang XJ, Pulsinelli WA: The therapeutic window in a rat model of reversible focal ischemia. Stroke 21:175, 1990
40. Kassell NF, Peerless SJ, Durward QJ et al: Treatment of ischemic deficits from vasospasm with

intravascular volume expansion and induced arterial hypertension. Neurosurgery 11:337, 1982
41. Kazda S, Hoffmeister F, Garthoff B, Towart R: Prevention of the postischaemic impaired reperfusion of the brain by nimodipine (BAY e 9736). Acta Neurol Scand [Suppl] 72:302, 1979
42. Kochhar A, Zivin JA, Lyden PD, Mazzarella V: Glutamate antagonist therapy reduces neurologic deficits produced by focal central nervous system ischemia. Arch Neurol 45:148, 1988
43. Komatsumoto S, Greenberg J, Hickey W, Reivich M: Effect of the ganglioside GM1 on neurologic function, electroencephalogram amplitude, and histology in chronic middle cerebral artery occlussion in cats. Stroke 19:1027, 1988
44. Lincoln NB, McGuirk E, Mulley GP et al: Effectiveness of speech therapy for aphasic stroke patients: a randomized controlled trial. Lancet 1:1197, 1984
45. Lipsey JR, Robinson RG, Pearlson GD et al: Nortriptyline treatment of post-stroke depression: a double-blind study. Lancet 1:297, 1984
46. Lodder J, van der Lugt PJM: Evaluation of the risk of immediate anticoagulant treatment in patients with embolic stroke of cardiac origin. Stroke 14:42, 1983
47. Mee E, Dorrance D, Lowe D, Neil-Dwyer G: Controlled study of nimodipine in aneurysm patients treated early after subarachnoid hemorrhage. Neurosurgery 22:484, 1988
48. Mohr JP, Dilanni M, Muschett JL et al: Nimodipine in acute ischemic stroke. Ann Neurol 26:124, 1989
49. Mori E, Tabuchi M, Yoshida T, Yamadori A: Intracarotid urokinase with thromboembolic occlusion of the middle cerebral artery. Stroke 19:802, 1988
50. Mori E, Yoneda Y, Ohksawa S et al: Double-blind, placebo-controlled trial of recombinant tissue plasminogen activator (rt-PA) in acute carotid stroke. Neurology (NY), suppl 1. 41:347, 1991
51. Olney JW, Labruyere J, Price MT: Pathological changes induced in cerebrocortical neurons by phencyclidine and related drugs. Science 244:1360, 1989
52. Paal G, Grossmann W, Kick J, Velho-Groneberg P: Dexamethasone and stroke—a one year follow-up study. (Oral presentation, Fourteenth World Congress of Neurology, New Delhi, October 27, 1989.)
53. Parikh RM, Robinson RG, Lipsey JR, Price TR: Nortriptyline treatment of post-stroke emotional lability: a double-blind study. Neurology (NY), suppl 1. 39:177, 1989
54. Park CK, Nehls DG, Graham DI et al: Focal cerebral ischaemia in the cat: treatment with the glutamate antagonist MK-801 after induction of ischaemia. J Cereb Blood Flow Metab 8:757, 1988
55. Pentoxifylline Study Group: Pentoxifylline (PTX) in acute ischemic stroke. Stroke 18:298, 1987
56. Pettigrew LC, Rosenbaum DM, Ostrow PT, Grotta JC: The effect of baclofen on regional glutamate levels in normal and ischemic brain. J Cereb Blood Flow Metab, suppl 1. 9:S304, 1989
57. Pickard JD, Murray GD, Illingworth R: Effect of oral nimodipine on cerebral infarction and outcome after subarachnoid hemorrhage: British aneurysm nimodipine trial. Br Med J 298:636, 1989
58. Picone CM, Grotta JC, Earls J et al: Immunohistochemical determination of calcium-calmodulin binding predicts neuronal damage after global ischemia. J Cereb Blood Flow Metab 9:805, 1989
59. Pulsinelli WA: Deafferentation of the hippocampus protects CA1 pyramidal neurons against ischemic injury. Stroke 16:144, 1985
60. Raichle ME: The pathophysiology of brain ischemia. Ann Neurol 13:2, 1983
61. Ramirez-Lassepas M, Cipolle RJ, Rodvold KA et al: Heparin-induced thrombocytopenia in patients with cerebrovascular ischemic disease. Neurology (NY) 34:736, 1984
62. Reding JR, Orta LA, Winter SW et al: Antidepressant therapy after stroke. Arch Neurol 43:763, 1986
63. Robinson RG, Price TR: Post-stroke depressive disorders: a follow-up study of 103 patients. Stroke 13:635, 1982
64. Rockoff MA, Marshall LF, Shapiro HM: High-dose barbiturate therapy in humans: a clinical review of 60 patients. Ann Neurol 6:194, 1979
65. Rockoff MA, Ropper AH: Treatment of intracranial hypertension. p. 21. In Ropper AH, Kennedy FK, Zervas NT (eds): Neurological and Neurosurgical Intensive care. University Park Press, Baltimore, 1983
66. Rosenbaum DM, Zabramski J, Frey J et al: Early treatment of ischemic stroke with a calcium antagonist. Stroke 22:437, 1991
67. Rothman SM, Olney JW: Glutamate and the pathophysiology of hypoxic-ischemic brain damage. Ann Neurol 19:105, 1986
68. Rothrock JF, Dittrich HC, McAllen S et al: Acute anticoagulation following cardioembolic stroke. Stroke 20:730, 1989
69. Scandinavian Stroke Study Group: Multicenter trial of hemodilution in acute ischemic stroke: results in the total patient population. Stroke 18:691, 1987
70. Shields RW Jr, Laureno R, Lachman T, Victor M: Anticoagulant-related hemorrhage in acute cerebral embolism. Stroke 15:426, 1984
71. Simon RP, Swan JH, Griffiths T, Meldrum BS: Blockade of NMDA receptors may protect against ischemic damage in the brain. Science 226:850, 1984
72. Sivenius J, Pyorala K, Heinonen O et al: The significance of intensity of rehabilitation of stroke—a controlled trial. Stroke 16:928, 1985
73. Solomon RA, Fink ME, Lennihan L: Prophylactic volume expansion therapy for the prevention of delayed cerebral ischemia after early aneurysm surgery. Arch Neurol 45:325, 1988
74. Steen PA, Newberg IA, Milde JH, Michenfelder JD: Nimodipine improves cerebral blood flow and neurologic recovery after complete cerebral ischemia in the dog. J Cereb Blood Flow Metab 3:38, 1983
75. Steinberg GK, Saleh J, Kunis D et al: Protective

effect of *N*-methyl-*d*-aspartate antagonists after focal cerebral ischemia in rabbits. Stroke 20:1247, 1989
76. Strand T, Asplund K, Eriksson S et al: Stroke unit care: who benefits?: comparisons with general medical care in relation to prognostic indicators on admission. Stroke 17:377, 1986
77. Swan JH, Meldrum BS: Early, not late, administration of NMDA receptor antagonists protects against selective ischaemic cell loss. J Cereb Blood Flow Metab, suppl 1. 9:S558, 1989
78. Tang AH: Protection from cerebral ischemia by U-50, 488E, a specific kappa opioid analgesic agent. Life Sci 37:1475, 1985
79. Tellez H, Bauer RB: Dexamethasone as treatment in cerebrovascular disease: a controlled study in intracerebral hemorrhage. Stroke 4:541, 1973
80. Thayer S, Murphy S, Miller R: Widespread distribution of dihydropyridine-sensitive calcium channels in the central nervous system. Mol Pharmacol 30:505, 1986
81. Trust Study Group: Randomized, double-blind, placebo-controlled trial of nimodipine in acute stroke. Lancet 336:1205, 1990
82. Vila EM, Guillen F, Villanueva JS et al: Placebo-controlled trial of nimodipine in the treatment of acute ischemic cerebral infarction. Stroke 21:1023, 1990
83. von Lubitz DKJE, Dambrosia JM, Kempski O, Redmon DJ: Cyclohexyl adenosine protects against neuronal death following ischemia in CA1 region of gerbil hippocampus. Stroke 19:1133, 1988
84. Wender D: Aphasic victim as investigator. Arch Neurol 46:91, 1989
85. Wentz RT, Weiss DG, Aten JL et al: Comparison of clinic, home, and deferred language treatment for aphasia: a Veterans Administration cooperative study. Arch Neurol 43:653, 1986
86. Whisnant JP: Discussion of progressing stroke: anticoagulant therapy. p. 182. In Milikan CH, Siekert RH, Whisnant JP (eds): Cerebral Vascular Diseases. Proceedings of the Third Research Conference. Grune & Stratton, Orlando, FL, 1961
87. Wieloch T, Harris RJ, Siesjo BK: Brain metabolism and ischemia: mechanism of cell damage and principals of protection. J Cereb Blood Flow Metab, suppl. 1. 2:S5, 1982
88. Yatsu FM, Hart RG, Mohr JP, Grotta JC: Anticoagulation of embolic strokes of cardiac origin: an update. Neurology (NY) 38:314, 1988
89. Young W, Flamm ES, Demopoulos HB et al: Naloxone ameliorates post-traumatic ischemia in experimental spinal contusion. J Neurosurg 55:209, 1981
90. Zivin JA, Fisher M, DeGirolami U et al: Tissue plaminogen activator reduced neurological damage after cerebral embolism. Science 230:1289, 1985

# 40
# *THROMBOLYTIC AND DEFIBRINOGENATING AGENTS FOR ISCHEMIC AND HEMORRHAGIC STROKE*

Thomas Brott

Acute thrombus formation or migration are the principal acute pathologic events for two-thirds or more of ischemic stroke patients angiographically studied within 6 hours of symptom onset.[42] Following acute rupture of a cerebral aneurysm, the resulting intrathecal clot is a principal determinant of delayed cerebral vasospasm.[47] With intracerebral hemorrhage (ICH), the acute bleeding and clot formation are principal determinants of patient mortality and morbidity.[13] Consequently, for ischemic and hemorrhagic stroke, the potential therapeutic role of thrombolytic and defibrinogenating agents has evoked considerable interest, particularly over the last 5 years.

For acute cerebral infarction, reviews of the experimental[110] and clinical[15,35,109,111] thrombolytic therapy investigations are available. For subarachnoid hemorrhage (SAH), a growing literature has been recently discussed.[44] For ICH, investigation of thrombolytic therapy has been modest.[91]

## THROMBOLYSIS FOR CEREBRAL INFARCTION

Following thrombolytic therapy for myocardial infarction,[81,122] the arterial recanalization rate has been 70 to 80 percent. Effective agents[81] include urokinase, single-chain urokinase-plasminogen activator (scu-PA), streptokinase, acylated plasminogen-streptokinase activator complex (APSAC), and tissue plasminogen activator (tPA). The mechanism of action for each of these agents differs,[24,81] but they all act directly or indirectly as plasminogen activators.

### Studies Prior to Computed Tomography

From 1958 to 1979, streptokinase,[6,80,85,86] urokinase,[1–3,14,48,59,60,84] thrombolysin,[22,87] fibrinolysin,[63,80,88,114] and plasmin[88] were studied as potential therapy for patients with acute ischemic stroke.

Treatment was usually given after a considerable delay following symptom onset, always several hours and sometimes several days. ICH was not adequately excluded, given that pretreatment computed tomography (CT) could not be performed. Hemorrhagic complications were probably increased by the anticoagulant therapy that often followed the thrombolytic regimen.

Clot lysis was documented for intravenous thrombolysin[22] and intravenous streptokinase.[85,86] Nonetheless, enthusiasm faltered following reports of discouraging clinical outcomes,[48,59,86] including often-fatal cerebral hemorrhage. One randomized study was completed:[86] 73 patients with progressive stroke were randomized to either streptokinase plus anticoagulation or to anticoagulation alone; 13 treated patients died, compared to 4 of the controls. Of the 10 treated patients examined postmortem, 3 had major intracerebral hemorrhage, and 1 had hemorrhagic infarction.

## Studies Following Availability of Computed Tomography

No blinded, randomized trials of thrombolytic therapy for acute cerebral infarction have been performed in the CT era. However, descriptions of the treatment of more than 400 acute stroke patients have been published. Urokinase,[4,18,50,58,90,98,103] streptokinase,[18,28,57,58,92,116] and tPA[16,19,120] have been tested. A phase I safety trial of APSAC is underway.

### Arterial Recanalization

Early clot lysis was documented for 50 percent of the stroke patients treated with intra-arterial streptokinase or urokinase (85 or 169) (Table 40-1)[28,34,58,90,116,120] following a variety of dosage regimens. Successful recanalization was accomplished in patients with cardiac embolic stroke, patients with atherothrombotic stroke, and patients with atheroembolic stroke—including patients with vertebrobasilar stroke.[58] The number of patients in any single study was too small to demonstrate or rule out a dose-effect response, or a relationship of patient age, gender, race, blood pressure, or medications to recanalization. Because of the limits of cerebral angiography, no information could be reported regarding thrombolysis within very small arteries or arterioles.

Patients treated early in the angiographic pilot study of Del Zoppo and colleagues[34] were more likely to have successful thrombolysis. Time from symptom onset to treatment was not clearly related to recanalization in the other angiographic studies.[28,58,90,116] In the setting of myocardial infarction, early treatment has facilitated clot lysis,[81] and fresh thrombi have been shown to be more susceptible to lysis than are older, well-organized thrombi.[49,69,99]

Large-volume thrombi were less likely to be lysed in the study of 22 patients treated with urokinase reported by Mori et al.[90] In the other angiographic studies, the volume of thrombus was not singled out as a negative predictor of thrombolysis.[28,34,58,116] Nonetheless, in a study of intravenous tPA without angiography,[118] the thrombi large enough to be visualized by the pretreatment CT (i.e., positive dense artery sign) were associated with lack of major clinical improvement and with the development of a large infarction-volume by CT, suggesting that recanalization was not achieved.

Angiographic information regarding recanalization rates with intravenous administration of streptokinase or urokinase is not available. Angiographic information is available for an ongoing open-label trial of intravenous tPA.[120] Of 57 patients who were found to have major arterial occlusions and who were treated within 8 hours of symptom-onset, 22 had partial or complete early recanalization (39 percent). This recanalization rate is similar to that shown to date for intra-arterial therapy (50 percent). The spon-

**TABLE 40-1. Recanalization Following Thrombolytic Therapy[a]**

| Agent | Time | Number Treated | Number (%) Recanalized | Stroke Type | Ref. |
|---|---|---|---|---|---|
| IA UK or SK | <2 wk (29 ≤ 24 h) | 43 | 19 (44) | Vertebrobasilar | 58 |
| IA UK or SK | 1–24 h (7.6 h mean) | 20 | 15 (75) | Carotid | 34 |
| IA UK | 50 min–12 h (4.5 h mean) | 22 | 10 (45) | MCA | 90 |
| IA SK | 30 min–3 wk | 12 | 12 (100) | Carotid | 116 |
| IA SK | 2 h–7 da | 15 | 7 (47) | Carotid (9) Vertebrobasilar (6) | 28 |
| IV tPA | ≤8 h | 57 | 22 (38) | Carotid Vertebrobasilar | 120 |
| Total | | 169 | 85 (50) | | |

*Abbreviations:* IA, intra-arterial; UK, urokinase; SK, streptokinase; IV, intravenous, tPA, tissue plasminogen activator; MCA, middle cerebral artery.

[a] Includes those studies with pre- and post-treatment angiography.

taneous recanalization rate without thrombolytic therapy has varied in clinical reports from 40 to 80 percent, but this rate has been determined in selected stroke patients studied with serial angiography over several days following symptom-onset.[29,30,43,66,108] The rate of spontaneous thrombolysis during the first hours after onset is not known.

Why is the reported rate of thrombolytic arterial recanalization so much lower for stroke than the recanalization rates of 60 to 70 percent or more reported for myocardial infarction?[81] In the stroke studies, many patients have been treated with lower doses of drug.[120] The time from symptom onset to the time of drug administration in the stroke angiographic studies has been hours longer than in the myocardial infarction studies. Furthermore, with the acutely occluded coronary artery, a fresh thrombus is present,[36] which is subject to the near-constant mechanical deformation resulting from the systolic contraction of the heart. With stroke, some of the thrombi could be older, better organized with more fibrin cross-linking, and so resistant to thrombolysis. Long, large-volume thrombi may be lodged quietly in the distal internal carotid artery and/or the middle cerebral stem,[42] disturbed only by arterial pulsation, with minimal surface area exposed to endogenous (or exogenous) thrombolytic substances.

## Clinical Benefit

No randomized trials of thrombolytic therapy for acute cerebral infarction have been completed since the introduction of CT scanning, and so clinical efficacy cannot be estimated with any accuracy. In the nonrandomized trials, clinical outcomes reported as "favorable," "excellent," or even "poor" cannot be adequately interpreted, particularly as no historical controls are available for comparison (in whom neurologic examinations were performed within the first hours after stroke onset). Recognizing these limitations, the pooled clinical results are considerably more encouraging than the results reported prior to the availability of CT.

Of the 342 patients reported for whom clinical information is provided, 124 (36 percent) showed major improvement.[16,28,34,50,58,90,92,103,116] Many of the responses could have been secondary to thrombolysis (Fig. 40-1). For patients with clinical and angiographic information provided, major improvement occurred in 32 of 63 with recanalization (51 percent) but occurred in only 3 of 49 without recanalization (6 percent) ($P$ = 0.000001, chi-square test).[28,34,58,90,116] This disparity cannot be readily explained by spontaneous improvement or by improvement related to patient selection (e.g., selecting patients experiencing transient ischemic attacks (TIAs)). For 31 of the 63 patients with early arterial recanalization, thrombolytic therapy failed with regard to clinical outcome (will successful thrombolysis, achieved within 2 to 6 hours, be too late for many stroke patients?).

Major improvement followed treatment of patients with cardiac embolic stroke and treatment of patients with large-vessel atherothrombotic stroke. Conclusions cannot be drawn regarding whether a particular patient profile will predict a positive (or negative) neurologic response to therapy. Comparisons of large numbers of randomized patients, treated compared to untreated, will be necessary.

Little solid information is available regarding patients with the clinical diagnosis of small-vessel occlusion. Limited numbers of such patients have been treated with thrombolytic therapy, and none have had pre- and post-treatment angiography. The pathophysiology of cerebral small-vessel distribution infarction is variable[53] and not clearly understood.[77] If the formation of a small-volume thrombus is an important acute event, then prompt thrombolytic therapy has potential to provide prompt recanalization, perhaps even in small doses.

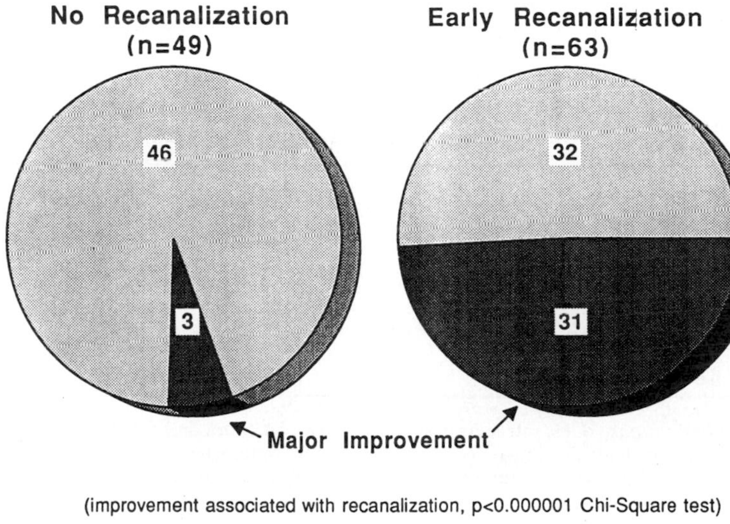


**Fig. 40-1.** In studies of thrombolytic therapy where pre- and post-treatment cerebral arteriography have been performed, major neurologic improvement has been associated with arterial recanalization (see text).

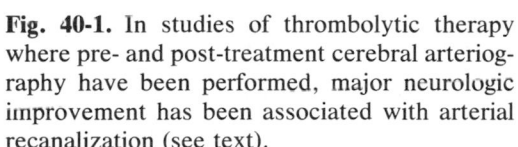

## Hemorrhagic Risk

Thrombolytic therapy is not innocuous (Table 40-2). The reported incidence of brain hemorrhage following treatment for ischemic stroke, with[17] or without reperfusion,[90] ranges from 0.7 to 56 percent.[16,35,58,90,103,116,120] In the absence of thrombolytic or anticoagulant therapy (or anticoagulants), the incidence of hemorrhagic conversion with hematoma formation has not been established. Okada et al.[95] recently reported three massive hematomas complicating acute infarction in 57 acute ischemic infarction patients (5 percent) who were not anticoagulated; the time of hematoma onset was not indicated. With thrombolytic therapy, brain hemorrhage has been reported for each of the agents tested as treatment for ischemic stroke. Brain hemorrhage has followed treatment of both vertebrobasilar stroke and carotid distribution stroke.

Five studies have been performed in which post-treatment CT scans were required[16,33,34,58,90,120] (Table 40-2), allowing detection of any hemorrhage, symptomatic or asymptomatic. ICH occurred in 19 of the 216 patients treated (9 percent). Ten of the ICH were symptomatic, and 8 were fatal (Fig. 40-2). Post-treatment angiography was performed in 14, and early arterial recanalization was demonstrated in 9; ICH occurred without reperfusion in 5 patients, each of whom was treated with intra-arterial urokinase.[58,90]

Potential risk factors for thrombolysis-related ICH include the thrombolytic agent used, route of administration, dose, time from stroke-onset to time of infusion, duration of infusion, patient age and blood pressure, concurrent anticoagulation, post-treatment fibrinogen concentration, infarction location, and site of initial acute thrombotic occlusion. Unfortunately, no conclusions can be drawn from the small number of ICHs that have occurred.[28,34,58,90,116] Increasing risk is likely to follow increasing doses, but confirmation (for tPA) awaits publication of details from two relatively large dose-escalation studies.[16,120] The lower incidence of ICH overall in those studies (5 percent) suggests the possibility that ICH risk may be lowered by administering therapy very early: 74 patients were treated in 90 minutes or less with 3 ICH,[16] and 57 were treated in 8 hours or less with 4 ICH.[120]

Preexisting ischemic brain injury is not necessary for the occurrence of thrombolysis-related ICH. At least one of the 17 hemorrhages complicating stroke treatment occurred outside the area of acute cerebral infarction.[16] With thrombolytic therapy (and heparin) for myocardial infarction, ICH into presumably uninjured brain has occurred in 0 to 5 percent of treated patients[31,70,112,117] and has had a mortality of 50 percent.[20,70,112,113] A systemic lytic state has been reported with some cases of ICH[20,90,113] but not in others.[70,112] The agent with the greatest fibrin specificity (tPA)[25,81] has not been safer with regard to ICH.[31,70,112] Consequently, ICH in many cases may be secondary to lysis of hemostatic plugs in previously damaged or acutely damaged cerebral blood vessels (Fig. 40-3), with or without a systemic lytic state. Concurrent heparin may increase risk for ICH,[102] particularly if the partial thromboplastin time is excessively prolonged.[70]

Unfortunately, distinguishing between intracerebral hematoma and hemorrhagic infarction is frequently impossible from the clinical information provided in the stroke therapy reports. Detailed clinical and radiographic descriptions are anticipated from the tPA dose-escalation studies. Preliminary results from the tPA Acute Stroke Study Group indicate 23 hemorrhagic infarcts in 57 patients.[120]

Major systemic hemorrhagic complications of thrombolytic therapy for stroke are infrequent. Only one fatal systemic hemorrhage has been reported in the thrombolytic studies performed since the introduction of CT (with the death resulting from a groin hematoma complicating cerebral angiography).[28]

## Potential Nonhemorrhagic Complications of Thrombolytic Therapy

### *Reperfusion Injury*

Reperfusion injury associated with edema[75] following presumed thrombolytic arterial recanalization has been suggested as the cause of death in two pa-

**TABLE 40-2. Intracerebral Hemorrhage Following Thrombolytic Therapy**[a]

| Thrombolytic Agent | Anticoagulant | No. Treated | No. ICH | No. with Recanalization | No. Fatal | Location | Ref. |
|---|---|---|---|---|---|---|---|
| IA UK or SK | Yes | 43 | 4 | 2 | 4 | 3 in pons | 58 |
| IA UK or SK | Yes | 20 | 4 | 4 | 0 | All in corpus striatum | 34 |
| IA UK | 6/22 | 22 | 4 | 1 | 1 | BG involved in all 4 | 90 |
| IV tPA | No | 74 | 3 | NS | 1 | Cerebellum, parietal lobe, thalamus | 16 |
| IV tPA | No | 57 | 4 | >2 | 3 | NS | 34, 120 |
| Total | | 216 | 19 | ≥9 | 9 | | |

*Abbreviations:* ICH, intracerebral hemorrhage; IA, intra-arterial; UK, urokinase; SK, streptokinase; IV, intravenous; BG, basal ganglia; NS, not specified; IV, intravenous; tPA, tissue plasminogen activator.

[a] Studies with post-treatment CT(s) required by protocol (distinguishing among hematoma, hemorrhagic transformation, or hemorrhagic infarction is difficult).

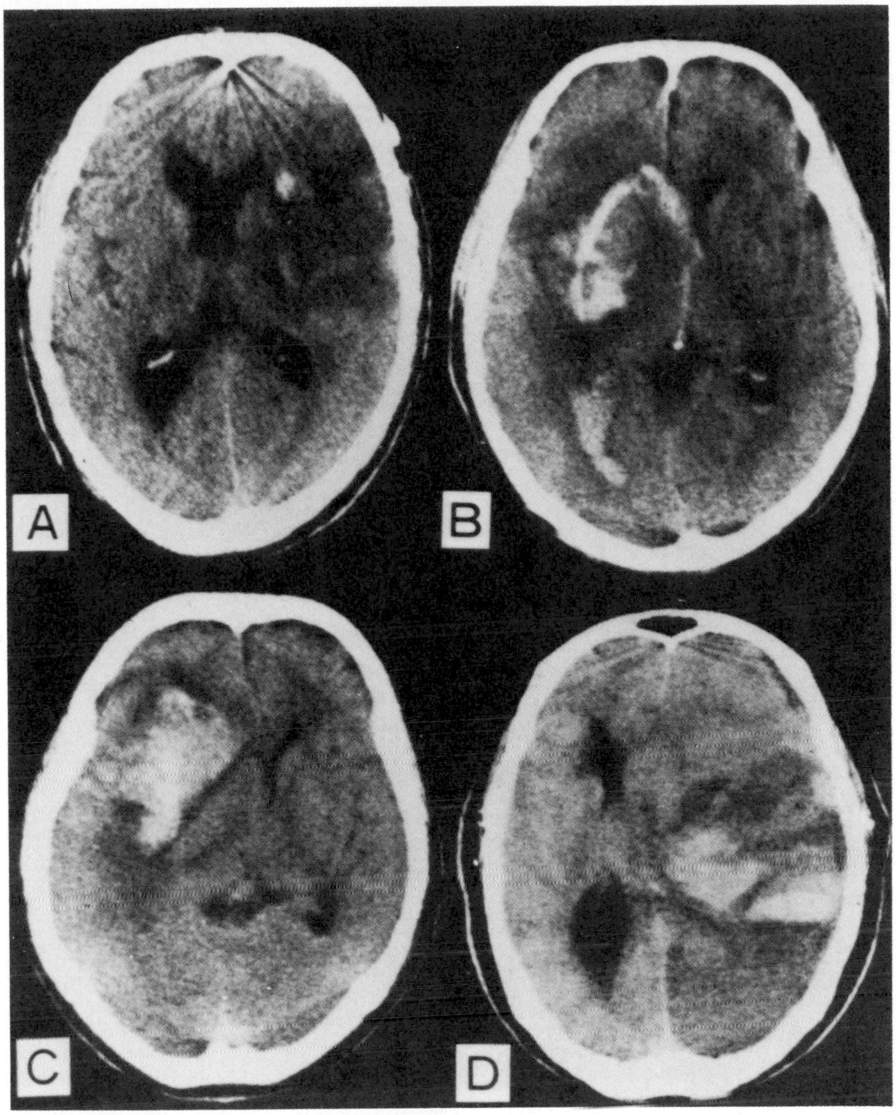


**Fig. 40-2.** Four examples of hemorrhagic change complicating thrombolytic therapy for ischemic stroke. The CT scans were obtained 24 hours after onset of the initial stroke symptoms in patients subsequently treated with intracarotid urokinase. (**A**) Small areas of hemorrhagic change predominantly at the margins of a sizeable left hemispheric infarction. (**B**) Area of hemorrhage in the right basal ganglia with penetration into the ventricles. (**C**) Hemorrhage in the right basal ganglia with displacement and shift of surrounding brain tissue. (**D**) Massive hematoma in the left hemisphere with dramatic mass effects. (From Mori et al,[90] with permission.)

tients,[73] without angiographic or pathologic confirmation. Nonhemorrhagic reperfusion injury has not been described in the studies summarized in Tables 40-1 and 40-2.

### *Arterial Reocclusion*

Arterial reocclusion after successful thrombolysis has not been documented for stroke patients, but the study designs of the trials reported were not adequate to detect reocclusion. Recurrent ischemia (with probably reocclusion) occurs in approximately 15 to 30 percent of patients treated with thrombolytic agents for acute myocardial infarction;[41,62] reocclusion has not been related to the type of artery originally occluded, nor to the morphology of any persistent post-treatment stenosis or thrombus.[41] Reocclusion may be less likely to occur in stroke patients. Many of the occlusions are embolic[42] with the acute thrombus lodged distally in a relatively normal vessel, overlying previously normal endothelium (vascular injury is the most potent stimulus for thrombus for-

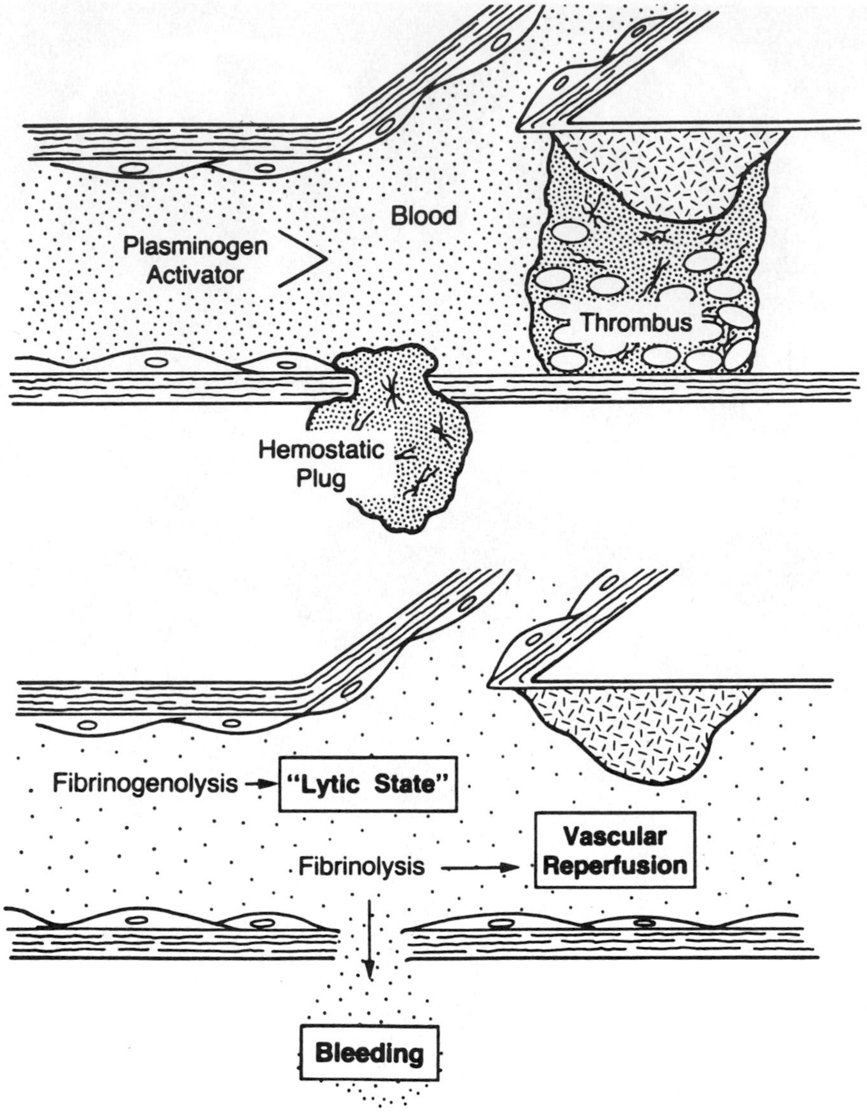


**Fig. 40-3.** The plasminogen activators act upon the surface of a pathologic thrombus, upon the surface of hemostatic plugs and thrombi sealing sites of previous vascular injury, and upon coagulation proteins within the plasma. Thrombolytic therapy may be a double-edged sword in that doses of a given agent potent enough for lysis of a pathologic thrombus may result in unwanted bleeding, secondary to lysis of protective hemostasic plugs or thrombi or secondary to a systemic lytic state. (From Marder and Sherry,[81] with permission.)

mation).[49] With myocardial infarction, the acute thrombus usually overlies a complex atherosclerotic plaque.[36]

### *Embolism from Incidental or Therapeutic Lysis*

Downstream systemic or brain embolism from incidental or therapeutic lysis of large thrombi could complicate thrombolytic treatment for stroke or for myocardial infarction. For example, patients with preexisting thrombus in the left atrium or the left ventricle could sustain distal embolization from fragments resulting from incidental intracardiac thrombolysis. This complication has yet to be reported.[31,61] In the stroke patient, therapeutic lysis of a proximal cerebral thrombus in a vascular territory with good collateral supply could occur, with the fragment(s) passing distally and occluding an end-arterial bed without good collaterals, resulting in a larger infarction and a greater neurologic deficit.

## Other Problems

### *Emergency Assessment of Vascular Anatomy*

The time window for effective stroke therapy may be quite small,[12,32,107] and older thrombi are more resistant to thrombolysis.[49,69,99] The risk of thrombolysis-related ICH may be lower with earlier treatment.[129] Rapid patient assessment is ideal.[10,42] Unfortunately, adding cerebral angiography to the necessary CT scan adds a minimum of 30 to 60 minutes before thrombolytic therapy can begin. Accordingly, studies requiring angiography may decrease the chances for therapeutic efficacy because of later treatment. If the delays do narrow the potential clinical advantage of thrombolytic therapy over no therapy, then randomized trials including angiography will require larger numbers for adequate sample size and statistical power. Eliminating pretreatment angiography has the disadvantage of delivering therapy "in the dark." No firm conclusions would be possible regarding the kind of stroke most (or least) likely to respond to thrombolytic therapy—a particularly important limitation, given the dangers of thrombolysis.

The solution would be the development of accurate, fast, noninvasive measures of cerebrovascular anatomy. Trancranial Doppler sonography (TCD),[89,101,126] magnetic resonance imaging (MRI) angiography,[124] and single photon emission tomography (SPECT)[40] can provide pre- and post-treatment cerebrovascular anatomic or physiologic information. Unfortunately, limitations regarding cost, availability, and the requirement for highly skilled technicians will probably limit development of these techniques for multihospital, around-the-clock stroke therapy trials. Using emergency brain CT for clues to thrombus localization has recently been described,[118] but this technique will likely be limited by low sensitivity and variable reliability.

### *Choice of Thrombolytic Agent*

To some degree the issue of the ideal thrombolytic agent[56] for stroke therapy is moot until a properly designed randomized trial demonstrates a clinical benefit for a particular thrombolytic regimen. Inspection of Tables 40-1 and 40-2 does not suggest an advantage of one agent over another with regard to safety or potential efficacy. With myocardial infarction, the question of the ideal agent is not clear.[81] Only now are head-to-head comparisons being carried out on a randomized basis.[122]

### *Dose of Thrombolytic Agent*

Currently used doses of urokinase or tPA may be inadequate for lysis of large volume thrombi.[33,90,118] The pace of thrombolysis correlates with the ratio of thrombus surface area to thrombus volume, and with the local concentration of the thrombolytic agent.[25,83,129] High doses of urokinase, streptokinase, or tPA might not be possible without excessive risk for post-treatment ICH. Useful information should come from the tPA Acute Stroke Study Group study as pre- and post-treatment angiograms will be available for all patients at each tPA dose-tier studied.[120]

### *Combination Therapy*

Numerous two-drug thrombolytic combinations[55,119,121] have been studied for myocardial infarction, and a degree of synergism has been suggested.[121] A clinical advantage for any one combination has not been established.

The role of platelets in fibrinolysis has been recently reviewed.[26] Combination of thrombolytic agents with antiplatelet drugs could be useful,[26] particularly as platelet activation may occur in humans following thrombolytic therapy.[71] The combination of streptokinase and aspirin for myocardial infarction was superior to streptokinase alone with respect to vascular mortality in the Second International Study of Infarct Survival (ISIS-2) trial.[26,67] No increased risk for ICH was observed. The addition of monoclonal antibodies to platelet aggregation receptors might also be of benefit.[26] In a monkey carotid artery model of platelet thrombus formation, Coller and colleagues[27] have studied the effects of murine monoclonal antibodies to the platelet aggregation receptor complex, GPIIb/IIIa. Minimum doses of antibody abolished thrombus formation without inducing a major prolongation of bleeding time; in 6 of 15 monkeys, abolition of thrombus formation was achieved with doses of antibody that did not abolish platelet aggregation.[27] Other novel agents that inhibit thrombus formation by platelets are under investigation.[26] For human stroke, single-agent clot lysis may eventually be superseded by combinations providing synergism of thrombolysis and platelet inhibition. In addition, regimens for arterial recanalization may be further complemented by agents providing neuronal protection.[51]

### *Improving Cerebral Arterial Recanalization Rates*

In cases where high doses of thrombolytic agent are judged to be necessary, superselective microcatheterization may be helpful by providing high concentrations of drug while minimizing systemic effects.[128] Mechanical manipulation of the thrombus may also be useful[68] by softening the proximal end of the thrombus and increasing drug-accessible surface area. If ultra-early therapy improves recanalization rates, then well-coordinated public education efforts will be warranted,[97] emphasizing the importance of seeking emergency attention for symptoms of stroke.

### *Minimizing Intracerebral Hemorrhage*

Experimentally, thrombolytic therapy has not been shown to significantly increase the risk of hematoma formation in the setting of experimental ischemic infarction,[78,79] yet hematoma formation complicates thrombolytic stroke therapy in 5 to 10 percent of stroke patients (Table 40-2). Perhaps the experimental models can be improved to resemble more closely the human clinical setting (e.g., investigating aged animals, manipulating blood pressure, simulating a lytic state), and so provide information useful in the design of human studies. Clinically, the absolute numbers of thrombolysis-related ICH have been small, but the consequences have been devastating (Table 40-2). Accordingly, when suspicions of a risk factor for ICH are raised, protocols may be modified on ethical grounds based on small numbers of ICH—numbers that may be too small to firmly establish the importance of that risk factor for any future general application of thrombolytic therapy.

As clinical outcome is more important than arterial recanalization, lower doses of drug may be preferable. For example, a low dose might be found with a significant thrombolytic effect but with a very low risk for ICH, low enough to justify treatment for a wide spectrum of stroke of patients. Such patients might include those over age 80, those with systolic blood pressures above 180 mmHg, or those with modest neurologic deficits. The risk of higher doses might be justified primarily for patients with severe deficits or with evidence for large-volume thrombi.

### *Laboratory Assessment of Thrombolysis*

In patients with stroke, laboratory tests of thrombolysis and coagulation have not yet been shown to be useful. With myocardial infarction, laboratory monitoring of thrombolytic therapy has been largely unrevealing.[81,102,113] A notable exception is the finding of a prolonged thrombolytic effect for tPA, 7 hours or longer after cessation of infusion.[38,54]

### *Thrombolytic Therapy for Dural Sinus Thrombosis*

Several reports[21,37,52,74,123,127] describing the use of systemic thrombolytic therapy for dural venous thrombosis have appeared. In addition, direct urokinase infusion has now been described in five patients,[9,104] and the clinical outcomes have been favorable. One patient was treated safely despite preurokinase bilateral venous hemorrhagic infarctions,[9] and a second patient developed major improvement despite a posturokinase hemorrhagic infarction.[104]

## DEFIBRINOGENATING AGENTS FOR CEREBRAL INFARCTION: ANCROD

Several snake venoms have been shown to degrade fibrinogen,[11] and one of these thrombinlike enzymes, ancrod, has been used as therapy for stroke. Ancrod[23] cleaves fibrinopeptide A but not fibrinopeptide B from circulating fibrinogen.[11] The polymer that forms from the altered fibrin contains only end-to-end bonding, without the usual cross-linking, and so this fibrin has reduced tensile strength and greater susceptibility to lysis by plasmin.[11] Following the administration of pharmacologic doses of ancrod, the concentration of fibrinogen promptly falls and blood viscosity decreases.[11,64,100] The concentration of fibrinogen-fibrin degradation products sharply rises, and the thrombolytic system is activated,[7,11] perhaps through the release of tissue plasminogen activator from vascular endothelial cells.[11]

Ancrod has been studied in two small controlled trials as therapy for acute cerebral infarction.[64,96] The results from each study suggested but did not establish improved outcome for the treated patients. Angiograms were not required, and so no direct evidence regarding arterial recanalization or thrombus inhibition was provided. Importantly, no significant hemorrhagic complications occurred, even in patients with prolonged hypofibrinogenemia (to concentrations of 50 to 100 mg% and lower).[64] A large multicenter, randomized therapeutic trial of ancrod is now underway in which treatment is initiated within 6 hours of symptom onset. The ancrod is continued over 6 days, with the fibrinogen concentration titrated to approximately 100 mg%.

Ancrod has also been investigated as therapy for 10 patients with subcortical arteriosclerotic encephalopathy.[100] The investigators obtained lowered fibrinogen concentration and lowered plasma viscosity over 1 month of treatment, as planned, but no clinical improvement was observed in the patients.

## INTRATHECAL THROMBOLYSIS FOR SUBARACHNOID HEMORRHAGE

The incidence of delayed-onset cerebral vasospasm following subarachnoid (SAH) correlates with the intrathecal blood visualized by CT scan.[39,47] The amount of clot correlates with the degree of clinical vasospasm, and the location of the clot correlates with the location of the vasospasm (as determined by cerebral angiography).[72] The pathophysiology of these correlations has been recently discussed.[44]

Early surgical clot removal has been reported to decrease the incidence of vasospasm,[115] but results have been inconsistent.[65] Unfortunately, thorough removal at the time of early aneurysm surgery is difficult to accomplish safely and so is not usually attempted.[44]

Several investigators have studied intrathecal administration of thrombolytic agents as a method of clot removal in animal models of subarachnoid hemorrhage (SAH).[5,45,46,106] In the baboon model of Findlay and Weir,[45,46] the placebo-treated animals have had persistent clot within the basal cisterns, angiographic findings of vasospasm, and diffuse ischemic injury at postmortem examination. Animals treated with tPA have had modest to major dissolution of the basilar clot, little radiographic or neurologic evidence of vasospasm, and minimal ischemic injury at postmortem.[45,46] At the time of intrathecal administration of the drug, resection of brain parenchyma and electrocautery have been performed to mimic some of the conditions of human aneurysmal SAH. Major complications of intrathecal thrombolytic therapy have not been encountered, a dose-effect has been identified with regard to clot dissolution, and significant effects upon systemic coagulation and thrombolysis have not been detected.

Investigation of intrathecal urokinase in humans following aneurysmal SAH has been carried out in small numbers of patients.[115,125] In North America, several phase I safety studies of intrathecal tPA are now in progress. Doses ranging from 5 to 50 mg are administered, either at the time of aneurysm clipping or via a preplaced intrathecal catheter 24 hours after surgical clipping. Early surgery and therapy are required, usually within 72 hours. No major complications have been described for the seven patients reported to date.[76]

## THROMBOLYSIS OF INTRACEREBRAL HEMATOMA

Stereotactic aspiration of clot as therapy for nontraumatic ICH has been evaluated,[8,93] but complete clot removal is often impossible.[94] In animal models of ICH, thrombolytic clot dissolution has been accomplished with urokinase in monkeys[105] and rabbits.[91] In humans, Matsumoto and Hondo[82] have reported treatment of 51 patients with spontaneous ICH, using urokinase. No complications were attributed to the urokinase instillations, although rebleeding occurred in two patients. A clinical benefit was not apparent.

## REFERENCES


1. Abe T: Oral urokinase: absorption, mechanisms of fibrinolytic enhancement and clinical effect on cerebral thrombosis. Folia Haematol 113:122, 1986
2. Abe T, Kazama M, Naito I et al: Clinical effect of urokinase (60,000 U/d) on cerebral infarction: comparative study by means of multicenter double-blind test. Blood and Vessel 12:342, 1981
3. Abe T, Kazawa M, Naito I et al: Clinical evaluation for efficacy of tissue culture urokinase (TCUK) on cerebral thrombosis by means of multicenter double-blind study. Blood and Vessel 12:321, 1981
4. Adachi K, Sahashi K, Fujii K et al: A significance of urokinase treatment in acute cerebral infarction: assessment from neurological signs and CT findings. J Aichi Med Univ Assoc 8:305, 1980
5. Alksne JF, Branson PJ, Bailey N: Modifications of experimental post-subarachnoid hemorrhage vasculopathy with intracisternal plasmin. Neurosurgery 23:335, 1988
6. Amias AG: Streptokinase, cerebral vascular disease—and triplets. Br Med J 1414, 1977
7. Apprill PG, Ashton J, Guerrero J et al: Ancrod decreases the frequency of cyclic flow variations and causes thrombolysis following acute coronary thrombosis. Am Heart J 113:898, 1987
8. Backlund EO, Holst H: Controlled subtotal evacuation of intracerebral haematomas by stereotactic technique. Surg Neurol 9:99, 1978
9. Barnwell SL, Halbach VV, Dowd CF et al: Endovascular thrombolytic therapy for dural sinus thrombosis. J Neurosurg 72:336A, 1990
10. Barsan WG, Brott TG, Olinger CP et al: Early treatment for acute ischemic stroke. (Editorial.) Ann Intern Med 111:449, 1989
11. Bell WB: Defibrinogenating enzymes. p. 886. In Colman RW, Hirsh J, Marder VJ, Salzman EW (eds): Hemostasis and Thrombosis. Lippincott, Philadelphia, 1987
12. Boisvert DP, Gelb AW, Tang C et al: Brain tolerance to middle cerebral artery occlusion during hypotension in primates. Surg Neurol 31:6, 1989
13. Broderick JP, Brott TG, Tomsick T et al: Ultra-early evaluation of intracerebral hemorrhage. J Neurosurg 72:195, 1990
14. Brooks J, Davis D, Devivo G: Blood hypercoagulability in acute cerebrovascular syndromes: its control with urokinase therapy. J Lab Clin Med 76:879, 1970
15. Brott TG: Thrombolysis and stroke in clinical practice: past, present and future. p. 189. In Sawaya R (ed): Fibrinolysis in the Neurosciences. Hanley and Belfus, Philadelphia, 1990
16. Brott TG, Haley EC, Levy D et al: Safety and potential efficacy of tissue plasminogen activator (tPA) for stroke, abstracted. Stroke 21:181, 1990
17. Bruckmann H, Ferbert A: Putaminal haemorrhage after recanalization of an embolic MCA occlusion treated with tissue plasminogen activator. Neuroradiology 31:95, 1989
18. Bruckmann HJ, Ringelstein EB, Buchner H et al: Vascular recanalizing techniques in the hind brain circulation. Neurosurg Rev 10:197, 1987
19. Buteux G, Jubault V, Suisse A et al: Local recombinant tissue plasminogen activator to clear cerebral artery thrombosis developing soon after surgery. Lancet 2:1143, 1988
20. Carlson SE, Aldrich MS, Greenberg HS et al: Intracerebral hemorrhage complicating intravenous tissue plasminogen activator treatment. Arch Neurol 45:1070, 1988
21. Castaigne P, Laplane D, Bousser MP: Superior sagittal sinus thrombosis. (Letter.) Arch Neurol 34:788, 1977
22. Clarke RL, Cliffton EE: The treatment of cerebrovascular thrombosis and embolism with fibrinolytic agents. Am J Cardiol 30:546, 1960
23. Cole CW, Bormanis J: Ancrod: a practical alternative to heparin. J Vasc Surg 8:59, 1988
24. Collen D: Molecular mechanisms of fibrinolysis and their application to fibrin-specific thrombolytic therapy. J Cell Biochem 33:77, 1987
25. Collen D, Strassen JM, Marafino J et al: Biological properties of human tissue-type plasminogen

activator obtained by expression of recombinant DNA in mammalian cells. J Pharmacol Exp Ther 231:146, 1984
26. Coller BS: Platelets and thrombolytic therapy. N Engl J Med 322:33, 1990
27. Coller BS, Folts JD, Smith SR et al: Abolition of in vivo platelet thrombus formation in primates with monoclonal antibodies to the platelet GPIIb/IIIa receptor: correlation with bleeding time, platelet aggregation, and blockade of GPIIb/IIIa receptors. Circulation 80:1766, 1989
28. Courtheoux P, Theron J, Derlon JM et al: In situ fibrinolysis in supra-aortic main vessels. J Neuroradiology 13:111, 1986
29. Dalal PM, Shah PM, Aiyar RR: Arteriographic study of cerebral embolism. Lancet 2:358, 1965
30. Dalal PM, Shah PM, Sheth SC et al: Cerebral embolism: angiographic observations on spontaneous clot lysis. Lancet 1:61, 1965
31. de Bono D: Problems in thrombolysis. p. 279. In Julian D, Kubler W, Norris RM et al (eds): Thrombolysis in Cardiovascular Disease. Marcel Dekker, New York, 1989
32. DeLey G, Weyne J, Demeester G et al: Experimental thromboembolic stroke studied by positron emission tomography: immediate versus delayed reperfusion by fibrinolysis. J Cereb Blood Flow Metab 8:539, 1988
33. Del Zoppo GJ: An open multicenter trial of rt-PA in acute stroke: safety and efficacy, abstracted. Thromb Haemost 62:27, 1989
34. Del Zoppo GJ, Ferbert A, Otis S et al: Local intraarterial fibrinolytic therapy in acute carotid territory stroke: a pilot study. Stroke 19:307, 1988
35. Del Zoppo GJ, Zeumer H, Harker LA: Thrombolytic therapy in stroke: possibilities and hazards. Stroke 17:595, 1986
36. DeWood MA: Prevalence total coronary occlusion during the early hours of transmural myocardial infarction. N Engl J Med 303:897, 1980
37. DiRocco C, Iannelli A, Leone G et al: Heparin-urokinase treatment in aseptic dural sinus thrombosis. Arch Neurol 38:431, 1981
38. Eisenberg PR, Sherman LA, Tiefenbrunn AJ et al: Sustained fibrinolysis after administration of tPA despite its short half-life in the circulation. Thromb Haemost 57:35, 1987
39. Eisentrout C, Tomsick TA, Tew JM: Computed tomography findings as a prognostic factor in subarachnoid hemorrhage for ruptured cerebral aneurysms, abstracted. Stroke 11:124, 1980
40. Ell P, Hocknell JML, Jarritt PH et al: A $^{99}Tc^{m}$-labelled radiotracer for the investigation of cerebral vascular disease. Nucl Med Commun 6:437, 1985
41. Ellis SG, Topol EJ, George BS et al: Recurrent ischemia without warning: analysis of risk factors for in-hospital ischemic events following successful thrombolysis with intravenous tissue plasminogen activator. Circulation 80:1159, 1989
42. Fieschi C, Argentino C, Lenzi GL et al: Clinical and instrumental evaluation of patients with ischemic stroke within the first six hours. J Neurol Sci 91:311, 1989
43. Fieschi C, Bozzao L: Transient embolic occlusion of the middle cerebral and internal carotid arteries in cerebral apoplexy. J Neurol Neurosurg Psychiatry 32:236, 1969
44. Findlay JM: Intrathecal thrombolytic therapy in the prevention of vasospasm following subarachnoid hemorrhage. p. 203. In Sawaya R (ed): Fibrinolysis in the Neurosciences. Hanley and Belfus, Philadelphia, 1990
45. Findlay JM, Weir BKA, Gordon P et al: Safety and efficacy of intrathecal thrombolytic therapy in a primate model of cerebral vasospasm. Neurosurgery 24:491, 1989
46. Findlay JM, Weir BKA, Kanamaru K et al: Intrathecal fibrinolytic therapy after subarachnoid hemorrhage: dosage study in a primate model and review of the literature. Can J Neurol Sci 16:28, 1989
47. Fisher CM, Kistler JP, Davis JM: The relation of cerebral vasospasm to subarachnoid blood visualized by computerized tomography, abstracted. Stroke 11:124, 1980
48. Fletcher AP, Alkjaersig N, Lew M: A pilot study of urokinase therapy in cerebral infarction. Stroke 7:135, 1976
49. Freiman DG: The structure of thrombi. p. 1136. In Colman RW, Hirsh J, Marder VJ et al (eds): Hemostasis and Thrombosis. 2nd Ed. Lippincott, Philadelphia, 1987
50. Fujishima M, Omae T, Tanaka K et al: Controlled trial of combined urokinase and dextran sulfate therapy in patients with acute cerebral infarction. Angiology 37:487, 1986
51. Gelmers HG, Gorter K, De Weerdt et al: A controlled trial of nimodipine in acute ischemic stroke. N Engl J Med 318:203, 1988
52. Gettelfinger DM, Kokmen E: Superior sagittal sinus thrombosis. Arch Neurol 34:2, 1977
53. Ghika J, Bogousslavsky J, Regli F: Infarcts in the territory of the deep perforators from the carotid system. Neurology (NY) 39:507, 1989
54. Grill HP, Brinker JA: Nonacute thrombolytic therapy: an adjunct to coronary angioplasty in patients with large intravascular thrombi. Am Heart J 118:662, 1989
55. Grines CL, Nissen SE, Booth DC et al: A new thrombolytic regimen for acute myocardial infarction using combination half dose tissue-type plasminogen activator with full dose streptokinase: a pilot study. J Am Coll Cardiol 14:573, 1989
56. Haber E, Quertermous T, Matsueda GR: Innovative approaches to plasminogen activator therapy. Science 243:51, 1989
57. Hacke W, Berg-Danner E, Zeumer H: Evoked potential monitoring during acute occlusion of the basilar artery and selective local thrombolytic therapy. Arch Psychiatr Nervenkr 232:541, 1982
58. Hacke W, Zeumer H, Ferbert A: Intraarterial thrombolytic therapy improves outcome in patients with acute vertebrobasilar occlusive disease. Stroke 19:1216, 1988
59. Hanaway J, Torack R, Fletcher AP et al: Intra-

cranial bleeding associated with urokinase therapy for acute ischemic hemispheral stroke. Stroke 7:143, 1976

60. Hass WK, Clauss RM, Goldberg AF: Special problems associated with surgical and thrombolytic treatment of strokes. Arch Surg 92:27, 1966
61. Held AC, Gore JM, Paraskos J et al: Impact of thrombolytic therapy on left ventricular mural thrombi in acute myocardial infarction. Am J Cardiol 62:310, 1988
62. Heras M, Chesebro JH, Thompson PL et al: Prevention of early and late rethrombosis and further strategies of coronary reperfusion. p. 203. In Julian D, Kubler W, Norris RM et al (eds): Thrombolysis in Cardiovascular Disease. Marcel Dekker, New York, 1989
63. Herndon RM, Meyer JS, Johnson JF et al: Treatment of cardiovascular thrombosis with fibrinolysin. Am J Cardiol 30:540, 1960
64. Hossman V, Heiss W, Besermeyer H et al: Controlled trial of ancrod in ischemic stroke. Arch Neurol 40:803, 1983
65. Inagawa T, Yamamoto M, Kamiya K: Effect of clot removal on cerebral vasospasm. J Neurosurg 72:224, 1990
66. Irino T, Taneda M, Minami T: Angiographic manifestations in postrecanalized cerebral infarction. Neurology (NY) 27:471, 1977
67. ISIS-2 (Second International Study of Infarct Survival) Collaborative Group: Randomized trial of intravenous streptokinase, oral aspirin, both, or neither among 17,187 cases of suspected acute myocardial infarction. Lancet 2:349, 1988
68. Jungreis CA, Wechsler LR, Horton JA: Intracranial thrombolysis via a catheter embedded in the clot. Stroke 20:1578, 1989
69. Kanamasa K, Watanabe I, Cercek B et al: Selective decrease in lysis of old thrombi after rapid administration of tissue-type plasminogen activator. JACC 14:1359, 1989
70. Kase CS, O'Neal AM, Fisher M et al: Intracranial hemorrhage after use of tissue plasminogen activator for coronary thrombolysis. Ann Intern Med 112:17, 1990
71. Kerins DM, Roy L, Fitzgerald GA et al: Platelet and vascular function during coronary thrombolysis with tissue-type plasminogen activator. Circulation 80:1718, 1989
72. Kistler JP, Crowell RM, Davis KR et al: The relation of cerebral vasospasm to the extent and location of subarachnoid blood visualized by CT scan: a prospective study. Neurology (NY) 33:424, 1983
73. Koudstaal PJ, Stibbe J, Vermeulen M: Fatal ischemic brain oedema after early thrombolysis with tissue plasminogen activator in acute stroke. Br Med J 297:1571, 1988
74. Krayenbuhl HA: Cerebral venous and sinus thrombosis. Clin Neurosurg 14:1, 1967
75. Kuroiwa T, Shibutani M, Okeda R: Blood-brain barrier disruption and exacerbation of ischemic brain edema after restoration of blood flow in experimental focal cerebral ischemia. Acta Neuropathol 76:62, 1988
76. Lamond R: Cisternal recombinant tPA administration in aneurysmal subarachnoid hemorrhage. J Neurosurg 72:336A, 1990
77. Landau WM: Au clair de lacune: holy, wholly, holey logic. Neurology (NY) 39:725, 1989
78. Lyden PD, Zivin JA, Clark WA et al: Tissue plasminogen activator-mediated thrombolysis of cerebral emboli and its effect on hemorrhagic infarction in rabbits. Neurology (NY) 39:703, 1989
79. Lyden PD, Zivin JA, Soll M et al: Intracerebral hemorrhage after experimental embolic infarction: anticoagulation. Arch Neurol 44:848, 1987
80. Malinovski I, Nikola IN: Embolism of the cerebral arteries. In Malinovski I, Nikola IN (eds): Anticoagulant and Thrombolytic Therapy in Surgery. CV Mosby, St. Louis, 1979
81. Marder VJ, Sherry S: Thrombolytic therapy: current status. N Engl J Med 23:1513, 1988
82. Matsumoto K, Hondo H: CT-guided stereotaxic evacuation of hypertensive intracerebral hematomas. J Neurosurg 61:440, 1984
83. Matsuo O, Rijken DC, Collen D: Comparison of the relative fibrinogenolytic, fibrinolytic and thrombolytic properties of tPA and urokinase in vitro. Thromb Haemost 45:225, 1981
84. Mazel MS, Riera R: Obstructive vascular disease treated by urokinase. Med Trial Tech Q 25:319, 1979
85. Meyer JS, Gilroy J, Barnhart ME et al: Anticoagulants plus streptokinase therapy in progressive stroke. JAMA 189:373, 1963
86. Meyer JS, Gilroy J, Barnhart ME et al: Therapeutic thrombolysis in cerebral thromboembolism: randomized evaluation of intravenous streptokinase. p. 200. In Siekert RG, Whisnant JP (eds): Cerebral Vascular Diseases. Grune & Stratton, Orlando, FL, 1965
87. Meyer JS, Herndon RM, Gotch F: Therapeutic thrombolysis. p. 160. In Millikan CH, Siekert W, Whisnant JP (eds): Cerebral Vasular Disease: Third Princeton Conference. Grune & Stratton, Orlando, FL, 1961
88. Meyer JS, Herndon RM, Johnson JF et al: Treatment of cerebrovascular thrombosis with plasmin and plasminogen activators. p. 373. In Millikan CH (ed): Cerebrovascular Disease. Williams & Wilkins, Baltimore, 1966
89. Mohr JP, Duterte DI, Oliveira VR et al: Recanalization of acute middle cerebral artery occlusion. Neurology (NY), suppl 1. 38:215, 1988
90. Mori E, Tabuchi M, Yoshida T et al: Intracarotid urokinase with thromboembolic occlusion of the middle cerebral artery. Stroke 19:802, 1988
91. Narayan KK, Narayan RK: Thrombolytic therapy of intracerebral hematomas. p. 198. In Sawaya R (ed): Fibrinolysis and the Central Nervous System. Hanley and Belfus, Philadelphia, 1990
92. Nenci GG, Gresele P, Taramelli M et al: Thrombolytic therapy for thromboembolism of vertebrobasilar artery. Angiology 34:561, 1983
93. Nizuma H, Shimizu Y, Yonemitxu T et al: Results of stereotactic aspiration in 175 cases of putaminal hemorrhage. Neurosurgery 24:814, 1989

94. Nizuma H, Suzuki J: Stereotactic aspiration of putaminal hemorrhage using a double track aspiration technique. Neurosurgery 22:432, 1988
95. Okada Y, Yamaguchi T, Minematsu K et al: Hemorrhagic transformation in cerebral embolism. Stroke 20:598, 1989
96. Olinger CP, Brott TG, Barsan WG et al: Use of ancrod in acute or progressing ischemic cerebral infarction. Ann Emerg Med 17:1208, 1988
97. O'Rourke MF, Ballantyne K, Thompson PL: Community aspects of coronary thrombolysis: public education and cost effectiveness. p. 309. In Julian D, Kubler W, Norris RM et al (eds): Thrombolysis in Cardiovascular Disease. Marcel Dekker, New York, 1989
98. Poeck K: Intraarterial thrombolytic therapy in acute stroke. Acta Neurol Belg 88:35, 1988
99. Rentrop KP, Feit F, Sherman W et al: Serial angiographic assessment of coronary artery obstruction and collateral flow in acute myocardial infarction. Circulation 80:1166, 1989
100. Ringelstein EB, Mauckner A, Schneider R et al: Effects of enzymatic blood defibrination in subcortical arterisclerotic encephalopathy. J Neurol Neurosurg Psychiatry 51:1051, 1988
101. Ringelstein EB, Zeumer H: The role of continuous-wave Doppler sonography in the diagnosis and management of basilar and vertebral artery occlusions, with special reference to its application during local fibrinolysis. J Neurol 228:161, 1982
102. Sane DC, Califf RM, Topol EJ et al: Bleeding during thrombolytic therapy for acute myocardial infarction: mechanisms and management. Ann Intern Med 111:1010, 1989
103. Sato Y, Mizoguchi K, Sato Y et al: Anticoagulant and thrombolytic therapy for cerebral embolism of cardiac origin. Kurume Med J 33:39, 1986
104. Scott JA, Pascuzzi RM, Hall PV et al: Treatment of dural sinus thrombosis with local urokinase infusion. J Neurosurg 68:284, 1988
105. Segal R, Dujovny M, Nelson D et al: Local urokinase treatment for spontaneous intracerebral hematoma. Clin Res 30:412A, 1982
106. Seifert V, Eisert WG, Stolke D et al: Efficacy of single intracisternal bolus injection of recombinant tissue plasminogen activator to prevent delayed cerebral vasospasm after experimental subarachnoid hemorrhage. Neurosurgery 25:590, 1989
107. Shiraishi K, Sharp FR, Simon RP: Sequential metabolic changes in rat brain following middle cerebral artery occlusion: a 2-deoxyglucose study. J Cereb Blood Flow and Metab 9:765, 1989
108. Sindermann F, Dichgans J, Bergleiter R: Occlusion of the middle cerebral artery and its branches: angiographic and clinical correlates. Brain 92:607, 1969
109. Sloan MA: Thrombolysis and stroke. Arch Neurol 44:748, 1987
110. Sloan MA: Thrombolytic therapy in experimental focal cerebral ischemia. In Sawaya R (ed): Fibrinolysis in the Neurosciences. Hanley and Belfus, Philadelphia, 1990
111. Sloan MA, del Zoppo GJ, Brott TG: Thrombolysis and stroke. In Julian DG, Kubler W, Norris RM et al (eds): Thrombolysis in Cardiovascular Disease. Marcel Dekker, New York, 1989
112. Sloan MA, Price TR, Randall AM et al: Intracerebral hemorrhage after rt-PA and heparin for acute myocardial infarction: the TIMI II pilot and randomized trial combined experience, abstracted. Stroke 21:182, 1990
113. Stump DC, Califf RM, Topol EJ et al: Pharmacodynamics of thrombolysis with recombinant tissue-type plasminogen activator: correlation with characteristics of and clinical outcomes in patients with acute myocardial infarction. Circulation 80:1222, 1989
114. Sussman BJ, Fitch TSP: Thrombolysis with fibrinolysin in cerebral arterial occlusion. JAMA 167:1705, 1958
115. Taneda M: Prevention of delayed ischemia by radical removal of subarachnoid clots immediately after rupture of cerebral aneurysms. p. 595. In Auer LM (ed): Timing of Aneurysm Surgery. Walter de Gruyter, Berlin, 1985
116. Theron J, Courtheoux P, Casasco A et al: Local intraarterial fibrinolysis in the carotid territory. AJNR 10:753, 1989
117. TIMI Operations Committee: Update from the thrombolysis in myocardial infarction trial. J Am Coll Cardiol 10:970, 1987
118. Tomsick T, Brott T, Barsan W et al: Thrombus localization with emergency cerebral computed tomography, abstracted. Stroke 21:180, 1990
119. Topol EJ, Ellis SG, Califf RM et al: Thrombolysis and Angioplasty in Myocardial Infarction (TAMI) 4 Study Group: combined tissue-type plasminogen activator and prostacyclin therapy for acute myocardial infarction. J Am Coll Cardiol 14:877, 1989
120. tPA Acute Stroke Study Group: An open multicenter study of the safety and efficacy of various doses of tPA in patients with acute stroke: a progress report, abstracted. Stroke 21:181, 1990
121. Van de Werf F, Collen D: Coronary thrombolysis by intravenous infusion of synergistic thrombolytic agents. p. 231. In Julian D, Kubler W, Norris RM et al (eds): Thrombolysis in Cardiovascular Disease. Marcel Dekker, New York, 1989
122. Verstraete M, Vaughan DE: Latest update in thrombolysis. p. 409. In Julian D, Kubler W, Norris RM et al (eds): Thrombolysis in Cardiovascular Disease. Marcel Dekker, NY, 1989
123. Vines FS, Davis DO: Clinical-radiological correlation in cerebral venous occlusive disease. Radiology 98:9, 1971
124. Wagle WA, Dumoulin CL, Souza SP et al: 3-DFT MR of carotid and basilar arteries. AJNR 10:911, 1989
125. Yoshida T, Ueki S, Takahashi A: Intrathecal irrigation with urokinase in ruptured cerebral aneuryms cases. Basic studies and clinical applications. Neurol Med Chir 24:987, 1985
126. Zanette EM, Fieschi C, Bozzao L et al: Comparison of cerebral angiography and transcranial doppler sonography in acute stroke. Stroke 20:899, 1989
127. Zeumer H: Vascular recanalizing techniques in

interventional neuroradiology. J Neurol 231:287, 1985
128. Zeumer H, Freitag HJ, Grzyska U et al: Interventional neuroradiology: local intraarterial fibrinolysis in acute vertebrobasilar occlusion: technical developments and recent results. Neuroradiology 31:336, 1989
129. Zivin JA: A perspective on the future of thrombolytic stroke therapy. p. 33. In Ginsberg MD and Dietrich WD (eds): Cerebrovascular Diseases. Raven Press, New York, 1989

# 41
# CARDIOGENIC BRAIN EMBOLISM: INCIDENCE, VARIETIES, TREATMENT

Jonathan Y. Streifler
Anthony J. Furlan
Henry J.M. Barnett

## DEFINITIONS

*Cerebral embolism* refers to an obstruction of a blood vessel in the brain by an embolus originating anywhere in the circulatory system. In the new National Institute of Neurological Disorders and Stroke (NINDS) classification,[239] *pathological* sources for arterial embolism include the heart, the great vessels (artery-to-artery), and other sources such as those that produce paradoxical embolism. *Clinically* artery-to-artery emboli are classified in the atherothrombotic category, distinctly different from the cardioembolic category.

*Cardiogenic brain embolism,* the subject of this chapter, refers only to an obstruction in the cerebral arteries by an embolus originating in the heart.

## FREQUENCY

A pooling of data from several clinical, epidemiologic and multicenter projects, although differing in criteria and extent of laboratory workup, indicates that 15 to 20 percent of all ischemic strokes are cardioembolic.[24,39,79,221] The prevalence of cardioembolic stroke in patients younger than 45 years of age is much higher, ranging from 23 to 36 percent.[4,18,40] This is explained mainly by the lower prevalence of atherothrombotic strokes in this age group, and despite the fact that some of the major cardiac conditions underlying cerebral emboli are more frequent in the elderly.[261] The most common cardiac conditions associated with cerebral emboli are listed in Table 41-1. Concomitant cerebrovascular atherosclerosis is found in so many older patients, that the mere presence of a potential cardioembolic source does not establish a cardiac-related stroke mechanism.

## GENERAL FEATURES OF CARDIOEMBOLIC STROKE

Traditionally, cardioembolic strokes are severe and disabling. They consist mainly of large cortical in-

**TABLE 41-1. Most Common Cardiac Conditions Associated with Cerebral Emboli**

| Source | Percent of All Cardiogenic Emboli |
|---|---|
| Nonvalvular atrial fibrillation | 45 |
| Acute myocardial infarction | 15 |
| Ventricular aneurysm | 10 |
| Rheumatic heart disease | 10 |
| Prosthetic cardiac valve | 10 |
| Others | 10 |

(Adapted from the Cerebral Embolism Task Force,[39] with permission.)

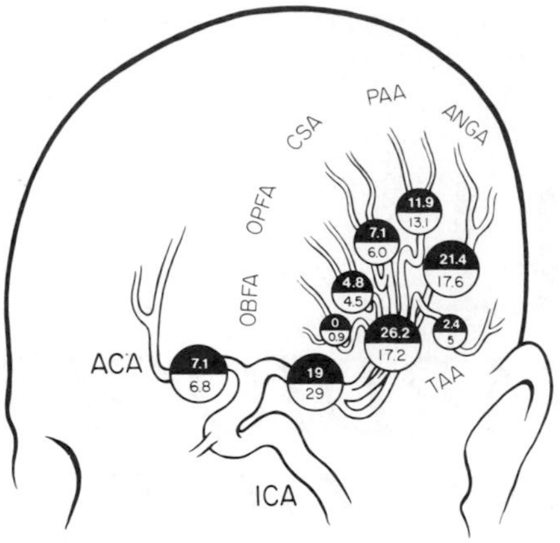


**Fig. 41-1.** "Balloon" catheters lodged in the branches of the internal carotid artery (ICA), in a proportion strikingly similar to the occlusion of branches of the anterior cerebral artery (ACA) and middle cerebral arteries. The lower numbers refer to the percentages of spontaneous occlusions, the upper to the percentages of the total "balloon emboli" that appear at these sites. The highest percentages of both were in the main middle cerebral trunk, the parietal arteries (PAA), and angular arteries (ANGA), with fewer in the central sulcus artery (CSA), operculofrontal artery (OPFA), temporal arteries (TAA), and orbitofrontal artery (OBFA). (Adapted from Gacs et al.,[88] with permission.)

farcts, some of which will undergo hemorrhagic transformation.[75,150] In a recent study, two-thirds of all massive cerebral infarctions were of cardiac embolic origin.[267] These features are commonly due to embolization of thrombus material or large vegetations, which constitute most of the cardiogenic emboli (Tables 41-1 and 41-2). Other cardiogenic emboli are smaller (Table 41-2); the associated cerebral events may be minor or transient with a small area of infarction,[108,128] or they may present as transient monocular blindness or a retinal infarction.[11,29,120,256]

The cerebral circulation absorbs 10 to 15 percent of the cardiac output,[170] and carotid artery blood flow accounts for approximately 90 percent of total cerebral blood flow.[103,104] The favorite sites for lodgment of cardiac emboli are the main trunk and branches of the middle cerebral artery (MCA). In a careful observational study, balloon emboli placed in the internal carotid artery favored the MCA location and lodged in the anterior cerebral artery only 7 percent of the time[88] (Fig. 41-1). About 10 percent of cerebral emboli enter the vertebral-basilar circulation, where they lodge mainly in the top of the basilar artery or in the main trunk or one of the branches of the posterior cerebral arteries.[35,194]

## CLINICAL DIAGNOSIS

Many historical and clinical features have been claimed to be relatively specific for an embolic stroke as opposed to a thrombotic one. These include the abrupt onset of a maximal deficit in an awake, usually active patient; headache, seizure, or diminished level of consciousness at the onset; and rapid improvement. Important additional features are a history of systemic embolism, the presence of a predisposing heart condition, a negative history of ipsilateral transient ischemic attacks (TIAs), and the involvement of more than one vascular area in the history or examination of the patient.[36,127,165,167,168]

**TABLE 41-2. Embolus Size (with Respect to Origin)**

| Large | Small |
|---|---|
| Ventricular thrombus (fibrin-rich) | Calcific material (valvular) |
| Atrial thrombus (fibrin-rich) | Small vegetations |
| | Platelet thrombi |
| Tumor material | Myxomatous material |
| Large vegetations | Septic material |

Based on recent studies,[23,133,207] the most specific criteria have been narrowed to (1) abrupt onset, (2) diminished level of consciousness at onset, (3) the history or presence of systemic embolism, and (4) the presence of a heart condition.

Emboli tend to occlude individual cortical branches and thus are frequently incriminated as the underlying cause in several distinct clinical syndromes, namely, isolated Wernicke's aphasia,[23,106] Broca's aphasia,[158] global aphasia without hemiparesis,[146] isolated hemianopia, and other features of the posterior cerebral artery syndromes.[23,74,194]

## CARDIAC EVALUATION

Historical information requires inquiry about rheumatic fever, recent or remote history of myocardial infarction, systemic embolism, and syncope or palpitations either in the past or at the onset of the stroke.

Physical examination must seek the presence of arrhythmia, cardiac valve dysfunction, cardiomegaly, cardiac failure, and any evidence of systemic embolization (petechiae, splinter hemorrhages, Roth's spots, visceral or limb ischemia).

Chest x-ray is used to help diagnose cardiomegaly or congestive heart failure.

A twelve-lead electrocardiogram (ECG) with a rhythm strip is used to detect an acute or old myocardial infarct and the nature of any dysrhythmia (e.g., atrial fibrillation, sick sinus syndrome). A 24-hour Holter monitor is recommended when the suspicion for a dysrhythmia is high and routine ECG is nondiagnostic.[209]

Echocardiography has a major role in the evaluation of patients suspected of a cardiac source for embolism. M-mode and particularly two-dimensional (2-D) echocardiography are excellent in showing the spatial and anatomic relationships of the heart, including valve configuration and movement, ventricular wall function, and the detection of masses in its cavities.[201,202]

Transesophageal echocardiography is superior for the evaluation of the left atrial appendage, the mitral valve apparatus, and the atrial septum.[192,200,232] It is also very sensitive in detecting atheromatosis of the aortic arch, which has recently been recognized as an occult source of systemic emboli.[200,252]

Doppler echocardiography is a useful technique for measuring the pressure gradient across a stenotic valve and thus estimating its severity. Color Doppler flow mapping is useful for estimating the degree of valvular regurgitation, and it provides a reasonable correlation with angiographic studies. Its greatest impact is in congenital heart diseases.[237] Contrast echocardiography is mainly used for the detection of intracardiac shunts.

It is beyond the scope of this chapter to provide more technical details and potential pitfalls of echocardiography; several recent reviews have been published.[71,201,202,232,237] It is excellent in the detection of left ventricular thrombi[61] (Fig. 41-2), mitral valve prolapse,[58,181,269] infective endocarditis,[171,182] patent foramen ovale,[145] atrial septal aneurysm,[229] cardiac myxoma,[156] and possibly left atrial thrombi.[235] It may detect very small valvular vegetations such as occur in nonbacterial thrombotic endocarditis[151] and may provide prognostic clues in many cardiac conditions (e.g., left atrial spontaneous echo contrast was found to be a good indicator for an increased thromboembolic risk in mitral valve disease[51]).

Other diagnostic techniques include ultrafast cardiac computed tomography (CT) scan, cardiac magnetic resonance imaging (MRI) and isotope-labeled platelet scintigraphy. These are relatively new and expensive, and further experience is needed before their role in the diagnosis of cardiac source of emboli can be ascertained.

Recently, an algorithm for a cardiac workup in patients with acute stroke has been suggested.[249] Extensive cardiac evaluation is considered mandatory for young stroke patients unless another pathogenesis is clear. For older patients, some advocate its use only if there is evidence of cardiac disease. The difficulty with this approach is that cerebral embolism may be

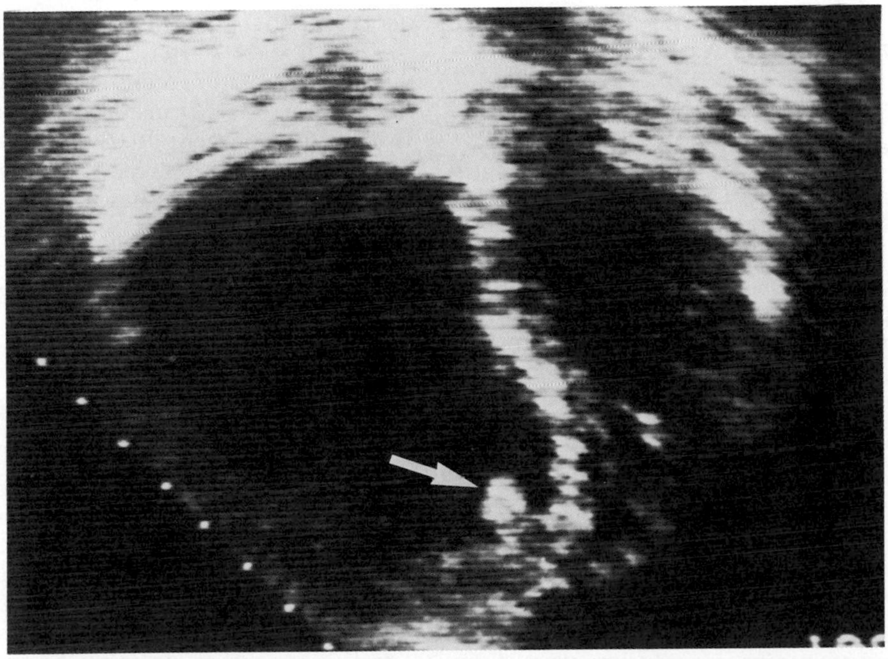

**Fig. 41-2.** Two-dimensional echocardiogram showing a mobile thrombus (*arrow*) within the left ventricle in a patient with dilated cardiomyopathy.

the presenting complaint in patients with cardiac disease not evident on history or physical examination.[120] Hence echocardiography should be considered in the workup of older patients with threatened or completed stroke in whom noncardiac mechanisms are inapparent.[40]

A retrospective analysis of 184 consecutive patients with focal cerebral ischemia admitted to our Intensive Stroke Research Unit illustrates the value of careful cardiac study.[209] There were 116 patients with stroke and 68 with transient ischemic attacks; cardiac disease was known by history and examination in 18.4 percent. An ECG detected cardiac disease in a further 14.1 percent: 3 additional patients with atrial fibrillation and 23 with silent myocardial infarction, predominantly in diabetics. Two-dimensional echocardiography, performed in approximately two-thirds of the patients, detected potential cardiac sources of emboli in a further 11.9 percent: 11 patients had dyskinetic segments, 6 had left ventricular thrombi, 1 had endocarditis, and 1 had global left ventricular dysfunction. All were monitored with continuous ECG recording for 48 hours: four instances of atrial fibrillation not previously suspected were detected. Approximately one-quarter of these patients underwent more prolonged ECG monitoring: two more with atrial fibrillation and one sick sinus syndrome were diagnosed. In summary, a number of these patients had potential sources of emboli not evident on history and examination: the majority (15.2 percent) were detected from the use of ECG monitoring and 2-D echocardiography.

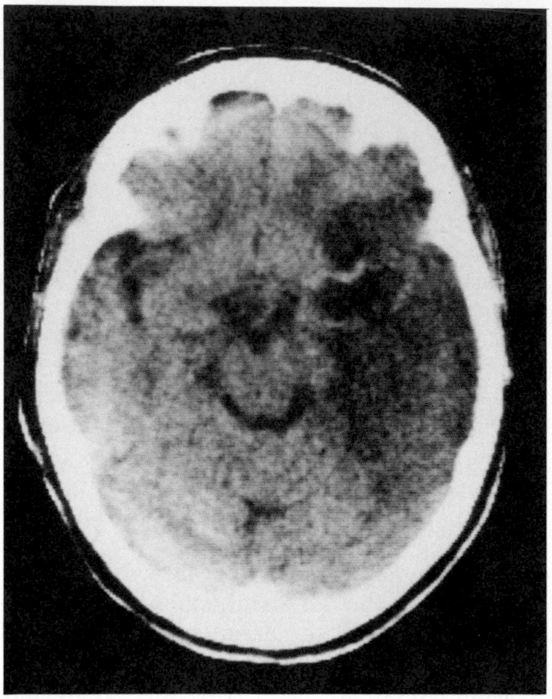

**Fig. 41-3.** A non-contrast scan demonstrating the left middle cerebral artery as a high-density structure along with nonhemorrhagic infarction in the distribution of the left middle and posterior cerebral arteries. (From Gacs et al.,[89] with permission.)

## RADIOLOGIC EVALUATION

### Brain Computed Tomography and Magnetic Resonance Imaging

Certain CT findings are fairly characteristic of embolic infarction: (1) the presence of a cortical infarct, especially in the distribution of the middle or posterior cerebral artery territories, (2) the demonstration of multiple infarcts in different territories, (3) an embolus visible in the middle cerebral artery ("hyperdense MCA sign") (Fig. 41-3), and (4) hemorrhage, usually deep within the infarct.[75,107,150] The disintegration of the original embolus and distal migration of embolic fragments results in hemorrhagic transformation.[39,75] The capillary walls, damaged by ischemia, are unable to bear the impact of the restored blood flow (Fig. 41-4). However, some instances of hemorrhagic transformation have been proved by autopsy with persistent occlusion of the main artery, suggesting that hemorrhagic transformation may result also from an early rise in perfusion pressure in the presence of efficient leptomeningeal collaterals.[183]

CT studies that have looked at hemorrhagic infarction immediately after stroke onset report a prevalence of 2 to 4 percent;[37,82] studies that included serial scans 2 to 4 days after the stroke onset report a prevalence of 10 to 20 percent.[38,107] A recent study[184] identified hemorrhagic transformation in 6.2 percent at 1 to 4 days, 27.5 percent at 10 days, and 40.6 percent at 1 month. This last figure is similar to the frequency reported in autopsy studies.[75,150] The majority of hemorrhagic transformations are clinically silent.

MRI can better identify multiple embolic infarcts in different territories,[266] adds no distinctive diagnostic features, but may be combined with MR angiography to identify MCA stem embolic occlusions.

### Cerebral Angiography

Isolated occlusion of the middle cerebral artery, the posterior cerebral artery, or one of their branches in the absence of atherosclerotic changes is highly suggestive of cardiogenic embolism. In a recent study where angiography was carried out within 6 hours of stroke onset, 15 of the 22 patients who had isolated intracranial occlusion demonstrated a well-defined cardiac source of emboli.[72] Spontaneous recanalization occurs in the majority of cases undergoing serial angiography.[184]

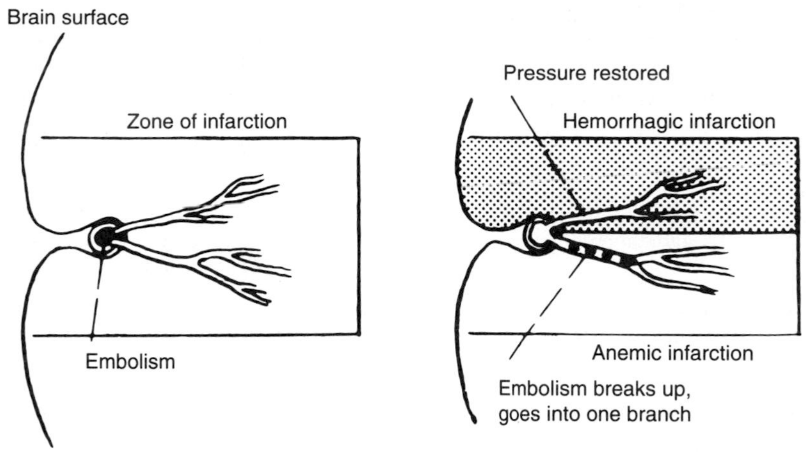


**Fig. 41-4.** Hypothetical mechanism of hemorrhagic transformation caused by distal migration of embolic fragments with reperfusion of infarcted tissue. (Adapted from Toole,[251] with permission.)

## CARDIAC DISEASES CAUSING CEREBRAL EMBOLISM

Intracardiac thrombi form in the presence of structural abnormalities of the heart valves or the walls of its chambers. They develop in the presence of dysrhythmias that cause stasis within the left atrium or in certain dyskinetic states of the left ventricle. Emboli may arise from valve vegetations, intracardiac tumors, or even from systemic veins when the embolic material traverses the heart through a patent foramen ovale or atrial septal defect (paradoxical embolism). Very rarely emboli arise from pulmonary veins or a pulmonary arteriovenous fistula. The mechanisms of these embolic phenomena are shown in Figure 41-5. The cardiac disorders associated with embolism and the location of the sources are listed in Table 41-3.

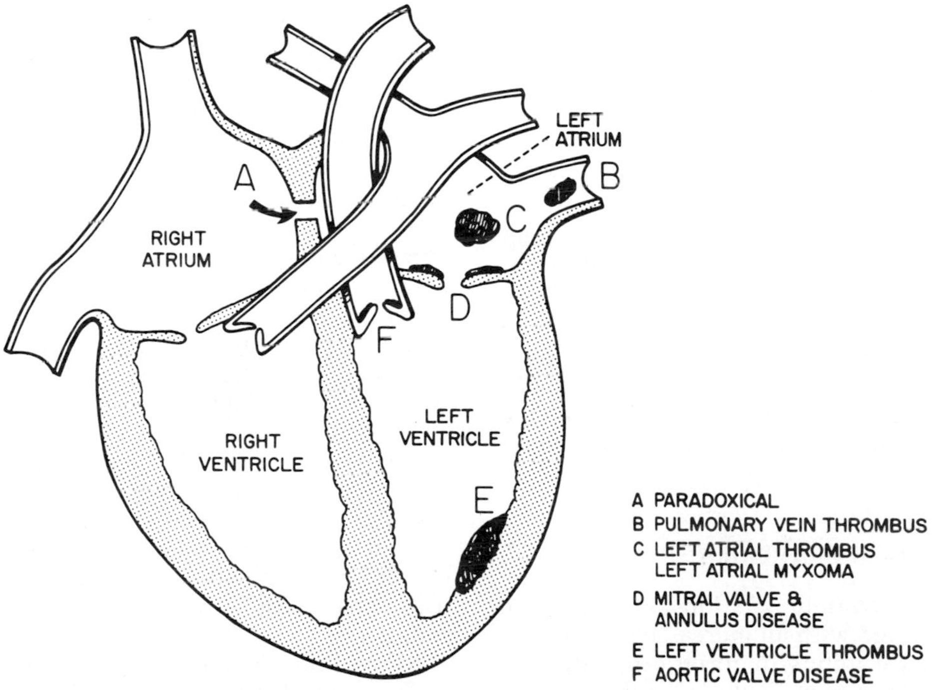


**Fig. 41-5.** A schematic representation of the heart showing the potential sites of origin of emboli.

**TABLE 41-3. Important Cardiac Sources for Cerebral Ischemia**

| Disorder | Location of Potentially Embolic Material |
|---|---|
| Myocardial infarction, recent, with endocardial damage | Endocardial surface left ventricle |
| Myocardial infarction, old, with akinetic segment or major aneurysmal dilation | Particularly apical, in left ventricle, trapped in trabeculae corneae cordis |
| Rheumatic mitral stenosis[a] | Auricle or dilated atrium |
| Rheumatic mitral regurgitation[a] | "Jet" lesions on atrial endocardium |
| Infective endocarditis | On the valve surface and at its attachment |
| Nonbacterial thrombotic endocarditis | On the valve surface |
| Libman-Sacks endocarditis | On the valve surface and less commonly on chordae tendineae, papillary muscles, and mural endocardium |
| Myxomatous degeneration (mitral valve prolapse)[a] | At atrial site of valve attachment, also on valve surface |
| Mitral annulus calcification[a] | Attached to valve surface[b] |
| Calcific aortic stenosis[a] | Calcification begins at base of cusp, but rarely extends to free edge |
| Prosthetic heart valve[a] | At site of attachment, also on surface of device |
| Cardiomyopathy | Atrium or ventricle, usually trapped in trabeculae corneae cordis |
| Atrial myxoma | Tumor usually attached to margin of septum secundum |
| Atrial fibrillation | Thrombus within the left atrium |
| Sick sinus syndrome | Thrombus within the left atrium |

[a] These are prone to infective endocarditis.
[b] In addition to thrombi, calcific material from the degenerative valve may break off as embolic material.
(Adapted and modified from Barnett,[270] with permission.)

## CARDIAC DYSRHYTHMIAS AND CEREBRAL EMBOLISM

The two abnormalities of cardiac rhythm most often associated with focal cerebral ischemia are atrial fibrillation and the sick sinus syndromes.

Diffuse *nonfocal* cerebral ischemia (i.e., syncope or Stokes-Adams attacks) may be caused by cardiac dysrhythmias that induce cerebral hypoperfusion. Reduction in cerebral perfusion is usually the result of complete heart block or paroxysmal tachyarrhythmia associated with a rapid ventricular rate of more than 180 beats per minutes (e.g., paroxysmal atrial tachycardia, ventricular tachycardia, or ventricular fibrillation). Focal cerebral ischemia is rare with such disturbances of cardiac rhythm. Of 290 patients requiring insertion of a pacemaker for cardiac arrhythmias, 4 had experienced focal cerebral ischemic symptoms, but in only 2 was the focal ischemia related to their cardiac rhythm disturbance.[208]

### Atrial Fibrillation

For many years atrial fibrillation (AF) has been known to be associated with an increased risk of cerebral emboli from thrombus material originating in the left atrium. Older reports included many patients with rheumatic heart disease and concomitant valvular disease carrying an independent risk. In the Framingham study[262] the presence of both carried a 17-fold increase in the risk of stroke as compared to normal controls.

In an autopsy study of 642 patients with atrial fibrillation of various causes, a left atrial thrombus was found in 15.8 percent as opposed to 1.7 percent in 642 age- and sex-matched controls. Left ventricular thrombus was encountered in 1 percent of patients with AF. Cerebral infarction occurred in 32.2 percent of the patients with AF and in only 11 percent of the controls. The frequency of cerebral infarction increased with the duration of fibrillation; the most common causes of AF were rheumatic and ischemic heart disease.[3]

Nonvalvular atrial fibrillation (NVAF) is the term commonly used to specify the group of patients in which the underlying cause is other than valvular disease. NVAF affects 2 to 5 percent of the general population over age 60[126,188] and, within this group, its prevalence increases steeply with advancing age.[126] NVAF is a major cause of cardioembolic stroke[36,39,168] as well as of massive cerebral infarction.[267] The presence of atrial fibrillation in acute stroke patients is associated with a worsened prognosis at 1 and 6 months.[34]

In the Framingham study,[262] NVAF carried a fivefold increased risk for stroke. The frequency of stroke varies depending on the populations under study: as low as 1.7 percent per year in an outpatient-based study in Olmsted County[55] and as high as 5 to 9 percent in inpatient-based studies.[73,217] For a group of nontreated patients with either chronic or intermittent AF, a 6 percent yearly risk of stroke has been suggested.[246]

NVAF is not a uniform group. The elderly, those with coexisting congestive heart failure or hypertension and those with a past history of stroke, harbor a higher stroke risk. Other risk factors include recent onset of arrhythmia, chronic forms (as opposed to paroxysmal), left ventricular wall abnormalities by echocardiogram, and the presence of left atrial enlargement.[32,77,246,261,263]

A subset of NVAF patients that carries a significantly lower risk of stroke includes patients younger than 60 years and without definable heart disease. This group of "lone atrial fibrillators" carries a yearly risk of stroke of less than 0.5 percent.[135,187]

Thyrotoxicosis, complicated by atrial fibrillation in 10 to 30 percent of patients,[62] accounts for only 2 to 5 percent of all NVAF cases.[195] Several reports, however, suggest that if provocative tests to reveal occult thyrotoxicosis are used, this figure may be as high as 30 percent.[62,78] Whether the risk of stroke in such patients is similar to or higher than other NVAF patients is controversial.[195,203]

Based on the accepted pathogenesis of stroke in most patients with NVAF (i.e., embolus originating from a left atrial thrombus), of antithrombotic treatment has been administered and evaluated in four randomized trials.[26,45,196,247] The first, a Danish trial (AFASAK),[196] indicated a benefit of warfarin over placebo, as well as over low-dose aspirin, with regard to all endpoint events (stroke, TIA, and systemic embolization). The rate of side effects necessitating withdrawal from the study in patients on conventional warfarin treatment was high. The patients in this trial tended to be elderly, with an average age of 74.2 years. The preliminary report from the North American Stroke Prevention in Atrial Fibrilation (SPAF) Study[247] indicated that both aspirin and warfarin are superior to placebo, but the benefit for aspirin was found only in patients under 75 years of age. This trial continues to seek an answer to the relative superiority, if any, of warfarin over aspirin. The dose of aspirin being tested is 325 mg/day, as compared with 75 mg/day in the Danish trial. Because major bleeding complicates conventional dosage of anticoagulation, especially in elderly, hypertensive patients,[149,217] and because a less intense anticoagulant regimen has been proven useful in other conditions (deep-vein thrombosis and prevention of pulmonary embolism) with fewer side effects,[114] the SPAF group is using a lower dose of warfarin (international normalized ratio (INR) 2.0 to 3.5) in their ongoing trial.[246]

The Boston Area Anticoagulation Trial for Atrial Fibrillation Study (BAATAF)[26] used even lower doses of warfarin (INR 1.5 to 2.7) and found it to be highly effective as compared to placebo (and possibly to aspirin casually taken by 46 percent of the placebo group). Bleeding complications were low; major bleeding occurred similarly in the control and treatment groups. The Canadian Atrial Fibrillation Anticoagulation Study (CAFA)[45] was prematurely terminated due to the publication of the positive results in the AFASAK and SPAF. It was the only double-blind study, and the target warfarin range was INR 2.0 to 3.0. This study also showed a beneficial effect of warfarin, though the difference was not statistically significant because of small numbers of outcome events in an abbreviated study. The relative risk reductions in the primary outcome events (ischemic stroke and systemic thromboembolism) for the four studies (AFASAK, SPAF, BAATAF, CAFA) were 60 percent, 81 percent, 86 percent, and 44.8 percent, respectively.

Analyses of these four trials may determine which subgroups benefit most and the required duration of antithrombotic therapy. The risk of stroke appears to be higher during the first 5 years after the onset of AF,[263] and it may be that very prolonged treatment yields a diminishing return. Long-term warfarin may not be justified in certain low-risk subgroups such as young patients with "lone AF." In such cases, aspirin may prove to be a reasonable alternative.

Anticoagulant therapy is strongly recommended in patients with AF secondary to mitral valve disease or dilated cardiomyopathy, in patients with NVAF who have documented systemic embolism, and probably in those with concomitant congestive heart failure. It is also recommended in patients with newly recognized thyrotoxicosis before a euthyroid state is reached, and before cardioversion in all patients.[62]

## Sick Sinus Syndrome

The term sick sinus syndrome (SSS) encompasses any form of sinus node depression, such as marked sinus bradycardia (less than 50 beats/min), sinus arrest, or sinoatrial block. The SSS occurs throughout life but is more common in older patients. It may be associated with ischemic heart disease, cardiomyopathies, and neuromuscular disease but is frequently idiopathic or degenerative in origin. The bradyarrhythmia is often associated with paroxysmal atrial tachyarrhythmia, including supraventricular tachycardia and atrial flutter or fibrillation. Such a combination is often referred to as the tachycardia-bradycardia syndrome.[115]

The clinical manifestations are mainly those produced by transient global cerebral ischemia (i.e., light-headedness and syncope). However, patients with SSS are at high risk for stroke, which is usually massive and presumably of cardiac embolic origin.[1,69,218]

Of a total of 56 patients with SSS, Rubenstein et al.[218] described 10 patients with focal cerebral ischemia, in 8 the bradycardia-tachycardia syndrome was present. Fairfax et al.[69] found a significantly higher incidence of embolism (predominantly cerebral) in 100 patients with the sick sinus syndrome, compared with 712 age- and sex-matched controls with chronic complete heart block. Their criteria for SSS were unexplained sinus bradycardia with a pulse less than 60 or recurrent sinus arrest with or without supraventricular tachyarrhythmias. Systemic and cerebral embolism occurred in 16 percent of these patients with SSS, compared to only 1.9 percent of those with chronic complete heart block ($P < 0.001$). Only 3 patients of 16 had purely systemic emboli, and in 13 the embolus was to the cerebral or retinal circulation with or without systemic embolism.

The only effective treatment for SSS is pacemaker implantation, yet the overall stroke rate is still high after pacing.[76] There are several types of pacemakers, and recent reports that analyzed the stroke rate with respect to the type of pacemaker used found a higher rate when ventricular demand pacemakers were used, as opposed to those of atrial demand, especially in the elderly.[76,222] Further analysis disclosed a much higher incidence of atrial fibrillation in the patients with ventricular pacemakers, an important factor that can partly explain the higher incidence of stroke in this group. In the majority of patients chronic AF appeared after pacer implantation. A causal factor may be the development of atrial enlargement in patients with the ventricular pacemaker, caused by atrial contraction against atrioventricular valves closed due to the retrograde ventriculoatrial conduction.[222] Thus, it seems that one of the measures for stroke prevention is to install an atrial demand pacemaker in all suitable candidates.[222]

Platelet antiaggregation agents may or may not provide protection against stroke and the role of anticoagulants has not been thoroughly assessed.[76]

## MYOCARDIAL INFARCTION

Acute myocardial infarction (AMI) is complicated by stroke in 2.5 percent of patients within 2 to 4 weeks of onset.[121,206] Most strokes occur in the presence of left ventricular thrombi (LVT)[121,245,258] (Fig. 41-6), believed to be the underlying cause for the cerebral embolism.

The presence of LVT is best detected with two-dimensional echocardiography; a specific, sensitive technique superior to cardiac ventriculography (Fig. 41-2).[201,202] By this technique, LVT were detected in 30 to 35 percent of a series of patients sustaining AMI, 2 to 11 days after its onset.[10,142,226,254]

Specific risk factors for LVT include the presence of a hypokinetic or akinetic segment of the ventricular wall and injury to the endocardial surface. These complications are more common in transmural, anterior wall infarcts and the combination of stasis and thrombogenicity enhances the formation of LVT.[10,86,121,179,258] Echocardiographic follow-up of relatively small numbers of patients with AMI, who had LVT but were treated in a "conservative" way (minidose heparin and aspirin), showed resolution of the thrombus in 80 percent of cases after 1 year, and at 2

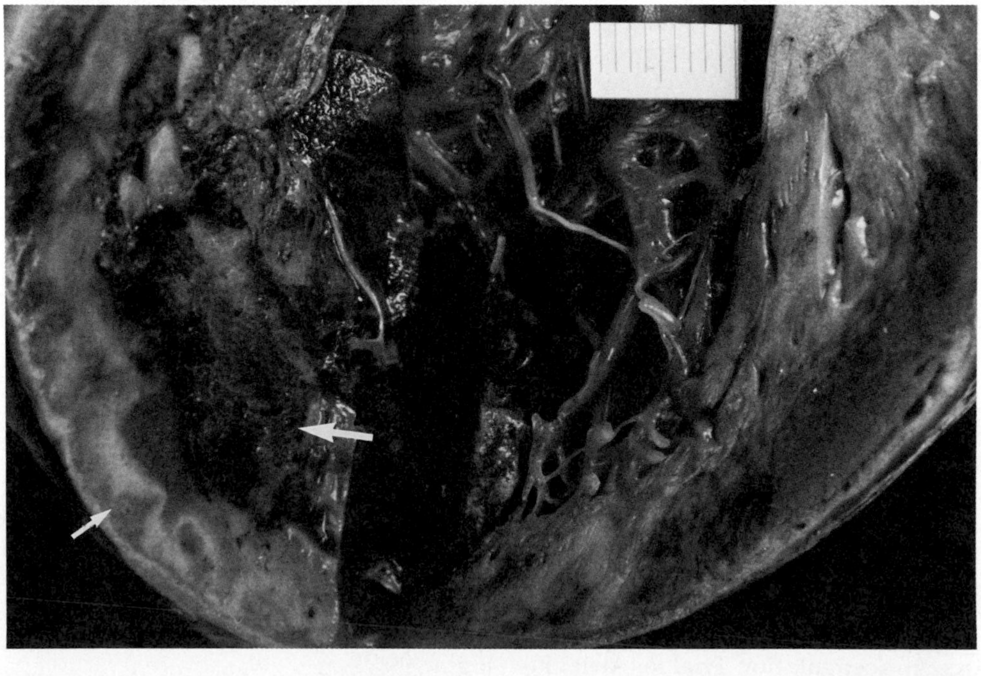

**Fig. 41-6.** Pathological specimen showing myocardial infarction (*small arrow*) with superimposed mural thrombosis (*large arrow*).

years a further disappearance in 20 percent was documented.[179] In another study,[141,142] where two-thirds of the patients with LVT were anticoagulated, about half the LVTs were resolved by the end of 12 weeks, regardless of treatment. In the anticoagulated group 93 percent showed either resolution or change in size or shape.[142]

The risk of clinical cerebral embolism in patients with LVT followed for up to 2 years is between 10 and 15 percent. The majority of strokes occur during the first 3 months, most within the first 10 days.[63,86,164] Risk factors for embolization include advanced age, as well as protrusion and mobility of the thrombotic mass in the left ventricle.[121,164]

In an autopsy study,[166] the prevalence of LVT as detected by echocardiography was confirmed, whereas nowadays that of cerebral and systemic embolization was higher than suspected clinically. Thrombi in the left heart were found in 35 percent of patients with a history of myocardial infarction. Patients with *acute* myocardial infarction had thrombi in the left side of the heart in 40 percent of instances, compared to only 26 percent in those with *healed* myocardial infarction. In patients with acute myocardial infarction with or without mural thrombi, cerebral and systemic arterial occlusions were detected in 35 percent and 21 percent, respectively. In patients with healed myocardial infarction, arterial occlusions were detected in 26 percent of patients with and in 28 percent of patients without mural thrombi.

LVT in healed myocardial infarction are usually associated with a persistent left ventricular dyskinesia or the presence of a left ventricular aneurysm. When these conditions have existed, LVT have been detected by echocardiography in almost half of the patients. The likelihood of emboli occurring has been variable.[86,144,245] In a recent study, where LVT were first detected at a mean of 32 months following an AMI, the embolic rate was 10 percent during 22 months of follow-up.[245]

Treatment to prevent stroke after AMI is still controversial.[40,63,86,179] Several controlled clinical trials demonstrated beneficial effects of anticoagulant therapy, yet the occurrence of hemorrhagic complications was high.[40] Recently, several large controlled studies have demonstrated much more favorable results. The first two studies, including 421 patients, clearly favored heparin anticoagulation. Both studies used subcutaneous (SC) heparin, 12,500 units every 12 hours for 10 days in patients with anterior AMI. The first study[254] compared this regimen to SC heparin in a dose that is given to prevent venous thrombosis (5,000 units bid). The incidence of LVT at day 10 was 11 percent in the high-dose group as opposed to 32 percent in the low-dose group. Nonhemorrhagic infarction occurred in 1 percent and 4 percent, respectively. In the second study,[226] the presence of LVT was evaluated by echocardiography before discharge. LVT were present in 36.5 percent of the controls who received no anticoagulation, as compared to 17.7 percent of the heparin-treated group. There were two embolic strokes in the control group as opposed to none in the treatment group.

A third study compared long-term warfarin therapy with placebo:[238] 1,214 patients entered the study at a mean of 27 days following the onset of AMI and were followed for an average of 37 months. The target warfarin range was 2.8 to 4.8 INR yet serious bleeding was noted in only 0.6 percent per year of the warfarin group. Stroke relative risk reduction was 55 percent, and death and reinfarction risk reductions were 24 and 34 percent, respectively.

Antiplatelet agents have usually,[122,141] but not always,[138] been found ineffective in the prevention/resolution of LVT and subsequent emboli. In one large multicenter trial, the stroke prevalence within 10 days of an AMI was reduced by half in those patients who were treated early with a 160-mg daily dose of aspirin as compared to placebo.[119]

Thrombolytic therapy is of short duration and is usually discontinued before the detection of LVT. Thus its role in prevention of LVT formation and subsequent stroke is uncertain.[40,63] The two most commonly used thrombolytic agents (i.e., streptokinase [SK] and alteplase (tissue plasminogen activator [tPA]) are associated with an increased rate of intracerebral hemorrhage.[204] With tPA the risk is lower, but the overall stroke rate is similar due to an apparent excess in ischemic strokes with the use of this agent.[118] Both SK and tPA may increase platelet aggregation, mainly by thrombin activation. This paradoxical hypercoagulable state is not inhibited by aspirin but can be reversed with heparin.[66] The latest large study[118] addressing this controversy compared the use of heparin to placebo subsequent to SK and tPA: heparin was started 12 hours after the administration of the thrombolytic agents. No additional benefit was detected from heparin with respect to stroke prevention or reinfarction, whereas the occurrence of major bleeding was somewhat higher.

The recommended treatment policy for patients with acute anterior transmural myocardial infarction includes the use of high-dose heparin, even if thrombolytic therapy is given initially.[63] Heparin should be given intravenously or subcutaneously in a dose sufficient to maintain a kaolin-cephalin coagulation time between 1.5 and 2.5 times the control. Echocardiography should be performed 5 to 7 days later to detect LVT. If no thrombus or wall motion abnormalities are found, heparin should be discontinued. If LVT or dyskinetic regions are present, warfarin may be started and continued under echocardiographic monitoring. Anticoagulant therapy should be discontinued after 3 to 6 months, even if LVT persists.[40,234]

Routine anticoagulation has not been recommended if LVT are detected in an aneurysmal sac at a time remote from AMI.[86] Instead, long-term anticoagulation has been recommended only in patients with cerebral insults attributed to persistent LVT.[40,234] However, this "conservative" approach must be reassessed following the results of the above-mentioned Oslo study.[238]

## Nonischemic Cardiomyopathies

This term is used to describe a heterogeneous, relatively rare group of cardiac conditions of different etiologies that result in progressive global cardiac dysfunction. Traditionally, the cardiomyopathies are divided into three types: dilated (formerly called congestive), hypertrophic, and restrictive. The latter is very rare in Western countries, whereas in the tropics it exists mainly as endocardial fibroelastosis. The hypertrophic type (also called idiopathic hypertrophic subaortic stenosis) is seldom associated with intracardiac thrombi or cerebral embolism unless atrial fibrillation coexists.[83,94]

## Dilated Cardiomyopathy

Differing causal conditions have been described in relation to this syndrome, including inflammatory processes (such as viral infections, Chagas disease, and other infectious agents), immunologic disorders, toxic agents (mainly alcohol and chemotherapeutic agents such as Adriamycin), nutritional deficiencies, and peripartum cardiomyopathy, as well as several forms of familial cardiomyopathies.[85,117] Unless a specific cause is identified, it is best to refer to most cases as idiopathic.

*Idiopathic dilated cardiomyopathy* (IDC) affects predominantly young men. It is a rare disease manifested by progressive heart failure, arrhythmia, or thromboembolism and its diagnosis is made by exclusion.[2,212,243] Prognosis is very poor and there is a high incidence of sudden death. Arrhythmias are common, either as nonsustained ventricular tachycardia or as chronic atrial fibrillation, which develops in 20 to 30 percent of the patients.[162,212] This arrhythmia and the high prevalence of left ventricular thrombi found in IDC, as well as in other types of dilated cardiomyopathies are believed to be the underlying cause for stroke and other embolic complications in these patients. In an autopsy study of 152 IDC patients,[212] ventricular thrombi or mural endocardial plaques (considered to be organized thrombi) were found in up to 78 percent of cases. The pathogenesis is believed to be chronic intracavitary stasis. Unlike patients after myocardial infarction there is no aneurysmal sac and thrombi tend to be relatively small and scattered throughout the cavity with a predilection for the apex where stasis is maximal[44,96,160] (Fig. 41-7). Echocardiography detects the presence of thrombi in 11 to 58 percent of patients with dilated cardiomyopathy (Fig. 41-2) yet it is not helpful for the detection of patients

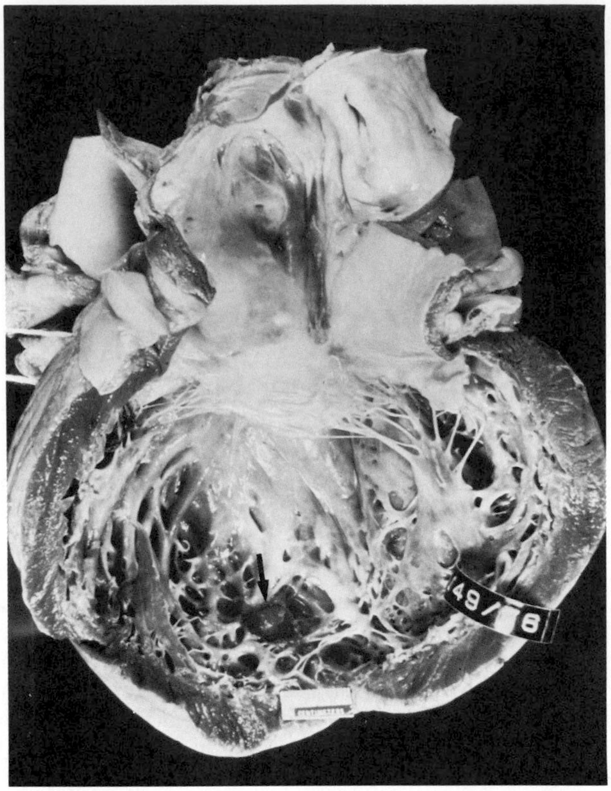

**Fig. 41-7.** Thrombus protruding (*arrow*) from trabeculae carneae cordis in patient with dilated cardiomyopathy. (From Barnett,[270] with permission.)

at high risk for stroke as no correlation has been found between the detection of thrombi and the presence of emboli.[44,96] The annual frequency of embolic complication varies between 1.4 and 3.5 percent in different series[44,85] depending on the presence or absence of anticoagulant therapy and probably also on the severity of the disease. Controversy exists regarding the importance of congestive heart failure, marked cardiac enlargement, and the presence of atrial fibrillation.[44,85,96]

The recommended empirical treatment to reduce the risk of embolization is long-term anticoagulation.[85,234] However, recently it has been reported that most patients do not receive this treatment.[160] This conservative approach may be due to the fact that the benefit of long-term anticoagulation has not been established convincingly or because of the higher risk for bleeding in such patients.[70,243] A plea for a prospective randomized trial of anticoagulation, including low-dose and minidose warfarin, has recently been published.[70]

Cerebral infarction is an uncommon complication in patients with inherited neuromuscular diseases who are prone to develop cardiomyopathies.[20] Cerebral embolization may occur, in several specific cardiomyopathies complicating systemic diseases such as sarcoidosis and amyloidosis.[210]

## VALVULAR HEART DISEASE

Recent years have witnessed a dramatic decline in the incidence of rheumatic heart disease. This has been offset by the recognition of an association between mitral valve prolapse and other less frequent valvular lesions and cerebral ischemia. Valvular disorders remain significant causes of embolic cerebral ischemia.

### Rheumatic Heart Disease

Clinical embolic events occur in about 20 percent of patients with rheumatic heart disease (RHD).[47,147] Embolism usually complicates mitral stenosis or mixed stenosis-regurgitation, whereas pure mitral regurgitation or aortic disease less frequently results in embolism.[47,50]

### Mitral Stenosis

Mitral stenosis is most frequently of rheumatic origin. Left atrial thrombi (Fig. 41-8) form in a large number of affected patients, particularly in the presence of atrial fibrillation or cardiac failure.[97] Left atrial thrombus is present in 15 to 17 percent of patients at autopsy, regardless of whether or not there has been a history of embolism.[47] Thrombi may develop in patients with only mild mitral stenosis,[230] explaining why embolism may be a presenting symptom of mitral stenosis. Thrombi may develop on "jet lesions" that can form on the wall of the left ventricle (Fig. 41-9). In patients with mitral stenosis the yearly frequency of all symptomatic emboli is about 4 percent; more than half are cerebral, but many asymptomatic systemic emboli and occasional asymptomatic cerebral emboli are found at postmortem. Recurrent embolism is common (30 to 75 percent), usually within 6 to 12 months[50,147,248] and the presence of atrial fibrillation increases the risk of embolism 4-fold.[47] The risk of embolism also increases with increasing duration of mitral stenosis.[216]

Surgical repair of mitral stenosis, either open or closed commissurotomy, also carries some risk of embolism. Percutaneous valvuloplasty—a technique that was only recently introduced—probably carries the same risk.[53,147,189]

Long-term anticoagulation is recommended for prophylaxis in patients with rheumatic mitral stenosis and coexistent atrial fibrillation as the combina-

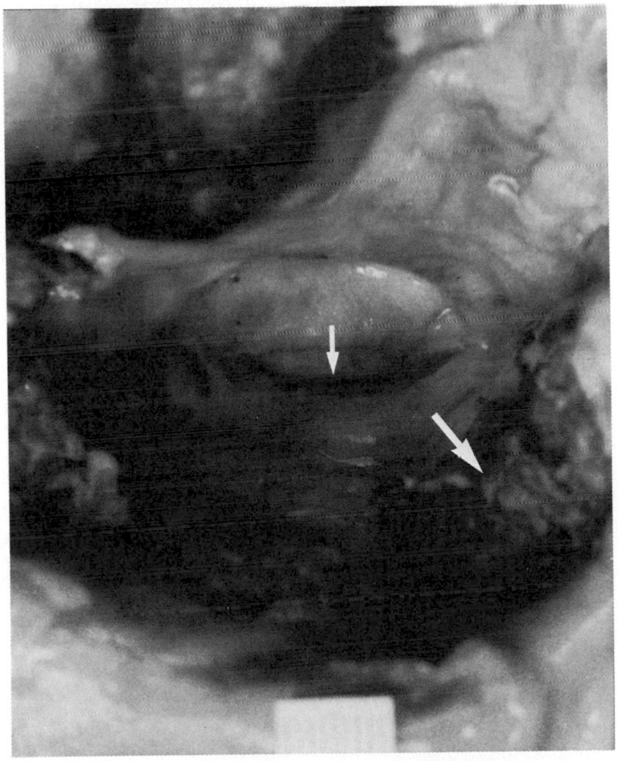

**Fig. 41-8.** Pathological specimen showing mitral stenosis (*small arrow*) and left atrial thrombus (*large arrow*).

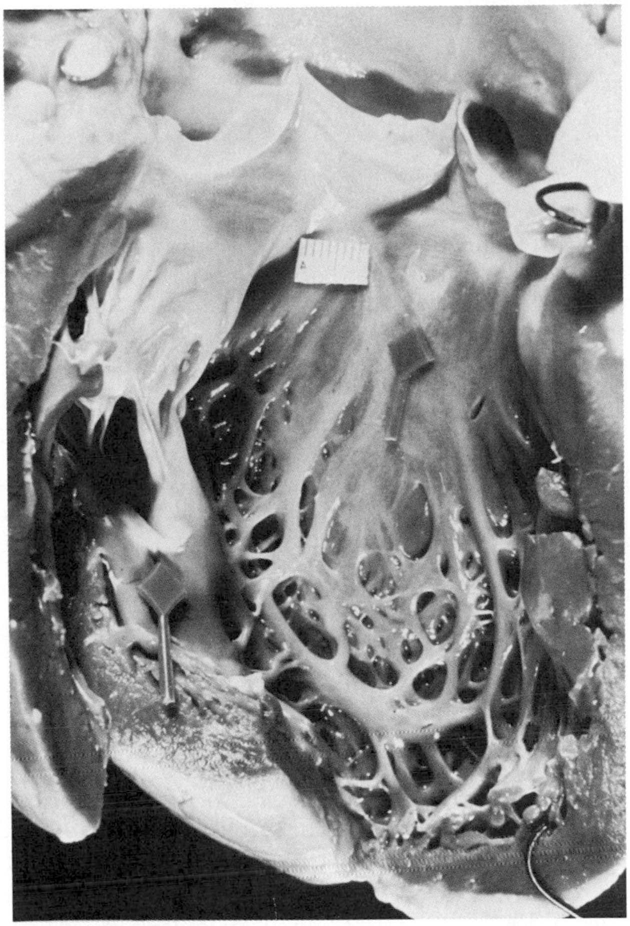

**Fig. 41-9.** Pathologic specimen showing mitral stenosis due to rheumatic heart disease with "jet lesions" (*arrows*) on the wall of the left ventricle.

tion of both carries a 17-fold increase in stroke risk compared with matched controls.[262] The embolic and recurrent embolic rates are notably reduced with long-term anticoagulation, although long-term therapy is not totally protective.[47,147,248]

## Mitral Regurgitation

Mitral regurgitation most commonly results from mitral valve prolapse or papillary muscle dysfunction in association with ischemic or rheumatic heart disease. When severe, the incompetence produces an ulcerated "jet lesion" on the atrial endocardial surface; left atrial thrombus may form there. This occurs in somewhat less than 10 percent of patients and almost invariably in the presence of atrial fibrillation.[244] Thromboembolism is a recognized complication of mitral regurgitation.[198] The incidence is low, even though atrial fibrillation is a common accompaniment particularly late in its course.[68,231]

## Aortic Stenosis

Isolated aortic stenosis is mainly caused by calcification of the valve cusps, a process observed predominantly in elderly people. Until recently this was considered a relatively benign disorder causing dizziness or syncope. Sudden death was an occasional complication. Most patients with cerebral embolism had multivalvular rheumatic disease or coexistent infective endocarditis.[139] With the introduction of echocardiography, Doppler, and catheterization it has become evident that calcific aortic stenosis may be responsible for more cerebral vascular insults than previously recognized.[53,113,128] Cerebral vascular complications occasionally occur with catheterization or percutaneous balloon valvuloplasty.

Calcific aortic stenosis is detected by echocardiography in about 1 percent of consecutive patients with either TIAs or strokes.[180,209] Emboli in these patients usually manifest as transient monocular blindness and retinal strokes.[29] The emboli are small, composed of calcium and detected by fundoscopy. Because of their small size they may produce no signs or symptoms elsewhere in the brain or in the systemic vasculature.[53] A relatively large autopsy study corroborates this hypothesis,[113] while another is not supportive.[139]

Larger emboli are usually caused by manipulation of the valve either by percutaneous balloon valvuloplasty or by the passage of a catheter.[128] After manipulation, some emboli are clinically silent and detected only by brain CT scan.[53]

Long-term antithrombotic therapy is not recommended in isolated aortic-stenosis. Antiplatelet agents may have a place in some symptomatic patients, although the evidence is based on speculation.[39,147]

## Mitral Annulus Calcification

Mitral annulus calcification (MAC) is a process of calcification that afflicts elderly people and is considered to be a degenerative aging process.[136,177,198] Apart from the coexistence of calcific aortic valve, MAC is frequently associated with coronary atherosclerosis, cardiac conduction disturbances, chronic atrial fibrillation, cardiomegaly, congestive heart failure, and carotid artery disease[8,84,136,174,177,180] (Fig. 41-10). Thus it is not surprising that MAC is associated with an increased risk of stroke.[8,56,174,180] Caseation of the ring and superimposed thrombus or endocarditis have been detected[148,199] (Fig. 41-11), and a few case reports have provided pathologic evidence of calcific embolic material in patients with MAC.[81,148,211] For the most part it is to be considered a marker of generalized calcific atherosclerosis, and it may not be an important cause of embolism.[39,84] The significance of this

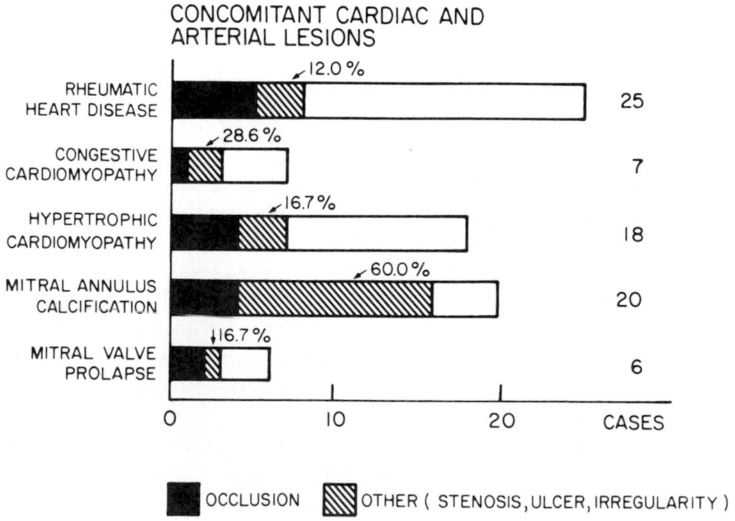


**Fig. 41-10.** A study of 76 patients with a variety of cardiac lesions in association with cerebral ischemic events. Cerebral angiography indicated highest percentage of concomitant potentially thromboembolic lesions in patients with mitral annulus calcification. (Courtesy of Dr. T. Irino, Osaka, Japan.)

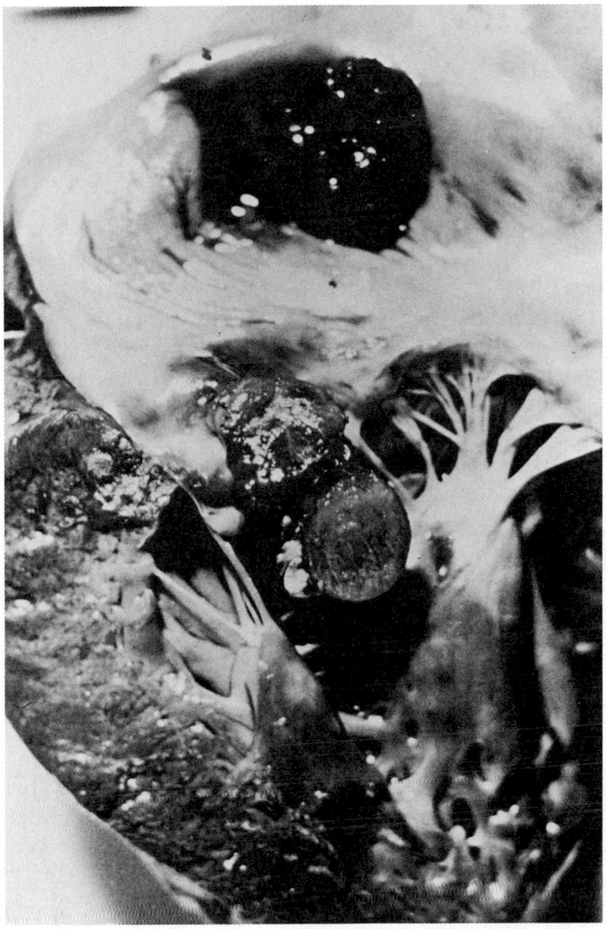

**Fig. 41-11.** Large thrombus attached to mitral annulus calcification: an incidental postmortem finding in an elderly patient. (From Pomerance,[199] with permission.)

lesion to stroke remains unsettled because it occurs in a population prone to progressive atheroma, and it is difficult to define which of the potential embolic mechanisms are operative in a given patient.

## Mitral Valve Prolapse

Mitral valve prolapse (MVP), first described by Barlow in 1963, is a common cardiac condition which has received considerable attention within the last 2 decades since the discovery that it may harbor several life-threatening complications.[54]

Classically, the diagnosis rests on the clinical findings of midsystolic click and late systolic murmur, and it is confirmed by the echocardiographic (M-mode, 2-D or both) demonstration of prolapse of the mitral leaflets into the left atrium during systole.[58] However, as MVP may produce no or ambiguous auscultatory findings on the one hand, and yet may be echocardiographically overdiagnosed (based on the less strict criteria of the past)[58] on the other, its prevalence has varied enormously. Even in more recent reports it varies between 3 and 13 percent[225,255] depending on the population under study. The usually accepted figure today is 4 percent.[58,157]

MVP is characterized pathologically by mucinous and fibromyxomatous degeneration of the leaflets and the chordae tendineae.[197] Usually an isolated finding, MVP may be an inherited disorder (autosomal dominant) and may be associated with other connective tissue disorders, including Marfan's and Ehlers-Danlos syndromes.[58]

Clinically, MVP is commonly silent or associated with nonspecific symptoms.[58] Several serious complications are known:[13,57,58,155] (1) infective endocarditis—the estimated risk is three to eight times higher than in the general population; (2) mitral regurgitation— MVP accounts for 38 to 64 percent of all cases of severe, pure mitral regurgitation; (3) serious arrhythmias; (4) sudden death (presumably arrhythmic); (5) nonbacterial thrombotic endocarditis (Fig. 41-12); and (6) cerebral and retinal ischemia.

Barnett[11] was the first to report the association between cerebral ischemic events and MVP, and subsequent reports followed.[14,102] Several studies have clearly demonstrated a significantly increased frequency of echocardiographically detectable MVP in patients under the age of 45 with cerebral ischemia, compared to simultaneously studied age- and sex-matched controls.[13,227]

There are several autopsy-proven cases of stroke in association with MVP.[27,46,93,228] In three cases, thrombus was present on the myxomatous mitral valve (Fig. 41-13). Several echocardiographic studies done on patients with MVP who sustained strokes reported the detection of left atrial masses, possibly thrombi, located in the angle formed by the posterior mitral leaflet and the posterior atrial wall, and even of a mobile mass, that was attached to the prolapsing leaflet.[99,178,214] It is important to ensure that this appearance is not produced merely by the folding of the redundant tissue of the degenerate leaflet. In other patients, embolic material resembling platelets and fibrin has been observed in the fundi[256] (Fig. 41-14). It is presumed that emboli of fibrin and platelets, originating from thrombotic deposits on the valve and its attachment play a major role in the causation of the cerebral ischemic events.[264]

Cerebral or retinal ischemia may be the presenting complaint and noncerebral systemic emboli have also been reported in patients with MVP.[27,93,120] Most cerebral events are mild strokes, TIAs, or recurrent amaurosis fugax.[120,132,256,264] Massive infarcts have been described, some reported when atrial fibrillation coexists.[228] Some patients have associated tachyarrhythmias or abnormalities of platelet activity.[227,264] Stroke associated with MVP has been described in women on oral contraceptive.[67]

Several reports detected the presence of MVP in more than 30 percent of young stroke patients;[25,137]

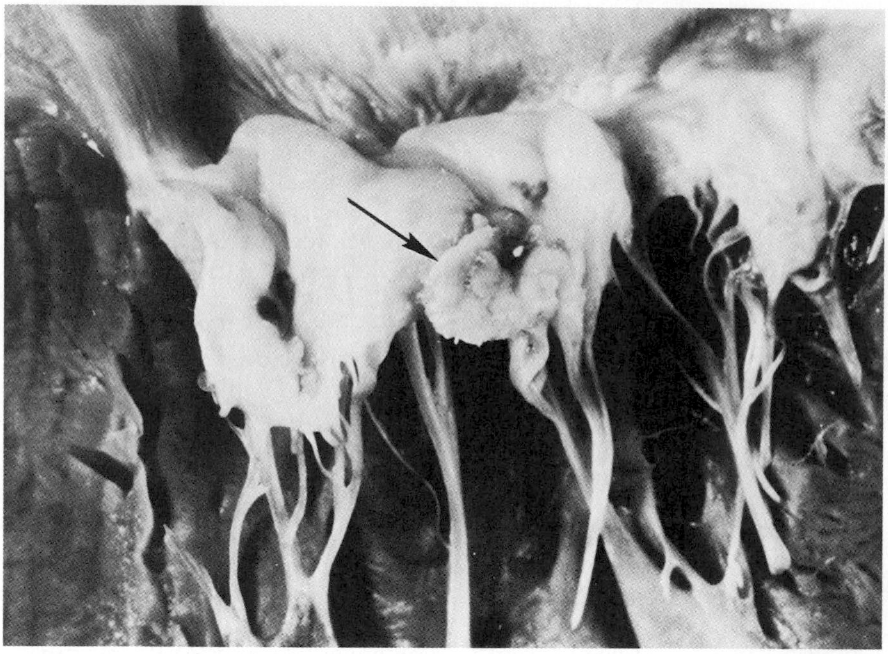

**Fig. 41-12.** Portion of posterior mitral valve leaflet, with largest vegetation (*arrow*) adherent to atrial surface near margin of closure. There is moderate, diffuse thickening of valve cusps. (From Bramlet et al.,[27] with permission.)

other studies claim that MVP was the putative cause in only 1.7 to 6 percent of similar patients.[15,65,100,176,215] The difference may be explained by the diligence with which complete cardiac studies are conducted, by the echocardiographic criteria used and by patient selection. By looking only at the data from young patients in whom the stroke remains unexplained despite an extensive search, figures are more consistent and indicate the presence of MVP in about 20 percent.[264] This is further supported by a recent study[130] that looked at this issue from another perspective: by comparing two groups of age-matched stroke patients with and without MVP but with similar attributes, a significant lack of stroke risk factors was found in the MVP group.

Considerable attention has been focused on the examination of patients with MVP to determine what features, if any, distinguish the majority who will follow a very benign course and the small minority who will suffer serious complications. According to echocardiographic criteria used in a retrospective study,[157] the group of patients with the classical form of MVP (i.e., thickening of the mitral valve leaflets and redundancy) was found to be at a higher risk for infective endocarditis (3 percent as compared to 0 percent in the nonclassical group), for moderate to severe mitral regurgitation (12 and 0 percent), and for the need for mitral valve replacement (6.6 and 0.7 percent). However, the frequency of stroke was similar (7.5 and 5.8 percent, respectively).

A prospective study on 237 patients with echocardiographically documented MVP followed for a mean of 6.2 years[181] disclosed two groups of patients. Those

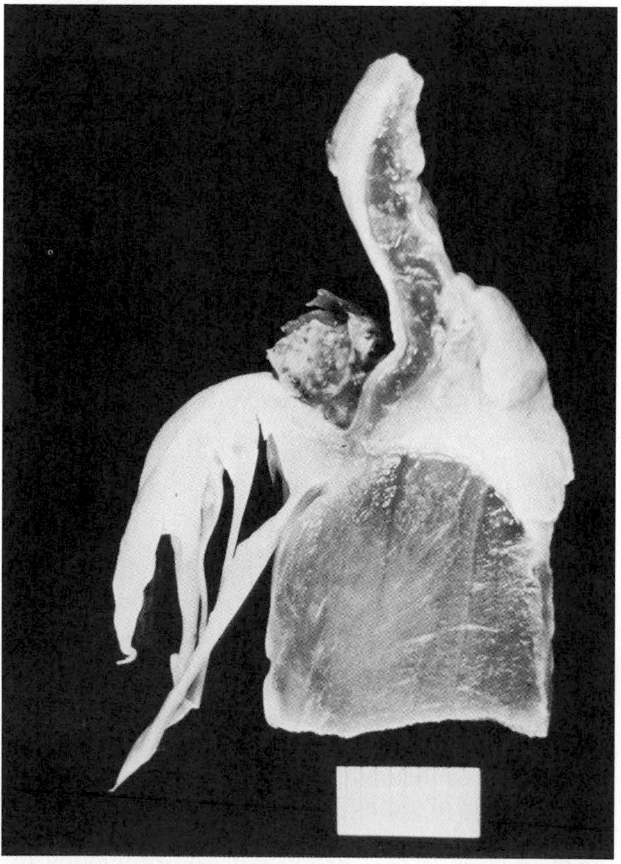

**Fig. 41-13.** Large thrombus attached to prolapsing mitral valve and its attachment to the left atrium. (From Barnett,[12] with permission.)

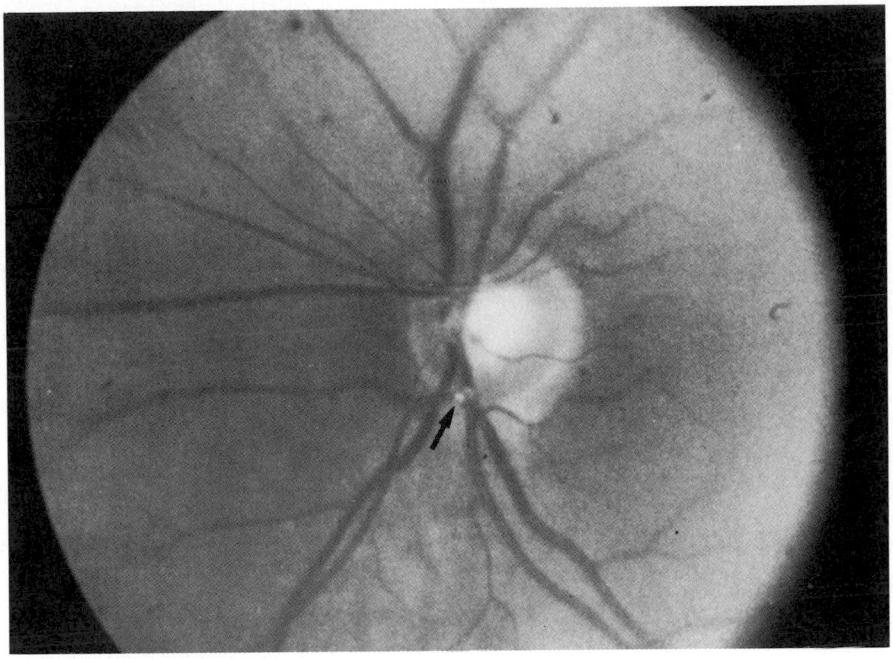

**Fig. 41-14.** Embolus (*arrow*) to the inferior branch of the central retinal artery in a patient with mitral valve prolapse. (From Watson,[256] with permission.)

with redundant mitral valve leaflets had a complication rate of 10.3 percent as compared to 0.7 percent in the "nonredundant" group. The complications included sudden death, infective endocarditis, and cerebral embolic events.

Demographic data indicate that men, and those patients over 45 years of age, are at increased risk of complications—mainly severe mitral regurgitation and infective endocarditis.[57,155]

Reliable predictors of stroke in populations with MVP have not been well defined. Overall, the stroke risk for those who harbor MVP and are followed in cardiac clinics is low, a fact that is discordant with the relatively high prevalence of MVP in younger stroke patients presenting to a neurology service.[7,125,173] The situation here is to be compared to cervical spondylosis. This condition is nearly ubiquitous in older patients and very few develop spastic paraparesis. On the other hand, among older subjects with slowly progressive spastic paraparesis, cervical spondylosis is the commonest cause.

Recurrence of cerebral ischemic events may occur; in one report the yearly stroke rate was 7 percent,[12] and in a recent review[264] recurrence has occurred in 20 percent of patients, mainly months or years apart and most patients had only recurrent TIAs or showed an almost complete recovery.

In summary, MVP is a common finding in the young, carries a benign course for most individuals, and is an unusual cause of stroke among those harboring MVP (the yearly incidence is 0.02 percent).[264] It should be considered as the underlying cause for stroke only if extensive search for other causes has been negative.

Prophylactic treatment is unwarranted in individuals with asymptomatic MVP. In patients where cerebral ischemia is attributed to MVP, aspirin therapy is recommended on empirical grounds, and only in treatment failures, when further events occur, should anticoagulants be used[147,264] for periods of 3 to 6 months, followed by aspirin therapy.

Guidelines for SBE prophylaxis as well as other conditions in the general management of certain subgroups of MVP patients have been published,[58] but are beyond the scope of this chapter.

## Prosthetic Heart Valve

Thromboembolism remains a major cause of morbidity and mortality complicating prosthetic valve implantation despite the introduction of new models of mechanical valves and bioprosthetic valves that have been especially designed to lessen thrombogenicity.[22,64,185,241] The majority of the thromboembolic events are cerebrovascular.[140,185,223]

There are many kinds of mechanical valves, all of which require life-long anticoagulation therapy to prevent thromboembolism.[90,241] Even with such treatment, patients with mechanical valves experience further embolic events at a rate comparable to nonanticoagulated patients with bioprosthetic valves. The rate of embolism in patients with mechanical mitral valves averages 3 to 4 percent per patient year of observation. In the aortic position, the rate is estimated to be lower—averaging 1.2 to 2.2 percent per year. When a bioprosthetic valve is inserted, long-term anticoagulation is not recommended when other risk factors are absent. The embolic rate for nonanticoagulated patients averages 2 to 4 percent per year and may be as low as 1.2 percent per patient year for the aortic bioprosthetic valve.[22,40,64]

In addition to the site and type of valve used, factors that influence the risk of arterial thromboembolism include the presence of atrial fibrillation, the first 3 postoperative months, left atrial thrombus, previous emboli, and the numbers of valves replaced.[64,112,185,241]

The presence of one or more of these risk factors usually requires the initiation of anticoagulant therapy; thus, as many as 80 percent of these patients will be anticoagulated[112] and exposed to the hazards of bleeding. The incidence of major hemorrhage complicating anticoagulant therapy is estimated at 1 to 2 percent per year.[147] and the combination of thrombotic and bleeding complications account for about 75 percent of valve-related complications in patients with mechanical valves and for about 50 percent of the complications in bioprosthetic valves.[22,64,185] The obvious need to reduce those risks has led to two different approaches:

1. A randomized trial was carried out in Europe, comparing the rate of *late* thromboembolic events in three different mechanical heart valve prostheses. The results showed a better outcome with the Bjork-Shiley valve.[140] Another study compared the latter with porcine bioprosthesis during a mean follow-up of 12 years:[22] survival with an *intact* valve was better with this mechanical valve, whereas bleeding complications were higher. There was no difference in thromboembolic events rate.
2. An attempt is being made to find a better equilibrium between activated procoagulants (initiated by the synthetic material of the prosthetic valve) and the anticoagulant—endogenous or exogenous (warfarin). In two recent prospective randomized studies high-intensity anticoagulation (international normalized ratio [INR] 2.5 to 40 or prothrombin time ratio 2.5) was compared to moderate intensity anticoagulation (INR 2.0 to 2.25 or prothrombin time ratio 1.5) in patients with bioprosthetic[253] and mechanical[223] valves. While the rate of thromboembolism remained similar, the risk of bleeding complications was significantly lower in those patients receiving the moderate dose.

Antiplatelet agents alone are much inferior to warfarin in adults with mechanical prosthetic valves and pose unacceptable risks of thromboembolism.[169] When using lower intensity of anticoagulation, some benefit may be gained by adding dipyridamole, a platelet inhibitor that does not alter the bleeding time.[42]

In children, because of the difficulty of controlling anticoagulation, several trials have used antiplatelet agents alone and claimed efficacy and safety.[191,259] This issue, however, remains controversial.[161] A recent study utilizing a medium-intensity anticoagulation in pregnant women disclosed a low incidence of thromboembolism or hemorrhage, yet the rate of fetal wastage and neonatal mortality was high.[224]

Prosthetic valve endocarditis is another complication and a potential source of cerebral embolism. Endocarditis has a yearly incidence of about 2.4 percent[48] in patients with prosthetic valves. Recently a much lower yearly incidence was reported (less than 1 percent).[22] The use of newer and more advanced valves may explain this difference. The occurrence of neurologic complications is higher with mechanical valves and when the prosthesis is in the mitral position.[131]

## Infective Endocarditis

The clinical spectrum of infective endocarditis (IE) has changed in many aspects during the last 25 years. At one time it was primarily a subacute infection on a preexisting rheumatic valvular disease caused by nonvirulent streptococcal species. With the declining incidence of rheumatic heart disease, its incidence has decreased yet the relative involvement of previously normal cardiac valves has increased and many cases are detected in young intravenous drug abusers.[116,129] Normal cardiac valves may become infected by virulent organisms, mainly *Staphylococcus aureus*, which is responsible for most cases of acute infective endocarditis.[116]

Neurologic complications contribute to the high mortality of infective endocarditis and the central nervous system becomes involved in several ways: ischemic and hemorrhagic strokes, multiple microemboli presenting as toxic encephalopathy, meningitis, pyogenic arteritis, mycotic aneurysm, and subarachnoid hemorrhage.[205]

Despite improved antibiotic and surgical therapy, the stroke rate continues to be high, averaging 15 to 20 percent of all IE.[108,205,220] This unchanged risk can be explained by the following: (1) The majority of strokes occur within the initial 48 hours of presentation and may herald the existence of IE.[108,220] (2) The risk and severity of embolism is higher when the offending organism is *Staphylococcus aureus* or epidermidis and with mechanical prosthetic valves,[52,108,131,220] all of which are more prevalent now.

The type and severity of the neurologic manifestations are determined in part by the size of the septic emboli, which are composed mainly of infected vegetations.[171] Attempts to predict the risk of embolism by echocardiographic detection of valvular vegetations have not proved to be totally reliable,[31,108] and the only measure proved to reduce the rate of stroke is early control of the infection by means of antibiotic therapy.[52,108,190]

As recurrent emboli seldom occur after the infection is controlled,[108,190] anticoagulants are not indicated for patients with native valve endocarditis.[108,147,190] It is normally recommended to continue anticoagulation in patients with prosthetic valve endocarditis unless an embolic stroke develops.[64,131,147,260] Anticoagulant therapy then poses the hazard of intracerebral bleeding. Intracerebral hemorrhages (ICH) occur in 7 percent of native valve endocarditis, mainly in intravenous drug abusers with uncontrolled *Staphylococcus aureus* infection and is presumably due to pyogenic arteritis.[108,109]

Mycotic aneurysm, an uncommon complication of IE may be responsible for the ICH. It occurs in all types of endocarditis, usually in distal branches of the middle cerebral artery. Aneurysms, which develop probably as a result of septic embolization to the vasa vasorum, usually are clinically silent and can heal with prolonged antibiotic treatment.[30,205] Rupture occurs unpredictably, and, as this carries a high mortality rate, an attempt must be made for their early detection. This complication should be sought in patients with focal neurologic findings, cerebrospinal fluid pleocytosis, and evidence of infarction or ICH on their CT scans.[30] Early four-vessel angiography is indicated in these patients. For those who require long-term anticoagulation, repeat angiography is recommended after completion of antibiotic therapy.[219]

Mural endocarditis is very rare but may occur either in the presence of a ventricular septal defect, with "jet lesions," with perforation of a cusp, or from rupture of a chordae tendinae in severely debilitated or immunosuppressed patients. The causative organism is usually *Candida albicans*,[236] whereas *Aspergillus* is commonly the underlying cause in patients with prior cardiovascular surgery.[265]

## Nonbacterial Thrombotic Endocarditis

Nonbacterial thrombotic endocarditis (NBTE) is the name commonly used to describe what was previously referred to as marantic, terminal, and verrucous endocarditis.

Although described in a vast range of disease processes, especially chronic and wasting ones,[33,152] NBTE is most common in patients with cancer: adenocarcinoma of the lung, pancreas, and prostate and hematologic malignancies predominating.[19,152,213]

Cerebral infarction is the second most common neuropathologic finding in patients dying of cancer, and within this group NBTE accounts for more than 25 percent.[98] Other cancer-related causes of symptomatic infarction include disseminated intravascular coagulopathy (DIC), septic emboli, tumor emboli, and cerebral venous and sinus thrombosis.

As the name implies, NBTE is a noninfectious type of endocarditis mainly found on previously normal cardiac valves, the mitral and aortic valves being the most commonly affected. The vegetations in NBTE are usually small and are composed of platelet and fibrin deposits (Fig. 41-15). The pathogenesis is still

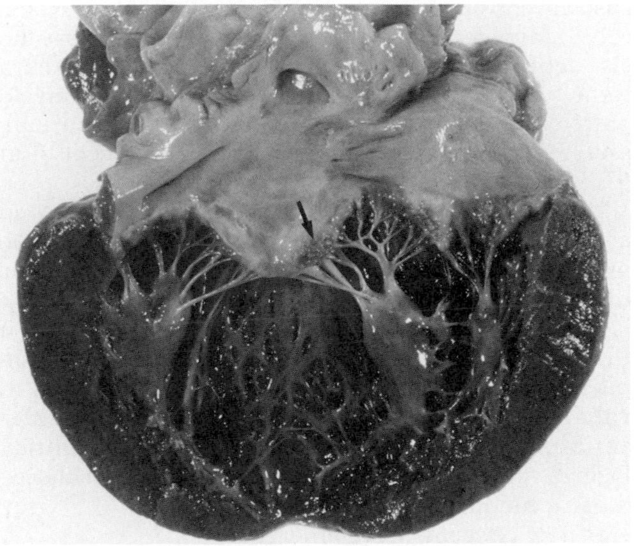

**Fig. 41-15.** Mitral valve vegetation of nonbacterial thrombotic endocarditis (*arrow*). (From Rogers et al.,[213] with permission.)

uncertain: a deranged valvular surface must precede the formation of NBTE and a hypercoagulable state is usually present. Whether the latter is a prerequisite for the formation of NBTE and what is the exact mechanism (DIC, tumor mucin, or procoagulant may be contibutory in individual patients) for this prothrombotic state is still debatable.[152,213]

Clinically, NBTE is underdiagnosed.[152,213] The main reasons are (1) NBTE is clinically silent in many cases; (2) significant cardiac murmurs are absent in the majority of cases; and (3) the vegetations are usually small and detection is difficult by both invasive and noninvasive techniques. Two-dimensional echocardiography in a relatively good diagnostic tool,[151] and early cerebral angiography may confirm the presence of multiple arterial branch occlusions reflecting brain emboli.[213] The clinical manifestations of NBTE are those of multiple systemic emboli with neurologic manifestations predominating, usually in the form of acute focal neurologic deficits, suggesting stroke. A diffuse form is suggestive of a metabolic encephalopathy. Embolic myocardial infarction is an occasional serious complication.[152,213]

Treatment is empirical. Most reports have been anecdotal and retrospective. Heparin anticoagulation may be beneficial, especially when there is a recognizable coagulopathy.[213]

## Systemic Lupus Erythematosus and Related Diseases

Systemic lupus erythematosus (SLE) is a multisystem autoimmune disease where neuropsychiatric manifestations are protean, but clinical cardiac disease is considered rare.[5,111] Central nervous system (CNS) involvement may manifest as delirium, psychosis, depression, altered consciousness, focal cerebral ischemia, cranial nerve dysfunction, chorea, myelopathy, and CNS infection.[5] Cerebral ischemia (usually recurrent episodes) occurs in 15 to 20 percent of all SLE patients.[59,87]

Until recently most of these CNS disorders were attributed to CNS vasculitis or vascular disorders other than embolism.[123] Atypical verrucous endocarditis (Fig. 41-16) or Libman-Sacks (L-S) endocarditis is a well-known and common pathologic finding in SLE patients earlier thought to have no clinical significance.[111] This endocarditis is not confined to valvular surfaces only, and has other features differentiating it from NBTE or rheumatic valvulitis.[80] From a reconsideration of the pathologic and echocardiographic findings in patients with SLE[49,59,87,91] several new concepts have emerged:

1. The etiology of strokes and maybe other CNS manifestation in SLE patients are often due to cardiac emboli (presumably originating from L-S endocarditis) with or without the presence of an antibody-mediated hypercoagulable state.
2. Clinically important valvular involvement in SLE is relatively frequent and sometimes requires surgery. This valvular involvement is different from (although perhaps the end stage of) L-S endocarditis, and is also associated with an increased risk for stroke. It is referred to as nonspecific (chronic) valvulitis mainly involving the mitral and aortic valves. Long-standing steroid treatment, known to facilitate scarring and calcification, may play a causal role.
3. Echocardiography is a useful tool in the detection and follow-up of valvular lesion in SLE patients.
4. A hypercoagulable state (induced mainly by antiphospholipid antibodies) is frequently found in SLE patients.[105] Its role in the pathogenesis of stroke in patients with or without cardiac lesion has yet to be determined. Antiphospholipid antibodies may predispose to L-S endocarditis.[9] This hypothesis is supported by recent reports of SLE patients that show a higher frequency of valvular lesions in those possessing antiphospholipid antibodies.[41,92]

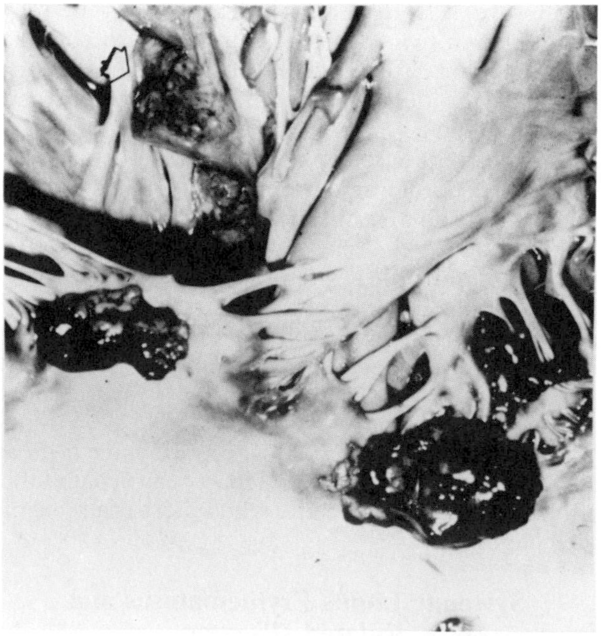

**Fig. 41-16.** Mitral valve area of opened left atrium and ventricle. There are several large vegetations involving both the valvular and the ventricular mural (*open arrow*) endocardium. (From Fox et al.,[80] with permission.)

Treatment is controversial. Anticoagulant therapy is recommended in patients who have sustained a stroke, as well as for stroke prevention in patients at high risk (i.e., with recognizable cardiac valvular lesion or previous TIA).[87,95,268]

Other autoimmune rheumatic diseases can cause central nervous system dysfunction through various mechanisms, including the presence of antiphospholipid antibodies and cardiac involvement. In Sjögren's syndrome, cardioembolic stroke may be attributed to coexistent cardiomyopathy.[186]

## Paradoxical Embolism

The name implies that an embolus originating in the venous system finds its way to lodge in the arterial tree, and implies the existence of right to left shunts. Possible shunts incriminated in the pathophysiology of paradoxical embolism include patent foramen ovale (PFO), atrial septal defect (ASD), and pulmonary arteriovenous fistula.[124,153,240]

Previously considered an unusual cause of cerebral embolism,[110,124,163] paradoxical embolism through a PFO has become a more popular explanation for strokes of unknown cause, especially in the young.[145,257] This concept needs to be examined critically.

PFO is found in about 30 percent of autopsies[101] (Fig. 41-17) and, recently, with the introduction of 2-D contrast echocardiography, a physiologic shunt was demonstrated in 10 to 18 percent of normal people by the use of this noninvasive technique.[145,154,257] By using a transesophageal color-coded Doppler echo, the detection of PFO may be improved.[172]

The presence of PFO by itself cannot explain the occurrence of cerebral embolism. Under normal conditions, the pressure in the right heart is lower than in the left side, the foramen ovale stays closed and there is no right to left shunt. In pathologic conditions where pulmonary hypertension exists, such shunts do occur[143] but in the healthy population such shunts may occur only transiently during Valsalva's maneuvers.[154]

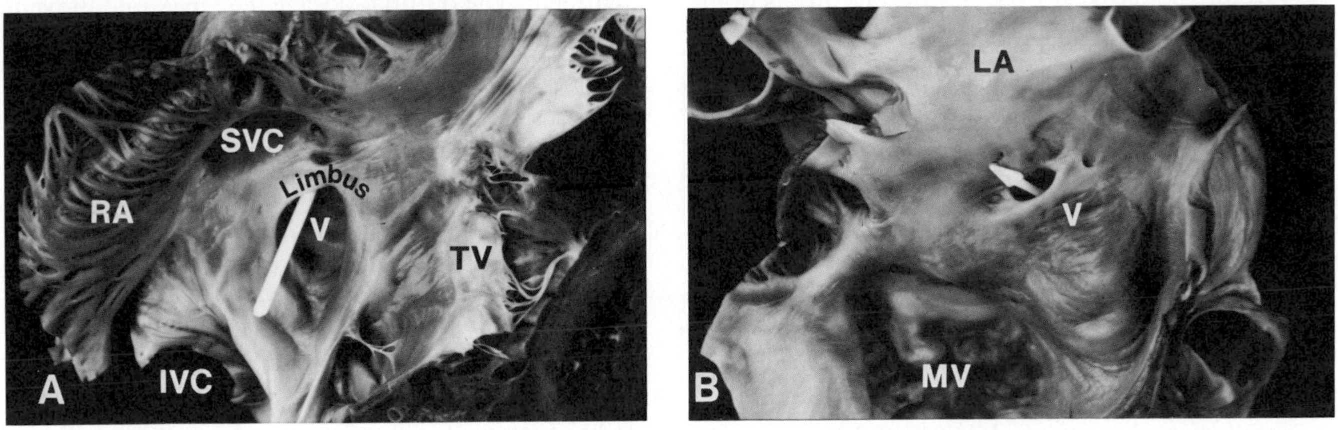


**Fig. 41-17.** Patent foramen ovale, shown in autopsy specimen from 85-year-old man. (**A**) Right atrial (RA) view shows a probe in foramen ovale, between limbus and valve (V) of fossa ovalis. (**B**) left atrial (LA) view shows same probe as in Fig. A exiting through ostium secundum, the prominent fenestration in the valve. Normally, when left atrial pressure exceeds right atrial pressure, the valve of the fossa ovalis impressed against the limbus and thereby closes the foramen ovale. IVC, inferior vena cava; MV, mitral valve; SVC, superior vena cava; TV, tricuspid valve. (From Hagen et al.,[101] with permission.)

A major difficulty in the acceptance of paradoxical embolism as the underlying mechanism for a substantial number of the strokes of unknown cause is the absence of venous thrombosis or signs of pulmonary embolism in most recent series.[124,145,257] In previous reports the presence of venous thrombosis was considered essential for the diagnosis.[163,250] In making more sweeping claims for its importance it is being assumed that there is an occult source, as occurs in cases of pulmonary embolism.[242]

The prevalence of PFO demonstrated by contrast echo was found to be much higher in young patients with stroke of unknown cause compared to control groups.[145,257] In the Lechat series[145] the authors referred to MVP as a risk factor only, whereas the PFO was claimed to be causal. There was no evidence for crural vein disease, or pulmonary embolism nor were the controls contemporary. Recently, transcranial Doppler has been used to clarify the potential cerebral embolic significance of a demonstrated shunt.[43]

Prophylactic treatment in this condition is an unsettled issue. In cases of proven venous thrombosis, the institution of anticoagulant therapy for several months, and other means of therapy, such as caval umbrellas, should be undertaken following the guidelines for the prevention of pulmonary emboli.[114] If the source of embolism is occult, a treatment regimen that includes a short course of anticoagulation followed by aspirin or aspirin alone may be sufficient.[21,145] In some patients closure of the PFO may be warranted.

## Congenital Heart Disease

Many congenital heart diseases are complicated by systemic or cerebral embolism. Mechanisms for embolization include cardiac dysrhythmia, paradoxical embolism, and bacterial endocarditis. The majority are in the cyanotic group in which the blood viscosity is high, and there is an increased tendency for venous thrombosis. Emboli are reported mainly in patients with the tetralogy of Fallot, ventricular or atrial septal defect, and transposition of the great vessels.[6,17] In a recent study in which 124 adults with cyanotic heart disease were followed for an average of 6.1 years, no clinical stroke was detected even in the presence of high hematocrit level.[193] In contrast, clinically silent atrial septal defect was incriminated as an underlying cause for stroke in young adults.[110] Atrial septal aneurysm, a rare congenital condition that is usually associated with an interatrial shunt and sometimes with mitral valve prolapse, has recently received attention as a possible cause for cardioembolic stroke.[16,60] Two-dimensional echocardiography preferably by the transesophageal route is the imaging technique of choice for the diagnosis of this defect.[229] Possible mechanisms include thrombus formation in the aneurysmal sac or paradoxical embolism.[16]

## Cardiac Myxoma

Cardiac myxoma, the most common primary heart tumor, is a rare tumor and a very rare cause of stroke. The tumor is usually benign and originates in the left atrium in 75 percent of cases. Primarily diagnosed in young and middle-aged adults, it may present with either constitutional, cardiac obstructive or embolic symptoms, alone or in combination. Obstructive symptoms are due mainly to an intermittent mitral stenosis. The constitutional symptoms are not specific and may mimic those arising in a variety of malignant, infectious, and immunologic diseases.[156]

Embolic manifestations occur in 20 to 45 percent of patients, sometimes as the first symptom. Although emboli may lodge in any part of the vascular bed, the central nervous system is involved in up to 50 percent of cases.[156] The embolic material consists mainly of myxomatous tissue, but occasionally only thrombotic material (originating from an adherent thrombus) can be found. In addition to multiple brain infarctions, tumor emboli cause cerebral aneurysms located on peripheral branches, which rarely rupture, presenting as an intracranial hemorrhage.[134,156]

Neurologic manifestations consist mainly of acute focal neurologic deficits that may be the initial presentation of the tumor.[134] As the tumor is friable, recurrent cerebral emboli are common prior to its surgical removal. These symptoms rarely recur following successful surgical removal.[134]

Diagnosis rests on the utilization of 2-D echocardiography. Cardiac CT or MRI can be added.[134,156] Therapy is surgical. Anticoagulation prior to surgery is not effective.[134]

### Cardiac Surgery

Many patients with the cardiac diseases described, of which the most prevalent is coronary artery disease, are subject to surgical procedures. Complicating systemic embolism occurs in all types of cardiac surgery including cardiopulmonary bypass (open heart) done for a variety of reasons, closed heart surgery (for other conditions), and heart transplantation.[175] As many as 5 percent of patients undergoing coronary artery bypass grafting are afflicted with a stroke.[28] Possible mechanisms include macroembolization of air, valve, and aortic atheroma debris, or left ventricular thrombus as well as microembolization of gas, fat, and aggregates of blood cells, platelets, and fibrin or particles of silicone or polyvinyl chloride tubing.[233]

When early heart surgery is performed as a result of cardioembolic stroke the risk of cerebral complication (mainly hemorrhage) is high (29 percent), particularly in the presence of infective endocarditis or large infarcts.[159]

## ACUTE TREATMENT OF NONSEPTIC CARDIOGENIC BRAIN EMBOLISM

In general, anticoagulant therapy is recommended for the prevention of nonseptic recurrent emboli in most cases of cardiogenic emboli. It is the therapy shown to be effective in most of these conditions.[40,234,268]

Specific treatment strategies were considered for each specific lesion where a special reference to the nature of the embolus was made (see below). There are, however, two problems that remain to be considered in view of the potential risk of anticoagulant therapy: (1) the optimal dose of anticoagulation to be used, and (2) the optimal time to start anticoagulant treatment. The optimal dosage (i.e., maximal prevention of recurrent emboli with minimal bleeding complications) is currently under intensive investigations for most of the cardiac sources. Generally speaking, a lower dose level of anticoagulation seems to suffice for most patients with emboligenic sources. As in the prevention of pulmonary emboli from deep-vein thrombosis[114] the newly recommended dose for warfarin treatment aims to prolong the prothrombin time to 1.5 times control (international normalized ratio between 2 and 3).[40] In the future it is expected that even lower doses may be shown to be adequate. In general, it is recommended to use heparin for the first few days and then to switch to warfarin.[234]

The optimal time to start treatment is still controversial,[234,268] and the physician faces a dilemma: the risk of recurrent emboli without treatment is about 12 percent during the first 2 weeks, and under early anticoagulant therapy it will drop to about 4 percent; yet the risk of therapy related to symptomatic brain hemorrhage and clinical worsening will be 5 percent for the same period.[39,234] This risk may be much higher in older patients, in those with large infarct size, with elevated blood pressure, and when bolus doses of heparin are given.[38,184] Such patients are excluded from the early treatment group. Keeping in mind that spontaneous hemorrhagic transformation mainly occurs within 48 hours after the stroke onset[107] and that anticoagulants may be hazardous in such patients because they may induce massive hematomas,[40,184] the following strategy is recommended: anticoagulant therapy should be withheld for 48 hours, and then, after obtaining a new CT scan, anticoagulation should be started in younger patients who have nonhemorrhagic infarcts of small or medium size. In other cases (i.e., elderly or hypertensive patients and those with large or hemorrhagic infarcts) it is wise to withhold treatment for 2 weeks.[40,234]

## REFERENCES


1. Abdon NJ, Zettervall O, Carlson J et al: Is occult atrial disorder a frequent cause of non-hemorrhagic stroke?—long-term ECG in 86 patients. Stroke 13:832, 1982
2. Abelmann WH, Lorell BH: The challenge of cardiomyopathy. J Am Coll Cardiol 13:1219, 1989
3. Aberg H: Atrial fibrillation. I. A study of atrial thrombosis and systemic embolism in a necropsy material. Acta Med Scand 185:373, 1969
4. Adams HP, Jr, Butler MJ, Biller J, Toffol GJ: Nonhemorrhagic cerebral infarction in young adults. Arch Neurol 43:793, 1986
5. Adelman DC, Saltiel E, Klinenberg JR: The neuropsychiatric manifestations of systemic lupus erythematosus: an overview. Semin Arthritis Rheum 15:185, 1986
6. Amitai Y, Blieden L, Shemtov A, Neufeld HN: Cerebrovascular accidents in infants and chil-

dren with congenital cyanotic heart disease. Isr J Med Sci 20:1143, 1984

7. Appelblatt NH, Willis PW, Lenhart JA et al: Ten to forty year follow-up of 69 patients with systolic click with or without apical late systolic murmur. Am J Cardiol 35:119, 1975
8. Aronow WS, Koenigsberg M, Kronzon I, Gutstein H: Association of mitral anular calcium with new thromboembolic stroke and cardiac events at 39-month follow-up in elderly patients. Am J Cardiol 1511, 1990
9. Asherson RA, Lubbe WF: Cerebral and valve lesions in SLE: association with antiphospholipid antibodies. J Rheumatol 15:539, 1988
10. Asinger RW, Mikell FL, Elsperger J, Hodges M: Incidence of left ventricular thrombosis after acute transmural myocardial infarction. N Engl J Med 305:297, 1981
11. Barnett HJM: Transient cerebral ischemia: pathogenesis, prognosis and management. Ann R Coll Physicians Surg Can 7:153, 1974
12. Barnett HJM: Embolism in mitral valve prolapse. Annu Rev Med 33:489, 1982
13. Barnett HJM, Boughner DR, Taylor WD, Cooper PE, Kostuk WJ, Nichol PM: Further evidence relating mitral-valve prolapse to cerebral ischemic events. N Engl J Med 302:139, 1980
14. Barnett HJM, Jones MW, Boughner DR, Kostuk WJ: Cerebral ischemic events associated with prolapsing mitral valve. Arch Neurol 33:777, 1976
15. Beattie BA, Biller J, Adams HP, Jr, Marsh III EE, Bruno A: Mitral valve prolapse is an uncommon cause of stroke in young adults, abstracted Neurology (NY), suppl 1. 39:S183, 1989
16. Belkin RN, Kisslo J: Atrial septal aneurysm: recognition and clinical relevance. Am Heart J 120:948, 1990
17. Berthrong M, Sabiston DC, Jr: Cerebral lesions in congenital heart disease: a review of one hundred and sixty-two cases. Bull Johns Hopkins Hosp 89:384, 1951
18. Bevan H, Sharma K, Bradley W: Stroke in young adults. Stroke 21:382, 1990
19. Biller J, Challa VR, Toole JF, Howard VJ: Nonbacterial thrombotic endocarditis: a neurologic perspective of clinicopathologic correlations of 99 patients. Arch Neurol 39:95, 1982
20. Biller J, Ionasescu V, Zellweger H et al: Incidence of cerebral infarction in inherited neuromuscular conditions. Stroke 18:805, 1987
21. Biller J, Johnson MR, Adams HP et al: Further observations on cerebral or retinal ischemia with right-left intracardiac shunts. Arch Neurol 44:740, 1987
22. Bloomfield P, Wheatley DJ, Prescott RJ, Miller HC: Twelve-year comparison of Bjork-Shiley mechanical heart valve with porcine bioprostheses. N Engl J Med 324:573, 1991
23. Bogousslavsky J, Cachin D, Regli F et al: Cardiac sources of embolism and cerebral infarction—clinical consequences and vascular concomitants: the Lausanne Stroke Registry. Neurology (NY) 41:855, 1991
24. Bogousslavsky J, Melle GV, Regli F: The Lausanne Stroke Registry: analysis of 1000 consecutive patients with first stroke. Stroke 19:1083, 1988
25. Bogousslavsky J, Regli F: Ischemic stroke in adults younger than 30 years of age. Arch Neurol 44:479, 1987
26. The Boston Area Anticoagulation Trial for Atrial Fibrillation Investigators: The effect of low-dose warfarin on the risk of stroke in patients with nonrheumatic atrial fibrillation. N Engl J Med 323:1505, 1990
27. Bramlet DA, Decker EL, Floyd WL: Nonbacterial thrombotic endocarditis as a cause of stroke in mitral valve prolapse. South Med J 75:1133, 1982
28. Breuer AC, Furlan AJ, Hanson MR: Central nervous system complications of coronary artery bypass graft surgery: prospective analysis of 421 patients. Stroke 14:682, 1983
29. Brockmeier LB, Adolph RJ, Gustin BW et al: Calcium emboli to the retinal artery in calcific aortic stenosis. Am Heart J 101:32, 1981
30. Brust JCM, Dickinson PCT, Hughes JEO, Holtzman RNN: The diagnosis and treatment of cerebral mycotic aneurysms. Ann Neurol 27:238, 1990
31. Buda AJ, Zotz RJ, Le Mire MS, Buch DS: Prognostic significance of vegetations detected by two-dimensional echocardiography in infective endocarditis. Am Heart J 112:1291, 1986
32. Cabin HS, Clubb KS, Hall C et al: Risk for systemic embolization of atrial fibrillation without mitral stenosis. Am J Cardiol 65:1112, 1990
33. Cammarosano C, Lewis W: Cardiac lesions in acquired immune deficiency syndrome (AIDS). J Am Coll Cardiol 5:703, 1985
34. Candelise L, Pinardi G, Morabito A: The Italian acute stroke study group: mortality in acute stroke with atrial fibrillation. Stroke 22:169, 1991
35. Caplan LR: Top of the basilar syndrome. Neurology (NY) 30:72, 1980
36. Caplan LR, Hier DB, D'Cruz I: Cerebral embolism in the Michael Reese Stroke Registry. Stroke 14:530, 1983
37. Cerebral Embolism Study Group: Immediate anticoagulation of embolic stroke: a randomized trial. Stroke 14:668, 1983
38. Cerebral Embolism Study Group: Cardioembolic stroke, immediate anticoagulation and brain hemorrhage. Arch Intern Med 147:636, 1987
39. Cerebral Embolism Task Force: Cardiogenic brain embolism. Arch Neurol 43:71, 1986
40. Cerebral Embolism Task Force: Cardiogenic brain embolism: the second report of the cerebral embolism task force. Arch Neurol, Jul 46:727, 1989
41. Chartash EK, Lans DM, Paget SA et al: Aortic insufficiency and mitral regurgitation in patients with systemic lupus erythematosus and the antiphospholipid syndrome. Am J Med 86:407, 1989
42. Chesebro JH, Adams PC, Fuster V: Antithrombotic therapy in patients with valvular heart

disease and prosthetic heart valves. J Am Coll Cardiol 8:41B, 1986
43. Chimowitz M, Nemec J, Marwick T et al: Transcranial Doppler ultrasound detects right to left cardiac or pulmonary shunts. Neurology (NY) 41:1902, 1991
44. Ciaccherie M, Castelli Q, Cecchi F et al: Lack of correlation between intracavitary thrombosis detected by cross-sectional echocardiography and systemic emboli in patients with dilated cardiomyopathy. Br Heart J 62:26, 1989
45. Connolly SJ, Laupacis A, Gent M et al: Canadian atrial fibrillation anticoagulation (CAFA) study. J Am Coll Cardiol 18:349–355, 1991
46. Cook AW, Bird TD, Spence AM et al: Myotonic dystrophy, mitral-valve prolapse, and stroke. Lancet 1:335, 1978
47. Coulshed N, Epstein EJ, McKendrick CS et al: Systemic embolism in mitral valve disease. Br Heart J 32:26, 1970
48. Cowgill LD, Addonizio VP, Hopeman AR: Prosthetic valve endocarditis. Curr Concepts Cardiol 11:623, 1986
49. Crozier IG, Li E, Milne MJ, Nicholls MG: Cardiac involvement in systemic lupus erythematosus detected by echocardiography. Am J Cardiol 65:1145, 1990
50. Daley R, Mattingly TW, Holt CL et al: Systemic arterial embolism in rheumatic heart disease. Am Heart J 42:566, 1951
51. Daniel WG, Nellessen U, Schroder W et al: Left atrial spontaneous echo contrast in mitral valve disease: an indicator for an increased thromboembolic risk. J Am Coll Cardiol 11:1204, 1988
52. Davenport J, Hart RG: Prosthetic valve endocarditis 1976–1987: antibiotics, anticoagulation, and stroke. Stroke 21:993, 1990
53. Davidson CJ, Skelton TN, Kisslo KB et al: The risk for systemic embolization associated with percutaneous balloon valvuloplasty in adults. Ann Intern Med 108:557, 1988
54. Davies NJ, Montague TJ: Mitral valve prolapse: The cardiac disease of the decade revisited. Ann R Coll Physicians Surg Can 22:307, 1989
55. Davis PH, Dambrosia JM, Schoenberg BS et al: Risk factors for ischemic stroke: a prospective study in Rochester, Minnesota. Ann Neurol 22:319, 1987
56. de Bono DP, Warlow CP: Mitral annulus calcification and cerebral or retinal ischemia. Lancet 2:383, 1979
57. Devereux RB, Hawkins I, Kramer-Fox R et al: Complications of mitral valve prolapse: disproportionate occurrence in men and older patients. Am J Med 81:751, 1986
58. Devereux RB, Kramer-Fox R, Kligfield P: Mitral valve prolapse: causes, clinical manifestations, and management. Ann Intern Med 111:305, 1989
59. Devinsky O, Petito CK, Alonso DR: Clinical and neuropathological findings in systemic lupus erythematosus: the role of vasculitis, heart emboli, and thrombotic thrombocytopenic purpura. Ann Neurol 23:380, 1988
60. Di Pasquale G, Andreoli A, Grazi P et al: Cardioembolic stroke from atrial septal aneurysm. Stroke 19:640, 1988
61. Domenicucci S, Bellotti P, Chiarella F et al: Spontaneous morphologic changes in left ventricular thrombi: prospective two-dimensional echocardiographic study. Circulation 75:737, 1987
62. Dunn M, Alexander J, de Silva R, Hildner F: Antithrombotic therapy in atrial fibrillation. Chest, suppl. 95:118S, 1989
63. Editorial: Left ventricular thrombosis and stroke following myocardial infarction. Lancet 335:759, 1990
64. Edmunds LH: Thrombotic and bleeding complications of prosthetic heart valves. Ann Thorac Surg 44:430, 1987
65. Egeblad H, Sorensen PS: Prevalence of mitral valve prolapse in younger patients with cerebral ischaemic attack: a blinded controlled study. Acta Med Scand 216:385, 1984
66. Eisenberg PR, Sherman LA, Jaffe AS: Paradoxic elevation of fibrinopeptide-A after streptokinase: evidence for continued thrombosis despite intense fibrinolysis. J Am Coll Cardiol 19:527, 1987
67. Elam MB, Viar MJ, Ratts TE, Chesney CM: Mitral valve prolapse in women with oral contraceptive-related cerebrovascular insufficiency. Arch Intern Med 146:73, 1986
68. Ellis LB, Ramirez A: The clinical course of patients with severe "rheumatic" mitral insufficiency. Am Heart J 78:406, 1969
69. Fairfax AJ, Lambert CD, Leatham A: Systemic embolism in chronic sinoatrial disorder. N Engl J Med 295:190, 1976
70. Falk RH: A plea for a clinical trial of anticoagulation in dilated cardiomyopathy. Am J Cardiol 65:914, 1990
71. Felner JM, Blumenstein BA, Schlant RC et al: Souces of variability in echocardiographic measurements. Am J Cardiol 45:995, 1980
72. Fieschi C, Argentino C, Lenzi GL et al: Clinical and instrumental evaluation of patients with ischemic stroke within the first six hours. J Neurol Sci 91:311, 1989
73. Fisher CM: Reducing risks of cerebral embolism. Geriatrics 34:59, 1979
74. Fisher CM: The posterior cerebral artery syndrome. Can J Neurol Sci 13:232, 1986
75. Fisher CM, Adams RD: Observations on brain embolism with special reference to hemorrhagic infarction. p. 17. In Furlan AJ (ed): The Heart and Stroke: Exploring Mutual Cardiovascular Issues. Springer-Verlag, New York, 1987
76. Fisher M, Kase CS, Stelle B, Mills RM, Jr: Ischemic stroke after cardiac pacemaker implantation in sick sinus syndrome. Stroke 19:712, 1988
77. Flegel KM, Shipley MJ, Rose G: Risk of stroke in nonrheumatic atrial fibrillation. Lancet 1:526, 1987
78. Forfar JC, Miller HC, Toft A: Occult thyrotoxicosis: a correctable cause of "idiopathic" atrial fibrillation. Am J Cardiol 44:9, 1979
79. Foulkes MA, Wolf PA, Price TR et al: The stroke

data bank: design, methods, and baseline characteristics. Stroke 19:547, 1988
80. Fox IS, Spence AM, Wheelis RF, Healey LA: Cerebral embolism in Libman-Sacks endocarditis. Neurology (NY) 30:487, 1980
81. Fulkerson PK, Beaver BM, Auseon JC, Graber HL: Calcification of the mitral annulus. Etiology, clinical associations, complication and therapy. Am J Med 66:967, 1979
82. Furlan AJ, Cavalier SJ, Hobbs RE et al: Hemorrhage and anticoagulation after nonseptic embolic brain infarction. Neurology (NY) 32:280, 1982
83. Furlan AJ, Craciun AR, Raju NR, Hart N: Cerebrovascular complications associated with idiopathic hypertrophic subaortic stenosis. Stroke 15:282, 1984
84. Furlan AJ, Cracuin AR, Salcedo E et al: Risk of stroke in patients with mitral annular calcification. Stroke 15:801, 1984
85. Fuster V, Gersh BJ, Giuliani ER et al: The natural history of idiopathic dilated cardiomyopathy. Am J Cardiol 47:525, 1981
86. Fuster V, Halperin JL: Left ventricular thrombi and cerebral embolism. N Engl J Med 320:392, 1989
87. Futrell N, Millikan C: Frequency, etiology, and prevention of stroke in patients with systemic lupus erythematosus. Stroke 20:583, 1989
88. Gacs G, Merei FT, Bodosi M: Balloon catheter as a model of cerebral emboli in humans. Stroke 13:39, 1982
89. Gacs G, Fox AJ, Barnett HJM, Viñuela F: CT visualization intracranial arterial thromboembolism. Stroke 14:756, 1983
90. Gadboys HC, Litwak RS, Niemetz J, Wisch N: Role of anticoagulants in preventing embolization from prosthetic heart valves. JAMA 202:134, 1967
91. Galve E, Candell-Riera J, Pigrau C et al: Prevalence, morphologic types, and evolution of cardiac valvular disease in systemic lupus erythematosus. N Engl J Med 319:817, 1988
92. Galve E, Ordi J, Candell-Riera J et al: Valvular heart disease in systemic lupus erythematosus. N Engl J Med 320:740, 1989
93. Geyer SJ, Franzini DA: Myxomatous degeneration of the mitral valve complicated by nonbacterial thrombotic endocarditis with systemic embolization. Am J Clin Pathol 72:489, 1979
94. Glancy DL, O'Brien KP, Gold HK, Epstein SE: Atrial fibrillation in patients with idiopathic hypertrophic subaortic stenosis. Br Heart J 32:652, 1970
95. Gorelick PB, Rusinowitz MS, Tiku M et al: Embolic stroke complicating systemic lupus erythematosus. Arch Neurol 42:813, 1985
96. Gottdiener JS, Gay JA, VanVoorhees L et al: Frequency and embolic potential of left ventricular thrombus in dilated cardiomyopathy: assessment by 2-dimensional echocardiography. Am J Cardiol 52:1281, 1983
97. Graef I, Berger AR, Bunim JJ, de la Chapelle CE: Auricular thrombosis in rheumatic heart disease. Arch Pathol 24:344, 1937
98. Graus F, Rogers LR, Posner JB: Cerebrovascular complications in patients with cancer. Medicine (Baltimore) 64:16, 1985
99. Gross CM, Nichols FT, von Dohlen TW, D'Cruz IA: Mitral valve prolapse and stroke: echocardiographic evidence for a missing causative link. J Am Soc Echo 2:94, 1989
100. Hachinski V, Norris JW: The Acute Stroke. p. 141. FA Davis, Philadelphia, 1985
101. Hagen PT, Scholz DG, Edwards WD: Incidence and size of patent foramen ovale during the first 10 decades of life: an autopsy study of 965 normal hearts. Mayo Clin Proc 59:17, 1984
102. Hanson MR, Conomy JP, Hodgman JR: Brain events associated with mitral valve prolapse. Stroke 11:499, 1980
103. Hardesty WH, Roberts B, Toole JF et al: Studies of carotid-artery blood flow in man. N Engl J Med 263:944, 1960
104. Hardesty WH, Whitacre WB, Toole JF et al: Studies on vertebral artery blood flow in man. Surg Gynecol Obstet 116:662, 1963
105. Harris EN, Gharavi AE, Hughes GRV: Antiphospholipid antibodies. Clin Rheum Dis 11:591, 1985
106. Harrison MJG, Marshall J: Wernicke aphasia and cardiac embolism. J Neurol Neurosurg Psychiatry 50:938, 1987
107. Hart RG, Easton JD: Hemorrhagic infarcts. Stroke 17:586, 1986
108. Hart RG, Foster JW, Luther MF, Kanter MC: Stroke in infective endocarditis. Stroke 21:695, 1990
109. Hart RG, Kagen-Hallet K, Joerns SE: Mechanisms of intracranial hemorrhage in infective endocarditis. Stroke 18:1048, 1987
110. Harvey JR, Teague SM, Anderson JL et al: Clinically silent atrial septal defects with evidence of cerebral embolization. Ann Intern Med 105:695, 1986
111. Hejtmancik MR, Wright JC, Quint R, Jennings FL: The cardiovascular manifestations of systemic lupus erythematosus. Am Heart J 68:119, 1964
112. Hetzer R, Topalidis T, Borst HG: Thromboembolism and anticoagulation after isolated mitral valve replacement with porcine heterografts. p. 172. In Cohn LH, Gallucci V (eds): Cardiac Prostheses. Yorke, New York, 1982
113. Holley KE, Bahn RC, McGoon DC, Mankin HT: Spontaneous calcific embolization associated with calcific aortic stenosis. Circulation 27:197, 1963
114. Hull R, Hirsh J, Jay R et al: Different intensities of anticoagulation in the long-term treatment of proximal venous thrombosis. N Engl J Med 307:1676, 1982
115. Hurst JW, Schlant RC, Rackley CE et al: The Heart: Arteries and Vein. 7th Ed. p. 506. McGraw-Hill, New York, 1990
116. Hurst JW, Schlant RC, Rackley CE et al: The Heart: Arteries and Vein. 7th Ed. p. 1230. McGraw-Hill, New York, 1990
117. Hurst JW, Schlant RC, Rackley CE et al:

The Heart: Arteries and Vein. 7th Ed. p. 1278. McGraw-Hill, New York, 1990
118. International Study Group: In-hospital mortality and clinical course of 20,891 patients with suspected acute myocardial infarction randomized between tissue plasminogen activator or streptokinase with or without heparin. Lancet 336:71, 1990
119. ISIS-2 (Second International Study of Infarct Survival) Collaborative Group: Randomized trial of intravenous streptokinase, oral aspirin, both, or neither among 17,187 cases of suspected acute myocardial infarction: ISIS-2. Lancet 2:349, 1988
120. Jackson AC, Boughner DR, Barnett HJM: Mitral valve prolapse and cerebral ischemic events in young patients. Neurology (NY) 34:784, 1984
121. Johannessen KA, Nordrehaug JE, von der Lippe G, Vollset SE: Risk factors for embolization in patients with left ventricular thrombi and acute myocardial infarction. Br Heart J 60:104, 1988
122. Johannessen KA, Stratton JR, Taulow E et al: Usefulness of aspirin plus dipyridamole in reducing left ventricular thrombus formation in anterior wall acute myocardial infarction. Am J Cardiol 63:101, 1989
123. Johnson RT, Richardson EP: The neurological manifestations of systemic lupus erythematosus. Medicine (Baltimore) 47:337, 1968
124. Jones HR, Jr, Caplan LR, Come PC et al: Cerebral emboli of paradoxical origin. Ann Neurol 13:314, 1983
125. Jones HR, Jr, Naggar CZ, Seljan MP, Downing LL: Mitral valve prolapse and cerebral ischemic events. A comparison between a neurology population with stroke and a cardiology population with mitral valve prolapse observed for five years. Stroke 13:451, 1982
126. Kannel WB, Abbott RD, Savage DD, McNamara PM: Epidemiologic features of chronic atrial fibrillation: the Framingham study. N Engl J Med 306:1018, 1982
127. Kannel WB, Dawber TR, Cohen MS et al: Vascular diseases of the brain: epidemiologic aspects: the Framingham study. Am J Public Health 55:1355, 1965
128. Kapila A, Hart RG: Calcific cerebral emboli and aortic stenosis: detection by computed tomography. Stroke 17:619, 1986
129. Kaye D: Changing pattern of infectious endocarditis. Am J Med, suppl. 6B:157, 1985
130. Kelly RE, Pina I, Lee SC: Cerebral ischemia and mitral valve prolapse: case-control study of associated factors. Stroke 19:443, 1988
131. Keyser DL, Biller J, Coffman TT, Adams HP, Jr: Neurologic complications of late prosthetic valve endocarditis. Stroke 21:472, 1990
132. Kimball RW, Hedges TR: Amaurosis fugax caused by a prolapsed mitral valve leaflet in the midsystolic click, late systolic murmur syndrome. Am J Ophthalmol 83:469, 1977
133. Kittner SJ, Sharkness CM, Price TR et al: Infarcts with a cardiac source of embolism in the NINCDS stroke data bank: historical features. Neurology (NY) 40:281, 1990
134. Knepper LE, Biller J, Adams HP, Bruno A: Neurologic manifestations of atrial myxoma. Stroke 19:1435, 1988
135. Kopecky SL, Gerah BJ, McGoon MD et al: The natural history of lone atrial fibrillation. N Engl J Med 317:669, 1987
136. Korn D, DeSanctis RW, Sell S: Massive calcification of the mitral annulus: a clinical pathological study of 14 cases. N Engl J Med 267:900, 1962
137. Kouvaras G, Bacoulas G: Association of mitral leaflet prolapse with cerebral ischemic events in the young and early middle-aged patient. Q J Med 55:387, 1985
138. Kouvaras G, Chronopoulos G, Souffras G et al: The effects of long-term antithrombotic treatment on left ventricular thrombi in patients after an acute myocardial infarction. Am Heart J 119:73, 1990
139. Kumpe CW, Bean WB: Aortic stenosis: a study of the clinical and pathologic aspects of 107 proved cases. Medicine (Baltimore) 27:139, 1948
140. Kuntze CE, Ebels T, Eijgelaar A, van der Heide JNH: Rates of thromboembolism with three different mechanical heart valve prostheses: randomized study. Lancet 1:514, 1989
141. Kupper AJF, Verheught FWA, Peels CH et al: Effect of low dose acetylsalicyclic acid on the frequency and haematologic activity of left ventricular thrombus in anterior wall acute myocardial infarction. Am J Cardiol 63:917, 1989
142. Kupper AJF, Verheught FWA, Peels CH et al: Left ventricular thrombus incidence and behavior studies by serial two-dimensional echocardiography in acute anterior myocardial infarction: left ventricular wall motion, systemic embolism and oral anticoagulation. J Am Coll Cardiol 13:1514, 1989
143. Lang I, Steurer G, Weissel M, Burghuber OC: Recurrent paradoxical embolism complicating severe thromboembolic pulmonary hypertension. Eur Heart J 9:678, 1988
144. Lapeyre AC III, Steele PM, Kazmier FJ et al: Systemic embolism in chronic left ventricular aneurysm: incidence and the role of anticoagulation. J Am Coll Cardiol 6:534, 1985
145. Lechat P, Mas JL, Lescault G et al: Prevalence of patent foramen ovale in patients with stroke. N Engl J Med 318:1148, 1988
146. Legatt AD, Rubin MJ, Kaplan LR et al: Global aphasia without hemiparesis: multiple etiologies. Neurology (NY) 37:201, 1987
147. Levine HJ, Pauker SG, Salzman EW: Antithrombotic therapy in valvular heart disease. Chest, suppl. 95:98S, 1989
148. Lin CS, Schwartz IS, Chapman I: Calcification of the mitral annulus fibrosus with systemic embolization. Arch Pathol Lab Med 111:411, 1987
149. Lodder J, Dennis MS, Van Raak L et al: Cooperative study on the value of long-term anticoagulation in stroke patients with nonrheumatic atrial fibrillation. Br Med J 296:1435, 1988
150. Lodder J, Krijne-Kubat B, Broekman J: Cerebral hemorrhagic infarction at autopsy: cardiac em-

bolic cause and the relationship to the cause of death. Stroke 17:626, 1986
151. Lopez JA, Fishbein MC, Seigel RJ: Echocardiographic features of nonbacterial thrombotic endocarditis. Am J Cardiol 59:478, 1987
152. Lopez JA, Ross RS, Fishbein MC, Siegel RJ: Nonbacterial thrombotic endocarditis: a review. Am Heart J 113:773, 1987
153. Loscalzo J: Paradoxical embolism: clinical presentation, diagnostic strategies, and therapeutic options. Am Heart J 112:141, 1986
154. Lynch JJ, Schuchard GH, Gross CM, Wann LS: Prevalence of right-to-left atrial shunting in a healthy population: detection by Valsalva maneuver contrast echocardiography. Am J Cardiol 53:1478, 1984
155. MacMahon SW, Roberts JK, Kramer-Fox R et al: Mitral valve prolapse and infective endocarditis. Am Heart J 113:1291, 1987
156. Markel ML, Waller BF, Armstrong WF: Cardiac myxoma: a review. Medicine (Baltimore) 66:114, 1987
157. Marks AR, Choong CY, Chir MBB et al: Identification of high-risk and low-risk subgroups of patients with mitral-valve prolapse. N Engl J Med 320:1031, 1989
158. Marsh III EE, Biller J, Tranel D et al: Etiology of stroke in broca's aphasia. Neurology (NY), suppl 1. 40:325, 1990
159. Maruyama M, Kuriyama Y, Sawada T et al: Brain damage after open heart surgery in patients with acute cardioembolic stroke. Stroke 20:1305, 1989
160. Maze SS, Kotler MN, Parry WR: Flow characteristics in the dilated left ventricle with thrombus. JACC 13:873, 1989
161. McGrath LB, Gonzalez-Levin L, Eldredge WJ et al: Thromboembolic and other events following valve replacement in a pediatric population treated with antiplatelet agents. Ann Thorac Surg 43:285, 1987
162. McKenna WJ, Alfonso F: Arrhythmias in the cardiomyopathies and mitral valve prolapse. p. 59. In Zipes DP, Rowlands DJ (eds): Progress in Cardiology. Lea and Febiger, Philadelphia, 1988
163. Meister SG, Grossman W, Dexter L, Dalen JE: Paradoxical embolism: diagnosis during life. Am J Med 53:292, 1972
164. Meltzer RS, Visser CE, Fuster V: Intracardiac thrombi and systemic embolization. Ann Intern Med 104:689, 1986
165. Meyer JS, Charney JZ, Rivera VM et al: Cerebral embolization: prospective clinical analysis of 42 cases. Stroke 2:541, 1971
166. Miller RD, Jordan RA, Parker RL, Edwards JE: Thromboembolism in acute and in healed myocardial infarction. II. Systemic and pulmonary arterial occlusion. Circulation 6:7, 1952
167. Millikan CH, Bauer RB, Goldschmidt J et al: A classification and outline of cerebrovascular disease: II. Stroke 6:564, 1975
168. Mohr JP, Caplan LR, Melski JW et al: The Harvard cooperative stroke registry: a prospective registry. Neurology (NY) 28:754, 1978
169. Mok CK, Boey J, Wang R et al: Warfarin versus dipyridamole-aspirin and pentoxifylline-aspirin for the prevention of prosthetic heart valve thromboembolism: a prospective randomized clinical trial. Circulation 72:1059, 1985
170. Mountcastle VB: Medical Physiology. 13th Ed. Vol. 2. Ch. 37. CV Mosby, St. Louis, 1974
171. Muggc A, Daniel WG, Frank G, Lichtlen PR: Echocardiography in infective endocarditis: reassessment of prognostic implications of vegetation size determined by the transthoracic and the transesophageal approach. J Am Coll Cardiol 14:631, 1989
172. Mugge A, Daniel WG, Klopper JW, Lichtlen PR: Visualization of patent foramen ovale by transesophageal color-coded Doppler echocardiography. Am J Cardiol 62:837, 1988
173. Naggar CZ, Pearson WN, Seljan MP: Frequency of complications of mitral valve prolapse in subjects aged 60 years and older. Am J Cardiol 58:1209, 1986
174. Nair CK, Thomson W, Ryschon K et al: Long-term follow-up of patients with echocardiographically detected mitral anular calcium and comparison with age- and sex-matched control subjects. Am J Cardiol 63:465, 1989
175. Nakatani T, Frazier OH, Lammermeier DE et al: Heterotopic heart transplantation: a reliable option for a select group of high-risk patients. J Heart Transplant 8:40, 1989
176. Nencini P, Inzitari D, Baraffi MC et al: Incidence of stroke in young adults in Florence, Italy. Stroke 19:977, 1988
177. Nestico PF, Depace NL, Morganroth J et al: Mitral annular calcification: clinical pathophysiology, and echocardiographic review. Am Heart J 107:989, 1984
178. Nichol P, Kertesz A: Two dimensional echocardiographic (2DE) detection of left atrial thrombus in patient with mitral valve prolapse and strokes. Circulation, suppl 11. 59/60:18, 1979
179. Nihoyannopoulos P, Smith GC, Maseri A, Foale RA: The natural history of left ventricular thrombus in myocardial infarction: a rationale in support of masterly inactivity. J Am Coll Cardiol 14:903, 1989
180. Nishide M, Irino T, Gotoh M et al: Cardiac abnormalities in ischemic cerebrovascular disease studied by two-dimensional echocardiography. Stroke 14:541, 1983
181. Nishimura RA, McGoon MD, Shub C et al: Echocardiographically documented mitral valve prolapse: long-term follow-up of 237 patients. N Engl J Med 313:1305, 1985
182. O'Brien JT, Geiser EA: Infective endocarditis and echocardiography. Am Heart J 108:386, 1984
183. Ogata J, Yutani C, Imakita M et al: Hemorrhagic infarct of the brain without a reopening of the occluded arteries in cardioembolic stroke. Stroke 20:876, 1989
184. Okada Y, Yamaguchi T, Minematsu K et al: Hemorrhagic transformation in cerebral embolism. Stroke 20:598, 1989
185. Olesen KH, Rygg IH, Wennevold A, Nyboe J: Long-term follow-up in 185 patients after mitral

valve replacement with the Lillehei-Kaster prosthesis: overall results and prosthesis-related complications. Eur Heart J 8:680, 1987
186. Olsen ML, Arnett FC, Rosenbaum D et al: Sjögren's syndrome and other rheumatic disorders presenting to a neurology service. J Autoimmun 2:477, 1989
187. Onundarson PT, Thorgeirsson G, Jonmundsson E et al: Chronic atrial fibrillation: epidemiologic features and 14 year follow-up: a case-control study. Eur Heart J 8:521, 1987
188. Ostrander LD, Brandt RL, Kjelsberg MO, Epstein FH: Electrocardiographic findings among the adult population of a total natural community, Tecumseh, Michigan. Circulation 31:888, 1965
189. Palacios I, Block PC, Brandi S et al: Percutaneous balloon valvotomy for patients with severe mitral stenosis. Circulation 75:778, 1987
190. Paschalis C, Pugsley W, John R, Harrison MJG: Rate of cerebral embolic events in relation to antibiotic and anticoagulant therapy in patients with bacterial endocarditis. Eur Neurol 30:87, 1990
191. Pass HI, Sade RM, Crawford FA, Hohn AR: Cardiac valve prostheses in children without anticoagulation. J Thorac Cardiovasc Surg 87:832, 1984
192. Pearson AC, Labovitz AJ, Tatineni S, Gomez CR: Superiority of transesophageal echocardiography in detecting cardiac source of embolism in patients with cerebral ischemia of uncertain etiology. J Am Coll Cardiol 17:66, 1991
193. Perloff JK, Rosove MH, Child JS, Wright GB: Adults with cyanotic congenital heart disease: hematologic management. Ann Intern Med 109:406, 1988
194. Pessin MS, Lathi ES, Cohen MB et al: Clinical features and mechanism of occipital infarction. Ann Neurol 21:290, 1987
195. Petersen P: Thromboembolic complications in atrial fibrillation. Stroke 21:4, 1990
196. Petersen P, Godtfredsen J, Boysen G: Placebo-controlled, randomized trial of warfarin and aspirin for prevention of thromboembolic complications in chronic atrial fibrillation.: The Copenhagen AFASAF study. Lancet 1:175, 1989
197. Pomerance A: Ballooning deformity (mucoid degeneration) of atrioventricular valves. Br Heart J 31:343, 1969
198. Pomerance A: Cardiac pathology and systemic murmurs in the elderly. Br Heart J 30:687, 1968
199. Pomerance A: Pathological and clinical study of calcification of the mitral valve ring. J Clin Pathol 23:354, 1970
200. Pop G, Sutherland GR, Koudstaal PJ et al: Transesophageal echocardiography in the detection of intracardiac embolic sources in patients with transient ischemic attacks. Stroke 21:560, 1990
201. Popp RL: Echocardiography. I. Medical progress. N Engl J Med 323:101, 1990
202. Popp RL: Echocardiography. II. Medical Progress. N Engl J Med 323:165, 1990
203. Presti CF, Hart RG: Thyrotoxicosis, atrial fibrillation, and embolism, revisited. Am Heart J 117:976, 1989, 1990
204. Price TR: Stroke in patients treated with thrombolytic therapy for acute myocardial infarction: the thrombosis in myocardial infarction clinical trial and a review of placebo-controlled trials. Stroke, suppl III. 21:8, 1990
205. Pruitt AA, Rubin RH, Karchmer AW, Duncan GW: Neurologic complications of bacterial endocarditis. Medicine (Baltimore) 57:329, 1978
206. Puletti M, Morocutti C, Borgia C et al: Acute myocardial infarction and brain. Ital J Neurol Sci 8:245, 1987
207. Ramirez-Lassepas M, Cipolle RJ, Bjork RJ et al: Can embolic stroke be diagnosed on the basis of neurologic clinical criteria? Arch Neurol 44:87, 1987
208. Reed RL, Siekert RG, Merideth J: Rarity of transient focal cerebral ischemia in cardiac dysrhythmia. JAMA 223:893, 1973
209. Rem JA, Hachinski VC, Boughner DR, Barnett HJM: Value of cardiac monitoring and echocardiography in TIA and stroke patients. Stroke 16:950, 1985
210. Rice GPA, Ebers GC, Newland F, Wysocki GP: Recurrent cerebral embolism in cardiac amyloidosis. Neurology (NY) 31:904, 1981
211. Ridolfi RL, Hutchins GM: Spontaneous calcific emboli from calcific mitral annulus fibrosus. Arch Pathol Lab Med 100:117, 1976
212. Roberts WC, Siegel RJ, McManus BM: Idiopathic dilated cardiomyopathy: analysis of 152 necropsy patients. Am J Cardiol 60:1340, 1987
213. Rogers LR, Cho ES, Kempin S, Posner JB: Cerebral infarction from nonbacterial thrombotic endocarditis: clinical and pathological study including the effects of anticoagulation. Am J Med 83:746, 1987
214. Rothbard RL, Nanda NC, Fleck G, Heinle RA: Mitral valve prolapse and stroke: detection of potential emboli by real-time two-dimensional echocardiography. Circulation, suppl 11. 59/60:99, 1979
215. Rothrock JF, Dittrich HC, Fleck P et al: Mitral valve prolapse and ischemic stroke in the young. Circulation 78:601, 1988
216. Rowe JC, Bland EF, Sprague HB, White PP: The course of mitral stenosis without surgery: ten- and twenty-year perspectives. Ann Intern Med 52:741, 1960
217. Roy D, Marchand E, Gagne P et al: Usefulness of anticoagulant therapy in the prevention of embolic complications of atrial fibrillation. Am Heart J 112:1139, 1986
218. Rubenstein JJ, Schulman CL, Yurchak PM, De Sanctis RW: Clinical spectrum of the sick sinus syndrome. Circulation 46:5, 1972
219. Salgado AV, Furlan AJ, Keys TF: Mycotic aneurysm, subarachnoid hemorrhage and indications for cerebral angiography in infectious endocarditis. Stroke 18:1057, 1987
220. Salgado AV, Furlan AJ, Keys TF et al: Neurological complications of native and prosthetic valve endocarditis: a 12-year experience. Neurology (NY) 39:173, 1989

221. Sandercock PAG, Warlow CP, Jone LN: Predisposing factors for cerebral infarction: the Oxfordshire community stroke project. Br Med J 298:75, 1989
222. Santini M, Alexidou G, Ansalone G et al: Relation of prognosis in sick sinus syndrome to age, conduction defects and modes of permanent cardiac pacing. Am J Cardiol 65:729, 1990
223. Saour JN, Sieck JO, Mamo LAR, Gallus AS: Trial of different intensities of anticoagulation in patients with prosthetic heart valves. N Engl J Med 322:428, 1990
224. Sareli P, England MJ, Berk MR et al: Maternal and fetal sequelae of anticoagulation during pregnancy in patients with mechanical heart valve prostheses. Am J Cardiol 63:1462, 1989
225. Savage DD, Garrison RJ, Devereaux RD et al: Mitral valve prolapse in the general population. I. Epidemiologic features: the Framingham Study. Am Heart J 106:571, 1983
226. The SCATI (Studio sulla Calciparina nell'angina e nella Trombosi Ventricolare nell'infarto) group: randomized controlled trial of subcutaneous calcium-heparin in acute myocardial infarction. Lancet 2:182, 1989
227. Scharf RE, Hennerici M, Bluschke V et al: Cerebral ischemia in young patients: is it associated with mitral valve prolapse and abnormal platelet activity in vivo? Stroke 13:454, 1982
228. Schnee MA, Bucal AA: Fatal embolism in mitral valve prolapse. Chest 83:285, 1983
229. Schneider B, Hanrath P, Vogel P, Meinertz T: Improved morphologic characterization of atrial septal aneurysm by transesophageal echocardiography: relation to cerebrovascular events. J Am Coll Cardiol 16:1000, 1990
230. Selzer A, Cohn KE: Natural history of mitral stenosis: a review. Circulation 45:878, 1972
231. Selzer A, Katayama F: Mitral regurgitation: clinical patterns, pathophysiology and natural history. Medicine (Baltimore) 51:337, 1972
232. Seward JB, Khandheria BK, Oh JK et al: Transesophageal echocardiography: technique, anatomic correlations, implementation, and clinical applications. Mayo Clin Proc 63:649, 1988
233. Shaw PJ, Bates D, Cartlidge NEF et al: Neurologic and neuropsychological morbidity following major surgery-comparison of coronary artery bypass and peripheral vascular surgery. Stroke 18:700, 1987
234. Sherman DG, Dyken ML, Fisher M et al: Antithrombotic therapy for cerebrovascular disorders, suppl. Chest 95:140S, 1989
235. Shrestha NK, Moreno FL, Narciso FV et al: Two-dimensional echocardiographic diagnosis of left atrial thrombus in rheumatic heart disease: a clinicopathologic study. Circulation 67:341, 1983
236. Silver MD: Infective endocarditis. p. 517. In Silver MD (ed): Cardiovascular Pathology. Churchill Livingstone, New York, 1983
237. Simpson IA, Camm AJ: Colour Doppler flow mapping: a new dimension for cardiac diagnosis. BMJ 300:1, 1990
238. Smith P, Arnesen H, Holme I: The effect of warfarin on mortality and reinfarction after myocardial infarction. N Engl J Med 323:147, 1990
239. Special Report from the National Institute of Neurological Disorders and Stroke: Classification of cerebrovascular diseases. III. Stroke 21:637, 1990
240. Stagaman DJ, Presti C, Rees C, Miller DD: Septic pulmonary arteriovenous fistula: an unusual conduit for systemic embolization in right-sided valvular endocarditis. Chest 97:1484, 1990
241. Stein PD, Kantrowitz A: Antithrombotic therapy in mechanical and biological prosthetic heart valves and saphenous vein bypass grafts. Chest 95:107S, 1989
242. Stein PD, Willis PW, DeMets: History and physical examination in acute pulmonary embolism in patients without preexisting cardiac or pulmonary disease. Am J Cardiol 47:218, 1981
243. Stevenson LW, Perloff JK: The dilated cardiomyopathies: clinical aspects. Cardiol Clin 6:187, 1988
244. Storer J, Lisan P, Delmonico JE, Jr, Bailey CP: Physiopathological concepts of mitral valvular disease: review of 225 cardiotomies. JAMA 155:103, 1954
245. Stratton JR, Resnick AD: Increased embolic risk in patients with left ventricular thrombi. Circulation 75:1004, 1987
246. Stroke Prevention in Atrial Fibrillation Investigators: Design of a multicenter randomized trial for the stroke prevention in atrial fibrillation study. Stroke 21:538, 1990
247. The Stroke Prevention in Atrial Fibrillation Study Group Investigators: Special report: preliminary report of the stroke prevention in atrial fibrillation study. N Engl J Med 322:863, 1990
248. Szekely P: Systemic embolism and anticoagulant prophylaxis in rheumatic heart disease. Br Med J 1:209, 1964
249. Tegeler CH, Downes TR: Cardiac imaging in stroke. Curr Concepts Cerebrovasc Dis Stroke 26:13, 1991
250. Thompson T, Evans W: Paradoxical embolism. Q J Med 23:135, 1930
251. Toole JF: Cerebrovascular Disorders. 4th Ed. p. 245. Raven Press, New York, 1990
252. Tunick PA, Culliford AT, Lamparello PJ, Kronzon I: Atheromatosis of the aortic arch as an occult source of multiple systemic emboli. Ann Intern Med 114:391, 1991
253. Turpie AGG, Gunstensen J, Hirsh J, Nelson H, Gent M: Randomized comparison of two intensities of oral anticoagulant therapy after tissue heart valve replacement. Lancet 1:1242, 1988
254. Turpie AGG, Robinson JG, Doyle DJ et al: Comparison of high-dose with low-dose subcutaneous heparin to prevent left ventricular mural thrombosis in patients with acute transmural anterior myocardial infarction. N Engl J Med 320:352, 1989
255. Warth DC, King ME, Cohen JM et al: Prevalence of mitral valve prolapse in normal children. J Am Coll Cardiol 5:1173, 1985

256. Watson RT: TIA, stroke and mitral valve prolapse. Neurology (NY) 29:886, 1979
257. Webster MWI, Smith HJ, Sharpe DN et al: Patent foramen ovale in young stroke patients. Lancet 2:11, 1988
258. Weinreich DJ, Burke JF, Pauletto FJ: Left ventricular mural thrombi complicating acute myocardial infarction: long-term follow-up with serial echocardiography. Ann Intern Med 100:789, 1984
259. Weinstein GS, Mavroudis C, Ebert PA: Preliminary experience with aspirin for anticoagulation in children with prosthetic cardiac valves. Ann Thorac Surg 33:549, 1982
260. Wilson WR, Geraci JE, Danielson GK et al: Anticoagulant therapy and central nervous system complications in patients with prosthetic valve endocarditis. Circulation 57:1004, 1978
261. Wolf PA, Abbott RD, Kannel WB: Atrial fibrillation: a major contributor to stroke in the elderly: the Framingham study. Arch Intern Med 147:1561, 1987
262. Wolf PA, Dawber TR, Thomas HE, Kannel WB: Epidemiologic assessment of chronic atrial fibrillation and risk of stroke: the Framingham study. Neurology (NY) 28:973, 1978
263. Wolf PA, Kannel WB, McGee DL: Duration of atrial fibrillation and imminence of stroke: the Framingham study. Stroke 14:664, 1983
264. Wolf PA, Sila CA: Cerebral ischemia with mitral valve prolapse. Am Heart J 113:1308, 1987
265. Woods GL, Wood RP, Shaw BW, Jr: Aspergillus endocarditis in patients without prior cardiovascular surgery: report of a case in a liver transplant recipient and review. (Abstract.) Rev Infect Dis 2:263, 1989
266. Yadav JS, Kinkel PR, Klee D et al: Small cerebral embolic infarctions: evaluation by magnetic resonance imaging. Neurology (NY) suppl 1. 39:160, 1989
267. Yamanouchi H, Tomonaga M, Shimada H et al: Nonvalvular atrial fibrillation as a cause of fatal massive cerebral infarction in the elderly. Stroke 20:1653, 1989
268. Yatsu FM, Hart RG, Mohr JP, Grotta JC: Anticoagulation of embolic strokes of cardiac origin: an update. Neurology (NY) 38:314, 1988
269. Zenker G, Erbel R, Kramer G et al: Transesophageal two-dimensional echocardiography in young patients with cerebral ischemic events. Stroke 19:345, 1988
270. Barnett HJM: Heart in ischemic stroke–a changing emphasis. p. 291. Barnett HJM (Ed): Neurologic Clinics. WB Saunders, Philadelphia, 1983.

# 42
# *THERAPY OF SECONDARY MEDICAL COMPLICATIONS OF STROKES*

Frank M. Yatsu
Thomas J. DeGraba
Sandra Hanson

Disabling neurologic deficits of strokes are devastating by taking away patients' independence and dignity; and for their physicians, the challenge is to optimize functional recovery and to establish realistic goals for meaningful activities of daily living (ADL). The task can be enormous, particularly when patients are more susceptible to developing serious secondary medical complications that adversely affect outcome. These secondary complications, the focus of this chapter, will be discussed under the following categories (Table 42-1): cardiovascular, pulmonary, excretory, nutritional, metabolic, psychiatric, immobility, and neurologic. Recent advances in acute stroke therapies and interventions to prevent stroke occurrence/recurrence, discussed in Chapter 39 on new acute stroke therapies, give greater hope to expectations that the incidence and devastation of strokes can be reduced even further, thereby minimizing concerns over secondary complications.[4,16,41] Nonetheless, until that time, these potential complications remain an ongoing threat to achieving optimum recovery, and require continued vigilance for intervention.

Neurologists may direct a stroke team or those caring for the strokes, but the most effective approach is a cooperative one, maximizing efficient communication between treating and consulting physicians and the nursing, nutrition, speech, occupational therapy, and rehabilitation staffs. For many of the secondary complications, as listed in Table 42-1, the specialist consultant, such as the cardiologist, neurosurgeon, pulmonologist, or urologist can assist in recommending specialized therapies or interventions to minimize complications and promote recovery.[25,35,47,63]

Efforts to minimize these multiple complications may be guided by the patient's likely prognosis. For example, a massive brain stem or hemispheric infarction resulting in stupor or coma may not warrant heroic measures. This widespread and gaining view acknowledges the realistic outcome of these patients, and concedes the ineluctable transition from life to death of lethal brain insults and can avoid the indignities of costly life support measures. Fully one-quarter of the stroke patients admitted to hospitals will have experienced lethal insults such as these.[98] On the

This work was supported by the Clayton Foundation for Research, Houston; and is dedicated to Professor Carlo Loeb of Genoa, Italy on the occasion of his retirement.

**TABLE 42-1. Medical and Neurologic Complications of Stroke**

| | |
|---|---|
| Cardiovascular and pulmonary functions | Cardiac arrhythmias, cardiac output, blood pressure stabilization, hypertension, congestive failure<br>Chronic obstructive pulmonary disease, pulmonary embolism, atelectasis, neurogenic pulmonary edema, pneumonia, intubation, tracheostomy |
| Nutritional and metabolic status | Intake and output, body weight, electrolytes and mineral metabolism<br>Salt and water metabolism: syndrome of inappropriate antidiuretic hormone secretion, central nervous system salt losing, salt retention |
| Excretory function | Bladder incontinence, "spastic bladder," hypotonicity/retention<br>Bowel: incontinence, constipation |
| Bed rest and immobility | Skin care: decubiti and sores contracture<br>Venous thrombosis and pulmonary emboli<br>Atelectasis |
| Psychiatric disorders | Depression<br>Confusional states: organic brain syndrome and sundowning |
| Neurologic complications | Seizures (general, partial)<br>Increased intracranial pressure<br>Coma/stupor<br>Cognitive defects and dementia |

other hand, patients with moderate or minimal neurologic deficits should be treated aggressively to avert secondary complications that may deny maximum recovery.

Stroke care, as a distinct medical condition requiring specialized intensive care units, has received increasing attention, particularly thrombolytic therapy and other interventions designed to minimize acute ischemic brain damage. Because of the necessity to monitor stroke patients under these circumstances to conduct frequent neurologic evaluations and for specialized interventions such as intracranial pressure recording, an argument has been made to treat these stroke patients in stroke intensive care units (stroke ICUs).[7,22,25,95] Although these arguments may appear reasonable, the major benefits of stroke ICUs have been in galvanizing interest in strokes and in heightening attention to nursing care with reduction in secondary problems due to decubitus ulcers and contractures in paralyzed limbs, but not in stroke outcome.[10,61]

In their community-based assessment of all 16 acute care hospitals in Cincinnati, Ohio, Brott and Reed[10] found that the 14 hospitals without specialized neurology/neurosurgery intensive care units were able, with conventional intensive care units, to manage acute strokes adequately and provide high-quality care. Specific areas of acute management which could be adequately handled in these units are in respiratory management (a Glasgow Coma Score of 5 or less is assumed to have increased intracranial pressure (ICP) and treated as such); cardiac care and fluid management (which require cardiac monitoring over the first 24 hours); blood pressure management; treatment of raised intracranial pressure (such as the elevation of the head to 30 degrees and use of mannitol as a dehydrating agent); and bedside assessment (for example, use of transcranial Doppler, electroencephalogram (EEG), or ICP monitoring). From this experience and others, acute strokes need not be segregated into a separate "stroke ICU." In fact, the presence of a separate stroke ICU has the potential hazard of creating a sense of medical isolation, which can be detrimental to the stroke patient's total care.

## CARDIOVASCULAR AND PULMONARY FUNCTIONS

Cardiovascular and pulmonary complications associated with strokes are due to (1) preexisting diseases, which can be aggravated by stroke; (2) stroke-induced cardiac arrhythmias and electrocardiographic (ECG) abnormalities; (3) neurogenic pulmonary edema; and (4) hypertension and the potential problems associated with its aggressive therapy.[2,9,15,39,48,49,54,55,66,68,89,97]

With preexisting cardiovascular and pulmonary diseases, strokes may worsen the underlying condition due to either neurologic deficits or secondary metabolic derangements.

It has been recognized for years that cerebral vascular events, such as subarachnoid hemorrhage, acute thromboembolic stroke, and cerebral hemorrhage have been associated with abnormalities on the electrocardiogram.[11,12,17,33] ECG abnormalities and acute cerebral vascular events were found in over 90 percent of patients in two large studies[17,30] as compared to approximately 40 percent in the age-sex match control population. The most common changes were QT prolongation (up to 45 percent), ST segment depression or T-wave inversion (35 to 50 percent), and U waves (up to 28 percent). Studies have also demonstrated a significant increase in cardiac arrhythmias with ectopic ventricular activity being the most common.[58,60] Myers et al.[58] noted that the occurrence of arrhythmias was independent of coexisting heart disease. The importance of the occurrence of these ECG abnormalities was highlighted by Lavy et al.,[50] who showed that the prognosis for patient survival was much worse in those patients with ischemic changes or arrhythmias on their ECG. In addition, it was noted that outcome was dependent upon ECG changes acquired during the acute stroke period rather than to preexisting heart disease.[50] Norris et al.[62] demonstrated, in a group of 230 patients with stroke, that serum CK-MB isoenzymes were elevated in 11 percent of the patients. This CK-MB elevation was correlated with evidence of acute myocardial ischemia by EKG and showed a 92 percent incidence of cardiac arrhythmias. Also of note was that the progressive ischemic changes on the ECG along with the timing of the CK-MB elevation indicated that the cardiac changes were most likely a result of and not the cause of the acute cerebral vascular event. Myers et al.[57] demonstrated that patients with ischemic infarcts and TIAs had an elevation of plasma norepinephrine levels versus a control population which was felt to be consistent with an increase in peripheral sympathetic activity producing cardiac abnormalities. Studies demonstrate[58] that elevated plasma norepinephrine concentration correlated with an increase in CK-MB (creatine kinase isoenzyme) but did not appear to correlate with an increase incidence of cardiac arrhythmias. Again, the significance of elevation of cardiac isoenzyme in the setting of acute cerebral vascular events have been shown to increase the mortality more than twofold (66 percent vs 30 percent) over those patients with normal cardiac enzymes.[17]

The etiology of these ECG changes and cardiac abnormalities may well represent a combination of factors. The existence of concomitant underlying coronary artery disease may likely play a role in the appearance of cardiac abnormalities and mortality.[50] Patients with severe coronary artery disease subjected to an elevation in sympathetic nervous stimulation due to an intracerebral event could clearly cause cardiac changes such as ischemia or arrhythmias due to increase myocardial oxygen demand. The theory which has gained most wide support is the belief that the discharge of catecholaminergic neurotransmitters into the systemic circulation in association with cerebral infarction, subarachnoid hemorrhage, and increased intracranial pressure, plus increased vagal traffic to the heart, provokes both hypertension and cardiac muscle damage.[59] In addition to the increase in myocardial contractility and heart rate in general, there is evidence that local discharge of the sympathetic nerve fibers within the ventricular muscle itself leads to a myofibrillar degeneration.[33] The subendocardial changes seen on autopsy studies correlate with elevation in cardiac enzymes and are histopathologically distinct from ischemic infarctions seen with coronary artery disease.[79]

In view of the evidence that cerebral vascular events cause serious arrhythmias, myocardial damage, and increase mortality secondary to these cardiac events, it is recommended that all patients with stroke be monitored for cardiac arrhythmias[97] in the first 24 to 72 hours after admission, and that serial cardiac isoenzymes are obtained on all patients with new ECG abnormalities. For cardiac output failure digitalis may be effective.[22]

Treatment modalities for these cardiac changes include beta-blockers to inhibit the catecholaminergic output, lidocaine for arrhythmias, and atropine for vagotonia. Type 1A arrhythmiatics, such as quinidine and procainamide, may prolong the QT interval and may not be appropriate in this setting.

It is well accepted that the greatest risk of mortality following a transient ischemic attack (TIA) or stroke is from cardiac causes.[29,90] It is estimated that 33 percent of patients with TIAs or stroke have symptomatic coronary artery disease.[13,42] Toole et al.[90] showed, in a 9-year follow-up study, that greater than 60 percent of all deaths in patients with TIAs resulted from myocardial infarctions. Others, as well, have echoed the findings that TIAs are not only a warning for future stroke, but point toward coronary artery disease and increased incidence of death due to myocardial infarction.[29,56] In light of the data of coronary artery disease existing in patients with thromboembolic stroke and TIA, a unified approach for cardiac monitoring and evaluation of coronary artery disease must be employed. In a prospective study of 506 patients[39] presenting with symptomatic extracranial cerebral vascular disease ($N = 288$) or asymptomatic carotid bruits ($N = 218$), 48 percent of those with clinical symptoms or EKG findings consistent with coronary artery disease and 16 percent with no suspicion of coronary artery disease, had severe coronary stenosis by angiography, warranting a revascularization procedure, or showed an inoperable lesion. The high prevalence of coronary artery disease suggests that patients with symptomatic coronary disease who have TIAs or stroke, requiring extracranial vascular surgery, should undergo coronary angiography. Patients without clinically apparent coronary artery disease should have cardiac screening including ECG stress test or a stress thallium. If these results are positive, coronary angiography should be performed to identify coronary stenosis requiring surgical intervention prior to carotidendarterectomy. Di Pasquale et al.[19] echoes the concept of cardiovascular evaluation. In a prospective study of 83 patients with TIAs or mild stroke without symptoms or ECG signs of ischemic heart disease, they demonstrated a 28 percent rate of coronary artery disease on exercise ECG tests and exercise thallium 201 myocardial scintigraphy. This is compared to a 6 percent rate of coronary artery disease seen in an age- and sex-matched control group with no clinical symptoms of cerebrovascular or coronary artery disease. Boucher et al.[8] demonstrated the predicted value of a stress thallium. It was shown that 8 of 16 patients with no clinical history of coronary artery disease, who had a positive stress thallium test, went on to have a myocardial infarction (MI) after their revascularization procedure for carotid occlusive disease. None of the 32 patients with normal stress thalamus had a MI after their operation. These data support the contention that presentation of cerebral ischemia should prompt an evaluation of the coronary system.

With pulmonary diseases such as chronic obstructive pulmonary disease (COPD), weakness of muscles of respiration due to hemiparesis, impairment of respiration due to brain stem lesions, and inadequate cough and gag leading to aspiration will embarrass and decompensate borderline pulmonary function. In addition, immobility of extremities due to paralysis with attendant stasis of blood and thrombosis can lead to multiple pulmonary emboli. In addition, atelectasis is a threat. Also, atelectasis secondary to immobility can lead to $O_2$ desaturation and thus lead to further hypoxic insult.

In patients with mildly impaired gag or swallowing, frequent suctioning and avoiding the supine position are indicated, but if gag and swallowing are seriously affected, either intubation or tracheostomy should be instituted to avoid the dangers of aspiration. In patients with unilateral brain stem lesions affecting the vagus nerve, specifically the dorsal motor nucleus, it is anticipated that the contralateral vagus nucleus will compensate to minimize dysphagia in several days or more. Under these circumstances, short-term intubation is justified.

Neurogenic pulmonary edema (NPE) occurs in association with dramatic insults to the central nervous system, such as massive subarachnoid hemorrhage, seizures or head trauma, although it has occurred with cerebral infarction.[21,74] Although NPE could occur from congestive heart failure resulting from massive and sustained hypertension secondary to catecholaminergic release, the most common mechanism is causing NPE is transudation of serum into lung alveoli.[88,91] In an analysis of 25 hemorrhagic stroke patients, 3 of whom experienced NPE, Touho et al.[91] measured pulmonary arterial pressure, pulmonary capillary wedge pressure, central venous pressure, cardiac index, systemic vascular resistance index, pulmonary vascular resistance index, and extravascular lung water using a double-indicator dilution method, the primary disorder with NPE is increased extravascular lung water. The defect is not explained

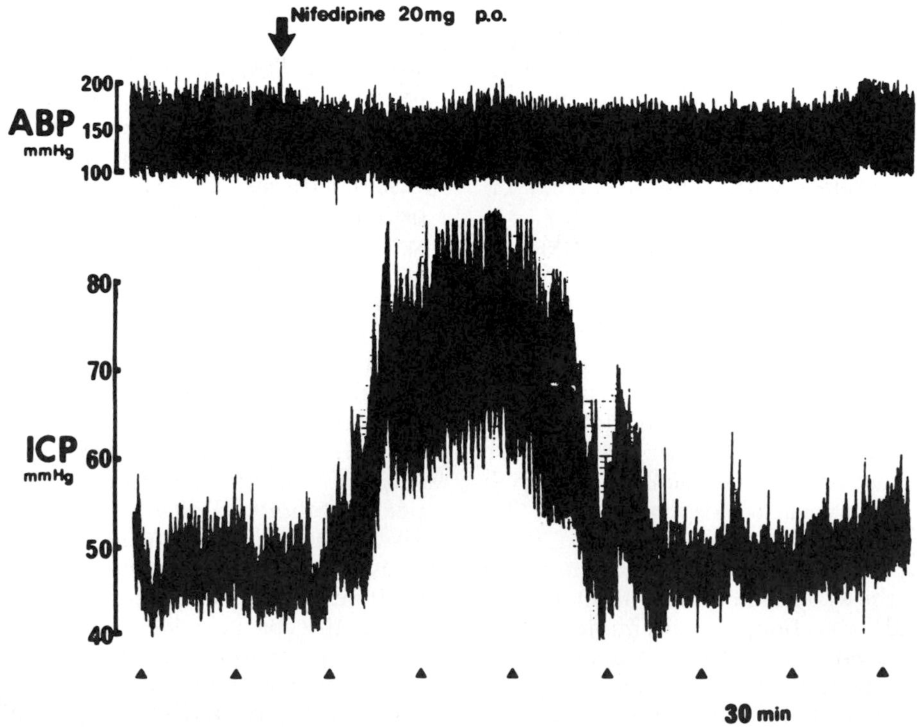


**Fig. 42-1.** Arterial blood pressure (ABP) and intracranial pressure (ICP) after administration of 20 mg sublingual nifedipine. This subject had marked elevation of ICP >40 mmHg. Note that a trivial reduction of ABP is associated with a dramatic, nearly 30 mmHg, rise in ICP. (From Hayashi et al.,[37] with permission.)

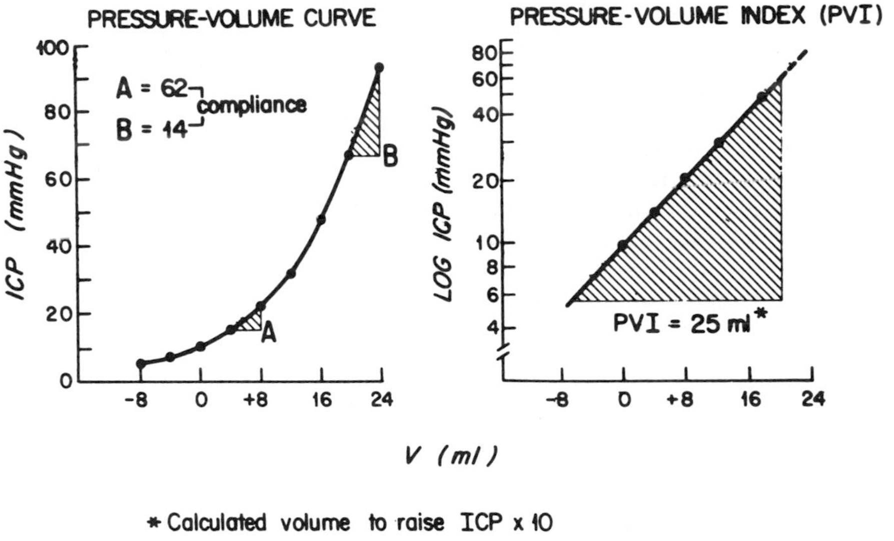


**Fig. 42-2.** The relationship between intracranial pressure (ICP) and volume (V) in normal adults. With increases in ICP, small increments in volume (e.g., from edema or hemorrhage) causes progressively greater increases in ICP. For example, with ICP at *A* of 17 mmHg, a volume (V) increase of 4 ml results in only an 8 mmHg rise in ICP, while with an initial ICP at *B* of 70 mmHg, a similar volume (V) increase of 4 ml provokes a 27 mmHg rise in ICP. Thus, compliance, or the change in ICP for any given increase in volume, is lower at reduced ICPs, such as at *A*, than at higher ones, such as at *B*. On the right-hand side of the figure is a semilogarithmic plot illustrating the pressure-volume index (PVI), the volume required to increase ICP by 1 log or 10 mmHg. (From Wechsler and Ropper,[95] with permission.)

by left ventricular failure, but by high permeability of water leading to pulmonary edema. Although α-adrenergic blockade, such as the use of phenoxybenzamine, has been advocated, institution of positive end-expiratory pressure suffices in clearing the patient of NPE.

Hypertension in acute strokes should not be treated unless to a modest degree of 10 to 15 percent reduction or if the patient has evidence of hypertensive encephalopathy.[10,18,32,99] One of the major reasons for not reducing blood pressure is to maintain necessary perfusion pressure of the cerebral circulation to ensure adequate tissue access to obligatory nutrients of oxygen and glucose. Strandgaard et al.[86] in their classic observation on cerebral blood flow in hypertensives noted that these individuals lose homeostatic control when the mean arterial pressure is reduced to below approximately 125 mmHg. More recently, Hayashi et al.[37] investigated stroke patients with increased intracranial pressure, using intraventricular recording devices, and found that hypotensive agents, such as calcium channel blockers, could produce a profound increase in intracranial pressure due to vasodilation, while only a trivial reduction in systemic arterial pressure occurred. These studies confirm the long-feared complication of hypotensive therapy in patients with strokes by compromising the perfusion pressure (see Figs. 42-1 and 42-2).

## NUTRITIONAL AND METABOLIC STATUS

Nutritional upkeep/balance and metabolic homeostasis are constantly threatened in stroke patients who may suffer inadequate intake of food and fluids because of sensorial depression, altered thirst mechanisms, or dysphagia.[65] For patients at risk of aspiration, either temporary nasogastric tube or percutaneous gastrostomy is indicated to ensure adequate nutrition and fluids. In some patients with severe dysphagia and sensorial depression in whom aspiration is a serious concern, early tracheostomy is justified to avert pneumonia. In patients who can handle secretions, but only marginally, the semi-Fowler's position with the head down and slightly turned will encourage pulmonary toilet to occur by gravity and minimize aspiration, particularly in conjunction with self or aid-administered suctioning.

Since most stroke patients will not have drunk fluids because of their disability, care should be taken to maximize their fluid balance with regular body weights and checks on intake and output. During hot weather when insensible fluid loss is greater, compensation for this loss must be calculated.

For severe strokes, such as massive subarachnoid hemorrhage, the syndrome of inappropriate antidiuretic hormone secretion (SIADH) may supervene; patients become confused and show symptoms of an organic brain syndrome. Checks of electrolytes will provide timely evaluation and intervention when the serum sodium begins to fall with evidence of a mismatch between serum and urine osmolality, suggestive of an increased secretion of antidiuretic hormone (ADH): free water is retained in the face, paradoxically, of hemodilution. In occasional cases of hyponatremia, the hyponatremia is not associated with volume expansion, but rather contraction and natriuresis can be accounted for by renal loss of sodium. For this condition, "cerebral salt wasting" has been applied, although the term is confusing, since it is inappropriately and synonymously used for SIADH. SIADH can be treated with fluid restriction by only compensating for insensible water loss, such as 800 cc per day; but the clinician is in the dilemma over concerns that hemoconcentration can provoke intravascular thrombosis and also hamper blood flow to the ischemic microcirculation surrounding a stroke. For severe hyponatremia below 115 mEq/L, coupled with evidence of sodium depletion and of sodium loss, infusion of sodium coupled with diuresis is indicated. However, the serum sodium should not be increased by more than 12 mEq/L per day, since restoration above this level is associated with pontine and extrapontine myelinolysis.

## EXCRETORY FUNCTIONS

Careful attention to bladder and bowel functions is a normal complement to concerns over hydration, nutrition and metabolic balance, especially in patients whose motor, sensory or mental disabilities do not allow them to communicate their needs for normal excretion. Stroke victims are frequently incontinent of both urine and feces due to loss of voluntary sphincter control or an inability to respond to sensations warning of either full rectum or bladder.[43] With brain stem and spinal cord strokes, both efferent and afferent pathways from bladder and rectum can be impaired, leading to either retention or incontinence.

For urinary retention, catheterization should be the last resort because of the hazards of urinary tract infections. For men, condom catheters can be used for overflow or autonomous bladders, but catheterization, either intermittent or constant indwelling, may be required to avert the potential dangers of hydroureters and hydronephrosis from urinary retention. For women, the problem of incontinence is complicated by the more ready occurrence of skin maceration from incontinence, which justifies catheterization until continence is restored.

Fecal incontinence occurs for both spinal cord and brain lesions, and the use of diapers with frequent changes can minimize skin maceration. Changing the diet to include more fiber will increase bulk to the stool as well. Constipation with fecal impaction can be a serious problem which is better treated by prevention with the use of enemas, rectal examinations, disempactions, and diet supplements with fiber.

## PSYCHIATRIC AND PSYCHOLOGICAL DISORDERS

Psychiatric and behavioral complications are common with strokes and are the result both of the patient's reaction to disabling neurologic deficits and of brain damage affecting brain areas provoking behavioral changes.[5] To an individual who has been healthy and independent, the inability to communicate, comprehend, ambulate, or remember easily lead to a reactive depression.[38] In addition, a variety of psychiatric and psychological disorders can occur resulting from neurotransmitter alterations or "chemical imbalances" due to damage to critical areas of brain. These disorders include not only depression, but mania, agitation, violence and range, and emotional lability.[70,85]

Moderate to severe depression is seen in a large percentage of stroke victims and yet many times goes undiagnosed and untreated.[24] In a series of reports on poststroke mood disorders, Robinson and colleagues[72] demonstrated that nearly one-half of all patients with thromboembolic or intracerebral hemorrhagic stroke developed clinically significant depression in the first 2 weeks. In a series of 103 acute stroke patients, 27 percent developed a major depression by DSM/III criteria and 20 percent developed less severe but nonetheless clinically significant minor depression (also classified dysthymic disorder by DSM/III). Of importance is that these depressive disorders persist for months if untreated. In a follow-up of the subgroup of patients with depression, Robinson found that approximately two-thirds remained depressed for 7 to 8 months. In addition, the prevalence of depression increased to 60 percent at 6 months after the stroke.[73] Therefore, if left untreated after stroke, depression can inhibit rehabilitation and recovery efforts commonly seen in the chronic stroke patient at 6 months to 2 years.[71]

The etiology of depressive syndromes quite naturally, at first glance, are believed due to the loss of motor function, communication skills, body image, and personal independence as well as confusional states and cognitive impairment. Benson reports that a major cause of poststroke depression is a result of a loss of linguist communications.[5] However, Robinson and colleagues[71,72] have observed that the severity of depression is not directly related to the degree of functional physical impairment or cognitive deficits. They found that depressive syndromes correlated closely with the location of the stroke lesion showing that 60 percent of patients with frontal lobe injury had major depression. The severity of depression was closely correlated with its proximity to the left frontal pole and was not associated with the degrees of Broca's aphasia, and therefore demonstrated the importance of the location of stroke in depression.[69] Some degree of depression, however, can be seen with strokes in any part of the brain, though clearly less frequent in posterior fossa strokes. It can also occur in right hemisphere infarct, though Robinson and colleagues believe that right-sided strokes are more commonly associated with mania.[70]

In addition to depressive disorders, other psychiatric syndromes complicate the poststroke patient's recovery including frustration, anger, emotional ability with inappropriate crying or laughing, as well as disconnection syndromes in which patients lose spatial or body orientation.[85] Symptoms of depression may be masked as psychosomatic symptoms commonly manifested as nonspecific head and face pain or limb or joint pain. In addition, inattention and apathy due to depression may be misinterpreted as dementia, so called "pseudodementia."[1]

Because the patient's response to all these factors and the degree of depression reflects the complexities of premorbid personality, successful handling of psychiatric and psychological disorders with strokes requires a team approach. The team can more successfully coordinate the entire evaluation and care of the patient, including neurologic, medical, psychological, psychiatric, nursing, and rehabilitative aspects. Surrounding the patient with familiar objects from home and with family members who are supportive, can minimize confusion, agitation and depression. Meaningful sensory stimuli, such as conversation, TV, reading, and so on, plus challenges by therapists, can motivate patients, but especially can minimize their sense of isolation and loss.[96]

Use of tricyclic antidepressants have been shown to be very effective in treating poststroke depression. Lipsey et al.[52] demonstrated that the use of nortriptyline is effective in treating depression and is well tolerated by patients over extended periods of time. It is recommended to avoid the sedative, anticholinergic or orthostatic side effects, that the patients are started on low doses of the tricyclic antidepressants once at night and slowly increased over a 2- to 3-week period of time. Beneficial effects generally take 2 to 3 weeks before becoming evident. It is always prudent, given the quinidinelike effects of nortriptyline, to obtain an ECG on patients prior to beginning the drug. Also care must be taken in patients with narrow angle glaucoma or urinary outlet obstruction before starting these drugs, which have anticholinergic effects. It is commonly believed that the deleterious effects of poststroke depression greatly outweighs mild anticholinergic side effects of these drugs.

Treatment for other psychiatric disturbances such as agitation, particularly "sundowning" at night may be treated with the major tranquilizers, such as haloperidol or thioridazine, though drug therapy for confusional states must be individualized and may actually exacerbate the symptoms.

## NEUROLOGIC DISORDERS

Major complications resulting from strokes, particularly ischemic strokes and intracerebral hemorrhage, include seizures, increased intracranial pressure, and significant cognitive impairment. Seizures, which occur most commonly with embolic strokes and intracerebral hemorrhage, must be controlled with anticonvulsants, rarely requiring pentobarbital coma.[14,45,53,67,84,87] Increased intracranial pressure, which can only be accurately determined with dural or intraventricular monitoring, should be controlled with hyperventilation and osmotic diuresis to avert potentially lethal herniation syndromes (see Fig. 42-2).[3,8,27,28,31,44,74–78,80–82] Cognitive deficits resulting from strokes can cause significant functional impairment due to sensory or interpersonal disabilities which will complicate recovery, adjustment and coping abilities of stroke victims. Importantly, cognitive deficits can render patients functionally demented by virtue of the critical area of brain affected.[85]

The occurrence of seizures in association with strokes is well-recognized.[6,20,34,36,40,46,51,64,83] In a review of 1,000 consecutive patients with strokes and TIAs, Kilpatrick et al.[46] assessed whether seizure occurrence correlated with stroke type, pathogenesis or outcome. They found that seizures occurred in 44 patients (4.4 percent), 10 of 65 (15 percent) due to lobar or extensive hemorrhage, 6 of 71 (9 percent) due to subarachnoid hemorrhage, 24 of 370 (1 percent) due to cortical infarction and 4 of 109 (4 percent) with transient ischemic attacks. Arteriovenous malformations were a frequent cause of hemorrhage associated with early seizures. Lacunar infarcts and deep hemorrhages were not associated with seizures. When seizures occurred, they took place within the first 24 hours after the stroke and tended to be partial seizures and were readily controlled with anticonvulsant medication. Interestingly, the occurrence of seizures was not associated with a higher mortality or worsened functional outcome. The favorable prognosis of late onset seizures due to strokes is further substantiated in a study by Fish et al.,[26] in which 29 such patients were followed for a period of nearly 5 years and excellent control with anticonvulsants was the rule.

Patients with strokes may display unique EEG findings, such as epileptiform discharges occurring either periodically as periodic lateralized epileptiform discharges (PLEDs) or as bilateral independent periodic transients (BIPLEDs) complicated by anoxia and/or infection. Also, nonperiodic spikes occur singly or bursts, sharp waves or sharp-and-slow waves contralateral to the acute stroke.[92]

The majority of early mortality in the first week following stroke can be attributed to the direct effect of the ischemic or hemorrhagic event,[84] with transtentorial herniation accounting for the greatest number of deaths within that time frame. During weeks 2 through 4, pulmonary emboli, a preventable disorder,[93] predominates as the principal factor in morbidity and mortality. Bronchopneumonia supervenes in the 2nd and 3rd months following stroke, while beyond 3 months the major cause of death is due to myocardial infarction.[29,56,90,93] It is well accepted that medical and or surgical intervention can significantly change the course and occurrence of each of these processes and makes the recognition of each critical.

## REFERENCES

1. Andrews K, Brocklehurst JC, Richards B, et al: The recovery of the severely disabled stroke patient. Rheumatol Rehabil 21:225, 1982
2. Barnett HJM: Heart in ischemic stroke—a changing emphasis. Neurol Clin 1:291, 1983
3. Beks JWF: Increased intracranial pressure. Clin Neurol Neurosurg 79:245, 1976
4. Bell RD et al: A novel treatment for ischemic intracranial hypertension in cats. Stroke 22:80, 1991
5. Benson DF: Psychiatric aspects of aphasia. Br J Psychiatry 123:555, 1973
6. Berger AR, Lipton RB, Lesser ML et al: Early seizures following intracerebral hemorrhage: implications for therapy. Neurology (NY) 38:1363, 1988
7. Bleck TP, Klawans HL: Neurologic emergencies. Med Clin North Am 70:1167, 1986
8. Boucher CA, Brewster DC, Darling RC et al: Determination of cardiac risk by dipyridamole-thallium imaging before peripheral vascular surgery. N Engl J Med 312:389, 1985
9. Breuer AC, Furlan AJ, Hanson MR et al: Central nervous system complications of coronary artery bypass graft surgery: prospective analysis of 421 patients. Stroke 14:682, 1983
10. Brott T, Reed RL: Intensive care for acute stroke in the community hospital setting: the first 24 hours. Stroke 20:694, 1989
11. Burch GE, Meyers R, Abildskov JA: A new electrocardiographic pattern observed in cerebrovascular accidents. Circulation 9:719, 1954
12. Byer E, Ashman R, Toth LA: Electrocardiogram with large, upright T-waves and long Q-T intervals. Am Heart J 33:796, 1947
13. Canadian Cooperative Study Group: A randomized trial of aspirin and sulfinpyrazone in threatened stroke. N Engl J Med 299:53, 1978
14. Cocita L, Favale E, Reni L: Epileptic seizures in cerebral arterial occlusive disease. Stroke 13:189, 1982
15. Cunha BA et al: Pneumonia syndromes: a clinical approach in the elderly. Geriatrics 45:49, 55, 1990
16. Dean JM, Rogers MC: Cerebral vascular diseases. Crit Care Clin 1:327, 1985
17. Dimant J, Grob D: Electrocardiographic changes and myocardial damage in patients with acute cerebrovascular accidents. Stroke 8:448, 1977
18. Dinsdale HB: Hypertensive encephalopathy. Neurol Clin 1:3, 1983
19. DiPasquale G et al: Cerebral ischemia and asymptomatic coronary heart disease: A prospective study of 83 patients. Stroke 17:1098, 1986.
20. Dodge PR, Richardson EP, Jr, Victor M: Recurrent convulsive seizures as a sequel to cerebral infarction: a clinical and pathological study. Brain 77:610, 1954
21. Drislane FW, Samuels MA: How cardiorespiratory problems are caused by neurologic disease. J Respir Dis 9:31, 1988
22. Eisenberg S, Madison L, Sensenbach W: Cerebral hemodynamic and metabolic studies in patients with congestive failure. Circulation 21:704, 1960
23. Escobedo F, Canetti V: Significance of the stroke intensive care unit. Adv Neurol 25:367, 1960
24. Feibel JH, Berk S, Joynt RJ: The unmet needs of stroke survivors. Neurology (NY) 29:592, 1979
25. Feigenson JS, McCarthy ML, Greenberg SD, Feigenson WD: Factors influencing outcome and length of stay in a stroke rehabilitation unit. Stroke 8:657, 1977
26. Fish DR, Miller DH, Roberts RC et al: The natural history of late-onset epilepsy secondary to vascular disease. Acta Neurol Scand 80:524, 1989
27. Fishman RA: Brain edema. N Engl J Med 293:706, 1975
28. Frank MS et al: Glycerol: a review of its pharmacology, pharmacokinetics, adverse reactions and clinical use. Pharmacotherapy 1:147, 1981
29. Goldner JC, Whisnant JP, Taylor WF: Long-term prognosis of transient cerebral ischemic attacks. Stroke 2:160, 1971
30. Goldstein D: The electrocardiogram in stroke with relationship to pathophysiological type and comparison with prior tracings. Stroke 10:253, 1979
31. Grady PA, Blaumanis OR: Cerebral venous blood gas tensions in elevated inracranial pressure. Stroke 17:946, 1986
32. Graham DI: Ischemic brain damage following emergency blood pressure lowering in hypertensive patients. Acta Med Scand, suppl. 678:61, 1982
33. Greenhoot JH, Reichenbach DD: Cardiac injury and subarachnoid hemorrhage: A clinical pathological and physiological correlation. J Neurosurg 30:521, 1969
34. Gupta SR, Naheedy MH, Elias D, Rubino FA: Postinfarction seizures: a clinical study. Stroke 19:1477, 1988
35. Hankey GJ et al: Complications of cerebral angiography for patients with mild carotid territory ischaemia being considered for carotid endarterectomy. J Neurol Neurosurg Psychiatry 53:542, 1990
36. Hauser WA, Ramirez-Lassepas M, Rosenstein R: Risk for seizures and epilepsy following cerebrovascular insults. Epilepsia 25:666, 1984

37. Hayashi M et al: Treatment of systemic hypertension and intracranial hypertension in cases of brain hemorrhage. Stroke 19:314, 1988
38. Hershey LA et al: Validation of cognitive and functional assessment instruments in vascular dementia. Int J Psychiatry Med 17:183, 1987
39. Hertzer NR, Young JR, Beven EG et al: Coronary angiography in 506 patients with extracranial cerebrovascular disease. Arch Intern Med 145:849, 1985
40. Horning CR et al: Epileptic seizures following ischemic cerebral infarction: Clinical picture, CT findings and prognosis. Eur Arch Psychiatr Neurol Sci 239:379, 1990
41. Ichord RN et al: Age-related differences in recovery of blood flow and metabolism after cerebral ischemia in swine. Stroke 22:626, 1991
42. Kannel WB, Wolf PA: Manifestations of coronary disease predisposing to stroke: the Framingham Study. JAMA 250:2942, 1983
43. Kendall AR, Karafin L: Classification of neurogenic bladder disease. Urol Clin North Am 1:37, 1974
44. Kennealy JA, McLennan JE, Loudon RG, McLaurin RL: Hyperventilation-induced cerebral hypoxia. Am Rev Respir Dis 122:407, 1980
45. Kieburtz K et al: Seizures following carotid endarterectomy. Arch Neurol 47:568, 1990
46. Kilpatrick CJ, Davis SM, Tress BM et al: Epileptic seizures in acute stroke. Arch Neurol 47:157, 1990
47. Knapp ME: Problems of rehabilitation of the hemiplegic patient. JAMA 169:224 1959
48. Kolin A, Norris JW: Myocardial damage from acute cerebral lesions. Stroke 15:990, 1984
49. Lacy PS, Earle AM: Central neural control of blood pressure and cardiac arrhythmias during subarachnoid hemorrhage in rats. Stroke 16:998, 1985
50. Lavy S, Yaar I, Melamed E, Stern S: The effect of acute stroke on cardiac functions as observed in an intensive care unit. Stroke 5:775, 1974
51. Lesser RP, Luders H, Dinner DS, Morris HH: Epileptic seizures due to thrombotic and embolic cerebrovascular disease in older patients. Epilepsia 26:622, 1985
52. Lipsey JR, Robinson RG, Pearlson GD et al: Nortriptyline treatment of post-stroke depression: a double-blind treatment trial. Lancet 297, 1984
53. Luhdorf K et al: Etiology of seizures in the elderly. Epilepsia 27:458, 1986
54. McMahon SM, Heyman A: The mechanics of breathing and stabilization of ventilation in patients with unilateral cerebral infarction. Stroke 5:518, 1974
55. Mikel HS, Yashes NV, Kempski O et al: Breathing 100% oxygen after global brain ischemia in Mongolian gerbils results in increased lipid peroxidation and increased mortality. Stroke 18:426, 1987
56. Muvronen A, Kaste M: Outcome of 314 patients with transient ischemic attacks. Stroke 13:24, 1982
57. Myers MG, Norris JW, Hachinski VC et al: Plasma norepinephrine in stroke. Stroke 12:200, 1981
58. Myers MG, Norris JW, Hachinski VC et al: Cardiac sequelae of acute stroke. Stroke 13:838, 1982
59. Norris JW: Effects of cerebrovascular lesions on the heart. Neurol Clin 1:87, 1983
60. Norris JW, Froggart GM, Hachinski VC: Cardiac arrhythmias in acute stroke. Stroke 9:394, 1978
61. Norris JW, Hachinski V: Acute stroke units: a reappraisal. Curr Concepts Cerebrovasc Dis 20:31, 1985
62. Norris JW, Hachinski VC, Myers MG et al: Serum cardiac enzymes in stroke. Stroke 10:548, 1979
63. Novak TA, Satterfield WT, Lyons K et al: Stroke onset and rehabilitation: time lag as a factor in treatment outcome. Arch Phys Med Rehabil 65:316, 1984
64. Olsen TS, Hogenhaven H, Thage O: Epilepsy after stroke. Neurology (NY) 37:1209, 1987
65. Pulsinelli WA, Levy DE, Sigsbee B et al: Increased damage after ischemic stroke in patients with hyperglycemia with or without established diabetes mellitus. Am J Med 74:540, 1983
66. Rem JA, Hachinski VC, Boughner DR, Barnett HJM: Value of cardiac monitoring and echocardiography in TIA and stroke patients. Stroke 16:950, 1985
67. Richardson EP, Jr, Dodge PR: Epilepsy in cerebral vascular disease. Epilepsia 3:49, 1959
68. Robin ED, Whaley RD, Crump CH, Travis DM: Alveolar gas tensions, pulmonary ventilation and blood pH during physiologic sleep in normal subjects. J Clin Invest 37:981, 1958
69. Robinson RG, Kobos KL, Starr LB et al: Mood disorders in stroke patients: importance of lesions location. Brain 107:81, 1984
70. Robinson RG, Morris PL, Federoff JP: Depression and cerebrovascular disease. (Discussion, p. 32.) J Clin Psychiatry, suppl. 51:26, 1990
71. Robinson RG, Price TR: Post-stroke depressive disorders: a follow-up of 103 outpatients. Stroke 13:635, 1982
72. Robinson RG, Starr LB, Kubos KL et al: A two year longitudinal study of post-stroke mood disorders: findings during the initial evaluation. Stroke 14:736, 1983
73. Robinson RG, Starr LB, Price TR: A two-year longitudinal study of mood disorders following stroke: prevention and duration at six months follow-up. Br J Psychiatry 144:256, 1984
74. Rockoff MA, Kennedy SK: Physiology and clinical aspects of raised intracranial pressure. p. 7. In Ropper AH, Kennedy S, Zervas NT (eds): Neurological and Neurosurgical Intensive Care. University Park Press, Baltimore, 1983
75. Ropper AH: Brain edema after stroke. Arch Neurol 41:26, 1984
76. Ropper AH: In favor of intracranial pressure monitoring and aggressive therapy in neurologic practice. Arch Neurol 42:1194, 1985
77. Ropper AH: Lateral displacement of the brain and level of consciousness in patients with an acute hemispheral mass. N Engl J Med 314:953, 1986
78. Ropper AH, O'Rourke D, Kennedy SK: Head position, intracranial pressure and compliance. Neurology (NY) 32:1288, 1982

79. Samuel MA: Neurogenic heart disease: a unifying hypothesis. Am J Cardiol 60:15J, 1987
80. Schrader H, Hall C, Zwetnow NN: Effects of prolonged supratentorial mass expansion on regional blood flow and cardiovascular parameters during the Cushing response. Acta Neurol Scand 72:283, 1985
81. Shaw GM, Alvord EC, Jr, Berry RG: Swelling of the brain following ischemic infarction with arterial occlusion. Arch Neurol 1:161, 1959
82. Shigemori M et al: Evaluation of brain dysfunction in hypertensive putaminal hemorrhage with multimodality evoked potentials. Stroke 18:72, 1987
83. Shinton RA, Gill JS, Melnick SC et al: The frequency, characteristics and prognosis of epileptic seizures at the onset of stroke. J Neurol Neurosurg Psychiatry 51:273, 1988
84. Silver FL, Norris JW, Lewis AJ, Hachinski VC: Early mortality following stroke: a prospective study. Stroke 15:492, 1984
85. Starkstein SE, Robinson RG: Affective disorders and cerebal vascular disease. Br J Psychiatry 154:170, 1989
86. Strangaard S, Olesen J, Skinhoj E et al: Autoregulation of brain circulation in severe arterial hypertension. Br Med J 1:507 1973
87. Sundaram MB: Etiology and patterns of seizures in the elderly. Neuroepidemiology 8:234, 1989
88. Theodore J, Robin ED: Pathogenesis of neurogenic pulmonary oedema. Lancet 2:749, 1975
89. Timaris PS: Aging of respiration. p. 303. In Timaris PS (ed): Physiological Basis of Geriatrics. Macmillan, New York, 1988
90. Toole JR, Yuson CP, Janeway R et al: Transient ischemic attacks: a prospective study of 225 patients. Neurology (NY) 28:746, 1978
91. Touho H et al: Neurogenic pulmonary edema in the acute stage of hemorrhagic cerebrovascular disease. Neurosurgery 25:762, 1989
92. Verma NP, Kooi KA: Contralateral epileptiform transients in stroke (CETS). Epilepsia 27:437, 1986
93. Viitanen M et al: Autopsy-verified causes of death after stroke. Acta Med Sand 222:401, 1987
94. Wallace JD, Levy LL: Blood pressure after stroke. JAMA 246:2177, 1981
95. Wechsler LR, Ropper AH: Management of stroke in the intensive care unit. Semin Neurol 6:324, 1986
96. Williams GO: Management of depression in the elderly. Primary Care 16:451, 1989
97. Wolf PA, Kannel WB, McGee DL et al: Duration of atrial fibrillation and imminence of stroke: the Framingham Study. Stroke 14:664, 1983
98. Yatsu FM, Becker C, McLeroy KR et al: Community hospital-based stroke programs: North Carolina, Oregon, and New York. I. Goals, Objectives, and Data Collection Procedures. Stroke 17:276, 1986
99. Yatsu FM, Zivin J: Hypertension in acute ischemic stroke: not to treat. Arch Neurol 42:999, 1985

# 43
# SURGERY FOR SYMPTOMATIC DISEASE DUE TO ARTERIOSCLEROSIS OF THE CAROTID ARTERY

James T. Robertson
Henry J.M. Barnett

## CAROTID ENDARTERECTOMY

The efficacy and appropriateness of carotid endarterectomy has sustained severe criticism by neurologists and physicians.[2,5,12,13,34,48,51,52] In 1984, carotid endarterectomy was the most commonly performed arterial vascular procedure. Approximately 107,000 cases were done in 1985, but severe criticism reduced the number of cases to approximately 70,000 in 1989.[12] Whisnant et al. estimated that approximately 35,000 new patients each year with carotid transient ischemia attack or recovered stroke with stenosis would be candidates for carotid endarterectomy.[49] If this estimate was correct, the number of carotid endarterectomies each year far exceeded the indications for the procedure in symptomatic patients. Approximately half the carotid endarterectomies were performed on asymptomatic patients.[5,21,25] In addition to projected excess number of procedures, the critics afforded evidence that the surgical risk was too high to justify the procedure and that antiplatelet therapy probably had an outcome better than surgical treatment.[2,7,13,19,23,36,46,48] The statement from the American College of Physicians, concerning the indications for carotid endarterectomy, concluded that surgical mortality rates of less than 1 percent and stroke-related morbidity of less than 3 percent for patients with transient ischemic attacks and stroke mortality plus stroke-related morbidity of less than 2 percent for patients with asymptomatic carotid artery disease were the values that must be matched to compete with available medical therapy.[36]

The numerous articles criticizing carotid endarterectomy have provoked a nihilistic attitude toward the surgical management of stroke prevention.[2,5,13,43] This is ironic, particularly since, simultaneously, the National Institutes of Health have funded two large, multicenter, controlled clinical trials to determine the optimal medical versus surgical management of patients with transient ischemic attacks and small strokes with carotid stenosis or ulceration and patients with asymptomatic carotid stenosis of 60 percent or more.[33,45] As a result, recruitment in these trials have been impaired. A recent consensus of a selected committee of neurologists, neurosurgeons, and vascular surgeons, recognizing the confusion and nihilistic attitude concerning indications for carotid endarterectomy recommended that the clinical trials be supported, but, in the interim, sustained the performance of carotid endarterectomy with low morbidity and mortality in selected patients with appropriate symptoms and a hemodynamic carotid lesion.[6] The limits were categorized by clinical presentation. The combined morbidity and mortality of the procedure should not exceed 3 percent for asymptomatic lesions, 5 percent for transient ischemic episodes, 7 percent for ischemic stroke, and 10 percent for recurrent carotid stenosis. In addition, the 30-day mortality rate from all causes related to endarterectomy should not exceed 2 percent. Concomitantly, ongoing quality audits should be performed in institutions where endarterectomy is being performed to ensure surgical adherence to these current suggested figures. The Committee exhorted that, until the results of the clinical trials are available, carotid endarterectomy should continue to be an established operative procedure for the care of patients with carotid atherosclerotic disease.

An exciting scientific landmark was announced on February 21, 1991 at the International Stroke Conference of the American Heart Association in San Francisco by Dr. H.J.M. Barnett, the Principal Investigator of the North American Symptomatic Carotid Endarterectomy Trial.[8,39] The interim analysis of approximately 600 patients who had been randomized either to medical or surgical therapy for transient ischemic attack or mild nondisabling stroke ipsilateral to a 70 to 90 percent narrowing of the internal carotid artery were unequivocally shown to be treated best by surgical therapy[32,39] (Fig. 43-1). The interim analysis showed that among these symptomatic patients with high-grade carotid stenosis (70 to 99 percent), carotid endarterectomy did indeed reduce the overall risk of fatal and nonfatal ipsilateral carotid stroke, despite any perioperative risk of any stroke or death from any cause. Including perioperative morbidity and mortality or its 32-day equivalent time in the medical group, over 26 percent of the medical group, but only 9 percent of the surgical patients, had experienced fatal or nonfatal ipsilateral at 24 months. This represents an absolute risk reduction of stroke in favor of surgery of 17 percent and a relative risk reduction of 65 percent. An exciting finding was that carotid endarterectomy was beneficial in the prevention of any stroke of any severity in any territory. Of great and supporting interest was the announcement of the European Study headed by Charles Warlow announcing a clear benefit for carotid endarterectomy in the same group of patients.[16] The answer is not available on the patients with stenoses from 30 to 69 percent who present with ipsilateral transient ischemic attacks or mild nondisabling stroke. Further accrual and follow-up will be necessary to answer how these patients are best treated. However, the interim secondary analysis did show that the degree of stenosis correlated extremely well with the risk reduction after surgery in symptomatic patients. This interim analysis points out the major scientific advantage of a prospective randomized clinical study in yielding a definitive uncontestable result. This was accomplished in slightly more than 600 properly medical versus surgical randomized patients.

The second study, the Asymptomatic Carotid Artery Study, is directed by Dr. James F. Toole, Principal Investigator, and now employs 34 centers contributing patients.[45] All of these patients have at least 60 percent blockage of the carotid artery by atherosclerosis, but are asymptomatic regarding the ipsilateral artery at the time of randomization. Since many centers operate on high-grade asymptomatic carotid artery stenosis patients, it is hoped that this study will enjoy more rapid recruitment and completion of its target of 1,500 patients randomized equally to medical and surgical therapy. Presently the study has enrolled 1,100 patients.

It has been estimated that the combined morbidity and mortality resulting from endarterectomy in all non-veterans hospitals in the United States could be 10 percent per year.[2] A recent review of cases performed at large or academic institutions revealed a 2.2 percent stroke rate and a mortality rate of 1.4 percent for a combined morbidity and mortality of 3.6 percent.[25] Surgery for asymptomatic carotid endarterectomy is safer carrying a combined morbidity and mortality of 2 percent or less.[45] There is little doubt that patient selection for endarterectomy plays an important role in surgical results. In this context, Sundt's grading of preoperative risk according to neurologic, medical, and angiographic status serves as an excellent example of the importance of patient selection.[25,42] Clearly, the clinical presentation, the patient's comorbidity and native stroke risk, and the angiographic findings are critical in patient selection and resulting morbidity and mortality. In Sundt's experience, the neurologically stable patients without other risk in grade 1 had a combined morbidity and mortality of less than 1 percent, whereas, without associated medical or angiographically determined risk, these patients had a combined morbidity and mortality of 8.5 percent.

The clinical settings where carotid endarterectomy is indicated are patients with at least a 50 percent carotid stenosis or a large ulcerated plaque with ipsilateral transient ischemic attacks, a reversible ischemic neurological deficit, or small stroke or selected cases of recurrent symptomatic carotid stenosis.[6,20,25,

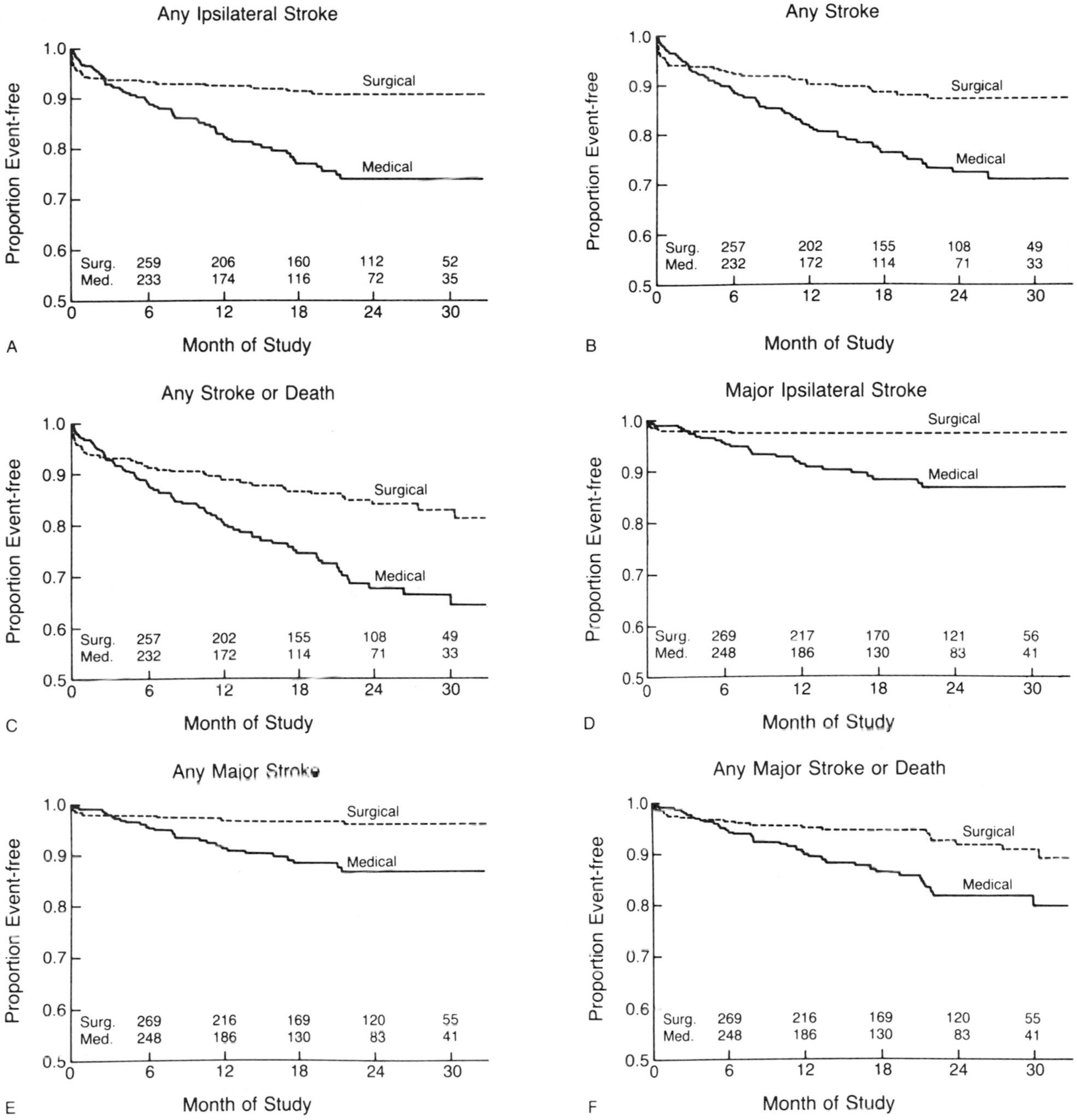


**Fig. 43-1. (A–F)** Survival curves for the treatment groups. These Kaplan-Meier survival curves show the probability of surviving six events indicating treatment failure after randomization. The number of patients who remained event-free in each treatment group is shown at 6-month intervals at the bottom of each graph; the numbers at time zero are 328 in the surgical group and 331 in the medical group. The curves of the groups differed significantly (by Mantel-Haenszel chi-square test, $P < 0.001$ for all events except "any major stroke or death," for which $P < 0.01$). (From NASCET,[32] with permission.)

[30,31,34,35,37,40] Individualized patients may require surgery for progressing stroke, progressive retina ischemia, acute carotid occlusion, symptomatic carotid stump syndrome, global cerebral ischemia due to multiple large-vessel occlusive disease, selected tandem lesions where the proximal stenosis is greater than the distal and in certain cases of symptomatic carotid dissection, and true or false aneurysm. The procedure is not indicated in patients presenting with vertebral basilar distribution transient ischemic attacks, multi-infarct dementia, patients with severe neurologic deficits, evidence of intracranial hemorrhage or large infarcts. Medical contraindications include the presence of congestive heart failure, a recent myocardial infarction, active angina, dementia, advanced malignancy, and uncertain diagnosis.[34,35,40]

## Preoperative Management and Evaluation

The physician must take whatever measures are necessary to ensure the carotid lesion is the cause of the patient's symptoms. The best surgical results are those patients operated on for true transient ischemic attacks or amaurosis fugax. Because evidence from postmortem and stroke registries report that 15 to 25 percent of ischemic events can be attributed to a cardiac embolic or dysrhythmic source, cardiac evaluation is essential.[2] Patients with active angina pectoris, a myocardial infarction, or congestive failure should be treated medically if at all possible. Since postoperative myocardial infarction is a leading cause of death after carotid endarterectomy, the patients must have adequate oxygenation and intravascular volume expansion before surgery. The immediate preoperative use of aspirin for platelet inhibition is recommended, even though rarely it will be necessary to administer platelet transfusion because of bleeding aggravated by aspirin therapy at surgery.[40] If the patient is having active transient ischemic attacks despite aspirin therapy, intravenous, continuous heparin therapy keeping the partial thromboplastin time at one and a half times control is recommended.[35] Platelet counts should be performed every third day, and if a thrombopenia occurs, heparin must be stopped to avoid a hypercoagulable syndrome. With short-term (less than 3 days) heparin therapy, the hypercoagulable syndrome is rare. Contraindications for heparin therapy must be followed. If the patient is severely hypertensive, every effort at control of the hypertension prior to surgery or heparin is mandated because of the increased risk of operating on patients with uncontrolled blood pressures in excess of 180/110 mmHg. Severe chronic obstructive pulmonary disease may be a contraindication to surgery. Preoperative management of pulmonary toilet in an effort to improve function is recommended. Uncontrolled diabetes mellitus must be regulated. Attention should be given to indications of renal insufficiency. If the patient is anemic and surgery felt to be urgent, then after appropriate studies to determine the cause, the anemia should be corrected prior to induction of general anesthesia. Careful attention to patient medication is indicated to be certain that appropriate drugs are not discontinued inadvertently.

## Prevention of Operative Complications

### *Preparation*

When the brain is presented with an ischemic insult, the cerebrovascular reactivity or cerebral autoregulation is impaired or lost. Thus the perfusion pressure of the brain depends on the systemic mean arterial pressure and, simultaneously, because of the loss of autoregulation, the brain is extremely vulnerable to sudden changes in systemic arterial pressure. The anesthesiologist must be aware of this liability in patients presenting for operation with ischemia and choose either Ethrane or Forane for general anesthesia or regional local anesthesia.[9,22,40] The operating table should be horizontal without head elevation and the head turned partially to the opposite side with modest elevation of the ipsilateral shoulder. Gentle prepping of the operative site avoids the possibility of dislodging emboli from a fragile carotid plaque.

A reverse S-shaped incision is preferred, in order to minimize postoperative wound contracture with discomfort and to afford wide exposure. The incision characteristically begins at the level of the mastoid and extends anteriorly along the anterior-medial border of the sternocleidomastoid muscle to about one to two finger-breadths above the sternal notch in the midline. Sharp dissection is essential. The use of a Shaw cutting cautery knife blade is preferred by many. After sectioning the platysma muscle vertically, the plane of dissection is anteromedial to the sternocleidomastoid muscle beginning inferiorly and proceeding superiorly. In the upper midportion of the incision, the transverse cervical nerve, which is responsible for the skin innervation medial to the incision and along the lower jaw, is divided. The external jugular vein is lateral to this incision and is preserved. The approach to the carotid sheath begins inferiorly along the anterior medial border of the sternocleidomastoid muscle and proceeds superiorly.

The carotid sheath is a fascial sheath formed by extensions of the deep cervical fascia and prevertebral fascia. The sheath contains the carotid artery, the jugular vein, and the vagus nerve. Inferiorly, along the common carotid artery, the carotid sheath is very well defined, and the thickened sheath overlying the common carotid is best opened vertically; this excision is extended superiorly up to the carotid bifurcation. The sheath is less well defined superiorly because of vascular branches. The sheath is preserved and tacked up with small sutures attached to the platysma. This allows subsequent closure of the sheath and also tends to elevate the carotid artery. The common carotid artery should be exposed inferiorly, if possible, to the point of a normal arterial wall. This may involve sectioning the omohyoid muscle. At the point where dissection of the common carotid artery begins, the patient is given intravenous heparin in a dose of 5,000 to 7,000 units. After 2 to 3 minutes, the patient is considered heparinized and the vascular surgical procedure can proceed.

### *Prevention of Embolization*

The major danger through this portion of the operation is embolization produced by excessive manipulation of the carotid bifurcation.[35,40] The surgeon must be intensely aware of the fragile nature of an atherosclerotic plaque, particularly with ulceration and/or intraluminal clot. Intraoperative embolization is a major cause of minor or major stroke as a result of the operation. Meticulously, the common carotid, and external and internal carotid arteries are exposed. The external jugular vein may require ligation superiorly as the posterior-superior lobe of the parotid gland is exposed. The common facial vein enters the jugular vein usually at the level of the bifurcation of the common carotid artery and routinely requires ligation and division. There may be numerous other branches that must be ligated and divided in order to adequately expose the targeted artery.

The available evidence strongly supports monitoring with electroencephalography to determine intraoperative episodes of ischemia produced by embolic or shunt occlusion and the necessity of a shunt.[34,38,40] During operation, if a major unexpected change occurs in the electroencephalogram (EEG), an embolus to the main trunk of the middle cerebral artery must be suspected. If this is a minor embolic episode, the change will frequently reverse, but if major, it may persist, and if it does, the routine recommended by Sundt includes ensuring heparinization is present by augmenting the original heparin dose if necessary and immediately giving intravenously 3 mg/kg thiopental or more, if necessary, to reach burst suppression of the electroencephalogram.[40] Subsequently, the endarterectomy should be completed as quickly as possible, and if the EEG change disappears or is minor, subsequently, the patient is allowed to awaken from anesthesia. If not, on-the-table arteriography is recommended, and if an embolus is found in the middle cerebral artery, either a middle cerebral embolectomy or extracranial, intracranial bypass surgery should be done.

Another option that has received clinical use, but a paucity of clinical published results, is the application of intravenous thromboplastin activator or another more common fibrinolytic drug such as streptokinase or urokinase. Spetzler[37] has reported the use of thromboplastin activator to reopen an internal carotid artery occluded at the carotid bifurcation intracranially with subsequent restoration of cerebral flow. This will require repeat arteriography. If these intra-arterial agents are used to dissolve the embolic clot the surgeon must be prepared to ensure hemostasis and prevent postoperative arterial bleeding.

If electroencephalographic monitoring is not performed, some surgeons routinely introduce an intra-arterial shunt.[35,41] The shunt may be employed as a straight common carotid to internal carotid shunt or else an externally looped shunt. Embolus as a result of shunt usage may be produced by intimal injury to the proximal common or distal internal carotid arteries or even dissection of the intima. The shunt may undergo occlusion during the procedure or emboli may be introduced into the shunt at the time of placement. Sundt emphasizes the unusual but recommended placement of the shunt first into the common carotid artery, making certain that any embolic material has been irrigated from the common carotid artery and the shunt allowed to bleed slightly and then placed into the internal carotid artery.[40] Most surgeons place the shunt into the internal carotid artery first and subsequently into the common carotid artery. The shunt should be presoaked in saline treated with heparin in a dose of 50 U/cc. In addition to preventing clotting, the wetting of the shunt prevents air bubbles from forming in the shunt at the time of placement.

At the time of the exposure of the common carotid artery, two Rummel tourniquets are placed around the proximal common carotid artery; on exposure of the external carotid artery, a Rummel tourniquet is placed around the proximal external carotid artery; a vascular loop is placed around the distal internal carotid artery; and the superior thyroid artery is usually occluded by looping an 0-silk suture around it and applying modest tension with a hemostat. This minor tension on the superior thyroid and external carotid arteries tends to displace the bifurcation inferiorly and elevate the carotid artery from the wound.

The internal carotid artery may be occluded with a Scoville aneurysm clip or with an 0-silk suture looped around the artery with a 4-0 suture through the loop to allow the loop to be loosened. Some surgeons use a small elastic vascular loop around the vessel, which is tightened by placing a vascular clip to complete the loop. This is frequently done at the time a shunt is inserted and helps secure the shunt distally.

Whether or not a proximal vascular clamp or the two Rummel tourniquets are used on the common carotid artery, every effort should be made to get proximal to the carotid plaque and apply these constricting devices on normal artery. The techniques used to occlude the distal internal carotid and external carotid arteries also emphasize the need to get distal to the atherosclerotic plaque and to minimize damage to the intima. Sundt is a strong advocate of the use of the soft-shoe Fogarty occlusive vascular clamp on the common carotid artery.[40] All of these efforts are designed not only to prevent damage of normal intima but to prevent fracturing of an atherosclerotic plaque with subsequent stenosis or subintimal dissection, or a site for thrombus formation with distal embolization postoperatively.

### *Endarterectomy Procedure*

The arteriotomy begins in the proximal common carotid artery and extends into the internal carotid artery. A #11 blade is used to open the common carotid artery at the site below the plaque, and then Potts scissors are used to incise the artery through the plaque into normal distal internal carotid artery. Obviously, the occluding clamps and/or loops are tightened prior to the arteriotomy. Some surgeons insist on removing the plaque from the internal carotid artery distally as the initial step. Others will immediately place a shunt in the internal and, subsequently, the common carotid artery or vice versa as described. Then the plaque is carefully dissected from the arterial wall using a blunt dissector, for example, a Penfield-4. When normal intima is reached in the common carotid artery, the intima is sharply dissected so as to allow no loose flap. The plaque is peeled from below upward to the external carotid artery where it is carefully dissected from the external carotid artery by intussusception. As this process proceeds up the external carotid artery, it is wise to release the occluding Rummel tourniquet temporarily to allow the plaque to be carefully removed and to ascertain the backflow from the external carotid artery. It is important to make certain the external carotid artery is left patent.[40] Subsequently, the plaque is peeled out of the internal carotid artery, and it usually will peel out quite smoothly distally. If the distal plaque is removed prior to insertion of a shunt, less distal artery need be exposed. On the other hand, if normal intima was exposed distal to the plaque prior to the insertion of the shunt, the plaque can quite easily be removed even with the shunt.

If the plaque peels out easily and leaves a distal smooth surface, no tacking sutures are necessary. If the distal intima remains quite thickened and infiltrated with plaque, it is necessary to remove this to the point of normal intima. The technique of nicking the more available thickened intima with the Potts scissors and peeling out the distal thickened intima circumferentially is recommended.[35] If there is any question about the distal intima being loose, it should be tacked down with 6-0 double-arm Prolene sutures proceeding from within the artery to the outer wall where the suture is tied. The suture should be placed vertically rather than horizontally to avoid constricting the lumen.

During the dissection of the plaque, the endarterectomy bed is frequently irrigated with heparin containing saline. This irrigation allows the identification of loose pieces of debris and plaque that must be meticulously removed from the endarterectomy site to prevent postoperative clotting. If a shunt has been used, it is helpful to place a 5- or 4-0 Prolene suture around the shunt to allow subsequent ease in removal of the shunt through the small remaining arteriotomy at the time of arterial closure. Other surgeons, to minimize migration of the shunt, will place 5- or 6-0, double-arm Prolene sutures around the shunt and through the arterial wall with a loose tie externally and remove this suture prior to shunt removal.

Once the vessel is meticulously cleaned, primary closure or closure with a fabric or vein patch ensues. The available evidence in the literature supports the use of a patch over primary closure.[21,25,26,40] There are clearly fewer postoperative carotid occlusions or ischemic events with the use of a patch. In addition, the incidence of restenosis is minimized, when compared to primary arterial closure.[10,15,25] Patching, whether fabric or vein is used, and meticulous placement of the suture to ensure a smooth patch are essential. A 6-0 Prolene suture is recommended as a running suture. Primary closure of the artery should also be effected using 6-0 Prolene suture. Just prior to closure, the shunt is removed, all vessels are allowed to flush, and subsequent primary closure is completed. Then the external carotid and common carotid arteries are opened and subsequently the internal artery is opened to minimize air or particulate embolization into the internal carotid artery system. If a fabric patch has been used and properly preclotted, bleeding is easily controlled by the application of Gelfoam and thrombin wrapped in a sheet of Surgicel to form a nice compressive pack. Additional arterial sutures may be needed if the initial suture technique did not ensure close and regular placement of the suture, allowing for site bleeding.

Meticulous attention to avoid damage to the running suture with placement of the additional sutures is necessary. Every effort must be made to avoid reversing the heparin for at least 20 minutes. Endarterectomy in animals with and without heparinization has shown after 10 minutes the use of heparin has usually protected the endarterectomy site, allowing a platelet coating without thrombus formation.[40] Longer use of heparin is probably more beneficial, and therefore every effort is made not to reverse the heparin. If bleeding is a problem after the first 10 to 20 minutes, the heparin may be reversed in stages. The half-life of operative heparin is approximately 60 minutes, and this should be taken into account at the time of heparin reversal with protamine hydrochloride. Generally, the heparin is reversed with 1 mg protamine for every 500 units of heparin.

The arterial wall is then palpated to determine the presence or absence of a thrill, which would indicate a loose intimal flap or some obstructive intraluminal mass. If a thrill is present, an arteriogram should be performed to determine the characteristics of the endarterectomy. If clot or debris if found inside the lumen, the vessel must be reoccluded and reopened, all debris removed, and closure reeffected.

If there is any question about the patency of the arterial system, an arteriogram should be performed. Operative ultrasound may be used, providing institutional expertise is available. Palpation of the superficial temporal artery should be reconfirmed; if that pulse is diminished or absent, the external carotid artery must be assumed to be partially or completely occluded. A clamp should be placed on the proximal external carotid artery, and distal occlusion of the internal carotid artery is achieved by the placement of Rummel tourniquets or vascular occluding clips or clamps; then the external carotid artery is opened, and almost invariably a dissected intima will be found, which should be removed and flow restored in the external carotid. At times, it is necessary to patch the external carotid artery to ensure an adequate lumen. This dissection of intima distal to the blind intussusception of the external carotid artery plaque is not unexpected. Patency of the external carotid artery is important to prevent an occluded stump as a source of embolic postoperatively and also to ensure adequate collateral circulation.

Prior to surgery, the surgeon should have determined whether or not the vessel had kinks or loops in it. After the endarterectomy, it is essential to remove any significant kinks or loops in the internal carotid artery system that are proximate or part of the operative field. These can be removed by resection and anastomosis with 6-0 Prolene suture and subsequent vein or fabric patching or plication of a short segment of the endarterectomized vessel.

### *Reconstruction of the Artery*

The overriding surgical principle must be reconstruction of the artery to ensure the optimal, unimpaired, well-directed arterial flow.[29] The overriding goal is to operate on the patient safely and not produce the stroke for which this prophylactic operation has been performed. Hertzer's comment, "few major operations are conceptually so simple, yet technically so unforgiving, as a carotid endarterectomy," must be remembered.[25] Rather than using confirmatory intraoperative arteriography, many surgeons are now using operative ultrasound to determine the patency and quality of the reconstructed artery. This noninvasive procedure deserves widespread consideration.

Subsequent to meticulous hemostasis, the wound is reconstructed, and, if feasible, the fascial sheath of the common carotid artery is resutured. Sundt uses a Teflon sheath around the distal common carotid artery and bifurcation after vein patching to prevent subsequent aneurysmal formation.[40] A Gore-Tex stint may be used around the internal carotid artery either to serve as an external support or to allow distal kinks to be lessened. Subsequent to absolute hemostasis the wound is closed.

### *Postoperative Hypertension*

From the point of restoration of flow, it is critical that the blood pressure be maintained at a level of approximately 150 mmHg systolic as a maximum. This may require the intravenous use of nitroprusside or nitroglycerin. The sudden restoration of high flow, particularly after the removal of a very tight stenosis and in the presence of heparin and/or aspirin, may produce intracerebral hemorrhage. The meticulous control of blood pressure is the major way of minimizing the hyperperfusion that often occurs following the removal of a high-grade stenosis. Sundt has shown flows to increase over 100 percent after a successful endarterectomy, particularly in patients presenting with a slow stroke syndrome, generalized cerebral ischemia, and multiple transient ischemic events.[40] Postoperative hypertension is a major treatable and preventable event. Smith has popularized the transcranial Doppler to monitor perioperatively for adequate collateral and hyperfusion.

The therapy of postoperative hypertension should begin at the point of restoration of flow and be maintained throughout the patient's hospital stay. Fortunately, the postoperative instability blood pressure usually disappears within 12 to 24 hours.

### *Postoperative Hypotension*

Postoperative hypotension may be as disastrous as postoperative hypertension. This instability of blood pressure in the postoperative state occurs in at least 50 percent of patients operated on under general anesthesia, but is quite unusual on patients operated on under regional anesthesia.[9,22] The instability of blood pressure is due to carotid sinus malfunction.[4] The carotid sinus is a major baroreceptor in normal individuals, and elevation in peripheral perfusion pressure results in stimulation of the receptor and the afferent of the receptor, the glossopharyngeal nerve, conducts the impulse to the medulla, which, through activation of the sympathetic or parasympathetic system, usually the latter produces a lowering of peripheral vascular tone and blood pressure and slowing of pulse rate. If the patient's peripheral blood pressure falls, the opposite occurs with activation of the sympathetic system. Patients with atherosclerosis of the carotid body often lose effective baroreceptor action.

Following endarterectomy, the carotid bulb can again distend, and the carotid sinus reflex can respond unduly actively, producing postoperative hypotension. On the other hand, as a result of the surgical procedure the reflex may be abolished, and postoperative hypotension occurs. The latter is more common than the former. Significant postoperative hypotension may produce cerebral ischemic complications and can best be treated by placing a patient in a Trendelenburg position, making certain that volume replacement is adequate because often these patients do not respond well to vasopressors.

In an effort to avoid postoperative hypotension many surgeons routinely section the innovation of the carotid sinus at surgery. Others consider restoration of carotid sinus activity as a bonus to aid in the subsequent management of previously hypertensive patients.

## Operative Damage to Nerves

The sensory branches of the cervical plexus, namely, the transverse cervical nerve and the greater auricular nerve and the cranial nerves, mandibular branch of the facial nerve, the vagus and its branches, the superior laryngeal and recurrent laryngeal nerves, the spinal accessory nerve, and the hypoglossal nerves may be damaged at the time of carotid endarterectomy.[17,27,29,40] In addition, damage to the cervical sympathetic chain may produce a complete Horner syndrome or in cases of high dissection of the internal carotid artery an incomplete Horner syndrome. The Cleveland Clinic report a complication rate for injury to the marginal mandibular nerve was 2 percent, the recurrent laryngeal nerve was 6 percent, the superior laryngeal nerve was 2 percent, and the hypoglossal nerve was 5 percent. Some degree of minor injury is probably more common. The sensory losses occurring with damage to the transverse cervical or greater auricular nerves, although annoying, do not produce the significant morbidity of the other cranial nerve injuries.

Meticulous surgical technique and knowledge of the anatomy with application of sharp dissection and routine use of the bipolar cautery will prevent all these complications, with the exception of the routine loss of the transverse cervical nerve in the carotid exposure preferred. Advocates of the transverse cervical incision argue that the transverse cervical nerve can be spared, so that the postoperative wound is more cosmetic, but the limits of exposure by this approach are a liability.

## Facial Nerve Injury

Total facial nerve paralysis is rare and only occurs when very high exposure of the carotid artery is required. In order to expose the internal carotid artery at C2 and above it is necessary to bring the incision anterior to the tragus of the ear and reflect the superficial lobe of the parotid superiorly and anteriorly and at times dislocate the jaw to allow access. In the process of this extensive dissection, traction on the main facial nerve trunk may produce a complete facial nerve paralysis. Otherwise the most common damage to the facial nerve is the mandibular branch, which usually occurs secondary to traction. Placing the major vertical traction on the posterior belly of the digastric or incising the deep fascia posteriorly along the sternocleidomastoid muscle will allow higher exposure and minimize traction on the mandibular and parotid aspects of the wound. Injury to the mandibular branch produces asymmetry of the mouth secondary to paralysis of the depressor of the lip. This is annoying to the patient in speech, and in eating the patient may bite the lower lip. Because it is usually a stretch injury and/or the facial nerve has numerous arborizations, the deficit usually clears within 3 months. In the rare annoying permanent cases of paralysis, plastic surgery may be required.

## Vagal Nerve Injury

Injury to the main trunk of the vagus nerve is rare.[16,27,40] The nerve usually runs posterior to the carotid artery between the carotid artery and the jugular vein and is covered by a separate fascial sheath. It may be injured in high exposure and by careless use of the cautery. Injury can be minimized by meticulous attention to anatomic detail and the use of the bipolar cautery. On occasion the vagus nerve may course anterior to the carotid artery on the right. In this circumstance the recurrent branch of the laryngeal nerve arises at the level of the carotid bifurcation and obviously either the vagus or the recurrent nerve may be easily sectioned. This complication must be avoided by being aware of its occurrence and not sectioning any nerve until its origin is determined. Thus the routine of always identifying the ansa hypoglossi and following the nerve proximally to its origin from the hypoglossal nerve prior to section. When an anterior vagus nerve is present, the nerve and its recurrent branch must be dissected and mobilized anteriorly and medially prior to the endarterectomy.

The recurrent branch of the laryngeal nerve is usually damaged by placing a self-retaining retractor deep to the level of trachea. The nerve arises at the root of the neck at about the level of C7–T1 and runs in front of the right subclavian artery. It runs below and behind the artery and then superiorly and medially behind the common carotid artery into the groove between the trachea and esophagus where it ascends to the lower border of the cricoid cartilage. It becomes the inferior laryngeal nerve and supplies intrinsic muscles of the larynx that control the vocal cord. Damage results in a unilateral vocal cord paralysis. This nerve is rarely if ever exposed during carotid endarterectomy and is usually damaged by traction.

The superior laryngeal nerve is a branch of the vagus nerve at the lower margin of the first cervical vertebra and runs posteriorly and medially to the internal and external carotid arteries. The nerve divides into an internal and external branch. The internal branch is responsible for the sensory supply of the epiglottis and the larynx above the vocal cords. The external branch is responsible for the motor supply to the cricothyroid muscle and the inferior pharyngeal constrictor. The nerve is covered by loose fascia posterior and medial to the carotid arteries and can best be seen just medial and deep to the carotid bifurcation. It is usually damaged by careless use of the cautery or direct posterior compression medial to the carotid bifurcation. Meticulous technique and the use of the bipolar cautery will minimize damage to this nerve. It also may be damaged by high exposure of the internal carotid artery at and above C1, so that in high dissection, the medial aspect of the vagus nerve must always be respected. Damage to the superior laryngeal nerve is very disabling because the patient not only has difficulty in swallowing but has loss of sensation in the right epiglottis and larynx, allowing food to migrate into the larynx, which produces aspiration and annoying coughing. This is particularly true at night.

## Spinal Accessory Nerve Injury

This motor nerve is rarely injured during carotid endarterectomy. In exiting the jugular foramen, the nerve lies superficial to the internal jugular vein and courses into the sternocleidomastoid muscle. The nerve is usually injured by misdirected exposure of the carotid artery into the posterior triangle of the neck or traction or cautery injury in superior exposures of the internal carotid artery. Damage results in complete paralysis of the sternocleidomastoid and trapezius muscles, which cause a dropped shoulder and discomfort in the neck and shoulder. If the nerve is sectioned and recognized, primary suture should be effected.

## Hypoglossal Nerve Injury

The hypoglossal nerve is totally responsible for the innervation of the tongue. Paralysis of the nerve produces slight impairment of speech and deviation of the tongue to the side of the paralysis with subsequent ipsilateral tongue atrophy. The descendens hypoglossi leave the nerve usually at its inferior curve and runs anterior and medial to the jugular vein and anterior to the carotid artery. Section of the descendens hypoglossi above the cervical branch, which forms the ansa cervicalis, produces no clinical syndrome. This branch, along with the cervical branch, is responsible for the motor supply of the deep strap muscles of the neck. As an external landmark the hypoglossal nerve usually runs at the level of the occipital artery. It is invariably crossed superiorly by the branch of the occipital artery to the sternocleidomastoid muscle. Occasionally, the nerve is crossed by an aberrant vein, and this vein may be closely adherent to the nerve. The nerve may be injured by direct traction or by the use of means other than bipolar cautery to remove a plexus of veins from around it, particularly superiorly. With an overlying vein, the nerve may be ligated and divided with the vein unless the nerve is meticulously and routinely exposed.

In order to avoid the use of the cautery or unnecessary traction or clamping, the branch to the sternocleidomastoid muscle must be routinely exposed, ligated, and divided. The nerve can then be displaced superiorly. If the hypoglossal nerve is sectioned, it should be sutured primarily. Otherwise, recovery of function can be anticipated within 3 months.

# Postoperative Complications

## Stroke or Transient Neurologic Deficit

If the patient awakens with a postoperative neurologic deficit, the surgeon is faced with the major catastrophe of the operation.[35,40] If the patient has a profound hemiplegia and aphasia and eye deviation to the side of the lesion, the prognosis is grave but not hopeless. Usually, a much less severe neurologic deficit is present. In the presence of a major deficit, the most likely cause is thrombosis of the internal carotid artery with or without distal embolization. The next most common cause is a distal internal carotid or middle cerebral artery embolus and, rarely, an intracerebral hemorrhage. In the face of an immediate significant deficit that is greater than a preoperative deficit, the patient should be given additional heparin to ensure heparinization, and the blood pressure should be elevated with vasopressors. Preparations should be made to immediately return the patient to the operating suite. Over the next few minutes, if the deficit is improving, therapy should be continued and arteriography planned. If the deficit is unimproved the patient should be returned to the operation suite and the wound reopened. If an excellent pulse is present in the carotid artery, an on-the-table arteriogram is performed. If the arteriogram reveals an arterial flap or partial clot thrombosis of the internal carotid artery, then appropriate vessel isolation and reopening of the vessel is indicated. If the thrombus is immediately available, it is removed and back-bleeding allowed. At this point, the mechanical cause of the thrombosis is usually identified as an intimal flap, and this is repaired.

Prior to restoration of flow an internal arteriogram is done by placing a #14-gauge intracatheter into the distal internal carotid artery and injecting 4 to 5 cc of contrasts to ensure that the distal internal carotid artery is patent and to determine whether there is an embolus in the middle cerebral artery. If the vessel is patent with or without the middle cerebral artery embolus, flow can be restored after reconstruction of the vessel. If an embolus exists in the intracranial carotid, the patient's blood pressure may be raised and back-bleeding allowed in the hope that the embolus will flush down the open artery. The arteriogram is repeated and if the distal internal carotid artery occlusion persists, then flow should not be restored, but preparation for a craniotomy should be carried out and embolectomy considered. Another consideration would be the use of intra-arterial thrombolytic agents and repeat arteriography to determine patency. If arterial patency can be achieved, the vessel is reconstructed and flow restored. If a middle cerebral artery embolus is present, flow should be restored by reconstruction of the artery and subsequent thrombolytic agents or craniotomy and embolectomy or extracranial-intracranial bypass surgery considered.

If, on opening the artery, no local thrombus is present and no backflow occurs, a Fogarty catheter should be passed distally to the level of the carotid canal and distended gently to remove distal thrombus. A distal thrombus without local operative thrombus would indicate distal intimal damage to the internal carotid artery, probably from dissection produced by shunting or intimal damage produced by forceful clamping. Not infrequently, on returning the patient to the operating room, the artery and arteriogram are normal. In this circumstance, it is presumed that either operative ischemia occurred despite monitoring or shunting or an embolus had occurred and dissolved. A distal branch or branches of the middle cerebral artery may be found to contain an embolus. Craniotomy with embolectomy, thrombolytic agents, or medical therapy may be the most satisfactory therapy. Generally, the prognosis with a distal embolus into the cortical arteries militates against surgical therapy.

Prevention of postoperative internal artery occlusion is best handled by the routine use of a vein or fabric patch. In Sundt's experience, 4 percent of the patients in whom the vessel had been closed primarily suffered a postoperative occlusion.[40] The literature reveals a postoperative occlusion in primary closure to range from 2 to 5 percent. A literature review and personal experience reveals the reconstructed primarily closed artery is more apt to have points of narrowing than the artery reconstructed by patch technique. Almost invariably, an internal carotid artery occlusion is secondary to technical factors that must be prevented by meticulous surgical technique.

Heparin-induced hypercoagulability may be responsible for postoperative thrombosis. This complication should be prevented by routine monitoring of platelet counts every third day in patients who are on constant heparinization and attempting to limit the heparinization to 3 to 4 days. Once this hypercoagulable state occurs, there is no definitive therapy.

Other factors in the prevention of postoperative occlusion at the operative site include the routine use of aspirin and not completely reversing the heparin after restoration of vessel flow. Also, operative and postoperative hypertension must be avoided.

If angiography demonstrates no cause for the neurologic deficit but shows evidence of a mass lesion, an intracerebral hemorrhage is present. If the arteriogram is normal, a postoperative computed tomography (CT) or magnetic resonance imaging scan is indicated to determine the presence of an intracerebral clot or infarction. If an intracerebral hemorrhage is seen, the patient's blood pressure should be maintained at a normal level. The heparin must be reversed with protamine hydrochloride. If the patient has received aspirin, platelet buttons given to reverse the aspirin effect is essential. Subsequently, surgical evacuation may be lifesaving. Unfortunately, when intracerebral hemorrhage occurs, it is often a massive bleed. If the hemorrhage is extensive and in the major hemisphere, no therapy is probably the most humane in view of the patient's dismal prognosis.

If arteriography confirms an external carotid artery occlusion and an embolus is seen in the internal carotid system or the arteriogram is otherwise normal, the probability is that an embolus arose from the external carotid artery. This patient should have the external carotid artery isolated from cerebral flow, opened, and a thrombectomy done and flow reconstituted, or, the patient should be heparinized for a week to 10 days to prevent additional embolization. If a common carotid artery occlusion is found, one can suspect an intimal lesion with dissection as the cause. This will necessitate extending the arteriotomy inferiorly to the clamp site with appropriate repair.

## Wound Hematoma and Carotid Suture Line Rupture

Postoperative hematoma with tracheal deviation, pain, and discomfort and an airway embarrassment is best treated by immediately opening the wound. In an emergency situation the wound must be opened in the bed, but, if possible, the patient should be returned to the operating room. If the hematoma is quite large and the patient maintaining his airway, after local preparation and drape, the wound should be opened under local anesthesia prior to intubation of the patient. Often the hematoma can be evacuated without the necessity of general anesthesia. If possible the rapid induction of general endotracheal anesthesia with respiratory paralysis and an attempt at intubation should be avoided because of major difficulty in placing an endotracheal tube without prior wound opening and partial clot evacuation. If intubation is required, the endotracheal tube probably should be left in place for 2 to 3 days to ensure that the airway is maintained.

On reopening the wound, the patient is frequently found to have either oozing from raw surfaces associated with aspirin therapy or an arterial or venous bleeder that requires ligation. The hematoma may also present with interference of swallowing and speech due to posterior dissection. The hematoma may extend into the mediastinum.

Rarely there is rupture of the suture line or graft used to close the carotid artery. An extreme emergency exists. The patient's death is imminent unless the airway can be maintained, the bleeding stopped, and shock treated. It may be necessary from a lifesaving standpoint to open the wound in the bed and occlude the carotid artery manually or with an available hemostat. If possible, the patient should be intubated and returned to surgery where the appropriate exposure and isolation of the carotid artery can be achieved. On rare occasions, the running suture will have been found to be broken. On other occasions, the patch graft may have torn. Whatever the cause, it must be repaired and the artery reconstituted.

A ruptured carotid suture line can be avoided by inspecting the arterial suture for areas of thinning and not nicking or knotting the suture in the process of wound closure. In addition, if Prolene is used, sutures should be tied with at least 6 to 7 knots and cut long.

Prevention of hematoma requires meticulous attention to hemostasis wound closure and the awareness of the liability of using aspirin or not reversing the heparin at closure of the artery. In addition, the meticulous control of blood pressure in the hypertensive patient is essential.

## Unusual Wound and Artery Complications

Postoperative wound infection is rare. Even in the face of a patch graft, providing the patient is neurologically intact, the wound should be opened, drained, and the appropriate organism identified and antibiotics given. The great danger is wound disruption secondary to infection or rejection of the graft used for angioplasty. The literature contains very little direction in the management of the wound with a patch graft that becomes infected. My single case healed without problem with the use of drainage and antibiotics.

On rare occasions, a false aneurysm will occur. This is most unusual with primary wound closure and usually occurs with angioplasty. It may be secondary to delayed incompetency of the vein graft or a low-grade infection of the fabric graft or partial delayed rupture of either one. The aneurysm usually presents with a mass in the neck or with episodes of transient ischemia or stroke. Rarely a 12th nerve palsy and mass are present. Surgical repair involves wide exposure with excision of the aneurysm and reconstruction of the artery either by patching or resection and grafting. If a graft is required, we prefer Gore-Tex tubing with end-to-end anastomosis between the common carotid and internal carotid arteries and implanting of the external carotid artery on an end-to-side anastomosis. If the common carotid origin is uninvolved in the aneurysmal process, an end-to-end anastomosis between the internal carotid artery may be possible.

## Ischemic Attacks

Dirrenberger and Deen have delineated the healing process after endarterectomy in a superb fashion.[40] They conclusively illustrate the benefit of operative heparinization and not reversing the heparin after arterial closure. The thrombogenicity of the endarteromized surface is fortunately short-lived. Immediately, the operative surface is quite thrombogenic, but after the first 20 minutes, it is less, and with heparin it is significantly less. The raw surface is covered by adhering platelets and fibrin. The period of thrombus formation does not exceed 6 to 8 hours. The protective platelet fibrin coat or the depletion of thromboplastin causes the surface to lose thrombogenicity.

Providing flow has been restored appropriately, postoperative embolization or occlusion of the carotid artery are usually events of the first few hours after surgical repair. However, ischemic events, whether they are transient ischemic attacks or reversible ischemic neurologic deficits, may occur up to the point of reendothelization of the arterial wall. This requires approximately a month. Other causes for delayed ischemic events include unrecognized arterial dissection or damage to the arterial wall secondary to vigorous clamping. An occluded external carotid artery may be the source emboli producing transient ischemic attacks.

Postoperative ischemic attacks or neurologic deficits are best managed by performing a CT scan of the head to exclude hemorrhage or infarction followed by an arteriogram. The status of the arterial tree will then determine whether operative or medical management is recommended.

## Hyperperfusion Syndromes

Hyperperfusion syndromes occur in patients operated on who have a high risk for carotid endarterectomy and who, after endarterectomy, have a marked increase in cerebral blood flow.[40] These patients often have paralysis of autoregulation ipsilateral to the surgery. There is a profound increase in intracranial flow postoperatively. This profound increase in intracranial flow can be determined by blood flow measurement or by serial transcranial Doppler measurement, preoperatively and postoperatively. When this syndrome occurs, the patient should have the blood pressure meticulously controlled in a low range of 120 to 130 mmHg systolic for several days.

The tremendous increase in flow frequently causes ipsilateral vascular headaches. In fact, ipsilateral headache is not uncommon following endarterectomy due to increased blood flow. Headache may be produced by carotid artery occlusion. If the patient's headache is better in the sitting position, it is most likely secondary to increased flow, whereas, if it is worse in the sitting position it may indicate carotid artery occlusion. The headaches are usually treated by analgesics. Aspirin and continued heparin should be avoided in patients with the hyperperfusion syndrome. Occasionally patients will have migraine variants. Migrainelike attacks usually occur in patients with documented increases in cerebral blood flow. The attacks usually involve visual scotomata in a visual field quadrant. No specific therapy is indicated.

Postoperative seizures may occur in patients with the hyperperfusion syndrome. The seizures usually occur about a week to 10 days following operation. The seizures are treated with Dilantin and usually they are short-lived. They may be difficult to control. A permanent seizure disorder is rare.

The most catastrophic complication occurring from hyperperfusion is intracerebral hemorrhage. Several authors have recorded the risk factors that contribute to the hyperperfusion syndrome. It is associated with advanced age, hypertensive disease, an unstable preoperative neurologic condition, a recent cerebral infarction, and the routine use of aspirin and heparin. The hemorrhage may be massive and fatal. It should be managed medically, if possible, by reversing the aspirin effect with the use of platelet transfusions, discontinuing heparin, and controlling the blood pressure to low normal.

### Myocardial Infarction, Dysrhythmia, or Congestive Heart Failure

The leading cause of death after endarterectomy is myocardial infarction, either immediate or, more often, delayed.[2,13,44] In view of the close association between arteriosclerotic heart disease and carotid atherosclerosis, every patient must be assumed to have coronary artery disease. Unstable angina, congestive heart failure, and significant cardiac arrhythmias are relative contraindications for carotid endarterectomy. They should be corrected or ameliorated as much as possible prior to surgery. All patients undergoing endarterectomy need adequate oxygenation and postoperative cardiac monitoring. Meticulous attention to avoid fluid overload or congestive heart is indicated. Maintenance of the patient on preoperative medication is frequently overlooked and may produce postoperative congestive heart failure or arrythmia.

There will be rare cases with the combination of multiple transient ischemic attacks associated with a significant carotid lesion and unstable angina or the development of unstable angina in the postoperative period. In the preoperative situation, simultaneous operation on the carotid artery and coronary arteries may be necessary; however, this invariably carries a higher morbidity than if the operations can be staged. The operation should be staged even if it means having the coronary artery team on call at the time of the endarterectomy. If the heart symptoms are critical, the coronary bypass procedure is done first.

### Recurrent Carotid Stenosis

Late recurrent stenosis is secondary to myointimal hyperplasia or atherosclerosis, usually the former. Recurrent stenosis occurs in 15 to 20 percent of surgical cases. It is symptomatic in only 2 to 3 percent. Reoperation is feasible but carries a significant greater risk than primary surgery. Recurrent stenosis may be prevented by routine patching of the arteriotomy.[10,15,40] Carotid eversion may also prevent this complication.[28]

### Summary

Criticism has appropriately focused a serious review of the indications for carotid endarterectomy. The prophylactic benefit of this operation depends on very low surgical morbidity and mortality. With symptomatic carotid stenosis (70 to 90 percent) surgery is over three times as effective in reducing stroke as medical therapy. This result is present within 3 months in the recent Symptomatic Carotid Therapy Trial. Recent literature would confirm the ever-increasing safety of the operation. This is due to meticulous selection of patients and improved perioperative and operative management of patients undergoing surgery. The qualifications of the surgeons have improved.

The increasing use of institutional audit may contribute to lower morbidity. The average surgeon does not record or review his surgical results. According to Hertzer "the stakes are so high and the margin for error is so low that carotid endarterectomy simply must be audited and reaudited at every hospital in which it is performed."[25] Evidence exists that audit has improved the surgical results, either through limiting the unqualified surgeon or forcing the qualified surgeon to understand the treacherous, unforgiving nature of poor surgical care and technique. With the cataloging of complications, evidence now exists as to their incidence, prevention, and management. Surgeons must continue to maintain combined morbidity and mortality for this procedure in the 3 percent range or under in the good-risk symptomatic or asymptomatic patient.

New angioplastic techniques are being employed with immediate apparent successful radiographic results.[44] Their future will require careful evaluation of risks and long-term benefits.[18]

## EXTRACRANIAL-INTRACRANIAL BYPASS SURGERY

The introduction of the operating microscope and the demonstration by Donaghy and Yasargil[11] that the superficial temporal branch of the external carotid artery could be successfully anastomosed to a cortical branch of the middle cerebral artery opened the exciting prospect that such a procedure might prevent a stroke or improve the restoration of function after ischemia. Anecdotal reports and case series without controls appeared. These optimistic claims and the apparent rational basis for the operation in adding new blood to the brain led to the learning of this type of skillful surgical technique by a number of surgeons. Pilot observation encouraged its consideration in stroke prevention, although the observations about improvement of stroke once it had occurred were sufficiently disappointing that the designing of a controlled trial for this application of the technique was less attractive. Because of the optimism that it might be of value in stroke prevention, a randomized controlled trial was conducted between 1976 and 1985. The results were disappointingly but overwhelmingly negative.[14] This randomized trial, which has become known as the EC/IC Bypass Study, admitted patients who had experienced transient ischemic attacks or minor nondisabling stroke in the internal carotid or middle cerebral artery territory within 3 months prior to randomization. They were stratified according to the radiologic site of the most distal le-

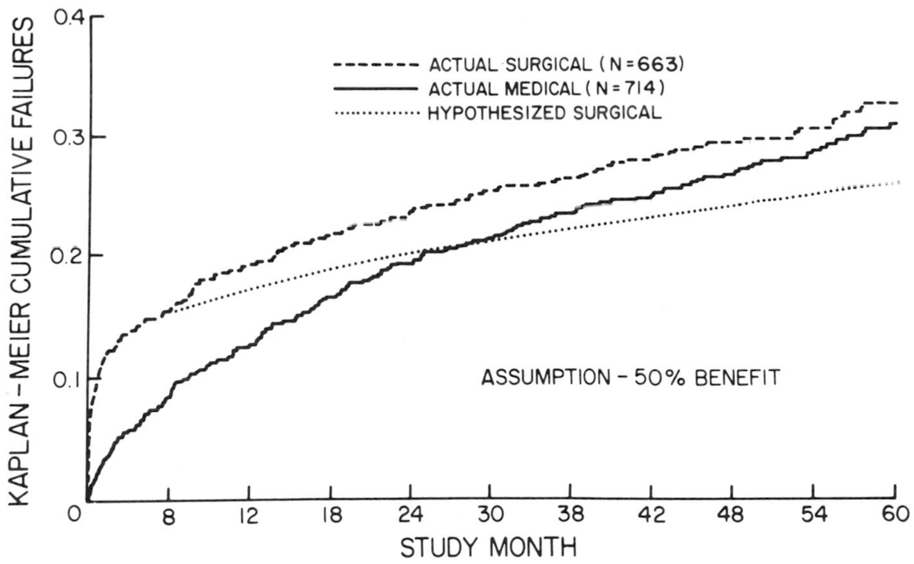


**Fig. 43-2.** Survival curves for the treatment groups. This Kaplan-Meier survival curve shows the probability of surviving free of stroke after randomization in the EC/IC Bypass Study contrasting the actual survival results with what would have been needed to demonstrate a significant benefit. At the time of randomization there were 663 patients in the surgical group and 714 in the medical group. If the procedure had contributed a 50 percent relative risk reduction, the survival line for the surgical patients would have been as supposed by the interrupted line.

sion: inaccessible internal carotid artery stenosis, internal carotid artery occlusion, and occlusion or stenosis of the main trunk of the middle cerebral artery.

Seventy-one collaborating centers located in North America, Europe, Japan, and Taiwan randomized 1,377 patients so that 663 patients received best medical care plus the anastomosis and 714 received only best medical care. The patency of the surgical anastomoses was higher than previously reported, reaching 94 percent in the North American centers, 97 percent in the European centers, and 98 percent in the Asian centers by postoperative arteriography. The 30-day perioperative major morbidity and mortality rates were the equivalent of the lowest that had been reported: 2.5 and 0.6 percent, respectively. No patients were lost, and the time of follow-up averaged 55.8 months.

The outcome events were stroke, stroke death, and any death. Particular interest focused on the prevention of stroke in the hemisphere in which the symptoms presented and for which the anastomosis was directed (Fig. 43-2).

From all analyses, no benefit was shown in stroke prevention. In none of the radiologic categories to which patients were randomized was the stroke-free survival better in the surgical group than in the comparable medical patients. It had been hoped and indeed some claimed after the results of the trial were reported that despite our findings some patients should have been shown to benefit from this procedure if they were afflicted with hemodynamic compromise as opposed to a lesion producing thromboembolic events. Routine and cerebral blood flow studies had not been able to establish this prior to the bypass study and subsequent studies by more sophisticated methods including positron emission tomography (PET) and single photon emission computed tomography (SPECT) have not identified patients in whom clinical benefit can be claimed.

The study included a majority of patients with internal carotid artery occlusion many of whom continued to have ischemic events after the occlusion had been verified. It included 74 patients with bilateral internal carotid artery occlusion and a small group with bilateral middle cerebral artery occlusion.[3,47] The study failed to show an expected benefit in these patients despite their severe hemodynamic compromise. There were 12 patients in the subgroup with bilateral carotid artery occlusion whose ischemic symptoms recurred with exercise and postural change. This hemodynamic symptom disappeared in the six patients treated surgically. In the patients assigned to the medical group, an equal number (six patients) had symptoms triggered by posture and exercise. Within 6 months, they too had ceased to experience these events. It would seem that the development of collateral circulation introduced sufficient new blood to the appropriate hemisphere that the symptoms disappeared spontaneously. If no control group had existed, it would have been very easy to have concluded erroneously that the disappearance of the symptoms was the direct result of surgery.

The functional status of the patients was evaluated on a functional status scale, which was calculated on each of the patients' 3-month follow-up in the post-randomization period. Those randomized to surgery experienced an improvement in their functional abilities (Fig. 43-3). It would have been tempting to assume that the cause of this improvement was the result of the operative procedure. Unfortunately for this conclusion there was similar and slightly more improvement in the functional status after randomization in the medically treated patients. Eventually, in both the medical and surgical groups, there was a decline in the functional status scale for patients beginning 2 years after randomization.[24]

The EC/IC Bypass Study was subjected to considerable criticism because it was alleged that a large number of the eligible patients in the participating centers had been subjected to the procedure without randomization and were operated on outside the study. The allegation was that the best patients had been diverted from the study and that the results were therefore not credible. Investigators in charge of this trial were able to determine that nine centers did not adhere to their agreement and operated on many patients outside the trial. Ten centers had a change of staff or lost interest in the trial. Fifty-two of the centers proved to be committed to the demanding standards of the protocol, and from them 87 percent of the patients came into the study. Repeating the analyses with and without the delinquent and the short-term centers did not alter the results derived from the analyses.[1]

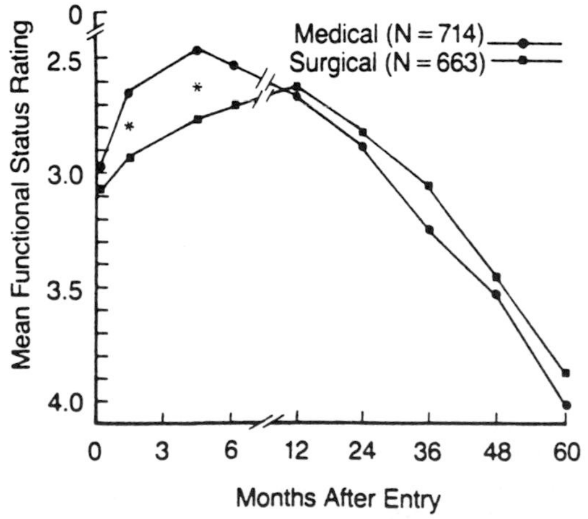


**Fig. 43-3.** Changes in functional status according to the 12-point scale, with lower numbers indicating better function in daily activities. Asterisks indicate $P < .01$. The early benefit from the surgical procedure, reflecting natural forces of improvement, coupled with medical care alone, could have been misconstrued and assigned to surgery had there been no control group. (From Haynes et al.,[24] with permission.)

Six years after the conclusion of the study, the following statements may be made with considerable certainty:

1. No convincing evidence exists that patients threatened with stroke from arteriosclerotic disease benefit from extracranial to intracranial anastomoses.
2. No randomized trial of patients with recent stroke has been conducted. Pilot observations make this an unlikely area for future studies.
3. Bypass surgery with posterior circulation anastomoses has proven hazardous and further studies in this area are difficult to justify.
4. Studies in the use of a variety of surgical bypass procedures for moyamoya disease are ongoing in Japan. The results will be watched with interest. This is a condition involving an obliterative process of the intracranial terminal branches of the internal carotid arteries. Although a rare disease, it might prove that a diversion of blood from the normal external carotid arteries to the internal carotid circulation will prove beneficial.
5. Surgeons have utilized bypass surgery when giant intracranial aneurysms or tumors involving a major intracranial artery are to be dealt with by permanently sacrificing the flow through these arteries. The observations reported to date encourage the continued use of bypass surgery under these circumstances. It is doubtful that a randomized clinical trial will ever be mounted to prove or disprove this strategy beyond doubt.
6. The EC/IC Bypass Study established the feasibility of conducting multicenter and interdisciplinary clinical trials evaluating potential surgical treatments for stroke prevention.

## REFERENCES

1. Barnett HJM, Fox A, Hachinski VC et al: Further conclusions from the extracranial-intracranial bypass trial. Surg Neurol 26:227, 1986
2. Barnett HPM, Plum F, Walton JN: Carotid endarterectomy—an expression of concern. Stroke 15:941, 1984
3. Bogousslvasky J, Wong W, Barnett HJM: Bilateral occlusion of the middle cerebral artery trunk. Stroke 17:1107, 1986
4. Bove EL, Fry WJ, Gross WS, Stanley JC: Hypotension and hypertension as consequences of baroreceptor dysfunction following carotid endarterectomy. Surgery 85:663, 1979
5. Brott TG et al: Changes patterns in the practice of carotid endarterectomy in a large metropolitan area. JAMA 255:2609, 1986
6. Callow AD, Kaplan LR, Correll JW et al: Carotid endarterectomy: what is its current status? Am J Med 85:835, 1988

7. Canadian Cooperative Study Group: A randomized trial of aspirin and sulfinpyrazone and threatened stroke. N Engl J Med 299:53, 1978
8. Clinical Alert: Benefit of endarterectomy for patients with high-grade stenosis of the internal carotid artery. NINDS News Release, Feb 27, 1991
9. Corson JD, Chang BB et al: The influence of anesthetic choice on carotid endarterectomy outcome. Arch Surg 122:807, 1987
10. Das MB, Hertzer NR, Ratliff NB et al: Recurrent carotid stenosis: a five year series of 65 re-operations. Ann Surg 202:2875, 1985
11. Donaghy RMP, Yasargil MG: Microvascular Surgery. Report of the First Conference, 1966. CV Mosby, St. Louis, 1967
12. Dyken ML: Carotid endarterectomy studies: a glimmering of science. Stroke 17:355, 1986
13. Dyken ML, Pokras R: The performance of endarterectomy for disease of the extracranial arteries of the head. Stroke 15:948, 1984
14. EC/IC Bypass Study Group: Failure of extracranial-intracranial arterial bypass to reduce the risk of ischemic stroke. N Engl J Med 313:1191, 1985
15. Edwards WH Jr et al: Recurrent carotid artery stenosis. Ann Surg 209:662, 1989
16. European Carotid Surgery Trialists' Collaborative Group: MRC European Surgery Trial: interim results for symptomatic patients with severe (70–99%) or with mild (0–29%) carotid stenosis. Lancet 337:1235, 1991
17. Evans WE, Mendelowitz DS, Liapisc J: Motor speech deficit following carotid endarterectomy. Ann Surg 196:461, 1982
18. Ferguson R: Getting it right the first time. AJNR 11:875, 1990
19. Fields WS, Lemak NA, Frankowski RF: Control trial of aspirin and cerebral ischemia. Stroke 8:301, 1977
20. Fields WS, Masleni K, Myer JS et al: Joint study of extracranial arterial occlusion: V. Progress report of prognosis following surgery or non-surgical treatment for transient cerebral ischemic attacks and cervical carotid artery lesions. JAMA 211:1993, 1970
21. Fode NC, Sundt TM, Robertson JT et al: Multicenter retrospective review of results in complication of carotid endarterectomy in1981. Stroke 17:370, 1986
22. Gabelman CG, Gann DS, Ashworth CJ, Carney WI: 100 consecutive carotid reconstructions: Local versus general anesthesia. Am J Surg, 145:477, 1983
23. Hass WK, Eastin JD, Adams HP et al: A randomized trial comparing ticlopidine hydrochloride with aspirin for the prevention of stroke in high-risk patients. N Engl J Med 321:501, 1989
24. Haynes RB, Mukherjee J, Sackett DL et al: Functional status changes following medical or surgical treatment for cerebral ischemia. JAMA 257:2043, 1987
25. Hertzer NR: Carotid endarterectomy—a crisis in confidence. (Presidential address.) J Vasc Surg 7:611, 1988
26. Hertzer NR et al: A prospective study of vein patch angioplasty during carotid endarterectomy: 3 yr. results for 801 patients in 917 operations. Ann Surg 206:628, 1987
27. Hertzer NR, Feldman BJ, Beven EG, Tucker HM: A prospective study of the incidence of injury to the cranial nerves during carotid endarterectomy. Surg Gynecol Obstet 151:781, 1980
28. Jones CE: Carotid eversion endarterectomy revisited. Am J Surg 157:323, 1989
29. Lusby RJ, Wylie EJ: Complications of carotid endarterectomy. Surg Clin North Am 63:1293, 1983
30. Merrick NJ, Fink A, Park RE, Brook RH: Derivation of clinical indications for carotid endarterectomy by an expert panel. Am J Public Health 77:187, 1987
31. Meyer FB, Sundt TM Jr, Piepgras DG et al: Emergency carotid endarterectomy for patients with acute carotid occlusion and profound neurologic deficits. Ann Surg 203:A2, 1986
32. NASCET Collaborators: Beneficial effect of carotid endarterectomy in symptomatic patients with high-grade carotid stenosis. N Engl J Med 325:445, 1991
33. North American Symptomatic Carotid Endarterectomy Study Group: Carotid endarterectomy: three critical evaluations. Stroke 18:987, 1987
34. Ojemann RG, Crowell RM: Cerebral Management of Cerebral Vascular Disease. Williams & Wilkins, Baltimore, 1983
35. Robertson JT, Auer NJ: Extracranial occlusive disease with carotid artery. p. 1559. In Youmans JR (ed): Neurological Surgery. Vol. 3. WB Saunders, Philadelphia, 1982
36. Sebul RD, Whisnant JP: Indications for carotid endarterectomy. Ann Intern Med 111:675, 1989
37. Spetzler RF: Internal carotid artery occlusion. In preparation.
38. Spetzler RF et al: Microsurgical endarterectomy under barbiturate protection: a prospective study. J Neurol Surg 65:63, 1986
39. Steering Committee of NASCET: North American Symptomatic Carotid Endarterectomy Trial: methods, patient characteristics and progress. Stroke 22:711, 1991
40. Sundt TM, Jr: Occlusive Cerebral Vascular Disease: Diagnosis and Surgical Management. WB Saunders, Philadelphia, 1987
41. Sundt TM, Jr et al: The risk-benefit ratio of intraoperative shunting during carotid endarterectomy: relevancy to operative and post-operative results in complications. Ann Surg 203:196, 1986
42. Sundt TM, Sandok BA, Whisnant JP: Carotid endarterectomy complications and pre-operative assessment of risk. Mayo Clin Proc 50:301, 1975
43. Theron J et al: New triple coaxial catheter system for carotid angioplasty with cerebral protection. AJNR 11:869, 1990
44. Till JS, Toole JF et al: Declining morbidity and mortality carotid endarterectomy. Stroke 18:823, 1987
45. Toole James F: The Asymptomatic Carotid Atherosclerosis Study. Public Health Service Grant, NINCDS-NS 22611, 1987
46. UK-TIA Study Group: United Kingdom Transient

Ischemic Attack Aspirin Trial: Interim results. Br Med J 296:316, 1988
47. Wade JPH, Wong W, Barnett HJM: Bilateral occlusion of the internal carotid arteries: presenting symptoms in 74 patients and a prospective study of 34 medically treated patients. Brain 110:667, 1987
48. Warlow C: Carotid endarterectomy: does it work? Stroke 15:1068, 1984
49. Whisnant JP, Fisher L, Robertson JT, Scheinberg P: Carotid endarterectomy decreased stroke and death in patients with transient ischemic attacks. Ann Neurol 22:72, 1987
50. Whisnant JP, Sandok BA, Sundt TM Jr: Carotid endarterectomy for unilateral carotid system transient cerebral ischemia. Mayo Clin Proc 58:171, 1983
51. Winslow CM et al: The appropriateness of carotid endarterectomy. N Engl J Med 318:721, 1988
52. Winslow CM, Solomon DH, Chassin MR et al: The appropriateness of carotid endarterectomy. N Engl J Med 318:721, 1988

# 44
# *CHANGING PERSPECTIVES IN ASYMPTOMATIC CAROTID STENOSIS*

J.W. Norris

Although auscultation of the head and neck for bruits has been practiced for many years, it is commonly omitted from routine physical examination because of the uncertainty of their significance. Early attempts at relating neck bruits to carotid angiographic findings could at best give only a rough idea of the correlation with underlying carotid stenosis due to the invasive nature of the procedures. Nevertheless, in one of the earliest documented studies, Javid et al.[23] in 1970 concluded that bruits often relate to the arteriographic appearances of carotid bifurcation stenosis, a risk factor for stroke, which might be prevented by carotid endarterectomy.

It was not for another 10 years that population studies with prospective follow-up indicated that the associated stroke risk is low, that the neck bruits were index lesions of diffuse atherosclerosis, and that the biggest threat to the patient was cardiac rather than cerebral events.[4,19,40]

Arterial bruits are due to turbulence of blood within the vessel, disturbing laminar flow. They are therefore found in a variety of conditions, including atherosclerotic plaques producing arterial stenosis, arterial kinks or coils, and when blood flow is abnormally high, such as in thyrotoxicosis or fevers. They may also be heard at a distance from a heart murmur when the vibrations from the abnormal valve are carried distally. They vary with posture and anxiety, and so change from time to time even with the same observer.

## NECK BRUITS

Most neck bruits indicate underlying pathology in the carotid artery[4] and, in general, signify an increased likelihood of stroke, since they imply carotid artery stenosis, although not necessarily on the same side.[20]

About 3 to 4 percent of the normal adult population have neck bruits[19,22] and this figure increases with the severity of stenosis but drops precipitously once the artery occludes. The prevalence of neck bruits increases with advancing age, reaching 8 percent of normal people over 75 years, 10 percent over 85, and 13 percent over 95. However, it is uncertain whether this increased prevalence of bruits is accompanied by an increased prevalence of stroke.[35]

Neck bruits localize poorly with the side of the carotid stenosis, being completely at random in some studies[20] but with some localizing value in others.[22] In one study,[7] using carotid Doppler-clinical correlation, there was a 64 percent incidence of underlying carotid stenosis ipsilateral to the neck bruit, and a 33 percent incidence on the contralateral "silent" side (Fig. 44-1).

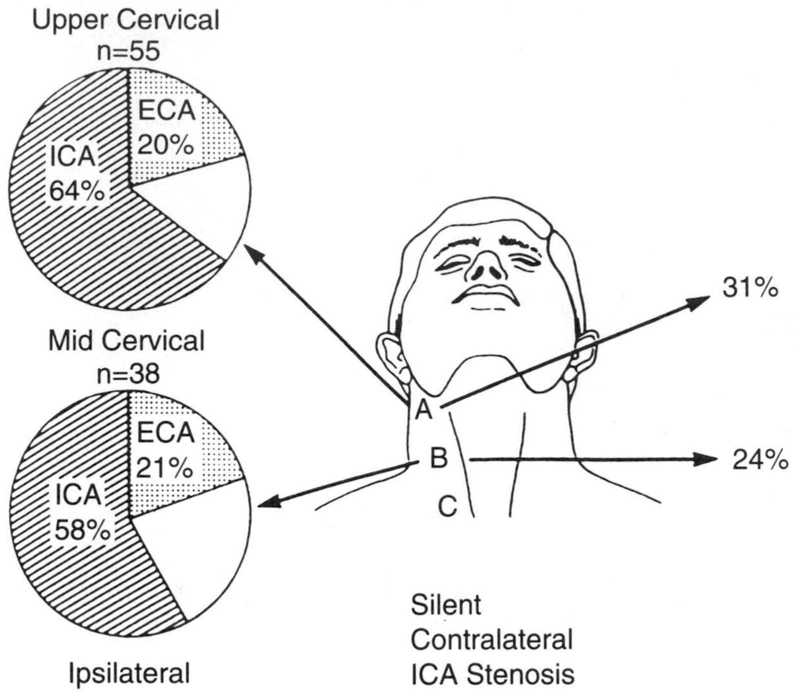


**Fig. 44-1.** Doppler findings in 93 patients with unilateral carotid bruits. ICA = internal carotid artery stenosis of at least 35 percent; ECA = external carotid artery stenosis. (From Chambers and Norris,[7] with permission.)

## OCULAR BRUITS

Ocular bruits were originally felt to indicate a contralateral carotid occlusion, rather than representing an intracranial arterial stenosis.[12,30] Later studies, with angiographic correlation, showed a variety of causes, including carotid siphon stenosis and periorbital lesions such as superficial angiomas or even Paget's disease. Intracranial causes of bruits over the eye include arteriovenous malformations and other vascular tumors such as meningiomas. Systemic illnesses with hyperdynamic circulatory states also produce ocular bruits.[27]

However, ocular bruits represented only a tiny fraction of head bruits heard in clinical practice, about 2 percent of all patients in our Doppler laboratory in Toronto.

## STROKE RISK OF ASYMPTOMATIC CAROTID LESIONS

The evaluated risk of ischemic cerebral events, whether transient ischemic attacks (TIAs) or stroke, depends on numerous factors. Retrospective reviews of medical records to determine whether patients had symptoms are of little value, and only prospective studies will be reported here. Also, the outcome of patients with neck bruits will be different from those with asymptomatic carotid stenosis.

In general, angiographic methods to evaluate the carotid arteries are unlikely to represent consecutive patients due to ethical considerations. Also, angiographic estimates of diameter relate poorly to ultrasound assessment of cross section. A 50 percent reduction of diameter corresponds to a 75 percent reduction of cross section, at which point the stenosis becomes hemodynamically significant;[11] stroke risk is directly correlated with the severity of carotid stenosis.[2,8,13,31,38] Duplex or B-mode imaging of carotid ulcers is notoriously inaccurate and therefore has no predictive value in relating arterial ulceration to stroke risk. However, Moore and colleagues[25] assessed the angiographic appearances of carotid ulceration and reported an increasing stroke risk with increasing depth of ulceration of the arterial wall.

Developments in noninvasive carotid imaging have facilitated a less biased evaluation of carotid bruits and carotid lesions, since carotid ultrasound can be used in consecutive patients without fear of complications.

The stroke risk in asymptomatic patients with neck bruits or carotid stenosis has been reviewed in detail by Hennerici et al.[16] In community studies of large populations, the annual stroke risk was about 1 percent (Table 44-1). The bruit was not necessarily related to the side of the stroke, and the strokes included

**TABLE 44-1. Annual Cerebral Event Rate and Death Rate in Prospective Studies Using Noninvasive Imaging**

| Ref. | *N* | Death (%) | TIA (%) | Stroke (%) | Ratio TIA : Stroke |
|---|---|---|---|---|---|
| 31 | 167 | ? | 4.0 | 4.0 | 3 : 2 |
| 8 | 500 | 4.0 | 4.0 | 1.7 | 3 : 1 |
| 16 | 339 | 7.0 | ? 3.0 | 1.0 | 4 : 1 |
| 2 | 242 | 9.8 | ? | 1.7 | 2 : 1 |
| 38 | 167 | 3.2 | 0.9 | 1.5 | 1 : 2[a] |

*Abbreviation:* TIA, transient ischemic attack.
[a] Follow-up by questionnaire.

**TABLE 44-2. Percent Annual Stroke Rate in 498 Patients with Asymptomatic Carotid Bruits**

| Carotid Stenosis (Doppler) (%) | Patients ($N = 498$) | Arteries ($N = 996$) |
|---|---|---|
| <35 | 0.9 | 0.4 |
| 35–50 | 0 | 0 |
| 50–75 | 0.9 | 0.6 |
| >75 | 5.5 | 2.8 |
| Overall rate | 1.7 | 0.6 |

(From Norris,[26] with permission.)

infarction, cerebral hemorrhage, or even subarachnoid hemorrhage.[19,40] These initial data brought a totally negative attitude to prophylactic carotid endarterectomy.

However, with the advent of noninvasive carotid imaging, it became clear that the side of the bruit was not necessarily the side of the stenosis, and that the overwhelmingly important factor was the degree of carotid stenosis. Although these prospective studies indicated a stroke risk of less than 1 percent per year, once the stenosis reached 75 percent, the annual risk rose closer to 5 percent (Table 44-2).[26] This is a critical figure, since it represents the stroke rate at which symptomatic patients are usually considered for carotid surgery,[39] so it could be a justifiable criterion for carotid surgery in asymptomatic patients.

Three trials have been launched randomizing patients with asymptomatic disease to receive either surgery or medical care. One trial has reported negative results.[6] Another has stopped entry, but the results are not yet available;[36] a third is ongoing.[1]

## OTHER VASCULAR RISKS

In the excellent, but now dated, survey of carotid surgery of asymptomatic carotid stenosis by Thompson and associates[34] in 1978, the major risk for carotid lesions was cardiac, not cerebrovascular; other fatal complications such as ruptured aortic aneurysm were also more critical. Later community studies confirmed a cardiac death rate of four to six times that of stroke,[16] so that it became clear that carotid bruits and carotid stenoses represent index lesions of more profound systemic arteriosclerosis than simply extracranial arterial disease. Even more relevant to the success of carotid surgery, the severity of stenosis relates to the risk of cardiac death. The very patients most likely to benefit from prophylactic carotid surgery are those most likely to die from myocardial infarction (Fig. 44-2).

Contralateral asymptomatic carotid stenosis in patients who have already undergone carotid surgery on the other side, have a similar annual stroke risk as

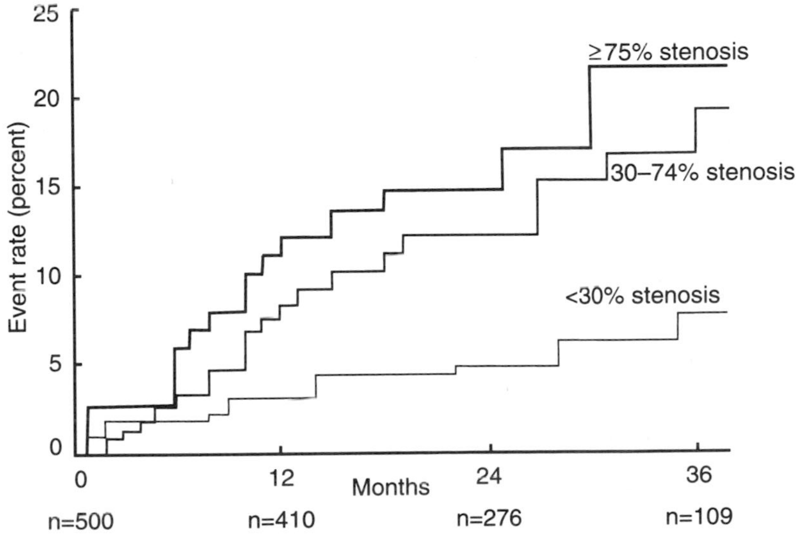


**Fig. 44-2.** Incidence of cardiac ischemic events in relation to the severity of carotid-artery stenosis on initial Doppler ultrasonography ($P < 0.0025$). (From Chambers and Norris,[8] with permission.)

those who are truly asymptomatic.[10] Hennerici et al.[16] termed these patients "pseudo-asymptomatic"; they should not be considered at equivalent risk to patients who have never experienced cerebral ischemic symptoms.

## TRANSIENT ISCHEMIC ATTACKS VERSUS STROKE AS THE INITIAL SYMPTOM

Levin et al.[24] were the first to point out the critical finding that in most cases TIAs precede the stroke in these asymptomatic patients. Many other prospective studies have confirmed this,[16] a finding unlikely to be discovered in retrospective studies, and even in prospective studies, if improperly monitored. However, it still leaves unanswered the management of those patients who experience a devastating or fatal stroke de novo.

## RISK PROFILE OF THE STROKE-SUSCEPTIBLE PATIENT

Clearly there is a group of patients with asymptomatic carotid lesions who are much more likely to experience morbidity and mortality than the rest. Only two factors have been identified for certain: the severity of carotid stenosis, and the speed of progression.

One of the earliest attempts to find a risk profile by Heyman et al.[19] noted that age and hypertension related to stroke outcome. Roederer et al.[31] measured the rate of progression of the arterial lesion and found that those with rapidly evolving stenoses were more stroke-prone (Fig. 44-3). A combination of severe carotid stenosis and rapid progression carries the highest risk of cerebral ischemic events[28] (Fig. 44-4).

Gender plays a curious role. Virtually all studies since Cutler[9] in 1967 found a higher incidence of neck bruits in women, yet women have fewer strokes. This was clearly illustrated in the study of Wiebers et al.[38] where stroke risk related directly to the degree of carotid stenosis evaluated by oculoplethysmography (OPG) (Fig. 44-5). Ford et al.,[13] investigating this dilemma, were unable to explain it, after ruling out other explanations such as different hematocrits, different caliber arteries, and different body habitus.

## FACTORS AFFECTING PROGRESSION OF CAROTID STENOSIS

It is common for each carotid artery to be involved to a different degree; sometimes one artery progresses rapidly to occlusion, while the other remains normal. Plaques are in a constant state of flux, and in the early stages, may appear and disappear over a few months, judging by the appearances on B-mode scanning.[17]

In the study in 1970 by Javid et al.,[23] progression of carotid stenosis was assessed over several years by carotid angiography. The authors concluded that local mechanical factors, not systemic (metabolic) factors, were the major influences on plaque growth, at least once the plaque is established.

Although information relating clinical symptoms to plaque pathology is scanty, Imparato et al.[21] have suggested that sudden enlargement or destruction of

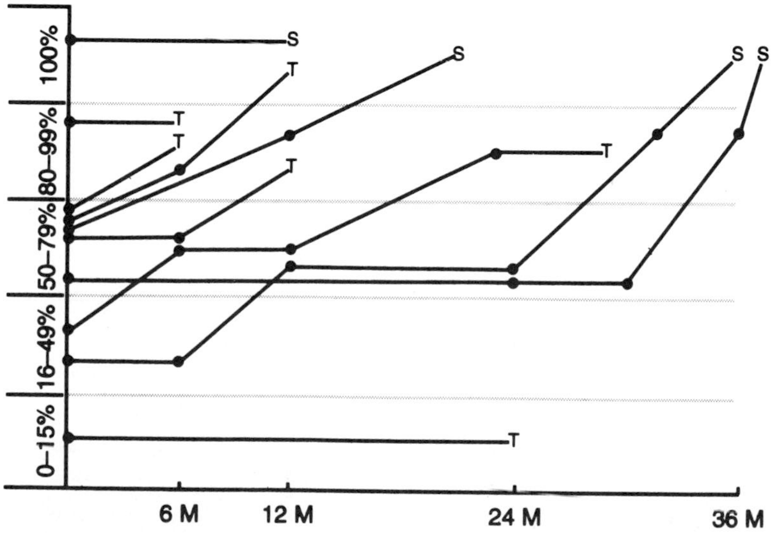


**Fig. 44-3.** Disease progression in symptomatic patients. Transient ischemic attacks (T) and stroke (S). (From Roederer et al.,[31] with permission.)

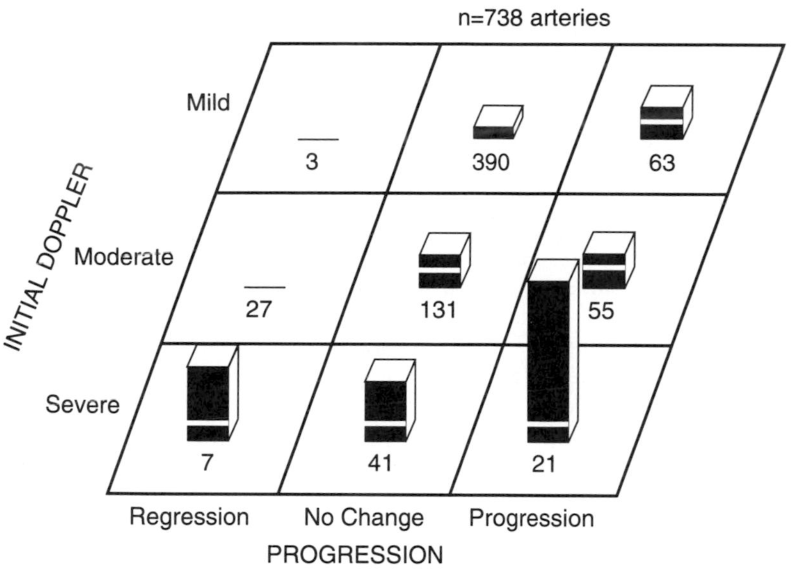


**Fig. 44-4.** Schema of risk ratio (log rank method) of occurrence of transient ischemic attack or stroke over 1 year, related to progression and severity of carotid stenosis. Numbers refer to arteries in each cell ($N = 738$). (From Norris and Bornstein,[28] with permission.)

plaques by intraplaque hemorrhage may play a pivotal role in symptomatology.

## IMPACT OF OUTCOME ON MANAGEMENT

Theoretically, since stroke risk increases with the degree of stenosis, so should the need for prophylactic surgery. However, the ultimate equation determining carotid endarterectomy is whether the surgical risks outweigh the spontaneous risks of stroke and death. The failure to establish a balance in favor of surgery has led to much concern, resulting in the launching of large, multicenter surgical trials on both sides of the Atlantic. This complex issue has been summarized and reviewed by Barnett.[3]

Meanwhile, alternative methods with great poten-

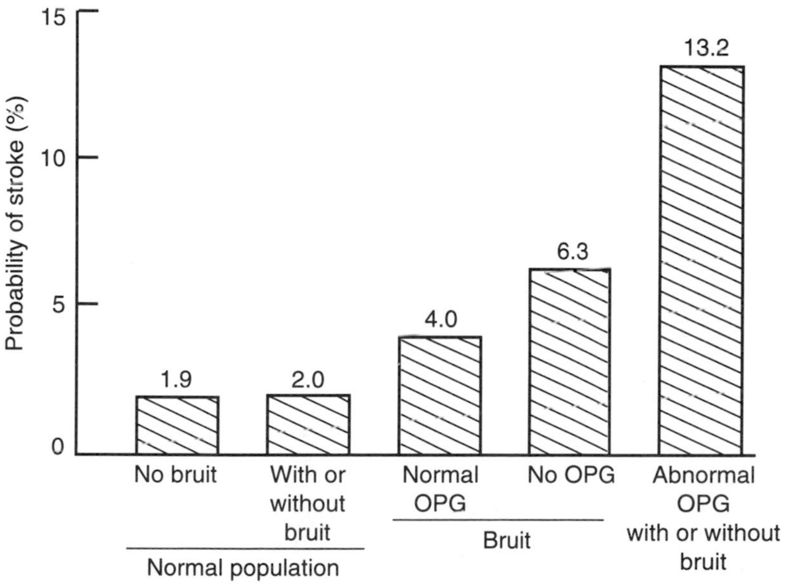


**Fig. 44-5.** Comparison of probability of stroke (given survival) over 4 years among patients with and without carotid bruit and abnormal oculoplethysmographic studies. (From Wiebers et al.,[38] with permission.)

tial are already beyond the experimental stage. Carotid angioplasty, using an expanding balloon during carotid angiography to crush the plaque and restore the lumen, is a promising new technique, which theoretically could replace carotid surgery.[33]

Surprisingly, so far, there have been few attempts to treat patients with asymptomatic carotid stenosis medically. So far, attempts at pharmacologic regression of carotid plaques in asymptomatic patients, (such as by aspirin and metoprolol) have met with failure.[29] There are theoretical hazards of using aspirin in these patients, where the drug might precipitate critical bleeding within the body of the plaque.[21] However, therapeutic regression of coronary atherosclerosis has been achieved,[5] establishing a precedent for pharmacologically induced regression of arterial stenosis elsewhere.

## CAROTID BRUITS AND GENERAL SURGERY

The discovery of a carotid bruit in an otherwise asymptomatic patient examined prior to surgery, particularly cardiac surgery, poses a dilemma. For many years it became routine practice in some centers to perform angiography and carotid endarterectomy prior to the surgical procedure if a stenosing carotid lesion was found, on the assumption that surgical hypotension could produce a hemodynamic stroke. A case for prophylactic carotid surgery in these circumstances is made by Hertzer et al.,[18] but an equally persuasive case against any such intervention is made by Furlan and Craciun.[14]

There are two possible explanations for the 2 to 3 percent stroke rate complicating cardiac surgery. Perioperative infarction might be hemodynamic, especially when a concomitant carotid stenosis is present, or from emboli due to debris released at open-heart surgery. However, most strokes occur in the absence of any underlying carotid stenosis and, in any case, usually occur days after the surgery.[15] Intracranial blood flow velocities measured during open-heart surgery are not affected by the presence of ipsilateral, severe, carotid stenosis.[37]

In the Cleveland Clinic study (probably the best published series), in patients who suffered a stroke prior to surgery, new perioperative strokes were due to worsening of the prior deficits and bore no relation to the presence of extracranial carotid stenosis.[32]

In the present state of knowledge, there seems no justification for performing staged prophylactic carotid surgery in patients with asymptomatic carotid stenosis, especially with the overwhelming evidence that strokes complicating open heart surgery are mainly embolic. The situation regarding noncardiac surgery (e.g., for cholecystectomy) is not so clear. Strokes complicating surgery are so rare (1 to 2 percent) that a randomized study to determine the answer would need more than a thousand patients, a formidable barrier to scientific prospective evaluation.

## CONCLUSION

Considerable data have now accumulated, detailing the vascular outcome of patients with asymptomatic carotid lesions. The major risk factors are established, but, carotid endarterectomy to prevent stroke became so controversial its practice diminished, both in symptomatic and asymptomatic patients. It is likely to resume now that some multicenter trials reveal promising results. Meanwhile, the advent of developing technology in carotid angioplasty could overtake direct surgical endarterectomy, and multicenter trials of drugs that might regress arterial plaques will also be instigated. Progress in research in the next few years will therefore prove critical to the management of these patients.

## REFERENCES

1. Asymptomatic Carotid Atherosclerosis Study Group: Study design for randomized prospective trial of carotid endarterectomy for asymptomatic atherosclerosis. Stroke 20:844, 1989
2. Autret A, Saudeau D, Bertrand PH et al: Stroke risk in patients with carotid stenosis. Lancet 1:888, 1987
3. Barnett HJM: Carotid endarterectomy: a challenge for scientific medicine. p. 171. In Norris JW, Hachinski VC (eds): Prevention of Stroke. Springer-Verlag, New York, 1991
4. Barnett HJM, Mohr JP, Yatsu FM: Asymptomatic carotid bruit or stenosis. p. 1207. In Barnett HJM, Mohr JP, Stein BM et al (eds): Stroke: Pathophysiology, Diagnosis, and Management. Vol. 2. Churchill Livingstone, New York, 1986
5. Brown G, Albers JJ, Fisher LD et al: Regression of coronary artery disease as a result of intensive lipid-lowering therapy in men with high levels of apolipoprotein B. N Engl J Med 323:1289, 1990
6. CASANOVA Study Group: Carotid surgery versus medical therapy in asymptomatic carotid stenosis. Stroke 22:1229, 1991
7. Chambers BR, Norris JW: Clinical significance of asymptomatic neck bruits. Neurology (NY) 35:742, 1985
8. Chambers BR, Norris JW: Outcome in patients with asymptomatic neck bruits. N Engl J Med 315:860, 1986
9. Cutler JL: Cerebrovascular disease in an elderly population. Circulation 36:394, 1967
10. Durward QJ, Ferguson GG, Barr HWK: The natural history of asymptomatic carotid bifurcation plaques. Stroke 13:459, 1982
11. Feussner JR, Matchar DB: When and how to study the carotid arteries. Ann Intern Med 109:805, 1988

12. Fisher CM: Cranial bruit associated with occlusion of the internal carotid artery. Neurology (NY) 7:299, 1957
13. Ford CS, Howard VJ, Howard G et al: The sex difference in manifestations of carotid bifurcation disease. Stroke 17:877, 1986
14. Furlan AJ, Craciun AR: Risk of stroke during coronary artery bypass graft surgery in patients with internal carotid artery disease documented by angiography. Stroke 16:797, 1985
15. Hart RG, Easton JD: Management of cervical bruits and carotid stenosis in preoperative patients. Stroke 14:290, 1983
16. Hennerici M, Hulsbomer H-B, Hefter H et al: Natural history of asymptomatic extracranial arterial disease. Brain 110:777, 1987
17. Hennerici M, Rautenberg W, Trockel U et al: Spontaneous progression and regression of small carotid atheroma. Lancet 1:1415, 1985
18. Hertzer NR, Loop FD, Beven EG: Management of coexistent carotid and coronary artery disease: a surgical viewpoint. p. 305. In Furlan AJ (ed): The Heart and Stroke. Springer-Verlag, New York, 1987
19. Heyman A, Wilkinson WE, Heyden S et al: Risk of stroke in asymptomatic persons with cervical arterial bruits: a population study in Evans County, Georgia. N Engl J Med 302:838, 1980
20. Howard VJ, Howard G, Harpold GJ et al: Correlation of carotid bruits and carotid atherosclerosis detected by B-Mode real-time ultrasonography. Stroke 20:1331, 1989
21. Imparato AM, Riles TS, Gorstein F: The carotid bifurcation plaque: pathologic findings associated with cerebral ischemia. Stroke 10:238, 1979
22. Ingall TJ, Homer D, Whisnant JP et al: Predictive value of carotid bruit for carotid atherosclerosis. Arch Neurol 46:418, 1989
23. Javid H, Ostermiller WE, Hengesh JW et al: Natural history of carotid bifurcation atheroma. Surgery 67:80, 1970
24. Levin SM, Sondheimer FK, Levin JM: The contralateral diseased but asymptomatic carotid artery: to operate or not?—an update. Am J Surg 140:203, 1980
25. Moore WS, Boren C, Malone JM et al: Natural history of nonstenotic, asymptomatic ulcerative lesions of the carotid artery. Arch Surg 113:1352, 1978
26. Norris JW: Management of asymptomatic neck bruits. Can J Cardiol 2:324, 1986
27. Norris JW: Head and neck bruits in stroke prevention. p. 103. In Norris JW, Hachinski VC (eds): Prevention of Stroke. Springer-Verlag, New York, 1991
28. Norris JW, Bornstein NM: Progression and regression of carotid stenosis. Stroke 17:755, 1986
29. Norris JW, Ziliotto C, Chambers BL et al: Failure of metoprolol and aspirin to regress carotid stenosis, abstracted. Neurology (NY), suppl. 40:415, 1990
30. Pessin MS, Paris W, Prager RJ et al: Ascultation of cervical and ocular bruits in extracranial occlusive carotid disease. Stroke 14:246, 1983
31. Roederer GO, Langlois YE, Jager KA et al: The natural history of carotid arterial disease in asymptomatic patients with cervical bruits. Stroke 15:605, 1984
32. Rorick MB, Furlan AJ: Risk of cardiac surgery in patient with prior stroke. Neurology 40:835, 1990
33. Theron J, Courtheoux P, Alachkar F et al: New triple coaxial catheter system for carotid angioplasty with cerebral protection. AJNR 11:869, 1990
34. Thompson JE, Patman RD, Talkington CM: Long-term outcome of patients having endarterectomy compared with unoperated controls. Ann Surg 188:308, 1978
35. van Ruiswyk J, Noble H, Sigmann P: The natural history of carotid bruits in elderly persons. Ann Intern Med 112:340, 1990
36. Veterans Administration Cooperative Study: Role of carotid endarterectomy in asymptomatic atherosclerosis. Stroke 17:534, 1986
37. von Reutern G-M, Hetzel A, Birnbaum D et al: Transcranial Doppler ultrasonography during cardiopulmonary bypass in patients with severe carotid stenosis or occlusion. Stroke 19:674, 1988
38. Wiebers DO, Whisnant JP, Sandok BA et al: Prospective comparison of a cohort with asymptomatic carotid bruit and a population-based cohort without carotid bruit. Stroke 21:984, 1990
39. Winslow CM, Solomon DH, Chassin MR et al: The appropriateness of carotid endarterectomy. N Engl J Med 318:721, 1988
40. Wolf PA, Kannel WB, Sorlie P et al: Asymptomatic carotid bruit and risk of stroke: the Framingham study. JAMA 245:1442, 1981

# 45
# *MEDICAL MANAGEMENT OF ANEURYSMAL SUBARACHNOID HEMORRHAGE*

Harold P. Adams, Jr.
Betsy B. Love

Subarachnoid hemorrhage accounts for 5 to 10 percent of all strokes[107,125] and has an incidence of 11 to 19.4/100,000.[57,90,150] Unlike other types of stroke, the incidence of subarachnoid hemorrhage is not declining.[150] The leading cause of subarachnoid hemorrhage, accounting for approximately 80 percent of cases, is rupture of an intracranial saccular aneurysm.[166,226] Patients with bleeding secondary to a ruptured saccular aneurysm have a different prognosis and present more complicated management problems than those with subarachnoid hemorrhage of other etiologies; therefore, this chapter will be restricted to the treatment of aneurysmal subarachnoid hemorrhage (SAH).

There is also evidence that care of patients with SAH not due to a ruptured aneurysm should differ from those who have an aneurysm. Outcomes are much better, rebleeding is infrequent, and delayed cerebral ischemia is uncommon.[160] Vigorous medical measures to lower the risk of rebleeding, vasospasm or ischemic stroke among patients with nonaneurysmal SAH are probably not indicated.[4] The group of patients with isolated perimesencephalic hemorrhage on CT have a particularly good prognosis, and these patients should be excluded from future clinical trials of SAH.[4]

Earlier diagnosis and better medical and surgical care may be reducing the mortality of SAH.[90] Yet despite advances in diagnosis and treatment, SAH is still a frequent cause of death or severe disability (Fig. 45-1). In population-based studies, the 30-day mortality of SAH is nearly 50 percent.[22,57,90,150,165,170,226] Most deaths occur within 1 week of the ictus; 10 percent die before reaching medical attention, and 25 percent die within 24 hours[57,115,159] (Fig. 45-1). Ljunggren et al.[115] noted that 17 percent of all patients with SAH were dead upon arrival to a hospital. Ruptured aneurysms are a leading neurologic cause of sudden death and often are found in medical examiner's cases. Reasons for sudden death include a large intraparenchymal hematoma, destruction of brain tissue, acute hydrocephalus, increased intracranial pressure, myocardial ischemia, cardiac arrhythmias, or acute respiratory failure.[70,81,83] In these cases, cranial computed tomography (CT) usually demonstrates massive intracerebral, intraventricular, or subarachnoid hemorrhage.[81] Intracranial pressure can be markedly elevated after SAH; resultant intracranial hypertension leads to in-

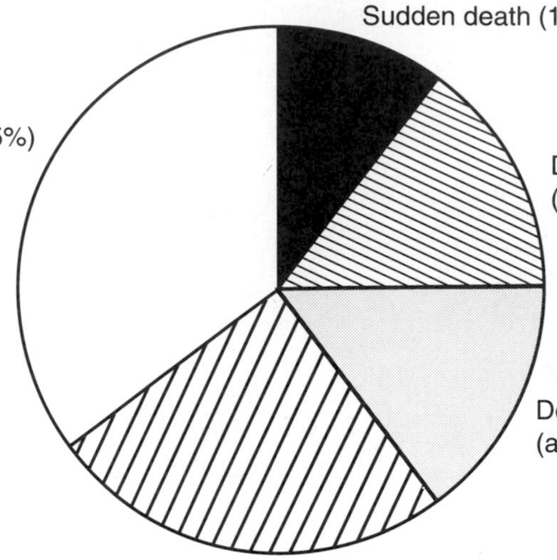


**Fig. 45-1.** Outcome after aneurysmal subarachnoid hemorrhage.

tracranial circulatory arrest and cerebral ischemia.[71] These moribund patients can have periodic or ataxic respirations, suggesting brain stem failure.[83] In these instances, survival is unlikely even with prompt medical care.

Even when terminally ill patients are excluded, the natural history of SAH is grim. The 3-month mortality among patients who reach a major medical center is approximately 25 percent.[7,93,163] The leading causes of death are sequelae of the initial hemorrhage, recurrent aneurysmal rupture, and vasospasm with ischemic stroke. Another 40 percent of hospitalized patients will have major neurologic residuals.[6,115,163,170] The chief reasons for neurologic impairment after SAH are consequences of initial aneurysmal rupture, vasospasm and ischemia, hydrocephalus, complications of surgery, and complications of medical management. Sequelae include cranial nerve palsies, monoparesis, hemiparesis, paraparesis, aphasia, mental status changes, and behavioral disorders or psychiatric disturbances that can hamper return to gainful employment or independence.[9,142,161,204,208]

Several factors that influence prognosis after SAH have been identified (Table 45-1). The two most important factors are the interval from SAH and the patient's level of consciousness. Most deaths and complications develop within 2 weeks of SAH; patients surviving this period without major complications have a generally favorable prognosis. Whisnant et al.[217] reported that the 60-day survival was 55 percent among patients seen within 24 hours of SAH and was 85 percent in patients surviving 2 weeks. Kassell et al.[93] reported favorable outcomes in 43 percent of patients first treated wihin 3 days of SAH, while favorable outcomes increased to 53 percent among patients admitted 4 to 7 days after SAH. Another study demonstrated that the 2-month mortality was 51 percent among patients seen within 3 days of SAH and was 13 percent among patients seen at 10 to 14 days.[11] The Cooperative Aneurysm Study reported a 3-month combined mortality and morbidity of 53 percent among patients treated within 3 days of SAH and of 44 percent among patients admitted on days 4 to 7.[7] When examining the possible usefulness of any intervention, the interval from SAH until treatment should be considered. The key test of any medical or surgical therapy is whether it improves outcome among acutely ill patients treated within the first few days after SAH.

Admitting level of consciousness is the most important clinical factor (Table 45-1). The 6-month mortality among comatose patients is 71 percent, while only 11 percent of initially alert patients will die during the same time period.[6] Other studies report an 11 to

**TABLE 45-1. Factors Predicting Less Favorable Outcome After Subarachnoid Hemorrhage**

*Clinical*

1. Admitting level of consciousness (coma)
2. Interval from subarachnoid hemorrhage (<3 days)
3. Age (>65)
4. Sex (women)
5. Prior hemorrhage or unrecognized warning leak
6. Presence of focal neurologic signs on admission
7. Presence of major comorbid diseases, including systemic hypertension

*Radiologic*

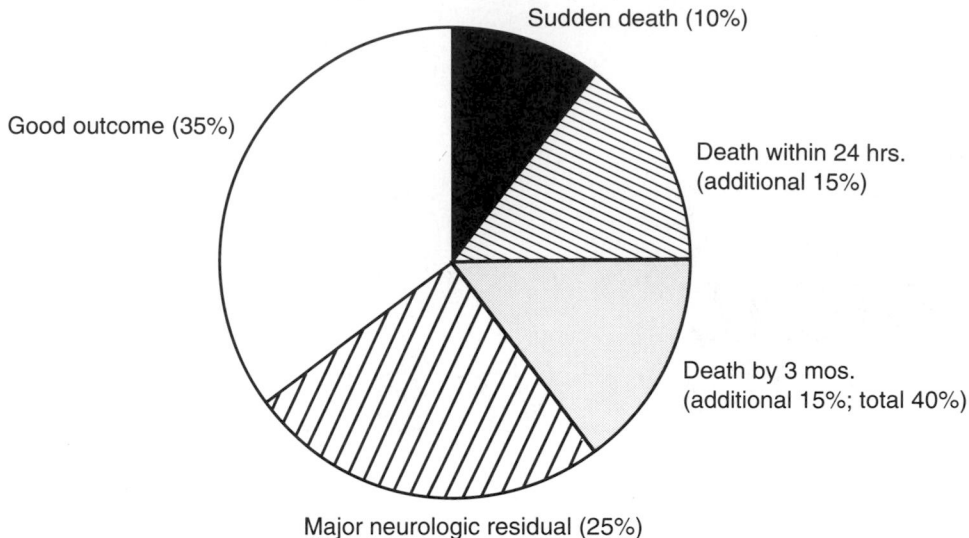

1. Abnormal CT scan
   - Local, thick collection or diffuse subarachnoid blood
   - Intracerebral or intraventricular blood
   - Mass effect
   - Hydrocephalus
2. Evidence of additional blood on sequential computed tomography
3. Vasospasm on arteriography
4. Anterior cerebral or vertebrobasilar aneurysm on arteriography
5. Giant aneurysm (25 mm or greater) on arteriography

30 percent mortality among good condition patients and an 80 to 85 percent mortality among poor condition patients.[21,217] Other clinical variables are less important. Neither the location nor the size of the aneurysm is a major determinant of prognosis, although giant aneurysms and those located on the basilar artery can present therapeutic dilemmas. Patients older than 65 years have a poorer prognosis than younger persons.[89] Patients who do not reach medical attention until after a second rupture of an aneurysm have a worse prognosis than those who have a single hemorrhage.[43] LeBlanc[111] reported the mortality by discharge with "warning leaks" was 52 percent compared to 23 percent among patients with a single hemorrhage.

Results of an initial CT examination also provide prognostic clues (Table 45-1). In general, CT results parallel clinical findings and are correlated with the time lag from SAH.[6] Patients with CT evidence of hydrocephalus, mass effect, intracerebral hematoma, intraventricular hemorrhage, or diffuse subarachnoid blood have a poorer prognosis than those who have a normal CT or who have a minimal amount of subarachnoid blood visualized.

Complications of SAH that can lead to death or disability are summarized in Table 45-2. For many years, attention has been directed at prevention of rebleeding or ischemic complications of cerebral vasospasm. These two conditions account for approximately 60 percent of the unfavorable outcomes.[216] Still, one-third of all patients who die or become disabled after SAH are injured primarily by the consequences of the initial hemorrhage. As management to prevent rebleeding and vasospasm improves, treatment of these complications will become increasingly important.[15,115] Early complications that may be manageable include hydrocephalus, convulsions, and cardiovascular events.

Therefore, goals of medical management are (1) to stabilize an acutely ill patient and treat early complications, (2) to prevent recurrent hemorrhage, and (3) to prevent vasospasm and cerebral ischemia. Treatment of SAH is complex and multifactorial; therapy aimed at prevention of one complication may aggravate management of another. For example, antifibrinolytic drugs may reduce the risk of rebleeding but may increase the risk of ischemic stroke. Conversely, successful management of one complication may leave the patient at risk for another; for example, prevention of early, fatal rebleeding may allow vasospasm to subsequently develop. Much of the care of patients with SAH is empirical or is based on anecdotal support. Several components of care have not been clinically tested; thus, many recommendations, including some in this chapter, are based on weak or conflicting scientific evidence.

**TABLE 45-2. Complications of Aneurysmal Subarachnoid Hemorrhage**

| |
|---|
| Neurologic |
| Intracerebral hematoma |
| Intraventricular hemorrhage |
| Cerebral edema |
| Hydrocephalus (acute, subacute, or chronic) |
| Recurrent hemorrhage |
| Vasospasm–cerebral ischemia |
| Seizures |
| Medical |
| Hypertension/hypotension |
| Myocardial infarction |
| Cardiac arrhythmias |
| Congestive heart failure |
| Adult respiratory distress syndrome |
| Pulmonary edema |
| Pneumonia |
| Atelectasis |
| Gastrointestinal bleeding |
| Anemia |
| Venous thromboembolism |
| Bleeding disorder |
| Hyponatremia/hypernatremia |
| Water loss |
| Hypokalemia |
| Complications of medical or surgical therapy |

## DIAGNOSIS OF ANEURYSMAL SUBARACHNOID HEMORRHAGE

The key to successful management of SAH is early treatment, which in turn is based on prompt and accurate diagnosis. Delayed recognition is a major problem. Approximately 10 percent of patients do not recognize the nature of their symptoms and do not quickly seek medical attention.[171] More bothersome is that physicians initially diagnose disorders other than SAH in 25 percent of cases.[1,5,49,95,171] In two series, physician misdiagnosis delayed treatment by an average of more than 4 days.[95,171] Unfortunately, misdiagnosis is most likely in the least seriously ill patient and this is the one most likely to be helped by early medical or surgical therapy.

## ACUTE MANAGEMENT OF SUBARACHNOID HEMORRHAGE

Patients with recent SAH are critically ill; their evaluation and treatment should be urgent. They should be transported to a medical center that has the capability to treat a patient with a ruptured aneurysm. Acute, potentially life-threatening, complications should be anticipated (Table 45-2). Personnel should closely monitor the patients and perform frequent measurements of vital signs, blood pressure, and neurologic status. Patients should have cardiac monitoring. Airway, breathing, and circulation should be supported, and, if necessary, supplemental oxygen, endotracheal intubation, or ventilatory assistance should be given. Intravenous access should be placed to expedite emergent administration of drugs. Normal saline or 0.45 saline can be given at a slow rate to maintain patency of the line.

**TABLE 45-3. Initial Diagnostic Evaluation of a Patient with a Suspected Subarachnoid Hemorrhage**

| |
|---|
| Complete blood count |
| Platelet count |
| Prothrombin time |
| Partial thromboplastin time |
| Serum glucose |
| Blood urea nitrogen |
| Serum creatinine |
| Serum electrolytes |
| Serum calcium |
| Liver function tests |
| Urinalysis |
| Electrocardiogram |
| Chest roentgenogram |
| Cranial CT (without contrast) |
| Cerebral arteriogram |
| *Optional, in selected cases* |
| Arterial blood gases |
| Contrast enhanced CT |
| Bleeding time |
| Cerebrospinal fluid |
| Magnetic resonance imaging |
| Transcranial Doppler |
| Electroencephalogram |
| Cerebral blood flow study |

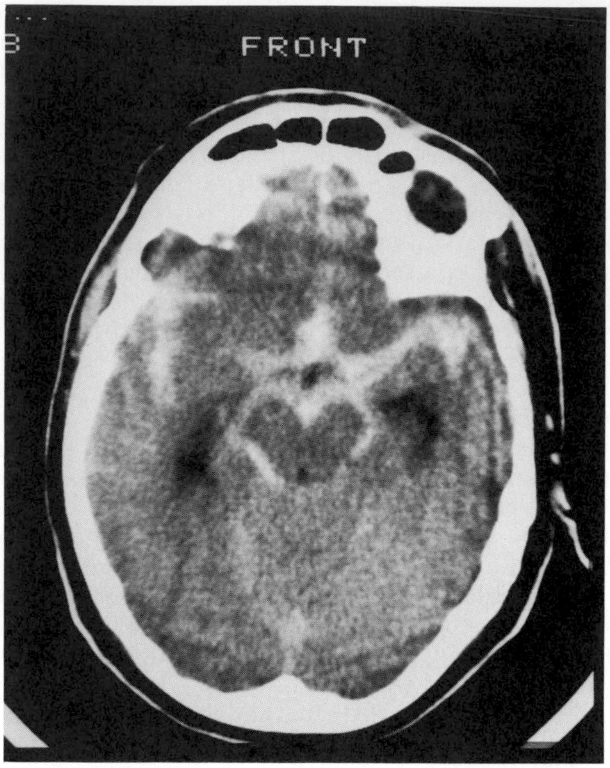


**Fig. 45-2.** Unenhanced computed tomography scan in patient with aneurysmal subarachnoid hemorrhage. Blood densities are noted in sylvian fissures and cisterns, interhemispheric fissure, basilar cistern, and circummesencephalic cistern. The temporal horns are dilated.

Evaluation should include CT, chest x-ray, electrocardiogram, and blood work (Table 45-3). CT will demonstrate subarachnoid blood and a number of other complications (Table 45-4; Figs. 45-2 to 45-5). When CT demonstrates intracranial bleeding, a lumbar puncture can be avoided. CT will be normal in approximately 10 percent of cases. If CT is negative, a cerebrospinal fluid (CSF) specimen should be obtained. While magnetic resonance imaging (MRI) may not be as good as CT for detecting acute subarachnoid blood, it may better demonstrate an aneurysm (Fig. 45-6). Once the diagnosis of SAH is confirmed, arteriography is required to demonstrate the presence and location of the aneurysm (Figs. 45-7 and 45-8). Both carotid circulations and the entire vertebrobasilar system should be visualized, although the sequence of arterial studies may be influenced by the CT findings.

**TABLE 45-4. Abnormalities Detected by Computed Tomography in Patients with Recent Subarachnoid Hemorrhage**

| Abnormality | Percentage |
|---|---|
| Subarachnoid blood | 85–92 |
| Focal, thin collection | |
| Focal, thick collection | |
| Diffuse, thin collection | |
| Diffuse, thick collection | |
| Intraventricular blood | 15–20 |
| Intracerebral blood | 15–20 |
| Subdural blood | 1–2 |
| Hydrocephalus | 10–20 |
| Mass effect | 5–8 |
| Ischemic lesion | 1–2 |
| Aneurysm[a] | 5 |
| Normal | 5–10 |

[a] Unenhanced computed tomography.

Patients should be admitted to a unit where monitoring equipment and neurologically trained nurses are available. Acute care is divided into general supportive efforts and treatment of specific complications.[2,18,33,52,146,178,211] For the first 24 hours, blood pressure, vital signs, and neurologic assessments should be measured hourly. After that time, examinations can be spaced farther apart in stable patients. Cardiac monitoring and, if necessary, continuous intra-arterial or noninvasive blood pressure monitoring should be extended for at least 24 to 48 hours after admission.

Forced bed rest is a traditional part of acute management of patients with recent SAH.[2,33,52,146,178,211] Visitors and external stimuli are restricted.[2,18,178,211] Passive range of motion exercises and frequent turning are performed. A water mattress or alternating pressure pneumatic bed can help reduce the risk of decubitus ulcers or atelectasis. Patients are assisted with self-care activities, such as bathing. Black et al.[20] demonstrated that external pneumatic calf compression will reduce the incidence of deep venous throm-

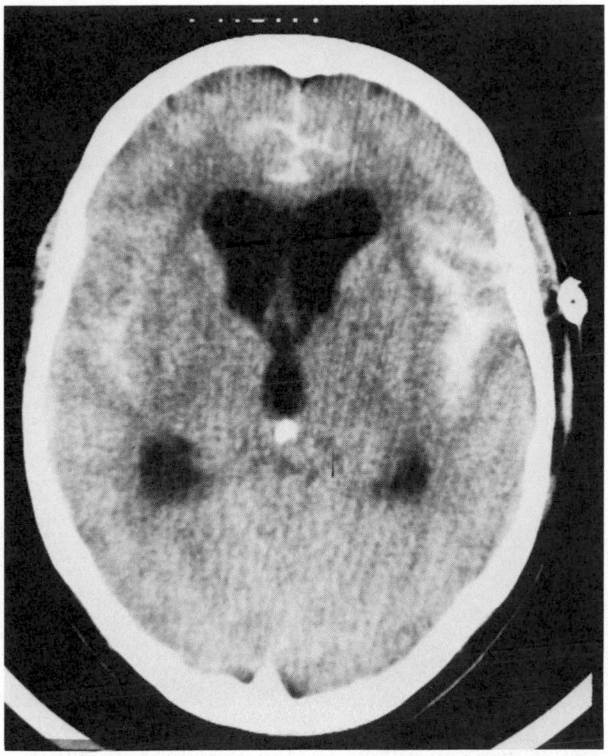

**Fig. 45-3.** Unenhanced computed tomography scan in patient with aneurysmal subarachnoid hemorrhage demonstrates blood densities in both sylvian fissures (a focal thick collection on the left) and blood in the interhemispheric fissure. Dilation of the third and lateral ventricles is noted.

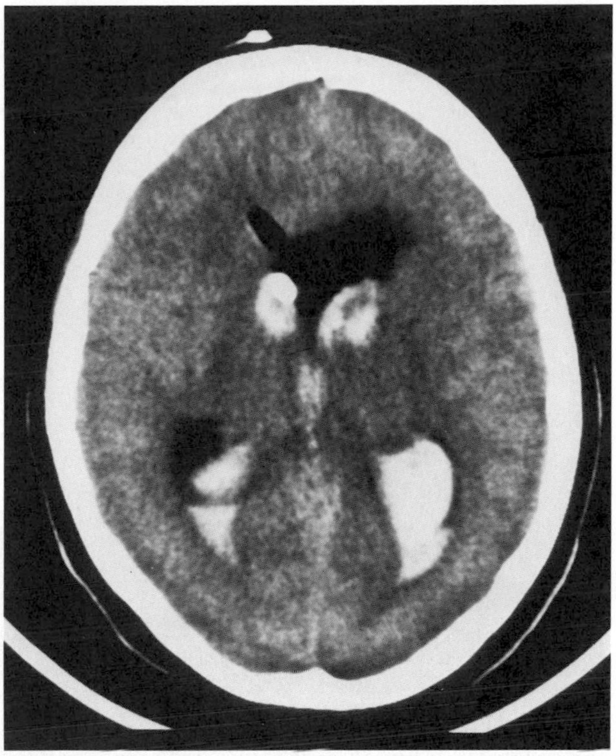

**Fig. 45-4.** Unenhanced computed tomography scan demonstrates an extensive intraventricular hemorrhage in a patient with a ruptured aneurysm. Density from a shunt is noted in the right frontal horn. A subtle blood density is noted in the interhemispheric fissure anteriorly and posteriorly.

bosis from 18 to 6 percent. Subcutaneous heparin for deep-vein thrombosis is usually avoided. Patients are not allowed to smoke. Gentle pulmonary toilet and nursing care to avoid pneumonia are important. One of the purposes of strict bed rest is to prevent rebleeding. In the late 1960s and early 1970s, the Cooperative Study of Intracranial Aneurysms and Subarachnoid Hemorrhage tested the value of forced bed rest.[137] The cumulative rebleeding rate among patients treated with bedrest during the first 14 days after SAH was greater than 25 percent.

During the first few days, intravenously administered drugs may be needed. Therefore, an intravenous access should be maintained with a slow infusion of normal saline. Fluid management and correction of electrolyte disturbances is described in more detail subsequently. Alert patients are given a soft, high-fiber diet supplemented by stool softeners.[2,18,178,211] Caffeinated and alcoholic beverages are avoided. Stuporous and comatose patients are not fed during the acute treatment period. If a patient is stable at 7 to 10 days after SAH and the airway is secured, then nasogastric feedings can be instituted. Parenteral hyperalimentation is usually not required. Multivitamins are added to the diet and intravenous fluids are given.

## Symptomatic Treatment

Patients can be confused or agitated as the result of brain injury, hydrocephalus, or increased intracranial pressure, or as a consequence of pain or nausea. Agitation may increase the risk of rebleeding or aggravate increased intracranial pressure or other acute complications. Control of pain or nausea may calm an otherwise irritable, combative patient. Sedatives can also be prescribed.[178,211] Regular administration of diazepam or phenobarbital may be useful in providing sedation; the usual starting dose is 5 mg of diazepam every 6 hours or phenobarbital 30 to 60 mg every 6 hours. In exceptional cases, haloperidol or a phenothiazine may be necessary.

The headache of SAH is intense and patients should be given ample medication to provide relief.[2,18,178,211] Most alert patients will require frequent doses of codeine, meperidine, or morphine to control pain. These drugs are usually given parenterally, in equianalgesic dosages that are administered to other patients with severe pain. If large doses of morphine are required, patients should be watched for evidence of respiratory depression. These medications can be combined with acetaminophen, hydroxyzine hydrochloride, or promethazine. Aspirin should be avoided because it

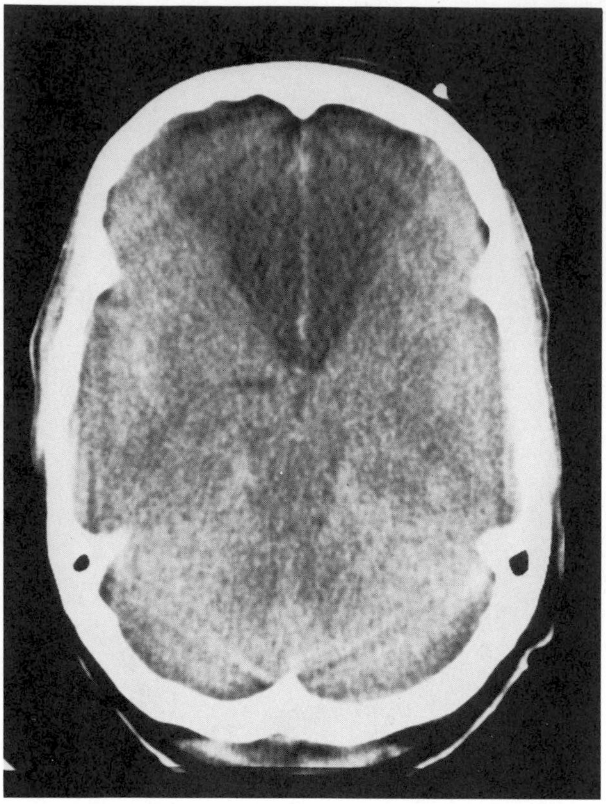

**Fig. 45-5.** Bilateral hypodensities in the distribution of both anterior cerebral arteries secondary to vasospasm in a patient with a ruptured anterior communicating artery aneurysm. Note the small amount of blood anteriorly in the interhemispheric fissure.

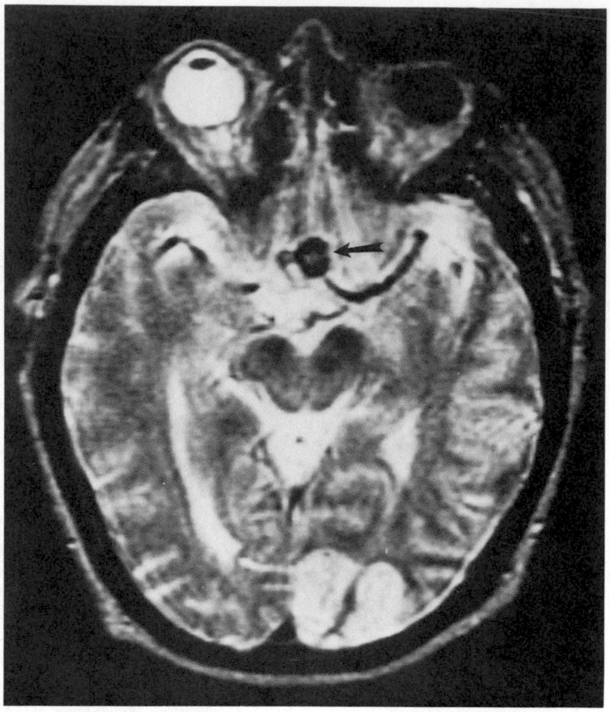

**Fig. 45-6.** T2-weighted magnetic resonance imaging in a patient with an anterior communicating artery aneurysm. A flow void is visualized (*arrow*).

prolongs the bleeding time. Some patients will have photophobia and phonophobia; a quiet, dark environment will help relieve some of these symptoms that may aggravate the headache. Sedation and sleep may help pain.

Severe nausea and intense vomiting are frequent and important complaints, particularly during the first 24 hours after SAH.[2,18,178,211] Patients should receive antiemetics such as trimethobenzamide (200-mg suppositories) or prochlorperazine (5 to 10 mg parenterally) to control these sympotoms.

## Anticonvulsants

Approximately 25 percent of patients will have seizures; most occur within the first 24 hours.[75,185] Hart et al.[75] noted that 63 percent of the seizures were at the time of aneurysmal rupture. Many "seizures" at the time of SAH are not truly epileptic but can represent transient decerebrate posturing secondary to increased intracranial pressure.[49,75] There is no correlation between epileptic seizures at the time of aneurysm rupture and the risk of rebleeding, early mortality, or major morbidity.[75,185] Although seizures after hospitalization are uncommon, they can be associated with recurrent hemorrhage. While physicians do prescribe anticonvulsants to a patient who has had a seizure as part of SAH, the prophylactic use of these drugs in patients who have not had seizures is controversial. No trial has tested the potential value of anticonvulsants in this group of patients. Because of the low rate of seizures after admission, Hart et al.[75] and Sundaram and Chow[185] doubted the need for routine administration of anticonvulsants to patients with recent SAH. However, others advise regular administration of either phenobarbital or phenytoin to reduce the risk of seizures.[2,33,178,211] The rationale for anticonvulsant treatment is that a seizure is a dangerous event in a patient with a recent SAH.

Pending a trial, the decision to prescribe anticonvulsants must be individualized. The benefit of anticonvulsants in seizure prophylaxis must be weighed against potential adverse reactions. The risk of major side effects to phenytoin and phenobarbital is so low that their administration during the first few weeks after SAH or until the aneurysm has been clipped seems prudent. Phenytoin is usually given orally in a dosage of 300 to 400 mg/day with adjustment of dosage based on serum levels and clinical responses. Phenobarbital is usually administered in a dosage of 120 to 240 mg/day and has the advantage of also providing sedation for agitated patients. If a patient is having convulsions, intravenous doses of anticonvulsants should be given.

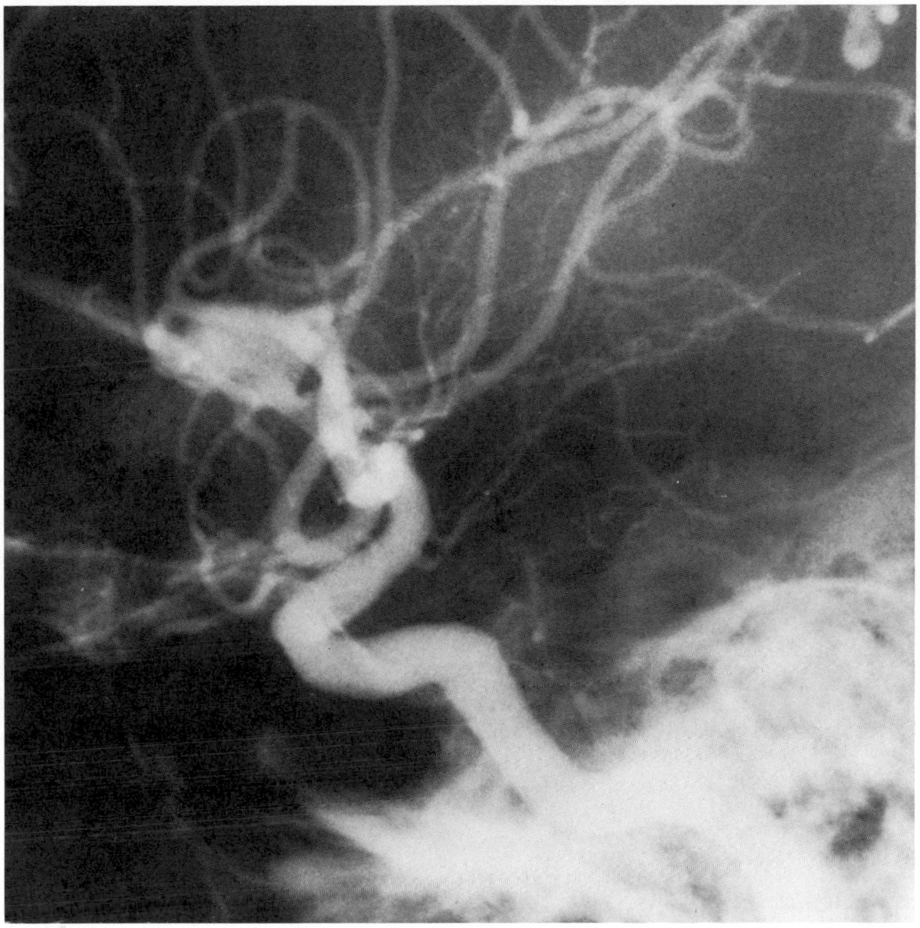

**Fig. 45-7.** Lateral view of a selective left carotid arteriogram demonstrating a large aneurysm of the anterior communicating and anterior cerebral arteries.

## Myocardial Ischemia and Cardiac Arrhythmias

Cardiac arrhythmias can be detected in almost all patients during the first few hours after SAH and in 20 percent arrhythmias are severe or life-threatening[37,45] (Table 45-5). Ventricular arrhythmias may be one of the causes of sudden death after SAH. Di Pasquale et al. noted torsade de pointes (a chaotic form of ventricular tachycardia with the QRS complexes varying between positive and negative polarity) in 3.8 percent of 132 patients who had Holter monitoring.[37] The severe arrhythmias were found in patients who had hypokalemia. Electrocardiographic changes that resemble those of acute myocardial ischemia are noted in 50 to 80 percent of all patients.[36,60,73,116,184] In fact, many patients with SAH have secondary myocardial ischemia. Subendocardial areas of focal ischemic necrosis are found among patients who had no history of coronary artery disease and who died of acute SAH.[105] Elevations of the cardiac isoenzymes of creatine kinase are also noted.[46,129]

SAH stimulates release of catecholamines by the posterior hypothalamus. Markedly elevated levels of norepinephrine can lead to hypokalemia, systemic hypertensive effects, left ventricular strain, coronary artery vasospasm or cardiac toxicity.[116] These effects can lead to myocardial ischemia or cardiac rhythm disturbances. Administration of a beta blocker such as propranolol may reduce the number and severity of cardiac sequelae.[44] In a small study, Neil-Dwyer et

**TABLE 45-5. Electrocardiographic Abnormalities After Subarachnoid Hemorrhage**

| |
|---|
| Prominent P waves |
| Prolonged or shortened P-R interval |
| Broad, inverted or flattened T waves |
| Q-T prolongation or shortening |
| ST segment elevation or depression |
| Prominent or inverted U waves |
| Pathological Q waves |
| S in $V_1$ and R in $V_5$ combined > 35 mm |
| Rhythm disturbances |

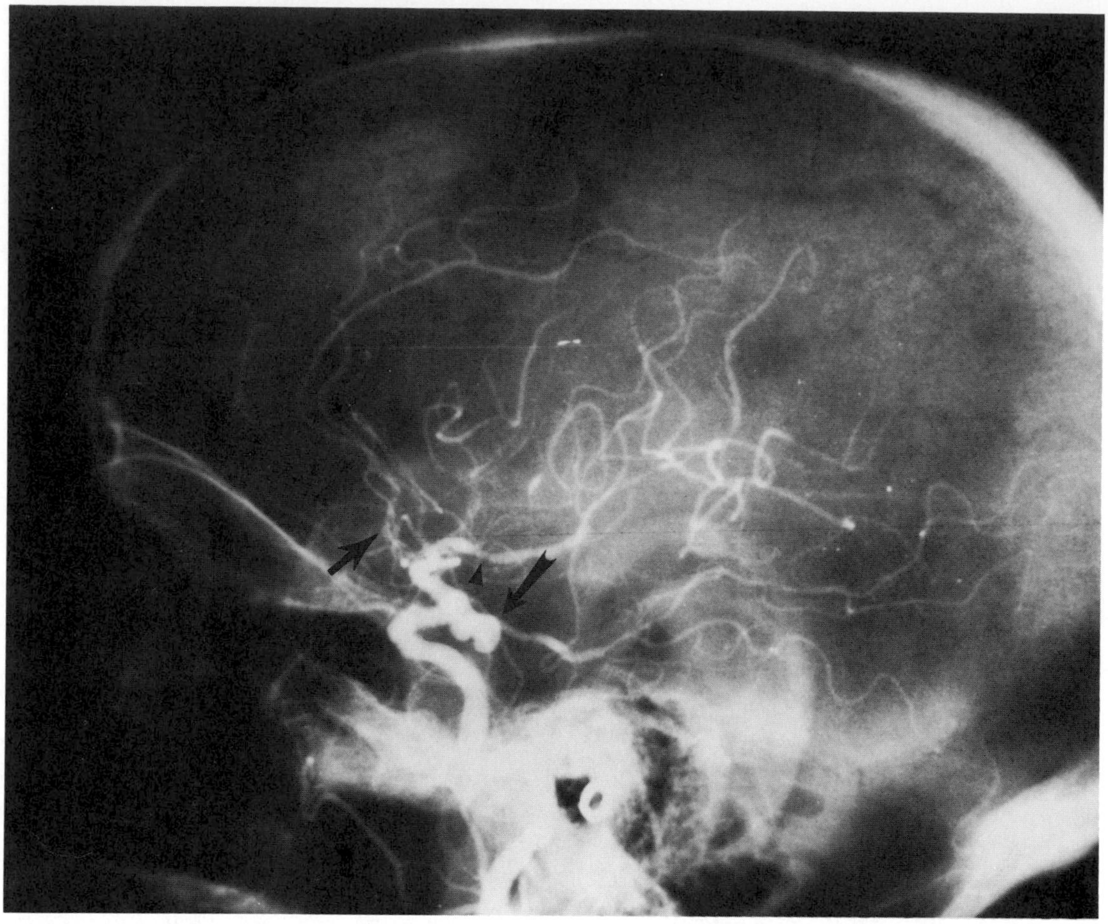

**Fig. 45-8.** A lateral view of the left carotid artery in a patient with a ruptured internal carotid artery aneurysm (*large arrow*). There is severe vasospasm with marked narrowing of the middle cerebral artery (*arrowhead*) and severe narrowing of the proximal anterior cerebral artery (*small arrow*).

al.[130] noted necrotic myocardial lesions in six patients who died after SAH and who had not taken propranolol and no necrotic lesions among six patients who died and who had been administered the drug. However, Marion et al.[116] concluded that there is insufficient evidence to support the routine use of propranolol. Further study of the potential value of a beta blocker or calcium channel blocker in reducing the cardiac sequelae of SAH is needed. A particularly vulnerable subgroup of patients may exist. Pending more definitive data, administration of these drugs should be decided on a case-by-case basis; there appears little reason to routinely administer drugs to all patients. Since the first 24 to 48 hours is the period of highest risk for cardiac complications, there is little justification to initiate routine administration of these drugs after that time period.

Neurogenic pulmonary edema is a rare but severe complication of SAH. It usually occurs in critically ill patients. Markedly increased extravascular lung water and intrapulmonary shunt lead to hypoxia. This complication has been frequently ascribed to increased sympathetic activity that leads to heart failure and vascular congestion. However, Touho et al.[194] suggest that high levels of vasogenic substances lead to increased permeability of pulmonary tissues. Treatment is difficult but includes oxygen and positive pressure ventilatory assistance.

## Antihypertensives

Arterial hypertension is commonly noted after SAH (Table 45-2). Arterial hypertension may result from elevated catecholamines and renins produced by hypothalamic disturbances.[116,131] Elevated intracranial pressure may induce arterial hypertension in an attempt to maintain adequate cerebral perfusion pressure. Elevated blood pressure may alleviate cerebral ischemic symptoms due to intracranial hypertension or vasospasm.[106] Arterial hypertension may also be secondary to seizures, vomiting, agitation, or pain. In addition, many patients have preexisting hypertension.

Hypertension after SAH is correlated with an increased rate of vasospasm and higher mortality.[39] Arterial hypertension also marks patients at high risk for recurrent hemorrhage. Treatment of hypertension is a traditional component of early management of SAH.[2,18,33,146,178,211] However, rapid or major reductions of blood pressure with secondary decline in cerebral perfusion pressure may be dangerous. Patients with vasospasm or increased intracranial pressure can have worsening of neurologic deficits or deterioration in level of consciousness in conjunction with a drop in blood pressure. In addition, some antihypertensive drugs (nitroglycerine, sodium nitroprusside, apresoline) are cerebrovasodilators. Resultant enlargement of the vascular bed might independently increase intracranial pressure.

Blood pressure often returns to normal levels after admission to the hospital and after symptoms such as pain are treated, and administration of an antihypertensive drug may be avoided. Patients with mild hypertension (mean arterial blood pressure less than 120 torr) should not receive antihypertensive drugs. Persons with a mean arterial blood pressure above 120 torr or a systolic blood pressure higher than 180 torr should be treated.[18] The therapeutic goal should be to reach blood pressure levels that are normal for the patient and to avoid hypotension. A reasonable target is a mean arterial blood pressure of 100 to 120 torr.

While alert patients with elevated arterial blood pressure can be given oral medications, parenteral drugs have the advantage of a prompt response. Antihypertensive drugs that were used prior to SAH are usually continued and should not be abruptly stopped. Short-acting antihypertensive drugs are desirable because of rapid resolution of partially desired effects. Because patients are often dehydrated or hyponatremic after SAH, diuretics should be avoided. Propranolol (20 to 40 mg every 6 hours), hydralazine (10 to 25 mg every 6 hours), or labetalol (200 to 400 mg/day) are the most frequently prescribed oral antihypertensives. Nimodipine or nicardipine may be found to be useful antihypertensive agents in patients with recent SAH. Patients who are unable to take oral medications or who are not responding to these agents may require parenteral hydralazine in a dosage of 10 to 25 mg every 4 to 6 hours. Patients with markedly elevated or unstable arterial pressures may warrant a continuous intravenous infusion of labetalol or sodium nitroprusside. The rate of the infusion is adjusted to the blood pressure response. These drugs should be given only if continuous intra-arterial or noninvasive blood pressure monitoring is also performed. The dosage of any antihypertensive drug must be individualized. Patients with SAH are often very sensitive to antihypertensive therapy and drops in blood pressure may be greater than expected.[26] Required doses may be less than those needed for other hypertensive emergencies.

Drug-induced hypotension might help prevent rebleeding. In a randomized trial, the Cooperative Aneurysm Study[134] compared drug-induced hypotension to bed rest. Vigorous administration of antihypertensives was associated with a 2-week mortality of 25 percent and a rebleeding rate of 20 percent. These rates were similar to those noted with bed rest. However, this study was performed more than 20 years ago and the antihypertensive drugs tested included diuretics, reserpine, and methyldopa. Newer antihypertensive drugs such as calcium channel blockers, selective beta blockers, or angiotensin converting enzyme inhibitors might be more effective and safer. Long-term administration of antihypertensive drugs has been proposed as an alternative to surgical clipping of the aneurysm for prevention of recurrent hemorrhage.[179] This approach has not gain widespread acceptance.

## Management of Electrolytes and Fluids

Disturbances in water and sodium balance occur in approximately one-third of patients.[218] Hyponatremia and volume depletion are correlated with a poor prognosis. These complications are most likely to occur in critically ill patients with large hemorrhages. Hyponatremia is associated with the subsequent development of hydrocephalus, vasospasm, and ischemic stroke. Severe hyponatremia can cause convulsions and is one of the reversible causes of coma after SAH.[128] The primary indication for rapid correction of hyponatremia is development of confusion or seizures in a patient without neurologic disease; however, this indication becomes blurred in patients with recent SAH. Conventional management of mild to moderate hyponatremia is fluid restriction. More vigorous treatment of hyponatremia consists of intravenous administration of hypertonic saline combined with a diuretic, such as furosemide, to prevent cardiac failure.

In the past, hyponatremia after SAH was usually attributed to inappropriate secretion of antidiuretic hormone and was treated with fluid restriction.[33,146,211] Recent evidence suggests that both sodium and water are lost after SAH.[118,132,182,218,219] Hyponatremia after SAH is not a simple dilutional problem that can be corrected solely by water restriction. Declines in plasma volume, red blood cell mass, and total blood volume occur.[132,182,219] A negative sodium balance results from the kidney's inability to conserve sodium (cerebral salt wasting).[38,132] The mechanism of water and sodium loss after SAH has not been explained. Recently, increased blood levels of atrial natriuretic factor have been implicated.[38,164] Levels of atrial natriuretic factor peak at 3 days after SAH and then fall by 7 days after the ictus.[38] Elevations in blood exceed those noted in CSF and are related to the severity of SAH.[164] The source of plasma and CSF atrial natriuretic factor is presumably the heart, not the brain.[164] Weinand et al.[210] suggested that interplay between antidiuretic hormone and atrial natriuretic factor may differ considerably between patients. Delineation of subgroups may have prognostic and therapeutic implications. Further research on the roles of antidiuretic hormone and atrial natriuretic factor in the water disorders after SAH is needed.

Fluid restriction to control hyponatremia and the development of cerebral edema after SAH has been attempted. In a randomized study, Nibbelink et al.[135] reported no improvement in mortality with strict fluid restriction. Restriction of fluids did not reduce problems with cerebral edema and was complicated by renal dysfunction. In addition, compliance with the strict fluid restriction was difficult to achieve.

Strict fluid restriction can be dangerous because it leads to contracted blood volume, increased blood viscosity, and hemoconcentration. These changes might increase the risk of cerebral ischemia in patients developing vasospasm after SAH. Wijdicks et al.[218] noted 21 infarctions among 26 patients who had fluid restriction to correct hyponatremia, and 6 infarctions in 18 patients who had hyponatremia but received normal volume of fluid. Solomon et al.[182] noted that 6 of 7 patients with symptomatic vasospasm had contracted red blood cell and total blood volumes. They concluded that volume status may be an important difference between asymptomatic and symptomatic vasospasm.

In contrast to previous attempts to restrict fluids, most patients are now given at least maintenance volumes of crystalloid and colloid solutions. The usual daily administration of liquids, including dietary and intravenous fluids, should be at least 2 to 3 liters. Additional fluids may be required, depending upon urinary or insensible water losses. Measurements of daily fluid intakes and losses expedite administration of supplemental fluids. Hypo-osmolar solutions should be avoided. If there is concern about the intravenous fluids inducing cardiac failure, a solution containing a low concentration of sodium can be used. Placement of a central venous pressure or pulmonary artery wedge pressure line to evaluate the cardiac status of patients given large volumes of fluids may improve safety. If the serum sodium does not normalize, a modest fluid restriction or infusion of a hyperosmolar solution can be instituted. Simultaneous use of diuretics should be avoided because they induce natriuresis as well as water loss. Volume expansion with both crystalloid and colloid fluids is now regularly given to patients with symptomatic vasospasm. This regimen is described in more detail subsequently.

Wijdicks et al.[220] administered 0.2 mg of fludrocortisone twice a day combined with daily fluid intake of at least 3 liters to 39 patients with recent SAH. Less severe declines in plasma volume and sodium balance were noted than in previously treated patients. Kassell et al.[97] used fludrocortisone or deoxycorticosterone acetate as adjunctive agents in managing symptomatic vasospasm. The addition of fludrocortisone to vigorous hydration may reduce severe water disturbances. This therapy warrants further testing.

Hypokalemia is often noted after SAH. It probably results from vomiting or can be secondary to elevated corticosteroids, renin, or catecholamines.[34] Hypokalemia has been associated with life-threatening cardiac arrhythmias after SAH.[37] It should be rapidly corrected.

## Management of Other Medical Complications

The acute neurologic event can cause hemorrhagic gastritis or stress gastric ulcers. Frequent vomiting or retching may lead to esophageal tears. These may lead to severe upper gastrointestinal bleeding. Patients should be given antacids every 4 to 6 hours in an effort to reduce the risk of these complications; dosages can be administered via a nasogastric tube placed in obtunded patients.[211] Ranitidine (150 mg orally twice a day) or cimetidine (400 mg orally twice a day) can also be given.

Obtunded patients are at risk for atelectasis, pulmonary hypoventilation, or aspiration pneumonia. Securing the airway, bronchopulmonary toilet and ventilatory assistance may be required. Other events such as renal failure, hepatic dysfunction, urinary tract infections, or other infections may also develop. Treatment of preexisting medical conditions should be continued.

## Treatment of Increased Intracranial Pressure

Decline in consciousness is the hallmark of increased intracranial pressure. Increased intracranial pressure results from a large intracerebral or intraventricular hematoma, mass effect of a secondary ischemic lesion, cerebral edema, or hydrocephalus. SAH also causes vasoparalysis and loss of autoregulation; dilated intracranial vessels will aggravate intracranial pressure. Intracranial pressure within a few minutes of aneurysmal rupture SAH is markedly elevated.[70,206] Intracranial pressure may equal mean arterial blood pressure and thus stop bleeding from the aneurysm, but it can also lead to intracranial circulatory arrest, inducing coma and possibly cerebral ischemia. A massive rise in intracranial pressure is one of the causes of sudden death after SAH and is probably one of the etiologies for several of the other acute complications, including cardiac arrhythmias. Prolonged and markedly elevated intracranial pressure can lead to cerebral ischemia and herniation. Increased intracranial pressure is directly related to death of comatose or critically patients. Prompt and aggressive management of increased intracranial pressure is the key to the acute treatment of patients with SAH.

Several medical and surgical measures to control intracranial hypertension may be attempted. In many patients, intracranial pressure monitoring is indicated; it will guide the timing of surgical or medical interventions.[42,162] Technological advances permit stereotactic placement of microscopic transducers in the brain or ventricles which accurately measure intracranial pressure. These measures are not accompanied by a prohibitively high rate of complications. Continuous intraventricular drainage combined with monitoring is an option, but this technique may be dangerous. Sudden reduction of intracranial pressure may precipitate recurrent rupture of an aneurysm by increasing transmural pressure.[207]

Treatment to control cerebral edema and increased intracranial pressure includes raising the head of the bed to promote venous drainage, fluid restriction, correction of hyponatremia, and prevention of hypoventilation and secondary hypercarbia. Intubation and hyperventilation are indicated when a patient is deteriorating. The most frequently prescribed medications are dexamethasone in daily doses of 16 to 24 mg or methylprednisolone, 90 to 120 mg/day. This therapy is controversial. There is no evidence that they are clinically useful in managing cerebral edema after intracranial hemorrhage.[191] While steroids might reduce the inflammatory reaction to blood in the subarachnoid space, theoretically diminishing headache, meningeal signs, and hydrocephalus, there is no evidence for these potential benefits. Use of steroids can be complicated by infections, gastrointestinal bleeding, and hyperglycemia. Because of the lack of established benefit in controlling intracranial hypertension and because of the many potential side effects, steroids should not be given.

Furosemide may reduce intracranial pressure by inhibiting production of CSF. It can be given in an acute emergency in a dose of 40 mg given intravenously and repeated as necessary. However, its diuretic effects can lead to electrolyte disturbances and hypovolemia. There are no studies testing its value in the management of recent SAH. While the administration of furosemide should be limited, it might be given as an adjunctive measure in rapidly deteriorating patients.

Mannitol is an osmotic agent that can be given intermittently to control increased intracranial pressure. The usual dose is 0.25 to 0.5 g/kg in a 20 percent concentration administered over 20 minutes.[119] A response is noted within minutes and the duration of action is approximately 4 to 6 hours. The drug can be repeated as needed. Larger doses of mannitol (1 g/kg) may be needed for a deteriorating patient. Secondary dehydration, hyperosmolarity, and a rebound increase in cerebral edema are possible complications of frequent doses of mannitol. If sequential doses of mannitol are required, urinary output should be compensated by intravenous fluids. Repeated measurements of serum electrolytes and osmolality should also be done. Measurement of central venous pressure or pulmonary wedge pressure will also improve safety of this treatment.

Barbiturates have been used to control intractable intracranial hypertension that complicates a number of acute neurologic diseases, including SAH. However, patients placed in a barbiturate-induced coma require costly and extensive supportive care, and there are no reports demonstrating efficacy of this regimen in patients with SAH.

Emergent surgical evacuation of a large hematoma may be needed to control intracranial hypertension or prevent herniation. Large intracerebral hematomas, usually in the basal ganglia and adjacent white matter are most frequent with ruptured internal carotid aneurysms or middle cerebral artery aneurysms.[23,144] Early surgical evacuation of the hematoma can be life-saving and should be offered for deteriorating patients.[23,144,190] Some patients can recover and return to independent activity. Patients who are in better clinical condition and with a ruptured middle cerebral artery aneurysm are most likely to benefit from a surgical approach.[190] Patients with a large hematoma, extensive intraventricular hemorrhage, or shift of midline structures on CT have the poorest postoperative outcomes.[144] Unfortunately, these are the patients most frequently referred to surgery. Operatively treated patients who are less severely damaged may have better outcomes. Surgical evacuation of a large hematoma should be a therapeutic option in any patient not responding to medical measures.

## Hydrocephalus

Hydrocephalus is an important complication of SAH that acutely leads to increased intracranial pressure or chronically leads to brain dysfunction. Heros[78] divided hydrocephalus after SAH into three categories: (1) acute—appearing within hours of aneurysmal rupture, (2) subacute—developing a few days after the ictus, and (3) delayed—ventricular dilatation noted weeks to years later. SAH is one of the leading causes of the syndrome of normal pressure hydrocephalus. Massive collections of blood can fill the ventricles, block the aqueduct of Sylvius, or obstruct the fourth ventricle. Subarachnoid collections can also fill the subarachnoid cisterns or coat the arachnoid villi. The prolonged presence of extensive subarachnoid clots is strongly associated with the appearance of hydrocephalus; thus, an intervention that prolongs the presence of these clots may promote development of hydrocephalus. Conversely, treatments that stimulate clot lysis may prevent hydrocephalus from developing.

Acute hydrocephalus is an important cause of massively increased intracranial pressure, and it requires treatment. It is usually associated with coma. Subacute hydrocephalus is a potential cause of a gradual decline in consciousness that occurs a few days after SAH. Intracranial pressure is more modestly elevated, and this pattern of hydrocephalus appears to be less serious than the acute ventricular dilation.[78] Symptoms of delayed hydrocephalus are a subacute dementia, gait apraxia, and bladder incontinence. Intracranial pressure is often not elevated.

Depending upon the criteria used for the diagnosis of hydrocephalus, its incidence has varied considerably between series. Based on CT evidence of ventricular enlargement, Black[19] diagnosed the presence of acute hydrocephalus in 63 percent of patients. Others have reported a frequency of 16 to 34 percent.[59,76,84,122,157,169,197,200] Recently, Graff-Radford et al.[68] reported that CT evidence of ventricular dilation was noted in 15 percent of 3,521 patients admitted to a hospital within 3 days of SAH. The frequency of symptomatic acute hydrocephalus is lower (13.2 percent).[68] Van Gijn et al.[197] noted depressed consciousness in 30 of 34 patients, while Hasen et al.[76] noted normal alertness in 25 of 91 patients within ventricular dilation. Besides a decline in consciousness, other symptoms of acute hydrocephalus include bilateral motor signs, miosis, and downward deviation of the eyes.[157,197] The rate of delayed communicating hydrocephalus after SAH is reported to be 7 percent.[197]

Acute hydrocephalus predicts increased mortality and morbidity after SAH.[19,197] In one series of 34 patients with acute hydrocephalus, 20 died.[197] Acute hydrocephalus has also been correlated with subsequent development of vasospasm.[19]

While acute hydrocephalus may spontaneously resolve,[76] most patients require placement of a temporary ventriculoperitoneal or ventriculocaval shunt.[78,108,169,190,200,227] Placement of a ventricular catheter may be difficult in a patient with a major intraventricular hemorrhage. Clots may occlude the catheter. Shunting is not always effective; in one series no patient recovered.[77] Hasan et al.[76] reported a high rate of shunt-related complications, including intracranial infections. Others have not reported similar rates.[23] A patient with subacute hydrocephalus can be observed, medically managed, and followed with sequential CT examinations. They can be treated with steroids, mannitol, or repeated lumbar puncture.[23] Placement of a shunt should be recommended in any patient with a depressed consciousness or progressively enlarging ventricles. Some patients will require only temporary placement of a shunt. If necessary, the shunt can later be made permanent.

## REBLEEDING

Recurrent hemorrhage is one of the two most feared complications of SAH. It is a leading cause of death or neurologic morbidity during the first 2 weeks after SAH and it is largely a fatal complication.[7,90] The mortality rate among patients who have rebleeding is approximatley twice that of patients with a single hemorrhage. Not infrequently an alert patient is seen in an emergency room because of a severe headache and is discharged only to return with a second cataclysmic hemorrhage. This scenario might be avoided by early diagnosis and treatment.

Preventing recurrent hemorrhage is one of the major goals of medical management. Torner et al.[193] found that the greatest risk period for rebleeding is during the first 24 hours after the ictus; rebleeding is noted in approximately 4 percent of patients during that period. In a Swedish series 9.6 percent of all patients admitted within 24 hours of SAH had very early rebleeding; most of these patients died.[85] This high rate of rebleeding has implications for the choice of medical or surgical treatment. Rebleeding may occur before a surgical team can be mobilized or before a drug may reach "therapeutic" levels in blood and CSF.

The cumulative rate of rebleeding during the first 2 weeks after SAH is approximately 15 to 25 percent.[21,150,163,193,217] Thereafter the rate of rebleeding declines quickly. The rate of rebleeding is 0.5 percent/day for the time period 10 to 30 days after SAH.[217] The rate of rebleeding after 1 month following SAH drops to 2 to 3 percent/year and persists at that level for at least the next 10 years.[193,217] Several clinical features identify persons at highest risk for early rebleeding.[193] The most important predictor is admitting level of consciousness. Patients in coma after a major SAH are at greatest risk of rebleeding. Rebleeding is also more common among older patients, women, and those with a systolic blood pressure above 170 torr.[203,222] The results of baseline CT do not consistently predict rebleeding.

Recurrent hemorrhage usually presents with a sudden change in neurologic condition with new headache and decline in consciousness. Extensor spasms or posturing may be an important early sign.[196] A convulsion that occurs during the acute period after SAH often marks a recurrent hemorrhage.[75] Rebleeding in a comatose patient may be overlooked and may be manifested only by a sudden change in respiratory pattern. Rebleeding should be sought in any patient who develops a new headache or suddenly worsens after SAH. The differential diagnosis of rebleeding is listed in Table 45-6. The clinical diagnosis of rebleeding may be incorrect in as many as one-third of

**TABLE 45-6. Differential Diagnosis of Neurologic Worsening After Subarachnoid Hemorrhage**

| |
|---|
| Recurrent hemorrhage |
| Vasospasm–cerebral ischemia |
| Hydrocephalus |
| Convulsions |
| Hyponatremia |
| Hypocalcemia |
| Hypotension |
| Hypoxia |
| Effects from drugs |

cases.[203] In one series of 62 patients with episodes of neurologic deterioration, 42 events were due to recurrent hemorrhage, but others were secondary to seizures, ischemia, or medical complications.[203] The diagnosis of rebleeding should not be made solely on clinical features, as this may lead to overdiagnosis.[196] Recurrent hemorrhage can be proved in most cases by the presence of additional blood on CT or in the CSF. CT is the best diagnostic study (Table 45-7). Van Crevel[196] pointed out that the CSF findings may be difficult to interpret.

Because there are no effective measures to ameliorate recurrent hemorrhage, treatment is aimed at prevention. Choices include prolonged bed rest, drug-induced hypotension, carotid ligation, antifibrinolytic drugs, and intracranial clipping of the aneurysm. The utility of forced bed rest and drug-induced hypotension in preventing rebleeding have been discussed previously.

Carotid ligation can be performed to prevent rebleeding from aneurysms of the distal internal carotid artery that cannot be approached by an intracranial operation. The purpose of this procedure is to reduce transmural pressure on the aneurysmal wall and thus lower the risk of recurrent rupture. Reducing perfusion may also predispose to thrombosis of the aneurysm. The rate of rebleeding is reduced by internal carotid ligation; the Cooperative Aneurysm Study noted that recurrent rupture occurred in 10.4 percent of 125 patients who had successful ligation.[148] Ligation of the internal carotid artery may be associated with infarction of the ipsilateral hemisphere. In the Cooperative Aneurysm Study, cerebral ischemic complications secondary to attempted or completed internal carotid ligation developed in 36.3 percent of patients.[148] Ligation of the common carotid artery rather than the internal carotid artery may lessen the risk of cerebral ischemia. Creation of an extracranial-intracranial arterial anastomosis may lower the risk of ischemia secondary to internal carotid ligation. Due to advances in intracranial operative techniques, development of invasive neuroradiologic procedures and persistent concerns about ischemic complications, carotid ligation is now rarely done. It should be limited to exceptional cases of large aneurysms in or near the cavernous sinus.

**TABLE 45-7. Diagnostic Studies That May Be Useful in the Evaluation of Patients with Neurologic Deterioration After Aneurysmal Subarachnoid Hemorrhage**

| Procedure | Reasons |
|---|---|
| Computed tomography | ? rebleeding, infarction edema, hydrocephalus |
| Electroencephalogram | ? convulsions |
| Transcranial Doppler | ? vasospasm |
| Cerebral blood flow study | ? vasospasm |
| Arteriography | ? vasospasm |
| Cerebrospinal fluid examination | ? rebleeding |
| Arterial blood gases | ? hypoxia, acidosis |
| Chest x-ray | ? pneumonia, pulmonary embolus, congestive heart failure |
| Electrocardiogram | ? arrhythmia, myocardial ischemia |
| Blood glucose | ? hyper-, hypoglycemia |
| Serum sodium | ? hyper-, hyponatremia |
| Serum calcium | ? hyper-, hypocalcemia |
| Serum magnesium | ? hyper-, hypomagnesemia |
| Cultures urine, blood, sputum | ? infection |
| Drug levels | ? excessive dosages: sedatives, anticonvulsants |

## Antifibrinolytic Therapy

Reports by Gibbs and O'Gorman[63] and by Mullan and Dawley[126] in the late 1960s stimulated study on the possible usefulness of antifibrinolytic drugs in the management of patients with recent SAH. At that time, early intracranial operations were not considered practical and medical management including drug-induced hypotension had not been shown to be useful in preventing rebleeding. A medical therapy before operation was needed to prevent rebleeding while the patient was recovering from the acute effects of the SAH.

The rationale for antifibrinolytic therapy is that the perianeurysmal clot formed by the initial hemorrhage can support the aneurysmal wall and prevent rerupture. Fibrinolytic activity of the CSF is stimulated after SAH, and enhanced lysis could lead to dissolution of this supportive clot.[55] This assumption has been challenged by Steinmetz and Grote,[183] who could not find increased CSF fibrinolytic activity. Rebleeding might be avoided if a drug could suppress antifibrinolytic activity and allow the clot to persist. Aminocaproic acid and tranexamic acid are the two drugs that have been most extensively studied. These drugs inhibit plasminogen activation of plasmin, thus stabilizing the fibrin clot. While antifibrinolytic drugs cross the blood-brain barrier, peak CSF levels are lower than plasma levels and are also delayed.[56,195] When given orally, levels in blood reach a maximal concentration in 2 hours.[117] Because of rapid renal clearance, frequent oral doses are required to maintain therapeutic levels. These drugs can also be given intravenously. If the drugs are given as a constant infusion without a loading bolus dose, a steady state in CSF can be reached in 36 hours. This means that the possible therapeutic level of the drug in CSF will not be achieved during the period of highest risk for recurrent hemorrhage. A 5-g intravenous loading dose of aminocaproic acid followed by constant infusion at a rate of 1 to 1½ g/h may permit rapid achievement of therapeutic levels.

Antifibrinolytic drugs are the subject of much controversy.[3,213] A number of small, uncontrolled studies or small, controlled trials give conflicting results.[13,28,29,54,61,102,120,176,199] These trials were reviewed by

Ramirez-Lassepas,[158] who noted numerous methodologic flaws and concluded that there was no evidence that antifibrinolytic drugs alter the natural history of SAH. In an independent critique, Vermeulen and Muizelaar[202] reached a similar conclusion.

A randomized, placebo-controlled trial of tranexamic acid in prevention of rebleeding in 479 patients seen within 3 days of SAH was performed in the Netherlands and United Kingdom.[201] This is the first large randomized trial of any single treatment in patients with recent SAH. Unfortunately, only 285 randomized patients were found to have arteriographic evidence of an intracranial aneurysm. Mortality was 28 percent among 130 patients with aneurysms, who were treated with tranexamic acid, and was 32 percent among 155 patients with aneurysms, who received placebo. This is not a significant difference. Rebleeding was significantly reduced to 9 percent with the use of tranexamic acid, compared to 24 percent with placebo. However, the positive effects in preventing rebleeding were negated by a significantly higher rate of ischemic stroke in the actively treated group (24 percent) compared to the placebo group (15 percent). Among the placebo-treated group, 51 percent of the deaths were secondary to rebleeding and 27 percent to ischemic stroke; among the patients given tranexamic acid, 23 percent of the deaths were due to recurrent hemorrhage and 45 percent were secondary to ischemic stroke. The reduction in mortality due to rebleeding being counteracted by increased mortality secondary to ischemia is similar to the results noted after early intracranial operation.

As a side project of the International Study on the Timing of Aneurysm Surgery, Kassell et al.[99] compared the results of treatment of 467 patients scheduled for delayed operation, who also received antifibrinolytic drugs, with 205 patients who did not receive either tranexamic acid or aminocaproic acid. While this was not a randomized trial, the two populations were very similar. Antifibrinolytic drugs reduced the 14-day rebleeding rate from 19.4 to 11.7 percent. However, ischemic deficits were more common with antifibrinolytic therapy, 32.4 percent versus 22.7 percent. The mortality rates at 30 days were similar between the two groups. Both studies demonstrated a lag in the therapeutic response of approximately 36 hours. This lag corresponds to the time required to achieve "therapeutic" CSF levels of tranexamic acid and aminocephalic acid.

There are major concerns about the safety of antifibrinolytic drugs. Although these critically ill patients are at bed rest for prolonged periods, the incidence of deep-vein thrombosis and pulmonary embolism is not high.[8] Oral administration of tranexamic acid can be accompanied by diarrhea. A fulminant myopathy, with rhabdomyolysis and myoglobinuria, may complicate prolonged administration (more than 2 weeks) of high doses of aminocaproic acid.[24,25,27,198] The myopathy may be secondary to intramuscular vascular occlusion and ischemia. Glick et al.[66] noted that high doses of aminocaproic acid can increase bleeding by its inhibitory effects on platelet function. This qualitative platelet defect can predispose to bleeding into the skin and other sites. It is possible that this qualitative platelet defect can explain some of the episodes of recurrent SAH. Antifibrinolytic drugs accentuate the development of hydrocephalus after SAH.[68,143,152] In the experience of Kassell et al.[99] the rate of hydrocephalus was increased from 6.8 to 13.5 percent with the administration of antifibrinolytic drugs. Graff-Radford et al.[68] noted a highly significant correlation between the preoperative use of antifibrinolytic drugs and the development of hydrocephalus; clinical hydrocephalus was diagnosed in 11.4 percent of 2,078 patients who did not receive this therapy and in 15.9 percent of 1,443 patients who did.

Cerebral ischemia is a possible side effect of antifibrinolytic therapy. Approximately 20 percent of 1,114 patients given either aminocaproic acid or tranexamic acid developed focal neurologic symptoms that could be attributed to ischemia.[8] Kassell et al.[99] and Vermeulen et al.[201] demonstrated that ischemic events negate the efficacy of antifibrinolytic therapy. The risk of ischemia with antifibrinolytic drugs markedly increases at approximately the seventh day after SAH. The increased risk of cerebral ischemia might be the result of (1) a persistent subarachnoid clot that induces vasospasm, (2) an intravascular change in coagulation that potentiates intra-arterial thrombosis or embolism, or (3) a change in blood viscosity. Recently, Beck et al.[17] noted that the combination of nicardipine and aminocaproic acid could be successfully given; the rates of rebleeding and ischemic stroke were very low.

Antifibrinolytic drugs are the only effective medical therapy in reducing the risk of early rebleeding after SAH. They remain an important part of the preoperative care of patients with SAH who are scheduled for delayed surgery. The established risks of antifibrinolytic therapy must be weighed against the benefits of preventing recurrent hemorrhage. While not proved, early bolus administration of drug followed by a constant intravenous maintenance infusion might prevent some instances of early rebleeding. Although the optimal dose is not established, most previous studies have used 24 to 36 g aminocaproic acid or 6 to 12 g tranexamic acid daily. The duration of therapy should be limited to 10 to 14 days, and the drug should be stopped 6 to 8 hours before surgery. Therapy should not be instituted in patients with delayed diagnosis because patients surviving 7 to 14 days after SAH have already passed the period of highest risk of rebleeding. There is little indication to give these drugs to patients with nonaneurysmal hemorrhages. This therapy should not be administered to a patient scheduled for early intracranial operation.

## Intracranial Operation

Surgery is an important component of overall management. Surgery may be required to clip an aneurysm to prevent rebleeding, to place a shunt to treat hydrocephalus, or to evacuate a life-threatening intracerebral hematoma. The indications for surgery to treat a hematoma or hydrocephalus have been discussed previously.

Most patients should have operative treatment of the aneurysm. Rare exceptions should be considered on a case-by-case basis. The age of the patient, seriousness of the neurologic injury, or the presence of serious comorbid diseases may weigh against an intracranial operation. While persons older than 60 may tolerate intracranial operation less well than younger persons, chronological age alone should not be a reason for not performing surgery. Amacher et al.[12] noted that good outcomes after operation occurred in 82 percent of persons younger than 60 and in 72 percent of older patients.

For most patients, the question should not be whether surgery should be done but rather when should surgery be performed. The optimal time for intracranial operation has not been established. In the past, early intracranial operation was complicated by high rates of mortality and morbidity. In a randomized trial, the Cooperative Aneurysm Study noted the mortality rates among patients operated on within or after 14 days of SAH were 44.5 and 23.2 percent, respectively.[67] Sundt and Whisnant[187] reported excellent results in 112 of 119 patients in good condition who were operatively treated within 30 days of SAH. The overall combined postoperative mortality and morbidity was 3.4 percent, and 7 percent of patients died or deteriorated before operation. Drake[41] concluded that delayed surgery was safe and associated with a low rate of postoperative complications. Delaying surgery until 10 to 14 days after SAH became a standard part of care. Postoperative results are much better with delayed operation.

However, delaying operation leaves the aneurysm untreated during the highest risk period for rebleeding. Surgeons rightly point out that overall management and not just postoperative results should be compared. The overall results of early medical care–delayed operation have not been satisfactory.[7,163,186] Arguments for early surgery (less than 3 days of SAH) are that operative clipping of the aneurysm eliminates the risk of recurrent hemorrhage and eases the treatment of vasospasm. The operation could be done before vasospasm has developed.[186] The primary reason for delayed surgery has been that delaying surgery allows the patient's condition to improve before being subjected to the risk of an intracranial operation.

New neurosurgical techniques, including the operating microscope, advances in neuroanesthesia, and improved perioperative care ease early intracranial operation. Several reports in the 1970s spurred reconsideration of very early intracranial operations (less than 3 days of SAH).[88,104,168] Since then, numerous surgeons have described generally favorable results with early intracranial operation.[21,86,94,114,188,214,225] Weir and Aronyk[214] noted better results with early operation in both good and poor condition patients. Kassell et al.[94] noted that the number of medical complications, the incidence of vasospasm and the length of hospitalization were reduced with early operation. Some investigators have suggested that lavage of the subarachnoid space at the time of early operation may prevent vasospasm or that operative clipping of the aneurysm will ease treatment of vasospasm.[94,188] However, Chyatte et al.[30] noted that the incidence of postoperative ischemia following early surgery is similar to preoperative ischemia noted with delayed surgery.

Several groups reported the results of early surgery combined with a variety of interventions, including treatment with calcium entry blockers or volume expansion, and monitoring with transcranial Doppler.[14,65,113,153,173,174,181] The results, in general, have been very favorable and investigators imply that early operation eliminates the risk of rebleeding and that adjunctive medical care has largely eliminated the risk of ischemic stroke. Juvela et al.[92] concluded earlier surgery was associated with a decline in the combined mortality due to rebleeding and surgery by 32 percent and in mortality of any cause by 21 percent. However, these improved results are largely compared to historical controls and several new interventions have been added simultaneously. It is not clear which measure is accounting for the improved results.

In a nationwide Japanese study, Nishimoto et al.[136] noted that mortality rates among patients operated on within 48 hours of SAH were not lower than those operated on later. While this was not a controlled study and included patients operated on to treat a major intracerebral hemorrhage, the mortality rate among patients in good condition operated on 24 to 48 hours after SAH was 44 percent. Only one study has tested timing of surgery. A small trial in Finland demonstrated improved outcomes with early operation.[139] While the trend favors early operation, the results are distorted by a simultaneous randomization to placebo or active treatment with calcium channel blocking drugs.

The influence of timing of surgery on outcome was examined in a large international epidemiologic study.[100,101] The International Study on the Timing of Aneurysm Surgery evaluated the outcomes of 3,521 patients hospitalized within 3 calendar days of SAH. At the time of admission, the surgeons stated the time of planned surgery. Patients were grouped into scheduled intervals of days 0 to 3, 4 to 6, 7 to 10, 11 to 14, and 15+ after SAH. While this was not a randomized trial, the large numbers assured that prognostic factors were similar in the early and delayed surgical populations.

Intracranial clipping of the aneurysm was done in approximately 92 percent of the 1,600 patients that had surgery planned for days 0 to 3. However, only 76 percent of persons with surgery planned for days 11 to 14 and 62 percent of those with operation planned for 15+ days after SAH actually underwent operation; many of these patients died or developed major complications that contraindicated operation. Among patients who had surgery, postoperative results were generally superior with delayed operation performed after day 10; good outcomes were noted in 77 percent of patients who had surgery on days 11 to 14 versus 66 percent of patients who had surgery on days 0 to 3. The rates of favorable outcomes among patients operated on each day during the 0- to 3-day interval were similar. The postoperative results were analogous regardless of the patient's age, sex, admitting level of consciousness, or location of the aneurysm. Inclusion of the unfavorable outcomes that occurred while awaiting operation demonstrates that the results of early operation are as good as early medical care and delayed operation. Approximately 62 percent of patients with surgery planned on days 11 to 14 and 63 percent of patients with surgery planned on days 0 to 3 had favorable outcomes. Patients with surgery planned on days 7 to 10 had a lower rate of unfavorable outcomes, which may be attributed to surgery at the time when vasospasm is at its worst.

Early surgery does not appear to be associated with a high rate of intraoperative complications such as rerupture of the aneurysm or marked cerebral edema. This study suggests that early operation reduces the mortality and morbidity related to rebleeding. However, the positive effects of prevention of recurrent hemorrhage are offset by vasospasm and cerebral ischemia. Early operation did not prevent the development of vasospasm. Early operation apparently did not sufficiently ease the management problems of patients with symptomatic vasospasm to lower morbidity or mortality from this complication.

Early operation (less than 3 days of SAH) appears to be useful, but the results are not so overwhelming that we can recommend early surgery for all cases. Early operation is not the standard of care. However, the possible benefit of early operation emphasizes the importance of early diagnosis. Several factors must be considered before recommending early surgery. Patients with large aneurysms or aneurysms in the posterior circulation may not be ideal candidates. Patients who are comatose, elderly, or have severe comorbid diseases may not tolerate an early intracranial operation. The entire team, including neuroradiologists, anesthesiologists, nurses, intensive care personnel, and operating room personnel, must be skilled in managing these critically ill patients and be readily available. Most importantly, the neurologic surgeon must have demonstrated success in operating on these acutely ill patients. If all these criteria are not met, the patient may not be best served by an early operation.

## VASOSPASM AND ISCHEMIC STROKE

Early intracranial operation and antifibrinolytic drugs have reduced the risk of recurrent hemorrhage. Yet these advances have not been accompanied by declines in mortality or morbidity primarily because of vasospasm-induced ischemic stroke. Brain infarctions now account for approximately one-third of all unfavorable outcomes after SAH.[98] Effective measures to prevent vasospasm or ischemic stroke are needed to improve the overall management of patients with SAH. In the 1950s, the term vasospasm was applied to the luminal narrowing following SAH, which was detected by arteriography. Abnormalities may be restricted to one artery or involve several vessels. Vasospasm does not complicate primary intracerebral or intraventricular hemorrhage. It is usually associated with ruptured aneurysms, although it can rarely follow subarachnoid bleeding from other sources. Autopsy examination of patients dying of acute vasospasm reveal morphologic changes in capillaries, veins, small arteries, and large arteries.[98] Changes include disruption of the internal elastic lamina, swelling of the media, smooth muscle necrosis, and infiltration of the adventitia by macrophages, lymphocytes, and plasma cells.[87] Smith et al.[180] noted endothelial desquamation, intimal proliferation, necrosis and fibrosis of the media, and intramural deposition of type V collagen. They concluded that the lumen of the vessel can remain constricted for weeks after SAH. On electron microscopy, degenerative changes in the tunica media and intima can persist for at least 2 weeks.[47]

The amount of blood in the subarachnoid space is correlated with the development of vasospasm.[31,32,79,98] A normal component of blood is presumably released at the time of SAH. This substance or a combination of factors, once liberated into the subarachnoid space, causes the vasospastic process. A large number of constituents of blood have been implicated in the pathogenesis of vasospasm, but no single substance has been established as the spasmogenic factor.[221] Vasospasm has been ascribed to a prolonged arterial contraction, a substance that inhibits vasodilation, an immunoreactive or inflammatory process, a mechanical phenomenon, or depressed arterial metabolism.[31,32,79,98,180] Findlay et al.[47] concluded that vasospasm is related to sustained contraction of the media associated with degenerative changes in both smooth muscle cells and endothelium. It is likely that vasospasm is the result of a complex multifactorial process. In the past, determining the etiology of vasospasm has been hampered by the lack of a clinically relevant animal model. Creation of a primate model that simulates the human condition should increase our understanding of vasospasm.[48]

The arterial narrowing caused by vasospasm impairs cerebral autoregulation and increases cerebral vascular resistance.[98] Declines in cerebral perfusion pressure and cerebral blood flow lead to brain ischemia.[31,79,98] A low mean arterial pressure, elevated intracranial pressure, or increased viscosity secondary to hemoconcentration or dehydration can aggravate the ischemic process. The end result is localized infarction in the arterial beds of the involved arteries. Infarctions are usually cortical and are in watershed regions between the anterior, middle, and posterior cerebral arteries.[69,82]

Major arterial narrowing at 1 week after SAH can be arteriographically demonstrated in approximately 70 percent of patients.[31,79,98] Vasospasm causes symptoms in approximately 20 to 30 percent of patients.[51,82] The severity of the arterial narrowing correlates with the likelihood of ischemic symptoms and an unfavorable outcome. The site of the ruptured aneurysm does not influence the development of vasospasm, but a frequent location for the narrowing is adjacent to the aneurysm and clot.[109] Vasospasm is most frequently seen in the distal portion of the internal carotid artery and proximal portions of the middle and anterior cerebral arteries. It can also be generalized or localized in an area of the brain remote from the aneurysm. Vasospasm is rarely detected within 48 hours of SAH, and it usually abates by 14 to 21 days.[109,215] It is usually at its peak severity and extent at 5 to 10 days after SAH.

Vasospasm is more likely to occur in women, patients in a poor neurologic condition, or patients with an abnormal electrocardiogram.[31,79,98,215] Acute hydrocephalus has also been correlated with vasospasm.[19,82] However, the extent of subarachnoid blood as demonstrated by an early CT examination is the most important forecaster of vasospasm.[40,50,58,103,124,145,167] A number of other abnormalities on CT may also have some prognostic significance, but they appear to be less important.[40]

Ischemic complications of vasospasm are most likely to occur among patients who have hyponatremia, dehydration, or hypotension. The symptoms of vasospasm usually begin insidiously.[31,79,82] Symptoms can wax and wane over several hours or evolve suddenly. Increased headache, low-grade fever, increased meningismus, seizures, and disturbances of consciousness are usually followed by the appearance of focal neurologic deficits that primarily reflect ischemia in the vascular beds of the anterior and middle cerebral arteries. Signs include mental status changes, abulia, akinesia, anosagnosia, aphasia, hemiparesis, paraparesis, or incontinence.[31,51,79,82] The ischemic process can proceed to infarction, leading to permanent neurologic residuals and hypodense lesions detected on CT.

The differential diagnosis of vasospasm as a cause of neurologic decline is the same as for rebleeding (Table 45-6). Alternative diagnoses should be excluded before vasospasm-induced ischemia is diagnosed; the recommended diagnostic studies are included in Table 45-7. Cerebral blood flow measurements will demonstrate local or generalized hypoperfusion. Sequential transcranial Doppler studies have been reported to be very useful.[35,175] The progressive narrowing of the lumen can be accompanied by increased velocity in the arteries.[175,224] The changes in velocity may precede the development of ischemic symptoms. Some authors advocate using the changes detected by transcranial Doppler as a guide for management.[175,224] While arteriographic demonstration of arterial narrowing is needed to establish a firm diagnosis of vasospasm, arteriography is not required to treat deteriorating patients for the presumptive diagnosis of delayed ischemic deficits secondary to vasospasm.

## Prevention and Treatment

A number of therapies that might prevent or reverse vasospasm have been examined in basic and clinical research studies. Summaries of these generally ineffective regimens have been outlined by Wilkins.[221,223]

Early intracranial operation with lavage of the subarachnoid space to remove the subarachnoid clots has been advocated.[140,209] The rationale is that removal of the clots might prevent the release of the substances that induce vasospasm. Mizukami et al.[123] reported the ability to remove most blood and that successfully treated patients developed no or mild vasospasm. However surgical removal of several isolated clots in a critically ill patient is difficult; much of the collected blood can be far from the surgical field. Extensive manipulation of the brain to remove the subarachnoid clots may also injure penetrating vessels, leading to ischemic deficits.[209] Despite promising preliminary studies, the International Study on the Timing of Aneurysm Surgery could not demonstrate any reduction in the incidence or severity of vasospasm.[101] It appears that vigorous lavage of the subarachnoid space is not a feasible way to prevent vasospasm in most patients. The intraoperative, intrathecal administration of a drug such as a calcium blocker, may prove to be effective.

Tani et al.[189] reported a favorable response with the use of OKY-1581, a selective antagonist of the thromboxane $A_2$ synthetase. Nizofenone is an agent that may protect against ischemia and the development of edema after SAH. A double-blind multicenter clinical trial in Japan reported modest improvement in favorable outcomes with treatment.[141] Further research on these two agents is needed to determine if they will add to the management of patients with vasospasm.

Shaw et al.[177] were unable to demonstrate any reduction in the severity of postoperative ischemic deficits with the administration of dipyridamole.

## Calcium Channel Blockers

Influx of extracellular calcium is an important component in sustaining contraction of smooth muscle and is a critical element in the process of cellular ischemia.[212] A calcium entry blocking drug that inhibits its entry might prevent vasospasm or its cerebral ischemic consequences.[74] The dihydropyridine derivatives nimodipine and nicardipine have received the most attention.[74,156] The pharmacokinetics of orally and intravenously administered nimodipine in patients with SAH have been evaluated.[205] Nimodipine reduces blood pressure but increases cerebral blood flow.[154] The area of increased blood flow is at the border zone of the ischemic lesion. Its hypotensive effects are dose-related.[110] The interactions between nimodipine or nicardipine and anesthetic agents in patients undergoing neurosurgical procedures have also been studied.[127]

Uncontrolled studies provide evidence that nimodipine may prevent ischemic stroke after SAH. These studies often combined early intracranial operation with a regimen of nimodipine given intrathecally, intravenously, and orally.[13,64,65,113,174] Nimodipine appears to reduce mortality after SAH, regardless of the timing of aneurysm surgery.[139] One study could not demonstrate any difference in outcomes among patients treated with nimodipine when compared to historical controls.[147] Grotenhuis et al.[71] treated six patients who had vasospasm with intracarotid injections of nimodipine and noted no response. In animal experiments, continuous intrathecal infusions of nimodipine have not been effective in preventing vasospasm.[112]

In a small randomized trial, Allen et al.[10] noted that orally administered nimodipine reduced the severity of ischemic deficits; 8 of 60 patients treated with placebo had moderate to severe ischemic strokes, while 1 of 56 nimodipine-treated patients had severe sequelae. This trial was criticized because only alert patients, those with the lowest risk of vasospasm, were enrolled and because there was little evidence to support the administered dose. This study did stimulate additional studies designed to test nimodipine's ability to prevent ischemia in patients who did not already have vasospasm.[91,121,138,149,151] Most have demonstrated a reduction in morbidity and mortality due to vasospasm but have not shown an effect in preventing vasospasm. Two studies have shown nimodipine's usefulness in preventing infarction in patients with established vasospasm.[91,151] The presumed mechanism of effectiveness is ameliorating cellular ischemia.

Nicardipine has the advantage over nimodipine of being more water-soluble, which eases problems in parenteral administration. A parenterally administered drug that has rapid effects may be very useful in critically ill patients. Flamm et al.[53] noted that a continuous intravenous large-dose infusion was accompanied by a much lower than expected rate of vasospasm and ischemic stroke. Results of pilot studies have prompted a randomized trial of nicardipine.

The preliminary results of one large randomized, placebo-controlled double-blind trial of nicardipine have been reported.[72] Nicardipine was given to 449 patients and 457 patients were in the control group. This trial permitted aggressive management of symptomatic vasospasm with drug-induced hypertension and hypervolemic hemodilution. At 3 months after SAH, the actively treated and control groups had similar rates of favorable and unfavorable outcomes. However, there was a 30 percent decline in the incidence of symptomatic vasospasm with the use of nicardipine. In addition, the administration of hypervolemic and hypertensive drugs was 26 percent greater among the control patients. The results suggest that nicardipine is useful in preventing ischemic sequelae of SAH, but the combination of aggressive volume expansion and drug-induced hypertension is also effective. These are additional data that support the use of calcium channel blockers supplemented by hypervolemic hemodilution and hypertension for prevention of ischemic stroke after SAH.

Patients with recently ruptured aneurysms should receive nimodipine as part of their general medical care. If the illness is not diagnosed until 10 to 14 days after SAH, the patient has already successfully survived the period of risk of ischemia, and nimodipine does not need to be prescribed. While several studies have prescribed nimodipine for up to 3 weeks after SAH, a shorter course (10 to 14 days) may be all that is needed. Nimodipine should not be discontinued for surgery. In the future, nicardipine may replace nimodipine. These drugs are generally safe and complications are few. As with all calcium entry blockers, hypotension is a potential side effect with both nimodipine and nicardipine.

## Prevention of Acute Ischemic Stroke

Infarction secondary to vasospasm is the leading cause of unfavorable outcomes among patients who are treated with early operation or antifibrinolytic drugs. No agent has been found to be effective in ameliorating the effects of acute ischemic stroke. Barbiturate-induced coma has been attempted in a group of seriously ill patients, but the results were not satisfactory.[96]

Increasing cerebral blood flow can ease ischemic symptoms and prevent permanent neurologic sequelae[62,97,155] (Table 45-8). Reduction in the diameter of the vascular lumen implies that the blood's rheologic characteristics will greatly influence flow. Severe losses of water and sodium will result in hemo-

**TABLE 45-8. Management Options in Treatment of a Patient with Symptomatic Vasospasm**

| |
|---|
| Treatment of increased intracranial pressure |
| Discontinue antihypertensive drugs |
| Discontinue antifibrinolytic drugs |
| Adequate oxygenation |
|   Ventilatory assistance? |
|   Supplemental oxygen? |
| Volume expansion |
|   Monitor with CVP or PAWP |
|   Goal is CVP = 10 mmHg or PAWP = 14–18 mmHg |
|   ECG monitoring |
|   Administer colloid solutions |
|     Plasmanate |
|     Albumin |
|     LMW dextran |
|     Hetastarch |
|   Administer crystalloid solutions |
|     Normal saline |
|   Fludrocortisone |
| Venesection |
|   Remove units of blood |
|   Simultaneous with fluid replacement |
|   Goal of hematocrit is 35–40% |
| Drug-induced hypertension |
|   Continuous invasive or noninvasive monitoring |
|   Elevate blood pressure 30–40 torr |
|   Titrate pressure to clinical response |
|     Dopamine |
|     Neo-Synephrine |
| Angioplasty |

concentration and dehydration, which in turn increase viscosity and reduce blood flow. The risk of ischemic complications of vasospasm is increased by hyponatremia and dehydration. Measures to prevent infarction by correcting the sodium and water losses should be initiated upon admission to the hospital. Strict fluid restriction is avoided and patients should receive at least 2 to 3 liters per day. Metabolic disorders that promote hyperosmolarity should be treated.

Autoregulation is also impaired by SAH and vasospasm; cerebral blood flow becomes pressure-dependent. Cerebral perfusion pressure is altered by changes in the mean arterial pressure and intracranial pressure. Improvement of venous drainage by proper positioning and elevation of the head, treatment of cerebral edema, and treatment of hydrocephalus will lower intracranial pressure and improve cerebral perfusion. If possible, antihypertensive drugs should be avoided. Deterioration in the neurologic condition should prompt an evaluation for the cause. After the diagnosis of symptomatic vasospasm is made, more aggressive treatment of increased intracranial pressure, including hyperventilation and mannitol, may be helpful. Antihypertensive and antifibrinolytic drugs should be discontinued.

Several investigators have reported that a combination of volume expansion and drug-induced hypertension will reverse the ischemic symptoms.[31,62,79,97,98,155] A proposed regimen is outlined in Table 45-8. Large volumes of both crystalloid and colloid solution are given. Venesection with removal of one or more units of blood to lower the hematocrit to the range of 35 to 40 percent has also been advocated. Adjunctive drugs help maintain the overhydrated state.[97] If an improvement is not observed following volume expansion, a vasopressor; most commonly, either dopamine or phenylephrine is added. The goal is to increase mean arterial pressure and thus increase cerebral perfusion pressure.

This is a very vigorous regimen that requires constant monitoring. Patients should be in an intensive care unit and have continuous arterial pressure, cardiac rhythm, and either central venous or, preferably, pulmonary artery wedge pressure monitoring. The desired target for central venous pressure is 10 mmHg and pulmonary artery wedge pressure is 14 to 18 mmHg. Continuous intracranial pressure monitoring is also often needed. Frequent laboratory assessments of electrolytes, serum osmolarity, blood gases, and blood counts are also required.

Investigators report neurologic improvement in many cases.[62,97] In some instances, neurologic deficits have reappeared when the therapy has been discontinued. Complications of this regimen include congestive heart failure, pulmonary edema, acute myocardial ischemia, cardiac arrhythmias, and rerupture of the aneurysm. In one series, rebleeding occurred in 3 of 16 patients whose aneurysms had not been operated on.[97] Hemorrhagic infarction can also complicate this therapy.[197] The use of low molecular weight dextran can be complicated by bleeding or anaphylaxis.[97]

## NEW THERAPIES

Several new interventions that may radically change the future management of SAH are being studied. For several years, interventional neuroradiologists have placed balloons into vessels to stimulate occlusions of large arteriovenous malformations and carotid-cavernous fistulas. This same technology is now being applied to intracranial saccular aneurysms. If an aneurysm can be obliterated by a balloon that is inserted via a small intraarterial catheter, the risks of a major intracranial operation might be avoided. Similarly, a prothrombotic or sclerosing agent might also be selectively infused into an aneurysm. Transluminal angioplasty has successfully and safely reversed vasospasm.[16,80,133] New drugs that protect the blood-brain barrier and limit pathologic changes in membranes may hold promise in patients with vasospasm.[228] Animal research suggests that intrathecal administration of a thrombolytic agent will expedite removal of the subarachnoid clots at the time of an intracranial operation and can prevent vasospasm.[48,172] All of these new interventions will need considerable testing before we will know whether they have a role in the management of SAH.

## CONCLUSIONS

Considerable progress is being made in the management of SAH. Medical and surgical measures that effectively prevent rebleeding and vasospasm appear to be reflected by a decline in the mortality and morbidity. There remains considerable room for improvement. We must increase our attention to the early diagnosis and acute care of these patients. New therapies are being tested that may further improve patient care.

## REFERENCES


1. Adams HP, Jr: Clinical manifestations and diagnosis of subarachnoid hemorrhage. Sem Neurol 4:304, 1984
2. Adams HP, Jr: Early management of the patient with recent aneurysmal subarachnoid hemorrhage. Stroke 17:1068, 1986
3. Adams HP, Jr: Antifibrinolytics in aneurysmal subarachnoid hemorrhage: do they have a role? Maybe. Arch Neurol 44:114, 1987
4. Adams HP, Jr, Gordon DL: Nonaneurysmal subarachnoid hemorrhage. Ann Neurol 29:461, 1991
5. Adams HP, Jr, Jergenson DD, Kassell NF, Sahs AL: Pitfalls in the recognition of subarachnoid hemorrhage. JAMA 244:794, 1980
6. Adams HP, Jr, Kassell NF, Torner JC: Usefulness of computed tomography in predicting outcome after aneurysmal subarachnoid hemorrhage: a preliminary report of the Cooperative Aneurysm study. Neurology 35:1263, 1985
7. Adams HP, Jr, Kassell NF, Torner JC et al: Early management of aneurysmal subarachnoid hemorrhage: a report of the Cooperative Aneurysm study. J Neurosurg 54:141, 1981
8. Adams HP, Jr, Nibbelink DW, Torner JC et al: Antifibrinolytic therapy in patients with aneurysmal subarachnoid hemorrhage. Arch Neurol 38:25, 1981
9. Alexander MP, Freedman M: Amnesia after anterior communicating artery aneurysm rupture. Neurology (NY) 34:752, 1984
10. Allen AS, Ahn HS, Preziosi TJ: Cerebral arterial spasm—a controlled trial of nimodipine in patients with subarachnoid hemorrhage. N Engl J Med 308:619, 1983
11. Alvord EC, Jr, Loeser JD, Bailey WL et al: Subarachnoid hemorrhage due to ruptured aneurysms: a simple method for estimating prognosis. Arch Neurol 27:273, 1972
12. Amacher AL, Ferguson GG, Drake CG et al: How old people tolerate intracranial surgery for aneurysm. Neurosurgery 1:242, 1977
13. Ameen AA, Illingworth R: Antifibrinolytic treatment in the pre-operative management of subarachnoid hemorrhage caused by ruptured intracranial aneurysm. J Neurol Neurosurg Psychiatry 44:220, 1981
14. Auer LM: Acute operation and preventive nimodipine improve outcome in patient with ruptured cerebral aneurysms. Neurosurgery 15:57, 1984
15. Ausman JI, Diaz FG, Malik GM et al: Current management of cerebral aneurysms: is it based on facts or myths? Surg Neurol 24:624, 1985
16. Barnwell SL, Higashida RT, Halbach VV et al: Transluminal angioplasty of intracerebral vessels for cerebral arterial spasm: reversal of neurological deficits after delayed treatment. Neurosurgery 25:424, 1989
17. Beck DW, Adams HP, Jr, Flamm ES et al: Combination of aminocaproic acid and nicardipine in treatment of aneurysmal subarachnoid hemorrhage. Stroke 19:63, 1988
18. Biller J, Godersky JC, Adams HP, Jr: Management of aneurysmal subarachnoid hemorrhage. Stroke 19:1300, 1988
19. Black PMcL: Hydrocephalus and vasospasm after subarachnoid hemorrhage from ruptured intracranial aneurysms. Neurosurgery 18:12, 1986
20. Black PMcL, Crowell RM, Abbott WM: External pneumatic calf compression reduces deep venous thrombosis in patients with ruptured intracranial aneurysms. Neurosurgery 18:25, 1986
21. Bolander HG, Kourtopoulos H, West KA: Retrospective analysis of 162 consecutive cases of ruptured intracranial aneurysms: total mortality and early surgery. Acta Neurochir 70:31, 1984
22. Bonita R, Beaglehole R, North JDK: Subarachnoid hemorrhage in New Zealand: an epidemiological study. Stroke 14:342, 1983
23. Brandt L, Sonesson B, Ljunggren B, Saveland H: Ruptured middle cerebral artery aneurysms with intracerebral hemorrhage in younger patients appearing moribund: emergency operation? Neurosurgery 20:925, 1987
24. Britt CW, Jr, Light RR, Peters BH, Schochet SS, Jr: Rhabdomyolysis during treatment with epsilon-aminocaproic acid. Arch Neurol 37:187, 1980
25. Brodkin HM: Myoglobinuria following epsilon-aminocaproic acid (EACA) therapy. J Neurosurg, 53:690, 1980
26. Brott T, MacCarthy EP: Antihypertensive therapy in stroke. p. 117. In Fisher M (ed): Medical Therapy of Acute Stroke. Marcel Dekker, New York, 1989
27. Brown JA, Wollmann RL, Mullan S: Myopathy induced by epsilon-aminocaproic acid. J Neurosurg 57:130, 1982
28. Chandra B: Treatment of subarachnoid hemorrhage from ruptured intracranial aneurysm with tranexamic acid: a double-blind clinical trial. Ann Neurol 3:502, 1978
29. Chowdhary VM, Sayed K: Comparative clinical trial of epsilon aminocaproic acid and tranexamic acid in the prevention of early recurrence of subarachnoid hemorrhage. J Neurol Neurosurg Psychiatry, 44:810, 1981
30. Chyatte D, Fode NC, Sundt TM, Jr: Early versus late intracranial aneurysm surgery in subarachnoid hemorrhage. J Neurosurg 69:326, 1988
31. Chyatte D, Sundt TM, Jr: Cerebral vasospasm

after subarachnoid hemorrhage. Mayo Clin Proc 59:498, 1984
32. Cook DA: The pharmacology of cerebral vasospasm. Pharmacology 29:1, 1984
33. Crowell RM, Zervas NT: Management of intracranial aneurysm. Med Clin N Am 63:695, 1979
34. Cruikshank JM, Neil-Dwyer G, Stott AW: Possible role of catecholamines, corticosteroids and potassium in production of electrocardiographic abnormalities associated with subarachnoid hemorrhage. Br Heart J 36:697, 1974
35. DeWitt LD, Wechsler LR: Transcranial Doppler. Stroke 19:915, 1988
36. Diamond T, Segal F: Subarachnoid hemorrhage masquerading electrocardiographically as acute myocardial infarction. Heart Lung 13:451, 1984
37. Di Pasquale G, Pinelli G, Andreoli A et al: Torsade de pointes and ventricular flutter-fibrillation following spontaneous cerebral subarachnoid hemorrhage. Int J Cardiol 18:163, 1988
38. Diringer M, Ladenson PW, Stern BJ et al: Plasma atrial natriuretic factor and subarachnoid hemorrhage. Stroke 19:1119, 1988
39. Disney L, Weir B, Grace M, Roberts P: Trends in blood pressure, osmolality and electrolytes after subarachnoid hemorrhage from aneurysms. Can J Neurol Sci 16:299, 1989
40. Doczi T, Ambrose J, O'Laoire S: Significance of contrast enhancement in cranial computed tomography after subarachnoid hemorrhage. J Neurosurg 60:335, 1984
41. Drake CG: Management of cerebral aneurysm. Stroke 12:273, 1981
42. Duff TA, Ayeni S, Levin AB, Javid M: Nonsurgical management of spontaneous intracerebral hematoma. Neurosurgery 9:387, 1981
43. Duffy GP: The "warning leak" in spontaneous subarachnoid hemorrhage. Med J Aust 1:514, 1983
44. Elliott HL, Campbell BC, Morgan I: Beta blockade in subarachnoid hemorrhage. Br Med J 2:1370, 1978
45. Estanol Vidal B, Badui Dergal E, Cesarman E et al: Cardiac arrhythmias associated with subarachnoid hemorrhage: prospective study. Neurosurgery 5:675, 1979
46. Fabinyi G, Hunt D, McKinley L: Myocardial creatine kinase isoenzyme in serum after subarachnoid hemorrhage. J Neurol Neurosurg Psychiatry 40:818, 1977
47. Findlay JM, Weir BKA, Kanamaru K, Espinosa F: Arterial wall changes in cerebral vasospasm. Neurosurgery 25:736, 1989
48. Findlay JM, Weir BKA, Steinke D et al: Effect of intracisternal thrombolytic therapy on subarachnoid clot and chronic vasopasm in a primate model of subarachnoid hemorrhage. J Neurosurg 69:723, 1988
49. Fisher CM: Clinical syndromes in cerebral thrombosis, hypertensive hemorrhage and ruptured saccular aneurysm. Clin Neurosurg 22:117, 1975
50. Fisher CM, Kistler JP, Davis JM: Relation of cerebral vasospasm to subarachnoid hemorrhage visualized by computerized tomographic scanning. Neurosurgery 6:1, 1980
51. Fisher CM, Roberson GH, Ojemann RG: Cerebral vasospasm with ruptured saccular aneurysm: the clinical manifestations. Neurosurgery 1:245, 1977
52. Flamm ES: Parasurgical treatment of aneurysms. Clin Neurosurg 24:240, 1976
53. Flamm ES, Adams HP, Jr, Beck DW et al: Dose-escalation study of intravenous nicardipine in patients with aneurysmal subarachnoid hemorrhage. J Neurosurg 68:393, 1988
54. Fodstad H: Antifibrinolytic treatment in subarachnoid hemorrhage. Present state. Acat Neurochir 63:233, 1982
55. Fodstad H, Nilsson IM: Coagulation and fibrinolysis in blood and cerebrospinal fluid after aneurysmal subarachnoid hemorrhage: effect of tranexamic acid (AMCA). Acta Neurochir 56:25, 1981
56. Fodstad H, Pilbrant A, Schannong M, Stromberg S: Determination of tranexamic acid (AMCA) and fibrin/fibrinogen degradation products in cerebrospinal fluid after aneurysmal subarachnoid hemorrhage. Acta Neurochir 58:1, 1981
57. Fogelholm R: Subarachnoid hemorrhage in middle-Finland: incidence, early prognosis and indications for neurological treatment. Stroke 12:296, 1981
58. Fraser J, Johnson S, Ray M, Robertson JT: Prediction of cerebral vasospasm with subarachnoid hemorrhage due to ruptured intracranial aneurysm by computed axial tomography. Neurosurgery 6:686, 1980
59. Galera R, Greitz T: Hydrocephalus in the adult secondary to the rupture of intracranial arterial aneurysms. J Neurosurg 32:634, 1970
60. Gascon P, Ley TJ, Toltzis RJ, Bonow RO: Spontaneous subarachnoid hemorrhage simulating acute transmural myocardial infarction. Am Heart J 105:511, 1983
61. Gelmers HJ: Prevention of recurrence of spontaneous subarachnoid hemorrhage by tranexamic acid. Acta Neurochir 52:45, 1980
62. Giannotta SL, McGillicuddy JE, Kindt GW: Diagnosis and treatment of postoperative cerebral vasospasm. Surg Neurol 8:286, 1977
63. Gibbs JR, O'Gorman P: Fibrinolysis in subarachnoid hemorrhage. Postgrad Med J 43:779, 1967
64. Gilsbach JM: Nimodipine in the prevention of ischaemic deficits after aneurysmal subarachnoid haemorrhage. Acta Neurochir 45:41, 1988
65. Gilsbach JM, Harders AG: Morbidity and mortality after early aneurysm surgery: a prospective study with nimodipine prevention. Acta Neurochir 96:1, 1989
66. Glick R, Green D, Tsao C-H et al: High dose ε-aminocaproic acid prolongs the bleeding time and increases rebleeding and intraoperative hemorrhage in patients with subarachnoid hemorrhage. Neurosurgery 9:398, 1981
67. Graf CJ, Nibbelink DW: Cooperative study on intracranial aneurysms and subarachnoid hem-

orrhage: report on a randomized treatment study. III. Intracranial surgery. Stroke 5:557, 1974

68. Graff-Radford NR, Torner JC, Adams HP, Jr, Kassell NF: Factors associated with hydrocephalus after subarachnoid hemorrhage: a report of the Cooperative Aneurysm study. Arch Neurol 46:744, 1989
69. Graham DI, MacPherson P, Pitts LH: Correlation between angiographic vasospasm, hematoma and ischemic brain damage following SAH. J Neurosurg 59:223, 1983
70. Grote E, Hassler W: The critical first minutes after subarachnoid hemorrhage. Neurosurgery 22:654, 1988
71. Grotenhuis JA, Bettag W, Fiebach BJO, Dabir K: Intracarotid slow bolus injection of nimodipine during angiography for treatment of cerebral vasospasm after SAH. J Neurosurg 61:231, 1984
72. Haley EC, Torner JC, Kassell NF, and participants. Cooperative randomized study of nicardipine in subarachnoid hemorrhage. Preliminary report. p. 519. In Sano K, Takakara K, Kassell NF, Sasaki T (eds): Cerebral Vasospasm. Proceedings of the Fourth International Conference on Cerebral Vasospasm. University of Tokyo Press, Tokyo, 1990
73. Harries AD: Subarachnoid hemorrhage and the electrocardiogram: a review. Postgrad Med J 57:294, 1981
74. Harris RJ, Branston NM, Symon L et al: The effects of a calcium antagonist, nimodipine, upon physiological responses of the cerebral vasculature and its possible influence upon focal cerebral ischaemia. Stroke 13:759, 1982
75. Hart RG, Byer JA, Slaughter JR et al: Occurrence and implications of seizures in subarachnoid hemorrhage due to ruptured intracranial aneurysms. Neurosurgery 8:417, 1981
76. Hasen D, Vermeulen M, Wijdicks EFM, et al: Management problems in acute hydrocephalus after subarachnoid hemorrhage. Stroke 20:747, 1989
77. Hayashi M, Kobayashi H, Kawano H et al: Cerebral blood flow and ICP patterns in patients with communicating hydrocephalus after aneurysm rupture. J Neurosurg 61:30, 1984
78. Heros RC: Acute hydrocephalus after subarachnoid hemorrhage. Stroke 20:715, 1989
79. Heros RC, Zervas NT, Varsos V: Cerebral vasospasm after subarachnoid hemorrhage: an update. Ann Neurol 14:599, 1983
80. Higashida RT, Halbach VV, Cahan LD et al: Transluminal angioplasty for treatment of intracranial arterial vasospasm. J Neurosurg 71:648, 1989
81. Hijdra A, van Gijn J: Early death from rupture of an intracranial aneurysm. J Neurosurg 57:765, 1982
82. Hijdra A, van Gijn J, Stefanko S et al: Delayed cerebral ischemia after aneurysmal subarachnoid hemorrhage: clinicoanatomic correlations. Neurology (NY) 36:329, 1986
83. Hijdra A, Vermeulen M, van Gijn J, van Crevel H: Respiratory arrest in subarachnoid hemorrhage. Neurology (NY) 34:1501, 1984
84. Hildebrandt G, Werner M, Kaps M, Busse O: Acute non-communicating hydrocephalus after spontaneous subarachnoid hemorrhage. Acta Neurochir 76:58, 1985
85. Hillman J, von Essen C, Leszniewski W, Johansson I: Significance of "ultra-early" rebleeding in subarachnoid hemorrhage. J Neurosurg 68:901, 1988
86. Hugenholtz H, Elgie R: Considerations in early surgery on good-risk patients with ruptured intracranial aneurysms. J Neurosurg 56:180, 1982
87. Hughes JT, Schianchi PM: Cerebral arterial spasm. A histological study at necropsy of the blood vessels in cases of subarachnoid hemorrhage. J Neurosurg 48:515, 1978
88. Hunt WE, Miller CA: The results of early operation for aneurysm. Clin Neurosurg 24:208, 1976
89. Inagawa T, Yamamoto M, Kamiya K, Ogasawara H: Management of elderly patients with aneurysmal subarachnoid hemorrhage. Clin Neurosurg 69:332, 1988
90. Ingall TJ, Whisnant JP, Wiebers DO, O'Fallon WM: Has there been a decline in subarachnoid hemorrhage mortality? Stroke 20:718, 1989
91. Jan M, Buchheit F, Tremoulet M: Therapeutic trial of intravenous nimodipine in patients with established cerebral vasospasm after rupture of intracranial aneurysm. Neurosurgery 23:154, 1988
92. Juvela S, Kaste M, Hillbom M: The effects of earlier surgery and shorter bedrest on the outcome in patients with subarachnoid haemorrhage. J Neurol Neurosurg Psychiatry 52:776, 1989
93. Kassell NF, Adams HP, Jr, Torner JC et al: Influence of timing of admission after aneurysmal subarachnoid hemorrhage on overall outcome: report of the Cooperative Aneurysm study. Stroke, 12:620, 1981
94. Kassell NF, Boarini DJ, Adams HP, Jr et al: Overall management of ruptured aneurysm: comparison of early and late operation. Neurosurgery 9:120, 1981
95. Kassell NF, Kongable GL, Torner JC et al: Delay in referral of patients with ruptured aneurysms to neurosurgical attention. Stroke 16:587, 1985
96. Kassell NF, Peerless SJ, Drake CG et al: Treatment of ischemic deficits from cerebral vasospasm with high dose barbiturate therapy. Neurosurgery 7:593, 1980
97. Kassell NF, Peerless SJ, Durward QJ et al: Treatment of ischemic deficits from vasospasm with intravascular volume expansion and induced arterial hypertension. Neurosurgery 11:337, 1982
98. Kassell NF, Sasaki T, Colohan ART, Nazar G: Cerebral vasospasm following aneurysmal subarachnoid hemorrhage. Stroke 16:562, 1985
99. Kassell NF, Torner JC, Adams HP, Jr: Antifibrinolytic therapy in the acute period following aneurysmal subarachnoid hemorrhage: preliminary observations from the Cooperative Aneurysm study. J Neurosurg 61:225, 1984

100. Kassell NF, Torner JC, Haley EC et al: The International Cooperative study on the timing of aneurysm surgery. I. Overall management results. J. Neurosurg 73:18, 1990
101. Kassell NF, Torner JC, Haley EC et al: The International Cooperative study on the timing of aneurysm surgery. II. Surgical results. J Neurosurg 73:34, 1990
102. Kaste M, Ramsay M: Tranexamic acid in subarachnoid hemorrhage: a double-blind study. Stroke 10:519, 1979
103. Kistler JP, Crowell RM, Davis KR et al: The relation of cerebral vasospasm to the extent and location of subarachnoid blood visualized by CT scan: a prospective study. Neurology (NY) 33:424, 1983
104. Kori S, Suzuki J: Early intracranial operation for ruptured aneurysms. Acta Neurochir 46:93, 1979
105. Koskelo P, Punsar S, Sipila W: Subendocardial hemorrhage and ECG changes in intracranial bleeding. Br Med J 1:1479, 1964
106. Kosnik EJ, Hunt WE: Postoperative hypertension in the management of patients with intracranial arterial aneurysms. J Neurosurg 45:148, 1976
107. Kunitz S, Gross C, Heyman A et al: The pilot stroke data bank: definition, design and data. Stroke 15:740, 1984
108. Kusske JA, Turner PT, Ojemann GA, Harris AB: Ventriculostomy for the treatment of acute hydrocephalus following subarachnoid hemorrhage. J Neurosurg 38:591, 1973
109. Kwak R, Niizuma H, Ohi T, Suzuki J: Angiographic study of cerebral vasospasm following rupture of intracranial aneurysms. I. Time of the appearance. Surg Neurol 11:257, 1979
110. Laursen J, Jensen F, Mikkelsen E, Jakobsen P: Nimodipine treatment of subarachnoid hemorrhage. Clin Neurol Neurosurg 90:329, 1988
111. LeBlanc R: The minor leak preceding subarachnoid hemorrhage. J Neurosurg 66:35, 1987
112. Lewis PJ, Weir BKA, Nosko MG et al: Intrathecal nimodipine therapy in a primate model of chronic cerebral vasospasm. Neurosurgery 22:492, 1988
113. Ljunggren B, Brandt L, Saveland H et al: Outcome in 60 consecutive patients treated with early aneurysm operation and intravenous nimodipine. J Neurosurg 61:864, 1984
114. Ljunggren B, Brandt L, Sundbarg G et al: Early management of aneurysmal subarachnoid hemorrhage. Neurosurgery 11:412, 1982
115. Ljunggren B, Saveland H, Brandt L, Zygmunt S: Early operation and overall outcome in aneurysmal subarachnoid hemorrhage. J Neurosurg 62:547, 1985
116. Marion DW, Segal R, Thompson ME: Subarachnoid hemorrhage and the heart. Neurosurgery 18:101, 1986
117. Markwardt F: Synthetic inhibitors of fibrinolysis: fibrinolytics and antifibrinolytics. Hand Exp Pharm 46:511, 1978
118. Maroon JC, Nelson PB: Hypovolemia in patients with subarachnoid hemorrhage: therapeutic implications. Neurosurgery 4:223, 1979
119. Marshall LF, Smith RW, Rausher LA, Shapiro HM: Mannitol dose requirements in brain-injured patients. J Neurosurg 48:169, 1978
120. Maurice-Williams RS: Prolonged antifibrinolysis: an effective non-surgical treatment for ruptured intracranial aneurysms:? Br Med J 1:945, 1978
121. Mee E, Dorrance D, Lowe D, Neil-Dwyer G: Controlled study of nimodipine in aneurysm patients treated early after subarachnoid hemorrhage. Neurosurgery 22:484, 1988
122. Milhorat TH: Acute hydrocephalus after aneurysmal subarachnoid hemorrhage. Neurosurgery 20:15, 1987
123. Mizukami M, Kawase T, Usami T, Tazawa T: Prevention of vasospasm by early operation with removal of subarachnoid blood. Neurosurgery 10:301, 1982
124. Mizukami M, Takemae T, Tazawa T et al: Value of computed tomography in the prediction of cerebral vasospasm after aneurysm rupture. Neurosurgery 7:583, 1980
125. Mohr JP, Caplan LR, Melski JW et al: The Harvard Cooperative Stroke Registry: a prospective registry. Neurology (NY) 28:754, 1978
126. Mullan S, Dawley J: Antifibrinolytic therapy for intracranial aneurysms. J Neurosurg 28:21, 1968
127. Muller H, Kafurke H, Marck P et al: Interactions between nimodipine and general anaesthesia: clinical investigations in 124 patients during neurosurgical operations. Acta Neurochir 45:29, 1988
128. Najim Al-Din AS, Jamieson DG: Reversible causes of altered consciousness after spontaneous subarachnoid hemorrhage. Br Med J 284:180, 1982
129. Neil-Dwyer G, Cruikshank J, Stratton C: B-blockers, plasma total creatine kinase and creatine kinase myocardial isoenzymes, and the prognosis of subarachnoid hemorrhage. Surg Neurol 25:163, 1986
130. Neil-Dwyer G, Walter P, Cruikshank JM et al: Effect of propranolol and phentolamine on myocardial necrosis after subarachnoid hemorrhage. Br Med J 2:990, 1978
131. Neil-Dwyer G, Walter P, Shaw HJH et al: Plasma renin activity in patients after a subarachnoid hemorrhage: a possible predictor of outcome. Neurosurgery 7:578, 1980
132. Nelson PB, Seif SM, Maroon JC, Robinson AG: Hyponatremia in intracranial disease: perhaps not the syndrome of inappropriate secretion of antidiuretic hormone (SIADH). J Neurosurg 55:938, 1981
133. Newell DW, Eskridge JM, Mayberg MR et al: Angioplasty for the treatment of symptomatic vasospasm following subarachnoid hemorrhage. J Neurosurg 71:654, 1989
134. Nibbelink DW: Considerations in the treatment of stroke: Cooperative Aneurysm study: antihypertensive and antifibrinolytic therapy follow-

ing subarachnoid hemorrhage from ruptured intracranial aneurysm. p. 155. In Whisnant JP, Sandok BA (eds): Cerebral Vascular Diseases. Grune & Stratton, New York, 1975
135. Nibbelink DW, Torner JC, Burmeister LF: Fluid restriction in combination with antifibrinolytic therapy. p. 307. In Sahs AL, Nibbelink DW, Torner JC (eds): Aneurysmal Subarachnoid Hemorrhage. Urban & Schwarzenberg, Baltimore, 1981, p. 307–330.
136. Nishimoto A, Veta K, Onbe H et al: Nationwide cooperative study of intracranial aneurysm surgery in Japan. Stroke 16:48, 1985
137. Nishioka H: Report of the Cooperative Study of Intracranial Aneurysms and Subarachnoid Hemorrhage. Section VII, Part I: Evaluation of conservative measurement of ruptured intracranial aneurysms. J Neurosurg 25:574, 1966
138. Ohman J, Heiskanen O: Effect of nimodipine on the outcome of patients after aneurysmal subarachnoid hemorrhage and surgery. J Neurosurg 69:683, 1988
139. Ohman J, Heiskanen O: Timing of operation for ruptured supratentorial aneurysms: a prospective randomized study. J Neurosurg 70:55, 1989
140. Ohta H, Ito Z, Yasui N, Suzuki A: Extensive evacuation of subarachnoid clot for prevention of vasospasm: effective or not? Acta Neurochir 63:111, 1982
141. Ohta T, Kikuchi H, Hashi K, Kudo Y: Nizofenone administration in the acute stage following subarachnoid hemorrhage: results of a multi-center controlled double-blind clinical study. J Neurosurg 64:420, 1986
142. Okawa M, Maeda S, Nukui H, Kawafuchi J: Psychiatric symptoms in ruptured anterior communicating aneurysms: social prognosis. Acta Psychiatr Scand 61:306, 1980
143. Park BE: Spontaneous subarachnoid hemorrhage complicated by communicating hydrocephalus: epsilon-aminocaproic acid as a possible predisposing factor. Surg Neurol 11:73, 1979
144. Pasqualin A, Bazzan A, Cavazzani P et al: Intracranial hematomas following aneurysmal rupture: experience with 309 cases. Surg Neurol 25:6, 1986
145. Pasqualin A, Rosta L, Da Pian R et al: Role of computed tomography in the management of vasospasm after subarachnoid hemorrhage. Neurosurgery 15:344, 1984
146. Peerless SJ: Pre- and postoperative management of cerebral aneurysms. Clin Neurosurg 26:209, 1979
147. Pellettieri L, Bolander H, Carlsson H, Sjolander U: Nimodipine treatment of selected good-risk patients with subarachnoid hemorrhage: no significant difference between present and historical controls. Surg Neurol 30:180, 1988
148. Perret GE, Nibbelink DW: Randomized treatment study: carotid ligation. p. 121. In Sahs AL, Nibbelink DW, Torner JC (eds): Aneurysmal Subarachnoid Hemorrhage. Urban and Schwarzenberg, Baltimore, 1981
149. Petruk KC, West M, Mohr G et al: Nimodipine treatment in poor-grade aneurysm patients. J Neurosurg 68:505, 1988
150. Phillips LH II, Whisnant JP, O'Fallon WM, Sundt TM, Jr: The unchanging pattern of subarachnoid hemorrhage in a community. Neurology (NY) 30:1034, 1980
151. Pickard JD, Murray GD, Illingworth R et al: Effect of oral nimodipine on cerebral infarction and outcome after subarachnoid haemorrhage: British aneurysm nimodipine trial. Br Med J 298:636, 1989
152. Pinna G, Pasqualin A, Vivenza C, DaPian R: Rebleeding, ischemia and hydrocephalus following antifibrinolytic treatment for ruptured cerebral aneurysms: a retrospective clinical study. Acta Neurochir 93:77, 1988
153. Popovic EA, Siu K: Ruptured intracranial aneurysms: a 12-month prospective study. Med J Aus 150:492, 1989
154. Pozzilli C, DiPiero V, Pantano P et al: Influence of nimodipine on cerebral blood flow in human cerebral ischaemia. J Neurol 236:199, 1989
155. Pritz MB, Giannotta SL, Kindt GW et al: Treatment of patients with neurological deficits associated with cerebral vasospasm by intravascular volume expansion. Neurosurgery 3:364, 1978
156. Przuntek H, V Baumgarten F, Mertens HG: Treatment of vasospasm due to subarachnoid hemorrhage with calcium entry blockers. Eur Neurol, suppl 1. 25:86, 1986
157. Raimondi AJ, Torres H: Acute hydrocephalus as a complication of subarachnoid hemorrhage. Surg Neurol 1:23, 1973
158. Ramirez-Lassepas M: Antifibrinolytic therapy in subarachnoid hemorrhage caused by ruptured intracranial aneurysm. Neurology 31:316, 1981
159. Reynolds AF, Shaw C-M: Bleeding patterns from ruptured intracranial aneurysms: an autopsy series of 205 patients. Surg Neurol 15:232, 1981
160. Rinkel GJE, Wijdicks EFM, Vermeulen M et al: The clinical course of perimesencephalic nonaneurysmal subarachnoid hemorrhage. Ann Neurol 29:463, 1991
161. Romner B, Sonesson B, Ljunggren B et al: Late magnetic resonance imaging related to neurobehavioral functioning after aneurysmal subarachnoid hemorrhage. Neurosurgery 25:390, 1989
162. Ropper AH, King RB: Intracranial pressure monitoring in comatose patients with cerebral hemorrhage. Arch Neurol 4:725, 1984
163. Ropper AH, Zervas NT: Outcome 1 year after SAH from cerebral aneurysm. Management morbidity, mortality and functional status in 112 consecutive good-risk patients. J Neurosurg 60:909, 1984
164. Rosenfeld JV, Barnett GH, Sila CA et al: The effect of subarachnoid hemorrhage on blood and CSF atrial natriuretic factor. J Neurosurg 71:32, 1989
165. Sacco RL, Wolf PA, Bharucha NE et al: Subarachnoid and intracerebral hemorrhage: natural history, prognosis and precursive factors in the Framingham study. Neurology (Cleveland) 34:847, 1984

166. Sahs AL: Preface: report of the Cooperative Study. In Sahs AL, Nibbelink DW et al (eds): Aneurysmal Subarachnoid Hemorrhage. Urban and Schwarzenberg, Baltimore, 1981
167. Sano H, Kanno T, Shinomiya Y et al: Prospection of chronic vasospasm by CT findings. Acta Neurochir 63:23, 1982
168. Sano K, Saito I: Timing and indication of surgery for ruptured intracranial aneurysms with regard to cerebral vasospasm. Acta Neurochir 41:49, 1978
169. Sastry Kolluri VR, Sengupta RP: Symptomatic hydrocephalus following aneurysmal subarachnoid hemorrhage. Surg Neurol 21:402, 1984
170. Saveland H, Sonesson B, Ljunggren B et al: Outcome evaluation following subarachnoid hemorrhage. J Neurosurg 64:191, 1986
171. Schievink WI, Van der Werf DJM, Hageman LM, Dreissen JJR: Referral pattern of patients with aneurysmal subarachnoid hemorrhage. Surg Neurol 29:367, 1988
172. Seifert V, Eisert WG, Stolke D, Goetz C: Efficacy of single intracisternal bolus injection of recombinant tissue plasminogen activator to prevent delayed cerebral vasospasm after experimental subarachnoid hemorrhage. Neurosurgery 25:590, 1989
173. Seifert V, Stolke D, Trost H-A: Timing of aneurysm surgery: comparison of results of early and delayed surgical intervention. Arch Psychiatr Neurol Sci 237:291, 1988
174. Seiler RW, Reulen HJ, Huber P et al: Outcome of aneurysmal subarachnoid hemorrhage in a hospital population: a prospective study including early operation, intravenous nimodipine and transcranial Doppler ultrasound. Neurosurgery 23:598, 1988
175. Sekhar LN, Wechsler LR, Yonas H et al: Value of transcranial Doppler examination in the diagnosis of cerebral vasospasm after subarachnoid hemorrhage. Neurosurgery 22:813, 1988
176. Sengupta RP, So SC, Villarejo-Ortega FJ: Use of epsilon-aminocaproic acid (EACA) in the preoperative management of ruptured intracranial aneurysms. J Neurosurg 44:479, 1976
177. Shaw MDM, Foy PM, Conway M et al: Dipyridamole and postoperative ischemic deficits in aneurysmal subarachnoid hemorrhage. J Neurosurg 63:699, 1985
178. Six EG, Clark JB, Early CB: Subarachnoid hemorrhage and intracranial aneurysms: a review of assessment and early management. Milit Med 148:497, 1983
179. Slosberg PS: Zero percent mortality due to recurrent hemorrhage in follow-up of medically treated ruptured single intracranial aneurysms: a 23-year study. Trans Am Neurol Assoc 104:180, 1979
180. Smith RR, Clower BR, Grotendorst GM et al: Arterial wall changes in early human vasospasm. Neurosurgery 16:171, 1985
181. Solomon RA, Fink ME, Lennihan L: Early aneurysm surgery and prophylactic hypervolemic hypertensive therapy for the treatment of aneurysmal subarachnoid hemorrhage. Neurosurgery 23:699, 1988
182. Solomon RA, Post KD, McMurtry JG III: Depression of circulating blood volume in patients after subarachnoid hemorrhage: implications for the management of symptomatic vasospasm. Neurosurgery 15:354, 1984
183. Steinmetz H, Grote E: The fibrinolytic activity of cerebrospinal fluid after subarachnoid hemorrhage. Neurol Res 5:59, 1983
184. Stober T, Kunze K: Electrocardiographic alterations in subarachnoid hemorrhage: correlation between spasm of the arteries of the left side of the brain and T inversion and QT prolongation. J Neurol 227:99, 1982
185. Sundaram MBM, Chow F: Seizures associated with spontaneous subarachnoid hemorrhage. Can J Neurol Sci 13:229, 1986
186. Sundt TM, Jr, Kobayashi S, Fode NC, Whisnant JP: Results and complications of surgical management of 809 intracranial aneurysms in 722 cases. J Neurosurg 56:753, 1982
187. Sundt TM, Jr, Whisnant JP: Subarachnoid hemorrhage from intracranial aneurysms: surgical management and natural history of disease. N Engl J Med 299:116, 1978
188. Taneda M: Effect of early operation for ruptured aneurysms on prevention of delayed ischemic symptoms. J Neurosurg 57:622, 1982
189. Tani E, Maeda Y, Fukumori T et al: Effect of selective inhibitor of thromboxane A2 synthetase on cerebral vasospasm after early surgery. J Neurosurg 61:24, 1984
190. Tapaninaho A, Hernesniemi J, Vapalahti M: Emergency treatment of cerebral aneurysms with large haematomas. Acta Neurochir 91:21, 1988
191. Tellez H, Bauer RB: Dexamethasone treatment in cerebrovascular disease. I. Controlled study in intracerebral hemorrhage. Stroke 4:541, 1973
192. Terada T, Komai N, Hayashi S et al: Hemorrhagic infarction after vasospasm due to ruptured cerebral aneurysm. Neurosurgery 18:415, 1986
193. Torner JC, Kassell NF, Wallace RB, Adams HP, Jr: Preoperative prognostic factors for rebleeding and survival in aneurysm patients receiving antifibrinolytic therapy: report of the Cooperative Aneurysm study. Neurosurgery 9:506, 9181
194. Touho H, Karasawa J, Shishido H et al: Neurogenic pulmonary edema in the acute stage of hemorrhagic cerebrovascular disease. Neurosurgery 25:762, 1989
195. Tovi D, Thulin CA: Ability of tranexamic acid to cross the blood-brain barrier and its use in patients with ruptured intracranial aneurysms. Acta Neurol Scand 48:257, 1972
196. van Crevel H: Pitfalls in the diagnosis of rebleeding from intracranial aneurysm. Clin Neurol Neurosurg 82:1, 1980
197. van Gijn J, Hijdra A, Wijdicks EFM et al: Acute hydrocephalus after aneurysmal subarachnoid hemorrhage. J Neurosurg 63:355, 1985
198. Vanneste JAL, van Wijngaarden GK: Epsilon-

aminocaproic acid myopathy. Eur Neurol 21:242, 1982.
199. Van Rossum J, Wintzen AR, Enotz LJ et al: Effect of tranexamic acid on rebleeding after subarachnoid hemorrhage: a double-blind controlled clinical trial. Ann Neurol 2:238, 1977
200. Vassilouthis J, Richardson AE: Ventricular dilation and communicating hydrocephalus following spontaneous subarachnoid hemorrhage. J Neurosurg 51:341, 1979
201. Vermeulen M, Lindsay KW, Murray GD et al: Antifibrinolytic treatment in subarachnoid hemorrhage. N Engl J Med 311:432, 1984
202. Vermeulen M, Muizelaar JP: Do antifibrinolytic agents prevent rebleeding after rupture of a cerebral aneurysm?—a review. Clin Neurol Neurosurg 82:25, 1980
203. Vermeulen M, van Gijn J, Hijdra A, van Crevel H: Causes of acute deterioration in patients with a ruptured intracranial aneurysm. J Neurosurg 60:935, 1984
204. Vilkki J, Holst P, Ohman J et al: Cognitive deficits related to computed tomographic findings after surgery for a ruptured intracranial aneurysm. Neurosurgery 25:166, 1989
205. Vinge E, Andersson KE, Brandt L et al: Pharmacokinetics of nimodipine in patients with aneurysmal subarachnoid hemorrhage. Eur J Clin Pharmacol 30:421, 1986
206. Voldby B: Pathophysiology of subarachnoid hemorrhage. Acta Neurochir 45:1, 1988
207. Voldby B, Envoldsen EM: Intracranial pressure changes following aneurysm rupture. 3. Recurrent hemorrhage. J Neurosurg 56:784, 1982
208. Volpe BT, Hirst W: Amnesia following the rupture and repair of an anterior communicating artery aneurysm. J Neurol Neurosurg Psychiatry 46:704, 1983
209. Wakabayashi T, Fujita S: Removal of subarachnoid blood clots after subarachnoid hemorrhage. Surg Neurol 21:553, 1984
210. Weinand ME, O'Boynick PL, Goetz KL: A study of serum antidiuretic hormone and atrial natriuretic peptide levels in a series of patients with intracranial disease and hyponatremia. Neurosurgery, 25:781, 1989
211. Weir B: Medical aspects of the preoperative management of aneurysms: a review. Can J Neurol Sci 6:441, 1979
212. Weir B: Calcium antagonists, cerebral ischemia and vasospasm. Can J Neurol Sci 11:239, 1984
213. Weir B: Antifibrinolytics in subarachnoid hemorrhage: Do they have a role? No. Arch Neurol 44:116, 1987
214. Weir B, Aronyk K: Management mortality and the timing of surgery for supratentorial aneurysms. J Neurosurg 54:146, 1981
215. Weir B, Grace M, Hansen J, Rothberg C: Time course of vasospasm in man. J Neurosurg, 48:173, 1978
216. Weir B, Rothberg C, Grace M et al: Relative prognostic significance of vasospasm following subarachnoid hemorrhage. Can J Neurol Sci 2:109, 1975
217. Whisnant JP, Phillips LH II, Sundt TM, Jr: Aneurysmal subarachnoid hemorrhage: timing of surgery and mortality. Mayo Clin Proc 57:471, 1982
218. Wijdicks EFM, Vermeulen M, Hijdra A, van Gijn J: Hyponatremia and cerebral infarction in patients with ruptured intracranial aneurysms: is fluid restriction harmful? Ann Neurol 17:137, 1985
219. Wijdicks EFM, Vermeulen M, Ten Haaf JA et al: Volume depletion and natriuresis in patients with a ruptured intracranial aneurysm. Ann Neurol 18:211, 1985
220. Wijdicks EFM, Vermeulen M, van Brummelen P, van Gijn J: The effect of fludrocortisone acetate on plasma volume and natriuresis in patients with aneurysmal subarachnoid hemorrhage. Clin Neurol Neurosurg 90:209, 1988
221. Wilkins RH: Attempted prevention or treatment of intracranial arterial spasm: a survey. Neurosurgery 6:198, 1980
222. Wilkins RH: Update: subarachnoid hemorrhage and saccular intracranial aneurysms. Surg Neurol 15:92, 1981
223. Wilkins RH: Attempts at prevention or treatment of intracranial arterial spasm: an update. Neurosurgery 18:808, 1986
224. Wilkins RH: Attempts at prevention and treatment of delayed ischaemic dysfunction in patients with subarachnoid haemorrhage. Acta Neurochir 45:36, 1988
225. Yamamoto I, Hara M, Ogura K et al: Early operation for ruptured intracranial aneurysms: comparative study with computed tomography. Neurosurgery 12:169, 1983
226. Yarnell P, Earnest MP: Primary non-traumatic intracranial hemorrhage: a municipal emergency hospital viewpoint. Stroke 7:608, 1976
227. Yasargil MG, Yonekawa Y, Zumstein B, Stahl HJ: Hydrocephalus following spontaneous subarachnoid hemorrhage: clinical features and treatment. J Neurosurg 39:474, 1973
228. Zuccarello M, Anderson DK: Protective effect of a 21-aminosteroid on the blood-brain barrier following subarachnoid hemorrhage in rats. Stroke 20:367, 1989

# 46 SURGERY OF INTRACRANIAL ANEURYSMS

Joseph M. Zabramski
Robert F. Spetzler

An aneurysm is defined as an abnormally circumscribed dilatation of an artery. In the cerebral circulation, most aneurysms take the form of thin-walled sacs protruding from the arteries of the circle of Willis or its major branches. With few exceptions these lesions make their presence known only after a rupture produces subarachnoid hemorrhage. More rarely, intracranial aneurysms present with the signs and symptoms of a mass lesion or are discovered incidentally when cerebral angiography, computed tomography (CT), or magnetic resonance (MR) imaging is performed for other diagnostic purposes (Figs. 46-1 and 46-2).

The modern history of intracranial aneurysms began with Charles Symonds, who, after suggesting that the diagnosis of subarachnoid hemorrhage could be made during life, investigated the matter at the request of his mentor, Harvey Cushing.[29] Symonds[139] not only coined the term *subarachnoid hemorrhage* and described the use of lumbar puncture for its diagnosis, but he also brought to the attention of the medical community, the relationship between this finding and rupture of intracranial aneurysms.

The introduction of cerebral angiography by Moniz[84] in 1927 allowed the diagnosis of ruptured cerebral aneurysm to be verified and the lesion to be accurately localized. By 1933, Dott[36] reported the clinical and angiographic findings of eight patients and the operative treatment of two of them. In 1937, Dandy[30] performed the first intracranial clipping of an aneurysm and with this bold approach opened the doors to the surgical therapy of intracranial aneurysms.

## INCIDENCE

Aneurysmal subarachnoid hemorrhage is a major health care problem. There are approximately 28,000 new cases each year in North America, based on a reported incidence rate of 12 cases per 100,000 population. In autopsy studies, about 5 percent of the population has been found to harbor intracranial aneurysms.[26,27,130] The incidence varies considerably from one report to another. One major cause of this variation is the lack of agreement about the size at which an arterial defect should be designated an aneurysm. If microaneurysms (2 mm or less) are considered, as many as 17 percent of routine autopsies can be expected to reveal intracranial aneurysms.[49] However, if only lesions larger than 4 mm are considered, the apparent incidence falls to less than 4 percent. The problem is further complicated by observations suggesting that the size of aneurysms is significantly underestimated during routine autopsy examinations. In an elegant study, McCormick and Acosta-Rua[78] demonstrated that perfusing unruptured aneursysm with saline under a pressure of 70 mmHg caused their size to increase by 30 percent to 60 percent.

Rupture of an intracranial aneurysm is the most common cause of subarachnoid hemorrhage: esti-

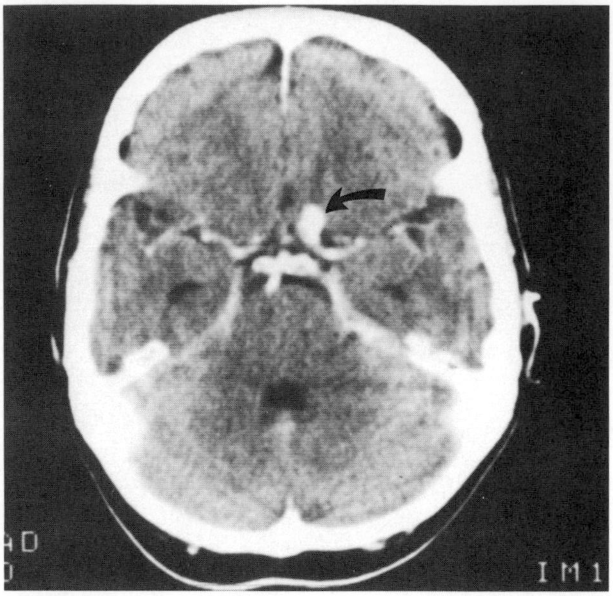

A

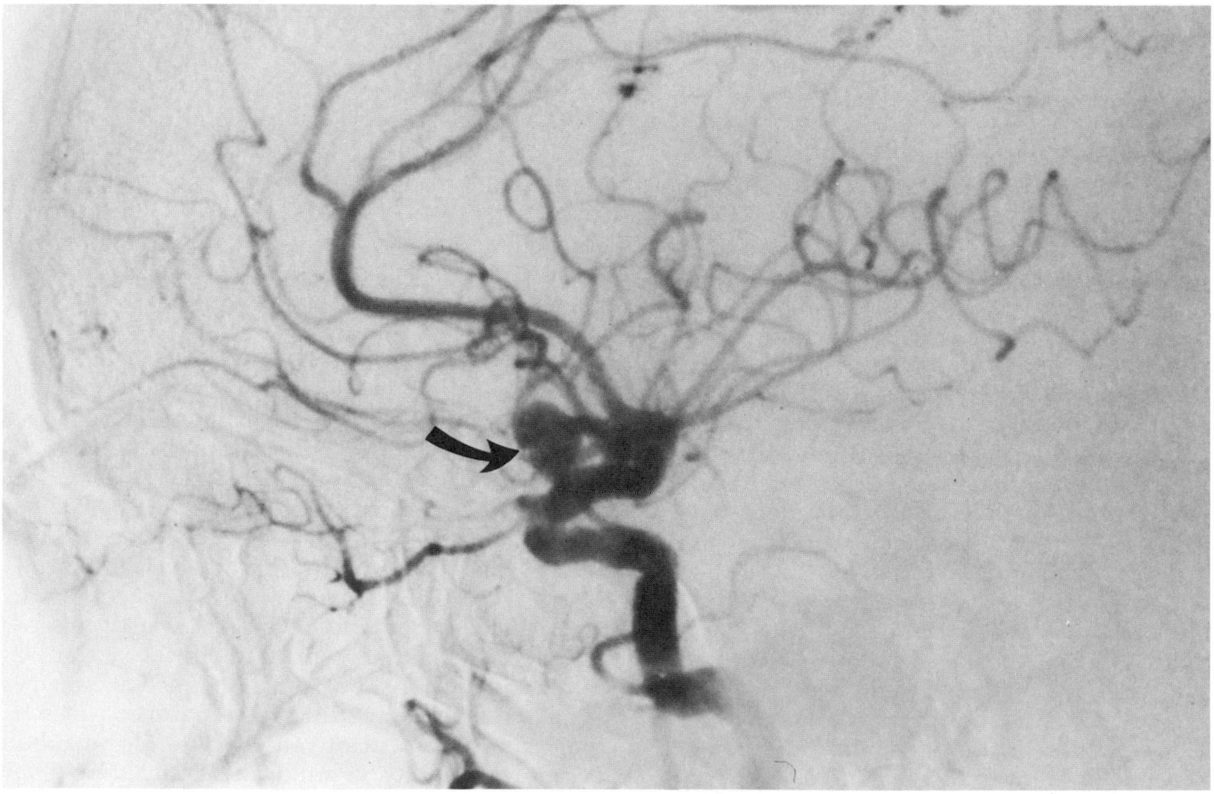

B

**Fig. 46-1.** A 55-year-old woman complained of persistent headache. (**A**) Computed tomography scan with contrast demonstrates an enhancing lesion (*arrow*) thought to be an aneurysm. (**B**) Left internal carotid angiogram in the same patient reveals an internal carotid artery aneurysm (*arrow*) measuring 8 mm at its greatest diameter. The aneurysm was electively clipped without complication.

mates based on the most recent data indicate that 80 to 90 percent of nontraumatic subarachnoid hemorrhage are a result of aneurysmal rupture.[58,135] The rupture of an intracranial aneurysm may also cause bleeding into the brain substance, the ventricular system, or the subdural space.

In the United States, the peak age for aneurysmal rupture is between 40 and 60 years of age.[75] In children and adolescents intracranial aneurysms are rare.[75,80,97] In studies based on routine postmortem examinations, the incidence of intracranial aneurysms increases with age and reaches a plateau in persons between the ages of 35 and 65 years.[55,77] When subarachnoid hemorrhage does occur in children, bleeding from an arteriovenous malformation (AVM) is usually the underlying cause: after the age of 20 years, hemorrhage is more likely to be the result of a ruptured aneurysm (Fig. 46-3).

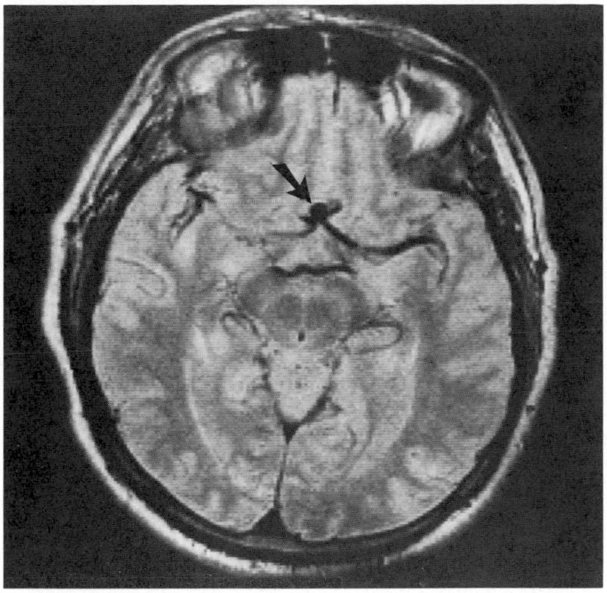

A

**Fig. 46-2.** A 34-year-old man had severe recurrent headaches after a motor vehicle accident. (**A**) Transverse T1-weighted magnetic resonance image through the base of the brain demonstrates a flow-related vascular defect consistent with an anterior communicating artery aneurysm (*arrow*). (**B**) Oblique view of the left common carotid artery angiogram reveals an approximately 6-mm anterior communicating artery aneurysm (*arrow*). The patient underwent elective clipping of the aneurysm without complication.

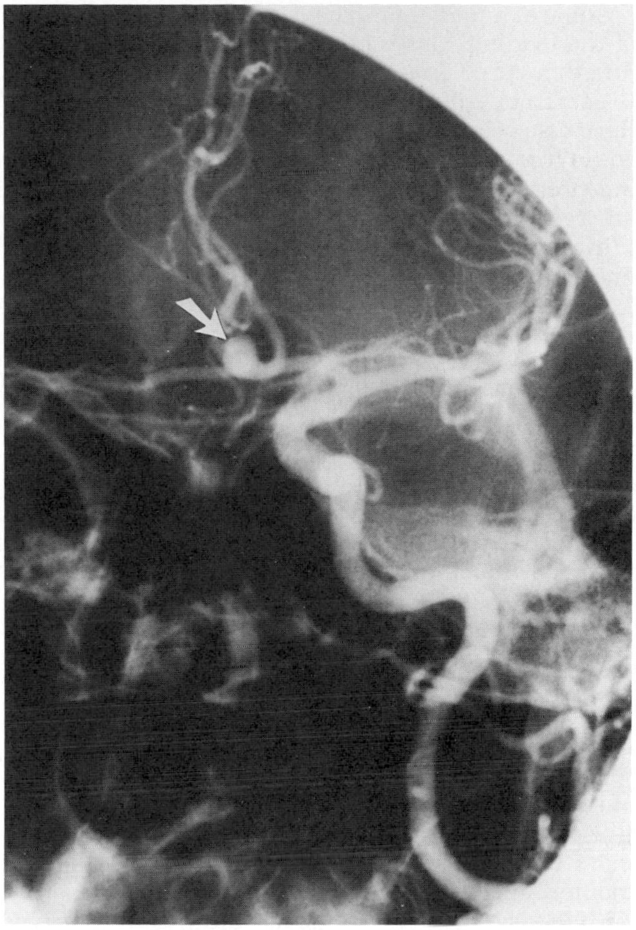

B

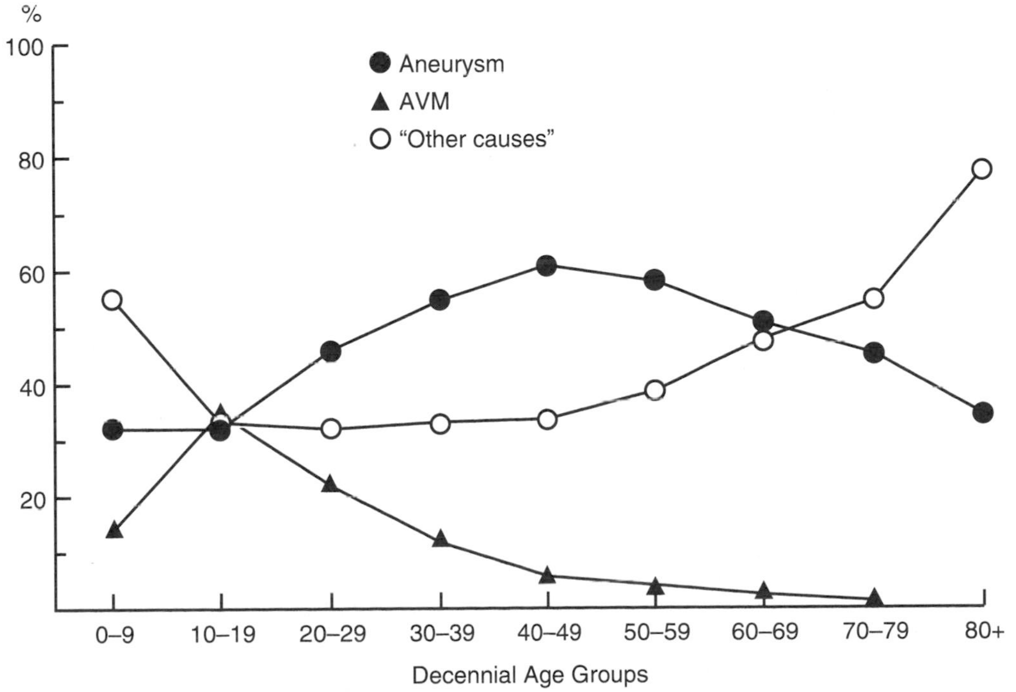


**Fig. 46-3.** Relative probability of major causes of subarachnoid hemorrhage in each decade of life. AVM, arteriovenous malformation. (From Sahs et al.,[110] with permission.)

Subarachnoid hemorrhage during pregnancy is one of the leading causes of maternal mortality in North America.[16,57,83] The incidence is reported to vary between 1 per 2,000 and 1 per 10,000 pregnancies, with the cause related to AVMs and aneurysms with about equal frequency.[83,106] AVMs tend to rupture early during pregnancy or during delivery, while aneurysms are reported to rupture most commonly during the third trimester, and only rarely during labor.[16,57,83] The evaluation and treatment of subarachnoid hemorrhage during pregnancy should be the same as if the patient were not pregnant. Craniotomy and clipping of the aneurysm are the most appropriate forms of therapy.[57,83,104] Prophylactic cesarean section has been recommended for the management of pregnant women with untreated aneurysms, but vaginal delivery with lumbar epidural anesthesia appears to be equally safe and effective and is therefore the method of choice.[57] Cesarean section is recommended if the mother is moribund and the child appears viable.

## DISTRIBUTION

The International Cooperative Study on the Timing of Aneurysm Surgery constitutes the most extensive series that has evaluated patients for the distribution of ruptured aneurysms. This study was the collaborative effort of 213 neurosurgeons at 68 medical centers in 15 countries. A total of 3,521 patients with documented aneurysmal subarachnoid hemorrhage were enrolled. In contrast to earlier studies of this type, most patients in this series underwent complete angiographic evaluation, including the posterior fossa vertebrobasilar system.

The distribution of ruptured aneurysms in these patients is presented in Table 46-1. The anterior communicating artery was the most common site of rupture, accounting for 34 percent of cases. It was followed by the internal carotid artery (30 percent) and middle cerebral artery distributions (22 percent). Aneurysms in the internal carotid artery distribution were most often encountered at the origin of the posterior communicating artery, followed by the carotid bifurcation and the origin of the ophthalmic artery. Aneurysms of the posterior circulation most commonly occurred at the basilar tip, followed by the vertebral origin of the posterior inferior cerebellar artery and the other basilar trunk branches. Overall, aneurysms of the vertebral and basilar artery systems composed 7.6 percent of the Cooperative Study series.

Multiple aneurysms are found in 20 to 30 percent of patients with aneurysmal subarachnoid hemorrhage.[3,88,96] When more than one aneurysm is discovered at angiography, the lesion responsible for the hemorrhage must be identified so that it can be treated first. In a retrospective analysis of 205 aneurysms in 69 patients, Nehls et al.[88] found that irregularity of contour was the most important factor identifying the site of rupture, although size and location were also helpful. When aneurysms were of similar size, the more irregular of the aneurysms was the site of rupture in 93.3 percent of cases. In fact, in only one instance did a larger, but less irregular, aneurysm rupture. When aneurysms have smooth walls, the largest and most proximal aneurysm was the one most likely to rupture. Finally, when all other factors were equal, the most frequent site of rupture was the posterior communicating artery, followed by the anterior communicating artery, the middle cerebral artery, and other internal carotid artery branch points. Focal spasm in the area of aneurysm is a rare but highly reliable angiographic sign for localizing the site of rupture. A CT scan can also help identify the aneurysm responsible for hemorrhage. Focal accumulations of subarachnoid blood (e.g., within the interhemispheric or sylvian fissures) are the most indicative signs (Fig. 46-4).

**TABLE 46-1. Distribution of Ruptured Aneurysms**

| Artery | No. of Cases | % |
|---|---|---|
| Internal carotid | | |
| Cavernous | 11 | 0.3 |
| Ophthalamic | 89 | 2.5 |
| Posterior communicating | 807 | 23.0 |
| Carotid bifurcation | 144 | 41.0 |
| Anterior cerebral | | |
| Proximal to anterior communicating | 59 | 1.7 |
| Anterior communicating | 1,184 | 34.0 |
| Distal to anterior communicating (A2) | 131 | 3.7 |
| Middle cerebral | | |
| Proximal to 1st main branch | 101 | 2.9 |
| At tri/bifurcation | 662 | 19.0 |
| Distal to tri/bifurcation | 23 | 0.7 |
| Posterior cerebral | | |
| P1 | 11 | 0.3 |
| P2 at posterior communicating | 10 | 0.3 |
| Distal posterior cerebral | 10 | 0.3 |
| Vertebral | | |
| Posterior inferior cerebellar | 88 | 2.5 |
| Vertebral junction | 18 | 0.5 |
| Basilar | | |
| Trunk at anterior inferior cerebellar | 7 | 0.2 |
| Bifurcation | 106 | 3.0 |
| Superior cerebellar | 16 | 4.5 |
| Other | 44 | 1.2 |
| Total | 3,521 | |

(Based on data from the International Cooperative Study on Timing of Aneurysm Surgery.)

## NATURAL HISTORY

Numerous retrospective studies have been conducted in an effort to elucidate the natural history of aneurysmal subarachnoid hemorrhage. Attempts to assemble a representative series have been hampered by the problems of evaluating patients who receive no treatment because of selection criteria and by the lack

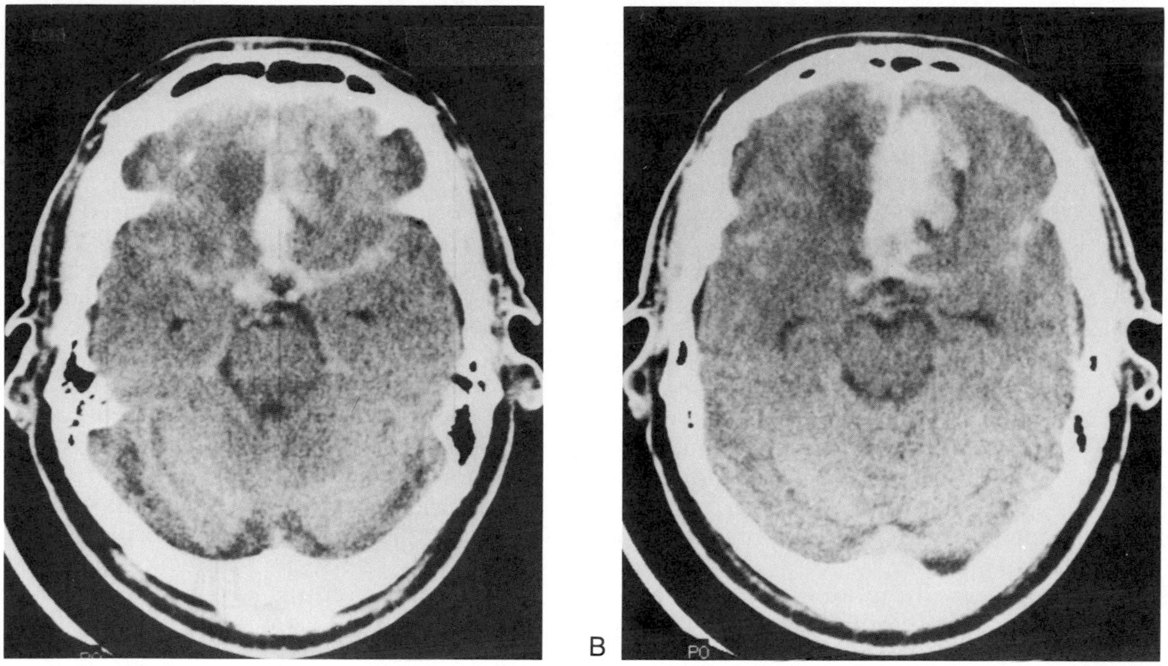

A B

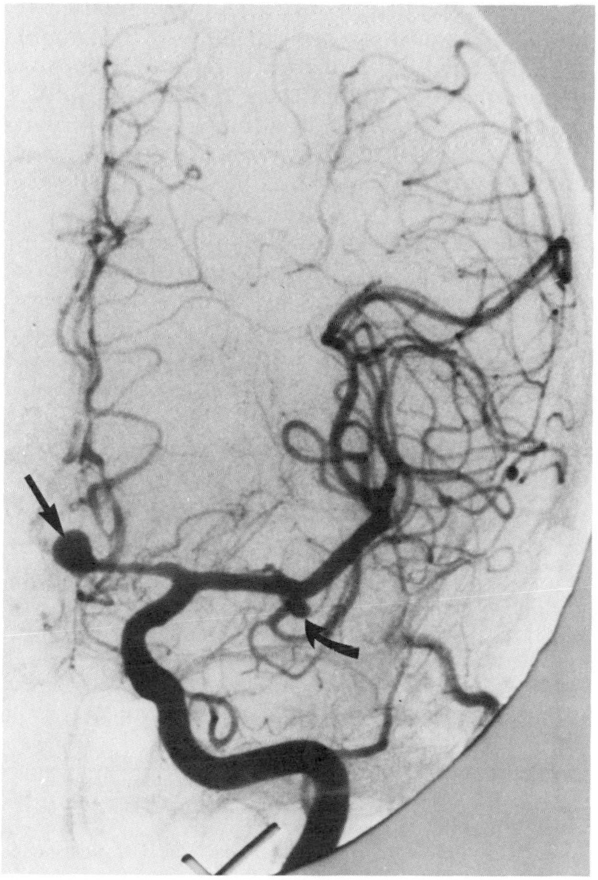

C

**Fig. 46-4.** A 56-year-old man presented with the sudden onset of severe headache, nausea, and photophobia. On evaluation in the emergency room, the patient was mildly lethargic and confused. (**A & B**) Basic head computed tomography scan images at two levels demonstrate a severe subarachnoid hemorrhage with a large collection of blood in the interhemispheric fissure. Subarachnoid hemorrhage in this distribution is nearly pathognomonic for rupture of an anterior communicating artery aneurysm. (**C**) Anteroposterior view of the left internal carotid artery angiogram reveals an approximately 7-mm anterior communicating artery aneurysm (*straight arrow*). Note also the small, incidental left middle cerebral artery aneurysm (*curved arrow*).

of angiographic evaluation in many historical studies. Despite these difficulties, various authors have collected valuable data that shed light on the factors affecting the prognosis of patients with ruptured aneurysms. The results of several population studies suggest that at least 15 percent of patients are found dead after the initial hemorrhage.[74,143] For patients who survive the acute hemorrhage, data from multiple Cooperative Studies suggest that the mortality rate during the first 2 weeks is 20 to 30 percent, with a morbidity of about 20 percent.[65,67,75] Rebleeding is a major cause of death and disability in the untreated patient. The risk of rebleeding during the first 2 weeks after hemorrhage is approximately 20 percent and increases to 33 percent at 1 month and 50 percent at 6 months.[61,65,75,108] Mortality from this second hemorrhage is 40 to 50 percent. The risk of rebleeding gradually diminishes, but does not go to zero. Approximately 3 percent of long-term survivors can be expected to rebleed annually.[61]

Even considering the limitations of the accumulated data, it is not unreasonable to estimate that there is a 45 percent mortality rate during the first year following rupture of an aneurysm, and a significant continuing threat of rebleeding thereafter. It becomes apparent, then, why so many treatment modalities have been applied in attempts to influence the unfavorable prognosis of these patients.

With regard to an individual patient's prognosis and chance of ultimate recovery, the most important factor appears to be the patient's clinical condition at the time treatment is begun. One of the systems most widely used in the grading of a patient's condition is the Hunt and Hess classification (Table 46-2). The scale heavily weighs the level of consciousness because this is the most important factor in predicting outcome. In discussing overall management outcome, patients are frequently divided into good (Hunt and Hess clinical grades I, II, and III) and poor grades (Hunt and Hess grades IV and V).

## PERIOPERATIVE MANAGEMENT

No discussion of the surgical treatment of patients with aneurysmal subarachnoid hemorrhage would be complete without reviewing perioperative management. The discussion here will be limited, however, as a thorough review of this topic is presented elsewhere in this volume.

**TABLE 46-2. Hunt and Hess Clinical Grading Scale**

| Group | Condition |
|---|---|
| 0 | Unruptured aneurysm |
| 1 | Asymptomatic or minimal headache and slight nuchal rigidity |
| 2 | Moderate or severe headache nuchal rigidity; no neurologic deficit other than cranial nerve palsy |
| 3 | Drowsiness, confusion, or mild focal deficit |
| 4 | Stupor, moderate to severe hemiparesis |
| 5 | Deep coma, decerebrate posturing, moribund appearance |

Perhaps no area of neurosurgery has undergone more rapid change than the management of patients with ruptured aneurysms. In 1983, when the original manuscript for this text was being prepared, early surgery in the patient with a ruptured aneurysm was considered controversial; antifibrinolytic agents were used routinely at many institutions to reduce the risk of rebleeding while patients awaited delayed surgery; and the first publications on the use of calcium antagonists and hypervolemic-hypertensive therapy for the treatment of vasospasm were appearing. Only 8 years later, early surgery for the clipping of ruptured aneurysms is the norm; intracisternal fibrinolytic agents (e.g., tissue plasminogen activator) are being studied for their ability to enhance the lysis of subarachnoid blood for the prevention of vasospasm; and calcium antagonists and hypervolemic-hypertensive therapy are part of the routine postoperative care at most institutions.

### General Care

The preoperative care of the patient with aneurysmal subarachnoid hemorrhage is directed toward minimizing the risk of recurrent hemorrhage and toward accelerating the patient's clinical recovery. Routine management should include admission to an intensive care unit, with cardiac monitoring and placement of an arterial line for the monitoring of blood pressure. Supportive care includes complete bed rest in a quiet room as well as sedation and pain medication as needed. For sedation and control of pain, we prefer small intravenous doses of morphine sulfate (1 to 4 mg/h), which has a short half-life, and can be readily reversed if necessary to evaluate apparent changes in mental status.

### Blood Pressure and Fluid Management

The decision of whether to treat hypertension, the choice of drugs, dosage schedules, and other elements of the management of blood pressure can be complex issues in the patient with aneurysmal subarachnoid hemorrhage. Hypertension may represent a response to increase intracranial pressure (ICP), pain, or anxiety. Blood pressure often returns to a normal range after the patient has been admitted to the hospital, and these problems have been addressed.

In general, we do not recommend treatment of hypertension in patients with systolic blood pressures under 160 mmHg. To control blood pressures above this level, we prefer one of the dihydropyridine class of calcium antagonists such as nimodipine or nicardipine. These agents have the advantage that while they lower systemic blood pressure, they tend to increase cerebral blood flow. Nimodipine is the only agent presently approved by the FDA for the prevention and treatment of delayed cerebral vasospasm and is thus started before other antihypertensives are instituted. Treatment with nimodipine (60 mg/4 h, orally) for the first 21 days after hemorrhage has been shown to significantly improve outcome and to decrease the incidence of delayed ischemic deficits in patients with ruptured aneurysms.[102] We routinely treat all patients with aneurysmal subarachnoid hemorrhage with nimodipine, beginning therapy soon after they are admitted to the intensive care unit. Occasionally patients are markedly sensitive to these agents, particularly the elderly and those on multiple antihypertensive medications. Therefore, we begin therapy with 30 mg (orally or via nasogastric tube) every 4 hours and increase this dose to 60 mg every 4 hours if the patient remains clinically stable. If blood pressure remains consistently above 160 mmHg before surgical clipping of the ruptured aneurysm, despite the initiation of therapy with nimodipine, small doses of labetolol or hydralazine-HCl can be given intravenously.

After the aneurysm is clipped, nimodipine is continued, but other antihypertensive agents are held for the first 2 weeks after hemorrhage (when patients are at greatest risk of vasospasm) unless systolic blood pressure exceeds 200 mmHg. Thereafter, routine medical management for hypertension is utilized. Careful monitoring of neurologic function is essential during the administration of antihypertensive agents. If the patient's clinical status deteriorates after receiving antihypertensive medication, vasospasm should be suspected and the blood pressure should be briskly returned to a previously well-tolerated level.

In patients who develop clinically symptomatic vasospasm, fluid therapy should be maximized and the blood pressure pharmacologically elevated. Our protocol for the management of symptomatic spasm is outlined in Table 46-3. It is important to recognize early symptoms of clinically significant vasospasm prior to the onset of severe ischemic deficits. Worsening headache, hyponatremia, and increasing lethargy 5 to 10 days after hemorrhage are the most frequent harbingers of vasospasm.

**TABLE 46-3. Hypervolemic-Hypertensive Protocol for Treatment of Symptomatic Vasospasm**

| |
|---|
| Swan-Ganz Catheter |
| Normal saline: 150 ml/h |
| Plasmanate: 100 ml/h prn |
| PAD > 12 mmHg |
| DDAVP: 1–2 ml intravenously Q6h |
| PRN urine output > 200 ml/h |
| (Hold for PAD > 16 mmHg, or serum sodium < 134 mEq/L) |
| Neosynephrine infusion (50 mg in 250 ml normal saline) |
| Titrate to maintain systolic blood pressure 180–220 mmHg and reverse ischemic deficits |
| (Hold for SVR > 1,500 dyn-s/m$^2$) |
| Dopamine infusion prn |
| Cardiac output < 5 L/min |
| 3% Sodium chloride sol'n: 30–50 ml/h |
| PRN serum sodium < 134 mEq/L |

*Abbreviations*: PAD, Pulmonary artery diastolic pressure; SVR, systemic vascular resistance.

**TABLE 46-4. Prophylactic Hypervolemic Fluid Therapy**

| |
|---|
| Low-Risk Vasospasm Protocol |
| (CT scan: little or no SAH) |
| Normal saline: 150 ml/h |
| Serum sodium level daily |
| Serum sodium < 134 mEq/L |
| Switch to high-risk protocol |
| |
| High-Risk Vasospasm Protocol |
| (CT scan: moderate or large SAH) |
| Swan-Ganz catheter |
| Normal saline: 150 ml/h |
| Plasmanate: 100 ml/h PRN |
| PAD < 8 mmHg |
| Serum sodium levels twice daily |
| 3% Sodium chloride sol'n: 30–50 ml/hr |
| PRN serum sodium level |
| < 134 mEq/L |
| (Hold for PAD > 16 mmHg) |

*Abbreviations*: SAH, subarachnoid hemorrhage; PAD, pulmonary artery diastolic pressure.

Fluid and electrolyte management and the treatment of vasospasm are reviewed in detail in Chapter 45 in this volume. In general, we use prophylactic hypervolemic therapy (Table 46-4) for all patients with aneurysmal hemorrhage during the initial 10 to 14 days after hemorrhage; intravenous fluid therapy is then gradually weaned in patients without clinical or transcranial Doppler evidence of spasm.

## Ventricular Drainage

Hydrocephalus is a constant threat in the patient with subarachnoid hemorrhage. When CT reveals evidence of hydrocephalus or intraventricular hemorrhage or when the patient has a depressed level of consciousness (i.e., Hunt and Hess grades III to V), an external ventriculostomy should be placed. If ICP is above 15 mmHg, the ventriculostomy is opened intermittently to drain at a level of 10 cm above the external auditory meatus. Cerebrospinal fluid (CSF) drainage at these levels maximizes cerebral perfusion and often improves clinical status by one to two grades on the Hunt and Hess Scale. Monitoring ICP is also useful in deciding whether to proceed with surgery in poor grade patients (Hunt and Hess grades IV and V; see section on Timing of Surgery in this chapter). Postoperatively, the drain is left open to constant drainage at 10 to 15 cm$H_2O$, until CSF output falls below 30 to 40 ml per shift, or until the 14th day after hemorrhage when the drain is progressively elevated in an attempt to wean the patient from the ventriculostomy. In our experience, approximately 30 percent of patients will require a CSF-shunting procedure.

Risk of infection from external ventriculostomy can be minimized by observing meticulous sterile technique, including a full surgical preparation, during placement of the catheter, prophylactic antibiotics (we prefer cefuroxime 1.5 g/8 h started immediately before placement of the catheter and continued until its removal), and tunneling the ventriculostomy catheter a minimum of 4 cm subcutaneously from the insertion site. Finally, it is important that the catheter be connected to a closed drainage system that does not require opening the system directly to air for zeroing or obtaining CSF samples.* CSF samples are obtained twice weekly on a routine basis for cell counts, Gram stain, and culture. Using this protocol, we have not found it necessary to change the ventriculostomy site every 2 to 3 days as some authors have recommended.[76,152] Indeed, we routinely leave ventricular drainage catheters in place as long as 2 to 3 weeks and have had only a 3 to 5 percent incidence of infection.

### Antifibrinolytic Therapy

Amicar and other antifibrinolytic agents that were once widely used to reduce the incidence of early rebleeding while patients awaited surgery (usually a period of 10 to 14 days) have fallen into disfavor. One reason for this change is that early clipping of aneurysms can be performed with modern microsurgical techniques without increasing the operative morbidity and mortality. More importantly, however, evidence from a number of studies has demonstrated that while therapy with antifibrinolytic agents significantly reduced the risk of early rebleeding by as much as 50 percent, their use was associated with an equally significant increase in the risk of ischemic complications.[43,66,144,145] In addition, the use of antifibrinolytic agents has been linked to an increased risk of hydrocephalus.[46,66,98,103] Overall, these studies fail to demonstrate any clear benefit associated with antifibrinolytic therapy, and this treatment can no longer be recommended. (For a more extensive review of this material, see Chapter 45 in this volume.)

## TIMING OF SURGERY FOR RUPTURED ANEURYSMS

The timing of surgery for the patient presenting with aneurysmal subarachnoid hemorrhage remains a controversial issue. Much of the debate arises from the failure of earlier authors to consider the historical developments in this field. Before the general introduction of the operating microscope in the early 1970s, the risks of early surgery after rupture of an aneurysm outweighed any potential benefit secondary to reduction in rebleeding from clipping. In the late 1970s and early 1980s, a small number of authors reported good outcomes in patients undergoing early surgery for ruptured aneurysms.[56,71,113,149] Simultaneously, the emphasis on the management of these patients shifted from operative morbidity and mortality rates to overall management outcome.

In a 1981 report, the Cooperative Aneurysm Study Group[1] analyzed the overall results of early medical management and delayed surgery for clipping of the ruptured aneurysm in 249 patients. The authors reported a favorable outcome in only 46 percent of patients with a mortality rate of 36.2 percent. Of patients admitted in good condition with a potential for complete recovery, only 55.7 percent had a favorable outcome, and 28.7 percent died. Other authors have reported similar results with an overall management mortality for delayed surgery between 40 and 60 percent.[39,63,81,107] As a result, early surgery was proposed by an increasing number of authors in an attempt to improve these disappointing figures.

This issue was addressed by the recently published International Cooperative Study on the Timing of Aneurysm Surgery.[67,68] Between January 1981 and June 1983, 3,521 patients who were hospitalized within 3 days of subarachnoid hemorrhage were enrolled in the cooperative multi-institutional protocol. This was an intention-to-treat study: when the patient was admitted, the surgeon stated the time of scheduled surgery. Results were analyzed on the basis of outcome assessed 6 months after hemorrhage. Intracranial operations were performed in 92 percent of patients who had surgery planned for days 0 to 3. However, 24 percent of the patients originally scheduled for surgery for 11 to 14 days after hemorrhage and 38 percent of those with surgery scheduled at 15+ days did not undergo clipping of their aneurysm. These patients died or had complications related to rebleeding and/or vasospasm that contraindicated surgery. Among alert patients, those operated on within 48 hours of rupture did as well as those undergoing surgery 2 weeks after hemorrhage. Early operation was not accompanied by a significantly higher rate of surgical complications than those associated with delayed operation. The overall results of management were almost identical in patients with surgery planned within 3 days of hemorrhage and in those with surgery scheduled for 11 to 14 days. The mortality was 20 percent, and 60 percent had good outcomes. Vasospasm was the major cause of death and poor outcome.

Early surgery eliminates the morbidity and mortality associated with rebleeding. In addition, with the aneurysm clipped, delayed ischemic deficits secondary to vasospasm can be treated more effectively and safely. In good-grade patients (Hunt and Hess grades I to III), multiple groups have reported that early surgery, the use of calcium antagonists, and hypervolemic-hypertensive therapy can reduce overall management mortality to 10 percent or less, with good outcomes in 75 percent or more of those who survive.[4–6,72,73,93,114,143]

* Becker External Drainage System, PS Medical, Goleta, CA 93117.

We reviewed our experience at the Barrow Neurological Institute from 1987 to 1990. Over this 3-year period, we operated early on all patients with documented aneurysmal subarachnoid hemorrhage, regardless of their clinical grade (excluding only patients without evidence of brain stem function). Early surgery (within 72 hours of hemorrhage) was performed in 90 patients. All patients were treated with aggressive fluid management, including hypervolemic-hypertensive therapy in those who developed evidence of cerebral vasospasm. At a 3-month follow-up, 81 percent of patients had good outcomes, 8 percent had poor outcomes, and 11 percent died. In good-grade patients (Hunt and Hess grades I to III), 88 percent had a good outcome, and only 7 percent died. In 23 poor-grade patients (Hunt and Hess grades IV and V), 56 percent had good outcomes and 26 percent died. Three patients had severe deficits, and one was vegetative.

Our experience parallels that reported in other recent series. Early surgery, combined with calcium antagonists and aggressive fluid management, improves survival and outcome. We now operate on all good-grade patients (Hunt and Hess grades I to III) regardless of the timing of presentation. When patients are referred on a delayed basis (4 or more days after hemorrhage) and are neurologically stable, we routinely maximize fluid-volume status and proceed with surgery; however, many surgeons will repeat angiography and delay operative clipping of the aneurysm if angiographic evidence of vasospasm is present. Although angiographic vasospasm may affect surgical outcome, its effect on overall management outcome is an issue that has not been addressed in clinical trials. When surgery is delayed because of angiographic evidence of vasospasm, patients are exposed to the risks of rebleeding. Furthermore, if the arterial spasm becomes clinically symptomatic, it cannot be treated safely in an aggressive fashion. Until this issue is more thoroughly studied, we think that angiographic evidence of spasm should not be considered an absolute contraindication to surgery. Special care should be taken in these patients to limit the risks of ischemic injury by preventing even mild intraoperative hypotension; reductions of systemic arterial pressure of more than 10 to 15 percent below postoperative levels should be avoided.

The decision of when and whether to operate on poor-grade patients (Hunt and Hess grades IV and V) after aneurysmal hemorrhage is much more controversial. Nevertheless, it is clear that occasional patients admitted in poor condition soon after hemorrhage will have a good outcome. Based on our experience in this population, we have developed a protocol for the selection of operative candidates based on CT scan data, ICP measurements, and angiographic findings (Fig. 46-5).[10] Briefly, all patients presenting with subarachnoid hemorrhage in grades IV

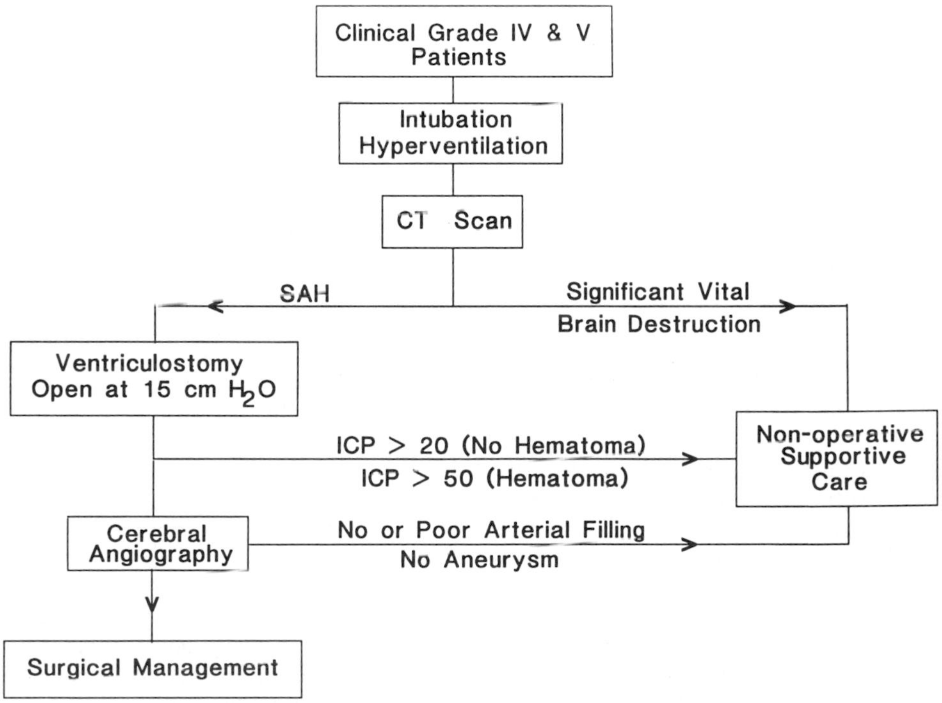


**Fig. 46-5.** Treatment algorithm for the management of poor-grade patients with aneurysmal subarachnoid hemorrhage. CT, computed tomography; SAH, subarachnoid hemorrhage; ICP, intracranial pressure. (Adapted from Bailes et al.,[10] with permission.)

and V have a ventriculostomy placed, except those who show radiographic evidence of irreversible brain destruction. For example, a large hematoma in the dominant basal ganglia would preclude active treatment. In addition, operative intervention is withheld for three reasons after ventriculostomy: (1) if ICP cannot be controlled below 20 $cmH_2O$ in the patient without hematoma, (2) if ICP is greater than 50 $cmH_2O$ in the patient with hematoma, or (3) if there is poor or absent intracranial filling on angiography. Once medically stable, the remaining patients have early surgery for aneurysm clipping and evacuation of any intracranial hematomas, irrespective of their neurologic examination. Postoperatively, patients are treated with calcium antagonists and aggressive hypervolemic-hypertensive therapy.

Certainly, patients in worse neurologic condition are expected to have a poorer outcome; however, clinical examination alone soon after aneurysmal hemorrhage is not a good criterion for predicting outcome.[10,53,101] In a prospective study that evaluated our protocol in 54 poor-grade patients, 35 patients (20 grade IV and 15 grade V) were selected for active treatment: 19 patients (54 percent) had a good outcome at 3 months and were independent for all activities of daily living; 4 patients (11 percent) were dependent for some activities but were not housebound; 4 patients were institutionalized with poor outcomes; and 8 patients (23 percent) died.[10] There were no survivors in the nonoperative group. Clearly, an aggressive surgical approach based on appropriate selection criteria is warranted in Grades IV and V patients.

While the decision tree outlined in Figure 46-5 is helpful in selecting patients for surgery, the decision of whether to operate on the poor-grade patient often rests on associated clinical variables. For example, most surgeons would clip a posterior communicating artery aneurysm in a young, Hunt and Hess grade 4 patient with a nondominant temporal lobe hematoma, whereas few would attempt intervention for a deep clot in the dominant hemisphere of an elderly Grade 4 patient with a carotid bifurcation aneurysm.

## MANAGEMENT OF MULTIPLE AND INCIDENTAL ANEURYSMS

Multiple aneurysms and aneurysms discovered incidentally are at risk of rupture. Attempts have been made to define a critical size (diameter) below which aneurysms should be observed. Wiebers et al.[151] reported 130 conservatively treated patients with unruptured aneurysms. During an average follow-up of 8.3 years, there were 15 hemorrhages, all in patients with aneurysms greater than 10 mm in diameter (mean diameter, 21.3 mm). Yet at the same institution, the mean size for ruptured aneurysms seen angiographically was 7.5 mm. To explain this discrepancy, the authors postulate that the critical size for aneurysm rupture is smaller if rupture occurs at or soon after the time of aneurysm formation. In an autopsy series, Crompton[28] found the critical size for aneurysm rupture to be 4 mm. Similarly, McCormick and Acosta-Rua[78] found 5 mm to be the critical size for rupture. In an analysis of angiograms from 1,093 patients with subarachnoid hemorrhage admitted to the Cooperative Aneurysm Study, Kassell and Torner[64] found that the median diameter for ruptured aneurysms was 7.0 mm. In contrast to the study by Wiebers et al.,[151] 71 percent of the aneurysms were smaller than 10 mm and 13 percent were less than 5 mm in diameter. In general, the data from the literature suggest that the critical size for rupture is between 4 and 7 mm.

Some controversy continues about the management of these lesions. A few authors recommend that unruptured aneurysms should not be operated on because the morbidity and mortality of surgery is higher than that associated with their natural history. However, a thoughtful analysis by van Crevel et al.[142] suggests otherwise. These authors used modern decision analysis techniques to compare the risks of nonoperative and operative treatment in patients with incidental aneurysms and calculated the break-even age at which patients with incidental aneurysms would no longer benefit from surgery (Fig. 46-6).[152] They pointed out that, when an aneurysm ruptures, the consequences are often devastating: population studies suggest that approximately 15 percent of patients are found dead after the initial hemorrhage, while 30 to 40 percent of those hospitalized die or have poor

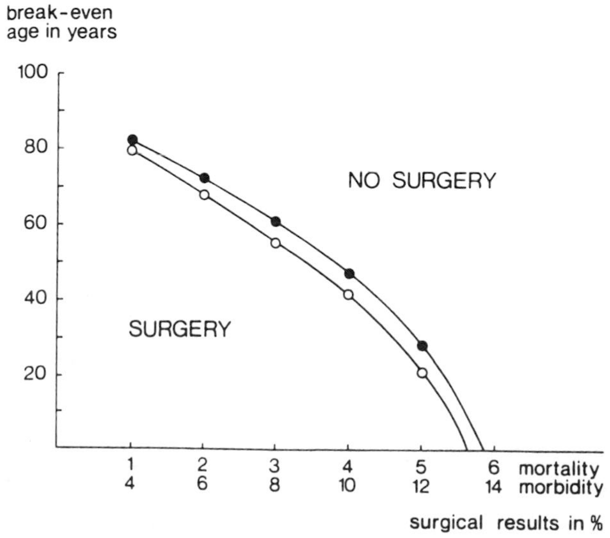


**Fig. 46-6.** Age of the patient at which surgery and no surgery have the same expected utility (break-even age) as a function of surgical morbidity and mortality. Patients are assumed to be good surgical candidates from a medical standpoint. Closed circles, females; open circles, males. (Adapted from van Crevel et al.,[142] with permission.)

outcomes.[23,67,74,102,142] A review of multiple studies reveals a risk of rupture for intact aneurysms of 1 to 2 percent per year.[31,61] Using these figures, the estimated combined morbidity and mortality for aneurysm rupture is 1.5 to 3 percent at 3 years, increasing to 2.5 to 5 percent at 5 years.

Microsurgical techniques and improvements in anesthesia have made the operative risks for the elective management of unruptured aneurysms extremely favorable. Samson et al.[112] reported no mortality and 6.3 percent morbidity in 49 patients. Salazar[111] had no mortality and 3.4 percent morbidity in his series. Drake[39] successfully clipped 289 intact aneurysms with no mortality and a morbidity of 1.7 percent.

These reports indicate that intact aneurysms are not benign lesions. In experienced hands, these lesions can be surgically treated with a combined morbidity and mortality less than that of their natural history over 3 to 5 years. If an aneurysm is accessible, and the patient is a good operative risk, then surgical treatment is the therapy of choice.

## MANAGEMENT OF MYCOTIC ANEURYSMS

Mycotic aneurysms develop as a result of infection in the arterial wall. The term "mycotic" was coined by Osler[95] in 1885, and, although it more properly refers to lesions caused by fungal infections, common usage through the years has applied the term mycotic to aneurysms produced by any infectious agent.

Mycotic aneurysms are caused by the extension of infection for emboli that lodge in the arterial lumen or within the vasa vasorum of the vessel wall. Once established, the ensuing infectious process leads to damage of the vessel wall and aneurysmal dilatation. The aneurysms are usually fusiform in shape, but saccular aneurysms do occur. Unlike congenital aneurysms, which are normally located at the proximal branching points of the circle of Willis, mycotic aneurysms typically are located more peripherally (Fig. 46-7).

Mycotic aneurysms constitute approximately 5 percent of cerebral aneurysms. They occur primarily as a complication of subacute bacterial endocarditis (SBE), but are also seen in patients with congenital heart disease and prominent right to left shunts. In patients who develop SBE, approximately 17 percent are reported to have symptoms of cerebral embolization. Clinical and pathologic studies have demonstrated the presence of mycotic aneurysms in approximately 4 percent of patients with SBE. Considering the embolic pathogenesis of these lesions, angiographic evaluation is recommended for patients with SBE and symptoms suggesting cerebral embolic events.

Patients who harbor an unruptured bacterial aneurysm(s) should be treated with high doses of the appropriate antibiotics, and the aneurysm should be followed with repeat angiography.[18,19,87] Because of the high morbidity and mortality associated with rupture of these lesions, angiography should be performed at weekly intervals during the initial stages of treat-

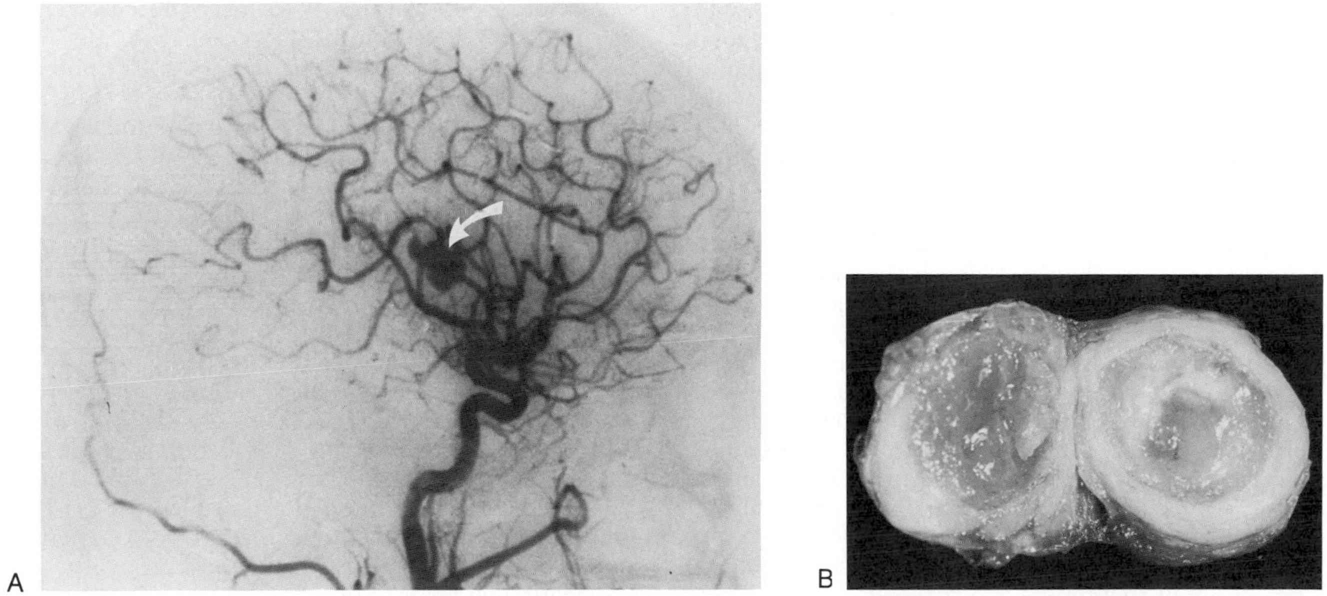


**Fig. 46-7.** (**A & B**) Angiographic and gross pathologic appearance of mycotic middle cerebral artery aneurysms (*arrow*) in a middle-aged male who presented with a history of left-hemisphere transient ischemic attacks, as well as with signs and symptoms of subacute bacterial endocarditis, including dyspnea, fever, chills, and a grade V/VI systolic ejection murmur.

ment. If the aneurysm thromboses or disappears, no further treatment is necessary. However, if the aneurysm enlarges or remains unchanged, it should be treated surgically. Insufficient experience is available to comment on whether fungal aneurysms can be treated successfully without surgery.

## GENERAL OPERATIVE CONSIDERATIONS

Although we strongly recommend the early clipping of ruptured aneurysms, we believe that surgery in these difficult cases is best performed by a well-rested, experienced team. At our institution, surgery is usually performed within 12 to 24 hours of admission. This short delay provides adequate time for complete angiographic evaluation and medical stabilization of the patient, including placement of a ventriculostomy if indicated. In our experience, many poor-grade patients will improve clinically during this period by as much as one to two grades on the Hunt and Hess Scale. The patient with an intracerebral or extra-axial hematoma who is deteriorating is an obvious exception and requires emergency surgical intervention.

The anesthesiologist should be experienced in the management of neurosurgical cases and familiar with the surgeon's preferences for intraoperative management (i.e., the use of mannitol and barbiturates; see the next section). They should assist with the operative positioning of the patient, including the padding of all pressure points. In all but the most urgent cases, surface electrodes are placed for the monitoring of EEG and somatosensory evoked potentials (Fig. 46-8). Before the patient is prepared for surgery, the edges of the operative field are draped with self-adhering plastic drapes (Fig. 46-8) that prevent moisture from solutions, blood, and intraoperative irrigation from interfering with scalp electrode function.

The advantage of an experienced scrub nurse who arranges the instrument table and hands the surgeon the appropriate instruments rapidly and efficiently cannot be overemphasized. The nurse should be positioned at the instrument table with unobstructed access to the surgeon's hands. A television monitor connected to a videocamera on the microscope should be visible to the nurse and the neuroanesthesiologist. The assisting surgeon is responsible for irrigating the operative field with a microirrigator composed of a 12-ml syringe attached to a slightly curved blunt-tipped needle. The surgeon should be comfortably positioned in a mobile chair with pedals for the microscope and bipolar readily accessible. Arm rests should be positioned to support the surgeon's forearms and wrists. Certainly, the quiet efficiency of an experienced operating room team is translated into lower morbidity and mortality for the patient.

### Anesthesia for Aneurysm Surgery

Advances in neuroanesthesia have markedly reduced the perioperative risks of intracranial surgery. Modern anesthetic management begins before the patient is transferred to the surgical suite with a complete review of the patient's history and current medical problems. In the alert patient, mild sedation can reduce stress and blood pressure fluctuations before the induction of anesthesia. Anesthesia is usually induced with a combination of agents with the goal of avoiding significant swings in blood pressure and heart rate. Hypotension in the clinically compromised patient may significantly reduce cerebral blood flow (CBF), while hypertension may increase the risk of recurrent aneurysmal hemorrhage. At our institution, a sedative such as midazolam (2 to 5 mg), combined with sodium thiopental (125 to 500 mg) and lidocaine (100 mg), is used for induction and is followed by complete neuromuscular blockade prior to any attempt at intubation. The patient is ventilated to maintain the end-tidal $P_{CO_2}$ between 30 and 40 torr until brain retraction is begun; it is then lowered to 25 torr. Anesthesia is maintained with a combination of inhalational agents such as isoflurane and nitrous oxide, while small intravenous doses of sufentanyl (or fentanyl in the patient with cardiac instability) are used to titrate blood pressure and heart rate within 10 percent of preoperative values. Mannitol (25 to 50 g) is delivered intravenously if the brain is not already slack when the dura is opened. Ventricular drainage and barbiturates (see next paragraph) are also valuable adjuncts in further reducing brain volume before retraction.

Previously, moderate systemic hypotension was routinely employed by most surgeons to reduce the risks of rupture during the dissection and clipping of aneurysms. This degree of hypotension would normally result in little or no change in CBF; however, in patients with aneurysmal subarachnoid hemorrhage, particularly those with a depressed level of consciousness or vasospasm, impaired cerebral autoregulation can lead to significant, generalized cerebral ischemia.[32,42,52,59,147] Most authors have abandoned the use of systemic hypotension in favor of short periods of temporary vessel occlusion to reduce the risk of premature aneurysm rupture or to control hemorrhage after rupture.[7,8,60,134] In general, temporary occlusion of the major intracranial vessels is well tolerated for 10 to 20 minutes.[8,60,79,134,136,138] Moderate hypothermia (34°C to 35°C), which is common under general anesthesia, also increases the brain's tolerance to ischemia. We routinely combine this degree of hypothermia with deep barbiturate anesthesia. Barbiturates are begun just prior to brain retraction: Thiopental is administered as a loading dose of 5 to 10 mg/kg of body weight followed by a continuous infusion titrated to produce 10 to 20 seconds of complete EEG

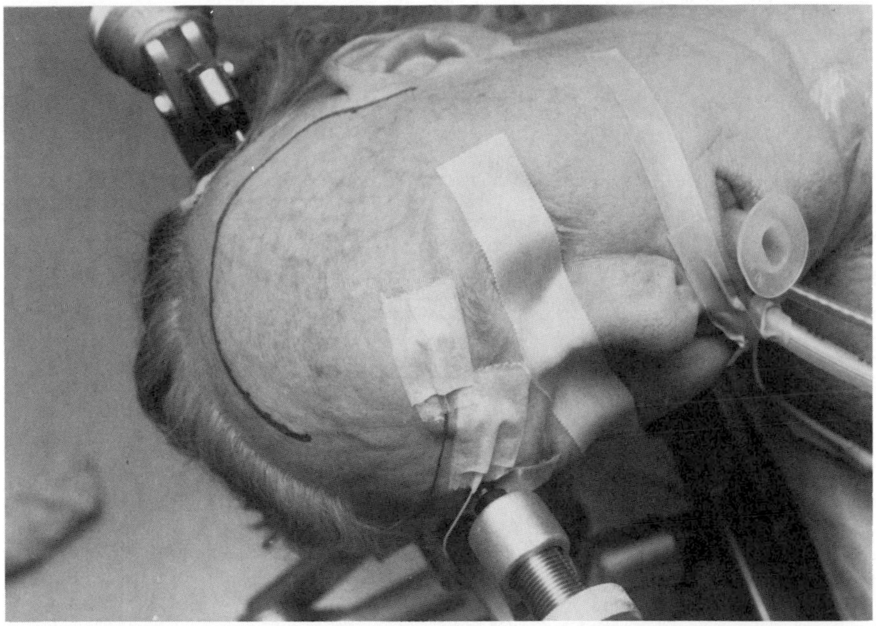
A

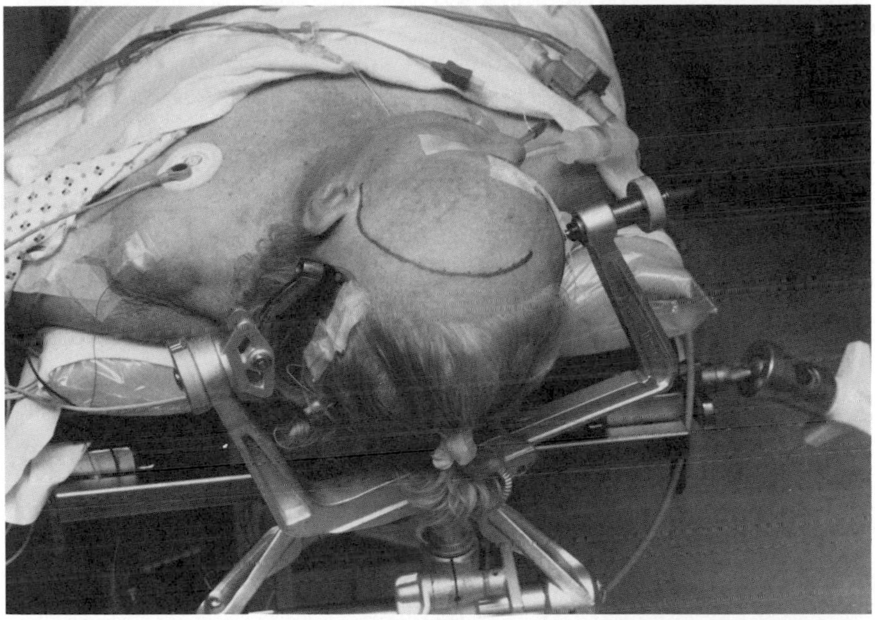
B

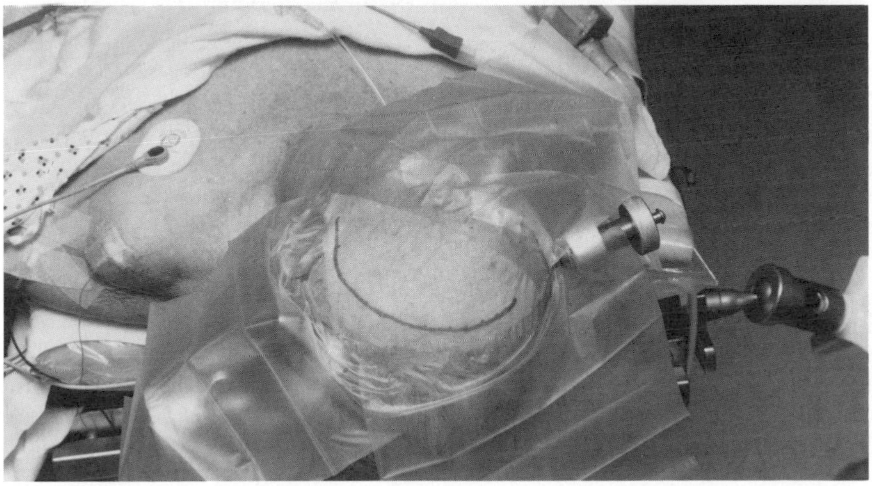
C

**Fig. 46-8.** (**A & B**) Intraoperative photographs demonstrating surface electrode lead placement for compressed spectral analysis monitoring of electroencephalogram activity and for median nerve somatosensory evoked potentials. The planned craniotomy incision has been outlined with a skin marker. (**C**) Self-adhering plastic drapes have been applied to the edges of the operative field to protect the leads from moisture.

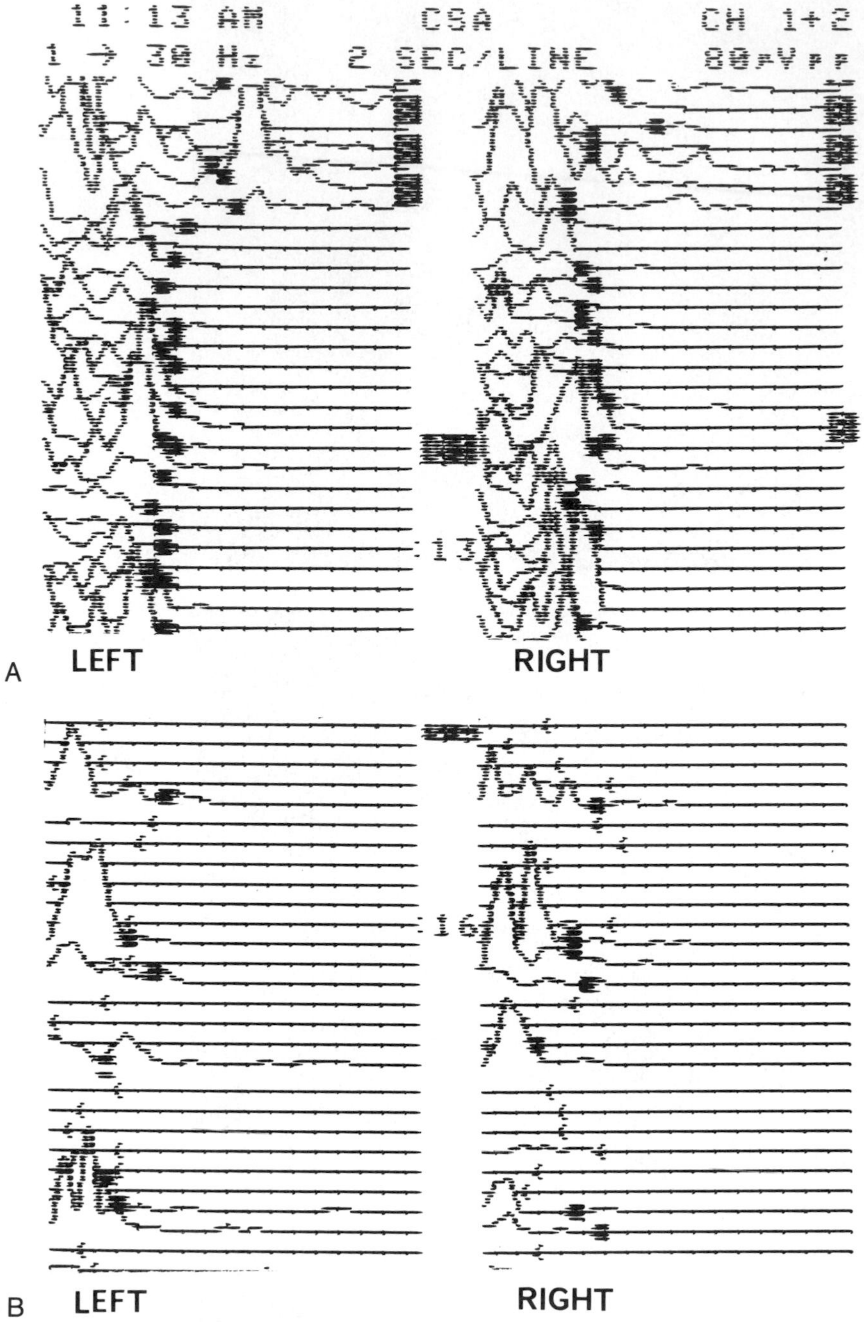


**Fig. 46-9.** Compressed spectral analysis (CSA) of electroencephalogram (EEG) activity during surgery for the elective aneurysm clipping in the patient presented in Figures 46-13 and 46-14. Compressed spectral analysis (**A**) before and (**B**) after induction of deep barbiturate coma with EEG burst suppression. Each line of the display represents a 2-second frequency spectrum analysis of EEG activity between 0 and 30 Hz. The flat lines represent periods of complete burst suppression.

burst suppression (Fig. 46-9). Blood pressure is maintained within 10 percent of preoperative values with small doses of ephedrine if necessary. Clinical and laboratory evidence suggests that barbiturates reduce the risk of ischemic injury during temporary vessel occlusion.[24,54,79,89,117–121]

## Direct Clipping of Aneurysms

The treatment of choice for most intracranial aneurysms is direct clipping of the neck. Aneurysms that are unsuitable for direct clipping can be approached in the various ways discussed below. Advances in mi-

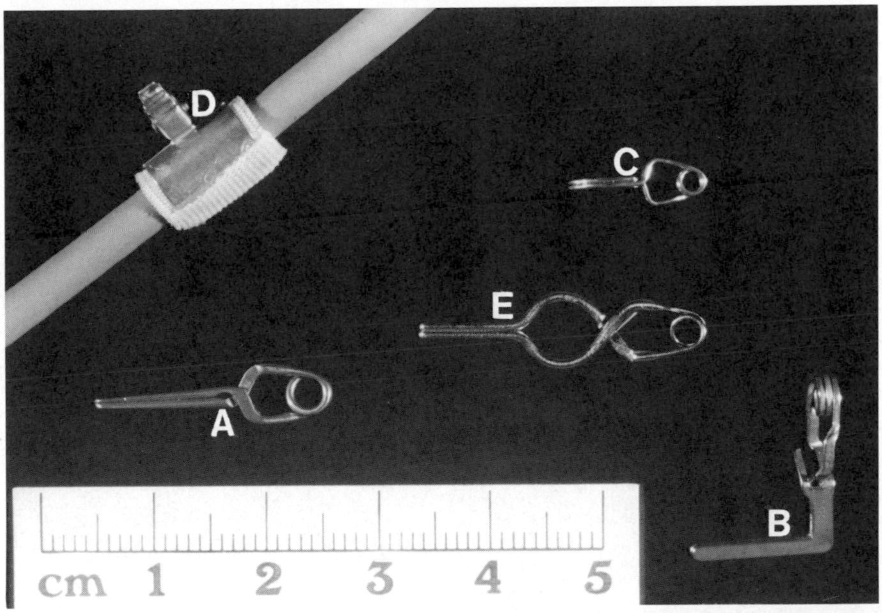


**Fig. 46-10.** Photograph of the types of aneurysm clips available to the surgeon. **A, B, C**: Clips with parallel blades in various shapes and sizes that are placed directly across the aneurysm neck. **D**: Circumferential clips that enclose the parent vessel completely and obliterate the aneurysm neck between the ends of the concave jaws. **E**: Clips that combine parallel jaws for obliterating the aneurysm neck with a proximal aperture through which an artery or nerve may pass.

crosurgical technique and the availability of a wide spectrum of aneurysm clips have increased the percentage of aneurysms suitable for direct neck obliteration.

Three types of spring-loaded clips are typically used (Fig. 46-10): (1) clips with parallel blades placed directly across the neck of the aneurysm come in all lengths, curves, and bayonet shapes; (2) circumferential clips that enclose the parent vessel to obliterate the aneurysm neck between the ends of the concave jaws; and (3) clips that combine the parallel, long, thin jaws of the first type with a proximal round aperture through which an artery or nerve may pass. These clips, in combination with the new thin appliers that allow rotation of the clip, permit accurate obliteration of the aneurysm neck even in narrow, awkward locations. Special clips with ultralow closing pressures designed to prevent intimal injury are also available for temporary vessel occlusion.

To treat aneurysms adequately, surgeons must have a large assortment of clips and appliers available so that the most appropriate instruments can be used for each individual case. Prior to the exposure of the aneurysm, the surgeon should select and have immediately available a minimum of three temporary vessel clips and one or two permanent aneurysm clips, in case of unexpected aneurysm rupture.

General principles involved in aneurysm surgery are briefly discussed. First and foremost, the operating room staff should be experienced with microsurgical technique and the use of the operating microscope. The brain should be protected (we prefer Telfa strips) and retracted gently. Care should be taken to keep the field moist with frequent irrigation. CSF drainage and mannitol can be used to facilitate brain retraction. The induction of barbiturate burst suppression when the dura is opened will also encourage brain relaxation, increase tolerance to ischemia, and afford a greater margin of safety in the event that temporary vessel occlusion is needed. Finally, and most importantly, should an aneurysm rupture, the impulse to react quickly and to attempt clip placement hurriedly should be resisted. Instead, a suction must be carefully and gently placed to permit controlled dissection of the aneurysm to continue. Frequently, hemorrhage from the ruptured dome can be controlled by gentle tamponade with a small cotton patty held in place with the sucker tip. At this point, temporary clips can be placed across the parent vessel(s) and dissection completed about the neck of the aneurysm. In our experience, temporary occlusion of major cerebral vessels under barbiturate protection is well tolerated for up to 10 to 20 minutes, assuming system and arterial pressure has been maintained in a normal range. With the neck of the aneurysm exposed, the surgeon should select the appropriate clip and apply it in an unhurried manner. If the clip is not satisfactorily placed, the reapplication of a different clip or the trial of an alternate clip applier should be attempted until perfect clip placement has been achieved. After the surgeon is satisfied that the clip has been appropriately placed, the dome of the aneurysm can be decompressed with a small needle to verify complete neck occlusion.

In certain broad-necked aneurysms, multiple clips may be necessary. The wide variety of fenestrated Sugita and Sunt-Keys clips are particularly adaptable to occlusion of an awkward aneurysm neck. Fenestrated, straight, or right-angle clips can be placed serially over the parent vessel to extend the length of neck occlusion (Fig. 46-11).

A

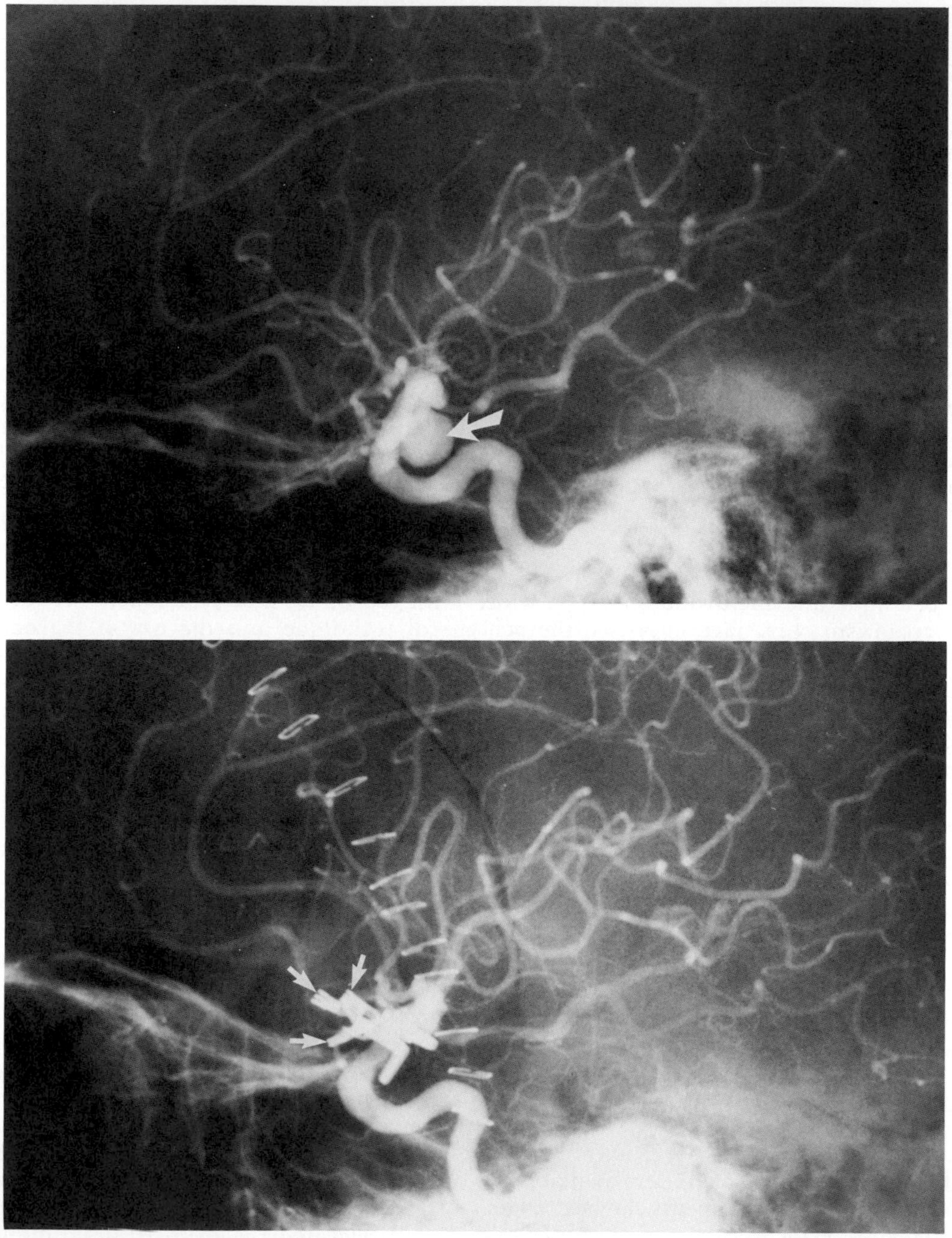

B

**Fig. 46-11.** A 53-year-old woman was referred for evaluation after experiencing transient ischemic attacks that affected the right upper extremity. (**A**) Lateral view of the left internal carotid artery angiogram demonstrating a large, left internal carotid artery aneurysm (*arrow*). Cardiac workup and extracranial vascular workup were negative for any other embolic source. (**B**) Lateral view of the postoperative left internal carotid artery angiogram demonstrating good clipping of the aneurysm. Note that a combination of three clips (*arrows*) has been used to obliterate the aneurysm neck.

## SPECIFIC OPERATIVE TECHNIQUES

### Aneurysms of the Anterior Circulation

The patient's head is positioned using three-point skeletal fixation with a Mayfield head-holder, rotated 45 degrees from midline, and inclined slightly toward the opposite shoulder. The skin incision is made from the posterior margin of the zygomatic process and carried forward and superiorly in a gently curving arc approximately 1 cm behind the hairline to the midline of the forehead (Fig. 46-12). The extension of the incision to midline has the advantage of allowing increased retraction of the scalp and muscle anteriorly, while avoiding extension of the incision into the non-

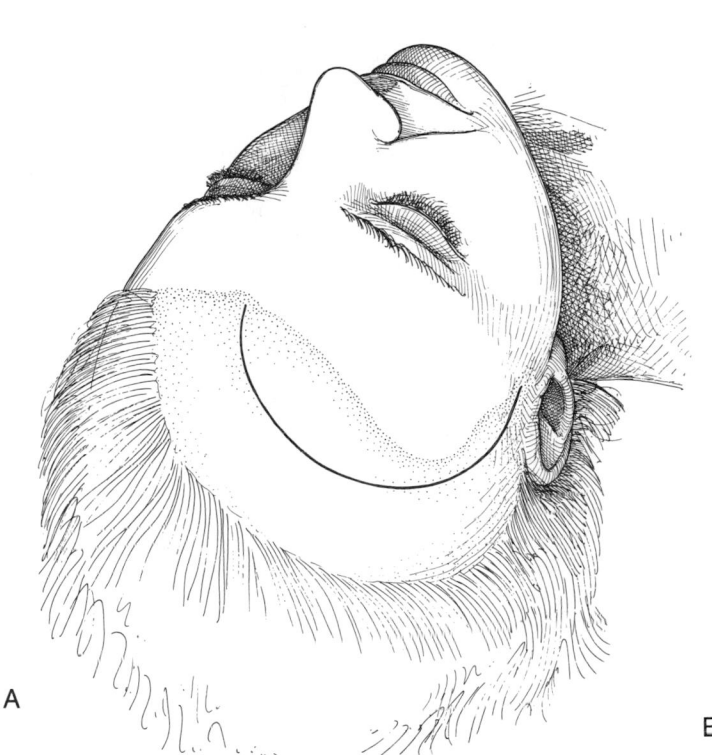

A

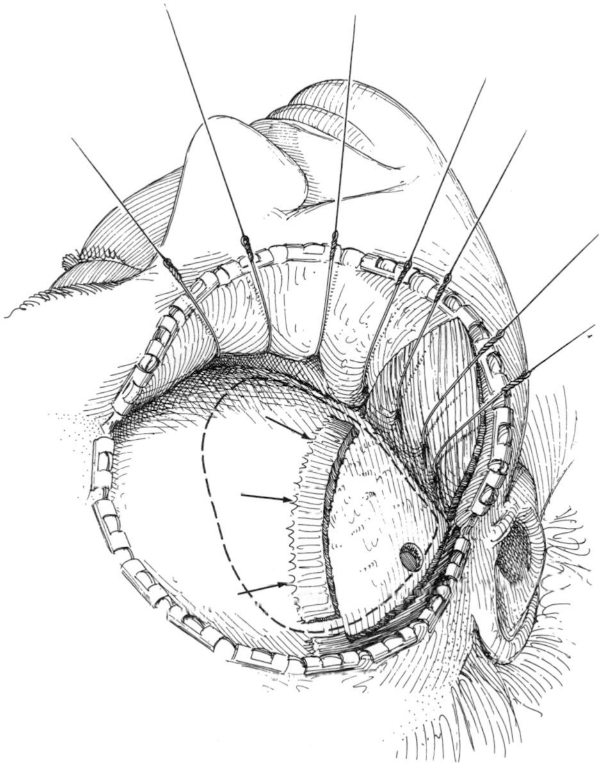

B

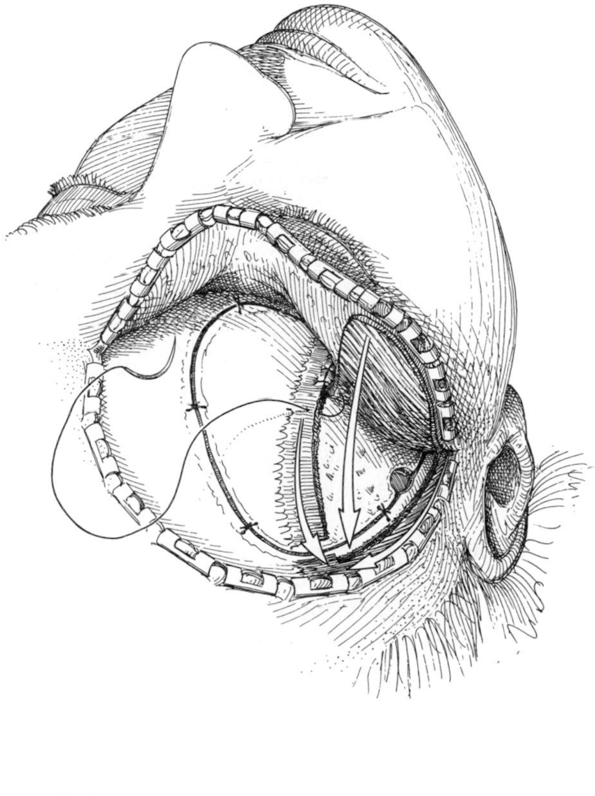

C

**Fig. 46-12.** Artist's drawings of the operative approach to anterior circulation aneurysms (see text for details). (**A**) Outline of incision for pterional craniotomy. (**B**) The scalp flap and underlying temporalis muscle have been elevated together with the exception of a small facial cuff along the insertion of the temporalis muscle (*arrows*). Fishhooks have been used to retract the scalp and temporalis muscle flaps. Note the outline for the planned bone flap, which is brought to the midpupillary line and as close to the frontal fossa floor as possible. (**C**) The intracranial portion of the procedure has been completed, and the bone flap has been replaced and firmly secured in position with multiple sutures. The cut edges of the temporalis fascia are being reapproximated with a running suture. This closure helps to ensure normal anatomic function of the temporalis muscle as well as to improve the postoperative cosmetic appearance of the temporal fossa region. (Adapted from Spetzler and Lee,[128] with permission.)

hair-bearing portion of the scalp, as is common when the incision stops at the midpupillary line. The scalp and underlying muscle are elevated together, with the exception of a small facial cuff along the insertion of the temporalis muscle (Fig. 46-12). This cuff is used during closure to firmly secure the temporalis muscle in its normal anatomic position, helping to reduce postoperative problems with temporal mandibular joint dysfunction and to improve the cosmetic appearance of the temporal fossa. The scalp and muscle are retracted with fishhooks attached to rubber bands, which are in turn secured to a Leyla bar (Fig. 46-13). A free frontotemporal bone flap is turned. The maximal amount of the lateral wall of the frontal fossa should be included in this free flap. The greater the bony exposure along the lateral wall of the frontal

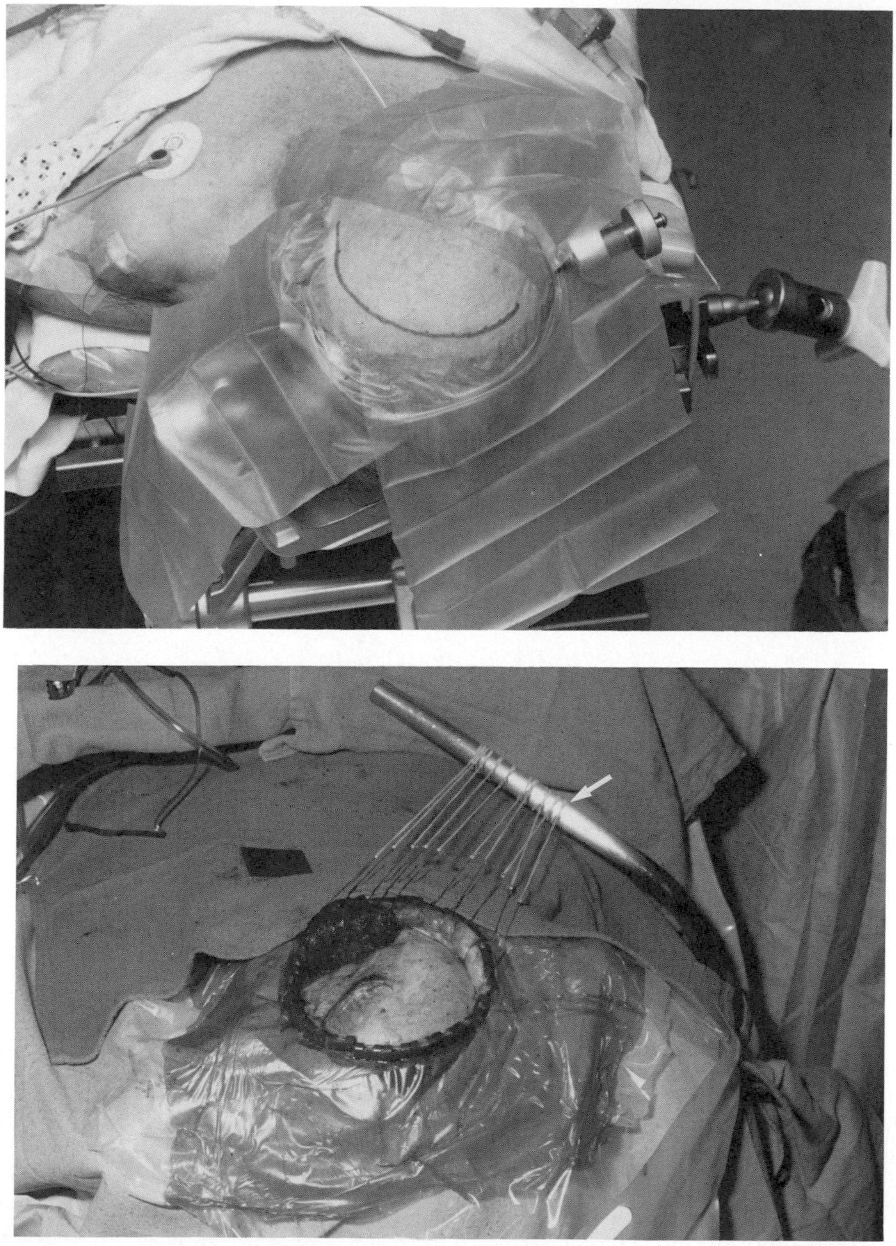

A

B

**Fig. 46-13.** The operative treatment of the incidental middle cerebral artery aneurysm in the 64-year-old woman discussed in Fig. 46-14 is depicted in serial photographs. (**A**) The patient has been positioned for a pterional craniotomy and the incision outlined. (**B**) The scalp flap has been turned, and the skin and muscle have been retracted using fishhooks attached to rubber bands, which are, in turn, secured to a Leyla bar (*arrow*). (*Figure continues.*)

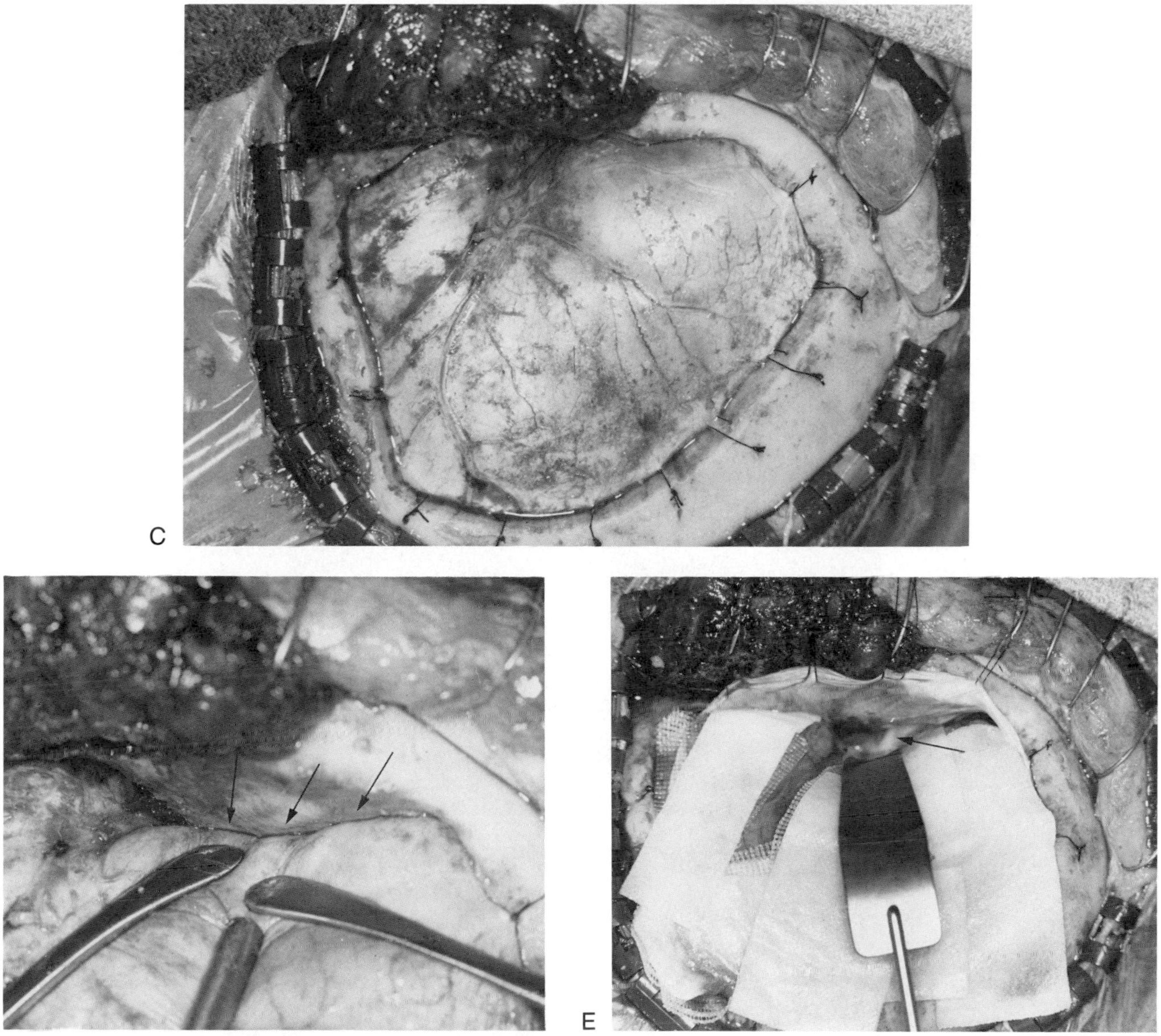

C D E

**Fig. 46-13** (*Continued*). (**C**) The craniotomy bone flap has been elevated and the underlying dura exposed. Dural tackup sutures have been placed at regular intervals around the margin of the bone flap to control bleeding. (**D**) The lateral bony wall of the frontal fossa and the sphenoid wing have been removed, using a high-speed drill to bring the dissection flat with the frontal fossa floor (*arrows*). This bony dissection minimizes the frontal lobe retraction necessary to visualize the aneurysm. (**E**) The dura has been opened, and the brain, which is covered with Telfa strips, is being gently elevated to expose the basal cisterns. The pristine white silhouette of the left optic nerve is faintly visible through the intact arachnoid membranes at the tip of the retractor blade (*arrow*). (*Figure continues.*)

F

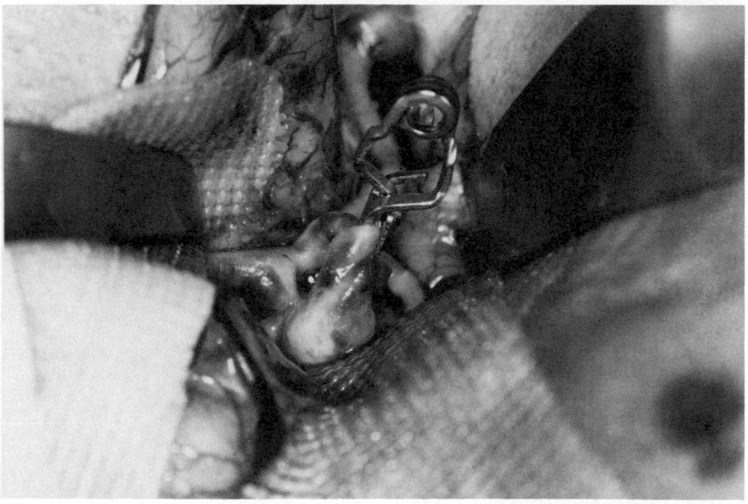
G

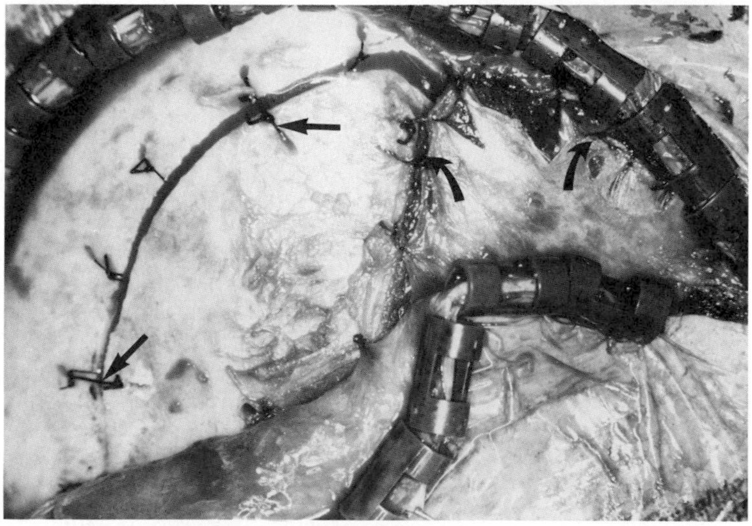
H

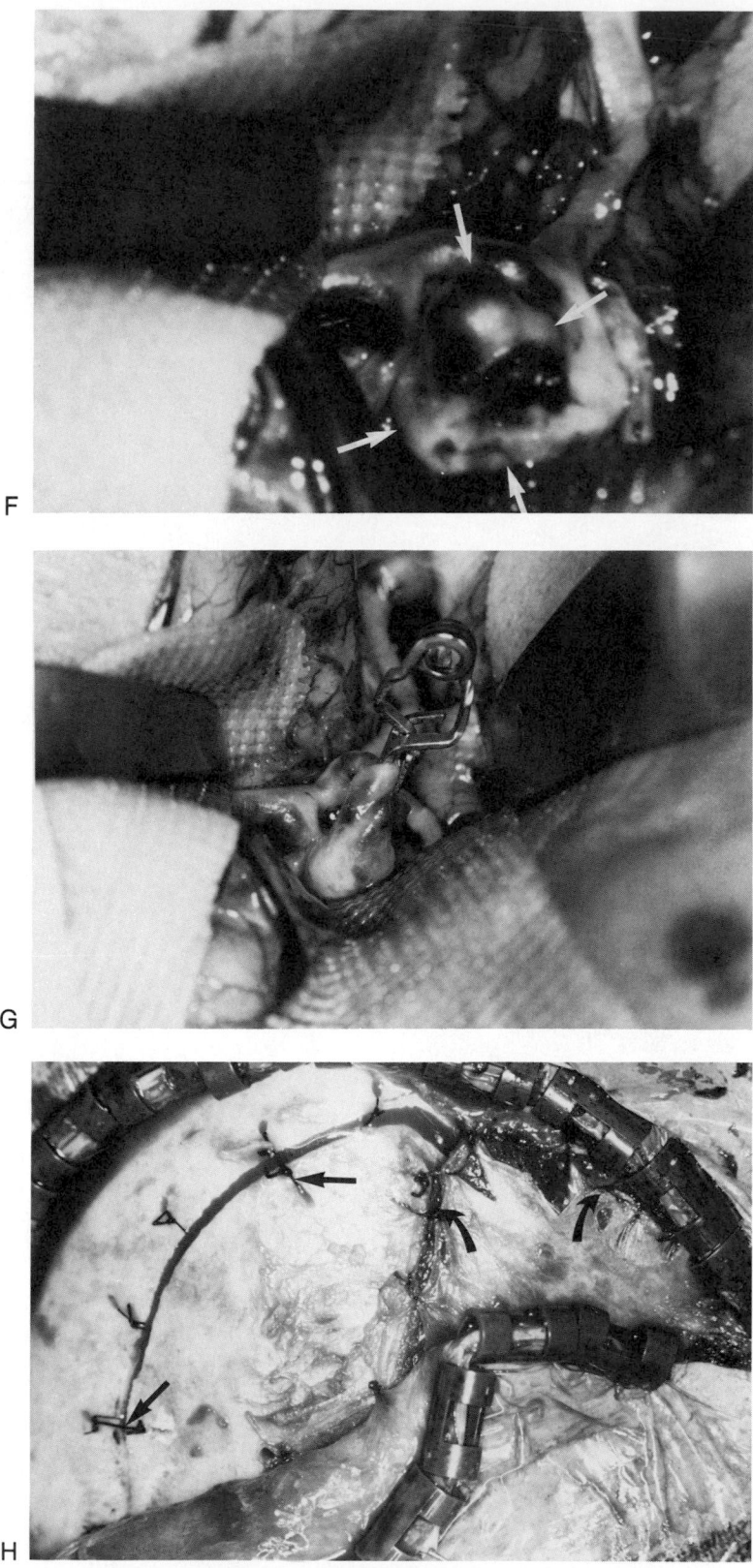

**Fig. 46-13** (*Continued*). (**F**) The sylvian fissure has been widely opened and the aneurysm at the middle cerebral artery bifurcation exposed (*arrows*). (**G**) The aneurysm has been dissected free from the surrounding vessels and the neck obliterated with a single clip. Note that the dome of the aneurysm has been punctured and collapsed to ensure that it no longer fills. (**H**) The craniotomy bone flap has been replaced and secured with heavy nylon sutures (*straight arrows*). The cut edges of the temporalis muscle have been reapproximated (*curved arrows*), and only the scalp closure remains to be completed.

fossa, the less retraction is necessary to expose the basal cisterns. We use a high-speed air drill* to complete bony resection of the lateral frontal wall, bringing it flush with the frontal fossa floor, and exposing the anterior superior margin of the temporal lobe (Fig. 46-13). The pterion is resected down to the anterior clinoid using the drill and small rongeurs. Drill holes should be placed at 2- to 3-cm intervals around the edges of the craniotomy for dural tackup sutures and for resecuring the bone flap later.

The dura is opened in a semilunar fashion and remains hinged along the floor of the frontal fossa, extending into the beginning of the temporal fossa. The dura is elevated and retracted with stay sutures over the muscle to provide maximum direct exposure. The brain should be covered to prevent drying and trauma from retractors and instruments; Telfa strips are a good choice and can be readily cut to different sizes. The frontal lobe is gently elevated with a self-retaining retractor. If necessary, another small, thin retractor can be placed over the temporal lobe at its junction with the sylvian fissure. If there is any resistance to retraction, measures to increase relaxation of the brain should be instituted as outlined above, including mannitol, barbiturates, and CSF drainage. In the patient without a ventricular catheter, retraction becomes easier once the basal cisterns are opened. Incising the arachnoid around the optic nerve and internal carotid artery provides a pathway for ample CSF drainage. The basal portion of the sylvian fissure is opened to complete exposure of the internal carotid artery. The need for further opening of the sylvian fissure is dictated by the type of aneurysm being approached, being least for anterior communicating artery aneurysms and greatest for those of the middle cerebral artery. By observing the proper arachnoid planes, the proximal middle cerebral artery and its major trunks can be exposed without dividing any arterial branches (Figs. 46-13 and 46-14).

The dissection and clipping of internal carotid artery and posterior communicating artery aneurysms are also greatly aided by opening the sylvian fissure widely. This is particularly true for carotid artery bifurcation aneurysms where the surgeon must take special care to avoid including any of the numerous small perforating arterial branches that arise from the proximal segments of the anterior cerebral and middle cerebral arteries.

The same general exposure is adequate for approaching anterior communicating artery aneurysms, except that only the basal portion of the sylvian fissure need be opened. The surgeon can elect to approach the anterior communicating artery aneurysm either directly through the resection of a small portion of the ipsilateral gyrus rectus or by following the proximal portion of the anterior cerebral artery to the communicating artery complex. The advantage of approaching through the gyrus rectus is that the small perforating arteries and recurrent Heubner's artery are exposed to much less risk of injury. The surgeon has to recognize the wide variability of the anatomy of the anterior communicating artery region. There may be two or more communicating arteries and even a plexiform arrangement. Indeed, the high incidence of variations from the normal anatomy in this region may contribute to the formation of aneurysms by producing turbulent flow patterns.

Paraclinoid and ophthalmic artery aneurysms that arise from the internal carotid artery as it exits the cavernous sinus are also approached in a similar manner. Complete exposure of the neck of the aneurysm for clipping frequently requires resection of the anterior clinoid process. The anterior clinoid process, along with the roof of the optic foramen can be safely removed using a diamond-tipped burr. The aneurysm and internal carotid artery are protected from the drill by reflecting a small flap of dura from the orbital roof.

## Pericallosal Aneurysms

Pericallosal aneurysms are relatively uncommon, composing only about 3 percent of aneurysms in most major series. An intrahemispheric approach is used for exposure. The bone flap should be sufficiently anterior to allow proximal control of the parent vessel prior to visualization of the aneurysm. A bifrontal sutar scalp incision located well behind the hairline provides good exposure. The scalp flap is reflected forward and inferiorly, and secured using the fishhook retractor system described above. The side of the craniotomy should be determined from the venous angiogram: the side with the greatest room between draining veins is selected. Tsutsumi et al.[140] have recently emphasized the complications associated with sacrificing bridging veins in the intrahemispheric approach to ruptured aneurysms in this area. It is relatively unimportant whether the approach is ipsilateral or contralateral. To minimize retraction of the frontal lobe, the bone flap should be carried across the sagittal sinus; the dura is then opened so that it remains hinged along the edge of the sinus and retracted with stay sutures to maximize midline exposure. The parent vessel is exposed proximally and followed until the aneurysm is identified. The aneurysm is clipped in the usual manner.

## Aneurysms of the Posterior Circulation

### Basilar Tip Aneurysms

Aneurysms involving the terminal portion of the basilar artery are responsible for approximately 3 percent of all aneurysmal subarachnoid hemorrhages. While once considered formidable, advances in mi-

* Midas Rex Institute Inc., 2929 Race, Fort Worth, TX 76111-9102.

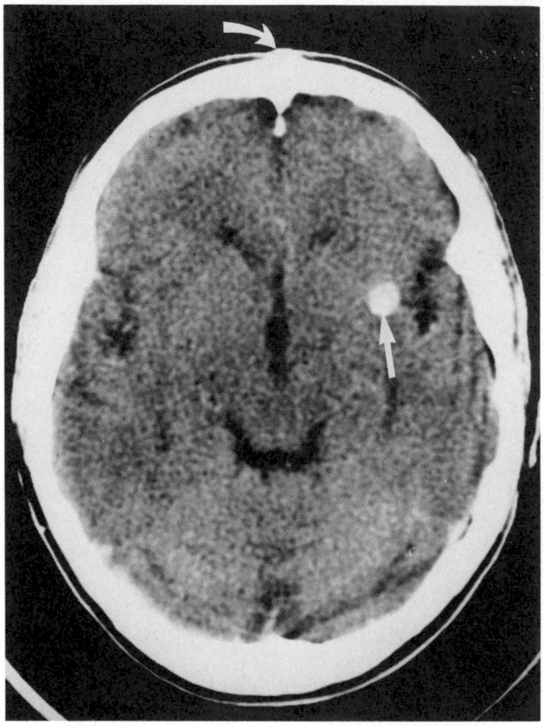

A

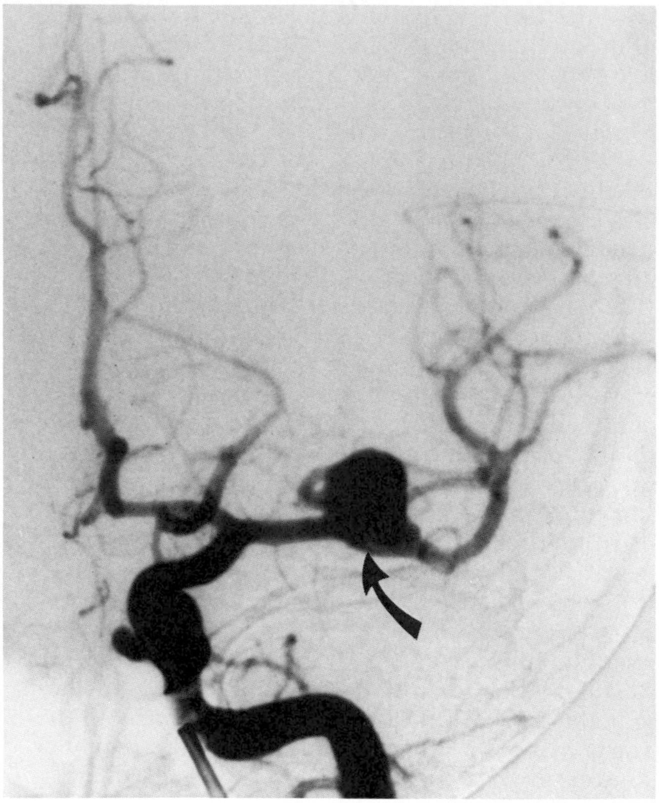

B

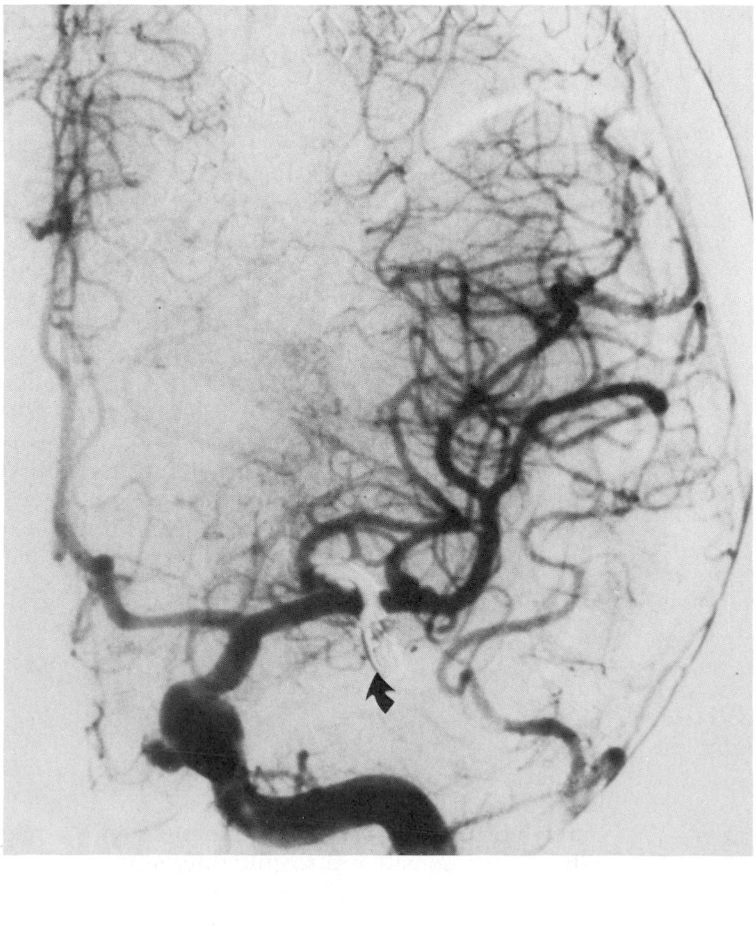

C

**Fig. 46-14.** A 64-year-old woman evaluated by a plastic surgeon for a slowly growing bony prominence in the midforehead. (**A**) Basic head computed tomography scan demonstrates an area of stippled calcification (*straight arrow*) in the left sylvian fissure consistent with a middle cerebral artery aneurysm. There was no history consistent with previous subarachnoid hemorrhage. Note also the small bony prominence (*curved arrow*) in the frontal region. (**B**) Anteroposterior view of the left internal carotid artery angiogram revealing a large left middle cerebral artery aneurysm (*arrow*). (**C**) Anteroposterior view of the postoperative angiogram demonstrating complete obliteration of the aneurysm from the cerebral circulation with no compromise of the parent vessels. A single, slightly curved clip (*arrow*) is faintly visible.

crosurgical technique and the availability of a wide variety of clips and slimline clip appliers has made the approach to the majority of these lesions routine at most major referral centers. For large or giant aneurysms of the basilar tip, the surgeon may need to consider hypothermic circulatory arrest as an adjunct in clipping; the indications for and rationale of this approach are discussed later in this section.

There are two general approaches to basilar tip aneurysms. The pterional approach as described above for anterior circulation aneurysms provides an excellent way to expose aneurysms of the basilar artery tip as well as those arising between the origin of the posterior cerebral and superior cerebellar arteries. After exposing the carotid artery, the sylvian fissure is widely opened and the posterior communicating artery is followed to the posterior cerebral artery and basilar tip. This approach is useful for small and medium-sized aneurysms, particularly those that point forward or straight up from the tip of the basilar artery. For large aneurysms and those that point back, we prefer the subtemporal exposure described below. It allows better visualization of the numerous perforating branches that arise and course behind the aneurysm to the brain stem. An otherwise excellent clipping that traps even one of these small perforators in the clip blades can cause serious neurologic deficits.

The subtemporal approach as first advocated by Drake provides excellent exposure to the distal segment of the basilar artery. To avoid injury to the dominant temporal lobe, the preferred approach is from the right side. A role is placed beneath the shoulder on the side of the surgical approach, and the head is rotated to a nearly horizontal plane. We use a modified pterional scalp incision with a slight posterior extension above the ear. The scalp flap and underlying temporalis muscle are elevated as described above, and retracted forward and down to maximize exposure of the temporal fossa. A second set of fishhooks attached to a Leyla bar are used to retract the inferior margins of the flap above the ear. A free bone flap is turned to allow full exposure of the frontal and temporal fossa. The craniotomy must be carried to the floor of the middle fossa to facilitate retraction and exposure. A high-speed drill is used to complete bony dissection, which usually includes partial resection of the zygomatic process. The importance of bony removal, despite entry into the mastoid air cells to become flush with the floor of the middle fossa, cannot be overemphasized (Fig. 46-15). Any lip of bone remaining above the middle fossa floor will require significantly more retraction of the temporal lobe and will increase the risk of temporal lobe ischemia or hemorrhage.

The operative approach to the basilar artery is beneath the anterior third of the temporal lobe. The temporal lobe should be covered with protective strips and retractors gently advanced to expose the tentorial edge and arachnoid of the prepontine cistern. If there is any resistance to retraction, measures to increase relaxation of the brain should be instituted as outlined above. Bridging veins from the temporal lobe tip can be coagulated and divided. The vein of Labbé should be identified as it courses beneath the free edge of the temporal lobe to enter the transverse sinus. Care must be taken to avoid stretching and tearing this important venous structure, because its sacrifice can be expected to lead to an extensive venous infarct. The 3rd cranial nerve and cerebral peduncle should be visible through the arachnoid at the tentorial edge. Depending on the location of the aneu-

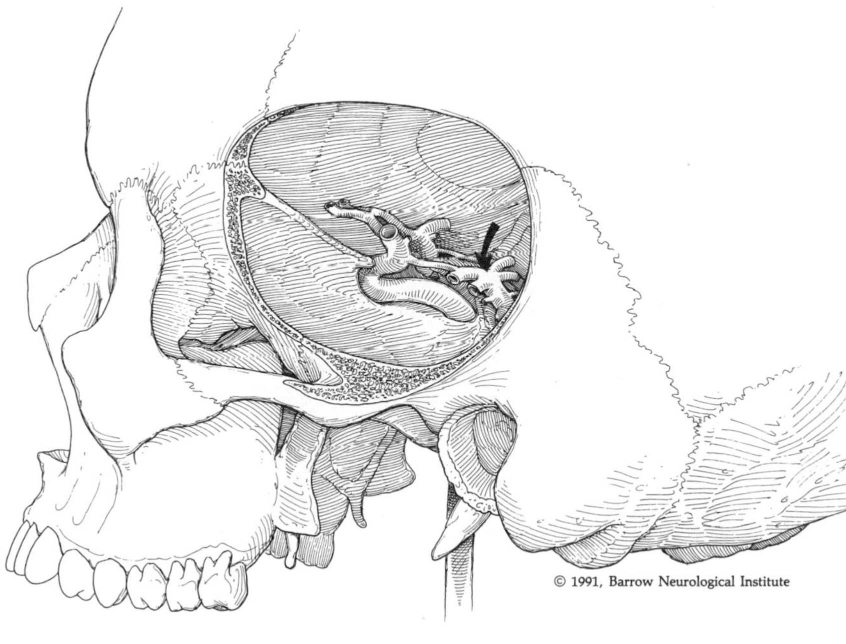


**Fig. 46-15.** Artist's sketch of the subtemporal exposure used for approaching aneurysms of the distal basilar artery (*arrow*), including those that arise at the level of the superior cerebellar artery and from the basilar tip. (© Barrow Neurological Institute, 1991.)

rysm, the surgeon may elect to open the arachnoid above or below the 3rd cranial nerve to enter the cistern. Leaving the arachnoid attachments intact on one side of the 3rd cranial nerve provides a natural system of retraction and helps minimize trauma to this delicate structure. The edge of the tentorium can be pulled back with a stay suture secured to the dura of the temporal fossa floor. If additional exposure is required, the tentorium can be incised and the cut edges retracted with stay sutures. It is important to identify the course of the 4th cranial nerve beneath the edge of the tentorium, if a tentorial incision is necessary.

The arachnoid can now be opened widely, and the superior cerebellar and posterior cerebral arteries can be identified. If the basilar artery is not already in view, these vessels can be followed proximally until their juncture with the basilar artery becomes visible. It is critical at this junction to expose the posterior cerebral artery and 3rd cranial nerve on the opposite side. Dissection needs to be sufficient to allow clipping of the aneurysm neck and to assure that the clip does not incorporate other neural or vascular structures. As noted above, perforating arteries arising from the proximal posterior cerebral artery trunk and from the distal basilar artery are numerous and important. Multiple trials of clips, with and without fenestrations, may be necessary to occlude the aneurysm neck safely.

## Midbasilar Aneurysms

Aneurysms located on the basilar artery at its midportion near the origin of the anterior inferior cerebellar artery or above the junction of the vertebral and basilar arteries are the most difficult to approach and to clip successfully. These are located in an obscure region of the posterior circulation, usually midline, and are equally difficult to reach from a standard posterior fossa or subtemporal approach. These aneurysms are best approached by a combined supra- and infratentorial approach, with exposure and ligation of the sigmoid sinus and cutting of the entire tentorium along its insertion into the petrous ridge (Fig. 46-16). This complex exposure is best accomplished by a team that includes an experienced neurosurgeon and an otolaryngologist with special interest in temporal bone anatomy.[2,124] This approach allows easy retraction of the cerebellum and provides exposure to the basilar artery from the direction of the 5th, 7th, and 8th cranial nerves above, or over the 9th, 10th, and 11th cranial nerves from below. Since it is difficult to have complete control of the parent vessel, the exposure offered by this technique is essential to obtaining a low morbidity and mortality.

If significant retraction is required to expose the basilar artery, inadequate bone removal may be the cause. Removal of even a few millimeters of bone laterally can dramatically improve exposure and reduce the need for retraction. Alternatively, the surgeon may find it beneficial to change the angle of approach from above to below, or vice versa. The aneurysm can usually be identified and manipulated by working around intervening cranial nerves. If necessary, the 9th cranial nerve and a few of the upper rootlets of the 10th cranial nerve can be sacrificed. If the aneurysm neck cannot be exposed for clipping, placement of a Hunterian ligature on the vertebral or basilar artery should be considered. This procedure, as practiced by Drake,[37] is useful in this small groups of patients.

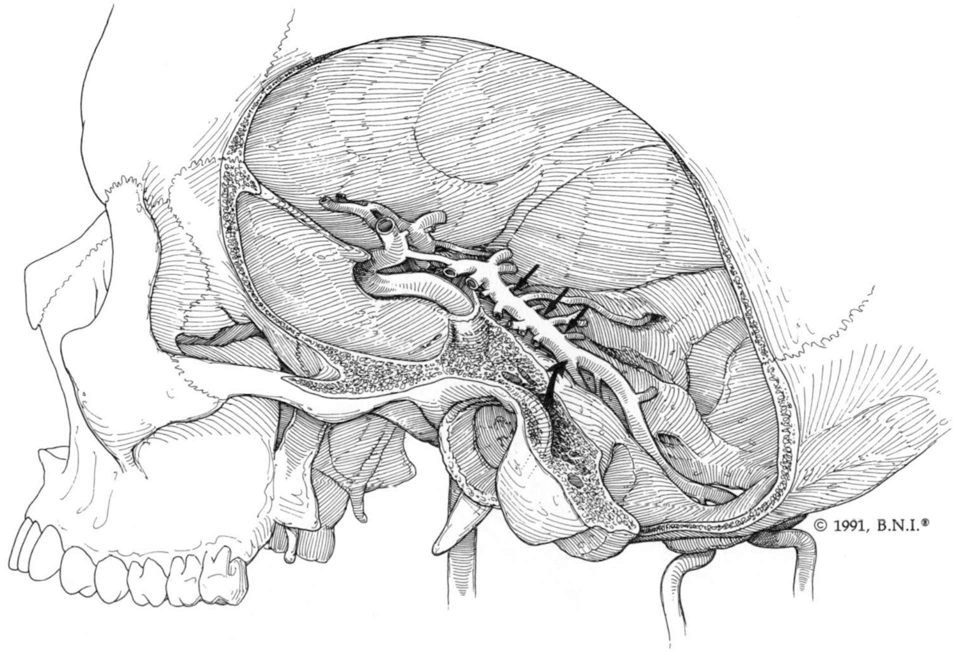


**Fig. 46-16.** Artist's sketch of the combined subtemporal-suboccipital exposure for approaching aneurysms of the midportion of the basilar artery (*straight arrows*) and the vertebrobasilar junction (*curved arrow*). (© Barrow Neurological Institute, 1991.)

### Vertebral Artery Aneurysms

Aneurysms of the vertebral artery typically arise at the origin of the posterior inferior cerebellar artery (PICA). They are relatively uncommon, accounting for only about 2 percent of the cases in major studies. Aneurysms along this intracranial segment of the vertebral artery are best exposed by a posterior fossa approach. For this approach, the patient is placed in a lateral decubitis, or park bench position, on the operating room table, and the head is fully flexed and turned 30 degrees from midline to the side of the lesion (Fig. 46-17). We prefer a hockey stick incision that allows lateral bone removal down to the foramen magnum and up to the transverse sinus as well as removal of the arch of C1. The arch of C1 is resected laterally to allow visualization of the vertebral artery as it enters the dural folds. The foramen magnum should be resected as far laterally as possible to the edge of the sigmoid sinus on the side of the aneurysm. The dura is opened in the midline and extended laterally in a cruciate fashion to the edges of the bony dissection. This approach exposes the vertebral artery through the cranial nerves from a lateral and inferior view. The vertebral artery is followed from its entry into the posterior fossa to the aneurysm, which may arise above, below, medial, or lateral to the origin of PICA. The neck is carefully dissected free and the aneurysm clipped in the usual fashion. Care must be taken to avoid compromise of PICA and the distal vertebral artery.

By extending the bony dissection to the sigmoid sinus and occipital condyle (Fig. 46-18), the surgeon can obtain sufficient exposure to approach the rare aneurysms of the vertebrobasilar junction. This so-called far-lateral suboccipital approach is well described in the literature.[48,50]

### Mycotic Aneurysms

The surgical approach to mycotic aneurysms, which most commonly involve the peripheral rather than proximal arterial branches, will require modification based on the exact location of the lesion. In general, however, the same principles apply as for the other aneurysms above, with the surgeon approaching the lesion for proximal vascular control prior to completing exposure of the lesion. Because of their propensity for deep sulcal branches, mycotic aneurysms may be difficult to locate. In such cases, the use of intraoperative ultrasound is helpful for selecting the appropriate sulcus to open. As discussed above, these aneurysms are commonly fusiform and involve the entire wall of the parent vessel. Obliteration of the aneurysm, therefore, frequently requires resection of the involved portion of the artery and microvascular reanastamosis or an extracranial-intracranial bypass.

## GIANT INTRACRANIAL ANEURYSMS

In the literature, the term giant aneurysm is reserved for lesions greater than 25 mm in diameter.[86] Giant aneurysms occur predominantly in females with a female-to-male ratio of about 3:1.[75,86,150] They most commonly occur in patients 30 to 60 years of age, the same age range at risk for aneurysms in general. The reported incidence of giant aneurysms varies, but they probably constitute no more than 5 percent of intracranial aneurysms.[75]

The patient with a giant aneurysm may present with signs and symptoms of a mass lesion. Chronic headache, visual impairment, oculomotor palsies, or progressive hemiparesis is common when the aneurysm arises in the anterior circulation[21,38,47,86,123,146,150]; other cranial nerve palsies and signs of brain stem compression may result from giant aneurysms of the vertebrobasilar system.[37,38,85] Embolic symptoms (i.e., transient ischemic attacks [TIAs] and stroke) have also been reported as many of these giant aneurysms contain extensive intramural thrombus.

Although it is generally believed that giant aneurysms seldom rupture, only a few studies in the literature support this notion. Our own experience and that of others suggest that from 30 to 80 percent of patients with giant aneurysms present with subarachnoid hemorrhage.[14,38,75,86,94,150] Some patients who present with mass effect or embolic symptoms have evidence of remote hemorrhage on MR imaging or at surgery.

The evaluation of the patient with a giant aneurysm should include both angiography and CT or MR imaging. Findings on CT or MR imaging may be pathognomonic for the diagnosis of giant aneurysms, demonstrating a large basal mass with a variable area of contrast filling associated with a partially enhancing intramural thrombus (Fig. 46-19). In other cases, more extensive thrombosis may result in a nonenhancing mass that can easily be mistaken for tumor. Because of intramural thrombus, the size of giant aneurysms is frequently underestimated when evaluated by angiography alone. The true size of these lesions can often be appreciated only by studying the CT scan or MR image.

From the few available reports in the literature, it appears that the prognosis for unoperated giant aneurysms is grim.[25,86] As many as 80 percent of patients die within a few years of diagnosis, either from subarachnoid hemorrhage or from increasing mass effect as the aneurysm continues to enlarge.

The management of giant intracranial aneurysms poses special problems. The neck of these lesions may become so wide that it incorporates the origins of adjacent branches making direct obliteration by clipping impossible. In other cases, calcification of the neck or partial thrombosis of the aneurysm makes attempts at clipping extremely hazardous. Finally,

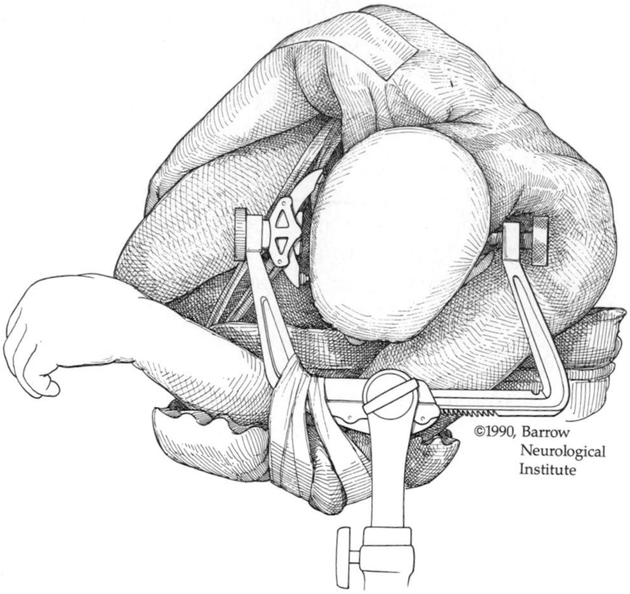


A

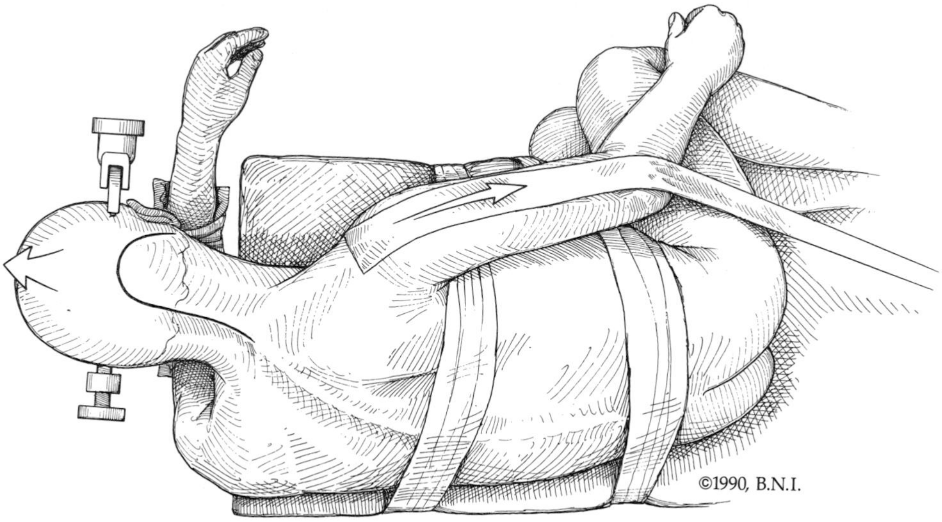


B

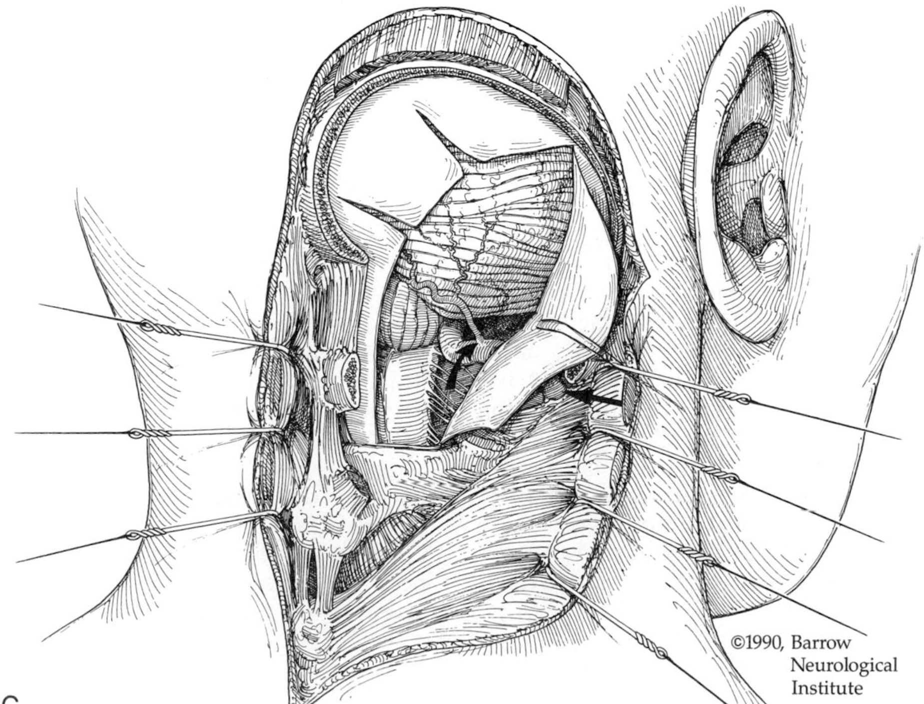


C

**Fig. 46-17.** Line drawings of the approach used for exposure of vertebral artery aneurysms. (**A**) The patient is placed in the park bench position, and care is taken to ensure proper padding of all pressure points. Note the cradle support for the lower arm. (**B**) Surgeon's view of the operative position. The incision for exposing the right vertebral artery is outlined. (**C**) The surgical exposure has been completed; the vertebral artery is visible extracranially as it exits the bony foramen of the 2nd cervical vertebra (*straight arrow*) and intradurally as it courses medially to give rise to the origin of the posterior inferior cerebellar artery (*curved arrow*). (From Spetzler and Grahm,[126] with permission; © Barrow Neurological Institute, 1990.)

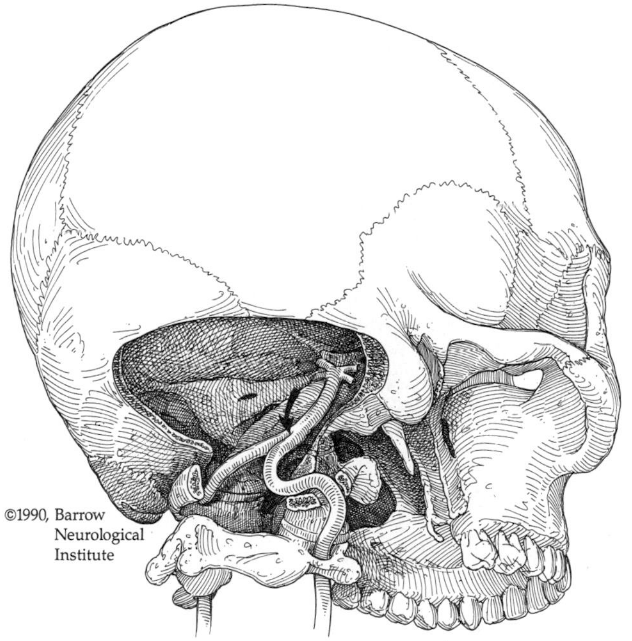


**Fig. 46-18.** Artist's sketch of the far lateral suboccipital exposure for visualization of aneurysms arising from the vertebrobasilar junction (*arrow*). (From Spetzler and Grahm,[126] with permission.)

the sheer size of the lesion combined with an awkward location may make it impossible to properly dissect the neck. A variety of surgical techniques have been developed to deal with these problems, including ligation or trapping procedures with or without microvascular bypass, partial resection of the aneurysm combined with direct microsurgical repair of the parent vessel, and clipping or direct repair under hypothermic circulatory arrest. The indications and basic principles of these techniques will be described below, along with references for the interested reader.

## Carotid Artery Ligation

Carotid artery ligation is performed to protect the aneurysm on the assumption that the reduction of arterial pressure and flow resulting from occlusion will decrease the likelihood of aneurysmal rupture and induce thrombosis of the sac. Physiologically this approach is supported by the prompt, immediate reduction in intravascular pressure that occurs distal to ligation of the internal carotid artery.[11,12,51,92] Serial angiographic studies have shown that carotid ligation can obliterate or reduce the size of giant aneurysms.[5,129,131] Because the risk of precipitating cerebral ischemia is considerable, simple carotid ligation has become a less favored alternative for the treatment of these lesions.

Cerebral infarction is a major immediate complication of carotid artery occlusion: approximately 10 to 20 percent of patients are unable to tolerate carotid artery occlusion.[69,90,92] In a series of 220 patients, Odom and Tindall[92] reported ischemic complications in 34 patients. Significantly, despite the immediate opening of the carotid artery after the onset of ischemia in this series, only 12 patients recovered completely.

Numerous techniques, including the Wada test, the measurement of carotid artery stump pressures, electroencephalographic monitoring, jugular venous blood sampling, gradual occlusion, and CBF measurements, have been proposed to help predict which patients can withstand permanent carotid occlusion. Many surgeons believe that gradual occlusion of the carotid artery is safer than acute occlusion, permitting the development of collateral blood flow; however, the results of the Cooperative Study on Aneurysms[90] failed to substantiate this assumption. Wada's test, which involves a trial occlusion of the carotid artery (most recently using endovascular balloon techniques)[44,148] as a test of adequate collateral circulation, reduces but does not eliminate ischemic complications as the onset of ischemic deficits is often delayed for hours to days. The majority of these delayed complications following carotid artery occlusion are most likely from embolic propagation rather than from low flow rates. However, there are clearly patients in whom the limited availability of collateral blood supplies markedly increases the risks of carotid occlusion.

Measurement of regional CBF with the carotid artery open and occluded may be of predictive value in selecting patients who can tolerate carotid occlusion.[41,82] Miller et al.[82] used a 25 percent reduction in CBF following occlusion of the carotid artery as their critical level; patients with reductions in CBF greater than 25 percent were rejected as candidates for carotid occlusion. Although this method resulted in the rejection of 20 percent of patients tested, the authors report that it virtually eliminated the incidence of perioperative ischemic complications following carotid artery occlusion.

It has long been recognized that carotid artery occlusion decreases the pressure in the distal internal carotid artery and causes the angiographic obliteration of some intracranial aneurysms. However, it does not completely protect the patient from the risk of rebleeding. Norlen and Olivecrona[91] reported a 10 to 15 percent incidence of death from recurrent subarachnoid hemorrhage in the long-term follow-up of patients undergoing carotid occlusion. In the report by the Cooperative Study, Nishioka[90] reported an 8 percent rebleeding rate on long-term follow-up of 1 to 6 years (mean, 3 years). Roski et al.[109] reported the results of long-term follow-up in 39 patients following carotid artery occlusion for the treatment of ruptured aneurysms, and noted repeat hemorrhage led to death in 8 percent. In this same study, the authors reported a 16 percent incidence of late TIAs and a 16.6 percent

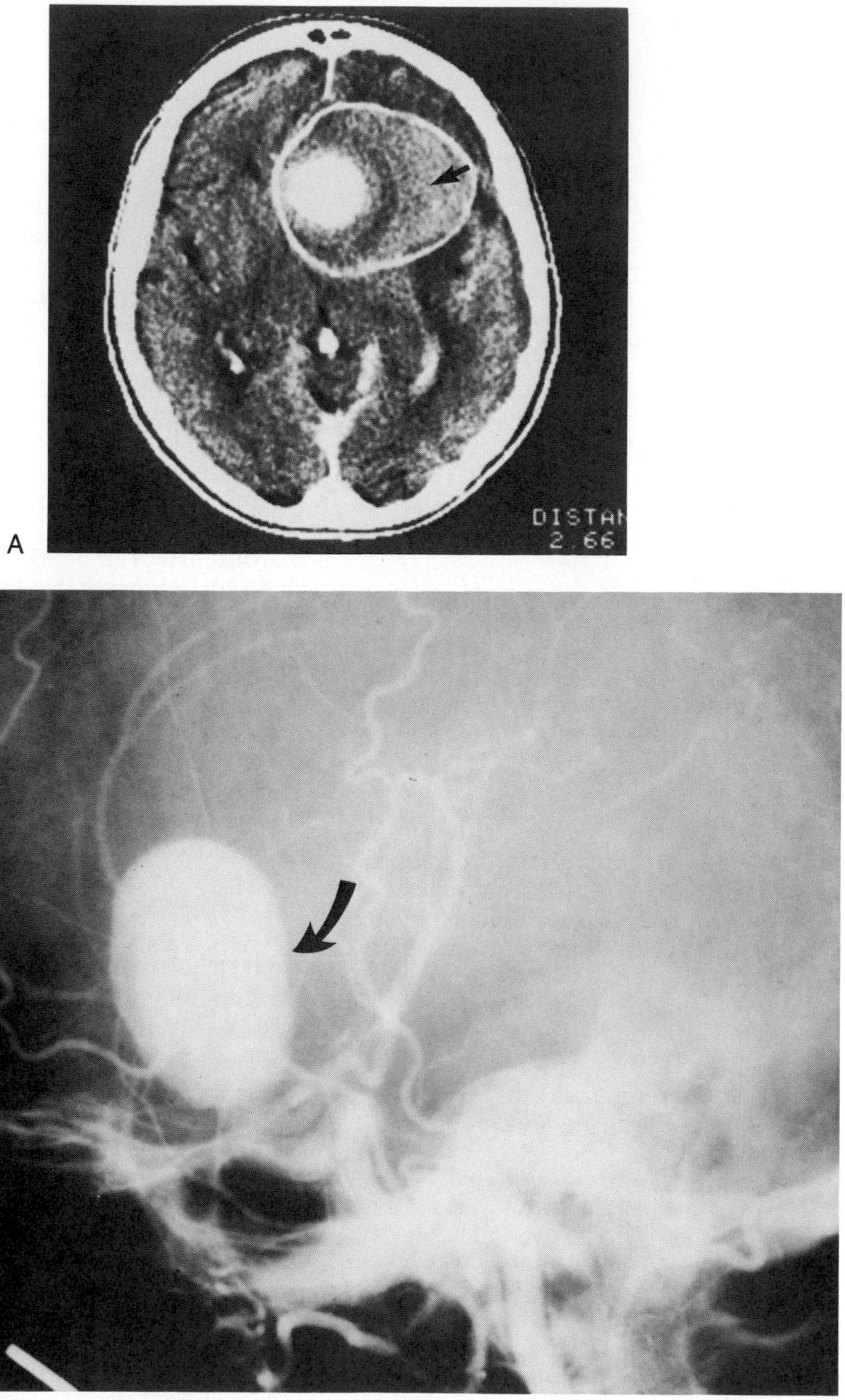


**Fig. 46-19.** A 56-year-old woman presented with dementia and progressive right-sided weakness. (**A**) Contrast-enhanced head computed tomography scan demonstrates a large, centrally enhancing mass with a thin rim of contrast bordering the lesion, producing the so-called target sign. This picture is nearly pathognomonic for a partially thrombosed giant aneurysm; the unenhancing portion of the mass (*arrow*) represents thrombus within the aneurysm dome. (**B**) Lateral view of the left internal carotid artery angiogram in the same patient confirms the diagnosis of a giant internal carotid artery aneurysm (*arrow*). Note that the size of the aneurysm is grossly underestimated by the angiogram (compare with the computed tomography scan), as only the central portion of the lesion fills with contrast.

incidence of delayed stroke ipsilateral to the side of internal carotid occlusion.

The above provides the rationale for our preference of utilizing an arterial bypass or venous jump graft in combination with trapping procedures for those aneurysms in which direct clipping or reconstruction is not possible.

## Direct Clipping

With modern microsurgical techniques, the majority of giant intracranial aneurysms can be directly clipped. Management often requires a combination of temporary trapping that permits decompression of the aneurysmal dome and even partial resection when the sac contains significant thrombus or the neck of the aneurysm is calcified. As discussed earlier, temporary vessel occlusion appears to be safe for 10 to 20 minutes, when the patient is under deep barbiturate anesthesia with burst suppression of EEG activity. To enhance the collateral blood supply, the patient should be kept normotensive to mildly hypertensive during temporary vessel occlusion.

Giant aneurysms involving the anterior circulation are approached initially in a standard fashion as described above with the goal of isolating the aneurysm neck. Care must be taken to ensure that all branches and adjacent vessels have been identified and dissected free from the neck before clipping is attempted. Often, one or two small branches may be firmly adherent to the aneurysm neck and resist attempts at dissection. If so, temporary clips should be applied to the parent vessel and major branches to trap the aneurysm. Any branches remaining adherent to the neck can then be safely dissected and the neck of the aneurysm clipped in a standard fashion. If preoperative studies demonstrate extensive thrombus within the aneurysm sac or the aneurysm is difficult to collapse, the dome can be opened sharply and thrombus removed manually or with an ultrasonic aspirator. Occasionally, it is necessary to perform a limited endarterectomy to permit clipping of the aneurysm neck without compromise of the parent vessel. If the surgeon is fully prepared and focused, the neck of the aneurysm can usually be decompressed and prepared for clipping within the safe period of temporary vessel occlusion defined above.

When giant aneurysms involve the supraclinoid portion of the internal carotid artery, proximal control of the artery can be obtained in the neck. Preoperative angiography should include views of the carotid bifurcation to assure that it is not significantly diseased. To aid in clipping, the aneurysm can be readily collapsed during temporary vessel occlusion by gentle aspiration of blood from a catheter placed in the cervical portion of the internal carotid artery.[13]

## Bypass Procedures

A small minority of giant aneurysms, particularly those involving the cavernous portion of the internal carotid artery, are best managed by combining a trapping procedure with an arterial bypass or venous jump graft.[9,132,137] Although a number of authors have demonstrated that dissection in the cavernous sinus for control of these aneurysms is possible, the risk of ischemic complications and cranial nerve deficits is significant.[33,35,62,99] Knowledge of the anatomy in this region has increased significantly in the last 5 years, primarily as a result of the management of skull base tumors.[100,114,115] Consequently, short venous jump grafts from the petrous portion of the carotid artery to its supraclinoid portion have replaced the much longer grafts from the cervical carotid that were previously necessary for a high-flow bypass (Fig. 46-20). These short venous grafts reduce the risks of late stenosis and offer markedly higher flow than the superficial temporal artery. Several groups have recently published descriptions of this procedure along with operative results.[32,45,125]

The patient is positioned for a frontotemporal craniotomy and the neck and leg on the operative side are prepared and draped. Although the saphenous vein in the lower leg is usually a satisfactory graft, the entire leg should be prepared for surgery as a precaution. After elevating the bone flap and completing resection of the lateral wall of the frontal and temporal fossae, an extensive extradural dissection is performed as described by Dolenc.[35] The dura is elevated from the frontal fossa floor, and the posterior lateral margin of the orbit and the anterior clinoid are resected with the aid of a high-speed drill. In the temporal fossa, the dura is carefully elevated and the meningeal artery and the greater petrosal nerve are identified and divided. Care must be taken to avoid traction on the greater petrosal nerve, which can lead to injury of the geniculate ganglion and facial nerve paresis. Using a diamond-tipped burr, the bone immediately inferior and lateral to the posterior margin of the foramen ovale is removed to expose the horizontal segment of the internal carotid artery. Typically, a 10- to 12-mm segment of the carotid artery can be isolated at this location. If this segment of the carotid artery is involved with the aneurysm or a sufficient length cannot be isolated for bypass, the internal carotid artery is dissected from the neck. The dura is now opened and the supraclinoid portion of the carotid artery is isolated. The carotid artery can usually be isolated proximal to the origin of the ophthalmic artery for trapping of the intracavernous aneurysm. Dissection of this portion of the carotid is aided by the previous resection of the anterior clinoid and by opening the dural ring that surrounds the vessel just proximal to its entry into the cavernous sinus.[34]

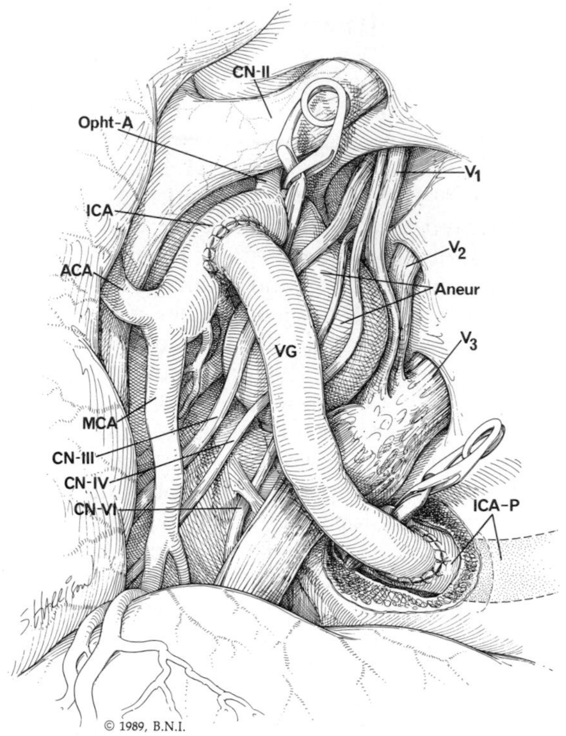


**Fig. 46-20.** Artist's sketch illustrating a vein graft (VG) from the petrous segment of the internal carotid artery (ICA-P) to the supraclinoid segment of the internal carotid artery (ICA) for the treatment of a giant aneurysm (Aneur) involving the cavernous segment of the internal carotid artery. Note that the aneurysm has been eliminated from the circulation by the placement of proximal and distal clips. The lateral wall of the cavernous sinus has been removed to display the course of the 3rd, 4th, and 6th cranial nerves (CN), and the 5th cranial nerve (V). Other labeled structures include the ophthalmic artery (Opht-A), anterior cerebral artery (ACA), middle cerebral artery (MCA), and the optic nerve (CN-II). (Adapted from Spetzler et al.,[125] with permission; © Barrow Neurological Institute, 1989.)

At this point the saphenous vein is harvested. For the short petrous-to-supraclinoid bypass, the saphenous vein below the knee is usually satisfactory; for the much longer cervical-to-supraclinoid bypass, we prefer the saphenous vein from the upper thigh and groin. To maximize long-term graft patency, the vein must not be injured when it is harvested and prepared for bypass.[22,70,105,131] With the patient under barbiturate burst-suppression, the aneurysm is trapped proximally and distally, and the venous bypass is performed (Fig. 46-20). Sufficient collateral blood flow is normally available through the anterior communicating and posterior communicating arteries to prevent ischemic injury during the period required to complete the bypass.

When giant aneurysms arise at the middle cerebral artery trifurcation, the neck often involves one of the

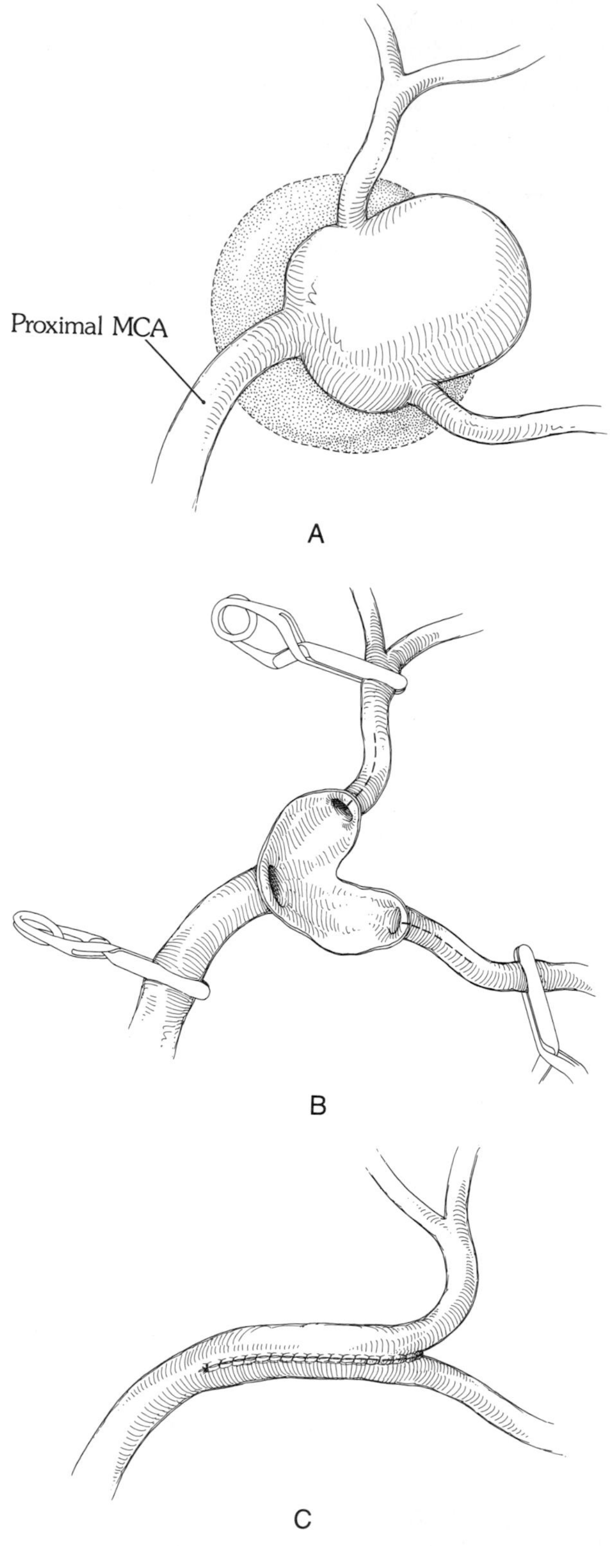


**Fig. 46-21.** (**A–C**) Line drawings illustrating the technique used to treat a giant middle cerebral artery (MCA) aneurysm that involves the origin of several major branches. The aneurysm is resected and the arterial wall is reconstructed using microvascular techniques. (From Bojanowski et al.,[20] with permission.)

major branches such that direct clipping becomes impossible without sacrificing the vessel. In such cases, the involved vessel can be divided at the time of the aneurysm clipping and reanastomosed to one of remaining intact trifurcation branches, or the aneurysm itself can be resected and the vessel wall directly reconstructed (Fig. 46-21).[19,130,132] Alternatively, an extracranial-intracranial arterial bypass can be performed (using the superficial temporal artery) to provide the needed collateral blood flow to the involved vessels.[9,132] Using such an approach, the surgeon can eliminate the majority of giant middle cerebral artery aneurysms from the circulation.

## Hypothermic Circulatory Arrest

The management of giant basilar artery aneurysms presents unusual problems because of their awkward location and because they cannot be directly controlled by temporary clipping. As discussed above, the aneurysms are surrounded by numerous small but highly important perforating branches that make accurate dissection and clipping of the neck paramount for a good outcome. A useful adjunct for the treatment of these lesions is total, hypothermic circulatory arrest. Several groups have reported improved results after using this technique in the treatment of giant intracranial aneurysms.[15,40,122,127,141] A multispecialty team is composed of a neurosurgeon, a cardiothoracic surgeon, a pump team, and an anesthesiologist with experience in both neurologic and cardiovascular surgery.

The aneurysm is initially exposed during a standard subtemporal approach as described above. Following exposure of the aneurysm neck, the patient is fully heparinized, the femoral artery and vein are cannulated, and extracorporeal circulation is initiated (Figs. 46-22 and 46-23). The patient is gradually cooled to a surface brain temperature of between 15 and 17°C. The pump is stopped and the blood is allowed to drain into the bypass pump reservoir, collapsing the aneurysm. Dissection about the neck of the aneurysm is completed, with care being taken to free all perforating vessels and major branches. If the aneurysm contains extensive thrombosis, it can be opened and partially evacuated to enable clipping of the neck. After clipping of the aneurysm, the pump is restarted and the patient is gradually rewarmed. The risk of intracerebral hematoma formation is minimized by avoiding any movement of the retractors after the patient has been heparinized and before he or she has been rewarmed and weaned from extracorporeal circulation and the heparin has been reversed. In addition, clotting factors and platelets are replenished by transfusing 1 to 2 units of autologous, fresh, whole blood that was removed during the initial exposure of the aneurysm. If necessary, the pump can be primed with 1 to 2 units of packed cells to maintain an adequate hemoglobin level.

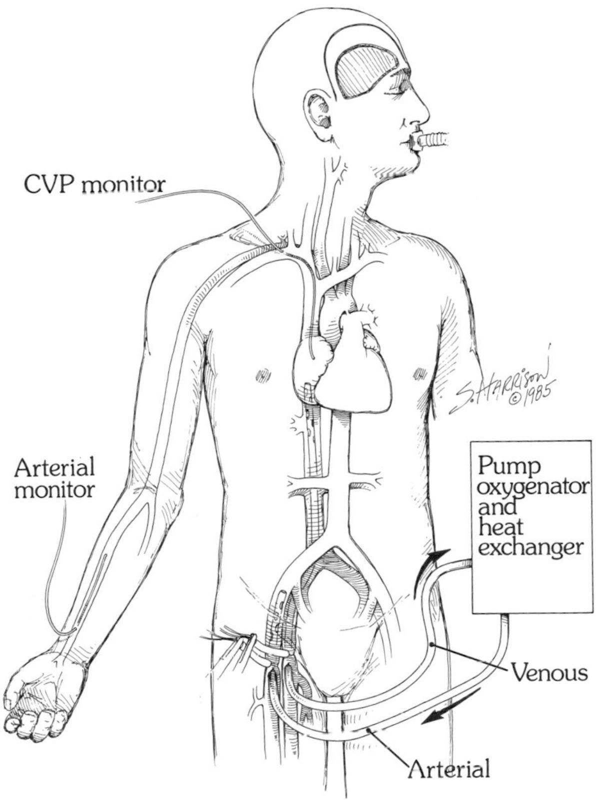


**Fig. 46-22.** Illustration of technique used to establish extracorporeal circulation during hypothermic circulatory arrest for intracranial aneurysms. The femoral artery and vein are cannulated in the groin and connected to the pump oxygenator and heat exchanger. This approach allows the cardiovascular and neurosurgical teams to work simultaneously as illustrated in Figure 46-23. CVP, central venous pressure. (From Spetzler et al.,[127] with permission.)

Using this technique, we have successfully clipped 18 giant basilar artery aneurysms (Fig. 46-24). There was one death in the postoperative period in a patient with a brain stem infarct for a mortality of 6 percent; transient deficits occurred in 8 patients and included 3rd cranial nerve palsies and mild hemiparesis. At a 6-month follow-up, 12 patients were independent with good outcomes, 4 patients had mild to moderate deficits requiring some assistance, and 1 patient had a poor outcome with severe cognitive impairment.

## SUMMARY

Advances in neuroanesthesia, the development of new microsurgical instruments, and the rapid evolution of microvascular techniques have dramatically reduced the operative morbidity and mortality associated with the surgical management of intracranial aneurysms. In patients with acute aneurysmal sub-

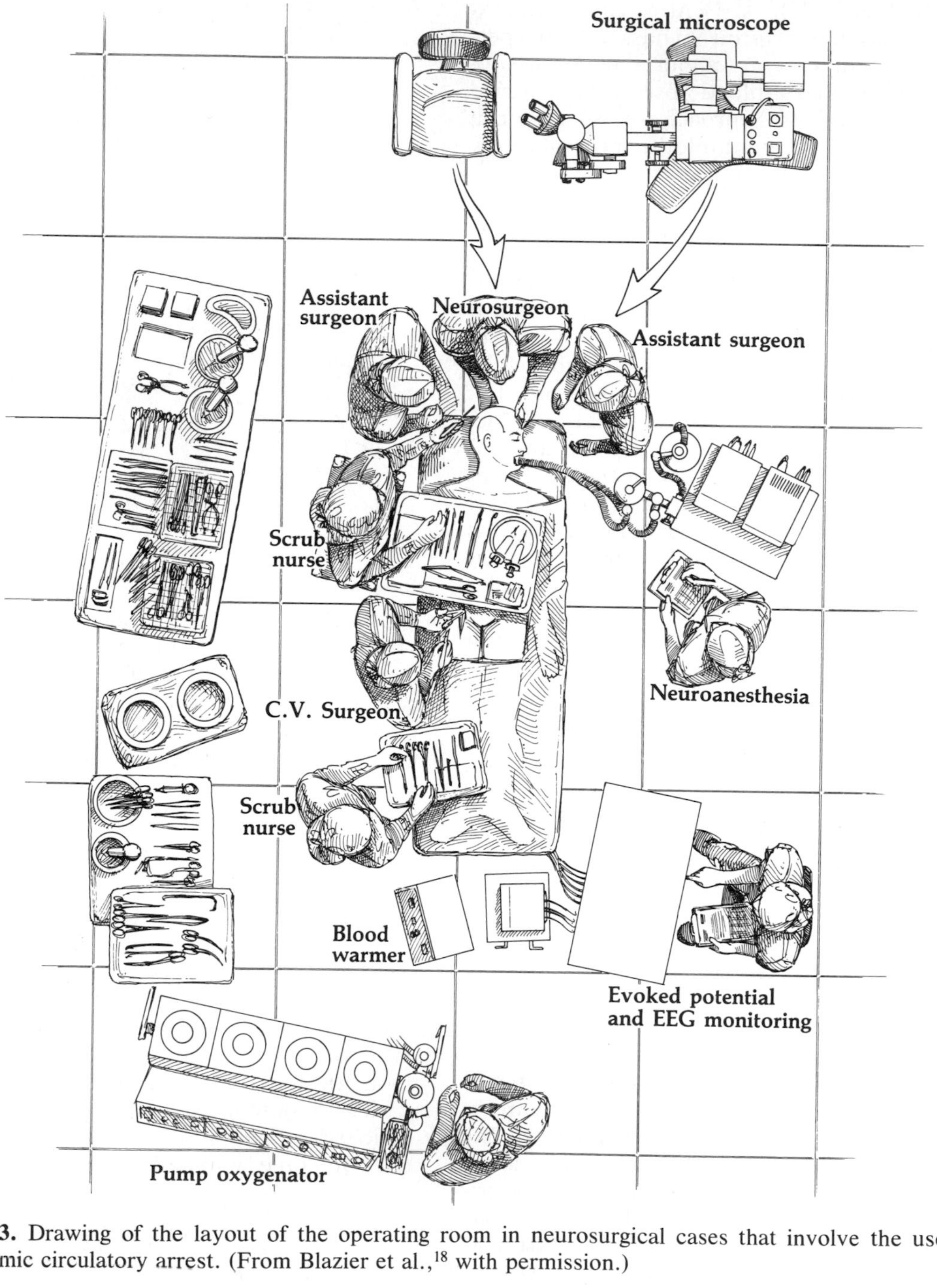


**Fig. 46-23.** Drawing of the layout of the operating room in neurosurgical cases that involve the use of hypothermic circulatory arrest. (From Blazier et al.,[18] with permission.)

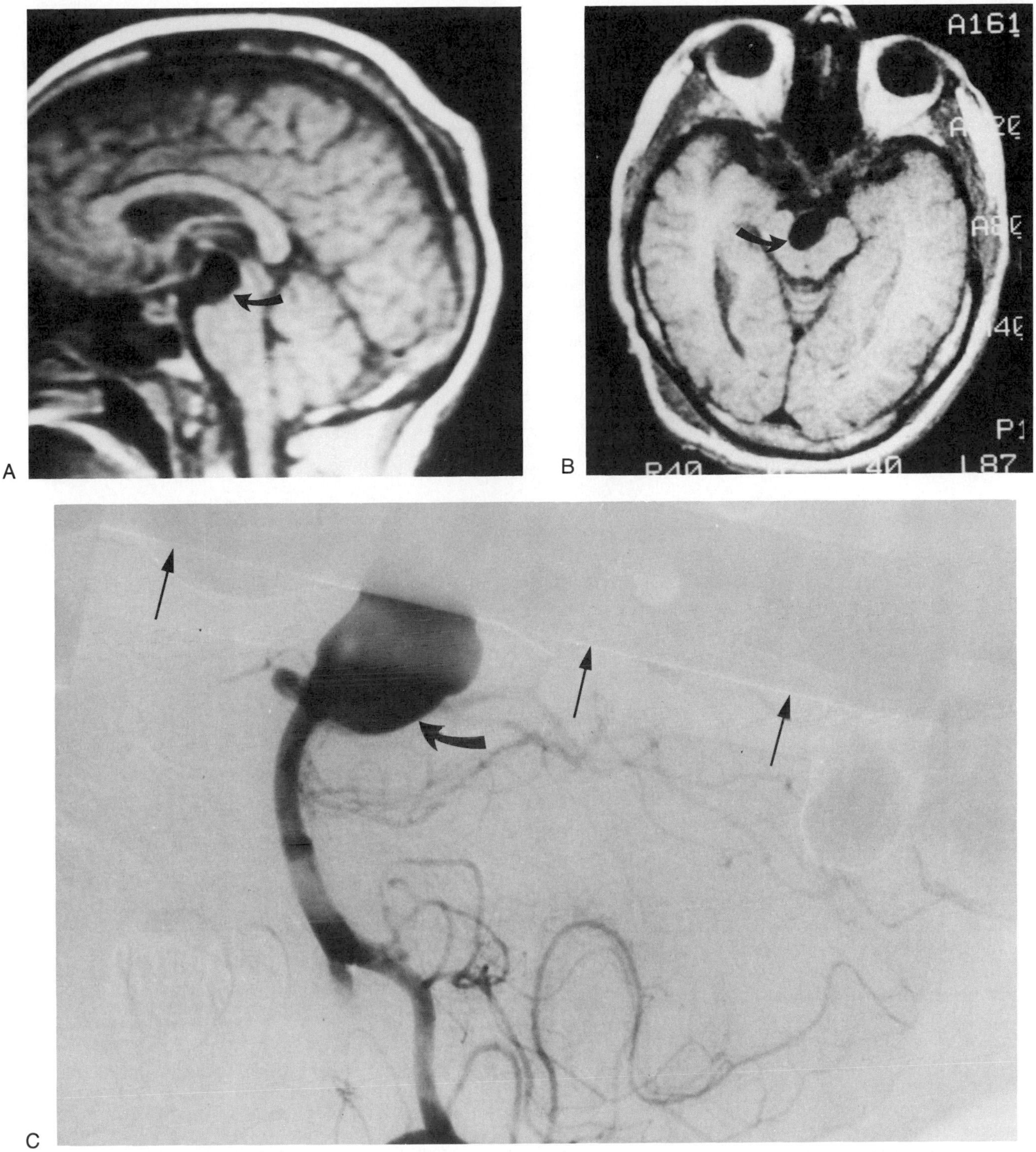


**Fig. 46-24.** A 51-year-old woman sustained a cervical spine fracture and mild head trauma in a motor vehicle accident. Magnetic resonance imaging of the head and neck was performed as part of her initial posttrauma evaluation. (**A & B**) Sagittal and transverse T1-weighted images revealed a giant, incidental basilar tip aneurysm (*arrows*). The cervical spine fracture was treated by immobilizing the patient with a halo vest and ring. (**C**) A lateral view of the vertebral artery angiogram confirmed the diagnosis of a giant basilar tip aneurysm (*curved arrow*). Artifact from the halo ring is apparent (*straight arrows*). On both the magnetic resonance images and the angiogram, the aneurysm dome angles up and back, distorting and displacing the brain stem. The cervical spine fracture healed without complication. Four months after her accident, the patient underwent clipping of the aneurysm under hypothermic circulatory arrest. The patient's recovery was quick and uneventful. (*Figure continues.*)

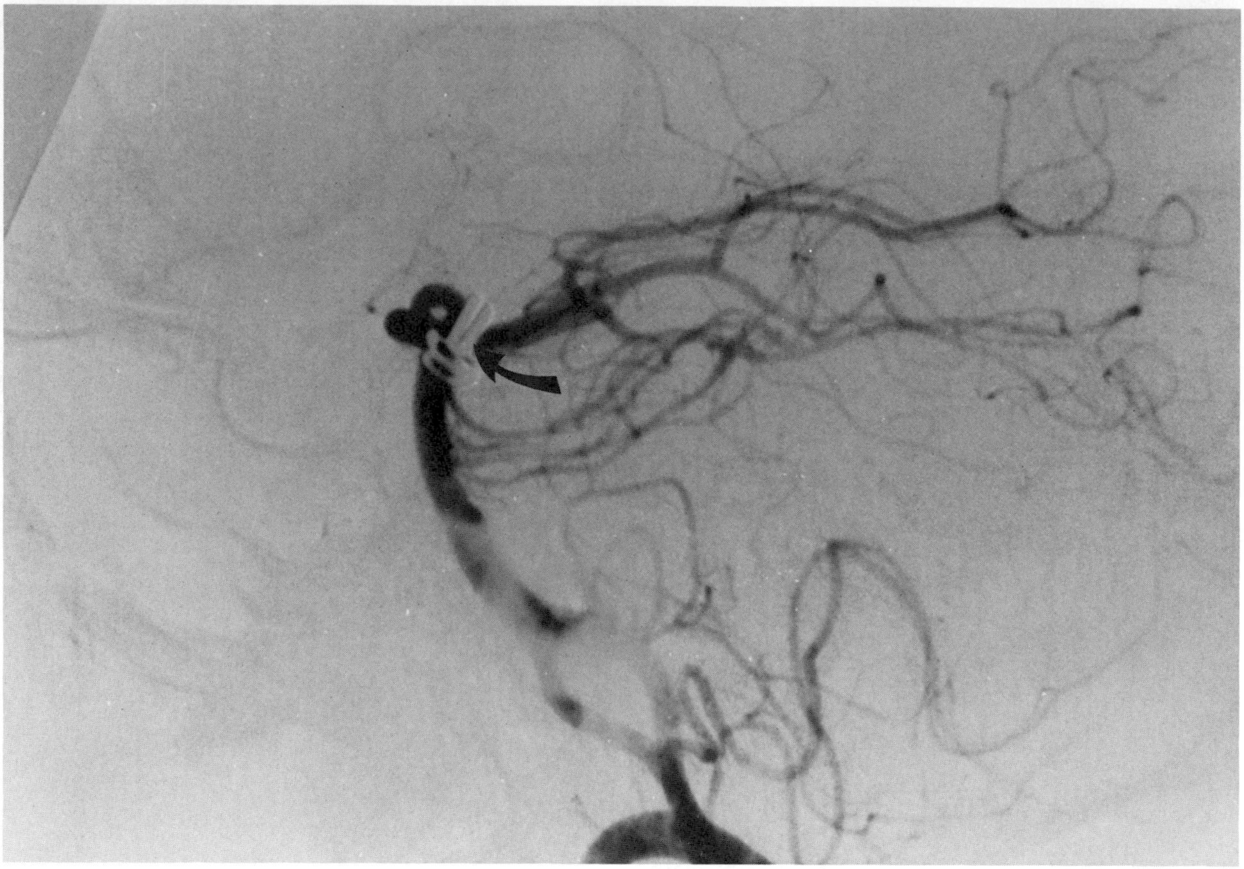

D

**Fig. 46-24** (*Continued*). (**D**) Lateral view of the postoperative vertebral angiogram reveals good clipping of the aneurysm with preservation of the normal branches. A single straight clip is faintly visible across the neck of the aneurysm (*arrow*).

arachnoid hemorrhage, early surgical intervention has now virtually eliminated the risk of rebleeding, while changes in perioperative management, including the use of hypervolemic-hypertensive therapy and calcium antagonist, have significantly blunted the devastating effect of vasospasm. In patients admitted to the hospital in good condition, early surgery and aggressive management have reduced morbidity and mortality to 10 to 20 percent. Ischemic deficits secondary to vasospasm remain the major cause of poor outcome in this group; several interesting new therapies are being evaluated in clinical trials and hold promise of further reducing morbidity and mortality.

## REFERENCES

1. Adams HP, Kassel NF, Torner JC et al: Early management of aneurysmal subarachnoid hemorrhage: a report of the Cooperative Aneurysm Study. J Neurosurg 54:141, 1981
2. Al-Mefty O, Fox JL, Rifai A et al: A combined infratemporal and posterior fossa approach for the removal of giant glomus tumors and chondrosarcomas. Surg Neurol 28:423, 1987
3. Andrews RJ, Spiegel PK: Intracranial aneurysms: age, sex, blood pressure, and multiplicity in an unselected series of patients. J Neurosurg 51:27, 1979
4. Auer LM: Acute operation and preventive nimodipine improve outcome in patients with ruptured cerebral aneurysms. Neurosurgery 15:57, 1984
5. Auer LM, Brandt L, Ebeling U et al: Nimodipine and early aneurysm operation in good condition SAH patients. Acta Neurochir (Wien) 82:7, 1986
6. Auer LM, Schneider GH, Auer T: Computerized tomography and prognosis in early aneurysm surgery. J Neurosurg 65:217, 1986
7. Ausman JI, Diaz FG, Malik GM et al: Current management of cerebral aneurysms: is it based on facts or myths? Surg Neurol 24:625, 1985
8. Ausman JI, Diaz FG, Malik GM et al: Management of cerebral aneurysms: further facts and additional myths. Surg Neurol 32:21, 1989
9. Ausman JI, Diaz FG, Sadasivan B et al: Giant intracranial aneurysm surgery: the role of microvascular reconstruction. Surg Neurol 34:8, 1990
10. Bailes JE, Spetzler RF, Hadley MN et al: Management morbidity and mortality of poor-

grade aneurysm patients. J Neurosurg 72:559, 1990
11. Bakay L, Sweet WH: Cervical and intracranial intra-arterial pressures with and without occlusion. Surg Gynecol Obstet 95:67, 1952
12. Bakay L, Sweet WH: Intra-arterial pressures in the neck and brain: late changes after carotid closure, acute measurements after vertebral closure. J Neurosurg 10:353, 1953
13. Batjer HH, Samson DS: Retrograde suction decompression of giant paraclinoidal aneurysms: technical note. J Neurosurg 73:305, 1990
14. Battaglia R, Pasqualin A, DaPian R: Italian Cooperative Study on Giant Intracranial Aneurysms. 1. Study design and clinical data. Acta Neurochir, suppl. (Wien) 42:49, 1988
15. Baumgartner WA, Silverberg GD, Ream AK et al: Reappraisal of cardiopulmonary bypass with deep hypothermia and circulatory arrest for complex neurosurgical operations. Surgery 94:242, 1983
16. Biller J, Adams HP, Jr: Cerebrovascular disorders associated with pregnancy. Am Fam Physician 33:125, 1986
17. Bingham WF: Treatment of mycotic intracranial aneurysms. J Neurosurg 46:428, 1977
18. Blazier CJ, Cavanaugh E, Antonioli L: Surgical treatment of complex cerebrovascular lesions utilizing hypothermia and circulatory arrest: nursing implications. Barrow Neurol Inst Q 5:33, 1990
19. Bohmfalk GL, Story JL, Wissinger JP et al: Bacterial intracranial aneurysm. J Neurosurg 48:369, 1978
20. Bojanowski WM, Spetzler RF, Carter LP: Reconstruction of the MCA bifurcation after excision of a giant aneurysm: technical note. J Neurosurg 68:974, 1988
21. Bokemeyer C, Frank B, Brandis A et al: Giant aneurysm causing frontal lobe syndrome. J Neurol 237:47, 1990
22. Boncheck LI: Prevention of endothelial damage during preparation of saphenous veins for bypass grafting. J Thorac Cardiovasc Surg 79:911, 1980
23. Bonita R, Thomson S: Subarachnoid hemorrhage: epidemiology, diagnosis, management, and outcome. Stroke 16:591, 1985
24. Branston NM, Hope DT, Symon L: Barbiturates in focal ischemia of primate cortex: effects on blood flow distribution, evoked potential, and extracellular potassium. Stroke 10:647, 1979
25. Bull J: Massive aneurysms at the base of the brain . Brain 92:535, 1969
26. Chason JL, Hindman WM: Berry aneurysms of the circle of Willis: results of a planned autopsy study. Neurology (NY) 8:41, 1958
27. Cohen MM: Cerebrovascular accidents: study of 201 cases. Arch Pathol 60:296, 1955
28. Crompton MR: Mechanism of growth and rupture in cerebral berry aneurysms. Br Med J 1:1138, 1966
29. Cushing H: Contributions to the clinical studies of intracranial aneurysms. Guys Hosp Rep 73:159, 1923
30. Dandy WE: Intracranial aneurysm of internal carotid artery cured by operation. Ann Surg 107:654, 1938
31. Dell S: Asymptomatic cerebral aneurysm: assessment of its risk of rupture. Neurosurgery 10:162, 1982
32. Dernbach PD, Little JR, Jones SC et al: Altered cerebral autoregulation and $CO_2$ reactivity after aneurysmal subarachnoid hemorrhage. Neurosurgery 22:822, 1988
33. Dolenc V: Direct microsurgical repair of intracavernous vascular lesions. J Neurosurg 58:824, 1983
34. Dolenc VV: A combined epi- and subdural direct approach to carotid-ophthalmic artery aneurysms. J Neurosurg 62:667, 1985
35. Dolenc V: Surgery of vascular lesions of the cavernous sinus. Clin Neurosurg 36:240, 1990
36. Dott NM: Intracranial aneurysms: cerebral arterioradiography: surgical treatment. Trans Med Chir Soc Edinb 47:219, 1932–33.
37. Drake CG: Ligation of the vertebral (unilateral or bilateral) or basilar artery in the treatment of large intracranial aneurysms. J Neurosurg 43:255, 1975
38. Drake CG: Giant intracranial aneurysms: experience with surgical treatment in 174 patients. Clin Neurosurg 26:12, 1979
39. Drake CG: Management of cerebral aneurysm. Stroke 12:273, 1981
40. Drake CG, Barr HKW, Coles JC et al: The use of extracorporeal circulation and profound hypothermia in the treatment of ruptured intracranial aneurysm. J Neurosurg 21:575, 1964
41. Erba SM, Horton JA, Latchaw RE et al: Balloon test occlusion of the internal carotid artery with stable xenon/CT cerebral blood flow imaging. AJNR 9:533, 1988
42. Fein JM, Lipow K, Marmarou A: Cortical artery pressure in normotensive and hypertensive aneurysm patients. J Neurosurg 59:51, 1983
43. Fodstad H: Antifibrinolytic treatment in subarachnoid haemorrhage: present state. Acta Neurochir 63:233, 1982
44. Fox AJ, Vinuela F, Pelz DM et al: Use of detachable balloons for proximal artery occlusion in the treatment of unclippable cerebral aneurysms. J Neurosurg 66:40, 1987
45. Fukushima T: Direct operative approach to the vascular lesions in the cavernous sinus: summary of 27 cases—Mt Fuji Workshop. Cerebrovas Dis 6:169, 1988
46. Graff-Radford NR, Torner JC, Adams HP, Jr et al: Factors associated with hydrocephalus after subarachnoid hemorrhage: a report of the Cooperative Aneurysm Study. Arch Neurol 46:744, 1989
47. Gross M: Giant middle cerebral aneurysm presenting as hemiparkinsonism. (Letter.) J Neurol Neurosurg Psychiatry 50:1075, 1987
48. Hammon WM, Kempe LG: The posterior fossa approach to aneurysms of the vertebral and basilar arteries. J Neurosurg 37:339, 1972
49. Hassler O: Morphological studies on the large cerebral arteries, with reference to aetiology of subarachnoid haemorrhage. Acta Psychiat Scand, suppl. 154:1, 1961

50. Heros RC: Lateral suboccipital approach for vertebral and vertebrobasilar artery lesions. J Neurosurg 64:559, 1986
51. Heyman A, Tindall GT, Finney WHM et al: Measurement of retinal artery and intracarotid pressures: following carotid artery occlusion with the Crutchfield clamp. J Neurosurg 17:297, 1960
52. Hitchcock ER, Tsementzis SA, Dow AA: Short- and long-term prognosis of patients with a subarachnoid hemorrhage in relation to intra-operative period of hypotension. Acta Neurochir (Wien) 70:235, 1984
53. Hochman MS: Reversal of fixed pupils after spontaneous intraventricular hemorrhage with secondary acute hydrocephalus: report of two cases treated with early ventriculostomy. Neurosurgery 18:777, 1986
54. Hoff JT, Pitts LH, Spetzler RF et al: Barbiturates for protection from cerebral ischemia in aneurysm surgery. Acta Neurol Scand, suppl. 64 56:158, 1977
55. Housepian EM, Pool JL: A systematic analysis of intracranial aneurysms from the autopsy file of the Presbyterian Hospital, 1914 to 1956. J Neuropathol Exp Neurol 17:409, 1958
56. Hugenholtz H, Elgie RG: Considerations in early surgery on good-risk patients with ruptured intracranial aneurysms. J Neurosurg 56:180, 1982
57. Hunt HB, Schifrin BS, Suzuki K: Ruptured berry aneurysms and pregnancy. Obstet Gynecol 43:827, 1974
58. Ingall TJ, Whisnant JP, Wiebers DO et al: Has there been a decline in subarachnoid hemorrhage mortality? Stroke 20:718, 1989
59. Ishii R: Regional cerebral blood flow in patients with ruptured intracranial aneurysms. J Neurosurg 50:587, 1979
60. Jabre A, Symon L: Temporary vascular occlusion during aneurysm surgery. Surg Neurol 27:47, 1987
61. Jane JA, Kassell NF, Torner JC et al: The natural history of aneurysms and arteriovenous malformations. J Neurosurg 62:321, 1985
62. Johnston I: Direct surgical treatment of bilateral intracavernous internal carotid artery aneurysms: case report. J Neurosurg 51:98, 1979
63. Kassell NF, Drake CG: Timing of aneurysm surgery. Neurosurgery 10:514, 1982
64. Kassell NF, Torner JC: Size of intracranial aneurysms. Neurosurgery 12:291, 1983
65. Kassell NF, Torner JC: The International Cooperative Study on Timing of Aneurysm Surgery—an update. Stroke 15:566, 1984
66. Kassell NF, Torner JC, Adams HP, Jr: Antifibrinolytic therapy in the acute period following aneurysmal subarachnoid hemorrhage: preliminary observations from the Cooperative Aneurysm Study. J Neurosurg 61:225, 1984
67. Kassell NF, Torner JC, Haley EC, Jr et al: The International Cooperative Study on the Timing of Aneurysm Surgery. 1. Overall management results. J Neurosurg 73:18, 1990
68. Kassell NF, Torner JC, Jane JA et al: The International Cooperative Study on the Timing of Aneurysm Surgery. 2. Surgical results. J Neurosurg 73:37, 1990
69. Landolt AM, Millikan CH: Pathogenesis of cerebral infarction secondary to mechanical carotid artery occlusion. Stroke 1:52, 1970
70. Lannerstad O, Dougan P, Bergqvist D: Effects of different graft preparation techniques on the acute thrombogenicity of autologous vein grafts: an experimental study in sheep. Eur Surg Res 19:395, 1987
71. Ljunggren B, Brandt L, Kagstrom E et al: Results of early operations for ruptured aneurysms. J Neurosurg 54:473, 1981
72. Ljunggren B, Brandt L, Saveland H et al: Outcome in 60 consecutive patients treated with early aneurysm operation and intravenous nimodipine. J Neurosurg 61:864, 1984
73. Ljunggren B, Saveland H, Brandt L et al: Early operation and overall outcome in aneurysmal subarachnoid hemorrhage. J Neurosurg 62:547, 1985
74. Ljunggren B, Saveland H, Brandt L et al: Aneurysmal subarachnoid hemorrhage: total annual outcome in a 1.46 million population. Surg Neurol 22:435, 1984
75. Locksley HB: Report on the Cooperative Study of Intracranial Aneurysms and Subarachnoid Hemorrhage. Sect. V, Part I: Natural history of subarachnoid hemorrhage, intracranial aneurysms and arteriovenous malformations: based on 6368 cases in the Cooperative Study. J Neurosurg 25:219, 1966
76. Mayhall CG, Archer NH, Lamb VA et al: Ventriculostomy-related infections: a prospective epidemiologic study. N Engl J Med 310:553, 1984
77. McCormick WF: Problems and pathogenesis of intracranial arterial aneurysms. p. 219. In Moossy J, Janeway R (eds): Cerebral Vascular Disease. Seventh Conference. Grune & Stratton, New York, 1971
78. McCormick WF, Acosta-Rua GJ: The size of intracranial saccular aneurysms: an autopsy study. J Neurosurg 33:422, 1970
79. McDermott MW, Durity FA, Borozny M et al: Temporary vessel occlusion and barbiturate protection in cerebral aneurysm surgery. Neurosurgery 25:54, 1989
80. Meyer FB, Sundt TM Jr, Fode NC et al: Cerebral aneurysms in childhood and adolescence. J Neurosurg 70:420, 1989
81. Milhorat TH, Krautheim M: Results of early and delayed operations for ruptured intracranial aneurysms in two series of 100 consecutive patients. Surg Neurol 26:123, 1986
82. Miller JD, Jawad K, Jennett B: Safety of carotid ligation and its role in the management of intracranial aneurysms. J Neurol Neurosurg Psychiatry 40:64, 1977
83. Minielly R, Yuzpe AA, Drake CG: Subarachnoid hemorrhage secondary to ruptured cerebral aneurysm in pregnancy. Obstet Gynecol 53:64, 1979
84. Moniz E: L'encéphalographie artérielle, son im-

portance dans la localisation des tumeurs cérébrales. Rev Neurol (Paris) 2:72, 1927
85. Morgan DW, Honan W: Lateral gaze palsy due to giant aneurysm of the posterior fossa. (Letter.) J Neurol Neurosurg Psychiatry 51:883, 1988
86. Morley TP, Barr HWK: Giant intracranial aneurysms: diagnosis, course, and management. Clin Neurosurg 16:73, 1969
87. Moskowitz MA, Rosenbaum AE, Tyler HR: Angiographically monitored resolution of cerebral mycotic aneurysms. Neurology (NY) 24:1103, 1974
88. Nehls DG, Flom RA, Carter LP et al: Multiple intracranial aneurysms: determining the site of rupture. J Neurosurg 63:342, 1985
89. Nehls DG, Todd MM, Spetzler RF et al: A comparison of the cerebral protective effects of isoflurane and barbiturates during temporary focal cerebral ischemia in primates. Anesthesiology 66:453, 1987
90. Nishioka H: Report of the Cooperative Study of Intracranial Aneurysms and Subarachnoid Hemorrhage. Sect. VIII, Part 1: Results of the treatment of intracranial aneurysms by occlusion of the carotid artery in the neck. J Neurosurg 25:660, 1966
91. Norlen G, Olivecrona H: Treatment of aneurysms of the circle of Willis. J Neurosurg 10:404, 1953
92. Odom GL, Tindall GT: Carotid ligation in the treatment of certain intracranial aneurysms. Clin Neurosurg 15:101, 1968
93. Ohman J, Heiskanen O: Timing of operation for ruptured supratentorial aneurysms: a prospective randomized study. J Neurosurg 70:55, 1989
94. Onuma T, Suzuki J: Surgical treatment of giant intracranial aneurysms. J Neurosurg 51:33, 1979
95. Osler W: Gulstonian lectures on malignant endocarditis. Lancet 1:393, 1885
96. Ostergaard JR, Hog E: Incidence of multiple intracranial aneurysms: influence of arterial hypertension and gender. J Neurosurg 63:49, 1985
97. Ostergaard JR, Voldby B: Intracranial arterial aneurysms in children and adolescents. J Neurosurg 58:832, 1983
98. Park BE: Spontaneous subarachnoid hemorrhage complicated by communicating hydrocephalus: epsilon amino caproic acid as a possible predisposing factor. Surg Neurol 11:73, 1979
99. Parkinson D: Carotid cavernous fistula: direct repair with preservation of the carotid artery: technical note. J Neurosurg 38:99, 1973
100. Paullus WS, Pait TG, Rhoton AL, Jr: Microsurgical exposure of the petrous portion of the carotid artery. J Neurosurg 47:713, 1977
101. Petruk KC, West M, Mohr G et al: Nimodipine treatment in poor-grade aneurysm patients: results of a multicenter double-blind placebo-controlled trial. J Neurosurg 68:505, 1988
102. Pickard JD, Murray GD, Illingworth R et al: Effect of oral nimodipine on cerebral infarction and outcome after subarachnoid haemorrhage: British aneurysm nimodipine trial. Br Med J 298:636, 1989
103. Pinna G, Pasqualin A, Vivenza C et al: Rebleeding, ischaemia and hydrocephalus following anti-fibrinolytic treatment for ruptured cerebral aneurysms: a retrospective clinical study. Acta Neurochir (Wien) 93:77, 1988
104. Pool JL: Treatment of intracranial aneurysms during pregnancy. JAMA 192:209, 1965
105. Puca A, Spetzler RF, Zabramski JM: Hydrostatic dilatation of autologous vein grafts: technical note. Neurosurgery 26:1071, 1990
106. Robinson JL, Hall CS, Sedzimir CB: Arteriovenous malformations, aneurysms, and pregnancy. J Neurosurg 41:63, 1974
107. Ropper AH, Zervas NT: Outcome 1 year after SAH from cerebral aneurysm: management morbidity, mortality and functional status in 112 consecutive good-risk patients. J Neurosurg 60:909, 1984
108. Rosenorn J, Eskesen V, Schmidt K et al: The risk of rebleeding from ruptured intracranial aneurysms. J Neurosurg 67:329, 1987
109. Roski RA, Spetzler RF, Nulsen FE: Late complications of carotid ligation in the treatment of intracranial aneurysms. J Neurosurg 54:583, 1981
110. Sahs A, Perret GE, Locksley HB, Nichioka H: Intracranial Aneurysms and Subarachnoid Hemorrhage. JB Lippincott, Philadelphia, 1969.
111. Salazar JL: Surgical treatment of asymptomatic and incidental intracranial aneurysms. J Neurosurg 53:20, 1980
112. Samson DS, Hodosh RM, Clark WK: Surgical management of unruptured asymptomatic aneurysms. J Neurosurg 46:731, 1977
113. Samson DS, Hodosh RM, Reid WR et al: Risk of intracranial aneurysm surgery in the good grade patient: early versus late operation. Neurosurgery 5:422, 1979
114. Saveland H, Ljunggren B, Brandt L et al: Delayed ischemic deterioration in patients with early aneurysm operation and intravenous nimodipine. Neurosurgery 18:146, 1986
115. Sekhar LN, Schramm VL Jr, Jones NF et al: Operative exposure and management of the petrous and upper cervical internal carotid artery. Neurosurgery 19:967, 1986
116. Sekhar LN, Schramm VL, Jr, Jones NF: Subtemporal-preauricular intratemporal fossa approach to large lateral and posterior cranial base neoplasms. J Neurosurg 67:488, 1987
117. Selman WR, Spetzler RF: Therapeutics for focal cerebral ischemia. Neurosurgery 6:446, 1980
118. Selman WR, Spetzler RF, Anton AH et al: Management of prolonged therapeutc barbiturate coma. Surg Neurol 15:9, 1981
119. Selman WR, Spetzler RF, Roessmann UR et al: Barbiturate-induced coma therapy for focal cerebral ischemia: effect after temporary and permanent MCA occlusion. J Neurosurg 55:220, 1981
120. Selman WR, Spetzler RF, Roski RA et al: Barbiturate coma in focal cerebral ischemia: relationship of protection to timing of therapy. J Neurosurg 56:685, 1982
121. Selman WR, Spetzler RF, Zabramski JM: In-

duced barbiturate coma. p. 343. In Wilkins RH, Rengachary SS (eds): Neurosurgery. New York: McGraw-Hill, 1985
122. Silverberg GD, Reitz BA, Ream AK: Hypothermia and cardiac arrest in the treatment of giant aneurysms of the cerebral circulation and hemangioblastoma of the medulla. J Neurosurg 55:337, 1981
123. Sonntag VKH, Yuan RH, Stein BM: Giant intracranial aneurysms: a review of 13 cases. Surg Neurol 8:81, 1977
124. Spetzler RF, Daspit CP, Pappas CTE: The combined supra- and infratentorial approach for lesions of the petrous and clival region: experience with 46 cases. J Neurosurg 76:588, 1992
125. Spetzler RF, Fukushima T, Martin N et al: Petrous carotid-to-intradural carotid saphenous vein graft for intracavenous giant aneurysm, tumor, and occlusive cerebrovascular disease. J Neurosurg 73:496, 1990
126. Spetzler RF, Grahm TW: The far-lateral approach to the inferior clivus and the upper cervical region: technical note. Barrow Neurol Inst 6:35, 1990
127. Spetzler RF, Hadley MN, Rigamonti D et al: Aneurysms of the basilar artery treated with circulatory arrest, hypothermia and barbiturate cerebral protection. J Neurosurg 68:868, 1988
128. Spetzler RF, Lee KS: Reconstruction of the temporalis muscle for the pterional craniotomy. J Neurosurg 73:636, 1990
129. Spetzler RF, Schuster H, Roski RA: Elective extracranial-intracranial arterial bypass in the treatment of inoperable giant aneurysms of the internal carotid artery. J Neurosurg 53:22, 1980
130. Stornelli SA, French JD: Subarachnoid hemorrhage—factors in prognosis and management. J Neurosurg 21:769, 1964
131. Sundt TM, Jr, Piepgras DG: Surgical approach to giant intracranial aneurysms: operative experience with 80 cases. J Neurosurg 51:731, 1979
132. Sundt TM Jr, Piepgras DG, Fode NC et al: Giant intracranial aneurysms. Clin Neurosurg 37:116, 1991
133. Sundt TM III, Sundt TM, Jr: Review article: principles of preparation of vein bypass grafts to maximize patency. J Neurosurg 66:172, 1987
134. Suzuki J: Temporary occlusion of trunk arteries of the brain during surgery. In Suzuki J (ed): Treatment of Cerebral Infarction. Springer-Verlag, New York, 1987
135. Suzuki S, Kayama T, Sakurai Y et al: Subarachnoid hemorrhage of unknown cause. Neurosurgery 21:310, 1987
136. Suzuki J, Kuak R, Okudaira Y: The safe time limit of temporary clamping of cerebral arteries in the direct surgical treatment of intracranial aneurysm under moderate hypothermia. p. 326. In Suzuki J (ed): Cerebral Aneurysms. Neuron, Tokyo, 1979
137. Symon L: Management of giant intracranial aneurysms. Clin Neurosurg 36:21, 1990
138. Symon L, Momma F, Murota T: Assessment of reversible cerebral ischaemia in man: intraoperative monitoring of the somatosensory evoked response. Acta Neurochir, suppl. (Wien) 42:3, 1988
139. Symonds CP: Spontaneous subarachnoid hemorrhage. Q J Med 18:93, 1924
140. Tsutsumi K, Shiokawa Y, Sakai T et al: Venous infarction following the interhemispheric approach in patients with acute subarachnoid hemorrhage. J Neurosurg 74:715, 1991
141. Uihlein A, MacCarty SC, Michenfelder JD et al: Deep hypothermia and surgical treatment of intracranial aneurysms: a five-year survey. JAMA 195:639, 1966
142. van Crevel H, Habbema JDF, Braakman R: Decision analysis of the management of incidental intracranial saccular aneurysms. Neurology (NY) 36:1335, 1986
143. Vapalahti M, Ljunggren B, Saveland H et al: Early aneurysm operation and outcome in two remote Scandinavian populations. J Neurosurg 60:1160, 1984
144. Vermeulen M, Lindsay KW, Murray GD et al: Antifibrinolytic treatment in subarachnoid hemorrhage. N Engl J Med 311:432, 1984
145. Vermeulen M, Muizelaar JP: Do antifibrinolytic agents prevent rebleeding after rupture of a cerebral aneurysm?—a review. Clin Neurol Neurosurg 82:25, 1980
146. Versavel M, Witmer JP, Matricali B: Giant aneurysm arising from the anterior cerebral artery and causing an isolated homonymous hemianopsia. Neurosurgery 22:560, 1988
147. Voldby B, Enevoldsen EM, Jensen FT: Cerebrovascular reactivity in patients with ruptured intracranial aneurysms. J Neurosurg 62:59, 1985
148. Weil SM, van Loveren HR, Tomsick TA et al: Management of inoperable cerebral aneurysms by the navigational balloon technique. Neurosurgery 21:296, 1987
149. Weir B, Aronyk K: Management mortality and the timing of surgery for supratentorial aneurysms. J Neurosurg 54:146, 1981
150. Whittle IR, Dorsch NW, Besser M: Giant intracranial aneurysms: diagnosis, management, and outcome. Surg Neurol 21:218, 1984
151. Wiebers DO, Whisnant JP, Sundt TM, Jr et al: The significance of unruptured intracranial saccular aneurysms. J Neurosurg 66:23, 1987
152. Wyler AR, Kelly WA: Use of antibiotics with external ventriculostomies. J Neurosurg 37:185, 1972

# 47
# SURGICAL DECISIONS IN VASCULAR MALFORMATIONS OF THE BRAIN

Bennett M. Stein

## MANAGEMENT DECISIONS

In order to determine the best management for a given disease process, there are certain basic facts that must be considered. These include a knowledge of the natural history of the disease process and the risk benefits statistics of the various forms of treatment. The problem in dealing with vascular malformations is compounded because of our lack of understanding of the natural history of the various vascular malformations, including arteriovenous malformations (AVMs), telangiectasias, and cavernous and venous malformations.[7,12,13,16,22,28,29,32,37,47,50,66,73,88,92,95,96,129,138,139] Therefore the liability of a "do nothing" course of action may not be fully appreciated by the medical community. Lack of information occurs because of the uncommon occurrence of these lesions, the fact that they often become apparent in young people but have a clinical course that may span decades.

In dealing with a relatively large group of patients who have had AVMs over the past 15 years, we have been able to review only a handful of them who have had sequential arteriography while their AVMs remain unmolested.[120,121] This group was culled primarily from a Veterans Administration Hospital population. The longest interval of follow-up was only 10 years. This small group of patients stressed the variability of these lesions, in that three remained the same, three got bigger, and three got somewhat smaller but did not disappear. The number of case reports documenting spontaneous obliteration of AVMs are few and anecdotal.[122,136] Most articles that speak of the natural history of vascular malformations are retrospective in nature.[12,29,32,37,88,95,96,129] Many of them are tainted by selection of patients based on age, history, size and location of malformations or deal with patients who have undergone tentative therapy. Obviously, such reviews give only a glimmer of the true nature of these disorders. Unfortunately, they are the best that we have and currently must be relied upon to provide the judgment for successful management of these problems.

The basic methods of therapy include the following alone or in combination: (1) surgery, (2) embolization, and (3) radiation: always with the option of leaving the lesion alone if risk of therapy appears great. There are strong advocates for each of these methods. My attitude is toward an aggressive approach, since I regard these lesions as inherently dangerous, occurring in a young and productive age group in which hemorrhage can be severely incapacitating or fatal.

The risks of surgery and embolization are self-evident at the time these procedures are performed, whereas the risks of radiotherapy may not be apparent for a number of years after the full course of treatment is rendered.[125] Similarly, the benefit of surgery is evident shortly after the performance of the procedure, since complete proven obliteration of the lesion is the aim and, when accomplished, implies cure of the patient. In terms of modification of a seizure disorder, the beneficial results of surgery may be difficult to determine. When embolization is utilized, rarely producing occlusion of the AVM, the benefits are not immediately apparent. It may take years if not decades of follow-up to determine the impact of this treatment on the incidence of recidivous hemorrhages, seizure disorders, or progressive neurologic deficits. In the case of radiotherapy, conventional or focused, the situation is even more nebulous. The changes that occur in an AVM and the surrounding normal brain effected by radiotherapy span years. Therefore, in the case of risk the answers may not be known for a number of years following the institution of radiotherapy. Proponents of radiation therapy stress that there is a high rate of AVM obliteration at the 2-year interval after therapy.[11,43,53,62,63,85,124,125] For example with AVMs under 3 cm, the expected obliteration rate approximates 85 percent. It is not known how long after this period the deleterious effects of radiotherapy may be observed.

Other factors that influence the natural history and therapy of these malformations include age, sex, social habits, and anatomic factors such as the size and location of the malformation and prior history. Reviewing our cases and considering that 15 percent of hemorrhages are silent, we feel that a history of hemorrhage is not a major factor in determining the future risk of a malformation. Other neurosurgeons with large series of AVMs, however, disagree and have expressed the opinion that a malformation that has previously hemorrhaged is more dangerous than one that has not.[25,37,60,96,140] Recent reviews of the problem indicate that the incidence of recurrent hemorrhage is 2 percent per year, and when measured in a young person the risk becomes intolerable.

The premise, therefore, that short-term follow-up will determine the risk after a treatment that is short of complete obliteration is false. Treatment that results in occlusion of portions of the malformation or of the feeding vessels, scarification and thickening of the walls of the vessels, or partial removal of the malformation falls short of complete obliteration of the malformation and therefore must stand the test of time over a considerable follow-up period and cannot be equated with cure.

## SURGERY

### Risk Considerations

Each patient with an AVM must be evaluated on an individual basis in reference to age, previous history, and size and location of the AVM. Locational designations include superficial or deep, hemispheric, basal ganglion, brain stem, posterior fossa, or medial hemisphere.[15,19,23,26,35,55,67,99,111–113,117,120,144,146,147]

In reference to age, a younger person not only is exposed over a large period to the natural risk from hemorrhage than an older person, but also will exhibit a better tolerance to surgery.[27] Since these AVMs frequently become apparent in the second, third, and fourth decades, it is this group that should be the focus of our concern. In general, patients over the age of 55 years are treated in a less aggressive fashion than younger patients. Other medical conditions such as cardiac abnormalities, presence of aneurysms, and systemic disease have to be considered in establishing risk.

The size of an AVM is considered another major factor in the operability of these lesions. A small lesion located in an accessible region of the brain, for example, the frontal pole, is relatively easy to remove and requires no adjuvant therapy[114,118,122,123] (Fig. 47-1). Larger lesions that involve more than one lobe or the posterior fossa and deep areas of the brain may be inoperable because of their great volume.[115] This would appear to run contrary to the theory that all tissue within the confines of a malformation is non-

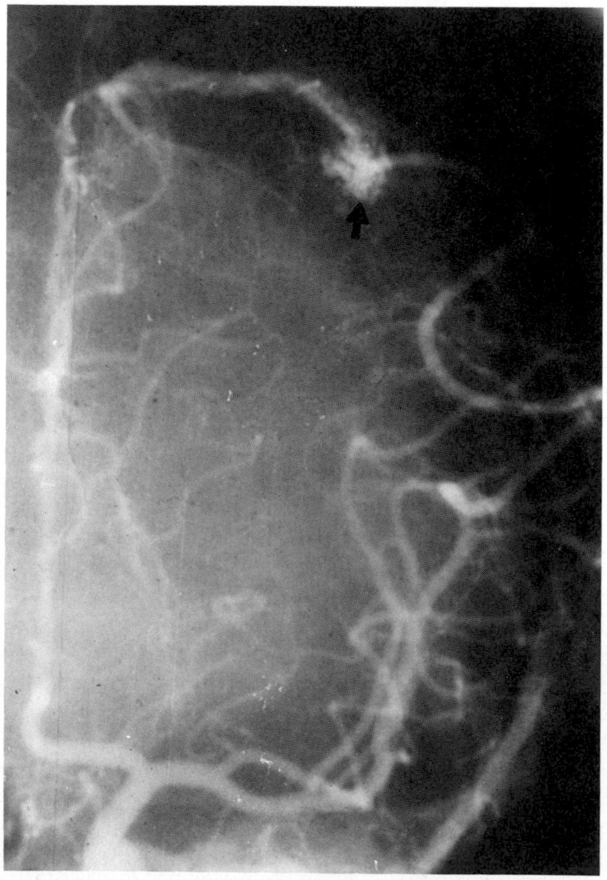

**Fig. 47-1.** Relatively small and circumscribed arteriovenous malformation (*arrow*) that presents no surgical challenge.

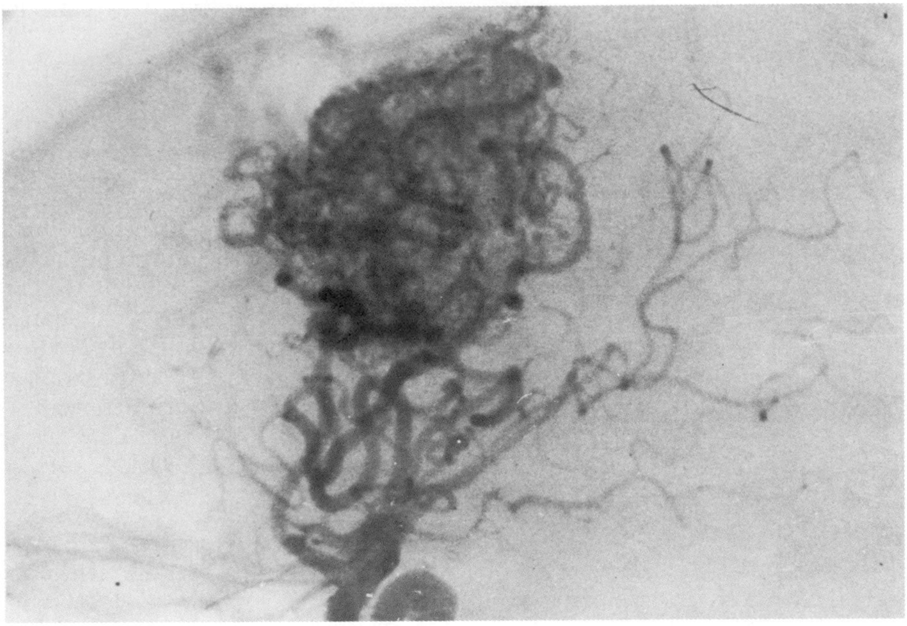

**Fig. 47-2.** Large arteriovenous malformation involving multiple lobes of eloquent brain. This is generally an inoperable lesion.

functional; not so: the technical difficulties encountered in attempting to remove massive malformations that span lobes of the brain are geometrically increased with size and will then preclude operative intervention (Fig. 47-2). The size and number of arterial to venous shunts must also be taken into account.[97,121,142]

The location of the malformation is one of the most important predictors of operability. Those lesions that are located superficially and in polar regions of the brain may be removed with relative ease.[1,24,25,110,118,140] Eloquent regions of the brain are often the site of AVMs. These may successfully be treated by experienced surgeons.[15,18,23,55,123,144] Malformations located in the diencephalon and basal ganglion are generally considered inoperable (Fig. 47-3), although there are rare reports of such lesions being removed.[35,113,131] Those malformations located in the brain stem—unless dissected by previous hemorrhage, reaching the surface of the brain stem, or lying in the cerebellopontine angle—are generally considered inoperable[23,111] (Fig. 47-4). Malformations located in obscure areas of the brain, such as the medial hemisphere, insula, roof of the third ventricle, and lateral ventricle, may be removed with some difficulty[112,117,146,147] (Fig. 47-5). Cerebellar lesions can be difficult to remove, since many of them are extensive with poorly defined borders. However, many can be removed and, considering the resiliency of cerebellar tissue, the long-term outlook can be excellent.[26,120]

The weight to be placed on the patient's history is debatable. We consider this factor the least important and approach AVMs regardless of history. Others have stated that a history of hemorrhage demands treatment, other factors being equal.

A detailed review of the arteriographic anatomy is

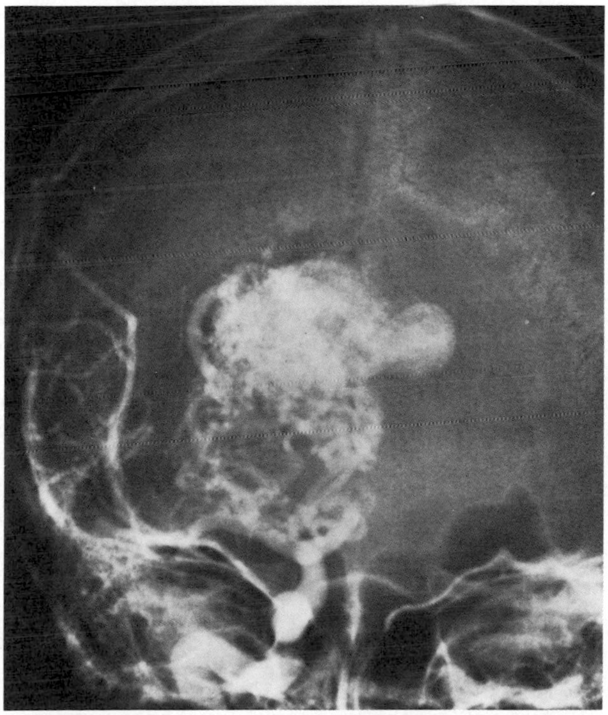

**Fig. 47-3.** Large arteriovenous malformation involving the diencephalic area. This is generally an untreatable problem.

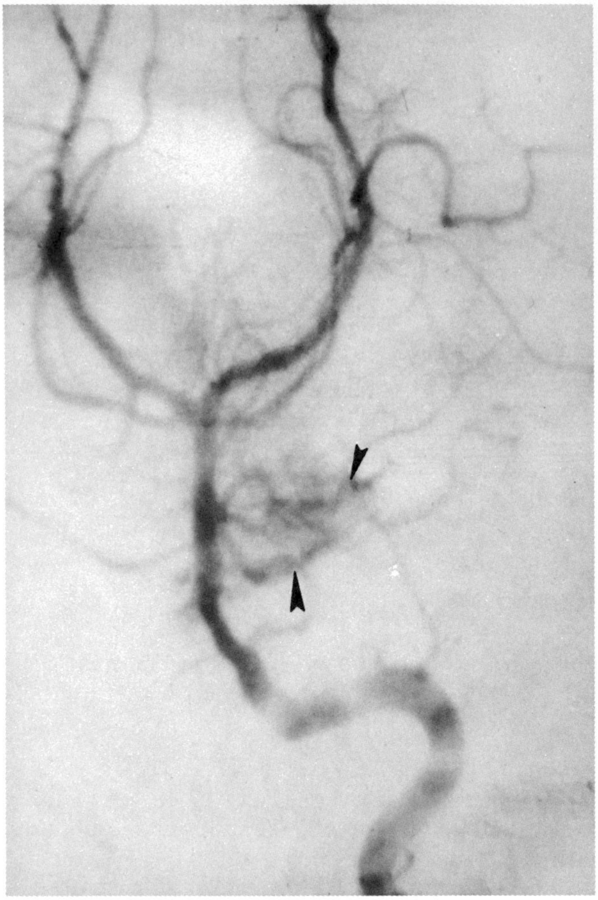

**Fig. 47-4.** Brain stem arteriovenous malformation (*arrows*) lying in pia of the brain stem. This lesion is potentially resectable.

invaluable in determining the exact course of the feeding arteries and draining veins, and this is further assisted by stereoscopic lateral angiograms. This materially aids the surgeon in the operative approach and design of the operation. The location of feeding arteries, the complexity and duplication of the draining venous system, and the discreteness of the malformation or definition of its borders are all factors that must be taken into consideration in a general fashion in determining the operability of a lesion. Magnetic resonance imaging (MRI) has been particularly useful in visualizing the configuration as well as relationship to border structures of an AVM.

In general, the determination of operability of a lesion must be made by a neurosurgeon and neurologist experienced in the management of a large number of AVM patients. The same principles expressed here have relevance to the other less common vascular malformations of the brain that have been previously categorized.

## Preoperative Adjuvant Procedures

We consider preoperative embolization, performed with a variety of substances, the most valuable adjuvant procedure to surgical resection of more complicated AVMs. This technique was introduced in a large number of cases by Luessenhop and Spence in 1960 and has since been refined by the neuroradiologist using transfemoral intravascular techniques to deliver the embolic material to the AVM.[10,20,45,133,143] The initial work of Luessenhop and Spence introduced the use of ceramic pellets, later changed to Silastic pellets, which could be introduced directly into the internal carotid circulation if this nourished the area of the AVM.[61] This early work has permitted a significantly long follow-up. The following conclusions were reached in recent articles, surveying over 200 patients:[59,60]

1. Recurrent hemorrhage rate and severity were not altered by embolization without obliteration of the AVM.
2. The safety of the procedure, both short term and long term, was verified.
3. Seizure disorder and progressive neurologic deterioration were often improved following successful embolization.
4. Surgery was facilitated by preoperative embolization.

Neuroradiologists using interventional techniques have continued to utilize particulate emboli in the preoperative treatment of these malformations.[60,108,133,143] The most popular emboli are made from Silastic, are spherical, and range in size from 1.5 mm to a maximum of 4 mm. The maximum is determined by the lumen of the largest catheter that can be directed via a transfemoral route to either the internal carotid or vertebral arteries. Other materials utilized are Gelfoam, isopropyl alcohol fragments, and liquids that polymerize to solids on contact with blood.

Liquid embolization has been carried out using small limited-leak balloon catheters, which are placed near the malformation.[20,51] The liquid that is injected through the catheter polymerizes and solidifies upon reaching the bloodstream. The most commonly used agent is bucrylate. The advantage of this technique is that it delivers the material directly to the AVM and fills the interstices. With refinement of intravascular catheters, it is possible to effectively deliver embolic material directly to the AVM. By this technique embolic material is placed into the AVM nidus with some overflow to the venous side, maximizing statis.[10,30,31,40,93,98,132,133,134] We have found that the placement of bucrylate into the AVM has prepared the patient best for surgical resection (Fig. 47-6).

We have found the greatest usefulness of embolization techniques as a preparation for surgery.[17,68,91,122,123,142] Embolization, in our estimation, reduces

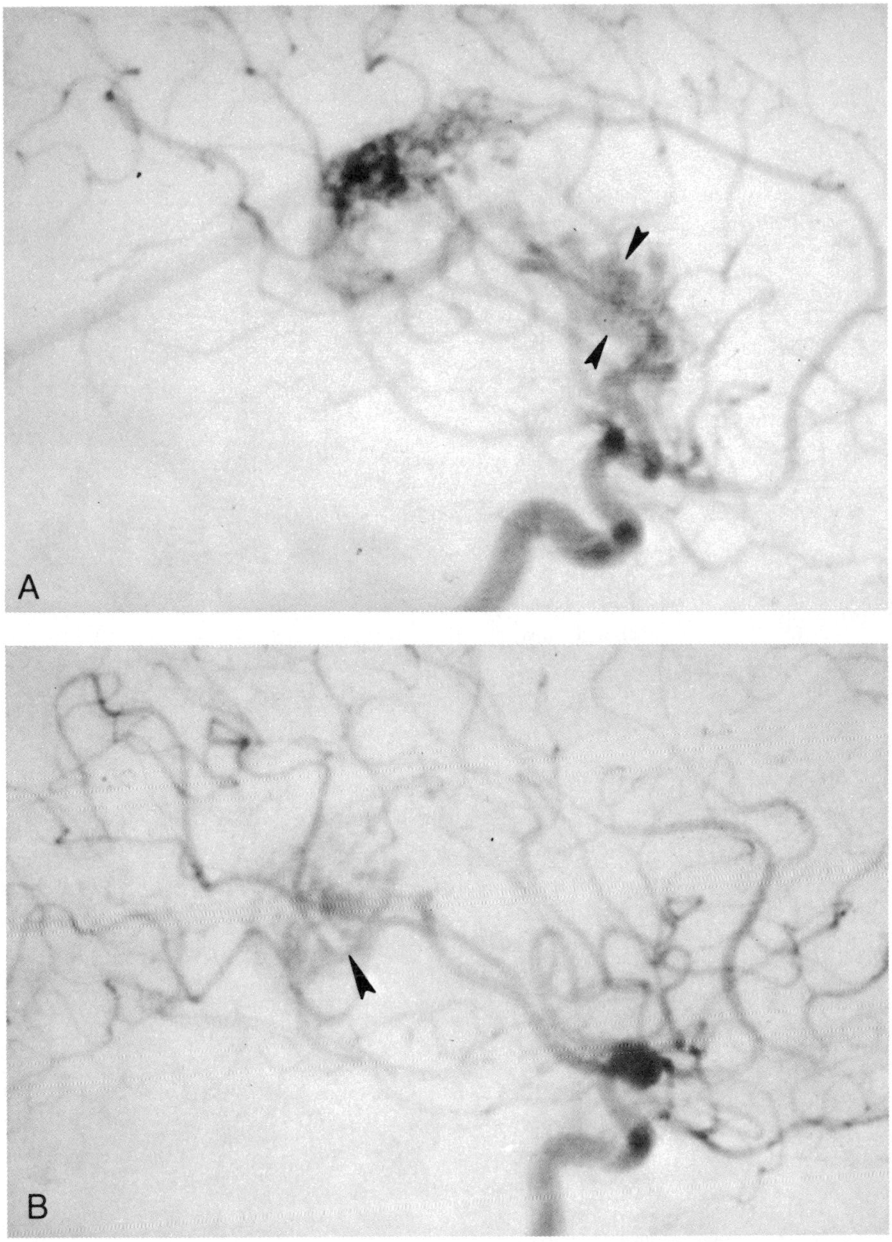

**Fig. 47-5.** (**A**) An arteriovenous malformation located within the anterior third ventricle (*small arrows*) following unsuccessful proton beam therapy. (**B**) Successful removal of the anterior third ventricular arteriovenous malformation. The second malformation (*large arrow*) was resected at a subsequent operation.

the size of the malformation and the blood flow and turgor within it, thereby facilitating the surgical procedure. Embolization may also eliminate deep feeding arteries that are relatively inaccessible or represent the final blood supply, an enigma to the surgeon working in the difficult margin around the malformation deep within the brain. Having already occluded arteries such as the lenticulostriate and branches of the posterior cerebral arteries allows the surgeon to approach this treacherous part of the operation with greater confidence (Fig. 47-7). Embolization also gradually reduces the shunt within the malformation, making the final removal of the shunt by surgery a less severe hemodynamic shock to the normal cerebral circulation. In order to be most effective in large AVMs, embolization may have to be carried out more than one time. This interruption of shunts in a gradual fashion addresses the issue of "perfusion pressure breakthrough."[116] This theory presumes that the sudden removal of a large artery to venous shunt throws

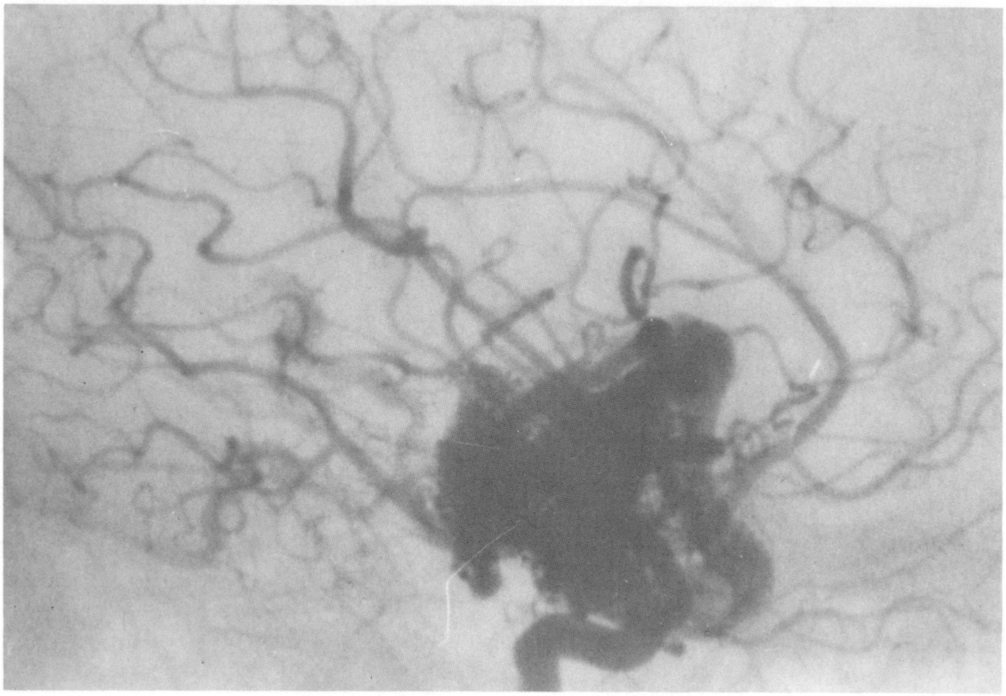

A

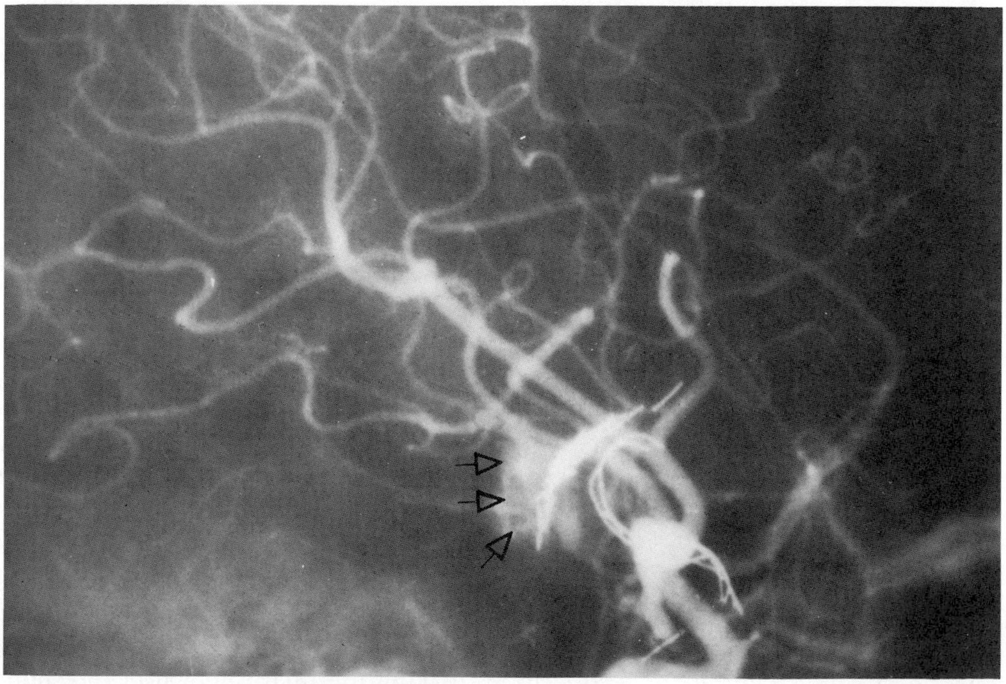

B

**Fig. 47-6.** (**A**) Lateral arteriogram showing a large temporal arteriovenous malformation. (**B**) Lateral angiogram of the same patient following successful endovascular embolization. The arteriovenous malformation has virtually disappeared. The contrast seen (*arrows*) is related to the endovascular material and does not represent residual arteriovenous malformation. The surgery was facilitated by this preoperative embolization.

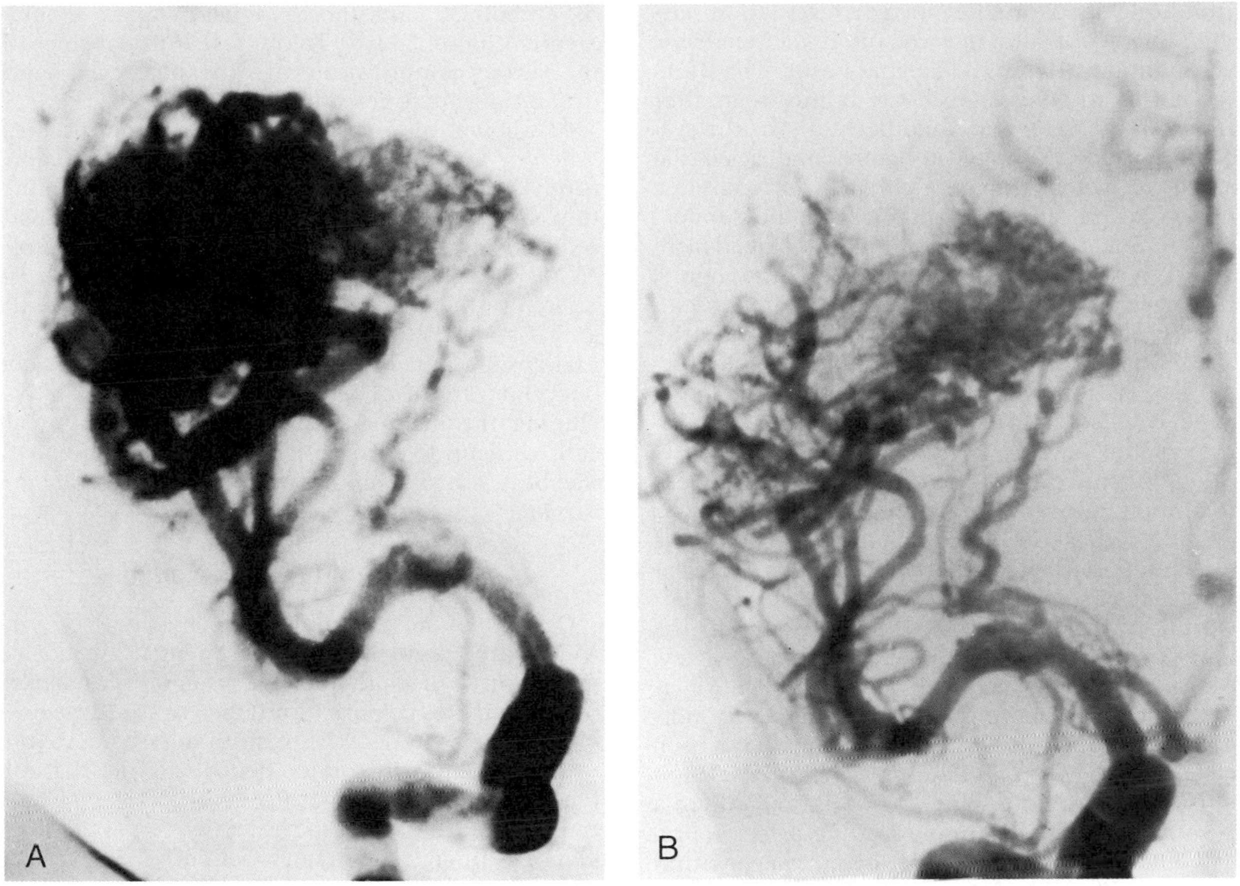


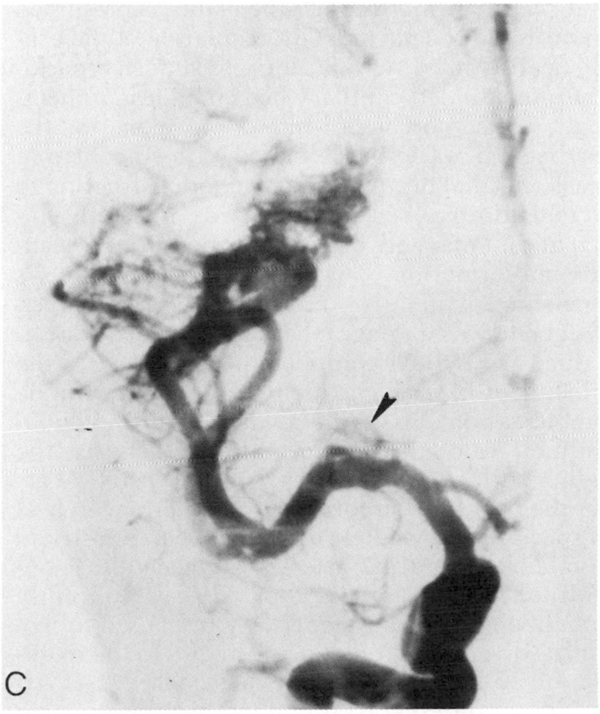


**Fig. 47-7.** (**A**) Large arteriovenous malformation of the frontotemporal region with deep and superficial arterial supply. (**B**) Elimination of much of the superficial blood supply to this malformation following embolization. (**C**) Elimination of the deep arterial supply to the malformation (*arrow*) by balloon-directed Silastic pellets.

an intolerable load on the normal circulation surrounding the AVM and may result in hemorrhage, edema, and infarction of the normal tissue. The situation is similar to congestive heart failure seen after removal of large artery to venous shunts in the systemic circulation. The suggested abnormalities in the major arteries nourishing an AVM with apparent loss of autoregulation or elastic qualities would support this theory. Successful embolization in a staged fashion permits a gradual reduction in these large shunts.

Complications from embolization are infrequent. When they occur, they are usually related to stray embolic material. A number of complications are recognized, for example, the material may traverse the fistula without being arrested and lodge in the capillary bed of the lung.[123] Fortunately, this is of little clinical significance, but when it occurs, the purpose of the embolization—obliteration of the fistula—is not served. If there is major venous occlusion, it is theoretically possible that the malformation could explode. In such cases, an apparently successful embolization may be followed within hours to days by the development of a parenchymal hematoma, in a few cases large enough to be fatal. This complication is rare.[56,59,133,134] Whether embolization causes hemorrhage is debatable, but three mechanisms have been suggested. First, the successful embolization is envisioned to result in acute temporary dilation, due to a rise in intraluminal pressure, in feeding arteries, presumably leading to their rupture; hemorrhage within hours would seem consistent with this explanation. Second, the shunting through the fistula is presumed to have altered the normal autoregulation of the otherwise healthy local vasculature, and sudden reperfusion into the dilated capillary bed could lead to hemorrhage or hemorrhagic infarction akin to the hemorrhagic diapedesis associated with embolism in otherwise normal brain.[51] Third, major obstruction to the venous drainage is incriminated.[1] Aberrant embolic material may lodge in arteries not directly feeding the malformation.[122] This complication, which is nothing short of an iatrogenic embolic stroke, is seen less frequently as angiographers have gained experience (Fig. 47-8). Such complications have led to the establishment of major guidelines for cases suitable for embolization. First, the feeding arteries should "mainline" into the malformation, such as the straighter surface branches of the middle cerebral artery or the posterior cerebral artery. Anterior cerebral and, especially, the acutely angulated lenticulostriate and thalamoperforating arteries are generally more difficult for reliable embolization. However, recently microballoon catheter systems have been used to successfully "divert" emboli at acute angles to the mainstream blood flow.[45,51,133,134] This has opened new vistas in the use of embolization, and even brain stem malformations may be embolized. Second, the flow of emboli to an AVM is favored by large diameters of the feeding arteries. The size ratio between the arteries to be embolized and those to be avoided should be greater than 4.5 : 1.[143] Taking all into consideration, the serious complication rate in experienced hands is in the range of 2 percent.

As shown by Luessenhop et al. and others,[10,17,30,45,59,134,142] embolization as a primary procedure is rarely successful in totally obliterating the malformation. Obviously, when the shunt becomes successfully reduced by a series of emboli, the "sink effect" of the AVM in drawing the pellets toward it decreases. Therefore there is a finite point when pellets will no longer go to the malformation and will enter the normal circulation. Theoretically, repeated injections of bucrylate afford a better opportunity of totally occluding the malformation; however, this is technically difficult to accomplish. Because of these factors, the best use of embolization is as an adjuvant to surgery.

## General Surgical Techniques

Operations on vascular malformations, especially AVMs, are complex procedures which are not commonly performed outside of large centers and are taxing not only to the patient but also to the surgeon. The immediate postoperative results may be devastating to the patient with major neurologic deficits, albeit temporary.[8,25,38,44,75,90,94,100,115,118,122,123,128,139,140] The initial impact, therefore, to the patient's psyche may be severe. Although the majority of patients have experienced the devastating effects of hemorrhage, there is a group of patients who live in peace with their AVMs, not realizing the potential hazard of their lesions. Even those patients who have experienced hemorrhage may have recovered fully and forgotten its devastating effects. Because many of these patients are intact neurologically and able to function in spite of their AVM at the time they consult the neurosurgeon, a discussion in depth about the implications of the malformation, the natural history, and the operative aims and risks should be carried out with the patient and his family prior to decision about treatment. The impact of the discussion is often disturbing to the patient, who is left in a quandary deciding what to do about a condition of which he knows little and fears even less, in the face of a dire prognostication by his physicians and the recommendation of a difficult and perhaps risky operation. This impact on the psyche has been noted to take its toll both before and after the operation, the latter in an anticlimactic state when the patient, fearing death or disablement, finds that he is intact and able to function.

Our team has elicited the help of a psychiatrist in interviewing patients prior to operative intervention and during the difficult postoperative period. In some of the patients psychological testing has been carried out prior to operation to determine their ability to withstand the stress and strains of decision making, the operation, and the postoperative convalescence.

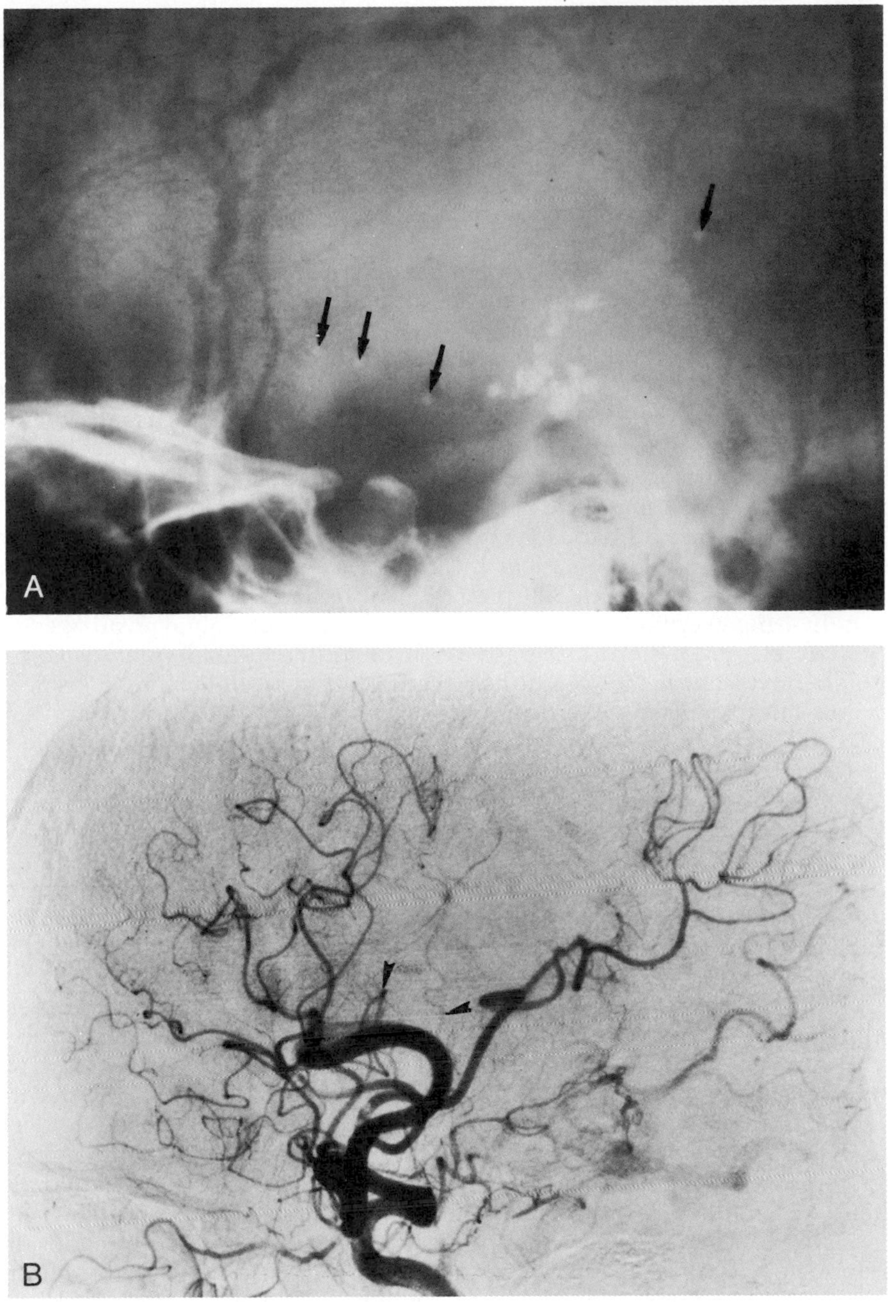


**Fig. 47-8.** (**A**) Aberrant emboli (*arrows*) during the course of successful reduction in an arteriovenous malformation. (**B**) These emboli block important branches of the middle cerebral artery (*arrows*). Although these aberrant emboli occluded major arteries, the neurologic deficit was short-lived.

Often it is beneficial to have the patients discuss their situation with other patients who have undergone surgical treatment of an AVM. For this purpose, there is a national support group composed of patients who are quite willing to discuss the situation with individuals teetering on the edge of what they consider the most important decision of their life. Frequently, there will be a patient who has already undergone operation for an AVM still in the hospital when a patient awaiting AVM surgery is admitted. It is extremely beneficial to have the preoperative patient discuss matters openly and freely with the patient who has already gone through the procedure in the hospital setting. Therefore a wide-ranging discussion should be carried out prior to the surgery, regarding all aspects of the disorder and the diagnostic and therapeutic modalities that are contemplated during the patient's hospitalization. I also encourage patients to take notes, develop questions, and review or seek second opinions. These points cannot be emphasized too greatly, for a patient who is well prepared for surgery, other therapeutic endeavors, and diagnostic procedures both pre- and postoperatively will be able to withstand and understand the operative procedure and get involved vigorously in any rehabilitation that may be required in the postoperative period. If the surgeon contemplates the possibility of residual postoperative defects that may require extensive rehabilitation therapy, the various effects of these defects should be explained in detail to the patient, discussing it in terms of the patients's lifestyle, career, and social activities. Our team includes the surgeon, neurologist, psychiatrist, and on occasion other patients in a setting conducive to thoughtful, unhurried, deliberate, and methodic reviews of the problem.

Following admission to the hospital, the patient is placed on Decadron (dexamethasone, Merck Sharp & Dohme) therapy, usually 4 mg every 6 h, antacids to cover the adverse gastric effects of steroid therapy, and an appropriate anticonvulsant if the patient has not already been on an anticonvulsant. We usually start patients on Dilantin therapy; should there be any hint of adverse reactions to this drug, we switch to phenobarbital. Appropriate loading doses must be given, since in many instances the patient is admitted to the hospital shortly prior to the contemplated operative procedure. One of the greatest concerns is for postoperative seizures, especially when operating on superficial supratentorial AVMs. If the patient cannot be loaded properly with Dilantin, then a boost of intravenous phenobarbital is given the morning of the surgery as part of the preparation. The usual dose is 120 mg given slowly intravenously. This can be repeated toward the end of the operation.

In most instances, the patients are not operated on in the acute throes of hemorrhage from an AVM.[99] Generally, we prefer to allow the hemorrhage to absorb and the patient to stabilize with decreased edema around the area of the hematoma cavity prior to operating and removing the AVM. In such cases, vigorous supportive measures and dehydrating agents are not needed, as most of these patients are in the middle decades, young and healthy, and have a normal cardiovascular system and cerebral circulation except for the dynamic changes associated with the AVM. The threat of recurrent hemorrhage is far less than seen in intracranial aneurysms, and therefore no special precautions are taken in these patients preoperatively to avert such recurrent hemorrhage.[95,96] Patients are allowed to carry out normal routine daily activities and are only sedated the night before and the morning of the operation.

In the operating room, the patient is placed on the operating table equipped with a heating blanket.[118] This prevents heat loss and adverse cooling of the patient during the long operative procedure. The anesthesia team sets up an intravenous catheter system and arterial line, usually in the radial artery, to monitor the blood pressure during induction. As with intracranial aneurysms, care must be taken that hypertensive levels of blood pressure are not developed during the induction of the patient. If the operation is to be in the sitting or semisitting position, then a central venous catheter is placed if feasible. This can be done after the patient is asleep in order to avoid the discomfort of such a procedure. This catheter may be used to measure the central venous pressure as well as aspirate any air that may enter the venous system. Following the placement of the arterial line, the patient is then induced, usually by intravenous anesthesia. The neuroanesthesia team of our service prefers the volatile anesthetic agent Forane or Fluothane, with the induction being carried out by thiopental sodium and a muscle relaxant.

After the intubation of the patient and establishment of anesthesia, the patient is turned on the side and a special spinal drainage catheter is inserted through the lumbar spine.[101] This utilizes a 14-gauge needle and an indwelling 5 French catheter. This is a ureteral type of catheter with a blunt tip and side holes. Its large size and multiple holes prevents any blockage of this catheter system during the positioning of the patient and the performance of the operation. Once an appropriate length of catheter has been placed into the spinal canal, the flow is checked and the catheter is stabilized by tape and brought out to the anesthesiologist. The patient is then positioned on the operating table. The various positions, depending upon the location and size of the malformation, will be discussed in detail. Generalities of the positioning include generous padding of the patient, especially over bony areas, again because of the length of the operation; rigid fixation of the head is carried out with a pin vise type of head-holder. The surface of the malformation should be placed as closely as possible to the horizontal or parallel to the floor. Also, the malformation should be as high as feasible above heart level in order to promote venous drainage and reduce the turgor within the malformation. In most patients, male and female, we remove only enough hair to perform a generous craniotomy around the malformation. For patients who are in the sitting position, a Doppler recorder is applied over the sternal region. Another heating blanket is then placed over the patient to ensure normothermia during the long operative procedure.

Special positions are used for malformations that are located in somewhat obscure areas.[117] For those malformations located high over the convexity or in the medial hemispheral region a sitting- or semisitting-slouch position is utilized so that the surgeon may work directly toward the malformation (Fig. 47-9). All the interhemispheric malformations may be approached by some version of the sitting position.

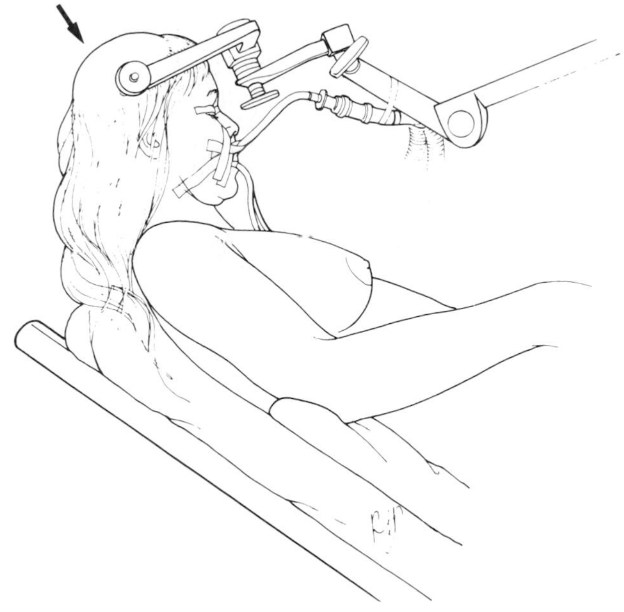

**Fig. 47-9.** Drawing of the sitting-slouch position used in the interhemispheric approach to medial hemisphere and deep midline arteriovenous malformations.

For those medially placed malformations that are in the region of the uncus or hippocampus, a subtemporal exposure or a sylvian fissure exposure may be utilized. In this case the patient is generally placed supine with the head extended in an attempt to place the malformation in the best perspective for the surgeon and as high as possible above the heart. The lateral or prone position is used for convexity, parietal, or occipital lesions. Those on the under surface or tentorial surface of the occipital lobe are approached best with the patient in a prone position. For posterior fossa operations the patient may be in either the sitting, lateral, or prone position.

Our anesthesia group has been monitoring cerebral blood flow by xenon and transcranial Doppler. This has been particularly useful in alerting us to potential serious circulatory changes during AVM removal.[9,58,79,82,83,87,104,148] The choice of an anesthetic agent is left up to the anesthesiologist; however, we prefer that the anesthesia agenda recognize the need for hypotension, often for prolonged periods, during the operative procedure. As with anesthetic agents, the choice of hypotensive drugs is left to the anesthesiologist. Prolonged periods of blood pressure reduction to 80 to 85 mmHg systolic may be required, and the anesthesiologist is cautioned to use agents which can be given for such prolonged periods of time. One must recognize that sustained administration of sodium nitroprusside may lead to cyanide buildup in the blood and even to poisoning in the rare case. Rarely is it necessary to lower blood pressure below 80 mmHg systolic for any prolonged period of time; however, short periods of greater hypotension under one-half hour, may be necessary to control deep bleeding from thin-walled vessels, especially in the periventricular area, to which so many AVMs extend. In this circumstance, blood pressure should be maintained between 70 and 80 mmHg systolic until the dissection is completed.

Brain relaxation is essential and this is accomplished by spinal drainage of cerebrospinal fluid, attention to the blood gases, especially the $P_{CO_2}$ level, which should be kept between 25 and 30 torr by proper ventilatory adjustments. Rarely should it be necessary to use large doses of dehydrating agents. If the brain is tight and requires vigorous measures for relaxation, the operation should be terminated as early as possible and recognition given to the fact that intracranial pressure is elevated and the patient further evaluated postoperatively, with reoperation carried out when feasible.

The following are some general principles applied to the removal of AVMs, especially those located in relatively accessible areas such as the convexities or polar regions of the cerebral hemispheres. The craniotomy should be generous and the dura opened widely so that the surface of the brain may be inspected. Landmarks are identified and correlated with angiogram analysis. Generally, the venous system on the surface of the brain provides the best road map as to the position of the AVM. Normal arteries course in and out in a tortuous fashion from gyri to sulci (Fig. 47-10). In, dealing with AVMs where the feeding arteries are enlarged and even more tortuous, the arteries may be difficult to identify at the margin of the malformation; however, the veins generally remain on the surface and can be correlated with the angiogram. In my estimation, the use of steroscopic angiograms evaluated in the operating room is invaluable in determining the exact configuration of the malformation. Although the malformation appears to reach the surface as seen in computed tomography (CT) scans and angiograms, in fact, the major portion of the malformation often lies just subcortical and the cortical appearance may not reflect the extent of the malformation under the surface (Fig. 47-11). It is important in such cases to violate as little of the cortex as possible, rather making a linear incision, removing a small amount of brain, and relying upon retraction of the relaxed brain to visualize the deeper portions of the malformation. Again, evaluation of the angiogram, MRI, and CT scan will give the surgeon a good indication as to what to expect.

In the initial phase of the operation, major superficial feeding arteries are sought; the large feeding arteries hidden in sulci may be especially difficult to visualize. It is important to anticipate how deep they are from the surface so that the sulci may be opened and the artery identified and sectioned. Cautery is used for the smaller arteries; cautery plus metallic clipping is used for the larger arteries as they are in-

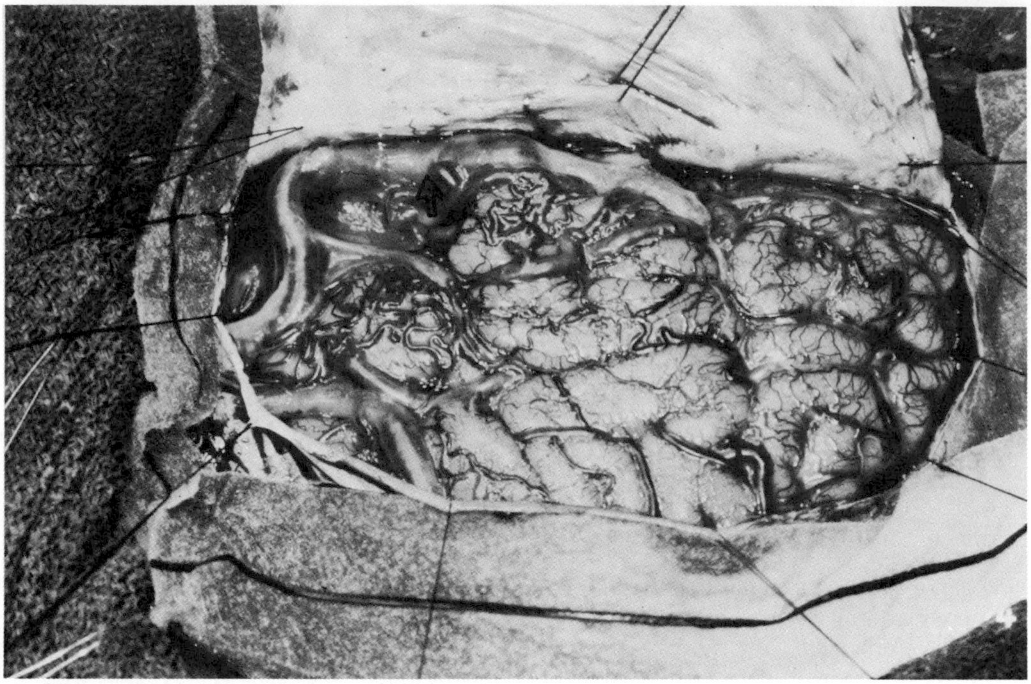

**Fig. 47-10.** Operative photograph showing a large cortical vein (*arrow*) visible as a definitive landmark guiding the surgeon in resection of an arteriovenous malformation.

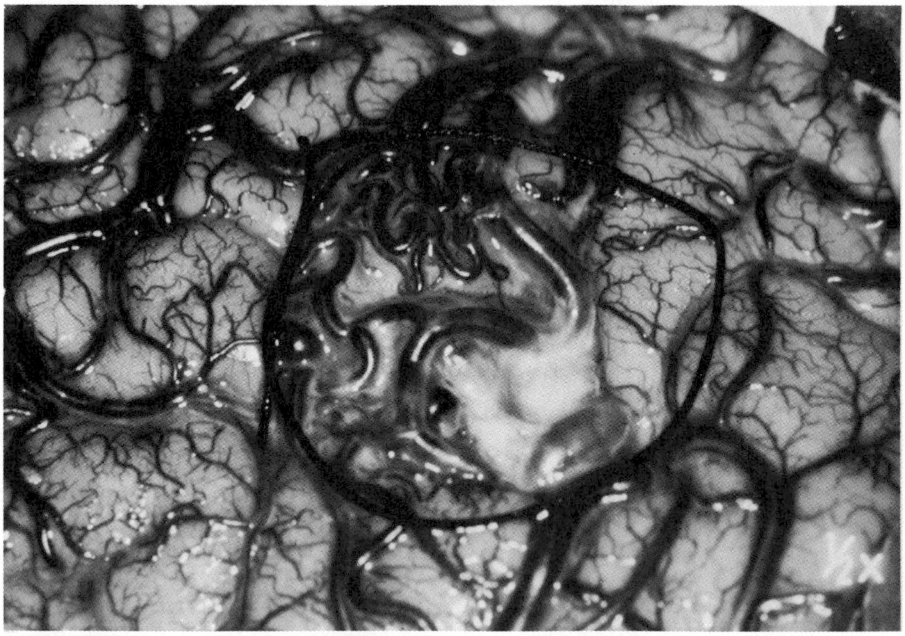

**Fig. 47-11.** Operative photograph with a silk suture designating the major portion of the malformation underlying the cortex and not visible on the cortex.

terrupted. By the use of bipolar cautery and microdissection under the microscope, the margin of the malformation as it approaches the surface of the brain is gradually circumscribed, with interruption of as many of the feeding arteries as possible. One large draining vein, either deep or superficial, particularly the largest vein, should be left until the final stage of the operation. To interrupt such a large draining system early will cause undue turgor within the malformation and greatly complicate the operative removal of these already treacherous lesions (Fig. 47-12).

Generally, there is a well-defined gliotic plane in which it is easy to dissect between the malformation and the normal brain. Tortuous coils of large corkscrew sinusoids may bulge into this interface and should be circumvented. When some of the major supply to the malformation has been secured, it is possible to gently coagulate, shrink back, and toughen these large venous channels on the periphery of the malformation, further simplifying the removal. However, it is generally impossible to shrink back major portions of the malformation in order to decompress it and attain greater working space between the malformation and the normal brain. This space is narrow and provided by removal of the gliotic area around the malformation and gentle retraction on the relaxed

**Fig. 47-12.** Drawings demonstrating the basic technique in the removal of an arteriovenous malformation. (**A**) Circumscription of the initial incision. (**B**) Securing of the deep arterial supply. (**C**) Final interruption of the major draining vein.

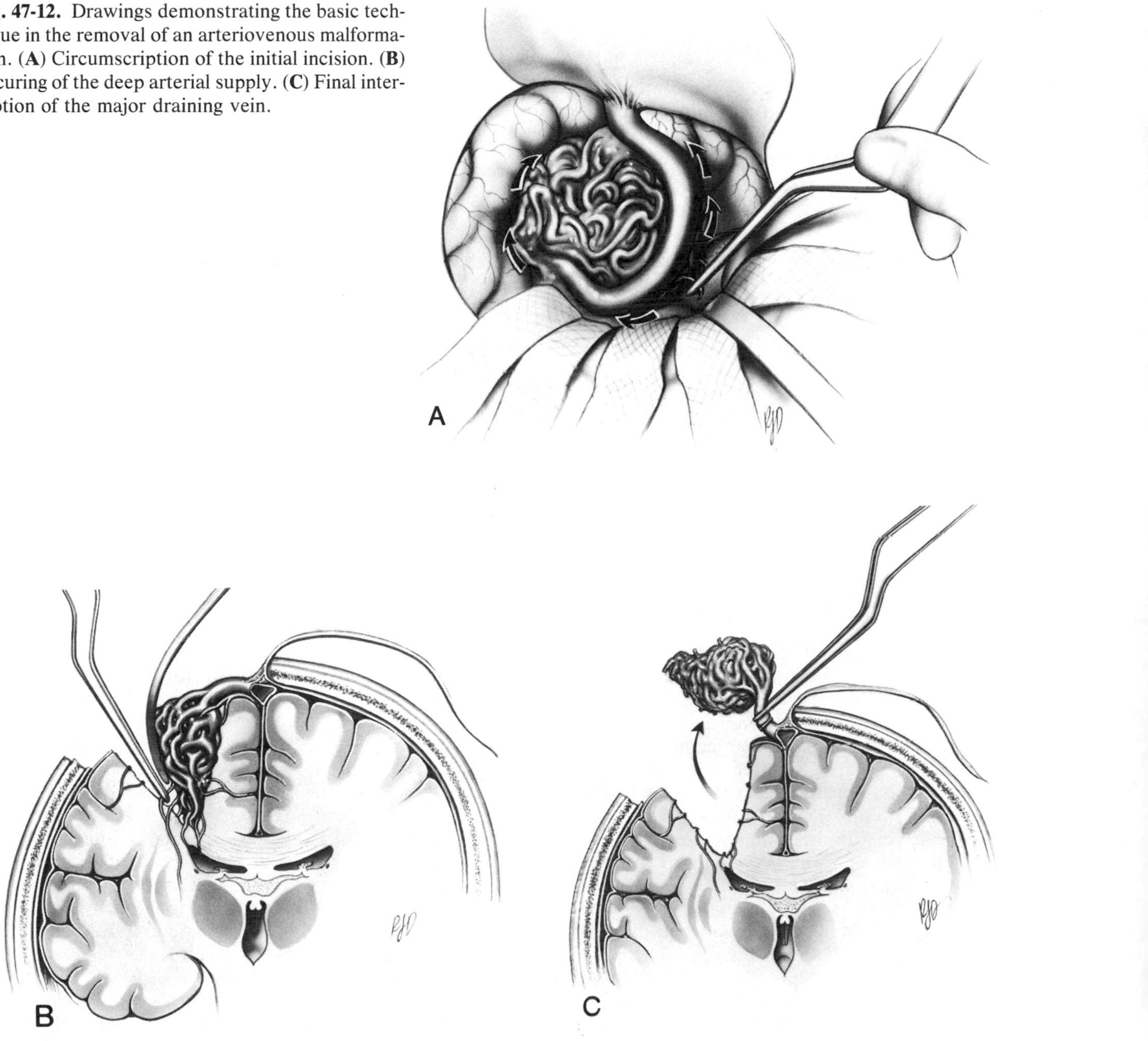

brain as the surgeon works deeper and deeper around the periphery of the malformation. Most of the large feeding arteries terminate in the malformation and may be interrupted at its margin. Others, enlarged and abnormally tortuous, may pass close by the malformation while giving large branches to the malformation. These primary arteries should not be interrupted; rather, their branches should be interrupted as the dissection is carried out. This type of arrangement may be anticipated from close scrutiny of the stereoscopic angiograms. In many cases, it may be necessary to dissect an artery in transit off the surface of a malformation. This requires microscopic dissection and exact control of the feeding vessels, with care being taken not to allow cautery to injure the primary vessel in transit.

Gradually, the dissected margin around the malformation is developed deeper and deeper as the surgeon works toward the deep apex of the malformation. In the vast majority of cases this apex will be found at the ependymal surface of the ventricle. Often there are secondary or primary draining veins at this apex that drain into the ependymal venous system. There may be arteries from the choroid plexus or anomalous periventricular arteries that enter deep portions of the malformation. In the white matter surrounding the malformation at its deeper extent are numerous small, thin-walled arteries carrying blood under high flow. These appear to be aberrant in the white matter and are extremely difficult to control by cautery or clipping because of the diaphanous nature of their walls and the cooling effect of the rapid blood flow on the cautery. These must be treated with great respect and their control is often assisted by hypotensive anesthesia. It is in this area, and not the surface, that the hypotension becomes invaluable. Similarly, the ependymal veins draining the malformation are also treacherous and must be secured, preventing massive hemorrhage into the ventricle and dispersion of blood throughout the cerebrospinal fluid with potential for hydrocephalus or vasospasm. When the choroid plexus supplies deeper portions of the malformation, the surgeon may find it extremely difficult to analyze and secure this blood supply. It appears to come from many different directions because of dual supply from the anterior and posterior choroidal arteries, which enter the choroid plexus in opposing directions. In many instances, it may be necessary to resect large portions of the choroid plexus that may be related to the deep portion of the malformation.

Preoperative embolization can be extremely useful in occluding some of the deep arterial supply to apex portions of the malformation. This materially assists the surgeon as this treacherous region deep in the brain along the narrow plane between the malformation and the normal brain is approached. When the major arterial supply has already been occluded by embolization, the task of removing the final segment of the malformation is made easier, although not simple. It should be restated that a primary large draining venous system should be left intact until every arterial feeder to the malformation has been secured. It also goes without saying that it is virtually impossible to remove larger malformations piecemeal; however, some of the small malformations measuring under 1 cm may be coagulated and removed piecemeal.

Following the successful resection of the malformation, hemostasis is tested, and residual fragments are searched for by allowing the blood pressure to come back to normotensive levels before hemostatic agents are placed around the area of resection and the wound closed. In some instances, elevation of the blood pressure from previously hypotensive levels to normotensive levels will lead to the disclosure of residual malformation in the periphery of an otherwise clean resection. Residual portions are identified by development of "vascular blisters," red veins in the white matter or the surface of the brain. Resection of this fragments must be accomplished; otherwise postoperative hemorrhage or other problems from residual malformation will plague the surgeon in the postoperative period. I prefer metallic clips only on large feeding arteries and draining veins and rely primarily on cautery. This leaves a cleaner wound that is easier to analyze by CT scan and postoperative angiography. Nothing specific is done with the cavity left by the removal of small or large AVMs. Any opening into the ventricular system should be covered as well as possible, usually with a sheet of Gelfoam, to prevent blood from mixing directly with the cerebrospinal fluid of the ventricle. The dura is closed and the bone flap and the rest of the would closed in the standard fashion. The patient is extubated and remains in a position similar to the one maintained during the operative procedure. This minimizes elevation of the intracranial venous pressure in the postoperative period and thereby reduces the risk of postoperative hemorrhage. The patient is monitored closely with intra-arterial blood pressure recording in the intensive care unit. In normotensive patients, we keep the systolic pressure below 120 mmHg, primarily through the use of beta blocking agents. To attain lower pressures in an awake young patient is near-impossible for a prolonged period.

The two greatest dangers in the postoperative period are hemorrhage and seizures. I have seen the latter occur as soon after the operative procedure as when the patient is being moved from the operating table to the stretcher. Postoperative clots are avoided or minimized by elevation of the head, maintenance of normotension, and minimization of Valsalva maneuvers or other maneuvers that will raise venous pressure. Some patients become extremely restless in the postoperative period, straining at restraints or attempting to dislodge their support systems. In such cases, it may be necessary to provide sedation, such as intravenous Valium, titrated to the patient's need. If there is any hint of something amiss, such as a patient who has wakened from the surgery relatively intact and subsequently deteriorates, a CT scan should be carried out immediately, searching for evidence of intracranial bleeding. I have found that the most likely time for a postoperative hemorrhage is within the first 12 to 24 hours. Delayed hemorrhaging after this period is extremely uncommon. If a postoperative clot is found, then the patient must be returned to the operating room and as much of the clot removed as possible. It may be extremely difficult to identify the bleeding source; however, residual malformation must be suspected in these cases. Often the surgeon has intuition, recalling an area that looked suspicious at the time of closure, but which was not pursued because of fatigue after a long operative procedure. It is here that one learns the lesson that inspection and evaluation of the wound at normotensive levels is as important as the time spent during removal of the AVM. It may be impossible to remove all of the clot in the second operation and perhaps unwise to remove the margin of the clot except in the areas that are under suspicion. The time necessary for postoperative arteriography is better spent operating on the patient, reducing the intracranial pressure by removing as much clot as possible and searching for residual portions of the malformation at the site of the bleeding point.

Postoperative seizures may be prevented in most cases by the appropriate use of anesthetic and anticonvulsant drugs. When Ethrane was used, it appeared to have an epileptogenic effect on those patients who were already sensitive. Some seizures are probably induced by changes in the cortical veins adjacent to the malformation. These changes are stasis, propagation of cortical vein thrombosis, and other dynamic changes that occur in blood flow within these important veins once the shunt has been removed. If the patient is properly loaded with anticonvulsants prior to surgery and given a boost of phenobarbital at the commencement and termination of the operation, then the incidence of postoperative seizures is markedly reduced. If the patient has a history of seizures, it is prudent to provide dual anticonvulsant coverage in the immediate intra- and postoperative periods. If the initial 12- to 24-hour postoperative period passes uneventfully, then the patient is mobilized as rapidly as possible.

Any neurologic deficits are treated as soon as applicable by intensive physiotherapy. On many occasions lesions that involve the sensory cortex of the parietal lobe will lead to severe paralysis because the patient has no stereognostic perception pertaining to these extremities. It is amazing how these patients may thus remain totally "paralyzed" for a week or 10 days and suddenly begin movement as their concept of the motor engram becomes viable again.

Postoperative arteriography is carried out in all cases. This is usually done in the week following operation. We have not done yearly or later arteriography and have had no cases of rebleeding when the immediate postoperative angiogram is negative. If a residual is seen it should be removed immediately.

A word should be said about postoperative deficits and their treatment. The surgeon will generally know whether the operation has gone well and whether the deficit will be a temporary one, perhaps lasting weeks, or whether the deficit is attributable to an intraoperative disaster and will be of a permanent nature. In any event the psychological impact of severe deficits, whether they are temporary or permanent, is unnerving to patients, even though they were coached about this prior to the operative procedure. Therefore encouragement and the early institution of vigorous rehabilitation are absolutely essential to these patients. Most of them are young and will work eagerly with a well-motivated therapist. Many of these deficits, especially the temporary ones, may be severe, with hemiplegia, hemisensory deficits, and other neurologic deficits of significant nature, depending upon the locus of the lesion. Because of the striking dynamic changes that occur in the cerebrovascular system following the resection of complicated AVMs, one may anticipate a high incidence of these temporary neurologic deficits postoperatively. In spite of the frequent occurrence of such deficits, there is marked improvement in almost all cases within days to weeks. These events suggest that the vascular changes responsible for these postoperative deficits are not on the basis of arterial occlusion with ischemic infarction but, rather, on the basis of venous stasis or infarction and brain edema, all reversible phenomena.

With removal of the AVM-associated shunts, there is decreased flow in the venous system with stasis and thrombosis. In addition, the vascular dynamics of not only the venous but arterial system lead to profound changes in intravascular pressure and flow resulting in brain edema, which is frequently observed on postoperative CT scans. Another consideration is arterial collateralization, which occurs rapidly in these young patients. The removal of large shunts and this collateral phenomenon provide a lush blood supply to the brain. It is presumed that these changes are wholly reversible and responsible for a rather unique course of events following the obliteration of an AVM. On the other hand, visual field defects that are complete postoperatively may or may not recover fully or even to a partial degree.[67] It is very difficult to predict the course of these deficits, since the visual system is so intimately involved with many of the malformations, including those that permeate the parietal area, as well as those located directly in or adjacent to the calcarine sulcus. Deficits related to cranial nerve or brain stem involvement by an AVM of the posterior focca may take much longer to resolve or may never resolve. Resolution is often predicated on the condition of these cranial nerves prior to the operative procedure. Severe cerebellar deficits postoperatively will almost always resolve, depending upon the extent of the involvement of the cerebellar structures, especially the deep nuclei.

## Vascular Changes Related to Obliteration of the Arteriovenous Malformation

It is a common observation that arteries at a distance from the malformation fill better immediately after the occlusion of the shunt, confirming some of the tenets of the theory of cerebral steal. However, less desirable effects also can occur, including acute cerebral edema, venous congestion, and, occasionally, frank hemorrhage. Using pulsed echo Doppler flowmeters and electromagnetic flow measurement with minature probes, Nornes et al.[82] studied the local hemodynamics of AVMs in 16 operated patients. A wide variation was found in the calculated flow in individual arteries, from as little as 3 ml/min to as much as 550 ml/min. The pressure of the arteries at their entrance into the AVM fistula was much reduced (40 to 77 mmHg) compared with systemic pressure, but on temporary occlusion an instant pressure rise to 55 to 95 mmHg occurred. On the venous side, the pressure fell to zero. The pressure drop along arteries leading to the fistula was greatest for the longer feeding arteries. These arteries also shared greater flow velocities and were of larger diameter. The cerebral perfusion pressure was estimated to be lowest in areas fed by these longer, more dilated arteries, whose final output was into the AVM fistula; these same arterial beds experienced the greatest increase in cerebral perfusion pressure after shunt occlusion and the highest incidence of postocclusion vasogenic edema. Presumably, these same arterial beds are more susceptible to "normal perfusion pressure breakthrough."[116] Very short feeding arteries did not show these effects.

A study of progressive postocclusive changes in the arterial networks has proved most instructive. Some feeding arteries undergo rapid reduction in size, but many take weeks to return to normal caliber. These slowly resolving changes suggest defective autoregulation not only within the malformations, but also in the large feeding arteries. This phenomenon may play a role in the perfusion pressure breakthrough theory and in the production of neurologic deficits in the post-treatment phase. In support of defective autoregulation are not only postobliteration ectasias in the feeding arteries, but the work of Nornes et al.[82,83] and others[4,6,9,33,41,76,97,104] who demonstrated many of the hemodynamic changes normally associated with autoregulation but lacking in AVMs. Dynamic studies in our laboratory have demonstrated a defective contractile response of large AVM nutrient arteries.[80] Young et al.,[148] recording blood flow during the removal of AVMs, have demonstrated a marked increase in blood flow, hyperemia, and presumed "congestion" of the brain around the AVM after removal. They have also confirmed the changes in intra-arterial and intravenous pressure that occur with AVM removal.[148] One of our cases is instructive (Fig. 47-13).

### *Case Study*

The patient was a 32-year-old right-handed man. He had a single focal motor seizure progressing to a grand mal convulsion initially involving the right side of the body, hand, arm, and face approximately 5 weeks prior to admission. Evaluation including a CT scan and angiogram demonstrated a left parietal AVM (Fig. 47-13A) and a proximal middle cerebral aneurysm (Fig. 47-13B). There was no evidence of hemorrhage. On 30 April 1984 total excision of the AVM without embolization was carried out (Fig. 47-13C). The major feeding artery was a middle cerebral branch that was markedly enlarged and went directly to the AVM. Postoperatively, the patient had no neurologic deficits and was discharged from the hospital 1 week after the surgery.

The patient was readmitted to the hospital on 1 June 1984, and, without a preliminary angiogram but with normal neurologic examination, the left middle cerebral artery aneurysm was uneventfully clipped. Hypotension to 80 mmHg systolic was used for 10 minutes, during the clip application. There was no evidence of cerebral vasospasm or evidence that this aneurysm had previously hemorrhaged. The patient was slow to awake from the operation, and it was noted that he was paretic on the right side. The arm, in fact, was flaccid and moved only to painful stimulation. He was not speaking and did not understand commands. A cerebral angiogram was immediately carried out. This showed marked vascular changes in the region of the AVM resection without residual AVM (Fig. 47-13D). The arteries proximal to the AVM showed ectasias and pooling of dye, indicating stasis of the contrast media and presumably blood in these vessels. The patient's blood pressure during this postoperative period fluctuated between 120 and 130 mmHg. Approximately 2 hours after the angiogram, he had a major seizure and was given appropriate intravenous anticonvulsants. He was also volume-expanded and his blood pressure was maintained at a hypertensive level of 140 to 150 mmHg systolic with a dopamine infusion: he had no further seizures. Within 24 hours after the operative procedure, he could squeeze the right hand weakly to command, but did not respond to other verbal commands, suggesting an improving dysphasia. The right lower extremity was markedly improved. Approximately 36 hours after the operation the patient was responding to verbal commands and the strength in the right arm was 80 percent normal. The dopamine drip was gradually reduced and the patient subsequently made a gradual improvement to full recovery.

Our theory is that ectatic changes persisted unexpectedly in the large feeding artery to the malforma-

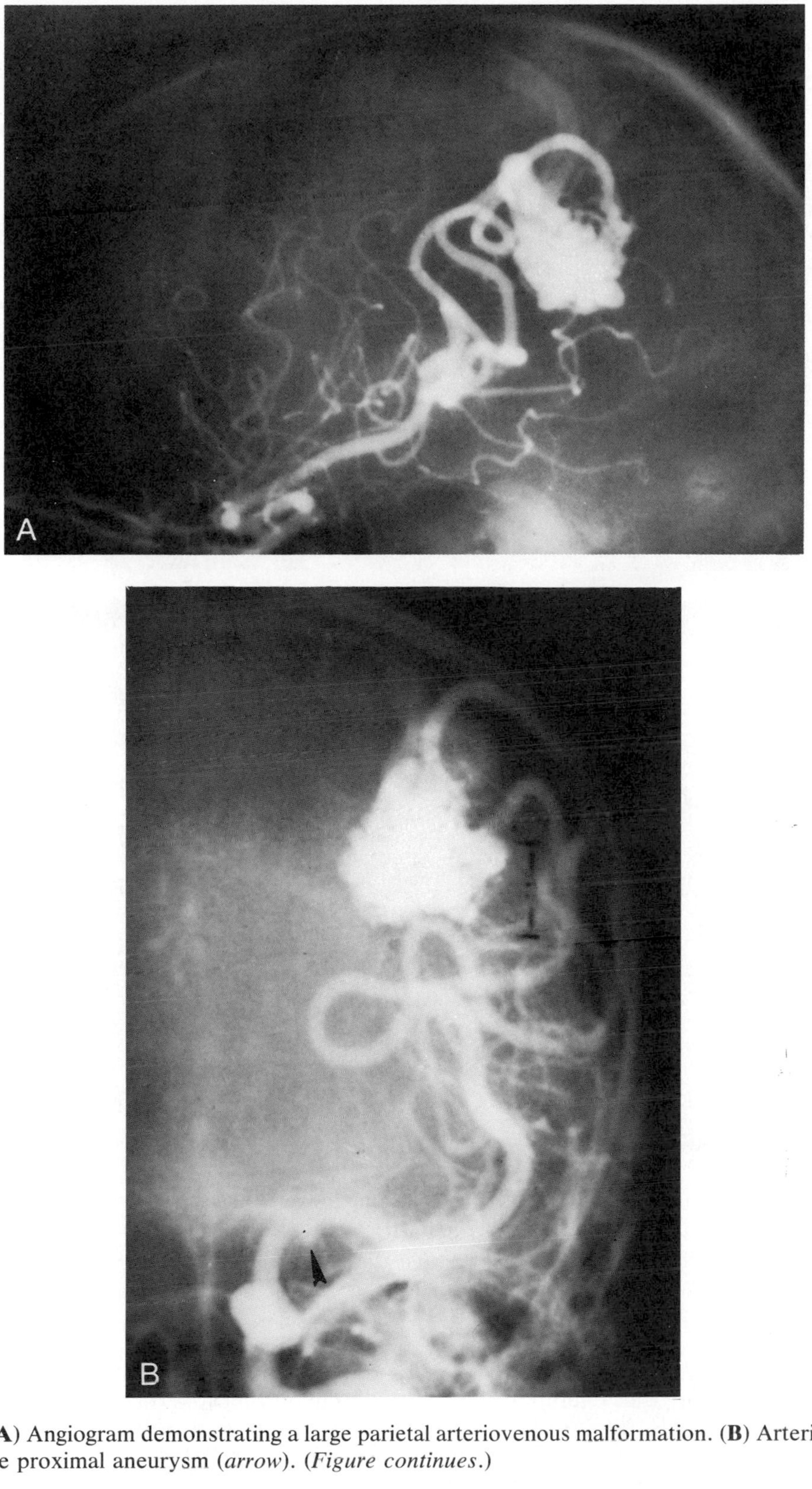


**Fig. 47-13.** (**A**) Angiogram demonstrating a large parietal arteriovenous malformation. (**B**) Arteriogram demonstrating the proximal aneurysm (*arrow*). (*Figure continues.*)

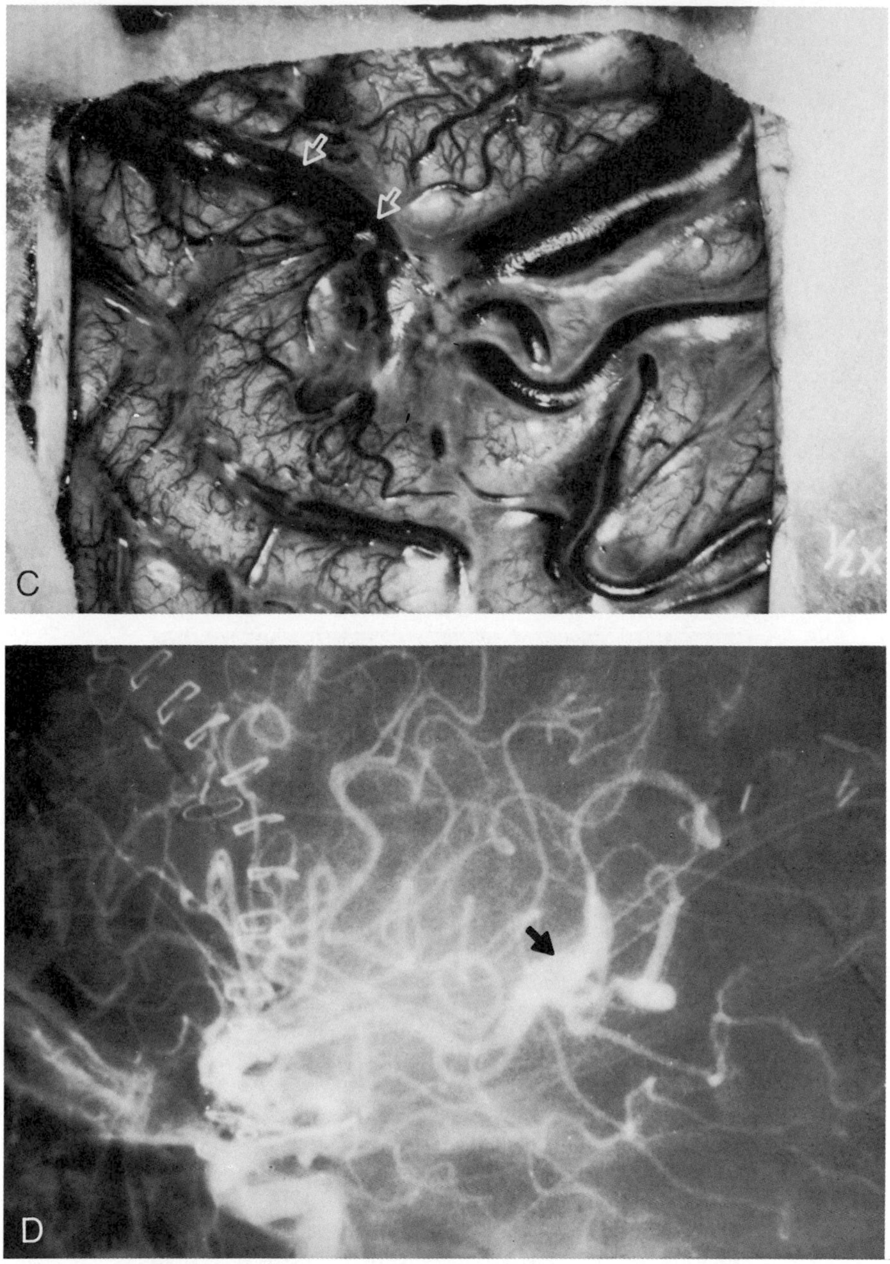


**Fig. 47-13** (*Continued*). **(C)** Operative photograph showing the large feeding artery (*arrows*) demonstrated by arteriography. **(D)** Arteriogram immediately following aneurysm surgery showing ectasia and stasis (*arrow*) within the middle cerebral artery previously supplying the arteriovenous malformation. The malformation had been resected 5 weeks previously.

tion, even after total removal. At the time of the second operative procedure for the clipping of the aneurysm, brief hypotension was used to a level of 80 mmHg for a period of approximately 10 minutes. With the background of the ectatic changes in the arteries nourishing the parietal temporal region, it would appear that some ischemia resulted and that these arteries were unable to autoregulate. The postoperative dysphasia and paresis cleared rapidly following the institution of volume expansion and hypertensive therapy. It is surprising that these vascular changes had not resolved at a period of 5 weeks from the initial operative procedure. There is strong suggestion that these large arterial feeders proximal to an AVM are abnormal in terms of their contractility and their ability to respond to physiologic changes in blood volume and blood pressure.[9,33,34,41,76,80]

## Postoperative Care

All AVM patients are monitored closely in a neurologic intensive care unit (ICU) setting for 24 to 72 hours postoperatively, depending on anticipated complications from surgery. Prevention and recognition of adverse circulatory changes or brain edema is paramount. Anticipation of these events can be gleaned from intraoperative observations and circulatory studies.[7,8,58,97,139] All the usual parameters are measured, including evaluation of cardiopulmonary function via Swan-Ganz catheter. The systolic blood pressure for 24 hours is maintained below 100 to 110 mmHg. Anemia is treated and intravenous fluids are limited. In cases of severe brain edema osmotherapy, steroids and, if necessary, intubation with respiratory control and barbiturate coma are instituted.[4]

## Postdischarge Care

Careful follow-up of the patient after discharge from the hospital is necessary in order to modify anticonvulsant drug regimes and encourage the patient in further rehabilitation therapy or direct the patient back into a normal sociological environment following these massive operations and psyche-wrenching problems. In our experience, if the malformation has been shown to be totally removed by postoperative arteriography, we have never seen a recurrence of the AVM. We have seen, however, on a number of occasions, CT scans performed for one reason or another months after successful removal of an AVM that suggest residual or recurrent malformation (Fig. 47-14). In all these cases, repeat arteriography has shown no residual malformation, leading us to assume that the CT scan can be fallaciously positive in the postoperative period. These changes are probably related to hyperemia, hyperperfusion, and gliosis around the resection and show up as "apparent vascular channels" on the postoperative CT scan. Therefore, in terms of false positive findings, I do not consider the CT scan a reliable way to evaluate the patient postoperatively. On the other hand, when scans are negative, this has been well correlated with negative postoperative arteriograms and, of course, the CT scan is invaluable in showing the gradual reduction of cerebral edema around the margins of the malformation and any changes in ventricular size.

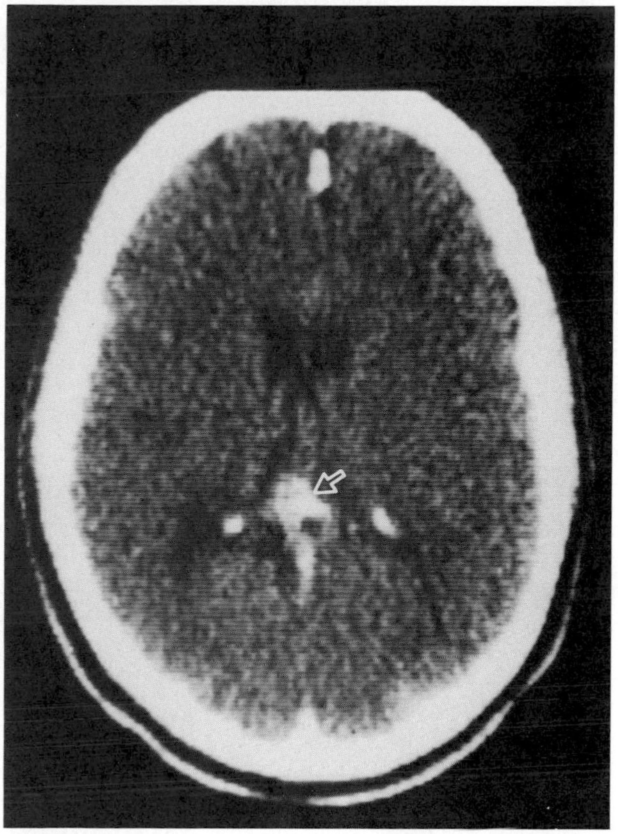

**Fig. 47-14.** A computed tomography scan with contrast performed 2 months following the removal of a posterior third ventricular arteriovenous malformation. This scan suggested residual arteriovenous malformation (*arrow*), which was shown by subsequent angiography not to be the case.

## Special Circumstances Related to the Location of Arteriovenous Malformations

### Posterior Fossa Arteriovenous Malformations

Posterior fossa AVMs deserve special consideration because of their rarity and high mortality and morbidity in terms of surgical resection or natural history.[15,23,26,111] These lesions are about 1/10 as common as supratentorial AVMs. They can be divided into the categories shown in Table 47-1 and Figure 47-15.

These lesions, even the larger ones, appear to have lower flow than their counterparts. They are much more difficult to visualize and analyze by angiography. The overlying bone structures, the lower flow in the vertebral system, and other factors make this analysis more difficult. Therefore these lesions cannot be approached with the anatomic precision that one utilizes in the supratentorial region. In my series of 40

**TABLE 47-1. Posterior Fossa Arteriovenous Malformation Categories[a]**

| |
|---|
| Cerebellar |
| Cerebellar hemisphere |
| Anterior vermis-midbrain |
| Posterior vermis-fourth ventricle |
| Brain stem |
| Intrinsic |
| Extrinsic |
| Cisternal-cerebellopontine angle |

[a] See also Figure 47-15.

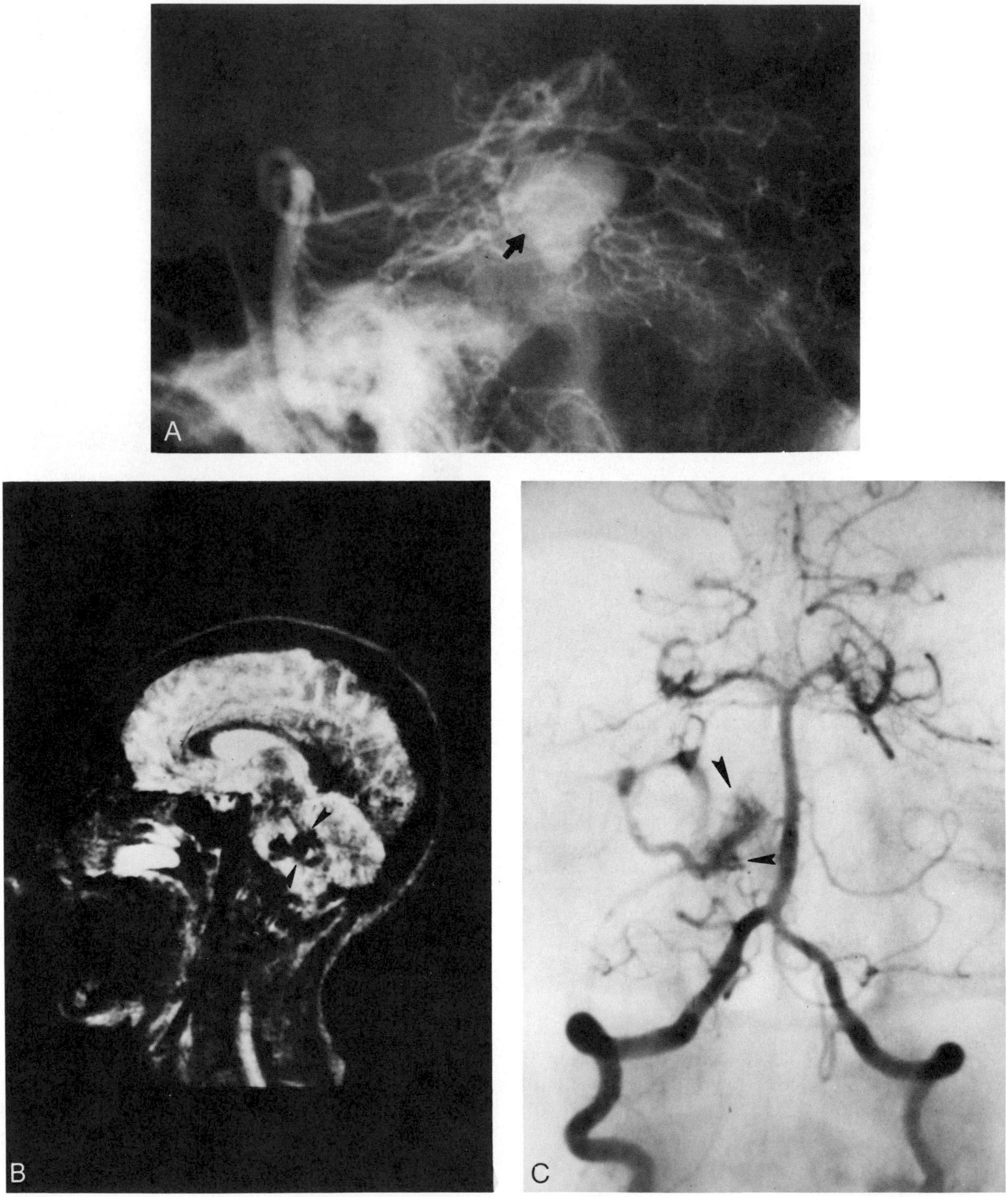


**Fig. 47-15.** Examples of posterior fossa arteriovenous malformations. (**A**) Large anterior cerebellar veris malformation associated with a venous aneurysm (*arrow*). (**B**) Nuclear magnetic resonance scan of brain stem arteriovenous malformation located within the substance of the brain stem (*arrows*) and unsuitable for surgical treatment. (**C**) Cerebellopontine angle arteriovenous malformation (*arrows*) commencing on the surface of the brain stem and extending deep (this arteriovenous malformation was resected).

posterior fossa malformations, the age distribution was the same as for other locations; however, virtually all these malformations presented with hemorrhage. In this aspect, these lesions are particularly treacherous because hemorrhages have led to severe brain stem compression and coma in many of the patients. When the lesions involve the cranial nerves, cranial nerve dysfunction may be permanent or prolonged. Similarly, those that involve the intrinsic structure of the brain stem may leave permanent damage as a result of hemorrhage.[15] There is very little margin of error or resiliency in the brain stem, as opposed to other portions of the brain. All these malformations must be approached with respect. Until recently it has been impossible to embolize these lesions and thereby reduce the shunt and turgor within the malformation prior to operative intervention. Currently, with the balloon-directed embolic technique, it is possible to embolize into the posterior inferior or anterior inferior cerebellar arteries, successfully reducing major arterial contributions to these malformations. The development of small mobile intravascular catheters has made it possible to successfully embolize these obscure malformations with liquid adhesives (Fig. 47-15).[133] It should be understood that these techniques are difficult and have the potential of creating devastating problems should the normal brain stem arteries be compromised in any way.

Operations on these malformations, as elsewhere, require wide exposure. The positioning of the patient is extremely important. For those malformations that lie in the hemispheral or posterior vermis region, the sitting position may be inappropriate, because it is necessary to elevate the cerebellum against gravity to visualize the feeding vessels from the posterior inferior or anterior inferior cerebellar arteries. Furthermore, although the sitting position is desirable in reducing venous tension within the malformation and adding a certain degree of hypotension, it can lead to devastating consequences when air embolism enters these high-flow systems. Also, it appears that induced hypotension may be counterproductive and in fact dangerous in those situations where a relative hypotension already exists. Clinical experience suggests that the removal of the shunt results in decrease in flow in the major sinuses of the posterior fossa and that this decrease in flow and resultant stasis are further compounded by the use of hypotension during the operative procedure. At least in one case, this has led to massive progressive thrombosis within these veins, with severe neurologic deficits. There is only one circumstance in which I routinely have the patient in the sitting position, and this is for lesions that are located in the anterior vermis adjacent to the midbrain region. Here the cerebellum falls away from the tentorium and a supracerebellar infratentorial approach may be used to great advantage, undermining and circumscribing the malformation while the feeding arteries, mostly the superior cerebellar and choroidal arteries, are identified and divided. The draining veins are generally to the straight sinus in the midline, and these can be avoided during the excision of most of the malformation. In other cases, the lateral or three-quarter prone position has been utilized, although this has the disadvantage of producing somewhat higher venous pressures; however, the ease for the surgeon, retraction of the cerebellum with the aid of gravity, and the avoidance of stasis in the sinuses are all advantageous.

Those malformations that involve the brain stem can only be analyzed at the time of surgery. Unfortunately, angiography is not sophisticated to the point where we can definitely determine how much of these malformations are intrinsic to the brain stem. Generally, they involve surface and superficial portions of the brain stem and can be dissected from these areas, since their feeding arteries come from pial branches of the major arteries of the posterior circulation. The venous drainage is also in the pia, and therefore these important vessels may be identified without entering the substance of the brain stem as the malformation is peeled away from the brain stem. Cranial nerve involvement is another matter. Here the feeding arteries may also supply the cranial nerves and the large draining veins may have affected the cranial nerves by contiguous pressure. In the postoperative period one may anticipate significant cranial nerve palsies. These are particularly bothersome when the 9th and 10th cranial nerves are involved. In such cases, even with unilateral involvement, patients have experienced difficulty in swallowing. This problem may last for months and must be managed by the placement of a nasogastric tube or gastrostomy. Tracheotomy over a prolonged period may also be necessary in such cases.

In a series of 40 posterior fossa malformations in my personal experience, the mortality rate has been 2 percent, and serious morbidity 12 percent (see later discussion on surgical management).

## Medial Hemisphere Arteriovenous Malformations

Medial hemisphere AVMs, often involving portions of the limbic system, comprise a surprisingly high percentage of AVMs—25 percent in my series.[117] In terms of surgical resection, these deserve special consideration. The location of these malformations can be categorized advantageously (Table 47-2). This categorization has the advantage of localizing the lesion and is a determinant in the surgical approach (Fig. 47-16). Those lesions located in the more anterior medial hemisphere region, involving the uncus and hippocampus, are approached through the sylvian fissure or through a subtemporal approach with varying degrees of resection of the inferior temporal gyrus. The malformations that are most difficult to reach are those located medial to the trigone of the lateral ven-

**TABLE 47-2. Medial Hemisphere Arteriovenous Malformation Regions**

| |
|---|
| Amygdaloid-uncus (anteromedial temporal) |
| Parahippocampal-fusiform gyrus (medial temporal) |
| Paratrigonal |
| Splenial-posterior third ventricle |
| Cingulate-medial hemisphere |

tricle. These may require a two-stage operation with an initial interhemispheric-parafalx approach followed by an infratemporal-tentorial approach to the residual portion of the malformation. Transcortical incisions via the temporoparietal region have also been recommended;[24] however, these have the disadvantage of not only violating eloquent areas of the brain, especially on the dominant side, but also reaching the malformation at its venous side, which often enters the ventricle, while the arterial supply is most distant from the surgeon. The approach is also relatively blind until the ventricular portion of the malformation is reached and requires a fair amount of retraction of eloquent areas of the brain. The surgeon is assisted when hemorrhage has occurred and there is softening or cavitation of the overlying white matter and cortex; however, in my experience, this has been uncommon. In most instances in my series, these difficult malformations have been managed by a parafalx-interhemispheric approach. The surgeon may reach almost as far as the peduncle of the midbrain to interrupt feeding arteries to these malformations located medial to the ventricular trigone. Those malformations located posterior at the splenium and involving the roof of the third ventricle as well as portions of the cingulate gyrus or the septal regions may be approached by a variety of interhemispheric approaches; the anteroposterior direction is dependent on the location of the malformation. The central area related to the rolandic draining veins and the motor and sensory strip should be spared any retraction.

The interhemispheric approaches, except for the most anterior ones, are effected with the patient in the sitting- or semisitting-slouch position (Fig. 47-9). This significantly reduces venous tension and gives the surgeon the most direct exposure of the surface of the malformation while facilitating control of the feeding arteries, whether they be from the anterior cerebral, posterior choroidal (medial and lateral), or the posterior cerebral arteries. The results of surgery have been excellent, which is ironic, considering the difficulty in removing these lesions and their often obscure location.

Those lesions lying in the diencephalic region may be approached by a variety of routes. Those located in relation to the lenticulostriate arteries, if separable from these arteries, may be approached through a sylvian fissure-splitting incision, with microsurgical removal of the lesion while preserving the important lenticulostriate arteries. The vast majority of thalamic lesions, however, are inoperable or, if operable,

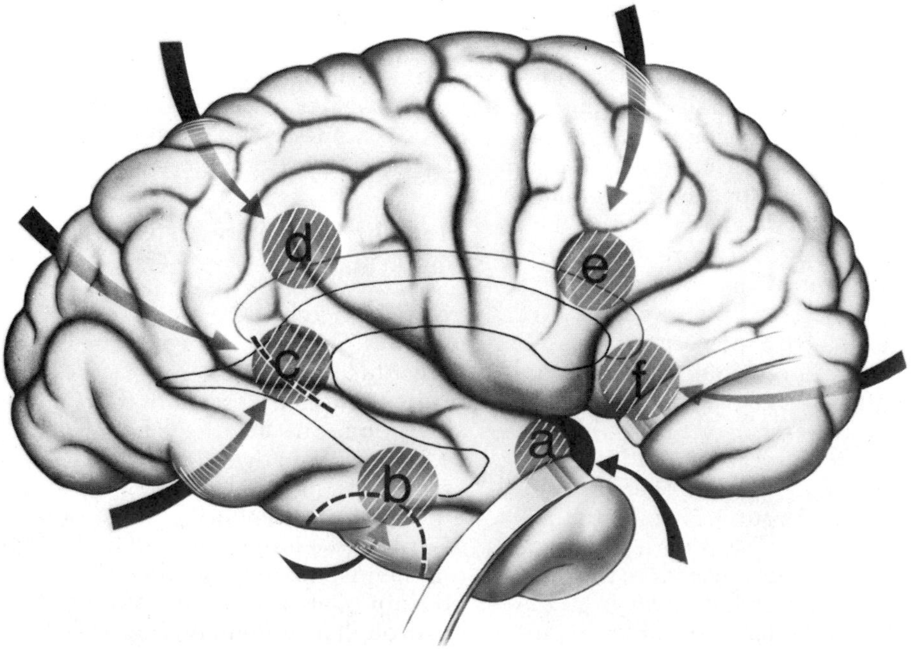


**Fig. 47-16.** Drawing of the various approaches to arteriovenous malformations of the medial hemisphere. These approaches are cataloged in Table 47-2.

are located in the more dorsal aspect of the thalamus or caudate nucleus, often entering the ventricular system. These may then be approached through the same interhemispheric approaches as used for medial hemisphere AVMs or by a route direct to the ventricular system. For those malformations located deep and involving the thalamus and roof of the third ventricle, the deep venous system, including the two important internal cerebral veins and the vein of Galen, should be and can be preserved in the successful removal of these lesions. These lesions are supplied primarily from major branches of the medial posterior choroidal arteries, and to a lesser extent from the lateral posterior choroidal arteries that enter into the glomus of the choroid plexus in the trigone of the lateral ventricle. It may take multiple attempts to remove these pesky and somewhat obscure malformations that involve regions of the thalamus. Their position is not easily identifiable when one observes the ependyma, even in cases of previous hemorrhage. The malformations seem to be somewhat diffuse and intertwined with portions of the thalamus.

We have found another interesting group of lesions located in the posterior corpus callosum, body of the caudate, and pulvinar region of the dominant hemisphere. Three such cases, all presenting with hemorrhages, were associated with profound recent memory deficits. These lesions have been discrete, and the structures involved were the body and tail of the caudate, portions of the corpus callosum, the left or dominant fornix, and small portions of the pulvinar (Fig. 47-17). We have not observed recent memory loss with similar lesions located in the nondominant hemisphere. The suggestion is that the aforementioned dominant hemisphere structures have some relation to the acquisition of memory.

## Aneurysms and Arteriovenous Malformations

In 10 to 15 percent of AVMs, there may be a tandem lesion of an aneurysm. This frequently occurs proximal to the AVM on the main feeding vessel. The decision as to which lesion should be treated first depends on which is symptomatic. In the face of a hemorrhage, the cause is usually the aneurysm, in which case this should be treated first and the AVM at a future date. If the site of hemorrhage is the AVM or the lesions are asymptomatic, then we prefer to remove the AVM first. There is then the possibility that the aneurysm will regress, and certainly with reduction of blood flow the aneurysm will be easier to treat. If the site of hemorrhage cannot be determined, then the aneurysm, on speculation, should be treated first. In some cases when the lesions are in proximity, it is possible to treat both at the same operation. In the case of tandem operations, 4 to 6 weeks should elapse between operations.[42,49]

## Intraoperative Angiography

Although some have recommended it, we have not found intraoperative angiography useful or practical.

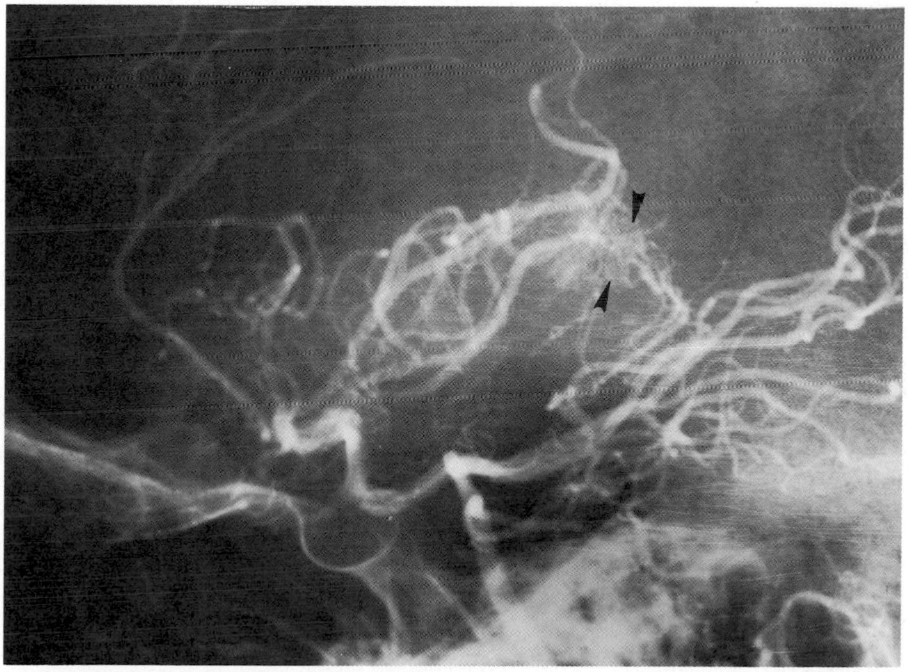

**Fig. 47-17.** Dominant hemisphere arteriovenous malformation (*arrows*) located in the region of the ventricular trigone, involving the caudate nucleus, fornix, and, to a lesser extent, the corpus callosum.

It is extremely difficult to obtain quality, and one must also consider the interference of various metallic retractors. This technique also requires prolonged intra-arterial catheterization and the prolongation of an already lengthy operation. Therefore we have not recommended or used this procedure, relying more on our experience, judgment, and view through the operating microscope as to the configuration and totality of removal of AVMs.

## Radiation Therapy for Arteriovenous Malformations: Proton Beam and Gamma Radiosurgery

The rationale for treating AVMs by focused radiation is based on the damaging effect of radiation on the vessels partaking in the AVM.[53,57,85,124,125,127,141] Regardless of the type of radiation utilized, the response of the vessel wall is the same. Early changes consist of subendothelial edema, fissuring of the walls, and microhemorrhage with resultant thrombosis secondary to changes in the vessel wall. The changes seen in the early phases after radiotherapy are minimal; however, long-term effects include the proliferation of endothelial cells with the deposition of a collagenous homogeneous material in the subendothelial region of the vessel wall. Medial thickening ensues, with fibrosis and, one hopes, occlusion of the lumen. The degree of occlusion or stenosis of the involved vessel depends on the diameter of the vessel. The alterations are obviously more impressive in small vessels than they are in the medium or large vessels, and more prominent in arteries than in the veins or the cavernous channels that occur within the confines of an AVM. Since the large sinuses or venous aneurysms so characteristic of an AVM contain little connective, elastic, or muscular tissue in the wall, there is little to be affected in these vessels, and therefore the effect in terms of obliteration of the lumen will be negligible.

The techniques of radiation therapy for AVMs have followed two basic patterns, the first recommended and utilized by Leksell and, subsequently, Steiner and colleagues employ stereotactically directed narrow beams of ionizing radiation from a $^{60}$Co gamma source emitting protons.[125] The other method utilized by Kjellberg et al.,[53] uses the stereotactic Bragg peak proton. This proton beam is designed to reach its peak or stop in a defined volume of tissue, presumably the AVM. Both methods use a stereotactic device and frame for the delivery of radiation. The proton beam technique requires a cyclotron and is not widely available. The details of the radiation technique and stereotactic and mechanical instrumentation are recorded in reports by many groups.[53,57,62,63,124,125,141] A large series of cases has been developed by both groups in which AVMs have been treated by radiosurgery, and follow-up, including CT scans and angiograms, has been performed at various times after the treatment. It must be realized that both these techniques require exotic instrumentation and are not widely available.

The criteria for the use of the techniques vary somewhat between these two major groups. Kjellberg et al.[53] have treated AVMs that are considered inaccessible to surgical resection, namely, those located centrally in eloquent areas of the brain or in the brain stem. Although they mention that those malformations under 3 cm respond better to proton beam radiation, they do not exclude larger lesions from treatment. Steiner et al.,[125] on the other hand, have been more discriminating and recommend that only those lesions under 3 cm be considered for radiosurgery. Both groups contemplate that radiation may be used in the future to be targeted specifically at major feeding arteries and not encompass the entire malformation. Steiner has suggested multiple radiation focuses targeting the large arteries of an AVM. The occlusion of these key vessels presumably will lead to occlusion of major portions of the AVM. If this methodology is successful, it may be realistic to treat, by radiosurgery, malformations larger than previously presumed possible. Furthermore, the use of embolization or surgery to reduce the arterial feeders and thereby the size of an AVM may also extend the use of radiosurgery. This method of treatment discounts the fact that most malformations hemorrhage from the large cavernous areas, which presumably would not be affected by this methodology, and also that treatments falling short of total obliteration of malformations have generally been regarded as ineffectual, based on past experience with embolization and selective surgical ligation of the feeding vessels. Another disadvantage of radiosurgery is the time frame as related to desired results. The effect of radiation is ongoing and therefore, even in the most successful cases, is slow to occlude the malformation, sometimes taking up to 2 or more years. Furthermore, the long-term effects of radiation are not known, since the follow-up of both groups is relatively short; only a few cases have been followed for a decade or more.

In the series of Steiner et al.,[125] 135 patients (the first treated in 1970) have been analyzed. Since good results appear to be related directly to the ability to include all the pathologic vessels within the radiation field, it is most appropriate to review their subgroup of 81 selected patients who were followed for 1 year with angiographic identification of the lesion. Total obliteration was obtained in 40 percent of those patients. In another group of 63 patients with a 2-year angiographic follow-up there was an 84 percent obliteration rate. In terms of complications, 4 of the 135 patients developed new neurologic deficits. These were apparently the result of delayed radiation necrosis. Radiation necrosis, however, appears to be related, as Kjellberg et al.[53] express, to the amount of radiation. In the series of Steiner et al.,[125] two patients had recurrent hemorrhage, but both of these hemorrhages were within a few months of the onset of radiation treatment, which could not be expected to be effective in this short time. In their entire group of AVMs, some of which were not satisfactorily radiated even though the time factors were appropriate, there were 8 cases out of 135 with recurrent hemorrhage. Steiner et al.[125] emphasize that the correct single dose of radiation is still not known.

Kjellberg et al.[53] record experience with over 400 patients and the use of proton beam therapy in the treatment of AVMs. Apparently, AVMs of all size and location have been treated with this methodology. The authors' figures are difficult to analyze; however, it appears that very few of the patients were followed long term. While they admit that the proton beam has no measurable effect on the AVM during the first year, there were 2 deaths among the first 75 patients treated, presumably due to hemorrhage from the AVM before it could be protected by the radiation. Similarly, there was a relatively low percentage of obliteration of the malformations—approximately 20 percent. The incidence of radiation necrosis and serious effects from this treatment is not detailed in the report of Kjellberg et al.,[53] but it appears to be higher in the initial portion of their series (in the range of 10 percent), when higher radiation doses were used, as compared to the latter portion of their series, when lower radiation doses were utilized.

With the proliferation of radiosurgery centers, practical application of this technique has narrowed to the use of the linear accelerator and the gamma knife.[62,141] Unfortunately long-term follow-up of matched cases has been lacking and undermines the credibility of the technique. It would appear that use of radiosurgery to treat the most favorable AVMs, those under 3 cm, results in an 85 percent obliteration rate with few short-term complications. Ironically, when such lesions are surgically accessible, and most are, surgery in experienced hands results in 100 percent obliteration with minimal complications. Unfortunately, in cases of larger AVMs, where surgical morbidity is significant, radiosurgery is not applicable because of the large doses of radiation required to obliterate these lesions. Although it is intriguing to speculate that these complex and treacherous lesions, in which surgical morbidity has been a major factor in the decision-making process, can be treated simply and painlessly by radiosurgery, a more extensive follow-up is required before this treatment can be embraced.[119] Currently, we reserve this treatment for those lesions that are totally inaccessible to embolization and surgical techniques, that is, primarily smaller lesions fed by small blood vessels and located in areas such as the central brain stem and diencephalon. One must also consider the possibility of serious irreversible side effects of radiation extended 10 or more years beyond the institution of treatment. It appears that we have little experience with this facet of radiotherapy, both in AVMs and benign tumors in which radiation has been utilized. The indiscriminate use of radiotherapy for other lesions located in more accessible regions of the brain and larger than the ones singled out by Steiner et al.[125] appears to be unjustified until further information relative to the long-term effect is available and unless surgery or other measures have been totally excluded from the treatment armamentarium.

## RESULTS OF SURGICAL MANAGEMENT

The following surgical results are based on a personal series of 350 operated cases of AVMs located in various parts of the brain. The problem presented by AVMs has been approached not only from the surgical viewpoint in this series but also as a team effort. This team includes a neurologist, a neuroradiologist, and a neuroanesthesiologist. The development of a team is consistent with our aim to treat these difficult lesions in the best way possible, including improvement in the surgical mortality and morbidity. This tribunal of physicians interested in AVMs selects patients for operation and rejects other patients who have malformations too large or located in inaccessible areas, which in our experience would result in a surgical morbidity and mortality rate too high to justify operation. Nevertheless, difficult malformations were not excluded if it was felt in each case, on the basis of past experience and location, that these could be resected with minimal surgical morbidity and mortality. Therefore 40 percent of the patients had malformations located in the dominant hemisphere and 45 percent of the patients had malformations located in eloquent portions of the brain, including the motor, sensory, and speech areas. An obscure group of malformations previously described, located on the medial hemisphere, comprised approximately 25 percent of the cases. Malformations located in the posterior fossa, which in our experience have a higher mortality and morbidity rate than those located elsewhere in the brain, comprised approximately 10 percent of the patients. The malformations had a wide spectrum of features, including (1) age of the patient, (2) size, (3) number and size of feeding arteries, and (4) direction and size of draining veins. All these factors were considered in determining operability.

The overall mortality was 1 percent in the series of personally operated AVMs. Morbidity is categorized as follows: (1) severe neurologic deficits such as hemiparesis, hemisensory loss, and speech deficits (2.5 percent); (2) moderate neurologic deficits that were not so severe as to impair the patient's functional activity but which limited daily living activities to a modest extent (3.5 percent); and (3) mild and nonlimiting neurologic deficits. In this last category fall primarily the various visual field defects that occurred in those lesions located in the optic radiations or the primary visual areas. These deficits range from hemianopias to quadrantopias or sector defects and after a period of time were compensated for by the patient so they did not compromise social or work activities. Visual field defects were seen in 12 percent of the patients. These were the mortality and morbidity figures we aimed for in determining whether a patient's AVM was operable. We feel that these figures justify a radical approach to selected AVMs.

In this series there were no recurrences of malformations that had been totally resected, as proved by a postoperative angiogram. In only one instance was a postoperative formal angiogram not performed because of extenuating circumstances on behalf of the patient. Additionally, there were no subsequent hemorrhages once the malformation had proved to be removed. In the series there were approximately 10 percent with aneurysms that occurred, for the most part, on proximal feeding arteries to the malformation. Not all these patients were treated by definitive surgery, that is, clipping of the aneurysm, and to date there has been no bleeding from the remaining aneurysm if it was left in place, which was the case in approximately 20 percent of those patients who had both aneurysms and AVM, the AVM having been resected.

## OUTCOME FROM CONSERVATIVE MANAGEMENT

Experience with conservative management in nonrandomized evaluations has been reported over many years. Troupp et al.[129] found neither the size nor the location of the AVM to have predictive value for rupture.

Few studies have yet appeared dealing with the natural history of unruptured AVMs. McCormick and colleagues' autopsy series[70–73] showed that only 12 percent of their cases had been symptomatic in life. In the few studies in which repeated angiograms have been done, roughly a third of AVMs have been found to enlarge, a third have remained static, and a third have shown regression[30,122,123] without any specific therapy. Whether such cases are exceptional and whether factors can be identified to predict the future course remain unknown at present.

As with intracranial aneurysms, steady advances in surgical technique have encouraged the more experienced surgeons to take on the more challenging cases. A recent series comparing surgical and conservative management is that of 145 cases reported by Guidetti and Delitala.[38] Based on their experience, these authors recommend surgery. Heros et al.[44] have recorded a similar experience.

## OTHER VASCULAR MALFORMATIONS

In this section we consider malformations that are more commonly seen by the neuropathologist than are AVMs, but which appear to be less commonly seen by the clinician.[70,73] These would include (1) cavernous malformations, (2) venous malformations, (3) telangiectasias, (4) vein of Galen malformations, (5) dural arteriovenous malformations, (6) carotid-cavernous fistulas, and (7) "cryptic malformations." These entities have been alternatively termed angiomas, which is a misnomer. There is no indication that any of these are neoplastic or have the capability of enlargement through proliferation; rather, the term *angioma* should be discarded in favor of *malformation*.

### Cavernous Malformations

Cavernous malformations of the brain, although occasionally incidental, are increasingly recognized as a heretofore obscure cause of seizures, hemorrhage, and progressive neurologic deficit. This apparently increased incidence can be attributed to the widespread use of contemporary and sophisticated imaging techniques. Although recognized on CT scan as a lesion without contrast, the appearance of cavernous malformations by MRI is virtually pathognomonic. Their nature of repeated small hemorrhages creates the MRI image of various stages of blood breakdown and thereby a variegated well-circumscribed lesion.[16,69,86,102,109,130,135]

Headaches may or may not be related, but the hemorrhages, when they do occur, are related to the malformation. These malformations are made up of a multitude of large cavernous vascular channels that can be identified neither as arteries nor as veins. Major portions are often thrombosed, and whatever portions are patent have such low-flow characteristics that they are generally not visible on angiograms, even with a prolonged venous phase and maximal injection of contrast agent. These lesions are most commonly seen in the cerebral hemispheres, where they may be superficial or deep and, in the latter case, paraventricular. In approximately 20 percent of cases, they are infratentorially located in the cerebellum or brain stem. In 5 percent of cases, they are found in the spinal cord. They generally appear as a dense contrast-enhancing area without mass effect. The larger ones may extend from the surface of the brain to the paraventricular region. In the spinal cord, they are intramedullary. Hemorrhages, when they occur, are rarely fatal and in most cases pursue a benign course with a low incidence of recidivous hemorrhage.

These lesions are commonly mistaken for intracranial tumors, but can be readily identified by the lack of mass effect. When exposed at surgery, they often appear larger than expected from the scan finding.[5] In some cases, the lesions may be encapsulated, with clefts at the margins, the result of old hemorrhage. Their resectability depends on the border between abnormal and normal, which, if indistinct, precludes excision. In most cases, symptomatic or asymptomatic, surgery is advised. This is based on the natural history. Many of the hemorrhages are presumed to be asymptomatic. In addition, the buildup of scar around the lesion from repeated hemosiderin deposition is felt to be a process leading to intractable seizures. Cavernous malformations of the brain stem generally have a more progressive and disastrous course. To date there is no evidence that radiosurgery plays a definitive role in the treatment of these lesions; in fact, it may be contraindicated.[54,137] One of our cases is illustrative (Fig. 47-18).

*Case History*

The patient, a 17-year-old right-handed woman at the time of operation, commenced having seizures 3 years prior to operation. These seizures were first petit mal in nature and culminated in a grand mal seizure, during which she collapsed and suffered a skull fracture. Following that seizure, which occurred 3 years prior to operation, she had imaging studies that showed a lesion present on non-contrast CT scan, slightly enhancing on contrast CT scan, and typical of a cavernous malformation on the MRI scan (Fig. 47-18). An arteriogram through all phases was normal. She was maintained on a therapeutic anticonvulsant regimen. She suffered no further seizures but maintained an abnormal electroencephalogram (EEG). Her neurologic examination was normal.

On 19 July 1990, operation was carried out with the total removal of a cavernous malformation (Fig. 47-18). At operation a large middle cerebral artery branch, identified as normal on the arteriogram, coursed intimately around the convexity surface of the malformation, giving small branches to it. These branches were not visualized as abnormal on the arteriogram. Postoperatively, the patient was maintained on anticonvulsants and was normal. One year postoperatively, the patient continues normal, and consideration is being given to stopping anticonvulsant medication.

## Venous Malformations

Venous malformations, also clinical curiosities, are turning up with a frequency that parallels the increasing use of CT and MRI scanning.[77,81,84,103,105 107] Again, the symptomatology, similar to that in cavernous malformations, is primarily reflected by seizure disorders, headaches, and, rarely, hemorrhage. In some cases, an associated cavernous malformation may be present in the vicinity of the venous malformation, explaining why, in some series of venous malformations, there was a 40 to 50 percent incidence of hemorrhage.[81,84,102,103,105] When hemorrhage has occurred, it has not been fatal, and often the patient recovered completely. These lesions may be located in any region of the brain, but have not been reported in the spinal cord. The CT scan and angiographic appearance are pathognomonic.[105] On the CT scan, there is generally a contrast-enhancing linear density representing the draining vein; a comparable image is seen by MRI scan. This appears in the white matter, but may extend to the cortical region. The angiogram, which is pathognomonic, shows a "caput medusae" arrangement of veins deep in the white matter, coalescing to a dilated venous channel, which passes through the white matter, usually toward the cortical surface. These are low-flow systems readily identified on the venous phase of the angiogram. There is no evidence of an arterial contribution to the lesion. At surgery, blood sampled from the draining vein is purely venous, with no evidence of arteriovenous shunting or elevated oxygen content. In most cases, especially those that do not present with hemorrhage, the approach should be conservative and surgery is not indicated. The dilemma arises when the lesion has hemorrhaged. The few cases that have been operated on, especially those located in the cerebellum, would indicate that the venous malformation represents an abnormal, probably congenital, but essential venous drainage for the deep white matter, subserving areas where surface veins are deficient.[107] In such cases, it may be impossible to remove the venous malformation, even if it has hemorrhaged, because of ensuing massive brain swelling due to the obliteration of the only venous drainage for that portion of the brain. Therefore even those venous malformations associated with hemorrhage should be treated with utmost caution and conservatism. It is comforting to note that the few data available on the natural history of these lesions suggest that recurrent hemorrhages are the exception rather than the rule. The following case is instructive (Fig. 47-19).

*Case Study*

The patient was a 24-year-old right-handed woman who was in excellent health until October 1983, when she developed a right cerebellar hemorrhage. This was operated on and the hemorrhage removed. Following the operation, a CT scan demonstrated the classic appearance of a venous malformation of the right cerebellar hemisphere. In a second operation, part of the malformation was removed, but a postoperative arteriogram still showed the characteristic findings of a venous malformation (Fig. 47-19A). Having fully recovered from the hemorrhage, she was referred to us, and in April 1984 a third operation was carried out on the right cerebellar hemisphere. There was evidence of old hemorrhage surrounding a tangle of veins that coalesced into a large single draining vein gaining the surface of the cerebellum and draining into the tentorium. Samples of blood from this vein indicated venous blood comparable to a peripheral venous sample. There was no evidence of arterial oxygenization of the blood in this vein. Temporary occlusion of this vein led to swelling of the cerebellar

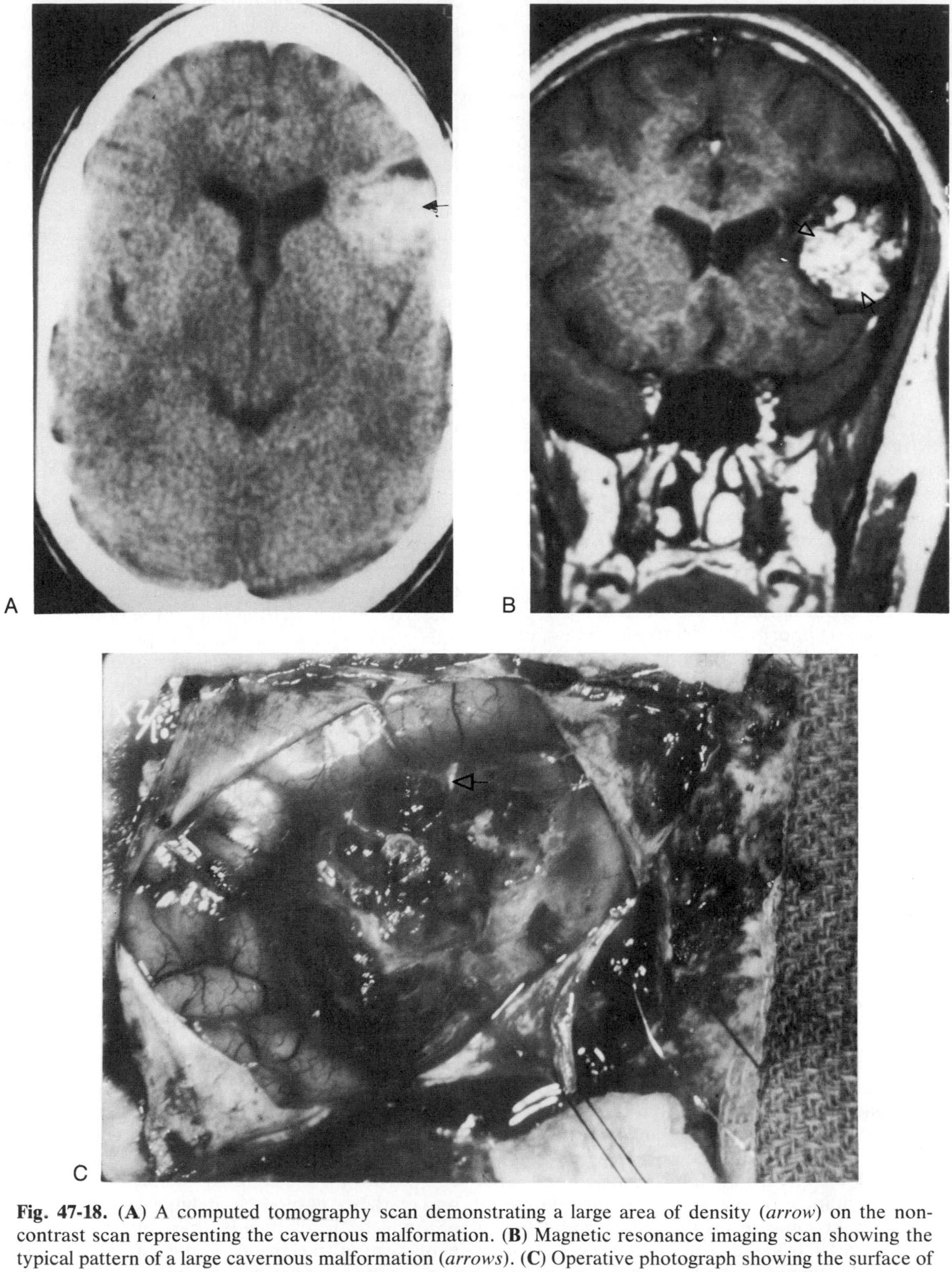


**Fig. 47-18.** (**A**) A computed tomography scan demonstrating a large area of density (*arrow*) on the non-contrast scan representing the cavernous malformation. (**B**) Magnetic resonance imaging scan showing the typical pattern of a large cavernous malformation (*arrows*). (**C**) Operative photograph showing the surface of the cavernous malformation and the middle cerebral branch coursing intimate to the malformation (*arrow*).

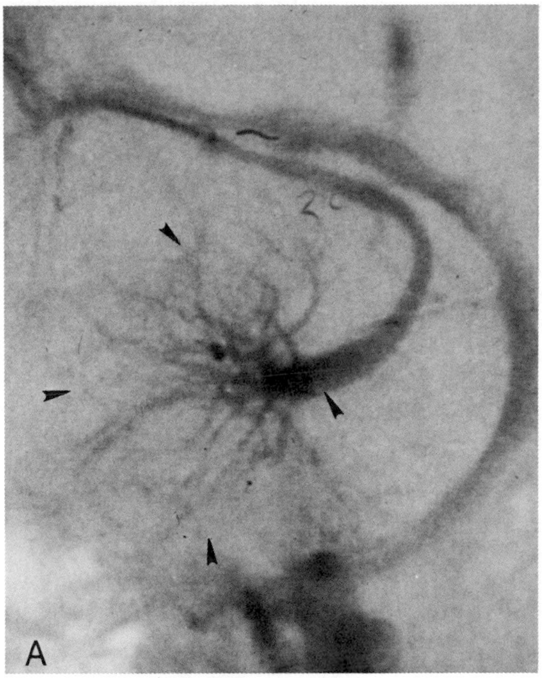


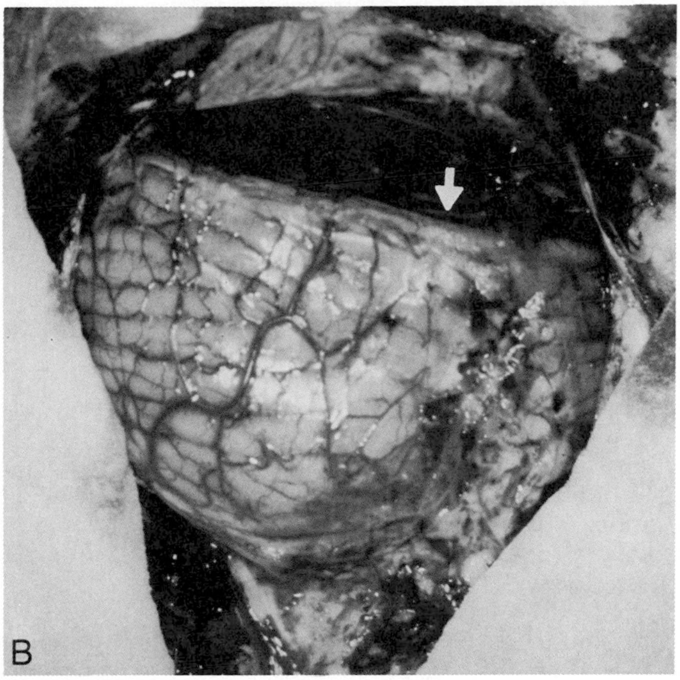


**Fig. 47-19.** Features of a venous malformation. (**A**) Posterior fossa angiogram showing the typical configuration of a venous malformation (*arrows*). (**B**) Operative photograph demonstrating the paucity of normal veins over the convexity of the right cerebellar hemisphere and the single large draining vein (*arrow*) representing the venous malformation.

hemisphere, and it was obvious that this was the only visible venous drainage for the posterior and superior surface of the right cerebellar hemisphere (Fig. 47-19B). The vein in the area of old hemorrhage was then coated with a scarifying material and the wound was closed.

It was presumed that the venous drainage of the right cerebellar hemisphere was anomalous, depending primarily on this enlarged vein for drainage of both the white matter and the cortex. The hemorrhage had occurred at a deep portion of the vein. We did not feel that part or all of this abnormal venous system could be obliterated without destroying important venous drainage. Five years after the surgery the patient was well, without recurrent hemorrhage, and an MRI showed no cavernous malformations.

## Telangiectasias

Telangiectasias are clinical curiosities that rarely lead to hemorrhage, but which can result in neurologic deficits.[28] These are not generally removed surgically, since their borders are ill defined and their significance uncertain. These lesions are frequently seen by the neuropathologist and may be associated with other lesions comprising the Rendu-Osler-Weber syndrome (Fig. 47-20).

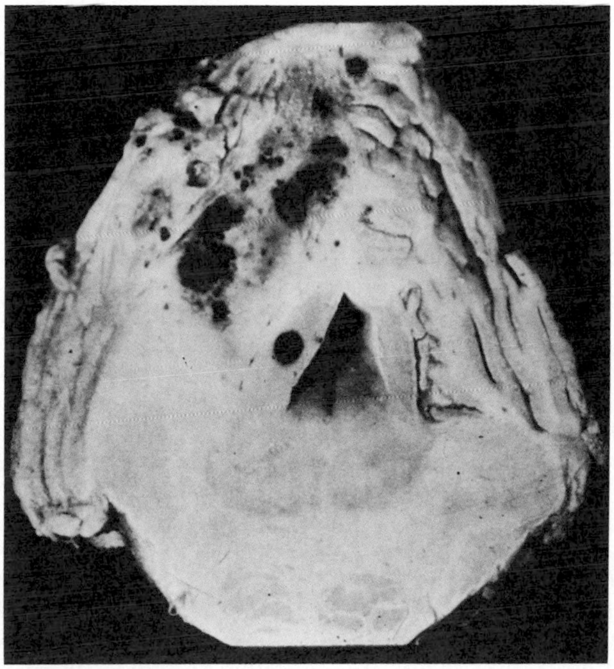

**Fig. 47-20.** Photograph showing a telangiectasia of the brain stem and cerebellum.

## Vein of Galen Malformations

Some malformations consist of arteriovenous connections in the region of the vein of Galen.[2,14,36,46,74] They are generally represented by large aneurysmal dilatations of the deep venous system in this region; in other instances, an AVM is the major component of the abnormality. In general, they act as a mass, with obstruction to the aqueduct, producing hydrocephalus. Uncommonly, they are associated with intracranial hemorrhage. These congenital lesions, unlike many of the other vascular malformations, become apparent in childhood, commonly in the form a rapid progressive hydrocephalus and also cardiac failure in the infant whose juvenile heart is unaccustomed to the high-flow arteriovenous shunts.

Patients with vein of Galen malformations may be divided into three groups: (1) those with direct arterial shunts to the vein of Galen, forming a large venous aneurysm, (2) those with a true AVM located in the posterior third ventricle and midbrain region, with veins draining into the vein of Galen and straight sinus, and (3) those with a combination of these two situations. The practical aspect of this categorization is that the first type of malformation is essentially a large artery to single vein shunt, whereas the second and third categories represent a true AVM, which forms the major portion of the malformation. This categorization has validity in terms of surgical approach and embolization.

### Clinical Presentation

The clinical presentation of these lesions is primarily related to the size of the shunt and the age of the patient; as reported by Amacher and Shillito,[2] it can be divided into four clinical patterns: (1) severe cardiac failure presenting within hours or days of birth, usually before the first week of life; (2) mild to moderate cardiac failure with increasing head size due to hydrocephalus, occurring around 6 months; (3) seizures and hydrocephalus occurring after the first year of life; and (4) subarachnoid hemorrhage in patients who have attained several years of age. It is significant that 64 percent of the patients become symptomatic before 2 years of age. In those infants who present with severe cardiac failure due to a large shunt and the major size of the aneursymal dilatation, there is little that can be done. The natural course is invariably fatal and therapeutic measures have generally been futile. These children are so young and their cardiac status so precarious that it has been impossible to use the appropriately sized catheter or amount of fluid required for embolization. Similarly, surgical procedures in this age group are generally fatal. If there is any way possible, and there rarely is, these children should be tided over by medical means directed at compensation for cardiac failure until they are older and better able to withstand the rigors of the various forms of treatment. In the older age group, with mild cardiac failure and signs of hydrocephalus, it is the hydrocephalus that often needs immediate attention. Hydrocephalus is generally due to the obstruction of the posterior third ventricle or aqueductal region and can be alleviated by the usual extracranial shunts. In patients with progressive cardiac failure, therapeutic endeavors designed to reduce or eliminate the arteriovenous shunts may be necessary. As a preliminary, CT scan evaluation and selective intracranial angiography are necessary. Arteriography will demonstrate the major arterial supply, which is generally from the posterior cerebral artery or its branches. In addition, there may be arterial supply of lesser importance from the anterior cerebral, middle cerebral, or superior cerebellar arteries.

### Embolization

Some of these malformations, depending upon the size of the shunt and the arteriographic anatomy, have been treated successfully by embolization.[45,74] Embolization, although not completely eliminating the shunt, has been effective in reducing it, ameliorating the abnormal cardiac failure. Hilal et al.[45] have been successful in utilizing the technique of Silastic pellet embolization.

### Surgical Approach

A promising technique reported by Mickle and Quisling[74] involves the placement of thrombogenic coils via the torcula into the malformation. Conversely, the open surgical approach is fraught with difficulties and a high morbidity and mortality.[14,145] As previously mentioned, the mortality rate for infants who present with severe cardiac decompensation within the first week or two of life has been prohibitive, and, for the most part, operation has been abandoned in this group. Operation becomes useful in those patients whose cardiac situation has been stabilized and who are better able to withstand an operative approach. The aim of the operation is to eliminate the arteriovenous shunts as much as possible, often totally, without injuring the blood supply to the normal structures, such as the midbrain, or interrupting the deep venous system. It is not necessary to excise the enlarged vein of Galen, as this will attenuate over time once the arterial contribution to it is eliminated.

The operation, because of hydrocephalus, is usually carried out with the patient in the prone position and may involve bilateral parietal craniotomies. Initially, the attack should be from the right side with a parietal craniotomy and retraction of the parietal lobe, with the greatest possible exposure of the dilated vein of Galen or AVM in this region. A supratentorial approach is preferred, since the majority of the malformation is located in this region, and it is difficult to work from the posterior fossa on the vascular supply that comes from the anterior cerebral or middle cerebral arteries. As the surgeon approaches the malformation from the right side, various arterial components are gradually eliminated by cautery and division. Subsequently, the remaining margins of the malformation are secured, either with the addition of a left parietal craniotomy or, in the modest- to smaller-sized malformations, entirely from the right side. Once the arterial contributions have been divided, the vein generally collapses, and it may be necessary to plicate it further in order to reduce its volume and thereby eliminate the mass effect created by this large distended vessel. Rarely, it is necessary to resect the entire malformation or veins. In fact, this may lead to venous congestion of the diencephalic region and high morbidity, if not mortality.

With this approach, the mortality of surgery in the older children with hydrocephalus and mild to moderate but stabilized cardiac failure has been in the range of 30 percent. This may seem somewhat high; however, the natural history of such lesions is universally dismal. The lowest mortality and morbidity have been experienced in older children who present with subarachnoid hemorrhage due to the malformation.

## Prognosis

Therefore malformations in the region of the vein of Galen in children represent a heterogeneous group of lesions ranging from single arteriovenous shunts with huge aneurysmal dilatations to true complex AVMs. The natural history and results of treatment have been uniformly dismal in those cases presenting with severe cardiac failure in the first few weeks of life. The best results are obtained in older children who present with none of the major complications of these malformations, such as cardiac failure or progressive hydrocephalus, but rather with a milder syndrome of subarachnoid hemorrhage. In this instance, the lesion can be excised as prophylaxis against future hemorrhage. In the intermediate group presenting with cardiac failure and hydrocephalus, but in the older child, the results of shunting procedures and interruption of feeding arteries have been reasonably encouraging.

## Dural Arteriovenous Malformations

The malformations that involve the dura are similar to those involving the brain in that they have major arterial supply with large venous drainage.[3,5,64,126] These venous channels may be extensive and usually empty into the major sinus. The malformations are generally modest in size, although small ones have been recorded as symptomatic and in some instances the size of the dural malformations can only be described as horrendous, being comprehensive and involving many of the major sinuses and much of one or both hemispheres. As cerebral AVMs, they appear to have a congenital origin. They are uncommon, comprising less than 10 percent of cerebral malformations. Their blood supply is most commonly from the external carotid or muscular branches of the vertebral artery, although on occasion they may be associated with cerebral AVMs and in these instances may be fed by the cerebral arteries (Fig. 47-21).

Dural AVMs may hemorrhage, often presenting with an acute subdural hemorrhage that may be severe and even fatal on occasion. Unlike their cerebral counterparts, they may also present with evidence of raised intracranial pressure, including papilledema, headaches, vomiting, and all of the manifestations of intracranial hypertension. These malformations, since they are often large and close to the skull, are more often producers of bruit than the cerebral malformations. Frequently, the patient's initial symptomatology is related to a noise in the ear. In children the massive shunting through the larger dural AVMs may lead to high-output cardiac failure, much as the situation seen with the vein of Galen malformations.

To summarize the clinical symptomatology, the AVMs of the dura, although associated with symptomatology similar to that of their cerebral counterparts, present with a different clinical spectrum; bruits, headaches, and signs of increased intracranial pressure are more common with dural malformations than with cerebral AVMs, whereas seizures and hemorrhage common with cerebral malformations tend to be uncommon with those located in the dura.

Dural malformations of the cranial cavity can be anatomically divided into those occurring supratentorially or in the anterior portion of the cranium, as opposed to those that are generally infratentorial or present in the posterior portion of the cranium. The former tend to drain into the sagittal sinus or the circular or cavernous sinuses, while the latter tend to drain into the posterior sagittal sinus or the straight or lateral sinuses, as well as the torcular region. The malformations can show diffuse small artery to major venous sinus shunting or may be associated with one or two major arteries shunting directly into large venous channels.

The diagnosis is often made from the clinical history; certainly the low incidence of hemorrhage would not lead one to suspect dural malformations as a major cause of intracranial hemorrhage. Definitive diagnosis is made by CT scan and either conventional or digital subtraction angiography. Because of the high flow of these systems and often comprehensive involvement of the dura, it may be difficult to define the location of shunts and detailed anatomy by conventional angiograms. In such cases, it may be necessary to use extra quantities of contrast agent and prolong the filming of the arterial and venous phases of the angiogram.

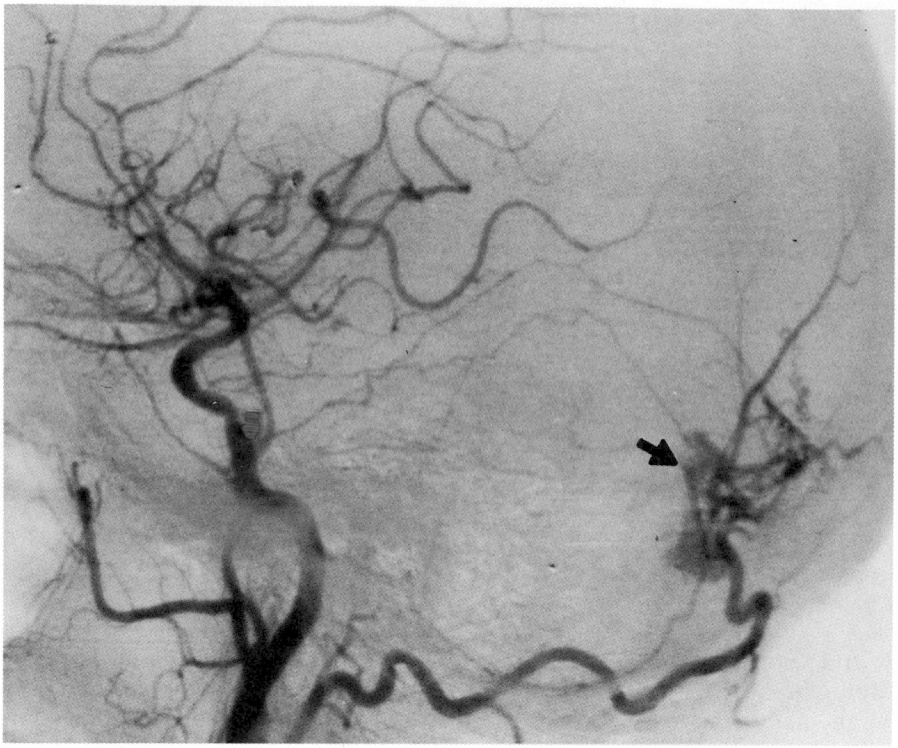

**Fig. 47-21.** Cerebral angiogram demonstrating a large dural malformation (*arrow*) and also a cerebral malformation somewhat masked by the features of the dural malformation.

## Surgical Approach

The treatment of these lesions can be more difficult than the treatment of their cerebral counterparts.[5,64,126] The reason for this is that these malformations tend to be diffuse and parasitize feeding arteries from many and varied dural surfaces. This makes complete obliteration of the lesion more difficult than the obliteration of a cerebral AVM. It is often necessary to remove all the dura surrounding the shunt into the major sinuses and even on occasion remove the major sinuses, which may lead to catastrophic problems, these channels being critical for normal venous drainage of the brain. However, unlike the case of cerebral AVMs, there have been many reports of spontaneous occlusion of dural AVMs during their natural course. This happens more frequently with those located in the anterior portion of the cranium than with those located posteriorly. Perhaps anteriorly the arterial supply is smaller in caliber and the sinuses into which the arteries flow are not as developed or as cavernous as those located in the posterior cranium. Obviously, it may be virtually impossible to locate and excise a dural malformation in the basal dura around such important structures such as the sella turcica, the clivus, cranial nerves, and the blood vessels related to these structures. Complicating the surgery even further is the fact that in some cases, there are both dural and cerebral malformations, interconnected and interdependent. Both must be removed at the time of surgery. The surgical procedures for the treatment of dural AVMs are primarily directed at those of smaller caliber and consist of cutting and resecting portions of the dura, especially the falx and tentorium.[126] This may be achieved with greater surgical efficiency in those lesions located in the posterior cranium; however, the dilemma occurs when the excision reaches the region of the major sinuses, such as the straight, sagittal, or lateral sinuses. In most instances, these cannot be sacrificed and must be left intact. It is often through the small remaining dural pedicle adjacent to these sinuses that the malformation acquires new collateral circulation and continues to be a problem. On other occasions, however, removal of the major feeders is related to spontaneous thrombosis of the residual feeding vessels and the fistula closes. This appears to be the case more frequently in those lesions located in the anterior cranium.

## Embolization

Embolization procedures have been particularly useful in the treatment of dural AVMs.[64] Selective catheterization of the proximal feeding arteries to these malformations can now be accomplished with great efficiency, especially with balloon catheters, which may then be inflated so as to block the distal flow of blood while a solidifying agent or particulate matter is injected distally into the malformation.

However, in some cases, such as those malformations located in and around the sella turcica, it may be impossible to direct the blocking agent into the small arteries directly supplying the malformation, and some of the material may be lost to other vessels comprising various branches of the extracranial circulation. In most instances, this will cause no problem. However, there have been cases of slough of the cutaneous or subcutaneous tissues. Of greater risk is the proximal migration of particulate matter or solidifying agents into the intracranial circulation. Such a complication can lead to catastrophic neurologic deficits due to cerebral embolization in a multitude of areas. Similarly, collaterals between distal branches of the external carotid circulation and the muscular branches of the vertebral artery may lead to embolization by solidifying substances into the posterior circulation. This has disastrous consequences in the distribution of the vertebral circulation, such as in the brain stem and occipital lobes. Therefore the embolization procedures cannot be taken lightly, and appropriate material must be used while the procedure is carried out by specialists who have had broad experience in techniques of embolization. When these criteria are met, it has been possible to successfully obliterate some of these dural malformations. There are many dural malformations fed by branches of critical arteries destined for the cerebral circulation, such as those malformations involving the tentorium, where the blood supply is through the meningohypophyseal trunk, a direct branch of the internal carotid artery. It is generally impossible to embolize into these lesions and those fed by muscular branches of the vertebral artery. On some occasions, it may be propitious to follow embolization by surgery in order to secure certain feeding vessels that cannot be successfully embolized.

## Risks of Therapy

As previously noted, in many cases therapeutic endeavors short of complete obliteration of the malformation may lead to relief of symptomatology such as bruits, headaches, and raised intracranial pressure. Since the incidence of hemorrhage, especially fatal or disabling hemorrhage, is low in these lesions, therapy short of complete success may be acceptable. The surgeon and the interventional neuroradiologist must realize this and be willing to stop short of total anatomic success, realizing that attempts at total obliteration often lead to a much higher complication rate from the therapeutic endeavors.

### Carotid-Cavernous Fistulas

Carotid-cavernous fistulas are in the true sense dural arteriovenous shunts.[21,39,48,52,65,78,89] However, as opposed to most vascular malformations involving the dura, these are anatomically direct single shunts between the internal carotid artery within the cavernous sinus and the various venous channels that make up the cavernous sinus. These fistulas are often associated with trauma, especially fractures through the base of the skull, that distort and lacerate the internal carotid artery, especially at the junction of small branches such as the artery to the cavernous sinus that lies directly within the cavernous sinus. In addition, these fistulas may develop spontaneously without any antecedent history of trauma. The symptom complex is generally classic and leads to the diagnosis in most cases. The symptomatology consists of injection of the sclera of the eye, the presence of dilated vessels around the eye and orbit, a pulsating exophthalamus, chemosis, ophthalmoplegia, and loss of vision in severe cases (Fig. 47-22), all this with a background of an annoying, persistent intracranial bruit. Extradural or intraorbital hemorrhage from these fistulas is extremely rare. The main threat is to the eye and to the patient's psyche because of the consistency of the bruit and the pain and discomfort associated with the ocular pathology.

The history of the therapy of these lesions is the history of neurosurgery, with ingenious attempts being made to stamp out these fistulas, and the degree of success with an intact patient is disturbingly low. Although the fistula is often a single channel between the internal carotid artery and the surrounding veins, attempts to occlude it with the major pressure difference between the artery and the sinus has led to the rapid development of collateral channels to feed the fistula. Therefore obliteration has often been extremely difficult without sacrifice of the internal carotid artery. Since the primary aim is to save the eye or reduce orbital symptomatology, one must also keep in mind the necessity of preserving the patient's vision. Similarly, measures short of total obliteration will only result in the return of the ocular symptomatology after a brief period of respite.

Parkinson,[89] in elegant anatomic studies, has detailed the anatomy of the carotid-cavernous sinus region, the basis of his study being surgical attempts to cure the fistula by direct intervention under extreme hypotension. His anatomic contributions have formed a foundation for current-day treatment. The treatment modalities fall into three major categories: (1) surgical intervention directed at the obliteration of the fistula and often the involved carotid artery, except for the direct technique developed by Parkinson; (2) techniques aimed at thrombosis of the venous side of the fistula; and (3) intravascular techniques developed by neuroradiologists whereby the carotid artery is occluded at the site of the fistula or the fistula itself is occluded with preservation of the carotid artery. A fourth endeavor might be mentioned, and this is the technique of intermittent manual occlusion of the internal carotid artery in the hopes of spontaneous remission of the fistula, which may occur in rare cases.

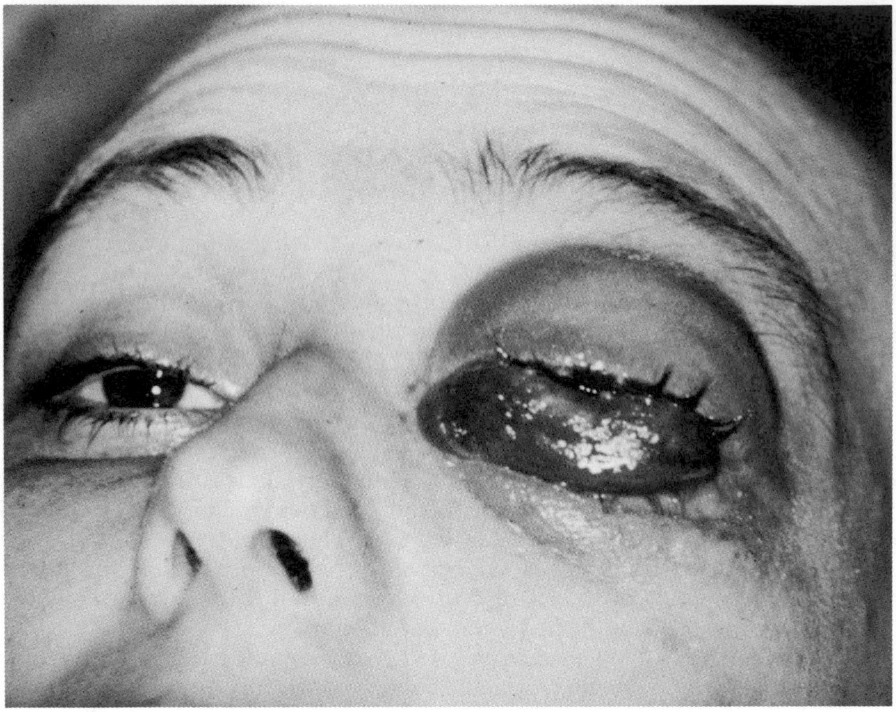

**Fig. 47-22.** Photograph demonstrating intense proptosis and chemosis secondary to a carotid-cavernous fistula.

## Surgical Intervention

The surgical approach, especially that of Parkinson, directly addresses the problem and has been successful in the hands of experienced neurosurgeons, such as Parkinson, but it is not for the faint of heart. It requires meticulous dissection of a high-pressure, high-flow system directly, albeit extreme hypotension and hypothermia have been utilized. It is a major operation and often requires cardiac arrest. In addition, during the stresses of the operation (time being a major factor) the delicate cranial nerves in this area must be preserved if the operation is to reach a successful conclusion with a resultant normal eye. The less direct approaches are the classic neurosurgical approaches and generally result in trapping of the internal carotid artery, especially in the area of the fistula. These operations are often multistaged, the first stage being to place a clip across the internal carotid artery, preferably between the ophthalamic artery and the cavernous sinus (not an easy task to preserve the ophthalamic artery), and then occluding the internal carotid artery in the neck, often preceded by embolization with particulate matter stuffing the internal carotid artery in the cavernous and petrous portions to ensure that all potential collaterals have been eliminated. This series of surgeries is laborious for both the surgeon and the patient. Although generally successful, this treatment may be associated with the risks attendant to the occlusion of a major artery of the cerebral circulation. On some occasions these fistulas are bilateral, and in these situations both internal carotid arteries cannot be occluded.

## Thrombosis Techniques

The technique of thrombosis of the venous portion of the fistula has been developed by Hosobuchi[48] and Mullan.[78] This requires the insertion of fine wires of different metallic content directly into the cavernous sinus. A study of the anatomy of the fistula and of the sinus allows the surgeon to place the wires free of the intracavernous structures of importance, such as the cranial nerves and the internal carotid artery. The coiling of these wires within the sinus, especially wires of a different composition, will provide a nidus for progressive thrombosis of the venous side of the fistula (Fig. 47-23). Unlike arteriovenous fistulas elsewhere, the buttressing effect of the dura prevents explosion of the fistula and thrombosis progresses within the venous side, generally with a smooth occlusion up to the lumen of the internal carotid artery. This procedure results in obliteration of the fistula in a high percentage of cases and preservation of the internal carotid artery. In Hosobuchi's series of 70 patients with a total of 81 fistulas, 11 of which were bilateral, the fistulas were obliterated in all except 3 cases.[48] In 5 patients the thrombosis extended to the internal carotid artery, with occlusion of that artery; 3 of these patients died and 2 developed a hemiparesis. Among the 67 survivors, none suffered significant

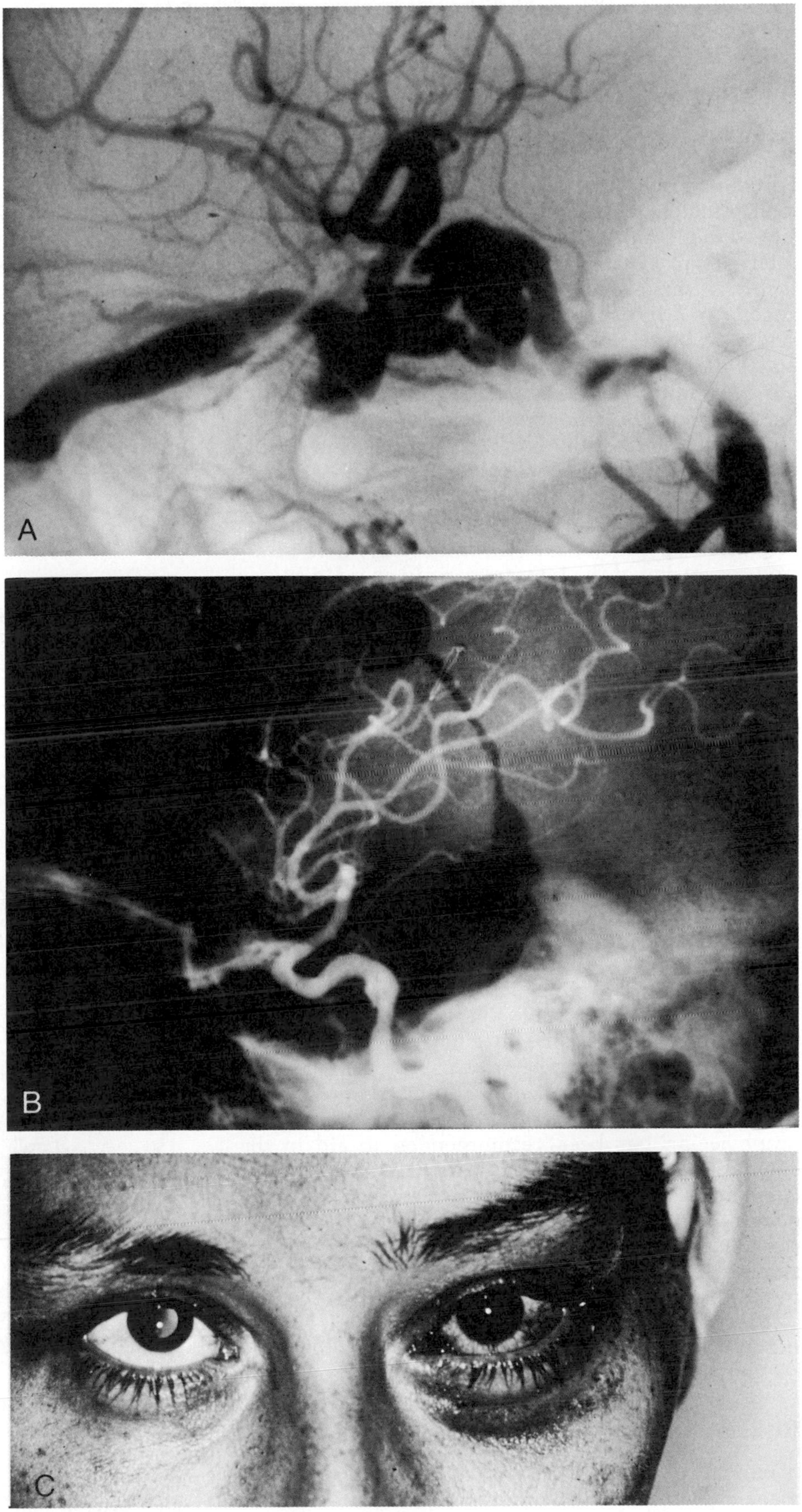


**Fig. 47-23.** Features of the electrothrombotic technique for carotid-cavernous fistula. (**A**) Cerebral angiogram showing the fistula. (**B**) Cerebral arteriogram demonstrating the obliteration of the fistula by the wire technique of Hosobuchi. (**C**) Regression of ocular abnormalities following obliteration of the fistula (same patient as in Fig. 47-22).

morbidity, and many of them showed improvement of extraocular palsies and of impaired vision.

## Intravascular Techniques

Intravascular techniques have now been developed by the interventional neuroradiologist.[21,39,52,65,108] Foremost among these procedures is the use of balloon catheters, either to be placed permanently at the site of the fistula, with occlusion and sacrifice of the internal carotid artery, or, more important, to be detached at the level of the fistula, with occlusion of the venous side but preservation of the internal carotid artery. Debrun et al.[21] have reported the use of detachable balloons filled with a solidifying material. There has been a high degree of success with this procedure and the benefit is the preservation of the carotid artery while the fistula is obliterated. However, the techniques are only successful in the hands of experienced interventional neuroradiologists, and there may be the hazard of deflation of the balloon and its migration up the internal carotid artery, with disastrous occlusion of the internal carotid or middle cerebral artery. Debrun et al.[21] used the detachable balloon in 17 cases with no mortality and only 1 significant morbidity. In all patients, the fistula was successfully occluded. Carotid artery flow was preserved in 12 of the 17 patients, and in the other 5 there were various degrees of occlusion of the internal carotid artery by the balloon. Viñuela et al.[134] have reviewed the treatment of these lesions by endovascular methods and emphasize that this method is now the treatment of choice. The approach may be either arterial (carotid artery) or venous (inferior petrossal sinus or superior ophthalmic vein).

## Intermittent Manual Occlusion of the Internal Carotid Artery

Finally, the conservative approach to carotid-cavernous fistulas has some merit, considering that a spontaneous disappearance rate of 5 percent exists in relation to these fistula. Intermittent compression of the internal carotid artery in the neck by the patient or physician has been recommended to aid in the spontaneous regression of these fistulas. In the milder cases, it may be necessary to take no action, since the ocular symptomatology is minimal and not life-threatening. In such cases, one can hope for either spontaneous regression or maintenance of a state of minimal symptomatology that is of no great distress to the patient. Valuable time is not lost while watching and evaluating such fistulas, as they will rarely pick up additional collateral circulation.

## Risks of Therapeutic Maneuvers

Whichever method is selected, it is important to place a premium on the preservation of the internal carotid artery and consider the degree of symptomatology in gauging the risks of the various therapeutic maneuvers. For example, it is difficult to justify a trapping procedure that entails obliteration of the internal carotid artery as well as external carotid artery with the result of glaucoma in the involved eye, even though the fistula has been eliminated. The glaucoma may progress to an ophthalmitis which results in the enucleation of that eye. The main purpose, of course, is to preserve vision and improve the eye, whereas in such an instance the eye is lost and there is a possible threat to the opposite eye from sympathetic ophthalmitis. In such a case the therapeutic endeavors carry a much higher risk than the natural history of the disease process.

# Cryptic Malformations

Cryptic malformations comprise a heterogeneous group, traditionally including any vascular anomaly that is visible either on CT scan or histologic evaluation but cannot be identified on angiograms[16,66,72] (Fig. 47-24). It is presumed that the nutrient vasculature is

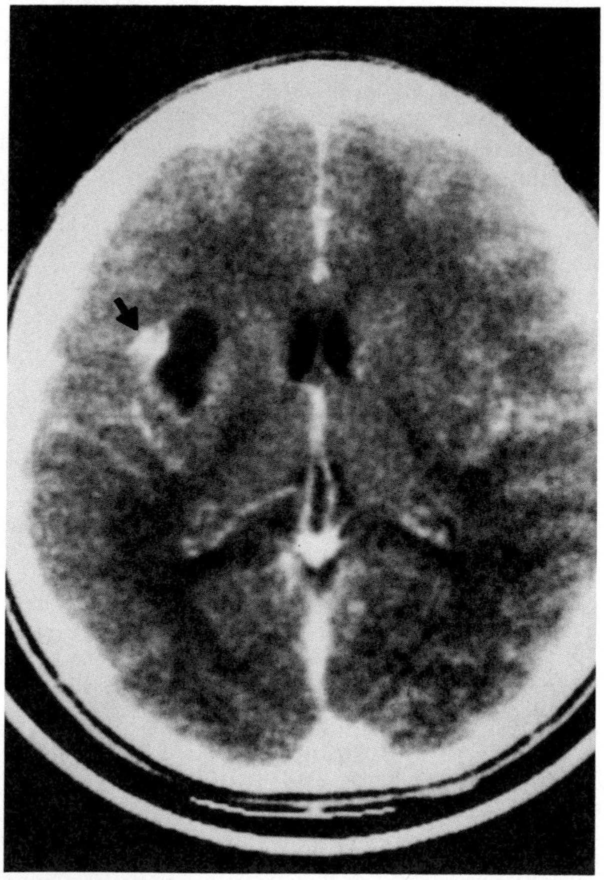

**Fig. 47-24.** A scan demonstrating a cryptic arteriovenous malformation (*arrow*) (the cause of encephalomalacia following hemorrhage). This was not demonstrable on arteriography. This malformation was successfully removed. Only a minute arterial supply to the malformation was observed at surgery.

too small to be observed on an angiogram. The lesions are generally discovered when an "apparently spontaneous" hematoma is evacuated from the brain. In the walls of the hematoma cavity, the surgeon may note a discrete nodule, which, when later examined by the neuropathologist, will be found to contain a mixture of thrombosed and patent vascular channels. In fact, the term "cryptic malformation" is a misnomer, since this category may embrace small AVMs, venous and cavernous malformations, as well as telangiectasias, which are not angiographically visible.

## REFERENCES


1. Amacher AL, Allock JM, Drake CG: Cerebral angiomas: the sequelae of surgical treatment. J Neurosurg 37:571, 1972
2. Amacher AL, Shillito J, Jr: The syndromes and surgical treatment of aneurysms of the great vein of Galen. J Neurosurg 39:89, 1973
3. Aminoff MJ: Vascular anomalies in the intracranial dura mater. Brain 96:601, 1973
4. Awad IA, LeBlanc R, Little JR: Blood flow measurements in intracranial arteriovenous malformations. p. 91. In Barrow DL (ed): Intracranial Vascular Malformations: Neurosurgical Topics. AANS Publications Committee, IL, 1990
5. Awad IA, Little JR: Dural arteriovenous malformations. p. 219. In Barrow DL (ed): Intracranial Vascular Malformations: Neurosurgical Topics. AANS Publications Committee, IL, 1990
6. Barnett GH, Little JR, Ebralium ZY et al: Cerebral circulation during arteriovenous malformation operation. Neurosurgery 20:836, 1987
7. Barrow DL: Intracranial Vascular Malformations: Neurosurgical Topics. AANS Publications Committee, IL, 1990
8. Batjer HH, Devous MD, Sr, Seibert GB et al: Intracranial arteriovenous malformation: relationship between clinical factors and surgical complications. Neurosurgery 24:75, 1989
9. Batjer HH, Purdy PD, Giller CA, Samson DS: Evidence of redistribution of cerebral blood flow during treatment for an intracranial arteriovenous malformation. Neurosurgery 25:599, 1989
10. Berenstein A, Kricheff II: Catheter and material selection for transarterial embolization. I. Technical considerations. II. Materials. Radiology 132:631, 1979
11. Betti OO, Munari C, Rosler R: Stereotactic radiosurgery with the linear accelerator: treatment of arteriovenous malformations. Neurosurgery 24:311, 1989
12. Brown RD, Jr, Wiebers DO, Forbes C et al: The natural history of unruptured intracranial arteriovenous malformations. J Neurosurg 68:352, 1988
13. Brown RD, Jr, Wiebers DO, Forbes GS: Unruptured intracranial aneurysms and arteriovenous malformations: frequency of intracranial hemorrhage and relationship of lesions. J Neurosurg 73:859, 1990
14. Bruce DA: Surgery of the vein of Galen arteriovenous malformation. Contemp Neurosurg 3:1, 1981
15. Chou SN, Erickson DL, Ortiz-uarez HJ: Surgical treatment of vascular lesions in the brain stem. J Neurosurg 42:23, 1975
16. Cohen HCM, Tucker WS, Humphreys RP, Perrin RJ: Angiographically cryptic histologically verified cerebrovascular malformations. Neurosurgery 10:704, 1982
17. Cromwell LD, Harris BA: Treatment of cerebral arteriovenous malformations: a combined neurosurgical and neuroradiological approach. J Neurosurg 52:705, 1982
18. DaPian R, Pasqualin A, Scienza R, Vivenza C: Microsurgical treatment of ten arteriovenous malformations in critical areas of the cerebrum. J Microsurg 1:305, 1980
19. DaPian R, Pasqualin A, Scienza R: Microsurgical treatment of juxtapeduncular angiomas. Surg Neurol 17:16, 1982
20. Debrun GM, Vinuela F, Fox A, Drake CG: Embolization of cerebral arteriovenous malformations with bucrylate: experience in 46 cases. J Neurosurg 56:615, 1982
21. Debrun GM, Vinuela F, Fox AJ et al: Indications for treatment and classification of 132 carotid-cavernous fistulas. Neurosurgery 22:285, 1988
22. Dias MS, Sekhar LN: Intracranial hemorrhage from aneurysms and arteriovenous malformations during pregnancy and the puerperium. Neurosurgery 27:855, 1990
23. Drake CG: Surgical removal of arteriovenous malformations from the brain stem and cerebellopontine angle. J Neurosurg 43:661, 1975
24. Drake CG: Cerebral arteriovenous malformations: considerations for and experience with surgical treatment in 166 cases. Clin Neurosurg 26:145, 1979
25. Drake CG: Arteriovenous malformations of the brain: the options for management. N Engl J Med 309:308, 1983
26. Drake CG, Friedman AH, Peerless SJ: Posterior fossa arteriovenous malformations. J Neurosurg 64:1, 1986
27. Epstein N, Epstein F: Arteriovenous malformation presenting as a first seizure in a 13-year-old child: surgical indications. Neurosurgery 7:391, 1980
28. Farrell DF, Forno LS: Symptomatic capillary telangiectasis of the brainstem without hemorrhage: report of an unusual case. Neurology (NY), 20:341, 1970
29. Forster DMC, Steiner L, Hakanson S: Arteriovenous malformations of the brain: a long-term clinical study. J Neurosurg 37:562, 1972
30. Fournier D, TerBrugge KG, Willinsky R et al: Endovascular treatment of intracerebral arteriovenous malformations: experience in 49 cases. J Neurosurg 75:228, 1991
31. Fox JL, Al Mefty O: Embolization of an arteriovenous malformation of the brain stem. Surg Neurol 8:7, 1977
32. Fults D, Kelly DL: The natural history of arteriovenous malformations of the brain: a clinical study. Neurosurgery 15:658, 1984

33. Garretson HD: Postoperative pressure and flow changes in the feeding arteries of cerebral arteriovenous malformations. Neurosurgery 4:544, 1979
34. Garretson HD: Intracranial arteriovenous malformations. p. 1448. In: Wilkins RH, Rengachary SS (eds): Neurosurgery. McGraw-Hill, New York, 1985
35. Garrido E, Stein BM: Removal of an arteriovenous malformation from the basal ganglion. J Neurosurg Psychiatry 41:992, 1978
36. Gold AP, Ransohoff J, Carter S: Vein of Galen malformation. Acta Neurol Scand, suppl. 40:1, 1964
37. Graf CJ, Perret G, Torner JC: Bleeding from cerebral arteriovenous malformations as part of their natural history. J Neurosurg 58:331, 1983
38. Guidetti B., DeLitala A: Intracranial arteriovenous malformations: conservative and surgical treatment. J Neurosurg 53:149, 1980
39. Halbach VV, Higashida RT, Hieshima GB, Hardin CW: Transvenous embolization of direct carotid-cavernous fistulas. ANJR 9:741, 1988
40. Halbach VV, Higashida RT, Yang P et al: Preoperative balloon occlusion of arteriovenous malformations. Neurosurgery 22:301, 1988
41. Hassler W, Steinmetz H: Cerebral hemodynamics in angioma patients: an intraoperative study. J Neurosurg 67:822, 1987
42. Hayashi S, Arimoto T, Itakura T et al: The association of intracranial aneurysms and arteriovenous malformation of the brain. J Neurosurg 55:971, 1981
43. Heros RC, Korosue K: Radiation treatment of cerebral arteriovenous malformations. N Engl J Med 323:127, 1990
44. Heros RC, Korosue K, Riebold P: Surgical excision of cerebral arteriovenous malformations: late results. Neurosurgery 26:570, 1990
45. Hilal SK, Sane P, Mawad ME et al: Therapeutic interventional radiologic procedures in neuroradiology. p. 1094. In Abrams (ed): Abrams Angiography: Vascular and Interventional Radiology. 3rd Ed. Little, Brown, Boston, 1983
46. Hoffman HJ, Chuang S, Hendrick EB et al: Aneurysms of the vein of Galen. J Neurosurg 57:316, 1982
47. Horton JC, Chambers WA, Lyons SL et al: Pregnancy and the risk of hemorrhage from cerebral arteriovenous malformations. Neurosurgery 27:867, 1990
48. Hosobuchi Y: Electrothrombosis of carotid-cavernous fistula. J Neurosurg 42:76, 1975
49. Hunt B, Suss RA, Samson D: Intracranial arteriovenous malformations associated with aneurysms. Neurosurgery 18:29, 1986
50. Jane J, Kassell N, Torner J, Winn HR: The natural history of ancurysms and arteriovenous malformations. J Neurosurg 62:321, 1985
51. Kerber CW: Use of balloon catheters in the treatment of cranial arterial abnormalities. Stroke 11:210, 1980
52. Kerber CW, Bank WO, Cromwell LD: Cyanoacrylate occlusion of carotid-cavernous fistula with preservation of carotid artery flow. Neurosurgery 4:210, 1979
53. Kjellberg RN, Hanamura T, Davis KR et al: Bragg-Peak proton beam therapy for arteriovenous malformations of the brain. N Engl J Med 309:269, 1983
54. Kondziolka D, Lunsford LD, Coffrey RJ et al: Stereotactic radiosurgery of angiographically occult vascular malformations: indications and preliminary experience. Neurosurgery 27:892, 1990
55. Kunc Z: Surgery of arteriovenous malformations in the speech and motor sensory regions. J Neurosurg 40:291, 1974
56. Kvam DA, Michelsen WJ, Quest DO: Intracerebral hemorrhage as a complication of artificial embolization. Neurosurg 7:491, 1980
57. Levy RP, Fabrikant JI, Frankel KA et al: Stereotactic heavy-charged-particle Bragg peak radiosurgery for the treatment of intracranial arteriovenous malformations in childhood and adolescence. Neurosurgery 24:841, 1989
58. Lindegaard K, Grolimund P, Aaslid R, Nornes H: Evaluation of cerebral AVMs using transcranial Doppler ultrasound. J Neurosurg 65:335, 1986
59. Luessenhop AJ, Presper JH: Surgical embolization of cerebral arteriovenous malformations through internal carotid and vertebral arteries: long-term results. J Neurosurg 42:443, 1975
60. Luessenhop AJ, Rosa L: Cerebral arteriovenous malformations. Indications for and results of surgery, and the role of intravascular techniques. J Neurosurg 60:14, 1984
61. Luessenhop AJ, Spence WT: Artificial embolization of cerebral arteries: report of use in a case of arteriovenous malformation. JAMA 172:1153, 1960
62. Lunsford LD: Treatment of arteriovenous malformations by radiosurgery. p. 179. In Barrow DL (ed): Intracranial Vascular Malformations: Neurosurgical Topics. AANS Publications Committee, IL, 1990
63. Lunsford LD, Flickinger J, Coffey RJ: Stereotactic gamma knife radiosurgery. Arch Neurol 47:169, 1990
64. Manaka S, Izawa M, Nawata H: Dural arteriovenous malformation treated by artificial embolization with liquid silicone. Surg Neurol 7:63, 1977
65. Manelfe C, Berenstein A: Treatment of carotid-cavernous fistulas by venous approach. J Neuroradiol 7:13, 1980
66. Margolis G, Odom GL, Woodhall B, Blon B: Role of small AVM in production of intracerebral hematomas. J Neurosurg 8:564, 1951
67. Martin NA, Wilson CB: Medial occipital arteriovenous malformations. J Neurosurg 56:798, 1982
68. Mawad M, Hilal S, Michelsen WJ et al: Occlusive vascular disease associated with cerebral arteriovenous malformations. Radiology 153:401, 1984
69. McCormick PC, Michelsen WJ: Management of intracranial cavernous and venous malformations. p. 197. In Barrow DL (ed): Intracranial Vascular Malformations: Neurosurgical Topics. AANS Publications Committee, IL, 1990

70. McCormick WF: The pathology of vascular ("arteriovenous") malformations. J Neurosurg 24:807, 1966
71. McCormick WF, Hardman JM, Boulter TR: Vascular malformations ("angiomas") of the brain with special reference to those occurring in the posterior fossa. J Neurosurg. 28:241, 1968
72. McCormick WF, Nofzinger JD: "Cryptic" vascular malformations of the central nervous system. J Neurosurg 24:865, 1966
73. McCormick WF, Rosenfield DB: Massive brain hemorrhage: a review of 144 cases and an examination of their causes. Stroke 4:946, 1973
74. Mickle JP, Quisling RG: The transtorcular embolization of vein of Galen aneurysms. J Neurosurg 64:731, 1986
75. Morello G, Broghi GP: Cerebral angiomas: a report of the 154 personal cases and a comparison between the results of surgical excision and conservative management. Acta Neurochir (Wien) 28:135, 1973
76. Morgan MK, Johnson I, Besser M et al: Cerebral arteriovenous malformations, steal and the hypertensive breakthrough threshold. J Neurosurg 66:563, 1987
77. Moritake K, Handa H, Mori K et al: Venous angiomas of the brain. Surg Neurol 14:95, 1980
78. Mullan S: Treatment of carotid-cavernous fistulas by cavernous sinus occlusion. J Neurosurg 50:131, 1979
79. Mullan S, Brown FD, Patronas NJ: Hyperemic and ischemic problems of surgical treatment of arteriovenous malformations. J Neurosurg 51:757, 1979
80. Muraszko K, Wang HH, Pelton G, Stein BM: A study of the reactivity of feeding vessels to arteriovenous malformations: correlation with clinical outcome. Neurosurgery 26:190, 1990
81. Nishizaki T, Tamaki N, Matsumoto S et al: Consideration of the operative indications for posterior fossa venous angiomas. Surg Neurol 25:441, 1986
82. Nornes H, Grip A: Hemodynamic aspects of cerebral arteriovenous malformations. J Neurosurg 53:456, 1980
83. Nornes H, Grip A, Wikeby P: Intraoperative evaluation of cerebral hemodynamics using directional Doppler technique. I. Arteriovenous malformations. J Neurosurg 50:145, 1979
84. Numaguchi Y, Kitamura K, Fukui M et al: Intracranial venous angiomas. Surg Neurol 18:193, 1982
85. Ogilvy CS: Radiation therapy for arteriovenous malformations: a review. Neurosurgery 26;5:725, 1990
86. Ogilvy CS, Heros RC, Ojemann RG et al: Angiographically occult arteriovenous malformations. J Neurosurg 69:350, 1988
87. Okabe T, Meyer JS, Okayasu H et al: Xenon-enhanced CT CBF measurements in cerebral AVMs before and after excision: contribution to pathogenesis and treatment. J Neurosurg 59:21, 1983
88. Ondra SL, Troupp H, George E, Schwav K: The natural history of symptomatic arteriovenous malformations of the brain: a 24-year follow-up assessment. J Neurosurg 73:387, 1990
89. Parkinson D: Carotid cavernous fistula: direct repair with preservation of the carotid artery: technical note. J Neurosurg 38:99, 1973
90. Parkinson D, Bachers G: Arteriovenous malformations: summary of 100 consecutive supratentorial cases. J Neurosurg 53:285, 1980
91. Pasqualin A, Scienza R, Cioffi F et al: Treatment of cerebral arteriovenous malformation with a combination of preoperative embolization and surgery. Neurosurgery 29:358, 1991
92. Paterson JH, McKissock W: A clinical survey of intracranial angiomas with special reference to their mode of progression and surgical treatment: a report of 110 cases. Brain 79:233, 1956
93. Patronas NJ, Marx WJ, Duda EE, Mullan JJ: Microvascular embolization of arteriovenous malformations: predicting success by cerebral angiography. Am J Neuroradiol 1:459, 1980
94. Pellettieri L: Surgical versus conservative treatment of intracranial arteriovenous malformations: a study in surgical decision-making. Acta Neurochir, suppl. (Wien) 29:1, 1979.
95. Perret G: The epidemiology and clinical course of arteriovenous malformations. p. 21. In Pia HW, Gleave JRW, Grote E, Zierski J (eds): Cerebral Angiomas: Advances in Diagnosis and Therapy. Springer-Verlag, New York, 1975
96. Perret G, Nishioka H: Report on the cooperative study of intracranial aneurysms and subarachnoid hemorrhage. VI. Arteriovenous malformations. J Neurosurg 25:467, 1966
97. Pertuiset B, Ancri D, Clergue F: Preoperative evaluation of hemodynamic factors in cerebral arteriovenous malformations for selection of a radical surgical tactic with special reference to vascular autoregulation disorders. Neurol Res 4:209, 1982
98. Pevsner PH, Doppman JL: Therapeutic embolization with a microballoon catheter. AJNR 1:171, 1980
99. Pia HW, Gleave JRW, Grote E et al: Cerebral Angiomas: Advances in Diagnosis and Therapy. p. 285. Springer Verlag, New York, 1975
100. Pool JL: Excision of cerebral arteriovenous malformations. J Neurosurg 29:312, 1968
101. Post KD, Stein BM: Technique for spinal drainage. Neurosurgery 4:255, 1979
102. Rigamonti D, Spetzler RF, Johnson PC et al: Cerebral vascular malformations. BNI Q 3:18, 1987
103. Rigamonti D, Spetzler RF, Drayer BP et al: Appearance of venous malformations on magnetic resonance imaging. J Neurosurg 69:535, 1988
104. Rosenblum BR, Bonner RF, Oldfield EH: Intraoperative measurement of cortical blood flow adjacent to cerebral AVMs using laser Doppler velocimetry. J Neurosurg 66:396, 1987
105. Rothfus WE, Albright AL, Casey KF et al: Cerebellar venous angiomas: "benign" entity? AJNR 5:61, 1984
106. Saito Y, Kobayashi N: Cerebral venous angiomas. Radiology 139:87, 1981
107. Senegor M, Dohrmann GJ, Wollman RL: Venous angiomas of the posterior fossa should be considered anomalous venous drainage. Surg Neurol 19:26, 1983

108. Serbinenko FA: Balloon catheterization and occlusion of major cerebral vessels. J Neurosurg 41:125, 1974
109. Simard JM, Garcia-Benjochea F, Ballinger WE et al: Cavernous angioma: a review of 126 collected and 12 new clinical cases. Neurosurgery 18:162, 1986
110. Sisti MB, Solomon RA, Stein BM: Stereotactic craniotomy in the resection of small arteriovenous malformations. J Neurosurg 75:40, 1991
111. Solomon RA, Stein BM: Management of arteriovenous malformations of the brain stem. J Neurosurg 64:857, 1986
112. Solomon RA, Stein BM: Surgical treatment of arteriovenous malformations that follow the tentorial ring. Neurosurgery 18:708, 1986
113. Solomon RA, Stein BM: Interhemispheric approach for the surgical removal of thalmocaudate arteriovenous malformations. J Neurosurg 66:345, 1987
114. Spetzler RF, Martin NA: A proposed grading system for arteriovenous malformations. J Neurosurg 65:476, 1986
115. Spetzler RF, Martin NA, Carter P et al: Surgical management of large AVMs by staged embolization and operative excision. J Neurosurg 67:17, 1987
116. Spetzler RF, Wilson CB, Weinstein P et al: Normal perfusion pressure breakthrough theory. Clin Neurosurg 25:651, 1978
117. Stein BM: Arteriovenous malformations of the medial cerebral hemisphere and the limbic system. J Neurosurg 60:23, 1984
118. Stein BM: General techniques for surgical removal of arteriovenous malformations. p. 143. In Wilson C, Stein BM (eds): Current Neurosurgical Practice. Intracranial Arteriovenous Malformations. Williams & Wilkins, Baltimore, 1984
119. Stein BM, Mohr JP, Sisti MB: Is radiosurgery all that it appears to be? (Letter to the Editor.) Arch Neurol 48:19, 1991
120. Stein BM, Solomon RA: Surgical approaches to posterior fossa arteriovenous malformations. Clin Neurosurg 37:353, 1991
121. Stein BM, Wolpert SM: Surgical and embolic treatment of cerebral arteriovenous malformations. Surg Neurol 7:359, 1977
122. Stein BM, Wolpert SM: Arteriovenous Malformations of the Brain. I. Current concepts and treatment. Arch Neurol 37:1, 1980
123. Stein BM, Wolpert SM: Arteriovenous malformations of the brain. II. Current concepts and treatment. Arch Neurol 37:69, 1980
124. Steinberg GK, Fabrikant JI, Marks MP et al: Stereotactic heavy-charged-particle Bragg-peak radiation for intracranial arteriovenous malformations. N Engl J Med 323:96, 1990
125. Steiner L, Leksell L, Forster DMC et al: Stereotactic radiosurgery in intracranial arteriovenous malformations. Acta Neurochir [Suppl] (Wien) 21:195, 1974
126. Sundt TM, Jr, Piepgras DG: The surgical approach to arteriovenous malformations of the lateral and sigmoid dural sinuses. J Neurosurg 59:32, 1983
127. Tognetti F, Andreoli A, Cuscini A, Testa C: Successful management of an intracranial arteriovenous malformation by conventional irradiation. J Neurosurg 63:193, 1985
128. Troupp H: Arteriovenous malformations of the brain: what are the indications for operation? p. 210. In Morley TP (ed): Current Controversies in Neurosurgery. WB Saunders, Philadelphia, 1976.
129. Troupp H, Marttila I, Halonen V: Arteriovenous malformations of the brain: prognosis without operation. Acta Neurochir 22:125, 1970
130. Vaquero J, Salazar R, Martinez P et al: Cavernomas of the central nervous system: clinical syndromes, CT scan diagnosis, and prognosis after surgical treatment in 25 cases. Acta Neurochir 85:29, 1987
131. Viale GL, Turtas S, Pau A: Surgical removal of striate arteriovenous malformations. Surg Neurol 14:321, 1980
132. Vinuela F, Dion JE, Fox AJ et al: Interventional neuroradiology for intracranial arteriovenous malformations. p. 169. In Barrow DL (ed): Intracranial Vascular Malformations: Neurosurgical Topics. AANS Publications Committee, IL, 1990
133. Vinuela FV, Dion J, Lylyk P, Duckweiler G: Update on interventional neuroradiology. AJR 153:23, 1989
134. Vinuela FV, Fox AJ, Pelz D et al: Angiographic follow-up of large cerebral AVMs incompletely embolized with isobutyl 2-cyanoacrylate. AJNR 7:919, 1986
135. Voigt K, Yasargil MG: Cerebral cavernous haemangiomas or cavernomas. Incidence, pathology, localization, diagnosis, clinical features and treatment: review of the literature and report of an unusual case. Neurochirurgia 19:59, 1976
136. Waltimo O: The relationship of size, density, and localization of intracranial arteriovenous malformations to the type of initial symptom. J Neurol Sci 19:13, 1973
137. Weil S, Tew JM, Steiner L: Comparison of radiosurgery and microsurgery for treatment of cavernous malformations of the brainstem, abstracted. J Neurosurg 72:713, 1990
138. Wilkins RH: Natural history of intracranial vascular malformations: a review. Neurosurgery 16:421, 1985
139. Wilson C, Stein BM: Intracranial Arteriovenous Malformations in Current Neurosurgical Practice. p. 1. Williams & Wilkins, Baltimore, 1984
140. Wilson CB, U HS, Dominque, J: Microsurgical treatment of intracranial vascular malformations. J Neurosurg 51:446, 1979
141. Winston KR, Lutz W: Linear accelerator as a neurosurgical tool for stereotactic radiosurgery. Neurosurgery 22:454, 1988
142. Wolpert SM, Stein BM: Catheter embolization of intracranial arteriovenous malformations as an aid to surgical excision. Neuroradiology 10:73, 1975
143. Wolpert SM, Stein BM: Factors governing the course of emboli in the therapeutic embolization of cerebral arteriovenous malformations. Radiology 131;1:125, 1979

144. Yamada S, Brauer FS, Knierim DS: Direct approach to arteriovenous malformations in functional areas of the cerebral hemisphere. J Neurosurg 72:418, 1990
145. Yasargil MG, Antic J, Lacha R et al: Arteriovenous malformations of vein of Galen: microsurgical treatment. Surg Neurol 6:195, 1976
146. Yasargil MG, Jain KK, Antic J et al: Arteriovenous malformations of the anterior and middle portion of the corpus callosum: microsurgical treatment. Surg Neurol 5:67, 1976
147. Yasargil MG, Jain KK, Antic J, Laciga R: Arteriovenous malformations of the splenium of the corpus callosum: microsurgical treatment. Surg Neurol 5:5, 1976
148. Young WL, Prohovnik I, Ornstein E et al: The effect of arteriovenous malformation resection on cerebrovascular reactivity to carbon dioxide. Neurosurgery 27:257, 1990

# 48

# *MANAGEMENT OF SPINAL VASCULAR MALFORMATIONS*

Paul C. McCormick
Bennett M. Stein

Spinal arteriovenous (AVMs) and cavernous malformations are the most commonly encountered spinal vascular malformations. While autopsy studies have described spinal venous malformations (angiomas) or capillary telangiectasia, these lesions rarely, if ever, require treatment. Spinal AVMs may be further classified into dural and intradural types according to the location of their nidus.

Management of spinal vascular malformations continues to evolve since the introduction of selective spinal angiography some 30 years ago. Since then, a better understanding of the anatomy and pathophysiology of these lesions, combined with contemporary imaging sophistication, endovascular capabilities, refined microsurgical techniques, and intraoperative spinal monitoring, has resulted in an increasing percentage of successful elimination of these treacherous lesions.

## ARTERIOVENOUS MALFORMATIONS

### Dural Fistula

The dural malformation (type I, long dorsal AVM) is the most common type of spinal AVM. This lesion accounts for about 75 percent of AVMs in most reported series.[1,7] Unlike true AVMs however, the nidus of this malformation is not a conglomeration of abnormally formed vessels, but rather a direct, probably acquired, arteriovenous fistula (Fig. 48-1). The fistula is typically located on the superior aspect of the dural root sleeve and consists of a direct communication between a radicular artery and a radicular vein. The absence of venous valves allows retrograde filling of the intradural venous system. Thus, the entire intradural component of the malformation is venous. Elevated intradural venous pressure caused by the fistula, probably in conjunction with an acquired or developmental abnormality of intradural venous drainage, contributes to the pathologic venous hypertension and progressive ischemia of the spinal cord. Thus, these lesions may share a similar etiology to the intracranial dural malformations that are frequently associated with dural venous sinus thrombosis. The dural fistula almost exclusively occurs in the lower thoracic and lumbar region in patients of middle and advanced years. Men are affected four times more commonly than women. The absence of associated metameric anomalies further attest to an acquired etiology. A relentless, progressive paraparesis, often punctuated by an exacerbation of symptoms with exercise or episodic worsening from venous thrombosis, is the well-known history of this lesion.

Treatment of the dural malformation is directed at elimination of the fistula. Stripping of the tortuous draining vein off the surface of the spinal cord is no longer advocated because it is unnecessary and may further comprise the venous drainage of the spinal

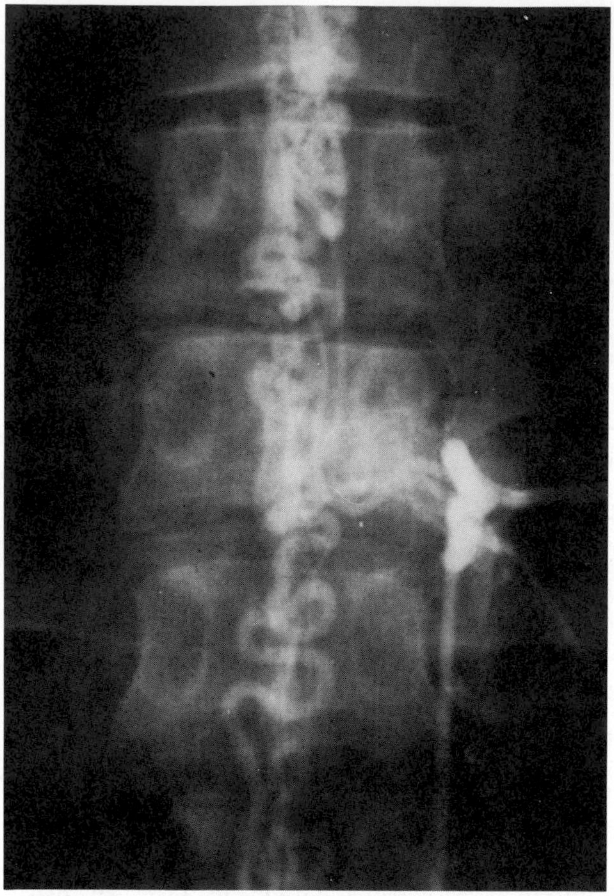

A

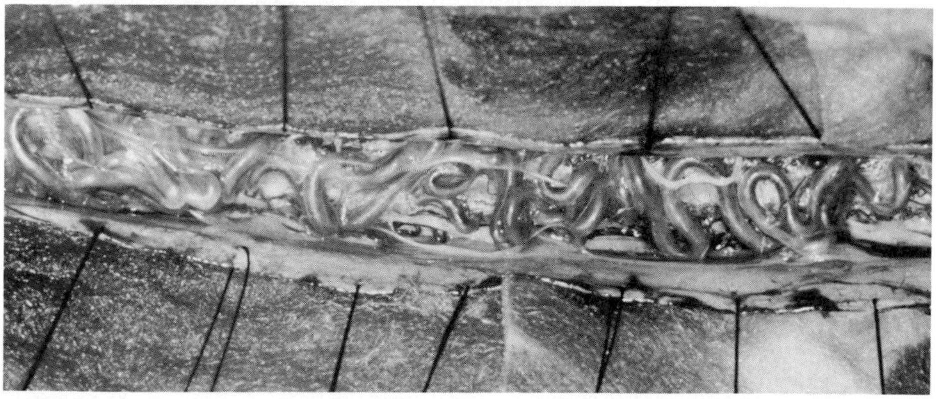

B

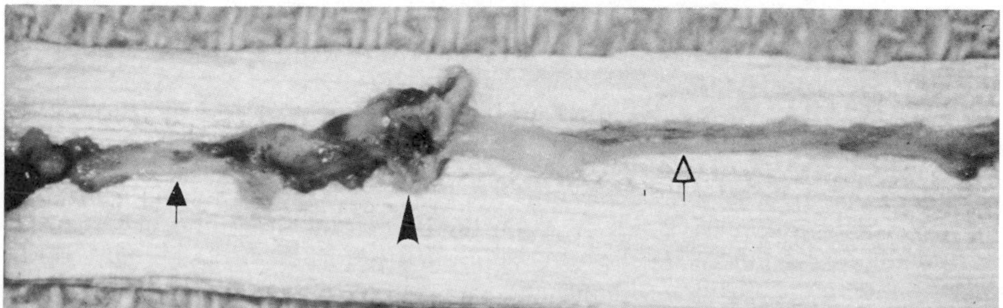

C

**Fig. 48-1.** (**A**) Selective spinal angiogram (right T10 intercostal artery injection) demonstrates typical single, long, coiled vessel, which represents engorged dorsal vein. (**B**) Operative photograph shows appearance of the tortuous vein on the dorsal surface of the spinal cord. (**C**) Photograph of excised specimen shows feeding artery (*closed arrow*), draining vein (*open arrow*), and intervening dural fistula (*arrowhead*). (*Figure continues.*)

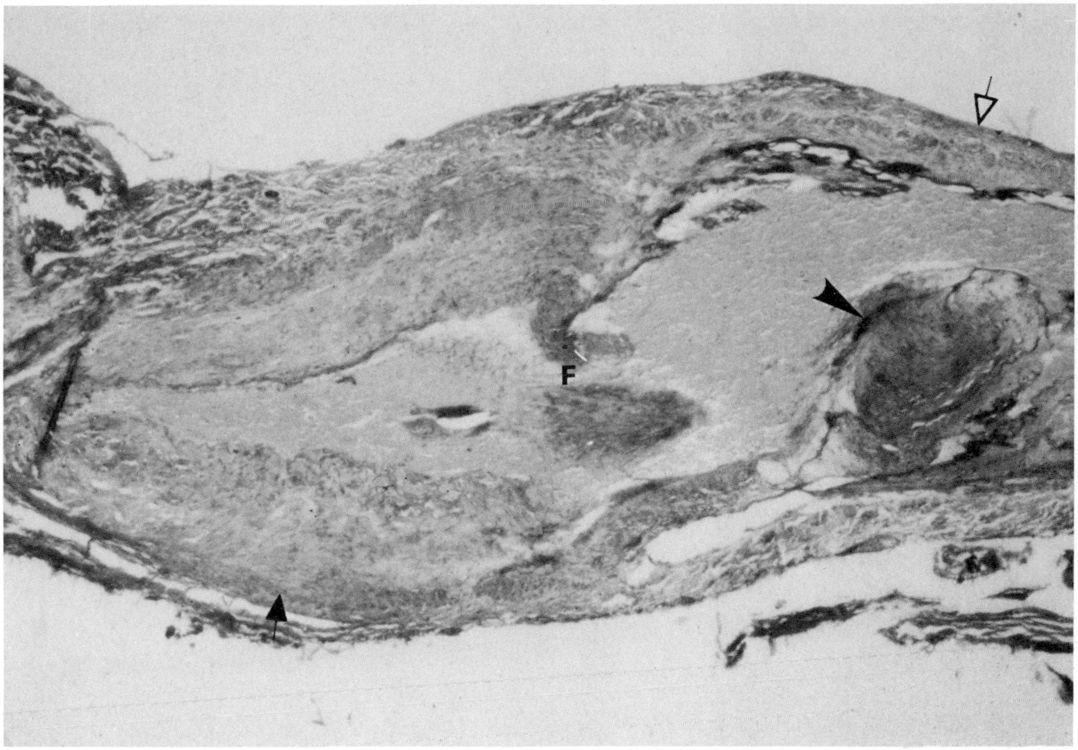


D

**Fig. 48-1** (*Continued*). (**D**) Photomicrograph of longitudinal section of Fig. C shows fistulous communication between thick-walled artery (*closed arrow*) and draining vein (*open arrow*). Note the intimal cushion (*arrowhead*), which is the morphologic consequence of direct arterial flow into a vein. The fistula site is also demonstrated.

cord. While endovascular embolization has been successful in blocking the fistula, the effects are usually short-lived because recanalization almost invariably occurs.[3] Surgical elimination of the fistula, therefore, represents the treatment of choice. This is a fairly simple procedure and may consist either of division of the draining vein near the dural root sleeve or excision of the dural root sleeve, which contains the fistula (Fig. 48-1).

Like most other progressive disorders of the spinal cord, outcome is most dependent on the immediate preoperative status. Significant return of neurologic function, which may be dramatic, can be anticipated in patients with mild to moderate deficit or with deficit of short duration. Fixed or long-standing deficits (i.e., several months to years) only rarely are affected by surgery. Thus, a premium is placed on early diagnosis and treatment of these lesions.

## Intradural Arteriovenous Malformations

Intradural arteriovenous malformations are further divided into glomus and juvenile types, and the rare direct arteriovenous fistula. These are true arteriovenous malformations, which are similar to their intracranial parenchymal counterparts. Their occasional association with metameric skin, bone, or other mesenchymal anomalies attest to their congenital origin. While dural fistulas occur almost exclusively in the thoracic and lumbar region, intradural malformations seem to occur in proportion to spinal cord vascular supply. Thus, cervical cord and lumbar enlargement/conus are the most common regions affected, while the thoracic cord is only rarely involved.

The glomus AVM is much more common in our experience. We reserve the term *juvenile AVM* to describe those huge-flow fistulous spinal malformations with vertebral and paraspinal involvement. These rare lesions typically present in childhood or adolescence with hemorrhage, pain, or a progressive neurologic deficit, which results from mechanical compression or arterial steal.[5] Cardiovascular abnormalities and an audible bruit are frequently present. Definitive therapy for these "juvenile" lesions is seldom possible although it has been reported when there has been definable nidus within the spinal cord.[6] More commonly, the entire transverse area of the spinal cord is contained within the interstices of the malformation. Partial treatment with endovascular techniques, however, may improve pain, cardiac symptoms, and neurologic deficit from arterial steal in some cases. These benefits are usually temporary, requiring repeat procedures at variable intervals.

A B

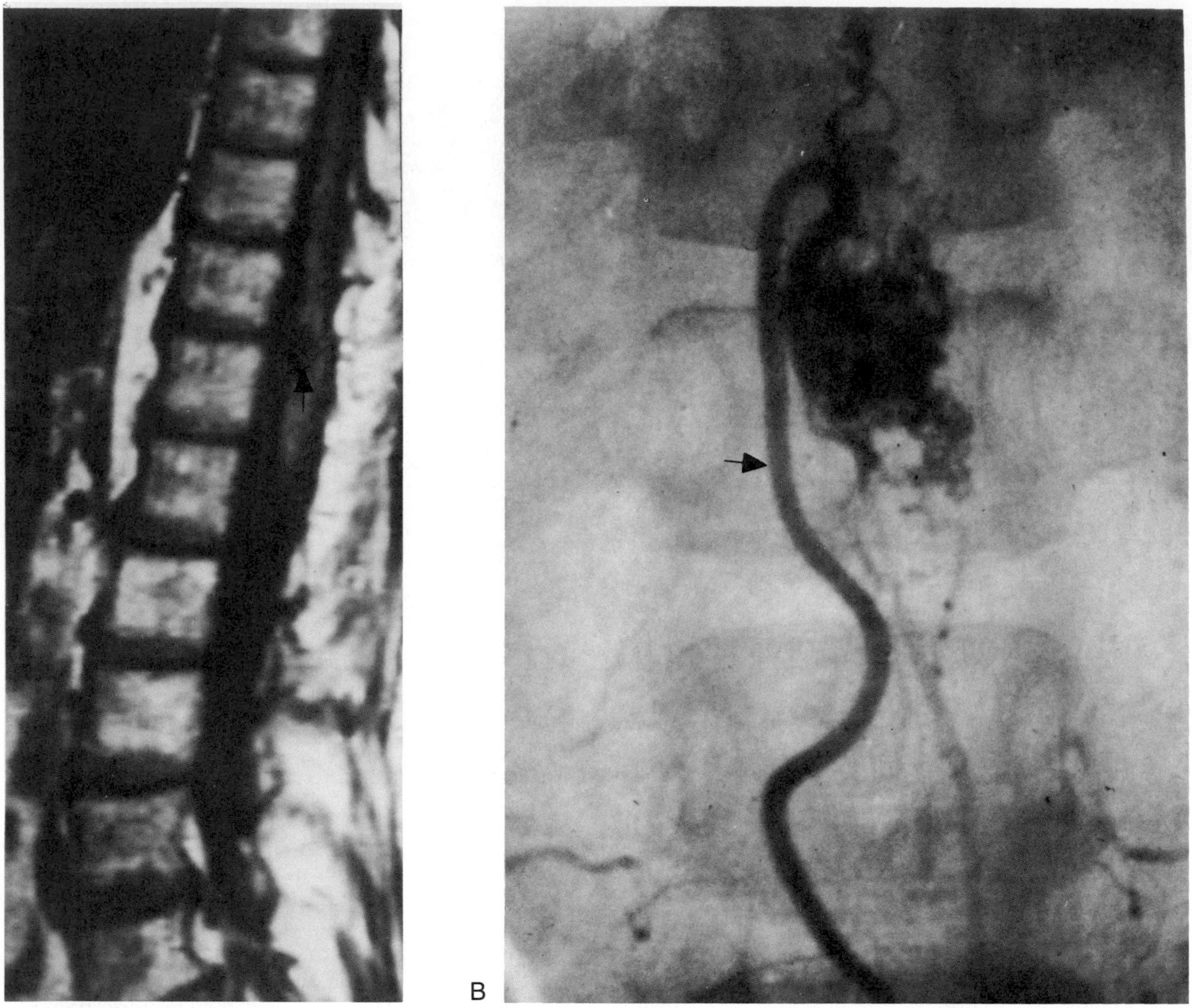

**Fig. 48-2.** (**A**) Sagittal magnetic resonance imaging in 56-year-old woman with acute onset of back pain, urinary dysfunction, and leg weakness, shows intramedullary arteriovenous malformation in ventral conus (*arrow*). (**B**) Initial selective spinal angiogram showed only one anterior medullary feeder arising from LL2 (*arrow*). Operative ligation of this feeder at its entry into the malformation was performed with gradual clinical improvement. At 1 year following surgery, urinary symptoms reappeared. (*Figure continues.*)

The glomus AVM is a high-flow lesion in comparison to the dural fistula, but generally has a slower shunt than seen with most intracranial AVMs. Exceptions to this exist, particularly in the cervical region. By definition, the glomus should have definable nidus, but this may not always be the case. The nidus may be intramedullary, pial, or both. The intramedullary nidus most commonly occupies the anterior portion of the spinal cord and invariably fills via an enlarged anterior spinal artery (Fig. 48-2). Aneurysmal dilations, which are usually venous, occur in about one-third of intradural AVMs, and in our experience is associated with a higher percentage of hemorrhagic presentation.

Angiography will typically reveal only one or at most two medullary arteries, which fill malformations located below the cervical spinal cord. This is probably a flow-related phenomenon, as other medullary feeders will be recruited if the major feeding vessel is occluded (Fig. 48-2). This is one reason for the failure of embolization to permanently treat the AVM.[3] Cervical glomus AVMs tend to be higher flow, with more feeding vessels demonstrated on angiography. This probably reflects the vascularity of

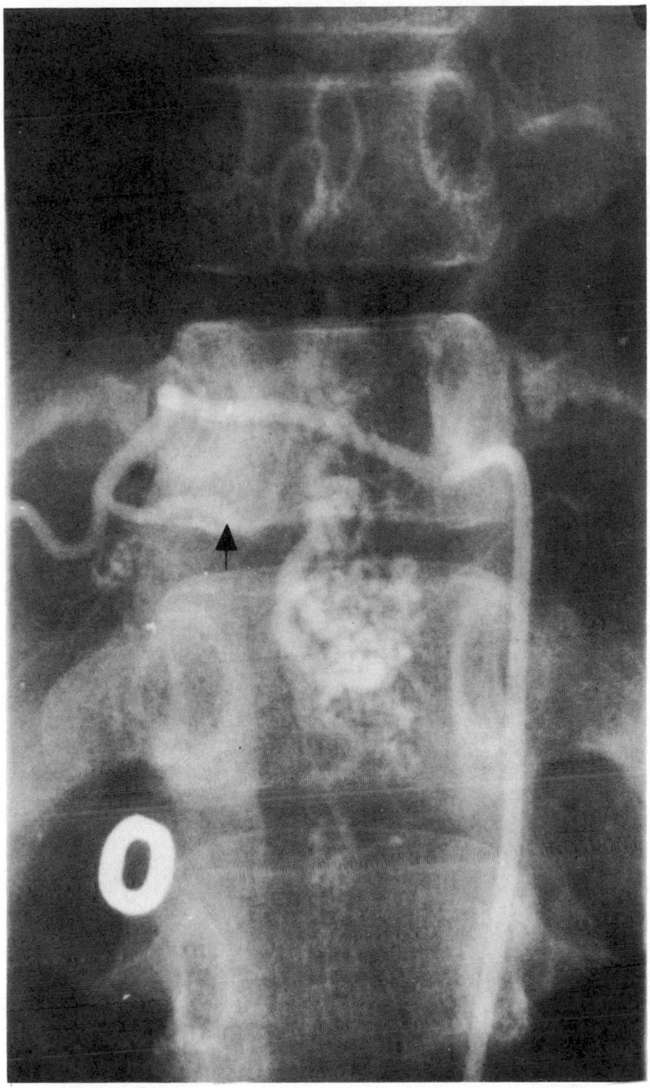

C

**Fig. 48-2** (*Continued*). (**C**) Repeat selective angiogram shows recurrence of arteriovenous malformation fed through RT11, which did not supply the arteriovenous malformation on angiographic injection 1 year earlier (*arrow*).

the cervical cord segment. Feeders may arise directly from the vertebral, thyrocervical, costocervical, deep cervical, and supreme intercostal arteries, as well as the descending limb of the anterior spinal artery.

A lateral or dorsolateral location is common for the pial glomus AVM, although a more ventral location is occasionally encountered. Pure dorsal lesions are usually encountered at the cervicomedullary junction. Pial malformations are supplied by circumferential pial branches from both the anterior and posterior spinal arteries as well as an occasional direct branch from the medullary artery. Deep penetrating branches from the anterior spinal system are invariably encountered if there are any intramedullary components to the malformation.

Intradural AVMs may present at any age, but the majority (about two-thirds) will become symptomatic during adolescence or early adult years.[5] An ictal event from subarachnoid or intramedullary hemorrhage or venous thrombosis appears to be the most frequent presentation, particularly in the younger patient or in the malformation with an aneurysmal dilation. Progressive neurologic deficit from arterial steal or mechanical compression is also common. Repeat hemorrhage is to be expected.

The neurologic consequence of a hemorrhagic presentation is variable. Purely subarachnoid hemorrhage may produce headache and meningeal irritation indistinguishable from subarachnoid hemorrhage of intracranial origin; even hydrocephalus may result. Sudden complete deficit from subarachnoid hemorrhage does occur, but is typically transitory and probably concussive in nature. Hematomyelia usually produces more devastating and permanent deficit.

## Management Considerations

The management of intradural spinal AVMs is difficult to standardize for several reasons. First, these are extremely rare lesions whose natural history is not well defined. Studies on the natural history of spinal AVMs are generally biased to reflect the progressive course of the much more commonly occurring dural fistula.[1,7] Second, these are potentially treacherous lesions whose initial or subsequent presentation may consist of a catastrophic event. Conversely, however, surgical or endovascular treatment of these lesions also carry significant risk of serious neurologic morbidity. Finally, although surgery is the cornerstone of treatment, the role of endovascular techniques as an adjunct to surgery or as primary treatment continues to evolve. Advances in catheter technology, electrothrombosis, rapidly polymerizing low-viscosity liquids, and precisely calibrated particular emboli, allow safer more distal vascular occlusion within the nidus. While these techniques have clearly been indispensable as adjuncts to surgical excision, they have also been utilized as primary treatment. Complete angiographic obliteration has been achieved in many cases. Long-term angiographic and clinical follow-up is needed to determine whether this obliteration is permanent or if recannulation occurs.[3] We have recently seen one patient who suffered repeat subarachnoid hemorrhage from a residual arteriovenous malformation 12 years following complete filling of the entire angioarchitecture of the AVM with liquid Silastic glue.

Determination of the operability of a spinal AVM hinges on the identification and characterization of the nidus. This may be easily identified on angiography with smaller, relatively slow-flow glomus AVMs with one or two medullary feeders, but can be very difficult in high-flow lesions whose early draining veins may obscure and overestimate the size of the nidus. For these lesions, embolization as an initial treatment is advisable. Magnetic resonance imaging (MRI) has become indispensable in defining the precise relationship to the spinal cord. High-quality sagittal and axial MRIs will define the precise relationship of the nidus to the spinal cord. This is extremely useful in selecting treatment options, planning operative strategies (i.e., myelotomy), and assessing the risk of intervention. The technique of operative removal of spinal AVMs requires adequate visualization, exposure, and meticulous microsurgical techniques. Although an intramedullary clot may assist the dissection, subarachnoid hemorrhage does not, so operative

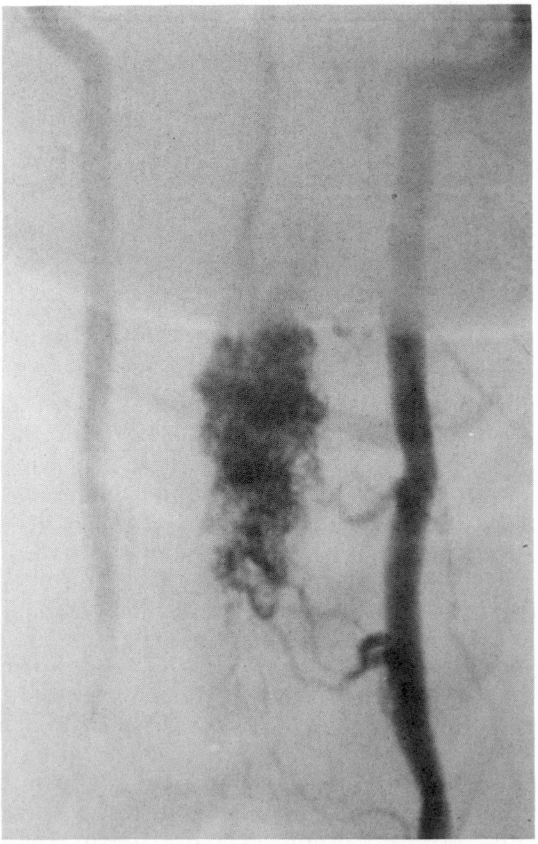
A

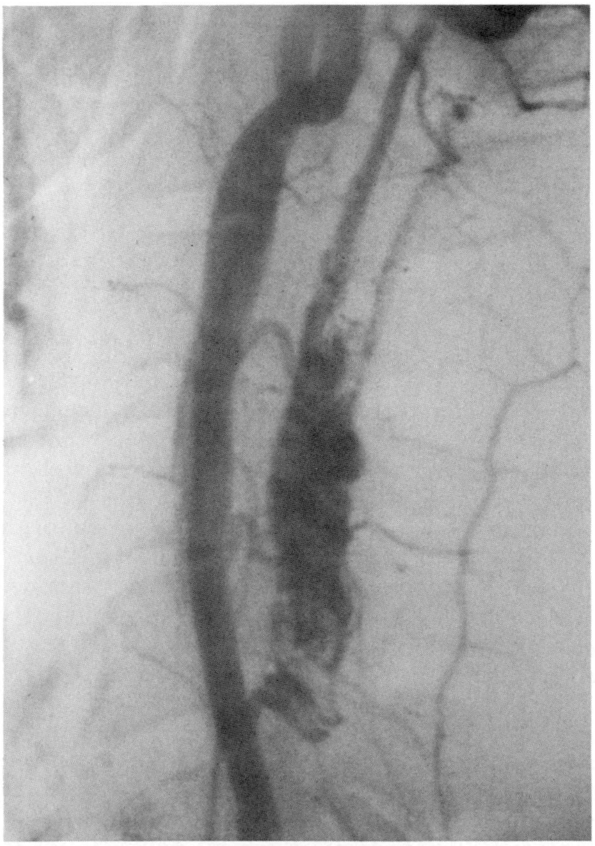
B

**Fig. 48-3.** (**A**) Anteroposterior view and (**B**) lateral view of cervical intramedullary arteriovenous malformation supplied through multiple medullary arteries off the vertebral artery. (*Figure continues.*)

intervention should be delayed, if possible following subarachnoid hemorrhage.

The prone position is adequate, although a three-quarter position may be useful for anteriorly placed lesions. An anterior transthoracic approach has also been described for removal of an anterior lesion. Somatosensory evoked potentials are routinely employed and are quite useful in assisting the removal of these vascular lesions. Following laminectomy and dural incision, the arachnoid is carefully dissected free from the underlying vessels and pia. Intermittent fine-needle intravascular pressure determination and/or Doppler sonography can help to distinguish artery from vein and assess the completeness of the resection. Superficial feeding arteries are cauterized and divided as they enter the malformation. The surgeon should resist the temptation to divide a large anterior medullary feeder along its ascending course. The descending limb of these ventrally placed feeders can be identified and divided near their entry into the malformation following dentate ligament section and gentle cord rotation from suture retraction on the proximal ligament stump.

The key to nidus dissection is to maintain the correct plane.[2] Entry into the nidus will cause troublesome bleeding and obscure planes. Conversely, a resection that is too wide increases the risk of neurologic deficit. The dissection should ideally take place right on the surface of the AVM. This will require myelotomy for intramedullary lesions. Gentle tension on the AVM with a suction dissector or bipolar forceps will identify small feeding arteries and draining veins, which are cauterized and divided. Larger draining veins are preserved as long as possible. Collateral cautery on the surface of the AVM will gradually shrink the nidus. The meticulous, often tedious, dissection continues systematically around the malformation until complete (Fig. 48-3). The remaining vein can then be cauterized and divided. Hemostasis must be carefully secured prior to wound closure.

In general, 80 to 90 percent good or excellent results with total excision (confirmed by angiography) can be anticipated. As with intramedullary tumors, outcome tends to relate to the cord level. The most favorable outcome is achieved with cervical lesions and followed by lumbar enlargement/conus malformations. Thoracic cord AVMs, although fortunately rare, present a much greater risk of operative morbidity.

C D

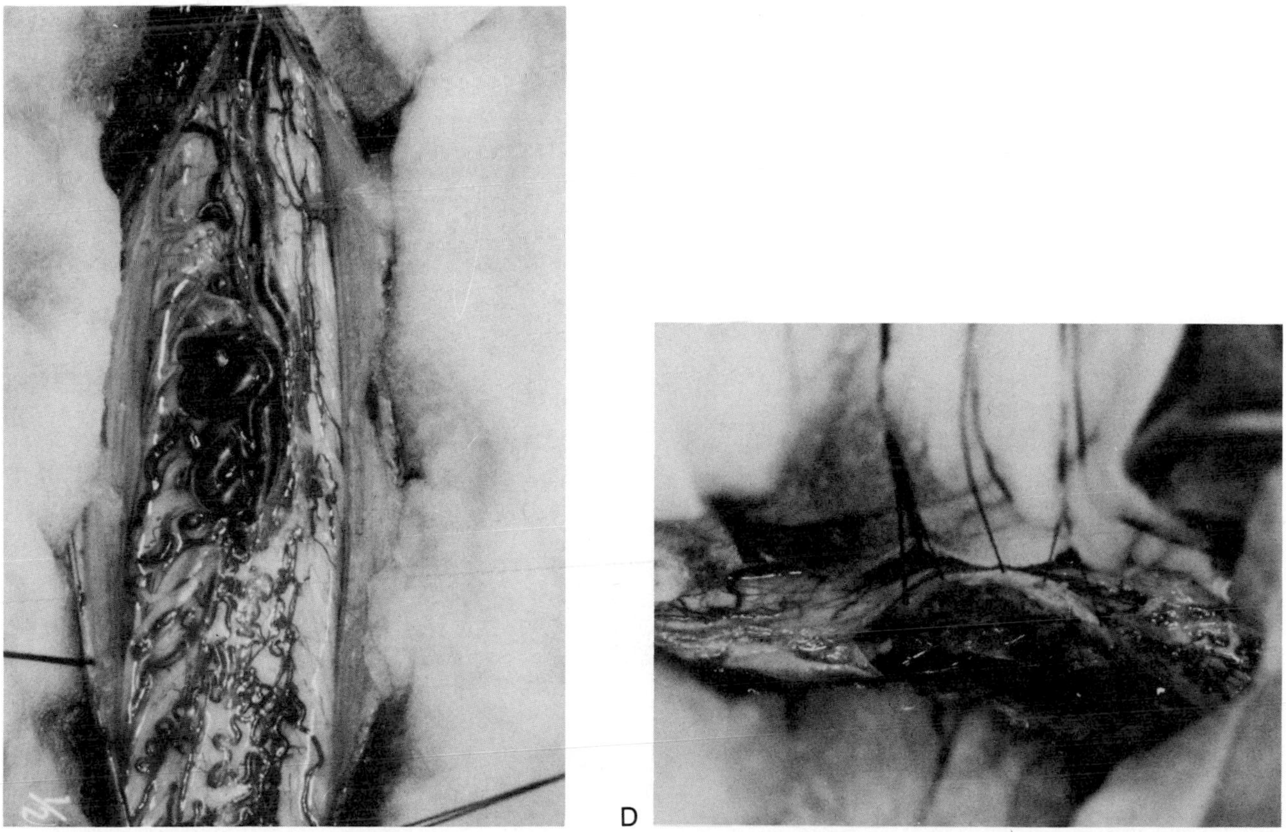

**Fig. 48-3** (*Continued*). (**C**) Intraoperative photograph shows feeding vessels and pial component of the nidus. (**D**) Operative photograph following complete resection of pial and intramedullary nidus.

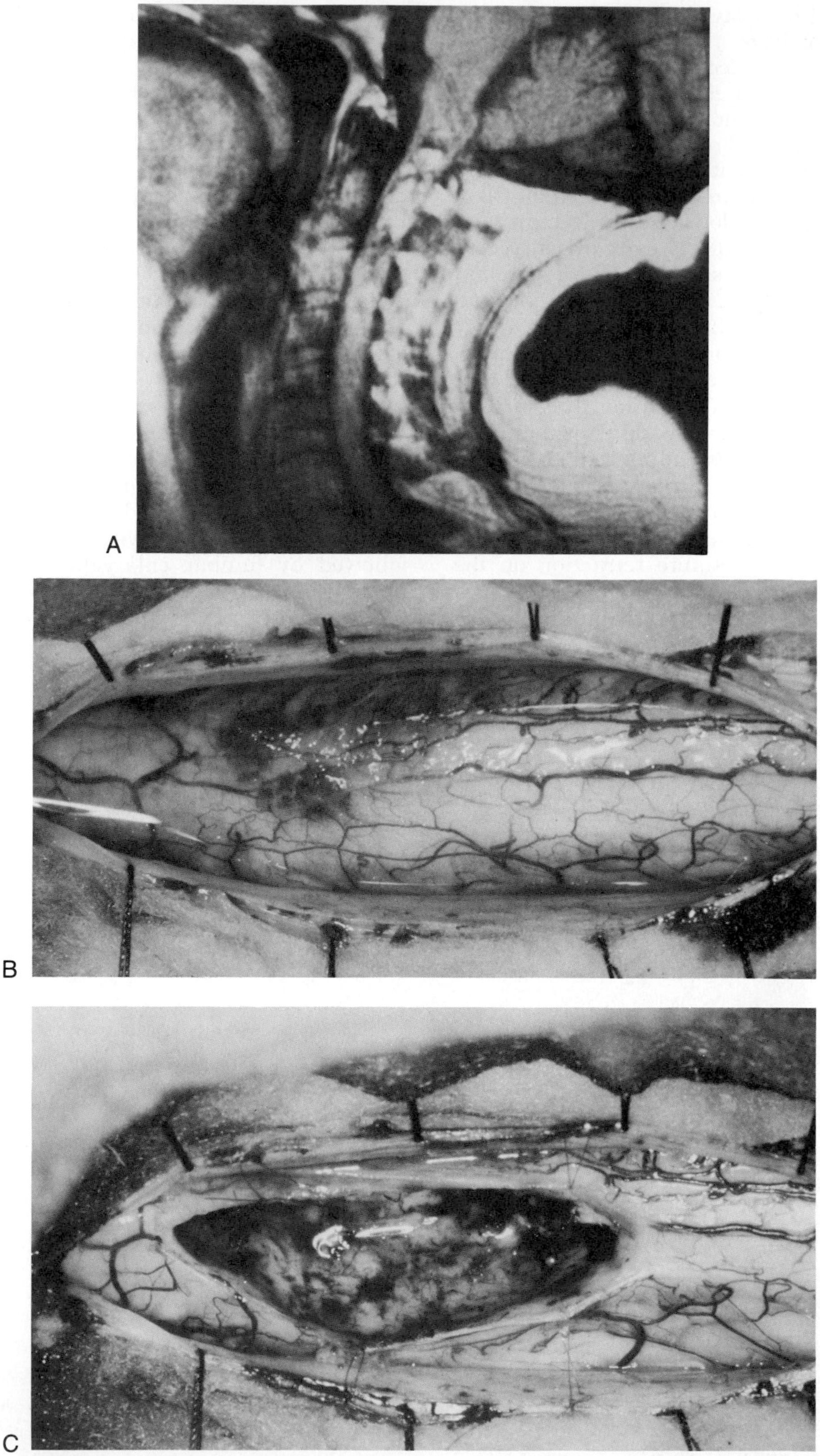


**Fig. 48-4.** (**A**) T1-weighted sagittal magnetic resonance imaging demonstrates intramedullary mass of upper cervical cord. The appearance is characteristic of a cavernous malformation. (**B**) Operative photograph clearly shows the cavernous malformation seen through the dorsal cord surface. (**C**) Operative photograph following complete resection of the cavernous malformation.

## Cavernous Malformations

Cavernous malformations are rare congenital lesions that may become symptomatic. They are occasionally multiple or familial in occurrence. About 10 percent of central nervous system cavernous malformations arise within the spinal cord. The characteristic histologic pattern of cavernous malformations is thin- or thick-walled vessels of capillary structure arranged in a sinusoidal network without intervening parenchyma.

Spinal cavernous malformations may produce an acute, recurrent, or progressive myelopathy. Prior to MRI, many patients were likely erroneously diagnosed as having multiple sclerosis, transverse myelitis, or associated myelopathic disorders. Acute and recurrent presentation probably result from hemorrhage. Unlike hematomyelia neurologic deficit may evolve over several hours or even days. It is rare for a hemorrhage from a cavernous malformation to produce complete paraplegia, although we witnessed this in one 15-year-old patient.[4] A progressive course is probably secondary to enlargement of the malformation, either from repeated internal hemorrhage, vessel dilation, or capillary budding. A neurotoxic effect of hemosiderin or compromise of surrounding microcirculation are alternative proposed mechanisms.

The diagnosis of cavernous malformation is made with MRI. The characteristic appearance consists of a central area of mixed signal intensity surrounded by a hypointense rim of hemosiderin (Fig. 48-4). Myelography followed by a computed tomography (CT) scan are often reported as normal even in the presence of significant deficit.[4] Angiography is unrevealing.

We believe that surgery should be considered for symptomatic lesions. Although cavernous malformations are unencapsulated, there is usually a plane of gliotic/hemosiderin-stained tissue that serves as an adequate dissection plane. Most patients will improve or stabilize following excision.[4] Occasionally, however, the malformation will be quite diffuse and unresectable.

## REFERENCES

1. Aminoff MJ, Logue V: The prognosis of patients with spinal vascular malformations. Brain 97:211, 1974
2. Cogen P, Stein BM: Spinal cord arteriovenous malformations with significant intramedullary components. J Neurosurg 59:471, 1983
3. Hall WA, Oldfield EH, Doppman JL: Recanalization of spinal arteriovenous malformations following embolization. J Neurosurg 70:714, 1989
4. McCormick PC, Michelsen WJ, Post KD et al: Cavernous malformations of the spinal cord. Neurosurgery 23:459, 1988
5. Rosenblum B, Oldfield EH, Doppman JL, et al: Spinal arteriovenous malformations: a comparison of dural arteriovenous fistulas and intradural AVMs in 81 patients. J Neurosurg 67:795, 1987
6. Spetzler RF, Zabramski JM, Flom RA: Management of juvenile spinal AVMs by embolization and operative excision. J Neurosurg 70:628, 1989
7. Tobin WD, Layton DD: The diagnosis and natural history of spinal cord arteriovenous malformations. Mayo Clin Proc 51:637, 1976

# 49
# *INTERVENTIONAL NEURORADIOLOGY*

Fernando Viñuela
Allan J. Fox

The progress of interventional neuroradiology as an alternative therapy for some intracranial congenital or acquired vascular lesions is associated with improvements in techniques of vascular superselective catheterization and navigation with microcatheters, microguidewires, and balloons. This therapeutic modality was primarily developed for the treatment of intracranial vascular lesions with high surgical morbimortality.

The goal of endovascular therapy is to obliterate congenital or acquired vascular abnormalities while sparing the blood supply of surrounding normal brain. This procedure may or may not be performed in conjunction with a neurosurgical procedure.

The technique of superselective embolization therapy involving the central nervous system has been developed by diagnostic neuroradiologists as an extension of techniques of catheterization and with the use of radiologic equipment for cerebrovascular verification. Vascular occlusive techniques include embolization with particles, balloons, and liquid agents (silicone, isobutylcyanoacrylate (IBCA), *n*-butylcyanoacrylate, etc.). These techniques must be performed by an experienced team composed of a neuroradiologist, neurosurgeon, neuroanesthesiologist, and vascular neurologist. They may carry an intrinsic risk of producing transient or permanent neurologic deficit if they are not handled properly.

The natural history of the disease, expectations of therapy, and potential complications associated with it must be discussed with patient and family as an introductory step before any type of therapy is performed.

## BRAIN ARTERIOVENOUS MALFORMATIONS

Cerebral arteriovenous malformations (AVMs) are the most common and extensively described vascular malformation of the central nervous system.[83] They occur anywhere in the central nervous system (CNS) and are said to be vascular hamartomas with an arteriovenous shunt of variable degree.[77,79] They are located in the brain parenchyma (pial AVMs), the dura mater (dural AVMs), or in both (mixed AVMs).[64]

Arteriovenous malformations may be supra- or infratentorial and are supplied from feeders arising from the internal carotid, external carotid, and/or vertebrobasilar systems, depending on their topography. They may be cortical or deep; the latter recruits blood supply from perforating arteries (lenticulostriate, thalamoperforators), and anterior and posterior choroidal arteries. The middle cerebral territory is the most frequently involved.

AVMs may be associated with aneurysms. This association was found in 6.7 percent of AVMs in a cooperative study[59] and in 9 percent of AVMs reported by Cronqvist and Troupp.[6] AVMs may also be associated with coarctation of the aorta and fibromuscular dysplasia.[68] Histologically, AVMs consist of a conglomerate of enlarged vessels of variable diameter and wall thickness. Vascular thrombosis and calcifications are not infrequent findings. The intervening brain tissue shows various degrees of edema, gliosis, demyelination, and calcifications.[79]

The clinical features of brain AVMs include SAH, seizures, progressive neurologic deficit, severe headaches, and mental deterioration. The natural history of the disease is unclear, and it is a source of controversy in the literature. Some reports claim that AVMs have a relatively benign long-term prognosis,[84] while others report a high morbimortality. Forster et al.[27] postulate that 10 to 17 percent of patients may die from a hemorrhage, and 40 to 50 percent may have deterioration of working capacity or become invalids over 20 to 40 years.

The choice of treatment of brain AVMs is based on the patient's clinical presentation and the size and topography of the lesion. Currently, the most effective treatment is complete surgical resection of the AVM nidus, although this approach may be restricted by the AVM size and involvement of brain eloquent areas.[22]

Endovascular embolization of brain AVMs was originally developed to facilitate final surgical resection of very large AVMs or as an alternative to surgery in those cases considered to be of great surgical risk. In some cases it is possible to obtain a complete obliteration of the AVM nidus by embolization alone and in AVMs involving brain eloquent areas (somatosensory, speech, basal ganglia, thalamus, diencephalon, mesencephalon, lower brain stem, cerebellar peduncles) incomplete AVM embolization may be complemented with radiotherapy of the residual AVM nidus.[5]

The goal of the endovascular therapist is to occlude the nidus of the AVM and its feeders as close as possible to it in order to preserve surrounding normal brain cortex. Endovascular occlusion of arterial feeders alone appears to be not as useful, since it stimulates enlargement of collaterals.[93] These collateral vessels are difficult to control surgically, and they mask the surgical plane of cleavage between the AVM nidus and surrounding brain cortex.

Luessenhop and Spence[57] introduced the use of particles to embolize brain AVMs. They used methyl methacrylate spheres delivered from the internal carotid or vertebral arteries in the neck. Later on, radiopaque silastic spheres were used in a similar fashion.[96] They were taken by the preferential flow toward the AVM and were impacted in the arterial feeders, without reaching the AVM nidus. Not unusually the change of flow dynamics diverted the spheres to normal cortical vessels. Angiographic follow-ups of AVMs embolized with these techniques showed recanalization of previously occluded AVM nidus due to the development of collateral circulation. Patronas et al.[67] reported that they could predict the efficacy of embolization of brain AVMs with silicone particles by analyzing the preembolization cerebral angiograms.

Postembolization transient neurologic deficits are commonly observed with this method of endovascular therapy. Complete functional recovery is observed in most cases.[95]

The detachable balloon technique was then developed by Serbinenko[80] and Debrun.[9] This method of embolization of brain AVMs is comparable to the proximal surgical or particulate obliteration of AVM feeders without occlusion of the AVM nidus. This methodology transfers the primary AVM supply to a prominent collateral circulation. This technique may be useful when the endovascular occlusion of the AVM feeders is immediately followed with final surgical resection.[35] The development of Silastic-calibrated leak balloons leading a flexible Silastic tubing was pioneered by Kerber[51] and Pevsner.[71] This system allowed safe navigation distal to the circle of Willis and selective catheterization of individual arterial feeders. The unpredictable behavior of the Silastic-calibrated leak balloon had an intrinsic risk of rupturing an arterial feeder by overinflation. Debrun et al.[12] developed a latex-calibrated leak balloon, and they postulated that the physical properties of this material made the latex balloon safer for cannulation and embolization of AVM feeders.

The selective catheterization of an AVM feeder is followed by a superselective angiogram and superselective Amytal test (injection of 30 mg Amytal).[89]

The superselective angiogram provides anatomic, dynamic, and functional information, not available in standard cerebral angiography[89] (Fig. 49-1). An AVM feeder may be differentiated into *primary* (only feeding AVM nidus) or *vessel en passage* (feeder also supplying normal brain distal to the AVM nidus). Superselective angiography also may identify arteriovenous fistulae associated to AVM nidus.[92] This association may be the source of sudden rupture of the AVM if the arteriovenous fistula is suddenly occluded by endovascular or surgical means.

The superselective injection of 30 mg amytal in an AVM feeder is performed with the patient awake and close clinical and electroencephalographic (EEG) monitoring. The Amytal injection may elicit transitory (1 to 3 minutes) clinical or EEG abnormalities if injected in a feeder also supplying normal cortex.[73,74] The use of this test appears to decrease iatrogenia in the embolization of AVM in or near cortical eloquent areas. The data obtained by endovascular Amytal test for the localization of brain eloquent areas correlate well with findings reported by Ojemann et al.[66] They used intraoperative stimulation mapping the dominant hemisphere to localize cortical sites essential for language. They concluded that there was a substantial variability in the localization of language function, and language cannot be reliably localized on anatomic criteria alone. Superselective amytal test in brain AVMs may depict a shift of functional cortex produced by the presence of an AVM nidus.[74]

More recently, the development of new microcatheters that do not need the lead of a calibrated leak balloon has decreased the possibility of damaging AVM feeders and has allowed the selection of multiple embolic materials.[15] The larger lumen of these microcatheters allows the delivery of particles as large as 500 $\mu$m in diameter, silk, and microcoils. Some of

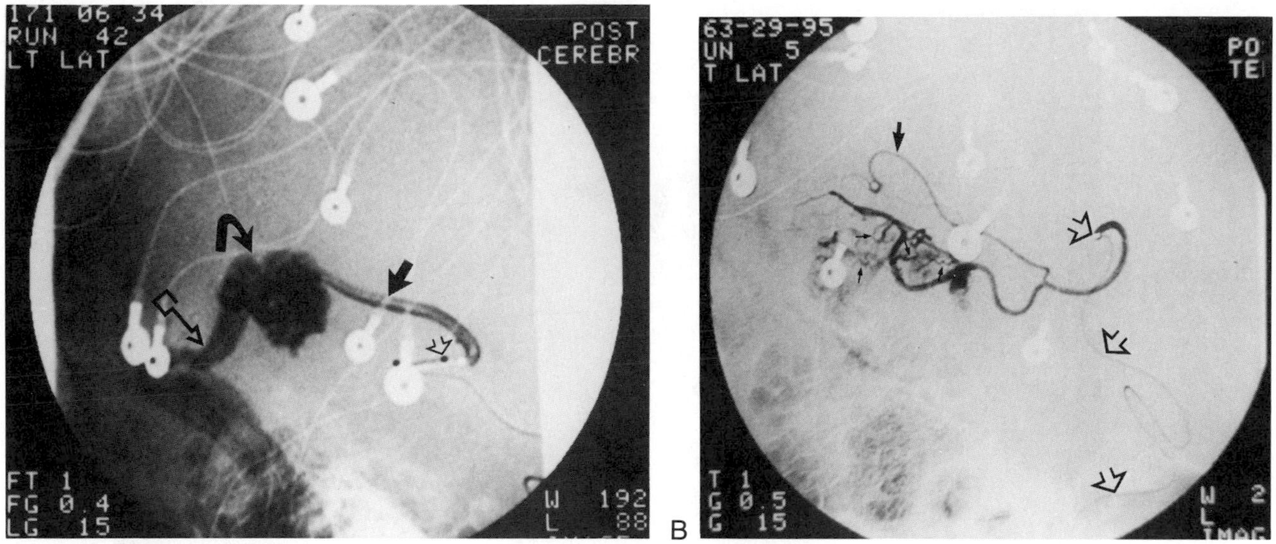


A B

**Fig. 49-1.** Preembolization superselective angiography. (**A**) Superselective angiogram of a primary feeder. The catheter tip (*open arrow*) is positioned in a posterior temporal feeder (*straight arrow*) only supplying the arteriovenous malformation nidus (*curved arrow*) and draining vein (*square arrow*). (**B**) Vessel en passage. The microcatheter (*open arrows*) is positioned in a posterior temporal artery that bifurcates in a normal superior temporal branch (*large straight arrow*) and in a feeder en passage. This artery supplies the arteriovenous malformation through small feeders while also supplying distal normal brain cortex (*small straight arrow*).

these microcatheters need a microguidewire to be advanced intracranially. The new generation of flow-guided microcatheters are less traumatic, though they have a smaller inner lumen, allowing only the injection of acrylic agents (isobutyl-2-cyanoacrylate, *n*-butylcyanoacrylate).[15]

The new generation of microcatheters also allows the monitoring of changes in intravascular pressure during embolization of a brain AVM (Fig. 49-2). The original technique was described by Duckwiler et al.[24] and Jungreis et al.[49] Prospective analysis of these data may provide useful information about postembolization local and regional intravascular pressure changes that may cause complications (postembolization vasogenic edema or hemorrhage related to normal perfusion pressure breakthrough).[82]

Complete occlusion of a brain AVM can be achieved by embolization alone (Fig. 49-3).[11] This mainly occurs in small AVMs fed by 1 to 3 pedicles.[93] In large or giant, multipediculate AVMs the purpose of the embolization is to reduce the size of the lesion and arteriovenous shunting as well as to promote progressive thrombosis of cortical veins associated with occluded portions of the AVM nidus[90] (Fig. 49-4). The preoperative embolization may be performed in the operative room[81] or in the radiology suite, using transfemoral techniques.[25,70]

A postembolization residual AVM in or near an eloquent area of the brain may be treated with different radiotherapeutic modalities.[5] Partial endovascular occlusion of large cortical AVMs may prevent progression of symptoms in patients with progressive neurologic deficit.[31] There is no evidence that partial embolization of an AVM presenting with intracranial hemorrhage or seizures changes its natural history. In selected cases, in which a substantial portion of the nidus of an AVM has been occluded, progressive thrombosis and complete obliteration of the lesion has been observed.[87]

Embolization of brain AVMs carries an intrinsic risk of transient or permanent neurologic deficit or death. Complications include gluing of the microcatheter in an AVM feeder, vasospasm, dissection, or rupture of an artery with intracranial hemorrhage, dissection of the vessels in the neck, intracranial emboli from coaxial catheters in the neck, postembolization ischemia, vasogenic edema or hemorrhage, and death.[11]

## ENDOVASCULAR THERAPY OF SPINAL ARTERIOVENOUS MALFORMATIONS

The incidence of spinal arteriovenous malformations ranges from 3.3 to 12.5 percent of spinal-occupying lesions, with an average of 8 to 10 percent.[14] Spinal AVMs may be isolated, most commonly affecting the middle and lower thoracic spinal cord.[61] Spinal

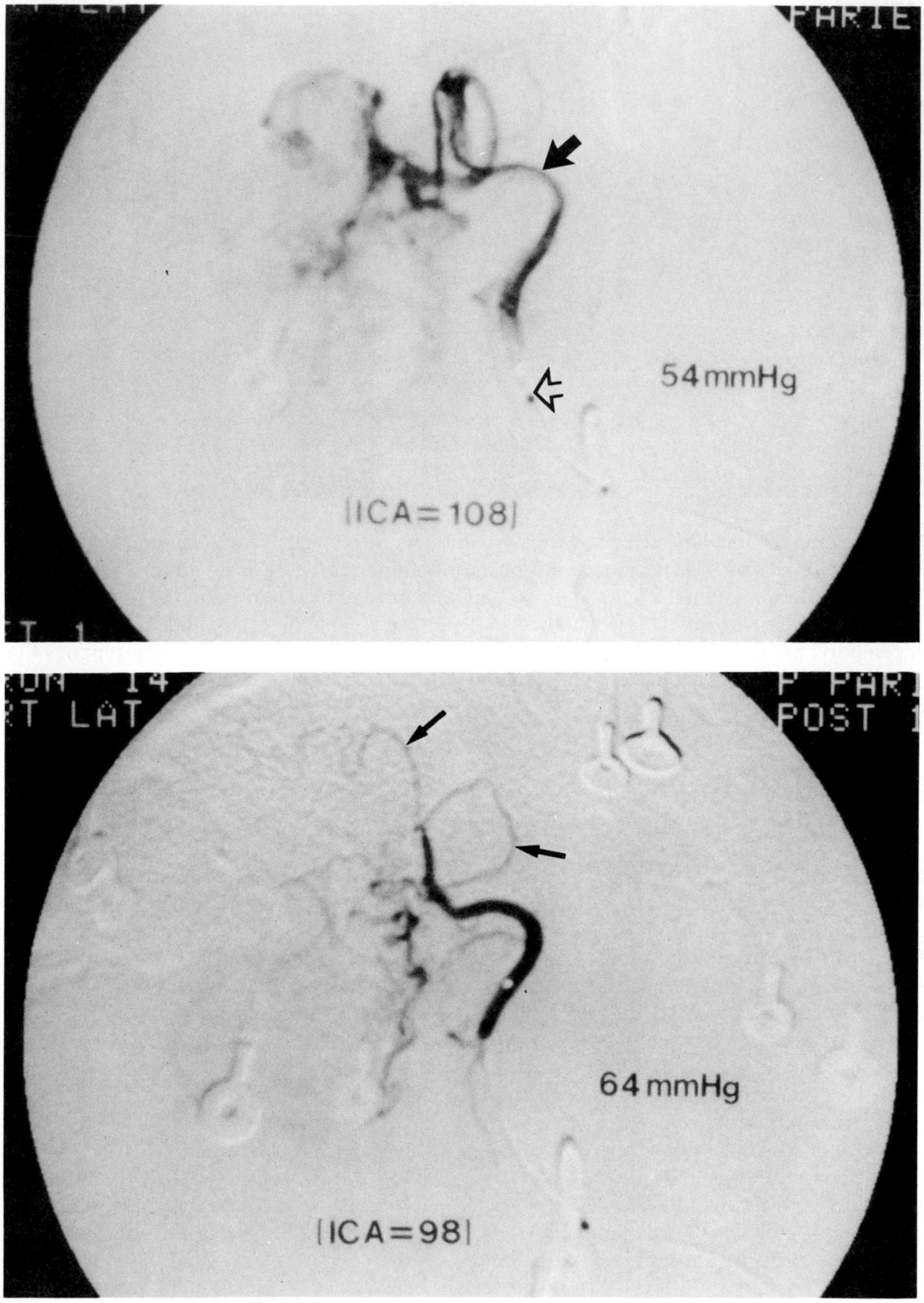


A

B

**Fig. 49-2.** Superselective intravascular pressure monitoring. (**A**) Preembolization pressure monitoring in an arteriovenous malformation feeder. The systemic mean pressure is 108 mmHg, while the mean pressure in the arteriovenous malformation feeder at the catheter tip (*open arrow*) is 54 mmHg. Angiogram shows the feeder (*arrow*) contribution to the lesion. (**B**) Postembolization simultaneous pressure monitoring showed an increase of 10 mmHg in the arteriovenous malformation feeder. Notice preservation of normal cortical branches (*arrows*) and complete obliteration of arteriovenous malformation feeders.

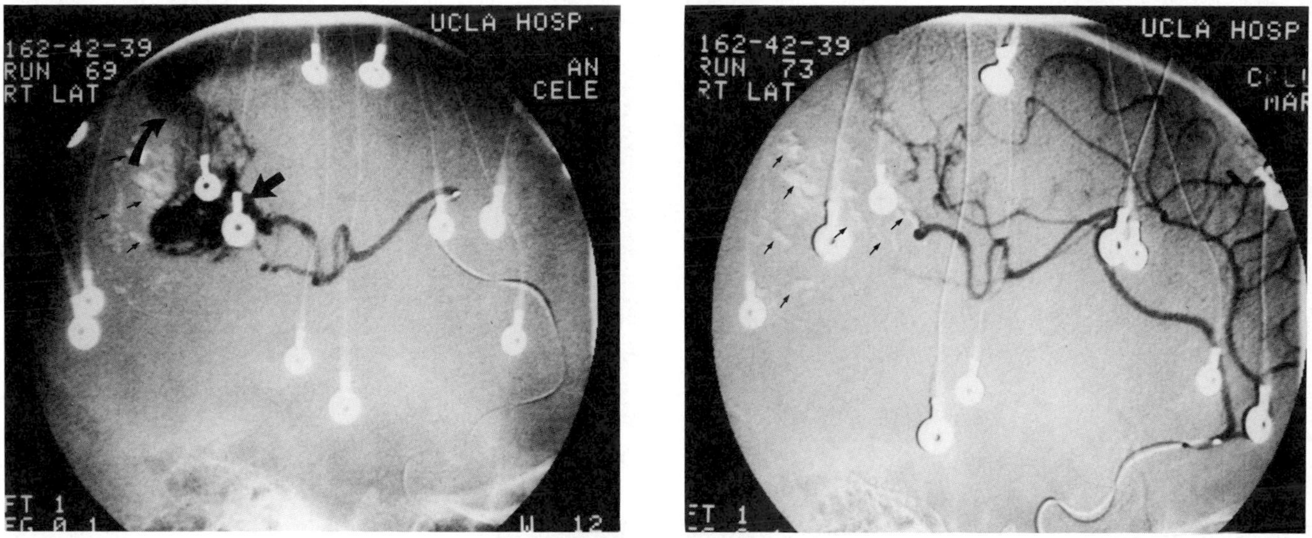


A B

**Fig. 49-3.** Complete arteriovenous malformation obliteration. (**A**) Preembolization pericallosal arteriogram shows a mesioparietal arteriovenous malformation nidus (*straight arrow*) and corresponding draining vein (*curved arrow*). Embolic material deposited in a previous embolization is noted (*small arrows*). (**B**) Immediate postembolization anterior cerebral arteriogram shows complete obliteration of the arteriovenous malformation nidus. A more widespread distribution of embolic material is noted (*small arrows*).

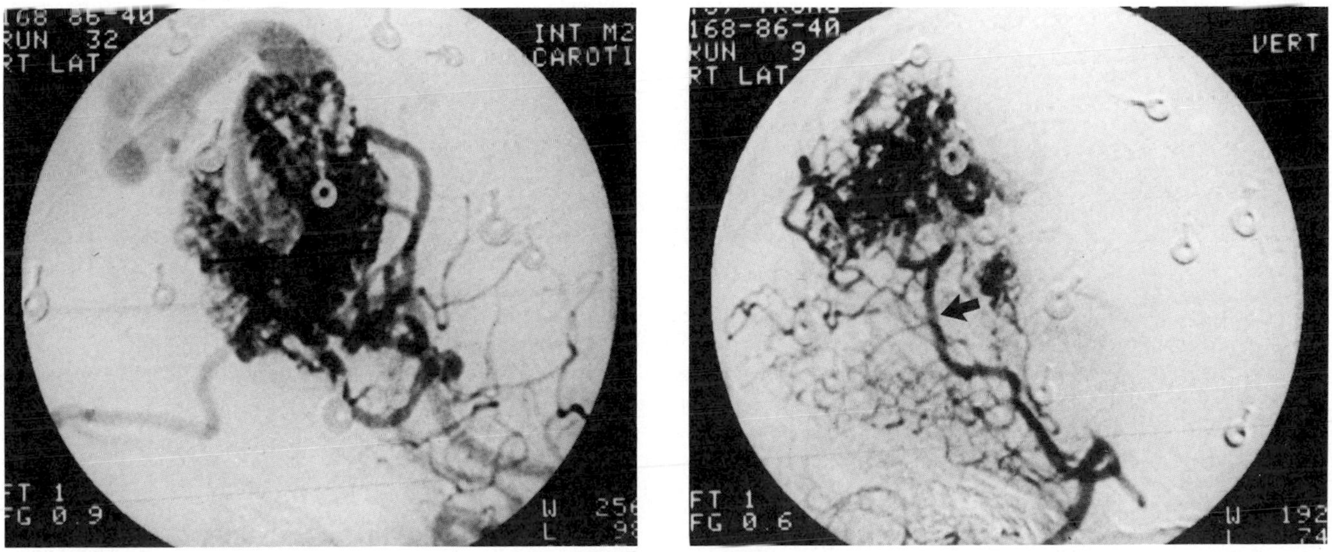


A B

**Fig. 49-4.** Presurgical embolization of large arteriovenous malformations. (**A**) Lateral right internal carotid angiogram shows a large parietal arteriovenous malformation supplied by several middle cerebral artery feeders. (**B**) Lateral right vertebral angiogram shows a large posterotemporal feeder (*arrow*) supplying the dorsal and posterior aspect of the AVM nidus. (*Figure continues.*)

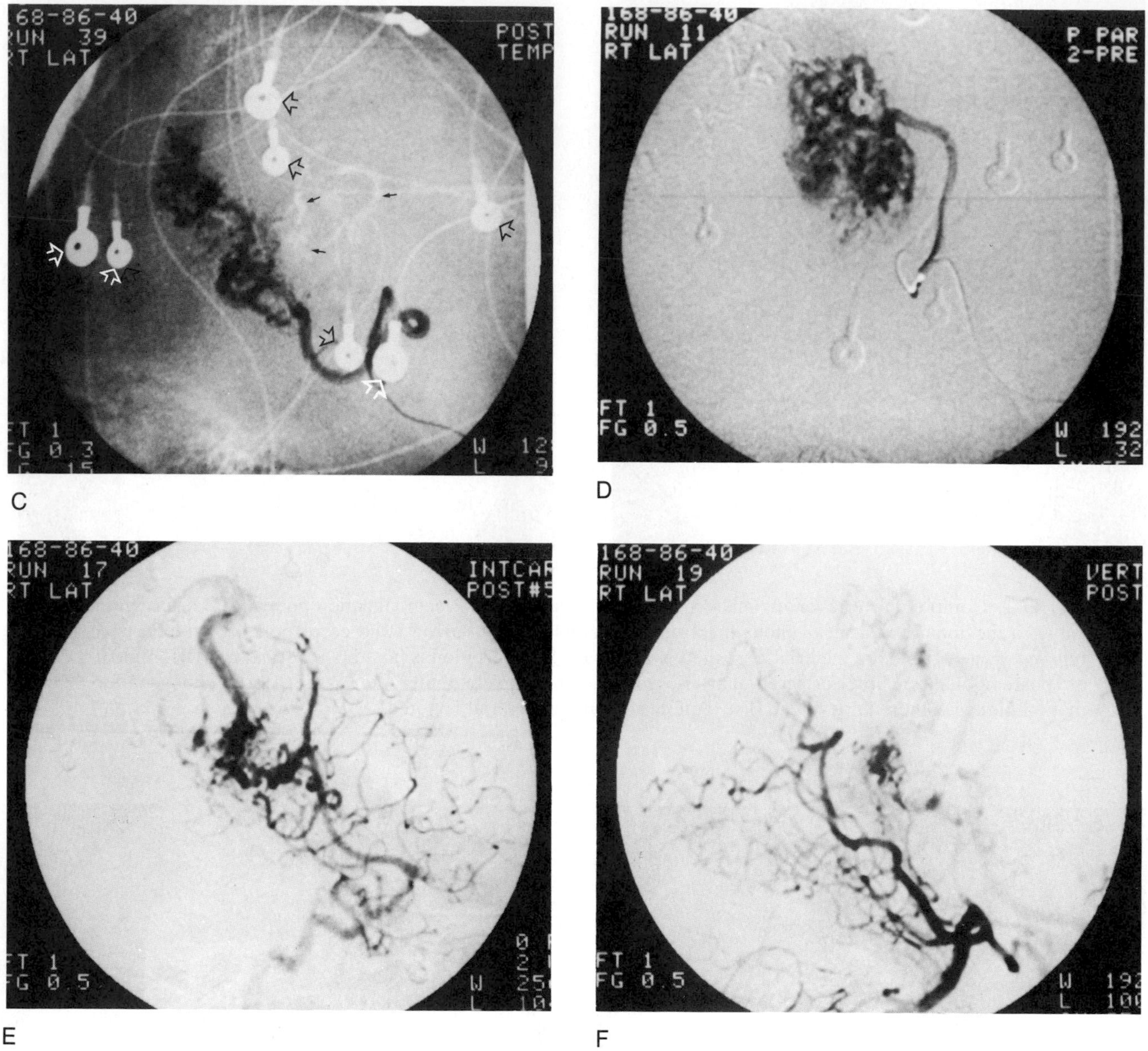


**Fig. 49-4** (*Continued*). (**C & D**) Examples of preembolization superselective angiogram of middle cerebral artery parietal feeders. (**E & F**) Immediate postembolization right internal carotid and vertebral angiograms show obliteration of most of the arteriovenous malformation nidus. Complete uneventful surgical resection of the residual arteriovenous malformation was performed 10 days postembolization.

pial AVMs represent the most frequent type of vascular malformation. Regional localization allows the identification of three main varieties: cervical AVMs (10 to 15 percent), cervicothoracic AVMs (20 to 30 percent), thoracolumbar and lumbosacral AVMs (50 percent), the majority being located below T8 to T10.[16] Spinal AVMs may be intramedullary, intradural-extramedullary, dural, or epidural.[17]

The clinical spectrum of spinal AVMs includes subarachnoid hemorrhage (10 to 30 percent of cases), spinal extradural and subdural hematomas, hematomyelia, spinal cord infarction, cord compression by a varix, and chronic progressive radiculomyelopathy.[4,53] As in the case of cerebral AVMs, endovascular or surgical treatment of spinal AVMs needs to be preceded by discussion of the natural history of the disease and pros and cons of therapy with the patient and family.

The first case of embolization of a spinal cord AVM was described by Doppman et al.[18] in 1971. Since then, this type of therapy has been performed alone or in conjunction with surgery. Embolization should be planned according to the size and topography of the vascular malformation (intramedullary, retromedullary, dural with pial venous drainage). Not infrequently spinal AVMs may be associated with extramedullary arteriovenous fistulae and aneurysms of the feeding vessels. This stresses the importance of an accurate angiographic assessment to define the feeding vessels, AVM nidus, draining veins, and blood supply to surrounding normal spinal cord.

Complete anatomic cure of spinal AVMs may be achieved by endovascular embolization alone. This is more often seen in spinal dural AVMs with pial venous drainage. The dural AVM is generally small, and it involves the dura mater lateral and inferior to the vertebral pedicle. The symptoms are produced by a generalized venous hypertension in the spinal cord from recruitment of perimedullary veins by the AVM.[50] IBCA appears to be the ideal embolic agent to be used with this type of spinal AVM.[62] Surgical excision of the residual AVM nidus may be attempted if the embolization is incomplete.

Riché et al.[75] reported their experience of embolization of spinal AVMs supplied by the anterior spinal artery. They described 21 patients treated by embolization alone, 6 treated with a combination of embolization and surgery, and 6 treated by surgery alone. They report excellent angiographic and clinical results in the cervical and dorsolumbar regions and mediocre results in the middorsal spinal cord. They explained these less than satisfactory results in the thoracic spine to the lack of sufficient collateral blood supply in this portion of the spinal cord.

The development of new microcatheters has improved the superselective catheterization of spinal AVM feeders, and recent reports in the literature point to marked improvement in clinical and morphologic results of embolization of intramedullary spinal AVMs[46,86] (Fig. 49-5). The morbidity of the procedure may be decreased by monitoring somatosensory-evoked potentials during the embolization[3] or by performing preembolization superselective Wada tests of AVM feeders.[19]

## ARTERIOVENOUS FISTULAS

An arteriovenous fistula (AVF) is an abnormal direct communication between an artery and a vein, bypassing the capillary system. Arteriovenous Fistulas (AVFs) may be congenital or acquired, and trauma is the most common of the latter. The most common AVFs amenable to embolization are carotid-cavernous (C/C) fistulas, vertebrovertebral fistulas, and AVFs involving branches of the external carotid artery.

The vein of Galen vascular malformation is the most common congenital intracranial AVF, though these AVFs may be found anywhere in the central nervous system (CNS).[91] They all pose a great therapeutic challenge.

The development of detachable balloons has revolutionized the therapy of AVFs. These balloons may be positioned in the venous side of the fistula via the affected artery, using a transfemoral approach.[9,80] Balloon embolization has become the treatment of choice in traumatic carotid-cavernous fistulas because of its excellent clinical results and low complication rate.[13] The most common approach is the transfemoral transarterial route. When the fistula and cavernous sinus are small, one balloon is sufficient to occlude the AVF (Fig. 49-6). In cases of laceration of the internal carotid artery and/or large cavernous sinus, it is necessary to deposit multiple detachable balloons in the cavernous sinus, and not infrequently the internal carotid artery needs to be occluded. Intravascular detachment of balloons in a traumatic C/C fistula may elicit technical complications, such as occlusion of the internal carotid artery, intracranial balloon migration by balloon early detachment or deflation, or development of arterial pseudoaneurysms by early balloon deflation.[13]

The transvenous embolization of traumatic carotid-cavernous fistulae was first described by Manelfe and Berenstein[60] and Debrun et al.[10] This approach may be used when the small size of the arterial laceration precludes the passage of the balloon from the arterial size. The inferior petrosal sinus is the most popular route. It may be catheterized by the transfemoral or transjugular approaches. An introducer is positioned in the jugular bulb pointing anteriorly and medially. The inferior petrosal sinus is then catheterized, using a microcatheter that is advanced into the cavernous sinus. This technique allows the use of detachable balloons, microcoils, or liquid agents at the fistula site[38] (Fig. 49-7).

The superior ophthalmic vein has also been used to reach the cavernous sinus in cases of traumatic carotid-cavernous fistulas. It may be exposed surgically in the orbit,[63] or it may be catheterized by transfemoral approach via an enlarged angular vein.[38]

The direct surgical exposure and embolization of the cavernous sinus may be used in those cases of failure of the transfemoral, arterial, or venous approaches.[48] Multiple embolic agents may be introduced in the cavernous sinus by direct intraoperative puncture (balloons, coils, silk, muscle, liquid agents).

For vertebrovertebral fistulas, the same technical approach applies as for traumatic carotid-cavernous fistulas.[33] Epidural varices associated with high-flow AVF in this region often compress the spinal cord or may be the source of hemorrhage. Vertebrovertebral AVFs are often difficult to treat because of the development of multiple feeders arising from ipsilateral and contralateral vertebral, ascending cervical, thyrocervical, and costocervical trunks as well as feeders from the external carotid artery.

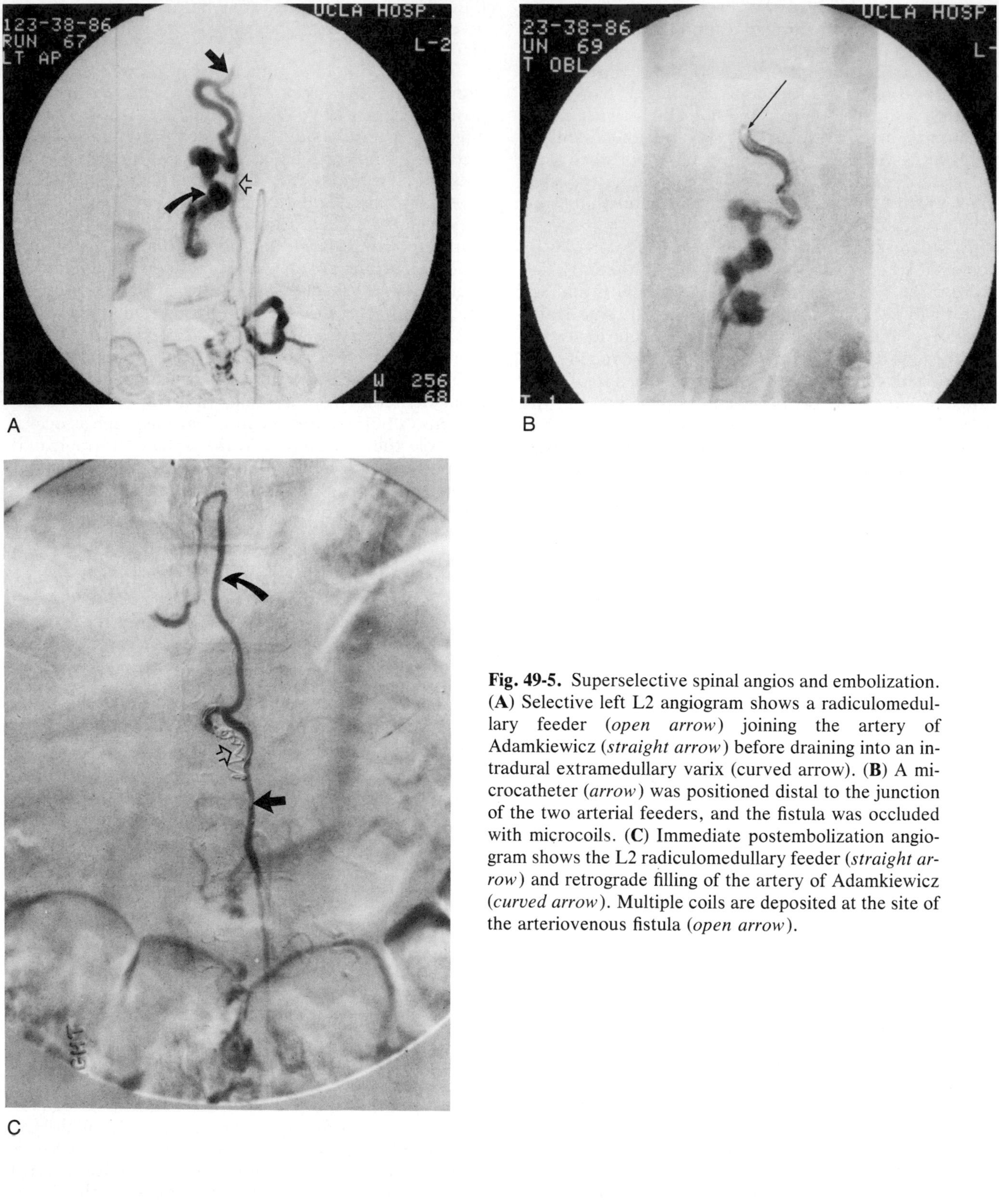


**Fig. 49-5.** Superselective spinal angios and embolization. (**A**) Selective left L2 angiogram shows a radiculomedullary feeder (*open arrow*) joining the artery of Adamkiewicz (*straight arrow*) before draining into an intradural extramedullary varix (curved arrow). (**B**) A microcatheter (*arrow*) was positioned distal to the junction of the two arterial feeders, and the fistula was occluded with microcoils. (**C**) Immediate postembolization angiogram shows the L2 radiculomedullary feeder (*straight arrow*) and retrograde filling of the artery of Adamkiewicz (*curved arrow*). Multiple coils are deposited at the site of the arteriovenous fistula (*open arrow*).

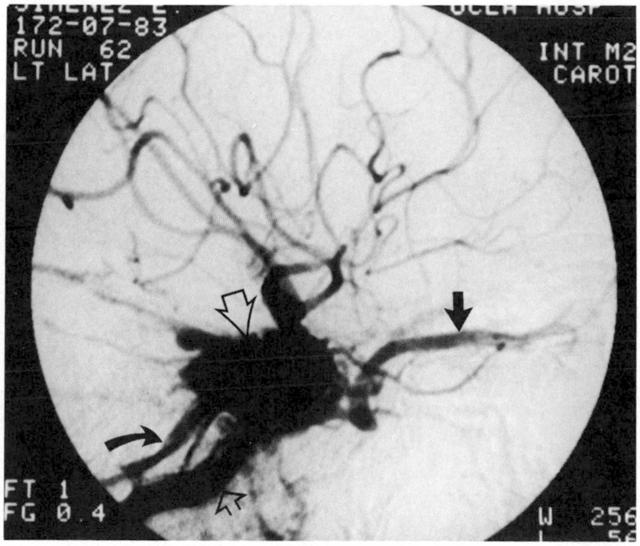


A

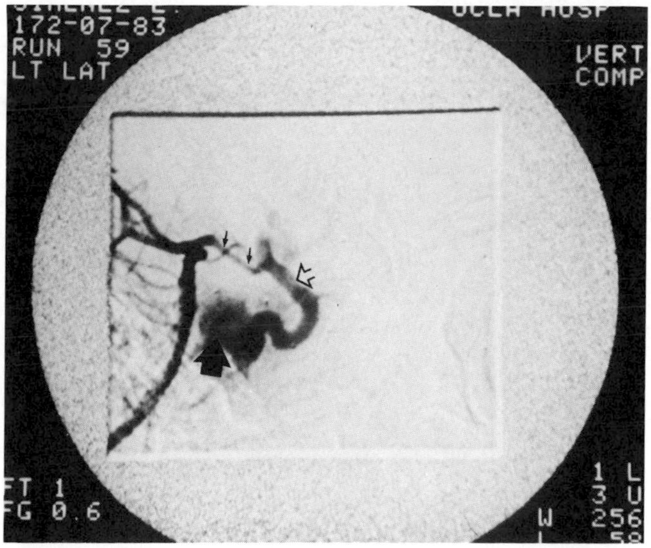


B

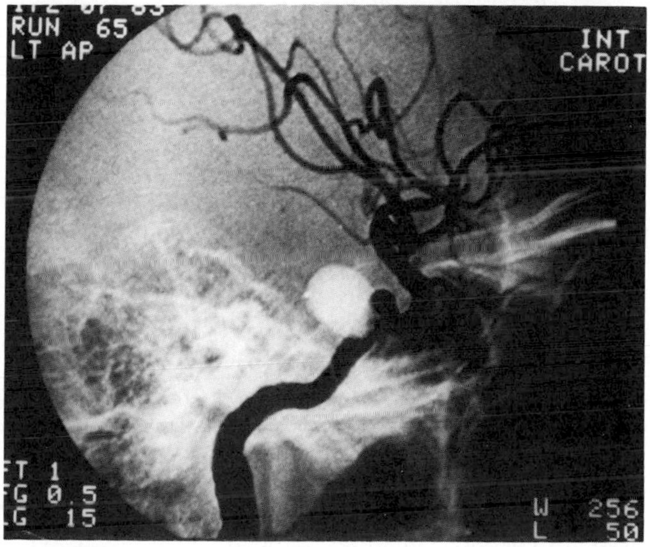


C

**Fig. 49-6.** Embolization of traumatic carotid-cavernous fistula. (**A**) Lateral left internal carotid angiogram shows the intrapetrous carotid (*open arrow*), and abnormal filling of the cavernous sinus (*triangle arrow*) draining into the superior ophthalmic vein (*straight arrow*) and inferior petrosal sinus (*curved arrow*). (**B**) Lateral left vertebral angiogram with compression of the left internal carotid artery in the neck shows retrograde filling of the ipsilateral posterior communicating artery (*small arrows*), supraclinoid carotid (*open arrow*), and the intracavernous fistula site (*large straight arrow*). (**C**) Immediate postembolization angiogram shows obliteration of the traumatic carotid-cavernous fistula by a single balloon with preservation of the lumen of the internal carotid artery.

Complex, spontaneous, or post-traumatic vertebrovertebral fistulas may be associated with vascular dysplasias, such as neurofibromatosis[7] or fibromuscular dysplasia.[40] In these cases it may be difficult to preserve the lumen of the vertebral artery because of the generalized dysplasia of this vessel.

An intracranial, congenital, or spontaneous AVF is a relatively rare vascular malformation that may be solitary or associated with other vascular abnormalities. Its clinical spectrum includes increased intracranial pressure produced by mass effect by a giant varix, intracranial hemorrhage, brain atrophy, or calcifications.[91]

The best known congenital AVF is the vein of Galen vascular malformation. Its clinical presentation varies with age and includes massive cardiac failure in neonates, moderate heart failure and hydrocephalus in infants and children, and seizures, hydrocephalus, and occasional subarachnoid hemorrhage (SAH) in adults.[1]

Yasargil[97] classifies vein of Galen vascular malformations into four types, depending upon angiographic findings: type I, direct arteriovenous fistulae in the wall of the vein of Galen varix with predominant blood supply from posterior choroidal and pericallosal arteries; type II, AVF in the wall of the varix with dominant participation of transmesencephalic and transdiencephalic feeders; type III, a combination of types I and II; and type IV, the dilated vein of Galen is only a draining ven from an arteriovenous

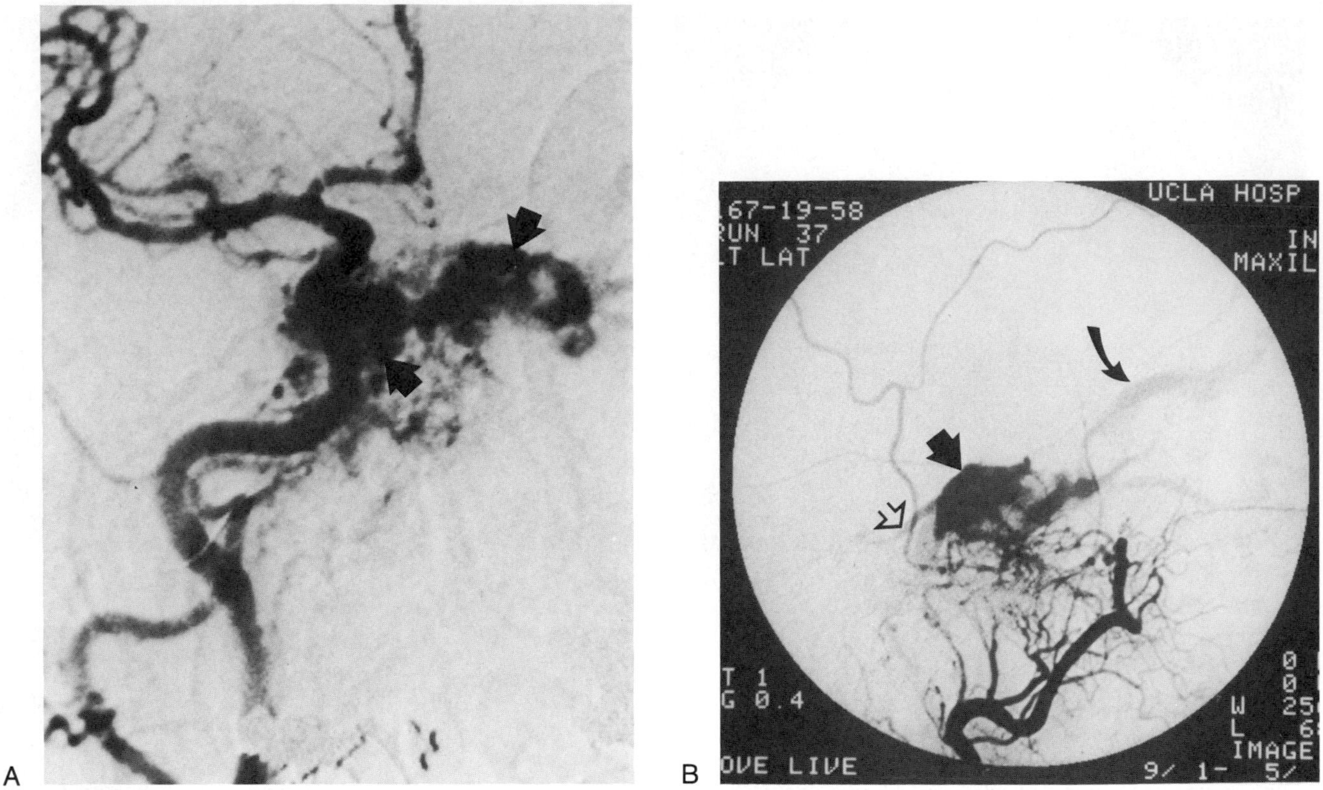


**Fig. 49-7.** Transvenous embolization of a carotid-cavernous fistula. (**A**) Right common carotid angiogram shows abnormal filling of right and left cavernous sinuses (*arrows*) due to a dural arteriovenous malformation of the right cavernous sinus. (**B**) Left external carotid angiogram shows several feeders supplying the dural arteriovenous malformation. Notice contrast material in the cavernous sinus (*straight arrow*) and drainage through the superior ophthalmic vein (*curved arrow*) and superior petrosal sinus (*open arrow*). (*Figure continues.*)

malformation involving diencephalon, mesencephalon, or cerebellum.

The surgical, transtorcular, transvenous embolization of this vascular malformation was popularized by Hanner and Quisling.[39] Staged, slow occlusion of the midline AVF is obtained with the deposit of Gianturco coils in the most anterior portion of the vein of Galen aneurysm. This progressive change in the arteriovenous shunting allows a better medical control of the concomitant hemodynamic changes observed in brain and heart.

Trasnfemoral, transarterial, or transvenous embolization of vein of Galen vascular malformations in neonates may also be done with excellent clinical and morphologic results. This technique also allows a progressive occlusion of intracranial high-flow AVF with liquid agents, microcoils, and silk. The use of a new generation of microcatheters allows a safe intracranial navigation in the neonate with the deposit of embolic material at the fistula site, as close as possible to the wall of the vein of Galen varix[20,56] (Fig. 49-8).

Giant intracranial varices related to spontaneous high-flow AVFs may be found in other areas of the CNS. They have a clinical presentation similar to the vein of Galen vascular malformation, though the congestive heart failure tends to be less severe. They also may be occluded by endovascular techniques alone or in combination with surgery[91] (Fig. 49-9).

## DURAL ARTERIOVENOUS MALFORMATIONS

Spontaneous dural arteriovenous malformations (AVMs) may be located anywhere in the dura mater but they are more common in the cavernous, lateral, sigmoid, and superior sagittal sinuses. They tend to affect the adult population, and they may be related to a partial or complete spontaneous occlusion of a dural sinus.[47]

The clinical presentation of dural AVMs includes intracranial bruit, increased intracranial pressure, and subarachnoid or intraparenchymal hemorrhage. The hemorrhage observed in dural AVMs is related to the rupture of an arterialized cortical vein recruited by the malformation more than the rupture of the dural AVM.[65]

**Fig. 49-7** (*Continued*). (**C**) A microcatheter was positioned in the inferior petrosal sinus (*curved arrow*) and its tip (*straight arrow*) is in the posterior aspect of the cavernous sinus. Notice contrast material filling the cavernous sinus (*open arrow*) and the superior ophthalmic vein (*triangle arrow*). Several microcoils were deposited in the right cavernous sinus. (**D**) Postembolization right common carotid angiogram shows complete obliteration of the dural arteriovenous malformation by the coils (*open arrows*) and preservation of the lumen of the intracavernous internal carotid artery.

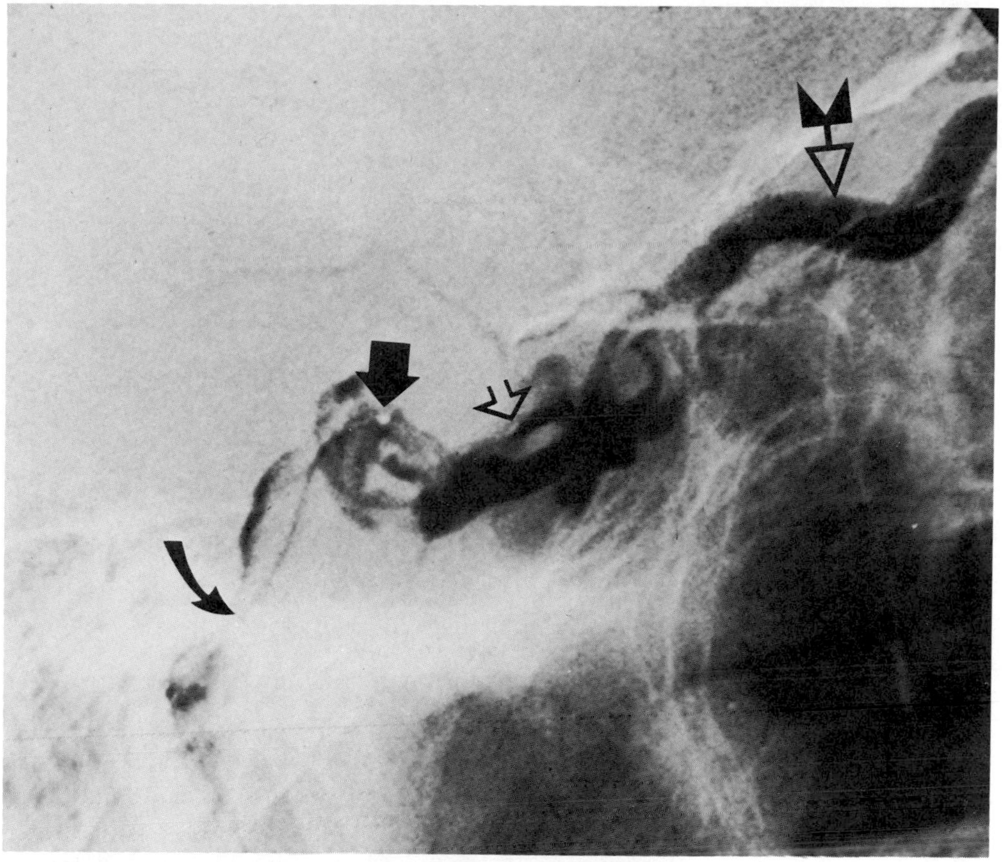

C

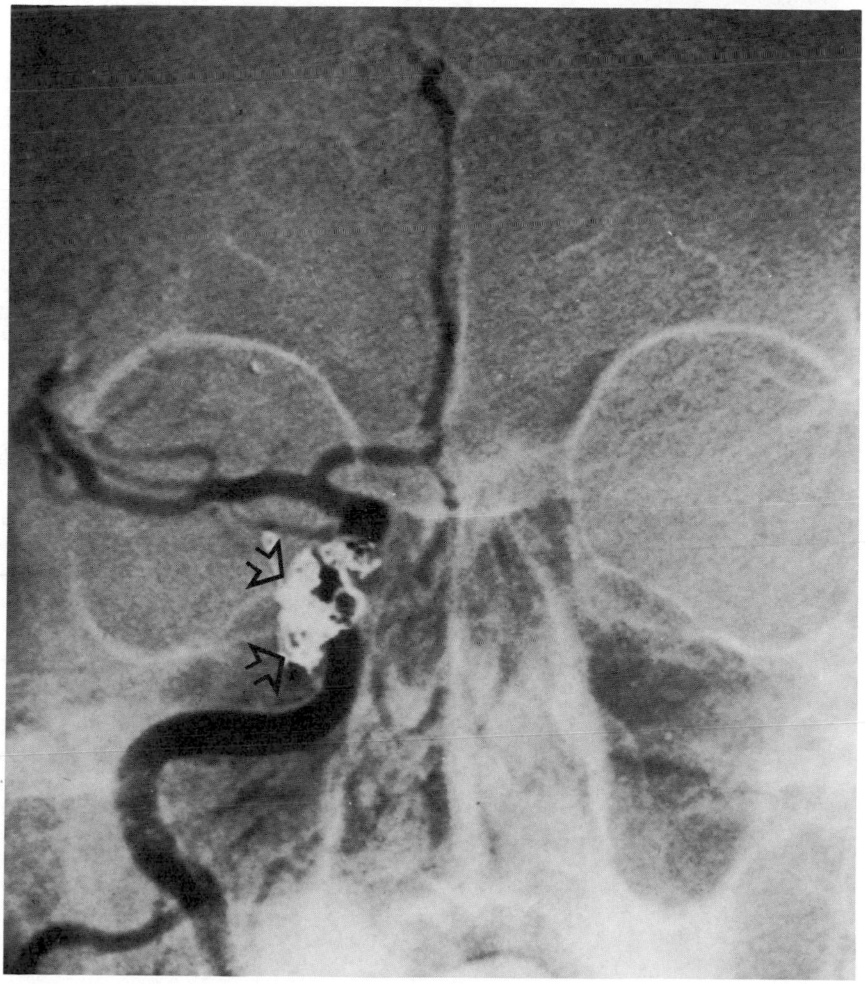

D

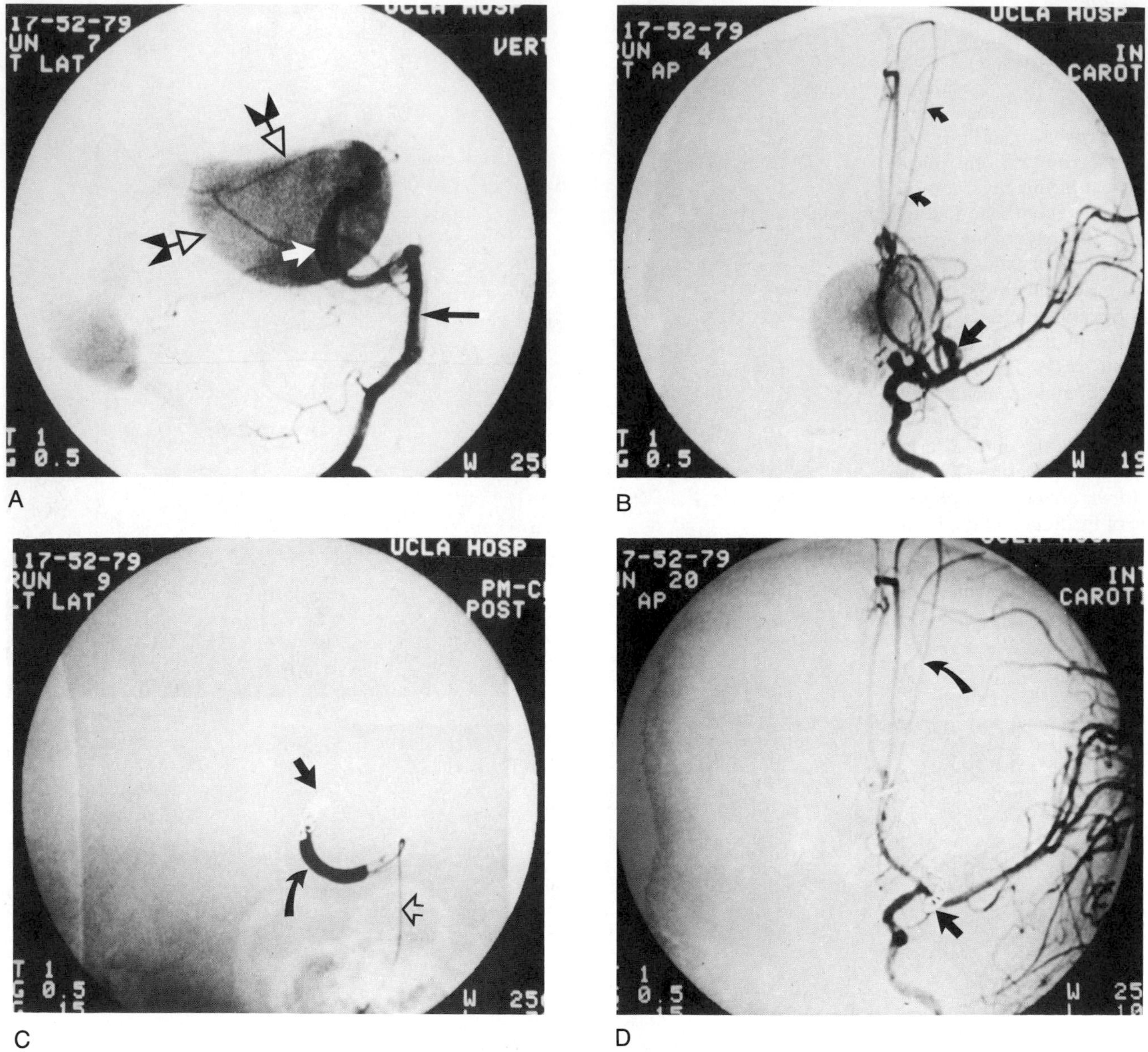


**Fig. 49-8.** Transfemoral embolization of a vein of Galen vascular malformation. (**A**) Lateral vertebral angiogram shows the basilar artery (*straight arrow*), and a fistulous connection between a posterior choroidal feeder (*white arrow*) and a vein of Galen aneurysm (*triangle arrows*). (**B**) Anteroposterior left internal carotid angiogram shows the posterior choroidal feeder previously described (*straight arrow*) and lesser participation from the left pericallosal artery (*curved arrows*). (**C**) Superselective postembolization angiogram shows the microcatheter in the basilar artery (*open arrow*), occlusion of the arteriovenous fistula with coils (*straight arrow*) and stagnant contrast material in the proximal posterior choroidal artery (*curved arrow*). (**D**) Postembolization left carotid angiogram shows the coils deposited in the left posterior choroidal feeder (*straight arrow*) and minor participation from the left pericallosal artery (*curved arrow*).

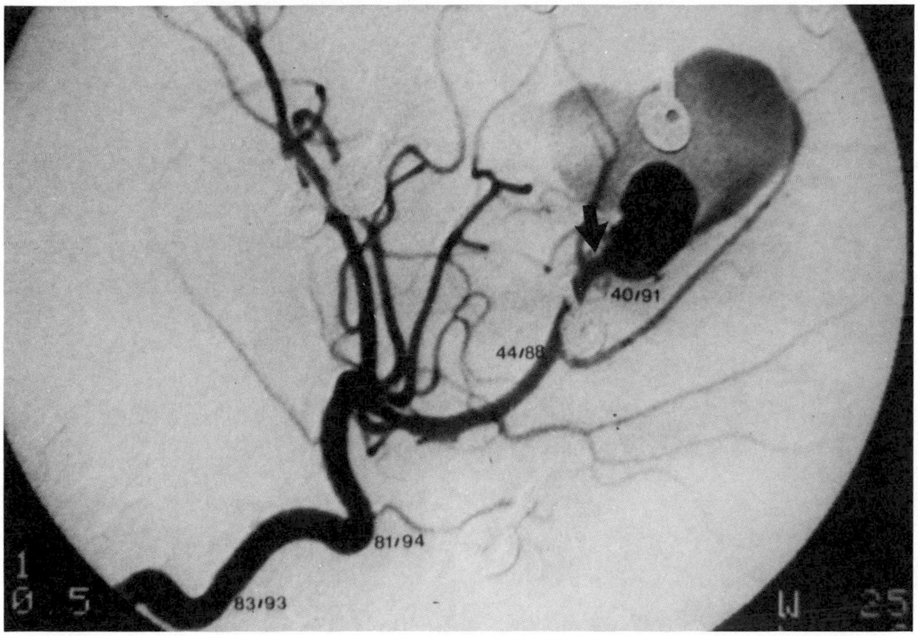


A

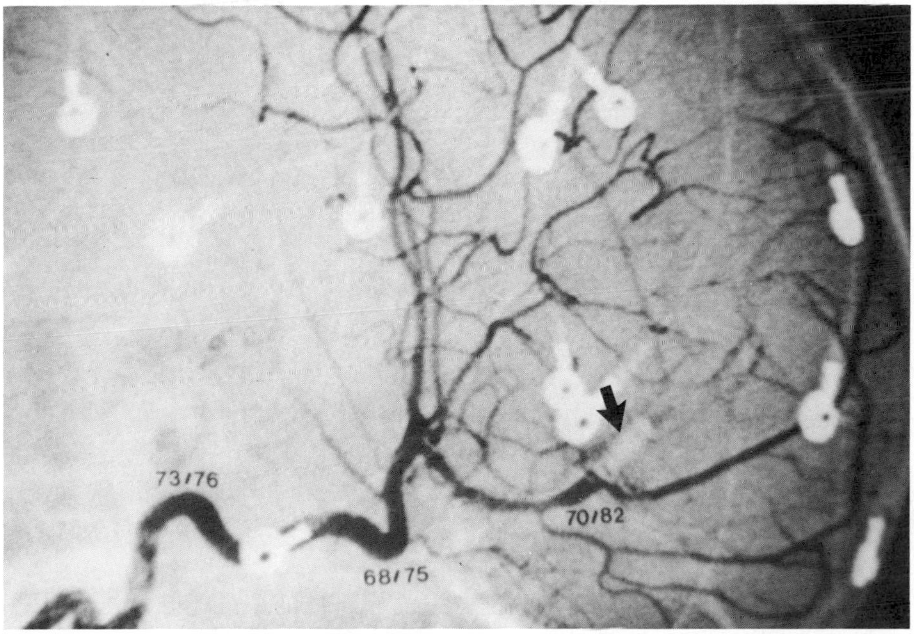


B

**Fig. 49-9.** Endovascular embolization of brain spontaneous arteriovenous fistula. (**A**) Lateral left internal carotid angiogram shows an arteriovenous fistula (*arrow*) between pericallosal artery and a mesiofrontal varix. Notice the median pressures in the anterior cerebral artery (44 mmHg) and at the fistula site (40 mmHg). (**B**) Immediate postembolization angiogram show obliteration of the arteriovenous fistula by a detachable balloon (*arrow*). Notice an immediate increase of 30 mmHg in the mean pressure at the fistula site.

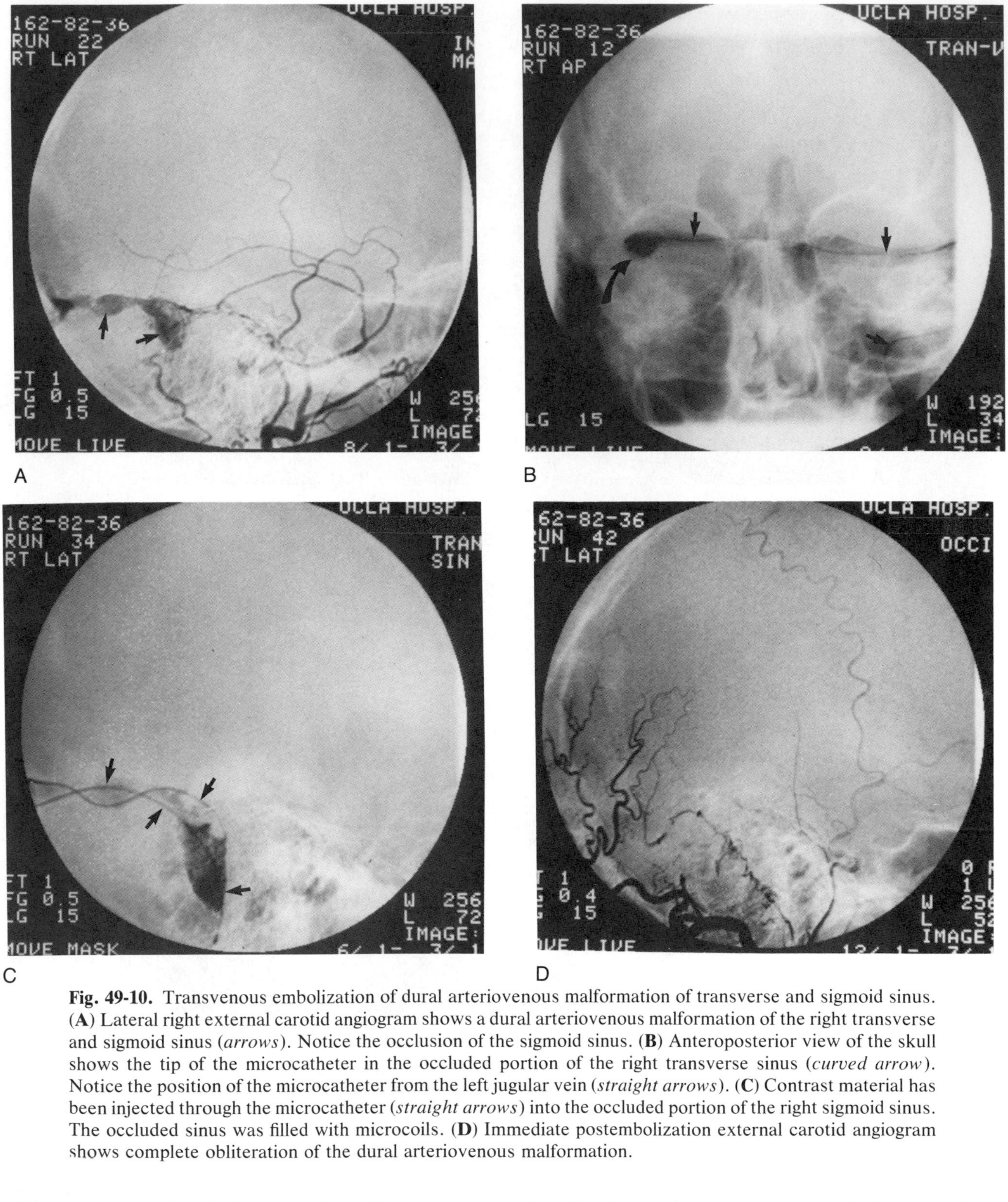


**Fig. 49-10.** Transvenous embolization of dural arteriovenous malformation of transverse and sigmoid sinus. (**A**) Lateral right external carotid angiogram shows a dural arteriovenous malformation of the right transverse and sigmoid sinus (*arrows*). Notice the occlusion of the sigmoid sinus. (**B**) Anteroposterior view of the skull shows the tip of the microcatheter in the occluded portion of the right transverse sinus (*curved arrow*). Notice the position of the microcatheter from the left jugular vein (*straight arrows*). (**C**) Contrast material has been injected through the microcatheter (*straight arrows*) into the occluded portion of the right sigmoid sinus. The occluded sinus was filled with microcoils. (**D**) Immediate postembolization external carotid angiogram shows complete obliteration of the dural arteriovenous malformation.

The transarterial embolization of dural AVMs usually achieves a satisfactory clinical result, though it seldom occludes the AVM completely. This technical challenge is related to the generous blood supply of the dura mater.[77] The transarterial occlusion of small distal feeders without concomitant obliteration of the AV shunting elicits development of myriad collaterals from ipsilateral and contralateral meningeal vessels (external carotid, internal carotid, and vertebral meningeal blood supply).

Halbach et al.[37] described complete obliteration of dural AVMs involving the cavernous and transverse sinuses by using the transvenous approach. Retrograde catheterization of the cavernous sinus or partially thrombosed transverse sinus may be achieved by using the microcatheters via transfemoral or transjugular routes. The dural AVMs and the involved sinus may be obliterated with the delivery of microcoils, silk, or liquid agents (Fig. 49-10).

Endovascular therapy of dural AVMs may cause complications such as blindness, stroke, and peripheral cranial nerve palsies.[72] These complications are related to untoward embolization of external carotid-internal carotid communications or neuromeningeal branches of the external carotid artery. These arteries supply cranial nerves when they pierce the dura at the skull base or within the cavernous sinus.[54]

## ENDOVASCULAR THERAPY IN HEAD AND NECK VASCULAR MALFORMATIONS AND TUMORS

The external carotid artery is the dominant route to embolize vascular tumors and malformations of the head and neck (capillary and cavernous hemangiomas of bone and soft tissue, cranial nerve schwannomas, glomus tumors, juvenile angiofibromas, meningiomas, arteriovenous malformations). A safe superselective catheterization of all branches of the external carotid artery using microcatheters and the awareness of potentially dangerous external-internal carotid collaterals have markedly decreased the morbidity of these procedures.[88]

The presurgical embolization of vascular tumors

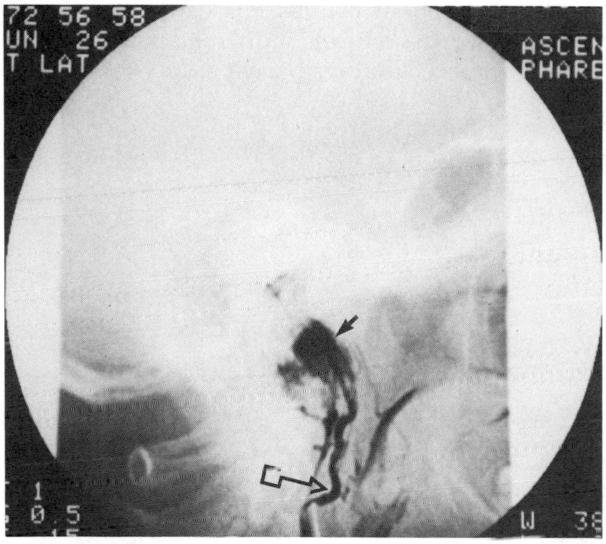


A

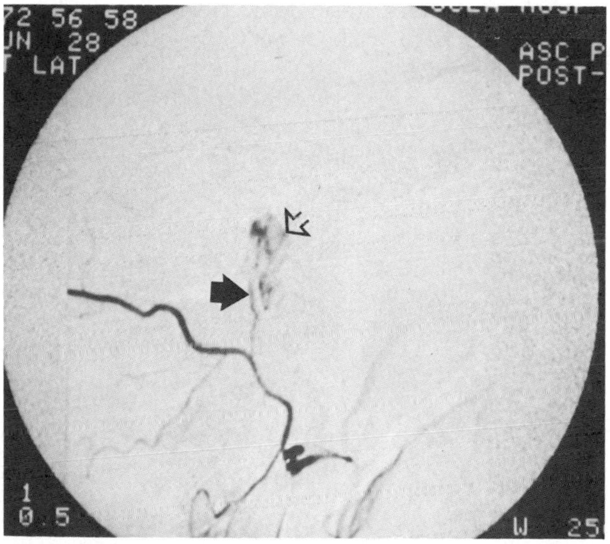


B

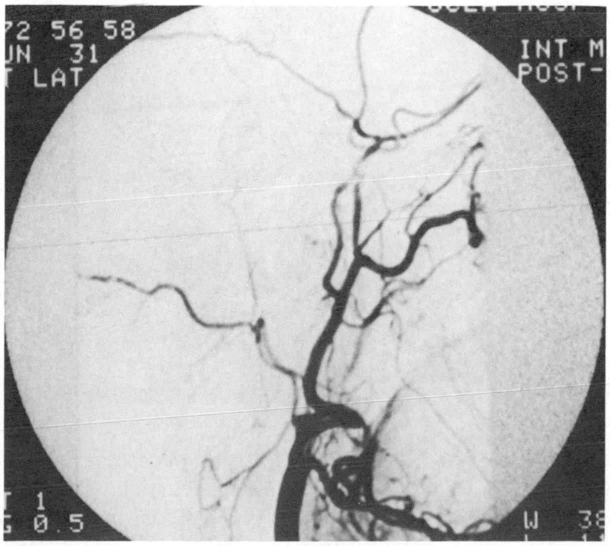


C

**Fig. 49-11.** Presurgical embolization of base of skull tumor. (**A**) Selective left ascending pharyngeal (*square arrow*) arteriogram shows a typical blushing from a small glomus jugulare (*straight arrow*). (**B**) Selective left occipital arteriogram shows tumor blush (*open arrow*) supplied by stylomastoid artery (*straight arrow*). (**C**) Postembolization left external carotid angiogram shows absence of tumor blush in the region of the left jugular fossa. The tumor was successfully resected without hemorrhagic complications.

such as chemodectomas (carotid body tumors, glomus vagale, glomus jugulare) and juvenile angiofibromas is now a standardized technique because it allows surgical removal of these rebellious vascular tumors with less blood loss and operative time.[94] It is possible to selectively catheterize individual tumor feeders and occlude the majority of the tumor bed with particles (polyvinal alcohol [PVA], 300 to 600 $\mu$m in diameter) (Fig. 49-11). Particles are preferred for lesions supplied by the middle meningeal, posterior auricular, or ascending pharyngeal arteries, because these arteries participate in the blood supply to several cranial nerves.[55] Delivery of the embolic material should be flow-directed and under fluoroscopic control in order to decrease the risk of embolization of intracranial circulation via external-internal carotid anastomosis.[52] Liquid agents such as acrylic material may be used in vascular malformations and fistulae or in those tumors with a fast arteriovenous shunting, when there is no risk of occluding blood supply to cranial nerves.[88]

The presurgical occlusion of the tumor bed has decreased the need for sacrificing the common carotid artery during surgery.[94] In cases of large, nonsurgical vascular tumors of the skull base, embolization of the tumor bed may be followed by radiotherapy of the residual tumor.

## CEREBRAL ANEURYSMS

Endovascular occlusive techniques using balloon catheter systems have also been applied to the treatment of intracranial aneurysms.[2,8,28,29,30,32,34,36,41–45,78,80] For most intracranial aneurysms, surgical clipping remains the treatment of choice.[69] The goal of obliterating aneurysms endovascularly and preserving the parent artery has been slower to be realized than for direct arteriovenous fistulas.[26] Because of some early problems[8] with such an approach, detachable balloons have been used for parent artery occlusion for

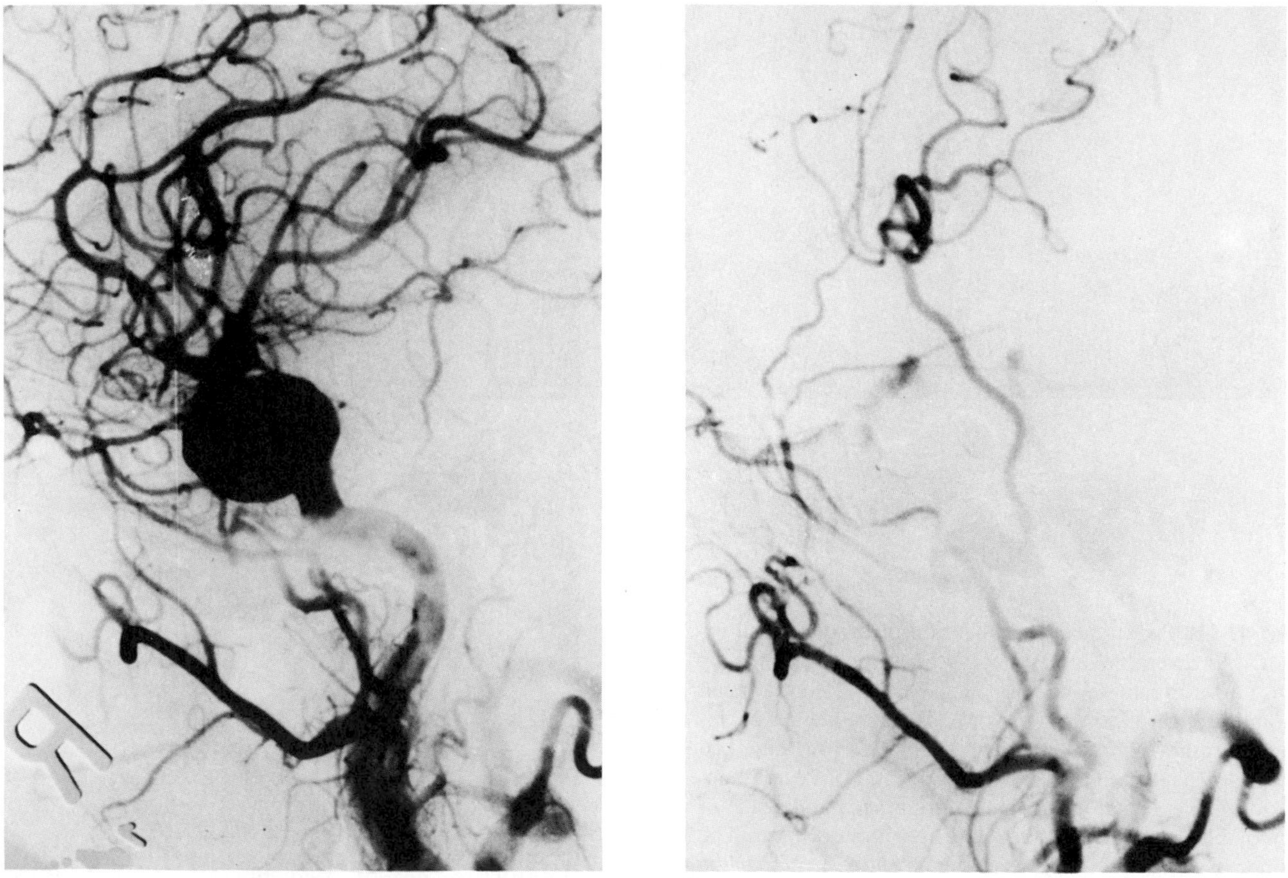

A B

**Fig. 49-12.** Balloon occlusion of carotid artery for cavernous aneurysm. (**A**) Lateral right carotid angiogram shows a cavernous carotid aneurysm. (**B**) Right carotid angiogram following unsuccessful balloon occlusion test and detachment of two balloons in the internal carotid artery below the aneurysm. The aneurysm and the artery have been isolated from the circulation. Collateral via superficial-to-middle cerebral bypass and retrograde ophthalmic collaterals are noted.

many unclippable aneurysms.[2,8,21,32] Following clinical, angiographic, and laboratory assessment of potential tolerance of arterial obliteration, the internal carotid or vertebral artery can be occluded by the percutaneous femoral cerebral catheterization technique with the patient awake. This technique is an alternative to surgical occlusion by ligation or Selverstone clamp. The procedure, when done under systemic heparinization, allows for a period of clinical monitoring following balloon inflation and prior to detachment. If the patient tolerates occlusion, the balloon is detached. A second balloon can be detached just proximal to the first for security. At the end of the procedure, heparinization is reversed and thrombosis allowed to take place, which most often obliterates the aneurysm as well as the carotid or vertebral artery. In cases where an artery is occluded for treatment of aneurysm below the level of the first major collateral (Fig. 49-12), complete aneurysm thrombosis will occur secondary to artery occlusion.[32] Where an artery is occluded for treatment of an aneurysm lying at or above the level of the first major collateral (Fig. 49-13), complete aneurysm thrombosis can be induced in more than half of cases[32] merely by change in flow patterns and turbulence. The approach to occlusion of parent arteries below an unclippable aneurysm stands as a convenient, safe alternative to other means of effecting arterial occlusion.[2,8,32] These procedures are carried out in awake patients merely as an extension of the angiographic procedure.

The treatment of intracranial aneurysms by endovascular approach preserving the parent vessels stands as a more elegant procedure.

Romadanov and Shcheglov[78] have used the detachable balloon approach as the primary therapy for a large series of intracranial aneurysms, the majority of

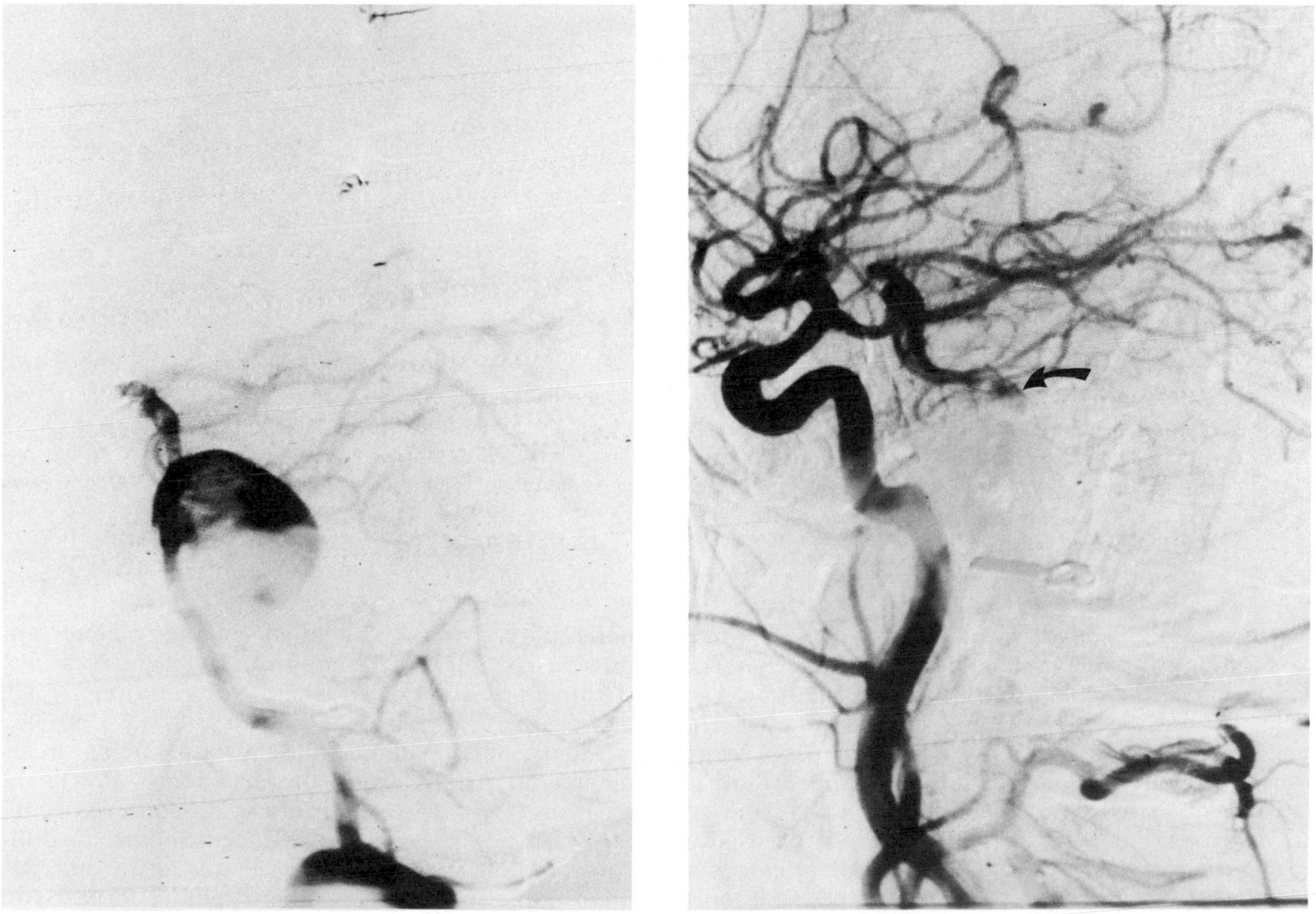

A B

**Fig. 49-13.** Proximal balloon occlusion of vertebral artery for large basilar aneurysm. (**A**) Lateral right vertebral angiogram following surgical exploration and occlusion of the left vertebral by clip. The large midbasilar aneurysm is well seen. (**B**) Immediately following balloon occlusion of the right vertebral at the C2-C3 level, right common carotid angiogram shows collaterals to the distal basilar with some continued filling of the basilar aneurysm (*curved arrow*). (*Figure continues.*)

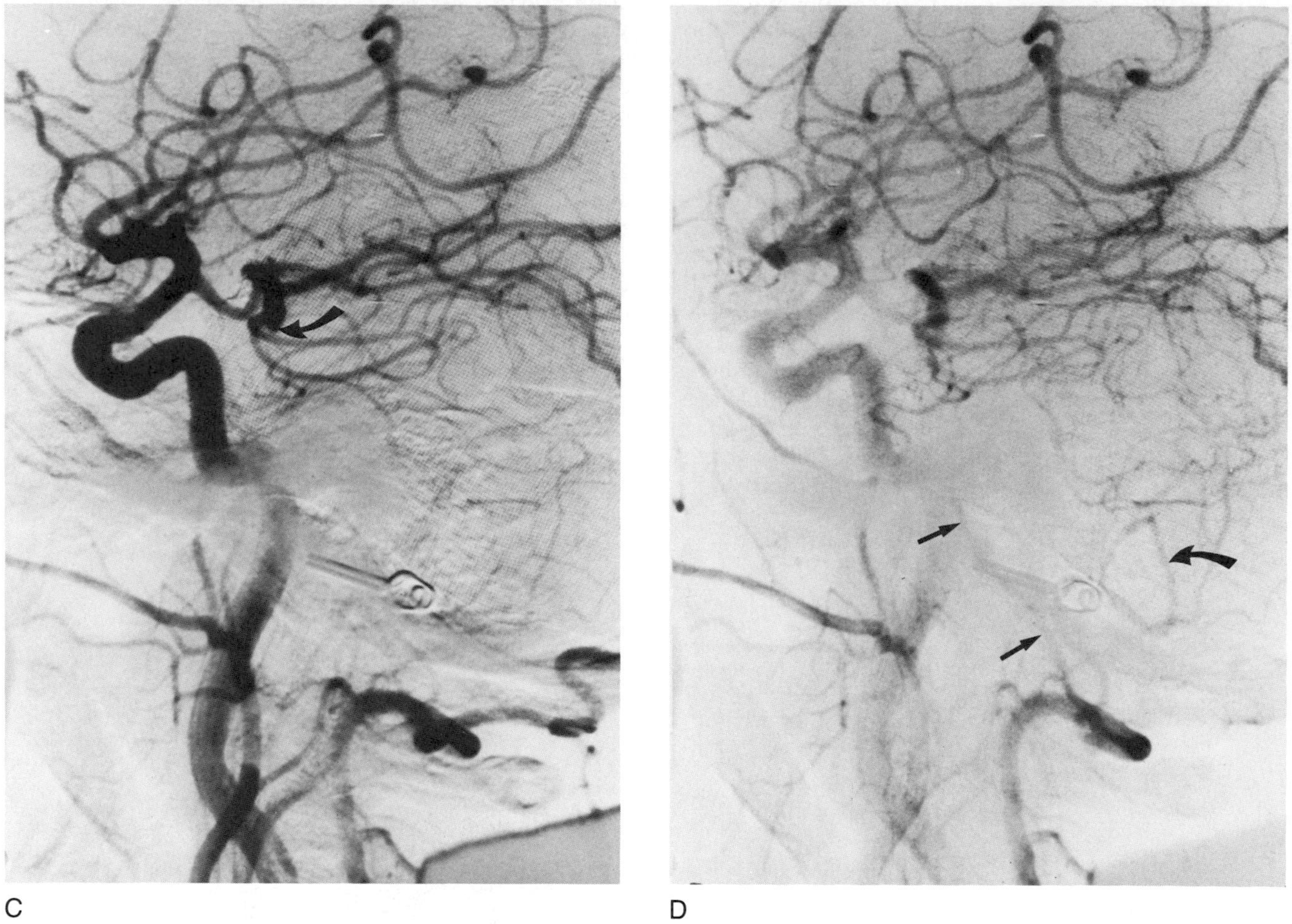


**Fig. 49-13** (*Continued*). (**C**) Late follow-up right carotid angiogram shows that the distal basilar artery (*curved arrow*) no longer supplies the aneurysm. (**D**) Later in the same angiogram as Fig. C, occipital collaterals reconstitute the right vertebral artery at C1, with antegrade flow up the basilar trunk (*arrows*) without aneurysm filling. The posterior inferior cerebellar artery (*curved arrow*) is also seen. This is an example of proximal occlusion, without trapping, leading to complete aneurysm thrombosis.

which would be considered surgically clippable. The vast majority of aneurysms treated in the Kiev series have been cold aneurysms with only a small number of aneurysms treated after having acutely bled. The largest series of aneurysms treated in the western world by endovascular approach with preservation of the parent vessels, in San Francisco,[36,41–44] consists only of cases that were surgically inaccessible because of the size or anatomy of the lesion and patients who were not candidates for general anesthesia. In both series, using local anesthesia, detachable balloons passed through the intracranial circulation, directed into the aneurysm, inflated with a polymerizing substance[34,85] and detached. The experience in hundreds of cases now has shown that most aneurysms can be potentially entered and filled by this balloon approach. The morbidity and mortality of endovascular treatment has included aneurysm rupture, stroke, and death.[42,43,45,78]

The use of detachable balloons for aneurysm treatment with parent artery preservation is slowly increasing (Fig. 49-14), with the main concerns being aneurysm rupture, especially in acute cases, the difficulty of filling the neck of wide-necked aneurysms, the migration of balloons into the thrombus in partially clotted giant aneurysms, and the potential of neck remnants[23,58] still filling. The development of new balloons, microcatheters, and alternative embolic materials such as microcoils (Fig. 49-15) promises to expand the endovascular therapy of aneurysms.

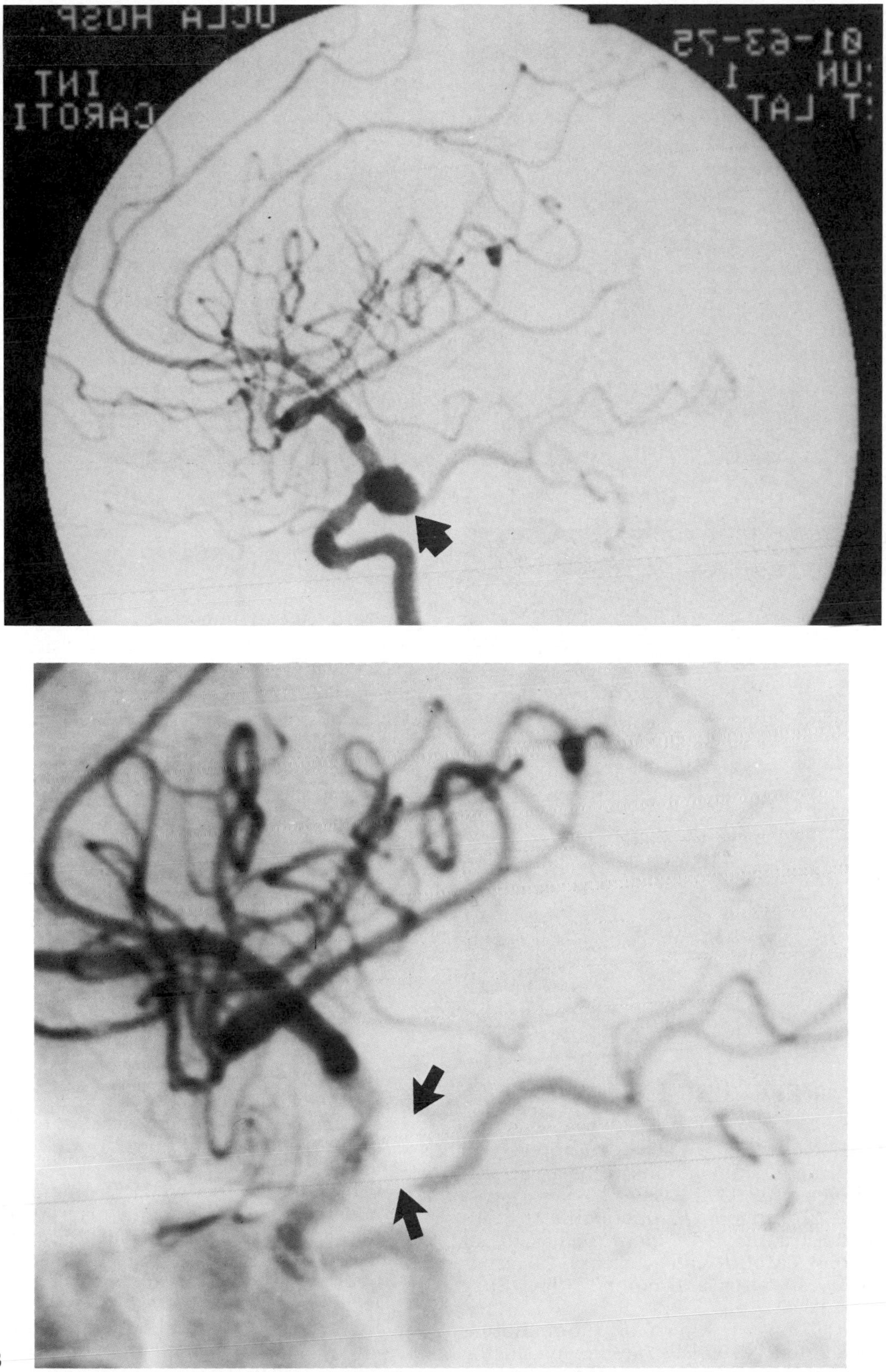

A

B

**Fig. 49-14.** Case of balloon in aneurysm with preservation of parent artery. (**A**) Lateral view of left internal carotid shows a middle-sized anterior communicating artery aneurysms (*arrow*). (**B**) Immediate postembolization angiogram shows complete obliteration of the aneurysm by detachable balloon (*arrows*). Notice the patency of the internal carotid and the posterior cerebral arteries.

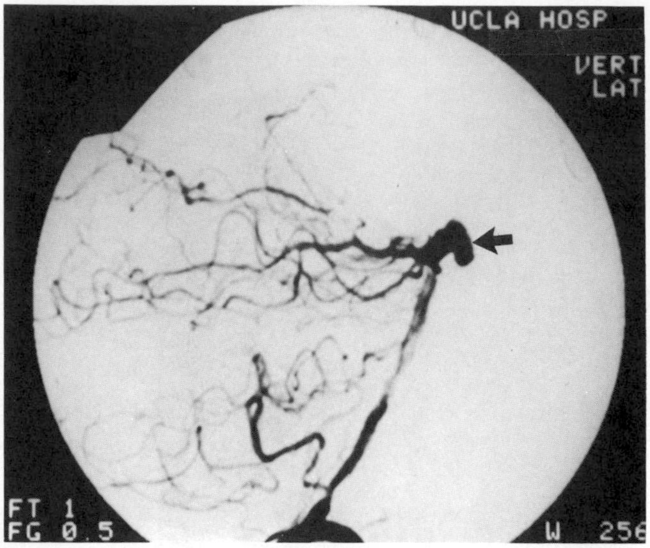


A

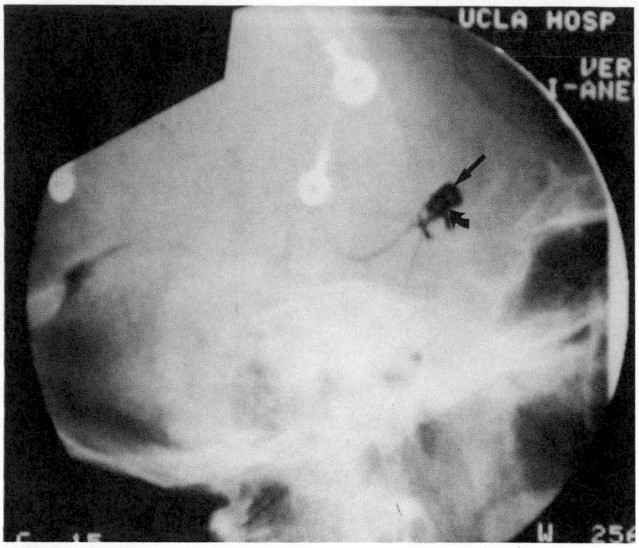


B

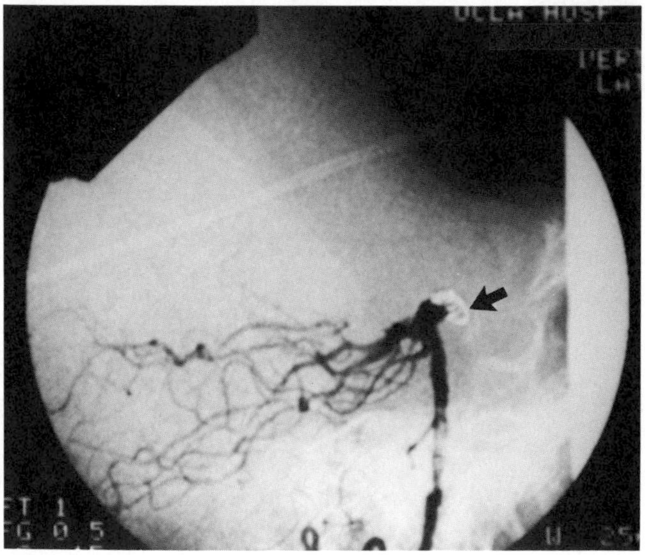

C

**Fig. 49-15.** Aneurysm occlusion with detachable microcoils. (**A**) Lateral view of vertebral angiogram shows a small basilar tip aneurysm growing anteriorly and inferiorly (*arrow*). (**B**) Superselective angiogram through a Tracker microcatheter shows the relationship between the dome of the aneurysm (*straight arrow*) to the osteum of the left posterior cerebral artery (*curved arrow*). (**C**) Postembolization angiogram shows complete obliteration of the aneurysm with detachable platinum microcoils (*straight arrow*).

## REFERENCES


1. Amacher AL, Shillito J, Jr: The syndromes and surgical treatment of aneurysms of the great vein of Galen. J Neurosurg 39:89, 1973
2. Berenstein A, Ransohoff J, Kupersmith M et al: Transvascular treatment of giant aneurysms of the cavernous carotid and vertebral arteries: functional investigation and embolization. Surg Neurol 21:3, 1984
3. Berenstein A, Young W, Ransohoff J: Somatosensory evoked potentials (SEP) monitoring during spinal angiography and its uses during therapeutic transvascular embolization. AJNR 3:96, 1982
4. Berestrand A, Hook O, Lidvall H: Vascular malformations of the spinal cord. Acta Neurol Scand 40:169, 1964
5. Betti OO, Munari C, Rosler R: Stereotactic radiosurgery with the linear accelerator: treatment of arteriovenous malformations. Neurosurgery 6:833, 1989
6. Cronqvist S, Troupp H: Intracranial arteriovenous malformations and arterial aneurysms in the same patient. Acta Neurol Scand 42:307, 1966
7. Deans WR, Bzoch S, Leibrock L et al: Arteriovenous fistula in patients with neurofibromatosis. Radiology 144:103, 1982
8. Debrun G, Fox A, Drake C et al: Giant unclippable aneurysms: treatment with detachable balloons. AJNR 2:167, 1981
9. Debrun G, Lacour P, Caron J: Detachable balloons and calibrated-leak balloons techniques in the treatment of cerebral vascular lesions. J Neurosurg 49, 635, 1978

10. Debrun J, Lacour P, Viñuela F et al: Treatment of 54 traumatic carotid cavernous fistulas. J Neurosurg 55:678, 1981
11. Debrun G, Viñuela F, Fox AJ et al: Embolization of cerebral arteriovenous malformations with bucylate: experience with 46 cases. J Neurosurg 56:615, 1982
12. Debrun GM, Viñuela FV, Fox AJ et al: Two different calibrated leak balloons: experimental work and application in humans. AJNR 3:407, 1982
13. Debrun GM, Viñuela F, Fox AJ et al: Indications for treatment and classification of 132 carotid-cavernous fistulas. Neurosurgery 22:285, 1988
14. Di Chiro G, Doppman J, Ommaya AK: Selective arteriography of arteriovenous aneurysms of spinal cord. Radiology 88:1065, 1967
15. Dion JE, Viñuela F, Lylyk P et al: Impact of recent technological advances on endovascular therapy of brain arteriovenous malformations and fistulas. Presented at the Annual Meeting of the Western Neuroradiological Society, Rancho Bernardo, CA, October 1988
16. Djindjian R: Neuroradiological examination of spinal cord angiomas. Handb Clin Neurol 12:631, 1972
17. Djindjian R, Favre C, Houdart L et al: Exploration angiographique des malformations vasculaires de la moelle épinère. Acta Radiol [Diagn] (Stockh) 5:145, 1966
18. Doppman JL, Di Chiro G, Ommaya AK: Percutaneous embolization of spinal cord arteriovenous malformations. J Neurosurg 34:48, 1971
19. Doppmann JL, Girton M, OldField EJ: Spinal Wada test. Radiology 161:319, 1986
20. Dowd CF, Halbach VV, Barnwell SL et al: Transfemoral venous embolization of vein of Galen malformations. AJNR 11:643, 1990
21 Drake CG: Giant intracranial aneurysms: experience with surgical treatment in 174 patients. Clin Neurosurg 26:12, 1979
22. Drake CG: Arteriovenous malformations of the brain: the options for management. N Engl J Med 309:308, 1983
23. Drake CG, Vanderlinden RG: The late consequences of incomplete surgical treatment of cerebral aneurysms. J Neurosurg 27:226, 1967
24. Duckwiler G, Dion J, Viñuela F et al: Intravascular microcatheter pressure monitoring: experimental results and early clinical evaluation. AJNR 11:169, 1990
25. Eskridge JM, Hartling RP: Preoperative embolization of brain AVMs using surgical silk and polyvinyl alcohol, abstracted. AJNR 10:882, 1989
26. Ferguson CG: Physical factors in the initiation, growth and rupture of human intracranial saccular aneurysms. J Neurosurg 37:666, 1972
27. Forster DMC, Steiner L, Hakanson S: Arteriovenous malformations of the brain: a long-term clinical study. J Neurosurg 37:562, 1972
28. Fox AJ, Drake CG: Aneurysm neck remnant following balloon embolization. J Neurosurg 67:321, 1987
29. Fox AJ, Drake CG: Endovascular therapy of intracranial aneurysms. AJNR 11:641, 1990
30. Fox AJ, Drake CG: Detachable balloon embolization for intracranial aneurysms. J Neurosurg 73:157, 1990
31. Fox AJ, Girvin JP, Viñuela F, Drake CG: Rolandic arteriovenous malformations: improvement in limb function by IBCA embolization. AJNR 6:575, 1985
32. Fox AJ, Viñuela F, Pelz DM, et al: Use of detachable balloons for proximal artery occlusion in the treatment of unclippable cerebral aneurysms. J Neurosurg 66:40, 1987
33. Fox AJ, Viñuela F, Pelz DM, Debrun GM: Vertebral and external carotid fistulas. Semin Interven Radiol 4:249, 1987
34. Goto K, Halbach VV, Hardin CW et al: Permanent inflation of detachable balloons with a low viscosity hydrophilic polymerizing system. Radiology 169:787, 1988
35. Halbach VV, Higashida RT, Hang P et al: Preoperative balloon occlusion of arteriovenous malformations. Neurosurgery 22:301, 1988
36. Halbach VV, Higashida RT, Hieshima GB: Treatment of intracranial aneurysms by balloon embolization therapy. Semin Interven Radiol 4:261, 1987
37. Halbach VV, Higashida RT, Hieshima GB et al: Transvenous embolization of dural AVMs. Presented at the Annual Meeting of the Western Neuroradiological Society, Rancho Bernardo, CA, October 1988
38. Halbach VV, Higashida RT, Hieshima GB, Hardin CW: Transvenous embolization of direct carotid-cavernous fistulas. AJNR 9:741, 1988
39. Hanner JS, Quisling RG: Gianturco coil embolization of vein of Galen aneurysms: technical aspects. Radiographics 8:935, 1988
40. Hieshima GB, Cahan LD, Mehringer CH et al: Spontaneous arteriovenous fistulas of cerebral vessels in association with the fibromuscular dysplasia. Neurosurgery 18:454, 1986
41. Hieshima GB, Higashida RT, Wapenski J et al. Balloon embolization of a large distal basilar aneurysm, case report. J Neurosurg 65:413, 1986
42. Higashida RT, Halbach VV, Cahan LD et al: Detachable balloon embolization therapy of posterior circulation intracranial aneurysms. J Neurosurg 71:512, 1989
43. Higashida RT, Halbach VV, Barnwell SL et al. Treatment of intracranial aneurysms with preservation of the parent vessel: results of percutaneous balloon embolization in 84 patients. AJNR 11:633, 1990
44. Higashida RT, Halbach VV, Dormandy B et al: Endovascular treatment of intracranial aneurysms using a new silicone microballoon device: technical considerations and indications for therapy. Radiology 174:687, 1990
45. Hodes JE, Fox AJ, Pelz DM, Peerless SJ: Rupture of aneurysms following balloon embolization. J Neurosurg 72:567–571, 1990
46. Horton JA, Latchan RE, Gold LH et al: Embolization of intramedullary arteriovenous malformations of the spinal cord. AJNR 7:113, 1986
47. Houser OW, Baker HL Jr, Rhoton AL, Jr et al: Intracranial dural arteriovenous malformations. Radiology 105:55, 1972

48. Isamat F, Ferrer E, Twose J: Direct intracavernous obliteration of high-flow carotid-cavernous fistulas. J Neurosurg 65:770, 1986
49. Jungreis CA, Horton JA, Hecht ST: Blood pressure changes in feeders to cerebral arteriovenous malformations during therapeutic embolization. AJNR 10:575, 1989
50. Kendall BE, Logue V: Spinal epidural angiomatous malformations draining into intrathecal veins. Neuroradiology 13:181, 1977
51. Kerber CW: Balloon catheter with a calibrated leak. Radiology 120:574, 1976
52. Kerber CW: Flow-controlled therapeutic embolization: a physiologic and safe technique. AJNR 1:77, 1980
53. Koeppen AH, Barron KD, Cox JF: Foix-Allojoanine syndrome. Acta Neuropathol 29:197, 1974
54. Lasjuanias P: Aspect angiographique de la vascularisation des nerfs craniens. Presented at the Congrès Annuel de la Societé Francaise de Neuroradiologie, Toulouse, France, May 1979
55. Lasjuanias PL: Craniofacial and upper cervical arteries: functional, clinical and angiographic aspects. Williams & Wilkins, Baltimore, 1981
56. Lasjuanias P, Terbrugee K, Chiu M et al: Pediatric surgical neuroangiography: a multicentre approach. Presented at the Symposium Neuroradiologicum, Stockholm, June 1986
57. Leussenhop AJ, Spence WT: Artificial embolization of cerebral arteries: report of use in a case of arteriovenous malformation. JAMA 172:1153, 1960
58. Lin T, Fox AJ, Drank CG: Regrowth of aneurysm sacs from residual neck following aneurysm clipping. J Neurosurg 70:556, 1989
59. Locksley HG: Report on the cooperative study of intracranial aneurysms and subarachnoid hemorrhage. Section II, Part I: Natural history of subarachnoid hemorrhage, intracranial aneurysms and arteriovenous malformations. J Neurosurg 25:19, 1966
60. Manelfe C, Berenstein A: Treatment of carotid-cavernous fistulas by venous approach. J Neuroradiol 7:13, 1980
61. McAllister VL, Kendall B, Bull JWD: Symptomatic vertebral hemangioma. Brain 98:71, 1975
62. Merland JJ, Reizine D: Treatment of arteriovenous spinal cord malformations. Semin Interven Radiol 4:281, 1987
63. Mu Huo Teng M, Yoo Guo W, Huang CHJ et al: Occlusion of arteriovenous malformations of the cavernous sinus via the superior ophthalmic vein. AJNR 9:539, 1988
64. Newton TH, Cronquist S: Involvement of dural arteries in intracranial arteriovenous malformations. Radiology 93:1071, 1969
65. Obrador S, Soto M, Silvela J: Clinical syndromes of arteriovenous malformations of the transverse-sigmoid sinus. J Neurol Neurosurg Psychiatry 38:436, 1975
66. Ojemann G, Ojemann J, Lettich E et al: Cortical language localization in left, dominant hemisphere: an electrical stimulation mapping investigation in 117 patients. J Neurosurg 71:316, 189
67. Patronas NJ, Marx WJ, Duda EE et al: Microvascular embolization of arteriovenous malformations: predicting success by cerebral angiography. AJNR 1:459, 1980
68. Pawbinskas AJ, Perloff D, Newton TH: Fibromuscular hyperplasia; an arterial dysplasia of increasing clinical importance. AJR 98:907, 1966
69. Peerless SJ, Drake CGT: Management of aneurysms of the posterior circulation. p. 1715. In Youmans JR (ed): Neurological Surgery. 2nd Ed. WB Saunders, Philadelphia, 1982
70. Pelz DM, Fox AJ, Viñuela F, Drake CC et al. Preoperative embolization of brain AVMs with isobutyl-2-cyanoacrylate. AJNR 9:757, 1988
71. Pevsner PH: Micro-balloon catheter for superselective angiography and therapeutic occlusion. AJR 128–225, 1977
72. Picard L, Bracard S, Moret J et al: Spontaneous dural arteriovenous fistulas. Semin Interven Radiol 4:219, 1987
73. Rauch RA, Viñuela F, Dion J et al: Preembolization functional evaluation in brain AVMs: the superselective amytal test. AJNR 13:303, 1992
74. Rauch RA, Viñuela F, Dion J et al: Pre-embolization functional evaluation in brain AVMs: the ability of superselective amytal test to predict neurologic dysfunction before embolization. AJN 13:309, 1992
75. Riché MC, Melki JP, Merland JJ: The current state of embolization of spinal cord vascular malformations via the anterior spinal artery. AJNR 4:378, 1983
76. Rodda RA, Calbert GD: Post-mortem arteriography of cerebral arteriovenous malformations. J Neurol Neurosurg Psychiatry 32:432, 1969
77. Roland J, Bernard C, Bracard S et al: Microvascularization of the intracranial dura mater. Surg Radiol Anat 9:43, 1987
78. Romodanov AP, Schcheglov VI: Intravascular occlusion of saccular aneurysms of the cerebral arteries by means of a detachable balloon cather. p. 25. In Krayenbuhl H (ed): Advances and Technical Standards in Neurosurgery. Vol. 9. Springer-Verlag, New York, 1982
79. Russel DJ: The pathology of spontaneous intracranial hemorrhage. Proc R Soc Med 47:689, 1954
80. Serbinenko FA: Balloon catheterization and occlusion of major cerebral vessels. J Neurosurg 41:125, 1974
81. Spetzler RF, Martin NA, Carter LP et al: Surgical management of large AVMs by staged embolization and operative excision. J Neurosurg 67:17, 1987
82. Spetzler RF, Wilson CB, Weinstein P et al: Normal perfusion pressure breakthrough theory. Clin Neurosurg 25:651, 1978
83. Stehbeus WE: Pathology of the cerebral blood vessels. St. Louis, CV Mosby, 1972
84. Svien HJ, McRae J: Arteriovenous anomalies of the brain. J Neurosurg 23:23, 1965
85. Taki W, Handa H, Yamagata S et al: Radio-opaque solidifying liquids for releasable balloon technique: a technical note. Surg Neurol 13:140, 1980
86. Thèron J, Cosgrove R, Melanson D, Ethier R: Spi-

nal arteriovenous malformations: advances in therapeutic embolization. Radiology 158:163, 1986

87. Viñuela F, Debrun G, Drake CG et al: Progressive thrombosis of brain arteriovenous malformations after embolization with isobutyl-2-cyanoacrylate. AJNR 4, 1233, 1983
88. Viñuela F, Debrun GM, Fox AJ: Detachable calibrated leak balloon for superselective angiography and embolization of dural arteriovenous malformations. J Neurosurg 1:817, 1983
89. Viñuela F, Debrun GM, Fox AJ et al: The role of the pre-embolization superselective angiogram in the treatment of brain arteriovenous malformations in isobutyl-2-cyanoacrylate. AJNR 7:919, 1986
90. Viñuela F, Dion J, Duckwiler G, Fox AJ et al: Endovascular embolization and surgery in brain AVMs. Experience with 101 cases. J Neurosurg 75:856, 1991
91. Viñuela F, Drake CG, Fox AJ, Pelz DM: Giant intracranial varices secondary to high-flow arteriovenous fistulae. J Neurosurg 66:198, 1987
92. Viñuela F, Fox AJ, Pelz DM: Identification of arteriovenous fistulae in cerebral AVMs: Important therapeutic implications. XIII Symposium Neuroradiologicum Stockholm June 23–28, 1986. Book of abstracts. 1G:149
93. Viñuela F, Fox AJ, Pelz D, Debrun G: Angiographic follow-up of large cerebral AVMs incompletely embolized with isobutyl-2-cyanoacrylate. AJNR 7:919, 1986
94. Ward PH, Liu C, Viñuela F, Bentson JR: Embolization: an adjunctive measure for removal of carotid body tumors. Laryngoscope 98:1287, 1988
95. Wolpert SM, Barnett FJ, Prager RJ: Benefits of embolization without surgery of cerebral arteriovenous malformations. AJNR 2:535, 1981
96. Wolpert SM, Stein BM: Factors governing the course of emboli in the therapeutic embolization of cerebral arteriovenous malformations. Radiology 131:125, 1979
97. Yasargil MG: AVM of vein of Galen region. p. 323. In Microneurosurgery. Vol. 3. Thieme, New York, 1988

# 50

# SPONTANEOUS BRAIN HEMORRHAGE: SURGICAL CONSIDERATIONS

Robert M. Crowell
Robert G. Ojemann
Christopher S. Ogilvy

Spontaneous brain hemorrhage is a rather common form of stroke. About 20 cases per 100,000 population occur annually. Brain hemorrhage and subarachnoid hemorrhage (10 per 100,000 per year) amount to about 15 percent of all strokes.

Although *evacuation of intracerebral hematoma* is one of the older neurosurgical procedures, the operation is undergoing major reevaluation in light of technological advances. Computed tomography (CT) now easily detects fresh brain hemorrhage, and magnetic resonance (MR) can sometimes give additional useful information. Classical surgical techniques for removal of clot are being supplemented (or supplanted) by stereotactic aspiration, facilitated by instillation of thrombolytic agents. Properly designed clinical trials have begun to demonstrate the specific situations in which clot removal can (or cannot) be of clinical benefit.

After the effects of acute hemorrhage are dealt with, the *risk of recurrent hemorrhage* requires assessment. CT and MR sometimes demonstrate the cause of hemorrhage, for example, aneurysm, cavernous angioma, or tumor. In questionable cases, angiography is warranted. Surgical correction of bleeding lesions is usually warranted to prevent recurrent hemorrhage. Guidelines for management are evolving, as experience with MR-depicted pathology and its natural history is accumulated.

## HISTORICAL PERSPECTIVE

In 1883 MacEwen[88] performed the first successful operation for intracerebral hematoma, thus making it one of the earliest neurosurgical procedures. Cushing,[33] in 1903, discussed the possibilities of surgical treatment in patients with intracerebral hematoma. Subsequently, numerous reports appeared describing evacuation of hematomas from the parenchyma of the brain. Bagley[9] stated in 1932 that the success of such procedures depended on the location of the hematoma within the brain. He suggested that evacuation of lobar lesions led to successful results, whereas removal of deep lesions led to unacceptable outcomes.

The treatment studies of McKissock[94] and Richardson[124–127] in the 1960s showed that many patients will also make a good recovery with medical therapy.[36] Subsequently, numerous studies attempted to define the role of surgery for brain hemorrhage. Surgery seems indicated as a lifesaving measure for the patient deteriorating with a large hematoma mass[32] and for some patients with cerebellar hematoma.[58] Beyond these concepts, it is not proven whether morbidity can be lessened by immediate or delayed removal of a hematoma. Recent controlled trials have failed to show benefit for evacuation of putaminal hemorrhage. Further controlled trials of various clinical situations will probably define indications for surgery.[97]

Computed tomography (CT) has revolutionized the management of patients with brain hemorrhage. CT has augmented development of criteria for medical and surgical management. Intensive medical therapy is guided by clinical and CT data, including continuous monitoring of intracranial pressure. Surgery is based on clinical status as well as size and location of hematoma on CT scan.

## ETIOLOGIES

Spontaneous brain hemorrhage may occur from many causes[26,40,44,45,93] (Fig. 50-1). Hypertension is often associated with hemorrhage into putamen, cerebellum, thalamus, or pons.[14,20,176] The source of bleeding in these cases seems to be microaneurysm or arteriolar necrosis. Such primary brain hemorrhages are usually distinguished from other causes by clinical and CT findings. For example, aneurysm (Fig. 50-2) and arteriovenous malformation may lead to intraparenchymal bleeding, but clinical features (age of the patient, history of hypertension or seizures) and CT changes (subarachnoid blood or draining veins) generally serve to distinguish them from primary brain hemorrhage. Intracranial tumors, especially melanoma and glioma, occasionally present with hemorrhage, but the CT signature is usually distinctive.[28,63,83,90,114,120,144] Rarely, abscess may lead to intraparenchymal bleeding.[64] Hemorrhagic infarction is often distinguished by its clinical features and CT appearance, but this may be underdiagnosed.[19,51] Patients on anticoagulation may occasionally have a

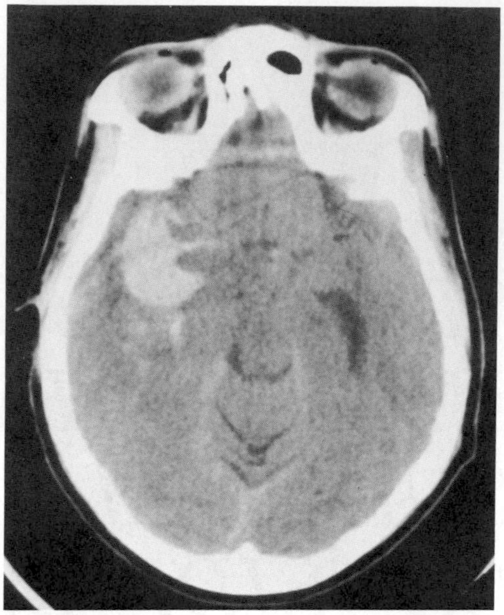

**Fig. 50-2.** Hemorrhage from posterior communicating artery-internal carotid artery aneurysm. Patient in coma with hemiplegia. Surgical clipping of aneurysm without angiography. Complete recovery.

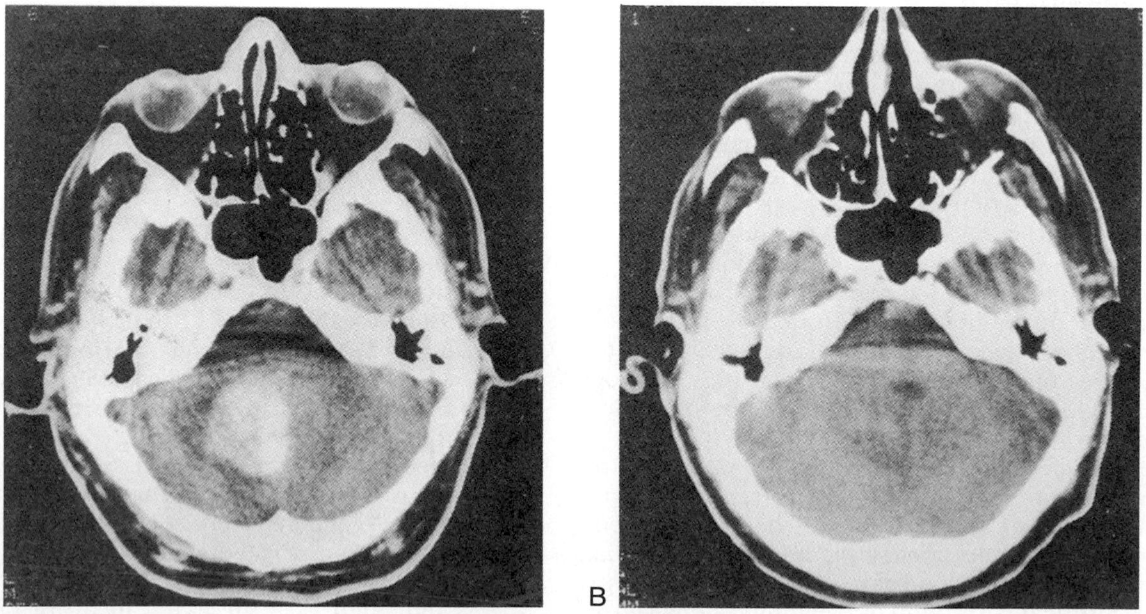

A B

**Fig. 50-1.** Cerebellar hemorrhage. (**A**) Computed tomography shows hematoma. (**B**) Computed tomography after stereotactic drainage. (From Mohadjer et al.,[99] with permission.)

brain hemorrhage,[81] generally in sites typical for hypertensive hemorrhage. In some instances, embolic infarction in anticoagulated patients may set the stage for more dramatic clinical manifestations due to bleeding into infarcted tissue. Endogenous coagulopathies, especially that caused by leukemia in the pediatric age group, may cause intraparenchymal hemorrhage.[2] In the elderly patient, amyloid angiopathy may be the cause of brain hemorrhage.[91,112] In some cases, vasculitis can be the cause of bleeding,[18,143] occasionally from exogenous agents such as cocaine or phenylpropanamine.[47] In a number of patients, especially those with a lobar hemorrhage, no source can be demonstrated despite extensive radiographic and pathologic studies.

The initial clinical effects from brain hemorrhage are due to direct destruction and displacement of local tissue.[4,131] CT and pathologic studies demonstrate tracking of blood along tissue planes, with displacement of tissue, especially white matter. The mechanism of later deterioration is less certain.[29] Serial CT studies have recently shown that rebleeding may be more frequent than previously suspected.[57] Edema and ischemic necrosis around the lesion probably are major factors. Experimental studies show decreased local cerebral blood flow.[103,104,128,129] In addition, hyperemia,[146] dysautoregulation, and blood-brain barrier disruption have been demonstrated.[73,76] Immune mechanisms and blood-derived toxins (such as glutamate and choline) may play a role in causing irreversible tissue damage.[97]

Resorption of the hematoma occurs over a course of months. The process is slow, because macrophage activity must occur along the edge of the mass. After a year, the hematoma site is converted to a slitlike cavity with orange-stained walls representing hemosiderin-laden macrophages.[17]

# EVALUATION

## Coagulation Studies

Routine coagulation studies should be performed in every case. These include prothrombin time (PT), partial thromboplastin time (PTT), and platelet count. The bleeding time should be estimated in patients receiving aspirin. Although these studies are usually normal, the occasional coagulopathy is detected and can be appropriately treated.

## Lumbar Puncture

There is no indication for a lumbar puncture (LP) in a patient suspected of having a brain hemorrhage. CT scan establishes the diagnosis noninvasively. In large hematomas, LP can cause transtentorial herniation, and in small hemorrhages, the cerebrospinal fluid (CSF) may be clear.[80]

## Computed Tomography

CT has dramatically altered management of brain hemorrhage.[5,52,55,75,89,119,138,163–165] Formerly, diagnosis of the condition was uncertain, and localization and sizing of lesions inferential. CT now routinely gives precise information about the localization, size, and configuration of parenchymal hemorrhage (Figs. 50-1 to 50-5; see Figs. 50-8 and 50-9). The presence and extent of subarachnoid hemorrhage and surrounding edema are depicted. CT also shows hydrocephalus, intraventricular hematoma, and ventricular compression or displacement. Information regarding volume of hematoma and involvement of posterior limb of internal capsule has been especially valuable in estimation of prognosis. Postoperative residual or recurrent hematoma can be detected.[35] CT occasionally suggests the etiology of hemorrhage, as, for example, by a calcified mass typical of giant aneurysm, a prominent draining vein suggestive of arteriovenous malformation (AVM), or an enhancing tumor mass.

Because it provides so much information with essentially no risk, CT is the study of choice for almost all patients suspected of brain hemorrhage. Only rarely does need for emergency surgery preclude CT evaluation. CT generally reduces need for potentially hazardous studies: LP and air studies are never indicated, and angiography only in selected cases.

Over several weeks, the high-density hematoma seen on CT scan gradually becomes isodense, and eventually develops a low-density appearance.[35,98] This apparently represents a change in photon absorption rather than actual resorption, as shown by CT-autopsy correlation. A few days to some months after hemorrhage, CT after contrast administration may show a ringlike enhancement around the hemorrhage, which represents edema or local ischemic infarction.[175]

## Magnetic Resonance Imaging

MR can readily image intraparenchymal hemorrhage, typically showing acute hematoma as bright signal on T2-weighted sequences.[25,153] The size of a hematoma may be overestimated on T2 sequences, since edema is also seen as bright signal; thus reference to T1-weighted images is needed to interpret the findings. As blood products decay over time, images of hematoma on T1- and T2-weighted sequences undergo a complex series of changes that have been characterized for acute, subacute, and chronic lesions.

For investigation of the source of hemorrhage, MRI can often be helpful (Fig. 50-3B). AVMs, giant (partially thrombosed) aneurysms, and cavernous angiomas have characteristic appearances.[105] Often tumors

A B
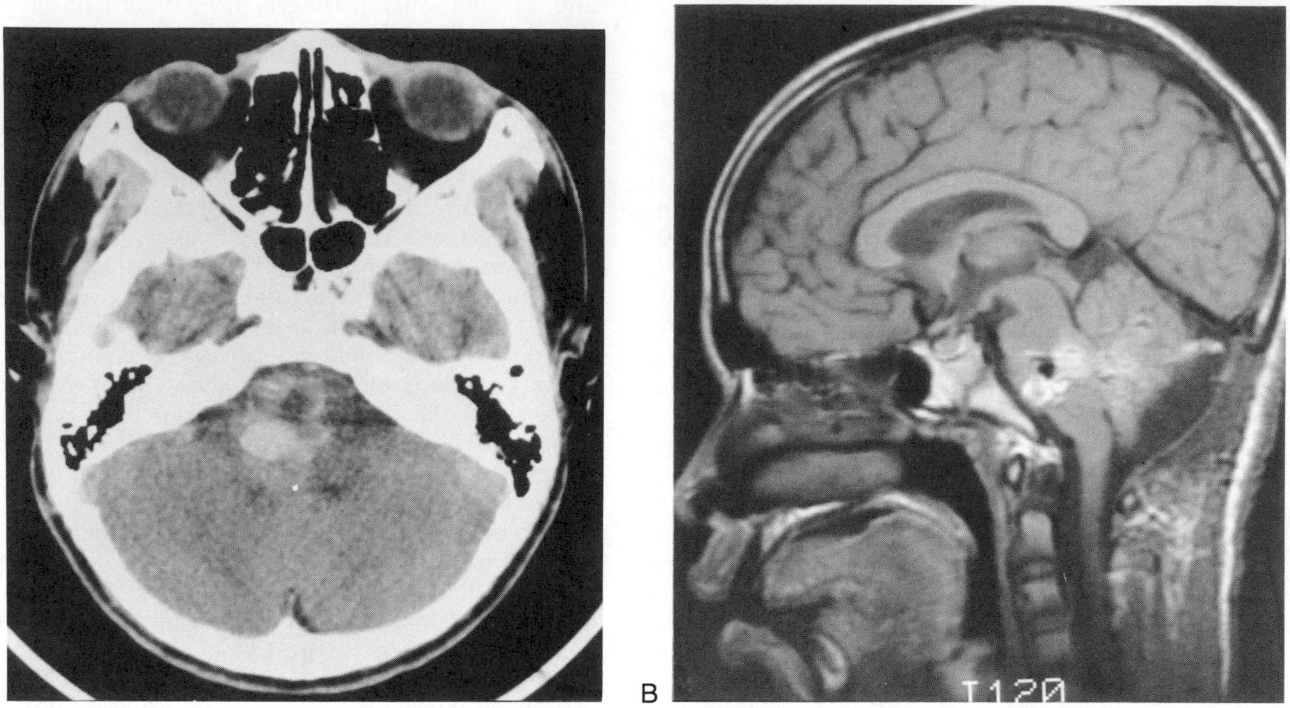


**Fig. 50-3.** Pontine hemorrhage from cavernous angioma. (**A**) Computed tomography shows hematoma. Patient in coma. Hematoma partially removed by emergency transvermian approach followed by clinical improvement. (**B**) Postoperative magnetic resonance imaging shows cavernous angioma. Reoperation with total excision of typical cavernous angioma. Recovery to minimal neurologic deficit.

can be identified by MRI, without and with gadolinium contrast enhancement. The combination of CT and MR often uncovers the cause of bleeding: CT is superior in detecting fresh clot and calcification, whereas MR is better in showing abnormal vessels and old blood products.

In some cases, MR angiography, done with phase contrast or two-dimensional time of flight techniques, may be helpful in evaluation of the etiology of hemorrhage. This is particularly true for sizable aneurysms and AVMs. However, clot and vessels are both bright, thus confusing the issue, and the detail is seldom sufficient to depict parent vessels precisely enough for surgery. Therefore, MRA is, so far, unable to supplant conventional angiography in the evaluation of brain hemorrhage of uncertain etiology.

### Angiography

In the typical hypertensive brain hemorrhage, angiography is rarely indicated.[66] In cases where hypertension is not the likely cause, particularly in lobar hemorrhage and in young people, when CT and MRI are nondiagnostic, angiography is indicated to determine if a vascular abnormality or tumor is present (Fig. 50-4B).[41,117,128] If angiography is negative, then repeat CT, MR, and angiography a few months later, after resolution of the mass effect, may permit visualization of AVM or tumor.

### Other Studies

While hematomas may be imaged by single-photon emission computed tomography (SPECT), photon emission tomography (PET),[39] or brain scanning, the clinical advantages of these studies have not been established. The role of monitoring of intracranial pressure has not been defined clearly.[116]

## INDICATIONS FOR SURGERY

Despite numerous series of medically and surgically treated patients with parenchymal hematoma, solid indications for surgery have not been established.[30,41,65,70,71,74,87,100,108,109,115,122,132,147] This statement holds for a range of surgical procedures, including open clot evacuation, stereotactic aspiration, and ventriculostomy. Even though some controlled prospective studies have been performed in the CT era, they are marred by small numbers, lack of adequate controls, and other design flaws. In the absence of adequate controlled studies, only broad guidelines for treatment can be suggested.

When a parenchymal hematoma threatens life, surgical removal of the lesion seems reasonable, especially in a young person with delayed deterioration. On the other hand, an elderly person with coma from onset and a huge dominant hemispheric clot is not a

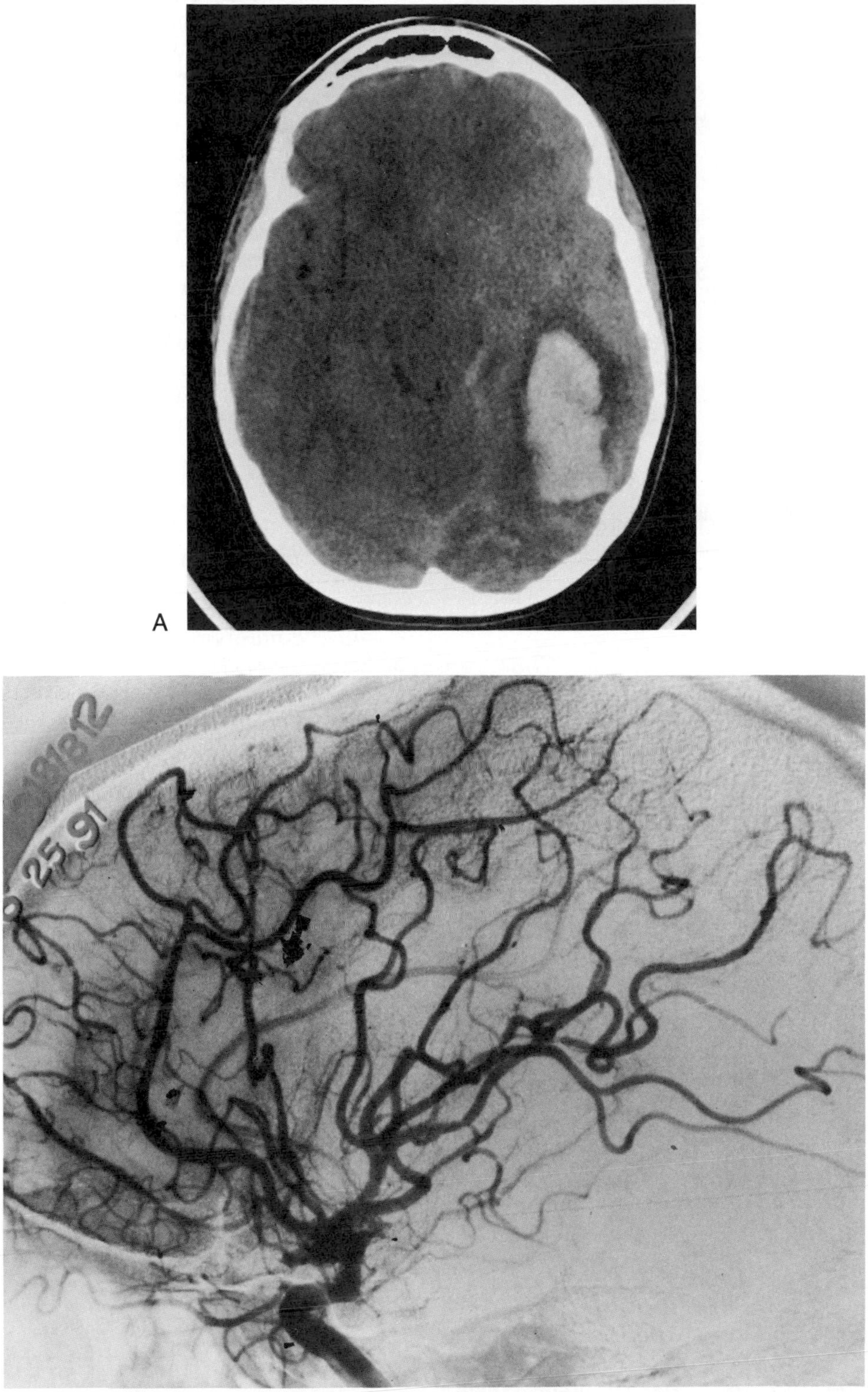

A

B

**Fig. 50-4.** Hemorrhage from vasculitis. (**A**) Computed tomography shows hematoma. (**B**) Vasculitis is demonstrated on angiography. Gradual deterioration with aphasia, hemiparesis, and obtundation. Surgical evacuation and steroid therapy with full recovery.

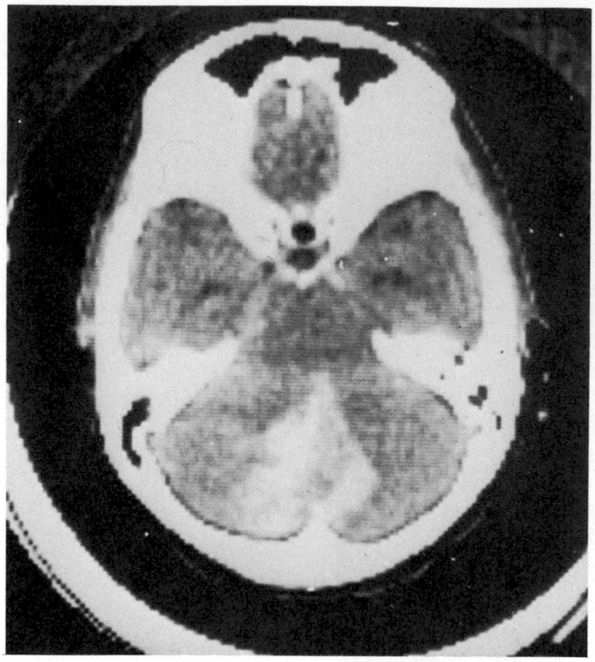

**Fig. 50-5.** Cerebellar hemorrhage. Large paravermian hematoma. Patient in coma. Awakened after surgical evacuation. Mild residual ataxia.

surgical candidate. Most cases lie in between these extremes, making decisions difficult. Although clear-cut indications are not yet available, clinical and CT guidelines for therapy are emerging. Some tentative indications can be offered; beginning with the most firmly established, they are as follows.

1. *Secondary deterioration* suggests reversibility of deficit in that function survived the initial hemorrhage (Fig. 50-4).[4,32] Recurrent hemorrhage appears to be an occasional cause of secondary deterioration. Medical therapy is usually ineffective in this setting. Further downhill progression, probably related to increased intracranial pressure, seems highly likely in such cases. As in 9 of 15 cases headed for almost certain death, surgery can be lifesaving to the deteriorating patient.[4,125] Operation seems especially appropriate for lesions extending into accessible lobar sites. Although data from modern controlled studies are unavailable, deterioration appears an eminently logical, fairly well-established, and widely accepted indication for surgery. Surgery is generally not recommended if there is massive hemorrhage with immediate loss of brain stem function and no response to medical therapy.
2. *Cerebellar hemorrhage* is a special management problem for which guidelines are available.[3] With hematoma near the brain stem, rapid and irreversible deterioration may take place without warning (Figs. 50-1 and 50-4). Surgical evacuation of these lesions is associated with low morbidity. To protect against abrupt deterioration, surgery is recommended for all lesions greater than 3 cm in diameter. Most smaller lesions have a benign course, and preliminary CT data have indicated that lesions smaller than 3 cm may be treated medically with good results. Large lesions may cause sudden coma even after 1 month, and removal should be considered whenever large clots are encountered. The role of sterotactic removal has been discussed.
3. *Diagnostic uncertainty* as to etiology sometimes requires exploratory operation.[13,107] CT, MRI, and angiography can generally identify tumors and AVMs, particularly if studies are repeated after mass effect has declined. However, if there is still a question, operation is occasionally warranted to establish the diagnosis of tumor, AVM, or cavernous angioma. This is particularly appropriate in the setting of recurrent hemorrhages with progressive deficit.
4. *Central hemorrhage* (medullary, pontine, and mesencephalic) may occasionally be evacuated with success (Fig. 50-3). This may be appropriate in a young patient with preserved brain stem function. In the case of thalamic and brain stem hemorrhage, a shunt procedure for acute hydrocephalus may be lifesaving.
5. *Stable persistent deficit* may or may not be improved by surgery. For moderate deficits, some authors suggest initial medical therapy.[128,131] If the deficits persist beyond 1 to 4 weeks, surgery may be offered on grounds that decompression may restore function to some marginal neurons, and surgery may hasten recovery and improve outcome,[125] as seen experimentally.[104] Reports of single cases and small series suggest that surgery may diminish late morbidity. Prospective clinical studies will be needed to evaluate the role of surgery for such patients. Benefits of early operation and delayed operation have been evaluated, but clear superiority of either approach has not been established. We have usually not recommended surgery in this setting, except when there is reasonable doubt as to the etiology (see above).
6. *Initial coma* has rarely been reversed by emergency operation.[87] Quality of survival has been fair at best, with all 4 survivors in a study of 21 cases requiring full-time care. Emergency operations in this setting seem rarely justified, even in a young person. Patients with clots greater than 85 cc in volume almost always succumb.

## SURGICAL TECHNIQUES

### Open Evacuation of Hematoma

The operation usually performed is a craniotomy with careful removal of the hematoma, exposed through a cortical incision, with the aid of loupes and headlight and taking care to avoid damage to the surrounding walls.[110] Some surgeons have advocated a microsurgical approach to inspect the cavity wall for a bleeding source,[160] but we have used this method only when studies suggest an unusual etiology.

Supratentorial hemorrhages are usually removed with the patient in a supine or semilateral position. Cerebellar hematomas are evacuated in the prone position, and an occipital ventricular tap relieves hydrocephalus. With the CT scan findings, there is usually no difficulty in localizing the hematoma. If there is a problem, the use of intraoperative ultrasound may help.

In the deteriorating patient, surgical treatment begins with maximum medical decompression. Mannitol, 100 g, is given intravenously. Intubation and hyperventilation are done. An arterial catheter is inserted, and blood pressure is controlled with sodium nitroprusside.

Often direct exposure to the hematoma is needed for its removal, because the clot is too firm to aspirate. A cortical incision is performed in an appropriate noneloquent gyrus (Fig. 50-6). For temporal or putaminal lesions, the anterior superior temporal gyrus is satisfactory, for parieto-occipital lesions, the superior parietal lobule; for frontal lesions, the superior frontal gyrus anterior to the motor strip; and for cerebellar lesions, a vermian or paramedian approach, depending on the lesion's location. A 2- to 3-cm cortisectomy is made with bipolar cautery and microscissors. Loupes and headlight permit satisfactory visualization. Deep exposure is greatly aided by self-retaining retractors (Fig. 50-7A). Evacuation of the hemorrhage is achieved with gentle suction and irrigation. Sometimes a tumor forceps can deliver a large, firm clot. Most of the hematoma is removed to achieve decompression, but the last adherent bits of clot may be left behind. This is done to avoid injury and bleeding from the walls of the cavity. Great care is taken to keep instruments, particularly the suction, away from this adjacent edematous white matter. Tissue suspicious of angioma or tumor warrants careful biopsy or excision.

Hemostasis is achieved with bipolar cautery. Surgicel is used to line the hematoma cavity. Hemostasis must be meticulous in order to avoid a recurrence. We

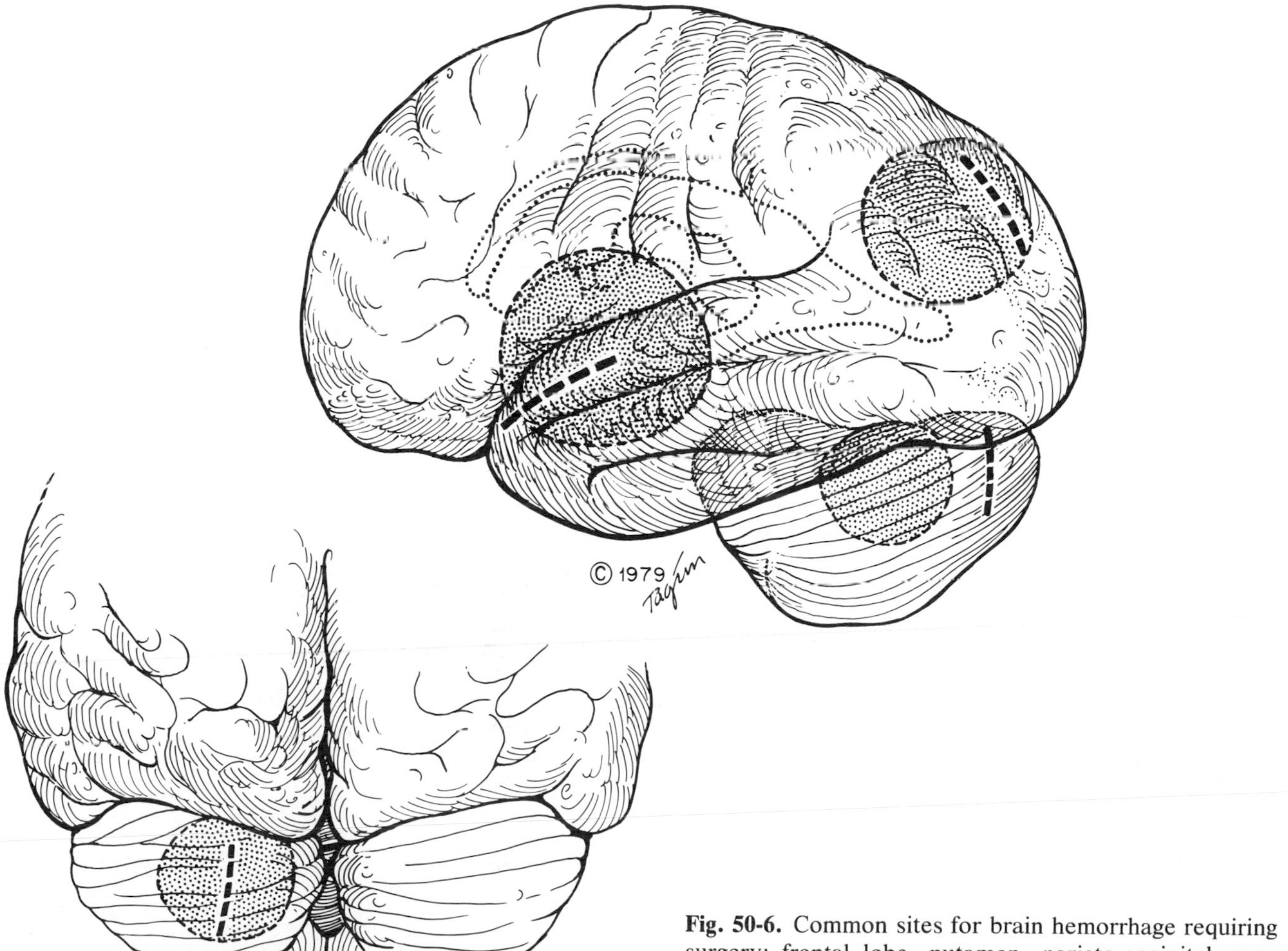


**Fig. 50-6.** Common sites for brain hemorrhage requiring surgery: frontal lobe, putamen, parieto-occipital area, and cerebellum. Cortical incisions are indicated.

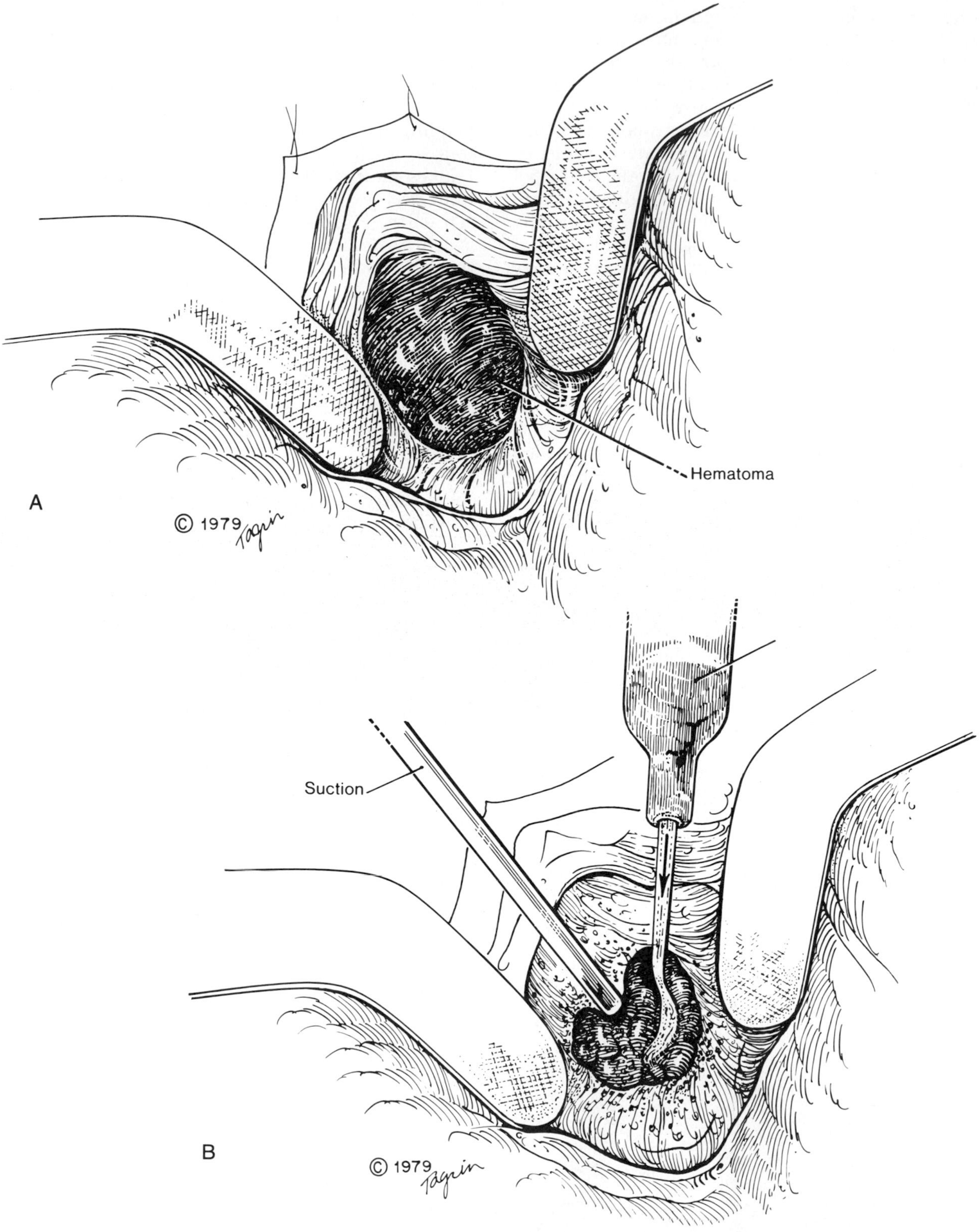


**Fig. 50-7.** Surgical technique for removal of brain hemorrhage. (**A**) Exposure of hematoma with self-retaining retractors. (**B**) Suction removal of hematoma. (*Figure continues.*)

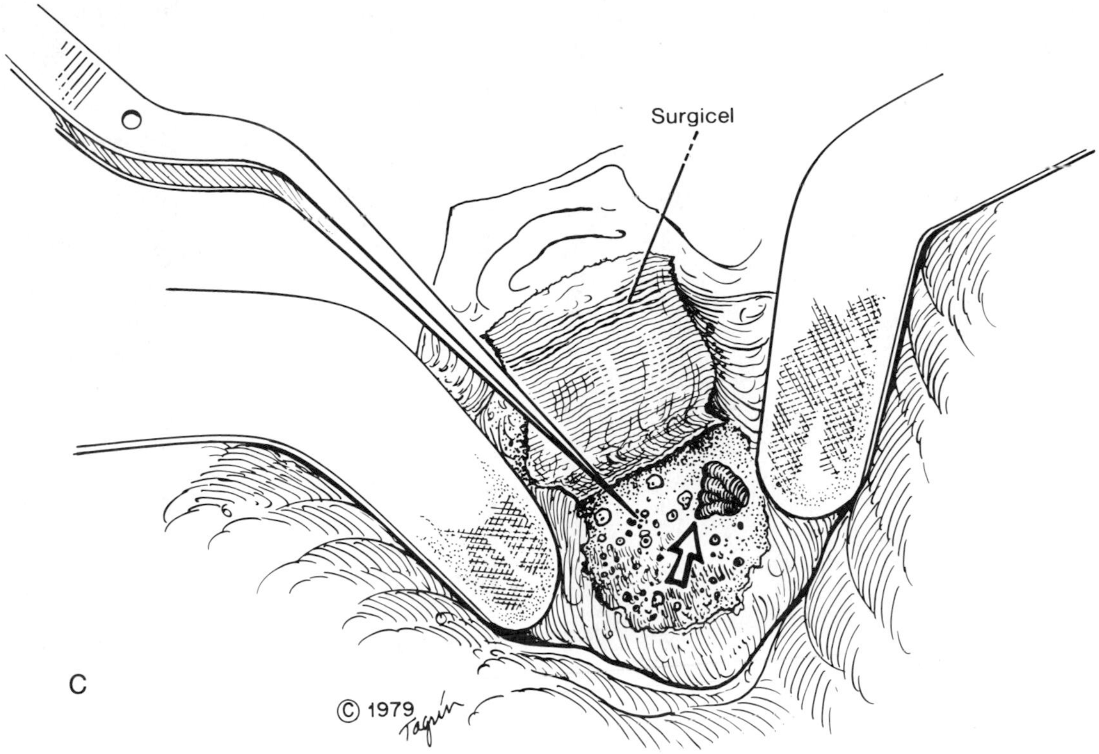


**Fig. 50-7** (*Continued*). (**C**) Hemostasis with bipolar cautery and Surgicel. Suspicious tissue (*arrow*) warrants biopsy.

raise blood pressure for 5 to 10 minutes to high-normal levels in order to check hemostasis. Additional bleeders have been noted and controlled in a number of cases. Great care must be taken to avoid hypertension, which could cause brain swelling. Closure is performed in routine fashion, usually without a drain. In some cases of cerebellar hemorrhage with hydrocephalus, a ventricular catheter may be left for a few days.

## Stereotactic Aspiration

Backlund and von Holst[8] first suggested stereotactic aspiration of intracerebral hematomas. Over the past decade a host of reports, especially from Japan, have appeared with results of stereotactic aspiration.[54,60–62,69] Postprocedure CT scans have shown impressive reductions in clot size, or even total removal (Fig. 50-1). Clinical results have been encouraging, with infrequent recurrent hemorrhage.

Thrombolytic agents have been added to stereotactic aspiration to permit greater clot removal.[99,169] Reports from Germany and Japan have been encouraging (Fig. 50-1).

A related technique is endoscopic clot aspiration, reported by Auer and colleagues.[7] This method utilizes intraoperative ultrasound to localize the hematoma.[130] An excellent controlled study in 100 cases showed a clear advantage for endoscopic evacuation over medical treatment. This method is not widely used, however, and results may be more operator-dependent than with stereotactic treatment.

In view of published results, stereotactic aspiration may be considered a reasonable alternative to open surgery when clot evacuation is warranted. In fact, this technique may even supplant craniotomy in the future.[97]

## Ventriculostomy

When hydrocephalus or intraventricular hemorrhage is symptomatic, ventricular drainage is often warranted (Fig. 50-8).[170] A standard ventricular drain is placed through a frontal bur hole, usually on the right side, but on the left if that ventricle seems more likely to drain satisfactorily. We use continuous drainage through a closed, sterile system, with the spillway set at 10 cm above the foramen of Monro. Within a few days, a decision is made regarding removal of the catheter or conversion to a ventriculoperitoneal shunt. Serial CT scans and a trial clamping of the drain may help make the decision. Antibiotics are given prophylactically while the drain is in place (oxacillin 1 g every 6 hours intravenously).

## Postoperative Care

Postoperative care must be meticulous in order to avoid recurrence. Blood pressure must be controlled, particularly as the anesthesia wears off.[67] Continuous

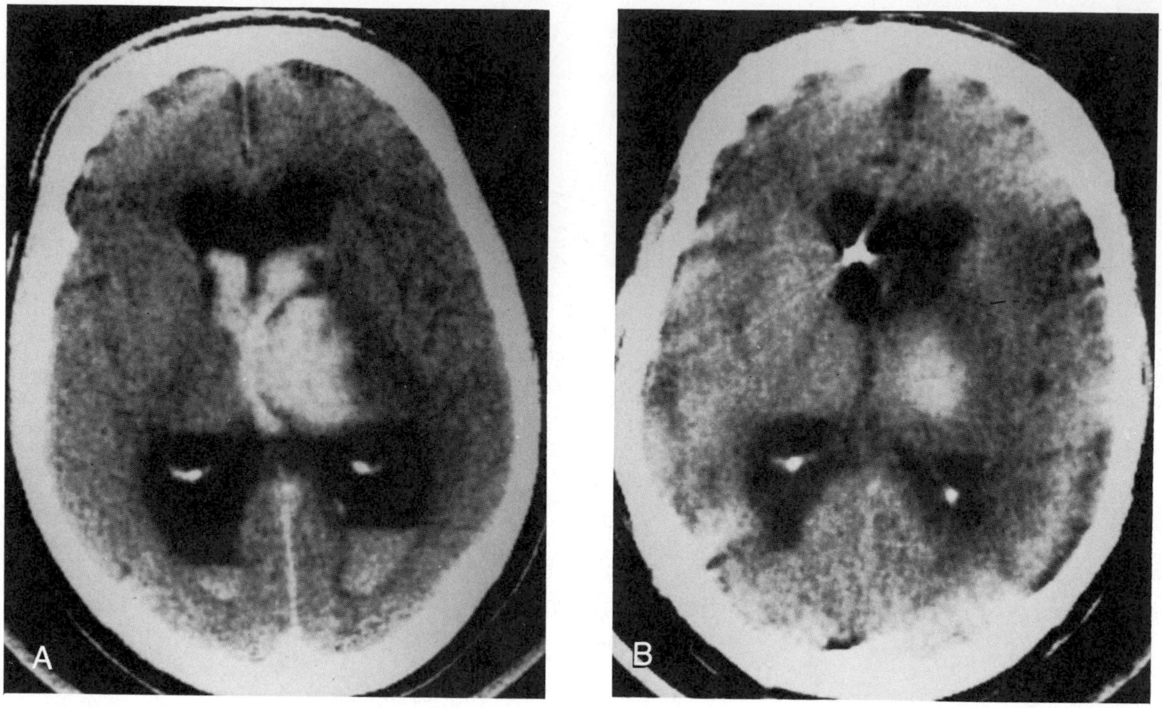


**Fig. 50-8.** Thalamic hemorrhage. (**A**) Computed tomography shows large hematoma extending into ventricular system with hydrocephalus. Patient in coma with fixed pupils. (**B**) Computed tomography after initial ventriculostomy and later ventriculoperitoneal shunt. Gradual improvement with residual left hemiparesis.

monitoring is done even during the transfer of the patient to the recovery room. Intravenous antihypertensive agents are given as needed to maintain the pressure in the normal range until oral agents can be substituted. Steroids are continued and then tapered approximately 1 week after surgery. If antithrombotic agents are indicated for other conditions (e.g., cardiac valve prosthesis), aspirin can be started after surgery with low risk of recurrence. Data are lacking, but warfarin probably can be resumed 1 month after surgery without risk of recurrent intraparenchymal bleeding. Serum electrolytes and osmolality are checked regularly during the early postoperative period. In case of neurologic deterioration, the CT is repeated in search of clot or hydrocephalus.

Other postoperative complications must be considered for avoidance. In an attempt to prevent deep venous thrombosis and potentially fatal pulmonary emboli, we use perioperative thigh high pneumatic compression boots and postoperative subcutaneous heparin (5,000 units bid).

To avert seizures, phenytoin (300 mg per day) is given to patients with supratentorial lesions. The anticonvulsant is tapered after 6 months, if an EEG shows no epileptiform activity. When hydrocephalus is symptomatic, a ventriculoperitoneal shunt may be necessary.

## SPECIFIC HEMORRHAGE LOCATIONS

### Putaminal Hemorrhage

The clinical syndrome is well-described.[45,59,111] Patients are characteristically up and active when they become ill. A hemiparesis develops and may progress to a hemiplegia accompanied in some patients by hemisensory loss, hemianopsia, dysphasia, or unawareness of the deficit, depending on the side involved. The hemorrhage may remain localized or it can track into the white matter of the frontal or temporal lobe, involve the internal capsule or rupture into the ventricle. The progression of symptoms may cease at any point or continue to coma and death within a few hours. In 27 consecutive patients, a smooth onset characterized 62 percent, while 30 percent developed symptoms so rapidly that observers felt the deficit was nearly maximal at onset.[111] None of the patients experienced fluctuation of the deficit. Headache affected only 14 percent at onset and only 28 percent at any time, leaving nearly 72 percent free of headache, even in the presence of substantial focal neurologic deficit.

In evaluation of CT scans in 24 patients with putaminal hemorrhage, three groups were defined.[59] In the first group, patients in coma were found to have massive hemorrhage and poor prognosis. Patients in the second group were alert with significant neurologic deficit and moderate-sized hematomas. Some made acceptable recoveries, but most were left with a substantial deficit. In the third group, mild deficits were found in relation to small hemorrhages. These patients generally made a good recovery. Whether surgery would have improved the outcome in groups 1 and 2 is not known.

Patients with small or moderate-sized hematomas in the putamen often make a good recovery either spontaneously or with medical management. When hematomas are larger than 3 cm in diameter, the initial treatment is usually medical, but if the patient develops progressive neurologic deficit or drowsiness despite medical treatment, then early surgical removal of the hematoma may be considered.[145,158]

In two major recent controlled studies of surgical evacuation of putaminal hemorrhages, no clear benefit was demonstrated.[11,68] However, stratification was not done regarding the initial mild deficit that progresses. We continue to consider this group for surgery.

### Thalamus

The classic features of thalamic hemorrhage are also well-described.[10,43,53] The initial deficit is hemisensory, and if the internal capsule becomes involved, motor weakness supervenes. Extension into the upper brain stem commonly leads to vertical gaze palsy, retraction nystagmus, skew deviation, loss of convergence, ptosis and miosis, anisocoria, or unreactive pupils. Dysphasia has been reported. Headache is rare. Compression of the third ventricle may cause hydrocephalus. In two reports of patients with thalamic hemorrhage, all died when the hematoma was greater than 3.3 cm on the CT scan, while patients harboring smaller hematomas recovered, but frequently with disability. There is no evidence to indicate whether direct surgery would be of benefit to patients with larger hematomas. In general, we have not operated on patients with thalamic hemorrhage except to treat hydrocephalus by emergency ventricular drainage or permanent ventricular peritoneal shunting (Fig. 50-8). The role of stereotactic operation is uncertain, but the less invasive nature of the procedure lends itself to such deep lesions.

### Lobar Hemorrhage

Ropper and Davis[128] have characterized the syndromes associated with lobar hemorrhage. Occipital hemorrhage (11 patients) caused severe pain around the ipsilateral eye and dense hemianopsia. Left temporal hemorrhage (7 patients) began with mild pain in or just anterior to the ear, fluent dysphasia with poor comprehension and relatively preserved repetition, and a partial hemianopic deficit. Patients with frontal hemorrhages (4 cases) had severe contralateral arm weakness, minimal leg and face weakness, and frontal headaches. Parietal hematomas (3 patients) began with anterior temporal headache and hemisensory disturbance. In these 26 patients, 8 (31 percent) were known to have had hypertension prior to hemorrhage, 14 (54 percent) had documentation of normal blood pressure, 2 (8 percent) were on anticoagulants, 2 (8 percent) had an AVM, and 1 (4 percent) a metastatic tumor. In another report of 22 patients with lobar hemorrhage, 45 percent were hypertensive, 14 percent had a metastatic tumor, 9 percent an AVM, 5 percent a blood dyscrasia, and in 27 percent the cause was unknown.[72] Amyloid angiopathy may be the source of bleeding in such patients.

In view of the varied etiologies, angiography is indicated in the evaluation of these lesions if the patient is stable.[72,172] If no etiology is discovered, the CT scan and angiography should be repeated some months after hemorrhage, when the effects of compression have subsided, because tumor or AVM may not have been seen on the initial study.

With a deteriorating patient and suspicion of aneurysm, emergency operation without angiography may be warranted (Fig. 50-2).

Most patients with spontaneous or hypertensive lobar hemorrhages will make a good recovery with medical treatment.[149,167] However, if the patients show signs of progressive neurologic deficit despite medical treatment, surgical removal of the hematoma is clearly indicated.[166,172]

### Intraventricular Hemorrhage

CT scan demonstrates the degree of intraventricular hemorrhage. Most such hematomas result from the rupture of a parenchymal hematoma into the ventricular system[76]; occasionally, primary intraventricular hemorrhage can occur. Although the traditional teaching has indicated a poor prognosis, intraventricular hemorrhage may be associated with a rather benign clinical course.[82,118,156] A review of 54 patients with intraventricular hemorrhage on the CT scan revealed an association with a number of disorders, such as hypertension, intracranial aneurysm, AVM, tumor, and coagulopathy.[82] In a report of 32 cases of hypertensive intracerebral hemorrhage, 63 percent had intraventricular rupture.[165] The guidelines for surgical treatment are the same as those suggested for parenchymal hematoma. Ventricular drainage is generally of limited value, because the catheter frequently becomes obstructed. Thrombolytic agents might be of value, but data are lacking. Occasionally, ventriculostomy can be lifesaving and is indicated for neurologic deterioration secondary to acute hydrocephalus. Patients surviving the acute phase often require a ventriculoperitoneal shunt.

## Cerebellar Hemorrhage

Frequently hemorrhages into the cerebellum lead to a life-threatening downhill course, which may be dramatically reversed by surgical intervention.[1,21,34,35,46,58,86,113,134] Since there is effective therapy, a patient suspected of having a cerebellar hemorrhage should have an immediate CT scan (Figs. 50-1 and 50-5).[120] The onset of the hemorrhage is usually sudden, with nausea, vomiting, and inability to stand or walk. In a series of 56 patients, headache was present in 75 percent, dizziness in 55 percent, and loss of consciousness at onset of 14 percent. Examination showed appendicular ataxia in 78 percent, facial palsy in 60 percent, and ipsilateral gaze palsy in 54 percent.[143] Cerebellar hemorrhage may occur in childhood.[48]

Cerebellar hematoma represents a special situation regarding treatment.[31] Deterioration due to brain stem compression is unpredictable, and it is important to treat the patient before compression causes alteration in the state of consciousness and an unstable clinical situation. In one report,[113] 10 of 12 patients who were alert or drowsy preoperatively survived operation, while only 4 of 16 who were stuporous or comatose before surgery lived. The relationship of the level of consciousness to prognosis and the importance of not delaying surgery in patients with acute cerebellar hematomas have been stressed in other reviews.[168,171] However, even for a patient in a deep coma, removal of the hematoma can result in good recovery, especially if the time interval between the development of the comatose state and surgery is short. In a report of 10 patients with cerebellar hematomas, six had a progressive course and all had hematomas 3 cm or greater on CT scan.[84] We generally recommend removal of hematomas that are larger than 3 cm in diameter if the patient is seen within the first week of hemorrhage. Patients seen later who have a stable neurologic course may be treated medically with close observation.

Patients with smaller lesions and no signs of brain stem compression are monitored carefully in the intensive care unit. Most patients with small hematomas have a benign course and may be treated medically with a good result.[56,84,95] On the other hand, once the patient shows signs of brain stem compression, deterioration can proceed abruptly. In this clinical setting, operation is indicated even if the hematoma is smaller than 3 cm. The hematoma is removed under direct vision via a suboccipital craniectomy. In addition, late deterioration has been reported as late as one month.[23] A few patients can be treated by ventricular drainage,[142] but this therapy alone does not relieve brain stem compression and may be followed by later deterioration. Ventricular drainage may be necessary after evacuation of the hematoma to treat persisting hydrocephalus.

## Mesencephalic Hemorrhage

In patients with mesencephalic hematoma, clinical features, including paralysis of vertical eye movements and a marked tendency to fall backward when standing, allow accurate localization of the lesion.[42,96,133] The etiology may be arteriovenous malformation or hypertension. Deterioration can result from extension of the hematoma mass. A subtemporal approach allows excellent exposure of the mesencephalon for evacuation of the hematoma, and a few successful cases have been reported.[37] Hydrocephalus can develop due to the obstruction of the aqueduct and can be successfully treated by ventriculoperitoneal shunting. The importance of initial close observation is emphasized with supportive care in the stable patient. Surgery is recommended for patients demonstrating evidence of deterioration from rebleeding or hydrocephalus.

## Pontine Hemorrhage

Hemorrhage into the pons is the most dramatic and least treatable of all brain hemorrhages.[17,49,155] A small hematoma often leads to immediate coma, rapid quadriplegia, with small, barely reactive pupils and extraocular movement disturbances. A "locked-in" syndrome occasionally results. Most patients do not survive the acute phase.

A few cases of successful removal of pontine hematomas have been reported (Fig. 50-3).[12,101] A review of 24 patients with pontine hemorrhage included 4 who had suboccipital craniotomy and several who had ventricular drainage.[133]

## Medullary Hemorrhage

Bulbar hemorrhage is almost always fatal.[27] In a quadriparetic young woman, we microsurgically removed a small hematoma from the medulla with good recovery. MR made the diagnosis, but no etiology was ever established.

# SPECIAL PATHOLOGIC ENTITIES

## Angiographically Occult Vascular Lesions

The histology of such lesions on excision is varied, including arteriovenous malformation, cavernous angioma, telengiectases, venous angioma, and tumor.[92,123,150] The risk of recurrent hemorrhage is probably likewise variable, but the threat is substantial for angiographically occult arteriovenous malformation or cavernous angioma. Occasionally such lesions occur in childhood.[38] The general diagnosis may be suspected on the basis of CT and MRI findings,[105,136] but specific diagnosis requires histologic analysis.[13]

When studies suggest an occult vascular lesion, if the pathology is accessible, generally excision is warranted.[85,102,159] For deep lesions (basal ganglia, thalamus, brain stem), initial careful follow-up is probably warranted, with surgical excision reserved for severe deficit, recurrent bleeding, or progressive neurologic deterioration (Fig. 50-3).[15,77–79,140,150,154,162,173] A particularly vexing concern is the lack of objective signs for radiographic follow-up of such lesions. The substantial rate of complications for occult lesions treated by radiosurgery suggests that excision is the preferred therapy, but some advocate radiosurgery.

## Angiitis

Inflammatory angiitis of the brain may present as spontaneous hemorrhage.[18,143] The diagnosis is established by angiography, which shows a beaded appearance of arteries. Precise etiology is unclear. Steroids may be helpful. Surgery may be dramatically beneficial for the hemorrhage (Fig. 50-4).

## Drug-Related Hemorrhage

Intravenous methamphetamine administration has been associated with cerebral angiitis and intracerebral hemorrhage.[174] Phencyclidine abuse may also lead to intraparenchymal hemorrhage.[16] There are reports of vasculitis and hemorrhage after phenylpropanolamine ingestion (diet pills).[47]

## Amyloid Angiopathy

Amyloid angiopathy may be the cause of spontaneous lobar hemorrhage.[91,112,151,152,157,161] The frequency is probably higher than previously accepted. The problem usually occurs in patients over 60 years of age, and may be associated with multiple hemorrhages. The diagnosis should be considered in lobar hemorrhage found in a normotensive elderly patient. If such a patient has had multiple hemorrhages, this diagnosis becomes the leading consideration. When amyloid angiopathy is suspected, efforts should be made to treat the patient medically, since surgery may be attended by severe hemorrhage. However, two recent reports suggest that careful operation can be carried out without further neurologic deterioration (Fig. 50-9). Care should be taken to avoid disturbing the cavity walls which may harbor fragile, amyloid-laden vessels.

## Anticoagulant Therapy

With widespread use of anticoagulants for treatment of cardiac and neurologic diseases, the number of patients with brain hemorrhage secondary to this cause has increased.[81] Most such cases are found to have either an excessively prolonged prothrombin time or a focal lesion such as an infarction to account for the bleeding. Such patients should be treated immediately with transfusion of fresh frozen plasma. In addition, vitamin K-1 is administered to restore normal coagulation. With these measures, operation can be safely performed. In one patient on warfarin and aspirin, we achieved solid hemostasis only with exchange transfusion of fresh blood atop fresh frozen plasma, vitamin K-1, and platelet administration.

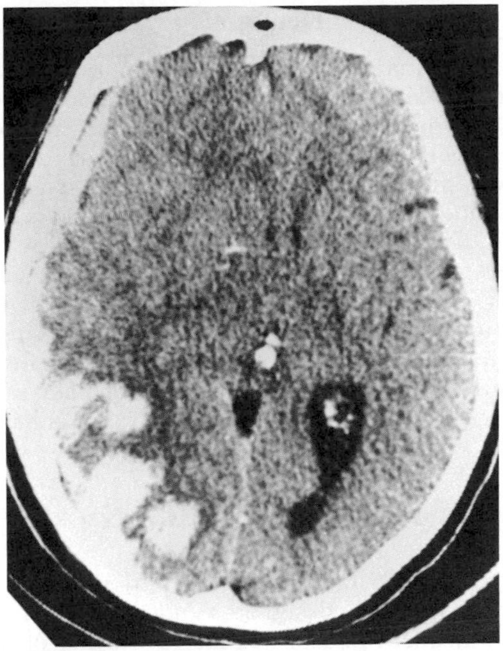

**Fig. 50-9.** Amyloid angiopathy with hemorrhage. Computed tomography scan shows multilobular lobar hemorrhage. Surgical removal led to fair recovery. Pathologic confirmation of amyloid angiopathy.

## Thrombocytopenia

This condition is diagnosed when the platelet count is lower than 80,000/mm$^3$. Intracerebral hemorrhage due to thrombocytopenia has been reported in idiopathic thrombocytopenic purpura and in a variety of secondary thrombocytopenias.[2,22,24] Usually the hemorrhage is intracerebral, but subdural hematoma has been reported. Surgery is hazardous if the platelet count is below 50,000 and is of concern with platelet counts in the 50,000 to 100,000 range. Platelet transfusions and corticosteroid therapy usually can achieve a hemostatic level. Guidelines for surgery are the same as in other conditions, once a hemostatic level of platelets can be achieved. Other hemorrhagic conditions, such as von Willebrand's disease, juvenile diabetic ketoacidosis,[6] and hepatic failure[106] have also been associated with brain hemorrhage.[3]

### Hemophilia

The great majority of hemophilia patients are deficient in factor VIII, a small number in factor IX, and an occasional patient in factor XI.[170] Brain hemorrhage usually is associated with mild head trauma. Any patient with hemophilia and a persistent headache should have a CT scan.[139] If hemorrhage is confirmed, then appropriate replacement therapy should be started immediately. To avoid spontaneous, intraoperative, or postoperative hemorrhage, it is necessary to maintain a level of at least 20 percent of the deficient factor with transfusions of the appropriate concentrate. If an operation is performed, replacement needs to be given until the incision is healed.

## FUTURE DIRECTIONS

The most important question is patient selection for surgery. A properly designed, randomized, controlled study is needed. Because of the variability of the illness, careful stratification must be done in search of subgroups which might benefit from surgery.[121,137,141] Some important factors are age, Glasgow Coma Scale, location of hematoma, volume of hematoma,[168] and involvement of crucial structures such as posterior limb of internal capsule.[50,135,148] The number of factors and existing experience suggest the study needs to be large, probably requiring multiple institutions. Stereotactic aspiration and thrombolysis would seem to be an attractive surgical technique for such a study, to minimize operative trauma and maximize technical reproducibility.

## ACKNOWLEDGMENTS

Thanks go to Dr. John Steichen for inclusion of Figures 2, 3 and 4 and to Dr. Richard Westmark for Figure 8. We acknowledge the excellent help of Edith Tagrin for the drawings and Julie Mann for typing the manuscript.

## REFERENCES

1. Acampora S, Guarniere L, Troisi F: Spontaneous intracerebellar hematoma: report of ten cases. Acta Neurochir (Wien) 66:83, 1982
2. Almani WS, Awid AS: Spontaneous intracranial bleeding in hemorrhagic diathesis. Surg Neurol 17:137, 1982
3. Almani WS, Awid AS: Spontaneous intracranial hemorrhage secondary to von Willebrand's disease. Surg Neurol 26:457, 1986
4. Arana-Iniquez R, Wilson E, Bastarrica E et al: Cerebral hematomas. Surg Neurol 6:45, 1976
5. Astarloa R, Jimenex-Scrig A, Gimeno A et al: Valor pronostico de la TAC en la hemorragia cerebral supratentorial cerebral hemorrhage: multivariate study in 114 patients. Arch Neurobiol (Madr) 52:234, 1989
6. Atluru VL: Spontaneous intracerebral hematomas in juvenile diabetic ketoacidosis. Pediatr Neurol 2:167, 1986
7. Auer LM, Deinsberger W, Niederkorn K et al: Endoscopic surgery versus medical treatment for spontaneous intracerebral hematoma: a randomized study. J Neurosurg 70:530, 1989
8. Backlund EQ, Von Holst H: Controlled subtotal evacuation of intracerebral hematomas by stereotactic technique. Surg Neurol 9:99, 1978
9. Bagley C: Spontaneous cerebral hemorrhage: discussion of four types, with surgical considerations. Arch Neurol Psychiatry 27:1133, 1932
10. Barraquer-Bordes L, Illa A, Escartin J et al: Thalamic hemorrhage: a study of 23 patients with diagnosis by computed tomography. Stroke 12:524, 1981
11. Batjer HH, Reisch JS, Allen BC et al: Failure of surgery to improve outcome in hypertensive putaminal hemorrhage: a prospective randomized trial. Arch Neurol 47:1103, 1990
12. Becker DH, Silverberg GD: Successful evacuation of an acute pontine hematoma. Surg Neurol 10:263, 1978
13. Becker DH, Townsend JJ, Kramer RA et al: Occult cerebrovascular malformations: a series of 18 histologically verified cases with negative angiography. Brain 102:249, 1979
14. Benes V, Koukoik F, Obrovska D: Two types of spontaneous intracerebral hemorrhage due to hypertension. J Neurosurg 37:509, 1972
15. Bertalanffy H, Gilsbach JM, Eggert HR et al: Microsurgery of deep-seated cavernous angiomas: report of 26 cases. Acta Neurochir (Wien) 108:91, 1991
16. Bessen HA: Intracranial hemorrhage associated with phencyclidine abuse. JAMA 248:585, 1982
17. Bewermeyer H, Hojer C, Szelies B et al: Die spontane Ponsblutung: eine Analyse von 38 Fallen. Nervenarzt 59:640, 1988
18. Biller J, Loftus CM, Moore SA: Isolated central nervous system angiitis first presenting as spontaneous intracranial hemorrhage. Neurosurgery 20:310, 1987
19. Bogousslavsky J, Regli F, Uske A et al: Early spontaneous hematoma in cerebral infarct: is primary cerebral hemorrhage overdiagnosed? Neurology (NY) 41:837, 1991
20. Brambilla GL, Sangiovanni G, Rainoldi F et al: Gli ematomi intracerebrali spontanei: trattamento e risultati a distanza. Minerva Med 77:1209, 1986
21. Brennan R, Bergland RM: Acute cerebellar hemorrhage: analysis of clinical findings and outcome in 12 cases. Neurology (NY) 27:527, 1977
22. Brenner B, Guilburd JN, Tatarsky I et al: Spontaneous intracranial hemorrhage in immune thrombocytopenic purpura. Neurosurgery 22:761, 1988
23. Brillman H: Acute hydrocephalus and death one month after nonsurgical treatment for acute cer-

ebellar hemorrhage: case report. J Neurosurg 50:374, 1979
24. Burrows RF, Caco CC, Kelton JG: Neonatal alloimmune thrombocytopenia: spontaneous in utero intracranial hemorrhage. Am J Hematol 28:98, 1988
25. Bydder GM, Steiner RE, Young IR et al: Clinical NMR imaging of the brain: 140 cases. Am J Neuroradiol 3:459, 1982
26. Calandre L, Arnal C, Ortega JF et al: Risk factors for spontaneous cerebral hematomas: case-control study. Stroke 17:1126, 1986
27. Calandre L, Felgueroso B, Bermejo F et al: Hematoma bulbar: presentaction de un caso con parada respiratoris y recuperacion espontanea. Arch Neurobiol (Madr) 49:95, 1986
28. Chee CP, Bailey IC, Refsum SE: Spontaneous massive haemorrhage into acoustic neuroma during anticoagulation therapy. Br J Neurosurg 1:489, 1987
29. Chen ST, Chen SD, Hsu CY et al: Progression of hypertensive intracerebral hemorrhage. Neurology (NY) 39:1509, 1989
30. Coraddu M, Nurchi GC, Floris F et al: Considerations about the surgial indication of the spontaneous cerebral haematomas. J Neurosurg Sci 34:35, 1990
31. Crowell RM, Ojemann RG: Cerebellar hemorrhage. p 135. In: WA Buchheit WA, Truex, Jr, RC (eds): Surgery of the Posterior Fossa. Raven Press, New York, 1979
32. Crowell RM, Ojemann RG: Surgery for brain hemorrhage. p. 233. In Moossy J, Reinmuth OM (eds): Cerebrovascular Diseases. New York, Raven Press, 1981
33. Cushing H: The blood pressure reaction of acute cerebral compression, illustrated by cases of intracranial hemorrhage. Am J Med Sci 125:1017, 1903
34. Dinsdale HB: Spontaneous hemorrhage in the posterior fossa. Arch Neurol 10:200, 1964
35. Dolinskas CA, Bilaniuk LT, Zimmerman RA et al: Computed tomography of intracerebral hematomas. I. Transmission CT observations on hematoma resolution. Am J Roentgenol Radium Ther Nucl Med 129:681, 1977
36. Duffy TA, Ayeni S, Levin AB, Javid M: Nonsurgical management of spontaneous intracerebral hematoma. Neurosurgery 9:387, 1981
37. Durward QJ, Barnett HJM, Barr HWK: Presentation and management of mesencephalic hematoma: report of 2 cases. J Neurosurg 56:123, 1982
38. el-Gohary EG, Tomita T, Gutierrez FA et al: Angiographically occult vascular malformations in childhood. Neurosurgery 20:759, 1987
39. Ericson K, von Holst H, Mosskin M et al: Positron emission tomography of cavernous haemangiomas of the brain. Acta Radiol [Diagn] (Stockh) 27:379, 1986
40. Espinosa Urrutia J: Hematomas intracerebrales espontaneous. Rev Med Panama 15:81, 1990
41. Fazio C: A neurologist's study of the problem concerning surgical treatment of spontaneous cerebral hemorrhage. Sci Med Ital 1:101, 1950
42. Fingerote RJ, Shuaib A, Brownell AK: Spontaneous midbrain hemorrhage. South Med J 83:280, 1990
43. Fisher CM: The pathologic and clinical aspects of thalamic hemorrhage. Trans Am Neurol Assoc 84:56, 1959
44. Fisher CM: The pathology and pathogenesis of intracerebral hemorrhage. p. 295. In Field WS (ed): Pathogenesis and Treatment of Cerebrovascular Disease. CC Thomas, Springfield, IL, 1961
45. Fisher CM: Clinical syndromes in cerebral hemorrhage. p. 295. In Fields WS (ed): Pathogenesis and Treatment of Cerebrovascular Disease. CC Thomas, Springfield, IL, 1961
46. Fisher CM, Picard EH, Polak A et al: Cerebellar hemorrhage: diagnosis and surgical treatment. J Nerv Ment Dis 140:38, 1965
47. Forman HP, Levin S, Stewart B et al: Cerebral vasculitis and hemorrhage in an adolescent taking diet pills containing phenylpropanolamine: case report and review of literature. Pediatrics 83:737, 1989
48. Freitas PE, Aquini MG: Spontaneous intracerebellar hematoma during childhood. Neurosurgery 21:103, 1987
49. Froment JC, Bascoulergue Y, Crouzet G et al: Apparently isolated, spontaneous haematomas of the brain stem: seven cases explored by CT and MRI. J Neuroradiol 16:38, 1989
50. Fukiishi Y, Arita S, Suzuki T: Predicting recovery of ambulatory function after hypertensive putaminal hemorrhage by multivariate analysis of acute-phase clinical data. Neurol Med Chir (Tokyo) 29:503, 1989
51. Garcia CA, Weisberg LA, McGarry PA et al: Spontaneous hemorrhage in previously ischemic (pale) cerebral infarcts. Comput Radiol 10:55, 1986
52. Godersky JC, Biller J: Diagnosis and treatment of spontaneous intracerebral hemorrhage. Compr Ther 13:22, 1987
53. Goto N, Kaneko M, Muraki M et al: Thalamic hemorrhage—a clinicoanatomic study. Neurol Med Chir (Tokyo) 22:24, 1982
54. Hayashi M, Hawegawa T, Kobayashi H et al: Aspiration of hypertensive intracerebral hematoma by stereotactic technique. Neurol Surg (Tokyo) 9:1365, 1981
55. Hayward RD, O'Reilly GVA: Computerized tomography and intracerebral hemorrhage. Am Heart J 93:126, 1977
56. Heiman TD, Satya-Murti S: Benign cerebellar hemorrhages. Ann Neurol 3:366, 1978
57. Herbstein DS, Schaumberg HH: Hypertensive intracerebral hematoma: an investigation of the initial hemorrhage and rebleeding using chormium $CR^{51}$-labeled erythrocytes. Arch Neurol 30:412, 1974
58. Heros RC: Cerebellar hemorrhage and infarction. Stroke 16:17, 1981
59. Hier DB, Davis KR, Richardson EP, Jr et al: Hypertensive putaminal hemorrhage. Ann Neurol 1:152, 1977
60. Higgins AC, Nashold BS: Stereotactic evacua-

tion of large intracerebral hematoma. Appl Neurophysiol 43:3, 1980
61. Hondo H, Matsumoto K, Tomida K, Shichijo F: CT-controlled stereotactic aspiration in hypertensive brain hemorrhage: six-month postoperative outcome. Appl Neurophysiol 50:233, 1987
62. Hondo H, Uno M, Sasaki K et al: Computed tomography controlled aspiration surgery for hypertensive intracranial hemorrhage: experience of more than 400 cases. Stereotact Funct Neurosurg 54–55:432, 1990
63. Husain MM, Metzer WS, Binet EF: Multiple intraparenchymal brain plasmacytomas with spontaneous intratumoral hemorrhage. Neurosurgery 20:619, 1987
64. Jamjoom AB, Atasoy M, Coakham HB: Spontaneous haemorrhage in a cerebellar abscess: a unique complication. Br J Neurosurg 4:231, 1990
65. Jensen G, Mosdal C, Sommer W: Sontane intracerebrale haematomer: en opgorelse over 54 opererede patienter. Ugeskr Laeger 148:2086, 1986
66. Jinkins JR: Current neuroradiological investigation of spontaneous hemorrhage into the craniospinal axis. Neurosurgery 18:664, 1986
67. Johnston JH, Beevers DG, Dunn FG et al: The importance of good blood pressure control in the prevention of stroke recurrence in hypertensive patients. Postgrad Med J 57:690, 1981
68. Juvela S, Heiskanen O, Poranen A et al: The treatment of spontaneous intracerebral hemorrhage: a prospective randomized trial of surgical and conservative treatment. J Neurosurg 70:755, 1989
69. Kandel EI, Peresedov VV: Stereotactic evacuation of spontaneous intracerebral hematomas. Stereotact Funct Neurosurg 54–55:427, 1990
70. Kaneko M, Tanaka K, Shimada T et al: Long-term evaluation of ultra-early operation for hypertensive intracerebral hemorrhage in 100 cases. J Neurosurg 58:838, 1983
71. Kanno T, Nagata J, Hoshino M et al: Evaluation of the hypertensive intracerebral hematoma based on the study of long-term outcome. II. A role of surgery in putaminal hemorrhage. No Shinkei Geka 14:1307, 1986
72. Kase CS, Williams JP, Wyatt DA, Mohr JP: Lobar intracerebral hematomas: clinical and CT analysis of 22 cases. Neurology (NY) 32:1146, 1982
73. Kawakami H, Kutsuzawa T, Uemura K et al: Regional cerebral blood flow in patients with hypertensive intracerebral hemorrhage. Stroke 5:207, 1974
74. Kawamura S, Ohta H, Suzuki A et al: Surgical indication and limitation in hypertensive intracerebral hemorrhage of the basal ganglia. No Shinkei Geka 14:1071, 1986
75. Kendall BE: Computed tomography in spontaneous intracerebral hematomas. Br J Radiol 51:563, 1978
76. Konig HJ: Zur Therapie und Prognose spontaner intrazerebraler Bluntungen mit Ventrikeleinbruch. Neurochirurgia (Stuttg) 29:75, 1986
77. Kumabe T, Suzuki M, Yoshimoto T et al: A case of cavernous angioma extended from the ventral part of the pons to the midbrain: subtemporal and trans-tentorial approach. No Shinkei Geka 16:1193, 1988
78. Kyoshima K, Nakazawa T, Nakasu S et al: Angiographically occult vascular malformations in the posterior fossa. Nippon Geka Hokan 58:257, 1989
79. LeDoux MS, Aronin PA, Odrezin GT: Surgically treated cavernous angiomas of the brain stem: report of two cases and review of the literature. Surg Neurol 35:395, 1991
80. Lee MX, Heaney LM, Jacobson RL, Klassen AC: Cerebrospinal fluid in cerebral hemorrhage and infarction. Stroke 6:638, 1975
81. Lieberman A, Hass WK, Rinto R et al: Intracranial hemorrhage and infarction in anticoagulated patients with prosthetic heart valves. Stroke 9:18, 1978
82. Little JR, Blomquist GA, Ethier R: Intraventricular hemorrhage in adults. Surg Neurol 8:143, 1977
83. Little JR, Dial B, Belanger G et al: Brain hemorrhage from intracranial tumor. Stroke 10:283, 1979
84. Little JR, Tubman DE, Ethier R: Cerebellar hemorrhage in adults: diagnosis by computerized tomography. J Neurosurg 48:575, 1978
85. Lobato RD, Perez C, Rivas JJ et al: Clinical, radiological, and pathological spectrum of angiographically occult intracranial vascular malformations: analysis of 21 cases and review of the literature. J Neurosurg 68:518, 1988
86. Locatelli D, Messina AL, Bonfanti N et al: Spontaneous cerebellar hemorrhage. Ital J Surg Sci 18:159, 1988
87. Luessenhop AJ, Shevlin WA, Ferrero AA et al: Surgical management of primary intracerebral hemorrhage. J Neurosurg 27:419, 1967
88. MacEwen W: An address on the surgery of the brain and spinal cord. Br Med J 2:302, 1888
89. Maiuri F, Corriero G, Passarelli F et al: CT indications for surgery and evaluation of prognosis in patients with spontaneous intracerebral haematomas. Br J Neurosurg 4:155, 1990
90. Mandybur TI: Intracranial hemorrhage caused by metastatic tumors. Neurology (NY) 27:650, 1977
91. Mandybur TI, Bates SRD: Fatal massive intracranial hemorrhage complicating cerebral amyloid angiopathy. Arch Neurol 35:246, 1978
92. Mason I, Aase JM, Orrison WW et al: Familial cavernous angiomas of the brain in an Hispanic family. Neurology (NY) 75:169, 1991
93. McCormick WF, Rosenfield DB: Massive brain hemorrhage: a review of 144 cases and an examination of their causes. Stroke 4:946, 1973
94. McKissock W, Richardson A, Taylor J: Primary intracerebral hemorrhage: a controlled trial of surgical and conservative treatment in 180 unselected cases. Lancet 2:221, 1961
95. McKissock W, Richardson A, Walsh L: Spontaneous cerebellar hemorrhage, a study of 34 con-

secutive cases treated surgically. Brain 83:1, 1960
96. Mehler MF, Ragone PS: Primary spontaneous mesencephalic hemorrhage. Can J Neurol Sci 15:435, 1988
97. Mendelow AD: Spontaneous intracerebral haemorrhage. (Editorial.) J Neurol Neurosurg Psychiatry 54:193, 1991
98. Messina AV, Chernik NL: Computed tomograph: the "resolving" intracerebral hemorrhage. Radiology 118:609, 1976
99. Mohadjer M, Eggert R, May J, Mayfrank L: CT-guided stereotactic fibrinolysis of spontaneous and hypertensive cerebellar hemorrhage: long-term results. J Neurosurg 73:217, 1990
100. Mosdal C, Jensen G, Sommer W et al: Spontaneous intracerebral haematomas: clinical and computertomographic findings and long-term outcome after surgical treatment. Acta Neurochir 83:92, 1986
101. Murphy MG: Successful evacuation of acute pontine hematoma. J Neurosurg 37:224, 1972
102. Nakagawa H, Furuta Y, Nakajima S et al: Surgical excision of familial cavernous angioma in the pontomedullary region—case report. Neurol Med Chir (Tokyo) 30:422, 1990
103. Nehls DG, Mendelow DA, Graham DI et al: Experimental intracerebral hemorrhage: progression of hemodynamic changes after production of a spontaneous mass lesion. Neurosurgery 23:439, 1988
104. Nehls DG, Mendelow DA, Graham DI et al: Experimental intracerebral hemorrhage: early removal of a spontaneous mass lesion improves late outcome. Neurosurgery 27:674, 1990
105. New PF, Ojemann RG, Davis KR et al: MR and CT of occult vascular malformations of the brain. AJR 147:985, 1986
106. Niizuma H, Suzuki J, Yonemitsu T et al: Spontaneous intracerebral hemorrhage and liver dysfunction. Stroke 19:852, 1988
107. Ogilvy CS, Heros RC, Ojemann RG et al: Angiographically occult arteriovenous malformations. J Neurosurg 69:350, 1988
108. Ojemann RG: Spontaneous brain hemorrhage: what treatment should we recommend? Stroke 14:467, 1983
109. Ojemann RG, Heros RC: Spontaneous brain hemorrhage. Stroke 14:458, 1983
110. Ojemann RG, Heros RC, Crowell RM: Surgical Management of Cerebrovascular Disease. 2nd Ed. Williams & Wilkins, Baltimore, 1987
111. Ojemann RG, Mohr JP: Hypertensive brain hemorrhage. Clin Neurosurg 23:220, 1975
112. Okazak H, Reagan R, Campbell RJ: Clinicopathologic studies of primary cerebral amyloid angiopathy. Mayo Clin Proc 54:22, 1979
113. Ott KH, Kase CS, Ojemann RG et al: Cerebellar hemorrhage: diagnosis and treatment: a review of 56 cases. Arch Neurol 31:160, 1974
114. Padt JP, Dereuk J, vander Eecken H: Intracerebral hemorrhage as initial symptom of a brain tumor. Acta Neurol Belg 73:241, 1973
115. Paillas JE, Alliez B: Surgical treatment of spontaneous intracerebral hemorrhage: immediate and long-term results in 250 cases. J Neurosurg 39:145, 1973
116. Papo I, Janny P, Caruselli G et al: Intracranial pressure time course in primary intracerebral hemorrhage. Neurosurgery 4:504, 1972
117. Pecker J, Ioualalen N, Brassier G et al: Place de l'arteriographie dans le diagnostic etiologique des hematomes intra-cerebraux spontanes. Neurochirurgie 32:281, 1986
118. Pia HW: The surgical treatment of intracerebral and intraventricular hematomas. Acta Neurochir (Wein) 27:149, 1972
119. Pineda A: Computed tomography in intracerebral hemorrhage. Surg Neurol 8:55, 1977
120. Pressman BD, Kirkwood JR, David DO: Posterior fossa hemorrhage: localization by computerized tomography. JAMA 232:932, 1975
121. Radberg JA, Olsson JE, Radberg CT: Prognostic parameters in spontaneous intracerebral hematomas with special reference to anticoagulant treatment. Stroke 22:571, 1991
122. Ransohoff J, Derby B, Kricheff I: Spontaneous intracerebral hemorrhage. Clin Neurosurg 18:247, 1971
123. Rapacki TF, Brantley MJ, Furlow TW et al: Heterogeneity of cerebral cavernous hemangiomas diagnosed by MR imaging. J Comput Assist Tomogr 14:18, 1990
124. Richardson A: The management of primary intracranial hemorrhage. Mod Trends Neurol 3:89, 1962
125. Richardson A: Surgical therapy of spontaneous intracerebral hemorrhage. p. 397. In Krayenbuhl H, Maspes PE, Sweet WH (eds): Progress in Neurological Surgery. Vol. 3. Year Book Medical Publications, Chicago, 1969
126. Richardson A: Surgical therapy of spontaneous intracerebral hemorrhage. Clin Neurosurg 18:247, 1971
127. Richardson A: Spontaneous intracerebral and cerebellar hemorhage. p. 210. In Russell RW (ed): Cerebral Arterial Disease. Churchill Livingstone, New York, 1976
128. Ropper A, Davis K: Lobar cerebral hemorrhage: acute syndromes in 26 cases. Ann Neurol 8:141, 1980
129. Ropper A, Zervas NT: Cerebral blood flow after experimental basal ganglia hemorrhage. Ann Neurol 11:266, 1980
130. Rubin JM, Dohrmann GJ: Use of ultrasonically guided probes and catheters in neurosurgery. Surg Neurol 18:143, 1982
131. Russell DS: The pathology of spontaneous intracranial hemorrhage. Proc R Soc Med 47:689, 1954
132. Sahuquillo J, Vilalta J, Sumalla J et al: Surgical vs. conservative treatment for spontaneous ICH. (Letter; Comment.) J Neurosurg 72:152, 1990
133. Sano K, Ochiai C: Brain stem hematomas: clinical aspects with reference to indications for treatment. p. 366. In Pia HW, Langmaid C, Zierski J (eds): Spontaneous Intracerebral Hematomas. Springer-Verlag, New York, 1980
134. Sano K, Yoshida S: Cerebellar hematomas. p. 348. In Pia HW, Langmaid C, Zierski J (eds):

Spontaneous Intracerebral Hematomas. Springer-Verlag, New York, 1980
135. Sasaki K, Matsumoto K: Relationship between motor disturbance and involvement of internal capsule in hypertensive thalamic hemorrhage. No Shinkei Geka 19:221, 1991
136. Schumacher M, Rossberg, Stoeter P: Differential Diagnose and Verlaufsuntersuchungen bei intracerebralen Blutungen. (CT Differential Diagnosis and Findings in Intracerebral Haemorrhage.) Arch Psychiatr Nervenkr 231:171, 1982
137. Schutz H, Bodeker RH, Damian M et al: Age-related spontaneous intracerebral hematoma in a German community. Stroke 21:1412, 1990
138. Scott WR, New PFJ, Davis KR, Schnur JA: Computerized axial tomography of intracerebral and intraventricular hemorrhage. Radiology 112:73, 1974
139. Seeler RA, Imana RB: Intracranial hemorrhage in patients with hemophilia. J Neurosurg 39:181, 1973
140. Seifert V, Gaab MR: Laser-assisted microsurgical extirpation of a brain stem cavernoma: case report. Neurosurgery 25:986, 1989
141. Senant J, Samson M, Proust B: Approache multi-factorielle due pronostic vital des hematomes intracerebraux spontanes. Rev Neurol 144:279, 1988
142. Shenkin HA, Zavala M: Cerebellar strokes: mortality, surgical indications and results of ventricular drainage. Lancet 2:429,1982
143. Shuangshoti S, Phunthumchinda K: Cerebral acute angiitides and extensive hemorrhages associated with clinically silent acute bacterial endocarditis. J Med Assoc Thai 70:523, 1987
144. Specht CS, Pinto-Lord C, Smith TW et al: Spontaneous hemorrhage in a mixed glioma of the cerebellum: case report. Neurosurgery 19:278, 1986
145. Suzuki J, Sato T: Grading and timing of operation in putaminal ICH. p. 274. In Pia HW, Langmaid C, Zierski J (eds): Spontaneous Intracerebral Hematomas. Springer-Verlag, New York, 1980
146. Suzuki R, Ohno K, Matsushima Y, Inaba Y: Serial changes in focal hyperemia associated with hypertensive putaminal hemorrhage. Stroke 19:322, 1988
147. Tedeschi G, Bernini FP, Cerillo A: Indication for surgical treatment of intracerebral hemorrhage. J Neurosurg 43:590, 1975
148. Thie A, Spitzer K, Lappe H et al: Prognostische Bedeutung initialer klinischer und apparativer Parameter bei spontanen intrazerebralen Blutungen. Fortschr Neurol Psychiatr 56:163, 1988
149. Troncale JA, Close D, Pham XD: Spontaneous hypertensive-arteriosclerotic intracerebral hemorrhage. J Fam Pract 29:243, 1989
150. Tung H, Giannotta SL, Chandrasoma PT et al: Recurrent intraparenchymal hemorrhages from angiographically occult vascular malformations. J Neurosurg 73:174, 1990
151. Tucker WJ, Bilbao J, Klodawsky H: Cerebral amyloid angiopathy and multiple intracranial hematomas. Neurosurgery 7:611, 1982
152. Tyler KL, Poletti CE, Heros RC: Cerebral amyloid angiopathy with multiple intracerebral hemorrhages. Neurosurgery 57:286, 1982
153. Uchino A, Ohnari N, Ohno M: Acute hypertensive intracranial hemorrhage: MR imaging at 1.5T. Nippon Igaku Hoshasen Gakkai Zasshi 49:1243, 1989
154. Uede T, Nonaka T, Takigami M et al: Cavernous malformation of the brain stem: clinical symptom and its surgical indication. No Shinkei Geka 19:27, 1991
155. Veerapen R: Spontaneous lateral pontine hemorrhage with associated trigeminal nerve root hematoma. Neurosurgery 25:451, 453, 1989
156. Verma A, Maheshwari MC, Bhargava S: Spontaneous intraventricular haemorrhage. J Neurol 234:233, 1987
157. Vinters HV, Gilbert JJ: Amyloid angiopathy: its incidence and complications in the aging brain. Stroke 12:118, 1981
158. Waga S, Miyazaki M, Okada M et al: Hypertensive putaminal hemorrhage: analysis of 182 patients. Surg Neurol 26:159, 1986
159. Wakai S: Angiographically occult vascular malformations (Letter.) J Neurosurg 74:527, 1991
160. Wakai S, Ueda Y, Inoh S et al: Angiographically occult angiomas: a report of thirteen cases with an analysis of the cases documented in the literature. Neurosurgery 17:549, 1985
161. Wattendorff AR, Bots GT, Went LN et al: Familial cerebral amyloid angiopathy presenting as recurrent cerebral hemorrhage. J Neurol Sci 55:121, 1982
162. Weil SM, Tew JM, Jr: Surgical management of brain stem vascular malformations. Acta Neurochir (Wien) 105:14, 1990
163. Weisberg L: Multiple spontaneous intracerebral hematomas: clinical and computed tomographic correlations. Neurology (NY) 37:897, 1981
164. Weisberg LA: Computerized tomograph in intracranial hemorrhage. Arch Neurol 36:422, 1979
165. Wiggins WS, Moody DM, Toole JF: Clinical and computerized tomographic study of hypertensive intracerebral hemorrhage. Arch Neurol 35:832, 1978
166. Yashon D, Kosnik EG: Chronic intracerebral hematoma. Neurosurgery 2:103, 1978
167. Yarnell P, Earnest MP: Primary non-traumatic intracranial hemorrhage: municipal emergency hospital viewpoint. Stroke 7:608, 1976
168. Yoshida H, Fujita H, Ohta K et al: Clinical study of hypertensive cerebellar hemorrhage: surgical indication and measurement of volume of hematoma. No Shinkei Geka 17:1105, 1989
169. Yoshida H, Komai N, Nakai E et al: Stereotactic evacuation of hypertensive cerebellar hemorrhage using plasminogen activator. No Shinkei Geka 17:421, 1989
170. Yoshida M, Hayashi T, Kuramoto S et al: Traumatic intracranial hematomas in hemophiliac children. Surg Neurol 12:115, 1979

171. Yoshida N, Kagawa M, Takeshita M et al: Grading and operative indication for hypertensive cerebellar hemorrhage. No Shinkei Geka 14:725, 1986
172. Yoshimoto H, Fujita H, Ohta K et al: Clinical study of hypertensive subcortical hemorrhage: surgical indication and long-term, functional prognosis. No Shinkei Geka 16:1465, 1988
173. Yoshimoto T, Suzuki J: Radical surgery on cavernous angioma of the brainstem. Surg Neurol 26:72, 1986
174. Yu Y, Cooper DR, Wellenstein DE et al: Cerebral angitis and intracerebral hemorrhage associated with methamphetamine abuse: case report. J Neurosurg 58:109, 1983
175. Zimmerman RD, Leeds NE, Naidich TP: Ring blush associated with intracerebral hematoma. Radiology 122:707, 1977
176. Zulch KJ: Pathologic aspects of cerebral accidents in arterial hypertension. Acta Neurol Belg 71:196, 1971

# 51
# *REHABILITATION OF THE STROKE SURVIVOR*

Glen E. Gresham

The essential goal of rehabilitation is the restoration of as much function as possible, trying to ensure that the performance levels achieved are the most optimal ones for each particular individual. All relevant functional parameters should be considered. For the stroke survivor, these usually include walking, other activities of daily living (ADL), several psychosocial dimensions, the living setting in the community and, when appropriate, return to work.

The specific process of medical rehabilitation is now formally established in many countries. In the United States, for example, the team approach and the professional components included therein (medicine, rehabilitation nursing, physical and occupational therapy, speech pathology, audiology, and psychosocial counseling) are not only customary but mandated for accreditation.[10,36] For stroke patients, the formalized rehabilitation process is applied in full, or in part; in a variety of clinical settings, including hospitals, free-standing rehabilitation centers, skilled nursing facilities, and the home.[18,23] In recent years, the various functional levels to be expected as outcomes for stroke survivors in medical rehabilitation programs have been studied and a variety of norms established.[3,16,17,19,25–28,30,39,44,47,59,60] While some differences of opinion exist regarding the relative value of specific rehabilitation techniques and programs, it is now expected that every physician and allied health professional caring for stroke survivors will give attention to functional parameters and try to facilitate each patient's ability to reach his or her full potential.

It is not the intent of this chapter to discuss in detail the various components of the currently established process for institutional medical rehabilitation in stroke. These are described in comprehensive reference volumes from the field of Rehabilitation Medicine.[2,8,11,24] The intent is, rather, to review the specific characteristics of stroke survivors that appear to be the basic determinants of functional potential and, in addition, to identify the various types of functional levels that stroke survivors are now expected to achieve (based on evidence from selected major studies published during the last 3 decades).

Each stroke survivor who becomes "medically stable" poses a challenge to the prognostic and care-planning skills of his or her physician. As the urgent issues of acute management are resolved, emphasis begins to shift to questions of long-term outcomes. These include the likelihood of survival, the various levels of function that each particular patient will be able to achieve, and the settings and services that will be most favorable for facilitating the achievement of those functional goals.

Each individual stroke survivor will eventually reach the point where his or her long-term potential for various types of function can be assessed in a rational manner. The time at which this occurs will vary, depending on the rate at which changing manifestations evolve. There is, however, good reason to begin this formulation early, since it can be modified as the situation changes and unnecessary delays and preventable complications can be avoided. Modern health care systems move swiftly (and expensively). It is no longer permissible to look upon stroke rehabilitation as a far-off process that can be deferred to some distant place and time. Cost factors, length of stay limitations, and other requirements make early and effective planning of the entire course of care a necessity.

There are, of course, basic components of good clinical care of the stroke patient that must be instituted very early, even before long-range functional potentials can be fully assessed. These include proper positioning, a regular schedule of turning, good skin care, early attention to possible removal of an indwelling catheter, establishment of a regular voiding and bowel evacuation pattern, and passive range of motion exercises. Failure to provide these basic elements of good stroke care greatly increases the risk of preventable complications that might impede further progress. Joint contractures, pressure sores, and ignored incontinence should not occur in the well-managed stroke patient. For physicians and nurses unfamiliar with these simple but essential basics of stroke care, consultation should be sought from knowledgeable sources, such as physiatrists, rehabilitation nurses, or others with specific training and experience in the functionally-oriented care of acute stroke patients.[8,11,12,24,34]

Once a program of knowledgeable bedside care is established as a complement to ongoing diagnostic and therapeutic maneuvers by the neurologist or other acute care physician, the basis is established for formulating a functional prognosis and designing a strategy to achieve it. As soon as the patient's condition stabilizes sufficiently, the latter can then be rapidly implemented. Should the patient not survive the acute episode, these elements of care will have added relatively little to the overall costs, and, as stressed previously, failure to provide them may jeopardize good functional outcomes if the patient lives.

**TABLE 51-1. Variables[a] that Must Be Assessed in Stroke[b] Survivors**

I. Intrinsic Characteristics of the Individual
- Demographic: age, sex, race, and marital status
- Precise neurologic deficit:
  - Motor (R hemiparesis; L hemiparesis; bilateral motor deficit; no motor deficit); degree of spasticity present
  - Sensory (hemisensory deficit or other)
  - Hemianopia
  - Speech problems (dysphasia, dysarthria)
  - Organic cognitive deficits
  - Other (e.g., cerebellar ataxia, cranial nerve palsies)
- Etiology of stroke (atherothrombotic brain infarct, hemorrhage)
- Comorbid processes (concurrent medical conditions that may affect survival or functional abilities)
- Psychosocial factors (premorbid personality, usual socialization patterns, affective state, and others)
- Educational level and other skills
- Vocational status
- Financial assets

II. Extrinsic Characteristics of the Individual's Environment
- Family constellation or significant others
- Physical environment of home
- Type of community (physical environment, resources, attitudes)
- Services available (medical, rehabilitative, ongoing)

[a] Specific variables, considered determinants of functional outcomes in stroke survivors, that should be assessed in each case.
[b] Stroke is defined as a fixed neurologic deficit, presumably of vascular origin, that persists for at least 48 hours.

## PROGNOSIS FOR FUNCTION IN STROKE SURVIVORS

A conceptual scheme for assessing the functional potential of each surviving stroke patient is a basic foundation for the rational management of the rehabilitation process. A suggested outline of the specific variables that should be considered is given in Table 51-1.

Characteristics of the stroke survivor, considered to be determinants of functional outcome, have been arbitrarily divided into "intrinsic" ones (that are considered inherent features of the patient) and "extrinsic" variables that make up the physical and social environmental setting in which the rehabilitation or functional enhancement process will occur. These variables from Table 51-1 can be amplified as follows.

The conventional demographic characteristics of age, sex, race, and marital status provide a basic template for formulating a functional prognosis for an individual stroke survivor. Age per se does not preclude good functional outcomes, but is associated with an increased probability of shorter survival, more comorbid processes, and adverse psychosocial conditions. Sex, race, and marital status, while not strong predictors of specific functional outcomes, are known to be of significance in survival generally and socioeconomic prospects, especially in later years.

The most powerful determinant of functional outcomes in stroke would appear to be the *specific neurological deficit.* While this may seem obvious, it is really not, since most of the studies of stroke outcomes treat stroke survivors as a homogenous entity. This is, of course, far from the case. For example, data from the Framingham Study,[33] drawn from a large community-based population, showed that of 148 long-term survivors of a documented completed stroke, only 67 had hemiparesis (34 left and 33 right), 4 had bilateral motor weakness, and 77 had no peripheral motor deficit at all (see Table 51-2). Thus, the frequent implicit assumption that permanent hemiparesis is the sine qua non of stroke is a less than complete appreciation of the total picture of stroke survivors. The fact is that stroke survivors manifest a variety of neurologic deficits that are not mutually exclusive, and each has some effect on the functional potential of that individual.

**TABLE 51-2. Neurologic Deficits Manifested by 148 Survivors of Documented Completed Stroke: The Framingham Study (April 1972 through March 1975)**

| Peripheral Motor Deficit | Hemisensory Defect | | Hemianopia | | Dysarthria | | Dysphasia | | All Patients | | |
|---|---|---|---|---|---|---|---|---|---|---|---|
| | Men | Women | Men | Women | Men | Women | Men | Women | Men | Women | Total |
| None | 4 | 1 | 3 | 2 | 1 | 2 | 7 | 6 | 31 | 46 | 77 |
| Left hemiparesis | 8 | 9 | 3 | 4 | 2 | 1 | 2 | 1 | 17 | 17 | 34 |
| Right hemiparesis | 5 | 5 | 2 | 2 | 8 | 7 | 5 | 5 | 16 | 17 | 33 |
| Bilateral | 2 | 2 | 1 | 2 | 1 | 1 | 1 | 0 | 2 | 2 | 4 |
| Total | 19 | 17 | 9 | 10 | 12 | 11 | 15 | 12 | 66 | 82 | 148 |

(From Gresham et al.,[33] with permission.)

As a beginning, the functional prognosis of a stroke patient requires a classification of the type of motor deficit (e.g., right hemiparesis, left hemiparesis, bilateral motor deficit, or no motor deficit), with some description of its severity and the degree of spasticity associated with it. Without this much diagnostic detail, speculation on eventual outcomes, such as walking or activities of daily living (ADL), has no fundamental rationale. In addition to the motor deficit, other aspects of the *precise neurologic deficit,* whenever present, must be appreciated. These include sensory deficits, hemianopia, speech problems (e.g., dysphasia, dysarthria), organic cognitive deficits, and any other concurrent abnormalities of either the central or peripheral nervous systems. Only a full appreciation of the entire neurologic deficit provides an adequate basis for projecting what that specific stroke survivor will eventually be able to accomplish in terms of function. As an obvious example, the patient with right hemiparesis alone will be likely to manage better than another person with similar motor deficit plus the added burden of dysphasia.

It would seem from the foregoing that currently available data should permit quantitative functional prognostication for at least walking and ADL from known constellations of complete neurologic deficits. Such is not the case, however. The reasons for this are many, but a major one is statistical. Most carefully done studies of stroke survivors involve, at most, a few hundred cases, and, while study populations of this magnitude may support inferences about major entities (such as right versus left hemiparesis, for instance), the addition of each new variable rapidly produces cells with very small numbers. For example, as shown in Table 51-2, out of 148 long-term stroke survivors in the Framingham Study, there were only 10 with concurrent right hemiparesis and dysphasia and only 11 with hemiparesis (either side) and coexistent heminanopia.[33] These orders of magnitude are even more noteworthy when it is remembered that the figures were derived from a cohort of 5,209 persons followed for over 20 years. In the future, more elaborate studies should enable greater precision in linking specific constellations of neurologic deficits with specific functional outcomes. For the present, however, the physician must rely heavily on thoughtful clinical judgment, realizing that the complete *precise neurological deficit* must be fully appreciated before meaningful prognostic thinking and rehabilitation program planning can begin.

Certain neurologic deficits, such as dysphasia, have an obvious negative impact on the future functional levels achievable by the stroke survivor. More subtle, but often more significant, are organic cognitive deficits that affect the patient's ability to learn (and hence benefit from rehabilitation services). Most medical rehabilitation workers are now oriented to using visual cues with patients with left cortical lesions and verbal cues with those with right cortical lesions. It is important, however, to utilize the most sophisticated psychometry readily available to gain as detailed a picture as possible of each stroke patient's specific residual cognitive abilities.[7]

Another host characteristic of importance to consider is etiology. Most of our current information about long-term functional outcomes in stroke has been derived from populations of stroke patients made up largely of survivors of atherothrombotic brain infarction (ABI). These accounted, for example, for 75 percent of the long-term stroke survivors in the Framingham Study Cohort.[33] This group is comprised largely of older persons, many with systemic cardiovascular disease, whose survival and functional outcome experience may not be fully relevant to other kinds of stroke patients (the younger person, for example, who has survived a bleeding saccular aneurysm), even when the specific neurologic deficits are the same.

Comorbidity is another crucial ingredient in functional prognosis that is frequently ignored. This important concept, elaborated and emphasized by Feinstein,[20] requires the assessment of all other concurrent conditions that may affect survival and functional outcomes and must, therefore, be included in prognostic formulation. Two types of comorbid conditions that are frequently found in stroke survivors are concurrent cardiovascular disease and other coexistent conditions that will affect specific functional outcomes. The frequency of the former was found to be significant in the Framingham subjects, as shown in Table 51-3.[33] Examples of the latter are concurrent chronic obstructive pulmonary disease (COPD), arthritis, or amputations, all of which will have much to do with the patient's eventual ability to walk, even though none are necessarily related to the stroke itself. Some forms of functional comorbidity, such as joint contractures or pressure sores, may be due to preventable complications. They must, however, be honestly included in the formulation of functional prognosis at the time the patient is to be mobilized.

Psychosocial factors play a significant role in determining functional outcomes in stroke. The generally high prevalence of psychosocial, even more than physical, disability in stroke survivors was well demonstrated in the Framingham Study[33] as shown in Table 51-4. It is, of course, always difficult to decide whether certain psychosocial characteristics of stroke survivors are among the determinants of functional outcomes or the outcomes themselves. An example of this is depression. Several studies have shown that there is an increased frequency of depression in stroke survivors,[4,15,52] as compared to other persons of the same age. It is, however, speculative as to how much is either reactive (to the overwhelming loss presented by the stroke) or unrelated (such as an involutional affective state that would have occurred in that individual anyway). Ongoing investigations are helping to clarify these interrelationships.[52] Meanwhile, it is important that clinicians take the time to include, in history-taking with stroke patients, such important psychosocial information as premorbid personality, usual socialization patterns, and current affective state as variables that must be considered in functional prognosis and dealt with in the management of care.

Other relevant characteristics of stroke patients, related to eventual outcomes, are educational level, other acquired skills, and premorbid vocational status. It is, of course, obvious that a stroke patient with severe dementia will benefit little from previous education or avocational skills. Conversely, the more intact person with no such personal assets may find no "quality" in his or her life. The need here, of course, is for the clinician to gather all of the relevant information so that knowledgeable guidance and appropriate referrals, in each individual case, can be provided.

The final "intrinsic" characteristic to be discussed, namely, financial status, could be regarded as part of the environmental setting. There is, however, such a range of individual differences in financial assets among stroke survivors who have similar environments and social supports, that it must be regarded as individual-specific. For example, a stroke patient with personal means has many immediate options in terms of living settings, equipment, and purchase of supportive services. At the other extreme, the already medically indigent patient, in the United States, has access to immediate federal payment for certain services (provided they are within guidelines) without the anguish and ambivalence of a "spenddown." The hapless middle person, not indigent but not well-off, may have the hardest time of all and require the most help in finding the really needed items and services at the most reasonable costs. In any event, no functional prognostication or long-term management plan is realistically complete without taking this variable into account. In the medical rehabilitation setting, social workers and other counselors provide invaluable help to patients and their physicians in evaluating and managing these problems.

The intrinsic characteristics of the stroke survivor, as previously discussed, are surely the prime determinants of what that patient will be able to accomplish in terms of life functions. There are, however, impor-

**TABLE 51-3. Frequency of 14 Documented Comorbid Disease Processes in 148 Stroke Survivors and 148 Stroke-Free Matched Controls: The Framingham Study (April 1972 through March 1975)**

| Type of Comorbid Disease[a] | Stroke Survivors | | Matched Controls | | |
|---|---|---|---|---|---|
| | *N* | % | *N* | % | *P* |
| Hypertension | 99 | 67 | 66 | 45 | <0.001 |
| Hypertensive cardiovascular disease[b] | 78 | 53 | 46 | 31 | <0.001 |
| Coronary heart disease | 47 | 32 | 30 | 20 | <0.05 |
| Other heart disease | 45 | 30 | 30 | 20 | <0.05 |
| Obesity | 33 | 22 | 18 | 12 | <0.05 |
| Diabetes mellitus | 32 | 22 | 15 | 10 | <0.02 |
| Arthritis | 32 | 22 | 18 | 12 | <0.05 |
| Left ventricular hypertrophy by ECG | 31 | 21 | 9 | 6 | <0.001 |
| Congestive heart failure | 26 | 18 | 7 | 5 | <0.001 |
| Chronic lung disease | 26 | 18 | 38 | 26 | NS |
| Peripheral vascular disease | 26 | 18 | 19 | 13 | NS |
| Cancer | 16 | 11 | 14 | 9 | NS |
| Intermittent claudication | 15 | 10 | 9 | 6 | NS |
| Extremity amputation | 3 | 2 | 0 | 0 | NS |
| Total number of subjects | 148 | 100 | 148 | 100 | |

[a] Not mutually exclusive categories.
[b] Includes cardiac enlargement by x-ray or ECG in hypertensive individual.
(From Gresham et al.,[33] with permission.)

**TABLE 51-4. Frequency of 9 Types of Functional Deficit in 148 Stroke Survivors and 148 Stroke-Free Matched Controls: The Framingham Study (April 1972 through March 1975)**

| Type of Functional Deficit[a] | Stroke Survivors *N* | Stroke Survivors % | Matched Controls *N* | Matched Controls % | *P* |
|---|---|---|---|---|---|
| Decreased vocational function | 93 | 63 | 54 | 36 | <0.001 |
| Decreased socialization outside the home | 87 | 59 | 42 | 28 | <0.001 |
| Limited in household tasks | 83 | 56 | 30 | 20 | <0.001 |
| Decrease in interests and hobbies | 70 | 47 | 30 | 20 | <0.001 |
| Decreased ability to use outside transportation | 65 | 44 | 19 | 13 | <0.001 |
| Decreased socialization at home | 64 | 43 | 41 | 28 | <0.01 |
| Dependent in ADL | 48 | 32 | 13 | 9 | <0.001 |
| Dependent in mobility | 32 | 22 | 9 | 6 | <0.001 |
| Not living at home (nursing home or other institutional setting) | 22 | 15 | 3 | 2 | <0.001 |
| Total number of subjects | 148 | 100 | 148 | 100 | |

[a] In descending order of frequency; not mutually exclusive categories.
[b] Dependent in ADL = Katz index score of C, D, E, F, G or other. (ADL, activities of daily living.)
(From Gresham et al.,[33] with permission.)

tant environmental factors that should not be ignored. Indeed, in the International Classification of Impairments, Disabilities, and Handicaps,[66] Wood and colleagues clearly distinguish the dimensions of impairment (such as the manifestations of a cerebral infarct), disability (such as problems in walking, ADL, and other specific activities), and handicap (inability to perform a social role, which is often influenced by environmental and societal factors extrinsic to the individual).[65]

Particular extrinsic factors that may profoundly affect eventual functional outcomes for stroke survivors include (but are not limited to) family constellation and/or significant others, the physical environment of the home, the type of community (physical environment, resources, and attitudes), and services available (medical, rehabilitative, and ongoing).

Regarding family constellation and/or significant others, it is readily apparent that motivation and opportunity for rapid reintegration into society of the stroke survivor will be, at least in part, related to the availability and enthusiasm of other people important to the patient.[5,6,14] With proper guidance, they can provide support, encouragement, and realistic help without falling into the traps of overprotectiveness (on the one hand) or thinly veiled rejection (on the other). Problems of the physical environment of the home, routine to medical rehabilitation teams, may be ignored by other care-givers. It is clear, for example, that the stroke survivor trained to ambulate in a well-lit, barrier-free environment may lose this skill if confronted by a combination of throw rugs, poorly lit steps, and complicated furniture arrangements.

Communities, of course, vary enormously in their basic hospitality to the handicapped. The physical environment can present either encouraging accessibility or formidable obstacles that overwhelm persons with mobility problems. The conventional concerns of "accessibility" are often oriented to the needs of wheelchair-bound, but actually younger, more cognitively intact persons (such as the spinal cord injured) who can often negotiate environments that the older, more frail, and easily confused stroke victim finds intimidating. Community resources are most variable and depend on many complicated determinants. It is vital to know what is available. For example, a community with "Meals on Wheels," transportation for the handicapped, and "Care-Ring" services could provide a whole new dimension of living to the handicapped stroke survivor trying to cope in another setting that lacked such resources. Attitudes, fortunately, are improving. In the past, they alone consigned many stroke survivors to sequestered and needlessly useless lives.

The final extrinsic factor to be considered is services available. The lack of total agreement over the merit of particular approaches to poststroke rehabilitation and long-term care should not be allowed to detract from the manifold accomplishments achieved by appropriate services rendered in a timely manner. The emphasis should be on ensuring that the specific services (medical, rehabilitative, and supportive) required by each stroke patient are obtained and continued until either maximum benefit has been achieved or it is concluded that they are clearly not providing the help hoped for. There has been a considerable amount of interesting research on the relative merits of various service combinations in the treatment of stroke survivors. Conventional medical rehabilitation has been shown to increase functional levels,[3,16,17,19,25,26,27,28,39,44,47,59] even after 12 months have elapsed after stroke onset.[44] Other studies have shown that gains achieved in medical rehabilitation programs are maintained for long periods of time,[25,47] supporting the basic cost-effectiveness of the service "package." Other studies suggest that alternative service groupings can serve stroke patients equally effectively.[21,53] In fact, newer evidence suggests that the timing and organization of rehabilitation services, rather than the total amount, may be the crucial determinant for success.[59,60] At the present state of knowledge, it seems reasonable to suggest that each stroke patient's constellation of needs be assessed and that these be matched, as rationally as possible, with specific services available in the community.

## LONG-TERM OUTCOMES IN STROKE

As previously noted, it is not yet possible to "plug in" the host characteristics of an individual stroke survivor and derive, through a formula, the specific profile of functional outcomes to be expected. It is, however, quite feasible to approximate this through an intellectual exercise combining careful observation and classification of the basic intrinsic and extrinsic characteristics of the patient (as discussed above) with a knowledge of the expected distribution of particular outcomes for stroke survivors generally. As noted above, most current research deals with stroke patients as a single group. This must be kept in mind when attempting to project outcomes for any one individual. There is, however, enough evidence available to enable the clinician, with an appreciation of what outcomes are to be expected in stroke survivors generally, to integrate this information with the characteristics of any individual patient in a formulation that will combine both rational prognosis and appropriate case management.

A suggested outline of outcome variables that have been studied in stroke survivors, is shown in Table 51-5. The list is by no means exhaustive, as each year sees new and interesting studies published that focus on an ever increasing number of important outcome variables. Experience suggests, however, that the variables shown in Table 51-5 are of unequivocal importance and should not be ignored.

**TABLE 51-5. Important Long-Term Outcome Variables That Have Been Studied in Survivors of Stroke**

| |
|---|
| Survival |
| Location or living setting (e.g., within an institution or independent in the community) |
| Walking (ambulation)—Considered independently or as a part of activities of daily living (ADL) |
| Activities of daily living (ADL)—Basic self-care, including feeding, toileting, dressing, transfers, mobility, bathing, and grooming |
| Instrumental activities of daily living (IADL) |
| Communication |
| Psychosocial function |
| Cognitive performance |
| Affect/mood; presence or absence of depression |
| Social integration: with family or significant others in wider community |
| Sexual function |
| Rewarding avocational pursuits |
| Vocational function |

### Survival

*Survival* is the variable basic to all other interest in the details of stroke outcomes. Early advocates of positive programs for stroke survivors, such as Rankin[51] and Adams[1] emphasized that, while stroke is indeed an entity of major mortality, nevertheless, significantly large numbers of victims survive with ongoing needs for many kinds of help and understanding. Thus, over the past 30 years, emphasis in medical thinking has shifted from a fatalistic preoccupation with high immediate and excess long-term mortality in stroke victims to include an appreciation of and an interest in the large number of stroke survivors who go on living in the general population. This has also led to an increasing sense of responsibility for identifying and meeting their needs.

Stroke remains an entity in which survival of the acute episode is less than 80 percent (at 30 days) and whose survivors are more likely to die, in each subsequent year, than their stroke-free counterparts of the same age.[54] In the Framingham cohort, however, overall 10-year survival after stroke was 35 percent, with much better rates for survivors of ABI without cardiovascular comorbidity.[54] There is, in addition, good evidence that the probability of survival after stroke is steadily increasing.[22] This, of course, offsets the declining incidence of stroke and continues to remind us that, for the forseeable future, a significant number of stroke survivors, many of them elderly, will be alive in the general population at any point in time, with needs that must be addressed. As acute neurologic care becomes more sophisticated, and the various nonneurologic causes of death in stroke survivors (cardiac, thromboembolic, infectious) are identified and better treated, the obvious effect will be a continuing or increasing number of persons who survive strokes and thus become candidates for rehabilitation and reintegration into the community. Ongoing sensitivity to their needs and provision of appropriate services to meet them is a fundamental responsibility of rehabilitation and long-term care providers.

### Location

*Location* or living setting (i.e., institutional or community) is an important outcome variable in stroke. In general, institutional living is regarded as more restrictive, less pleasant, and much more expensive than community living (at least in the United States). It was, therefore, of interest when we found that only 15 percent of long-term stroke survivors in the Framingham cohort were living in an institutional setting.[33] This frequency was compared to others determined in Norway,[49] Australia,[61] and Rochester, Minnesota.[46,64] The latter tended to be somewhat higher, but this was deemed attributable to a difference in the number and desirability of institutional settings available, rather than simple greater ability to manage in the community. Finally, interesting recent research suggests that specific host characteristics, such as gender, increase the risk of institutionalization after stroke.[41]

## Walking

Unlike many impairments, stroke does not usually destroy the ability to walk. This is due, largely, to a predilection for involvement of the distribution of the middle cerebral artery. Independent ambulation, with or without an assistive device but not requiring help from another person, was observed in 78 percent of long-term stroke survivors in the Framingham Study[33] (see Table 51-4). Other studies, with highly selected institutional populations (e.g., patients referred for rehabilitation services in various types of programs), have found frequencies for eventual independent ambulation ranging from 52[39] to 87 percent.[60] Since the Framingham Study data were derived from a large, carefully followed community cohort, the 78 percent frequency is considered to be reasonably reflective of what should be expected as an overall long-term outcome.

With the awareness that four out of five long-term stroke survivors should eventually be able to walk independently, the clinician is better equipped to approach the assessment and management of each individual patient. For each patient who proves not to be progressing toward independent ambulation, the reasons should be obvious. In addition, if the constraints appear to be in any way remediable, an obligation exists to ensure that the patient receives the needed services and equipment.

Stroke survivors who are treated in a conventional medical rehabilitation setting (whether it be a hospital, a free-standing clinic, a skilled nursing facility, or a home program) will have had the benefit of physiatric assessment and a program of physical therapy. As such, the issues of preserving range of motion, muscle strengthening, improving coordination, gait training, prescription and provision of the most appropriate ankle-foot orthosis and walking aid, as well as the knowledgeable management of increasing spasticity will all have been systematically addressed. Patients managed in other settings, however, may have unfulfilled service needs that should be recognized. Finally, those who have walked well in a sheltered institutional setting may decompensate if discharged abruptly and without preparation into an inhospitable environment.

Only after all reasonable efforts have proved fruitless and the reasons for the stroke survivor's remaining unable to walk are clear, should the managing clinician settle for a wheelchair or a lesser level of mobility. It is important to remember that the average stroke survivor, in spite of having suffered a serious illness and an initially overwhelming impairment, can and does walk independently, thus achieving a degree of independence in mobility that is quite compatible with continuing a relatively normal pattern of daily life.

## Activities of Daily Living

The ADL spectrum of functional parameters has received a considerable amount of study and is the best known and most standardized set of outcome variables in stroke. Formally designated as an Index Medicus category in 1968, ADL comprises the daily functions that an individual must be able to perform in order to get along without another person carrying out daily personal care services (with all the expense and loss of personal autonomy that this implies).

It is not surprising that a high percentage of studies regarding ADL outcomes in stroke has appeared in the medical rehabilitation literature. Rehabilitation Medicine has always emphasized maximization of independence in personal care activities as the first step in returning the impaired individual to a meaningful life in the community. Indeed, independence in ADL is the dividing line between those persons who might manage on their own and those who will continue to require either an institutional setting or extended personal care services in the home. For a stroke survivor, for example, the achievement of independence in ADL makes a life of autonomy and manageable costs in a community setting a possibility, unless he or she requires constant supervision because of dementia or emotional disorders. Thus, ADL independence is a major goal toward which the stroke survivor labors, aided by knowledgeable health care, rehabilitation, and human service professionals.

The specific functional variables that comprise ADL are now quite well delineated. Table 51-6 lists the 11 generally agreed-upon variables as ascertained by Donaldson and co-workers in their 1973 study.[13] For stroke survivors, it is now widely understood that the important ADL outcome parameters include dressing (upper and lower body; indoor and outdoor garments; and both putting on and taking off clothing), ambulation (already covered above in terms of walking, and including wheelchair mobility where walking is not possible), bathing (autonomy is highly dependent on the type of setting available), feeding, transfers, toileting (both bladder and bowel), and grooming (e.g., combing hair, shaving, and applying makeup). Other variables, such as bed activities, are useful for assessing progress from postictal helplessness to maximal independence, but the seven variables listed above comprise the basic requirements for being able to leave the institutional setting and manage without direct and daily personal care services.

Because of the multiplicity of ADL outcome variables, there has been a major investigative effort since the 1960s to achieve a composite, overall expression of the level of independence in ADL, utilizing some

**TABLE 51-6. Variables Used in Scoring Independence in ADL by Three Standard Indexes**

| ADL Variable | Katz Index of ADL (1963) | Barthel Index (1965) | Kenny Self-Care Evaluation (1965) | Frequency of Use in 25 Published ADL Scales |
|---|---|---|---|---|
| 1. Dressing | + | + | + | 1.00 (all) |
| 2. Ambulation | + | + | + | 0.96 |
| 3. Bathing | + | + | + | 0.92 |
| 4. Feeding | + | + | + | 0.88 |
| 5. Transfers | + | + | + | 0.72 |
| 6. Toileting | + | + | + | 0.72 |
| 7. Grooming | 0 | + | + | 0.68 |
| 8. Wheelchair activities | 0 | + | + | 0.64 |
| 9. Elevation | 0 | + | + | 0.48 |
| 10. Continence | + | + | 0 | 0.44 |
| 11. Bed activities | 0 | + | + | 0.36 |

*Abbreviation*: ADL, activities of daily living.
(From Gresham et al.,[32] with permission.)

type of classification such as an ordinal scale.[40,45,58] The advantages of such an approach include not only the greater ease of managing a single overall expression of ADL independence in documenting a patient's progress (as opposed to a number of separate component ratings), but also the opportunity such instruments provide to use aggregate data for both investigative and administrative purposes.[13,31]

One of the first major studies to use a standardized functional assessment instrument to assess objectively the ADL independence of a group of stroke survivors was published by Katz et al. in 1966.[39] They studied 138 elderly patients who had survived a first stroke for 30 days and had been referred to a geriatric rehabilitation hospital. They found that 43 percent of these stroke survivors were independent in ADL, as measured by the Katz Index of ADL,[40] at the end of two years. In the 1970s, Gresham and co-workers used the same instrument to classify levels of ADL independence in 148 long-term survivors of stroke in the Framingham Study and 148 stroke-free controls matched for age and sex (see Table 51-4).[33] The frequencies found were 68 percent and 91 percent in the stroke survivor and control groups, respectively. This not only helped to establish the level of ADL independence to be expected in stroke survivors, but documented the fact, previously implied, that these levels were truly related to stroke and not just to advanced age. Since the Katz Index of ADL was used as the classification instrument in both studies, it could be inferred that the differences in frequencies found were due to basic differences in the groups studied (i.e., an elderly institutional, as opposed to a middle-aged community population), rather than to disparate methodologies.

Other investigators, using other instruments, have found frequencies of ADL independence in stroke survivors that are generally within this range of from slightly less than half to about two-thirds. For example, in Feigenson's large series published in 1977, 54 percent of stroke patients were independent in ADL, as measured by the Burke Stroke Time-Oriented Profile (BUSTOP), at the time of discharge from a Stroke Rehabilitation Unit.[16,19] Other documented frequencies of ADL independence include 45 and 62 percent, respectively, in medical and stroke unit patients 16 weeks after admission, in the study by Wade et al.[60]

These various investigations, using rigorous methodologic approaches, have been able to establish a norm for ADL independence as an outcome variable in stroke. The documentation that this can be achieved in two out of three otherwise unselected long-term stroke survivors[33] is a powerful argument against the fatalistic, "do-nothing" approach to stroke patients and a source of encouragement to the efforts of those that feel the rewards of independent function warrant an ongoing positive emphasis in the clinical management of stroke survivors.

Another source of normative data on ADL outcomes in stroke is the work of Granger and associates.[25–28] Building upon the earlier work of Moskowitz and McCann,[47,48] Barthel and Mahoney,[45] Wylie,[67] and others, they have carried out an elaborate series of studies of outcomes in stroke, using adapted versions of the PULSES Profile[48] and the Barthel Index,[45] as incorporated into the Long-Range Evaluation Summary (LRES).[29]

Initially, these studies looked at 164 stroke patients discharged from a hospital stroke unit and found that higher discharge Barthel Scores, reflecting greater independence in ADL, were positively correlated with returning home, as opposed to requiring an institutional environment.[27]

In subsequent studies of this and other populations, the interrelationships between Barthel Index scores, as a measure of independence in ADL, and other variables (both initial characteristics and other outcomes) were explored. In 1979, Granger, Albrecht, and Hamilton published their widely recognized paper in which their formalized functional assessment approach was used to study a random sample of 658 patients in the ten-center Comprehensive Service

Needs Study.[25] Medical rehabilitation patients from the 10 centers were evaluated at admission to medical rehabilitation, at discharge, and at follow-up 2 years after discharge. For the 134 patients in this group with focal cerebral disorders, the mean Barthel Index scores were 34, 71, and 72 for the three points in time, respectively. Thus, as one of the many contributions of these studies, another major step was taken toward the generation of normative ADL data for several types of medical rehabilitation patients, including stroke survivors. In addition, the data documented that the ADL scores of the focal cerebral disorder group did indeed increase during medical rehabilitation and, very importantly, were maintained after discharge. The early commitment and consistent adherence to the use of these specific functional assessment instruments has been a major methodologic strength of this series of studies by Granger and co-workers. In so doing, they have made it easier for others to understand better the ways in which their data were derived and to compare their findings with those of other investigators and documenters of clinical programs using the same instruments.

The choice of the Barthel Index, as the most useful way to classify independence in ADL, was made by Granger and colleagues for a number of reasons. These include comprehensiveness in terms of component variables, numerical scoring, the ability to retain subscores for each variable, and the fact that a maximum score of 100 on the Barthel Index means that the individual can get along without attendant care (even though independent living may still be precluded by other factors). This is conceptually consonant with the current process of medical rehabilitation, in which the "maximum benefit" of inpatient physical restoration is usually synonomous with reaching the highest achievable level of independence in ADL.

The use of the Barthel Index by Wylie and Granger,[25–28,67] the PULSES Profile by Moskowitz and Granger,[25–27,47] the Katz Index of ADL by Katz and Ford,[39] Gresham et al., and others,[33] the BUSTOP by Feigenson et al.,[16,17,19] and the Kenny Self-Care Evaluation by Anderson et al[3] illustrates the methodologic heterogeneity that has characterized research in the ADL outcomes of stroke. This obviously leads to the issue of comparability of data.

A study by Gresham, Phillips, and Labi compared the relative merits of the Katz Index of ADL, the Barthel Index, and the Kenny Self-Care Evaluation in terms of scoring ADL independence in stroke.[32] By using the Donaldson ADL Evaluation Form,[13] which contains all the data needed for all three instruments, administered on the 148 stroke survivors in the Framingham Study, they found that there was no statistically significant difference in the overall prevalence ratios of perfect ADL independence as determined by each (see Table 51-7). Differences in sensitivity (the Kenny Self-Care Evaluation being the most sensitive and the Katz Index of ADL the least) previously noted by Donaldson, Wagner, and Gresham were again demonstrated. In light of these findings, it seems hopeful that a more methodologically unified and sophisticated approach for studying ADL outcomes in stroke will soon be a reality.[37,42] With greater understanding of the magnitude and determinants of specific ADL deficits in stroke survivors should come the new research ideas and innovative clinical interventions that will promote greater independence and, in so doing, lower the costs of ongoing care.

For example, it might be argued that better technology should be able to increase ADL independence in stroke survivors above the two-thirds maximum level currently documented. The work of both Granger[26] and Feigenson[16,17,19,28] suggests that the most prevalent ADL deficits of stroke survivors are not related to bowel and bladder problems (where better adaptive equipment is less likely to be helpful) but to areas such as dressing, transfers, and mobility where technological advances could conceivably make a difference. It is hoped that such improvement will soon occur. For now, the two out of three frequency of ADL independence stands as the group norm for long-term survivors of stroke.

## Instrumental Activities of Daily Living

Instrumental activities of daily living (IADL) have been less intensively studied than personal ADL but are of great importance in formulating prognoses and care plans for survivors of stroke. These activities, such as homemaking and shopping, represent an ex-

**TABLE 51-7. Frequency of Independence in ADL[a,b]**

| Instrument | Frequency of Full Independence in ADL (%) | Ref. |
|---|---|---|
| Barthel Index | 35.1 | 45 |
| Katz Index of ADL | 39.2 | 40 |
| Kenny Self-Care Evaluation | 41.9 | 58 |

*Abbreviation*: ADL, activities of daily living.
[a] As determined simultaneously by three different instruments in 148 long-term stroke survivors in the Framingham Study cohort. Independence = a perfect score.
[b] $N = 148$. Frequencies are not significantly different as determined by the Z test.
(From Gresham et al.,[32] with permission.)

tension of ADL skills into more complex areas that are important in independent living. Such skills obviously depend on cognitive, emotional, and environmental factors, as well as physical competence in motor skills. They comprise the next step, in terms of assessment and helping, from independence in personal self-care towards truly autonomous living patterns. A useful elaboration of IADL is found in the long-range evaluation system (LRES) of Granger.[29]

As with personal ADL, instrumental ADL is the particular professional purview of the occupational therapists who comprise a vital part of the regular medical rehabilitation team.

## Communication

Communication is a variable of great importance to stroke survivors whose neurologic deficit includes such problems as dysphasia and dysarthria. As seen in Table 51-2, 27 (18 percent) and 23 (16 percent) of the 148 long-term stroke survivors in the Framingham cohort were found to have dysphasia and dysarthria, respectively. Residual frequencies of such magnitude emphasize the importance of carrying out adequate assessments and establishing plans for enhancement of communication skills for stroke survivors with these problems.

This is best performed by experienced speech pathologists. By combining structured functional assessment of overall communication skills[55–57,63] with audiometric screening and good clinical judgment, the speech pathologist can both adequately describe the precise deficit and suggest the most feasible method of overall communication for each individual patient. The shift in emphasis from speech alone to overall communication is a significant development that is well described by Sarno.[56]

As with physical therapy services for mobility, and occupational therapy for ADL, the presence of the speech pathologist on the conventional rehabilitation team facilitates early and coordinated attention to the communication needs of stroke patients.

## Psychosocial Function

Psychosocial function comprises a number of outcome variables of great complexity and importance in stroke survivors. It has been clearly documented that the overall psychosocial disability manifested by long-term stroke survivors exceeds anything that could be explained by physical limitations alone[33] (see Table 51-4). Labi et al.[43] showed that physically restored stroke survivors still had significant excess psychosocial dysfunction.[43] As stated previously, it is frequently difficult to determine how much of this dysfunction is due to organic deficits from the stroke per se and how much to other factors.

The details and determinants of this problem are beginning to be better understood. As noted previously, Feibel and Springer,[15] Robinson et al., [52] and Binder[4] have documented an increased amount of depression in stroke survivors and, in so doing, identify a clinical entity that can be evaluated and possibly successfully treated by the patient's physician or an appropriate consultant.

The assessment of cognitive function in the stroke patient is vitally important but often elusive.[7] A sensible beginning would appear to be the consistent use of a simple screening instrument for dementia.[50] These are well known to geriatricians and are nicely summarized by Kane and Kane.[38] Physicians not wishing to rely on such an instrument can always draw their own conclusions from interviewing the patient in greater depth. Whatever the avenue to awareness, the identification of specific cognitive dysfunction in the stroke survivor immediately raises the possibility that conventional rehabilitation services, which rely so heavily on learning by the patient for their success, may be facing unusual difficulties and a decreased likelihood for achievement. It is better to face these possibilities directly rather than to continue in a round of unsuccessful rehabilitation programs that end up frustrating both patient and provider.

In practical terms, it is often difficult for the primary physician to find appropriate cognitive assessment consultants and therapists for his or her stroke patients. While most large centers offer expertise in neuropsychology and other forms of psychometry, many primary physicians may legitimately elect to settle for less sophisticated services that are readily available in the patient's own community. Formalized rehabilitation settings will uniformly address the psychosocial dimension in stroke patients, many with great methodologic sophistication. In the last analysis, however, the primary physician will have to decide how much cognitive dysfunction exists and how it should be approached.

Cognitive remediation is currently a very active field of investigation, greatly stimulated by the present "epidemic" of traumatic closed head injuries.[35] While much is being learned about cerebral dysfunction, it is important for physicians to remember that findings from brain-injured groups with multiple deficits may not be uniformly applicable to stroke survivors whose cerebral lesions are usually more discrete.

While affective states and cognitive function are important components of the psychosocial disability of stroke survivors, many of the problems are situational, interpersonal, and/or related to family dynamics. Many talented investigators have begun to explore these problems in depth.[5,6,14] Meanwhile, established medical rehabilitation programs all have psychosocial counselors (i.e., psychiatrists, psychologists, social workers, or rehabilitation counselors) who are attuned, by training and experience, to the specific problems of the physically handicapped. They can be expected to provide more knowledgeable and realistic help to the stroke survivor than can mental health professionals without such experience.

### Sexual Function

Physicians working with stroke survivors should be familiar with the fact that such persons continue to have sexual identities, needs, and capabilities. Since the specific organs involved in sexual activity are bilaterally innervated, there is no physiologic reason why unilateral stroke per se should permanently impair sexual capabilities. Recently, a number of formal studies have begun to look more specifically at sexual function in stroke survivors.[4,9,12] Their findings suggest that more information and understanding on sexual matters from health care professionals would be helpful to stroke survivors.

### Rewarding Avocational Pursuits

Since classical medical rehabilitation began with the concept that returning handicapped people to work would generate more funds from taxes than were expended for rehabilitation services, it is understandable that only recently has the emphasis in stroke rehabilitation been extended to include "quality of life." The simple facts are that a large number of persons who survive strokes are already retired because of age, and some others are eager to exercise the option to retire that is presented by a major, disabling illness such as stroke (not to mention the great number of homemakers whose great contributions are not reflected in terms of tax revenues). It is, therefore, increasingly obvious that a life of good quality, for most stroke survivors, will have to be achieved outside the workplace. It is therefore, incumbent upon physicians and other health professionals interested in stroke survivors, to support and facilitate creative and useful programs that can offer participation and meaning. For many stroke patients and their families, the Stroke Clubs (sponsored by the American Heart Association and other agencies) provide a helpful means of reentry into community activities.

### Vocational Function

It is important to remember that many individual stroke survivors can and do return to work.[2,33,62] The fact that they are not always in the majority does not dim the glow of their individual achievements. As previously addressed, however, some stroke survivors will not *wish* to rejoin the work force. Many will be already retired, some will welcome a means for early retirement, and others will face the familiar financial disincentives (loss of disability income and related health insurance benefits) that encourage many handicapped Americans to shy away from employment possibilities.

Weisbroth[62] and others have shown that programs of vocational rehabilitation services can help many stroke survivors to reenter the work force. Again, conventional medical rehabilitation programs will routinely consider this possibility. Other providers should remember that, if the possibility of return to work exists, the patient should be referred to the state vocational agency (in most states, the Division of Vocational Rehabilitation or the Office of Vocational Rehabilitation) where programs of assessment, training, and placement are available for appropriate candidates.

## SUMMARY

In spite of increased mortality, significant numbers of stroke survivors will live on in the community, and health and human services providers have a responsibility to meet their needs. A thorough assessment of each individual's problems and strengths is basic to planning the appropriate program of care. In general, four out of five long-term stroke survivors will walk, two out of three will be independent in ADL, and fewer than two out of ten will require an institutional living setting. Psychosocial problems will exceed purely physical ones and persist after maximum physical restoration has occurred. Although a minority of stroke survivors will return to work due to age and other factors, a good quality of life is a legitimate goal for each. Conventional medical rehabilitation programs, in a variety of settings, will systematically address all of these facets and work toward the coordinated remediation of all deficits found. For patients in settings where conventional medical rehabilitation programs are not available, alternative forms of service provision have been shown to be effective as well. Research, using objective functional assessment techniques, has documented that stroke patients, as a group, do improve in functional levels during the postacute, or "rehabilitative" phase and that this improvement is maintained.

## REFERENCES

1. Adams GF, Merrett JD: Prognosis and survival in the aftermath of hemiplegia. Br Med J: 309, 1961
2. Anderson TP: Rehabilitation of patients with completed stroke. p. 583. In Kottke FJ, Stillwell GK, Lehmann JF (eds): Krusen's Handbook of Physical Medicine and Rehabilitation. WB Saunders, Philadelphia, 1982
3. Anderson TP, Boureston N, Greenberg FR, Hildyard VG: Predictive factors in stroke rehabilitation. Arch Phys Med Rehabil 55:545, 1974

4. Binder LM: Emotional problems after stroke. Stroke 15:174, 1984
5. Bishop DS: Behavioural Problems and the Disabled: Assessment and Management. Williams & Wilkins, Baltimore, 1980
6. Bishop DS, Epstein NB, Keitner GI et al: Stroke: Morale, family functioning, health status and functional capacity. Arch Phys Med Rehabil 67:84, 1986
7. Boller F: Strokes and behavior: Disorders of higher cortical functions following cerebral disease. Curr Concepts Cerebrovasc Dis Stroke, Jan–Feb, 1981
8. Brandstater ME, Basmajian JV: Stroke Rehabilitation. Williams & Wilkins, Baltimore, 1987
9. Bray GP, DeFrank RS, Wolf TL: Sexual functioning in stroke survivors. Arch Phys Med Rehabil 62:286, 1981
10. Commission on Accreditation of Rehabilitation Facilities (CARF): Standards Manual for Facilities Serving People with Disabilities. p. 39. Tuscon, Az, 1983
11. De Lisa JA: Rehabilitation Medicine: Principles and Practice. Lippincott, Philadelphia, 1988
12. Dittmar SS: Rehabilitation Nursing: Process and Application. CV Mosby, St. Louis, 1989
13. Donaldson SW, Wagner CC, Gresham GE: A unified ADL evaluation form. Arch Phys Med Rehabil 54:175, 1973
14. Evans RL, Northwood LK: Social support needs in adjustment to stroke. Arch Phys Med Rehabil 64:61, 1983
15. Feibel JH, Springer CJ: Depression and failure to resume social activities after stroke. Arch Phys Med Rehabil 63:276, 1981
16. Feigenson JS, McCarthy ML, Greenberg SD, Feigenson WD: Factors influencing outcome and length of stay in a stroke rehabilitation unit. 2. Comparison of 318 screened and 248 unscreened patients. Stroke 8:657, 1977
17. Feigenson JS, McCarthy ML, Meese PD et al: Stroke rehabilitation. I. Factors predicting outcome and length of stay—an overview. NY State J Med 77:1426, 1977
18. Feigensón JS, McDowell FH: Stroke rehabilitation: alternatives for health care delivery. NY State J Med 80:752, 1980
19. Feigenson JS, McDowell FH, Meese P et al: Factors influencing outcome and length of stay in a stroke rehabilitation unit. 1. Analysis of 248 unscreened patients—medical and functional prognostic indicators. Stroke 8:651, 1977
20. Feinstein AR: Clinical Judgement. Williams & Wilkins, Baltimore, 1967
21. Feldman DJ, Lee PR, Unterecker J et al: A comparison of functionally oriented medical care and formal rehabilitation in the management of patients with hemiplegia due to cerebrovascular disease. J Chronic Dis 15:297, 1962
22. Garraway WM, Whishnant JP, Drury I: The changing pattern of survival following stroke. Stroke 14:699, 1983
23. Gibson CJ: Epidemiology and patterns of care of stroke patients. Arch Phys Med Rehabil 55:398, 1974
24. Goodgold J: Rehabilitation Medicine, CV Mosby, St. Louis, 1988
25. Granger CV, Albrecht GL, Hamilton BB: Outcome of comprehensive medical rehabilitation: Measurement by PULSES profile and the Barthel index. Arch Phys Med Rehabil 60:145, 1979
26. Granger CV, Dewis LS, Peters NC et al: Stroke rehabilitation: analysis of repeated Barthel index measures. Arch Phys Med Rehabil 60:14, 1979
27. Granger CV, Greer DS, Liset E et al: Measurement of outcomes of care for stroke patients. Stroke 6:34, 1975
28. Granger CV, Hamilton BB, Gresham GE: The stroke rehabilitation outcome study. 1. General description. Arch Phys Med Rehabil 69:506, 1988
29. Granger CV, McNamara MA: Functional assessment utilization: the long-range evaluation system (LRES). p. 99. In Granger CV, Gresham GE (eds): Functional Assessment in Rehabilitation Medicine. Williams & Wilkins, Baltimore, 1984
30. Granger CV, Sherwood CC, Greer DS: Functional status measures in a comprehensive stroke program. Arch Phys Med Rehabil 58:555, 1977
31. Gresham GE, Labi MLC: Functional assessment instruments currently available for documenting outcomes in rehabilitation medicine. p. 65. In Granger CV, Gresham GE (eds): Functional Assessment in Rehabilitation Medicine. Williams & Wilkins, Baltimore, 1984
32. Gresham GE, Phillips TF, Labi MLC: ADL status in stroke: relative merits of three standard indexes. Arch Phys Med Rehabil 61:355, 1980
33. Gresham GE, Phillips TF, Wolf PA et al: Epidemiologic profile of long-term stroke disability: the Framingham Study. Arch Phys Med Rehabil 60:487 1979
34. Holt NB, Hicks D (eds): Comprehensive Rehabilitation Nursing. McGraw-Hill, New York, 1981
35. Jennett B, Teasdale G: Management of Head Injuries. FA Davis, Philadelphia, 1981
36. Joint Commission on Accreditation of Hospitals (JCAH): Accreditation Manual for Hospitals, 1984. p. 159. Rehabilitation Programs/Services. 1984
37. Jongbloed L: Prediction of function after stroke: a critical review. Stroke 17:765, 1986
38. Kane RA, Kane RL: Assessing the Elderly: A Practical Guide to Measurement. Lexington Books, Lexington, MA, 1981
39. Katz S, Ford AB, Chinn AB, Newill VA: Prognosis after strokes. II. Long-term course of 159 patients. Medicine (Baltimore) 45:236, 1966
40. Katz S, Ford AB, Moskowitz RW et al: Studies of illness in the aged: the index of ADL: a standardized measure of biological and psychosocial function. JAMA 185:914, 1963
41. Kelly-Hayes M, Wolf PA, Kannel WB et al: Factors influencing survival and the need for institutionalization following stroke: the Framingham Study. Arch Phys Med Rehabil 69:415, 1988
42. Labi MLC, Gresham GE: Some research applications of functional assessment instruments used in rehabilitation medicine. p. 86. In Granger CV, Gresham GE (eds): Functional Assessment in Re-

habilitation Medicine. Williams & Wilkins, Baltimore, 1984
43. Labi MLC, Phillips TF, Gresham GE: Psychosocial disability in physically restored long-term stroke survivors. Arch Phys Med Rehabil 61:561, 1980
44. Lehmann JF, DeLateur BJ, Fowler RS, Jr et al: Stroke: does rehabilitation affect outcome? Arch Phys Med Rehabil 56:375, 1975
45. Mahoney FJ, Barthel DW: Functional evaluation: the Barthel index. Md St Med J 14:61, 1965
46. Matsumoto N, Whishnant JP, Kurland LT, Okazaki H: Natural history of stroke in Rochester, Minnesota, 1955 through 1969: an extension of a previous study, 1945 through 1954. Stroke 4:20, 1973
47. Moskowitz E, Lightbody FEH, Freitag NS: Long-term follow-up of the post-stroke patient. Arch Phys Med Rehabil 53:167, 1972
48. Moskowitz E, McCann CB: Classification of disability in the chronically ill and aging. J Chronic Dis 5:342, 1957
49. Petlund CF: Prevalence and invalidity from stroke in Aust-Agder County of Norway. Universitetsforlaget, Oslo, 1970
50. Pfeiffer E: Short portable mental status questionnaire for assessment of organic brain deficit in elderly patients. Am Geriatr Soc 23:433, 1975
51. Rankin J: Cerebral vascular accidents in patients over the age of 60. II. Prognosis. Scott Med J 2:200, 1957
52. Robinson RG, Starr LB, Price TR: A two-year longitudinal study of post-stroke mood disorders: prevalence and duration at six months follow-up. Br J Psychiatry 144:256, 1984
53. Rogoff JB, Cooney DV, Kutner B: Hemiplegia: a study of home rehabilitation. J Chronic Dis 17:539, 1964
54. Sacco RL, Wolf PA, Kannel WB, McNamara PM: Survival and recurrence following stroke. The Framingham study. Stroke 13:290, 1982
55. Sarno JE, Sarno MT, Levita E: Evaluating language improvement after completed stroke. Arch Phys Med Rehabil 52:73, 1971
56. Sarno MT: Functional measurement in verbal impairment secondary to brain damage. p. 210. In Granger CV, Gresham GE (eds): Functional Assessment in Rehabilitation Medicine. Williams & Wilkins, Baltimore, 1984
57. Sarno MT, Levita E: Natural course of recovery in severe aphasia. Arch Phys Med Rehabil 52:175, 1971
58. Schoening HA, Anderegg L, Bergstrom D et al: Numerical scoring of self-care status of patients. Arch Phys Med Rehabil 46:689, 1965
59. Smith ME, Garraway WM, Smith DL, Akhtar AJ: Therapy impact on functional outcome in a controlled trial of stroke rehabilitation. Arch Phys Med Rehabil 63:21, 1982
60. Wade DT, Skilbeck CE, Langton Hewer R: Predicting Barthel ADL score at 6 months after an acute stroke. Arch Phys Med Rehabil 64:24, 1983
61. Wallace DC: A study of the natural history of cerebral vascular disease. Med J Aust 1:90, 1967
62. Weisbroth S, Esibill N, Zuger RR: Factors in the vocational success of hemiplegic patients. Arch Phys Med Rehabil 52:441, 1971
63. Wertz RT, Weiss DG, Aten JL et al: Comparison of clinic, home and deferred language treatment for aphasia: a Veterans Administration Cooperative Study. Arch Neurol 43:653, 1986
64. Whishnant JP, Fitzgibbons JP, Kurland LT, Sayre GP: Natural history of stroke in Rochester, Minnesota, 1945 through 1954. Stroke 2:11, 1971
65. Wood PHN, Badley EM: People with Disabilities. Monograph No. 12. World Rehabilitation Fund, New York, 1980
66. World Health Organization: International Classification of Impairments, Disabilities, and Handicaps. World Health Organization, Geneva, 1980
67. Wylie CM: Measuring end results of rehabilitation of patients with stroke. Public Health Rep 82:893, 1967

# Index

Page numbers followed by f indicate figures; those followed by t indicate tables.

## A

## B

## C

## E

## F

## G

## M

# N

## S

## T

## W